Neuropsychological Assessment

NEUROPSYCHOLOGICAL ASSESSMENT

Fourth Edition

Muriel D. Lezak
Diane B. Howieson
David W. Loring

with
H. Julia Hannay
Jill S. Fischer

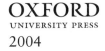

OXFORD
UNIVERSITY PRESS
2004

OXFORD
UNIVERSITY PRESS

Oxford   New York
Auckland   Bangkok   Buenos Aires   Cape Town   Chennai
Dar es Salaam   Delhi   Hong Kong   Istanbul   Karachi   Kolkata
Kuala Lumpur   Madrid   Melbourne   Mexico City   Mumbai   Nairobi
São Paulo   Shanghai   Taipei   Tokyo   Toronto

Published by Oxford University Press, Inc.
198 Madison Avenue, New York, New York, 10016
http://www.oup.com

Oxford is a registered trademark of Oxford University Press

Library of Congress Cataloging-in-Publication Data
Neuropsychological assessment /
Muriel D. Lezak . . . [et al.].—4th ed.
p. cm.   Previous ed. cataloged under: Lezak, Muriel Deutsch.
Includes bibliographical references and index.
ISBN 0-19-511121-4
1. Neuropsychological tests.
I. Lezak, Muriel Deutsch. Neuropsychological assessment.
II. Lezak, Muriel Deutsch.
RC386.6.N48L49 2004   616.8′0475—dc22   2003190065

9 8 7 6 5 4 3 2

Printed in the United States of America
on acid-free paper

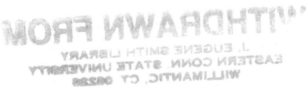

*To our patient spouses who gave us
their loving support when we really needed it.*

Preface

From the 1983 publication of the second edition of this book to 1995 when the third edition was issued, the already swollen river of new knowledge and techniques in the neurosciences in general—in neuropsychology in particular—grew into a torrent. Since 1995, that torrent continues to mount at such a rapid rate that it threatens to inundate the individual neuroscience-based researcher or practitioner with more important new data and evolving examination and treatment techniques than any conscientious person can absorb, much less incorporate into practice or research.

In our review of the literature, two aspects of neuropsychology's evolutionary path came to our attention. Unlike previous editions, we find a geographic expansion in authorship: No longer do virtually all of the authors come from North America or Europe; rather, important contributions now come from all the continents (except Antarctica—as yet). The other evolutionary trend is that fewer articles and books have single authorship; most now are collaborative efforts. *Neuropsychological Assessment-4* is no exception.

When the first edition of this book appeared in 1976, the goal of providing a satisfactory knowledge base and acquainting the reader with almost all of the neuropsychological assessment techniques was reasonable. Today this goal cannot be achieved: one can anticipate that in the weeks between the time we send this edition off to be printed and the time it becomes available to the public, new research findings and changes in significant theoretical concepts and technical innovations will have made some parts of this book outdated or controversial, and will have created important omissions in other parts. Moreover, in perusing the ever-growing flood of books, journals, newsletters, and advertisements in neuropsychology and related neurosciences, we have had to acknowledge the impossibility of presenting all the research, theories, and examination techniques rele-

vant to neuropsychological assessment. This has altered the goal for this book from giving our readers an exhaustive coverage of neuropsychology and its related fields to providing a broad but necessarily and selectively restricted range of the information that is currently relevant and necessary for understanding and undertaking neuropsychological assessment.

Although its size has increased, the organization of this book remains the same as in the third edition. The first eight chapters offer an empirically based, conceptual foundation for understanding the critical elements of neuropsychological assessment: who, when, why, and—in general terms—how. These chapters should also serve as an information resource as we have attempted to provide as extensive and current a set of references as feasible. Chapter sequences for the test compendium remain the same. Like its predecessor, this fourth edition of *Neuropsychological Assessment* has an updated Appendix containing names and addresses of test publishers. We regret the absence of an Author Index, but so many authors will have so many citations that such an index has lost its usefulness.

If some readers are curious about how a single-authored book became a team product, they may wish to know that, yes we did distribute topics—sometimes chapters, sometimes chapter sections, and in the case of Chapter 7, we allotted diseases to one another. Although most assignments were the responsibility of just one of us, a few had two or more authors. We believe the book has benefitted from this collaborative effort. We hope our readers do too.

Portland, Oregon	M. D. L.
Portland, Oregon	D. B. H.
Washington, D.C.	D. W. L.
Houston, Texas	H. J. H.
Winnetka, Illinois	J. S. F.

Acknowledgments

As both clinical and research neuropsychologists, we owe our greatest debt to neuropsychology's grand pioneers who enabled the felicitious melding of neurocognitive, clinical, and measurement psychology, behavioral neurology, and neuropsychiatry which we practice and rely on for research today. Those who have died must be remembered and honored for their contributions to the development of our profession. Each of them has at least several of their works cited here. Outstanding among those we have known are D. Frank Benson, Mihai Botez, Nelson Butters, Laird Cermak, Patricia Goldman-Rakic, Harold Goodglass, Dorothy Gronwall, Henri Hécaen, Charles Matthews, Freda Newcombe, Oscar Parsons, Justine Sergent, Aaron Smith, and Joseph Wepman.

We want to acknowledge the many important and creative contributions by Arthur Benton, his personal contributions that came as guidance, support, and mentoring of several of us, and a very practical one—for without Dr. Benton's encouragement this book would not exist. Others who have contributed time and thought to this edition are Robert Butler, Bruce Hermann, Merrill Hiscock, Glenn Larrabee, Gregory Lee, Kim Meador, Fenwick Nichols, Audrey Sherman, and our always stimulating and challenging Portland colleagues in the 2nd Wednesday Neuropsychology Case Conference.

Also thanks to our editor, Jeffrey House: although he couldn't keep us on schedule, he did prod us to completion and put us in the care of a most patient and effective production editor, Leslie Anglin. Thank you for all your help, Leslie.

M. D. L.
D. B. H.
D. W. L.

Contents

I | THEORY AND PRACTICE OF NEUROPSYCHOLOGICAL ASSESSMENT

1 | The Practice of Neuropsychological Assessment

Imaging is not enough.

Mortimer Mishkin, 1988

Clinical neuropsychology is an applied science concerned with the behavioral expression of brain dysfunction. It owes its primordial—and often fanciful—concepts to those who, since earliest historic times, puzzled about what made people do what they did and how. These were the philosophers, physicians, scientists, artists, tinkerers, and dreamers who first called attention to what seemed to be linkages between body (not necessarily brain) structures and people's common responses to common situations as well as their behavioral anomalies (Castro-Caldas and Grafman, 2000; Finger, 1994, 2000; C.G. Gross, 1998; L.H. Marshall and Magoun, 1998). In the 19th century the idea of controlled observations became generally accepted, thus providing the conceptual tool with which the first generation of neuroscientists laid out the basic schema of brain–behavior relationships that hold today (Benton, 2000; Benton [collected papers in L. Costa and Spreen, 1985, *passim*]; Boring, 1950; M. Critchley and Critchley, 1998; Hécaen et Lanteri-Laura, 1977; Stringer, Cooley, and Christensen, 2002; N.J. Wade and Brozek, 2001).

In the first half of the 20th century, war-damaged brains gave the chief impetus to the development of clinical neuropsychology. The need for screening and diagnosis of brain injured and behaviorally disturbed servicemen during the first World War and for their rehabilitation afterward created large-scale demands for neuropsychology programs (e.g., K. Goldstein, 1995 [1939]; Homskaya, 2001; see references in Luria, 1973b; Poppelreuter, 1990 [1917]; W.R. Russell [see references in Newcombe, 1969]). The second World War and then the wars in east Asia and the Mideast promoted the development of many talented neuropsychologists and of increasingly sophisticated examination and treatment techniques.

While clinical neuropsychology can trace its lineage directly to the clinical neurosciences, psychology contributed the two other domains of knowledge and skill that are integral to the scientific discipline and clinical

practices of neuropsychology today. Educational psychologists, beginning with Binet (with Simon, 1908) and Spearman (1904), initially developed tests to capture that elusive concept "intelligence." Following these pioneers, mental measurement specialists produced a multitude of examination techniques to screen recruits for the military and to assist educational evaluations; some of these techniques—such as Raven's Progressive Matrices, the Wechsler Intelligence Scales, and the Wide Range Achievement Tests—have been incorporated into the neuropsychological test canon (Boake, 2002). Society's acceptance of educational testing led to a proliferation of large-scale, statistics-dependent testing programs that provided neuropsychology with an understanding of the nature and varieties of mental abilities from a normative perspective. Educational testing has also been the source of ever more reliable measurement techniques and statistical tools for test standardization and the development of normative data, analysis of research findings, and validation studies (Anastasi and Urbina, 1997; Mayrhauser, 1992; McFall and Townsend, 1998). Clinical psychologists and psychologists specializing in personality and social behavior research borrowed from and further elaborated principles and techniques found in educational testing, giving neuropsychology this important assessment dimension (Cripe, 1997; G.J. Meyer et al., 2001).

Psychology's other critical contribution to neuropsychological assessment comes primarily from experimental studies of cognitive functions in both humans and other animals. In its early development, human studies of cognition mainly dealt with normal subjects—predominantly college students who sometimes earned course credits for their cooperation. Animal studies and clinical reports of brain injured persons, especially soldiers with localized wounds and stroke patients, generated much of what was known about the alterations and limitations of specific cognitive functions when one part of the brain is missing or compromised. In the latter half of the 20th century, many experimental psychologists became aware of the wealth of information about cognitive functions to be gained from studying brain injured persons, especially those with localized lesions (e.g., G. Cohen et al., 2000; Gazzaniga, 2000a, *passim;* Rapp, 2001; Tulving and Craik, 2000, *passim*). Similarly, neuroscientists have become aware of the usefulness of cognitive constructs and psychological techniques when studying brain–behavior relationships (Feinberg and Farah, 2003, *passim;* Fuster, 1995; Luria, 1966; 1973b; Margolin, 1992; Mesulam, 2000, *passim*). Now in the 21st century, neuropsychologists and other neuroscientists have the further advantage of dynamic imaging techniques which, by opening windows into brain processing, further refine our understanding of the neural foundations of behavior (Frackowiak, Friston, et al., 1997; Gazzaniga, 2000a, *passim;* Rugg, 1997). Knowledge from these studies provides neuropsychologists with the neurologically meaningful psychological constructs necessary for the analysis and comprehension of the uniquely and often anomalously multifaceted behavioral presentations of their patients.

When doing assessments, clinical neuropsychologists typically address a variety of questions with awareness of both the neurological and psychological import of their patients' behaviors and with respect for and interest in their patients' very disparate capacities. The diversity of problems and persons presents an unending challenge to examiners who want to satisfy the purposes for which the examination was undertaken and still evaluate patients at levels suited to their capacities and limitations. In this complex and expanding field, few facts or principles can be taken for granted, few techniques would not benefit from modifications, and few procedures will not be bent or broken as knowledge and experience accumulate. The practice of neuropsychology calls for flexibility, curiosity, inventiveness, and empathy even in the seemingly most routine situations (B. Caplan and Shechter, 1995). Moreover, even seemingly routine neuropsychological assessments hold the promise of new insights into the workings of the brain and the excitement of discovery.

The rapid evolution of neuropsychological assessment in recent years reflects a growing sensitivity among clinicians generally to the practical problems of identification, assessment, care, and treatment of brain impaired patients. Psychologists, psychiatrists, and counselors ask for neuropsychological assistance in identifying those candidates for their services who may have underlying neurological disorders. Neurologists and neurosurgeons request behavioral evaluations to aid in diagnosis and to document the course of brain disorders or the effects of treatment (e.g., Grabowski et al., 2002). A fruitful interaction is taking place between neuropsychology and gerontology that enhances the knowledge and clinical applications of each discipline (see Chapter 8, pp. 294–301).

Child neuropsychology has developed hand in hand with advances in the study of mental retardation, learning disabilities, and children's behavior problems. As this text concerns neuropsychological issues relevant to adults, we refer the interested reader to the current child neuropsychology literature (V. Anderson et al., 2001; Baron, Fennell, and Voeller, 1995; Pennington, 2002; C. Reynolds and Fletcher-Janzen, 1997; Sattler, 2001a,b; L.T. Singer and Zeskind, 2001; Teeter and Semrud-Clikeman, 1997; Yeates, Ris, and Taylor, 2000). Adults whose cognitive and behavioral problems stem from developmental disorders or childhood onset conditions may also be in need of a neuropsychological evaluation. Although they are more likely to be seen in clinics or by neuropsychologists specializing in the care of adults, the preponderance of the literature on their problems can be found in books and articles dealing with child neuropsychology. Thus, readers interested in developmental conditions such as attentional deficit hyperactivity disorder, spina bifida, or hydrocephalus arising from a perinatal incident, or in residuals of childhood meningitis or effects of cancer treatment of children, for example, are referred to the developmental literature.

When this book first appeared, much of the emphasis in clinical neuropsychology was on assessing behavioral change. In part this occurred because so much of the demand on neuropsychology had been for assistance with diagnostic problems. Moreover, since many patients seen by neuropsychologists were considered too limited in their capacity to benefit from behavioral training programs and counseling, these kinds of treatment did not seem to offer practical options for their care. Yet, as one of the clinical sciences, neuropsychology has been evolving naturally: assessment tends to play a predominant role while these sciences are relatively young; treatment techniques develop as diagnostic categories and etiological relationships are defined and clarified and the nature of the patients' disorders become better understood. Today, treatment planning and evaluation have become not merely commonplace but often necessary considerations for neuropsychologists performing assessments.

Any of six different purposes may prompt a neuropsychological examination: *diagnosis; patient care—*including questions about management and planning; *treatment-1: identifying treatment needs,* individualizing treatment programs, and keeping abreast of patients' changing treatment requirements; *treatment-2: evaluating treatment efficacy; research,* both theoretical and applied; and now in the United States and to a lesser extent elsewhere, *forensic questions* are frequently referred to neuropsychologists (Prigatano and

Pliskin, 2003, *passim*). Each purpose calls for some differences in assessment strategies. Yet many assessments serve two or more purposes, requiring the examiner to integrate the strategies in order to gain the needed information about the patient in the most focused and succinct manner possible.

1. *Diagnosis.* Neuropsychological assessment can be useful in discriminating between psychiatric and neurological symptoms, in identifying a possible neurological disorder in a nonpsychiatric patient, in helping to distinguish between different neurological conditions, and in providing behavioral data for localizing the site—or at least the hemisphere side—of a lesion. However, the use of neuropsychological assessment as a diagnostic tool has diminished while its contributions to patient care and treatment and to understanding behavioral phenomena and brain function have grown. This shift is due at least in part to the development of noninvasive neurodiagnostic techniques which are both highly sensitive and reliable for many diagnostic purposes (e.g., neuroimaging [see Bigler, 1996; Frith and Friston, 1997; Papanicolaou, 1998] and electrophysiological techniques [Andreassi, 1995; Daube, 1996; Frackowiak, Friston, et al., 1997; Kutas and Dale, 1997]; see also pp. 15–17]. Thus, accurate diagnosis, including localization of a lesion, is often achieved by means of the neurologist's examination and laboratory devices.

Still, conditions remain in which even the most sensitive laboratory analyses may not be diagnostically enlightening, such as toxic encephalopathies (e.g., Anger, 1990; Morrow, 1998), Alzheimer's disease and related dementing processes (e.g., Derrer et al., 2002; Filley and Cullum, 1993; Kaye, Swihart, Howieson, et al., 1997; O'Rourke, Tuokko, Hayden, and Beattie, 1997; Visser, Scheltens, Verhey, et al., 1999; Welsh-Bohmer et al., 2003), and mild traumatic brain injury (TBI) (e.g., T.L. Bennett and Raymond, 1997b; Bigler, 1999; Cullum and Thompson, 1997; Ricker and Zafonte, 2000; Reitan and Wolfson, 1999; N.R. Varney and Varney, 1995). In these conditions the neuropsychological findings can be diagnostically crucial.

Even when the site and extent of a brain lesion have been shown on imaging, the image will not identify the nature of residual behavioral strengths and the accompanying deficits: for this neuropsychological assessment is needed. It has been known for decades that despite general similarities in the pattern of brain function sites, these patterns will differ more or less between people (see pp. 32, 85). These kinds of difference are demonstrated nicely by Bigler (2001a) who describes three cases with localized lesions that appeared quite similar on neuroimaging though each had a distinctively different psychosocial outcome. Moreover, cognitive assessment can document mental abilities that are inconsistent with anatomic findings, as for example the 101-year-old nun whose test scores were high but whose autopsy showed "abundant neurofibrillary tangles and senile plaques, the classic lesions of Alzheimer's disease" (Snowdon, 1997). Markowitsch and Calabrese (1996), too, discuss instances in which patients' level of functioning exceeded expectations based on neuroimaging. Thus, neuropsychological techniques will most likely continue to be an essential part of the neurodiagnostic apparatus.

Although limited in its applications as a primary diagnostic tool, neuropsychological assessment can aid in prediction—whether it be the outcome of a diagnosed condition (Bendixen and Benton, 1996; E.D. Richardson, Varney, Roberts et al., 1997; S.B. Rourke and Grant, 1999; Trenerry, 1996), the likelihood that a neuropathological condition will be manifested (Boll, 1985; Ingraham and Aiken, 1996), or the practical consequences of a particular kind of brain impairment (Burgess, Alderman, Evans, et al., 1998; Cahn, Sullivan, Shear, et al., 1998; van Gorp, Baerwald, Ferrando, et al., 1999). As one example of its many purposes, the neuropsychological examination of postcoma traumatic brain injury (TBI) patients in the early stages following their return to consciousness or cessation of posttraumatic amnesia is prognostic of their eventual outcome (Lucas, 1998; Newcombe, 1985; S.R. Ross, Millis, and Rosenthal, 1997). In persons at risk for Huntington's disease, the earliest evidence of illness may show up as subtle alterations in neuropsychological status best observed by refined assessment techniques (Campodonico, Aylward, Codori, et al., 1998; T. Diamond et al., 1992).

Screening is another aspect of diagnosis. Until quite recently, screening was a rather crudely conceived affair, typically dedicated to identifying "brain damaged" patients from among a diagnostically mixed population such as might be found in long-term psychiatric care facilities. Little attention was paid to either base rate issues or the prevalence of conditions in which psychiatric and neurologic contributions were mixed and interactive (e.g., C.G. Watson and Plemel, 1978; Mapou, 1988, and A. Smith, 1983, p. 467, discuss this issue). Yet screening has a place in neuropsychological assessment when used in a more refined manner to identify persons most likely at risk for some specified condition or in need of further diagnostic study, and where brevity is required—whether because of the press of patients who may benefit from neuropsychological assessment (D.N. Allen, Sprenkel, Heyman, et al., 1998 or because the patient's condition may preclude a lengthy assessment (S. Walker, 1992) (also see Chapter 6, p. 150).

2. *Patient care and planning.* Whether or not diagnosis is an issue, many patients are referred for detailed information about their cognitive status, behavioral alterations, and personality characteristics—often with questions about their adjustment to their disabilities—so that they and the people responsible for their well-being may know how the neurological condition has affected their behavior. At the very least the neuropsychologist has a responsibility to describe the patient as fully as necessary for intelligent understanding and care.

Descriptive evaluations may be employed in many ways in the care and treatment of brain injured patients. Precise descriptive information about cognitive and emotional status is essential for careful management of many neurological disorders. Rational planning usually depends on an understanding of patients' capabilities and limitations, the kinds of psychological change they are undergoing, and the impact of these changes on their experiences of themselves and on their behavior.

A 55-year-old right-handed management expert with a bachelor's degree in economics was hospitalized with a stroke involving the left frontoparietal cortex three months after taking over as chief executive of a foundering firm. He had been an effective troubleshooter, who devoted most of his waking hours to work. In this new post, his first as chief, his responsibilities called for abilities to analyze and integrate large amounts of information, including complex financial records and sales and manufacturing reports; creative thinking; good judgment; and rebuilding the employees' faltering morale. Although acutely he had displayed right-sided weakness and diminished sensation involving both his arm and leg, motor and sensory functions rapidly returned to near normal levels and he was discharged from the hospital after 10 days. Within 5 months he was walking 3 1/2 miles daily, he was using his right hand for an estimated 75% of activities, and he felt fit and ready to return to work. In questioning the wisdom of this decision, his neurologist referred him for a neuropsychological examination.

This bright man achieved test scores in the *high average* to *superior* ability ranges yet his performance was punctuated by lapses of judgment (e.g., when asked what he would do if he was the first to see smoke and fire at the movies he said, "If you're the first—if it's not a dangerous fire try to put it out by yourself. However, if it's a large fire beyond your control you should immediately alert the audience by yelling and screaming and capturing their attention"; when directed to write what was wrong with a picture portraying two persons sitting comfortably out in the rain, he listed seven different answers, such as, "Right-hand side of rain drops moves [sic] to right on right side of pict. [sic]," but completely overlooked the central problem). Impaired self-monitoring appeared in his rapid performance of a task requiring the subject to work quickly while keeping track of what has already been done (*Figural Fluency Test*)—he worked faster than

most but left a trail of errors; in assigning numbers to symbols from memory (*Symbol Digit Modalities Test*) without noting that he gave the same number to two different symbols only inches apart; and in allowing two small errors to remain on a page of arithmetic calculations done without a time limit. Not surprisingly, he had word finding difficulties which showed up in his need for phonetic cueing to retrieve six words on the *Boston Naming Test* while not recalling two even with cueing; this problem also appeared in discourse; for example, he stated that a dog and a lion were alike in being "both members of the animal factory, I mean animal life." On self-report of his emotional status (*Beck Depression Inventory, Symptom Check List-90-R*) he portrayed himself as having no qualms, suffering no emotional or psychiatric symptoms.

In interview the patient assured me [mdl] that he was ready to return to a job that he relished. As his work has been his life, he had no "extracurricular" interests or activities. He denied fatigue or that his temperament had changed, insisting he was fully capable of resuming all of his managerial duties.

It was concluded that the performance defects, though subtle, could be serious impediments at this occupational level. Moreover, lack of appreciation of these deficits plus the great extent to which this man's life—and sense of dignity and self-worth—were bound up in his work suggested that he would have difficulty in understanding and accepting his condition and adapting to it in a constructive manner. His potential for serious depression seemed high.

The patient was seen with his wife for a report of the examination findings with recommendations and to evaluate his emotional situation in the light of both his wife's reports and her capacity to understand and support him. With her present, he could no longer deny fatigue since it undermined both his efficiency and his good nature, as evident in her examples of how his efficiency and disposition were better in the morning than later in the day. She welcomed learning about fatigue as his untypical irritability and cognitive lapses had puzzled her. With his neurologist's permission, he made practical plans to return to work—for half-days only, and with an "assistant" who would review his actions and decisions. His need for this help became apparent to him after he was shown some of his failures in self-monitoring. At the same time he was given encouraging information regarding his many well-preserved abilities. (Judgmental errors were not pointed out: While he could comprehend the concrete evidence of self-monitoring errors, it would require more extensive counseling for a man with an impaired capacity for complex abstractions to grasp the complex and abstract issues involved in evaluating judgments. Moreover, learning that his stroke had rendered him careless and susceptible to fatigue was enough bad news for the patient to hear in one hour; to have given more discouraging information than was practically needed at this time would have been cruel and probably counterproductive.)

An interesting solution was worked out for the problem of how to get this self-acknowledged workaholic to accept a four-hour work day: If he went to work in the morning, his wife was sure he would soon begin stretching his time limit to five and six or more hours. He therefore agreed to go to work after his morning walk or a golf game and a midday rest period so that, arriving at the office after 1 PM, he was much less likely to exceed his half-day work limit.

Ten months after the stroke the patient reported that he was on the job about 60 hours per week and had been told he "was doing excellent work." He described a mild naming problem and other minor confusions. He also acknowledged some feelings of depression in the evening and a sleep disturbance for which his neurologist began medication.

In many cases the neuropsychological examination can answer questions concerning patients' capacity for self-care, reliability in following a therapeutic regimen, ability not merely to drive a car but to handle traffic emergencies (Brouwer and Withaar, 1997; Haikonen et al., 1998; Lundqvist, Alinder, Alm, et al., 1997) or appreciation of money and of their financial situation (Cahn, Sullivan, Shear, et al., 1998). When all the data of a comprehensive neuropsychological examination—the patient's history, background, and present situation; the qualitative observations; and the quantitative scores—are taken together, the examiner should have a realistic appreciation of how the patient reacts to deficits and can best compensate for them, and whether and how retraining could be profitably undertaken (A.-L. Christensen and Caetano, 1996; Diller, 2000; Sohlberg and Mateer, 2001).

The relative sensitivity and precision of neuropsychological measurements make them well suited for following the course of many neurological diseases (Heaton, Grant, Butters, et al., 1995; Wild and Kaye, 1998). Data from successive neuropsychological examinations repeated at regular intervals can provide reliable indications of whether the underlying neurological condition is changing, and if so, how rapidly and in what ways (e.g., Salmon, Heindel, and Lange, 1999). Parenté and Anderson (1984) used repeated testing to ascertain whether brain injured candidates for rehabilitation could learn well enough to warrant cognitive retraining. Freides (1985) recommended repeated testing to evaluate performance inconsistencies in patients with attentional deficits. Deterioration on repeated testing can identify a dementing process early in its course (J.C. Morris, McKeel, Storandt, et al., 1991; Paque and Warrington, 1995). Repeated testing may also be used to measure the effects of surgical procedures, medical treatment, or retraining.

A single, 27-year-old, highly skilled logger with no history of psychiatric disturbance underwent surgical removal of a right frontotemporal subdural hematoma resulting from a car accident. Twenty months later his mother brought him, protesting but docile, to the hospital. This alert, oriented, but poorly groomed man complained of voices that came from his teeth, explaining that he received radio waves and could "communicate to their source." He was emotionally flat with sparse speech and frequent 20- to 30-second response latencies that occasionally disrupted his train of thought. He denied depression and sleeping or eating disturbances. He also denied delusions or hallucinations, but during an interview pointed out Ichabod Crane's headless horseman while looking across the hospital lawn. As he became comfortable, he talked more freely and revealed that he was continually troubled by delusional ideation. His mother complained that he was almost completely reclusive, without initiative, and indifferent to his surroundings. He had some concern about being watched, and once she had heard him muttering, "I would like my mind back."

Most of his neuropsychological test scores were below those he had obtained when examined 6 1/2 months after the injury. His only scores above *average* were on two tests of well-learned verbal material: background information and reading vocabulary. He received scores in the *low average* to *borderline defective* ranges on oral arithmetic, visuomotor tracking, and all visual reasoning and visuoconstructive—including drawing—tests. Although his verbal learning curve was considerably below *average,* immediate verbal span and verbal retention were within the *average* range. Immediate recall of designs was *defective.*

Shortly after he was hospitalized and had completed the 20 month examination, he was put on trifluoperazine (Stelazine), 15 mg h.s., continuing this treatment for a month while remaining under observation. He was then reexamined. The patient was still poorly groomed, alert, and oriented. His reaction times were well *within normal limits.* Speech and thinking were unremarkable. While not expressing strong emotions, he smiled, complained, and displayed irritation appropriately. He reported what hallucinating had been like and related the content of some of his hallucinations. He talked about doing physical activities when he returned home but felt he was not yet ready to work.

His test scores 21 months after the injury were mostly in the *high average* to *superior* ranges. Much of his gain came from faster response times which enabled him to get full credit rather than partial or no credit on timed items he had completed perfectly but slowly the previous month. Although puzzle constructions (both geometric designs and objects) were performed at a *high average* level, his drawing continued to be of *low average* quality (but better than at 20 months). All verbal memory tests were performed at *average* to *high average* levels; his visual memory test response was without error, gaining him a *superior* rating. He did simple visuomotor tracking tasks without error and at an *average* rate of speed; his score on a complex visuomotor tracking task was at the 90th percentile.

In this case, repeated testing provided documentation of both the cognitive repercussions of his psychiatric disturbance and the effects of psychotropic medication on his cognitive functioning. This case demonstrates the value of repeated testing, particularly when one or another aspect of the patient's behavior appears to be in flux. Had testing been done only at the time of the second examination, a very distorted impression of the patient's cognitive status would have been gained. Fortunately, since the patient was in a research project, the first examination data were available to cast doubt on the validity of the second set of tests, performed when he was acutely psychotic, and therefore the third examination was given as well.

Brain impaired patients must have factual information about their functioning to understand themselves and to set realistic goals, yet their need for this information is often overlooked. Most people who sustain brain injury or disease experience changes in their self-awareness and emotional functioning; but because they are on the inside, so to speak, they may have difficulty appreciating how their behavior has changed and what about them is still the same (Prigatano and Schacter, 1991, *passim*). These misperceptions tend to heighten what mental confusion may already be present as a result of altered patterns of neural activity.

Distrust of their experiences, particularly their memory and perceptions, is a problem shared by many brain damaged persons, probably as a result of even very slight disruptions and alterations of the exceedingly complex neural pathways that mediate cognitive and other behavioral functions. This distrust seems to arise from the feelings of strangeness and confusion accompanying previously familiar habits, thoughts, and sensations that are now experienced differently and from newly acquired tendencies to make errors (T.L. Bennett and Raymond, 1997a; Lezak, 1978b. See also Skloot, 2003, for a poet's account of this experience). The self-doubt of the brain injured person, often referred to as "perplexity," is usually distinguishable from neurotic self-doubts about life goals, values, principles, and so on, but can be just as painful and emotionally crippling. Three years after undergoing a left frontal craniotomy for a parasagittal meningioma, a 45-year-old primary school teacher described this problem most tellingly:

Perplexity, the not knowing for sure if you're right, is difficult to cope with. Before my surgery I could repeat conversations verbatim. I knew what was said and who said it. . . . Since my surgery I don't have that capability anymore. Not being able to remember for sure what was said makes me feel very insecure.

Careful reporting and explanation of psychological findings can do much to allay the patient's anxieties and dispel confusion. The following case exemplifies both patients' needs for information about their psychological status and how disruptive even mild experiences of perplexity can be.

An attractive, unmarried 24-year-old bank teller sustained a brain concussion in a car accident while on a skiing trip in Europe. She appeared to have improved almost completely,

with only a little residual facial numbness. When she came home, she returned to her old job but was unable to perform acceptably although she seemed capable of doing each part of it well. She lost interest in outdoor sports although her coordination and strength were essentially unimpaired. She became socially withdrawn, moody, morose, and dependent. A psychiatrist diagnosed depression, and when her unhappiness was not diminished by counseling or antidepressant drugs, he administered electroshock treatment, which gave only temporary relief.

While waiting to begin a second course of shock treatment, she was given a neuropsychological examination at the request of the insurer responsible for awarding monetary compensation for her injuries. This examination demonstrated a small but definite impairment of auditory span, concentration, and mental tracking. The patient reported a pervasive sense of unsureness which she expressed in hesitancy and doubt about almost everything she did. These feelings of doubt had undermined her trust in many previously automatic responses, destroying a lively spontaneity that was once a very appealing feature of her personality. Further, like many postconcussion patients, she had compounded the problem by interpreting her inner uneasiness as symptomatic of "mental illness," and psychiatric opinion confirmed her fears. Thus, while her cognitive impairment was not an obstacle to rehabilitation, her bewildered experience of it led to disastrous changes in her personal life. A clear explanation of her actual limitations and their implications brought immediate relief of anxiety and set the stage for sound counseling.

The concerned family, too, needs to know about their patient's condition in order to respond appropriately (D.N. Brooks, 1991; Camplair et al., 2003; Lezak, 1988a, 1996; Proulx, 1999). Family members need to understand the patient's new, often puzzling, mental changes and what may be their psychosocial repercussions. Even quite subtle defects in motivation, in abilities to plan, organize, and carry out activities, and in self-monitoring can compromise patients' capacities to earn a living and thus render them socially dependent. Moreover, many brain impaired patients no longer fit easily into family life as irritability, self-centeredness, impulsivity, or apathy create awesome emotional burdens on family members, generate conflicts between family members and with the patient, and strain family ties, often beyond endurance (Lezak, 1978a, 1986b; L.M. Smith and Godfrey, 1995).

3. *Treatment-1: Treatment planning and remediation.* Today, much more of the work of neuropsychologists is involved in treatment or research on treatment (Vanderploeg, 1998). Rehabilitation programs for cognitive impairments and behavioral disorders arising from neuropathological conditions now have access to effective behavioral treatments based on neuropsychological knowledge and tested by neuropsychological techniques (for examples from many parts of the world see:

A.-L. Christensen and Uzzell, 2000; Pélissier, Barat, and Mazaux, 1991; Ponsford, 1995; Prigatano, 1999; Stuss, Winocur, and Robertson, 1999; B.A. Wilson and McLellan, 1997).

In the rehabilitation setting, the application of neuropsychological knowledge and neuropsychologically based treatment techniques to individual patients creates additional assessment demands: Sensitive, broad-gauged, and accurate neuropsychological assessment is necessary for determining the most appropriate treatment for each rehabilitation candidate with brain dysfunction (Allain et al., 1995; T.L. Bennett, 2001; Raskin and Mateer, 2000; Sloan and Ponsford, 1995; Sohlberg and Mateer, 2001). In addressing the behavioral and cognitive aspects of patient behavior, these assessments will include both delineation of problem areas and evaluation of the patient's strengths and potential for rehabilitation. In programs of any but the shortest duration, repeated assessments will be required to appreciate the patient's changing needs and competencies and adapt programs and goals correspondingly. Since rehabilitation treatment and care is often shared by professionals from many disciplines and their subspecialties, such as psychiatrists, speech pathologists, rehabilitation counselors, occupational and physical therapists, and visiting nurses, a current and centralized appraisal of patients' neuropsychological status enables these treatment specialists to maintain common goals and understanding of the patient. In addition, it can give an often more important analysis of how patients fail that will tell the therapist how patients might improve their performances in problem areas (e.g., Greenwald and Rothi, 1998; B.A. Wilson, 1986).

A 30-year-old lawyer, recently graduated in the top ten percent of his law school class, sustained a ruptured right anterior communicating artery aneurysm. Surgical intervention stopped the bleeding but left him with memory impairments that included difficulty in retrieving stored information when searching for it and very poor prospective memory (i.e., remembering to remember some activity originally planned or agreed upon for the future, or remembering to keep track of and use needed tools such as memory aids). Other deficits associable to frontal lobe damage included diminished emotional capacity, empathic ability, self-awareness, spontaneity, drive, and initiative-taking; impaired social judgment and planning ability; and poor self-monitoring. Yet he retained verbal and academic skills and knowledge, good visuospatial and abstract reasoning abilities, appropriate social behaviors, and motor function.

Following repeated failed efforts to enter the practice of law, his wife placed him in a recently organized rehabilitation program directed by a therapist whose experience had been almost exclusively with aphasic patients. The program emphasized training to enhance attentional functions and to compensate for memory deficits. This trainee learned how to keep a memory diary and notebook, which could support him through most of his usual activities and responsibilities; and he was appropriately drilled in the necessary memory and note-taking habits. What was overlooked was the overriding problem that it did not occur to him to remember what he needed to remember when he needed to remember it. (When his car keys were put aside where he could see them with instructions to get them when the examination was completed, at the end of the session he simply left the examining room and did not think of his keys until he was outside the building and I [mdl] asked if he had forgotten something. He then demonstrated a good recall of what he had left behind and where.)

One week after the conclusion of this costly eight-week program, while learning the route on a new job delivering in-house mail, he laid his memory book down somewhere and never found it again—nor did he ever prepare another one for himself despite an evident need for it. An inquiry into the rehabilitation program disclosed a lack of appreciation of the nature of frontal lobe damage and the needs and limitations of persons with brain injuries of this kind.

The same rehabilitation service provided a virtually identical training program to a 42-year-old civil engineer who had incurred severe attentional and memory deficits as a result of a rear-end collision in which the impact to his car threw his head forcibly back onto the head rest. This man was keenly and painfully aware of his deficits, and he retained strong emotional and motivational capacities, good social and practical judgment, and abilities for planning, initiation, and self-monitoring. He too had excellent verbal and visuospatial knowledge and skills, good reasoning ability, and no motor deficits. For him this program was very beneficial as it gave him the attentional training he needed and enhanced his spontaneously initiated efforts to compensate for his memory deficits. With this training he was able to continue doing work that was similar to what he had done before the accident, only on a relatively simplified level and a slower performance schedule.

4. *Treatment-2: Treatment evaluation.* With the ever-increasing use of rehabilitation and retraining services must come questions regarding their worth (Kashner et al., 2003). These services tend to be costly, both monetarily and in expenditure of professional time. Consumers and referring clinicians need to ask whether a given service promises more than can be delivered, or whether what is produced in terms of the patient's behavioral changes has psychological or social value and is maintained long enough to warrant the costs. Here again, neuropsychological assessment can help answer these questions (Sohlberg and Mateer, 1989; Trexler, 2000; Vanderploeg, 1998; see also Diller and Ben-Yishay, 2003; Kaszniak and Bortz, 1993; Ricker, 1998; and B.A. Wilson and Evans, 2003, for a discussion of the cost-effectiveness of neuropsychological evaluations of rehabilitation patients).

Neuropsychological evaluation can often best demonstrate the effects—both positive and negative—

of surgical (e.g., B.D. Bell and Davies, 1998, temporal lobectomy for seizure control; M.F. Newman et al., 2001, coronary artery bypass surgery; Vingerhoets, Van Nooten, and Jannes, 1996, open-heart surgery) or brain stimulation (e.g., Moretti et al., 2002a, to treat Parkinson's disease; Vallar, Rusconi, and Bernardini, 1996, to improve left visuospatial awareness) treatments of brain disorders and associated conditions. Testing for drug efficacy and side effects also requires neuropsychological assessment data (Meador, Loring, Hulihan, et al., 2003; C.M. Ryan and Hendrickson, 1998). Examples of these kinds of testing programs can be found for medications for many different conditions such as cancer (C.A. Meyers, Scheibel, and Forman, 1991), HIV (human immunodeficiency virus) (Llorente, van Gorp, et al., 2001), seizure control (Kelland and Lewis, 1996), attentional deficit disorders (Riordan, Flashman, Saykin, et al., 1999), multiple sclerosis (Fischer, Priore, et al., 2000), hypertension (Jonas et al., 2001), and psychiatric disorders: "difficulties with concentration, memory, and more complicated *executive* cognitive functions occur . . . secondary to many medications used to treat neurologic and other medical illnesses . . . modern neuropsychologic testing has allowed extensive batteries . . . to better define the [cognitive] deficits of individual patients" (Roy-Byrne and Fann, 1997, p. 967).

5. *Research*. Neuropsychological assessment has been used to study the organization of brain activity and its translation into behavior, and to investigate specific brain disorders and behavioral disabilities (this book, *passim*; see especially Chapters 2, 3, 7, and 8). Research with neuropsychological assessment techniques also involves their development, standardization, and evaluation. The precision and sensitivity of neuropsychological measurement techniques make them valuable tools for studying both the large and small—and sometimes quite subtle—behavioral alterations that are the externally and objectively observable manifestations of underlying brain pathology.

The practical foundations of clinical neuropsychology are also based to a large measure on neuropsychological research (see Hannay, Bieliauskas, et al., 1998: Houston Conference on Specialty Education and Training in Clinical Neuropsychology, 1998). Many of the tests used in neuropsychological evaluations—such as those for arithmetic or for visual memory and learning—were originally developed for the examination of normal cognitive functioning and recalibrated for neuropsychological use in the course of research on brain dysfunction. Other assessment techniques—such as certain tests of tactile identification or concept formation—were designed specifically for research on

normal brain dysfunction. Their subsequent incorporation into clinical use attests to the very lively exchange between research and practice. This exchange works especially well in neuropsychology because clinician and researcher are so often one and the same.

Neuropsychological research has also made crucial contributions to the study of normal behavior and brain functions. The following areas of inquiry afford only a partial glimpse into these rapidly expanding knowledge domains. Neuropsychological assessment techniques provide the data for interpreting brain mapping studies (e.g., Frackowiak, Friston, Frith et al., 1997, *passim;* Gold, Berman, Randolph, et al., 1996; S.C. Johnson et al., 2001; A.C. Roberts, Robbins, and Weiskrantz, 1998, *passim*). Cognitive status in normal aging has been tracked by neuropsychological assessments repeated over the course of years and even decades (e.g., Malec, Smith, Ivnik, et al., 1997; Snowdon, 1997; Tranel, Benton, and Olson, 1997). The roles that demographic characteristics play in the expression of mental abilities are often best delineated by neuropsychological findings (e.g., Ardila, Ostrosky-Solis, et al., 2000; Kempler, Teng, Dick, et al., 1998; Kimura, 1999; Vanderploeg, Axelrod, et al., 1997; Ylikoski, Ylikoski, Erkinjuntti, et al., 1998). Increasingly precise analyses of specific cognitive functions have been made possible by neuropsychological assessment techniques (e.g., Dollinger, 1995; Schretlen, Pearlson, Anthony, et al., 2000; Troyer, Moscovitch, and Winocur, 1997).

6. *Forensic Neuropsychology*. Neuropsychological assessment undertaken for legal proceedings has become quite commonplace in personal injury actions in which monetary compensation is sought for claims of bodily injury and loss of function (Heilbronner and Pliskin, 2003; McCaffrey, Williams, Fisher, and Laing, 1997; Nemeth, 1993; Sweet, 1999a). Although the forensic arena may be regarded as requiring some differences in assessment approaches, most questions referred to a neuropsychologist will either ask for a diagnostic opinion (e.g., "Has this person sustained brain damage as a result of . . . ?") or a description of the subject's neuropsychological status (e.g., "Will the behavioral impairment due to the subject's neuropathological condition keep him from gainful employment? Will treatment help to return her to the workplace?"). Usually the referral for a neuropsychological evaluation will include (or at least imply) both questions (e.g., "Are the subject's memory complaints due to . . . , and if so, how debilitating are they?"). In such cases, the neuropsychologist attempts to determine whether the claimant has sustained brain impairment which is associable to the injury in question. When the claimant is brain impaired, an evaluation of the type and amount

of behavioral impairment sustained is intrinsically bound up with the diagnostic process. In such cases the examiner typically estimates the claimant's rehabilitation potential along with the extent of any need for future care. Not infrequently the request for compensation may hinge on the neuropsychologist's report.

In criminal cases, a neuropsychologist may assess a defendant when there is reason to suspect that brain dysfunction contributed to the misbehavior or when there is a question about mental capacity to stand trial. The case of the murderer of President Kennedy's alleged assailant remains as probably the most famous instance in which a psychologist determined that the defendant's capacity for judgment and self-control was impaired by brain dysfunction (J. Kaplan and Waltz, 1965). Interestingly, the possibility that the defendant, Jack Ruby, had psychomotor epilepsy was first raised by Dr. Roy Schafer's interpretation of the psychological test findings and subsequently confirmed by electroencephalographic (EEG; i.e., brain wave) studies. At the sentencing stage of a criminal proceeding, the neuropsychologist may also be asked to give an opinion about treatment or potential for rehabilitation of a convicted defendant.

Use of neuropsychologists' examination findings, opinions, and testimony in the legal arena has engendered what, from some perspectives, seems to be a whole new industry dedicated to unearthing malingerers and exaggerators whose poor performances on neuropsychological tests make them appear to be cognitively impaired—or more impaired, in cases where impairment may be mild. To this end, a multitude of examination techniques and new tests have been devised (Chapter 20; also see J.S. Hayes, Hilsabeck, and Gouvier, 1999; Pankratz, 1998; Vickery et al., 2001). Whether the problem of malingering and symptom exaggeration in neuropsychological examinations is as great as the proliferation of techniques for identifying faked responding would suggest remains unanswered. Certainly, when dealing with forensic issues the examining neuropsychologist must be alert to the possibility that claimants in tort actions or defendents in criminal cases may—deliberately or unwittingly—perform below their optimal level; but the examiner must also remain mindful that for most examinees their dignity is a most prized attribute that is not readily sold. Moreover, base rates of malingering or symptom exaggeration probably vary with the population under study: TBI patients in a general clinical population would probably have a lower rate than those referred by defense lawyers who have an opportunity to screen claimants—and settle with those who are unequivocally injured—before referring the questionable cases for further study (e.g., Fox, et al., 1995; see Stanczak et al.,

2000, for a discussion of subject-selection biases in neuropsychological research; Ruffalo, 2003, for a discussion of examiner bias).

Usually a neuropsychological examination serves more than one purpose. Even though the examination may be initially undertaken to answer a single question such as a diagnostic issue, the neuropsychologist may uncover vocational or family problems, or patient care needs that have been overlooked, or the patient may prove to be a suitable candidate for research. Integral to all neuropsychological assessment procedures is an evaluation of the patient's needs and circumstances from a *psychological* perspective that considers quality of life, emotional status, and potential for social integration. When new information that has emerged in the course of an examination raises additional questions, the neuropsychologist will enlarge the scope of inquiry to include newly identified issues, as well as those stated in the referral.

Should a single examination be undertaken to serve several purposes—diagnosis, patient care, and research—a great deal of data may be collected about the patient and then applied selectively. For example, the examination of patients complaining of immediate memory problems can be conducted to answer various questions. A diagnostic determination of whether immediate memory is impaired may only require finding out if they can recall significantly fewer words of a list and numbers of a series than the slowest intact adult. To understand how they are affected by memory dysfunction, it is important to know the number of words they can recall freely and under what conditions, the nature of their errors, their awareness of and reactions to their deficit and its effect on their day-to-day activities. Research might involve studying immediate memory in conjunction with blood sugar levels or brain wave tests, or comparing the performance of these memory impaired persons to that of patients with other kinds of memory complaints.

THE VALIDITY OF NEUROPSYCHOLOGICAL ASSESSMENT

A question that has been repeatedly raised about the usefulness and validity of neuropsychological assessments concerns its "ecological" validity. *Ecological validity* typically refers to how well the neuropsychological assessment data predict future behavior or behavioral outcomes. These questions have been partially answered—almost always affirmatively—in research that has examined relationships between neuropsychological findings and ultimate diagnoses, e.g., the detection of dementia (Bondi, Salmon, Galasko, et al., 1999;

G.J. Meyer et al., 2001), between neuropsychological findings and imaging data (E.D. Bigler, 2001b), and between neuropsychological findings and employability for example (see also Sbordone and Long, 1996; B.A. Wilson, 1993).

Most recently very specific studies on the predictive accuracy of neuropsychological data have appeared for a variety of behavioral conditions: Prediction of treatment outcome for substance abuse patients rested significantly on Digit Span Backward and the Beck Depression Inventory (Teichner et al., 2001). Hanks and colleagues (1999) found that measures of executive function (Letter-Number Sequencing, Controlled Oral Word Assocation Test, Trail Making Test-B, Wisconsin Card Sorting Test) along with story recall (Logical Memory) "were strongly related to measures of functional outcome 6 months after rehabilitation" of patients with spinal cord injury, orthopedic disorders, or TBI (p. 1030). HIV$^+$ patients' employability varied with their performances on tests of memory, cognitive flexibility, and psychomotor speed (van Gorp, Baerwald, Ferrando, et al., 1999). Neuropsychological test findings that correlated significantly with the functional deficits of multiple sclerosis were on the California Verbal Learning Test–long delay free recall, the Paced Auditory Serial Addition Test, the Symbol Digit Modalities Test, and two recall items from the Rivermead Behavioral Memory Test (Higginson et al., 2000).

Several aspects of the very practical prediction of ability to perform activities of daily living (ADL) have been explored (A. Baird, Podell, et al., 2001; Cahn, Sullivan, et al., 1998; Cahn-Weiner, Boyle, and Malloy, 2002). Deloche and his coworkers (1996) report a strong relationship between scores on an arithmetic test battery and those on an ADL questionnaire. The Hooper Visual Organization Test above all, but also the Boston Naming Test and immediate recall of Logical Memory and Visual Reproduction were predictive of safety and independence in several activity domains (E.D. Richardson, Nadler, and Malloy, 1995). A comparison of rehabilitation inpatients who fail and those who do not showed that the former made more perseverative errors on the Wisconsin Card Sorting Test and performed more poorly on the Stroop and Visual Form Discrimination tests (Rapport, Hanks, et al., 1998). The problem of predicting driving competency was addressed by J.E. Meyers, Volbrecht, and Kaster-Bundgaard (1999), who reviewed the data from several hundred examination protocols of persons referred for neuropsychological assessment. They report that discriminant function analysis was 94.4% accurate in identifying competence and noncompetence in driving.

A number of studies have looked at TBI outcome predictions. S.R. Ross and his colleagues (1997) report that two tests, the Rey Auditory Verbal Learning Test and the Trail Making Test together and "in conjunction with age significantly predicted psychosocial outcome after TBI as measured by patient report" (p. 168). A review of studies examining work status after TBI found that a number of neuropsychological tests were predictive, especially "measures of executive functions and flexibility" (p. 23); specifically named tests were the Wisconsin Card Sorting Test, a dual—attention and memory—task, the Trail Making Test-B, and the Tinker Toy Test; findings on the predictive success (for work status) of memory tests varied considerably (Crépeau and Scherzer, 1993). Another study of TBI patients' return to work found that, "Neuropsychological test performance is related to important behavior in outpatient brain-injury survivors" (p. 382), and further noted that, "no measures of trauma severity contributed in a useful way to this prediction (of employment/unemployment)" (p. 391) (M.L. Bowman, 1996). T.W. Teasdale and colleagues (1997) also documented the validity of tests—of visuomotor speed and accuracy and complex visual learning given before entry into rehabilitation—as predictors of return to work after rehabilitation.

WHAT CAN WE EXPECT OF NEUROPSYCHOLOGICAL ASSESSMENT AT THE BEGINNING OF THIS NEW CENTURY?

In the 1995 edition of this book, the question was asked, "What might the future hold for neuropsychological assessment?" From neuropsychology's past history it was easy to predict correctly that there would be a continuing proliferation of tests, batteries, nontest assessment approaches, and technical refinements for many of these assessment tools. Moreover, what was predicted in 1995 appears to be valid today: i.e., if present trends augur the future, we can expect more and more varied applications of neuropsychological assessment in both clinical and theoretical research in medicine, the neurosciences, education, and the social sciences as well (e.g., see Cacioppo, Berntson, et al., 2002).

Some specific trends predicted in 1995 will certainly continue into the future. Concerns about the validity of test and battery based interpretations and predictions have been addressed by many researchers using a variety of techniques applied to an even wider variety of tests. For example, some studies provide new norms or examine the validity of tests of very specific aspects of such functions as visual memory (Barr, Chelune,

Hermann, et al., 1997; Paolo, Tröster, and Ryan, 1998a,b); concept formation and mental flexibility (Holtz, Gearhart, and Watson, 1996; Kozel and Meyers, 1998; Upton and Thompson, 1999), and verbal abilities (Ruff, Light, Parker, and Levin, 1996; Warrington, 1997). Other studies have analyzed the components of tests (e.g., *Line Bisection:* Luh, 1995; *Money Road-Map Test:* Vingerhoets, Lannoo, and Bauwens, 1996; *Wisconsin Card Sorting Test:* Greve, Ingram, and Bianchini, 1998). Still other studies have focussed on the neuropsychological and statistical bases of test batteries (e.g., the *CANTAB Battery:* Robbins, James, Owen, et al., 1998; the *Halstead-Reitan Battery:* Dikmen, Heaton, Grant, and Temkin, 1999; the *Wechsler Adult Intelligence Scale-III:* Kreiner and Ryan, 2001; J.J. Ryan and Paolo, 2001).

Computerized assessment programs have been proliferating and may be on the verge of assuming a dominant place in the neuropsychological assessment repertory. The advantages and disadvantages of computerized assessment have been reviewed, with recommendations and cautions (e.g., K.M. Adams and Heaton, 1987; Bleiberg et al., 2000; Gonzalez et al., 2003; Larrabee and Crook, 1996). Guidelines for the appropriate and ethical computerization of neuropsychological assessments, first published in 1987, are valid today and should be reviewed by anyone contemplating the introduction of computerized programs into their examination procedures (see Matthews, 1991). However, a perusal of recently published articles, books, and test publishers' catalogues suggests that, by and large, most clinicians and research examiners continue to rely primarily on clinical assessment techniques with some use of specialized computer programs (e.g., for the *Category Test,* the *Continuous Performance Test,* the *Wisconsin Card Sorting Test*). Thus, while their development continues, computerized tests have a more adjunctive than central role in the practice of clinical neuropsychology. However, their use for large-scale research and study programs is increasing (Anger, Rohlman, and Storzbach, 1999; Anger, Storzbach, et al., 1998; Bowler, Thaler, et al., 1990).

By 1995, the need to develop appropriate assessment techniques and test norms for older age groups had become urgent. That need has been well-satisfied since then in books (e.g., Nussbaum, 1997; Tuokko and Hadjistavropoulos, 1998; Woodruff-Pak, 1997) and in journals. It is now rare for an issue of any of the most popular neuropsychology journals to appear that does not contain at least one article dealing with some aspect of the aging brain, its competencies, and its vicissitudes.

One measure of the degree to which neuropsychology has become an accepted and valued partner in both clinical and research enterprises is its dispersion to cultures other than Western European, and its applications to language groups other than those for which tests were originally developed. At the beginning of the 21st century, neuropsychology is facing new challenges to its usefulness posed by the need for both greater cross-cultural sensitivity (Nell, 1999; Pontón and León-Carrión, 2001; Shepard and Leathem, 1999) and more language-appropriate tests (see Chapter 6, pp. 313–314). The increase in demands for neuropsychological assessment of persons with limited or no English language background has been the impetus for developing instruments written in the patient's language and standardized on persons in that patient's culture and language group; use of interpreters is only a second-best partial solution (Artioli y Fortuny and Mullaney, 1998; LaCalle, 1987). In the United States and Mexico, test developers and translators have begun to respond to the need for Spanish language tests with appropriate standardization (e.g., Acevedo et al., 2000; Ardila, 2000b; Pontón and León-Carrión, 2001; Stricks, Pittman, Jacobs, et al., 1998; Taussig, Mack, and Henderson, 1996). Studies providing norms and analyses of tests in Chinese reflect the increasing application of neuropsychological assessment in the Far East (Chan and Poon, 1999; Hua, Chang, and Chen, 1997; Lu and Bigler, 2000). These are good beginnings, as a next important goal for neuropsychological assessment should be the dissemination of research-based language- and culture-appropriate neuropsychological examination techniques and skills.

While real progress has been made over the last few decades in understanding cognitive and other neuropsychological processes and how to assess them, further knowledge is needed for tests and testing procedures to be sufficiently organized and standardized that assessments may be reliably reproducible, practically valid, and readily comprehensible. The range of disorders and disease processes, the variation in the presentation of each across individuals, the overlapping presentations of disorders and diseases, their pharmacologic and other treatments, and the interaction between the effects of these disorders make it unlikely that any "one size fits all" battery can be developed or should even be contemplated. Reitan noted as early as 1964 that, "We may be able to accumulate large enough groups [for normative purposes] within the next 20 years, but we would hope by that time the results might have lost their significance at least partially through obsoletion of the test battery." However, today's knowledge about the neuropathological and psychological entities that are the subject of neuropsychology together with the increasingly sensitive statistical techniques for test evaluation should lead to some simplification and generalization in examination procedures.

One means of achieving such a goal while retaining the flexibility appropriate for the great variety of persons and problems dealt with in neuropsychological assessment could be a series of relatively short fixed batteries designed for use with particular disorders and diseases and specific deficit clusters (e.g., visuomotor dysfunction, short-term memory disorders). Neuropsychologists in the future would then have at their disposal a set of test modules and perhaps structured interviews (each containing several tests) that can be upgraded as knowledge increases and that can be applied in various combinations to answer particular questions and meet specific patients' needs.

2 | Basic Concepts

If our brains were so simple that we could understand them, we would be so simple that we could not.

Anonymous [from dwl]

EXAMINING THE BRAIN

The usual clinical approach to the study of brain functions has, historically, been the neurological examination, which includes extensive study of the brain's chief product—behavior. The neurologist examines the strength, efficiency, reactivity, and appropriateness of the patient's responses to commands, questions, discrete stimulation of particular neural subsystems, and challenges to specific muscle groups and motor patterns. The neurologist also examines body structures, looking for such evidence of brain dysfunction as swelling of the retina or atrophied muscles due to insufficient neural stimulation. In the neurological examination of behavior, the clinician reviews behavior patterns generated by neuroanatomical subsystems, measuring patients' responses in relatively coarse gradations or noting their absence.

Following the development of scanning techniques, beginning in the mid-1970s, imaging has become a critical part of the diagnostic workup for most patients. *Computerized tomography* (*CT*) and *magnetic resonance imaging* (*MRI*) techniques reconstruct different densities and constituents of internal structures into clinically useful shadow pictures of the intracranial anatomy (Beauchamp and Bryan, 1997; R.O. Hopkins, Abildskov, et al., 1997; Hurley et al., 2002).

Neuropsychological assessment is another method of examining the brain by studying its behavioral product. Since the subject matter of neuropsychological assessment is behavior, it relies on many of the same techniques, assumptions, and theories as does psychological assessment. Also like psychological assessment, neuropsychological assessment involves the *intensive* study of behavior by means of interviews and standardized scaled tests and questionnaires that provide relatively precise and sensitive indices of behavior. The distinctive character of neuropsychological assessment lies in a conceptual frame of reference that takes brain function as its point of departure. Regardless of whether a behavioral study is undertaken for clinical or research

purposes, it is neuropsychological so long as the questions that prompted it, the central issues, the findings, or the inferences drawn from them ultimately relate to brain function. Like neurology, the findings are interpreted within the clinical context of the patient's presentation and other observations (see Chapter 5).

Direct observation of the fully integrated functioning of living human brains will probably always be impossible, although many rapidly evolving technological advances are bringing us closer to this goal (D'Esposito and Postle, 2002; Heeger and Ress, 2002). These newer examinations techniques rely upon indirect, typically noninvasive, methods. Originally developed for clinical examinations, these techniques are also used by cognitive neuroscientists and neuropsychologists to examine correlates of virtually all aspects of behavior in both patient populations and healthy subjects (e.g., see Gazzaniga, 2000, *passim*; Hugdahl and Davidson, 2003, *passim*).

The earliest instruments for studying brain function that continue to be in use are electrophysiological (e.g., see Daube, 2002, *passim*). These include *electroencephalography* (*EEG*), *electrodermal activity,* and *evoked* and *event-related potential* (*EP, ERP*). EEG frequency and patterns not only are affected by many brain diseases but have also been used to study aspects of cognition; e.g., high frequency has been associated with attentional activity for decades (Sheer and Schrock, 1986; Oken and Chiappa, 1985). Some investigators now hypothesize that it documents conscious awareness by demonstrating integrated neural activity across distributed cerebral regions (Crick and Koch, 1998; Meador, Ray, Echauz et al., 2002). *Magnetoencephalography* (the magnetic cousin of the EEG that records magnetic rather than electrical fields) has also been increasingly used to examine brain functions in patients and healthy volunteers alike (Reite, Cullum, et al., 1993; Reite, Teale, and Rojas, 1999).

Electrodermal activity (with components such as skin conductance level and galvanic skin response) reflects autonomic nervous system functioning, provides a measure of emotional response (Bauer, 1998; Critchley, 2002; Zahn and Mirsky, 1999), and has demonstrated recognition in the absence of conscious perception (Tranel and Damasio, 2000). Both EP and ERPs have demonstrated hemispheric specialization (Papanicolaou,

Moore, Deutsch, et al., 1988; Papanicolaou, Moore, Levin, and Eisenberg, 1987) and processing speed and efficiency (J.J. Allen, 2002; Picton et al., 2000; Zappoli, 1988).

The large volumes of data generated by these techniques may be quantified and analyzed using a variety of statistical methods. Quantified data may then be displayed on a stylized head or brain image or MRI, a practice that is often referred to as *brain mapping* (F.H. Duffy, Iyer, and Surwillo, 1989; Nuwer, 1989). Numerous technological and methodological problems in this practice, however, lead to a high rate of erroneous interpretations. Thus, whether EEG/EP brain mapping techniques should be employed in routine clinical assessments of many different kinds of patients has become a controversial issue (Nuwer, 1997).

Other noninvasive methods that permit the study (and visualization) of ongoing brain activity (Friedland, 1990; Oder et al., 1996) are often collectively called *functional brain imaging*. These techniques have proven useful for exploring both normal brain functioning and the nature of specific brain disorders (Buckner, 2000; Pincus and Tucker, 2003, *passim*; P. Zimmerman and Leclercq, 2002). Neuropsychologists interested in these methods should become familiar with the many assumptions and methodological concerns about them (see Papanicolaou, 1999, for a review).

Regional cerebral blood flow (*rCBF*), one of the older functional brain imaging techniques, reflects the brain's metabolic activity indirectly as changes in the magnitude of blood flow in different brain regions. rCBF provides a relatively inexpensive means for visualizing and recording brain function (D.J. Brooks, 2001; Deutsch et al., 1988; Nobler, Mann, and Sackeim, 1999; Nobler, Olvet, and Sackeim, 2002; Risberg, 1989). *Positron emission tomography* (*PET*) visualizes brain metabolism directly as glucose radioisotopes emit decay signals, their quantity indicating the level of brain activity in a given area (Oder et al., 1996; J.C. Patterson and Kotrla, 2002; C. Price and Friston, 2003). PET not only contributes valuable information about the functioning of diseased brains but has also become an important tool for understanding normal brain activity (Aguirre, 2003; Cabeza and Nyberg, 2000; George et al., 2000; Reiman et al., 2000; Rugg, 2002; Tzourio et al., 1995). *Single photon emission computed tomography* (*SPECT*) is similar to PET but less expensive and involves a contrast agent that is readily available. Comparison of interictal and ictal SPECT scans in epilepsy surgery candidates has been valuable for identifying seizure onset (So, 2000). In studies of cognition and other forms of behavior, these procedures typically compared data obtained during an activation task of interest (e.g., verbalizations) to data from a resting or other control state. The contribution of the activation task is inferred from the differences between the two task conditions.

However, each of these procedures has limitations. For example, PET applications are limited by their dependence on radioisotopes that must be generated in a nearby cyclotron and have only a short half-life (J.C. Patterson and Kotrla, 2002) and by their cost (Reiman et al., 2000). SPECT generally does not have the necessary temporal and spatial resolution for use in activation studies of cognition. Moreover, many studies using these methods to investigate brain–behavior relationships report group findings rather than for individuals, thus limiting their clinical application.

Functional magnetic resonance imaging (*fMRI*) has already produced an impressive number of studies, and this can be expected to increase at an ever expanding rate. In addition to the many current clinical applications of motor and language mapping, fMRI has become a popular method for investigating traditional psychological processes such as time perception (S.M. Rao, Mayer, and Harrington, 2001), semantic processing (Bookheimer, 2002), emotional processing (M.S. George et al., 2000; R.C. Gur, Schroder, et al., 2002), response inhibition (Durston et al., 2002), face recognition (Joseph and Gathers, 2002), somatosensory processing (Meador, Allison, Loring et al., 2002), sexual arousal (Arnow et al., 2002), and many others. More than the other procedures discussed, fMRI will greatly affect neuropsychology as well as cognitive neuroscience in general, in part due to its widespread use.

The clinical need to identify cerebral language and memory dominance in neurosurgery candidates led to the development of invasive techniques such as the *Wada test* (intracarotid injection of amobarbital for temporary pharmacological inactivation of one side of the brain) and electrical cortical stimulation mapping to minimize the surgical risk to these functions (Loring, Meador, Lee, and King, 1992; Branch, Milner, and Rasmussen, 1964; Ojemann, Cawthon, and Lettich, 1990; Penfield and Rasmussen, 1950). Not only have these procedures significantly reduced cognitive morbidity following epilepsy surgery, but they have also greatly enhanced our knowledge of brain–behavior relationships. Atypical language representation, for example, alters the expected pattern of neuropsychological findings, even in the absence of large cerebral pathology (Loring, Strauss, et al., 1999).

These procedures have impediments in that they are invasive and afford only a limited range of assessable behavior due to the restrictions on patient response in an operating theater and the short duration of medication effects. Generalizability of data obtained by this technique is further limited by the atypical functioning of these patients' diseased or damaged brains.

Many of the same questions addressed by the Wada test and cortical stimulation mapping in patients may be answered in studies of healthy volunteers using such noninvasive techniques as *transcranial magnetic stimulation* (C.M. Epstein et al., 1999; L.C. Robertson and Rafal, 2000), *functional transcranial Doppler* (Knecht et al., 2000), *magnetoencephalography/magnetic source imaging* (Papanicolaou et al., 2001; Simos, Breier et al., 1999; Simos, Castillo, et al., 2001), and *fMRI* (J.R. Binder, Swanson, et al., 1996; Desmond et al., 1995; Detre et al., 1998; W.D. Gaillard et al., 2000; Jokeit et al., 2001).

"BRAIN DAMAGE" AND "ORGANICITY"

Throughout the 1930s and 40s and well into the 50s, most clinicians treated "brain damage" or brain dysfunction as if it were a unitary phenomenon— "organicity." The determination of whether a patient was "organic" was often the reason for neuropsychological consultation. It was well recognized that brain damage resulted from many different conditions and had different effects (Babcock, 1930; Klebanoff, 1945) and that certain specific brain–behavior correlates, such as the role of the left hemisphere in language functions, appeared with predictable regularity. Yet much of the work with "brain damaged" patients was based on the assumption that organicity was characterized by one central and therefore universal behavioral defect (K. Goldstein, 1939; Yates, 1954). Even so thoughtful an observer as Teuber could say in 1948 that, "Multiple-factor hypotheses are not necessarily preferable to an equally tentative, heuristic formulation of a general factor—the assumption of a fundamental disturbance . . . which appears with different specifications in each cerebral region. In fact, the assumption of a fundamental disturbance may have definite advantages at the present state of knowledge" (pp. 45–46).

The early formulations of brain damage as a unitary condition that is either present or absent were reflected in the proliferation of single function tests of "organicity" that were evaluated, in turn, solely in terms of how well they distinguished "organic" from psychiatric patients or normal control subjects (e.g., Klebanoff, 1945; Spreen and Benton, 1965; Yates, 1954). The "fundamental disturbance" of brain damage, however, turned out to be exasperatingly elusive. Despite many ingenious efforts to devise a test or examination technique that would be sensitive to organicity per se— a neuropsychological litmus paper, so to speak—no one behavioral phenomenon could be found that was shared by all brain injured persons but by no one else. This one-dimensional approach to neuropsychological

assessment continues to show up occasionally in the literature and in clinical assumptions.

In neuropsychology's next evolutionary stage, "brain damage" was still treated as a unitary phenomenon but was given measurable extension. The theoretical basis for this position had been provided by Karl Lashley in his *Law of Mass Action* and *Principle of Equipotentiality* (1929). Lashley knew that even in rats certain functions, such as visual discrimination, were predictably compromised by lesions involving well-defined cortical areas of the brain. However, his experiments with rats led him to conclude that by and large the effectiveness of an animal's behavior and the extent to which its cortex was intact were directly correlated regardless of the site of damage, and that the contributions of different parts of the cortex were interchangeable.

In their once popular paper, L.F. Chapman and Wolff (1959) reviewed the literature on localization of function, presented data on their patients, and concluded, with Lashley, that sheer extent of cortical loss played a greater role in determining the amount of cognitive impairment than did the site of the lesion. "Brain damage" (or "organicity" or "organic impairment"— the terms varied from author to author but the meaning was essentially the same) took on a one-dimensionality and lack of specificity similar to that of the concept "sick." Neither "brain damage" nor "sickness" has etiological implications; neither implies the presence or absence of any particular symptoms or signs, nor can predictions or prescriptions be made on the basis of either term. Still, "brain damage" as a unitary but measurable condition remains a vigorous concept, reflected in the many test and battery indices, ratios, and quotients that purport to represent some quantity or relative degree of neurobehavioral impairment.

Advances in diagnostic medicine, with the exception of certain cases with mild or questionable cognitive impairment, have changed the typical referral question to the neuropsychologist from one that attempts to determine if the patient has neurologic disease or not. In most cases, the presence of "brain damage" has been clinically established and often verified radiologically. However, the *behavioral* repercussions of brain damage vary with the nature, extent, location, and duration of the lesion; with the age, sex, physical condition, and psychosocial background and status of the patient; and with individual neuroanatomical and physiological differences (see Chapters 3, 7, and 8). Not only does the pattern of neuropsychological deficits differ with different lesion characteristics and locations, but two persons with similar pathology and lesion sites may have distinctly different neuropsychological profiles (DeBleser, 1988; Howard, 1997; Luria, 1970). In contrast, patients with damage at different sites may present similar deficits (Naeser, Palumbo, et al., 1989). Thus, although "brain damage" may be useful as an organizing concept for a broad range of behavioral disorders, when dealing with individual patients the concept of brain damage only becomes meaningful in terms of specific behavioral dysfunctions and their implications regarding underlying brain pathology.

CONCERNING TERMINOLOGY

The experience of wading through the older neuropsychological literature shares some characteristics with exploring an archaeological dig into a long-inhabited site. Much as the archaeologist finds artifacts that are both similar and different, evolving and discarded, so a reader can find, scattered through the decades, descriptions of the various neuropsychological disorders in terms (usually names of syndromes or behavioral anomalies) no longer in use and forgotten by most, terms that have evolved from one meaning to another, and terms that have retained their identity and currency pretty much as when first coined. Moreover, not all earlier terms given to the same neuropsychological phenomena over the past ten decades have been supplanted or fallen into disuse so that even the relatively recent literature may contain two or more expressions for the same or similar observations (e.g., see p. 33 for current aphasia terms, pp. 26, 34–35 for varieties of "working memory"). This rich terminological heritage can be very confusing, as Newcombe and Ratcliffe (1989) point out in their discussion of the terminological problems attendant on the study of disorders of visuospatial analysis. (See also Lishman's [1997] discussion of the terminological confusion surrounding "confusion," for example, and other common terms that are variously used to refer to mental states, to well-defined diagnostic entities, or to specific instances of abnormal behavior.)

In this book we have made an effort to use only terms that are currently widely accepted. Some still popular but poorly defined terms have been replaced by simpler and more apt substitutes for some of the classical terminology. For example, in order to distinguish those constructional disorders that have been called "constructional apraxia" from the neuropsychologically meaningful concept of praxis, which "in the strict sense, refers to the motor integration employed used to execute complex learned movements" (Strub and Black, 2000). We follow Strub and Black's lead by maintaining a terminological distinction between these functional classes. Thus we use "constructional defects" or "constructional impairment" to refer to these kinds of disorders; the term "apraxia" is reserved for the special class of dysfunctions characterized by a breakdown in the direction or execution of complex motor acts. "Apraxia" has problems of its own as different investigators define and use such terms as "ideational apraxia," "ideomotor apraxia," and "ideokinetic apraxia" in confusingly different ways (compare, for example, Hécaen and Albert, 1978; Heilman and Rothi, 2003; Walsh and Darby, 1999; M. Williams, 1979). Kimura and Archibald (1974) suggested that the forms of apraxia that have been called "ideational, ideomotor, ideokinetic, and so on" do not relate to "behaviorally different phenomena, but [to] disturbances at different points in a hypothetical sequence of cognitive events involved in making a movement." Rather than attempt to reconcile the many disparities in the use of these terms and their definitions, we call these disturbances simply "apraxias" (see also Hanna-Pladdy and Rothi, 2001).

DIMENSIONS OF BEHAVIOR

Behavior may be conceptualized in terms of three functional systems: (1) *cognition*, which is the information-handling aspect of behavior; (2) *emotionality*, which concerns feelings and motivation; and (3) *executive functions*, which have to do with how behavior is expressed. Components of each of these three sets of functions are as integral to every bit of behavior as are length and breadth and height to the shape of any object. Moreover, like the dimensions of space, each one can be conceptualized and treated separately. The early Greek philosophers were the first to conceive of a tripartite division of behavior, postulating that different principles of the "soul" governed the rational, appetitive, and animating aspects of behavior. Present-day research in the behavioral sciences tends to support the philosophers' intuitive insights into how the totality of behavior is organized. These classical and scientifically meaningful functional systems lend themselves well to the practical observation, measurement, and description of behavior and constitute a framework for organizing behavioral data generally.

In neuropsychology, the cognitive functions have received more attention than the emotional and control systems. This is partly because the cognitive defects of brain injured patients can figure so prominently in their symptomatology; partly because they can be so readily conceptualized, measured, and correlated with neuroanatomically identifiable systems; and partly because the structured nature of most medical and psychological examinations does not provide much opportunity for subtle emotional and control deficits to become evident.

However, brain damage rarely affects just one of these systems. Rather, the disruptive effects of most brain lesions, regardless of their size or location, usually involve all three systems (Lezak, 1994).

For example, Korsakoff's psychosis, a condition most commonly associated with severe chronic alcoholism, has typically been described only in terms of cognitive dysfunctions; e.g., "The characteristic feature of Korsakow's [sic] syndrome is a certain type of amnesia. The patient has a gross defect of memory for recent events so that he has no recollection of what has happened even half an hour previously. He is disoriented in space and time and he fills the gaps in his memory by confabulation, that is, by giving imaginary accounts of his activities" (Walton, 1994; see also Squire, 1987; Tranel and Damasio, 2002). Yet chronic Korsakoff patients also exhibit profound changes in affect and executive, or control, functions that may be more crippling and more representative of the psychological devastations of this disease than the memory impairments.

Patients with this condition tend to be emotionally flat, to lack the impulse to initiate activity, and, if given a goal requiring more than an immediate one- or two-step response, to be unable to organize, set into motion, and carry through a plan of action to reach it (Heindel, Salmon, and Butters, 1991). Everyday frustrations, sad events, or worrisome problems, when brought to their attention, will arouse a somewhat appropriate affective response, as will a pleasant happening or a treat; but the arousal is only transitory, subsiding with a change in topic or distraction such as someone entering the room. When not stimulated from outside or by physiological urges, these responsive, comprehending, often well-spoken and well-mannered patients sit quite comfortably doing nothing, not even attending to a TV or nearby conversation. When they have the urge to move, they walk about aimlessly. Even those who talk about wanting to visit a relative, for instance, or call a lawyer, make no effort to do so, although doors are unlocked and the public telephone is in full view.

The behavioral defects characteristic of many patients with right hemisphere damage also reflect the involvement of all three systems. It is well known that these patients are especially likely to show impairments in such cognitive activities as spatial organization, integration of visual and spatial stimuli, and comprehension and manipulation of percepts that do not readily lend themselves to verbal analysis. Right hemisphere damaged patients may also experience characteristic emotional dysfunctions such as an indifference reaction (ignoring, playing down, or being unaware of mental and physical disabilities and situational problems), uncalled-for optimism or even euphoria, inappropriate emotional responses and insensitivity to the feelings of others, and loss of the self-perspective needed for accurate self-criticism, appreciation of limitations, or making constructive changes in behavior or attitudes (Cummings and Mega, 2003; Cutting, 1990; Gainotti, 1972). Furthermore, despite strong, well-expressed motivations and demonstrated knowledgeability and capability, impairments in the capacity to plan and organize complex activities and thinking immobilize many of the same right hemisphere damaged patients who have difficulty performing visuospatial tasks (Brownell and Martino, 1998; Lezak, 1994).

Behavior problems may also become more acute and the symptom picture more complex as secondary reactions to the specific problems created by the brain injury further involve each system. Additional repercussions and reactions may then occur as the patient attempts to cope with succeeding sets of reactions and the problems they bring.

The following case of a man who sustained relatively minor brain injuries demonstrates some typical interactions between impairments in different psychological systems.

A middle-aged clerk, the father of teenaged children, incurred a left-sided head injury in a car accident and was unconscious for several days. When examined three months after the accident, his principal complaint was fatigue. His scores on cognitive tests were consistently *high average* (between the 75th and 90th percentiles). The only cognitive difficulty demonstrated in the psychological examination was a slight impairment of verbal fluency exhibited by a few word-use errors on a sentence-building task. This verbal fluency problem did not seem grave, but it had serious implications for the patient's adjustment.

Because he could no longer produce fluent speech automatically, the patient had to exercise constant vigilance and conscious effort to talk as well as he did. This effort was a continuous drain on his energy so that he fatigued easily. Verbal fluency tended to deteriorate when he grew tired, giving rise to a vicious cycle in which he put out more effort when he was tired, further sapping his energy at the times he needed it the most. He felt worn out and became discouraged, irritable, and depressed. Emotional control too was no longer as automatic or effective as before the accident, and it was poorest when he was tired. He "blew up" frequently with little provocation. His children did not hide their annoyance with their grouchy, sullen father, and his wife became protective and overly solicitous. The patient perceived his family's behavior as further proof of his inadequacy and hopelessness. His depression deepened, he became more self-conscious about his speech, and the fluency problem frequently worsened.

COGNITIVE FUNCTIONS

> Cognitive abilities (and disabilities) are functional properties of the individual that are not directly observed but instead are *inferred* from . . . behavior. . . . All behavior (including neuropsychological test performances) is multiply determined: a patient's failure on a test of abstract reasoning may not be due to a specific impairment in conceptual thinking but to attention disorder, verbal disability, or inability to discriminate the stimuli of the test instead.
> *Abigail B. Sivan and Arthur L. Benton, 1999*

The four major classes of cognitive functions have their analogues in the computer operations of input, storage, processing (e.g., sorting, combining, relating data in various ways), and output. Thus, (1) *receptive functions* involve the abilities to select, acquire, classify, and integrate information; (2) *memory and learning* refer to information storage and retrieval; (3) *thinking* concerns the mental organization and reorganization of information; and (4) *expressive functions* are the means through which information is communicated or acted upon. Each functional class comprises many discrete activities—such as color recognition or immediate memory for spoken words. Although each function constitutes a distinct class of behaviors, normally they work in close, interdependent concert. Despite the seeming ease with which the classes of cognitive functions can be distinguished conceptually, more than merely interdependent, they are inextricably bound together—different facets of the same activity. A.R. Damasio, H. Damasio, and Tranel (1990) describe the memory (information storage and retrieval) components of visual recognition. They also call attention to the role that thinking (concept formation) plays in the seemingly simple act of identifying a visual stimulus by name. Both practical applications and theory-making benefit from our ability to differentiate these various components of behavior.

Generally speaking, within each class of cognitive functions a division may be made between those functions that mediate verbal/symbolic information and those that deal with data that cannot be communicated in words or symbols, such as complex visual or sound patterns. These subclasses of functions differ from one another in their neuroanatomical organization and in their behavioral expression while sharing other basic neuroanatomical and psychometric relationships within the functional system.

The identification of discrete functions within each class of cognitive functions varies with the perspective and techniques of the investigator. Examiners using simple tests that elicit discrete responses can study highly specific functions. Multidimensional tests call for complex responses and thus measure broader and more complex functions. Verbal functions enter into verbal test responses. Motor functions are demonstrated on tests involving motor behavior. When practical considerations of time and equipment limit the functions that can be studied or when relevant tests are not administered, the examiner may remain ignorant of the untested functions or how their impairment contributes to a patient's deficits (Finger et al., 1988; Teuber, 1969). Although different investigators may identify or define some of the narrower subclasses of functions differently, they agree on the major functional systems and the large subdivisions.

However, these functional divisions are, to some extent, conceptual constructions that help the clinician understand what goes into the typically very complex behaviors and test responses of their brain damaged patients. Discrete functions described here and in Chapter 3 rarely occur in isolation; but rather contribute to the much more commonly seen larger patterns of dysfunction due to damage to a "continuous, graded functional[ly]" organized cerebral cortex (E. Goldberg, 1995).

Academic psychology studies attentional functions within the framework of cognitive psychology. However, attentional functions differ from the functional groups listed above in that they underlie and, in a sense, maintain the activity of the cognitive functions. To carry the computer analogy a step further, attentional functions serve somewhat as command operations, calling into play one or more cognitive functions. For this reason, they are classified as *mental activity variables* here (see pp. 33–35).

Neuropsychology and the Concept of Intelligence: Brain Function Is Too Complex To Be Communicated in a Single Score

> General intelligence is as valid as the "strength of soil" concept is for plant growers. It is not wrong but archaic.
>
> *J.P. Das, 1989*

Cognitive activity was originally attributed to a single function, *intelligence.* Early investigators treated the concept of intelligence as if it were a unitary variable which, like physical strength, increased at a regular rate in the course of normal childhood development (Binet and Simon, 1908; Terman, 1916) and decreased with the amount of brain tissue lost through accident or disease (L.F. Chapman and Wolff, 1959; Lashley, 1938). As refinements in testing and data-handling techniques have afforded greater precision and control over observations of cognitive activity, it has become evident that the behavior measured by "intelligence" tests involves specific cognitive and executive functions (Ardila, 1999a; Feinberg and Farah, 2003a; Frackowiak, Friston, Frith, 1997; Rains, 2002; see also Chapter 3).

Neuropsychological research has contributed significantly to the redefinition of the nature of "intelligence" (Gazzaniga, 2000, *passim;* Kolb and Wishaw, 1996; Mesulam, 2000b). One of neuropsychology's earliest findings was that the summation scores (i.e., "intelligence quotient" ["IQ"] scores) on standard intelligence tests do not bear a predictably direct relationship to the size of brain lesions (Hebb, 1942; Maher, 1963). When a discrete brain lesion produces deficits involving a broad range of cognitive functions, these functions may be affected in different ways. Abilities most directly served by the damaged tissue may be destroyed; associated or dependent abilities may be depressed or distorted, while some others may appear to be heightened or enhanced (e.g., see p. xx).

Differences in the vulnerability of specific mental abilities also characterize the effects of deteriorating brain disease (e.g., Filley, 2001; Mesulam, 2000a; Parks, Zec, and Wilson, 1993; see Chapter 7, *passim*). Not only are some functions disrupted in the early stages while others may remain relatively intact for years, but the affected functions also deteriorate at different rates. Differential deterioration of diverse psychological functions also occurs in aging (see pp. 296–300). Moreover, citing the lateral frontal lobes as the seat of "intelligence" because they are involved in various abstraction and conceptualizing tasks (J. Duncan et al., 2000) does not identify a cerebral locus for "intelligence" but rather illustrates one of the many different definitions of intelligence and is a nice example of circular reasoning. In sum, neuropsychological studies have not found a general cognitive or intellectual function, but rather many discrete ones that work together so smoothly in the intact brain that cognition is experienced as a single, seamless attribute.

From a neuropsychological perspective, Piercy (1964) defined intelligence as a "tendency for cerebral regions subserving different intellectual functions to be proportionately developed in any one individual. According to this notion, people with good verbal ability will tend also to have good non-verbal ability, in much the same way as people with big hands tend to have big feet" (p. 341). The performance of most adults on cognitive ability tests reflects both this tendency for test scores generally to converge around the same level and for some test scores to vary in differing degrees from the central tendency (Carroll, 1993; J.D. Matarazzo and Prifitera, 1989; Neisser et al., 1996). J.R. Flynn (1987, 1999), finding significant increases in large group "IQ" scores from generation to generation (the "Flynn effect"), concluded that these increases reflected changing environmental factors, presumably the same factors that contribute to intraindividual score convergence.

In cognitively intact adults, specialization of interests and activities and singular experiences contribute to intraindividual differences (Halpern, 1997). Socialization experiences, personal expectations, educational limitations, emotional disturbance, physical illness or handicaps, and brain dysfunction tend to magnify intraindividual test differences to significant proportions (e.g., see A.S. Kaufman, McLean, and Reynolds, 1988; Razani et al., 2001; Suzuki and Valencia, 1997).

Thus, the unitary concept of intelligence has only limited application in neuropsychological assessment. The concept of intelligence may seem to justify the practice of using the level of a cognitively impaired patient's best educational or vocational achievement or performance on an "intelligence" test as a best indicator of premorbid functioning—against which to compare current activities, observations, and test performances (see Chapter 4). However, psychologists have defined the concept of intelligence in so many different ways as to have lost what central meaning it originally had in philosophical discourse (Ardila, 1999a; Garcia, 1981). "Cognitive abilities" or "mental abilities" are the terms we will use when referring to those psychological functions dedicated to information reception, processing, and expression, and to executive functions—the abilities necessary for metacognitive control and direction of mental experience.

"IQ" and other summation or composite scores

> The term IQ is bound to the myths that intelligence is unitary, fixed, and predetermined. . . . As long as the term IQ is used, these myths will complicate efforts to communicate the meaning of test results and classification decisions.
>
> *D.J. Reschly, 1981*

"IQ" refers to a derived score used in many test batteries designed to measure a hypothesized general ability, intelligence. Because of the multiplicity of cognitive functions assessed in these batteries, IQ scores are not useful in describing cognitive test performances. IQ scores obtained from such tests represent a composite of performances on different kinds of items, on different items in the same tests when administered at different levels of difficulty, on different items in different editions of test batteries bearing the same name, or on different batteries contributing different kinds of items (Anastasi and Urbina, 1997; M.H. Daniel, 1997). If nothing else, the variability in sources from which the scores are derived should lead to serious questioning of their meaningfulness. Such composite scores are often good predictors of academic performance, which is not surprising given their heavy loading of school-type and culturally familiar items. Yet they represent so many different kinds of more or less confounded functions as to be conceptually meaningless (Lezak, 1988b).

In neuropsychological assessment in particular, IQ scores are often unreliable indices of neuropathic deterioration. Specific defects restricted to certain test modalities, for example, may give a totally erroneous impression of significant intellectual impairment when actually many cognitive functions may be relatively intact and lower total scores are a reflection of impairment of specific functional modalities. Conversely, IQs may obscure selective defects in specific tests (A. Smith, 1966, p. 56). Leatham (1999) illustrates this point with the case of a postencephalitic man who "could not learn anything new" but achieved an IQ score of 128.

In fact, any derived score based on a combination of scores from two or more measures of different abilities results in loss of data. Should the levels of performance for the combined measures differ, the composite score—which will be somewhere between the highest and the lowest of the combined measures—will be misleading (Lezak, 2002). Averaged scores on a Wechsler Intelligence Scale battery provide just about as much information as do averaged scores on a school report card. Students with a four-point average can only have had an A in each subject; those with a zero grade point average obviously failed all subjects. Excluding these extremes, it is impossible to predict a student's performance in any one subject. In the same way, it is impossible to predict specific disabilities and areas of competency or dysfunction from averaged ability test scores (e.g., "IQ" scores). Thus composite scores of any kind have no place in neuropsychological assessment.

"IQ" may also stand for the concept of intelligence; e.g., in statements like "IQ is a product of genetic and environmental factors." It may refer to the idea of an inborn quantity of mental ability residing within each person and demonstrable through appropriate testing; e.g., "Harry is a good student, he must have a high IQ" (Lezak, 1988b). Moreover, interpretations of IQ scores in terms of what practical meaning they might have can vary widely, even among professionals, such as high school teachers and psychiatrists, whose training should have provided a common understanding of these scores (L. Wright, 1970).

S.E. Folstein (1989) called attention to how, in the United States, current use of IQ scores contributes further misery to already tragic situations. She explained that many patients with Huntington's disease whose mental abilities have deteriorated beyond the point that they can continue working will still perform sufficiently well on enough of the tests in Wechsler Intelligence Scale batteries to achieve an IQ score above 70, the number selected by the Social Security Disability Insurance (SSDI) agency as separating those able to work from those too mentally impaired for competitive employment. Thus, SSDI may refuse benefits to cognitively disabled persons simply on the grounds that their IQ score is too high, even when appropriate assessment reveals a pattern of disparate levels of functioning that preclude the patient from earning a living. Similar problems affect severely injured *traumatic brain injury (TBI)* patients who have been refused benefits because their summed test score is too high, even though they lack the judgment, social graces, self-control, mental flexi-

bility, memory and attentional abilities, and stamina to hold down even a routine kind of job.

One must never misconstrue a normal intelligence test result as an indication of normal intellectual status after head trauma, or worse, as indicative of a normal brain; *to do so would be to commit the cardinal sin of confusing absence of evidence with evidence of absence* [italics, mdl]. (Teuber, 1969)

In sum, "IQ" as a score is inherently meaningless and not infrequently misleading as well. "IQ"—whether concept, score, or catchword—has outlived whatever usefulness it may once have had and should be discarded.

Unfortunately, other summary scores also obscure actual test performances. Probably the most venerable of these summary scores is the Digit Span score which, in the Wechsler batteries (Wechsler Intelligence Scales for Adults [p. 649]; Wechsler Memory Scales [p. 481]), includes not only both forward and reversed span scores—each examining different aspects of short-term auditory memory and attention (see pp. 351–352)—but further confounds the data by adding a reliability measure (i.e., two trials at each span length).

Combined scores such as the "Index Scores" in Wechsler batteries may also obscure important information obtainable only by examining discrete scores. The Wechsler Adult Intelligence Scale-III (WAIS-III) features several Index Scores which are compilations of scores of individual tests that load on the same factor *in large-scale population* studies (The Psychological Corporation, 1997). However, in the individual case, large differences between the discrete test scores can illuminate core problems which would be submerged by the summation Index Score (see p. 653).

CLASSES OF COGNITIVE FUNCTIONS

As more is learned about how the brain processes information, it becomes more difficult to make theoretically acceptable distinctions between the different functions involved in human information processing. In the laboratory, precise discriminations between sensation and perception may depend upon whether incoming information is processed by analysis of superficial physical and sensory characteristics or through pattern recognition and meaningful associations. The fluidity of theoretical models of perception and memory in particular becomes apparent in the admission of A.R. Damasio, Tranel, and Damasio (1989) that "We have no way of distinguishing what might be conceived of as the higher echelons of perception from the lower echelons of recognition. . . . [T]here is no definable point of demarcation between perception and recognition" (p. 317).

Further, studies of perception without awareness, such as *blindsight* (Weiskrantz, 1986) or covert face recognition in *prosopagnosia* (defective face recognition) (Farah, 2001; J.E. McNeil and Warrington, 1993) indicate how perception and awareness each depend upon intercellular networks in which information is transferred in both parallel and serial processing networks (Farah, O'Reilly, and Vecera, 1993; Fuster, 2003; Pashler, 1998).

Efforts to conceptualize memory functions come up against this same kind of theoretical problem. "Memory research in cognitive neuroscience has literally exploded within the past few years, leaving clinical neurologists and psychologists with a complex array of fragmented perspectives on memory, a variety of subdivisions of mnestic capacities, and a bundle of rivaling or just redundant 'models' and 'network' hypotheses" (Helmstaedter and Kurthen, 2001).

Rather than entering theoretical battlegrounds on ticklish issues that are not material to most practical applications in neuropsychology, we shall discuss these functions within a conceptual framework that has proven useful in psychological assessment generally and in neuropsychological assessment particularly.

Receptive Functions

Entry of information into the central processing system proceeds from sensory stimulation, i.e., *sensation*, through *perception*, which involves the integration of sensory impressions into psychologically meaningful data, and thence into memory. Thus, light on the retina creates a visual *sensation; perception* involves encoding the impulses transmitted by the aroused retina into a pattern of hues, shades, and intensities recognized as a daffodil in bloom.

Neuroscientists have discovered that the components of sensation can be splintered into ever smaller receptive units. The Nobel Prize winning research of Hubel and Weisel (1962, 1968) demonstrated that neurons in the visual cortex are arranged in columns that respond preferentially to stimuli at specific locations and at specific orientations. How discrete these subsystems may be is shown by the report of A.R. Damasio, Damasio, and Tranel (1990) that, "when fragments of a face are presented in isolation, for example, eyes or mouth, different neurons respond to different fragments."

Sensory reception

Sensory reception involves an arousal process that triggers central registration leading to analysis, encoding, and integrative activities. The organism receives sensation passively, shutting it out only, for instance, by holding the nose to avoid a stench. Even in soundest slumber, a stomach ache or a loud noise will rouse the sleeper. However, sensations are rarely experienced in themselves, and perceptions depend greatly on attentional factors (Meador, Allison, et al., 2002; Meador, Ray et al., 2001). Most sensory data enter neurobehavioral systems as perceptions already endowed with previously learned meanings (Forde and Humphreys, 1999; Goodale, 2000; Shiffrin and Schneider, 1977). Neuropsychological assessment and research focus primarily on the five traditionally recognized senses: sight, hearing, touch, taste, and smell. Berthoz (2000) calls attention to other senses such as movement, space, balance, and effort.

Perception and the agnosias

Perception involves active processing of the continuous torrent of sensations as well as their inhibition or filtering from consciousness. This processing comprises many successive and interactive stages. Those that deal with the simplest physical or sensory characteristics, such as color, shape, or tone, come first in the processing sequence and serve as foundations for the more complex, "higher" levels of semantic and visuoconceptual processing that integrate sensory stimuli with one another at each moment, successively, and with the organism's past experience (Fuster, 2003; A. Martin, Ungerleider, and Haxby, 2000; Rapp, 2001, *passim*).

Normal perception in the healthy organism is a complex process engaging many different aspects of brain functioning (Coslett and Saffran, 1992; Goodale, 2000; Löwel and Singer, 2002). Like other cognitive functions, the extensive cortical distribution and complexity of perceptual activities make them highly vulnerable to brain injury. Perceptual defects resulting from brain injury can occur through loss of a primary sensory input such as vision or smell and also through impairment of specific integrative processes. Although it may be difficult to separate the sensory from the perceptual components of a behavioral defect in some severely brain injured patients, sensation and perception each has its own functional integrity. This can be seen clearly when perceptual organization is maintained despite very severe sensory defects or when perceptual functions are markedly disrupted in patients with little or no sensory deficit. The nearly deaf person can readily understand speech patterns when the sound is sufficiently amplified, whereas some brain damaged persons with keen auditory acuity cannot make sense out of what they hear.

The perceptual functions include such activities as awareness, recognition, discrimination, patterning, and orientation. Impairments in perceptual integration appear as disorders of recognition, the *agnosias* (literally, no knowledge). Teuber (1968) clarified the distinction between sensory and perceptual defects by defining agnosia as "a normal percept stripped of its meanings." Moreover, "True agnosia . . . relates to the whole perceptual field, whether right or left," in contrast to unilateral imperception phenomena where the patient is unaware of sensations or events on only one side (see pp. 66–67). Since a disturbance in any one perceptual activity may affect any of the sensory modalities as well as different aspects of each one, a catalogue of discrete perceptual disturbances can be quite lengthy. Benson (1989) listed six different kinds of visual agnosias. Bauer and Demery (1993) identified three distinctive auditory agnosias, and M. Williams (1979) described another three involving various aspects of body awareness.

This list could be expanded, for within most of these categories of perceptual defect there are functionally discrete subcategories; e.g., Heilman and Valenstein (2003) list 25 in the index, and the *INS Dictionary of Neuropsychology* (Loring, 1999) defines 14. For instance, loss of the ability to recognize faces (*prosopagnosia* or *face agnosia*), one of the visual agnosias, may be manifested in at least two different forms: inability to recognize familiar faces and inability to recognize unfamiliar faces, which usually do not occur together (Benton, 1980; De Haan, 2001; Warrington and James, 1967b). Moreover, prosopagnosia can occur with or without intact abilities to recognize associated characteristics such as a person's facial expression, age, and sex (Tranel, Damasio, and Damasio, 1988) and thus lends itself to subcategories. A.R. Damasio (1990) suggested that the highly discrete dissociations that can occur within the visual modality (e.g., inability to recognize a person's face with intact recognition for the same person's gait) or between categories presented visually (e.g., man-made tools vs. natural objects; printed words vs. multidigit numbers) reflect the processing characteristics of the neural systems that form the substrates of knowledge (e.g., Riddoch and Humphreys, 2001). The fine degree to which brain organization is specialized becomes apparent in patients with similarly placed lesions who can identify inanimate objects but not animate ones, or comprehend words that are abstract better than those that are concrete (Warrington and Shallice, 1984).

Rather than offering a list of the many different forms that agnosias can take, E. Goldberg (1990) organized the various agnosias into two major categories: *associative agnosias* arise from a breakdown in one or more aspects of the patient's information store or "generic" knowledge and *apperceptive agnosias* are due to higher level perceptual disturbances. The specific content of an agnosic disorder depends on individual variations in the specific functions involved in a lesion site.

Memory

If any one faculty of our nature may be called more wonderful than the rest, I do think it is memory. There seems something more speakingly incomprehensible in the powers, the failures, the inequalities of memory, than in any other of our intelligences. The memory is sometimes so retentive, so serviceable, so obedient—at others, so bewildered and so weak—and at others again, so tyrannic, so beyond control!—We are to be sure a miracle every way—but our powers of recollecting and forgetting, do seem peculiarly past finding out.

Jane Austen, Mansfield Park, *1814 (1961)*

Memory is a cortical network, an array of connective links formed by experience between neurons of the neocortex . . . the function of cortical neurons in memory derives exclusively from their being part of such networks.

Joaquin M. Fuster, 1995

Central to all cognitive functions and probably to all that is characteristically human in a person's behavior is the capacity for memory, learning, and intentional access to this knowledge store. Memory frees the individual from dependency on physiological urges or situational happenstance for pleasure seeking; dread and despair do not occur in a memory vacuum. Severely impaired memory isolates patients from emotionally or practically meaningful contact with the world about them and deprives them of a sense of personal continuity, rendering them passive and helplessly dependent. Mildly to moderately impaired memory has a disorienting effect.

How many memory systems?

Perhaps the most important recent contribution to the evolution of our understanding of memory has been the demonstration that, with other mammals, we have a number of distinctly different systems that serve our memories (Squire and Knowlton, 2000). Intimations of a dual nature of memory have cropped up in the literature since the 1960s, when B. Milner (1962, 1965) and Corkin (1968) demonstrated that the now famous patient, H.M., could learn and retain some new skills despite profound amnesia (literally, no memory). Ever since surgery for epilepsy had unexpectedly left him with no hippocampus (paired structures necessary for learning about objects, ideas, and the course of one's life), H.M. has had memory deficits that severely compromise access to previously learned information as well as a complete inability to learn new information or recall ongoing events. The possibility of more memory systems, each with its own relatively discrete neurotransmitters or neuroanatomic underpinnings, may also be entertained (Mayes, 2000a; Schacter, Wagner, and Buckner, 2000).

A functional duality of memory systems, so vividly demonstrated in amnesic patients and patients with degenerative disorders (e.g., see N. Butters and Stuss, 1989) has provided the basis for conceptualizing memory functions in terms of two long-term storage and retrieval systems: a *declarative* system, or *explicit memory* which deals with facts and events and is available to consciousness, and a *nondeclarative* or *implicit* system which is "nonconscious" (Squire and Knowlton, 2000). However, depending on one's perspective, the count of systems or kinds of memory varies. In a clinical perspective, Mayes (2000a) divides declarative memory into *semantic* (fact memory) and *episodic* (autobiographic memory), and nondeclarative memory into *item-specific implicit memory* (*ISIM*) and *procedural*—also implicit—memory (see also Baddeley, 2002). This classification gives four long-term storage systems plus one system for *short-term* (what Mayes calls *working*) memory which is supported by neuroimaging studies (Schacter, Wagner, and Buckner, 2000). As of July 25, 2002, Tulving (2002b) had counted "134 different named types of memory."

While the dual system classification remains at the core of most other ways of conceptualizing memory systems and subsystems, some variations have been offered. For example, in listing long-term storage systems by their neuroanatomic sites, "thought to be especially important for each form of declarative and nondeclarative memory," Squire and Zola (1996) raise the count of systems to six by adding *classical conditioning* (two systems, one for emotional and one for skeletal responses) and *reflex learning*, while merging semantic and episodic memory into one declarative system and not including short-term memory in their count. However, for clinical purposes, the dual system conceptualization—into declarative (explicit) and nondeclarative (implicit) memory with its major subsystems—provides a useful framework for observing and understanding patterns of memory competence and deficits presented by our patients. The discussion of memory here generally follows the dual system framework of Baddeley (2002) and Mayes (2000a).

Declarative (explicit) memory

Most memory research and theory has focused on abilities to learn about and remember information, objects, and events. This is the kind of memory that patients refer to when complaining of memory problems, that teachers address for most educational activities, that is the "memory" of common parlance. It has been described as "the mental capacity of retaining and reviving impressions, or of recalling or recognizing previous experiences . . . act or fact of retaining mental impressions" (J. Stein, 1966) and, as such, always involves awareness (Moscovitch, 2000). Referring to it as "explicit memory," Demitrack and his colleagues (1992) point out that declarative memory involves "a conscious and intentional recollection" process.

Stages of memory processing

Despite the plethora of theories about stages (R.C. Atkinson and Shiffrin, 1968; G.H. Bower, 2000; R.F. Thompson, 1988) or processing levels (S.C. Brown and Craik, 2000; Craik, 1979), for clinical purposes a three-stage or elaborated two-stage model of declarative memory provides a suitable framework for conceptualizing and understanding dysfunctional memory (Balota et al., 2000; McGaugh, 1966; Parkin, 2001). Moreover, clinically, three kinds of memory are distinguishable. Two are succeeding stages of *short-term storage* (see also Baddeley, 2002; Loring, 1999; R.C. Petersen and Weingartner, 1991, for discussions of memory terminology). Recent research has questioned whether short-term storage is a distinct memory function as considerable evidence indicates that it is essentially one aspect of the consolidation process (Fuster, 2003; Parkin, 2001). However for clinical purposes it remains a useful concept (e.g., Baddeley, 2002).

1. *Registration,* or *sensory, memory* holds large amounts of incoming information briefly (on the order of seconds) in *sensory store* (Balota et al., 2000; Vallar and Papagno, 2002). It is neither strictly a memory function nor a perceptual function but rather a selecting and recording process by which perceptions enter the memory system. Registration involves the programming of acquired sensory response patterns (perceptual tendencies) in the recording and memorizing center of the brain (Nauta, 1964). The first traces of a stimulus may be experienced as a fleeting visual image (*iconic memory,* lasting up to 200 msec) or auditory "replay" (*echoic memory,* lasting up to 2,000 msec), indicating early stage processing in terms of sensory modality (Fuster, 1995; Koch and Crick, 2000). The affective, set (perceptual and response predisposition), and attention-focusing components of perception play an integral role in the registration process (Brain, 1969; S.C. Brown and Craik, 2000; Markowitsch, 2000). Either information being registered is further processed as short-term memory or it quickly decays.

2a. *Immediate memory,* the first stage of *short-term*

memory (STM) storage, temporarily holds information retained from the registration process. While theoretically distinguishable from attention, in practice, short-term memory may be equated with simple immediate span of attention (Baddeley, 2000; Howieson and Lezak, 2002; see pp. 34, 350–351). Immediate memory represents neuronal activation in which the relevant perceptual components have been integrated (Doty, 1979; Mishkin and Appenzeller, 1987). It serves "as a limited capacity store from which information is transferred to a more permanent store" and also "as a limited capacity retrieval system" (Fuster, 1995; see also Squire, 1986). Having shown that immediate memory normally handles about seven bits of information at a time, give or take two, G.A. Miller (1956) observed that this restricted holding capacity of "immediate memory impose[s] severe limitations on the amount of information that we are able to perceive, process, and remember." Immediate memory is of sufficient duration to enable a person to respond to ongoing events when more enduring forms of memory have been lost (Talland, 1965a; Victor et al., 1971). It typically lasts from about 30 seconds up to several minutes.

Although immediate memory is usually conceptualized as a unitary process, Baddeley (1986, 2002) shows how it may operate as a set of subsystems "controlled by a limited capacity executive system," which together is *working memory*. It is hypothesized that working memory consists of two subsystems, one for processing language—the "phonological loop"—and one for visuospatial data—"the visuospatial sketch pad" (see also Vallar and Papagno, 2002). The functions of working memory are "to hold information in mind, to internalize information, and to use that information to guide behavior without the aid of or in the absence of reliable external cues" (Goldman-Rakic, 1993, p. 15; see also Andrade, 2001; Fuster, 2003).

R.D. Morris and Baddeley (1988) suggested that a *primary memory* component of short-term storage can be differentiated from working memory in that the former is highly attention dependent, dissipating rapidly with distraction. Early stage Alzheimer patients and patients with frontal lobe lesions, for example, may demonstrate a relatively intact working memory but a very fragile primary memory.

Numerous studies have supported Hebb's (1949) insightful hunch that information in immediate memory is temporarily maintained in *reverberating neural circuits* (self-contained neural networks that sustain a nerve impulse by channeling it repeatedly through the same network) (Dudai, 1989; Fuster, 1995; McGaugh et al., 1990, *passim;* Rosenzweig and Leiman, 1968; Shepherd, 1998). It appears that, if not converted into a more stable biochemical organization for longer last-ing storage, the electrochemical activity that constitutes the immediate memory trace spontaneously dissipates and the memory is not retained. For example, only the rare reader with a "photographic" memory will be able to recall verbatim the first sentence on the preceding page although almost everyone who has read this far will have just seen it.

2b. *Rehearsal* is any repetitive mental process that serves to lengthen the duration of a memory trace (S.C. Brown and Craik, 2000). With rehearsal, a memory trace may be maintained for hours. Rehearsal increases the likelihood that a given bit of information will be permanently stored but does not ensure it (Baddeley, 1986).

2c. Another kind of short-term memory may be distinguished from immediate memory in that it lasts from an hour or so to one or two days—longer than a reverberating circuit could be maintained by even the most conscientious rehearsal efforts, but not yet permanently fixed as learned material in long-term storage (Fuster, 1995; Rosenzweig and Leiman, 1968; Tranel and Damasio, 2002). This may be evidence of an intermediate step "in a continuous spectrum of interlocked molecular mechanisms of . . . the multistep, multichannel nature of memory" (Dudai, 1989).

3. *Long-term memory (LTM)* or *secondary memory*—i.e., *learning*, the acquisition of new information—refers to the organism's ability to store information. Long-term memory is most readily distinguishable from short-term memory in amnesic patients, i.e., persons unable to retain new information for more than a few minutes without continuing rehearsal. Although amnesic conditions may have very different etiologies (see Chapter 7, *passim*), they all have in common a relatively intact short-term memory capacity with significant long-term memory impairments (Baddeley and Warrington, 1970; O'Connor and Verfaellie, 2002; Parkin, 2001).

The process of storing information as long-term memory, *consolidation,* may occur quickly or continue for considerable lengths of time without requiring active involvement (Lynch, 2000; Mayes, 1988; Squire, 1987). *Learning* implies consolidation—what is learned is consolidated. "Consolidation best refers to a hypothesized process of reorganization within representations of stored information, which continues as long as information is being forgotten" (Squire, 1986, p. 241). Memory acquisition and retention result from the interaction of multiple networks distributed through time and space. Many theories of memory consolidation propose a gradual transfer of memory that requires processing from hippocampal and medial temporal lobe structures to the neocortex for longer term storage (Kapur and Brooks, 1999).

"Learning" often implies effortful or attentive activity on the part of the learner. Yet when the declarative memory system is intact, much information is also acquired without directed effort, by means of *incidental learning* (Dudai, 1989; Kimball and Holyoak, 2000). Incidental learning tends to be susceptible to impairment with some kinds of brain damage (S. Cooper, 1982; C. Ryan, Butters, Montgomery, et al., 1980). Much of the information in the long-term storage system appears to be organized on the basis of meaning and associations, whereas in the short-term storage system it is organized in terms of contiguity or of sensory properties such as similar sounds, shapes, or colors (G.H. Bower, 2000; Craik and Lockhart, 1972). However, Baddeley (1978) observed that rote repetition and association built on superficial, relatively meaningless stimulus characteristics can lead to learning too.

Long-term memory storage involves a number of processes occurring at the cellular level. These include neurochemical alterations in the *neuron* (nerve cell), neurochemical alterations of the *synapse* (the point of interaction between nerve cell endings) that may account for differences in the amount of neurotransmitter released or taken up at the synaptic juncture, elaboration of the dendritic (branching out) structures of the neuron to increase the number of contacts made with other cells (Fuster, 1995; D. Johnston and Amaral, 1998; Levitan and Kaczmarek, 2002; Löwel and Singer, 2002; Lynch, 2000), and perhaps *pruning* or *apoptosis* (programmed cell death) of some connections with disuse (Edelman, 1989; Huttenlocher, 2002). There is no single local site for stored memories; instead, memories involve neuronal contributions from many cortical and subcortical centers (Fuster, 1995; Markowitsch, 2000; Penfield, 1968; Thatcher and John, 1977), with "different brain systems playing different roles in the memory system" (R.F. Thompson, 1976). Encoding, storage, and retrieval of information in the memory system appear to take place according to both principles of association (Levitan and Kaczmarek, 2002; McClelland, 2000) and "characteristics that are unique to a particular stimulus" (S.C. Brown and Craik, 2000, p. 98). Breakdown in the capacity to store or retrieve material results in distinctive memory disorders.

Recent and *remote* memory are clinical terms that refer, respectively, to *autobiographical memories* stored within the last few hours, days, weeks, or even months and to older memories dating from early childhood (e.g., Strub and Black, 2000; see also Neisser and Libby, 2000). In intact persons it is virtually impossible to determine where recent memory ends and remote memory begins, for there are no major discontinuities in memory from the present to early wisps of infantile rec-

ollection. Recent memory and remote memory become meaningful concepts when dealing with problems of *amnesia* (literally, no memory), periods for which there is no recall, in contrast to memory impairments which may involve specific deficits. Then remote memory becomes recall of information stored prior to the amnesic episode or state.

Amnesia

When registration or storage processes are impaired by disease or accident, acquisition of new information or recall of old may range from spotty to nonexistent (Kapur, 1988a; T.M. Lee et al., 2002; O'Connor and Verfaellie, 2002; Tulving, 2002a; Zola-Morgan, 2003). The nature of these deficits is largely determined by lesion site, as memory impairments can result from injuries to many different parts of the brain (Bogen, 1997). Temporary disruption of these processes, which often follows head injury or *electroconvulsive therapy* (*ECT*) for psychiatric conditions, obliterates memory for the period of impairment (Cahill and Frith, 1995; Y. Stern and Sackeim, 2002). Destruction of these capacities results in a permanent memory vacuum from the time of onset of the disorder.

The inability or impaired ability to remember one's life events beginning with the onset of a condition is called *anterograde amnesia*. Patients with anterograde amnesia are, for most practical purposes, unable to learn and have defective recent memory. The kind and severity of the memory defect vary somewhat with the nature of the disorder (Kopelman, Stanhope, and Kingsley, 1999; O'Connor and Verfaellie, 2002; Y. Stern and Sackeim, 2002).

Loss of memory for events preceding the onset of brain injury, most often due to trauma, is called *retrograde amnesia*. It tends to be relatively short (30 minutes or less) with TBI but can be extensive (E. Goldberg and Bilder, 1986). When retrograde amnesia occurs with brain disease, loss of one's own history and events may go back years and even decades (M.S. Albert, Butters, and Brandt, 1981; N. Butters and Cermak, 1986; Corkin, Hurt, et al., 1987) and typically follows a temporal gradient in which newer memories are more vulnerable to loss than older ones (M.S. Albert, Butters, and Levin, 1979; Beatty, Salmon, Butters, et al., 1988; Kapur, Millar, et al., 1998; Squire, Clark, and Knowlton, 2001). The dissociation of anterograde and retrograde memory problems in patients with memory disorders has shown that the anatomical structures involved in new learning and in retrieval of old memories are different (E. Goldberg, Antin, et al., 1981; Markowitsch, 2000). Hippocampal damage is implicated in the defective storage processes of anterograde amnesia (see pp. 50–51). The retrieval problems of retrograde amnesia have been associated with diencephalic lesions, most specifically with nuclei in the mammillary bodies and/or the thalamus (see p. 46) and interconnecting pathways (N. Butters and Stuss, 1989; Markowitsch, 2000; Y. Stern and Sackeim, 2002), and also with other subcortical structures and cortical regions (Nyberg and Cabeza, 2000).

Long-enduring retrograde amnesia that extends back for years or decades is usually accompanied by an equally prominent anterograde amnesia; these patients neither recall much of their history nor learn much that is new. For a dense retrograde amnesia to occur on an organic basis with learning ability remaining fully intact is relatively rare (E. Goldberg, Antin, et al., 1981; Kopelman, 1987a).

A 52-year-old machine maintenance man complained of "amnesia" a few days after his head was bumped in a minor traffic accident. He knew his name but denied memory for any personal history preceding the accident while registering and retaining postaccident events, names, and places normally. This burly, well-muscled fellow moved like a child, spoke in a soft—almost lisping—manner, and was only passively responsive in interview. He was watched over by his woman companion who described a complete personality change since the accident. She reported that he had been raised in a rural community in a southeastern state and had not completed high school. With these observations and this history, rather than begin a battery of tests, he was hypnotized.

Under hypnosis, a manly, pleasantly assertive, rather concrete-minded personality emerged. In the course of six hypnotherapy sessions the patient revealed that, as a prize fighter when young he had learned to consider his fists to be "lethal weapons." Some years before the accident he had become very angry with a brother-in-law who picked a fight and was knocked down by the patient. Six days later this man died, apparently from a previously diagnosed heart condition; yet the patient became convinced that he had killed him and that his anger was potentially murderous. Just days before the traffic accident, the patient's son informed him that he had fathered a baby while in service overseas but was not going to take responsibility for baby or mother. This enraged the patient who reined in his anger only with great effort. He was riding with his son when the accident occurred. A very momentary loss of consciousness when he bumped his head provided a rationale—amnesia—for a new, safely ineffectual personality to evolve, fully dissociated from the personality he feared could murder his son. Counseling under hypnosis and later in his normal state helped him to learn about and cope with his anger appropriately.

Aspects and elements of declarative memory

Recall vs. recognition. The effectiveness of the memory system also depends on how readily and completely information can be retrieved. Information retrieval is *remembering,* which may occur through *recall* involving an active, complex search process (S.C. Brown and Craik, 2000; Mayes, 1988). The question, "What is the capital of Oregon?" tests the recall function. When a like stimulus triggers awareness, remembering takes place through *recognition.* The question "Which of the following is the capital of Oregon: Albany, Portland, or Salem?" tests the recognition function. Retrieval by recognition is much easier than free recall for both intact and brain impaired persons (N. Butters, Wolfe, Granholm, and Martone, 1986; M.K. Johnson, 1990). On superficial examination, retrieval problems can be mistaken for learning or retention problems, but the nature of an apparent learning problem can be determined by appropriate testing techniques (H.S. Levin, 1986; see pp. 414–415).

Elements of declarative memory. The many different kinds of memory function become apparent in pathological conditions of the brain (Shimamura, 1989; Stuss and Levine, 2002; Van der Werf et al., 2000; Verfaellie and O'Connor, 2000). Besides the overriding distinctions between short-term and long-term memory, patients may display deficits that are specific to the nature of the information to be learned, i.e., *material specific.* Such deficits are specific to either verbal or nonverbalized information (Buckner, 2000; Jones-Gotman, 1991a; B. Milner, 1974), or to motor skill learning (Corkin, 1968; Mayes, 2000b), cutting across sensory modalities. Further, a similar distinction is made for *modality specific* memory, which depends on the specific sensory modality of testing, and is most often identified when examining working memory (Conant et al., 1999; Fastenau, Conant, and Lauer, 1998).

Brain disease affects different kinds of memories in long-term storage differentially so that a motor speech habit, such as organizing certain sounds into a word, may be wholly retained while rules for organizing words into meaningful speech are lost (H. Damasio and Damasio, 1989; Geschwind, 1970). Stored memories involving different sensory modalities, knowledge categories, and output mechanisms are also differentially affected by brain disease (Farah, Hammond, et al., 1989; K. Patterson and Hodges, 1995). For example, recognition of printed words or numbers may be severely impaired while speech comprehension and picture recognition remain relatively intact. Differences between what learned information is affected or not by brain disease may be so fine that access to one category of words is retained while words in a similar category are lost, e.g., proper names relating to specific people vs. proper names with a general referent (Warrington and McCarthy, 1987; see also A.R. Damasio, 1990; Warrington and Shallice, 1984), living vs. nonliving things (E. Strauss, Semenza, et al., 2000), or memory for landmarks vs. route recall (Schacter and Nadel, 1991). Thus, some very focal brain lesions reveal that large material-specific categories, such as semantic or spatial memory, break down into ever more discrete subsystems following the parallel fragmentation of perceptual processes into the same material-specific subsystems, and that the content categories of both memory and perception are differentially vulnerable to brain damage (Schacter, 1990a; Shelton and Caramazzo, 2001).

Another distinction can be made between *episodic* or *event* memory, also called *declarative* memory, and *semantic memory* (Mayes, 1988; Tulving, 1985, 2000; Wheeler, 2002). The former refers to memories of one's own experiences and is therefore unique and localizable in time and space. Semantic memory, i.e., what is learned as knowledge, is "timeless and spaceless," as, for instance, the alphabet or historical data unrelated to a person's life. The clinical meaningfulness of this distinction becomes evident in patients whose posttraumatic or postencephalitic retrograde amnesia may extend back weeks and even years, although their fund of information, language usage, and practical knowledge may be quite intact (Warrington and McCarthy, 1988).

Yet another distinction, between *automatic* and *effortful* memory, rests on whether learning involves active, effortful processing or passive acquisition (Balota, Dolan, and Duchek, 2000; Hasher and Zacks, 1979; M.K. Johnson and Hirst, 1991). Clinically, the difference between automatic and effortful memory commonly shows up in a relatively normal immediate recall of digits or letters that is characteristic of many brain disorders (e.g., head trauma, Alzheimer's dementia, multiple sclerosis), a recall that requires little processing in contrast to reduced performance on a task requiring effort, such as reciting a string of digits in reverse, a phenomenon that also appears with advanced age. That these are distinctive memory processes is shown by facilitation of the effortful task when the dopamine neurotransmitter system is stimulated with no corresponding improvement in the automatic memory task (R.P. Newman et al., 1984).

In selected patient groups, other kinds of memory that can be distinguished from the usual categories of declarative memory have been identified. *Source memory* (K.J. Mitchell and Johnson, 2000; Schacter, Harbluk, and McLachlan, 1984; Shimamura, 2002) or *contextual memory* (J.R. Anderson and Schooler, 2000; Parkin, 2001; Schacter, 1987) refers to knowledge of where or when something was learned, i.e., the contextual information surrounding the learning experience. Source memory may be a form of incidental memory.

Prospective memory is a recently distinguished capacity that involves both the "what" knowledge of de-

clarative memory and executive functioning. It is the ability "to remember to do something at a particular time" (Baddeley, Harris, et al., 1987; see Brandimonte et al., 1996, *passim*; Shimamura, Janowsky, and Squire, 1991). The importance of prospective memory becomes apparent in those patients with frontal lobe injuries whose memory abilities in the classical sense may be relatively intact but whose social dependency is due, at least in part, to their inability to remember to carry out previously decided upon activities at designated times or places (Sohlberg and Mateer, 2001; see p. 81). For example, it may not occur to them to keep appointments they have made, although when reminded or cued it becomes obvious that this information was not lost but rather was not recalled when needed.

Nondeclarative (implicit) memory

The knowledge and skills in nondeclarative memory have been defined as "knowledge that is expressed in performance without subjects' phenomenal awareness that they possess it" (Schacter, McAndrews, and Moscovitch, 1988). Two subsystems are clinically relevant: *procedural memory* and *priming* or *perceptual learning* (Baddeley, 2002; Mayes, 2000b; Squire and Knowlton, 2000). *Classical conditioning* is also considered a form of nondeclarative memory (Squire and Knowlton, 2000). Different aspects of implicit memory and learning activities are processed within neuroanatomically different systems (Fuster, 1995; Heindel, Salmon, et al., 1989; Squire and Knowlton, 2000; Tranel and Damasio, 2000).

Procedural, or *skill memory*, includes motor and cognitive skill learning and perceptual, "how to," learning; *priming* refers to a form of cued recall in which, without the subject's awareness, prior exposure facilitates the response; and classical conditioning (Mayes, 1988; Squire, 1987). Two elements common to these different aspects of memory are their preservation in most amnesic patients (Ewert et al., 1989; Martone, Butters, Payne, et al., 1984; O'Connor and Verfaillie, 2002) and that they are acquired or used without awareness or deliberate effort (Graf et al., 1984; Nissen and Bullemer, 1987).

Aspects of procedural memory have always been available through our observations of patients who remember nothing of ongoing events and little of their past history yet retain abilities to walk and talk, dress and eat, etc.; i.e., their well-ingrained habits that do not depend on conscious awareness remain intact (Fuster, 1995; Gabrieli, 1998; Mayes, 2000b). Mishkin and Petri (1984) considered procedural memory "a habit system." Moreover, procedural memory has been repeatedly demonstrated in intact subjects taught unusual skills, such as reading inverted type (Kolers, 1976) or learning the sequence for a set of changing locations (Willingham et al., 1989). Now that procedural memory has been not just identified but well-studied, it holds some promise for specific kinds of rehabilitative interventions for memory impaired patients (Donaghy and Williams, 1998; Farina et al., 2002; Glisky et al., 1986).

Forgetting

Some loss of or diminished access to information—both recently acquired and stored in the past—occurs continually as normal *forgetting*. Normal forgetting rates differ with such psychological variables as personal meaningfulness of the material and conceptual styles, as well as with age differences and probably some developmental differences. Normal forgetting differs from amnesic conditions in that only amnesia involves the inaccessibility or nonrecording of large chunks of personal memories.

What the process(es) of normal forgetting might be is still unclear. The Freudian view hypothesized that nothing is lost from memory and the problem lies in faulty or repressed retrieval processes. However, systematic research has shown that forgetting really happens and that what is forgotten is lost from memory through disuse or interference by more recently or vividly learned information or experiences (Mayes, 1988; Squire, 1987). Perhaps most important of these processes is "autonomous decay . . . due to physiologic and metabolic processes with progressive erosion of synaptic connections" (G.H. Bower, 2000). Fuster (1995) points out that initial "poor fixation of the memory" accounts for some instances of forgetting. This becomes most apparent in clinical conditions in which attentional processes are so impaired that passing stimuli (in conversation or as events) are barely attended to and weakly stored, if it all (Howieson and Lezak, 2002).

What seems likely is that normally both kinds of processes are operative: psychodynamic suppression or repression of some unwanted or unneeded memories takes place along with organic dissolution of others. Forgetting proceeds more rapidly with certain neurobehavioral conditions, e.g., Alzheimer's disease (Dannenbaum et al., 1988), amnesia (Isaac and Mayes, 1999), frontotemporal dementia (Pasquier et al., 2001), aging (Tombaugh and Hubley, 2001), and vascular dementia (Vanderploeg, Yuspeh, and Schinka, 2001).

Thinking

Thinking may be defined as any mental operation that relates two or more bits of information explicitly (as in making an arithmetic computation) or implicitly (as in judging that this is bad, i.e., relative to that) (Fuster, 2003). A host of complex cognitive functions is subsumed under the rubric of thinking, such as computation, reasoning and judgment, concept formation, abstracting and generalizing, ordering, organizing, planning, and problem solving (see Sohlberg and Mateer, 1989).

The nature of the information being mentally manipulated (e.g., numbers, design concepts, words) and the operation (e.g., comparing, compounding, abstracting, ordering) define the category of thinking. Thus, "verbal reasoning" comprises several operations done with words; it generally includes ordering and comparing, sometimes analyzing and synthesizing (e.g., Cosmides and Tooby, 2000). "Computation" may involve operations of ordering and compounding done with numbers (Dehaene, 2000; Fasotti, 1992), and distance judgment involves abstracting and comparing ideas of spatial extension.

The concept of "higher" and "lower" mental processes originated with the ancient Greek philosophers. This concept figures in the hierarchical theories of brain functions and mental ability factors in which "higher" refers to the more complex mental operations and "lower" to the simpler ones. Thinking is at the high end of this scale. The degree to which a concept is *abstract* or *concrete* also determines its place on the scale. For example, the abstract idea "a living organism" is presumed to represent a higher level of thinking than the more concrete idea "my cat Pansy;" the abstract rule "file specific topics under general topics" is likewise considered to be at a higher level of thinking than the instructions "file 'fir' under 'conifer,' file 'conifer' under 'tree.'"

The higher cognitive functions of abstraction, reasoning, judgment, analysis, and synthesis tend to be relatively sensitive to diffuse brain injury, even when most specific receptive, expressive, or memory functions remain essentially intact (Knopman and Selnes, 2003; Mesulam, 2000a). They may also be disrupted by any one of a number of lesions in functionally discrete areas of the brain at lower levels of the hierarchy (Gitelman, 2002). Thus the higher cognitive functions tend to be more "fragile" than the lower, more discrete functions. Conversely, higher cognitive abilities may remain relatively unaffected in the presence of specific receptive, expressive, and memory dysfunctions (E. Goldberg, 2001; Pincus and Tucker, 2003; Teuber et al., 1951; Wepman, 1976; for case examples, see Ogden, 1996).

Problem solving can take place at any point along the complexity and abstraction continua. The simplest issues of daily living call upon it, such as inserting tooth brushing into the morning routine or determining what to do when the soap dish is empty. Einstein did the same in his efforts to account for light distortions in the solar system. Problem solving involves executive functions (see pp. 35–37, and Chapter 16) as well as thinking, since a problem first has to be identified. Patients with executive disorders can look at an empty soap dish without recognizing that it presents a problem to be solved and yet be able to figure out what to do once the problem has been brought to their attention.

Unlike other cognitive functions, thinking is not tied to specific neuroanatomical systems, although the disruption of feedback, regulatory, and integrating mechanisms can affect complex cognitive activity more profoundly than other cognitive functions (Luria, 1966). "There is no . . . anatomy of the higher cerebral functions in the strict sense of the word. . . . Thinking is regarded as a function of the entire brain that defies localization" (Gloning and Hoff, 1969).

Arithmetic concepts and operations, however, are basic thinking tools that can be disrupted in quite specific ways by more or less localized lesions (Denburg and Tranel, 2003; Fasotti, 1992; Grafman and Rickard, 1997). Their vulnerability to different lesion loci has revealed at least three distinctive aspects to arithmetic activity; each, when impaired, gives rise to a specific kind of *acalculia* (literally, no counting) (E. Goldberg, 1990; Grafman, 1988; Spiers, 1987): (1) appreciation and knowledge of number concepts (acalculias associated with verbal defects); (2) ability to organize and manipulate numbers spatially as in long division or multiplication of two or more numbers (*spatial dyscalculia*); and (3) ability to perform arithmetic operations (*anarithmetria*). Neuroimaging studies have further fractionated components of number processes in showing associations of specific components with different cerebral regions (Dehaene, 2000; Gitelman, 2002).

As with other cognitive functions, the quality of any complex operation will depend in part on the extent to which its sensory and motor components are intact at the central integrative (cortical) level (E. Goldberg, 1990; Riddoch and Humphreys, 2001). For example, patients with certain somatosensory perceptual defects tend to do poorly on reasoning tasks involving visuospatial concepts (Farah, 2003a; Teuber, 1959); patients whose perceptual disabilities are associated with lesions in the visual system are more likely to have difficulty solving problems involving visual concepts (B. Milner, 1954; Tranel, 2002). Verbal defects tend to have more obvious and widespread cognitive consequences than defects in other functional systems because task instructions are frequently verbal, self-regulation and self-critiquing mechanisms are typically

verbal, and ideational systems—even for nonverbal material—are usually verbal (Luria, 1973a).

Expressive Functions

Expressive functions, such as speaking, drawing or writing, manipulating, physical gestures, facial expressions or movements, make up the sum of observable behavior. Mental activity is inferred from them.

Apraxia

Disturbances of purposeful expressive functions are known as *apraxias* (literally, no work) (Liepmann, [1900] 1988). The apraxias typically involve impairment of learned voluntary acts despite adequate motor innervation of capable muscles, adequate sensorimotor coordination for complex acts carried out without conscious intent (e.g., articulating isolated spontaneous words or phrases clearly when volitional speech is blocked, brushing crumbs or fiddling with objects when intentional hand movements cannot be performed), and comprehension of the elements and goals of the desired activity. Given the complexity of purposeful activity, it is not surprising that apraxia occurs with disruption of pathways at different stages (initiation, positioning, coordination, and/or sequencing of motor components) in the evolution of an act or sequential action (Grafton, 2002; Heilman and Rothi, 2003; Roy and Square, 1985).

Apraxic disorders may appear when pathways have been disrupted that connect the processing of information (e.g., instructions, knowledge of tools or acts) with centers for motor programming or when there has been a breakdown in motor integration and executive functions integral to the performance of complex learned acts (De Renzi, Faglioni, and Sorgato, 1982; Luria, 1966, 1973b). Thus, when asked to show how he would use a pencil, an apraxic patient who has adequate strength and full use of his muscles may be unable to organize finger and hand movements relative to the pencil sufficiently well to manipulate it appropriately. He may even be unable to relate the instructions to hand movements although he understands the nature of the task (Geschwind, 1975; Heilman and Rothi, 2003). "[T]he hallmark of apraxia is the appearance of well-executed but incorrect movements" (Bogen, 1993).

Apraxias tend to occur in clusters of disabilities that share a common anatomical pattern of brain damage (Dee et al., 1970; Geschwind, 1975). For example, apraxias involving impaired ability to perform skilled tasks on command or imitatively and to use objects appropriately and at will are commonly associated with lesions near or overlapping speech centers, and they typically appear concomitantly with communication disabilities (Heilman and Rothi, 2003; Kertesz, 1996; Meador, Loring, Lee, et al., 1999). A more narrowly defined relationship between deficits in expressive speech (Broca's aphasia, see pp. 33, 77–78) and facial apraxia further exemplifies the anatomical contiguity of brain areas specifically involved in verbal expression and facial movement (Kertesz, 1996; Kertesz and Hooper, 1982; Verstichel et Cambier, 1996), even though these disorders have been dissociated in some cases (Heilman and Rothi, 2003). Apraxia of speech, too, may appear in impaired initiation, positioning, co-ordination, and/or sequencing of the motor components of speech (Square-Storer and Roy, 1989). These problems can be mistaken for or occur concurrently with defective articulation (*dysarthria*). Yet language (symbol formulation) deficits and apraxic phenomena often occur independently of one another (Haaland and Flaherty, 1984; Heilman and Rothi, 2003; Roy, 1983).

Constructional disorders

Constructional disorders, often classified as apraxias, are actually not apraxias in the strict sense of the concept. Rather, they are disturbances "in formulative activities such as assembling, building, drawing, in which the spatial form of the product proves to be unsuccessful without there being an apraxia of single movements" (Benton, 1969a). They are more often associated with lesions of the nonspeech hemisphere of the brain than with lesions of the hemisphere that is dominant for speech (De Renzi, 1997b), and they frequently appear with defects of spatial perception (Benton, 1973, 1982). Just as constructional disorders and those involving space perception tend to go together but can each be present as a relatively isolated impairment, so the different constructional disorders may appear in relative isolation. Thus, some patients will experience difficulty in performing all constructional tasks; others who make good block constructions may consistently produce poor drawings; still others may copy drawings well but be unable to do free drawing, etc. Certain constructional tasks, such as clock drawing, are useful bedside examination procedures as the multiple factors required for success (planning, spatial organization, motor control, etc.) make simple construction tasks sensitive to cognitive impairments resulting from a variety of conditions (M. Freedman, Leach, et al., 1994; Strub and Black, 2000; Tuokko, Hadjistavropoulos et al., 1992).

Aphasia

Defects of symbol formulation, the *aphasias* and *dysphasias* (literally, no speech and impaired speech, re-spectively) were traditionally considered to be apraxias, for the end product of every kind of aphasic or language disturbance is expressive, appearing as defective or absent speech or defective symbol production (F.L. Darley, 1967; Poeck, 1983). An influential older classification of aphasic disorders defined auditory and visual agnosias for symbolic material as receptive aphasias and defined verbal apraxias as expressive aphasias (Brodal, 1981). With expansion and refinements in the systematic observation and treatment of aphasic disturbances, this simplistic two-part classification has lost its usefulness (Benson and Ardila, 1996; Mazzucchi, 2000). Today most investigators identify many more types of aphasia (e.g., Benson, 1993 [ten types]; A.R. Damasio and Damasio, 2000 [eight types]; Kertesz, 2001 [ten types]; Verstichel et Cambier, 1996 [nine types]). Some investigators describe a variety of subtypes as well (e.g., E. Goldberg, 1989; Goodglass, Kaplan, and Barresi, 2000; Luria, 1973b) or decry the usual typologies as having outlived both their usefulness and much contradictory new data (A. Basso, 2003; D. Caplan, 2003; Caramazza, 1984; Howard, 1997).

Analysis of the discrete patterns of defective language processing that can occur with circumscribed brain lesions have identified component processes necessary for normal speech and suggest a regularity in their neuroanatomical correlates (Crosson, 1985; A.R. Damasio and Damasio, 2000; H. Damasio and Damasio, 1989; Naeser, 1982). Broad patterns of correlation between types of language dysfunction and neuroanatomical structures appear with sufficient regularity to warrant the development of aphasia typologies (A.R. Damasio and Damasio, 2000; Geschwind, 1970, 1972; Kertesz, 2001). However, the presentation of aphasic symptoms also varies enough from patient to patient and in individual patients over time that clear distinctions do not hold up in many cases (M.P. Alexander, 2003; Howard, 1997). Thus, it is not surprising that the identification of aphasia *syndromes* (sets of symptoms that occur together with sufficient frequency as to "suggest the presence of a specific disease" or site of damage [Geschwind and Strub, 1975]) is complicated both by differences of opinion as to what constitutes an aphasia syndrome and differences in the labels given those symptom constellations that have been conceptualized as syndromes. The major subdivisions named in much of the literature are presented in Table 2.1, p. 33. It is of interest to note that only four aphasia syndromes are identified by all the authors named in Table 2.1; if all syndromes named in these references were included, the list would be considerably longer.

Several different ways of comprehending the aphasias have been suggested. Benson's (1993) format classifies each of eight relatively common types of aphasia on the basis of whether the patient can repeat what is

TABLE 2.1 Most Commonly Defined Aphasic Syndromes

Aphasia Type	DISTINGUISHING SYNDROME FEATURES				
	Fluency	Comprehension	Repetition	Naming	Other Names
Broca's*	Poor	Good	Poor	Poor	Expressive, motor
Wernicke's*	Good	Poor	Poor	Poor	Receptive, sensory
Global*	Poor	Poor	Poor	Poor	—
Conduction*	Good	Good	Poor	Good	—
Anomic	Good	Good	Good	Poor	Amnesic, semantic
Transcortical motor	Poor	Good	Good	Poor	—
Transcortical	Good	Poor	Good	Poor	—
Subcortical	Fair to good	Variable	Variable	Variable	—

For syndrome descriptions see Benson, 1993; A.R. Damasio and Damasio, 2000; Goodglass and Kaplan, 1983a; Kertesz, 2001; Verstichel et Cambier, 1996.
*Denotes syndromes named in all the above references.

heard. In his schema, the most common aphasia syndromes, except anomic aphasia, are characterized by "abnormal repetition;" *transcortical aphasias* (in which receptive and expressive speech areas remain connected but are isolated from other brain areas necessary for normal speech and language)—which differ from one another in degree of fluency and comprehension—plus anomic aphasia make up the "normal repetition" grouping. Another categorization of the aphasias discriminates between defects in linguistic components of speech such as loss of word meaning (semantic deficits) and agrammatic speech (syntactic deficits) (Saffran, 2003; Marin and Gordon, 1979). Yet another organization format rests on the degree to which the "language-processing systems" are anatomically near or involved with sensory or motor systems (Dronkers et al., 2000; E. Goldberg, 1990). However, Poeck (1983) pointed out that "the syndromes of aphasia . . . are, to a large extent, artifacts produced by the vascularization of the language area" (p. 84). It is possible to define aphasia syndromes because of the large interindividual similarities in brain organization and arterial distribution, which, Poeck estimated, hold for "about 80%" of aphasic patients.

Like other kinds of cognitive defects, language disturbances usually appear in clusters of related dysfunctions. "Impairment of any of the cerebral systems essential to language processes is usually reflected in more than one language modality; conversely impairment of any modality often reflects involvement of more than one process" (Schuell, 1955, p. 308). Thus, *agraphia* (literally, no writing) and *alexia* (literally, no reading) only rarely occur alone. They are most often found together and in association with other language disturbances, typically appearing as impairment rather than total loss of function and in many different forms (Coslett, 2003; Kertesz, 2001; Roeltgen, 2003). In contrast to alexia, which denotes reading defects in persons who could read before the onset of brain damage or disease, *dyslexia* typically refers to developmental disorders in otherwise competent children who do not make normal progress in reading (Coltheart, 1987; Galaburda, 2001; Lovett, 2003). Developmental dysgraphia differs from agraphia on the same etiological basis (Ellis, 1982). Language disturbances may also occur in confusional states arising from metabolic or toxic disorders rather than from a focal brain lesion (Chédru and Geschwind, 1972).

Mental Activity Variables

These are behavior characteristics that concern the efficiency of mental processes. They are intimately involved in cognitive operations but do not have a unique behavioral end product. They can be classified roughly into three categories: *level of consciousness, attentional functions,* and *activity rate.*

Consciousness

The concept of consciousness has eluded a universally acceptable definition (R. Carter, 2002; Dennett, 1991; Farah, 2001). Thus it is not surprising that efforts to identify its neural substrate system and neurobiology are still at the hypothesis-making stage (e.g., Koch and Crick, 2000; Metzinger, 2000, *passim*). Consciousness generally concerns the level at which the organism is receptive to stimulation or is awake. The words "conscious" or "consciousness" are also often used to refer to *awareness* of self and surroundings and in this sense can be confused with "attention." To maintain a clear distinction between "conscious" as indicating an awake state and "conscious" as the state of being aware of something, we will refer to the latter concept as "awareness" (Merikle et al., 2001; Sperry, 1984; Weiskrantz, 1997). In the sense used in this book, specific aspects of awareness can be blotted out by brain damage, such as awareness of one's left arm or some implicit skill memory (Farah, 2000; Schacter, McAndrews, and

Moscovitch, 1988). Awareness can even be divided, with two awarenesses coexisting, as experienced by "split-brain" patients (Baynes and Gazzaniga, 2000; Kinsbourne, 1988; Loring, Meador, and Lee, 1989). Yet consciousness is also a general manifestation of brain activity that may become more or less responsive to stimuli but has no separable parts.

Level of consciousness ranges over a continuum from full alertness through drowsiness, somnolence, and stupor, to coma (Plum and Posner, 1980; Strub and Black, 2000; Trzepacz et al., 2002). Even slight depressions of the alert state may significantly affect a person's mental efficiency, leading to tiredness, inattention, or slowness. Levels of alertness can vary in response to organismic changes as in metabolism, circadian rhythms, fatigue level, or other organic states (e.g., tonic changes) (Stringer, 1996; van Zomeren and Brouwer, 1987). Variations in brain electrophysiology measured by such techniques as electroencephalography and evoked potentials are seen with altered levels of consciousness (Andreassi, 1995; Daube, 2002; Frith and Dolan, 1997). Although disturbances of consciousness may accompany a functional disorder, they usually reflect pathological conditions of the brain (Lishman, 1997; Strub, 1996b; Trzepacz et al., 2002).

Attention

Attention refers to several different capacities or processes that are related aspects of how the organism becomes receptive to stimuli and how it may begin processing incoming or attended-to excitation (whether internal or external) (Parasuraman, 1998). Showing how widely divergent definitions of attention may be are Mirsky's (1989) placement of attention within the broader category of "information processing" and Gazzaniga's (1987) conclusion that "the attention system . . . functions independently of information processing activities and [not as] . . . an emergent property of an ongoing processing system." Many investigators seem most comfortable with one or more of the characteristics that William James (1890) and others ascribed to attention (e.g., see Leclercq, 2002; Pashler, 1998; Parasuraman, 1998). These include its two aspects, "reflex" (i.e., automatic processes) and "voluntary" (i.e., controlled processes). On the basis of a large-scale factor analysis, Spikman, Kiers, and their collaborators (2001) called them "Stimulus-driven Reaction" and "Memory-driven Action," respectively, especially noting that the subject's *control* is a primary characteristic of the latter. Other characteristics of attention that have been identified are its finite resources and the capacities both for disengagement to shift focus and for responsivity to either sensory or semantic stimulus characteristics. An-

other kind of difference between attentional activities has to do with whether it is sustained *tonic attention* as occurs in *vigilance* or it shifts responsively as *phasic attention,* which orients the organism to changing stimuli.

Most investigators conceive of attention as a system in which processing occurs sequentially in a series of stages within different brain systems involved in attention (Butter, 1987; Luck and Hillyard, 2000). This system appears to be organized in a hierarchical manner in which the earliest entries are modality specific while late-stage processing—e.g., at the level of awareness—is supramodal (Butter, 1987; Posner, 1990). Disorders of attention may arise from lesions involving different points in this system (L.C. Robertson and Rafal, 2000; Rousseaux et al., 2002).

A salient characteristic of the attentional system is its *limited capacity* (Lavie, 2001; Pashler, 1998; Posner, 1978; van Zomeren and Brouwer, 1994). Only so much processing activity can take place at a time, such that engagement of the system in processing one attentional task calling on controlled attention can interfere with a second task having similar processing requirements. Thus, one may be unable to concentrate on a radio newscast while closely following a sporting event on television yet can easily perform an automatic (in this case, highly overlearned) attention task such as driving on a familiar route while listening to the newscast.

Attentional capacity varies not only between individuals but also within each person at different times and under different conditions. Depression or fatigue, for example, can temporarily reduce it in intact adults (Landrø, Stiles, and Sletvold, 2001; P. Zimmerman and Leclercq, 2002); old age (Parasuraman and Greenwood, 1998; Van der Linden and Collette, 2002) and brain injury may reduce attentional capacity more lastingly (L.C. Robertson and Rafal, 2000; Rousseaux, Fimm, and Cantagallo, 2002; van Zomeren and Brouwer, 1994).

Simple immediate span of attention—how much information can be grasped at once—is a relatively effortless process that tends to be resistant to the effects of aging and of many brain disorders. It may be considered a form of working memory but is an integral component of attentional functioning (Howieson and Lezak, 2002). Four other aspects of attention are more fragile and thus often of greater clinical interest (Leclercq, 2002; Mateer, 2000; Posner, 1988; Van der Linden and Collette, 2002; van Zomeren and Brouwer, 1994). (1) *Focused* or *selective attention* is probably the most studied aspect and the one people usually have in mind when talking about attention. It is the capacity to highlight the one or two important stimuli or ideas being dealt with while suppressing awareness of competing distractions. It is commonly referred to as *concentration.* Sohlberg and Mateer (1989) additionally distinguished between focused and selective attention by attributing the "ability to respond discretely" to specific stimuli to the focusing aspect of attention and the capacity to ward off distractions to selective attention. (2) *Sustained attention,* or *vigilance,* refers to the capacity to maintain an attentional activity over a period of time. (3) *Divided attention* involves the ability to respond to more than one task at a time or to multiple elements or operations within a task, as in a complex mental task. It is thus very sensitive to any condition that reduces attentional capacity. (4) *Alternating attention* allows for shifts in focus and tasks.

While these different aspects of attention can be demonstrated by different examination techniques, even discrete damage involving a part of the attentional system can create alterations that affect more than one aspect of attention. Underlying many patients' attentional disorders is *slowed processing,* which can have broad-ranging effects on attentional activities (Gronwall and Sampson, 1974; Ponsford, 1995; Saffran, Dell, and Schwartz, 2000; van Zomeren and Brouwer, 1994).

Patients with brain disorders associated with slowed processing—certain traumatic brain injuries and multiple sclerosis, for example—often complain of "memory problems," although memory assessment may demonstrate minimal if any diminution in their abilities to learn new or retrieve old information. On questioning, the examiner discovers that these "memory problems" typically occur when the patient is bombarded by rapidly passing stimuli. These patients miss parts of conversations (e.g., a time or place for meeting, part of a story). Many of them also report misplacing objects as an example of their "memory problem." What frequently has happened is that on entering the house with keys or wallet in hand they are distracted by children or a spouse eager to speak to them or by loud sounds or sight of some unfinished chore. With no recollection of what they have been told or where they set their keys, they and their families naturally interpret this as a "memory problem" rather than one of slowed processing speed which also makes difficult the processing of multiple simultaneous stimuli. When the true nature of this problem is appreciated, patients and families can alter ineffective methods of exchanging messages and conducting activities, with beneficial effects on the patient's "memory." (Howieson and Lezak, 2002)

Impaired attention and concentration are among the most common mental problems associated with brain damage (Leclercq, Deloche, and Rousseaux, 2002; Lezak, 1978b, 1989). When attentional deficits occur, all the cognitive functions may be intact and the person may even be capable of some high level performances, yet overall cognitive productivity suffers from inattentiveness, faulty concentration, and consequent fatigue (e.g., Stuss, Ely, Hugenholtz, et al., 1985, Stuss, Stethem, Hugenholtz, et al., 1989).

Activity rate

Activity rate refers to the speed at which mental activities are performed and to speed of motor responses. Behavioral slowing is a common characteristic of both aging and brain damage (see Chapter 7 and pp. 297–298). Motor response slowing is readily observable and may be associated with weakness, poor coordination, or—in testing writing or tracing speed—a prior hand or arm injury. Slowing of mental activity shows up most clearly in delayed reaction times and in longer than average total performance times in the absence of a specific motor disability. It can be inferred from *patterns* of mental inefficiency, such as reduced auditory span plus diminished performance accuracy plus poor concentration, although each of these problems can occur on some basis other than generalized mental slowing. Slowed processing speed appears to contribute significantly to the benign memory lapses of elderly persons (Luszcz and Bryan, 1999; D.C. Park et al., 1996; Salthouse, 1991a).

EXECUTIVE FUNCTIONS

The executive functions consist of those capacities that enable a person to engage successfully in independent, purposive, self-serving behavior. They differ from cognitive functions in a number of ways. Questions about executive functions ask *how* or *whether* a person goes about doing something (e.g., Will you do it and, if so, how and when?); questions about cognitive functions are generally phrased in terms of *what* or *how much* (e.g., How much do you know? What can you do?). So long as the executive functions are intact, a person can sustain considerable cognitive loss and still continue to be independent, constructively self-serving, and productive. When executive functions are impaired, the individual may no longer be capable of satisfactory self-care, of performing remunerative or useful work independently, or of maintaining normal social relationships regardless of how well-preserved the cognitive capacities are—or how high the person scores on tests of skills, knowledge, and abilities. Cognitive deficits usually involve specific functions or functional areas; impairments in executive functions tend to show up globally, affecting all aspects of behavior. However, executive disorders can affect cognitive functioning directly in compromised strategies to approaching, planning, or carrying out cognitive tasks, or in defective monitoring of the performance (P.W. Burgess et al., 1998; E. Goldberg, 2001; Lezak, 1982a; Ogden, 1996, *passim*).

For example, a young woman who survived a head-on collision displayed a complete lack of motivation with inability to initiate almost all behaviors including eating and drinking, leisure or housework activities, social interactions, sewing (which she had once done well), or reading (which she can still do with comprehension). Although new learning ability is virtually nonexistent and her constructional abilities are significantly impaired, her cognitive losses are relatively circumscribed in that verbal skills and much of her background knowledge and capacity to retrieve old information—both semantic and episodic—are fairly intact. Yet she performs these cognitive tasks—and any other activites—only when expressly directed or stimulated by others, and then external supervision must be maintained for her to complete what she began.

Many of the behavior problems arising from impaired executive functions are apparent even to casual or naive observers. For experienced clinicians, these problems can serve as hallmarks of significant brain injury (Lezak, 1996). Among them are signs of a defective capacity for self-control or self-direction such as emotional lability or flattening, a heightened tendency to irritability and excitability, impulsivity, erratic carelessness, rigidity, and difficulty in making shifts in attention and in ongoing behavior. Deterioration in personal grooming and cleanliness may also distinguish these patients.

Other defects in executive functions, however, are not so obvious. The problems they occasion may be missed or not recognized as neuropsychological by examiners who see patients only in the well-structured inpatient and clinic settings in which psychiatry and neurology patients are ordinarily observed (Lezak, 1982a). Perhaps the most serious of these problems, from a psychosocial standpoint, are impaired capacity to initiate activity, decreased or absent motivation (*anergia*), and defects in planning and carrying out the activity sequences that make up goal-directed behaviors (Lezak, 1989; Luria, 1966; Sohlberg and Mateer, 2001; Walsh and Darby, 1999). Patients without significant impairment of receptive or expressive functions who suffer primarily from these kinds of control defects are often mistakenly judged to be malingering, lazy or spoiled, psychiatrically disturbed, or—if this kind of defect appears following a legally compensable brain injury—exhibiting a "compensation neurosis" that some interested persons may believe will disappear when the patient's legal claim has been settled.

How crippling defects of executive functions can be is vividly demonstrated by the case of a hand surgeon who had had a hypoxic (*hypoxia*: insufficient oxygen) episode during a cardiac arrest that occurred in the course of minor facial surgery. His cognitive abilities, for the most part, were not greatly affected, but initiating, self-correcting, and self-regulating behaviors were severely compromised. He also displayed some difficulty with new learning—not so much that he lost track of the date or could not follow sporting events from week to week but enough to render his memory, particularly prospective memory, unreliable for most practical purposes.

One year after the anoxic episode, the patient's scores on Wechsler Intelligence Scale tests ranged from *high average* (75th percentile) to *very superior* (99th percentile), except on Digit Symbol, performed without error but at a rate of speed that placed this performance low in the *average* score range. His Trail Making Test speed was *within normal limits* and he demonstrated good verbal fluency and visual discrimination abilities—all in keeping with his highest educational and professional achievements. On the basis of a clinical psychologist's conclusion that these high test scores indicated "no clear evidence of organicity" and a psychiatric diagnosis of "traumatic depressive neurosis," the patient's insurance company denied his claim (pressed by his guardian brother) for disability payments. Retesting six years later, again at the request of the brother, produced the same pattern of scores.

The patient's exceptionally good test performance belied his actual behavioral capacity. Seven years after the hypoxic episode, this 45-year-old man who had had a successful private practice was working for his brother as a delivery truck driver. This youthful-looking, nicely groomed man explained, on questioning, that his niece bought all of his clothing and even selected his wardrobe for important occasions such as this examination. He knew neither where nor with what she bought his clothes, and did not seem to appreciate that this ignorance was unusual. He was well mannered and pleasantly responsive to questions but volunteered nothing spontaneously and made no inquiries in an hour-and-a-half interview. His matter-of-fact, humorless manner of speaking remained unchanged regardless of the topic.

When asked, the patient reported that his practice had been sold but he did not know to whom, for how much, or who had the money. This once briefly married man who had enjoyed years of affluent independence had no questions or complaints about living in his brother's home. He had no idea how much his room and board cost or where the money came from for his support, nor did he exhibit any curiosity or interest in this topic. He said he liked doing deliveries for his brother because "I get to talk to people." He had enjoyed surgery and said he would like to return to it but thought that he was too slow now. When asked what plans he had, his reply was, "None."

His sister-in-law reported that it took several years of rigorous rule setting to get the patient to bathe and change his underclothes each morning. He still changes his outer clothing only when instructed. He eats when hungry without planning or accommodating himself to the family's plans. If left home alone for a day or so he may not eat at all, although he fixes himself coffee. In seven years he has not brought home or asked for any food, yet he enjoys his meals. He spends most of his leisure time in front of the TV. Though once an active sports enthusiast he has made no plans to hunt or fish in seven years, but he enjoys these sports when taken by relatives.

Because the patient's brother runs his own business, he is able to keep the patient employed. He explained that he can give his brother only routine assignments that require no judgment, and these only one at a time. As the patient finishes each assignment, he calls into his brother's office for the next one. Although he knows that his brother is his guardian, the patient has never questioned or complained about his legal status. When the brother reinstituted suit for the patient's disability insurance, the company again denied the claim in the belief that the high test scores showed he was capable of returning to his profession. It was only when the insurance adjustor was reminded of the inappropriateness of the patient's life-style and the unlikelihood that an experienced, competent surgeon would contentedly remain a legal dependent in his brother's household for seven years that the adjustor could appreciate the psychological devastation the surgeon had suffered.

PERSONALITY/EMOTIONALITY VARIABLES

Some personality or emotional change usually follows brain injury (Greve et al., 2001; Koponen et al., 2002; Max et al., 2001). Some changes tend to occur as fairly characteristic behavior patterns that relate to specific anatomical sites (e.g., Baribeau and Roth, 1996; Davidson and Irwin, 2002; Gainotti, 1972, 1989; Lishman, 1997; Ruckdeschel-Hibbard et al., 1986). Among the most common direct effects of brain injury on personality are emotional dulling, disinhibition, diminution of anxiety with associated emotional blandness or mild euphoria, and reduced social sensitivity. Heightened anxiety, depressed mood, and hypersensitivity in interpersonal interactions may also occur (Blumer and Benson, 1975; Ghika-Schmid and Bogousslavsky, 2001; K. Goldstein, 1939; D.J. Stein and Hugo, 2002).

Profound personality changes frequently follow brain injury or occur with brain disease. These seem to be not so much a direct product of the illness as patients' reactions to their experiences of loss, chronic frustration, and radical changes in life style. Consequently, depression is probably the most common single emotional characteristic of brain damaged patients generally, with pervasive anxiety following closely behind (J.F. Jackson, 1988; Lezak, 1978b). When mental inefficiency (i.e., attentional deficits typically associated with slowed processing and diffuse damage) is a prominent feature, obsessive-compulsive traits frequently evolve (Lezak, 1989; D.J. Stein and Hugo, 2002). Some other common behavior problems of brain injured people are irritability, restlessness, low frustration tolerance, and apathy (Galbraith, 1985; Heilman, Blonder, et al., 2000, 2003).

Few brain damaged patients experience personality changes that are simply either direct consequences of the brain injury or secondary reactions to impairment and loss. For the most part, the personality changes, emotional distress, and behavior problems of brain damaged patients are the product of extremely complex interactions involving their neurological disabilities, present social demands, previously established behavior patterns, and ongoing reactions to all of these (Gainotti, 1993). When brain injury is mild, personality and the capacity for self-awareness usually remain fairly intact so that emotional and characterological alterations for the most part will be reactive and adaptive (compensatory) to the patients' altered experiences of themselves. As severity increases, so do organic contributions to personality and emotional changes. With severe damage, little may remain of the premorbid personality and of reactive capabilities and responses.

Some brain injured patients display emotional instability characterized by rapid, often exaggerated affective swings, a condition called *emotional lability*. Three kinds of lability associated with brain damage can be distinguished.

1. The emotional ups and downs of some labile patients result from weakened controls and lowered frustration tolerance. This is often most pronounced in the acute stages of their illness and when they are fatigued or stressed. Their emotional expression and their feelings are congruent, and their sensitivity and capacity for emotional response are intact. However, emotional reactions, particularly under conditions of stress or fatigue, will be stronger and may last longer than was usual for them premorbidly (R.S. Fowler and Fordyce, 1974).

2. A second group of labile patients have lost emotional sensitivity and the capacity for modulating emotionally charged behavior. They tend to overreact emotionally to whatever external stimulation impinges on them. Their emotional reactivity can generally be brought out in an interview by abruptly changing the subject from a pleasant topic to an unpleasant one and back again, for these patients will beam or cloud up with each topic change. When left alone and physically comfortable, they typically seem emotionless (M.R. Bond, 1984; Prigatano, 1987).

3. A third group of labile patients differs from the others in that their feelings are generally appropriate, but brief episodes of strong affective expression—usually tearful crying, sometimes laughter—can be triggered by even quite mild stimulation. This is the *pseudobulbar state* (Heilman, Blonder, et al., 2003; Lieberman and Benson, 1977; R.G. Robinson and Starkstein, 2002). It results from structural lesions that involve the frontal cortex and connecting pathways to lower brain structures. This condition has been most usually observed with left-sided anterior damage (House et al., 1990). The feelings of patients with this condition are frequently not congruent with their appearance, and they generally can report the discrepancy. Because they tend

to cry with every emotionally arousing event, even happy or exciting ones, family members and visitors see them crying much of the time and often misinterpret the tears as evidence of depression. Sometimes the bewildered patient comes to the same mistaken conclusion and then really does become depressed. These patients can be identified by the frequency, intensity, and irrelevancy of their tears or guffaws; the rapidity with which the emotional reaction subsides; and the dissociation between their appearance and their stated feelings (B.W. Black, 1982; Heilman, Blonder, et al., 2003; Pino e Melo and Bogousslavsky, 2001).

Although most brain injured persons tend to undergo adverse emotional changes, for a few, brain damage seems to make life more pleasant. This can be most striking in those emotionally constricted, anxious, overly responsible people who become more easygoing and relaxed as a result of a pathological brain condition. A clinical psychologist wrote about himself several years after sustaining significant brain damage marked by almost a week in coma and initial right-sided paralysis:

People close to me tell me that I am easier to live with and work with, now that I am not the highly self-controlled person that I used to be. My emotions are more openly displayed and more accessible, partially due to the brain damage which precludes any storing up of emotion, and partially due to the maturational aspects of this whole life-threatening experience. . . . Furthermore, my blood pressure is amazingly low. My one-track mind seems to help me to take each day as it comes without excessive worry and to enjoy the simple things of life in a way that I never did before. (Linge, 1980)

However, their families may suffer instead. The following case illustrates this kind of personality change.

A young Vietnam veteran lost the entire right frontal portion of his brain in a land mine explosion. His mother and wife described him as having been a quietly pleasant, conscientious, and diligent sawmill worker before entering the service. When he returned home, all of his speech functions and most other cognitive abilities were intact. He was completely free of anxiety and thus without a worry in the world. He had also become very easygoing, self-indulgent, and lacking in both drive and sensitivity to others. His wife was unable to get him to share her concerns when the baby had a fever or the rent was

due. Not only did she have to handle all the finances, carry all the family and home responsibilities, and do all the planning, but she also had to see that her husband went to work on time and that he did not drink up his paycheck or spend it in a shopping spree before getting home on Friday night. For several years his wife tried to cope with the burdens of a carefree husband. She finally left him after he had ceased working and had begun a pattern of monthly drinking binges that left little of his considerable compensation checks.

One significant and relatively common concomitant of brain injury is a changed sexual drive (Boller and Frank, 1981; Foley and Sanders, 1997a,b; Perrigot et al., 1991; Wiseman and Fowler, 2002; Zasler, 1993). A married person who has settled into a comfortable sexual activity pattern of intercourse two or three times a week may begin demanding sex two and three times a day from the bewildered spouse. More frequently, the patient loses sexual interest or capability (Askin-Edgar et al., 2002; L.M. Binder, Howieson, and Coull, 1987; Bolderini et al., 1991; Lechtenberg, 1999; S. Newman, 1984). This leaves the partner feeling unsatisfied and unloved, adding to other tensions and worries associated with cognitive and personality changes in the patient (Lezak, 1978a; Zasler, 1993). For example, some brain damaged men are unable to achieve or sustain an erection, or they may have ejaculatory problems secondary to nervous tissue damage (D.N. Allen and Goreczny, 1995; Bray et al., 1981; Foley and Sanders, 1997b). Patients who become crude, boorish, or childlike as a result of brain damage no longer are welcome bed partners and may be bewildered and upset when rejected by their once affectionate mates. Younger persons brain damaged before experiencing an adult sexual relationship may not be able to acquire acceptable behavior and appropriate attitudes. Adults who were normally functioning when single often have difficulty finding and keeping partners because of cognitive limitations or social incompetence resulting from their neurological impairments. For all these reasons, the sexual functioning of many brain damaged persons will be thwarted (Griffith et al., 1990). Although some sexual problems diminish in time, for many patients they seriously complicate the problems of readjusting to new limitations and handicaps by adding another strange set of frustrations, impulses, and reactions.

3 | The Behavioral Geography of the Brain

So much is now known about the brain—and yet so little. The structure of the brain is well visualized with current technology and minute details of cell structure can be seen with electron microscopy. Even structural changes in the neuron associated with learning have been photographed (Eichenbaum and Cohen, 2001; Engert and Bonhoeffer, 1999). Neuronal pathways have been traced to and from major regions of the brain (for some pathway examples, see Markowitsch, 2000, for memory; Frackowiak et al., 1997, chap. 5, for the somatosensory system; Lichter and Cummings, 2001, *passim,* for frontal-subcortical circuitry; Rolls, 1999, for emotions; Shepherd, 1998, for a review of synaptic circuits; Spencer, 2000b, chap. 1, for neurotoxicity; and Steinmetz et al., 2001, for connections underlying learning).

With the remarkable developments in functional neuroimaging, investigators are exploring the complex interaction of regions of the brain during specific experiences and behaviors through measurement of brain blood flow or metabolism (for some imaging examples of complex behaviors, see Andreasen, 2001, for sensory and motor activation in controls and psychiatric patients; Driver and Baylis, 1998, for an assortment of visual responses; Frackowiak et al., 1997 for reading, higher cortical processes including emotions, and varieties of memory, in chaps. 13, 14, 15; Haxby, Courtney, and Clark, 1998, for different aspects of active attention; and Lumer, 2000, for visuoperceptual discriminations). The combination of functional neuroimaging with methods for detecting the temporal order of brain activation in multiple brain regions, such as electroencephalography (EEG) and magnetoencephalography (MEG) (Andreassi, 1995; Daube, 2002), allows for an understanding of the sequence in which brain regions are put "on line" during a mental task.

This beginning understanding of the complexities of brain activation lays the foundation for a neuroscience-based revision of the big questions self-conscious humans have asked for centuries: What is the neural (anatomic, physiologic) nature of consciousness (e.g., R. Carter, 2002; Dehaene, 2002, *passim;* L. Weiskrantz, 1997)? What are the relative contributions and interactions of

genotype and experience (e.g., P.R. Huttenlocher, 2002; B.F. Pennington, 2002). What are the neuroanatomic bases of "self" (Metzinger, 2000, *passim,* 2003, *passim*)?

New technology has supported many traditional beliefs about the brain and challenged others. The long-held belief that neurons do not proliferate after early stages of development has been shaken by considerable evidence showing that new neurons are produced in the adult brains of a number of mammalian species, perhaps playing a role in brain injury repair and new learning (H.S. Levin and Grafman, 2000; Sohlberg and Mateer, 2001; D.G. Stein et al., 1995). In the past few years it has been shown that adult-produced neurons are found in the dentate gyrus of the hippocampus and neocortex in the monkey (Gould, Reeves, Fallah et al., 1999; Gould, Reeves, Graziano, and Gross, 1999), and the hippocampal formation of the human is capable of generating neurons throughout life (Eriksson et al., 1998). The implications of these findings for human aging and diseases are unknown.

In addition, the roles of many brain regions are far more complex than previously thought. The basal ganglia and cerebellum, once believed to be motor control centers, are now being appreciated for their influences on cognition and psychiatric disorders (Barlow, 2002; Crosson, Moore, and Wierenga, 2003; D.M. Jacobs, Levy, and Marder, 1997; Lichter and Cummings, 2001, *passim*). Even the motor cortex appears to play an active role in processing abstract learned information (A.F. Carpenter et al., 1999).

This chapter presents a brief (and necessarily superficial) sketch of some of the structural arrangements in the human central nervous system that are intimately connected with behavioral function. This sketch is followed by a review of anatomical and functional interrelationships that appear with enough regularity to have psychologically meaningful predictive value. More detailed information on neuroanatomy and its behavioral correlates is available in such standard references as Afifi and Bergman (1998), Hendelman (2000), and Nolte (1999). A.R. Damasio and Tranel (1991), Mesulam (2000c), and Tranel (2002) provide excellent reviews of brain–behavior relationships. Reviews of the brain correlates for a variety of neuropsychological disorders can be found in Feinberg and Farah (2003a), Heilman and Valenstein (2003), Kolb and Whishaw (1996), Naugle, Cullum, and Bigler (1997), and Yudofsky and Hales (2002).

The role of physiological and biochemical events in behavioral expression adds another important dimension to neuropsychological phenomena. Most of the work in these areas is beyond the scope of this book. Readers wishing to learn how biochemistry and neurophysiology relate to behavioral phenomena can consult Andreassi (1995), Cacioppo et al. (2000), Shepherd (1998), and P.F. Smith and Darlington (1996).

BRAIN PATHOLOGY AND PSYCHOLOGICAL FUNCTIONS

> There is no localizable single store for the meaning of a given entity or event within a cortical region. Rather, meaning is achieved by widespread multiregional activation of fragmentary records pertinent to a given stimulus and according to a combinatorial code specific or partially specific to the entity . . . the meaning of an entity, in this sense, is not stored anywhere in the brain in permanent fashion; instead it is re-created anew for every instantiation.
>
> *Daniel Tranel and Antonio R. Damasio, 2000*

The relationship between brain and behavior is exceedingly intricate and frequently puzzling. Our understanding of this fundamental relationship is still very limited, but the broad outlines and many details of the correlations between brain and behavior have been sufficiently well explained to be clinically useful. Any given behavior is the product of a myriad of complex neurophysiological and biochemical interactions involving the whole brain. Complex acts, such as swatting a fly or reading this page, are the products of countless neural interactions involving many, often far-flung sites in the neural network; their neuroanatomical correlates are not confined to any local area of the brain (Luria, 1966; Sherrington, 1955; see also Fuster, 2003; Parks, Levine, and Long, 1998).

Yet discrete psychological activities such as the perception of a pure tone or the movement of a finger can be disrupted by *lesions* (localized abnormal tissues changes) involving approximately the same anatomical structures in most human brains. Additionally, one focal lesion may affect many functions when the damaged neural structure is involved with more or less different functions thus producing a neurobehavioral *syndrome,* a cluster of deficits that tend to occur together with some regularity (Benton, 1977b [1985]; Bogousslavsky and Caplan, 2001, *passim;* H. Damasio

and Damasio, 1989; E. Goldberg, 1995). This disruption of complex behavior by brain lesions occurs with such consistent anatomical regularity that inability to understand speech, to recall recent events, or to copy a design, for example, can often be predicted when the site of the lesion is known (Benton, 1981[1985]; Filley, 1995; Geschwind, 1979; Rapp, 2001; Strub and Black, 2000). Knowledge of the *localization of dysfunction,* as this correlation between damaged neuroanatomical structures and behavioral functions may be called, also enables neuropsychologists and neurologists to make educated guesses about the site of a lesion on the basis of abnormal patterns of behavior. However, similar lesions may have quite dissimilar behavioral outcomes (Bigler, 2001b). Markowitsch (1984) described the limits of prediction: "[a] straightforward correlation between a particular brain lesion and observable functional deficits is . . . unlikely . . . as a lesioned structure is known not to act on its own, but depends in its function on a network of input and output channels, and as the equilibrium of the brain will be influenced in many and up to now largely unpredictable ways by even a restricted lesion" (p. 40).

Moreover, localization of dysfunction cannot imply a "push-button" relationship between local brain sites and specific behaviors as the brain's processing functions take place at multiple levels (e.g., encoding a single modality of a percept, energizing memory search, recognition, attribution of meaning) within complex, integrated, interactive, and often widely distributed systems. Thus lesions at many different brain sites may alter or extinguish a single complex act (Luria, 1973b; Nichelli, Grafman, et al., 1994; Sergent, 1988b), as can lesions interrupting the neural pathways connecting areas of the brain involved in the act (Geschwind, 1965; Tranel and Damasio, 2000). E. Miller (1972) reminded us that,

> It is tempting to conclude that if by removing a particular part of the brain we can produce a deficit in behavior, e.g., a difficulty in verbal learning following removal of the left temporal lobe in man, then that part of the brain must be responsible for the impaired function. . . . [T]his conclusion does not necessarily follow from the evidence as can be seen from the following analogy. If we were to remove the fuel tank from a car we would not be surprised to find that the car was incapable of moving itself forward. Nevertheless, it would be very misleading to infer that the function of the fuel tank is to propel the car. (pp. 19–20)

THE CELLULAR SUBSTRATE

The nervous system makes behavior possible. It is involved in the reception, processing, storage, and transmission of information within the organism and in the organism's exchanges with the outside world. It is a dynamic system in that its activity modifies its performance, its internal relationships, and its capacity to mediate stimuli from the outside.

The brain has two types of cells. *Neurons* conduct nerve impulses that transmit information in the brain and throughout the nervous system. Estimates of the number of nerve cells (neurons) in the brain range from "ten thousand million" (10 billion) (Beaumont, 1988b) to as much as 10^{12} (Strange, 1992). *Glia,* ten to 50 times more numerous than neurons, are supporting brain cells that lack the ability to transmit information (Kandel et al., 2000; Levitan and Kaczmarak, 2002). Their functions are not fully understood, but they are thought to have nutritional and scavenger functions and to release growth factors. *Astrocytes* are one major type of glial cell with an additional role as a component of the *blood–brain barrier* which prevents some substances in the blood from entering into brain cells (P.A. Stewart, 1997). Another major type of glial cell are *oligodendroglia,* which also form *myelin,* the substance of axonal sheaths (see below).

Nerve cells vary in shape and function (Levitan and Kaczmarek, 2002). Most have a cell body, multiple branching *dendrites* that receive stimulation from other neurons, and an *axon* that carries the electrical nerve impulse (called *action potential*). Although the neuron has only one initial segment of axon, the axon may branch to produce collateral segments. Axons vary in length. Long axons have myelin sheaths that provide insulation for high-speed conduction of nerve impulses (Andreassi, 1995; Kandell et al., 2000; Victor and Ropper, 2001).

When well-nourished and adequately stimulated, tiny transmission organs at the neuronal tips proliferate abundantly, providing the human nervous system with an astronomical multiplicity of points of interaction between nerve cells, the *synapses* (Shepherd and Koch, 1998). S. Green (1987) estimates that within the brain a single neuron may have direct synaptic contact with as many as several thousand other neurons. Extrapolating from neuronal and synaptic densities in cat cortex, Shepherd and Koch (1998) calculate that there "must be" approximately 10 billion cells in the human cortex alone, which would give rise to 60 trillion (60 × 10^{12}) synapses. The stimulation of a neuron can have either an excitatory or inhibitory effect. The postsynaptic cell computes its excitatory and inhibitory inputs and either fires a nerve impulse or not. Alterations in spatial and temporal excitation patterns in the brain's circuitry can add considerably more to its dynamic potential as stimulation applied to a neural pathway heightens that pathway's sensitivity and increases the efficacy with which neuronal excitation may be transmitted through its synapses (Engert and Bonhoeffer, 1999; Koch and Segev, 2000; McAllister Usrey, et al., 2002; Toni et al., 1999). Long-lasting synaptic modifications are called *long-term potentiation* and *long-term depression* (Fuster, 1995; Lynch, 2000; McGaugh, Weinberger, and Lynch, 1995, *passim*). Together these mechanisms of synaptic modification provide the neural potential for the variability and flexibility of human behavior (Levitan and Kaczmarek, 2002; Rolls and Treves, 1998; Shepherd, 1998, *passim*).

Nerve cells do not touch one another at synapses. Communication between neurons is made primarily through the medium of *neurotransmitters,* chemical agents generated within and secreted by stimulated nerve cells. These substances can bridge synaptic gaps between nerve cells to activate receptor neurons (E.S. Levine and Black, 2000; D.A. McCormick, 1998; P.G. Nelson and Davenport, 1999). The discovery of more than 100 neurotransmitters (National Advisory Mental Health Council, 1989) gives some idea of the possible range of selective activation between neurons as each neurotransmitter can bind to and thus activate only those receptor sites with the corresponding molecular conformation, and a single neuron may produce and release more than one of these chemical messengers (Hökfelt et al., 1984; Levitan and Kaczmarek, 2002). The key transmitters implicated in neurologic and psychiatric diseases are acetylcholine, dopamine, norepinephrine, serotonin, glutamate, and gamma-aminobutyric acid (Andreasen, 2001; Wilcox and Gonzales, 1995).

When a nerve cell is injured or diseased, it may stop functioning and the circuits to which it contributed will then be disrupted. Some circuits may eventually reactivate as damaged cells resume functioning or alternative patterns involving different cell populations take over (see pp. 293–294, regarding brain injury and neuroplasticity). When a circuit loses a sufficiently great number of neurons, the broken circuit can neither be reactivated nor replaced. In general, when a human neuron dies, it is not replaced, except in the capacity of the dentate gyrus of the human hippocampus to generate new neurons (Eriksson et al., 1998). Evidence of the generation of new neurons in response to injury or disease is still lacking.

During development neurons initiate a process—*apoptosis*—that kills them to enhance the organization of specific neuronal pathways, a process called *pruning* (Rakic, 2000; Yuan, 2000; Yuan and Yankner, 2000). Diseases of the nervous system may result from the apoptotic process or other forms of cell death which is normally prevented in the healthy adult state by neurotrophic factors (Leist and Nicotera, 1997; Raff, 1998; McAllister, Usrey, et al., 2002).

THE STRUCTURE OF THE BRAIN

The brain is an intricately patterned complex of small and delicate structures. Three major anatomical divisions of the brain succeed one another along the brain stem: the *hindbrain,* the *midbrain,* and the *forebrain* (see Figs. 3.1 and 3.2; for detailed graphic displays, see also Montemurro and Bruni, 1988; Netter, 1983). Structurally, the brain centers that are lowest are the most simply organized. The brain's forward development is characterized by a pronounced tendency for increased anatomical complexity and diversity culminating in the huge, elaborate structures at the brain's front end, the *cerebrum* or *cerebral hemispheres* (since most cerebral structures are laterally paired). The brain's functional organization parallels its structural development as functional complexity increases from the lower brain stem up through its succeeding parts. By and large, lower brain centers mediate simpler, more primitive functions while the forward (top in humans) part of the brain, the cerebral cortex (see p. 52ff), mediates the highest functions.

Within the brain are four fluid-filled pouches, or *ventricles,* through which *cerebrospinal fluid (CSF)* flows (Schmidley and Maas, 1990; see also Netter, 1983, pp. 30–31). The most prominent of the pouches, the lateral ventricles, are a pair of horn-shaped reservoirs situated inside the cerebral hemispheres, running from front to back and curving around into the temporal lobe (see Fig. 3.3, p. 42). The third ventricle is situated in the midline in the *diencephalon* ("between-brain")

(see Figs. 3.3 and 3.6, p. 49). The fourth lies within the brain stem. Cerebrospinal fluid is produced by specialized tissues within all of the ventricles but mostly in the lateral ventricles. The cerebrospinal fluid serves as a shock absorber and helps to maintain the shape of the soft nervous tissue of the brain. Obstruction of the flow of cerebrospinal fluid in adults can create the condition known as *normal pressure hydrocephalus (NPH)* (see pp. 256–257). In conditions in which brain substance deteriorates, the ventricles enlarge to fill in the void. Thus, the size of the ventricles can be an important indicator of the brain's status.

In addition, an elaborate network of blood vessels maintains a rich supply of nutrients to the extremely oxygen-dependent brain tissue (Golanov and Reis, 1997; Hudetz, 1997; Powers, 1990). The cerebral blood supply comes from three major arterial distributions (Fig. 3.4; see Sokoloff, 1997; Tatu et al., 2001). The site of disease or damage to arterial circulation determines the area of the brain cut off from its oxygen supply and, to a large extent, the neuropathologic consequences (see Figs. 3.1 and 3.7, 3.12, pp. 53, 64; pp. 63–85 for a review of cerebral lobes and their functions; pp. 194–202 for pathologies arising from cerebrovascular disorders). The anterior and middle cerebral arteries branch from the internal carotid artery. The anterior division supplies the anterior frontal lobe and *medial* (toward the midline) regions of the brain. The middle cerebral artery feeds the lateral temporal, parietal, and posterior frontal lobes and sends branches deep into subcortical regions. The posterior circulation

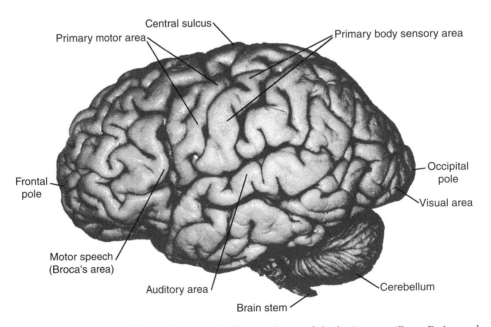

FIGURE 3.1 Lateral view of the cerebrum, cerebellum, and part of the brain stem. (From DeArmond, Fusco, and Dewey, 1976)

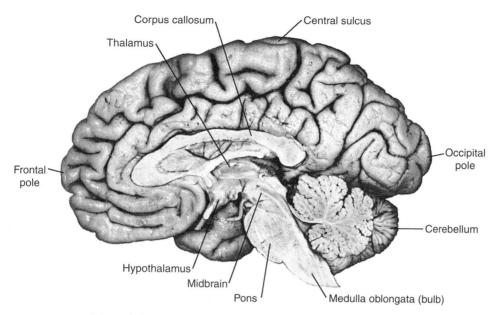

FIGURE 3.2 Medial view of the brain. (From DeArmond, Fusco, and Dewey, 1976)

originates from the vertebral arteries, which join to form the basilar artery. They provide blood to the brain stem and cerebellum. The basilar artery divides into the posterior cerebral arteries and supplies the occipital cortex and medial and inferior regions of the temporal lobe.

The Hindbrain

The medulla oblongata

The lowest part of the brain stem is the hindbrain, and its lowest section is the *medulla oblongata* or *bulb* (see Figs. 3.2 and 3.5, p. 45). The corticospinal tract, which runs down it, crosses the midline here so that each cerebral hemisphere has motor control over the opposite side of the body. The hindbrain is the site of basic life-maintaining centers for nervous control of respiration, blood pressure, and heartbeat. Significant injury to the bulb generally results in death. The medulla contains *nuclei* (clusters of functionally related nerve cells) involved in movements of mouth and throat structures necessary for swallowing, speech, and such related activities as gagging and control of drooling. Damage to lateral medullary structures can result in sensory deficits (J.S. Kim et al., 1997).

The reticular formation

Running through the bulb from the upper cord to the diencephalon is the *reticular formation*, a network of intertwined and interconnecting nerve cell bodies and

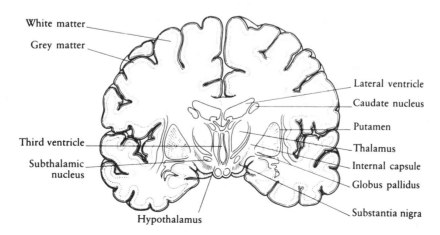

FIGURE 3.3 Coronal (vertical) section of the human brain "taken roughly through the ears" showing diencephalic and other subcortical cerebral structures. (From Strange, 1992)

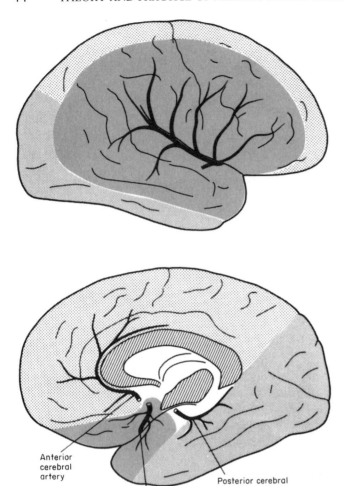

Anterior
cerebral
artery

Posterior cerebral
artery

Middle cerebral artery

FIGURE 3.4 The parts of the brain supplied with blood from the main arterial branches. (From P. Brodal, 1992)

fibers that enter into or connect with all major neural tracts going to and from the brain (see Figs. 3.5, p. 45 and 3.17, p. 77). The reticular formation is not a single functional unit but contains many nerve centers, i.e., nuclei. These nerve centers mediate important and complex postural reflexes, contribute to the smoothness of muscle activity, and maintain muscle tone. The reticular formation, from about the level of the lower third of the pons (see below and Figs. 3.2 and 3.5) up to and including diencephalic structures, is also the site of the *reticular activating system* (*RAS*), which is the part of the network that controls wakefulness and alerting mechanisms that ready the individual to react (S. Green, 1987; Mirsky, 1989). The RAS modulates attention through its arousal of the cerebral cortex (Mesulam, 2000b; Parasuraman, Warm, and See, 1998; Van Zomeren and Brouwer, 1994). The intact functioning of this network is a precondition for conscious behavior since it arouses the sleeping or inattentive or-

ganism (G. Roth, 2000). Brain stem lesions involving the RAS give rise to sleep disturbances and to global disorders of consciousness and responsivity such as drowsiness, somnolence, stupor, or coma.

The pons

The *pons* is high in the hindbrain (Figs. 3.2 and 3.5, pp. 42, 45). It contains major pathways for fibers running between the cerebral cortex and the cerebellum (see below), which is attached to the brain stem. Together, the pons and cerebellum correlate postural and *kinesthetic* (muscle movement sense) information, refining and regulating motor impulses relayed from the cerebrum at the top of the brain stem. Lesions of the pons may cause motor, sensory, and coordination disorders (L.R. Caplan, 2001; Chung and Caplan, 2001).

The cerebellum

The *cerebellum* is at the posterior base of the brain (Figs. 3.1, 3.2, 3.5). In addition to reciprocal connections with vestibular and brain stem nuclei, the *hypothalamus* (see p. 47), and the spinal cord, it has strong connections with the motor cortex and contributes to motor control through influences on programming and execution of actions. Cerebellar damage is commonly known to produce problems of fine motor control, coordination, and postural regulation (Barlow, 2002). Dizziness (*vertigo*) and jerky eye movements may also accompany cerebellar damage.

It is becoming increasingly evident that the cerebellum has a variety of nonmotor functions involving all aspects of behavior (Schmahmann, 2003). Highly organized neural pathways from both lower and higher areas of the brain project through the pons to the cerebellum (Llinás and Walton, 1998; Schmahmann and Sherman, 1998). The cerebellum projects through the thalamus to the same cortical areas from which it receives input, including frontal, parietal, and superior temporal cortices (Botez, Gravel, Attig, and Vezina, 1985; Schmahmann and Sherman, 1998). Through its connections with these cortical areas and with subcortical sites, cerebellar lesions can disrupt abstract reasoning, verbal fluency, visuospatial abilities, attention, emotional modulation (Botez, Lalonde, and Botez-Marquard, 1996; Middleton and Strick, 2000a; Schmahmann and Sherman, 1998), and planning and time judgment (Dow, 1988; Ivry and Fiez, 2000; MacLean, 1991). The cerebellum is also involved in linguistic processing (H.C. Leiner et al., 1989), word generation (Raichle, 2000), set shifting (Le et al., 1998), working memory (Desmond et al., 1997), and memory and learning (Nyberg, 1998)—especially habit forma-

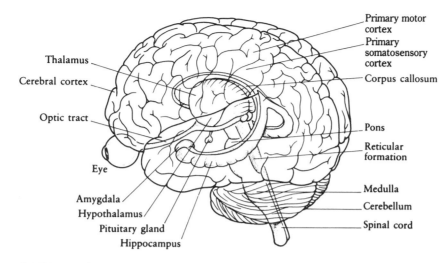

FIGURE 3.5 Diagram showing the hippocampus in relation to the rest of the brain. (From Strange, 1992)

tion (Eichenbaum and Cohen, 2001; H.C. Leiner et al., 1986; R.F. Thompson, 1988). Moreover, speed of information processing slows with cerebellar lesions (Botez, Gravel, et al., 1985). Some disruptions may be transient (Botez et al., 1985; Botez-Marquard, Leveille, and Botez, 1994; Schmahmann and Sherman, 1998). Personality changes and psychiatric disorders have also been linked to cerebellar dysfunction (Andreasen, 2001; P. Martin and Albers, 1995; J. Parvizi et al., 2001).

The Midbrain

The *midbrain (mesencephalon)*, a small area just forward of the hindbrain, includes the major portion of the reticular activating system. Its functioning may be a prerequisite for conscious experience (Parvizi and Damasio, 2001). It also contains both sensory and motor correlation centers (see Fig. 3.2). Auditory and visual system processing that takes place in midbrain nuclei contributes to the integration of reflex and automatic responses. Midbrain lesions have been associated with specific movement disabilities such as certain types of tremor, rigidity, and extraneous movements of local muscle groups. Even impaired memory retrieval has been associated with damage to midbrain pathways projecting to structures in the memory system (E. Goldberg, Antin, Bilder, et al., 1981; Hommel and Besson, 2001).

The Forebrain: Diencephalic Structures

The most forward part of the brain has two subdivisions. The *diencephalon* ("between-brain") comprises a set of structures, including correlation and relay centers, that evolved at the *anterior*, or most forward, part

of the brain stem. These structures are almost completely embedded within the two halves of the *forebrain*, the *telencephalon*.

The thalamus

From a neuropsychological viewpoint, the most important of the diencephalic structures are the *thalamus* and the *hypothalamus* (see Figs. 3.2, 3.3, p. 43, 3.5 and 3.6, p. 49). The thalamus is a small, paired, somewhat oval structure lying along the right and left sides of the third ventricle. Each half of the thalamus consists of eleven nuclei or more, depending on whether minor or peripheral structures are distinguished or included in the count. The two halves are matched approximately in size, shape, and position to corresponding nuclei in the other half. Most of the anatomic interconnections formed by these nuclei and many of their functional contributions are known. Nevertheless, growing understanding of how complex are the fine circuitry, feedback loops, and many functional systems in which the thalamus is enmeshed, and of the interplay between its neurophysiological processes, its neurotransmitters, and its structures encourages speculation and requires caution when interpreting research findings (Steriade et al., 1990).

A complete description of the complex connections of the many thalamic nuclei with cortical, brainstem, and limbic system (see pp. 49–51) structures is beyond the scope of this book. The basic organization and highlights are presented instead.

Thalamic nuclei have extensive reciprocal connections with the cortex that are topographically organized (S.M. Sherman and Koch, 1998). Sensory nuclei serve as major sensory relay centers for all senses except smell and project to primary sensory cortices (see pp. 53–54). Body sensations in particular may be degraded or lost with damage to appropriate thalamic nuclei (L.R. Caplan, 1980; Graff-Radford, Damasio, et al., 1985), with an associated impairment of the ability to make tactile discriminations and identification of what is felt (*tactile object agnosia*) (Caselli, 1991; Bauer and Demery, 2003). Although pain sensation typically remains intact or is only mildly diminished, with some kinds of thalamic damage it may be heightened to an excruciating degree (A. Barth et al., 2001; Brodal, 1981; Clifford, 1990). Other thalamic nuclei are relay pathways for vision, hearing, and taste (J.S. Kim, 2001). Still other areas are relay nuclei for limbic structures. Motor nuclei receive input from the cerebellum and the basal ganglia and project to the motor association cortex. As the termination site for the ascending RAS, it is not surprising that the thalamus has important arousal and sleep-producing functions (S. Green, 1987; J. Newman, 1997; Steriade et al., 1990) and that it alerts—activates and intensifies—specific processing and response systems (Crosson, 1992; LaBerge, 2000; Mesulam, 2000b). Its involvement in attention shows up in diminished awareness of stimuli impinging on the side opposite the lesion (*unilateral inattention*) (Heilman, Watson, and Valenstein, 2003; Ojemann, 1984; Posner, 1988).

The thalamus also plays a significant role in regulating higher-level brain activity (S.M. Sherman and Koch, 1998). The *dorsomedial nucleus* is of particular interest because of its established role in memory and its extensive reciprocal connections with the prefrontal cortex (Graff-Radford, 2003; Mesulam, 2000b). It also receives input from the temporal cortex, *amygdala* (see pp. 49–50), hypothalamus, and other thalamic nuclei (Afifi and Bergman, 1998). That the dorsomedial nuclei of the thalamus participate in memory functions has been known ever since lesions here were associated with the memory deficit of Korsakoff's psychosis (von Cramon et al., 1985; Victor, Adams, and Collins, 1971; see pp. 262–265). In most if not all cases of memory impairment associated with the thalamus, lesions have extended to the *mammillothalamic tract* (Graff-Radford, 2003; Markowitsch, 2000; Verfaellie and Cermak, 1997). The mammillothalamic tract connects the *mammillary bodies* (small structures at the posterior part of the hypothalamus involved in information correlation and transmission [Brodal, 1981; Crosson, 1992]) to the thalamus which sends projections on a pathway to the prefrontal cortex and medial temporal lobe (Fuster, 1994; Markowitsch, 2000).

Two kinds of memory impairments tend to accompany thalamic lesions: (1) Learning is compromised (anterograde amnesia), possibly by defective encoding, which makes effective retrieval difficult if not impossible (N. Butters, 1984a; Mayes, 1988; Ojemann, Hoyenga, and Ward, 1971); possibly by a diminished capacity of learning processes to free up readily for succeeding exposures to new information (defective *release from proactive inhibition*) (N. Butters and Stuss, 1989; Parkin, 1984). A rapid loss of newly acquired information may also occur (Stuss, Guberman, et al., 1988), although usually when patients with thalamic memory impairment do learn they forget no faster than do intact persons (Parkin, 1984). (2) Recall of past information is defective (retrograde amnesia), typically in a *temporal gradient* such that recall of the most recent (premorbid) events and new information is most impaired, and increasingly older memories are increasingly better retrieved (N. Butters and Albert, 1982; Kopelman, 2001). Montaldi and Parkin (1989) suggest that these two kinds of memory impairment are different aspects of a breakdown in the use of context (encoding), for retrieval depends on establishing and maintaining "contextual relations among existing memories." Errors made by an unlettered file clerk would provide an analogy for these learning and retrieval deficits: Items filed randomly remain in the file cabinet but cannot be retrieved by directed search, yet they may pop up from time to time, unconnected to any intent to find them (see also Hodges, 1995).

Amnesic patients with bilateral diencephalic lesions, such as Korsakoff patients, tend to show disturbances in time sense and the ability to make temporal discriminations that may play a role in their prominent retrieval deficits (Graff-Radford, Tranel, et al., 1990; Squire, Haist, and Shimamura, 1989). Characteristically, memory-impaired patients with thalamic or other diencephalic lesions lack appreciation of their deficits, in this differing from many other memory-impaired persons (Mesulam, 2000b; Parkin, 1984; Schacter, 1991). In a review of 61 cases of adults with thalamic lesions, mostly resulting from stroke, half had problems with concept formation, flexibility of thinking, or executive functions (Van der Werf et al., 2000).

Differences in how the two halves of the brain process data, so pronounced at the highest—cortical—level, first appear in thalamic processing of sensory information (A. Barth et al., 2001; J.W. Brown, 1975). In its lateral asymmetry, thalamic organization parallels cortical organization in that left thalamic structures are implicated in verbal activity, and right thalamic structures in nonverbal aspects of cognitive performance. For example, patients who have left thalamic lesions or who are undergoing left thalamic electrostimulation have not lost the capacity for verbal communication but may experience dysnomia and other language disruption (Crosson, 1992; Graff-Radford,

Damasio, et al., 1985; M.D. Johnson and Ojemann, 2000). This pattern is not considered to be a true aphasia, but rather has been described as a "withering" of language functioning that sometimes leads to mutism. Apathy, confusion, and disorientation characterize this behavior pattern (J.W. Brown, 1974; see also D. Caplan, 1987; Mazaux and Orgogozo, 1982). Patients with left thalamic lesions may achieve lower scores on verbal tests than patients whose thalamic damage is limited to the right side (Graff-Radford, Damasio, et al., 1985; Vilkki, 1979). Language deficits do not appear with very small thalamic lesions, suggesting that observable language deficits at the thalamic level require destruction of more than one pathway or nucleus, as would happen with larger lesions (Wallesch, Kornhuber, et al., 1983).

Neuroimaging studies have shown that right thalamic regions are involved in identifying shapes or locations (LaBerge, 2000). Patients who have right thalamic lesions or who undergo electrostimulation of the right thalamus can have difficulty with face or pattern recognition and pattern matching (Fedio and Van Buren, 1975; Vilkki and Laitinen, 1974, 1976), maze tracing (Meier and Story, 1967), and design reconstruction (Graff-Radford, Damasio, et al., 1985). Heilman, Watson, and Valenstein (2003) provide graphic evidence of patients with right thalamic lesions who displayed left-sided inattention characteristic of patients with right-sided—particularly right posterior—cortical lesions (the "neglect syndrome"; see pp. 72–73). This phenomenon may also accompany left thalamic lesions, although unilateral inattention occurs more often with right-sided damage (Posner, 1988; Velasco et al., 1986; Vilkki, 1984). Although some studies have suggested that unilateral thalamic lesions lead to modality-specific memory deficits (Graff-Radford, Damasio, et al., 1985; M.D. Johnson and Ojemann, 2000; Stuss, Guberman, et al., 1988), conflicting data leave this question unresolved (N. Kapur, 1988b; Rousseaux et al., 1986).

Alterations in emotional capacity and responsivity tend to accompany thalamic damage, typically as apathy, loss of spontaneity and drive, and affective flattening, emotional characteristics that are integral to the Korsakoff syndrome (O'Connor et al., 1995; Schott et al., 1980; Stuss, Guberman, et al., 1988). Yet disinhibited behavior and emotions occasionally appear with bilateral thalamic lesions (Graff-Radford, Tranel, et al., 1990). Transient manic episodes may follow right thalamic infarctions, with few such reactions—or strong emotional responses—seen when the lesion is on the left (Cummings and Mega, 2003; Starkstein, Robinson, Berthier, et al., 1988). These emotional and personality changes in diencephalic amnesia patients re-

flect how intimately interlocked are the emotional and memory components of the limbic system.

The other limbic system structures that have been specifically implicated in impairment of the recording and consolidation processes of memory are the mammillary bodies and the *fornix* (a central forebrain structure that links the hippocampal and the mammillothalamic areas of the limbic system) (N. Butters and Stuss, 1989; Markowitsch, 2000; Tanaka et al., 1997; Warrington and Weiskrantz, 1982). Massive anterograde amnesia and some retrograde amnesia can result from diffuse lesions involving the mammillary bodies and the thalamus (Graff-Radford, Tranel, et al., 1990; Kopelman, 2002; Squire, Haist, and Shimamura, 1989). Recording of ongoing events may be impaired by lesions of the fornix (Grafman, Salazar, et al., 1985; Mayes, 2000b; Ojemann, 1966; Warrington and Weiskrantz, 1982).

The hypothalamus

Although it takes up less than one-half of one percent of the brain's total weight, the *hypothalamus* regulates such important physiologically based drives as appetite, sexual arousal, and thirst (Netter, 1983; Rolls, 1999; C.B. Saper, 1990). It receives inputs from many brain regions and coordinates autonomic and endocrine functions. Behavior patterns having to do with physical protection, such as rage and fear reactions, are also regulated by hypothalamic centers. Depending on the site of the damage, lesions to hypothalamic nuclei can result in a variety of symptoms, including obesity, disorders of temperature control, and diminished drive states and responsivity (F.G. Flynn et al., 1988). Mood states may also be affected by hypothalamic lesions (Andreason, 2001; Shepherd, 1994; Wolkowitz and Reus, 2001). Damage to the mammillary bodies in the posterior hypothalamus disrupts memory processing (Tanaka et al., 1997).

The Forebrain: The Cerebrum

The basal ganglia

The *cerebrum,* the most recently evolved, most elaborated, and by far the largest brain structure, has two hemispheres that are almost but not quite identical mirror images of each other (see Figs. 3.5, p. 45 and 3.7, p. 53). Within each *cerebral hemisphere,* at its base, are situated a number of nuclear masses known as the *basal ganglia* ("ganglion" is another term for "nucleus"). In most nomenclatures the basal ganglia refer to the *caudate, putamen,* and *globus pallidus* (see Figs. 3.3, 3.6, 3.17, pp. 45, 49, 77). In some sources, the basal ganglia include the amygdala, *subthalamic nucleus, substantia nigra,* and other subcortical structures (see Figs. 3.5 and 3.17, pp. 45, 77). The cerebral cortex projects directly to the caudate and putamen, and the globus pallidus and substantia nigra project back to the cerebral cortex through the thalamus. In addition to the motor cortex, the basal ganglia have reciprocal connections with at least nine other cortical areas, including subdivisions of the premotor, oculomotor, prefrontal (dorsolateral and orbitofrontal), and inferotemporal cortices (Middleton and Strick, 2000a, b; Rolls, 1999). Somatotopic representation of specific body parts (e.g., hand, foot, face) within basal ganglia structures overlap, are similar for different individuals, and are unlike the pattern of cortical body part representation (Maillard et al., 2000).

"Figuratively speaking, the *neostriatum* (caudate and putamen) can be considered as part of the system which translates cognition into action" (Divac, 1977; see also Brunia and Van Boxtel, 2000; Passingham, 1997). The basal ganglia influence all aspects of motor control, and movement disorders may be the most common and obvious symptoms of basal ganglia damage (Crosson, Moore, and Wierenga, 2003). They are not motor nuclei in a strict sense, as damage to them gives rise to various motor disturbances but does not result in paralysis. The movement disorders associated with basal ganglia disease have been thoroughly described, but what these nuclei contribute to the motor system is less well understood (Haaland and Harrington, 1990; Thach and Montgomery, 1990). In general, diseases of the basal ganglia are characterized by abnormal involuntary movements at rest. The particular effects vary with the specific site of injury. These nuclei also play an important role in the acquisition of habits and skills (Jog et al., 1999; see also Blazquez et al., 2002; Graybiel and Kubota, 2003).

Much of the understanding of the influence of the basal ganglia on movement and other aspects of behavior has been obtained by studying patients with *Parkinson's disease* and *Huntington's disease* (see pp. 225–227, 234–236). Parkinson's disease, primarily occuring with depletion of the neurotransmitter *dopamine* in the neostriatum due to degeneration of the substantia nigra, results in poverty of movement. It is interesting to note that difficulties in starting activities and in altering the course of ongoing activities characterize both motor and mental aspects of this disease (R.G. Brown, 2003). Huntington's disease, which develops with loss of neurons in the caudate nucleus, is characterized by excessive motor activity. Huntington patients, like Parkinson patients, appear to have trouble initiating cognitive processes (Brandt and Butters, 1996) and control over cognitive functions as well as

movements is impaired (Richer and Chouinard, 2003). In both conditions, many cognitive abilities are impaired and emotional disturbances may be prominent.

The neostriatum appears to be a key component of the procedural memory system (Fuster, 1995; Mishkin and Appenzeller, 1987; Knowlton et al., 1996), perhaps serving as a procedural memory buffer for established skills and response patterns and participating in the development of new response strategies (skills) for novel situations (Saint-Cyr and Taylor, 1992). With damage to the basal ganglia, cognitive flexibility—the ability to generate and shift ideas and responses—is reduced (Lawrence et al., 1999; Mendez, Adams, and Lewandowski, 1989). Hemispheric lateralization becomes apparent with unilateral lesions, both in motor disturbances affecting the side of the body contralateral to the lesioned nuclei and in the nature of the concomitant cognitive disorders (L.R. Caplan, Schmahmann, et al., 1990). Several different types of aphasic and related communication disorders have been described in association with left-sided lesions (Cummings and Mega, 2003). In some patients, lesions in the left basal ganglia alone or in conjunction with left cortical lesions have been associated with defective knowledge of the colors of familiar objects (Varney and Risse, 1993). Symptoms tend to vary in a fairly regular manner with the lesion site (M.P. Alexander, Naeser, and Palumbo, 1987; Basso, Della Sala, and Farabola, 1987; A.R. Damasio, Damasio, and Rizzo, 1982; Tanridag and Kirshner, 1985), paralleling the cortical aphasia pattern of reduced output with anterior lesions, reduced comprehension with posterior ones (Crosson, 1992; Naeser, Alexander, et al., 1982). Left unilateral inattention accompanies some right-sided basal ganglia lesions (Bisiach and Vallar, 1988; Ferro, Kertesz, and Black, 1987; L.R. Caplan, Schmahmann, et al., 1990; Vallar and Perani, 1986; Villardita et al., 1983).

Dramatic and disruptive personality changes may occur in Huntington's disease as basal ganglia degeneration proceeds (see pp. 227, 235–236). Moreover, alterations in basal ganglia circuits involved with nonmotor areas of the cortex have been implicated in a wide variety of neuropsychiatric disorders including schizophrenia, obsessive-compulsive disorder, depression, Tourette's syndrome, autism, and attention deficit disorders (D.J. Stein and Hugo, 2002; Middleton and Strick, 2000b; M.A. Taylor, 1999). Emotional flattening with loss of drive resulting in more or less severe states of inertia can occur with bilateral basal ganglia damage (Bhatia and Marsden, 1994; Laplane et al., 1984; Strub, 1989). These *anergic* (unenergized, apathetic) conditions resemble those associated with some kinds of frontal damage and further emphasize the interrelationships between the basal ganglia and the frontal lobes. Mood differences have shown up in new stroke patients with lateralized basal ganglia lesions, in that more patients with left-sided damage were depressed than those with right-sided involvement (Starkstein, Robinson, Berthier, et al., 1988).

The *nucleus basalis of Meynert* is a small basal forebrain structure lying partly within and partly adjacent to the basal ganglia (N. Butters, 1985; H. Damasio and Damasio, 1989). It is an important source of the cholinergic neurotransmitters implicated in learning. Loss of neurons here occurs in degenerative dementing disorders in which memory impairment is a prominent feature (Fuster, 1995; J.D. Rogers et al., 1985).

The Limbic System

The *limbic system* includes, among other structures, the amygdala and two phylogenetically old regions of cortex: the cingulate gyrus and the hippocampus (Dudai, 1989; Markowitsch, 2000; Papez, 1937; see also Figs. 3.5, p. 45 and 3.6). Its components are embedded in structures as far apart as the reticular activating system in the brain stem and olfactory nuclei underlying the forebrain. These structures have important roles in emotion, motivation, and memory (Damasio, 1994; Markowitsch, 2000; Mesulam, 2000b; Don M. Tucker, Derryberry, and Luu, 2000). The intimate connection between memory and emotions is illustrated by Korsakoff patients with severe learning impairments who retain emotionally laden words better than neutral ones

(J. Kessler et al., 1987). This same phenomenon has been observed in some anergic TBI (traumatic brain injury) patients whose condition implicates limbic damage and whose responsiveness and learning ability increase when emotionally stimulated. Disturbances in emotional behavior occur in association with seizure activity involving these structures (see pp. 76, 322).

The amygdala

This small structure is located deep in the anterior part of the temporal lobe (Fig. 3.5, p. 45). Consisting of a number of nuclei with differing input and output pathways, it has connections with the cerebral cortex, hippocampus, basal ganglia, thalamus, hypothalamus, and brain stem nucei. It plays important roles in emotional processing and learning (Bechara, Damasio, Damasio, and Lee, 1999; Rolls, 1999; Sarter and Markowitsch, 1985) and in the modulation of attention (Eichenbaum and Cohen, 2001).

Not surprisingly, given its rich hypothalamic interconnections, the amygdala is intimately involved with vegetative and protective drive states, movement patterns, and associated emotional responses. It has direct connections with the primitive olfaction centers (*olfactory bulbs*) (A.R. Damasio, 2001; Shepherd and Greer, 1998; see Fig. 3.5). Damage to the amygdala's interconnecting structures (e.g., the posterior septum lying between the hemispheres in front of the anterior commissure) has been associated with both hypersexuality

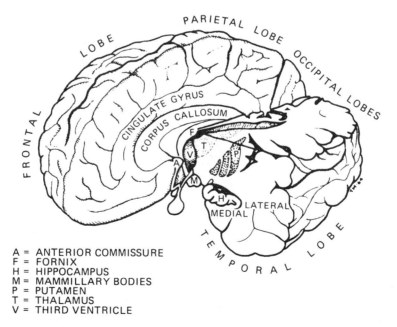

A = ANTERIOR COMMISSURE
F = FORNIX
H = HIPPOCAMPUS
M = MAMMILLARY BODIES
P = PUTAMEN
T = THALAMUS
V = THIRD VENTRICLE

FIGURE 3.6 Cutaway perspective drawing of a human brain showing the spatial relationships of most of the regions and structures thought to be related to general memory function. (The putamen is shown only as a landmark for readers familiar with the brain.) (From Ojemann, 1966)

and diminished aggressive capacity (Brodal, 1981; Gorman and Cummings, 1992). Semiautomatic visceral activities, particularly those concerned with feeding (e.g., chewing, salivating, licking, and gagging) and with the visceral components of fear reactions, are affected by stimulation or ablation of the amygdala. This small structure may also be necessary for processing facial expressions of fear (Adolphs and Damasio, 2000; Rolls, 1999). Seizure activity and experimental stimulation of the amygdala provoke visceral responses associated with fright and mouth movements involved in feeding.

Removal of the amygdala from both hemispheres can have a "taming" effect on humans and other animals alike, with loss of the ability to make emotionally meaningful discriminations between stimuli (Cahill and McGaugh, 1998; Killcross, 2000; J. Rosen and Schulkin, 1998; Pincus and Tucker, 2003). Amygdalectomized humans become apathetic showing little spontaneity, creativity, or affective expression (Aggleton, 1993; G.P. Lee, Bechara, Adolphs, et al., 1989). In addition, the ability to make social interpretations of facial expressions is impaired in patients with bilateral amygdala lesions (Adolphs et al., 1998). Amygdala dysfunction has been implicated in autism (Baron-Cohen, 1995; Baron-Cohen et al., 2000).

The amygdala provides an emotional "tag" to memory traces (Doty, 1990; Rolls, 1990; Sarter and Markowitsch, 1985). With its connections to the orbitofrontal cortex, the amygdala appears to be necessary for learning to associate sensory stimuli with reward (Rolls and Treves, 1998). Information about rewards and emotions is sent from the amygdala to the hippocampus. Material learned by amygdalectomized patients tends to be retained, but they become more dependent on context and external structure for learning new material, for retrieval generally, and for maintaining directed attention and tracking than prior to surgery (R. Anderson, 1978). The amygdala may play an important role in memory consolidation by influencing neuroplasticity in other brain regions (McGaugh, 2000), although much remains speculative. Its specialized memory functions appear to involve object recognition (Mishkin and Appenzeller, 1987). Bilateral destruction of the amygdala in humans does not produce a prominent amnesic disorder (G.P. Lee, Meador, Smith, et al., 1988; Markowitsch, Calabrese, Wurker, et al., 1994; I.F. Small et al., 1977). However, lesions in the amygdala and nearby temporal cortex contribute to the severity of memory deficits associated with hippocampal damage (Jernigan, Ostergaard, and Fennema-Notestine, 2001). Amygdalectomized patients are slow to acquire a mind set, but once it is established it becomes hard to dislodge; yet performance on standard measures of mental abilities (e.g., Wechsler Intelligence

Scale tests) remains essentially unchanged (R. Andersen, 1978).

The *Klüver-Bucy syndrome* follows bilateral destruction of the amygdala and *uncus* (the small hooked front end of the inner temporal lobe fold). This is a rare condition that can occur with disease (e.g., herpes encephalitis [see pp. 275–276]) or trauma. These placid patients lose the capacity to learn and to make perceptual distinctions, they eat excessively and indiscriminately, and they may become hypersexual, often indiscriminately so (Cummings and Mega, 2003; Hayman et al., 1998; Trimble, Mendez, and Cummings, 1997).

The cingulate cortex

The *cingulate gyrus* is located in the medial aspects of the hemispheres above the corpus callosum (Fig. 3.6). It has important influences on attention, response selection, and emotional behavior (Brunia and Van Boxtel, 2000; Chelazzi and Corbetta, 2000; Rolls, 1999). Anterior and posterior portions have different projections and roles. Together with the lateral prefrontal cortex, the anterior cingulate cortex controls behavior by detecting errors and signaling the occurrence of conflicts during information processing. These functions are critical for the regulation of behavior according to self-determined intentions. The relative contribution of the two structures is a matter of debate (J.D. Cohen et al., 2000; Gehring and Knight, 2000). Lesions of the anterior cingulate cortex interfere with selective attention, response competition monitoring, and self-initiated behavior (R.A. Cohen et al., 1999; Danckert et al., 2000; Devinsky, Morrell, and Vogt, 1995; Posner and Rothbart, 1998). The anterior cingulate is also involved in pain perception (Rolls, 1999). Whereas the anterior cingulate receives projections mainly from the amygdala, the posterior cingulate receives most projections from the hippocampus (see below) and is part of the neural pathway for memory (Desgranges et al., 1998; Mesulam, 2000b).

The hippocampus

A major component of the memory system, the *hippocampus* runs within the inside fold of each temporal lobe for much of its length (Figs. 3.5 and 3.6, pp. 45, 46). Converging evidence from lesion studies, epilepsy surgery, and functional imaging studies points to its primary role in normal learning and retention. The hippocampus is well-designed for rapid association of information from many different cortical areas (Eichenbaum and Cohen, 2001; D. Johnston and Amaral, 1998; O'Keefe and Nadel, 1978). The hippocampus has been identified as one site of interaction between the perception and the memory systems with a particular role in spatial memory (Mishkin and Appenzeller, 1987; Zola and Squire, 2000). Only sensorimotor skill learning and simple forms of conditioning take place in other brain centers (Buckner and Tulving, 1995; Corkin, 1968; Eichenbaum and Cohen, 2001; Mayes, 2000b; Squire and Knowlton, 2000).

The hippocampus has been described as using a "snapshot" type of processing to remember a scene or episode with its unique elements and contextual features (Rolls and Treves, 1998). The hippocampus can later activate retrieval of the whole representation when a small part of the representation occurs (McClelland, 1994; Rolls and Treves, 1998). Two-way information between many areas of the cortex and the hippocampus goes through the *entorhinal cortex* as information about rewards and emotions travels from the amygdala to the hippocampus. A second pathway for outputs from the hippocampus to the cortex goes by way of the *fornix* and thalamus (Fig. 3.6).

The hippocampus and adjacent areas of the temporal lobe are critical for learning, i.e., the formation of new memories (Ogden, 1996, chap. 3; Rempel-Clower et al., 1996; Zola and Squire, 2000; see pp. 75–76). It has been suggested that the hippocampus processes new memories by assigning each experience an index corresponding to the areas of the neocortex which, when activated, reproduce the experience or memory (Alvarez and Squire, 1994; Schacter, 1998). The hippocampal index typically includes information about events and their context, such as when and where they occurred as well as emotions and thoughts associated with them. The index corresponding to a particular memory, such as a conversation or other activity, is crucial for activating the memory until the neocortex consolidates the memory by linking all the features of the experience to one another. After consolidation, direct neocortical links are sufficient for storing the memory (Schacter, Norman, and Koutstaal, 1998). Old memories do not appear to be stored in the hippocampus; rather, storage is probably distributed throughout the cortex (Fuster, 1995; Rempel-Clower et al., 1996; Rolls and Treves, 1998).

Bilateral damage to the hippocampus can produce severe anterograde amnesia (Rempel-Clower et al., 1996; Tulving and Markowitsch, 1998). The cortical regions adjacent to the hippocampus, the entorhinal cortex, parahippocampus, and other perirhinal cortices provide major input to the hippocampus. When lesions of the hippocampus extend into these regions, the severity of the memory impairment worsens and the likelihood of extensive retrograde amnesia increases (K.S. Graham and Hodges, 1997; J.M. Reed and Squire,

1998). Damage to the hippocampus and adjacent areas of the temporal lobe is responsible for the memory impairment so prominent in mild Alzheimer's disease (Cotman and Anderson, 1995; Jack et al., 1999; Kaye, Swihart, Howieson, et al., 1997). Disturbances in emotional behavior occur in association with seizure activity involving the hippocampus as well as the amygdala and uncus (Heilman, Blonder, et al., 2003; Pincus and Tucker, 2003; Wieser, 1986).

Unilateral destruction of the hippocampus can result in lateralized processing differences. Loss of the left hippocampus impairs verbal memory, and destruction of the right hippocampus results in defective recognition and recall of "complex visual and auditory patterns to which a name cannot readily be assigned" (B. Milner, 1970, p. 30; see also A.R. Damasio, 2001; Jones-Gotman, 1987). For example, London taxi drivers recalling familiar routes showed right hippocampal activation on PET scans (Maguire et al., 1997). However, rote verbal learning may be more vulnerable to left hippocampal disease than learning meaningful material (a story) (Saling et al., 1993). Story recall appears to be affected—but to a lesser degree than rote learning—by damage to either the right or left hippocampus. Additionally, learning unrelated as opposed to related word pairs is disproportionately impaired with left, rather than right, hippocampal disease (A.G. Wood et al., 2000).

Intracerebral conduction pathways

> The mind depends as much on white matter as on its gray counterpart.
>
> *Christopher M. Filley, 2001*

Much of the bulk of the cerebral hemispheres is *white matter,* consisting of densely packed conduction fibers that transmit neural impulses between cortical points within a hemisphere (*association fibers*), between the hemispheres (*commissural fibers*), or between the cerebral cortex and lower centers (*projection fibers*). Lesions in cerebral white matter sever connections between lower and higher centers or between cortical areas. White matter lesions are found in many dementing disorders and appear to be specifically associated with attentional impairments (Filley, 2001; Junqué et al., 1990).

The *corpus callosum* is the great band of commissural fibers connecting the two hemispheres (see Figs. 3.2, 3.5, and 3.6, pp. 42, 45, 49). Other interhemispheric connections are provided by some smaller bands of fibers. Interhemispheric communication maintained by the corpus callosum and other commissural fibers enforces integration of cerebral activity between the two hemispheres (Banich, 1995; Trevarthen, 1990; E. Zaidel, Clarke, and Suyenobu, 1990).

The corpus callosum is organized with a great deal of regularity (Brodal, 1981; J.M. Clarke et al., 1998; Witelson, 1995). Fibers from the frontal cortex make up its anterior portion. The posterior portion consists of fibers originating in the posterior cortex. Fibers from the visual cortex at the posterior pole of the cerebrum occupy the posterior end portion of the callosum. Midcallosal areas contain a mixture of fibers coming from both anterior and posterior regions. Studies of sex differences in overall size of the corpus callosum have produced inconsistent results (Bishop and Wahlstein, 1997; H.L. Burke and Yeo, 1994; Davatzikos and Resnick, 1998; Salat et al., 1997; Witelson, 1989; E. Zaidel, Aboitiz, et al., 1995). Some studies have found that the corpus callosum tends to be larger in nonright-handers (Cowell et al., 1993; Habib, Gayraud, Oliva, et al., 1991; Witelson, 1985).

Surgical section of the corpus callosum cuts off direct interhemispheric communication (Baynes and Gazzaniga, 2000; Bogen, 1985; Seymour et al., 1994). When examined by special neuropsychological techniques (see E. Zaidel, Zaidel, and Bogen 1990), patients who have undergone section of commissural fibers (*commissurotomy*) exhibit profound behavioral discontinuities between perception, comprehension, and response, which reflect significant functional differences between the hemispheres. Probably because direct communication between two cortical points occurs far less frequently than indirect communication relayed through lower brain centers, especially the thalamus and the basal ganglia, these patients generally manage to perform everyday activities quite well, including tasks involving interhemispheric information transfer (J.J. Myers and Sperry, 1985; Sergent, 1990, 1991b; E. Zaidel, Clarke, and Suyenobu, 1990) and emotional and conceptual information not dependent on language or complex visuospatial processes (Cronin-Golomb, 1986). In noting that alertness remains unaffected by commissurotomy and that emotional tone is consistent between the hemispheres, Sperry (1990) suggested that both phenomena rely on bilateral projections through the intact brain stem.

Some persons with *agenesis of the corpus callosum* (a rare congenital condition in which the corpus callosum is insufficiently developed or absent altogether) are identified only when some other condition brings them to a neurologist's attention, as they normally display no neurological or neuropsychological defects (L.J. Harris, 1995; E. Zaidel, Iacoboni, et al., 2003) other than slowed motor performances, particularly of bimanual tasks (Lassonde et al., 1991). However, persons with congenital agenesis of the corpus callosum also tend to be generally slowed on perceptual and language tasks involving interhemispheric communication,

and some show specific linguistic and/or visuospatial deficits (Jeeves, 1990, 1994; see also E. Zaidel and Iacoboni, 2003). In some cases, problems with higher order cognitive processes such as concept formation, reasoning, and problem solving with limited social insight have been observed (W.S. Brown and Paul, 2000). The functional disconnection between hemispheres and the effects of surgical hemispheric disconnection have been demonstrated by the same kinds of testing techniques (Bogen, 1985; Jeeves, 1990; E. Zaidel, 1990).

The cerebral cortex

The cortex of the cerebral hemispheres, the convoluted outer layer of gray matter composed of nerve cell bodies and their synaptic connections, is the most highly organized correlation center of the brain (see Figs. 3.1 and 3.2), but the specificity of cortical structures in mediating behavior is neither clear-cut nor circumscribed (R.C. Collins, 1990; Frackowiak, Friston, et al., 1997, Part Two). Predictably established relationships between cortical areas and behavior reflect the systematic organization of the cortex and its interconnections. Now modern visualizing techniques display what thoughtful clinicians had suspected: multiple cortical and subcortical areas are involved to some degree in the mediation of complex behaviors (Fuster, 1995; Mesulam, 2000b) and specific brain regions are typically multifunctional (Lloyd, 2000). The boundaries of functionally definable cortical areas, or *zones*, are vague. Cells subserving a specific function are highly concentrated in the primary area of a zone, thin out, and overlap with other zones as the perimeter of the zone is approached (E. Goldberg, 1989, 1995; Polyakov, 1966). Cortical activity at every level, from the cellular to the integrated system, is maintained and modulated by complex feedback loops that in themselves constitute major subsystems, some within the cortex and others involving subcortical centers and pathways as well. "Processing patterns take many forms, including *parallel*, *convergent* [integrative], *divergent* [spreading excitation], *nonlinear*, *recursive* [feeding back onto itself] and *iterative*" (H. Damasio and Damasio, 1989, p. 71). Even those functions that are subserved by cells located within relatively well-defined cortical areas have a significant number of components distributed outside the local cortical center (Brodal, 1981; Paulesu, Frackowiak, and Bottini, 1997).

THE CEREBRAL CORTEX AND BEHAVIOR

Cortical involvement appears to be a prerequisite for awareness of experience (Fuster, 1995; Köhler and Moscovitch, 1997; G. Roth, 2000). Patterns of functional localization in the cerebral cortex are broadly organized along two spatial planes. The *lateral plane* cuts through *homologous* (in the corresponding position) areas of the right and left hemispheres. The *longitudinal plane* runs from the front to the back of the cortex, with a relatively sharp demarcation between functions that are primarily localized in the forward portion of the cortex and those whose primary localization is behind the *central sulcus* or *fissure of Rolando*.

Lateral Organization

Lateral symmetry

The two cerebral hemispheres are nearly symmetrical. The primary sensory and motor centers are homologously positioned within the cerebral cortex of each hemisphere in a mirror-image relationship. With certain exceptions, such as the visual and auditory systems, the centers in each cerebral hemisphere predominate in mediating the activities of the *contralateral* (other side) half of the body (see Fig. 3.7). Thus, an injury to the primary *somesthetic* or *somatosensory* (sensations on the body) area of the right hemisphere results in decreased or absent sensation in the corresponding left-sided body part; an injury affecting the left motor cortex results in a right-sided weakness or paralysis (*hemiplegia*).

Point-to-point representation on the cortex. The organization of both the primary sensory and primary motor areas of the cortex provides for a point-to-point representation of the body. The amount of cortex identified with each body portion or organ is proportional to the number of sensory or motor nerve endings in that part of the body rather than to its size. For example, the areas concerned with sensation and movement of the tongue or fingers are much more extensive than the areas representing the elbow or back.

The visual system is also organized on a contralateral plan, but it is one-half of each *visual field* (the entire view encompassed by the eye) that is projected onto the contralateral visual cortex (see Fig. 3.7). Fibers originating in the right half of each retina, which registers stimuli in the left visual field, project to the right visual cortex; fibers from the left half of the retina convey the right visual field image to the left visual cortex. Thus, destruction of either eye leaves both halves of the visual field intact. Destruction of the right or the left primary visual cortex or of all the fibers leading to either side results in blindness for that side of both visual fields (*homonymous hemianopia*). Lesions involving a portion of the visual projection fibers or visual cortex result in circumscribed *field defects*, such as areas of blindness (*scotoma*, pl. *scotomata*) within the visual field of one or both eyes, depending on whether the lesion involves the visual pathway before or after its fibers cross on their route from the retina of the eye to the visual cortex. The precise point-to-point arrangement of projection fibers from the retina to the visual cortex permits especially accurate localization of lesions within the primary visual system (Sterling, 1998). Visual recognition is mediated by (at least) two different systems, each with different pathways involving different parts of the cortex (Goodale, 2000; Mesulam, 2000b; see Fig. 3.14, p. 68). One system processes visuospatial analysis, and one is dedicated to pattern analysis and object recognition; movement perception may involve a third system (Iwata, 1989; Zihl et al., 1983).

Some patients with brain injuries that do not impair visual acuity or recognition complain of blurred vision or degraded percepts, particularly with sustained activity, such as reading, or when exposure is very brief (Hankey, 2001; Sergent, 1984; Zihl, 1989). These problems reflect the complexity of an interactive net-

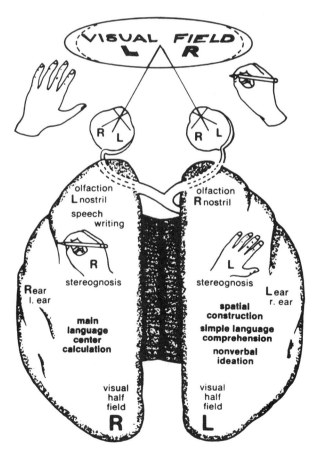

FIGURE 3.7 Schematic diagram of visual fields, optic tracts, and the associated brain areas, showing left and right lateralization in humans. (From Sperry, 1984)

work system in which the effects of lesions resonate throughout the network, slowing and distorting multiple aspects of cerebral processing with these resultant visual disturbances.

A majority of the nerve fibers transmitting auditory stimulation from each ear are projected to the primary auditory centers in the opposite hemisphere; the remaining fibers go to the *ipsilateral* (same side) auditory cortex. Thus, the contralateral pattern is preserved to a large degree in the auditory system too. As a result of this mixed projection pattern, destruction of one of the primary auditory centers does not result in loss of hearing in the contralateral ear. A point-to-point relationship between sense receptors and cortical cells is also laid out on the primary auditory cortex, with cortical representation arranged according to pitch, from high tones to low ones.

Destruction of a primary cortical sensory or motor area results in specific sensory or motor deficits but generally has little effect on the higher cortical functions. For instance, an adult-onset lesion limited to the primary visual cortex produces loss of visual awareness (cortical blindness, blindsight; see p. 66) while reasoning ability, emotional control, and even the ability for visual conceptualization may remain intact (Farah, 2003b; Güzeldere et al., 2000; Weiskrantz, 1986). Some mild decrements in movement speed and strength of the hand on the same side as lesions in the motor cortex have been reported (Smutok et al., 1989; see also Cramer, Finklestein, Schaechter et al., 1999, for a discussion of ipsilateral and bilateral motor control).

Association areas of the cortex. Cortical representation of sensory or motor nerve endings in the body takes place on a direct point-to-point basis, but stimulation of the *primary* cortical area gives rise only to meaningless sensations or nonfunctional movements (Brodal, 1981; Luria, 1966). Modified and complex functions involve the cortex adjacent to primary sensory and motor centers (E. Goldberg, 1989, 1990; Passingham, 1997; Paulesu et al., 1997). Neurons in these *secondary* cortical areas integrate and refine raw percepts or simple motor responses. *Tertiary* association or overlap zones are areas peripheral to functional centers where the neuronal components of two or more different functions or modalities are interspersed. The posterior association cortex, in which supramodal integration of perceptual functions takes place has also been called the *multimodal* (Pandya and Yeterian, 1990) or *heteromodal* (Mesulam, 2000b; Strub and Black, 1988) cortex. These processing areas are connected in a "stepwise" manner such that information-bearing stimuli reach the cortex first in the primary sensory centers. They then pass through the cortical

association areas in order of increasing complexity, interconnecting with other cortical and subcortical structures along the way to frontal and limbic system association areas and finally expression in action, thought, and feeling (Arciniegas and Beresford, 2001; Mesulam, 2000b; Pandya and Yeterian, 1990, 1998). These projection systems have both forward and reciprocal connections at each step in the progression to the frontal lobes; and each sensory association area makes specific frontal lobe connections which, too, have their reciprocal connections back to the association areas of the posterior cortex (Rolls, 1998).

Unlike damage to primary cortical areas, a lesion involving association areas and overlap zones typically does not result in specific sensory or motor defects; rather, the behavioral effects of such damage will more likely appear as a pattern of deficits running through related functions or as impairment of a general capacity (E. Goldberg, 1989, 1995). Thus, certain lesions that are implicated in drawing distortions also tend to affect the ability to do computations on paper; lesions of the auditory association cortex do not interfere with hearing acuity per se but with the appreciation of patterned sounds.

Asymmetry between the hemispheres

A second kind of organization across the lateral plane differentiates the two hemispheres with respect to the localization of primary cognitive functions and to significant qualitative aspects of behavior processed by each of the hemispheres. Although no two human brains are exactly alike in their structure, in most people the right frontal area is wider than the left and the right frontal pole protrudes beyond the left while the reverse is true of the occipital pole: the left occipital pole is frequently wider and protrudes further posteriorly than the right but the central portion of the right hemisphere is frequently wider than the left (Damasio and Geschwind, 1984; Jänke and Steinmetz, 2003). Men show greater degrees of frontal and occipital asymmetry than women (Bear, Schiff, et al., 1986). These asymmetries exist in fetal brains (de Lacoste et al., 1991; Weinberger, Luchins, et al., 1982; Witelson, 1995). The left *Sylvian fissure*, the fold between the temporal and frontal lobes, is larger than the right in most people (Witelson, 1995), even in newborns (Seidenwurm et al., 1985). Much attention has focused on the asymmetry of the posterior portion of the superior surface of the temporal lobe, the *planum temporale*. This region, which is involved in auditory processing, is larger on the left side in most right-handers (Beaton, 1997; E. Strauss, LaPointe, et al., 1985). Differences in the neurotransmitters found in each hemisphere have also been associated with differences in hemisphere function (Berridge et al., 2003; Direnfeld et al., 1984; Glick et al., 1982; R.G. Robinson and Starkstein, 2002) and sex (Arato et al., 1991). These differences may have an evolutionary foundation, for they have been found in primates and other animals (Corballis, 1991; Geschwind and Galaburda, 1985; Nottebohm, 1979). The lateralized size differential in primates is paralleled in some species by left lateralization for vocal communication (MacNeilage, 1987).

Lateralized cerebral differences may also occur at the level of cellular organization (B. Anderson et al., 1999; Galuske et al., 2000; Gazzaniga, 2000b; Peled et al., 1998). As early as 1963, Hécaen and Angelergues, on careful review of the neuropsychological symptoms associated with lesions of the right or left hemisphere, speculated that neural organization might be more closely knit and integrated on the left, more diffuse on the right. In accounting for findings that the spatial performance of right hemisphere damaged patients is adversely affected by lesions occurring anywhere in a fairly wide area while only those left hemisphere damaged patients with relatively severe damage to a well-defined area show impaired performance on spatial tasks, De Renzi and Faglioni (1967), too, hypothesized more diffuse representation of functions in the right hemisphere and more focal representation in the left. A similar conclusion follows from findings that patients with right hemisphere damage tend to have a reduced capacity for tactile discrimination and sensorimotor tasks in both hands while those with left hemisphere damage experience impaired tactile discrimination only in the contralateral hand (Hom and Reitan, 1982; Semmes, 1968), although contradictory data have been reported (Benton, 1972). Hemispheric bias extends to fine motor control, but differs from the usual perceptual bias in that left hemisphere damage is associated with bilateral motor response deficits, and damage to the right produces only contralateral impairment (Haaland, Cleeland, and Carr, 1977; Harrington and Haaland, 1991a; Jason, 1990; Okuda et al., 1995). Moreover, lesions outside the right hemisphere's sensorimotor area can contribute to motor deficits, but in the left hemisphere motor deficits occur only with lesions involving the sensorimotor area (Haaland and Yeo, 1989).

Additional data supporting a hypothesis that the right hemisphere is more diffusely organized than the left have been provided by evidence that visuospatial and constructional disabilities of patients with right hemisphere damage do not differ significantly regardless of the extensiveness of damage (Kertesz and Dobrowolski, 1981). Hammond (1982) reports that damage to the left hemisphere tends to reduce acuity of time discrimination more than right-sided damage, suggest-ing that the left hemisphere has a capacity for finer temporal resolution than the right. Also, the right hemisphere does not appear to be as discretely organized as the left for visuoperceptual and associated visual memory operations (Fried et al., 1982; Wasserstein, Zappula, Rosen, and Gerstman, 1984). Kolb and Whishaw (1996, pp. 204–207) offer several interpretations of these observations.

Functional specialization of the hemispheres. The supramodal nature of hemisphere specialization shows up in a number of ways: One is the organization of the left hemisphere for "linear" processing of sequentially presenting stimuli such as verbal statements, mathematical propositions, and the programming of rapid motor sequences. The right hemisphere is superior for "configurational" processing required by material that cannot be described adequately in words or strings of symbols, such as the appearance of a face or three-dimensional spatial relationships (Bogen, 1969a,b; Carlesimo and Caltagirone, 1995; Lezak, 1994; Swithenby et al., 1998). The two hemispheres process global/local or whole/detail information differently (L.C. Robertson and Rafal, 2000; Rossion et al., 2000), what Delis, Kiefner, and Fridlund (1988) refer to as the level of hierarchical analysis. When asked to copy or read a large-scale stimulus such as the shape of a letter or other common symbol composed of many different symbols in small scale (see Fig. 3.8), patients with left hemisphere disease will tend to ignore the small bits and interpret the large-scale figure; those whose lesions are on the right are more likely to overlook the big symbol but respond to the small ones. This can be interpreted as indicating a left hemisphere superiority in processing detailed information, a right hemisphere predilection for large-scale or global percepts.

Yet another processing difference between the hemispheres has to do with stimulus familiarity, as the right hemisphere appears to be best suited to handling novel information while the left tends to be more adept with familiar material such as "well-routinized codes" (E. Goldberg, 1990; E. Goldberg and Costa, 1981). Other studies have associated the right hemisphere with early, less detailed stages of processing, which may also be those that emerge first in the course of development, leaving the left hemisphere to perform later stage op-

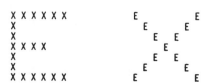

FIGURE 3.8 Examples of global/local stimuli.

erations on more detailed features (Bouma, 1990; Sergent, 1984, 1988a).

However, laboratory studies of normal subjects and "split brain" patients have shown that which hemisphere processes what depends on the relative weighting of many variables (Beaumont, 1997). In addition to underlying hemispheric organization, these include the nature of the task (e.g., modality, speed factors, complexity), the subject's set of expectancies, prior experiences with the task, previously developed perceptual or response strategies, and inherent subject variables such as sex and handedness (Bouma, 1990; Bryden, 1978; Kuhl, 2000; S.C. Levine, 1995). Thus, in these subjects the degree to which hemispheric specialization occurs at any given time is a relative phenomenon rather than an absolute one (Hellige, 1995; L.C. Robertson, 1995; Sergent, 1991a; E. Zaidel, Clarke, and Suyenobu, 1990). Moreover, it is important to recognize that normal behavior is a function of the whole brain with important contributions from both hemispheres entering into every activity and emotional state. Only laboratory studies of intact or split brain subjects or studies of persons with lateralized brain damage demonstrate the differences in hemisphere function.

The most obvious functional difference between the hemispheres is that the left hemisphere in most people is *dominant* for speech (i.e., language functions are primarily mediated in the left hemisphere) and the right hemisphere predominates in mediating complex, difficult-to-verbalize stimuli. Absence of words does not make a stimulus "nonverbal." Pictorial, diagrammatic, or design stimuli—sounds, sensations of touch and taste, etc.—may be more or less susceptible to verbal labeling depending on their meaningfulness, complexity, familiarity, potential for affective arousal, and other characteristics such as patterning or number. Thus, when classifying a wordless stimulus as verbal or nonverbal, it is important to take into account how readily it can be verbalized.

For most people the left hemisphere is the primary mediator of verbal functions (Indefrey and Levelt, 2000), including reading and writing, understanding and speaking, verbal ideation, verbal memory, and even comprehension of verbal symbols traced on the skin. The left hemisphere also mediates the numerical symbol system. Moreover, left hemisphere lateralization extends to control of posturing and of sequencing hand and arm movements, and of the musculature of speech, although bilateral structures are involved. Processing the linear and rapidly changing acoustic information needed for speech comprehension is better with the left than the right hemisphere (Beeman and Chiarello, 1998; Howard, 1997; J. Schwartz and Tallal, 1980).

Males show a stronger left hemisphere lateralization for phonological processing than females (Shaywitz et al., 1995; E. Zaidel, Aboitiz, et al., 1995).

Right hemisphere language capacities have been demonstrated for comprehension of speech and written material. One significant contribution is the appreciation and integration of relationships in verbal discourse and narrative materials (Beeman and Chiarello, 1998, *passim;* Delis, Wapner, et al., 1983; Kiehl et al., 1999), which is a capacity necessary for enjoying a good joke (Beeman, 1998; H. Gardner, 1994). The right hemisphere also appears to provide the possibility of alternative meanings, getting away from purely literal interpretations of verbal material (Bottini et al., 1994; Brownell and Martino, 1998; Fiore and Schooler, 1998). Following commissurotomy, when speech is directed to the right hemisphere, much of what is heard is comprehended so long as it remains simple (Baynes and Eliassen, 1998; Searleman, 1977). Although functional imaging studies show a preponderance of left cerebral activity in reading (C.J. Price, 1997), not surprisingly, given its visuospatial components, reading also engages the right hemisphere, activating specific areas (Banich and Nicholas, 1998; Gaillard and Converso, 1988; Huettner et al., 1989; Indefrey and Levelt, 2000; Ornstein et al., 1979). In contrast to the ability for rapid, automatic processing of printed words by the intact left hemisphere, the healthy right hemisphere takes a slower and generally inefficient letter by letter approach (C. Burgess and Lund, 1998; Chiarello, 1988), which may be useful when word shapes have unfamiliar forms (Banich and Nicholas, 1998). The right hemisphere appears to have a reading lexicon (Bogen, 1997; Coslett and Saffran, 1998), but the more verbally adept left hemisphere normally blocks access to it so that the right hemisphere's knowledge of words becomes evident only through laboratory manipulations or with left hemisphere damage (Landis and Regard, 1988; Landis, Regard, et al., 1983). The right hemisphere seems to be sensitive to speech intonations (Borod, Bloom, and Santschi-Haywood, 1998; Ivry and Lebby, 1998), and is necessary for voice recognition (Van Lancker, Kreiman, and Cummings, 1989).

Less can be said for the verbal expressive capacities of the right hemisphere since they are quite limited, as displayed—or rather, not displayed—by split brain patients who make few utterances in response to right brain stimulation (Baynes and Gazzaniga, 2000; E. Zaidel, 1978). The right hemisphere appears to play a role in organizing verbal production conceptually (Brownell and Martino, 1998; Joanette et al., 1990), with specific temporal and prefrontal involvement in comprehending story meanings (Nichelli, Grafman, et al., 1995). It may be necessary for meaningfully expressive speech intonation (*prosody*) (Borod, Bloom, and Santschi-Haywood, 1998; Filley, 1995; E.D. Ross, 2000). The right hemisphere contributes to the maintenance of context-appropriate and emotionally appropriate verbal behavior (Brownell and Martino, 1998; Joanette et al., 1990), although this contribution is not limited to communications but extends to all behavior domains (Lezak, 1994). That the right hemisphere has a language capacity can also be inferred in aphasic patients with left-sided lesions who showed improvement from their immediate post-stroke deficits accompanied by measurably heightened right hemisphere activity (Frackowiak, 1997; B.T. Gold and Kertesz, 2000; Heiss et al., 1999; Murdoch, 1990; Papanicolaou et al., 1988).

The right hemisphere has also been erroneously called the "minor" or "nondominant" hemisphere because the often subtle character of right hemisphere disorders led early observers to believe that it played no specialized role in behavior.[1] However, although limited linguistically, the right hemisphere is "fully human with respect to its cognitive depth and complexity" (J. Levy, 1983).

The right hemisphere dominates the processing of information that does not readily lend itself to verbalization. This includes the reception and storage of visual data, tactile and visual recognition of shapes and forms, perception of spatial orientation and perspective, and copying and drawing geometric and representational designs and pictures. The left hemisphere seems to predominate in metric distance judgments (Hellige, 1988; McCarthy and Warrington, 1990), while the right hemisphere has superiority in metric angle judgments (Benton, Sivan, et al., 1994; Mehta and Newcombe, 1996). Thus both hemispheres contribute to processing spatial information, with some differences in what they process most efficiently (Banich, 1995; Sergent, 1991b). Arithmetic calculations (involving spatial organization of the problem elements as distinct from left hemisphere–mediated linear arithmetic problems involving, for instance, stories or equations with an $a + b = c$ form [Dehaene, 2000]) have a significant right hemisphere component (Grafman and Rickard, 1997; H.S. Levin, Goldstein, and Spiers, 1993). Some aspects of musical ability are also localized on the right, as are abilities to recognize and discriminate nonverbal sounds (Bauer, 1993; Bauer and McDonald, 2003).

The right hemisphere has bilateral involvement in somatosensory sensitivity and discrimination. It may be superior in distinguishing odors (Zatorre and Jones-Gotman, 1990).

Data from a variety of sources suggest right hemisphere dominance for spatial attention specifically, if not attention generally: Patients with compromised right hemisphere functioning tend to have diminished awareness of or responsiveness to stimuli presented to their left side; reaction times mediated by the right hemisphere are faster than those mediated by the left; and the right hemisphere is activated equally by stimuli from either side in contrast to more exclusively contralateral left hemisphere activation (Heilman and Van Den Abell, 1980; Heilman, Watson, and Valenstein, 2003; Meador, Loring, Lee, et al., 1988; Mesulam, 2000b). However, other studies suggest that neither hemisphere has an attentional advantage, but rather that each hemisphere directs attention contralaterally (Mirsky, 1989; Posner, 1990), and that they are equally capable of detecting stimuli (Prather et al., 1992). The right hemisphere appears to direct attention to far space while the left hemisphere directs attention to near space (Heilman, Chatterjee, and Doty, 1995). The appearance of right hemisphere superiority for attention in some situations may stem from its ability to integrate complex, nonlinear information rapidly.

Facial recognition studies exemplify the processing differences underlying many aspects of hemisphere specialization. When pictured faces are presented normally to each field separately they are processed more rapidly when presented to the left field/right hemisphere than to the right field/left hemisphere; but no right hemisphere advantage appears when faces are inverted (Tovée, 1996). "It seems that, in the right hemisphere, upright faces are processed in terms of their feature configuration, whereas inverted faces are processed in a piecemeal manner, feature by feature. . . . In the left hemisphere, both upright and inverted faces seem to be processed in a piecemeal manner." (pp. 134–135)

Cognitive alterations with lateralized lesions. Time-bound relationships of sequence and order characterize many of the functions that are vulnerable to left hemisphere lesions (Harrington and Haaland, 1991a, 1992). The most obvious cognitive defect associated with left hemisphere damage is aphasia (Feinberg and Farah, 2003b; Wernicke, 1874/1977). This complex of disorders reflects a very basic underlying capacity of the left hemisphere that is not dependent on hearing, as deaf persons who sign can develop an aphasia for their nonauditory language in the areas associated with aphasia in hearing persons (Bellugi et al., 1983; Poizner et al., 1990). Other left hemisphere disorders include verbal memory or verbal fluency deficits, concrete

---

[1]Because the left hemisphere is usually dominant for speech in both right- and left-handed persons (see pp. 305–306), it became customary to refer to it as the "dominant" hemisphere before the dominant functions of the right hemisphere were appreciated (Benton, 1972). The most common pattern, in which the left and right hemispheres predominate for verbal and nonverbal functions, respectively, is generally assumed in writing about the hemispheres today and will be assumed here.

thinking, specific impairments in reading or writing, and impaired arithmetic ability characterized by defects or loss of basic mathematical concepts of operations and even of number (Grafman and Rickard, 1997; Delazer and Bartha, 2001). Patients with left hemisphere damage may make defective constructions largely because of tendencies toward simplification and difficulties in drawing angles, but they also may display deficits in visuospatial orientation and short-term recall (Mehta et al., 1989). Their ability to perform complex manual—as well as oral—motor sequences may be impaired (Harrington and Haaland, 1992; Meador, Loring, Lee et al., 1999; Schluter et al., 2001).

The diversity of behavioral disorders associated with right hemisphere damage continues to thwart efforts to devise a neat classification system for them (S. Clarke, 2001; Cutting, 1990; Feinberg and Farah, 2003c; Filley, 1995). Pimental and Kingsbury (1989) reviewed syndrome classifications offered by other writers and proposed one of their own with seven major classes encompassing 18 lower level categories, of which some contain further subclasses of symptoms. The many different presentations of right hemisphere dysfunction may be understood as determined in large part by the specific area(s) of damage in terms of gradients of cortical specialization (E. Goldberg, 1989, 1995; see p. 65). No attempt to include every kind of impairment reported in the literature will be made here. Rather, the most prominent features of right hemisphere dysfunction will be described, with more detailed presentations in the sections on the functional organization of the cerebral cortex.

Patients with right hemisphere damage may be quite fluent, even verbose (Brookshire, 1978; Cutting, 1990; Rivers and Love, 1980), but illogical and given to loose generalizations and bad judgment (Stemmer and Joanette, 1998). They are apt to have difficulty ordering, organizing, and making sense out of complex stimuli or situations, and thus many display planning defects and some are no longer able to process the components of music. These organizational deficits can impair appreciation of complex verbal information so that verbal comprehension may be compromised by confusion of the elements of what is heard, by personalized intrusions, by literal interpretations, and by a generalized loss of gist in a morass of details (Beeman and Chiarello, 1998, *passim*). Their speech may be uninflected and aprosodic, paralleling their difficulty in comprehending speech intonations (E.D. Ross, 2003). These patients are vulnerable to difficulty in maintaining a high level of alertness (Ladavas et al., 1989), which may be akin to the association of right hemisphere lesions with *impersistence*—the inability to sustain facial or limb postures (Pimental and Kingsbury, 1989b). Perceptual deficits, particularly left-sided

inattention phenomena and those involving degraded stimuli or unusual presentations, are not uncommon (McCarthy and Warrington, 1990). The visuospatial perceptual deficits that trouble many patients with right-lateralized damage can affect different cognitive activities (Farah and Feinberg, 2003b, *passim;* Vuilleumier, 2001). Arithmetic failures are most likely to appear in written calculations that require spatial organization of the problems' elements (Grafman and Rickard, 1997; see Fig. 3.16, p. 72). Visuospatial and other perceptual deficits show up in these patients' difficulty copying designs, making constructions, and matching or discriminating patterns or faces. Patients with right hemisphere damage may have particular problems with spatial orientation and visuo-spatial memory such that they get lost, even in familiar surroundings, and can be slow to learn their way around a new area. Their constructional disabilities may reflect both their spatial disorientation and defective capacity for perceptual or conceptual organization. Stereoscopic vision may be affected (Benton and Hécaen, 1970). Their reaction times are slowed.

The painful efforts of a right hemisphere stroke patient to arrange plain and diagonally colored blocks according to a pictured pattern (Fig. 3.9a, p. 59) illustrate the kind of solutions available to a person in whom only the left hemisphere is fully intact. This glib 51-year-old retired salesman constructed several simple 2 × 2 block design patterns correctly by verbalizing the relations. "The red one (block) on the right goes above the white one; there's another red one to the left of the white one." This method worked so long as the relationships of each block to the others in the pattern remained obvious. When the diagonality of a design obscured the relative placement of the blocks, he could neither perceive how each block fit into the design nor guide himself with verbal cues. He continued to use verbal cues, but at this level of complexity his verbalizations only served to confuse him further. He attempted to reproduce diagonally oriented designs by lining up the blocks diagonally (e.g., "to the side," "in back of") without regard for the squared (2 × 2 or 3 × 3) format. He could not orient any one block to more than another single block at a time, and he was unable to maintain a center of focus to the design he was constructing.

On the same task, a 31-year-old mildly dysphasic former logger who had had left hemisphere surgery involving the visual association area had no difficulty until he came to the first 3 × 3 design, the only one of the four nine-block designs that lends itself readily to verbal analysis. On this design, he reproduced the overall pattern immediately but oriented one corner block erroneously. He attempted to reorient it but then turned a correctly oriented block into a 180° error. Though dissatisfied with this solution, he was unable to localize his error or define the simple angulation pattern (Fig. 3.9b).

As illustrated in Figure 3.9, the distinctive processing qualities of each hemisphere become evident in the mediation of spatial relations. Left hemisphere processing

Design 6

Design 7

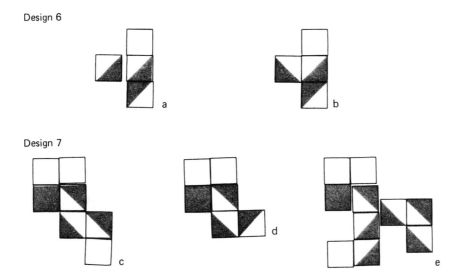

FIGURE 3.9a Attempts of a 51-year-old right hemisphere stroke patient to copy pictured designs with colored blocks. (*a*) First stage in the construction of a 2 × 2 chevron design. (*b*) Second stage: the patient does not see the 2 × 2 format and gives up after four minutes. (*c*) First stage in construction of 3 × 3 pinwheel pattern (see below). (*d*) Second stage. (*e*) Third and final stage. This patient later told his wife that he believed the examiner was preparing him for "architect school."

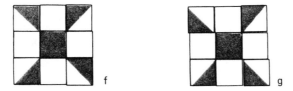

FIGURE 3.9b Attempts of a 31-year-old patient with a surgical lesion of the left visual association area to copy the 3 × 3 pinwheel design with colored blocks. (*f*) Initial soluation: 180° rotation of upper left corner block. (*g*) "Corrected" solution: upper left corner block rotated to correct position and lower right corner rotated 180° to incorrect position.

tends to break the visual percept into details that can be identified and conceptualized verbally in terms of number or length of lines, size and direction of angles, etc. In the right hemisphere the tendency is to deal with the same visual stimuli as spatially related wholes. Thus, for most people, the ability to perform such complex visual tasks as the formation of complete impressions from fragmented percepts (the closure function), the appreciation of differences in patterns, and the recognition and remembering of faces depends on the functioning of the right hemisphere. Together the two processing systems provide recognition, storage, and comprehension of discrete and continuous, serial and simultaneous, detailed and holistic aspects of experience across at least the major sensory modalities of vision, audition, and touch.

Although greatly oversimplified, this model has clinical value. Loss of tissue in a hemisphere tends to impair its particular processing capacity. When a lesion has rendered lateralized areas essentially nonfunctional, the intact hemisphere may process activities normally handled by the damaged hemisphere (W.H. Moore, 1984; Papanicolaou et al., 1988; Fig. 3.9a is an example of this phenomenon). Moreover, a diminished contribution from one hemisphere may be accompanied by augmented or exaggerated activ-

ity of the other when released from the inhibitory or competitive constraints of normal hemispheric interactions (Lezak, 1994; Novelly et al., 1984; Shimizu et al., 2000; Starkstein and Robinson, 1997). This phenomenon appears in the verbosity and overwriting of many right hemisphere damaged patients (Cutting, 1990; Lezak and Newman, 1979; Yamadori et al., 1986; see Fig. 3.10, p. 60). The functional difference between hemispheres also appears in the tendency for patients with left-sided damage to be more accurate in remembering large visually presented forms than the small details making up those forms; but when the lesion is on the right, recall of the details is more accurate than recall of the whole composed figure (Delis, Robertson, and Efron, 1986) (see Fig. 3.8, p. 55). These examples suggest that one hemisphere's function is enhanced when the other hemisphere is impaired. In an analogous manner, patients with left hemisphere disease tend to reproduce the essential configuration but leave out details when copying drawings (see Fig. 3.11, p. 61), and they may perform some visuoperceptual tasks better than intact subjects (Y. Kim et al., 1984; Wasserstein, Zappulla, Rosen, et al., 1987).

Memory and learning also show hemispheric differences. Loss of the left hippocampus and nearby corti-

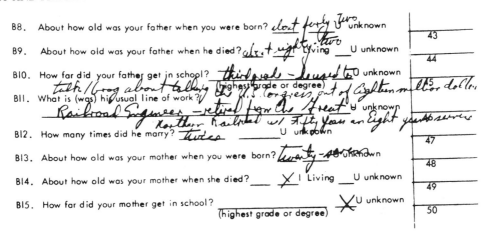

FIGURE 3.10 Overwriting (hypergraphia) by a 48-year-old college-educated retired police investigator suffering right temporal lobe atrophy secondary to a local right temporal lobe stroke.

cal areas impairs verbal memory, and destruction of the right hippocampus results in defective recognition and recall of "complex visual and auditory patterns to which a name cannot readily be assigned" (B. Milner, 1970, p. 30; see also Abrahams et al., 1997; Jones-Gotman, Zatorre, Olivier, et al., 1997; R.G. Morris, Abrahams, and Polkey, 1995; Pillon, Bazin, Deweer, et al., 1999; Sass, Buchanan, Kraemer, et al., 1995).

The subjects for most studies of memory and the temporal lobe are patients who have had portions of one or both temporal lobes excised, usually for seizure control. These studies show that memory deficits with temporal lobe lesions also differ according to the side of the lesion (G.P. Lee, Loring, and Thompson, 1989; B. Milner, 1972; R.G. Morris, Abrahams, and Polkey, 1995; Pillon, Bazin, Deweer, et al., 1999; M.L. Smith, 1989). Impaired verbal memory appears with surgical resection of the left temporal lobe (Seidenberg, Hermann, et al., 1998) and nonverbal (auditory, tactile, visual) memory disturbances accompany right temporal lobe resection. With left temporal lobectomies, deficits have been found for different kinds of verbal memory, including episodic (both short-term and learning), semantic, and remote memory (Frisk and Milner, 1990; Loring and Meador, 2003b; M.L. Smith, 1989). These patients also lag behind normal controls in learning de-

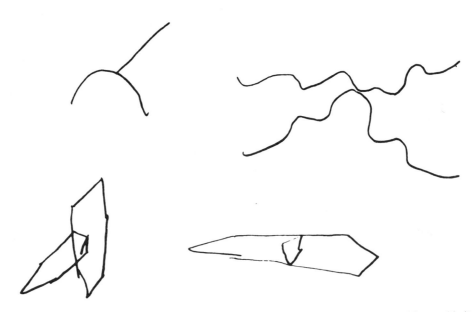

FIGURE 3.11 Simplification and distortions of four Bender-Gestalt designs by a 45-year-old assembly line worker with a high school education. These drawings were made four years after he had incurred left frontal damage in an industrial accident.

signs, although once learned their retention is good, unlike patients with right temporal lesions, who fail both aspects of this memory task (Jones-Gotman, 1986). Reduced access to verbal labeling may explain the left temporal patients' slowed learning. Learning manual sequences becomes more difficult following left but not right temporal lobectomy (Jason, 1987). Cortical stimulation of the anterior left temporal cortex interferes with verbal learning without affecting speech, while stimulation of the posterior left temporal cortex is more likely to result in retrieval (word finding) problems and *anomia* (literally, no words) (Fedio and Van Buren, 1974; Ojemann, 1978). Lesions in different areas of the left temporal lobe differentially affect the degree and nature of impairment in immediate auditory recall of tones or digits (W.P. Gordon, 1983).

Memory deficits documented for patients with right temporal lobectomies and other temporal lobe lesions involve designs, faces, melodies, and spatial formats such as those used in maze learning (e.g., Abrahams et al., 1997). In short, these patients display memory impairments when perceptions or knowledge cannot be readily put into words (B.E. Shapiro, Grossman, and Gardner, 1981; M.L. Smith, 1989). This left–right difference has been found in brain activation studies comparing the effect of stimulus material on temporal lobes (Dolan et al., 1997; Ojemann, 1978) and on the prefrontal cortex's role in memory (A.C. Lee et al., 2000; K.B. McDermott, Ojemann, et al., 1999; A.D. Wagner et al., 1998). However, current evidence suggests that the relationship between the type of material (verbal vs. nonverbalizable) to be learned or modality of stimulus input and hemisphere involvement is not simple. Functional neuroimaging data demonstrate that both hemispheres may be activated by a verbal memory task (Buckner et al., 1998; S.C. Johnson et al., 2001).

Emotional alterations with lateralized lesions. The complementary modes of processing that distinguish the cognitive activities of the two hemispheres extend to emotional behavior as well (Bear, 1983; Borod, Bloom, and Santschi-Haywood, 1998; Gainotti, 1984, 2000; Gainotti, Caltagirone, and Zoccolotti, 1993; Heilman, Blonder, et al., 2003). The configurational processing of the right hemisphere lends itself most readily to the handling of the multidimensional and alogical stimuli that convey *emotional tone,* such as facial expressions (Benowitz, Bear, et al., 1983; Borod, Haywood, and Koff, 1997; Ivry and Lebby, 1998; Moreno et al., 1990) and voice quality (Blumstein and Cooper, 1974; Joanette et al., 1990; Ley and Bryden, 1982). The analytic, bit-by-bit processing of the left hemisphere deals best with the words of emotion. A

face distorted by fear and the exclamation "I'm scared to death" both convey affective meaning, but the meaning of each is normally processed well by only one hemisphere (Hansch and Pirozzolo, 1980; Safer and Leventhal, 1977). Thus, patients with right hemisphere damage tend to experience relative difficulty in discerning the emotional features of stimuli, whether visual or auditory, with corresponding diminution in their emotional responsivity (Adolphs and Damasio, 2000; Borod, Cicero et al., 1998; Cicone et al., 1980; Ruckdeschel-Hibbard et al., 1986; Van Lancker and Sidtis, 1992). While impairments in affective recognition appear to be supramodal, deficits in recognizing different kinds of affective communication (e.g., facial expressions, gestures, prosody) can occur independently of one another (Bowers et al., 1993). Patients with such deficits are limited in both their comprehension and their enjoyment of humor (H. Gardner 1994; H. Gardner et al., 1975). Patients with left hemisphere lesions have less difficulty appreciating facial expressions and voice intonation, and most are normally responsive to uncaptioned cartoons but do as poorly as right hemisphere patients when the stimulus is verbal (see also Heilman, Scholes, and Watson, 1975). Self-reference processing and self-evaluation appear to have mostly right hemisphere involvement (J.P. Keenan et al., 2000), although both hemispheres contribute to processing of aspects of personal information (Kircher et al., 2001).

Differences in emotional expression can also distinguish patients with lateralized lesions (Borod, 1993; Etcoff, 1986). Right hemisphere–lesioned patients' range and intensity of affective intonation are frequently inappropriate (Borod, Koff, Lorch, and Nicholas, 1985; Borod, St. Clair, et al., 1990; Joanette et al., 1990; B.E. Shapiro and Danly, 1985). In the controversy over whether their facial behavior is less expressive than that of persons with left hemisphere damage or of normal control subjects, Brozgold and colleagues (1998) and Montreys and Borod (1998) say it is while Pizzamiglio and Mammucari (1989) say it is not. The preponderance of research on normal subjects indicates heightened expressiveness on the left side of the face (Borod, Kent, et al., 1988; Dopson et al., 1984; Sackeim, Gur, and Saucy, 1978). These findings are generally interpreted as indicating right hemisphere superiority for affective expression.

There is disagreement as to whether right hemisphere damaged patients experience emotions any less than other people. Some studies have found reduced autonomic responses to what would normally be an emotional stimulus (Gainotti, 1997). However, given their impaired appreciation of emotionally charged stimuli, this may raise a chicken–egg question concerning what is the fundamental deficit here. Others, myself [mdl] included, have observed strong—but not necessarily appropriate—emotional reactions in patients with right-lateralized damage, leading to the hypothesis that their experience of emotional communications and their capacity to transmit the nuances and subtleties of their own feeling states differ from normal affective processing (Barbizet, 1974; Lezak, 1994; Morrow, Vrtunski, et al., 1981; E.D. Ross and Rush, 1981), leaving them out of joint with those around them.

Hemispheric differences have been reported for the emotional and even personality changes that may accompany brain injury (Gainotti, 1993; Prigatano, 1987; Sackeim, Greenburg, et al., 1982). Patients with left hemisphere lesions can exhibit a *catastrophic reaction* (extreme and disruptive transient emotional disturbance). The catastrophic reaction may appear as acute—often disorganizing—anxiety, agitation, or tearfulness, disrupting the activity that provoked it. Typically, it occurs when patients are confronted with their limitations, as when taking a test (Prigatano, 1987; R.G. Robinson and Starkstein, 2002). They tend to regain their composure as soon as the source of frustration is removed. Anxiety is also a common feature of left hemisphere involvement (Gainotti, 1972; Galin, 1974). It may show up as undue cautiousness (Jones-Gotman and Milner, 1977) or oversensitivity to impairments and a tendency to exaggerate disabilities (Keppel and Crowe, 2000). Yet, despite tendencies to be overly sensitive to their disabilities, many patients with left hemisphere lesions ultimately compensate for them well enough to make a satisfactory adjustment to their disabilities and living situations (Tellier et al., 1990).

In contrast, patients whose injuries involve the right hemisphere are less likely to be dissatisfied with themselves or their performances than are those with left hemisphere lesions (Keppel and Crowe, 2000) and less likely to be aware of their mistakes (McGlynn and Schacter, 1989). They are more likely to be apathetic (Andersson et al., 1999), to be risk takers (L. Miller, and Milner, 1985), and to have poorer social functioning (Brozgold et al., 1998). At least in the acute or early stages of their condition, they may display an *indifference reaction*, tending to deny or make light of the extent of their disabilities (Gainotti, 1972; Pimental and Kingsbury, 1989). In extreme cases, patients are unaware of such seemingly obvious defects as crippling left-sided paralysis or slurred and poorly articulated speech. In the long run these patients tend to have difficulty making satisfactory psychosocial adaptations, with those whose lesions are anterior being most maladjusted in all areas of psychosocial functioning (Tellier et al., 1990).

What can be considered an experimental model of these changes stems from use of the *Wada technique* of intracarotid injections of sodium amytal for pharmacological inactivation of one side of the brain to evaluate lateralization of function before surgical treatment of epilepsy (Jones-Gotman, 1987; Rausch and Risinger, 1990; Wada and Rasmussen, 1960). The emotional reactions of these patients tend to differ depending on which side is inactivated (Ahern et al., 1994; Davidson and Henriques, 2000; G.P. Lee, Loring, et al., 1990; Nebes, 1978). Patients whose left hemisphere has been inactivated are tearful and tell of feelings of depression more often than their right hemisphere counterparts, who are more apt to laugh and feel euphoric. In the same vein, Regard and Landis (1988) found that pictures exposed to the left visual field were disliked and those to the right were liked. Since the emotional alterations seen with some stroke patients and in lateralized pharmacological inactivation have been interpreted as representing the tendencies of the disinhibited intact hemisphere, some investigators have hypothesized that each hemisphere is specialized for positive (the left) or negative (the right) emotions, suggesting relationships between the lateralized affective phenomena and psychiatric disorders (e.g., Flor-Henry, 1986; G.P. Lee, Loring, et al., 1990).

However, studies of depression in stroke patients have produced inconsistent results (A.J. Carson et al., 2000; Sato et al., 1999; Singh et al., 2000). Shimoda and Robinson (1999) found that hospitalized stroke patients with the greatest incidence of depression were those with left anterior hemisphere lesions. At short-term follow-up (3–6 months), proximity of the lesion to the frontal pole and lesion volume correlated with depression in both right and left hemisphere stroke patients. At long-term follow-up (1–2 years), depression was significantly associated with right hemisphere lesion volume and proximity of the lesion to the occipital pole. Moreover, the incidence of depression in patients with left hemisphere disease dropped over the course of the first year (R.G. Robinson and Manes, 2000). Impaired social functioning was most evident in those patients who remained depressed. Consistent with these findings are reports of a higher incidence of depression in patients with anterior lesions 2–4 months poststroke (J.S. Kim and Choi-Kwon, 2000; Singh et al., 2000) and with right hemisphere lesions at six months poststroke (MacHale et al., 1998). Women are more likely to be depressed in the acute stages of a left hemisphere stroke than men (Paradiso and Robinson, 1998).

Gainotti, Caltagirone, and Zoccolotti (1993) suggest that the emotional processing tendencies of the two hemispheres are complementary: "The right hemisphere seems to be involved preferentially in functions of emotional arousal, intimately linked to the generation of the autonomic components of the emotional response, whereas the left hemisphere seems to play a more important role in functions of intentional control of the emotional expressive apparatus" (pp. 86–87). These authors hypothesize that language development tends to override the left hemisphere's capacity for emotional immediacy while, in contrast, the more spontaneous and pronounced affective display characteristic of right hemisphere emotionality gives that hemisphere the appearance of superior emotional endowment.

The differences in presentation of depression in right and left hemisphere damaged patients would seem to support this hypothesis. With left hemisphere damaged patients, depression seems to reflect awareness of deficit; the more severe the deficit and acute the patient's capacity for awareness, the more likely it is that the patient will be depressed. As awareness of deficit is often muted or lacking with right hemisphere lesions (K. Carpenter et al., 1995; Meador, Loring, Feinberg, et al., 2000; Pederson, Jorgensen, Nakayama, et al., 1996), these patients tend to be spared the agony of severe depression particularly early in the course of their condition. When the lesion is on the right, the emotional disturbance does not seem to arise from awareness of defects so much as from the secondary effects of the patient's diminished self-awareness and social insensitivity. Patients with right hemisphere lesions who do not appreciate the nature or extent of their disability tend to set unrealistic goals for themselves or to maintain previous goals without taking their new limitations into account. As a result, they frequently fail to realize their expectations. Their diminished capacity for self-awareness and for emotional spontaneity and sensitivity can make them unpleasant to live with and thus more likely to be rejected by family and friends than are patients with left hemisphere lesions. Depression in patients with right-sided cortical damage may take longer to develop than it does in patients with left hemisphere involvement since it is less likely to be an emotional response to immediately perceived disabilities than to a more slowly evolving reaction to their secondary consequences. When depression does develop in patients with right-sided disease, however, it can be more chronic, more debilitating, and more resistive to intervention.

These descriptions of differences in the emotional behavior of right and left hemisphere damaged patients reflect observed tendencies that are not necessary consequences of unilateral brain disease (Gainotti, 1993). Neither are the emotional reactions reported here associated only with unilateral brain lesions. Mourning reactions naturally follow the experience of personal loss of a capacity whether it be due to brain injury, a lesion lower down in the nervous system, or amputation of a body part. Inappropriate euphoria and self-satisfaction may accompany lesions involving other than right hemisphere areas of the cortex (McGlynn and Schacter, 1989). Further, premorbid personality colors the quality of patients' responses to their disabilities. Thus, the clinician should never be tempted to predict the site of damage from the patient's mood alone.

While knowledge of the asymmetrical pattern of cerebral organization adds to the understanding of many cognitive and emotional phenomena associated with unilateral lesions or demonstrated in laboratory studies of normal subjects or commissurotomized patients, it is inappropriate to generalize these findings to the behavior of persons whose brains are intact (Sergent, 1984; Springer and Deutsch, 1989). In normal persons, the functioning of the two hemispheres is tightly yoked by the corpus callosum so that neither can be engaged without significant activation of the other (Lezak, 1982b). As much as cognitive styles and personal tastes and habits might seem to reflect the processing characteristics of one or the other hemisphere, these qualities appear to be integral to both hemispheres (Arndt and Berger, 1978; Sperry et al., 1979). "In the normal intact state, the conscious activity is typically a unified and coherent bilateral process that spans both hemispheres through the commissures" (Sperry, 1976). Even when the hemispheres have been surgically separated, the "brain works as a single and unified organism" (Sergent, 1987).

Advantages of hemisphere interaction. Simple tasks in which the processing capacity of one hemisphere is sufficient are performed faster and with more advantage than if both hemispheres are engaged (Belger and Banich, 1998; Ringo et al., 1994). However, very few tasks rely exclusively on one hemisphere. Interaction between the hemispheres also has important mutually enhancing effects. Complex mental tasks such as reading, arithmetic, and word and object learning are performed best when both hemispheres can be actively engaged (Belger and Banich, 1998; Gaillard, 1990; Huettner et al., 1989; Moscovitch, 1979; A. Rey, 1959; Weissman and Banich, 2000). Other mutually enhancing effects of bilateral processing show up in the superior memorizing and retrieval of both verbal and configurational material when simultaneously processed (encoded) by the verbal and configurational systems (B. Milner, 1978; Moscovitch, 1979); in enhanced cognitive efficiency of normal subjects when hemispheric activation is bilateral rather than unilateral (J.M. Berger and Perret, 1986; J.M. Berger, Perret, and Zimmermann, 1987); and in better performances of visual tasks by commissurotomized patients when both hemispheres participate than when vision is restricted to either hemisphere (Sergent, 1991a,b; E. Zaidel, 1979).

The cerebral processing of music illuminates the differences in what each hemisphere contributes, the complexities of hemispheric interactions, and how experience can alter hemispheric roles. The left hemisphere tends to predominate in the processing of sequential and discrete tonal components of music (Botez and Botez, 1996; Breitling et al., 1987; Gaede et al., 1978). Inability to use both hands to play a musical instrument (*bimanual instrument apraxia*) has been reported with left hemisphere lesions that spare motor functions (Benton, 1977a). The right hemisphere predominates in melody recognition and in melodic singing (H.W. Gordon and Bogen, 1974; Kumkova, 1990; Samson and Zatorre, 1988; Yamadori et al., 1977). Its involvement with chord analysis is generally greatest for musically untrained persons (Gaede et al., 1978). Training can alter these hemispheric biases so that, for musicians, the left hemisphere predominates for melody recognition (Bever and Chiarello, 1974; Messerli, Pegna, and Sordet, 1995), tone discrimination (Mazziota et al., 1982; Shanon, 1981), and musical judgments (Shanon, 1980, 1984). Moreover, intact, untrained persons tend not to show lateralized effects for tone discrimination or musical judgments (Shanon, 1980, 1981, 1984). Taken altogether, these findings suggest that while cerebral processing of different components of music is lateralized with each hemisphere predominating in certain aspects, both hemispheres are needed for musical appreciation and performance (Bauer and McDonald, 2003).

The bilateral integration of cerebral function is most clearly exhibited by creative artists, who typically have intact brains. Excepting singing, harmonica playing, and the small repertoire of piano pieces written for one hand, making music is a two-handed activity. Moreover, for instruments such as guitars and the entire violin family, the right hand performs those aspects of the music that are mediated predominantly by the right hemisphere, such as expression and tonality, while the left hand interprets the linear sequence of notes best deciphered by the left hemisphere. Right-handed artists do their drawing, painting, sculpting, and modeling with the right hand, with perhaps an occasional assist from the left. Thus, by its very nature, the artist's performance involves the smoothly integrated activity of both hemispheres. The contributions of each hemisphere are indistinguishable and inseparable as the artist's two eyes and two ears guide the two hands or the bisymmetrical speech and singing structures that together render the artistic production.

Longitudinal Organization

Although no two human brains are exactly alike in their structure, all normally developed brains share the same major distinguishing features (see Fig. 3.12). The external surface of each half of the cerebral cortex is wrinkled into a complex of ridges or convolutions called *gyri* (sing., *gyrus*), which are separated by two deep fissures and many shallow clefts, the *sulci* (sing., *sulcus*). The two prominent fissures and certain of the major sulci divide each hemisphere into four lobes, the occipital, parietal, temporal, and frontal lobes. (For detailed delineations of cortical features and landmarks, see Brodal, 1981; Kolb and Whishaw, 1996; Mesulam, 2000b.)

The *central sulcus* divides the cerebral hemispheres into anterior and posterior regions. Immediately in front of the central sulcus lies the precentral gyrus which contains much of the *primary motor* or *motor*

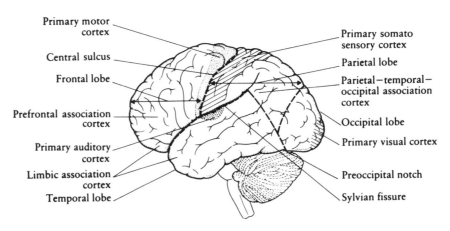

FIGURE 3.12 The lobe divisions of the human brain and their functional anatomy. (From Strange, 1992)

projection area. The entire area forward of the central sulcus is known as the *precentral* or *prerolandic* area. The bulk of the *primary somesthetic* or *somatosensory projection* area is located in the gyrus just behind the central sulcus. The area behind the central sulcus is also known as the *retrorolandic* or *postcentral* area.

Certain functional systems have primary or significant representation on the cerebral cortex with sufficient regularity that the lobes do provide a useful anatomical frame of reference for functional localization, much as a continent provides a geographical frame of reference for a country. However, because the lobes were originally defined solely on the basis of their gross appearance, some functionally definable areas overlap two and even three lobes. For example, the boundary between the parietal and occipital lobes is arbitrarily defined by a minor sulcus, the *parieto-occipital sulcus,* lying in what is now known to be an overlap zone for visual and spatial functions.

A two-dimensional organization of cortical functions lends itself to a schema that offers a framework for conceptualizing cortical organization. The posterior parts of the cortex behind the central sulcus are primarily involved in the analysis, coding, and storage of information, while the area anterior to the central sulcus is involved in the formation of intentions and programs for behavior (Luria, 1970). That is, information analyzed by the retrorolandic cortex is sent to prerolandic regions for planning and action. Prerolandic areas also receive information from subcortical areas regarding past experiences and emotions, which is used in decision making about actions. The actual interweaving of different functional components complicates this simple model as the right hemisphere has some involvement with verbal functions, some nonverbal behavior is mediated by the left cortex, and neural pathways between anterior and posterior regions ensure other extensive interactions.

FUNCTIONAL ORGANIZATION OF THE POSTERIOR CORTEX

Primary sensory areas are located in the posterior cortex. The primary visual cortex is located on the occipital lobes at the most posterior portion of the cerebral hemisphere (see Fig. 3.12, p. 64). The postcentral gyrus, at the most forward part of the parietal lobe, contains the primary sensory (somatosensory) projection area. The primary auditory cortex is located on the uppermost fold of the temporal lobe close to where it joins the parietal lobe. Kinesthetic and vestibular functions are mediated by areas low on the parietal lobe near the occipital and temporal lobe boundary regions. Sensory

information undergoes extensive associative elaboration through reciprocal connections with other cortical and subcortical areas (Kolb and Whishaw, 1996; Mesulam, 1998).

No clear-cut demarcations exist among any of the functions localized on the posterior cortex. Rather, although the primary centers of the major functions served by the posterior cerebral regions are relatively distant from one another, secondary association areas gradually fade into tertiary overlap, or heteromodal, zones in which auditory, visual, and body-sensing components commingle.

As a general rule, the character of the defects arising from lesions of the association areas of the posterior cortex varies according to the extent to which the lesion involves each of the sense modalities. Any disorder with a visual component, for example, may implicate some occipital lobe involvement. If a patient with visual agnosia also has difficulty estimating close distances or feels confused in familiar surroundings, then parietal lobe areas serving spatially related kinesthetic and vestibular functions may also be affected. Knowledge of the sites of the primary sensory centers and of the behavioral correlates of lesions to these sites and to the intermediate association areas enables the clinician to infer the approximate location of a lesion from the patient's behavioral symptoms (see E. Goldberg, 1989, 1990, for a detailed elaboration of this functional schema).

The Occipital Lobes and Their Disorders

The visual pathway travels from the retina through the *lateral geniculate nucleus* of the thalamus to the primary visual cortex. A lesion anywhere in the path between the lateral geniculate and primary visual cortex can produce a homonymous hemianopia (see p. 53). Lesions of the primary visual cortex result in discrete blind spots in the corresponding parts of the visual fields but do not alter the comprehension of visual stimuli or the ability to make a proper response to what is seen.

Blindness and associated problems

The nature of the blindness that accompanies total loss of function of the primary visual cortex, and the patient's response to it, varies with the extent of involvement of subcortical or associated cortical areas. Some visual discriminations may take place at the thalamic level, but the cortex is necessary for the conscious experience of visual phenomena (Celesia et al., 1991; Koch and Crick, 2000; Weiskrantz, 1986). Although it is rare for damage or dysfunction to be restricted to the primary visual cortex, when this does occur bilaterally the patient appears to have lost the capacity to distinguish forms or patterns while remaining responsive to light and dark, a condition called *cortical blindness* (Barton and Caplan, 2001; Luria, 1966). Patients may exhibit visually responsive behavior without experiencing vision, a phenomenon called *blindsight* (Farah, 2003b; Weiskrantz, 1986, 1996; Zeki, 1997). This phenomenon suggests that limited information in the blind visual field may project through alternate pathways to visual association areas. Total blindness due to brain damage appears to require large bilateral occipital cortex lesions (Barton and Caplan, 2001), and some patients have had destruction of thalamic areas as well as the visual cortex or the pathways leading to it (Teuber, 1975). In *denial of blindness* due to brain damage (*visual anosognosia*), patients lack appreciation that they are blind and attempt to behave as if sighted, making elaborate explanations and rationalizations for difficulties in getting around, handling objects, etc. (Redlich and Dorsey, 1945; Feinberg, 2003). Denial of blindness, sometimes called *Anton's syndrome,* may occur with several different lesion patterns; but typically the lesions are bilateral and involve the occipital lobe (Goldenberg, Mullbacher, and Nowak, 1995; McGlynn and Schacter, 1989). Such denial appears to be associated with disruption of corticothalamic connections and breakdown of sensory feedback loops.

Visual agnosias and other visual distortions

Lesions involving the visual association areas of the occipital lobes give rise to *visual agnosias,* or visual distortions (Benson, 1989; A.R. Damasio, Tranel, and Rizzo, 2000; Farah, 2003b; E. Goldberg, 1990; Mazaux, Dehail, et al., 1999). Only rarely do visuoperceptual disturbances result from lesions of other lobes or subcortical structures without occipital cortical damage as well. More often, impairments of visual awareness or visual recognition are associated with disturbances of other perceptual modalities; for example, when lesions in parietal regions extend to the occipital lobe disorders of visuospatial functions may occur.

Visual agnosia refers to a variety of relatively rare visual disturbances in which some aspect(s) of visual perception is defective in persons who can see and who are normally knowledgeable about information coming through other perceptual channels (Benson, 1989; A.R. Damasio, Tranel, and Damasio, 1989; Farah, 1999; Lissauer, [1888] 1988). They typically occur with bilateral occipital lesions (Vuilleumier, 2001).

In *apperceptive visual agnosia,* patients cannot synthesize what they see (M. Grossman, Galetta, and D'Esposito, 1997; see also Humphreys, 1999). They

may indicate awareness of discrete parts of a word or a phrase, or recognize elements of an object without organizing the discrete percepts into a perceptual whole. Drawings by these patients are fragmented: bits and pieces are recognizable but are not put together. They cannot recognize an object presented in unconventional views, such as recognizing an object usually seen from the side (e.g., a teapot) but now viewed from the top (Davidoff and Warrington, 1999). These patients often display general cognitive deterioration as well (Bauer, 1993). Patients with *associative visual agnosia* (or *visual object agnosia*) can perceive the whole of a visual stimulus, such as a familiar object, but cannot recognize it although they may be able to identify it by touch, sound, or smell (Ogden, 1996; see also Farah and Feinberg, 2003a). The examiner can distinguish visual object agnosia from a naming impairment by asking the patient who cannot name the object to give any identifying information, such as what function it has.

Simultaneous agnosia, or *simultanagnosia*—also known as *Balint's syndrome*—appears as an inability to perceive more than one object or point in space at a time (Bauer, 1993; A.R. Damasio, Tranel, and Rizzo, 2000; Rafal, 1997a). This extreme perceptual limitation impairs these patients' ability to move about; they get lost easily, and even reaching for something in their field of vision becomes difficult (L.C. Robertson and Rafal, 2000). Some workers highlight abnormalities in control of eye movements, resulting in difficulty in shifting visual attention from one point in the visual field to another (Pierrot-Deseilligny, 2001; Tranel and Damasio, 2000), but L.R. Robertson and Rafal (2000) discuss it in terms of reduced access to "spatial representations that normally guide attention from one object to another in a cluttered field." Both explanations appear to be valid, as patients with Balint's syndrome have difficulty directing their gaze *and* shifting from a fixation point (Barton and Caplan, 2001; Benson, 1989; Rizzo and Robin, 1990). *Color agnosia,* the inability to appreciate differences between colors or to relate colors to objects in the presence of intact color vision, may occur in association with other visual agnosias (Gloning et al., 1968; Lennie, 2001), particularly color naming and recognition defects (A.R. Damasio, Tranel, and Rizzo, 2000). However, in describing five patients with occipital lesions, each presenting a different pattern of visual agnosia, Warrington (1986b) demonstrated that agnosic color, shape, and location deficits are fully dissociable. Inability to comprehend pantomimes (*pantomime agnosia*), even when the ability to copy them remains intact, has been reported with lesions confined to the occipital lobes (Rothi, Mack, and Heilman, 1986).

Some visual agnosias are particularly associated with right- or left-sided damage (see Chaves and Caplan, 2001). *Associative visual agnosia* usually occurs with lesions of the left occipitotemporal region (De Renzi, 2000). Patients with lesions in the left occipital cortex and its subcortical connections may have a reading problem that stems from defects of visual recognition, organization, and scanning rather than from defective comprehension of written material, which usually occurs only with parietal damage or in aphasia (R.B. Friedman et al., 1993; Köhler and Moscovitch, 1997). Defective color naming frequently accompanies this kind of reading disability and is also typically associated with damage to the left occipital lobe or to underlying white matter containing visual system pathways (Benson, 1989; A.R. Damasio and Damasio, 1983). Beauvois and Saillant (1985) identified an *optic aphasia for colors* in which "the functional interactions between verbal and visual representations" are impaired. One form of *acalculia* (literally, "no counting"), a disorder that Grewel (1952) considered a primary type of impaired arithmetic ability in which the calculation process itself is affected, may result from visual disturbances of symbol perception associated with left occipital cortex lesions.

Visual inattention refers to imperception of stimuli. Material in one visual field—usually the left—can be seen but remains unnoticed unless the patient's attention is drawn to it (Chaves and Caplan, 2001; see Fig. 3.13). This form of visual inattention, also known as *unilateral sensory* or *spatial neglect,* typically occurs when there is right parietal lobe involvement as well as occipital lobe damage. Right occipital lesions are less likely to give rise to inattention. The so-called "visual inattention" associated with occipital lobe damage is similar to simultaneous agnosia in that the patient spontaneously perceives only one thing at a time. It differs from simultaneous agnosia in that the patient will see more than one object if others are pointed out; this is not the case in a true simultaneous agnosia.

Other visuoperceptual anomalies associated with occipital lesions include achromatopsia (loss of color vision in one or both visual half-fields), astereopsis (loss of stereoscopic vision), metamorphopsias (visual distortions), monocular polyopias (double, triple, or more vision in one eye), optic allesthesia (misplacement of percepts in space), and palinopsia (perseverated visual percept) (Barton and Caplan, 2001; Benson, 1989; A.R. Damasio, 1988; Zihl, 1989). These are very rare conditions but of theoretical interest as they may provide clues to cortical organization and function. Lesions associated with these conditions tend to involve the parietal cortex as well.

Prosopagnosia

Some workers report that another kind of visual agnosia, *prosopagnosia* (inability to recognize faces), occurs only when the cortex on the undersides of the occipital and temporal lobes is damaged bilaterally (A.R. Damasio, 1985; Geschwind, 1979; Mesulam, 2000b, p. 337), although other investigators have observed this phenomenon when the damage is restricted to the right hemisphere (De Renzi, 1997a; De Renzi, Perani, Carlesimo et al., 1994; Landis, Cummings, et al., 1986; Vuilleumier, 2001). It can present with just occipital lesions, but often temporal lobe lesions and sometimes parietal damage accompany the lesions (e.g., see A.R. Damasio, 1985; Tranel, Damasio, and Damasio, 1988). In normal subjects, only *ventromedial* areas (at the base of the brain toward the midline of the posterior right hemisphere) are specifically activated during a face recognition task (G. McCarthy, 2000; Sergent, Ohta, and MacDonald, 1992).

Difficulty in discriminating and matching unfamiliar faces may accompany left as well as right hemisphere lesions (Benton, 1980; Benton, Sivan, Hamsher, et al., 1994), although impairment tends to be greater when the lesion is on the right (Sergent, 1989). It is less frequent among patients with left hemisphere damage, affecting only aphasic patients who have comprehension defects at about the same rate of occurrence for all patients with right hemisphere damage. Capitani et al. (1978) reported that among patients unable to recognize unfamiliar faces, those with parietal rather than occipital lobe involvement were significantly more error prone on a color discrimination task, with the right-lesioned patients making almost twice as many errors as those whose lesions were on the left.

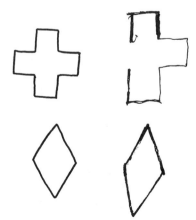

FIGURE 3.13 Example of inattention to the left visual field by a 57-year-old college graduate with a right parieto-occipital lesion.

Oliver Sacks richly described the extraordinary condition of prosopagnosia for familiar faces in his book *The Man who Mistook His Wife for a Hat* (1987). Like many prosopagnosics, his patient suffered visual agnosia on a broad scale, with inability to recognize faces as just one of many recognition deficits. This defect may show up whenever these patients must use vision to make a specific identification of an item in a category of objects or creatures, e.g., a bird watcher unable to identify birds or a farmer unable to recognize specific animals he once knew by name (A.R. Damasio, 1985).

Characteristic hemisphere processing differences show up in face recognition performances of patients with unilateral occipital lobe lesions (A.R. Damasio, Tranel, and Rizzo, 2000). Left occipital lesioned patients using right hemisphere processing strategies form their impressions quickly but may make semantic (i.e., naming) errors. With right occipital lesions, recognition proceeds slowly and laboriously in a piecemeal manner, but is often successful. A.R. Damasio, Damasio, and Tranel (1990) described other problems of perceptual fragmentation that can appear with prosopagnosia.

Reports on prosopagnosia in the literature indicate that it is about four times more common in men than in women, a finding that may reflect sex differences in cerebral organization (Mazzucchi and Biber, 1983; see pp. 301–303). Although impaired recognition of both familiar and unfamiliar faces is often treated as a single condition, these two forms of prosopagnosia can occur separately and thus their cerebral organization differs (D.R. Malone et al., 1982; R.A. McCarthy and Warrington, 1990). Some patients with this condition can appreciate the facial expressions, age, and sex of faces they may not recognize (A.R. Damasio, Tranel, and Rizzo, 2000). Lesions in occipital sites can result in the most flagrant and circumscribed face recognition deficits, but storage and processing also appear to take place at many other cortical and subcortical sites. Inability to recognize familiar faces may result from inaccessibility of memory traces for known faces stored in other brain regions (Carlesimo and Caltagirone, 1995). Thus the neuroanatomic model for face recognition suggests a pattern for the "multiple representation of visual stimuli" generally (A.R. Damasio, Damasio, and Tranel, 1990) and of information from the other sensory modalities as well (C.G. Phillips et al., 1984).

Two visuoperceptual systems

Another anatomic dimension that differentiates visual functions has to do with a *dorsal* (top side of the cerebrum)–*ventral* (under side) distinction (see Fig. 3.14). Two now well-identified visual systems have separate pathways with different cortical loci (Barton and Ca-

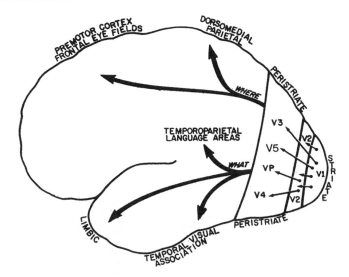

FIGURE 3.14 Organization of the two major visual pathways in the human brain. (From Mesulam, 2000b)

plan, 2001; Goodale, 2000; Mesulam, 2000b). One runs dorsally from the occipital to the parietal lobe. This parieto-occipital pathway is involved with spatial analysis, providing for spatial orientation: it gives visual "where" information. The temporo-occipital pathway, which takes a ventral route from the occipital lobe, conveys information about shapes and patterns, the "what" of visual perception. In clarifying their different contributions, D.N. Levine and his colleagues (1985) note that damage to either pathway can result in spatial disorientation but for different reasons: with damage to the dorsal pathway, patients will experience visual disorientation; when the damage involves the ventral pathway, "patients lose their way because they cannot recognize landmarks." Many of these latter patients have difficulty with face and object recognition (Hermann, Seidenberg, et al., 1993).

The Posterior Association Cortex and Its Disorders

Association areas in the parieto-temporo-occipital region are situated just in front of the visual association areas and behind the primary sensory strip (see Fig. 3.12, p. 64). They run from the *longitudinal fissure*, sometimes called the *sagittal fissure* (the deep cleft separating the two hemispheres) laterally into the areas adjacent to and just above the temporal lobe where temporal, occipital, and parietal elements commingle. These association areas include much of the parietal and occipital lobes and some temporal association areas. Functionally they are the site of cortical integration for all behavior involving vision, touch, body awareness and spatial orientation, verbal comprehension, localization in space, abstract and complex cognitive functions of mathematical reasoning, and the formulation of logical propositions that have their conceptual roots in basic visuospatial experiences such as "inside," "bigger," "and," or "instead of." It is within these areas that intermodal sensory integration takes place, making this region "an association area of association areas" (Geschwind, 1965) or "heteromodal association cortex" (Mesulam, 2000b) or "multimodal sensory convergence areas" (Heilman, 2002).

A variety of *apraxias* (inability to perform learned purposeful movements) and agnosias have been ascribed to parieto-temporo-occipital lesions. Most of them have to do with verbal or with nonverbal stimuli but not with both and thus are asymmetrically localized. A few occur with lesions in either hemisphere.

Defects arising from posterior lesions in either hemisphere

Constructional disorders are among the predominantly parietal lobe disabilities that appear with lesions on either side of the midline (F.W. Black and Bernard, 1984; De Renzi, 1997b), reflecting the involvement of both hemispheres in processing spatial information (Sergent, 1991a,b). They involve impairment of the "capacity to draw or construct two or three dimensional figures or shapes from one and two dimensional units" (Strub and Black, 2000). They seem to be closely associated with perceptual defects (Pillon, 1981a,b; Sohlberg and Mateer, 2001). Constructional disorders take different forms depending on the hemispheric side of the lesion (Consoli, 1979; Cutting, 1990; Walsh and Darby, 1999; Warrington, James, and Kinsbourne, 1966). Left-sided lesions are apt to disrupt the programming or ordering of movements necessary for constructional activity (Hécaen and Albert, 1978). Visuospatial defects associated with impaired understanding of spatial relationships or defective spatial imagery tend to underlie right hemisphere constructional disorders (Pillon, 1979). Diagonality in a design or construction can be particularly disorienting to patients with right hemisphere lesions (B. Milner, 1971; Warrington, James, and Kinsbourne, 1966). Defects in copying designs appear in the drawings of patients with left hemisphere lesions as simplification and difficulty in making angles, and in the drawings of patients with right-sided involvement as a tendency to a counterclockwise tilt (rotation), fragmented percepts, irrelevant overelaborativeness, and inattention to the left half of the page or the left half of elements on the page (Diller and Weinberg, 1965; Ducarne and Pillon, 1974; Warrington, James, and Kinsbourne, 1966). (See Fig. 3.15a,b for freehand drawings of left and right hemisphere damaged patients showing typical hemispheric defects.) As-

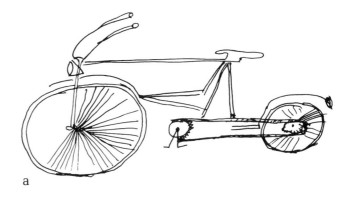

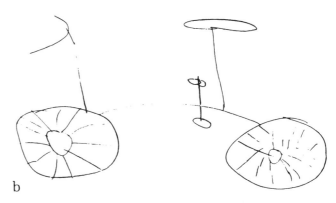

FIGURE 3.15a This bicycle was drawn by the same 51-year-old retired salesman who constructed the block designs of Figure 3.9 (*a–e*). This drawing demonstrate that neglect of the left visual field is not due to carelessness as the patient painstaking provided details and was very pleased with his performance. *b:* This bicycle was drawn by a 24-year-old college graduate almost a year after he received a severe injury to the left side of his head. He originally drew the bike without pedals, adding them when asked, "How do you make it go?"

sembling puzzles in two- and three-dimensional space may be affected by both right and left hemisphere lesions (E. Kaplan, 1988; E. Kaplan, Fein, et al., 1991).

Some studies have not shown any difference in the frequency with which left and right hemisphere damaged patients have constructional disorders (e.g., Arena and Gainotti, 1978; F.W. Black and Bernard, 1984; Dee et al., 1970); others (Belleza et al., 1979; Y. Kim et al., 1984; Warrington, James, and Maciejewski, 1986) have reported more constructional disabilities among right brain damaged patients. Although Arena and Gainotti (1978) attribute differences in findings to the number of aphasic patients included in the left hemisphere damaged samples, other differences between the studies may also account for the apparently conflicting findings. For example, Benton (1984) used a difficult three-dimensional construction task while Arena and Gainotti (1978) had their patients copy relatively simple geometric designs. Another factor is time since injury. When examined six months after stroke, a left hemisphere group showed more improvement and better performance than a right hemisphere group (Sunderland, Tinson, and Bradley, 1994).

The integration of sensory, motor, and attentional signals that takes place within the posterior parietal cortex enables the direction and shifting of attention and response which are prerequisites for effectively dealing with space (J.F. Stein, 1991; see also Farah, Wong, et al., 1989; Mesulam, 1983). One identified function mediated in the parietal lobes is the ability to disengage attention in order to be able to reengage it rapidly and correctly: parietal lobe damage significantly slows the disengagement process (L.C. Robertson and Rafal, 2000), with the greatest slowing occurring when the lesion is on the right (Morrow and Ratcliff, 1988; Posner et al., 1984; Roy, Reuter-Lorenz, Roy, et al., 1987).

A short-term memory disorder, associated with lesions in that portion of the parietal lobe lying just above the posterior temporal lobe (the *inferior parietal lobule*), reflects the usual auditory/visual lateralization pattern (N. Butters, Samuels, et al., 1970; Mayes, 2000b; Vallar and Papagno, 2002). Thus, with left-sided lesions in this area, the number of digits, tones (W.P. Gordon, 1983), or words (Risse et al., 1984) that can be recalled immediately upon hearing them is abnormally low; patients with right-sided lesions here show reduced short-term recall for geometric patterns. Direct cortical stimulation studies (Mayes, 1988; Ojemann, 1980; Ojemann, Cawthon, and Lettich, 1990) and functional imaging (C.R. Clark et al., 2000) have also implicated this region in short-term memory.

Hécaen (1969) associated difficulties in serial ordering with impairment of the parieto-temporo-occipital area of both the left and right hemispheres. Perception of the temporal order in which stimuli are presented is much more likely to be impaired by left than right hemisphere lesions involving the posterior association areas (Carmon and Nachson, 1971; von Steinbüchel et al., 1999), except when the stimulus array also includes complex spatial configurations, for then the patients with right hemisphere lesions do worse than those with left-sided lesions (Carmon, 1978). Disruption of the sequential organization of speech associated with left hemisphere lesions may result in the language formulation defects of aphasia. Right-sided lesions of the parieto-temporo-occipital area appear to interfere with the comprehension of order and sequence so that the patient has difficulty seeing or dealing with temporal relationships and is unable to make plans (Milberg, Cummings, et al., 1979).

Damage to the crossed optic radiations underlying either parietal cortex results in loss of vision in the con-

tralateral lower visual field quadrant (Barton and Caplan, 2001; Pearlman, 1990). Lesions in either hemisphere involving the somatosensory association areas posterior to the postcentral gyrus can produce a *tactile agnosia* or *astereognosis* (inability to identify an object by touch) to the body side opposite the lesion (Caselli, 2003). Some patients with right-sided lesions here may experience bilateral astereognosis (Vuilleumier, 2001). Sensitivity to the size, weight, and texture of hand-held objects is also diminished contralaterally by these lesions (A.R. Damasio, 1988). Left-sided inattention appears to exacerbate the problem and, with severely reduced left hand sensitivity, bilateral tactile agnosia may appear (Caselli, 1991). Semmes' (1968) findings that right hemisphere lesions may be associated with impairment of shape perception in both hands have received support (e.g., Boll, 1974), but a high incidence of bilateral sensory defects has also been noted among patients with unilateral lesions of either hemisphere (B. Milner, 1975). Parietal lesions in either hemisphere may disrupt the guidance of movements insofar as they depend on somatosensory contributions (Jason, 1990).

Other neuropsychological abnormalities historically associated with just one side of the cortex do show up with lesions on the unexpected side in right-handed patients. In the succeeding pages, those that are typically associated with a hemispheric side will be presented in accord with their characteristic lateralization, with significant exceptions noted.

Defects arising from left posterior hemisphere lesions

The posterior language areas are situated at the juncture of the temporal and parietal lobes. Fluent aphasia and related symbol-processing disabilities are generally the most prominent symptoms of left parieto-temporo-occipital lesions. This form of aphasia is usually characterized by incomprehension, jargon speech, *echolalia* (parrotted speech), and apparent lack of awareness of the communication disability. It commonly follows cortical damage within this area where "the great afferent systems" of audition, vision, and body sensation overlap (M.P. Alexander, 2003; Benson, 1988; A.R. Damasio and Damasio, 2000; Dronkers et al., 2000; see pp. 32–33). W.R. Russell (1963) pointed out that even very small cortical lesions in this area can have widespread and devastating consequences for verbal behavior. Howard (1997) offers an interpretation of imaging data, noting that language capabilities are more widespread and occur in less well-delineated cortical areas than is assumed in classical localization theory (see also Kertesz and Gold, 2003).

Communication disabilities arising from lesions in the left parieto-temporo-occipital region may involve impaired or absent recognition or comprehension of the semantic—and logical—features of language (Bachman and Albert, 1988; Howard, 1997; E. Goldberg, 1990; McCarthy and Warrington, 1990). Lesions overlapping both the parietal and occipital cortex may give rise to reading defects (R.B. Friedman et al., 1983). Writing ability can be disrupted by lesions in a number of cortical sites (Luria, 1966), mostly on the left and often in the posterior association cortex (Roeltgen, 2003). The nature of the writing defect depends on the site and extent of the lesion (Roeltgen, 2003). In many cases the defects of written language reflect the defects of a concomitant aphasia or apraxia (Bub and Chertkow, 1988; Luria, 1970).

Apraxias characterized by disturbances of nonverbal symbolization, such as gestural defects or inability to demonstrate an activity in pantomime or to comprehend pantomimed activity, are usually associated with lesions involving language comprehension areas and the overlap zone for kinesthetic and visual areas of the left hemisphere, occurring less often with anterior lesions (Haaland and Yeo, 1989; Heilman and Rothi, 2003; Jason, 1990; Kareken et al., 1998; Meador, Loring, Lee, et al., 1999). Defective ability to comprehend gestures has been specifically associated with impaired reading comprehension in some aphasic patients, with constructional disorders in others (Ferro, Santos, et al., 1980). Impairments in sequential hand movements are strongly associated with left parietal lesions (Haaland and Yeo, 1989). Apraxias often occur with aphasia and may be obscured by or confused with the language disorder. De Renzi, Motti, and Nichelli (1980) observed that while 50% of patients with left-sided lesions were apraxic, so too were 20% of those damaged on the right, although right-lesioned patients had milder deficits. That apraxia and aphasia can occur separately implicates different but anatomically close or overlapping neural networks (Heilman and Rothi, 2003; Kertesz, Ferro, and Shewan, 1984).

Like writing, arithmetic abilities depend on intact cortex at several sites (Rosselli and Ardila, 1989; Rickard et al., 2000; Spiers, 1987). Acalculia is most common and most severe with lesions of the left posterior cortex (Dehaene, 2000; Grafman and Rickard, 1997) and pure *agraphia* (inability to write) may also result from lesions in this area (Schomer, Pegna, et al., 1998). This area contributes to knowledge of arithmetic operations (Langdon and Warrington, 1997; Warrington, 1982) such that lesions here may disrupt computational operations in patients who can make reasonable quantity estimates. Left posterior lesions may also involve defective number reading and writing (H.S. Levin, Goldstein, and Spiers, 1993) or errors due to spatial disorientation (Grafman, 1988; Grafman, Passafiume, et al., 1982; Walsh and Darby, 1999).

Acalculia and agraphia generally appear in association with other communication disabilities. When they occur with left–right spatial disorientation and an inability to identify one's own fingers, to orient oneself to one's own fingers, to recognize or to name them (*finger agnosia*), the symptom cluster is known as *Gerstmann's syndrome* (Gerstmann, 1940, 1957) and the lesion is likely to involve the left parieto-occipital region. Acalculia associated with finger agnosia typically disrupts such relatively simple arithmetic operations as counting or ordering numbers. The frequency with which these individual symptoms occur together reflects an underlying cortical organization in which components involved in the different impaired acts are in close anatomical proximity. Other deficits—including aphasia—are also frequently associated with one or more of these symptoms (Benton, 1977b; Denburg and Tranel, 2003). Moreover, both finger agnosia and right–left disorientation can be present when cortical damage is on the right (Benton, 1977b [1985]; Denburg and Tranel, 2003). Thus, rather than achieving the stature of a syndrome with an underlying functional unity (e.g., Orgogozo, 1976), the symptoms identified by Gerstmann may best be understood together as a "cluster" which may provide valuable localizing information (Geschwind and Strub, 1974).

Agnosias arising from left hemisphere lesions just anterior to the visual association area may appear as disorientation of either extrapersonal or personal space and are likely to have either a symbolic or left–right component (Benton, 1973 [1985]; E. Goldberg, 1990). Not only may disorders of extrapersonal or personal space occur separately, but different kinds of personal space deficits and disorientations can be distinguished (Lishman, 1997; Newcombe and Ratcliff, 1989). However, visuospatial perception tends to remain accurate (Belleza et al., 1979).

Disabilities arising from left hemisphere lesions tend to be more severe when the patient is also aphasic. Although all of these disturbances can occur in the absence of aphasia, it is rare for any of them to appear as the sole defect.

Defects arising from right posterior hemisphere lesions

A commonly seen disorder associated with the right parietal lobe is impaired constructional ability (Benton, 1967 [1985]; De Renzi, 1997b; Farah, 2003a). Vestibular and oculomotor disorders, defective spatial orientation, or impaired visual scanning contribute to the constructional disability. A right hemisphere *dyscalculia* shows up on written calculations as an inability to manipulate numbers in spatial relationships, such as us-

CALCULATIONS

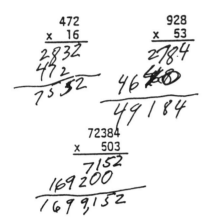

FIGURE 3.16 Example of spatial dyscalculia by the traumatically injured pediatrician described on pp. 80–81 whose reading inattention is shown in Figure 10.7. Note neglect of the 6 on the left of the problem in the upper left corner; errors on left side of bottom problem which appear to be due to more than simple neglect; labored but finally correct working out of problem in middle right side of page. This test was taken with no time limit.

ing decimal places or "carrying," although the patient retains mathematical concepts and the ability to do problems mentally (Denburg and Tranel, 2003; see Fig. 3.16). Spatial (or visuospatial) dyscalculia is frequently associated with constructional deficits (H.S. Levin, Goldstein, and Spiers, 1993; Rosselli and Ardila, 1989) and seems to follow from more general impairments of spatial orientation or organization. *Apraxia for dressing,* in which the patient has difficulty relating to and organizing parts of his body to parts of his clothing, may accompany right-sided parietal lesions (Damasio, Tranel, and Rizzo, 2000; Hier, Mondlock, and Caplan, 1983a,b; Pimental and Kingsbury, 1989). It is not a true apraxia but rather symptomatic of spatial disorientation coupled, in many instances, with left visuospatial inattention (Poeck, 1986; see below). Other performance disabilities of patients with right parietal lobe involvement are also products of a perceptual disorder, such as impaired ability to localize objects in left hemispace (Mesulam, 2000b). For example, the chief complaint of a middle-aged rancher with a right parieto-occipital lesion was difficulty in eating because his hand frequently missed when he put it out to reach the cup or his fork overshot his plate.

Many of the perceptual disorders arising from lesions of the right posterior association cortex are related to the phenomenon of inattention or *sensory neglect,* the tendency for decreased or absent awareness of events presented to the half of the body contralateral to the hemisphere side of the lesion that is not the result of a sensory defect (Bisiach and Vallar, 1988; S. Clarke, 2001; Heilman, Watson, and Valenstein, 2003; Mesulam, 2000b; Rafal, 1997b). The most common lesion site for chronic inattention is the temporoparietal cortex, with severity of the deficit directly related to lesion size. Kertesz and Dobrowolski (1981) observed left-sided inattention occurring more prominently among patients whose lesions involved the area around the central sulcus (including posterior frontal and some temporal lobe tissue) than among patients whose lesions were confined to the parietal lobe; yet Vallar and Perani's studies (1986, 1987) implicated the parietal lobe as the most common lesion site associated with inattention. Egelko, Gordon, and their colleagues (1988) noted that each of the three posterior lobes could be involved, with "a lack of specificity in the relationship between the regions of right neuroanatomic damage and visual–spatial inattention."

A few left hemisphere damaged patients experience this problem (Köhler and Moscovitch, 1997), usually during the acute stage of their illness (Colombo et al., 1976). Inattention has been reported in association with lesions on either side when patients with lateralized brain damage are given tasks too difficult for them to perform; for example, auditory letter matching elicited inattention from left hemisphere lesioned patients, while on a difficult visual discrimination task both right- and left-lesioned patients displayed inattention (Leicester et al., 1969). When inattentive patients were primed with a picture displayed to the neglected field, the amount of time they took to make a lexical decision was significantly shortened when the picture and word were semantically related, indicating that processing was taking place unconsciously in the impaired field (McGlinchey-Berroth et al., 1993). Inattention can occur in any perceptual modality but rarely involves all of them (S. Clarke, 2001; Umilta, 1995).

Inattention may be manifested in a number of ways. It may occur as a relatively discrete and subtle disorder apparent only to the examiner. When stimulated bilaterally with a light touch to both cheeks or fingers wiggled in the outside periphery of each visual field simultaneously, inattentive patients tend to ignore the stimulus on the left (*double simultaneous stimulation*), although they have no apparent difficulty noticing the stimuli when presented one at a time. This form of inattention has been variously called *sensory inattention, sensory extinction, sensory suppression,* or *perceptual rivalry* (Walsh and Darby, 1999). Visual extinction is frequently associated with other manifestations of inattention in patients with right-sided lesions, but these two phenomena can occur separately (Barbieri and De Renzi, 1989; S. Clarke, 2001). They are often accompanied by similar deficits in the auditory or tactile modalities, and by left nostril extinction for odors (Bellas et al., 1988). Although technically differentiable and bearing different names, extinction and inattention are probably two aspects of the same pathological process (Bisiach, 1991; Mesulam, 2000; Rafal, 2000). In this book, "inattention" refers to all aspects of unilaterally depressed awareness.

Although usually presenting as one syndrome, inattention for personal and extrapersonal space do not always occur together (Bisiach, Perani, et al., 1986). In its more severe forms, inattention for personal space may amount to a complete agnosia for the half of space or for the half of the patient's body opposite the side of the lesion (*hemisomatognosia*). Mild inattention to one's own body may appear as simple negligence: the patient with right-sided damage rarely uses the left hand spontaneously, may bump into objects on the left, or may not use left-side pockets. In more extreme cases, usually associated with left hemiplegia, patients may appear completely unaware of the left half of the body, even to the point of denying left-side disabilities (*anosognosia*) or being unable to recognize that the paralyzed limbs belong to them (Cutting, 1990; Feinberg, 2003). Most cases of anosognosia involve the inferior parietal cortex, but it can occur with purely subcortical lesions or with frontal damage (Bisiach and Geminiani, 1991). S.W. Anderson and Tranel (1989) found that all of their patients with impaired awareness of physical disabilities also lacked awareness of their cognitive defects. Anosognosia creates a serious obstacle to rehabilitation as these patients typically see no need to exert the effort or submit to the discomforts required for effective rehabilitation.

In left visuospatial inattention, not only may patients not attend to stimuli in the left half of space, but they may also fail to draw or copy all of the left side of a figure or design and tend to flatten or otherwise diminish the left side of complete figures (see Figs. 3.13; 10.9). When copying written material, the patient with unilateral inattention may omit words or numbers on the left side of the model, even though the copy makes less than good sense (see Chapter 10, Fig. 10.8, p. 385). Increasing the complexity of the drawing task increases the likelihood of eliciting the inattention phenomenon (Pillon, 1981a). In reading, words on the left side of the page may be omitted although such omissions alter or lose the meaning of the text (Mesulam, 2000b; see Chapter 10, Fig. 10.7, p. 384). This form of visual imperception typically occurs only when the right parietal damage extends to occipital association areas. Left visual inattention is frequently, but not necessarily, accompanied by left visual field defects, most usually a left homonymous hemianopsia. Some patients with obvious left-sided inattention, particularly those with visual inattention, display a gaze defect such that they do not spontaneously scan the left side of space, even when spoken to from the left. These are the patients who begin reading in the middle of a line of print when asked to read and who seem unaware that the words out of context of the left half of the line make no sense. Most such right hemisphere damaged patients stop reading on their own, explaining that they have "lost interest," although they can still read with understanding when their gaze is guided. Even in their mental imagery, some of these patients may omit left-sided features (Bisiach and Luzzatti, 1978; Meador, Loring, Bowers, and Heilman, 1987).

A 45-year-old pediatrician sustained a large area of right parietal damage in a motor vehicle accident. A year later he requested that his medical license be reinstated so he could resume practice. He acknowledged a visual deficit which he attributed to loss of sight in his right eye and the left visual field of his left eye and for which he wore a little telescopic monocle with a very narrow range of focus. He claimed that this device enabled him to read. He had been divorced and was living independently at the time of the accident, but since then he has stayed with his mother. He denied physical and cognitive problems other than a restricted range of vision which he felt would not interfere with his ability to return to his profession.

On examination he achieved scores in the *superior* to *very superior* range on tests of old verbal knowledge although he performed at only *average* to *high average* levels on conceptual verbal tasks. Verbal fluency (the rapidity with which he could generate words) was just *low average*, well below expectations for his education and verbal skills. On written tests he made a number of small errors, such as copying the word bicycle as "bicyclicle," Harry as "Larry," and mistrust (on a list immediately below the word displease, which he copied correctly) as "distrust." Despite a *very superior* oral arithmetic performance, he made errors on four of 20 written calculation problems, of which two involved left spatial inattention (see Fig. 3.16). Verbal memory functions were well *within normal limits*.

On visuoperceptual and constructional tasks, his scores were generally *average* except for slowing on a visual reasoning test which dropped his score to *low average*. In his copy of a set of line drawn designs (see Chapter 14, Fig. 14.1, p. 533), left visuospatial inattention errors were prominent as he omitted the left dot of a dotted arrowhead figure and the left side of a three-sided square. Although he recalled eight of the nine figures, on both immediate and delayed recall trials, he continued to omit the dot and forgot the incomplete figure altogether. On Line Bisection, 13 of 19 "midlines" were pushed to the right. On an oral reading task arranged to be sensitive to left-side inattention, in addition to misreading an occasional word he omitted several words or phrases on the left side of the page (see Fig. 10.7, p. 384) whether reading with or without his monocle. Essentially the performances did not differ.

In a follow-up interview he acknowledged unawareness of the inattention problem, but then reported having had both inattention and left-sided hemiparesis immediately after the accident. In ascribing his visuoperceptual problems to compromised vision, this physician demonstrated that he had been unaware of their nature. Moreover, despite painstaking efforts at checking and rechecking his performances—as was evident on the calculation page and other paper-and-pencil tasks—he did not self-monitor effectively, another aspect of not being aware of his deficits. The extent of his anosognosia and associated judgmental impairments became apparent when he persisted in his ambition to return to medical practice after being informed of his limitations.

Visuospatial disturbances associated with lesions of the parieto-occipital cortex include impairment of topographical or spatial thought and memory (Benson, 1989; De Renzi, 1997b; Newcombe and Ratcliff, 1989). Some workers identify temporo-occipital sites as the critical lesion area for object recognition (Dolan et al., 1997; Habib and Sirigu, 1987; Landis, Cummings, Benson, and Palmer, 1986). Another problem is perceptual fragmentation (Denny-Brown, 1962). A severely left hemiparetic political historian, for instance, when shown photographs of famous people he had known, named bits and pieces correctly, e.g., "This is a mouth . . . this is an eye," but was unable to organize the discrete features into recognizable faces. Warrington and Taylor (1973) also related difficulties in perceptual classification, specifically, the inability to recognize an object from an unfamiliar perspective, to right parietal lesions (see also McCarthy and Warrington, 1990). Appreciation of facial expressions may also be impaired (Adolphs and Damasio, 2000).

The Temporal Lobes and Their Disorders

Temporal cortex functions: information processing and lesion-associated defects

The primary auditory cortex is located on the upper posterior transverse folds of the temporal cortex (*Heschel's gyrus*), for the most part tucked within the *Sylvian fissure* (see Figs. 3.1 and 3.12, pp. 42, 64). This part of the superior temporal gyrus receives input from the *medial geniculate nucleus* of the thalamus. Much of the temporal lobe cortex is concerned with hearing and related functions, such as auditory memory storage and complex perceptual organization.

The superior temporal cortex and adjacent areas are critical for central auditory processing (Mesulam, 2000b; Vuillemier, 2001). The auditory pathways transmit information about sound in all parts of space to both hemispheres through major contralateral and mi-

nor ipsilateral projections (see Fig. 3.7, p. 53). The condition of cortical deafness occurs with bilateral destruction of the primary auditory cortices, but most cases with severe hearing loss also have subcortical lesions (Bauer and McDonald, 2003). Patients whose lesions are limited to the cortex are typically not deaf but their auditory recognition will be deficient (Kolb and Whishaw, 1996). Thus "cortical deafness" is a misnomer as these patients retain some hearing capacity (Coslett, Brashear, and Heilman, 1984; Hécaen and Albert, 1978).

The importance of the temporal lobes to central auditory processing becomes evident following surgical removal of either anterior temporal lobe (Efron and Crandall, 1983; Efron, Crandall, et al., 1983). In these patients, dominance for tonal pitch becomes heightened for sound heard ipsilateral to the lobectomy relative to diminished dominance on the contralateral side. This operation impairs the ability to discriminate and focus on one sound in the midst of many—the "cocktail party" effect—again for the side opposite the lesioned lobe. Cortical association areas of the left temporal lobe mediate the perception of such verbal material as word and number and voice recognition (B. Milner, 1971; Van Lancker, Cummings, et al., 1988). The farther back a lesion occurs on the temporal lobe, the more likely it is to produce alexia and verbal apraxias.

Polster and Rose (1998) describe disorders of auditory processing that parallel those of visual processing. *Pure word deafness* is an inability to comprehend spoken words despite intact hearing, speech production, reading ability, and recognition of nonlinguisitic sounds which occurs mostly with left temporal lesions. *Auditory agnosia* is an inability to recognize auditorily presented environmental sounds independent of any deficit in processing spoken language and is primarily associated with a right temporal lobe lesion. However, lesion localization is variable from case to case and often these conditions involve bilateral lesions (Bauer and McDonald, 2003). *Phonagnosia* is an inability to recognize familiar voices which may develop with a lesion in the right parietal lobe. Anatomically distinct "what" and "where" systems, also analogous to the visual processing system, have been described (Clarke, Bellman, Meuli et al., 2000; Rauschecker and Tian, 2000).

Considerable interindividual variability exists for the aphasias and associated language and other cognitive disorders, both with respect to anatomic differences in functionally relevant sites and with respect to differences in anatomic lesion patterns which, together, make the identification of deficit sites a matter of frequency of occurrence (M.P. Alexander, 2003; Dronkers et al., 2000). Any individual case is likely to deviate from the common frequency patterns (D. Caplan, 1987; De Bleser, 1988; Ojemann, 1980). Interindividual variability holds true for most other cortical functions, but few have been mapped as often or as carefully as the language functions.

Perhaps the most crippling of the communication disorders is *Wernicke's aphasia* (also called *sensory, fluent,* or *jargon aphasia;* see Chapter 2, Table 2.1, p. 33) since these patients can understand little of what they hear, although motor production of speech remains intact (Benson, 1993; A.R. Damasio and Geschwind, 1984; A.R. Damasio and Damasio, 2000; Dronkers et al., 2000). Many such patients prattle grammatically and syntactically correct nonsense. The auditory incomprehension of patients with lesions in Wernicke's area does not extend to nonverbal sounds for they can respond appropriately to sirens, squealing brakes, and the like. Moreover, these patients are frequently anosognosic, neither appreciating their deficits nor aware of their errors, and thus unable to self-monitor, self-correct, or benefit readily from therapy (Lebrun, 1987; Rubens and Garrett, 1991).

Lesions in the left temporal lobe may disrupt retrieval of words which, when severe, can seriously disrupt fluent speech (*dysnomia*) (A.R. Damasio and Damasio, 2000; Fuster, 1999; Indefrey and Levelt, 2000; Kremin, 1988). Anatomically separate regions tend to process words for distinct kinds of items, such as animals or tools (A. Martin, Wiggs, Ungerleider, and Haxby, 1996).

Many patients with a naming disorder find it hard to remember or comprehend long lists, sentences, or complex verbal material; and their ability for new verbal learning may be greatly diminished or even abolished. After left temporal lobectomy, patients tend to perform complex verbal tasks somewhat less well than prior to surgery, verbal memory tends to worsen (Ivnik, Sharbrough, and Laws, 1988), and they do poorly on tests that simulate everyday memory skills (Ivnik, Malec, Sharbrough, et al., 1993). What they do recall tends to be confounded with their associations, appearing as intrusion errors in their responses (Crosson, Sartor, et al., 1993).

Patients with cortical lesions of the right temporal lobe are unlikely to have language disabilities. These patients may have trouble organizing complex data or formulating multifaceted plans (Fiore and Schooler, 1998). Impairments in sequencing operations (Canavan et al., 1989; Milberg et al., 1979) have also been associated with right temporal lobe lesions. Temporal lobe damage may result in some form of *amusia* (literally, no music), particularly involving receptive aspects of musicianship such as the abilities to distinguish tones, tonal patterns, beats, or timbre, often but not necessarily with resulting inability to enjoy music or to sing or hum a tune or rhythmical pattern (Alajouanine, 1948; Benton, 1977a; Samson and Zatorre, 1988; Shankweiler, 1966). Odor perception may require in-

tact temporal lobes (Eskenazi et al., 1986; Jones-Gotman and Zatorre, 1988) and is particularly vulnerable to right temporal lesions (Abraham and Mathai, 1983; Martinez et al., 1993).

The temporal lobes also contain some components of the visual system (Eichenbaum and Cohen, 2001) including the crossed optic radiations from the upper quadrants of the visual fields, so that temporal lobe damage can result in a visual field defect (Barton and Caplan, 2001; Kolb and Whishaw, 1996). Damage in ventral posterior portions of the temporal cortex can produce a variety of visuoperceptual abnormalities, such as deficits in visual discrimination and visual word and pattern recognition that occur without deficits on visuospatial tasks (Fedio, Martin, and Brouwers, 1984; Kolb and Whishaw, 1996; B. Milner, 1958). This pattern of impaired object recognition with intact spatial localization appeared following temporal lobectomies that involved "the anterior portion of the occipitotemporal object recognition system" (Hermann, Seidenberg, et al., 1993). Left–right asymmetry follows the verbal–nonverbal pattern of the posterior cortex.

The olfactory cortex is located in the medial temporal lobe near the tip and involves the uncus. It receives its input from the olfactory bulb at the base of the frontal lobe.

Memory in the temporal lobes and associated disorders

Along with the limbic system (pp. 49–51), many regions of the temporal lobes are critical for normal learning and retention (see Fig. 3.6, p. 49). Lesions of the left temporal lobe disrupt verbal memory and right temporal lobe lesions interfere with memory for many different nonverbal tasks (Tranel and Damasio, 2002; Jones-Gotman, Zatorre, Olivier, et al., 1997; Markowitsch, 2000). In some cases lesions of the temporal neocortex may impair learning and retention by disconnecting the hippocampus from cortical input (Jones-Gotman et al., 1997).

Cortical regions appear to be organized for long-term storage of memories (Fuster, 1999). Awake patients undergoing brain surgery report vivid auditory and visual recall of previously experienced scenes and episodes upon electrical stimulation of the exposed temporal lobe cortex (Gloor et al., 1982; Penfield, 1958). Nauta (1964) speculated that these memories involve widespread neural mechanisms and that the temporal cortex and, to a lesser extent, the occipital cortex play roles in organizing the discrete components of memory for orderly and complete recall. Information involving each modality appears to be stored in the association cortex adjacent to its primary sensory cortex (A.R.

Damasio, Damasio, and Tranel, 1990; Killackey, 1990; A. Martin, Haxby, Lalonde, et al., 1995). Thus, retrieval of visual information is impaired by lesions of the visual association cortex of the occipital lobe, impaired retrieval of auditory information follows lesions of the auditory association cortex of the temporal lobe, and so on. Some patients with cortical lesions have shown selective deficits in retrieving highly specific types of information, such as items in certain categories but not others (Gabrieli, 1998; A. Martin et al., 1997). This finding suggests that cortical representation of knowledge is highly organized. Loss of facts, knowledge of objects, and meaning of words have been reported with selective damage to the inferolateral temporal gyri of one or both temporal lobes, with sparing of the hippocampal and parahippocampal gyri (K.S. Graham and Hodges, 1997). Thus, while the hippocampus and medial limbic structures are involved in the processing of newly learned information that has not yet consolidated, the temporal cortex appears to house old learned information.

A variety of emotional disorders are common with temporal as well as limbic lesions, including anxiety, delusions, and mood disorders (Heilman, Blonder, et al., 2000; Trimble et al., 1997). Abnormal electrical activity of the brain associated with *temporal lobe epilepsy (TLE)* typically originates within the temporal lobe. Specific problems associated with temporal lobe epilepsy include alterations of mood, obsessional thinking, changes in consciousness, hallucinations, and perceptual distortions in all sensory modalities including pain, and stereotyped, often repetitive and meaningless motor behavior that may comprise quite complex activities (Filley, 1995; Schomer, O'Connor, et al., 2000; G.J. Tucker, 2002). Other names for these disturbances are *psychomotor epilepsy* and *psychomotor* or *complex partial seizures* (Pincus and Tucker, 2003; see p. 322 for a fuller discussion of the cognitive and personality/ emotional features of temporal lobe epilepsy).

THE PRECENTRAL (ANTERIOR) CORTEX: FRONTAL LOBE DISORDERS

In the course of the brain's evolution, the frontal lobes developed most recently to become its largest structures. It was only natural for early students of brain function to conclude that the frontal lobes must therefore be the seat of the highest cognitive functions. Thus, when Hebb reported in 1939 that a small series of patients who had undergone surgical removal of frontal lobe tissue showed no loss in IQ score on a standard intelligence test, he provoked a controversy. In his comprehensive review of the literature on the psychologi-

cal consequences of frontal lobe lesions, Klebanoff (1945) noted the seemingly unresolvable discrepancies between studies reporting on the cognitive status of patients with frontal lobe lesions. He found that since Fritsch and Hitzig ([1870] 1969) first reported mental deterioration in patients with traumatic frontal lesions, more authors had described cognitive deficits in patients with frontal lobe damage than denied the presence of such deficits in their patients.

The large number of World War II missile wound survivors and the popularity of psychosurgery on the frontal lobes for treatment of psychiatric disorders in the 1940s and 1950s ultimately provided enough cases of frontal brain damage to eliminate speculative misconceptions about frontal lobe functions. We know now that many cognitive and social behaviors may be disrupted by frontal lobe damage. Hebb's observations were limited both by his use of structured tests that primarily measured old learning and well-established skills rather than abilities to solve unfamiliar problems or exercise judgment, for example, and by his choice of summed IQ scores for his comparison criteria rather than subtest scores or qualitative aspects of the patient's performance. It may be that the frontal lobes are the closest neural representation of popular notions of "intelligence" or Spearman's *g* because of their important role in contributing to success on diverse cognitive tasks (J. Duncan et al., 2000). The three major divisions of the frontal lobes differ functionally although each is involved more or less directly with behavior output (Fig. 3.17; E. Goldberg, 1990; Pandya and Barnes, 1987; Stuss and Benson, 1986; Stuss, Eskes, and Foster, 1994; see H.C. Damasio, 1991, for a detailed delineation of the anatomy of the frontal lobes and Pandya and Yeterian, 1998, for diagrams of interconnections within the frontal lobes and with other regions of the brain).

Precentral Division

The most posterior, precentral, division lies in the first two ridges in front of the central sulcus. This is the primary motor cortex, which mediates movement (not isolated muscles) and as such has important connections with the cerebellum, the basal ganglia, and the motor divisions of the thalamus. Lesions here result in (weakness) *paresis* or paralysis of the corresponding body parts (Eslinger and Reichwein, 2001; Mesulam, 2000b). Inside the fold of the frontal and temporal lobes formed by the Sylvian fissure is the primary taste cortex (Pritchard, 1999).

Premotor Division

Situated just anterior to the precentral area, the *premotor* and *supplementary motor* areas have been iden-

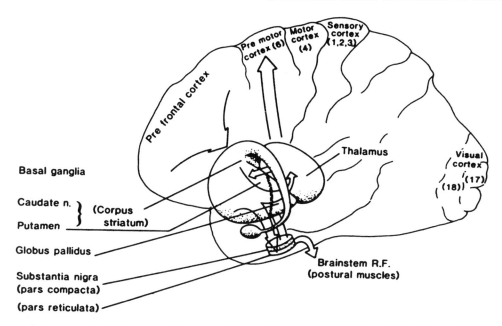

FIGURE 3.17 The three subdivisions of the frontal lobes with their most prominent subcortical connections indicated. (From J.F. Stein, 1985)

tified as the site in which the integration of motor skills and learned action sequences takes place (A.R. Damasio and Anderson, 2003; Eslinger and Geddes, 2001; Kolb and Whishaw, 1996; Nilsson et al., 2000). Premotor areas participate in afferent/efferent loops with the basal ganglia and thalamus; the looped interconnections are probably targeted to specific sites on both cortical and subcortical structures (Middleton and Strick, 2001; Passingham, 1997). Lesions here do not result in loss of the ability to move, but rather disrupt the integration of the motor components of complex acts, producing discontinuous or uncoordinated movements and impaired motor skills, and may also affect limb strength (Jason, 1990; Mesulam, 2000b). The supplemental motor area appears to mediate preparatory arousal to action at a preconscious stage in the generation of movement; thus lesions in this area may disrupt movement initiation as well (J.W. Brown, 1987). The ability to copy rapidly executed hand movements may be associated with right- or left-sided lesions in this area (Jason, 1986). Left premotor cortex has been implicated in the motor planning aspect of rapid word generation (Condon et al., 1997).

In the left hemisphere, lesions in the portion of the motor association area that mediates the motor organization and patterning of speech may result in speech disturbances that have as their common feature disruption of speech production with intact comprehension. These deficits may range in severity from total suppression of speech (D. Caplan, 1987; Eslinger and Reichwein, 2001; Jonas, 1987) to mild slowing and re-

duced spontaneity of speech production (Stuss and Benson, 1984, 1990). Other alterations in speech production may include stuttering, poor or monotonous tonal quality, or diminished control of the rate of speech production. Luria (1966, 1970; see also Dronkers et al., 2000) described a motor pattern apraxia of speech (*oral apraxia*) which may include difficulty imitating simple oral gestures in connection with lesions in this area, although this condition can also occur with somewhat more posterior lesions (Tognola and Vignolo, 1980). Patients with this condition display disturbances in organizing the muscles of the speech apparatus to form sounds or in patterning groups of sounds into words. This may leave them incapable of fluent speech production, although their ability to comprehend language is not necessarily impaired. Closely associated with this *supplemental motor area* mediating speech mechanisms are those involved in the initiation and programming of fine hand movements (Jonas, 1987; Vuilleumier, 2001), so it is not surprising that severe agraphia can follow lesions here (D. Caplan, 1987; Roeltgen, 1997). The anterior language center, *Broca's area,* is lower on the lateral slope of the prefrontal cortex (Benson, 1988, 1993; Broca, 1865, in Berker, Berker, and Smith, 1986; A.R. Damasio and Geschwind, 1984) (see Fig. 3.1, p. 42). It serves as "the final common path for the generation of speech impulses" (Luria, 1970, p. 197). Lesions to this area give rise to *Broca's,* or *efferent, motor aphasia* (see Chapter 2, Table 2.1, p. 33), which involves defective symbol formulation as well as a breakdown in the orderly production of speech. Verbal learning can be compromised by lesions in this region (Risse et al., 1984).

Lesions in corresponding areas on the right may contribute to fragmented or piecemeal *modus operandi*, reflected most clearly in impairments of perceptual organization and of planning (see example, p. 134). *Expressive amusia* or *avocalia* (inability to sing) has been seen with lesions of either frontal lobe but occurs most often in association with aphasia when lesions are on the left (Benton, 1977a; Botez and Botez, 1996). Other activities disturbed by lesions involving the right premotor area include diminished grip strength for both men and women (Leonard et al., 1988) and *motor impersistence* (reduced ability to maintain a motor act, such as eye closure or tongue protrusion) (Ben-Yishay, Diller, Gerstman, and Haas, 1968; Eslinger and Reichwein, 2001; Kertesz, Nicholson, Cancelliere, et al., 1985).

Prefrontal Division

The cortex and underlying white matter of the frontal lobes is the site of interconnections and feedback loops between the major sensory and motor systems, linking and integrating all components of behavior at the highest level (Fuster, 1995; Kolb and Whishaw, 1996; Middleton and Strick, 2001a,b; Pandya and Barnes, 1987). Pathways carrying information about the external environment from the posterior cortex—of which about 60% comes from the heteromodal association cortex and only 25% from secondary association areas (Strub and Black, 1988)—and information about internal states from the limbic system converge in the anterior portions of the frontal lobes, the *prefrontal cortex*. Thus, the anterior frontal lobes are where already correlated incoming information from all sources—external and internal, conscious and unconscious, memory storage and visceral arousal centers—is integrated and enters ongoing activity (Dubois, Pillon, et Sirigu, 1994; Fuster, 2003). "The human prefrontal cortex attends, integrates, formulates, executes, monitors, modifies, and judges all nervous system activities" (Stuss and Benson, 1987). Perecman (1987) refers to it as "the seat of consciousness." G.A. Miller and his colleagues (1960) called it the "organ of civilization," a definition that speaks to the fragility of complex behavioral patterns and socially acquired attitudes in the damaged brain (Eslinger, 1998b; E. Goldberg and Bilder, 1987) and to its central role in the normal experience of self (Frith, 1998; Stuss, 1991b). In modern jargon, E. Goldberg (2001) refers to it as "the brain's CEO."

Lesions of the frontal lobes tend not to disrupt cognitive functions as obviously as do postcentral lesions.

Rather, frontal lobe damage may be conceptualized as disrupting reciprocal relationships between the major functional systems—the sensory systems of the posterior cortex; the limbic-memory system with its interconnections to subcortical regions involved in arousal, affective, and motivational states; and the effector mechanisms of the motor system. Nauta (1971) characterized frontal lobe disorders as "derangement of behavioral programming." Fuster (1994) drew attention to a breakdown in the temporal organization of behavior with frontal lobe lesions, resulting both in deficient integration of immediate past experience (situational context) with ongoing activity and in defective planning. Frontal lobe disorders involve *how* a person responds, which can certainly affect the "*what*," the content of the response. Frontal lobe patients' failures on test items are more likely to result from an inappropriate approach to problems than from lack of knowledge or from perceptual or language incapacities *per se*. For example, patients with frontal lobe damage (almost always involving the right frontal lobe) occasionally will call item one on the Hooper Visual Organization Test "a duck" (see Chapter 10, Fig. 10.19, p. 400) and demonstrate that they understand the instructions (to figure out what the cut-up drawings would represent if put together) by answering items two and three correctly. In such cases, the completed "flying duck" shape of the top piece in item one appears to be a stronger stimulus than the directions to combine the pieces. These patients demonstrate accurate perception and facility and accuracy in naming or writing but get stalled in carrying out all of an intentional performance—in this case by one strong feature of a complex stimulus. Others (e.g., Luria, 1966; Ochsner and Schacter, 2000; Stuss and Benson, 1984, 1987; Walsh and Darby, 1999) have called attention to the dissociation between what these patients say or appear to see or comprehend and what they do or seem to feel.

Prefrontal subdivisions

The prefrontal portion of the frontal lobes is also subdivided, with different functions (or rather, different behavioral disorders associated with specific lesion sites) mediated in different cortical regions (Fuster, 1995; Pandya and Barnes, 1987; Stuss and Benson, 1984; Walsh and Darby, 1999; Walsh, 1991). Typically, three major subdivisions are identified, each with connections to different thalamic nuclei (Brodal, 1981; Mayes, 1988; Pribram, 1987) as well as interconnections with other cortical and subcortical structures. Most of these are two-way connections with neural pathways projecting both to and from prefrontal cortex (Strub and Black, 2000).

Defects in the control, regulation, and integration of cognitive activities tend to predominate in patients with *dorsolateral* lesions, i.e., when the lesion is on the top or outer sides—the convexity—of the frontal lobes. According to Goldman-Rakic (1998), the dorsolateral prefrontal cortex has a generic function—"on-line" processing of information or working memory in the service of a wide range of cognitive functions. This process occurs through multiple neural circuits to relevant sensory, motor, and limbic areas that integrate attention, memory, motor, and possibly affective dimensions of behavior. The *medial regions* (also called *cingulate* or *limbic cortex*) are located on the sides of the lobes between the hemispheres. Lesions here or subcortical lesions that involve pathways connecting the cortex between and just under the hemispheres with the drive and affective integration centers in the diencephalon are most apt to affect emotional and social behavior by dampening or nullifying altogether capacities for emotional experience and for drive and motivation (Barrash et al., 2000; A.R. Damasio and Van Hoesen, 1983). The degree to which emotions and drive are compromised tends to be highly correlated, suggesting that affect and drive are two sides of the same coin: Frontally damaged patients with loss of affective capacity will have low drive states, even for such basic needs as food or drink; with only mildly muted emotionality, life-sustaining drives will remain intact but sexual interest may be reduced, along with interest in initiating and maintaining social or vocational activities.

The *orbital* (*basal, ventral*) frontal cortex plays a key role in impulse control and in regulation and maintenance of set and of ongoing behavior (P. Malloy, Bihrle, et al., 1993; Stuss, Benson, Kaplan, et al., 1983). In healthy persons this region is involved in the expression of aggressive behavior (Pietrini et al., 2000). Damage here can give rise to disinhibitions and impulsivity, with such associated behavior problems as aggressive outbursts and sexual promiscuity (Eslinger, 1999a; Grafman, Schwab, et al., 1996). Lesions here also can disrupt a patient's ability to be guided by future consequences of their actions (Bechara, Damasio, Damasio, and Anderson, 1994) and lead to poor decisions (Bechara, Damasio, Damasio, and Lee, 1999). Left-sided traumatic damage to this area has been associated with prolonged unconsciousness (Salazar, Martin, and Grafman, 1987). Frontal lobe disturbances thus tend to have repercussions throughout the behavioral repertoire (Luria, 1973a; Stuss, Gow, and Hetherington, 1992).

Because the structures involved in the primary processing of olfactory stimuli are situated at the base of the frontal lobes, odor discrimination is affected by orbitofrontal lesions—in both nostrils when the lesion is on the right but only in the left nostril with left-sided lesions (Eslinger, Damasio, and Van Hoesen, 1982; Zatorre and Jones-Gotman, 1991). Thus, impaired odor detection frequently accompanies the behavioral disorders associated with orbitofrontal damage (Eslinger, 1999b; P. Malloy, Bihrle, et al., 1993; Stuss, 1993; Varney and Menefee, 1993). Diminished odor discrimination may also occur with lesions in the limbic system nuclei lying within the temporal lobes and with damage to temporal lobe pathways connecting these nuclei to the orbitofrontal olfactory centers. This effect typically appears with right but not left temporal pathway lesions (Martinez et al., 1993). Temporal lobe connections to the orbitobasal forebrain are further implicated in cognitive functioning. Patients with lesions here are similar to patients with focal temporal lobe damage in displaying prominent modality-specific learning problems along with some less severe diminution in reasoning abilities (Salazar, Grafman, Schlesselman, et al., 1986).

Lateralization of frontal functions

Although lateralization of cognitive activity is less frequently described in patients with frontal damage, many of the usual distinctions between left and right hemisphere functions obtain here too. As noted above, decreased verbal fluency and impoverishment of spontaneous speech tend to be associated with left frontal lobe lesions, although mildly depressed verbal fluency can occur with right frontal lobe lesions (R.W. Butler, Rorsman, et al., 1993; Frisk and Milner, 1990; Laine, 1988; Perret, 1974). Other verbal problems associated with left anterior damage involve the organization of language and include disrupted and confused narrative sequences, simplified syntax, incomplete sentences and clauses, descriptions reduced to single words and distorted by misnaming and perseveration, and a general impoverishment of language with mutism as the extreme case (M.P. Alexander, Benson, and Stuss, 1989; Kaczmarek, 1984, 1987). Stuss and Benson (1990) emphasize that prefrontal language problems arise from self-regulatory and organizing deficits that are "neither language nor cognitive problems" (p. 43) but are the product of impaired executive functions. Patients with left frontal lesions do poorly in learning sequential manual positions and in generating different finger positions (gestural fluency), although both left and right frontal lesions can compromise the ability to make meaningful gestures, such as the sign for hitchhiking (Jason, 1985a, 1987). Deficits in making spatial analyses, including orientation and rotation problems, can occur with left frontal lesions (Y. Kim et al., 1984) but also may appear with right anterior lesions (e.g., Lezak, 1989).

Constructional deficits have been noted in patients with right frontal lobe lesions who have difficulty with the motor rather than the perceptual components of the task (Benton, 1968). The ability to invent unique designs (design fluency) is depressed with right anterior lesions (Jones-Gotman, 1991a; Jones-Gotman and Milner, 1977). Expressive language problems also affect patients with right frontal damage (Kaczmarek, 1984, 1987). Their narrative responses too may show a breakdown in internal structure related to poor overall organization of the material. Stereotyped expressions are relatively common. The prosodic quality of speech may be muted or lost (Frisk and Milner, 1990). Picture descriptions may be faulty, mostly due to misinterpretations of elements but also of the picture as a whole. Perhaps most important, as it compromises their capacity to adapt to their disabilities, is a tendency for defective evaluation of their condition (Kaczmarek, 1987). Other kinds of impaired evaluations have also been noted in these patients, such as inaccurate estimations of prices (M.L. Smith and Milner, 1984) and of frequency of events (M. L. Smith and Milner, 1988). Stuss and colleagues have stressed the importance of the right frontal lobe in emotional expression, modulation, and appreciation (Shammi and Stuss, 1999; Stuss and Alexander, 1999; Stuss, Gow, and Hetherington, 1992). In addition, the right prefrontal cortex may be a preferential component in self-recognition and self-evaluation (H.P. Keenan et al., 2000).

In recent years several overall differences in cognitive features of the left and right prefrontal lobes have been described. B. Milner and Petrides (1984) suggested that the left prefrontal cortex is important for control of self-generated plans and strategies and the right is important for monitoring externally ordered events. Using different cognitive tasks, E. Goldberg, Podell, and Lovell (1994) found a similar distinction. In particular, they suggest that the left prefrontal system is responsible for guiding cognitive selection by working memory–mediated internal contingencies, while the right prefrontal system makes selections based on external environmental contingencies. While their data support this lateralization in men, women did not show a lateralized effect.

Many investigators have found differential prefrontal cortex involvement based on the type of memory process under consideration. Left prefrontal activation occurs with verbal learning and verbal working memory (Buckner and Tulving, 1995; Nyberg and Cabeza, 2000). A number of studies have shown that the left prefrontal cortex is primarily involved in encoding and the right is preferentially activated during retrieval (Haxby, Ungerleider, Horwitz, et al., 1996; Owen, Milner, et al., 1996; Shallice, Fletcher, Frith, et al., 1994;

Tulving, Kapur, Craik, et al., 1994; Ragland, Gur, et al., 2000). However, this dichotomy has been challenged and it is likely that differences in the roles of the left and right hemispheres depend on the particular memory demands as well as the type of stimulus to be learned (Iidaka et al., 2000; S. Kapur et al., 1995; Klingberg and Roland, 1998; A. Martin, Wiggs, and Weisberg, 1997). Mesulam (2000b) notes left/right differences in working memory paralleling the common verbal/spatial lateralization pattern. Autobiographical memory, too, may preferentially engage networks within the right frontotemporal region (G.R. Fink et al., 1996; J.P. Keenan et al., 2000).

Prefrontal cortex and attention

The prefrontal cortex is among the many structures involved in attention. Significant frontal activation takes place during selective attention activities in intact subjects (Mesulam, 2000b; Swick and Knight, 1998). Prefrontal cortex mediates the capacity to make and control shifts in attention (Mirsky, 1989). Luria (1973a) observed that it "*participates decisively in the higher forms of attention,*" for example, in "*raising the level of vigilance,*" in selectivity, and in maintaining a set (see also van Zomeren and Brouwer, 1990). The prefrontal cortex and anterior cingulate appear to be engaged when subjects must concentrate on solving new problems but not when attention is no longer required because the task has become automatic (Passingham, 1997, 1998). Thus attentional functions are frequently impaired with frontal lobe lesions (Luria, 1973a; Stuss and Benson, 1984). These patients may be sluggish in reacting to stimuli, unable to maintain an attentional focus (Stuss, 1993), or highly susceptible to distractions. Vendrell and his colleagues (1995) specifically implicate the right prefrontal cortex as important for sustained attention.

Patients with frontal lesions frequently have difficulty when divided attention is required, such as performing two tasks at once (Baddeley, Della Sala, Papagno, and Spinnler, 1996). Functional neuroimaging studies also support the view that the prefrontal cortex is involved in dual task performance but not when either task is performed separately (D'Esposito et al., 1995). Working memory tasks (those that require temporary storage and manipulation of information in the brain) depend on the frontal lobes (Braver et al., 1997; Dubois, Levy, Verin, et al., 1995; Fuster, 1999; Goldman-Rakic, 1993; Rypma and D'Esposito, 1999; B.E. Swartz et al., 1995).

Problems with both working memory, and short-term memory appear to be due at least in part to the poor ability of frontal patients to withstand interference to what they may be attempting to keep in mind, whether from the environment or from their own associations (Fuster, 1985; Kapur, 1988b; Knight and Grabowecky, 2000; Stuss, 1991a; Swick and Knight, 1998). Jonides and Smith (1997) identify two multifaceted components of working memory: one involves temporary storage of information in specific modalities with its component processes (e.g., transformation into other codes, storage, rehearsal) and the other involves the processes treating the (temporarily) stored information, such as time tagging, sequencing, prioritizing, etc.

Left visuospatial inattention can occur with right anterior lesions (Heilman, Watson, and Valenstein, 2003; Mesulam, 2000b; see also Chapter 9, Fig. 9.8, p. 348) but is much less common with frontal than with parietal involvement (Bisiach and Vallar, 1988; Rizzolatti and Camarda, 1987; Vallar and Perani, 1987). Heilman, Watson, and Valenstein (2003) suggest that frontal inattention may be associated with arousal and intentional deficits. Others have interpreted this problem as reflecting involvement with one of the multiple sites in the visuoperceptual network (Mesulam, 2000b; Rizzolatti and Gallese, 1988; S. Stein and Volpe, 1983). Some patients with frontal lesions seem stuporous unless actively stimulated. Others can be so distractible as to be hyperactive. Still other patients with frontal damage may show little or no evidence of attentional disturbances, leaving open to conjecture the contributions of subcortical and other structures in the attention impaired patients.

Prefrontal cortex and memory

Memory disorders have long been associated with prefrontal lesions. However, when carefully examined, these patients typically do not have a disorder of the memory system, but rather they have disorders of one or more functions that facilitate memory.

The phenomenon of frontal amnesia demonstrates how inertia and executive disorders in particular can interfere with cognitive processes (Stuss and Benson, 1984, 1986; Walsh, 1987). Patients with frontal amnesia, when read a story or a list of words, may seem able to recall only a little if any of what they heard and steadfastly assert they cannot remember. Yet, when prompted or given specific questions (such as, "Where did the story take place?" rather than "Begin at the beginning and tell me everything you can remember"), they may produce some responses, even quite full ones, once started. The same patients may be unable to give their age although they know the date, their year of birth, and how to solve formally presented subtraction problems. What they cannot do, in each of these examples, is spontaneously undertake the activity that

will provide the answer—in the first case, selecting the requested information from memory and, in the second case, identifying a solution set for the question and acting on it. Not being able to remember to remember (*prospective memory*) creates serious practical problems for these patients—forgetting to go to work, to keep appointments, even to bathe or change clothes as needed (Cockburn, 1996a). Frontal amnesia problems constitute one of the most serious obstacles to the remediation of the behavioral problems associated with frontal lobe damage; for if it does not occur to trainees to remember what they were taught or supposed to do (or not do), then whatever was learned cannot be put to use.

A 35-year-old mechanic sustained compound depressed fractures of the "left frontal bone" with cortical lacerations when a "heavy . . . machine exploded in his face." Following intensive rehabilitation he was able to return home where he assumed household chores and the daytime care of his three-year-old son. He reported that he can carry out his duties if his wife "leaves me a note in the morning of some of the things she wants done, and if she didn't put that down it wouldn't get done because I wouldn't think about it. So I try to get what she's got on her list done. And then there's lists that I make up, and if I don't look at the list, I don't do anything on it."

Two years after the accident and shortly before this interview, this man's verbal performances on the Wechsler tests were mostly within the *average* range excepting a *borderline defective* score on Similarities (which calls on verbal concepts); on the predominantly visual tests his scores were at *average* and *high average* levels. All scores on formal memory testing (Wechsler Memory Scale–Revised) were at or above the mean for his age, and 4 of the 13 listed on the Record Form were more than one standard deviation above the mean.

The frontal lobes facilitate memory in a variety of ways. They provide structure to stimulus encoding (Fletcher et al., 1998). Thus, some of these patients' memory problems may be related to diminished capacity to integrate temporally separated events (Fuster, 1980, 1985), such as difficulty in making recency judgments (B. Milner, 1971; Petrides, 1989), and to poor recall of contextual information associated with what they may remember (impaired source memory) (Janowsky, Shimamura, and Squire, 1989). They may recall a fragment of memory but be unable to situate the memory in its appropriate context for time and place. Patients with frontal lesions tend not to order or organize what they learn, although with appropriate cueing adequate recall can be demonstrated (Jetter et al., 1986), which may account for their proportionately better performances on recognition than on recall formats where retrieval strategies are less needed (Janowsky, Shimamura, Kritchevsky, and Squire, 1989).

The frontal lobes are necessary for criterion setting and monitoring during retrieval of memories, particularly on difficult tasks (Fletcher, Shallice, Frith, et al., 1998; Incisa della Rocchetta and Milner, 1993; Schacter, Norman, and Koustaal, 1998). Failure in these functions can lead to poor recall or false memories (Schacter, 1999a, *passim;* Schacter, Norman, Koustaal, et al., 1998). Stuss and Benson (1987) showed how diminished control can affect the behavior of patients with prefrontal damage: they may be fully aware of what should be done, but in not doing it at the appropriate time, they appear to have forgotten the task (impaired prospective memory) (see also Glisky, 1996).

Patients with lesions in the medial basal region of the frontal lobes or with subcortical lesions in adjacent white matter may suffer a true amnestic condition that is pronounced and often accompanied by spontaneous and florid confabulation (M.P. Alexander and Freedman, 1984; A.R. Damasio, 2001; P. Malloy, Bihrle, et al., 1993; Rapcsak, Kaszniak, Reminger, et al., 1998; Stuss, Alexander, et al., 1978).

A 60-year-old retired teacher who had had a stroke involving the medial basal region of her left frontal lobe complained of back pain due to lifting a cow onto a barn roof. Five days later she reported having piloted a 200-passenger plane the previous day.

Prefrontal cortex and cognitive functions

Cognitive impairment associated with destruction or disconnection of frontal lobe tissue usually does not appear as a loss of specific skills, information, or even reasoning or problem-solving ability (Teuber, 1964). In fact, patients with frontal lobe lesions often do not do poorly on those formal ability tests in which another person directs the examination, sets the pace, starts and stops the activity, and makes all the discretionary decisions (Brazelli et al., 1994; Lezak, 1982a; Stuss, Benson, Kaplan, et al., 1983). The closed-ended questions of common fact and familiar situations and the well-structured puzzles with concrete solutions that make up standard tests of cognitive abilities are not likely to present special problems for many patients with frontal lobe injuries (Tranel, 2003). Perseveration or carelessness may depress a patient's scores somewhat but usually not enough to lower them significantly. Cognitive defects associated with frontal lobe damage tend to show up most clearly in the course of daily living and are more often observed by relatives and co-workers than by a medical or psychological examiner in a standard interview. Common complaints about such patients concern apathy, carelessness, poor or unreliable judgment, poor adaptability to new situations, and blunted social sensibility (Eslinger, Grattan, and Geder,

1995; Lezak, 1989; Lishman, 1997; R.S. Parker, 2001). However, these are not cognitive deficits in themselves but defects in processing one or more aspects of behavioral integration and expression.

Frontal lobe syndromes include many behavioral disorders (Grafman and Litvan, 1999; Sohlberg and Mateer, 2001; Stuss and Benson, 1986) which are differentiable both in their appearance and in their occurrence (Burgess and Shallice, 1994; Varney and Menefee, 1993). Patients with prefrontal damage show an information processing deficit that reduces their sensitivity to novel stimuli and may help explain the stimulus-bound phenomenon (Daffner et al., 2000; R.T. Knight, 1984). Difficulty with working memory and impulsivity may interfere with learning or with performing tasks requiring delayed responses (B. Milner, 1971; R.J.J. Roberts and Pennington, 1996). Defective abstract thinking and sluggish response shifts can result in impaired mental efficiency (Janowsky, Shimamura, Kritchevsky, and Squire, 1989; Sohlberg and Mateer, 2001; Stuss and Benson, 1984). Diminished capacity for behavioral or mental flexibility can greatly limit imaginative or creative thinking (Eslinger and Grattan, 1993). It can also constrain volition and adaptive decision making (E. Goldberg and Podell, 2000). These defects may be aspects of *stimulus boundedness* which, in its milder forms, appears as slowing in shifting attention from one element in the environment to another, particularly from a strong stimulus source to a weak or subtle or complex one, or from a well-defined external stimulus to an internal or psychological event. Patients who are severely stimulus-bound may have difficulty directing their gaze or manipulating objects; when the condition is extreme, they may handle or look at whatever their attention has fixed upon as if their hands or eyes were stuck to it, literally pulling themselves away with difficulty. Others, on seeing usable objects (an apple, a fork), may irresistibly respond to them: e.g., eat the apple; go through eating motions with a fork, regardless of the appropriateness of the behavior for the situation—what Lhermitte (1983) termed "utilization behavior." In describing these kinds of behavior defects as "environmental dependency syndrome" and a pathological kind of "imitation behavior," Lhermitte (1986), with his colleagues (1986), called attention to the degree to which these patients are driven by environmental stimuli (see also S. Archibald et al., 2001).

Perseveration, in which patients repeat a movement, or an act or activity involuntarily, often unwittingly, is a related phenomenon, but the stimulus to which they seem bound is one that they themselves generated (E. Goldberg, 2001; E. Goldberg and Bilder, 1987; Hauser, 1999; Na et al., 1999; Sandson and Albert, 1987). Yet these patients often ignore environmental cues so that their actions are out of context with situational demands and incidental learning is reduced (Vilkki, 1988). They may be unable to profit from experience, perhaps due to insufficient reactivation of autonomic states that accompanied emotionally charged (pleasurable, painful) situations (A.R. Damasio, Tranel, and Damasio, 1990), and thus can only make poor, if any, use of feedback or reality testing (Le Gall, Joseph, and Truelle, 1987; Rolls, 1998; Sohlberg and Mateer, 2001).

With prefrontal damage, a tendency for a dissociation can occur between language behaviors and ongoing activity so that patients are less apt to use verbal cues (such as subvocalization) to direct, guide, or organize their ongoing behavior with resultant perseveration, fragmentation, or premature termination of a response (K.H. Goldstein, 1948; Luria and Homskaya, 1964; Shallice, 1982; Vilkki, 1988). However, fragmentation or disorganization of premorbidly intact behavioral sequences and activity patterns appears to be the underlying problem for these patients (Truelle, Le Gall, et al., 1995; M.F. Schwartz et al., 1993; see also Grafman, Sirigu, et al., 1993). Activities requiring abilities to make and use sequences or otherwise organize activity are particularly prone to being compromised by prefrontal lesions (Canavan et al., 1989; Messerli et al., 1979; Stuss and Benson, 1984; Zalla et al., 2001), possibly due to reduced ability to refocus attention to alternative response strategies (Della Malva et al., 1993; Godefroy and Rousseaux, 1997; B. Levine, Stuss, Milberg, et al., 1998; Robbins, 1998; Satish et al., 1999). For example, copying hand position sequences, especially when rapid production is required, is affected by frontal lobe lesions (Jason, 1986; Truelle, Le Gall, et al., 1995; Petrides, 1989). Thus planning—which Goel and Grafman refer to as "anticipatory sequencing"—and problem solving, which require intact sequencing and organizing abilities, are frequently impaired in these patients (D. Carlin et al., 2000; Goel, Grafman, Tajik, et al., 1997; Goel and Grafman, 2000; Koechlin et al., 1999; R.G. Morris, Miotto, Feigenbaum, et al., 1997; Pillon 1981b; Shallice and Burgess, 1991a; Vilkki, 1988). Defective self-monitoring and self-correcting are common problems with prefrontal lesions (Stuss and Benson, 1984; Walsh and Darby, 1999).

Even when simple reaction time is intact, responses to complex tasks may be slowed (Le Gall, Joseph and Truelle, 1987). The frontal lobes have also been implicated in defects of time sense including recency judgments and time-span estimations and, in patients with bilateral frontal lobe damage, orientation in time (Benton, 1968; M.A. Butters, Kasniak, et al., 1994; B. Mil-

ner, Corsi, and Leonard, 1991). These patients may make erroneous and sometimes bizarre estimates of size and number (Shallice and Evans, 1978). Practical and social judgment is frequently impaired. With all of these impediments to cognitive competency, it follows that patients with frontal lobe lesions show little of the imagination or innovative thinking essential to creativity (Zangwill, 1966).

Behavior problems associated with prefrontal damage

Practical and social judgment problems are frequently observed in patients with prefrontal damage (Dimitrov et al., 1996). In fact, social disability is often the most debilitating feature of these patients (Eslinger, Grattan, and Geder, 1995; Lezak, 1989; Lezak and O'Brien, 1988, 1990; see also Macmillan's, 2000, collection of stories, reports, and observations of Phineas Gage). Behavior disorders associated with prefrontal damage tend to be supramodal. Similar problems may occur with lesions involving other areas of the brain, but in these instances they are apt to be associated with specific cognitive, sensory, or motor disabilities. The behavioral disturbances associated with frontal lobe damage can be roughly classified into five general groups with considerable overlap.

1. *Problems of starting* appear in decreased spontaneity, decreased productivity, decreased rate at which behavior is emitted, or decreased or lost initiative. In its milder forms, patients lack initiative and ambition but may be able to carry through normal activities quite adequately, particularly if these activities are familiar, well-structured, or guided.

A 37-year-old experienced railway brakeman was slammed onto his forehead when his train suddenly lurched. After a few weeks' recuperation he returned to his job and continued to work satisfactorily. However, he had ceased to engage in activities with his family, no longer made weekend or social plans, and spent all of his leisure time playing the same computer game. His interest in food was negligible and he had ceased initiating sexual activity.

More severely affected patients are apt to do little beyond routine self-care and home activities. To a casual or naive observer, and often to their family and close associates, these patients appear to be lazy. Many can "talk a good game" about plans and projects but are actually unable to transform their words into deeds. An extreme dissociation between words and deeds has been called *pathological inertia* which can be seen when a frontal lobe patient describes the correct response to a task but never acts it out. Severe problems of starting appear as apathy, unresponsiveness, or mutism, and often are associated with superior medial damage (Eslinger, Grattan, and Geder, 1995; Sohlberg and Mateer, 2001).

A railway crossing accident severely injured a 25-year-old schoolteacher who became totally socially dependent. She ate only when food was set before her so she could see it. The only activities she initiated were going to the bathroom and going to bed to sleep, both prompted by body needs. Yet on questioning she reported plans for Christmas, for a party for her aunt.

2. *Difficulties in making mental or behavioral shifts*, whether they are shifts in attention, changes in movement, or flexibility in attitude, come under the heading of *perseveration* or *rigidity*. Perseveration refers specifically to repetitive prolongation or continuation of an act or activity sequence, or repetition of the same or a similar response to various questions, tasks, or situations. In the latter sense it may be described as stereotypy of behavior. Perseveration may also occur with lesions of other lobes, but then it typically appears only in conjunction with the patient's specific cognitive deficits (E. Goldberg and Tucker, 1979; Walsh and Darby, 1999). In frontal lobe patients, perseveration tends to be *supramodal*—to occur in a variety of situations and on a variety of tasks. Perseveration may sometimes be seen as difficulty in suppressing ongoing activities or attention to prior stimulation. On familiar tasks it may be expressed in repetitive and uncritical perpetuation of a response that was once correct but becomes an uncorrected error under changed circumstances or in continuation of a response beyond its proper end point. Perseveration may occur as a result of lesions throughout the frontal lobes but particularly with dorsolateral lesions (Eslinger, Grattan, and Geder, 1995; Walsh, 1991). Frontal lobe patients may exhibit rigidity in their behavior and thinking without perseveration. Since behavioral and attitudinal patterns of rigidity characterize some neurologically intact people, rigidity alone does not give sufficient grounds for suspecting frontal lobe damage.

3. *Problems in stopping*—in braking or modulating ongoing behavior—show up in impulsivity, overreactivity, disinhibition, and difficulties in holding back a wrong or unwanted response, particularly when it may either have a strong association value or be part of an already ongoing response chain. They have difficulty delaying gratification of reward. These problems frequently come under the heading of "loss of control," and these patients are often described as having "control problems." The lesion is often orbital (Bechara, Damasio, and Damasio, 2000; Eslinger et al., 1995).

4. *Deficient self-awareness* results in an inability to perceive performance errors, to appreciate the impact one makes on others, to size up a social situation appropriately, and to have empathy for others (Eslinger, Grattan, and Geder, 1995; Prigatano, 1991c; Prigatano and Schacter, 1991, *passim;* Schacter, 1990b; Stuss, Gow, and Hetherington, 1992). When frontal damage occurs in childhood, the social deficits can be profound and may include impairments in acquiring social conventions and moral reasoning (S.W. Anderson, Bechara, Damasio, et al., 1999; S.W. Anderson, Damasio, Tranel, and Damasio, 2000). Defective self-criticism is associated with tendencies of some frontal lobe patients to be euphoric and self-satisfied, to experience little or no anxiety, and to be impulsive and unconcerned about social conventions. The very sense of self—which everyday experience suggests is intrinsic to human nature—turns out to be highly vulnerable to frontal lobe damage (Stuss, 1991b; Stuss and Alexander, 2000). Failure to respond normally to emotional and social reinforcers may be a fundamental deficit leading to inappropriate behavior (Rolls, Hornak, Wade, and McGrath, 1994). Impaired self-awareness and social behavior often result from lesions of the orbital cortex and related limbic areas (Sarazin et al., 1998).

A 38-year-old former truck driver and athlete sustained a frontal injury in a motor vehicle accident. Although his cognitive test scores (on Wechsler ability and memory tests) eventually improved to the *average* range, he was unable to keep a job. Repeated placements failed because he constantly talked to coworkers, disrupting their ability to work. Eventually he was tried in a warehouse job that would take advantage of his good strength and physical abilities and put limited demands on cognitive skills and social competence. However, he wanted to show his co-workers that he was the best by loading trucks faster than anyone else. His speed was at the expense of safety. When he could not be persuaded to use caution, he was fired.

5. *A concrete attitude* or loss of the abstract attitude (K. Goldstein, 1944, 1948) is also common among patients with frontal lobe damage. This appears in an inability to dissociate oneself from one's immediate surrounds in a literal attitude in which objects, experiences, and behavior are all taken at their most obvious face value. The patient becomes incapable of planning and foresight or of sustaining goal-directed behavior. This defect, which is also identified as loss or impairment of abstract attitude, is not the same as impaired ability to form or use abstract concepts. Although many patients with frontal lobe lesions do have difficulty handling abstract concepts and spontaneously generate only concrete ones, others retain high-level conceptual abilities despite a day-to-day literal-mindedness and loss of perspective.

CLINICAL LIMITATIONS OF FUNCTIONAL LOCALIZATION

Symptoms must be viewed as expressions of disturbances in a system, not as direct expressions of focal loss of neuronal tissue.

A. L. Benton, 1981

A well-grounded understanding of functional localization strengthens the clinician's diagnostic capabilities so long as the limitations of its applicability in the individual case are taken into account. Common patterns of behavioral impairment associated with such well-understood neurological conditions as certain kinds of cerebrovascular accidents tend to involve the same anatomical structures with predictable regularity. For example, stroke patients with right arm paralysis due to a lesion involving the left motor projection area of the frontal cortex will generally have an associated Broca's (motor or expressive) aphasia. Yet, the clinician will sometimes find behavioral disparities between patients with cortical lesions of apparently similar location and size: some ambulatory stroke victims whose right arms are paralyzed are practically mute; others have successfully returned to highly verbal occupations. On the other hand, aphasics may present with similar symptoms, but their lesions vary in site or size (De Bleser, 1988; Basso, Capitani, Laiacona, and Zanobio, 1985). In line with these clinical observations, cortical mapping by electrode stimulation (Ojemann, 1979) and neuroimaging techniques (Mazziota, Toga, et al., 1997) demonstrates a great deal of interindividual variability in cortical patterning. Examples from functional imaging studies show that many different areas of the brain may be engaged during a cognitive task (see Frackowiak, Friston, Frith, et al., 1997, *passim*; Gazzaniga, 2000a, *passim*). For even the relatively simple task of telling whether words represent a pleasant or unpleasant concept, the following areas of the brain showed increased activation: left superior frontal cortex, medial frontal cortex, left superior temporal cortex, posterior cingulate, left parahippocampal gyrus, and left inferior frontal gyrus (K.B. McDermott, Ojemann, et al., 1999).

Other apparent discontinuities between a patient's behavior and neurological status may occur when a pattern of behavioral impairment develops spontaneously and without physical evidence of neurological disease. In such cases, "hard" neurological findings (e.g., such positive physical changes on neurological examination as primitive reflexes, unilateral weakness, or spasticity) or abnormal laboratory results (e.g., protein in the spinal fluid, brain wave abnormalities, or radiological anomalies) may appear in time, for instance, as a tumor grows or as arteriosclerotic changes block more blood vessels. Occasionally a suspected brain abnormality may be demonstrated only on postmortem examination, and even then correlative tissue changes may not always be found (A. Smith, 1962a). Moreover, well-defined brain lesions have shown up on neuroimaging (Chodosh et al., 1988) or at autopsy of persons with no symptoms of brain disease (Crystal, Dickson, et al., 1988; Phadke and Best, 1983).

The uncertain relation between brain activity and human behavior obligates the clinician to exercise care in observation and caution in prediction, and to take nothing for granted when applying the principles of functional localization to diagnostic problems. However, this uncertain relation does not negate the dominant tendencies to regularity in the functional organization of brain tissue. Knowledge of the regularity with which brain–behavior correlations occur enables the clinician to determine whether a patient's behavioral symptoms make anatomical sense, to know what subtle or unobtrusive changes may accompany the more obvious ones, and to guide the neurosurgeon or neuroradiologist in further diagnostic procedures.

4 | The Rationale of Deficit Measurement

One distinguishing characteristic of neuropsychological assessment is its emphasis on the identification and measurement of psychological—cognitive and behavioral—deficits, for it is primarily in deficiencies and dysfunctional alterations of cognition, emotionality, and self-direction and management (i.e., executive functions) that brain disorders are manifested behaviorally. Neuropsychological assessment is also concerned with the documentation and description of preserved functions—the patient's behavioral competencies and strengths. In assessments focused on delineating neuropsychological dysfunction—whether for the purpose of making a diagnostic discrimination, evaluating legal competency or establishing a legal claim, identifying rehabilitation needs, or attempting to understand a patient's aberrant behavior—the examiner still has an obligation to patients and caregivers to identify and report preserved abilities and behavioral potentials.

Yet brain damage always implies behavioral impairment. Even when psychological changes after a brain injury or concomitant with brain disease are viewed as improvement rather than impairment, as when there is a welcome increase in sociability or relief from neurotic anxiety, a careful assessment will probably reveal an underlying loss.

A 47-year-old postal clerk with a bachelor's degree in education boasted of having recently become an "extrovert" after having been painfully shy most of his life. His wife brought him to the neurologist with complaints of deteriorating judgment, childishness, untidiness, and negligent personal hygiene. The patient reported no notable behavioral changes other than his newfound ability to approach and talk with people.

On examination, although many cognitive functions tested at a *superior* level, in accord with his academic history and his wife's reports of his prior functioning, the patient performed poorly on tests involving immediate memory, new learning, and attention and concentration. The discrepancy between his best and poorest performances suggested that this patient had already sustained cognitive losses. A precociously developing Alzheimer-type dementia was suspected.

In some patients the loss, or deficit, may be subtle, becoming apparent only on complex judgmental tasks or under emotionally charged conditions. In others, behavioral evidence of impairment may be so slight or ill-defined as to be unobservable under ordinary conditions; only patient reports of vague, unaccustomed, frustrations or uneasiness suggest the possibility of an underlying brain disorder.

A 55-year-old dermatologist received a blow to the head when another skier swerved onto him, knocking him to the ground so hard that his helmet was smashed on the left side. Shortly thereafter he sought a neuropsychological consultation to help him decide about continuing to practice as he fatigued easily, had minor memory lapses, and noticed concentration problems. This highly educated man gave lower than expected performances on tests of verbal abstraction (Similarities), visual judgment (Picture Completion), and verbal recall (story and list learning), and performances were significantly poorer than expected when structuring a drawing (R-O Complex Figure) and on visual recall. Additionally, subtle deficits appeared in word searching hesitations, several instances of loss of instructional set, tracking slips when concentrating on another task, and incidental learning problems which also suggested some slowed processing as delayed recall was considerably better than immediate recall. These lower than expected scores and occasionally bungled responses appeared to reflect mild acquired impairments which together were experienced as memory problems and mental inefficiency.

A year later, he requested a reexamination to confirm his impression that cognitive functioning had improved. He reported an active winter of skiing which validated his feeling that balance and reflexes were normal. However, he had noticed that he missed seeing some close-at-hand objects which—when pointed out—were in plain view and usually on his left side; but he reported no difficulty driving nor did he bump into things. He wondered whether he might have a visual inattention problem. On testing, reasoning about visually presented material (Picture Completion) was now in the *superior* range although he had long response times, and verbal learning had improved to almost normal levels. Visual recall remained *defective*, but delayed visual recognition was *within normal limits*. However, on a visual scanning task (*Woodcock-Johnson III-Cog* [*WJ-III Cog*], *Pair Cancellation*), he made eight omission errors on the left side of the page and three on the right (see Fig. 10.1, p. 376). When last year's eight operation errors on printed calculation problems (Fig. 4.1, p. 87) were reviewed, it became apparent that left visuospatial inattention had obscured his awareness of the operation sign on the left of these problems, and that he continued to have a mild form of this problem. It was suspected that he had sustained a mild contre coup in the accident: mild because his acute self-awareness distinguished him from patients with large and/or deep right parietal lesions, contre coup because left visuospatial inattention implicates a right hemisphere lesion in a right-handed man.

Although the effects of brain disorders are rarely confined to a single behavioral dimension or functional system, the assessment of psychological deficit has focused on cognitive impairment for a number of reasons. First, some degree of cognitive impairment accompanies almost all brain dysfunction and is a diagnostically significant feature of many neurological disorders. Moreover, many of the common cognitive defects—aphasias, failures of judgment, lapses of memory, etc.—are likely to be noticed by the casual observer and to interfere most obviously with the patient's capacity to function independently.

In addition, psychologists are better able to measure cognitive activity than any other kind of behavior, except perhaps simple psychophysical reactions and sensorimotor responses. Certainly, cognitive behavior—typically as mental abilities, skills, or knowledge—has been systematically scrutinized more times in more permutations and combinations and with more replications and controls than has any other class of behavior. Out of all these data have evolved numerous reliable and well-standardized techniques for identifying, defining, grading, measuring, and comparing the spectrum of cognitive functioning. Intelligence testing and educational testing provide the neuropsychologist with a ready-made set of operations and a well-defined frame of reference that can be fruitfully applied to deficit measurement (Lezak, 1988c). The deficit measurement paradigm can be used with other behavioral impairments such as personality change, reduced mental efficiency, or defective executive functioning. However, personality measurement, particularly of brain impaired individuals, has not yet achieved the community of agreement nor the levels of reliability or predictability that are now taken for granted when measuring cognitive functions. Furthermore, in clinical settings impairments in efficiency and executive functions are usually evaluated on the basis of their effect on specific cognitive activities or personality characteristics rather than studied in their own right.

In the following discussion, any mention of a test will refer only to individual tests, not batteries (such as the Wechsler Intelligence Scales [WIS]) or even those test sets, such as Digits Forward and Digits Backward, that custom has led some to think of as a single test. This consideration of individual tests comes from demonstrations of the significant intertest variability in patient performances, the strong association of different patterns of test performance with different kinds of brain pathology, the demographic and other factors which contribute to the normal range of intraindividual test score variations, and the specificity of the brain–behavior relationships underlying many cognitive functions (e.g., see Grant and Adams, 1996, *passim;* Mesulam, 2000b; Naugle, Cullum, and Bigler, 1998). This knowledge of intraindividual variations in test performances does not support the popular concept of "intelligence" as a global—or near-global—phenomenon which can be summed up in a single score (Ardila, 1999a), nor does it support summing scores on any two or more tests that measure different functions, such as combining the scores of the WIS for adults (WIS-A) Block Design test which involves abstract visual analysis and visuospatial conceptualization and WIS-A Picture Completion test which not only has

CALCULATIONS

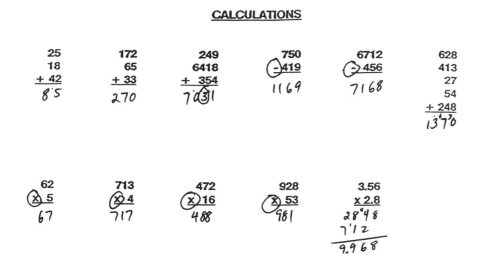

FIGURE 4.1 Calculations test errors (circled) made by a 55-year-old dermatologist with a contre coup from striking his head on the left. Note neglect of operation signs on subtraction and multiplication problems.

no visuospatial component and requires no manipulation by the subject but has a considerable verbal weighting and calls on the ability to draw upon acculturated experience, together with a third—also quite different test— Matrix Reasoning (The Psychological Corporation, 1997).

COMPARISON STANDARDS FOR DEFICIT MEASUREMENT

The concept of behavioral deficit presupposes some ideal, normal, or prior level of functioning against which the patient's performance may be measured. This level, the *comparison standard,* may be *normative* (derived from an appropriate population) or *individual* (derived from the patient's history or present characteristics), depending on the patient, the behavior being evaluated, and the assessment's purpose(s). Neuropsychological assessment uses both normative and individual comparison standards for measuring deficit, as appropriate for the function or activity being examined and the purpose of the examination. Examiners need to be aware of judgmental biases when estimating premorbid abilities (Kareken, 1997).

Normative Comparison Standards

The population average

The normative comparison standard may be an *average* or middle (*median*) score. For adults, the normative standard, or "norm," for many measurable psychological functions and characteristics is a score representing the average or median performance of some more or less well-defined population, such as white women or college graduates over 40. For many cognitive functions, variables of age and education or vocational achievement may significantly affect test performance. With test developers' growing sophistication, these variables are increasingly taken into account in establishing test norms for adults. The measurement of children's behavior is concerned with abilities and traits that change with age, so the normative standard may be the average age or grade at which a given trait or function appears or reaches some criterion level of performance (e.g., Binet et Simon, 1908). Because of the differential rate of development for boys and girls, children's norms are best given separately for each sex.

Since so many tests have been constructed for children in education and training programs, normative standards based on either average performance level or average age when performance competence first appears are available for a broad range of cognitive behaviors: from simple visuomotor reaction time or verbal mimicry to the most complex activities involving higher mathematics, visuospatial conceptualization, or sophisticated social judgments (Anastasi and Urbina, 1997; see, e.g., normative tables in Woodcock-Johnson III [Woodcock, McGrew, and Mather, 2001c]). Norms based on averages or median scores have also been derived for social behaviors, such as frequency of church attendance or age for participation in team play; for vocational interests, such as medicine or truck driving; or for personality traits, such as assertiveness or hypochondria.

In neuropsychological assessment, population norms are most useful in evaluating basic cognitive functions that develop throughout childhood. They can be distinguished from complex mental abilities or academic skills when examined as relatively pure functions. Many tests of memory, perception, and attention and those involving motor skills fall into this category (e.g., see Dodrill, 1999; J.M. Williams, 1997). *Typically, performances of these capacities do not distribute normally;* i.e., the proportions and score ranges of persons receiving scores above and below the mean are not statistically similar as they are in normal distributions (e.g., see Benton, Sivan, Hamsher, et al., 1994; Johnstone, Slaughter, et al., 1997; Stuss, Stethem, and Pelchat, 1988). Moreover, the overall distribution of scores for these capacities tends to be skewed in the substandard direction as a few persons in any randomly selected sample can be expected to perform poorly, while nature has set an upper limit on such aspects of mental activity as processing speed and short-term storage capacity. Functions most suited to evaluation by population norms also tend to be age dependent, particularly from the middle adult years onward, necessitating the use of age-graded norms (Baltes and Graf, 1996; Lezak, 1987a); and education too contributes to performance on these tests (e.g., Mitrushina, Boone, and D'Elia, 1999, *passim*).

Population norms may be applicable to tests that are relatively pure (and simple) measures of the function of interest (e.g., see Hannay, 1986): As the number of different kinds of variables contributing to a measure increases, the more likely will that measure's distribution approach normality (Siegel, 1956). The distributions of the WIS-A summed IQ scores (for the Verbal Scale [VSIQ], the Performance Scale [PSIQ], and both scales together, i.e., the Full Scale [FSIQ]) or scores on tests involving a complex of cognitive functions (e.g., Raven's Progressive Matrices) demonstrate this statistical phenomenon.

Species-wide performance expectations

The norms for some psychological functions and traits are actually species-wide performance expectations for adults, although for infants or children they may be age or grade averages. This is the case for all cognitive functions and skills that follow a common course of development, that are usually fully developed long before adulthood, and that are taken for granted as part and parcel of the normal adult behavioral repertoire. Speech is a good example. The average two-year-old child speaks in two- and three-word phrases. The ability to communicate verbally most needs and thoughts is expected of four and five year olds. Seventh- and eighth-grade children can utter and comprehend word groupings in all the basic grammatical forms and their elaborations. Subsequent speech development mainly involves more variety, elegance, abstractness, or complexity of verbal expression. Thus, the adult norm for speech is the intact ability to communicate effectively by speech, which all but a few adults can do. Some other skills that almost all neurologically intact adults can perform are counting change, drawing a recognizable person, and using simple construction tools or cooking utensils. Each of these skills is learned, improves with practice, has a common developmental history for most adults, and is sufficiently easy that its mastery or potential mastery is taken for granted. Anything less than an acceptable performance in an adult raises the suspicion of impairment.

Many species-wide capacities, although not apparent at birth, are manifested relatively early and similarly in all intact persons. Their development appears to be essentially maturational and relatively independent of social learning, although training may enhance their expression and aging may dull it. These include capacities for motor and visuomotor control and coordination; basic perceptual discriminations—e.g., of color, pattern, and form; of pitch, tone, and loudness; and of orientation to personal and extrapersonal space. Everyday life rarely calls upon the pure expression of these capacities. Rather, they are integral to the complex behaviors that make up the normal activities of children and adults alike. Thus, in themselves these capacities are usually observed only by deliberate examination.

Other species-wide normative standards involve components of behavior so rudimentary that they are not generally thought of as psychological functions or abilities. Binaural hearing, or the ability to localize a touch on the skin or to discriminate between noxious and pleasant stimuli, are capacities that are an expected part of the endowment of each human organism, present at birth or shortly thereafter. These capacities are not learned in the usual sense, nor, except when impaired by accident or disease, do they change over time and with experience. Some of these species-wide functions, such as fine tactile discrimination, are typically tested in the neurological examination (e.g., Perkin, 1998; Strub, 1996a).

Neuropsychological assessment procedures that test these basic functions possessed by all intact adults usually focus on discrete acts or responses and thus may identify the defective components of impaired cognitive behavior (e.g., A.-L. Christensen, 1979; Luria, 1999). However, examinations limited to discrete components of complex functions and functional systems provide little information about how well the patient can perform the complex behaviors involving component defects. Moreover, when the behavioral concomitants of brain damage are mild or subtle, particularly when associated with widespread or diffuse rather than well-defined lesions, few if any of these rudimentary components of cognitive behavior will be demonstrably impaired on the basis of species-wide norms.

Customary standards

A number of assumed normative standards have been arbitrarily set, usually by custom. Probably the most familiar of these is the visual acuity standard: 20/20 vision does not represent an average but an arbitrary ideal, which is met or surpassed by different proportions of the population, depending on age. Among the few customary standards of interest in neuropsychological assessment is verbal response latency—the amount of time a person takes to answer a simple question—which has normative values of one or two seconds for informal conversation in most Western cultures.

Applications and limitations of normative standards

Normative comparison standards are useful for most psychological purposes, including the description of cognitive status for both children and adults, for educational and vocational planning, and for personality assessment. In the assessment of persons with known or suspected adult-onset brain pathology, however, normative standards are appropriate only when the function or skill or capacity that is being measured is well within the capability of all intact adults and does not vary greatly with age, sex, education, or general mental ability. Thus, the capacity for meaningful verbal communication will be evaluated on the basis of population norms. In contrast, vocabulary level, which correlates highly with both social class and education (Heaton, Ryan, et al., 1996; Sattler, 2001a; P.E. Vernon, 1978), needs an individual comparison standard.

When it is known or suspected that a patient has suffered a decline in cognitive abilities that are normally distributed in the adult population, a description of that patient's functioning in terms of population norms (i.e., by standard test scores) will, in itself, shed no light on the extent of impairment unless there was documentation of premorbid cognitive levels (in school achievement tests or army placement examinations, for example). For premorbidly dull patients, *low average* scores would not indicate a significant drop in the level of examined functions. In contrast, an *average* score would represent a deficit for a person whose premorbid ability level had been generally *superior* (see pp. 148–149 for a statistical interpretation of ability categories). Moreover, comparisons with population averages do not add to the information implied in standardized test scores, for standardized test scores are themselves numerical comparisons with population norms. Thus, when examining patients for adult-onset deficits, only by comparing present with prior functioning can the examiner identify real losses.

The first step in measuring cognitive deficit in an adult is to establish—or estimate, when direct information is not available—the patient's premorbid performance level for all of the functions and abilities being assessed. For those functions with species-wide norms, this task is easy. Adults who can no longer name objects or copy a simple design or who appear unaware of one side of their body have an obvious deficit. For normally distributed functions and abilities for which the normative standard is an average, however, *only an individual comparison provides a meaningful basis for assessing deficit.* A population average is not an appropriate comparison standard since it will not necessarily apply to the individual patient. By definition, one-half of the population will achieve a score within the *average* range on any well-constructed psychological test which generates a normal distribution of scores; the remainder perform at many different levels both above and below the *average* range. Although an *average* score may be, statistically, the most likely score a person will receive, statistical likelihood is a far cry from the individual case.

Individual Comparison Standards

As a rule, *individual comparison standards* are called for whenever a psychological trait or function that is normally distributed in the intact adult population is evaluated for change. This rule applies to both deficit measurement and the measurement of behavioral change generally. When dealing with functions for which there are species-wide or customary norms—such as finger-tapping rate or accuracy of auditory discrimination—normative standards are appropriate for deficit measurement. Yet even these kinds of abilities change with age and at some performance levels differ for men and women thus requiring some demographic norming.

The use of individual comparison standards is probably most clearly exemplified in *rate of change* studies,

which depend solely on intraindividual comparisons. Here the same set of tests is administered three times or more at spaced intervals, and the differences between chronologically sequential pairs of test scores are compared. In child psychology the measurement of rate of change is necessary for examining the rate of development. Rate of change procedures also have broad applications in neuropsychology. Knowledge of the rate at which the patient's performance is deteriorating can contribute to the accuracy of predictions of the course of a degenerative disease (e.g., see B.E. Levin, Tomer, and Rey, 1992; A.J. Thompson, 1998). For purposes of rehabilitation, the rate at which cognitive functions improve following cerebral insult may not only aid in predicting the patient's ultimate performance levels but also provide information about the effectiveness of rehabilitative efforts (van Balen et al., 2002; Leclercq and Sturm, 2002). Further, rate of change studies contribute to understanding the long-range effects of brain injury on mental abilities.

THE MEASUREMENT OF DEFICIT

For most abilities that distribute normally in the population at large, determination of deficits rests on the comparison between what can be assumed to be the patient's characteristic premorbid level of cognitive functioning as determined from historical data (including old test scores when available) and the obtained test performances (scores plus qualitative features). Thus, much of clinical neuropsychological assessment involves *intraindividual* comparisons of the abilities and skills under consideration.

Direct Measurement of Deficit

Deficit can be assessed directly when there are normative comparison standards against which the behavior in question can be compared. The extent of the discrepancy between the level of performance expected for an adult and the level of the patient's performance (which may be given in terms of the age at which the average child performs in a comparable manner) provides one measure of the amount of deficit the patient has sustained. For example, the average six-year-old will answer 22 to 26 items correctly on the Verbal Comprehension test of the WJ-III Cog. The test performance of an adult who completed high school but can do no better could be reported as being "at the level of a six-year-old" on word knowledge.

Direct deficit measurement using individual comparison standards can be a simple, straightforward operation: The examiner compares premorbid and current examples of the behavior in question and evaluates the discrepancies. Hoofien, Vakil, and Gilboa's (2000) study of cognitive impairment following brain injuries (mostly due to trauma) illustrates this procedure. They compared the scores that army veterans made on tests taken at the time of their induction into service with scores obtained on the Wechsler Adult Intelligence Scale–Revised (WAIS-R) postinjury approximately 13 years later. The findings of this direct comparison provided unequivocal evidence of cognitive impairment.

The direct method using individual comparison standards requires the availability of premorbid test scores, school grades, or other relevant observational data. In many cases, these will be nonexistent or difficult to obtain. Therefore, more often than not, the examiner must use indirect methods of deficit assessment from which individual comparison standards can be inferred.

Indirect Measurement of Deficit

In indirect measurement, the examiner compares the present performance with an *estimate* of the patient's original ability level. This estimate may be drawn from a variety of sources. It is the examiner's task to find meaningful and defensible estimates of the pretraumatic or premorbid ability levels to serve as comparison standards for each patient.

Methods of indirect measurement

Different methods of inferring the comparison standard for each patient have been applied with varying degrees of success (Axelrod, Vanderploeg, and Schinka, 1999; M.R. Basso, Bornstein, Roper, and McCoy, 2000; Crawford, 1992; Hoofien, Vakil, and Gilboa, 2000; Johnstone, Slaughter et al., 1997; also see U.S. Congress, Office of Technology Assessment, 1987, pp. 282–283). Historical and observational data are obvious sources of information from which estimates of premorbid ability may be drawn directly. Estimates based on these sources will be more or less satisfactory depending on how much is known of the patient's past, and whether what is known or can be observed is sufficiently characteristic to distinguish this patient from other people. For example, if all that an examiner knows about a brain injured, cognitively impaired patient is that he was a logger with a ninth-grade education and his observed vocabulary and interests seem appropriate to his occupation and education, then the examiner can only estimate a barely *average* ability level as the comparison standard. If the patient had been brighter than most, could reason exceptionally well, could tell stories cleverly, or had been due for a promotion to supervisor, this information would prob-

ably not be available to the examiner, who would then have no way of knowing from history and observations alone just how bright this particular logger had been.

Premorbid ability estimates inferred from historical and observational data alone may be spuriously low. Moreover, some patient self-reports may run a little high (Greiffenstein, Baker, and Johnson-Greene, 2002). Yet the need for accurate estimates has increasingly become apparent, especially in evaluating complaints of mental deterioration in older persons (Yuspeh et al., 1998). In response to this need, neuropsychologists have devised a number of distinctive methods for making these estimates. The most commonly used techniques for indirect assessment of premorbid ability rely on cognitive test scores, on extrapolation from current reading ability, on demographic variables, or on some combination of these. In reviewing these methods it is important to appreciate that, without exception, the comparison standard for evaluating them has been the three WIS-A IQ scores or just the FSIQ. That the FSIQ as a criterion has its own problems becomes apparent when subjects' cognitive functioning is not impaired, for then, when the estimate is derived only from the several highest Wechsler test scores, the average of all test scores (i.e., the FSIQ) will of necessity be lower than the derived estimate (excepting, of course, when the test score range covers no more than two points) (see p. 99 for an example). Moreover, the FSIQ will necessarily underrepresent the premorbid level of functioning when patients have cognitive compromise in areas tested by the WIS-A.

Mental ability test scores for estimating premorbid ability. A common feature of techniques based on test scores is that the premorbid ability level is estimated from the scores themselves. For many years a popular method for estimating premorbid ability level from test performance used a vocabulary score as the single best indicator of original intellectual endowment (Yates, 1954). This method was based on observations that many cognitively deteriorating patients retained old, well-established verbal skills long after recent memory, reasoning, arithmetic ability, and other cognitive functions were severely compromised. Moreover, of all the Wechsler tests, Vocabulary correlates most highly with education, which also can be a good indicator of premorbid functioning (Heaton, Ryan, et al., 1996; Johnstone, Slaughter, et al., 1997; Tremont et al., 1999). A well-known example of this method is the *Shipley Institute of Living Scale (SILS)* (Shipley and Burlingame, 1941; Zachary, 1986; see pp. 669–670), which contains a multiple-choice (testing recognition rather than recall) vocabulary section and verbal reasoning items. It was expected that mentally deteriorated persons would show marked discrepancies between their vocabulary and reasoning scores. A recent large-scale study (889 persons 60–94 years old) dispensed with the reasoning items: "WAIS-R Equivalent FSIQ" scores, calculated for the upper range (19–40) of SILS Vocabulary scores alone, are offered as estimates of premorbid ability in dementia examinations (Yuspeh et al., 1998).

D. Wechsler and others used the same principle to devise "deterioration ratios," which mostly compared scores on vocabulary and other verbally weighted scores with performance on tests sensitive to attentional deficits and visuomotor slowing (see pp. 655–656). On the assumption that certain cognitive skills will hold up for most brain damaged persons, McFie (1975)—and, more recently, Krull and his colleagues (1995)—proposed that the sturdiest tests in Wechsler's scales are Vocabulary and Picture Completion, both involving verbal skills. The average of the scores, or the highest score of the two should one of them be markedly depressed, becomes the estimated premorbid IQ score (McFie, 1975) when evaluated with demographic data (Krull et al., 1995, see p. 95; also see Axelrod, Vanderploeg, and Schinka, 1999). Vanderploeg and Schinka (1995) point out the obvious when observing that Verbal scale tests predict VSIQ best and that Performance scale tests predict PSIQ best. Combining the individual WAIS-R tests with demographic variables (age, sex, race, education, occupation) in a series of regression equations, Information and Vocabulary emerged as the best estimates of VSIQ and FSIQ and Block Design, Picture Completion, and Object Assembly gave the best estimates of PSIQ.

Larrabee, Largen, and Levin (1985) found that other Wechsler tests purported to be resilient (e.g., Information and Picture Completion) were as vulnerable to the effects of dementia as those Wechsler regarded as sensitive to mental deterioration. Moreover, the Similarities test, which Wechsler (1958) listed as vulnerable to brain dysfunction, held up best (in both WAIS and WAIS-R versions) when given to neuropsychologically impaired polysubstance abusers (J.A. Sweeney et al., 1989). Vocabulary and related verbal skill scores sometimes do provide the best estimates of the general premorbid ability level. However, vocabulary tests such as Wechsler's, which require oral definitions, tend to be more vulnerable to brain damage than verbal tests that can be answered in a word or two, require only recognition, or call on practical experience. Further, many patients with left hemisphere lesions suffer deterioration of verbal skills which shows up in relatively lower scores on more than one test of verbal function. Aphasic patients have the most obvious verbal disabilities; some are unable to use verbal symbols at all. Some patients with left hemisphere lesions are not technically aphasic, but their verbal fluency is sufficiently depressed that vocabulary scores do not provide good comparison standards.

Word reading tests for estimating premorbid ability. In attempting to improve on vocabulary-based methods of estimating the cognitive deterioration of patients with diffusely dementing conditions, H.E. Nelson (1982; H.E. Nelson and Willison, 1991) and Crawford (with Parker and Besson, 1988; Crawford, Parker, Stewart, et al., 1989; Crawford, Deary, et al., 2001) proposed that scores on the *National Adult Reading Test (NART)* can reliably estimate the comparison standard, i.e., premorbid ability level. The NART requires oral reading of 50 phonetically irregular words, varying in frequency of use (see Table 13.9, p. 524). Of course, this technique can only be used with languages, such as English, in which the spelling of many words is phonetically irregular. In essence, these word reading tests provide an estimate of vocabulary size.

Correlations of NART-generated IQ score estimates with the WAIS and the WAIS-R (British version) FSIQ have run in the range of .72 (H.E. Nelson, 1982) to .81 (Crawford, Parker, Stewart et al., 1989). Correlations with the VSIQ are a little higher, while those with the PSIQ are considerably lower. A revision of the NART (NART-R UK) substituted new items for eight words that had not been scored reliably (Crawford, 1992). The correlation of the IQ score estimate generated by this form of the NART with the WAIS-R FSIQ score was .77. The NART and the British version of the WAIS-R were given to 179 77-year-olds who, at age 11, had taken a "group mental ability test" (presumably paper-and-pencil administration) (Crawford, Deary, et al., 2001). A correlation of NART estimates with the 66-year-old IQ scores ($r = .73$) showed that the late estimates were in the same range as the early test scores.

The *North American Adult Reading Test (NAART)*[1] (Blair and Spreen, 1989; Spreen and Strauss, 1998) was developed for U.S. and Canadian patients. This 61-word list contains 35 of the original NART words (see Table 4.1, p. 93). While the NAART scores correlate reasonably well with the WAIS-R VSIQ ($r = .83$), correlation with the FSIQ ($r = .75$) leaves a great deal of unaccounted variance, and the correlation with the PSIQ ($r = .40$) is too low to be useful as a general indicator of premorbid ability (Spreen and Strauss, 1991). It is of interest that for this verbal skill test the mean number of words correctly pronounced steadily increased from 36.7 ± 6.7 at ages 16–29 to approximately 43 ± 8.4 at

---

[1]Pronunciation guide and conversion (to IQ score estimates) formulas are in Spreen and Strauss (1998), p. 76.

TABLE 4.1 *North American Adult Reading Test (NAART): Word List*

Debt	Placebo	Detente	Sidereal
Debris	Procreate	Impugn	Abstemious
Aisle	Psalm	Capon	Beatify
Reign	Banal	Radix	Gaoled
Depot	Rarefy	Aeon	Demesne
Simile	Gist	Epitome	Syncope
Lingerie	Corps	Equivocal	Ennui
Recipe	Hors d'oeuvre	Reify	Drachim
Gouge	Sieve	Indices	Cidevant
Heir	Hiatus	Assignate	Epergne
Subtle	Gauche	Topiary	Vivace
Catacomb	Zealot	Caveat	Talipes
Bouquet	Paradigm	Superfluous	Synecdoche
Gauge	Facade	Leviathan	
Colonel	Cellist	Prelate	
Subpoena	Indict	Quadruped	

From Spreen and Strauss (1998)

ages 40–59 to 45.8 ± 8.4 at 70+ (Spreen and Strauss, 1998, p. 80).

The *AMNART* is a 45-word "American version" of the NART which proved sensitive to the developing semantic deficits of patients with early Alzheimer-type dementia (Storandt, Stone, and LaBarge, 1995). Mayo norms have been published for 361 healthy persons in 11 age ranges from 56 to 97 (Ivnik, Malek, Smith, et al., 1996). A recent 50-word version of the NART, the *American National Reading Test (ANART)* was developed to be more appropriate for the ethnically heterogeneous U.S. population (Gladsjo, Heaton, et al., 1999). It shares 28 words with the NAART. The ANART enhanced premorbid estimates for predominantly verbal tests to a limited degree, but made no useful contribution to estimates of either the PSIQ or scores of other tests with relatively few verbal components.

A short form of the NART (*Short NART*) was recommended for subjects who fail more than five of the first twenty-five items (Beardsall and Brayne, 1990), particularly those who fail many and are thus confronted with repeated failures. For subjects who pronounced between twelve and twenty of the first 25 NART words correctly, a procedure enables the examiner to estimate a full NART score; lower scores are assumed to be no different from what the total score would be if the entire word list had been given. While IQ score estimates obtained by this method correlated with NART estimates with "virtually equivalent" accuracy, these correlations left a considerable unexplained variance (23%–31%) and produced a small

number of very discrepant estimates of ability as defined by the WIS-A IQ scores (Crawford, Allan, Jack, et al., 1991). Baddeley, Emslie, and Nimmo-Smith (1988) simplified even further Nelson's relatively simple reading pronunciation task in a word recognition test (identifying which of a pair of letter groups is a real word). The level of difficulty at which the patient begins to fail consistently serves as an indicator of premorbid general ability.

A technique developed to be sensitive to anterior lesions, the *Homophone Meaning Generation Test (HMGT)*, has been applied to the problem of estimating the degree to which a patient is impaired (Crawford and Warrington, 2002). The task, which requires a shift in cognitive set, asks the subject for other meanings for a set of eight homophones (e.g., *pear*–pair, pare; *sight*–site, cite) (Warrington, 2000, see p. 629). Noting that the HMGT correlated at a statistically significant level with the NART ($r = .605$), Crawford and Warrington (2002) devised a formula[1] which, by evaluating the discrepancy between the HMGT raw score and the NART estimated premorbid score, will presumably provide a best estimate of "the severity of cognitive deficits."

The *Reading* test of the *Wide Range Ability Test (WRAT-READ)* was developed on the same principle as the NART tests, using more to less frequently appearing words—although not all WRAT-READ words are phonetically irregular—to evaluate reading level (Wilkinson, 1993; see p. 525). Studies of its effectiveness in estimating premorbid mental ability have produced findings similar to those for the NART and its variants (Johnstone and Wilhelm, 1996; Kareken et al., 1995). In comparisons of NART-R and WRAT-READ, Wiens, Bryan, and Crossen (1993) reported that the former test best estimated their cognitively intact subjects whose FSIQ scores were in the 100–109 range while consistently overestimating those whose FSIQ scores fell below 100 and underestimating the rest; WRAT-READ's estimations were more accurate in predicting lower FSIQ scores but underestimations of *average* and better FSIQ scores were even greater than for the NART-R. For neurologically impaired patients, a comparison of NAART and WRAT-READ found that while both "are appropriate estimates of premorbid verbal intelligence," NAART had standardization and range limitations while WRAT-READ provided a better estimate of the lower ranges of the VSIQ making WRAT-READ more applicable to the population "at higher risk for TBI" (Johnstone, Callahan, et al., 1996).

[1]To use this formula, Crawford invites clinicians to download the computer program (http: www.psyc.abdn.ac.uk/homedir/jcrawford/HMGT.htm).

Correlations between these word reading tests and the criterion tests (mostly WIS-A IQ scores) tend to be directly related to education level (Crawford, Stewart, Garthwaite, et al., 1988; Johnstone, Slaughter, et al., 1997; Maddrey et al., 1996; Storandt, Stone, and LaBarge, 1995; Stebbins, Wilson, et al., 1990). Some studies that took age into account dealt with subjects in the early to middle adult years with insignificant NART/NAART x age correlations resulting (e.g., Blair and Spreen, 1989; Wiens, Bryan, and Crossen, 1993). However, when subjects' age range extends across several age cohorts into old age, age effects emerge (Crawford, Stewart, Garthwaite, et al., 1988; Spreen and Strauss, 1998). Yet, although age effects reached significance ($r = -.18$) for a wide range subject sample (ages 17–88), when the much stronger correlations for education ($r = .51$) and social class ($r = -.36$) were partialled out, the very small age effects were nullified (Crawford, Stewart, Garthwaite, et al., 1988). Kareken and his colleagues (1995) reported significant correlations between race (whites, African Americans) and all three WAIS-R IQ scores and WRAT-READ scores. They questioned whether "quality of education may be a mitigating factor," but did not consider the pronunciation differences between "Black English" and standard American English (see pp. 313–314).

By and large, the findings of studies on this technique have shown that when attempting to predict VSIQ and FSIQ scores of *cognitively intact* persons from their reading level, these tests are fairly accurate (Crawford, 1992; Crawford, Deary, et al., 2001; J.J. Ryan and Paolo, 1992; Spreen and Strauss, 1998; Wiens, Bryan, and Crossen, 1993). Regardless of which Wechsler edition is used, correlations between NART/NAART or WRAT-READ scores and VSIQ tend to be highest, FSIQ correlations are typically a little lower but still account for a large portion of the variance, while PSIQ correlations are too low for the reading test scores to be predictive of anything. Moreover, the greater the actual IQ score deviation from 100, the more discrepant estimates by the NART or one of its variants: "there is truncation of the spread of predicted IQs on either end of the distribution leading to unreliable estimates for individuals at other than average ability levels" (Spreen and Strauss, 1998, pp. 80–81).

Furthermore, reading test scores do tend to decline when given to dementing patients (Crawford, Millar, and Milne, 2001; Johnstone, Callahan, et al., 1996; Storandt, Stone, and LaBarge, 1995) but typically less than IQ scores (Maddrey et al., 1996). This method has been questioned as underestimating the premorbid ability of dementia patients—the degree of underestimation being fairly directly related to the severity of dementia—(Stebbins, Wilson et al., 1990), of mildly demented patients with linguistic deficits (Stebbins, Gilley, et al., 1990), and of those more severely demented (Spreen and Strauss, 1991). For 20 elderly and neurologically impaired patients whose mean education was 8.8 ± 3.07 years, all three WAIS-R IQ scores (77.80 to 82.65) were significantly lower than NART estimates (from 93.05 to 95.25) (J.J. Ryan and Paolo, 1992). Yet, despite "mild" declines in NART-R scores, Maddrey and his colleagues (1996) recommend its use for dementing patients, even those whose deterioration is "more advanced."

Correlations of the NART with the three Wechsler IQ scores were a little lower for an English speaking South African population than for U.K. subjects. This discrepancy suggests that a language test standardized on one population may not work as well with another in which small differences in language have developed over time (Struben and Tredoux, 1989; see pp. 313–314).

Demographic variables for estimating premorbid ability. One problem with word-reading scores is their vulnerability to brain disorders, especially those involving verbal abilities; one advantage of demographic variables is their independence from the patient's neuropsychological status at the time of examination. In questioning the use of test score formulas for estimating premorbid ability (specifically, WIS-A FSIQ scores), R.S. Wilson, Rosenbaum, and Brown (1979; also in Rourke, Costa, et al., 1991) devised the first formula using demographic variables (age, sex, race, education, and occupation) to make this estimation. This formula predicted only two-thirds of 491 subjects' WAIS FSIQ scores within a ten-point error range; most of the larger prediction errors occurred at the high and low ends of their sample, overpredicting high scores and underpredicting low ones (Karzmark, Heaton, et al., 1985; also in Rourke, Costa, et al., 1991). Exaggerated estimations at the distribution extremes were also reported by F.C. Goldstein, Gary, and Levin (1986; also in Rourke, Costa, et al., 1991), although Wilson's formula provided "an adequate" fit to WAIS data for the 69 neurologically unimpaired subjects.

Recognizing the need for ability estimates geared to the WAIS-R, Barona, Reynolds, and Chastain (1984) elaborated on Wilson's work by incorporating the variables of geographic region, urban–rural residence, and handedness into the estimation formula. They devised three formulas for predicting each of the WAIS-R IQ scores. These authors did not report the amount and extent of prediction errors produced by their formulas but cautioned that, "where the premorbid Full Scale IQ was above 120 or below 69, utilization of the formuli [*sic*] might result in a serious under- or over-estimation, respectively" (p. 887). Other studies evaluating both the Wilson and the Barona estimation procedures found that at best they misclassified more than one-half of the patients (Silverstein, 1987), or "both formulas perform[ed] essentially at chance levels" (Sweet, Moberg, and Tovian, et al., 1990). Perez and her colleagues (1996) suggested that this formula—and its 1986 elaboration by Barona and Chastain—was useful for premorbid ability estimates but obtained VSIQ and FSIQ correlations in the .48 to .52 range for the control group. Yet for classifying subjects on the basis of the size of differences between estimated and obtained scores, the original Barona procedure identified 76.7% of the neurologically impaired patients and 90% of control subjects; an elaboration of the Barona procedure (Barona and Chastain, 1986) improved classification to 80% and 95% of patients and control subjects, respectively. Helmes (1996) applied the 1984 Barona equations in a truly large-scale study (8,660 randomly selected elderly Canadians—excluding three women in their 100s). The three IQ score means of each 5-year group calculated from this formula were within one point of 100 with few exceptions, suggesting that this formula produced reasonably accurate estimates. Main effects for sex and education were significant. However, another study comparing estimation techniques found that the 1984 Barona method generated the lowest correlation of estimated FSIQ with actual FSIQ ($r = .62$) (Axelrod, Vanderploeg, and Schinka, 1999).

A set of equations developed on British demographic data gave even less accurate estimates of WAIS (British) scores, predicting just 50% of the variance for FSIQ and VSIQ scores and only 30% for the PSIQ score (Crawford, Stewart, Cochrane, et al., 1989). In a later study of the predictive value of demographic variables, Crawford and Allan (1997) found that occupation provided the best estimate of the three WAIS-R IQ scores with correlations of $-.65$, $-.65$, and $-.50$ for FSIQ, VSIQ, and PSIQ, respectively. It is noteworthy that occupation and education correlated relatively highly ($r = .65$). When age and education were added in, the multiple regression results accounted for 53%, 53%, and 32% of the variance for the three IQ scores, respectively. As in most other studies, the contribution of age was neglible. This demographic formula joins word reading tests in not predicting PSIQ effectively.

Demographic variables combined with test scores for estimating premorbid ability. Further efforts to improve estimates of premorbid ability have generated formulas that combine word recognition test scores with demographic variables. In studies of normal subjects, while demographic variables accounted for 50% of the FSIQ score variance (Crawford, Stewart,

Cochrane, et al., 1989; Crawford, Stewart, Parker, et al., 1989) and NART scores alone predicted 66% of the variance, the FSIQ score variance based on a combination of these variables was 73% (Crawford, Stewart, Parker, et al., 1989). Strong relationships showed up between scores generated by equations combining NART scores with demographic variables and scores on individual WAIS tests: the greatest factor loadings were on the highly verbal tests (in the .76–.89 range), with almost as strong relationships (.71 and .72) occurring between the equation-generated scores and the Block Design and Arithmetic tests, respectively (Crawford, Cochrane, Besson, et al., 1990). These workers interpreted the findings as indicating that an appropriate combination of the NART score and demographic variables provides a good measure of premorbid general ability. However, another study examining different subject groups (e.g., Korsakoff's syndrome, Alzheimer's disease) found that NART (and NART-R) alone correlated better with WIS-A FSIQ than did either of two demographic formulas, nor did combining NART and demographic data enhance NART estimates (Bright et al., 2002).

Other attempts to enhance the accuracy of premorbid estimations from current test performance involve WIS-A tests. Krull and his colleagues (1995) devised the *Oklahoma Premorbid Intelligence Estimation (OPIE)*, using Vocabulary and Picture Completion scores of the WAIS-R standardization population along with age, education, occupation, and race data. They generated formulas for predicting VSIQ, PSIQ, and FSIQ, evaluating the accuracy of their formulas against the (presumably) cognitively intact WAIS-R standardization population on which they were developed. Not surprisingly, the predicted and actual correlations were high ($r = .87$, $.78$, $.87$ for V-, P-, and FSIQ scales, respectively). OPIE formulas were then developed to predict FSIQ using raw scores for Vocabulary, Picture Completion, both of these tests, or the raw score for whichever of these two tests had the highest non-age-corrected scaled score (BEST method) for subjects in the authors' patient data base (J.G. Scott et al., 1997). FSIQ predictions made by the the BEST formula most closely approximated the normative distribution's mean and standard deviation, a finding interpreted as indicating that the BEST method gave the best estimation. The formula using both Vocabulary and Picture Completion scores produced the least appropriate FSIQ approximations.

Because different patients will make their highest score(s) on different WIS-A tests, Vanderploeg and Schinka (1995) developed tables—which take demographic data of age, sex, race, education, and occupation into account—for estimating the three WAIS-R IQ scores from the 11 WAIS-R tests. They too used the WAIS-R standardization data to generate their 33 regression formulas, three for each WAIS-R test. Presumably, when the obtained IQ score is significantly below the expected IQ score level for a test, a deficit may be inferred.

Comparisons between methods for estimating premorbid ability. With so many estimation procedures to choose from, it is natural to wonder which works best. M.R. Basso, Bornstein, and their colleagues (2000), after testing the Barona, revised Barona, OPIE, and BEST-3, concluded that none of the methods based on regression formulas were satisfactory. They pointed out that the phenomenon of regression to the mean affected all these methods, most significantly the Barona (i.e., purely demographic) methods. Scores at the extremes of the IQ range were most vulnerable to estimation errors. The prediction accuracy of other studies (see below) tends to vary with the demographic characteristics of the samples tested.

For each of the three WIS-A IQ scores, Kareken and his colleagues (1995) compared formulas that included parental education level and race with WRAT-R reading scores to estimations derived from the original Barona (et al., 1984) equation. Using "healthy young adults," these workers reported that while the average discrepancy between these two estimates was "moderate," the reading + parental education technique generated both higher scores and a broader range of estimated scores—broader than did Barona estimates or the actual score range. Since correlations between the two methods indicated shared variances of only moderate size (for V-, P-, and FSIQ scores, $r = .46, .61,$ and $.55$, respectively), the authors concluded that each method "tap[s] different aspects of variance."

When estimates of impairment due to TBI and derived from WRAT-R reading scores were compared with impairment estimates based on education level, the latter method produced larger impairment estimates for the WAIS-R FSIQ score and also for two noncognitive tests: Grip Strength and Finger Tapping (Johnstone, Slaughter, et al., 1997). The reading score impairment estimations exceeded those predicted by education level on each of the two trials of the Trail Making Test. The authors wisely conclude that "different methods of estimating neuropsychological impairment > produce very different results" and suggest that neither of these methods is appropriate for estimating premorbid levels of motor skills.

A comparison of five methods for predicting premorbid ability level used as a criterion how closely the estimated FSIQ of brain impaired patients approximated the actual FSIQ score of matched control subjects (J.G. Scott et al., 1997). Four methods were based on a combination of WIS-A test scores and demographic data: three OPIE variants and a procedure using the OPIE equation that generated the highest score (BEST-3); a fifth was the purely demographically based Barona (et al., 1984) procedure. The demographically based method produced the smallest discrepancy between the clinical sample and the matched control group, and although it had the highest rate of group classification (based on estimated − obtained scores), all five methods had "an equal degree of overall classification accuracy." The Barona score had the lowest correlation by far with the subjects' actual FSIQ scores ($r = .62$; all others were in the .84 to .88 range). The authors point out discrepancies between these findings and those of previous studies in concluding that the four methods using OPIE equations were "equally effective," while expressing puzzlement over the Barona method's history of good performance in predicting FSIQ scores and in classifying subjects.

Also comparing the Barona and OPIE methods for estimating premorbid intelligence with two reading tests (NAART, WRAT-3), S.L. Griffin and her coworkers (2002) report that the Barona method was least useful, overestimating WAIS-R "below average" and "average" FSIQ scores and underestimating those in the "above average" ranges. OPIE overestimated the "average" FSIQ scores, NAART overestimated "below average" and "average" FSIQ, and the WRAT-R underestimated both "below average" and " above average" FSIQ.

With premorbid ability scores for 54 neurologically impaired patients, Hoofien, Vakil, and Gilboa (2000) evaluated two estimation procedures. BEST-10 utilizes the highest ten predicted test scores generated from Vanderploeg and Schinka's (1995) 30 prediction equations (the Hebrew WAIS-R has no Vocabulary test) which included age, sex, race, premorbid occupation, and premorbid education. BEST-2, based on which of the Information or Picture Completion test scores is highest, integrates into its score the same demographic variables. For predictive validity, the current WAIS-R FSIQ score correlated significantly with the premorbid transformed IQ score ($r = .63$); BEST-10's correlation was virtually identical, and BEST-2's correlation was a little lower ($r = .58$); concurrent validity correlations were, as expected, considerably higher (BEST-2 $r = .86$, BEST-10 $r = .85$). When comparing paired differences between the transformed premorbid IQ score, the postmorbid WAIS-R FSIQ, and the two BEST methods, the postmorbid FSIQ for these patients was 19.04 points lower than their premorbid scores, BEST-2 estimations were 5.39 points below premorbid IQ scores, but BEST-10 was only 2.07 points lower than the original test scores. BEST-10 premorbid estimations had fewer (8) instances of IQ score differences of 15 or greater than did BEST-2 with 13 such instances. These data suggest that BEST-10 may provide a better estimate of premorbid ability than BEST-2. The authors suggest that estimation procedures using best performances have higher predictive accuracy than those constructed on assumptions regarding "hold" tests. However, Hoofien and his colleagues (2000) warn against a purely "mechanical" application of the BEST-10 method, observing that some isolated skills or abilities can lead to an undeservedly high estimate. For such cases they recommend both the inclusion of demographic data for its "balancing effect" and clinical judgment. These authors further note that the large differences between the predictive validity correlations and those for concurrent validity cast serious question on estimation methods validated on current test scores.

Although none of these methods satisfies the clinical need for a reasonably accurate estimate of premorbid ability, all of them show the value of extratest data and the penalties paid for restricting access to any particular kind of information when seeking the most suitable comparison standards for a cognitively impaired patient.

THE BEST PERFORMANCE METHOD

A simpler method utilizes test scores, other observations, and historical data. This is the *best performance method*, in which the level of the best performance—whether it be the highest score or set of scores, nonscorable behavior not necessarily observed in a formal testing situation, or evidence of premorbid achievement—serves as the best estimate of premorbid ability. Once the highest level of functioning has been identified, it becomes the standard against which all other aspects of the patient's current performance are compared.

The *best performance method* rests on a number of assumptions that guide the examiner in its practical applications. Basic to this method is the assumption that, *given reasonably normal conditions of physical and mental development, there is one performance level that best represents each person's cognitive abilities and skills generally.* This assumption follows from the well-documented phenomenon of the transituational consistency of cognitive behavior. According to this assumption, the performance level of most normally developed, healthy persons on most tests of cognitive functioning probably provides a reasonable estimate of their performance level on most other cognitive tasks (see B.D. Bell and Roper, 1998, for a discussion of this phenomenon at the *high average* ability level; Dodrill, 1999, gives an example at the *low average* level). This as-

sumption allows the examiner to estimate a cognitively impaired patient's premorbid general ability level from one or, better yet, several current test scores while also taking into account other indicators such as professional achievement or evidence of a highly developed skill.

Intraindividual differences in ability levels may vary with a person's experience and interests, perhaps with sex and handedness, and perhaps on the basis of inborn talents and deficiencies. Yet, by and large, persons who perform well in one area perform well in others; and the converse also holds true: a dullard in arithmetic is less likely to spell well than is someone who has mastered calculus. This assumption does not deny its many exceptions, but rather speaks to a general tendency that enables the neuropsychological examiner to use test performances to make as fair an estimate as possible of premorbid ability in *neurologically impaired persons* with undistinguished school or vocational careers. A corollary assumption is that *marked discrepancies between the levels at which a person performs different cognitive functions or skills probably give evidence of disease, developmental anomalies, cultural deprivation, emotional disturbance, or some other condition that has interfered with the full expression of that person's cognitive potential.* An analysis of the WAIS-R normative population into nine average score "core" profiles exemplifies this assumption as only one profile, accounting for 8.2% of this demographically stratified sample, shows a variation of as much as 6 scaled score points, and one that includes 6.2% of the sample shows a 5-point disparity between the average high and low scores (McDermott et al., 1989). The rest of the scatter discrepancies are in the 0–4 point range.

Another assumption is that *cognitive potential or capacity of adults can be either realized or reduced by external influences; it is not possible to function at a higher level than biological capacity will permit.* Brain injury—or cultural deprivation, poor work habits, or anxiety—can only depress cognitive abilities (A. Rey, 1964). An important corollary to this assumption is that, *for cognitively impaired persons, the least depressed abilities may be the best remaining behavioral representatives of the original cognitive potential* (Axelrod, Vanderploeg, and Schinka, 1999; Hoofien, Vakil, and Gilboa, 2000; Krull et al., 1995; J.G. Scott et al., 1997).

The phenomenon of overachievement (people performing better than their general ability level would seem to warrant) appears to contradict this assumption; but in fact, overachievers do not exceed their biological limitations. Rather, they expend an inordinate amount of energy and effort on developing one or two special skills, usually to the neglect of others. Academic overachievers generally know their material mostly by rote and cannot handle the complex mental operations or highly abstract concepts enjoyed by people at *superior* and *very superior* ability levels.

A related assumption is that *few persons consistently function at their maximum potential,* for cognitive effectiveness can be compromised in many ways: by illness, educational deficiencies, impulsivity, test anxiety, disinterest—the list could go on and on. A person's performance of any task may be the best that can be done at that time but still only indicates a floor, not the ceiling, of the level of abilities involved in that task. Running offers an analogy: no matter how fast the runner, the possibility remains that she could have reached the goal even faster, if only by a fraction of a second.

Another related assumption is that *within the limits of chance variations, the ability to perform a task is at least as high as a person's highest level of performance of that task.* It cannot be less. This assumption may not seem to be so obvious when a psychologist is attempting to estimate a premorbid ability level from remnants of abilities or knowledge. In the face of a generally shabby performance, examiners may be reluctant to extrapolate an estimate of *superior* premorbid ability from one or two indicators of superiority, such as a demonstration of how to use a complicated machine or the apt use of several abstract or uncommon words, unless they accept the assumption that prerequisite to knowledge or the development of any skill is the ability to learn or perform it. A patient who names Grant as president of the United States during the Civil War and says that Greece is the capital of Italy but then identifies Einstein and Marie Curie correctly is demonstrating a significantly higher level of prior intellectual achievement than the test score suggests. The poor responses do not negate the good ones; the difference between them suggests the extent to which the patient has suffered cognitive deterioration.

It is also assumed that *a patient's premorbid ability level can be reconstructed or estimated from many different kinds of behavioral observations or historical facts.* Material on which to base estimates of original cognitive potential may be drawn from interview impressions, reports from family and friends, test scores, prior academic or employment level, school grades, army rating, or an intellectual product such as a letter or an invention. Information that a man had earned a Ph.D. in physics or that a woman had designed a set of complex computer programs is all that is needed to make an estimate of *very superior* premorbid intelligence, regardless of present mental dilapidation. Except in the most obvious cases of unequivocal high achievement, the estimates should be based on information from as many sources as possible to minimize the likelihood that significant data have been overlooked, resulting in an underestimation of the patient's premorbid ability level.

Verbal fluency can be masked by shyness, or a highly developed graphic design talent can be lost to a motor paralysis. Such achievements might remain unknown without careful testing or painstaking inquiry.

The value of the best performance method depends on the appropriateness of the data on which estimates of premorbid ability are founded. This estimation method places on the examiner the responsibility for making an adequate survey of the patient's accomplishments and residual abilities. This requires sensitive observation with particular attention to qualitative aspects of the patient's test performance; good history taking, including—when possible and potentially relevant—contacting family, friends, and other likely sources of information about the patient such as schools and employers; and enough testing to obtain an overview of the patient's cognitive abilities in each major functional domain.

The best performance method has very practical advantages. Perhaps most important is that a broad range of the patient's abilities is taken into account in identifying a comparison standard for evaluating deficit. By looking at the whole range of cognitive functions and skills for a comparison standard, examiners are least likely to bias their evaluations of any specific group of patients, such as those with depressed verbal functions. Moreover, examiners using this method are not bound to one battery of tests or to tests alone for they can base their estimates on nontest behavior and behavioral reports as well. For patients whose general functioning is too low or too spotty for them to complete a standardized adult test, or who suffer specific sensory or motor defects, children's tests or tests of specific skills or functions used for career counseling or job placement provide opportunities to demonstrate residual cognitive abilities.

In general, the examiner should not rely on a single high test score for estimating premorbid ability unless history or observations provide supporting evidence. The examiner also needs to be alert to overachievers whose highest scores are generally on vocabulary, general information, or arithmetic tests, as these are the skills most commonly inflated by parental or school pressure on an ordinary student. Overachievers frequently have high memory scores too. They do not do as well on tests of reasoning, judgment, original thinking, and problem solving, whether or not words are involved. One or two high scores on memory tests should not be used for estimating the premorbid ability level since, of all the cognitive functions, memory is the least reliable indicator of general cognitive ability. Dull people can have very good memories; some extremely bright people have been notoriously absent-minded.

It is rare to find only one outstandingly high score in a complete neuropsychological examination. Usually even severely impaired patients produce a cluster of relatively higher scores in their least damaged area of functioning so that the likelihood of overestimating the premorbid ability level from a single, spuriously high score is slight. The examiner is much more likely to err by underestimating the original ability level of the severely brain injured patient who is unable to perform well on any task.

In criticizing this method for systematically producing overestimates of premorbid ability, Mortensen and his colleagues (1991) give some excellent examples of how misuse of the best performance method can result in spurious estimates. Most of their "best performance" estimates were based solely on the highest score obtained by *normal control subjects* on a WIS-A battery. What they found, of course, was that the highest score among tests contributing to a summation score (i.e., an IQ score) is always higher than the IQ score since the IQ score is essentially a mean of all the scores, both higher and lower. Therefore, in cognitively intact subjects, the highest WIS-A test score is not an acceptable predictor of the WIS-A IQ score. Moreover, in relying solely on the highest score, the Mortensen study violated an important directive for identifying the best performance: that *the estimate should take into account as much information as possible about the patient and not rely on test scores alone.* In most cases, the best performance estimate will be based on a cluster of highest scores. Thus, developing a comparison standard using this method is not a simple mechanical procedure but calls upon clinical judgment and sensitivity to the many different conditions and variables that can influence a person's test performances.

THE DEFICIT MEASUREMENT PARADIGM

Once the comparison standard has been determined, whether directly from population norms, premorbid test data, or historical information, or indirectly from current test findings and observation, the examiner may assess deficit. This is done by comparing the level of the patient's present cognitive performances with the expected level—the comparison standard. Discrepancies between the expected level and present functioning are then evaluated for statistical significance (see pp. 148–149, 153–154). A statistically significant discrepancy between expected and observed performance levels for any cognitive function or activity represents a cognitive deficit.

This comparison is made for each test score. For each comparison where premorbid test scores are not available, the comparison standard is the estimate of original ability. By chance alone, a certain amount of variation (scatter) between test scores can be expected for even the most normal persons. Although these chance variations tend to be small (Cronbach, 1984), they can vary with the test instrument and with different scoring systems (see p. 652 for a discussion of the use of age-graded scores in interpreting WIS-A data). If significant discrepancies occur for more than one test score, a pattern of deficit may emerge. By comparing any given pattern of deficit with patterns known to be associated with specific neurological or psychological conditions, the examiner may be able to identify etiological and remedial possibilities for the patient's problems. When differences between expected and observed performance levels are not statistically significant, deficit cannot be inferred on the basis of just a few higher or lower scores.

For example, it is statistically unlikely that a person whose premorbid ability level was decidedly better than *average* cannot solve fourth- or fifth-grade arithmetic problems on paper or name at least 16 animals in one minute. If the performance of a middle-aged patient whose original ability is estimated at the *high average* level fails to meet these relatively low performance levels, then an assessment of impairment of certain arithmetic and verbal fluency abilities can be made with confidence. If the same patient performs at an *average* level on tests of verbal reasoning and learning, that discrepancy is not significant even though performance is somewhat lower than expected. These somewhat lowered scores need to be considered in any overall evaluation in which significant impairment has been found in other areas. However, when taken by themselves, *average* scores obtained by patients of *high average* mental competence do not indicate impairment, since they may be due to normal score fluctuations. In contrast, just *average* verbal reasoning and learning scores achieved by persons of estimated original *very superior* endowment do represent a statistically significant discrepancy, so that in exceptionally bright persons, *average* scores indicate deficit.

Identifiable patterns of cognitive impairment can be demonstrated by the deficit measurement method. Although the discussion here has focussed on assessment of deficit where a neurological disorder is known or suspected, this method can be used to evaluate the cognitive functioning of psychiatrically disabled or educationally or culturally deprived persons as well because the evaluation is conducted within the context of the patient's background and experiences, taking into account historical data and the circumstances of the patient's present situation (Gollin et al., 1989; W.G. Rosen, 1989). The evaluation of children's cognitive disorders follows the same model (Hynd and Willis, 1987; Sattler, 2001a; E.M. Taylor, 1959). It is of use not only as an aid to neurological or psychiatric diagnosis but also in educational and rehabilitation planning.

5 | The Neuropsychological Examination: Procedures

Psychological testing is a . . . process wherein a particular scale is administered to obtain a specific score. . . . In contrast, psychological assessment is concerned with the clinician who takes a variety of test scores, generally obtained from multiple test methods, and considers the data in the context of history, referral information, and observed behavior to understand the person being evaluated, to answer the referral questions, and then to communicate findings to the patient, his or her significant others, and referral sources.

G.J. Meyers, S.E. Finn, L.D. Eyde, et al., 2001

Two rules should guide the neuropsychological examiner: (1) *treat each patient as an individual*; (2) *think about what you are doing.* Other than these, the enormous variety of neurological conditions, patient capacities, and examination purposes necessitates a flexible, open, and imaginative approach. General guidelines for the examination can be summed up in the injunction: *Tailor the examination to the patient's needs, abilities, and limitations,* and to special examination requirements. By adapting the examination to the patient rather than the other way around, the examiner can answer the examination questions most fully at the least cost and with the greatest benefit to the patient.

The neuropsychological examination can be individually tailored in two ways. Examiners can select tests and examination techniques for their appropriateness to the patient and for their relevancy to those diagnostic or planning questions that prompted the examination and that arise during its course. They can also apply these assessment tools in a sensitive and resourceful manner by adapting them to suit the patient's condition and enlarging upon them to gain a full measure of information.

CONCEPTUAL FRAMEWORK OF THE EXAMINATION

Purposes of the Examination

Neuropsychological examinations may be conducted for any of a number of purposes: to aid in diagnosis; to help with management, care, and planning; to evaluate the effectiveness of a treatment technique; to pro-

vide information for a legal matter; or to do research. In many cases, an examination may be undertaken for more than one purpose. In order to know what kind of information should be obtained in the examination, the examiner must have a clear idea of the reasons for which the patient is being seen.

Although the reason for referral usually is the chief purpose for examining the patient, the examiner needs to evaluate its appropriateness. Since most referrals for neuropsychological assessment come from persons who do not have expertise in neuropsychology, it is not surprising that many of their questions are poorly formulated or beside the point. Thus, the referral may ask for an evaluation of the patient's capacity to return to work after a stroke or head injury when the patient's actual need is for a rehabilitation program and an evaluation of competency to handle funds. Frequently, the neuropsychological assessment will address several issues, each important to the patient's welfare, although the referral may have been concerned with only one. Moreover, few referrals are explicit enough to suggest a focus for the examination or are sufficiently broad to define its scope. A request for differential diagnosis between neurologically based and "functional" behavior disorders, for example, would rarely ask the examiner to give tests sensitive to frontal lobe dysfunction. The need to give such tests has to be determined by the examiner from the history, the interview, and the patient's performance in the course of the examination. In the final analysis, the content and direction of any neuropsychological examination that is adapted to the patient's needs and capacities must be decided by the examiner.

Examination Questions

The purpose(s) of the examination should determine its overall thrust and the general questions that need to be asked. The examiner will probably also address specific questions: about the level of performance of a particular skill—e.g., spelling when the patient mentions a loss from premorbid status; or about which impaired functions may account for the defective performance of a complex activity—e.g., whether spelling deficits are due to a phonological impairment, defective recall of irregular words, or other disorder (see McCarthy and Warrington, 1990). Examination questions fall into one of two categories. *Diagnostic questions* concern the nature of the patient's symptoms and complaints in terms of their etiology and prognosis; i.e., they ask whether the patient has a neuropsychologically relevant condition and, if so, what it is. *Descriptive questions* inquire into the characteristics of the patient's condition; i.e., they ask how the patient's problem is expressed. Within these two large categories are specific questions that may each be best answered through somewhat different approaches.

Diagnostic questions

Diagnostic questions are typically asked when patients are referred for a neuropsychological evaluation following the emergence of a cognitive or behavioral problem without a known etiology. Questions concerning the nature or source of the patient's condition are always questions of *differential diagnosis*. Whether implied or directly stated, these questions ask which of two or more diagnostic pigeonholes suits the patient's behavior best. In neuropsychology, diagnostic categorization can consist of coarse screening to distinguish the probable "neurological impairment" from a "psychiatric or emotional disturbance," fine discriminations between cognitive deterioration due to onset of a dementing process or to a growing tumor, or even finer discriminations such as those between the behavioral effects of a specific focal lesion and the effects of a lesion that may have encroached on an adjacent part of the brain. In large part, diagnostic evaluations depend on syndrome analysis (Heilman and Valenstein, 2003; Mesulam, 2000c; Stringer, 1996). The behavioral consequences of many neurological conditions have been described and knowledge about an individual patient (history, appearance, interview behavior, test performance) can be compared to these well-described conditions. In other cases, an unusual presentation might be analyzed on the basis of a theoretical understanding of brain–behavior relationships (e.g., Farah and Feinberg, 2000; Ogden, 1996; Walsh, 1995).

In looking for neuropsychological evidence of brain disease, the examiner may need to determine whether the patient's level of functioning has deteriorated. Thus, a fundamental question will be, "How good was the patient at his or her best?" When the etiology of a patient's probable brain dysfunction is unkown, risk factors for brain diseases should be taken into account, such as predisposing conditions for vascular disease, exposure to environmental toxins, recent occurrence of a blow to the head, or presence of substance abuse. Differential diagnosis can sometimes hinge on data

from the personal history, the nature of the onset of the condition, and circumstances surrounding its onset. In considering diagnoses the examiner needs to know whether anyone in the family had a condition similar to the patient's, how fast the condition is progressing, and the patient's mental attitude and personal circumstances at the time problems emerged. Another important diagnostic question asks whether the pattern of deficits exhibited by the patient fits a known or reasonable pattern of brain disease—or fits one pattern better than another. More specific diagnostic questions will ask which particular brain functions are compromised, which are intact, and how the specific deficits might account for the patient's behavioral anomalies.

The diagnostic process involves the successive elimination of alternative possibilities, or hypotheses (see also pp. 112–113). The examiner formulates the first set of hypotheses on the basis of the referral question, information obtained from the history or informants, and the initial impression of the patient. Each diagnostic hypothesis is tested by comparing what is known of the patient's condition (history, appearance, interview behavior, test performance) with what is expected for that particular diagnostic classification. As the examination proceeds, the examiner can progressively refine general hypotheses (e.g., that the patient is suffering from a brain disorder) into increasingly specific hypotheses (e.g., that the disorder most likely stems from a progressive dementing condition; that this progressive disorder is more likely to be an Alzheimer's type of dementia, multi-infarct dementia, or normal pressure hydrocephalus).

Neuropsychologists do not make a neurological diagnosis, but they may provide data and diagnostic formulations that contribute to the diagnostic conclusions. Neuropsychological findings assume particular diagnostic importance when neither a neurological nor a psychiatric evaluation can account for behavioral aberrations.

Descriptive questions

In cases where a diagnosis is established, many referral questions call for behavioral descriptions. Questions about specific capacities frequently arise in the course of vocational and educational planning. They become especially important when planning involves withdrawal or return of normal adult rights and privileges, such as a driving license or legal competency. In these cases, questions about the patient's competencies may be at least as important as those about the patient's deficits, and the neuropsychological examination may not be extensive, but rather will focus on the relevant skills and functions.

The effectiveness of remediation techniques and rehabilitation programs depends in part on accurate appraisals of what the candidate patient can and cannot do (Ponsford, 1995, *passim;* Prigatano, 1999; Sohlberg and Mateer, 2001). Foremost, rehabilitation workers must know how aware the patients are of their condition and the patients' capacity to incorporate new information and skills (Eslinger, Grattan, and Geder, 1995; Prigatano, 1991b). For example, a learning-based program for a postanoxic patient whose learning ability is virtually nonexistent will necessarily fail, although certain kinds of patterned drilling may reduce some of the patient's care needs (Mazaux, Giroire, et al., 1991). As the sophistication of these programs increases along with limitations on their financial coverage, accurate and appropriate behavioral descriptions can reduce much of the time spent in figuring out a suitable program for the patient. Competent assessment can enable rehabilitation specialists to set realistic goals and expend their efforts efficiently (Ponsford, 1995; Wrightson and Gronwall, 1999).

Longitudinal studies involving repeated measures over time are conducted when monitoring the course of disease progression, assessing improvement from an acute event such as head injury or stroke, or documenting treatment effectiveness. In such cases, a broad range of functions usually comes under regular neuropsychological review. An initial examination, consisting of a full-scale assessment of each of the major functions in combinations of input and output modalities, is sometimes called a *baseline study,* for it provides the first set of data against which the findings of later examinations will be compared. Regularly repeated full-scale assessments give information about the rate and extent of improvement or deterioration and about relative rates of change between functions.

Most examinations address one or more questions concerning the presence of a brain disorder, the estimation of the original potential or premorbid level of functioning, and the status of current cognitive functioning. Many examinations also generate one or two questions relevant to the specific case. Few examinations should have identical questions and procedures. An examiner who does much the same thing with almost every patient may not be attending to the implicit part of a referral question, to the patient's needs, or to the aberrations that point to specific defects and particular problems.

CONDUCT OF THE EXAMINATION

Foundations

The examiner's background

The knowledge base in medicine, psychology, other health related disciplines, and the basic sciences is ex-

panding at an increasing rate. Clinicans are thus becoming more and more specialized since their practice incorporates a smaller portion of clinical and research knowledge. It is harder than ever to be a well-rounded clinician. When seeing a patient for the first time or an established patient with new complaints and sometimes old ones, the examiner must conduct a thorough, up-to-date interview that can provide information pertinent to the diagnosis and treatment of the disorder as well as the interaction of various disorders and treatments. Clinicians cannot help but bring their own biases and preconceptions to the diagnostic process which may be based on out-of-date knowledge, experiences and views that are relevant for one population but not another, and even personal life events. Clinicians therefore have an ethical responsibility to update their knowledge and to be aware of their professional biases and of the impact of these and their personal experiences on the diagnostic process. Since a clinician can be an expert only in a relatively small area of knowledge, it is important to try to "know what you do not know" and thus, when to refer to someone with that knowledge.

In conducting neuropsychological assessments, in order to know what questions to ask, how particular hypotheses can be tested, or what clues or hunches to pursue, a strong background in neuropathology is necessary, including familiarity with neuroanatomy and neurophysiological principles. The neuropsychological examiner's background in cognitive psychology should include an understanding of the complex, multifaceted, and interactive nature of the cognitive functions; and in clinical psychology, the competent examiner requires knowledge of psychiatric syndromes and of test theory and practice. Even to know what constitutes a neuropsychologically adequate review of the patient's mental status requires a broad understanding of brain function and its neuroanatomical correlates. Moreover, the examiner must have had enough clinical training and supervised "hands on" experience to know what extratest data (e.g., personal and medical history items, school grades and reports) are needed to make sense out of any given set of observations and test scores, to weigh all of the data appropriately, and to integrate them in a theoretically meaningful and practically usable manner. These requirements are spelled out in detail in the Policy Statement of the Houston Conference on Specialty Education and Training in Clinical Neuropsychology (Hannay, Bieliauskas, Crosson, et al., 1998, pp. 160–165). Reference to further information can be found in the most recent report of Division 40 (Clinical Neuropsychology), American Psychological Association (Eubanks, 1997; see also Bush and Drexler, 2002, *passim;* J. T. Barth, Pliskin, et al., 2003).

The patient's background

In neuropsychological assessment, few if any single bits of information are meaningful in themselves. A test score, for example, takes on diagnostic or practical significance only when compared with other test scores, with academic or vocational accomplishments or aims, or with the patient's interview behavior. Even when the examination has been undertaken for descriptive purposes only, as after a head injury, it is important to distinguish a low test score that is as good as the patient has ever done from a similarly low score when it represents a significant loss from a much higher premorbid performance level. Thus, in order to interpret the examination data properly, each bit of data must be evaluated within a suitable context (Strub and Black, 1988; Vanderploeg, 1994; Walsh and Darby, 1999) or it may be misinterpreted. A study by Perlick and Atkins (1984), for example, showed how changes in a patient's reported age led clinicians to differ in their diagnostic impressions, as they are more likely to suspect dementia in elderly patients and depression in middle-aged ones, although the presented data were identical in each instance except for the attributed ages.

The relevant context will vary for different patients and different aspects of the examination. Usually, therefore, the examiner will want to become informed about many facets of the patient's life. Some of this information can be obtained from the referral source, from records, from hospital personnel working with the patient, or from family, friends, or people with whom the patient works. Patients who can give their own history and discuss their problems reasonably well will be able to provide much of the needed information. Having a broad base of data about the patient will not guarantee accurate judgments, but it can greatly reduce errors. Moreover, the more examiners know about their patients prior to the examination, the better prepared will they be to ask relevant questions and choose tests that are germane to the presenting problems.

Context for interpreting the examination findings may come from any of four aspects of the patient's background: (1) social history, (2) present life circumstances, (3) medical history and current medical status, and (4) circumstances surrounding the examination. Sometimes the examiner has information about only two or three of them. Korsakoff patients, for example, cannot give a social history or tell much about their current living situation. However, with the aid of informants and records, as possible, the examiner should inquire into each of these categories of background information. The practise of *blind analysis*—in which the examiner evaluates a set of test scores without benefit of history, records, or ever having seen the patient—may be useful for teaching or reviewing a case but is particularly inappropriate as a basis for clinical decisions.

1. Social history. Information about the patient's educational and work experiences may be the best source of data about the patient's original cognitive potential. Unexpected relationships do occur, such as when someone of low educational background performs well above the *average* range on cognitive tests. Social history will often show that these bright persons had few opportunities or little encouragement for more schooling. Military service history may contain important information, too. Military service gave some blue-collar workers their only opportunity to display their natural talents. A discussion of military service experiences may also unearth a head injury or illness that the patient had not thought to mention to a less experienced or less thorough examiner. When reviewing educational and work history, attention should be paid to how work and school performance relate to the medical history and other aspects of the social history.

A 45-year-old longshoreman, admitted to the hospital for seizures, had a long history of declining occupational status. He had been a fighter pilot in World War II, had completed a college education after the war, and had begun his working career in business administration. Subsequent jobs were increasingly less taxing mentally. Just before his latest job he had been a foreman on the docks. Angiographic studies displayed a massive *arteriovenous malformation (AVM)* that presumably had been growing over the years. Although hindsight allows us to surmise that his slowly lowering occupational level reflected the gradual growth of this space displacing lesion, it was only when his symptoms became flagrant that his occupational decline was appreciated as symptomatic of the neuropathological condition.

Knowledge of the socioeconomic status of the patient's family of origin as well as current socioeconomic status is often necessary for interpreting cognitive test scores—particularly those measuring verbal skills, which tend to reflect the parents' social class as well as academic achievement (Sattler, 2001a). The examiner usually needs to find out the highest socioeconomic status the patient had attained or the predominant adult socioeconomic status. In most cases, the examiner should also ask about the patient's school and work history and the occupational level and education of parents, siblings, and other important family members. Educational and occupational background may also influence patients' attitudes about their symptoms. Those who depend largely on verbal skills in their occupation become very distressed by a mild word finding problem, while others who are not accustomed to relying much on verbal skills may be much less disturbed by the same kind of impairment or may even be able to disregard it.

The patient's marital history may provide relevant information, including the obvious issues of number of spouses (or companions), length of relationship(s), and the nature of the dissolution of each significant alliance. The marital history may tell a great deal about the patient's long-term emotional stability, social adjustment, and judgment. It may also contain historical landmarks reflecting neuropsychologically relevant changes in social or emotional behavior.

Information about the present spouse's health, socioeconomic background, current activity pattern, and appreciation of the patient's condition is frequently useful for understanding the patient's behavior (e.g., anxiety, dependency) and is imperative for planning and guidance. The same questions need to be asked about whoever is the most significant person in an unmarried patient's life. Knowledge about the patient's current living situation and of the spouse's or responsible relative's condition is important both for understanding the patient's mood and concerns—or lack of concern—about the examination and the disorder that prompted it, and for gauging the reliability of the informant closest to the patient.

Other aspects of the patient's background should also be reviewed. When antisocial behavior is suspected, the examiner will want to inquire about confrontations with the law. A review of family history is obviously important when a hereditary condition is suspected. Moreover, awareness of family experiences with illness and family attitudes about being sick may clarify many of the patient's symptoms, complaints, and preoccupations.

If historical data are the bricks, then chronology is the mortar needed to reconstruct the patient's history meaningfully. For example, the fact that the patient has had a series of unfortunate marriages is open to a variety of interpretations. In contrast, a chronology-based history of one marriage that lasted for two decades, dissolved more than a year after the patient was in coma for several days as a result of a car accident, and then was followed by a decade filled with several brief marriages and liaisons suggests that the patient may have sustained a personality change secondary to the head injury. Additional information that the patient had been a steady worker prior to the accident but since has been unable to hold a job for long gives additional support to that hypothesis (e.g., for the classic example of a good worker whose head injury made him unemployable, see Macmillan's *An Odd Kind of Fame. Stories of Phineas Gage*, 2000). As another example, an elderly patient's complaint of recent mental slowing suggests a number of diagnostic possibilities: that the slowing followed the close occurrence of widowhood, retirement, and change of domicile should alert the diagnostician to the likelihood of depression.

2. Present life circumstances. When inquiring about the patient's current life situation, the examiner should go beyond factual questions about occupation, income and indebtedness, family statistics, and leisure activities to find out the patient's views and feelings about them. The examiner needs to know how long a working patient has held the present job, what changes have taken place or are expected at work, whether the work is enjoyed, and whether there are problems on the job. The examiner should attempt to learn about the quality of the patient's family life and such not uncommon family concerns as troublesome in-laws, acting-out adolescents, and illness or substance abuse among family members. New sexual problems can appear as a result of brain disease, or old ones may complicate the patient's symptoms and adjustment to a dysfunctional condition. Family problems, marital discord, and sexual dysfunction can generate so much tension that symptoms may be exacerbated or test performance adversely affected.

3. Medical history and current medical status. Information about the patient's medical history will usually come from a treating physician, a review of medical charts when possible, and reports of prior examinations as well as the patient's reports. When enough information is available to integrate the medical history with the social history, the examiner can often get a good idea of the nature of the condition and the problems created by it. Discrepancies between patients' reports of health history and the current medical condition or what medical records or physicians have reported may give a clue to the nature of their complaints or to the presence of a neuropsychological disorder. Medication records may prove significant in understanding the patient's functioning.

Some aspects of the patient's health status that are not infrequently overlooked in the usual medical examination may have considerable importance for neuropsychological assessment. These include visual and auditory defects that may not be documented or even examined when the patient is young and the defects are mild or when the patient is old or has other sensory deficits, motor disabilities, or mental changes. In addition, sleeping and eating habits may be overlooked in a medical examination, although impaired sleep and poor eating habits can be important symptoms of depression; increased sleep, childish or very limited food preferences, or an insatiable appetite may be symptomatic of brain disease.

4. Circumstances surrounding the examination. The test performance can be evaluated accurately only in light of the reasons for referral and the relevance of the examination to the patient. For example, does the patient stand to gain money or lose a custody battle as a result of the examination? May a job or hope for early retirement be jeopardized by the findings? Only by knowing what the patient believes may be gained or lost as a result of the neuropsychological evaluation can the examiner appreciate how the patient perceives the examination.

Procedures

Patients' cooperation in the examination process is extremely important, and one of the neuropsychologist's main tasks is to enlist such cooperation.

A.-L. Christensen, 1989

Referral

The way patients learn of their referral for neuropsychological assessment can affect how they view the examination, thus setting the stage for such diverse responses as cooperation, anxiety, distrust, and other attitudes that may modify test performance (J.G. Allen et al., 1986; Bennett-Levy, Klein-Boonschate, et al., 1994). Ideally, referring persons explain to patients, and to their families whenever possible, the purpose of the referral, the general nature of the examination with particular emphasis on how this examination might be helpful or, if it involves a risk, what that risk might be, and the patient's choice in the matter. Neuropsychologists who work with the same referral source(s), such as residents in a teaching hospital, a neurosurgical team, or a group of lawyers, can encourage this kind of patient preparation. When patients receive no preparation and hear they are to have a "psychological" evaluation, some may come to the conclusion that others think they are emotionally unstable or crazy.

Often it is not possible to deal directly with referring persons. Rather than risk a confrontation with a poorly prepared and negativistic or fearful patient, some examiners routinely send informational letters to new patients, explaining in general terms the kinds of problems dealt with and the procedures the patient can anticipate (see Kurlychek and Glang, 1984; J. Green, 2000, for examples of such a letter).

When to examine

Sudden onset conditions; e.g., trauma, stroke. Within the first few weeks or months following a sudden onset event, a brief examination may be necessary for several reasons: to ascertain the patient's ability to comprehend and follow instructions; to evaluate competency when the patient may require a guardian; or to determine whether the patient can retain enough new information to begin a retraining program.

As a general rule, formal assessment should not be undertaken during the acute or postacute stages. During this period—typically up to the first six to twelve weeks following the event—changes in the patient's neuropsychological status can occur so rapidly that information gained one day may be obsolete the next. Moreover, fatigue overtakes many of these early stage patients very quickly and, as they tire, their mental efficiency plummets making it impossible for them to demonstrate their actual capabilities. Both fatigue and awareness of poor performances can feed the depressive tendencies experienced by many neuropsychologically impaired patients. Additionally, as transient neuropsychological disturbances set in motion by the pathologic event may not yet have cleared up, many patients continue to be mentally sluggish for several months after the event, which also keeps them from performing up to their potential. Patients who were aware of doing poorly when examined when their deficits were most pronounced may be reluctant to accept a reexamination for fear of reliving that previously painful situation.

Following the postacute stage, when the patient's sensorium has cleared and stamina has been regained—usually some time within the third to sixth month after the event—an initial comprehensive neuropsychological examination can be given. In cases of minor impairment or rapid improvement, the goal may be to see if the patient can return soon to previous activities and, if so, whether temporary adaptations—such as reduced hours or a quiet environment—will be required (e.g., see Wrightson and Gronwall, 1999). When impairment is more severe, typical early assessment goals will be to identify specific remediation needs and the residual capacities that can be used for remediation; to make an initial projection about the patient's ultimate levels of impairment and improvement—and psychosocial functioning, including education and career potential; and to reevaluate competency when it had been withdrawn earlier.

Long-term planning for training and vocation when these seem feasible, or for level of care of patients who will probably remain socially dependent, can be done sometime within one to two years after the event. A relatively short examination, focusing mainly on potential problem areas, may suffice for older patients who are close to or in retirement, for then the purpose of the examination is to evaluate needs for further therapy, care, and counseling for patient and family. Most younger persons will benefit from a comprehensive neuropsychological examination.

Evolving conditions, e.g., degenerative diseases, tumor. Early in the course of an evolving condition when neurobehavioral problems are first suspected, the neuropsychological examination can contribute significantly to diagnosis (Bondi, Salmon, and Kaszniak, 1996; Chen et al., 2001; Derrer, Howieson, et al., 2001; Gómez-Isla and Hyman, 2003; see also pp. 212–213). Repeated examinations may then become necessary for a variety of reasons: When seeking a definitive diagnosis and early findings were vague and perhaps of psychological rather than neurological origin, a second examination six to eight months after the first may answer the diagnostic questions. With questions of dementia, after twelve to eighteen months the examination is more likely to be definitive (J.C. Morris, McKeel, Storandt, et al., 1991). In evaluating rate of decline as an aid to counseling and rational planning for conditions in which the rate of deterioration varies considerably between patients, such as multiple sclerosis or Huntington's disease, examinations at one to two year intervals can be useful. Timing for evaluations of the effects of treatment will vary according to how long the treatment takes and whether it is disruptive to the patient's mental status, such as treatments by chemotherapy, radiation, or surgery for brain tumor patients.

Initial planning

The neuropsychological examination proceeds in stages. In the first stage, the examiner plans an overall approach to the problem. The hypotheses to be tested and the techniques used to test them will depend on the examiner's initial understanding and evaluation of the referral questions and on the accompanying information about the patient.

Preparatory interview

The initial interview and assessment make up the second stage. Here the examiner tentatively determines the range of functions to be examined, the extent to which psychosocial issues or emotional and personality factors should be explored, the level—of sophistication, complexity, abstraction, etc.—at which the examination should be conducted, and the limitations set by the patient's handicaps. Administrative issues, such as fees, referrals, and formal reports to other persons or agencies, should also be discussed with the patient at this time.

The first 15–20 minutes of examination time are usually used to evaluate the patient's capacity to take tests and to ascertain how well the purpose of the examination is understood. The examiner also needs time to prepare the patient for the assessment procedures and to obtain consent. This interview may take longer than 20 minutes, particularly with anxious or slow patients,

those who have a confusing history, or those whose misconceptions might compromise their intelligent cooperation. The examiner may spend the entire first session preparing a patient who fatigues rapidly and comprehends slowly, reserving testing for subsequent days when the patient feels comfortable and is refreshed. On questioning 129 examinees—mostly TBI and stroke patients—following their neuropsychological examination, Bennett-Levy, Klein-Boonschate, and their colleagues (1994) found that the participation of a relative in interviews, both introductory and for feedback, not only provided more historical information but helped clarify issues for the patient.

At least seven topics must be covered with competent patients before testing begins if the examiner wants to be assured of their full cooperation.[1] (1) *The purpose of the examination:* Do they know the reasons for the referral, and do they have questions about it? (2) *The nature of the examination:* Do patients understand that the examination will be primarily concerned with cognitive functioning and that being examined by a neuropsychologist is not evidence of craziness? (3) *The use to which examination information will be put:* Patients must have a clear idea of who will receive a report and how it may be used. (4) *Confidentiality:* Competent patients must be reassured not only about the confidentiality of the examination but also that they have control over their privacy except (i) when the examination has been conducted for litigation purposes and all parties to the dispute may have access to the findings, (ii) when confidentiality is limited by law (e.g., reported intent of harm to self or a stated person), or (iii) when insurance companies paying for the examination are entitled to the report. (5) *Feedback to the patient:* Patients should know before the examination begins who will report the test findings and, if possible, when. (6) *A brief explanation of the test procedures:* Many patients are very reassured by a few words about the tests they will be taking.

I'll be asking you to do a number of different kinds of tasks. Some will remind you of school because I'll be asking questions about things you've already learned or I'll give you arithmetic or memory problems to do, just like a teacher. Others will be different kinds of puzzles and games. You may find that some things I ask you to do are fun and some seem silly; some of the tests will be very easy and some may be so difficult you won't even know what I'm talking about or showing you; but all of them will help me to understand better how your brain is working, what you are doing well, what difficulties you are having, and how you might be helped.

---

[1]In the United States, examining clinicians providing health-care services are now required by the Health Information Privacy Protection Act (HIPPA) to review items 1–5 with their patients or patients' guardians.

(7) *How the patient feels about taking the tests:* This can be the most important topic of all, for unless patients feel that taking the tests is not shameful, not degrading, not a sign of weakness or childishness, not threatening their job or legal status or whatever else may be a worry, they cannot meaningfully or wholeheartedly cooperate. Moreover, the threat can be imminent when a job, or competency, or custody of children is at stake. It is then incumbent upon the examiner to give patients a clear understanding of the possible consequences of noncooperation as well as full cooperation so that they can make a realistic decision about undergoing the examination. In addition, (8) *when the patient is paying for the services,* the (estimated in some cases) amount, method of payment, etc. should be agreed upon before the examination begins.

Following principles for ethical assessment—and now, in the United States, following the law—the neuropsychologist examiner will want to obtain the patient's informed consent before beginning the examination (Johnson-Greene et al., 1997; Macciocchi, 2000). While the patient's cooperation following a review of these seven—or eight—points would seem to imply informed consent, many patients for whom a neuropsychological examination is requested have a limited or even no capacity to acquiese to the examination. Others take the examination under various kinds of legal duress, such as inability to pursue a personal injury claim, threat of losing the right to make financial or medical decisions, or the risk of receiving a more severe punishment when charged with a criminal act. Moreover, the examiner can never guarantee that something in the examination or the findings will not distress the patient (e.g., a catastrophic reaction, identification of an early dementing process), nor is the examiner able to predict *a priori* that such an event may occur during the examination or such an outcome. Thus, in neuropsychology, informed consent is an imperative goal to approach as closely as possible. In the individual case, the neuropsychologist examiner must be cognizant of any limitations to realizing this goal and able to account for any variations from standards and requirements for informed consent.

Ideally, the introductory interview includes both the patient and a significant other person, enabling the examiner to identify consistencies and discrepancies in reported problems. Reports by collateral sources can offer important clues to the patient's insight and the disabilities the neuropsychologist will want to investigate. Both the patient and the accompanying person should be questioned about when and how the problems began and changes in problems over time.

The patient has an important role in this process: to provide accurate and detailed information, sometimes information that the clinician did not think to ask. I always ask patients if there is anything else that I should know about their life or current events that might be helpful [hjh].

A patient whose mental functioning is impaired may not be able to take an active, effective role in the interview. In such cases it may be necessary for a family member or close friend to participate. The patient and others need to feel free to express their opinions and to question the assumptions or conclusions voiced by the clinician. When this occurs the clinician must heed what is said since faulty assumptions and the conclusions on which they are based can lead to misdiagnosis and inappropriate treatment, sometimes with negligible but sometimes with important consequences.

The examiner can also conduct a brief mental status examination (MSE; see Chapter 18 for a detailed description) in this preliminary interview. The patient's contribution to the preliminary discussion will give the examiner a fairly good idea of the level at which to conduct the examination. When beginning the examination with one of the published tests that has a section for identifying information that the examiner is expected to fill out, the examiner can ask the patient to answer the questions of date, place, birth date, education, and occupation on the answer sheets, thereby getting information about the patient's orientation and personal awareness while doing the necessary record keeping. In asking for the date, be alert to the patient wearing a watch that shows the date. Ask these patients not to look at their watch when responding to date questions. (I ask patients to sign and date—again without checking their watch—all drawings, thus obtaining several samples of time orientation [mdl]).

Patients who are not competent may be unable to appreciate all of the initial discussion. However, the examiner should make some effort to see that each topic is covered within the limits of the patient's comprehension and that the patient has had an opportunity to express concerns about the examination, to bring up confusing issues, and to ask questions.

Observations

Observation is the foundation of all psychological assessment. The contribution that psychological—and neuropsychological—assessment makes to the understanding of behavior lies in the evaluation and interpretation of behavioral data that, in the final analysis, represent observations of the patient.

Indirect observations consist of statements or observations made by others or of examples of patient behavior. The latter typically consist of letters or notes, constructions, or art forms created by the patient but could also include pictures of a TV screen the patient smashed or of a neatly groomed flower bed. Verbal reports may be the most common means by which family members, caregivers, teachers, and others convey their observations of the patient. However, grades, work proficiency ratings, and other scores and notes in records are also behavioral descriptions obtained by observational methods, although presented in a form that is more or less abstracted from the original observations.

The psychological examination offers the opportunity of learning about patients through two kinds of *direct observation*. Informal observations, which can be made from the moment the patient appears, provide invaluable information about almost every aspect of patient behavior: how they walk, talk, respond to new situations and new faces—or familiar ones, if this is the second or third examination—and leave-taking. Patients' habits of dressing and grooming become apparent, as do more subtle attitudes about people generally, about themselves and the people in their lives specifically. Informal observation can focus on patients' emotional status to find out how and when they express their feelings and what is emotionally important to them. The formal—test-based—examination provides a different kind of opportunity for informal observation, for here examiners can see how patients deal with prestructured situations in which the range of available responses is restricted, while observing their interaction with activities and requirements familiar to the examiner.

Psychological tests provide formalized observational techniques. They are simply a means of enhancing (refining, standardizing) our observations. They can be thought of as extensions of our organs of perception—the "seven-league boots" of clinical behavioral observation. If we use them properly, as extensions of our observational end-organs, like "seven-league boots" they enable us to accomplish much more with greater speed. When tests are misused as substitutes for rather than extensions of clinical observation, they can obscure our view of the patient much as seven-league boots would get in the way if worn over the head. (Lezak, 1987a, p. 46)

Nontest observations, such as those obtained during an interview, can be systematized, either as an informal mental status examination or following one of the many standardized mental status formats (see Chapter 18). Some clinicians have drafted guidelines as an aid to systematizing their nontest observations and to guard against overlooking some important area (e.g., Brooks, Truelle, et al. 1994; Murrey, 2000a; Spreen and Strauss, 1998; Strub and Black, 2000).

Test selection

Selection of tests for a particular patient or purpose will depend on a number of considerations. Some have to do with the goal(s) of the examination, some involve aspects of the tests, and then there are practical issues that must be addressed.

1. The examination goals. The goal(s) of the examination will obviously contribute to test selection. A competency evaluation may begin and end with a brief mental status rating scale if it demonstrates the patient's incompetency. At the other extreme, appropriate assessment of a premorbidly bright young TBI candidate for rehabilitation may call for tests examining every dimension of cognitive and executive functioning to determine all relevant areas of weakness and strength. For most people receiving a neuropsychological assessment, evaluation of their emotional status and how it relates to neuropathology and/or their psychosocial functioning is a necessary component of the examination.

2. Validity and reliability. Tests of cognitive abilities are getting better at both meeting reasonable criteria for validity and reliability and having appropriate norms. Many useful examination techniques that evolved out of clinical experience or research now have published score data from at least small normal control groups (Mitrushina, Boone, and D'Elia, 1999; Spreen and Strauss, 1998).

Validity is the degree to which the accumulated evidence supports the specific interpretations that the test's developers, or users, claim (Retzlaff and Gibertini, 1994; Anastasi and Urbina, 1997). However, the tests used by neuropsychologists rarely measure one cognitive skill or behavior so that different interpretations show up in the literature. For example, the well-scaled and normed Visual Reproduction test of the Wechsler Memory Scale–Revised (which is almost identical with its newer version in the Wechsler Memory Scale-III) may be much more a measure of visuospatial reasoning and analysis than of memory (Leonberger et al., 1991), yet others have documented a prominent visual construction component (Chelune, Bornstein, and Prifitera, 1990). These findings make it a questionable test for neuropsychological assessment, as it neither appears to do what it purports to do nor, because of its memory components, does well what it apparently does best (see also Teng, Wimer, et al., 1989 for this confound in a similar visual "memory" test). Thus, not all tests used by neuropsychologists will meet all validity criteria, for even after years of use, what many of the most popular tests measure remains unclear (Dodrill, 1997; see also pp. 136–138). Moreover, validity will vary with the use to which a test is put: A test with good predictive validity when used to discriminate patients with Alzheimer's disease from elderly depressed persons may not identify which young TBI patients are likely to benefit from rehabilitation (Heinrichs, 1990).

Besides the usual validity requirements to ensure that a test measures the brain functions or mental abilities it purports to measure, two kinds of evidence for validity hold special interest for neuropsychologists: *Face validity*, the quality of appearing to measure what the test is supposed to measure, becomes important when dealing with easily confused or upset patients who are thus more likely to reject tasks that seem nonsensical to them. This kind of reluctance has been particularly noted in elderly patients who will willingly tackle a test that appears relevant to their needs (Cunningham, 1986; Mahurin and Pirozzolo, 1986). *Predictive validity*, especially as it applies to practical, "real-life" situations, is a much sought-after test attribute which has been increasingly realized despite its somewhat elusive nature (see pp. 11–12).

Reliability of a test—the regularity with which it generates the same score under similar retest conditions or the regularity with which different parts of a test produce similar findings—can be ascertained only with normal control subjects. When examining brain damaged patients with cognitive deficits, test reliability becomes an important feature: repeated test performances by cognitively intact persons must be similar if that test can measure with any degree of confidence the common kinds of change that characterize performances of brain impaired persons (i.e., improvement, deterioration, instability, fatigue effects, diurnal effects, etc.). In choosing a test for neuropsychological assessment, the test's vulnerability to the vagaries of the testing situation must also be taken into account. For example, differences in the speed at which the examiner reads a story for recall can greatly affect the amount of material a patient troubled by slowed processing retains (Shum, Murry, and Eadie, 1997).

Reliability of test performances by patients with brain disorders may become practically nonexistent, given the changing course of most of these disorders and the vulnerability of many brain impaired patients to daily—sometimes even hourly—alterations in their level of mental efficiency (e.g., Bleiberg et al., 1997). In fact, because neuropsychological assessment is so often undertaken to document differences—improvement after surgery, for example, or further deterioration when dementia is suspected—the most useful tests can be those most sensitive to fluctuations in patient performances.

Moreover, many "good" tests that do satisfy the usual statistical criteria for reliability may be of little value for neuropsychological purposes. Test batteries that generate summed or averaged scores based on a clutch of discrete tests provide another example of good reliability (the more scores, the more reliable their sum) of a score that conveys no neuropsychologically relevant information unless it is either so low or so high that the level of the contributing scores is obvious (Lezak, 1988b; Walsh, 1995; see pp. 21–22).

3. Sensitivity and specificity. A test's *sensitivity* or *specificity* for particular conditions makes it more or less useful, depending on the purpose of the examination (L. Costa, 1988; Mapou, 1988; see also pp. 149–150). For general screening, as when attempting to identify persons whose mentation is abnormal for whatever reason, a sensitive test such as Wechsler's Digit Symbol will be preferred. However, since poor performance on this test can result from a variety of conditions—including a carpal tunnel syndrome or inferior education—such a test will be of little value to the examiner hoping to delineate the precise nature of a patient's deficits. Rather, for understanding the components of a cognitive deficit, tests that examine specific, relatively pure, aspects of neuropsychological functions—i.e., that have high specificity—are needed (Mapou, 1995; McCarthy and Warrington, 1990; Teng, Wimer, et al., 1989). Many sensitive examination techniques have evolved out of clinical experience or research, and while they are effective at eliciting abnormal phenomena in impaired patients, they have not been standardized on a large scale or even on small groups (Luria, 1966).

A test sensitive to unilateral inattention, when given to 100 randomly chosen normal adult control subjects, will prove both reliable and valid, for the phenomenon is unlikely to be elicited at all. Yet giving the same test to patients with documented left visuospatial inattention may elicit the phenomenon in only some of the cases, and if given more than once soon after onset of the pathological condition, might prove highly unreliable as patients' responses to this kind of test can vary from day to day.

4. Parallel forms. Perhaps more than any other area of psychological assessment, neuropsychology requires instruments designed for repeated measurements as so many examinations of persons with known or suspected brain damage must be repeated over time—to assess deterioration or improvement, treatment effects, and changes with age or other life circumstances (Freides, 1985). As yet, few commercially available tests have parallel forms suitable for retesting or come in a format that withstands practice effects reasonably well. McCaffrey, Duff, and Westervelt (2000a,b) have addressed this problem by publishing test–retest data for most of the tests in more or less common use by neuropsychologists. While such tables do not substitute for parallel forms, they do provide the examiner with a rational basis for evaluating retest scores.

5. Time and costs. Not least of the determinants of test selection are the practical ones of administration time (which should include scoring and report writing time as well) and cost of materials (Lezak, 2002). Prices put some tests out of reach of many neuropsychologists; when the cost is outrageously high for what is offered, the test deserves neglect. There may be a few neuropsychological functions or mental abilities that cannot be assessed by relatively inexpensive means even if the examiner shops around, reproduces tests in the public domain, and is imaginative in applying the tests that are available and affordable; but I do not know which they might be [mdl]. Barncord and Wanlass (1999) offer an "ecological" solution to the large amounts of paper consumed by neuropsychological examinations, suggesting use of "plastic sheet protectors . . . and fine-tipped washable markers" which would be applicable to such tests as the Trail Making Test and Symbol Digit Modalities Test. This would save not only paper but money as well. Barncord and Wanlass note that this technique would be applicable only when a complete record is not required. For clinical purposes, even when litigation is not an issue, the complete record is important for documenting patient errors—or absence of errors [mdl].

Administration time becomes an increasingly important issue as neuropsychological referrals grow while agency and institutional money to pay for assessments does not keep pace or may be shrinking. Moreover, patients' time is often valuable or limited: many patients have difficulty getting away from jobs or family responsibilities for lengthy testing sessions; those who fatigue easily may not be able to maintain their usual performance level much beyond two hours. These issues of patient time and expense and of availability of neuropsychological services together recommend that examinations be kept to the essential minimum.

6. Nonstandardized assessment techniques. Occasionally a patient presents an assessment problem for which no well-standardized test is suitable (B. Caplan and Shechter, 1995). Improvising appropriate testing techniques can then tax the imagination and ingenuity of any conscientious examiner. Sometimes a suitable test can be found among the many new and often experimental techniques reported in the literature. Some of them are reviewed in this book. These experimental techniques are often inadequately standardized, or they may not test the functions they purport to test. Some may be so subject to chance error as to be undependable. Patient data of others may be insufficient for judging the test's utility. However, these experimental and relatively unproven tests may be useful in themselves or as a source of ideas for further innovations. Rarely can clinical examiners evaluate an unfamiliar test's patient and control

data methodically, but with experience they can learn to judge reports and manuals of new tests well enough to know whether the tasks, the author's interpretation, the reported findings, and the test's reliability are reasonably suitable for their purposes. When making this kind of evaluation of a relatively untried test, clinical standards need not be as strict as research standards.

A 38-year-old court reporter, an excellent stenographer and transcriber, sustained bilateral parietal bruising (seen on magnetic resonance imaging) when the train she was on derailed with an abrupt jolt. She had been sleeping on her side on a bench seat when the accident occurred. She was confused and disoriented for the next several days. When she tried to return to work, along with the more common attentional problems associated with TBI, she found that she had great difficulty spelling phonetically irregular words and mild spelling problems with regular ones. To document her spelling complaints, she was given an informal spelling test comprising both phonologically regular and irregular words. Evaluation of her responses—39% misspellings—was consistent with other reports of well-educated patients with *lexical agraphia* (Beauvois and Dérousné, 1981; Roeltgen, 2003; see Fig. 5.1). Since the issue concerned proportion of misspellings of com-

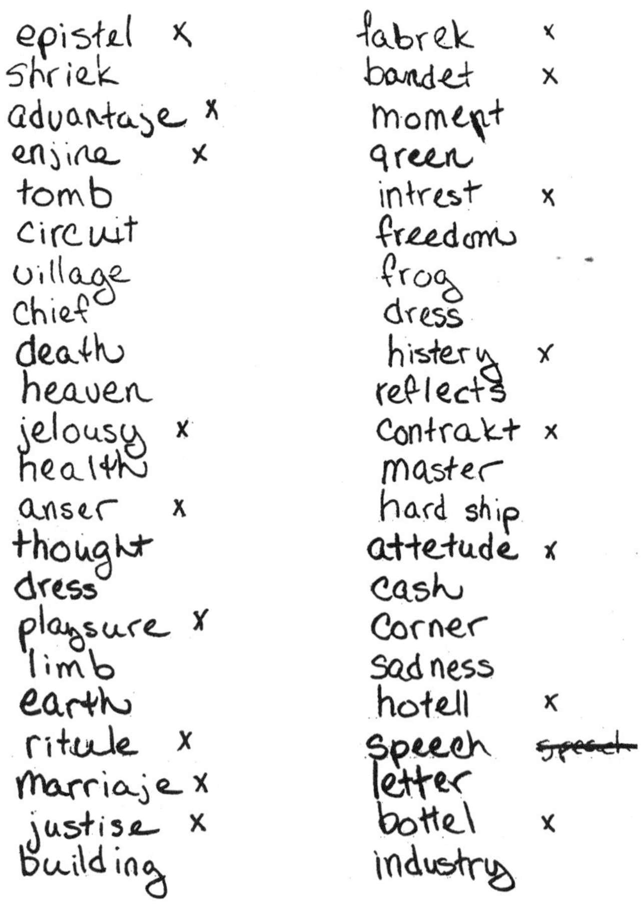

FIGURE 5.1 An improvised test for lexical agraphia.

mon words and the difference between phonetically regular and irregular words and not the academic level of spelling, this was an instance in which an informal test served well to document the patient's problem.

Beginning with a basic test battery

Along with the examination questions, the patient's capacities and the examiner's test repertory determine what tests and assessment techniques will be used. In an individualized examination, the examiner rarely knows exactly which tests will be given before the examination has begun. Many examiners start with a basic battery that touches upon the major dimensions of cognitive behavior (e.g., *Attention, Visuoperception and visual reasoning, Memory and Learning, Verbal functions and academic skills, Construction, Concept formation, Self-regulation [executive functions] and motor ability, and Emotional status*). They then drop some tests or choose additional tests as the examination proceeds. The patient's strengths, limitations, and specific handicaps will determine how tests in the battery are used, which must be discarded, and which require modifications to suit the patient's capabilities. As the examiner raises and tests hypotheses regarding possible diagnoses, areas of cognitive dysfunction or competence, and psychosocial or emotional contributions to the behavioral picture, it usually becomes necessary to go beyond a basic battery and use techniques relevant to this patient at this time.

When redundancy in test selection is avoided, such a battery of tests will generally take three to four hours when given by an experienced examiner. They can usually be completed in one session, depending on the subject's level of cooperation and stamina, but can be given in two sittings—preferably on two different days, if the patient fatigues easily.

This book reviews a number of paper-and-pencil tests that patients can take by themselves. These tests may be given by clerical or nursing staff; some of them may have computerized administrations available. Some of these tests were developed as timed tests: time taken can provide useful information. However, sometimes it is more important to find out what the patient can do regardless of time, and the test can be taken either untimed or the person proctoring the test can note how much was done within the time limit but allow the patient to proceed to the end of the test.

When working with outpatients who come from a distance or may have tight time schedules, it is often impractical to expect them to spend another several hours on the paper-and-pencil tests. Responsible patients who are fairly intact may take the paper-and-pencil materials home and mail them back or return them at a later appointment. Irresponsible, immature,

easily confused, or disoriented and poorly motivated patients should be given the paper-and-pencil tests under supervision, as should patients whose families tend to be protective or overly helpful. The examiner may also deem it necessary to supervise the paper-and-pencil testing in some cases under litigation.

In deciding when to continue testing with more specialized assessment techniques or to discontinue, it is important to keep in mind that a *negative* (i.e., *within normal limits*, not abnormal) performance does not rule out brain pathology; it only demonstrates which functions are at least reasonably intact. However, when a patient's test and interview behavior are *within normal limits*, the examiner cannot continue looking indefinitely for evidence of a lesion that may not be there. Rather, a good history, keen observation, a well-founded understanding of patterns of neurological and psychiatric dysfunction, and common sense should tell the examiner when to stop—or to keep looking.

Test selection for research

Of course, when following a research protocol, the examiner is not free to exercise the flexibility and inventiveness that characterize the selection and presentation of test materials in the clinical situation. For research purposes, the prime consideration in selecting examination techniques is whether they will effectively test the hypotheses or demonstrate the phenomenon in question (e.g., see Fischer, Priore, et al., 2000). Other important issues in putting together a research battery include practicality, time, and the appropriateness of the instruments for the population under consideration. Since the research investigator cannot change instruments or procedures in midstream without losing or confounding data, selection of a research battery requires a great deal of care. In developing the *Minimal Assessment of Cognitive Function in Multiple Sclerosis (MACFIMS)*, the working group noted the importance of flexibility to allow for supplanting the less satisfactory tests with newly developed tests that may be more suitable (Fischer, Rudick, et al., 1999).

Just as a basic battery can be modified for individuals in the clinical examination, so too tests can be added or subtracted depending on research needs. Moreover, since a research patient may also be receiving clinical attention, tests specific for the patient's condition can be added to a research battery as the patient's needs might require.

A note on ready-made batteries

The popularity of ready-made batteries attests to the need for neuropsychological testing and to a lack of knowledge among neuropsychologically inexperienced psychologists about how to do it (Lezak, 2002; Sweet,

Moberg, and Westergaard, 1996). The most popular batteries extend the scope of the examination beyond the barely minimal neuropsychological examination (which may consist of one of the WIS-A batteries, a drawing test, and parts or all of a published memory battery). They offer reliable scoring methods for gross diagnostic screening (see Chapter 17). Ready-made batteries can be invaluable in research programs requiring well-standardized tests.

When batteries are used as directed, most patients undergo more testing than is necessary but not enough to satisfy the examination questions specific to their problems. Also, like most psychological tests, ready-made batteries are not geared to the patient's handicaps. The patient with a significant perceptual or motor disability may not be able to perform major portions of the prescribed tests, in which case the functions normally measured by the unusable test items remain unexamined. However, batteries do acquaint the inexperienced examiner with a variety of tests and with the importance of evaluating many different behaviors when doing neuropsychological testing. They can provide a good starting place for some newcomers to the field, who may then expand their test repertory and introduce variations into their administration procedures as they gain experience and develop their own point of view.

Orsini, Van Gorp, and Boone (1988) pointed out that unless examiners feel free to introduce new assessment techniques into their testing repertory, they cannot take advantage of new knowledge and new developments in the cognitive neurosciences (see also, Lezak, 2002). By the same token, it is easier for some examiners to continue to use questionable or outmoded tests or scoring techniques when they seem validated by being part of a ready-made battery (e.g., see pp. 506–507 for a discussion of the Aphasia Screening Test, which the author—Joseph Wepman—repudiated in the 1970s). A ready-made battery may also seem to confer neuropsychological competence on its users, giving false complacency to naive examiners, particularly if it is popular and has accrued a long reference trail. However, no battery can substitute for knowledge—about patients, medical and psychological conditions, the nature of cognition and psychosocial conduct, and how to use tests and measurement techniques. Batteries do not render diagnostic opinions or behavioral descriptions, clinicians do; and without the necessary knowledge, clinicians cannot form reliably valid opinions, no matter what battery they use (see W.G. Snow, 1985).

Hypothesis testing

This stage of the examination usually has many steps. It begins as the data of the initial examination answer initial questions, raise new ones, and may shift the focus from one kind of question to another or from one set of impaired functions that at first appeared to be of critical importance in understanding the patient's complaints to another set of functions. Hypotheses can be tested in one or more of several ways: by bringing in the appropriate tests (see below), by testing the limits, and by seeking more information about the patient's history or current functioning. It may also involve changes in the examination plan, in the pace at which the examination is conducted, and in the techniques used. Changes in the procedures and shifts in focus may be made in the course of the examination. At any stage of the examination the examiner may decide that more medical or social information about the patient is needed, that it would be more appropriate to observe rather than test the patient, or that another person should be interviewed, such as a complaining spouse or an intact sibling, for adequate understanding of the patient's condition. This flexible approach enables the examiner to generate multistage, serial hypotheses for identifying subtle or discrete dysfunctions or to make fine diagnostic or etiologic discriminations.

Without knowing why a patient has a particular difficulty, the examiner cannot predict the circumstances in which it will show up. Since most neuropsychological examination techniques in clinical use elicit complex responses, the determination of the specific impairments that underlie any given lowered performance becomes an important part of many neuropsychological evaluations. This is usually done by setting up a general hypothesis and testing it in each particular condition.

If, for example, the examiner hypothesizes that a patient's slow performance on the Block Design test of one of the Wechsler Intelligence Scales (WIS-A) was due to general slowing, all other timed performances must be examined to see if the hypothesis holds. A finding that the patient is also slow on all other timed tests would give strong support to the hypothesis. It would not, however, answer the question of whether other deficits also contributed to the low Block Design score. Thus, to find out just what defective functions or capacities entered into the impaired performance requires additional analyses. This is done by looking at the component functions that might be contributing to the phenomenon of interest in other parts of the patient's performance (e.g., house drawing, design copying, for evidence of a problem with construction; other timed tests to determine whether slowing occurs generally) in which one of the variables under examination plays no role and all other conditions are equal. When the patient does well on the task used to examine the alternative variable (e.g., visuospatial construction), the hypothesis that the alternative variable also contributes to the phenomenon of interest can be rejected. If the patient performs poorly on the second task as well as the first, then the hypothesis that poor performance on the first task is multiply determined cannot be rejected.

This example illustrates the method of *double dissociation* for identifying which components of complex cognitive activities are impaired and which are preserved (E. Goldberg, 2001, p. 52; Weiskrantz, 1991; see also p. 153).

These conceptual procedures can lead to diagnostic impressions and to the identification of specific deficits. In clinical practice, examiners typically do not formalize these procedures or spell them out in detail but apply them intuitively. Yet, whether used wittingly or unwittingly, this conceptual framework underlies much of the diagnostic enterprise and behavioral analysis in individualized neuropsychological assessment.

Selection of additional tests

The addition of specialized tests depends on continuing formulation and reformulation of hypotheses as new data answer some questions and raise others. Hypotheses involving differentiation of learning from retrieval, for instance, will dictate the use of techniques for assessing learning when retrieval is impaired. Finer-grained hypotheses concerning the content of the material to be learned—e.g., meaningful vs. meaningless or concrete vs. abstract or the modality in which it is presented—will require different tests, modifications of existing tests, or the innovative use of relevant materials in an appropriate test format (Fantie and Kolb, 1991). Every function can be examined across modalities and in systematically varied formats. In each case the examiner can best determine what particular combinations of modality, content, and format are needed to test the pertinent hypotheses.

The examination of a 40-year-old unemployed nursing assistant illustrates the application and value of a hypothesis-testing approach. While seeing a psychiatrist for a sleep disorder, she complained of difficulty learning and remembering all the medical procedures she had to perform. She had attempted suicide by carbon monoxide poisoning three years earlier. The attempt was aborted when she had to urinate. She reported that on leaving the car she found she had temporarily lost control of her limbs. She worked only sporadically after this. The question of a residual memory impairment due to hypoxia prompted the referral for a neuropsychological assessment. On the basis of this information, the planned examination focused on memory and learning.

In the interview preceding testing, she reported that her mind seemed to have "slowed down" and she "often felt disoriented," so much so that she had become dependent on her husband to take her to unfamiliar places. She also reported two head injuries, one as a child when a boulder struck her head without loss of consciousness. More recently, while hyperventilating, she fell on an andiron and was "knocked out."

Although she had difficulty subtracting serial threes, she performed well on every verbal and visual memory test (consonant trigrams, Digit Span, story recall, Auditory-Verbal Learning Test [AVLT], and recall trials of the Symbol Digit Modalities Test and the Complex Figure Test). She did have a decreased immediate recall span on the first (I) and interference (B) trials of the AVLT, a deficit implicating span of attention under conditions of stimulus overload rather than memory. The original hypothesis of memory disorder was not supported. However, her performances called for another hypothesis to be tested: Despite *average* scores on verbal skill tests and a *high average* performance on a visual reasoning task (Picture Completion), her Block Design scores were in the *low average* range and her copy of the Complex Figure was *defective* due to elongation, one omitted line, and poor detailing (although both recall trials were at an *average* level). These poor performances, taken with her complaints of spatial disorientation, suggested a visuospatial problem. To explore this hypothesis, further testing was required. The originally planned examination, which had included a test of verbal retrieval (Boston Naming Test) and one for sequential learning (Serial Digit Learning), was halted and other tests specific for visuospatial deficits were given, including the Location and Copy subtests of the MacQuarrie Test for Mechanical Ability, Judgment of Line Orientation, the Hooper Visual Organization Test, and a free drawing of a house. Scores on these tests ranged from *low average* to *borderline defective*, and the house drawing was childishly crude with a markedly distorted attempt at perspective. Thus a deficit pattern emerged that contrasted with her excellent memory and learning abilities and the *high average* Picture Completion performance.

As this patient seemed neither depressed nor unduly anxious in this examination, her somewhat histrionic emotional displays and complaints about having been ill-served by her parents did not appear to be contributing to her cognitive deficits; rather, the experiences of disorientation she reported could be a factor contributing to the stress for which she sought psychiatric help, and visuospatial deficits could contribute to difficulty assimilating the range of medical assistant procedures. No conclusive etiology for her attentional and visuospatial problems could be developed from the available history, although, given her reports of head injury, TBI was a likely candidate.

Concluding the examination

The final stage, of course, has to do with concluding the examination as hypotheses are supported or rejected, and the examiner answers the salient diagnostic and descriptive questions or explains why they cannot be answered (e.g., at this time, by these means). When it appears that assessment procedures are making patients aware of deficits or distressing patients because they assume—rightly or wrongly—that they performed poorly, the examiner can end the examination with a relatively easy task, leaving the patient with some sense of success (Nancy R. Bryant, personal communication, 1999 [mdl]). The conclusions should also lead to recommendations for improving or at least making the most of the patient's condition and situation and for whatever follow-up contacts may be needed.

The examination is incomplete until the findings have been reported. Ideally, two kinds of reports are provided: one as oral feedback to patients and whoever they choose to hear it; the other one written for the referral source and, if the examination is performed in an institution such as a hospital, for the institution's records.

The interpretative interview. A most important yet sometimes neglected part of the neuropsychological examination is the follow-up interview to provide patients with an understanding of their problems and how their neuropsychological status relates to their future, including recommendations on how to ameliorate or compensate for their difficulties. Feedback generally is most useful when patients bring their closest family member(s) or companion(s), as these people almost always need understanding of and seek guidance for dealing with the patient's problems. This interview should take place after the examiner has had time to review and integrate the examination findings (which include interview observations) with the history, presenting problems, and examination objectives. Patients who have been provided an interpretation of the examination findings are more likely to view the examination experience positively than those not receiving it (Bennett-Levy, Klein-Boonschate, et al., 1994).

By briefly describing each test, discussing the patient's performance on it, indicating that individuals who have difficulty on some test might experience a particular everyday problem, and asking if that is the case for the patient, the clinician can elicit useful validating information. This interview can also help patients understand the events that brought them to a neuropsychological examination. The interpretive interview can in itself be part of the treatment process, a means of allaying some anxieties, conveying information about strengths as well as weaknesses to the patient, and providing future directions for further diagnostic procedures if necessary or for treatment. A lack of validation of the clinician's interpretation of the patient's performance(s) may lead the clinician in a new direction. In either case, useful information has been obtained by the clinician, while the patient has been given the opportunity to gain insight into the nature of the presenting problems or—at the very least—to understand why the various tests were given and what to do next. Often counseling will be provided in the course of the interpretive interview, usually as recommendations to help with specific problems. For example, for

patients with a reduced auditory span, the examiner may tell the patient, "When unsure of what you've heard, ask for a repetition, or repeat or paraphrase the speaker (giving examples of how to do this and explaining paraphrasing as needed). Moreover, in a dispute over who said what in the course of a family conversation, your recall is probably the incorrect one." For the family members the examiner advises, "Speak slowly and in short phrases, pause between phrases, and check on the accuracy of what the patient has grasped from the conversation."

Occasionally, in reviewing the examination data, the examiner will discover some omissions—in the history, in following to completion a line of hypothesis testing—and will use some of this interview time to collect the needed additional information. In this case, and sometimes when informal counseling has begun, a second or even a third interpretive interview will be necessary.

Most referral sources—physicians, the patient's lawyer, a rehabilitation team—welcome having the examiner do this follow-up interview. In some instances, such as referral from a clinician already counseling the patient or treating a psychiatric disorder, referring persons may want to review the examination findings with their patients themselves. Neuropsychological examiners need to discuss this issue with referring clinicians so that patients can learn in the preparatory interview who will report the findings to them. Some other referrals, such as those made by a personal injury defense attorney, do not offer a ready solution to the question of who does the follow-up: An examiner hired by persons viewed by the patient as inimical to his or her interests is not in a position to offer counsel or even, in some instances, to reveal the findings. In these cases the examiner can ask the referring attorney to make sure that the patient's physician or the psychologist used by the patient's attorney receive a copy of the report with a request to discuss the findings, conclusions, and recommendations with the patient. This solution is not always successful. It is an attempt to avoid what I call "hit-and-run" examinations in which patients are expected to expose their frailties in an often arduous examination without receiving even an inkling of how they did, what the examiner thought of them, or what information came out that could be useful to them in the conduct of their lives [mdl].

Written reports. Like the examination, the written report needs to be appropriate for the circumstances. A brief bedside examination may require nothing more than a chart note. A complex diagnostic problem on which a patient's employment or legal status depends would require a much more thorough and explanatory report, always geared to the intended audience (see Armengol et al., 2001, for report-writing guidelines and samples of reports on a variety of cases for different situations).

An aid to test selection: a compendium of tests and assessment techniques, chapters 9–20

In the last 12 chapters of this book, most tests of cognitive functions and personality in common use, and many less common tests, are reviewed. These are tests and assessment techniques that are particularly well suited for clinical neuropsychological examination. Clinical examiners can employ the assessment techniques presented in these chapters for most neuropsychological assessment purposes in most kinds of work settings. Most of these tests have been standardized or used experimentally so that reports of the performances of control subjects are available (see Heaton, Grant, and Matthews, 1991; Mitrushina, Boone, and D'Elia, 1999; Spreen and Strauss, 1998). However, the normative populations and control groups for many of these tests may differ from individual patients on critical variables such as age, education, or cultural background, requiring caution and a good deal of "test-wiseness" on the part of the examiner who attempts to extrapolate from unsuitable norms.

PROCEDURAL CONSIDERATIONS IN NEUROPSYCHOLOGICAL ASSESSMENT

Testing Issues

Order of test presentation

The order of presentation of tests in a battery has not been shown to have appreciable effects on performance (Cassel, 1962). Neuger and his colleagues (1981) noted a single exception to this rule when they gave a battery containing many different tests. A slight slowing occurred on a test of manual speed, Finger Tapping, when administered later in the day. No important effects appeared when both WAIS-III and the Wechsler Memory Scale-III (WMS-III) batteries were given in different order; the most pronounced score difference was on Digit-Symbol Coding when the WAIS-III was given last, an effect that could be due to fatigue (Zhu and Tulsky, 2000). The examiner who is accustomed to a specific presentation sequence may feel somewhat uncomfortable and less efficient if it is varied. In an examination tailored to the patient's needs, the examiner varies the testing sequence to ensure the patient's maximum productivity (e.g., see Benedict, Fischer, et al., 2002). For example, tests that the examiner suspects will be difficult for a particular patient can be given at the beginning of a testing session when the patient is least fatigued; or a test that has taxed or discouraged the patient can be followed by one on which the patient can relax or feel successful. The latest revisions of the WIS-A (WAIS-R, Wechsler, 1981; WAIS-III, Wechsler, 1997a–c) alternate verbal tests with visuoperceptual or construction tests as a standard procedure. This presentation sequence increases the likelihood that a test that is easy for the patient follows one that was difficult so that the patient need not experience one failure after another.

Another consideration in sequencing the tests is the need to keep the patient busy during the interval preceding delayed trials on learning tests. A format which makes the most economical use of examination time varies succeeding tasks with respect to modalities examined and difficulty levels while filling in these delay periods. The choice of these interval tasks should rest in part on whether high or low levels of potential interference are desired: if the question of interference susceptibility is important, the examiner may select a vocabulary or verbal fluency test as an interference test for word list learning; otherwise, selection of a word generating task should be avoided.

Testing the limits

Knowledge of the patient's capacities can be extended by going beyond the limits of the test set by the standard procedures.

The WIS-A oral Arithmetic questions provide a good example. When patients fail the more difficult items because of an auditory span, concentration, or mental tracking problem—which becomes obvious when patients ask to have the question repeated or repeat question elements incorrectly—the examiner still does not know whether they understand the problem, can perform the calculations correctly, or know what operations are called for. If the examiner stops at the point at which these patients fail the requisite number of items without further exploration, any conclusion drawn about the patient's arithmetic ability is questionable. In cases like this, arithmetic ability can easily be tested further by providing pencil and paper and repeating the failed items. Some patients can do the problems once they have written the elements down, and still others do not perform any better with paper than without it but provide written documentation of the nature of their difficulty.

Testing the limits does not affect the standard test procedures or scoring. It is done only after the test or test item in question has been completed according to standard test instructions. This method not only preserves the statistical and normative meaning of the test scores but it also can afford interesting and often important information about the patient's functioning.

For example, a patient who achieves an arithmetic score in the *borderline defective* ability range on the standard presentation of the test and who solves all the problems quickly and correctly at a *superior* level of functioning after writing down the elements of a problem, demonstrates a crippling auditory span or mental tracking problem with an intact capacity to handle quite complex computational problems as long as they can be seen. From the test score alone, one might conclude that the patient's competency to handle sizeable sums of money is questionable; on the basis of the more complete examination of arithmetic ability, the patient might be encouraged to continue bookkeeping and other arithmetic-dependent activities.

Testing the limits can be done with any test. The limits should be tested whenever there is suspicion that an impairment of some function other than the one under consideration is interfering with an adequate demonstration of that function. Imaginative and careful limit testing can provide a better understanding of the extent to which a function or functional system is impaired and the impact this impairment may have on related functional systems (R.F. Cohen and Mapou, 1988). Much of the special testing done with handicapped patients is a form of testing the limits (see B. Caplan and Shechter, 1995; pp. 118–120).

A limit-testing procedure has been formalized for the WIS battery (the *WAIS-R as a Neuropsychological Instrument* [WAIS-RNI]) (E. Kaplan, Fein, et al., 1991). While WIS-A tests are the subject matter for the techniques Kaplan and her colleagues have devised, these techniques can serve as models for expanded assessments generally (see also E. Kaplan, 1988).

Practice effects

The effects of repeated examinations have been studied in both normal subjects and brain damaged patients (McCaffrey, Duff, and Westervelt, 2000a,b). In the former and many of the latter, an overall pattern of test susceptibility to practice effects emerges. By and large, tests that have a large speed component, require an unfamiliar or infrequently practiced mode of response, or have a single solution—particularly if it can be easily conceptualized once it is attained—are more likely to show significant practice effects (M.R. Basso, Bornstein, and Lang, 1999; Bornstein, Baker, and Douglass, 1987; McCaffrey, Ortega, et al., 1993). This phenomenon appears on the WIS-A tests as the more unfamiliar tasks on the Performance Scale show greater practice effects than do the Verbal Scale tests (Cimino, 1994). It has also been seen in PET studies as shifts in activation patterns with repeated practise of a task (Démonet, 1995). The problem of practice effects is particularly important in memory testing since repeated

testing with the same tests leads to learning of the material in all but seriously memory-impaired patients (Benedict and Zgaljardic, 1998; Lezak, 1982c; B.A. Wilson, Watson, et al., 2000).

Numerous studies have also shown a general test-taking benefit in which enhanced performance may occur after repeated examinations, even with different test items (Benedict and Zgaljardic, 1998; B.A. Wilson, Watson, et al., 2000). The patient appears to learn how to approach the task more effectively, i.e., has acquired a test-taking set, or "test-wiseness." For many tests—particularly those with strong ceiling effects, such as digit span—the greatest practice effects are likely to occur between the first and second examinations (Benedict and Zgaljardic, 1998; Ivnik, Smith, Lucas, et al., 1999; Ivnik, Smith, Malec, et al., 1995; Rapport, Axelrod, et al., 1997). To bypass this problem, a frequently used research procedure provides for two or more baseline examinations before introducing an experimental condition (Fischer, 1999; McCaffery and Westervelt, 1995).

When a brain disorder renders a test, such as Block Design, difficult to conceptualize, the patient is unlikely to improve with practice alone (Diller, Ben-Yishay, et al., 1974). Improvements attributable to practice tend to be minimal, but this varies with the nature, site, and severity of the lesion and with the patient's age. B.A. Wilson, Watson, and their colleagues (2000) point out that test characteristics also determine whether brain injured patients' performances will improve with repetition. McCaffery, Duff, and Westervelt's (2000a,b) comprehensive and well-organized review of the hundreds of studies using repeated testing of both control and specified patient groups makes clear which tests are most vulnerable to practice effects and which patient groups tend to be least susceptible.

Except for single solution tests and others with a significant learning component, large changes between test and retest are not common among normal persons (Dikmen, Machamer, et al., 1990; McCaffery, Duff, and Westervelt, 2000a,b). On retest, WIS-A test scores have proven to be quite robust (Matarazzo, Carmody, and Jacobs, 1980; see McCaffery, Duff, and Westervelt, 2000a). For example, only 10% of the individual test scores obtained by 29 normal young adults on the WAIS changed more than two scaled score points in either direction on retest after a 20-week interval. Yet changes of three or more points occurred with sufficient frequency to lead the authors to caution against making inferences on the basis of any single score change "*in isolation*" (Matarazzo, Carmody, and Jacobs, 1980). These data illustrate how scores in the individual case may not follow group trends. Moreover, score stability when examined in healthy subjects can vary with the nature of the test: verbal knowledge and skills tend to be most stable over a period of years; retention scores show the greatest variability (Ivnik, Smith, Malec, et al., 1995).

Age differentials with respect to tendencies to practice effects have been reported, but no clear pattern emerges. On WIS-A tests some authors note a greater tendency for practice effects among younger subjects (Shatz, 1981), and some find little difference between younger (25–54) and older (75+) age groups, except for a significant effect for Digit Span (J.J. Ryan, Paolo, and Brungardt, 1992). Moreover, on one test of attention (Paced Auditory Serial Addition Test), a practice effect emerged for the 40–70 age range with little effect for ages 20–39; and another (Trail Making Test B) produced a U-shaped curve with greatest effects in the 20s and 50s and virtually none in the 30s and 40s (Stuss, Stethem, and Poirier, 1987). Practice effects occurred for adults 65–79 years old on the WMS-R Logical Memory test administered once a year for 4 years but not for subjects 80 and older (Hickman, Howieson, et al., 2000). Mitrushina and Satz (1991) found that unlike younger adults, those 75 years and older did not benefit from yearly repeated testing on a battery of tests. In both these studies, age-related decline may have offset practice effects. Moreover, in diseases that occur with aging, such as Alzheimer's disease, the impact of age and the disease may be compounded resulting in no practice benefits for these patients (D.B. Cooper et al., 2001).

Absence of practice effects on tests when the effect is expected, such as memory tests, may also be clinically meaningful. For example, for patients who have undergone temporal lobectomy, retest scores at levels similar to preoperative scores may reflect an actual decrement in learning ability, and a small decrement after surgery may indicate a fairly large loss in learning ability (Chelune, Naugle, et al., 1991). When a dementing condition is suspected, progression of even mildly lowered scores on tests typically vulnerable to practice effects suggests a deteriorating process (R.G. Knight, 1992).

The number of tests with alternate forms is limited because of the need to produce tests with demonstrated interform reliability. If alternate forms do not have an equal level of difficulty, then changing forms may introduce more unwanted variance than practice effects (see Benedict and Zgaljardic, 1998).

Use of technicians

Reliance on technicians to administer and score tests expanded with the use of commercially available batteries, particularly the Halstead-Reitan Battery (HRB) (DeLuca, 1989). Some neuropsychologists base their reports entirely on what the technician provides in terms of scores and observations. Most neuropsychologists who use technicians have them give the routine tests; the neuropsychologist conducts the interviews and additional specialized testing as needed, writes reports, and consults with patients and referral sources.

The advantages of using a technician are obvious: Saving time enables the neuropsychologist to see more patients. In research projects, in which immutable test selection judgments have been completed before any subjects are examined and qualitative data are usually irrelevant, having technicians do the assessments is typically the best use of everyone's time and may contribute to objective data collection (NAN Policy and Planning Committee, 2000b). Moreover, as technicians are paid at one-third or less the rate of a neuropsychologist, a technician-examiner can reduce costs at savings to the patients or a research grant. When the technician is a sensitive observer and the neuropsychologist has also conducted a reasonably lengthy examination with the patient, the patient benefits in having been observed by two clinicians, thus reducing the likelihood of important information being overlooked.

However, there are disadvantages as well. They will be greatest for those who write their reports on the basis of "blind analysis," as these neuropsychologists cannot identify testing errors, appreciate the extent to which patients' emotional status and attitudes toward the examination colored their test performances, or have any idea of what might have been missed in terms of important qualitative aspects of performance or problems in major areas of cognitive functioning that a hypothesis-testing approach would have brought to light. In referring to the parallel between blind analysis in neuropsychology and laboratory procedures in medicine, John Reddon observed that "some neuropsychologists think that a report can be written about a patient without ever seeing the patient because Neuropsychology is only concerned with the brain or CNS. . . . Urine analysts or MRI or CT analysts do not see their patients before interpreting their test results so why should neuropsychologists?" He then answered this question by pointing out that neuropsychological assessment is not simply a medical procedure but requires "a holistic approach that considers the patient as a person . . . and not just a brain that can be treated in isolation" (Reddon, personal communication, 1989 [mdl]). Moreover, insensitive technicians who generate test scores without keeping a record of how the patient performs, or whose observations tend to be limited by inadequate training or lack of experience, can only provide a restricted data base for those functions they examine. Prigatano (2000) points out that when most of the patient's contact is with a technician who simply tests in a lengthy examination, and the neuropsychologist—who has seen the patient only briefly, if at all—seems more interested in the test scores than in the patient, the patient is more likely to come away unhappy about the examination experience.

The minimal education and training requirements for technicians are spelled out in the report of the Division 40 (American Psychological Association) Task Force on Education, Accreditation, and Credentialing (1989; Bornstein, 1991) and have been further elaborated in an American Academy of Clinical Neuropsychology policy statement (1999) on "use of nondoctoral level personnel in conducting clinical neuropsychological evaluations." "These psychometric technicians, psychometrists, and other psychologist-assistants, as well as trainees enrolled in formal educational and training programs" typically hold nondoctoral degrees in psychology or related fields. Their role has been clearly defined as strictly limited to administering and scoring tests under the supervision of a licensed neuropsychologist whose responsibility it is to select and interpret the tests, do the clinical interviews, and communicate the examination findings appropriately (American Academy of Clinical Neuropsychology, 1999; see also McSweeny and Naugle, 2002; NAN Policy and Planning Committee, 2000b).

Examining Special Populations

Patients with sensory or motor deficits

Visual problems. Many persons referred for neuropsychological assessment will have reduced visual acuity or other visual problems that could interfere with their test performance. Defective visual acuity is common in elderly persons and may be due to any number of problems—such as blurring, *presbyopia* (age-related far-sightedness), cataract, and corneal disorders—and frequently to some combination of them (Godwin-Austen and Bendall, 1990; Matjucha and Katz, 1994; E. Wallace et al., 1994). M. Cohen and colleagues (1989) documented defective convergence—which is necessary for efficient near vision—in 42% of traumatically brain injured patients requiring rehabilitation services. These authors noted that other visual disturbances were also common after head injury, mostly clearing up during the first postinjury year.

A visual problem that can occur after a head injury, stroke, or other abrupt insult to the brain, or that may be symptomatic of degenerative disease of the central nervous system, is eye muscle imbalance resulting in double vision (*diplopia*). Patients may not see double at all angles or in all areas of the visual field and may experience only slight discomfort or confusion with the head tilted a certain way. For others the diplopia may compromise their ability to read, write, draw, or solve intricate visual puzzles altogether. Young, well-motivated patients with diplopia frequently learn to suppress one set of images and, within one to three years, become relatively untroubled by the problem. Other patients report that they have been handicapped for years by what may appear on examination to be a minor disability. Should the patient complain of visual problems, the examiner may want a neurological or ophthalmological opinion before determining whether the patient can be examined with tests requiring visual acuity.

Persons over the age of 45 need to be checked for visual competency as many of them will need reading glasses for fine, close work. Those who use reading glasses should be reminded to bring them to the examination. Not infrequently, hospitalized patients will not have brought their glasses with them. Examiners in hospital settings in particular should keep reading glasses with their testing equipment.

Hearing problems. Although most people readily acknowledge their visual defects, many who are hard-of-hearing are secretive about auditory handicaps. It is not unusual to find hard-of-hearing persons who prefer to guess what the examiner is saying rather than admit their problem and ask the examiner to speak up. It is also not unusual for persons in obvious need of hearing aids to reject their use, even when they own aids that have been fitted for them. Sensitive observation can often uncover hearing impairment, as these patients may cock their head to direct their best ear to the examiner, make a consistent pattern of errors in response to the examiner's questions or comments, or ask the examiner to repeat what was said. When hard-of-hearing patients come for the examination without hearing aids, the examiner must speak loudly, clearly, and slowly, and check for receptive accuracy by having these patients repeat what they think they have heard.

Patients coming for neuropsychological assessment are more likely to have hearing loss than the population at large. Along with cognitive and other kinds of deficits, hearing impairments can occur as a result of brain damage. Moreover, defective hearing increases with advancing age so that many patients with neurological disorders associated with aging will also have compromised hearing (E. Wallace et al., 1994; M. Vernon, 1989). Diminished sound detection is not the only problem that affects auditory acuity. Some patients who have little difficulty hearing most sounds, even soft ones, find it hard to discriminate sounds such as certain consonants. A commonly used but crude test of auditory acuity involving rattling paper or snapping fingers by the patient's ear will not identify this problem which can seriously interfere with accurate cognitive testing (Schear, Skenes, and Larson, 1988).

Lateralized sensory deficits. Brain impaired patients with lateralized lesions will have reduced vision or hearing on the side opposite the lesion with little awareness that they have such a problem. This is particularly true for patients who have *homonymous field cuts* (loss of vision in the same part of the field of each eye) or in whom nerve damage has reduced auditory acuity or auditory discrimination functions in one ear only. Their normal conversational behavior may give no hint of the deficit, yet presentation of test material to the affected side makes their task more difficult (B. Caplan, 1985).

The neuropsychologist is often not able to find out quickly and reliably whether the patient's sight or hearing has suffered impairment. Therefore, when the patient is known to have a lateralized lesion, it is a good testing practice for the examiner to sit either across from the patient or to the side least likely to be affected. The examiner must take care that the patient can see all of the visually presented material and the examiner should speak to the ear on the side of the lesion. Patients with right-sided lesions, in particular, may have reduced awareness of stimuli in the left half of space so that all material must be presented to their right side. Use of vertical arrays for presenting visual stimuli to these patients should be considered (B. Caplan, 1988; B. Caplan and Shechter, 1995).

Motor problems. Motor deficits do not present as great an obstacle to standardized and comprehensive testing as sensory deficits since most all but constructional abilities can be examined when a patient is unable to use either hand. Many brain injured patients with lateralized lesions will have use of only one hand, and that may not be the preferred hand. One-handed performances on construction or drawing tests tend to be a little slowed, particularly when performed by the nonpreferred hand. In one study, neurologically intact subjects using the nonpreferred hand in drawing tasks tended to make no more errors than with the preferred hand, although left-handed distortion errors were notably greater than those made by the right hand (Dee and Fontenot, 1969). Yet another study found that intact right-handed subjects tended to perform visuomotor tasks more accurately with their left than their right hands, "presumably because they were being more attentive and cautious" when using the nonpreferred hand (Y. Kim et al., 1984).

Meeting the challenge of sensory or motor deficits. Neuropsychological assessment of patients with sensory or motor deficits presents the problem of testing a variety of functions in as many modalities as possible with a more or less restricted test repertory. Since almost all psychological tests have been constructed with physically able persons in mind, examiners often have to find reasonable alternatives to the standard tests the physically impaired patient cannot use, or they have to juggle test norms, improvise, or, as a last resort, do without (B. Caplan and Shechter, 1995).

Although the examination of patients with sensory or motor disabilities is necessarily limited insofar as the affected input or output modality is concerned, the disability should not preclude at least some test evaluation of any cognitive function or executive capacity not immediately dependent on the affected modality. Of course, blind patients cannot be tested for their ability to organize visual percepts, nor can patients with profound facial paralysis be tested for verbal fluency; but patients with these deficits can be tested for memory and learning, arithmetic, vocabulary, abstract reasoning, comprehension of spatial relationships, a multitude of verbal skills, and other abilities.

Published tests that can be substituted for those ordinarily given are available for most general functions. Deaf patients can be given printed tests or the examiner can write out what is normally spoken; questions can be read to blind patients. For verbal and mathematical functions, there are many printed and orally administered tests of arithmetic skills, vocabulary, and abstract reasoning in particular that have useful norms. Other common tests of verbal functions, such as tests of background information, common sense reasoning and judgment, and verbal (reading) comprehension, do not have fully standardized counterparts in the other modality, whether it be visual or auditory. For some of these, similar kinds of alternative tests are available although formats, norms, or standardization populations may differ. For example, language responses of deaf patients are slower when signed than when spoken (A.B. Wolff et al., 1989).

There are fewer ready-made substitutes for tests involving pictures or designs although some test parallels can be found, and the clinician may be able to invent others. The *haptic* (touch) modality lends itself most readily as a substitute for visually presented tests of nonverbal functions. For example, to assess concept formation of blind patients, size, shape, and texture offer testable dimensions. To test pattern learning or searching behavior, tactile mazes may be used in place of visual mazes. Three-dimensional block constructions will test constructional functions of patients who cannot see painted designs or printed patterns. Even so, it is difficult to find a suitable nonvisual alternative for perceptual organization tests such as the Hooper Visual Organization Test or Picture Arrangement, for a visuoconstructive task such as drawing a house or a bicycle, or for many other tests requiring vision. However, for sighted patients, even older ones or those whose near vision is below average, acuity does not seem to contribute importantly to performance on the visually presented WIS-A tests and others in general use (Schear and Sato, 1989; Storandt and Futterman, 1982).

The patient with a movement disorder presents similar challenges. Visuoperceptual functions in these patients can be relatively easily tested since most tests of these functions lend themselves to spoken answers or pointing. However, drawing tasks requiring relatively fine motor coordination cannot be satisfactorily evaluated when the patient's preferred hand is paralyzed or spastic. Even when only the nonpreferred hand is involved, some inefficiency and slowing on other construction tasks will result from the patient's inability to anchor a piece of paper with the nonpreferred hand or to turn blocks or manipulate parts of a puzzle with two-handed efficiency. After discussing some of the major issues in assessing patients with movement disorders (e.g., Huntington's disease, Parkinson's disease, cerebellar dysfunction), Stout and Paulsen (2003) identify the motor demands and suggest possible adaptations for a number of tests in most common use.

Some tests have been devised specifically for physically handicapped people. Most of them are listed in test catalogues or can be located through local rehabilitation services. One problem that these substitute tests present is normative comparability; but since this is a problem in any substitute or alternative version of a standard test, it should not dissuade the examiner if the procedure appears to test the relevant functions. Another problem is that alternative forms usually test many fewer and sometimes different functions than the original test. For example, multiple-choice forms of design copying tests obviously do not measure constructional abilities. What may be less obvious is the loss of the data about the patient's ability to organize, plan, and order responses. Unless the examiner is fully aware of all that is missing in an alternative battery, some important functions may be overlooked.

The severely handicapped patient

When mental or physical handicaps greatly limit the range of response, it may first be necessary to determine whether the patient has enough verbal comprehension for formal testing procedures. A set of questions and commands calling for one-word answers and simple gestures will quickly give the needed information. Those that are simplest and most likely to be answered are given first to increase the likelihood of initial success. Questions calling for "yes" or "no" answers will not be useful when patients with impaired speech cannot sound out the difference between "uh-huh" and "unh-unh" clearly, nor is it easy for weak or

tremulous patients to nod or waggle their heads with distinct precision. However, when patients can say "yes" and "no" distinctly, a series of questions calling for these responses can assess many aspects of cognitive functioning since significantly more than 50% must be correct to exceed random responding (McMillan, 1996a; McMillan and Herbert, 2000).

A speaking patient might be asked the following kinds of questions:

What is your name?
What is your age?
Where are you now?
What do you call this (hand, thumb, article of patient's clothing, coin, button, or safety pin)?
What do you do with a (pen, comb, matches, key)?
What color is (your tie, my dress, etc.)?
How many fingers can you see (two or three trials)?
How many coins in my hand (two or three trials)?
Say the alphabet; count from one to twenty.

Patients who do not speak well enough to be understood can be examined for verbal comprehension and ability to follow directions.

Show me your (hand, thumb, a button, your nose).
Give me your (left, right [the nonparalyzed]) hand.
Put your (nonparalyzed) hand on your (left, right [other]) elbow.

Place several small objects (button, coin, etc.) in front of the patient with a request.

Show me the button (or key, coin, etc.).
Show me what opens doors. How do you use it?
Show me what you use to write. How do you use it?
Do what I do (salute; touch nose, ear opposite hand, chin in succession).

Place several coins in front of the patient.

Show me the quarter (nickel, dime, etc.).
Show me the smallest coin.
Give me (three, two, five) coins.

Patients who can handle a pencil may be asked to write their name, age, where they live, and to answer simple questions calling for "yes," "no," short word, or simple number answers; and to write the alphabet and the first twenty numbers. Patients who cannot write may be asked to draw a circle, copy a circle drawn by the examiner, copy a vertical line drawn by the examiner, draw a square, and imitate the examiner's gestures and patterns of tapping with a pencil. Word recognition can be tested by asking the patient to point to one of several words printed on a word card or piece of paper that is the same as a spoken word (e.g., "cat": cat, dog, hat), or that answers a question (e.g., "Which do you wear on your head?"). Reading comprehension can be tested by printing the question as well as the answers or by giving the patient a card with printed instructions such as, "If you are a man (or "if it is morning"), hand this card back to me; but if you are a woman (or "if it is afternoon"), set it down." The Boston Diagnostic Aphasia Examination (Goodglass and Kaplan, 1983b) and other tests for aphasia contain similar low-level questions that can be appropriate for nonaphasic but motorically and/or mentally handicapped patients. Adamovich and her colleagues (1985) describe a variety of tasks for low level assessment of nonspeaking patients.

Patients who respond to most of these questions correctly are able to comprehend and cooperate well enough for formal testing. Patients unable to answer more than two or three questions probably cannot be tested reliably. Their behavior is best evaluated by rating scales (see Chapter 18, *passim*).

A case report of a 22-year-old woman rendered quadriplegic and anarthric by a traffic TBI was dependent on a feeding tube to live, and considered to be in a vegetative state (McMillan, 1996a). Euthanasia was considered, but first the court required a neurobehavioral examination. It was found that she could press a button with her clenched right hand. She was instructed in a pattern of holding or withholding the button press for "yes" and "no" respectively. With this response capacity in place, she was given a set of questions of the order, "Is your sister's name Lydia?" "Is your sister's name Lucy?", with correct "yes" responses randomized among the "no" responses. By this technique, cognitive competency was established, which allowed further exploration into her feelings, insight into her condition, and whether she wanted to live. She did, and continued to want to live at least for the next several years, despite her report of some pain and depression. (McMillan and Herbert, 2000)

The severely brain damaged patient

With few exceptions, tests developed for adults have neither items nor norms for grading the performance of severely mentally impaired adults. On adult tests, the bottom 1% or 2% of the noninstitutionalized adult population can usually pass the simplest items. These items leave a relatively wide range of behaviors unexamined and are too few to allow for meaningful performance gradations. Yet it is as important to know about the impairment pattern, the rate and extent of improvement or deterioration, and the relative strengths and weaknesses of the severely brain damaged patient as it is for the less afflicted patient.

For patients with severe mental deficits, one solution is to use children's tests (e.g., see E.M. Taylor, 1959: despite its age, this book contains many tests applicable to very impaired adults). Tests developed for children examine many functions in every important modality as well as providing children's norms for some

tests originally developed for adults (for example, the *Developmental Test of Visual-Motor Integration* or the *Snijders-Oomen Nonverbal Intelligence Test [SON-R 5¹/₂–17]*). Most of the *Woodcock-Johnson III Tests of Cognitive Abilities* extend to those younger than 2 years, all go to prekindergarten levels, and almost all have norms going to adult levels. When given to retarded adults, children's tests require little or no change in wording or procedure. At the lowest performance levels, the examiner may have to evaluate observations of the patient by means of developmental scales.

Some simple tests and tests of discrete functions were devised for use with severely impaired adults. Tests for elderly patients suspected of having deteriorating brain diseases are generally applicable to very defective adults of all ages (K.J. Christensen, Multhaup, et al., 1991a; Fuld, 1980; Fuld, Masur, et al., 1990; Mattis, 1988; Saxton, McGonigle-Gibson, et al., 1990; Saxton and Swihart, 1989; and the CERAD battery, J.C. Morris, Heyman, Mohs, et al., 1989). A.-L. Christensen's (1979) systematization of Luria's neuropsychological investigation techniques gives detailed instructions for examining many of the perceptual, motor, and narrowly defined cognitive functions basic to complex cognitive and adaptive behavior. These techniques are particularly well suited for patients who are too impaired to respond meaningfully to graded tests of cognitive prowess but whose residual capacities need assessment for rehabilitation or management. Their clinical value lies in their flexibility, their focus on qualitative aspects of the data they elicit, and their facilitation of useful behavioral descriptions of the individual patient. Observations made by means of Luria's techniques or by means of the developmental scales and simple tests that enable the examiner to discern and discriminate functions at low performance levels cannot be reduced to numbers and arithmetic operations without losing the very sensitivity that examination of these functions and good neuropsychological practice requires.

Elderly persons

Psychological studies of elderly people have shown that, with some psychometrically important exceptions, healthy and active people in their seventies and eighties do not differ greatly in skills or abilities from the generations following them (Howieson, Holm, and Kaye, 1993; Tranel, Benton, and Olson, 1997; see also pp. 296–300, *passim*). However, the diminished sensory acuity, motor strength and speed, and particularly, flexibility and adaptability that accompany advancing age are apt to affect the elderly person's test performance adversely (Bondi, Salmon, and Kaszniak, 1996). These age-related handicaps can result in spuriously low scores and incorrect conclusions about the cognitive functioning of older persons (Birren and Schaie, 1989, *passim;* Lindley, 1989). I.K. Krauss (1980) offered guidelines for evaluating the older worker's capacity to continue employment that can apply to neuropsychological assessment of the elderly as well. Among them are recommendations that print be large and of high contrast; that answer sheets, which typically add a visual search dimension to whatever else is being tested, be eliminated; that tests have as high face validity as possible; and that norms be appropriate.

When examining elderly people, the clinician needs to determine whether their auditory and visual acuity is adequate for the tests they will be taking and, if not, to make every effort to correct the deficit or assist them in compensating for it (Lezak, 1986; Schear and Skenes, 1991; M. Vernon, 1989). Some conditions that can adversely affect a person's neuropsychological status are more common among the elderly. These include fatigue, central nervous system side effects due to medication, and lowered energy level or feelings of malaise associated with a chronic illness (Lawton, 1986). A review of the patient's recent health history should help the examiner to identify these problems so that testing will be appropriate for the patient's physical capacities and test interpretation will take such problems into account.

A pattern of slowly paced speech using words of low complexity, called "Elderspeak" has been recommended to clinicians working with older persons (L.C. McGuire et al., 2000). This should come easily to sensitive examiners who have already been modifying their speech patterns for their more severely impaired patients. Although McGuire and her colleagues recommend "Elderspeak" when important information is given to older persons—and by implication, when examining them—the examiner must judge when it is appropriate and when a sophisticated and alert patient would feel demeaned by such simplified speech.

Since age-related slowing affects the performance of timed tasks, the examiner who is interested in how elderly patients perform a given timed task can administer it without timing (e.g., see Storandt, 1977). Although this is not a standardized procedure, it will provide the qualitative information about whether they can do the task at all, what kinds of errors they make, how well they correct them, etc. This procedure will probably answer most of the examination questions that prompted use of the timed test. Since older persons are also apt to be more cautious (Schaie, 1974), this too may contribute to performance slowing. When the examiner suspects that patients are being unduly cautious, an explanation of the need to work quickly may help them perform more efficiently.

Often the most important factor in examining elderly persons is their cooperation (Aiken, 1980; Holden, 1988b). With no school requirements to be met, no jobs to prepare for, and usually little previous experience with psychological tests, retired persons may very reasonably not want to go through fatiguing mental gymnastics that may well make them look stupid to the youngster in the white coat sitting across the table. Particularly if they are not feeling well or are concerned about diminishing mental acuity, elderly persons may view a test as a nuisance or an unwarranted intrusion into their privacy. Thus, explaining to elderly persons the need for the examination and introducing them to the testing situation will often require more time than with younger people. When the patient is ill or convalescing, the examiner needs to be especially alert to signs of fatigue and sensitive to testing problems created by an unusually short attention span or increased distractibility. It has been suggested that some of these problems can be avoided by examining elderly people with familiar materials such as playing cards or popular magazines, and designing tasks that are obviously meaningful and nonthreatening (Holden, 1988b; Krauss, 1980).

When examinee and examiner speak different languages

Migration—of refugees, of persons seeking work or rejoining their displaced families—has brought millions of people into cultures and language environments foreign to them. When understanding or treatment of a brain disorder would benefit from neuropsychological assessment, the examiner must address a new set of issues if the patient is to be treated appropriately.

Translators and interpreters. In many big cities with relatively large populations of foreign language speakers, medical centers provide interpreters, e.g., in our medical center, besides Spanish and Russian, translators are available for several Asian languages and the common European ones [dbh, mdl]. Metropolitan court systems also will have a pool of interpreters available. However, even when the interpreter can provide a technically accurate rendition of test questions and patient responses, slippages in the interpreter's understanding of what is actually required or some of our terms of art can result in an inadequate or biased examination, especially when the examiner's language is the interpreter's second—or even third—language (see pp. 313, 314).

Ideally, when working with an interpreter, the examiner reviews the assessment procedures, including intentional and idiomatic aspects of the wording of instructions and test questions, so that the interpreter has a practical idea of the normal response expectations for any item or test. In practice, this can rarely be accomplished because of time and cost limitations. Thus, when working with a neuropsychologically naive interpreter who is also unfamiliar with tests and test culture, the examiner must be on the lookout for unexpected aberrations in the patient's responses as these could indicate translation slippage in one or the other direction. Slippages may be easiest to recognize on such tests as Wechsler's Arithmetic, Digit Span or Block Design tests, or word fluency, confrontation naming, or design copying tests in which little cultural bias enters into the task and most people in most cultures are equipped to respond appropriately given the correct instructions.

Some tests will be more susceptible to cultural bias than others: Wechsler's Comprehension and Picture Arrangement tests, for example, both require fairly subtle social understandings to achieve a high score; a request to draw a bicycle is asking for failure from a refugee raised in a hill village—but may be an effective way of examining an urban Chinese person. Still, for a Spanish language battery developed for Hispanics of Latin American background or birth in the United States, education turned out to be an overriding variable despite efforts to make the tests culture-compatible (Pontón, Satz, et al., 1996). All tests were affected, both word-based and predominantly visual ones, including Block Design, the Complex Figure Test, and a test of fine motor dexterity. Lowest correlations with education occurred where least expected—on the WHO-UCLA Auditory Verbal Learning Test (Maj, D'Elia, et al., 1993).

Examiners need also be aware that bilingualism can alter normal performance expectations (Ardila, 2000a). A group of community living Spanish–English speakers performed speed and calculation tasks better in their first language (Ardila, Rosselli, Ostrosky-Solis, et al., 2000), but bilinguals' production on a semantic fluency task fell below that of monolinguals and their own phonetic fluency (Rosselli, Ardila, Ostrosky-Solis, et al., 2000). Adults fully fluent in their second language performed memory and learning tasks at the same level as monolingual subjects; but those who were weaker in their second language had lower rates of learning and retention (J.G. Harris, Cullum, and Puente, 1995).

Clinicians practising independently or in smaller communities may not have access to trained interpreters and thus face a dilemma: to examine, however crudely, or to refer to someone who can provide for translation or who speaks the patient's language. Nonverbal tests are available for examining these patients, but they require the subject to have an understanding of Western culture and at least a modicum of formal education, which makes these tests unsuitable for use with many migrants throughout the world. These tests have typically been developed to examine the mental abilities of children but, with age ranges into the late teens, they are applicable to adults (e.g., Bracken and McCallum, 1998; Hammill et al.; P.J. Tellegen et al., 1998). Artiola i Fortuny and Mullaney (1998) point out the ethical hazards when an examiner has only a superficial knowledge of the patient's language. They advise examiners not well-grounded in a language to get an interpreter or make an appropriate referral. La-Calle (1987) warns against casual interpreters, usually family members or friends, who may be ill-equipped to translate accurately or protective of the patient.

Cultural factors

The patient's cultural background should be considered when planning and interpreting assessment data (see pp. 310–312). Awareness of cross-cultural influences and bias becomes essential for the assessment of people who come from cultural backgrounds other than those of a test's developers and original standardization population (Ardila, 1995; Loewenstein, Arguelles, et al., 1994; Perez-Arce, 1999). A leading assessment problem is the lack of well-standardized, culturally relevant tests for minority groups. One approach to the problem is to use tests that show the least cross-cultural differences (e.g., Levav et al., 1998; Maj et al., 1993). Other workers have focused on the need to develop tests and normative data appropriate for distinct cultural groups (e.g., D.M. Jacobs et al., 1997; Mungas and Reed, 2000; Rey et al., 1999).

Common Assessment Problems with Brain Disorders

The mental inefficiency that often prompts a referral for neuropsychological assessment presents both conditions that need to be investigated in their own right and obstacles to a fair assessment of cognitive abilities. Thus the examiner must not only document the presence and nature of mental inefficiency problems but must attempt to get as full a picture as possible of the cognitive functions that may be compromised by mental inefficiency.

Attentional deficits

Attentional deficits can obscure the patient's abilities in almost every area of cognitive functioning. Their effects tend to show up in those activities that provide little or no visual guidance and thus require the patient to perform most of the task's operations mentally. While some patients with attentional deficits will experience difficulty in all aspects of attention, the problems of many other patients will be confined to only one or two of them.

Reduced auditory span. Many patients have a reduced auditory attention span such that they only hear part of what was said, particularly if the message is relatively long, complex, or contains unfamiliar or unexpected wording. These are the patients who, when given a 23-syllable request to subtract a calculated sum from "a half-dollar," subtract the correct sum correctly from a dollar, thus giving an erroneous response to the question and earning no credit. When asked to repeat what they heard, these patients typically report, "a dollar," the "half" getting lost in what was for them too much verbiage to process at once. Their correct answers to shorter but more difficult arithmetic items and their good performances when given paper and pencil will further demonstrate the attentional nature of their error.

Mental tracking problems. Other patients may have mental tracking problems; i.e., difficulty juggling information mentally or keeping track of complex information. They get confused or completely lost performing complex mental tracking tasks such as serial subtraction, although they can readily demonstrate their arithmetic competence on paper. These problems often show up in many repetitions on list-learning or list-generating tasks when patients have difficulty keeping track of their ongoing mental activities, e.g., what they have already said, while still actively conducting a mental search.

Distractibility. Another common concomitant of brain impairment is distractibility: some patients have difficulty shutting out or ignoring extraneous stimulation, be it noise outside the testing room, test material scattered on the examination table, or a brightly colored tie or flashy earrings on the examiner. This difficulty may exacerbate attentional problems and increase the likelihood of fatigue and frustration. Distractibility can interfere with learning and cognitive performances generally (Aks and Coren, 1990). The examiner may not appreciate the patient's difficulty, for the normal person screens out extraneous stimuli so automatically that most people are unaware that this problem exists for others. To reduce the likelihood of interference from unnecessary distractions, the examination should be conducted in what is sometimes referred to as a "sterile environment." The examining room should be relatively soundproof and decorated in quiet colors, with no bright or distracting objects in sight. The examiner's clothing too can be an unwitting source of distraction. Drab colors and quiet patterns or a lab coat are recommended apparel for testing. The examining table should be kept bare except for materials needed for the test at hand.

Clocks and ticking sounds can be bothersome. Clocks should be quiet and out of sight, even when test instructions include references to timing. A wall or desk clock with an easily readable second indicator, placed out of the patient's line of sight, is an excellent substitute for a stopwatch and frees the examiner's hands for note taking and manipulation of test materials. An efficient way to use a watch or regular clock for unobtrusive timing is to pay attention only to the second marker, noting in seconds the times at which a task was begun and completed. Minutes are marked with a slash. Total time is then 60 sec for each slash plus the number of seconds between the two times. For example, $53 \ // \ 18 = ([60 - 53] + 18) + 120 = 145$ seconds. The examiner can count times under 30 seconds with a fair degree of accuracy by making a dot on the answer sheet every 5 seconds.

Street noises, a telephone's ring, or a door slamming down the hall can easily break an ongoing train of thought in many brain damaged patients. If this occurs in the middle of a timed test, the examiner must decide whether to repeat the item, count the full time taken—including the interruption and recovery—count the time minus the interruption and recovery time, do the item over using an alternate form if possible, skip that item and prorate the score, or repeat the test again another day. Should there not be another testing day, then an alternate form is the next best choice, and an estimate of time taken without the interruption is a third choice. A prorated score is also acceptable.

A record of the effects of interruptions due to distractibility on timed tasks gives valuable information about the patient's efficiency. Comparisons between *efficiency* (performance under standard conditions) and *ability* (performance under optimal conditions) are important for understanding both competencies and deficits, as well as for rehabilitation and vocational planning (Corkin, Growdon, Desclos, and Rosen, 1989; Gronwall and Sampson, 1974). The actual effect of the distraction, whether it be in terms of increased response time, lowered productivity within the allotted time, or more errors, should also be noted and reported. Moreover, Nemec's (1978) identification of differences in susceptibility to auditory-verbal or visual pattern distractors in left and right hemisphere damaged patients, respectively, has practical implications for testing in terms of the kinds of distractors most likely to disturb a particular patient.

The sensitive examiner will document attention lapses and how they affect the patient's performance generally and within specific functional domains. Whenever possible, these lapses need to be explored, usually through testing the limits, to clarify the level of the patient's actual ability to perform a particular kind of task and how the attentional problem(s) interferes.

Memory disorders

Many problems in following instructions or correctly comprehending lengthy or complex test items read aloud by the examiner seem to be due to faulty memory but actually reflect attentional deficits. However, memory disorders too can interfere with assessment procedures.

Defective working memory. A few patients have difficulty retaining information, such as instructions on what to do, for more than a minute or two. They may fail a task for performing the wrong operation rather than because of inability to do what was required. This problem can show up on tasks requiring a series of responses. For example, on the Picture Completion test of the WIS-A battery, rather than continuing to indicate what is missing in the pictures, some patients begin reporting what they think is *wrong;* yet if reminded of the instructions, many will admit they forgot what they were supposed to do and then proceed to respond correctly. If not reminded, they would have failed on items they could do perfectly well, and the low score—if interpreted as due to a visuoperceptual or reasoning problem—would have been seriously misleading. Similar instances of forgetting can show up on certain tests of the ability to generate hypotheses (e.g., Category Test, Wisconsin Card Sorting Test, and Object Identification Task) in which patients who have figured out the response pattern that emerges in the course of working through a series of items subsequently forget it as they work through the series. In these latter tasks the examiner must note when failure occurs after the correct hypothesis has been achieved as these failures may indicate defective working memory.

Defective retrieval. A not uncommon source of poor scores on memory tests is defective retrieval. Many patients with retrieval problems learn well but are unable to recall at will what they have learned. When learning is not examined by means of a recognition format or by cueing techniques, a naive examiner can easily misinterpret the patient's poor showing on free recall as evidence of a learning problem. Perhaps more than any other sin against patients committed by naive and inadequately trained examiners is that of mistaking defective retrieval for a learning disorder.

Fatigue

Patients with brain disorders tend to fatigue easily, particularly when an acute condition occurred relatively recently (Lezak, 1978b; van Zomeren and Brouwer, 1990). Easy fatigability can also be a chronic problem in some conditions, such as multiple sclerosis (R.H. Paul et al., 1998b), Parkinson's disease (Karlsen et al., 1999) and, of course, chronic fatigue syndrome (Tiersky et al., 1997). Once fatigued, the patients take longer to recuperate than do normal persons.

The cognitive effects of fatigue have been studied in association with a variety of medical conditions including cancer (Cull et al., 1996; C.A. Meyers, 2000a,b), chemotherapy (Caraceni et al., 1998; P.B. Jacobsen et al., 1999; Valentine et al., 1998), respiratory disease (P.D. White et al., 1998), and post-polio syndrome (Bruno et al., 1993). When associated cognitive impairments have been found, they involve sustained attention, concentration, reaction time, and processing speed (Groopman, 1998; Tiersky et al., 1997). Several research groups have studied people after fatigue-producing exercise or sleep deprivation. In one study, healthy young males had slower choice reaction times following heavy exercise compared to lighter exercise (Fery and Ferry, 1997). Four administrations of the Paced Auditory Serial Addition Test (PASAT) (pp. 364–365), chosen because it requires mental exertion, were given within three hours to patients whose condition tends to make them fatigue-prone (S.K. Johnson et al., 1997). Patient groups performed consistently below control level, with chronic fatigue and depressed patients showing significant fatigue effects despite intervening rest periods. Studies of sleep deprivation have found deficits in hand–eye coordination (D. Dawson and Reid, 1997), psychomotor vigilance (Dinges et al., 1997), executive function (Fluck and File, 1998), psychomotor speed and accuracy, and visuospatial reasoning and recall (Verstraeten et al., 1996).

However, some studies report no association between complaints of fatigue and neuropsychological impairment (e.g., Schagen et al., 1999; C.E. Schwartz et al., 1996) or an association with one condition (chronic fatigue syndrome) but not with others (multiple sclerosis, depression; S.K. Johnson et al., 1997). Stuss, Stethem, Hugenholtz, and their colleagues (1989) reported that TBI patients performing reaction time tasks for 90 minutes did not show fatigue effects, regardless of injury severity. Complaints of poor concentration and memory in some patients may be related to mood disorders (Cull, Hay, et al., 1996) or fatigue-related distress (C.E. Schwartz et al., 1996) rather than associated fatigue. TBI patients with complaints of mental fatigue were compared with controls on a divided attention task under conditions of increasing attentional demands, with no differences appearing between the two groups (H. Riese, Hoedemaeker, Brouwer, et al., 1999).

Many brain impaired patients will tell the examiner when they are tired, but others may not be aware themselves or may be unwilling to admit fatigue. Therefore, the examiner must be alert to such signs as slurring of speech, an increased droop on the paralyzed side of the patient's face, motor slowing increasingly apparent as the examination continues, or restlessness. Patients who are abnormally susceptible to fatigue are most apt to be rested and energized in the early morning and will perform at their best at this time. Even the seemingly restful interlude of lunch may require considerable effort from a debilitated patient and increase fatigue. Physical or occupational therapy is exhausting for many postacute patients. Therefore, in arranging test time, the patient's daily activity schedule must be considered if the effects of fatigue are to be kept minimal. When necessary, the examiner may insist that the patient take a nap before being tested. For patients who must be examined late in the day, in addition to requesting that they rest beforehand, the examiner should recommend that they have a snack.

Some patients fatigue so quickly that they can only work for brief periods. Their examination may continue over days if their performance begins to suffer noticeably after 10–15 minutes of concentrated effort. On occasion, a patient's fatigue may require the examiner to stop testing in the middle of a test in which items are graduated in difficulty or arranged to produce a learning effect. When the test is resumed, the examiner must decide whether to start from the beginning and risk overlearning or pick up where they left off, taking a chance that the patient will have lost the response set or forgotten what was learned on the first few items.

Pain

Certain pain syndromes are common in the general population, particularly headache and back pain. Many patients with traumatic brain injury experience pain whether from headaches or bodily injuries, and pain may result from other brain disorders such as thalamic stroke, multiple sclerosis, or disease involving cranial or peripheral nerves.

Patients with pain often have reduced attentional capacity, processing speed, and psychomotor speed (Grigsby, Rosenberg, and Busenbark, 1995). When comparing TBI patients with and without pain complaints and TBI noncomplainers with neurologically intact chronic pain patients, those complaining of pain tended to perform more poorly (see R.P. Hart, Martelli, and Zasler, 2000, for a review of recent studies). Deficits in learning and problem solving too occur in some neurologically intact pain patients (Blackwood, 1996; Jorge et al., 1999), and their cognitive deficits may be exacerbated by emotional distress (Iezzi et al., 1999; Kewman et al., 1991; S. Thomas et al., 2000). Heyer and his colleagues (2000) found both process-

ing speed and problem solving reduced in cognitively intact elderly patients the day after spinal surgery; poorer performances correlated with higher scores on a pain scale. Grigsby and his coworkers (1995) hypothesized that pain may disrupt speed-dependent cognitive functions. Understanding performance deficits by patients with pain may be confounded with the effects of pain medication (Banning and Sjøgren, 1990).

However, the presence of pain does not necessarily affect cognitive functioning negatively (B.D. Bell et al., 1999; J.E. Meyers and Diep, 2000). Performances by chronic pain patients on tests of attentional functions, memory, reasoning, and construction were directly related to their general activity level, regardless of extent of emotional distress (S. Thomas et al., 2000). While pain reduced cognitive functioning in some patients (P. Sjøgren, Olsen, et al., 2000), it may heighten "working memory" (PASAT performance, pp. 364–365) in others (P. Sjøgren, Thomsen, and Olsen, 2000).

The interpretation of the relationship between pain and cognitive dysfunction is complicated by a variety of symptoms that are often highly associated with pain and may be key factors in this relationship, including anxiety, depression, sleep disturbance, and emotional distress (Cripe, Maxwell, and Hill, 1995; Jorge et al., 1999). Cripe and his colleagues (1995) further point out that the chronicity of the problem (neurologic symptoms, pain, and/or emotional distress) may be a relevant factor in the patient's behavior as "neurologically impaired patients . . . might experience more acute emotional distress in the acute phase of their illness" than at later stages (p. 265). Women, particularly those who tend to be fearful, experience lower pain thresholds compared to men (Keogh and Birkby, 1999).

R.P. Hart, Martelli, and Zasler (2000) stress the importance of attempting to minimize the effects of pain on test performance when chronic pain is one of the patient's presenting complaints. They suggest postponing neuropsychological assessment until aggressive efforts aimed at pain reduction have been tried. In cases where pain treatment is not successful, they offer a variety of suggestions. It may be possible to alter physical aspects of the testing situation to ensure optimal comfort. Frequent breaks allowing the patient to move about, brief "stand up and stretch breaks," or short appointments may be helpful. Pain assessment scales may indicate the degree of suffering experienced by the patient, and mood assessment scales and symptom checklists may help clarify the role of emotional factors in the patient's experience of pain. Cripe (1996b) cautions against using inventories designed to assist in psychiatric diagnosis (e.g., the Minnesota Multiphasic Personality Inventory [MMPI]) to identify patients for whom pain is a significant problem. Measures of the patient's ability to muster and sustain effort may provide insight into the role of low energy and fatigue associated with pain. When patients report that their pain is in the moderate to intense range, interpretation of test scores that are below expectation requires consideration of the role of pain on test performance.

Performance inconsistency

It is not unusual for patients with cerebral impairments to report that they have "good days" and "bad days," so it should not be surprising to discover that in some conditions the level of an individual's performances can vary noticeably from day to day (Bleiberg et al., 1997) and even hour to hour (A. Smith, 1993), especially with lapses of attention (Stuss, Pogue, et al., 1994; van Zomeren and Brouwer, 1990). The Stuss group found no relationship between the extent of performance fluctuations on a graded set of reaction time tests and TBI severity, nor did they find consistency in how individual patients performed on different days (see also Stuss, Stethem, Hugenholtz, et al., 1989).

Performance variability may be most obvious in patients with seizure disorders, as seizure frequency, severity, duration, and after effects can greatly influence performance in the hours or days just before or after a seizure episode (Freides, 1985). Alterations in alertness, fatigue levels, and sense of well-being are not uncommon in many other conditions as well (Fischer, 2003). Nespoulous and Soum (2000), noting that in aphasic patients "variability is the rule," recommend giving the patient different kinds of test to aid in determining the conditions under which the patient can sustain or lose performance stability. This recommendation presupposes that performance variability reflects to some extent a coherent dysfunction pattern. Repeated examinations using—in so far as possible—tests that are relatively resistant to practice effects will help to identify best performance and typical performance levels in patients with these kinds of ups and downs.

Motivation

The motivational capacity of some brain impaired patients, particularly those with damage to the limbic system or prefrontal areas, may be diminished or lost (Stuss, Van Reekum, and Murphy, 2000; see also pp. 49–51, 79, 83). This condition often reflects the patient's inability to formulate meaningful goals or to initiate and carry out plans. Behaviorally, motivational defects appear as more or less pervasive and crippling apathy (Lezak, 1989; Walsh and Darby, 1999). Because of their general lack of involvement and a behavioral presentation that Lishman (1973) calls "sluggishness,"

such patients may perform significantly below their capacities unless cajoled or goaded or otherwise stimulated to perform. On the other hand, a monetary incentive did not improve the cognitive performances of college students with histories of mild TBI whose motivational capacity was essentially intact (Orey et al., 2000; see also pp. 765, 766).

Anxiety, stress, and distress

It is not unusual for the circumstances leading to a neuropsychological examination to have been experienced as anxiety-producing or stressful. Persons involved in litigation frequently admit to anxiety and other symptoms of stress (Gasquoine, 1997a; Murrey, 2000b). Patients who have acquired neuropsychological and other deficits altering their ability to function normally in their relationships and/or their work and living situations have been going through significant and typically highly stressful and anxiety-producing life changes (T.H. Holmes and Rahe, 1967). Negative expectations about one's potential performance or abilities can affect the test performance (Suhr and Gunstad, 2002). Moreover, the examination itself can be a source of anxiety (Bennett-Levy, Klein-Boonschate, et al., 1994).

A 60-year-old minister appeared anxious during memory testing. He had requested a neuropsychological examination because he was no longer able to recall names of his parishioners, some of whom he had known for years. He feared that an examination would reveal Alzheimer's disease, yet he realized that he had to find out whether this was the problem.

High anxiety levels may result in such mental efficiency problems as slowing, scrambled or blocked thoughts and words, and memory failure (Buckelew and Hannay, 1986; G.D. King et al., 1978; J.E. Mueller, 1979; Sarason et al., 1986); they enhance distractibility (Eysenck, 1991) and are exacerbated by depression (Kizilbash et al., 2002, see p. 128). High levels of test anxiety have been shown to affect adversely performance on many different kinds of mental ability tests (C. Fletcher et al., 1998; Minnaert, 1999; Musch and Broder, 1999; Oliver, 1999). Specific memory dysfunction in some combat survivors (Yehuda et al., 1995) and exacerbation of cognitive deficits following TBI (Bryant and Harvey, 1999a,b; McMillan, 1996b) have been associated with posttraumatic stress disorder (see also p. 175). However, these effects—and posttraumatic stress disorder—are far from common responses to difficult situations (M. Bowman, 1997). Some studies found that anxiety and emotional distress (in TBI patients, Gasquoine, 1997b; in "healthy men," Waldstein et al., 1997; in open-heart surgery candidates, Vingerhoets, De Soete, and Jannes, 1995) and "emotional disturbances" (in psychiatric patients without brain damage as well as TBI patients, Reitan and Wolfson, 1997b) do not appear to affect cognitive performances. When anxiety contributes to distractibility, anxiety effects may be reduced by instructions that help to focus the examinee's attention on the task at hand (Sarason et al., 1986) or by tasks which so occupy the subject's attention as to override test anxiety (J.H. Lee, 1999).

Depression and frustration

Depression is associated with many brain disorders and may be due to any combination of "neuroanatomic, neurochemical, and psychosocial factors" (Rosenthal, Christensen, and Ross, 1998; Sweet, Newman, and Bell, 1992; see pp. 329–331, 332–333). It can interfere with the motivational aspects of memory in that the patient simply puts less effort into the necessary recall. Prospective memory may be particularly vulnerable to this aspect of a depressed mental state (Hertel, 2000). Moreover, depression and frustration are often intimately related to fatigue in many ill patients, with and without brain disorders (Akechi et al., 1999); and the pernicious interplay between them can seriously compromise the patient's performance (Kaszniak and Allender, 1985; Lezak, 1978b). Fatigue-prone patients will stumble more when walking, speaking, and thinking and become more frustrated, which in turn drains their energies and increases their fatigue. This results in a greater likelihood of failure and leads to more frustration and eventual despair. Repeated failure in exercising previously accomplished skills, difficulty in solving once easy problems, and the need for effort to coordinate previously automatic responses can further contribute to the depression that commonly accompanies brain disorders. After a while, some patients quit trying. Such discouragement usually carries over into their test performances and may obscure cognitive strengths from themselves as well as the examiner.

When examining brain injured patients it is important to deal with problems of motivation and depression. Encouragement is useful. The examiner can deliberately ensure that patients will have some success, no matter how extensive the impairments. Frequently the neuropsychologist may be the first person to discuss the patient's feelings and particularly to give reassurance that depression is natural and common to people with this condition and that it may well dissipate in time. Many patients experience a great deal of relief and even some lifting of their depression by this kind of informational reassurance.

The examiner needs to form a clear picture of a depressed patient's state at the time of testing, as a mild depression or a transiently depressed mood state is less likely to affect test performance than a more severe one. Depression can—but will not necessarily—interfere with performance due to distracting ruminations (Sarason et al., 1986) and/or response slowing (Kalska et al., 1999) and, most usually, some learning deficits (Goggin et al., 1997; D.A. King and Caine, 1996; Rosenstein, 1998). However, cognitive performances by most depressed patients, whether brain damaged or not, may not be affected by the depression (Reitan and Wolfson, 1997b; Rohling et al., 2002), and even major depression may not add to neuropsychological impairments (Crews et al., 1999; J.L. Wong, Wetterneck, and Klein, 2000). In TBI patients, depressive effects on cognition tend to appear as very mild diminution of "visual attention and psychomotor skills," but the more severely injured the patient, the less likely will there be such effects (E.M.S. Sherman et al., 2000). However, when depression is compounded by anxiety, learning efficiency was compromised for a large sample of noninjured Vietnam veterans (Kizilbash et al., 2002). Sweet and his colleagues (1992) caution examiners not to use mildly depressed scores on tests of attention or memory as evidence of a brain disorder in depressed patients, but rather to look for other patterns of disability or signs of dysfunction.

Patients in litigation

Providing evaluations for legal purposes presents special challenges. Because the findings in forensic cases are prepared for nonclinicians, the conclusions should be both scientifically defensible and expressed or explained in lay terms. Moreover, at least the major portion of the examination procedures should have supporting references available (see Daubert v. Merrell Dow Pharmaceuticals, 509 US 579 [1993]). Fulfilling these requirements may be difficult because of the nature of the patient's impairment. The most important data may be behavioral or qualitative, such as apathy or changes in comportment associated with frontal lobe injuries, and thus appear "subjective." In these cases, conclusions can be supported by information obtained from persons close to the patient, such as a spouse or intimate friend, and should be explainable in terms of known brain–behavior relationships and reports in the literature rather than deviant test scores. The following discussion summarizes assessment issues and does not cover testifying as an expert witness, court proceedings, or other legal issues (for a full discussion, see Murrey, 2000a).

When a psychologist is retained to examine a person involved in litigation, this arrangement may alter the examiner's duties to the patient as well as the rules of confidentiality (L.M. Binder and Thompson, 1995). Examiners may be asked to have an observer during the examination. Having a third party present can change the climate of the examination by making the patient self-conscious, inducing the patient to perform in a manner expected by the observer, or producing the possibility of distractions that normally would not exist (McCaffrey, Fisher, et al., 1996; McSweeny, Becker, et al., 1998). Kehrer and her colleagues (2000) found "a significant observer effect . . . on tests of brief auditory attention, sustained attention, speed of information processing, and verbal fluency." These workers recommend "caution . . . when any observer is present (including trainees)." For these reasons, the National Academy of Neuropsychology (NAN) Policy and Planning Committee (2000a) strongly recommends that third party observers be excluded from the examination. Additionally, the NAN committee pointed out that having a nonpsychologist present violates test security, which is also a concern of test publishers.

In my experience [mdl], if the examiner is adamant about not allowing an observer into the examining room and explains the reasons for protecting the subject and the test materials from an invasive intrusion, most lawyers will usually agree to these requirements and, if the issue must be adjudicated, the court will usually support this protection. If not, the examiner must decide whether to accede to this request or not; and if not, the examiner must be willing to relinquish this case to another who would accept such an intrusion (see also McCaffrey, Fisher, et al., 1996). Although recording the examination on tape may seem to be a realistic alternative to having an observer present, test security is necessarily compromised by such an arrangement and the possibly distractive effects of taping on the patient are unknown.

Often, forensic evaluations are lengthy due to the perceived need to be thorough. It is particularly important in injury cases that the premorbid status of the patient be established with as much evidence as possible. The examiner should have an understanding of the base rates of the neurobehavioral symptoms relevant to the case at hand (Lees-Haley, 1997; Rosenfeld et al., 2000; Yedid, 2000b).

In choosing tests, preference should be given to well-known ones with appropriate normative data and, as much as possible, known rates of error. As is true for clinical evaluations, when performance below expectation is observed on one test, the reliability of the finding should be assessed using other tests requiring similar cognitive skills. Every effort should be made to understand discrepancies so that spurious findings can be distinguished from true impairment. Emotional problems frequently complicate the patient's clinical picture. The patient's emotional and psychiatric status should be assessed in order to appreciate potential contributions of depression, anxiety, or psychotic thinking to test performance.

When performance below expectation is observed, the examiner should assess the patient's motivation and cooperation and, most notably, the possibility that the subject has wittingly (i.e., malingering) or unwittingly exaggerated present symptoms or introduced imagined ones (Yedid, 2000a). Intentionally feigning or exaggerating symptoms typically occurs in the context of potential secondary gain, which may be financial or psychological (e.g., perpetuating a dependency role) (Pankratz, 1998).

Tests have been developed to measure response bias and, especially, deliberate malingering (see Chapter 20). However, the determination of malingering or other response bias must be based on overall clinical evaluation (Frederick et al., 1994). Alternative explanations for poor performance on these tests should be considered, such as anxiety, perplexity, fatigue, misunderstanding of instructions, or fear of failure. Moreover, for some patients—and especially with some tests—poor performance may only reflect a significant memory or perceptual disorder. Estimates of base rates of malingering vary from clinician to clinician but average around 17% in the forensic setting, about 10% in some clinical settings (Rosenfeld et al., 2000). When base rates are this low, the positive predictive accuracy of tests can be unacceptably low, so caution is advised in interpreting scores of malingering tests.

Most tests of motivation examine one or another aspect of memory because of the prevalence of memory complaints in patients who have had any kind of damage to the brain. Tests of motivation involving other cognitive domains are scarce, although data from research studies suggest models (see Pankratz, 1983, 1998).

Neuropsychological evaluations may be requested to provide evidence for competency determinations, which are made by the court. The purpose of the evaluation and the consequences of impaired performance should be explained to the examinee. Although the risk of antagonizing some people exists, they need to understand that it is important for them to give their best effort in the examination. Test selection should be based on the particular competency in question (see p. 700ff for a discussion of tests for competency). Most competency judgments require that the person has good reality contact, general orientation to time, memory for pertinent personal information, and intact reasoning and judgment including appreciation of one's condition, situation, and needs. Competency evaluations in criminal cases may involve assessing culpable state of mind or competency to stand trial. The former requires assessment of a defendant's intent to do something wrong while the latter involves assessing whether a defendant is able to understand the nature of the charges and assist in the defense of the case.

The same person may be examined by more than one psychologist within a short period of time when attorneys are seeking to make their case as convincing as possible or when opposing attorneys each request an examination. Since practice effects can be substantial, the second psychologist will want to know which tests have already been given so that alternate tests may be selected, or areas of underrepresentation at the first examination may be appropriately explored. When this information is not available, the examiner needs to ask the patient if the test materials are familiar, and if so, arrange to see the previous examination's data before preparing a report. Interpretation of repeated tests is more accurate if their practice effects are known (McCaffery, Duff, and Westervelt, 2000a,b).

Neuropsychologists are bound to provide an objective evaluation and to present the findings and conclusions in an unbiased manner. Awareness of the pressures in the forensic setting can help them avoid bias (Van Gorp and McMullen, 1997).

MAXIMIZING THE PATIENT'S PERFORMANCE LEVEL

The goal of testing is always to obtain the best performance the patient is capable of producing.
S.R. Heaton and R.K. Heaton, 1981

It is not difficult to get a brain damaged patient to do poorly on a psychological examination, for the quality of the performance can be exceedingly vulnerable to external influences or changes in internal states. All an examiner need do is make these patients tired or anxious, or subject them to any one of a number of distractions most people ordinarily do not even notice, and their test scores will plummet. In neuropsychological assessment, the difficult task is enabling the patient to perform as well as possible.

Eliciting the patient's maximum output is necessary for a valid behavioral assessment. Interpretation of test scores and of test behavior is predicated on the assumption that the demonstrated behavior is a representative sample of the patient's true capacity in that area. Of course, it is unlikely that all of a person's ability to do something can ever be demonstrated; for this reason many psychologists distinguish between a patient's level of test performance and an estimated ability level. The practical goal is to help patients do their best so that the difference between what they can do and how they actually perform is negligible.

Optimal versus Standard Conditions

In the ideal testing situation, both *optimal* and *standard* conditions prevail. Optimal conditions are those that enable patients to do their best on the tests. They differ from patient to patient, but for most brain injured patients they include freedom from distractions, a nonthreatening emotional climate, and protection from fatigue. Standard conditions are prescribed by the test-maker to ensure that each administration of the test is as much like every other administration as possible so that scores obtained on different test administrations can be compared. To this end, many test-makers give detailed directions on the presentation of their test, including specific instructions on word usage, handling the material, etc. Highly standardized test administration is necessary when using norms of tests that have a fine-graded and statistically well standardized scoring system, such as the Wechsler Intelligence Scale tests. By exposing each patient to nearly identical situations, the standardization of testing procedures also enables the examiner to discover the individual characteristics of each patient's responses.

Normally, there need be no conflict between optimal and standard conditions. When brain impaired patients are tested, however, a number of them will be unable to perform well within the confines of the standard instructions.

For some patients, the difficulty may be in understanding the standard instructions. Instructional problems can occur on memory tests with concrete-minded or poorly inhibited brain injured patients. When given a list of numbers or words, some patients are apt to begin reciting the items one right after the other as the examiner is still reading the list. Additional instructions must be given if the patient is to do the test as originally conceived and standardized. In these cases, patients' immediate repetition may spoil the ready-made word or number series. When giving these kinds of memory tests, it is helpful to have a substitute list handy, particularly if the examiner does not plan to see the patient at a later date. Otherwise, the identical list can be repeated later in the examination, with the necessary embellishments to the standard instructions.

To provide additional information on immediate memory and allow the examiner to verify comprehension of test questions, the examiner can ask patients to repeat the question when erroneous responses sound as if they have forgotten or misheard elements of the question. It is particularly important to find out what patients understood or retained when their response is so wide of the mark that it is doubtful they were answering the question the examiner asked. In such cases, subtle attention, memory, or hearing defects may emerge; or if the wrong answer was due to a chance mishearing of the question, the patient has an opportunity to correct the error and gain the credit due.

Many other comprehension problems of these kinds are peculiar to brain injured patients. A little more flexibility and looseness in interpreting the standard procedures are required on the examiner's part to make the most of the test and elicit the patient's best performance. "The same words do not necessarily mean the same thing to different people and it is the meaning of the instructions which should be the same for all people rather than the wording" (M. Williams, 1965, p. xvii).

The examination of these patients can pose still other problems. Should a patient not answer a question for 30 seconds or more, the examiner can ask the patient to repeat it, thus finding out if lack of response is due to inattention, forgetting, slow thinking, uncertainty, or unwillingness to admit failure. When the patient has demonstrated a serious defect of attention, immediate memory, or capacity to make generalizations, it is necessary to repeat the format each time one of a series of similar questions is asked. For example, if the patient's vocabulary is being tested, the examiner must ask what the word means with every new word, for the subject may not remember how to respond without prompting at each question.

Scoring questions arise when the patient gives two or more responses to questions that have only one correct or one best response. When one of the patient's answers is correct, the examiner should invite the patient to decide which answer is preferred and then score accordingly.

Timing presents even greater and more common standardization problems than incomprehension in that both brain impaired and elderly patients are likely to do timed tests slowly and lose credit for good performances. Many timing problems can be handled by testing the limits. With a brain damaged population and with older patients (Storandt, 1977), many timed tests should yield two scores: the score for the response within the time limit and another for the performance regardless of time (e.g., see Corkin, Growdon, Desclos, and Rosen, 1989).

Nowhere is the conflict between optimal and standard conditions so pronounced or so unnecessary as in the issue of emotional support and reassurance of the test-taking patient. For many examiners, standard conditions have come to mean that they have to maintain an emotionally impassive, standoffish attitude toward their patients when testing. The stern admonitions of test-makers to adhere to the wording of the test manual and not tell the patient whether any single item was passed have probably contributed to the practice of coldly mechanical test administration.

From the viewpoint of any but the most severely regressed or socially insensitive patient, that kind of test experience is very anxiety-provoking. Almost every patient approaches psychological testing with a great deal of apprehension. Brain injured patients and persons suspected of harboring a brain tumor or some insidious degenerative disease are often frankly frightened. When confronted with an examiner who displays no facial expression and speaks in an emotionally toneless voice, who never smiles, and who responds only briefly and curtly to the patient's questions or efforts at conversation, patients generally assume that they are doing something wrong—failing or displeasing the examiner—and their anxiety soars. Such a threatening situation can compromise some aspects of the test performance. Undue anxiety certainly will not be conducive to a representative performance (Bennett-Levy, Klein-Boonschate, et al., 1994).

Fear of appearing stupid may also prevent impaired patients from showing what they can do. In working with patients who have memory disorders, the examiner need be aware that in order to save face many of them say they cannot remember not only when they cannot remember but also when they can make a response but are unsure of its correctness. When the examiner gently and encouragingly pushes them in a way that makes them feel more comfortable, most patients who at first denied any recall of test material demonstrate at least some memory.

Although standard conditions do require that the examiner adhere to the instructions in the test manual and give no hint regarding the correctness of a response, these requirements can easily be met without creating a climate of fear and discomfort. A sensitive examination calls for the same techniques the psychologist uses to put a patient at ease in an interview and to establish a good working relationship. Conversational patter is appropriate and can be very anxiety-reducing. The examiner can maintain a relaxed conversational flow with the patient throughout the entire test session without permitting it to interrupt the administration of any single item or task. The examiner can give continual support and encouragement to the patient without indicating success or failure by smiling and rewarding the patient's *efforts* with words such as "Good," "Fine," and "You're doing well" or "You're really trying hard!" Examiners who distribute praise randomly and not just following correct responses are no more giving away answers than if they remained stonily silent throughout (M.B. Shapiro, 1951). However, the patient feels comforted, reassured about doing something right and pleasing—or at least not displeasing—the examiner.

The examiner who has established this kind of warmly supportive atmosphere can discuss with patients their strengths, weaknesses, and specific problems as these appear in the course of the examination. Interested, comfortable patients will be able to provide the examiner with information about their functioning that they might otherwise have forgotten or be unwilling to share. They will also be receptive to the examiner's explanations and recommendations regarding the difficulties that they are encountering and are exploring with the examiner. The examination will have been a mutual learning and sharing experience.

When Optimal Conditions Are Not Best

Some patients who complain of significant problems attending, learning, and responding efficiently in their homes or at work perform well in the usual protective examination situation. Their complaints, when not supported by examination findings, may become suspect or be interpreted as signs of some emotional disturbance brought on or exacerbated by a recent head injury or a chronic neurologic disease. Yet the explanation for the discrepancy between their complaints and their performance can lie in the calm and quiet examining situation in which distractions are kept to a minimum. This contrasts with their difficulties concentrating in a noisy machine shop or buzzing busy office, or keeping thoughts and perceptions focused in a shopping mall with its flashing lights, bustling crowds, and piped-in music from many—often conflicting—sources. Of course an examination cannot be conducted in a mall. However, the examiner can usually find a way to test the effects of piped-in music or distracting street or corridor noises on a patient's mental efficiency. Those examiners whose work setting does not provide a sound-proofed room with controlled lighting and no interruptions may not always be able to evoke their patients' best performance, but they are likely to learn more about how the patients perform in real life.

Talking to Patients

With few exceptions, examiners will communicate best by keeping their language simple. Almost all of the concepts that professionals tend to communicate in technical language can be conveyed in everyday words. It may initially take some effort to substitute "find out about your problem" for "differential diagnosis" or "loss of sight in the left half of each of your eyes" for "left homonymous hemianopsia" or "difficulty thinking in terms of ideas" for "abstract conceptualization." Examiners may find that forcing themselves to word these concepts in their native tongue may add to their understanding as well. Exceptions to this rule may be those brain damaged patients who were originally well endowed and highly accomplished, for whom complex ideation and an extensive vocabulary came naturally, and who need recognition of their premorbid status and reassurance of residual intellectual competencies. Talking

at their educational level conveys this reassurance and acknowledges their intellectual achievements implicitly and thereby even more forcefully than telling them.

Now for some "don'ts." Don't "invite" patients to be examined, to take a particular test or, for that matter, to do anything they need to do. If you invite people to do something or ask if they would care to do it, they can say "no" as well as "yes." Once a patient has refused you have no choice but to go along with the decision since you offered the opportunity. Therefore, when patients must do something, tell them what it is they need to do as simply and as directly as you can.

I have a personal distaste for using expressions such as "I would like you to . . . " or "I want you to . . . " when asking patients to do something [mdl]. I feel it is important for them to undertake for their own sake whatever it is the clinician asks or recommends and that they not do it merely or even additionally to please the clinician. Thus, I tell patients what they need to do using such expressions as, "I'm going to show you some pictures and your job is to . . . " or, "When I say 'Go,' you are to. . . . "

My last "don't" also concerns a personal distaste, and that is for the use of the first person plural when asking the patient to do something: "Let's try these puzzles" or "Let's take a few minutes' rest." The essential model for this plural construction is the kindergarten teacher's directive, "Let's go to the bathroom." The usual reason for it is reluctance to appear bossy or rude. Because it smacks of the kindergarten and is inherently incorrect (the examiner is not going to take the test nor does the examiner need a rest from the testing), sensitive patients may feel they are being demeaned.

CONSTRUCTIVE ASSESSMENT

Every psychological examination can be a personally useful experience for the patient. Patients should leave the examination feeling that they have gained something for their efforts, whether it was an increased sense of dignity or self-worth, insight into their behavior, or constructive appreciation of their problems or limitations.

When patients feel better at the end of the examination than they did at the beginning, the examiner has probably helped them to perform at their best. When they understand themselves better at the end than at the beginning, the examinations were probably conducted in a spirit of mutual cooperation in which patients were treated as reasoning, responsible individuals. It is a truism that good psychological treatment requires continuing assessment. By the same token, good assessment will also contribute to each patient's psychological well-being.

6 | The Neuropsychological Examination: Interpretation

H. JULIA HANNAY AND MURIEL D. LEZAK

THE NATURE OF NEUROPSYCHOLOGICAL EXAMINATION DATA

The basic data of psychological examinations, like any other psychological data, are behavioral observations. In order to get a broad and meaningful sample of the patient's behavior from which to draw diagnostic inferences or conclusions relevant to patient care and planning, the psychological examiner needs to have made or obtained reports of many different kinds of observations, including historical and demographic information.

Different Kinds of Examination Data

Background data

Background data are essential for providing the context in which current observations can be best understood. In most instances, accurate interpretation of the patient's examination behavior and test responses requires at least some knowledge of the developmental and medical history, family background, educational and occupational accomplishments (or failures), and the patient's current living situation and level of social functioning. The examiner must take into account a number of patient variables when evaluating test performances, including sensory and motor status, alertness cycles and fatigability, medication regimen, and the likelihood of drug or alcohol dependency. An appreciation of the patient's current medical and neurological status can guide the examiner's search for a pattern of neuropsychological deficits.

The importance of background information in interpreting examination observations is obvious when evaluating a test score on school-related skills such as arithmetic and spelling or in the light of a vocational history that implies a particular performance level (e.g., a journeyman millwright must be of at least *average* ability but is more likely to achieve *high average* or even better scores on many tests; to succeed as an ex-

ecutive chef requires at least *high average* ability but, again, many would perform at a *superior* level on cognitive tests). However, motivation to reach a goal is also important: professionals can be of *average* ability while an individual with exceptional ability might be a shoe clerk. The contributions of such background variables as age or education to test performance has not always been appreciated in the interpretation of many different kinds of tests, including those purporting to measure neuropsychological integrity (e.g., Reitan and Wolfson, 1995b; D. Wechsler, 1997a,b—no education data for computed scores on any tests).

Behavioral observations

Naturalistic observations can provide extremely useful information about how the patient functions outside the formalized, usually highly structured, and possibly intimidating examination setting. Psychological examiners rarely study patients in their everyday setting, but reports from nursing personnel or family members may help set the stage for evaluating examination data or at least raise questions about what the examiner observes or should look for.

The value of naturalistic observations may be most evident when formal examination findings alone would lead to conclusions that patients are more or less capable than they actually are (Capitani, 1997; Newcombe, 1987). Such an error is most likely to occur when the examiner confounds observed *performance* with *ability*. For example, many people who survive even quite severe head trauma in moving vehicle accidents ultimately achieve scores that are within or close to the *average* ability range on most tests of cognitive function (B. Crosson, Greene, et al., 1990; H.S. Levin, Grossman, et al., 1979; Stuss, Ely, et al., 1985). Yet, by some accounts, as few as one-third of them hold jobs in the competitive market as so many are troubled by problems of attention, temperament, and self-control (M.L. Bowman, 1996; Cohadon et al., 2002;

133

Hoofien et al., 1990; Lezak and O'Brien, 1990). The behavioral characteristics that compromise their adequate and sometimes even excellent cognitive skills are not elicited in the usual neuropsychiatric or neuropsychological examination. However, they become painfully apparent to anyone who is with these patients as they go about their usual activities—or, in many cases, inactivities. In contrast, there is the shy, anxious, or suspicious patient who responds only minimally to a white-coated examiner but whose everyday behavior is far superior to anything the examiner sees; and also patients whose coping strategies enable them to function well *despite* significant cognitive deficits (B.A. Wilson, 2000; R.L. Wood, 1986).

How patients conduct themselves in the course of the examination is another source of useful information. Their comportment needs to be documented and evaluated as attitudes toward the examination, conversation or silence, the appropriateness of their demeanor and social responses, can tell a lot about their neuropsychological status as well as enrich the context in which their responses to the examination proper will be evaluated.

Test data

> In a very real sense there is virtually no such thing as a neuropsychological test. Only the method of drawing inferences about the tests is neuropsychological.
> *K.W. Walsh, 1992*

Testing differs from these other forms of psychological data gathering in that it elicits behavior samples in a standardized, replicable, and more or less artificial and restrictive situation (Anastasi and Urbina, 1997; B.F. Green, 1981; S.M. Turner et al., 2001). Its strengths lie in the approximate sameness of the test situation for each subject, for it is the sameness that enables the examiner to compare behavior samples between individuals, over time, or with expected performance levels. Its weaknesses too lie in the sameness, in that psychological test observations are limited to the behaviors occasioned by the test situation.

To apply examination findings to the problems that trouble the patient, the psychological examiner extrapolates from a limited set of observations to the patient's behavior in real-life situations. Extrapolation from the data is a common feature of other kinds of psychological data handling as well, since it is rarely possible to observe a human subject in every problem area. Extrapolations are likely to be as accurate as the observations on which they are based are pertinent, precise, and comprehensive, as the situations are similar, and as the generalizations are apt.

A 48-year-old advertising manager with originally superior cognitive abilities sustained a right hemisphere stroke with minimal sensory or motor deficits. He was examined at the request of his company when he wanted to return to work. His verbal skills in general were high average to superior, but he was unable to construct two-dimensional geometric designs with colored blocks, put together cut-up picture puzzles, or draw a house or person with proper proportions (see Fig. 6.1). The neuropsychologist did not observe the patient on the job but, generalizing from these samples, she concluded that the visuoperceptual distortions and misjudgments demonstrated on the test would be of a similar kind and would occur to a similar extent with layout and design material. The patient was advised against retaining responsibility for the work of the display section of his department. Later conferences with the patient's employers confirmed that he was no longer able to evaluate or supervise the display operations.

In most instances examiners rely on their common-sense judgments and practical experiences in making test-based predictions about their patients' real-life functioning. Studies of the *predictive validity* and *ecological validity* of neuropsychological tests show that many of them have a good predictive relationship with a variety of disease characteristics (e.g. 202, 222) and practical issues (see pp. 11–12).

Quantitative and Qualitative Data

Every psychological observation can be expressed either numerically as quantitative data or descriptively as qualitative data. Each of these classes of data can constitute a self-sufficient data base as demonstrated by two different approaches to neuropsychological as-

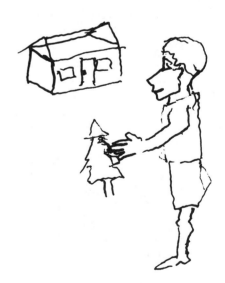

FIGURE 6.1 House-Tree-Person drawings of the 48-year-old advertising manager described in the text (size reduced to one-third of original).

sessment. An actuarial system developed by Ralph Reitan (Reitan, 1966; Reitan and Wolfson, 1993) and elaborated by others (e.g., Heaton, Grant, and Matthews, 1991; Moses, Pritchard, and Adams, 1996) exemplifies the quantitative method. It relies on scores, derived indices, and score relationships for diagnostic predictions. Practitioners using this method may have a technician examine the patient so that, except for an introductory or closing interview, their data base is in numerical, often computer-processed, form. At the other extreme is a clinical approach built upon richly detailed observations without objective standardization (A.-L. Christensen, 1979; Luria, 1966, 1973b). These clinicians documented their observations in careful detail, much as neurologists or psychiatrists describe what they observe. Both approaches have contributed significantly to the development of contemporary neuropsychology. Together they provide the observational frames of reference and techniques for taking into account, documenting, and communicating the complexity, variability, and subtleties of patient behavior.

Although some studies suggest that reliance on actuarial evaluation of scores alone provides the best approach to clinical diagnosis (Dawes et al., 1989), this position has not been consistently supported in neuropsychology (Cimino, 1994; Heaton, Grant, Anthony, and Lehman, 1981; Leli and Filskov, 1984; Ogden-Epker and Cullum, 2001). Nor is it appropriate for many—perhaps most—assessment questions in neuropsychology, as only simple diagnostic decision-making satisfies the conditions necessary for actuarial predictions to be more accurate than clinical ones: (1) that there be only a small number of probable outcomes (e.g., left cortical lesion, right cortical lesion, diffuse damage, no impairment); (2) that the prediction variables be known (which limits the amount of information that can be processed by an actuarial formula to the information on which the formula was based); and (3) that the data from which the formula was derived be relevant to the questions asked (Pankratz and Taplin, 1982).

Proponents of actuarial evaluations overlook the realities of neuropsychological practice in an era of advanced neuroimaging technology: most assessments are not undertaken for diagnostic purposes but to describe the patient's neuropsychological status. Even in those instances in which the examination is undertaken for diagnostic purposes the issue is more likely to concern diagnostic discrimination requiring consideration of a broad range of disorders—including the possibility of more than one pathological condition being operative—than making a decision between three or four discrete alternatives. Moreover, not infrequently diagnosis involves variables that are unique to the individual case and not necessarily obvious to a naive observer or

revealed by questionnaires, variables for which no actuarial formulas have been developed or are ever likely to be developed (J.T. Barth, Ryan, and Hawk, 1992). It is also important to note that the comparisons in most studies purporting to evaluate the efficacy of clinical versus actuarial judgments are not presenting the examiners with real patients with whom the examiner has a live interaction, but rather with the scores generated in the examination—and just the scores, without even descriptions of the qualitative aspects of the performance (e.g., Faust, Hart, and Guilmette, 1988; Faust, Hart, Guilmette, and Arkes, 1988; Leli and Filskov, 1984).

Quantitative data

The number is not the reality, it is only an abstract symbol of some part or aspect of the reality measured. The number is a reduction of many events into a single symbol. The reality was the complex dynamic performance.

Lloyd Cripe, 1996a (p. 191)

Scores are summary statements about observed behavior. Scores may be obtained for any set of behavior samples that can be categorized according to some principle. The scorer evaluates each behavior sample to see how well it fits a predetermined category and then gives it a place on a numerical scale (Anastasi and Urbina, 1997).

A commonly used scale for individual test items has two points, one for "good" or "pass" and the other for "poor" or "fail." Three-point scales, which add a middle grade of "fair" or "barely pass," are often used for grading ability test items. Few item scales contain more than five to seven scoring levels because the gradations become so fine as to be confusing to the scorer and meaningless for interpretation. Scored tests with more than one item produce a summary score that is usually the simple sum of the scores for all the individual items. Occasionally, test-makers incorporate a correction for guessing into their scoring systems so that the final score is not just a simple summation.

Thus, a final test score may misrepresent the behavior under examination on at least two counts: It is based on only one narrowly defined aspect of a set of behavior samples, and it is two or more steps removed from the original behavior. "Global," "aggregate," or "full-scale" scores calculated by summing or averaging a set of test scores are three to four steps removed from the behavior they represent.

Summary index scores based on item scores that have had their normal range restricted to just two points representing either pass or fail, or "within normal limits" or "brain damaged," are also many steps removed from the original observations. Thus "index scores," which are based on various combinations of scores on two or more—more or less similar—tests suffer the same problems as any other summed score in that they too obscure the data. One might wonder why index scores should exist at all: if the tests entering into an index score are so similar that they can be treated as though they examined the same aspects of cognitive functioning, then two tests would seem unnecessary. On the other hand, if each of two tests produces a different score pattern or normative distribution or sensitivity to particular kinds of brain dysfunction, then the two are different and should be treated individually so that the differences in patient performances on these tests can be evident and available for sensitive test interpretation.

The inclusion of test scores in the psychological data base satisfies the need for objective, readily replicable data cast in a form that permits reliable interpretation and meaningful comparisons. Standard scoring systems provide the means for reducing a vast array of different behaviors to a single numerical system (see pp. 141–143). This standardization enables the examiner to compare the score of any one test performance of a patient with all other scores of that patient, or with any group or performance criteria.

Completely different behaviors, such as writing skills and visual reaction time, can be compared on a single numerical scale: one person might receive a high score for elegant penmanship but a low one on speed of response to a visual signal; another might be high on both kinds of tasks or low on both. Considering one behavior at a time, a scoring system permits direct comparisons between the handwriting of a 60-year-old stroke patient and that of school-children at various grade levels, or between the patient's visual reaction time and that of other stroke patients of the same age.

Problems in the evaluation of quantitative data

> To reason—or do research—only in terms of scores and score-patterns is to do violence to the nature of the raw material.
>
> *Roy Schafer, 1948*

When interpreting test scores it is important to keep in mind their artificial and abstract nature. Some examiners come to equate a score with the behavior it is supposed to represent. Others prize standardized, replicable test scores as "harder," more "scientific" data at the expense of unquantified observations. Reification of test scores can lead the examiner to overlook or discount direct observations. A test-score approach to psychological assessment that minimizes the importance of qualitative data can result in serious distortions in the

interpretations, conclusions, and recommendations drawn from such a one-sided data base.

To be neuropsychologically meaningful, a test score should represent as few kinds of behavior or dimensions of cognitive functions as possible. The simpler the test task, the clearer the meaning of scored evaluations of the behavior elicited by that task. Correspondingly, it is often difficult to know just what functions contribute to a score obtained on a complex, multidimensional test task without appropriate evaluation based on a search for commonalities in the patient's performances on different tests, hypotheses generated from observations of the qualitative features of the patient's behavior, and the examiner's knowledge of brain–behavior relationships and how they are affected by neuropathological conditions (Milberg, Hebben, and Kaplan, 1996; Walsh and Darby, 1999).

If a score is overinclusive, as in the case of summed or averaged test battery scores, it becomes virtually impossible to know just what behavioral or cognitive characteristic it represents. Its usefulness for highlighting differences in ability and skill levels is nullified, for the patient's behavior is hidden behind a hodgepodge of cognitive functions and statistical manipulations (J.M. Butler et al., 1963; A. Smith, 1966, 1983). N. Butters (1984b) illustrated this problem in reporting that the "memory quotient" (MQ) obtained by summing and averaging scores on the Wechsler Memory Scale (WMS) was the same for two groups of patients, each with very different kinds of memory disorders based on very different neuropathological processes. His conclusion that "reliance on a single quantitative measure of memory . . . for the assessment of amnesic symptoms may have as many limitations as does the utilization of an isolated score . . . for the full description of aphasia" (p. 33) applies to every other kind of neuropsychological dysfunction as well. The same principle of multideterminants holds for single test scores too as similar errors lowering scores in similar ways can occur for different reasons (e.g., attentional deficits, language limitations, motor slowing, sensory deficits, slowed processing, etc.).

Further, the range of observations an examiner can make is restricted by the test. This is particularly the case with multiple-choice paper-and-pencil tests and those that restrict the patient's responses to button pushing or another mechanized activity that limits opportunities for self-expression. A busy examiner may not stay to observe the cooperative, comprehending, or docile patient manipulating buttons or levers or taking a paper-and-pencil test. Multiple-choice and automated tests offer no behavior alternatives beyond the prescribed set of responses. Qualitative differences in these test performances are recorded only when there are frank aberrations in test-taking behavior, such as qualifying statements written on the answer sheet of a personality test or more than one alternative marked on a single-answer multiple-choice test. For most paper-and-pencil or automated tests, how the patient solves the problem or goes about answering the question remains unknown or is, at best, a matter of conjecture based on such relatively insubstantial information as heaviness or neatness of pencil marks, test-taking errors, patterns of nonresponse, erasures, and the occasional pencil-sketched spelling tryouts or arithmetic computations in the margin.

In addition, the fine-grained scaling provided by the most sophisticated instruments for measuring cognitive competence is not suited to the assessment of many of the behavioral symptoms of cerebral neuropathology. Defects in behaviors that have what can be considered "species-wide" norms, i.e., that occur at a developmentally early stage and are performed effectively by all but the most severely impaired school-aged children, such as speech and dressing, are usually readily apparent. Quantitative norms generally do not enhance the observer's sensitivity to these problems nor do any test norms pegged at adult ability levels when applied to persons with severe defects in the tested ability area. Using a finely scaled vocabulary test to examine an aphasic patient, for example, is like trying to discover the shape of a flower with a microscope: the examiner will simply miss the point. Moreover, behavioral aberrations due to brain dysfunction are often so highly individualized and specific to the associated lesion that their distribution in the population at large, or even in the brain impaired population, does not lend itself to actuarial prediction techniques (W.G. Willis, 1984).

The evaluation of test scores in the context of direct observations is essential when doing neuropsychological assessment. For many brain impaired patients, test scores alone give relatively little information about the patient's functioning. The meat of the matter is often how a patient solves a problem or approaches a task rather than what the score is. "There are many reasons for failing and there are many ways you can go about it. And if you don't know in fact which way the patient was going about it, failure doesn't tell you very much" (Walsh and Darby, 1999). There can also be more than one way to pass a test.

A 54-year-old sales manager sustained a right frontal lobe injury when he fell as a result of a heart attack with several moments of cardiac arrest. On the Hooper Visual Organization Test, he achieved a score of 26 out of a possible 30, well within the *normal* range. However, not only did his errors reflect perceptual fragmentation (e.g., he called a cut-up broom a "long candle in holder"), but his correct responses were also fragmented (e.g., "wrist and hand and fingers" instead of the usual response, "hand;" "ball stitched and cut" instead of "baseball").

Another patient, a 40-year-old computer designer with a seven-year history of multiple sclerosis, made only 13 errors on the Category Test (CT), a number considerably lower than the 27 error mean reported for persons at his very high level of mental ability (Mitrushina, Boone, and D'Elia, 1999). (His scores on the Gates-MacGinitie Vocabulary and Comprehension subtests were at the 99th percentile; WAIS-R Information and Arithmetic age-graded scaled scores were in the *very superior* and *superior* ranges, respectively.) On two of the more difficult CT subtests he figured out the response principle within the first five trials, yet on one subtest he made 4 errors after a run of 14 correct answers and on the other he gave 2 incorrect responses after 15 correct answers. This error pattern suggested difficulty keeping in mind solutions that he had figured out easily enough but lost track of while performing the task. Nine repetitions on the first five trials of the Auditory Verbal Learning Test and two serial subtraction errors unremarked by him, one on subtracting "7s" when he went from "16" to "19," the other on the easier task of subtracting 3s when he said "23, 21," further supported the impression that this graduate engineer "has difficulty in monitoring his mental activity . . . and [it] is probably difficult for him to do more than one thing at a time." (K. Wild, personal communication, 1991)

This latter case also illustrates the relevance of education and occupation in evaluating test performances since, by themselves, all of these scores are well *within normal limits,* none suggestive of cognitive dysfunction. Axelrod and Goldman (1996) describe two hypothetical cases that achieve many of the same scores but for very different reasons.

Then consider two patients who achieve the same score on the WIS-A Arithmetic test but may have very different problems and abilities with respect to arithmetic. One patient performs the easy, single operation problems quickly and correctly but fails the more difficult items requiring two operations or more for solution because of an inability to retain and juggle so much at once in his immediate memory. The other patient has no difficulty remembering item content. She answers many of the simpler items correctly but very slowly, counting aloud on her fingers. She is unable to conceptualize or perform the operations on the more difficult items. The numerical score masks the disparate performances of these patients. As this test exemplifies, what a test actually is measuring may not be what its name suggests or what the test maker has claimed for it: while a test of arithmetic ability for some persons with limited education or native learning ability, the WIS-A Arithmetic's oral format makes it a test of attention and short-term memory for most adults, a feature that is now recognized by the test maker (Wechsler, 1997a); see also pp. 602–604, 652). Walsh (1992) called this long-standing misinterpretation of what Arithmetic was measuring, "The Pitfall of Face Validity."

The potential for error when relying on test scores alone is illustrated in two well-publicized studies on the clinical interpretation of test scores.

Almost all of the participating psychologists drew erroneous conclusions from test scores faked by three preadolescents and three adolescents, respectively (Faust, Hart, and Guilmette, 1988; Faust, Hart, et al., 1988). Although the investigators used these data to question the ability of neuropsychological examiners to detect malingering, their findings are open to two quite different interpretations: (1) *Valid interpretations of neuropsychological status cannot be accomplished by reliance on scores alone.* Neuropsychological assessment requires knowledge and understanding of *how* the subject performed the tests, of the circumstances of the examination—*why, where, when, what for*—and of the subject's appreciation of and attitudes about these circumstances. The psychologist/subjects of these studies did not have access to this information and apparently did not realize the need for it. (2) *Training, experience, and knowledge are prerequisites for neuropsychological competence.* Of 226 mailings containing the children's protocols that were properly addressed, only seventy-seven (34%) "usable ones" were returned; of the adolescent study, again only about one-third of potential judges completed the evaluation task. The authors made much of the 8+ years of practice in neuropsychology claimed by these respondent-judges, but they note that in the child study only "about 17%" had completed formal postdoctoral training in neuropsychology, and in the adolescent study this number dropped to 12.5%. They do not report how many diplomates of the American Board of Professional Psychology in Neuropsychology participated in each study. (Bigler [1990b] found that only one of 77 respondents to the child study had achieved diplomate status!); nor do they explain that any psychologist can claim to be a neuropsychologist with little training and no supervision. An untrained person can be as neuropsychologically naive in the 8th or even the 16th year of practice as in the first. Those psychologists who were willing to draw clinical conclusions from this kind of neuropsychological numerology may well have been less well-trained or knowledgeable than the greater number of psychologists who actively declined or simply did not send in the requested judgments. (I was one who actively declined [mdl].)

Qualitative data

Qualitative data are direct observations. In the formal neuropsychological examination these include observations of the patient's test-taking behavior as well as test behavior per se. Observations of patients' appearance, verbalizations, gestures, tone of voice, mood and affect, personal concerns, habits, and idiosyncrasies can provide a great deal of information about their life situation and overall adjustment, as well as attitudes toward the examination and the condition that brings them to it. More specific to the test situation are observations of patients' reactions to the examination itself, their approach to different kinds of test problems, and their expressions of feelings and opinions about how they are performing. Observations of the manner in which they handle test material, the wording of test responses, the nature and consistency of errors and successes, fluctuations in attention and perseverance, emotional state, and the quality of performance from moment to moment as they interact with the examiner and with the different kinds of test material are the qualitative data of the test performance itself (Milberg, Hebben, and Kaplan, 1996; Walsh and Darby, 1999).

Limitations of qualitative data

Distortion or misinterpretation of information obtained by direct observation results from different kinds of methodological and examination problems. All of the standardization, reliability, and validity problems inherent in the collection and evaluation of data by a single observer are ever-present threats to objectivity (Spreen and Risser, 2003, p. 46). In neuropsychological assessment, the vagaries of neurological impairment compound these problems. When the patient's communication skills are questionable, examiners can never be certain that they have understood their transactions with the patient—or that the patient has understood them. Worse yet, the communication disability may be so subtle and well masked by the patient that the examiner is not aware of communication slips. There is also the likelihood that the patient's actions will be idiosyncratic and therefore unfamiliar and subject to misunderstanding. Some patients may be entirely or variably uncooperative, many times quite unintentionally.

Moreover, when the neurological insult does not produce specific defects but rather reduces efficiency in the performance of behaviors that tend to be normally distributed among adults, such as response rate, recall of words or designs, and ability to abstract and generalize, examiners benefit from scaled tests with standardized norms. The early behavioral evidence of a deteriorating disease and much of the behavioral expression of traumatic brain injury or little strokes can occur as a quantifiable diminution in the efficiency of the affected system(s) rather than as a qualitative distortion of the normal response. This can be a prominent feature of conditions of rapid onset, such as trauma, stroke, or certain infections, particularly after the acute stages have passed and the first vivid and highly specific symptoms have dissipated. In such cases it is often difficult if not impossible to appreciate the nature or extent of cognitive impairment without recourse to quantifiable examination techniques that permit a relatively objective comparison between different functions. It is true that as clinicians gain experience with many patients from different backgrounds, representing a wide range of abilities, and suffering from a variety of cerebral insults, they are increasingly able to estimate or at least anticipate the subtle deficits that show up as lowered scores on tests. This sharpening of observational talents reflects the development of internalized norms based on clinical experience accumulated over the years.

Blurring the line between quantitative and qualitative evaluations

Efforts to systematize and even enhance observation of how subjects go about failing—or succeeding—when tested have produced a potentially clinically valuable hybrid: quantification of the qualitative aspects of test responses (Poreh, 2000). Glozman (1999) shows how the examination procedures considered to be most qualitative can be quantified and thus adaptable for retest comparisons and research. She developed a six-point scale ranging from 0 (no symptoms) to 3 (total failure), with half-steps between 0 and 1 and 2 to document relatively subtle differences in performance levels.

Other neuropsychologists have developed systems for scoring qualitative features. Joy, Fein, Kaplan, and Freedman (2001) demonstrate this hybrid technique in their analysis of Block Design (WIS-A) performances into specific components that distinguish good from poor solutions. Based on their observations they devised a numerical rating scheme and normed it on a large sample of healthy older (50–90 years) subjects, thus providing criteria for normal ranges of error types for this age group. Joy and his colleagues emphasize that the purely quantitative "pass–fail" scoring system does not do justice to older subjects who may copy most but not quite all of a design correctly.

Quantified qualitative errors provide information about lateralized deficits that scores alone cannot give. Quantifying broken configuration errors on Block Design discriminated seizure patients with left hemisphere foci from those with foci on the right as the latter made more such errors ($p = .008$) although the raw score means for these two groups were virtually identical (left, 26.6 ± 12.4; right, 26.4 ± 12.8) (Zipf-Williams et al., 2000). Perceptual fragmentation (naming a picture part) on the Hooper Visual Organization Test was a problem for more right than left hemisphere stroke patients, while the reverse was true for failures in providing the correct name of the picture (Nadler, Grace, et al., 1996; see p. 400).

Methods for evaluating strategy and the kinds of error made in copying the Complex Figure have been available for decades (see pp. 542–547). Their score distributions, relationships to recall scores, interindividual variability, and correlates with executive function measures were evaluated by Troyer and Wishart (1997)

who recommended that, although not all had satisfactory statistical properties, examiners "may wish to select a system appropriate for their needs."

Integrated data

The integrated use of qualitative and quantitative examination data treats these two different kinds of information as different parts of the whole data base. Test scores that have been interpreted without reference to the context of the examination in which they were obtained may be objective but meaningless in their individual applications. Clinical observations unsupported by standardized and quantifiable testing, although full of import for the individual, lack the comparability necessary for many diagnostic and planning decisions. Descriptive observations flesh out the skeletal structure of numerical test scores. Each is incomplete without the other. The value of taking into account all aspects of a test performance was exemplified in a study comparing the accuracy of purely score-based predictors of lateralization with accuracy based on score profiles plus qualitative aspects of the patient's performance (Ogden-Epker and Cullum, 2001). Accuracy was greatest when qualitative features entered into performance interpretation.

Common Interpretation Errors

1. If this, then that: the problem of overgeneralizing

Kevin Walsh (1985) described a not uncommon interpretation error made by examiners who overgeneralize their findings. He gives the example of two diagnostically different groups (patients with right hemisphere damage and those with chronic alcoholism) generating one similar cluster of scores, a parallel that led some investigators to conclude that chronic alcoholism somehow shriveled the right but not the left hemisphere (see p. 261). At the individual case level, dementia patients as well as chronic alcoholics can earn depressed scores on the same WIS tests that are particularly sensitive to right hemisphere damage. If all that the examiner attends to is this cluster of low scores, then diagnostic confusion can result. The logic of this kind of thinking "is the same as arguing that because a horse meets the test of being a large animal with four legs [then] any newly encountered large animal with four legs must be a horse" (E. Miller, 1983).

2. Failure to demonstrate a reduced performance: the problem of false negatives

The absence of low scores or other evidence of impaired performance is expected in intact persons but will also occur when brain damaged patients have not been given an appropriate examination (Teuber, 1969).

3. Confirmatory bias

This is the common tendency to "seek and value supportive evidence at the expense of contrary evidence" when the outcome is [presumably] known (Wedding and Faust, 1989).

A neuropsychologist who specializes in blind analysis of Halstead-Reitan data reviewed the case of a highly educated middle-aged woman who claimed neuropsychological deficits as a result of being stunned when her car was struck from the rear some 21 months before she took the examination in question. In the report on his analysis of the test scores alone the neuropsychologist stated that, "The test results would be compatible with some type of traumatic injury (such as a blow to the head), but they could possibly have been due to some other kind of condition, such as viral or bacterial infection of the brain." After reviewing the history he concluded that although he had suspected an infectious disorder as an alternative diagnostic possibility, the case history that he later reviewed provided no evidence of encephalitis or meningitis, deemed by him to be the most likely types of infection. He thus concluded that the injury sustained in the motor vehicle accident caused the neuropsychological deficits indicated by the test data. Interestingly, the patient's medical history showed that complaints of sensory alterations and motor weakness dating back almost two decades were considered to be suggestive of multiple sclerosis; a recent MRI scan added support to this diagnostic possibility.

4. Misuse of salient data: over- and underinterpretation

Wedding and Faust (1989) made the important point that a single dramatic finding (which could simply be a normal mistake; see Roy, 1982) may be given much greater weight than a not very interesting history that extends over years (such as steady employment) or base rate data. On the other hand, a cluster of a few abnormal examination findings that correspond with the patient's complaints and condition may provide important evidence of a cerebral disorder, even when most scores reflect intact functioning. Gronwall (1991) illustrated this point with mild head trauma as an example, as many of these patients perform at or near premorbid levels except on tests sensitive to attentional disturbances. If only one or two such tests are given, then a single abnormal finding could seem to be due to chance when it is not.

5. Underutilization of base rates

Base rates are particularly relevant when evaluating "diagnostic" signs or symptoms (Duncan and Snow,

1987). When a sign occurs more frequently than the condition it indicates, relying on that sign as a diagnostic indicator "will always produce more errors than would the practice of completely disregarding the sign(s)" (Wedding and Faust, 1989; see also Palmer, Boone, Lesser, et al., 1998). Another way of viewing this issue is to regard any sign that can occur with more than one condition as possibly suggestive but never pathognomonic. Such signs can lead to potentially fruitful hypotheses but not to conclusions. Thus, slurred speech rarely occurs in the intact adult population and so is usually indicative of some problem; but whether that problem is multiple sclerosis, a relatively recent right hemisphere infarct, or acute alcoholism—all conditions in which speech slurring can occur—must be determined by some other means.

EVALUATION OF NEUROPSYCHOLOGICAL EXAMINATION DATA

Qualitative Aspects of Examination Behavior

Two kinds of behavior are of special interest to the neuropsychological examiner when evaluating the qualitative aspects of a patient's behavior during the examination. One, of course, is behavior that differs from normal expectations or customary activity for the circumstances. Responding to Block Design instructions by matter-of-factly setting the blocks on the stimulus cards is obviously an aberrant response that deserves more attention than a score of zero alone would indicate. Satisfaction with a blatantly distorted response or tears and agitation when finding some test items difficult also should elicit the examiner's interest, as should statements of displeasure with a mistake unaccompanied by any attempt to correct it. Each of these behavioral aberrations may arise for any number of reasons. However, each is most likely to occur in association with certain neurological conditions and thus can also alert the examiner to look for other evidence of the suspected condition.

Regardless of their possible diagnostic usefulness, these aberrant responses also afford the examiner samples of behavior that, if characteristic, tell a lot about how patients think and how they perceive themselves, the world, and its expectations. The patient who sets blocks on the card not only has not comprehended the instructions but also is not aware of this failure when proceeding—unselfconsciously?—with this display of very concrete, structure-dependent behavior. Patients who express pleasure over an incorrect response are also unaware of their failures but, along with a distorted perception of the task, the product, or both, they demonstrate self-awareness and some sense of a scheme of things or a state of self-expectations that this performance satisfied.

The second kind of qualitatively interesting behaviors deserves special attention whether or not they are aberrant. Gratuitous responses are the comments patients make about their test performance or while they are taking the test, or the elaborations beyond the necessary requirements of a task that may enrich or distort their drawings, stories, or problem solutions, and usually individualize them. The value of gratuitous responses is well recognized in the interpretation of projective test material, for it is the gratuitously added adjectives, adverbs, or action verbs, flights of fancy whether verbal or graphic, spontaneously introduced characters, objects, or situations, that reflect the patient's mood and betray his or her preoccupations. Gratuitous responses are of similar value in neuropsychological assessment. The unnecessarily detailed spokes and gears of a bike with no pedals (see Fig. 6.2) tell of the patient's involvement with details at the expense of practical considerations. Expressions of self-doubt or self-criticism repeatedly voiced during a mental examination may reflect perplexity or depression and raise the possibility that the patient is not performing up to capacity (Lezak, 1978b).

In addition, patient responses gained by testing the limits or using the standard test material in an innovative manner to explore one or another working hypothesis have to be evaluated qualitatively. For example, on asking a patient to recall a set of designs ordinarily presented as a copy task (e.g., Wepman's variations of the Bender-Gestalt Test), the examiner will look for systematically occurring distortions—in size, angulation, simplifications, perseverations—that, if they did not occur on the copy trial, may shed some light on the patient's visual memory problems. In looking for systematic deviations in these and other drawing characteristics that may reflect dysfunction of one or more behavioral systems, the examiner also analyzes the patient's self-reports, stories, and comments for such qualities as disjunctive thinking, appropriateness of vocabulary, simplicity or complexity of grammatical constructions, richness or paucity of descriptions, etc.

Test Scores

Test scores can be expressed in a variety of forms. Rarely does a test-maker use a *raw* score—the simple sum of correct answers or correct answers minus a portion of the incorrect ones—for in itself a raw score communicates nothing about its relative value. Instead, test-makers generally report scores as values of a scale based on the raw scores made by a *standardization population* (the group of individuals tested for the purpose of obtaining normative data on the test). Each score then becomes a statement of its value relative to all other scores on that scale. Different kinds of scales provide more or less readily comprehended and statistically well-defined standards for comparing any one score with the scores of the standardization population. The most widely used scale is based on the *standard score.*

Standard scores

The usefulness of standard scores. The treatment of test scores in neuropsychological assessment is often a more complex task than in other kinds of cognitive evaluations because test scores can come from many different sources. In the usual cognitive examination, generally conducted for purposes of academic evaluation or career counseling, the bulk of the testing is done

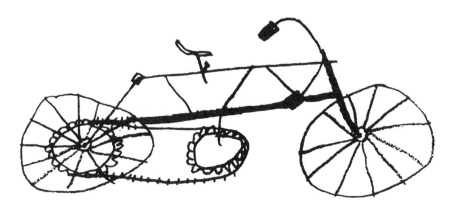

FIGURE 6.2 This bicycle was drawn by a 61-year-old retired millwright with a high school education. Two years prior to the neuropsychological examination he had suffered a stroke involving the right parietal lobe. He displayed no obvious sensory or motor deficits, and was alert, articulate, and cheerful but so garrulous that his talking could be interrupted only with difficulty. His highest WAIS scores, Picture Completion and Picture Arrangement, were in the *high average* ability range.

with one test battery, such as one of the WIS-A batteries or the Woodcock-Johnson Tests of Cognitive Ability. Within these batteries the scores for each of the individual tests are on the same scale and standardized on the same population so that test scores can be compared directly.

On the other hand, no single test battery provides all the information needed for adequate assessment of most patients presenting neuropsychological questions. Techniques employed in the assessment of different aspects of cognitive functioning have been developed at different times, in different places, on different populations, for different ability and maturity levels, with different scoring and classification systems, and for different purposes. Taken together, they are an unsystematized aggregate of more or less standardized tests, experimental techniques, and observational aids that have proven useful in demonstrating deficits or disturbances in some cognitive function or activity. These scores are not directly comparable with one another.

To make the comparisons necessary for evaluating impairment, the many disparate test scores must be convertible into one scale with identical units. Such a scale can serve as a kind of test users' *lingua franca*, permitting direct comparison between many different kinds of measurements. The scale that is most meaningful statistically and that probably serves the intermediary function between different tests best is one de-

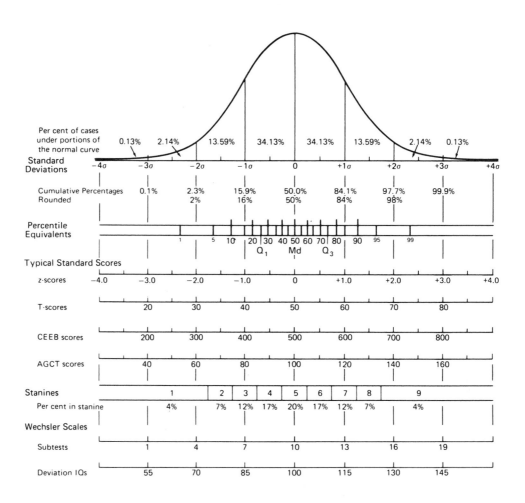

NOTE: *This chart cannot be used to equate scores on one test to scores on another test. For example, both 600 on the CEEB and 120 on the AGCT are one standard deviation above their respective means, but they do not represent "equal" standings because the scores were obtained from different groups.*

FIGURE 6.3 The relationship of some commonly used test scores to the normal curve and to one another. AGCT, Army General Classification Test; CEEB, College Entrance Examination Board. (Reprinted from the *Test Service Bulletin* of The Psychological Corporation, 1955).

rived from the normal probability curve and based on the standard deviation unit (SD) (Anastasi and Urbina, 1997) (see Fig. 6.3, p. 142).

The value of basing a common scale on the standard deviation unit lies primarily in the statistical nature of the standard deviation as a measure of the spread or dispersion of a set of scores (X_1, X_2, X_{-3}, etc.) around their mean (M). Standard deviation units describe known proportions of the normal probability curve (note on Fig. 6.3, "Percent of cases under portions of the normal curve"). This has very practical applications for comparing and evaluating psychological data in that the position of any test score on a standard deviation unit scale, in itself, defines the proportion of people taking the test who will obtain scores above and below the given score. Virtually all scaled psychological test data can be converted to standard deviation units for intertest comparisons. Furthermore, a score based on the standard deviation, a *standard score,* can generally be estimated from a *percentile,* which is the most commonly used nonstandard score in adult testing.

The likelihood that two numerically different scores are significantly different can also be estimated from their relative positions on a standard deviation unit scale. This use of the standard deviation unit scale is of particular importance in neuropsychological testing, for evaluation of test scores depends upon the significance of their distance from one another or from the comparison standard. Since direct statistical evaluations of the difference between scores obtained on different kinds of tests are rarely possible, the examiner must use estimates of the ranges of significance levels based on score comparisons. In general, differences of two standard deviations or more may be considered significant, whereas differences of one to two standard deviations suggest a trend; although M.J. Taylor and Heaton (2001) accept scores falling at -1 SD as indicating deficit.

Kinds of standard scores. Standard scores come in different forms but are all translations of the same scale, based on the mean and the standard deviation. The *z-score* is the basic, unelaborated standard score from which all others can be derived. The *z*-score represents, in standard deviation units, the amount a score deviates from the mean of the population from which it is drawn.

$$z = \frac{X - M}{s}$$

The mean of the normal curve is set at zero and the standard deviation unit has a value of one. Scores are stated in terms of their distance from the mean as mea-

sured in standard deviation units. Scores above the mean have a positive value; those below the mean are negative. Elaborations of the z-score are called *derived scores.* Derived scores provide the same information as do *z*-scores, but the score value is expressed in scale units that are more familiar to most test users than z-scores. Test-makers can assign any value they wish to the standard deviation and mean of their distribution of test scores. Usually, they follow convention and choose commonly used values. (Note the different means and standard deviations for tests listed in Fig. 6.3.) When the standardization populations are similar, all of the different kinds of standard scores are directly comparable with one another, the standard deviation and its relationship to the normal curve serving as the key to translation (see Fig. 6.3).

Estimating standard scores from nonstandard scores. Since most published standardized tests today use a standard score format for handling the numerical test data, their scores present little or no problem to the examiner wishing to make intertest comparisons. However, there are still a few test-makers who report their standardization data in percentile or IQ score equivalents. In these cases, standard score approximations can be estimated. Unless there is reason to believe that the standardization population is not normally distributed, a standard score equivalent for a percentile score can be estimated from a table of normal curve functions. Table 6.1 gives z-score approximations, taken from a normal curve table, for 21 percentiles ranging from 1 to 99 in five-point steps. The z-score that best approximates a given percentile is the one that corresponds to the percentile closest to the percentile in question.

Exceptions to the use of standard scores

Standardization population differences. In evaluating a patient's performance on a variety of tests, the examiner can only compare scores from different tests when the standardization populations of each of the

TABLE 6.1 Standard Score Equivalents for 21 Percentile Scores Ranging from 1 to 99

Percentile Score	z-Score	Percentile Score	z-Score	Percentile Score	z-Score
99	+2.33	65	+0.39	30	−0.52
95	+1.65	60	+0.25	25	−0.68
90	+1.28	55	+0.13	20	−0.84
85	+1.04	50	0	15	−1.04
80	+0.84	45	−0.13	10	−1.28
75	+0.68	40	−0.25	5	−1.65
70	0.52	35	−0.39	1	−2.33

tests are identical or at least reasonably similar, with respect to both demographic characteristics and score distribution (Anastasi and Urbina, 1997; Axelrod and Goldman, 1996; Mitrushina, Boone, and D'Elia, 1999; see Chapter 2). Otherwise, even though their scales and units are statistically identical, the operational meanings of the different values are as different as the populations from which they are drawn. The restriction becomes obvious should an examiner attempt to compare a vocabulary score obtained on a WIS-A test, which was standardized on cross-sections of the general adult population, with a score on the Graduate Record Examination (GRE), standardized on college graduates. A person who receives an *average* score on the GRE would probably achieve scores of one to two standard deviations above the mean on WIS-A tests, since the average college graduate typically scores one to two standard deviations above the general population mean on tests of this type (Anastasi, 1965). Although each of these mean scores has the same z-score value, the performance levels they represent are very different.

Test-makers usually describe their standardization populations in terms of sex, race, age, and/or education. Intraindividual comparability of scores may differ between the sexes in that women tend to do less well on advanced arithmetic problems and visuospatial items and men are more likely to display a verbal skill disadvantage (see pp. 303–304). Education, too, affects level of performance on different kinds of tests differentially, making its greatest contribution to tasks involving verbal skills, stored information, and other school-related activities, but affects test performances in all areas (see pp. 315–317). Significant differences between major racial groups have not been consistently demonstrated in the score patterns of tests of various cognitive abilities or in neuropsychological functioning (Faulstitch, McAnulty, et al., 1987; A.S. Kaufman, McLean, and Reynolds, 1988; P.E. Vernon, 1979; see also Manly, Jacobs, Touradji, et al., 2002). Vocational and regional differences between standardization populations may also contribute to differences between test norms. However, vocational differences generally correlate highly with educational differences, and regional differences tend to be relatively insignificant compared with age and variables that are highly correlated with income level, such as education or vocation.

Age can be a very significant variable when evaluating test scores of older patients (see pp. 296–301 and Chapters 9–16, *passim*). In patients over 50, the normal changes with age may obscure subtle cognitive changes that could herald an early, correctable stage of a tumor or vascular disease. The use of age-graded scores puts the aging patient's scoring pattern into sharper focus. Age-graded scores are important aids to differential diagnosis in patients over 50 and are essential to the evaluation of test performances of patients over 65. Although not all tests an examiner may wish to use have age-graded norms or age corrections, enough are available to determine the extent to which a patient might be exceeding the performance decrements expected at a given age.

Children's tests. Some children's tests are applicable to the examination of patients with severe cognitive impairment or profound disability. Additionally, many good tests of academic abilities such as arithmetic, reading, and spelling have been standardized for child or adolescent populations. The best of these invariably have standard score norms that, by and large, cannot be applied to an adult population because of the significant effect of age and education on performance differences between adults and children.

Senior high school norms are the one exception to this rule. On tests of mental ability that provide adult norms extending into the late teens, the population of 18-year-olds does not perform much differently than the adult population at large (e.g., see D. Wechsler, 1955, 1981, 1997a), and four years of high school is a reasonable approximation of the adult educational level. This exception makes a great number of very well-standardized and easily administered paper-and-pencil academic skill tests available for the examination of adults, and no scoring changes are necessary.

All other children's tests are best scored and reported in terms of mental age (MA), which is psychologically the most meaningful score derived from these tests. Most children's tests provide mental age norms or grade level norms (which readily convert into mental age). Mental age scores allow the examiner to estimate the extent of impairment, or to compare performance on different tests or between two or more tests administered over time, just as is done with test performances in terms of standard scores. When test norms for children's tests are given in standard scores or percentiles for each age or set of ages the examiner can convert the score to a mental age score by finding the age at which the obtained score is closest to a score at the 50th percentile or the standard score mean. Mental age scores can be useful for planning educational or retraining programs.

Small standardization populations. A number of interesting and potentially useful tests of specific skills and abilities have been devised for studies of particular neuropsychological problems in which the standardization groups are relatively small (often under 20) (e.g., Talland, 1965a). Standard score conversions are inappropriate if not impossible in such cases. When there is a clear relationship between the condition under study and a particular kind of performance on a given test, there is frequently a fairly clear-cut separation between patient and control group scores. Any given patient's score can be evaluated in terms of how closely it compares with the score ranges of either the patient or the control group reported in the study.

Nonparametric distributions

It is not uncommon for score distributions generated by a neuropsychologically useful test to be markedly skewed—often due to ceiling (e.g., digit span) or floor (e.g., Trail Making Test) effects inherent in the nature of the test (Retzlaff and Gibertini, 1994). For these tests—including many of those used in neuropsychological assessment—standard scores, which theoretically imply a distribution base that reasonably approximates the parametric ideal of a bell-shaped curve, are of questionable value as, with skewing, the weight of scores at the far end of a distribution becomes greatly exaggerated, resulting in overblown standard deviations (Lezak and Gray, 1991). When this occurs, standard deviations can be so large that even performances that seemingly should fall into the abnormal range appear to be *within normal limits*. The Trail Making Test provides an instructive example of this statistical phenomenon.

Heaton, Grant, and Matthews (1986, reported in Mitrushina, Boone, and D'Elia, 1999, p. 58) thoughtfully provided score ranges and median scores along with means and standard deviations of a normative population. Their 20–29 year group's average score was 86 ± 39 sec but the range of 47" to 245" with a median score of 76 indicates that many more subjects performed below than above the mean and that the large standard deviation—swollen by a few very slow responders—brings subjects under the umbrella of *within normal limits* who—taking as much as 124" (i.e., < -1 SD) to complete Trails B—do not belong there.

Benton showed the way to resolve the problem of skewed distributions by identifying the score at the 5th percentile as the boundary for abnormality—i.e., *defective* performance (see Benton, Sivan, Hamsher, et al., 1994). Benton and his coworkers use percentiles to define degrees of competency on nonparametric test performances which also avoids the pitfalls of trying to fit nonparametric data into a Procrustean parametric bed.

Reporting Scores

The practice of reporting test performances in terms of scores can be confusing and misleading, particularly since most recipients of test reports are teachers, guidance counselors, physicians, and lawyers who lack

training in the niceties of psychometrics. One important source of faulty communication is variability in the size of assigned standard deviations (see Fig. 6.3, note how the Army General Classification Test [AGCT] and Wechsler Deviation IQ scores differ at different levels). Thus, a score of 110 is at the 75th %ile (at the low edge of the *high average* range) when $SD = 15$, but when $SD = 10$ the same score will be at approximately the 67th %ile (within the *average* range). Unless the persons who receive the test report are statistically sophisticated and knowledgeable about the scaling idiosyncrasies of test makers, it is unlikely that they will notice or appreciate these kinds of discrepancies.[1]

Another difficulty in reporting scores lies in the statistically naive person's natural assumption that if one measurement is larger than another, there is a difference in the quantity of whatever is being measured. Unfortunately, few persons unschooled in statistics understand measurement error; they do not realize that two different numbers need not necessarily stand for different quantities but may be chance variations in the measurement of the same quantity. Laymen who see a report listing a WIS-A Similarities score of 9 and an Arithmetic score of 11 are likely to draw the probably erroneous conclusion that the subject does better in mathematics than in verbal reasoning. Since most score differences of this magnitude are chance variations, it is more likely that the subject is equally capable in both areas.

Further, there has been a tendency, both within school systems and in the culture at large, to reify test scores (Lezak, 1988b). In many schools, this has too often resulted in the arbitrary and rigid sorting of children into different parts of a classroom, into different ability level classes, and onto different vocational tracks. In its extreme form, reification of test scores has provided a predominant frame of reference for evaluating people generally. It is usually heard in remarks that take some real or supposed IQ score to indicate an individual's personal or social worth. "Sam couldn't have more than an 'IQ' of 80," means that the speaker thinks Sam is socially incompetent. "My Suzy's 'IQ' is 160!" is a statement of pride.

Although these numerical metaphors presumably are meaningful for the people who use them, the meanings are not standardized or objective, nor do they bear any necessary relationships to the meaning test-makers define for the scores in their scoring systems. Thus, the communication of numerical test scores, particularly if the test-taker has labeled them "IQ" scores, becomes

[1]A discussion was prompted by Freides' (1993) opinion that scores should be appended to reports. The pros and cons of this proposal appear in Freides (1995), R. Matarazzo (1995), and Naugle and McSweeney (1995, 1996). The decision regarding score reporting remains the neuropsychologist's except, of course, when required to release them by court order.

an uncertain business since the examiners have no way of knowing what kind of meaning their readers have already attached to mental test scores.

One way to avoid the many difficulties inherent in test score reporting is to write about test performances in terms of the commonly accepted classification of ability levels (D. Wechsler, 1958, 1981, 1997a). In the standard classification system, each ability level represents a statistically defined range of scores. Both percentile scores and standard scores can be classified in terms of ability level (see Table 6.2).

Test performances communicated in terms of ability levels have generally accepted and relatively clear meanings. When in doubt as to whether such classifications as *average, high average,* and so on make sense to the reader, the examiner can qualify them with a statement about the percentile range they represent, for the public generally understands the meaning of percentiles. For example, in reporting Wechsler test scores of 12 and 13, the examiner can say, "The patient's performance on [the particular tests] was within the *high average* ability level, which is between the upper 75th and 91st percentiles, approximately."

One caveat to the use of percentiles should be mentioned. The terms *percent* (as in percent correct) and *percentile* (rank) are not interchangeable and sometimes not clearly distinguished conceptually by the public.

When being deposed, a lawyer essentially made the statement "Mr. X performed at the 50th percentile on this test and you said that was an *average* performance. If I'd got 50% on any test in school that would have been considered poor performance."

What the lawyer failed to realize is that *percent correct* on a test is related to variables such as the difficulty of the items and the test-taker's knowledge and psychological and physical state at the time of administration. If a test is easy, 80% correct could be the 50th %ile with half of the class scoring at this level or above. If a test is difficult, 25% correct could be at the 50th %ile with only one half of the class making 25% or more correct responses. *Percentile (rank)* refers to the position of the score in the distribution of scores. On every test, regardless of the test and test-taker variables, the 50th percentile is always the middle score (or median [*Mdn*]) in the distribution.

Converting scores to ability levels also enables the examiner to report clusters of scores that may be one or two—or, in the case of tests with fine-grained scales, several—score points apart but that probably represent a normal variation of scores around a single ability level. Thus, in dealing with the performance of a patient who receives scores of 8, 9, or 10 on each Wechsler test involving verbal skills, the examiner can report that, "The patient's verbal skill level is *average.*" Significant performance discrepancies can also be readily noted. Should a patient achieve *average* scores on verbal tests but *low average* to *borderline defective* scores on constructional tasks, the examiner can note both the levels of the different clusters of test scores and the likelihood that discrepancies between these levels approach or reach significance.

INTERPRETING THE EXAMINATION DATA

Examination data can be used for diagnostic decision-making, treatment, and planning purposes in several ways. Issues arise with respect to choice of tests, norms, criteria for impairment, and sensitivity/specificity data. Additionally, *screening techniques* are used in some clinical situations to determine whether a defect due to brain dysfunction is likely to be present; screening test findings need to be carefully evaluated by the clinician. A *pattern approach* to test score analysis can provide diagnostically useful information as well as greater efficacy than simple screening techniques in identifying organically impaired persons. *Integrated interpretation* takes into account test signs of brain damage and test score patterns in conjunction with the qualitative aspects of the examination. Each of these issues and approaches will be discussed below.

Evaluation Issues

Norms

Most tests of a single cognitive function, ability, or skill do not have separate norms for age, sex, education, etc. A few widely used tests of general mental abilities take into account the geographic distribution of their standardization population; the rest are usually standardized on local people. Tests developed in Minnesota will have Minnesota norms; New York test-makers use a

TABLE 6.2 Classification of Ability Levels

Classification	z-Score	Percent Included	Lower Limit of Percentile Range
Very superior	+2.0 and above	2.2	98
Superior	+1.3 to 2.0	6.7	91
High average	+0.6 to 1.3	16.1	75
Average	±0.6	50.0	25
Low average	−0.6 to −1.3	16.1	9
Borderline	−1.3 to −2.0	6.7	2
Retarded	−2.0 and below	2.2	—

big city population; and British tests are standardized on British populations. Although this situation results in less than perfect comparability between the different tests, in most cases the examiner has no choice but to use norms of tests standardized on an undefined mixed or nonrandom adult sample. Experience quickly demonstrates that this is usually not a serious hardship, for these "mixed-bag" norms generally serve their purpose. "I sometimes determine *SD* units for a patient's score on several norms to see if they produce a different category of performance. Most of the time it doesn't make a significant difference. [If] it does then [one has] to use judgment [hjh]." Certainly one important normative fault of many single-purpose tests is that they lack discriminating norms at the population extremes. Different norms, derived on different samples in different places, and sometimes for different reasons, can produce quite different evaluations for some subjects resulting in false positives or false negatives, depending on the subject's score, condition, and the norm against which the score is compared (Kalechstein et al., 1998; Lezak, 2002).

Thus, finding appropriate norms for each patient is still a challenge for clinicians. Many neuropsychologists collect a variety of norms over the years from the research literature [e.g., hjh, mdl]. The situation has improved to some degree in recent years with the publication of collections of norms for many but not all of the most favored tests (Mitrushina, Boone and D'Elia, 1999; Spreen and Strauss, 1998). However, there are times when none of these norms really applies to a particular person's performance on a specific test. In such cases, the procedure involves checking against several norm samples to see if there is a reasonable degree of consistency across norms. When the data from other tests involving a different normative sample but measuring essentially the same cognitive or motor abilities are not in agreement, this should alert the clinician about a problem with the norms for that test as applied to this individual. This problem with norms is very important in forensic cases, for example, when the choice of norms can introduce interpretation bias (van Gorp and McMullen, 1997). The final decision concerning the selection of norms requires clinical judgment.

A large body of evidence clearly indicates that demographic variables—especially age and education—are related to performance (and sex and race on some tests) (see data presented in Chapters 9–16, *passim*). Yet some have argued against the use of demographically based norms and suggest that test score adjustment may invalidate the raw test scores (Reitan and Wolfson, 1995b). This argument is based on findings that test performance was significantly related to age and education for normal subjects but not to age and

barely for education in a brain damaged group. However, a reduction in the association between demographics and performance is to be expected on a statistical basis for brain damaged individuals.

Suppose that variable X is significantly related to variable Y in the normal population. If a group of individuals is randomly selected from the population, the relationship between variables X and Y will continue to be present in this group. Add random error to one of the variables, for instance Y, and the relationship between X and (Y + random error) will be reduced. Now apply this reasoning to an example bearing on the argument against use of demographic score adjustments. Age is related to performance on a memory test in the normal population. Some individuals, a random sample from the normal population, have a brain disorder and are asked to take the memory test. The effects of their brain dysfunction on memory performance introduces random error, given that brain dysfunction varies in the cause, location, severity, and effects on each person's current physiology, psychiatric status, circumstances, motivation, etc. As a result, the statistical association between age and memory test performance is likely to be reduced.

If aspects of the brain damage itself had been held constant in the Reitan and Wolfson (1995b) study that prompted questioning about use of demographic variables, perhaps the associations would have been quite significant in the brain damaged group too (Vanderploeg, Axelrod, and Sherer, 1997). If younger individuals had more severe brain damage than older ones or more educated individuals had greater brain damage than less educated ones, the age–education relationships could be small or insignificant. In short, changes in these relationships do not invalidate the use of demographically based norms. Since premorbid neuropsychological test data are rare, demographically based norms aid test interpretation. Without demographically appropriate norms, the false positive rate for older or poorly educated normal individuals tends to increase (Bornstein, 1985, 1986a; Prigatano and Parsons, 1976; also see pp. 315–316). Some false negative findings can be expected (J.E. Morgan and Caccappolo-van Vliet, 2001). Yet, if a test consistently produces many false negatives or false positives with particular demographic combinations, this problem requires reevaluation of norms or demographic scoring adjustments.

At this time, relatively few normative samples include all of the demographic variable combinations that may be pertinent to measurement data on a particular ability or behavior. Those few samples in which all relevant demographic variables have been taken into account typically have too few subjects for dependable interpretation in the individual case.

Impairment criteria

Neuropsychologists generally use a criterion for suggesting that overall performance on a particular test is impaired, but it is not necessarily explicitly stated and is unlikely to appear in reports. Once test data have been reliably scored and appropriate norms have been chosen to convert scores to standard scores and percentiles, the clinician needs to determine if performance on individual tests is impaired or not and whether the pattern of performance is consistent with the background and any neurologic, psychiatric, and/or other medical disorders. Sometimes, when poor performance does not represent an acquired impairment, simple questions about a person's abilities may elicit information that confirms lifelong difficulty in these areas of cognitive or motor ability. A poor performance may also indicate that the person was not motivated to do well or was anxious, depressed, or hostile to the test-taking endeavor rather than impaired.

Estimates of premorbid level of patient's functioning become important in determining whether a given test performance represents impairment (see pp. 90–91, 99). In some cases such estimates are relatively easy to make because prior test data are available from school, military, medical, psychological, or neuropsychological records. At other times, the current test data are the primary source of the estimate. A change from this estimate, perhaps 1, 1.5, or 2 SDs lower than the premorbid estimate, may be used as the criterion for determining the likelihood that a particular test performance is impaired. A test score that appears to represent a 1 SD change from premorbid functioning may not be a statistically significant change but may indicate an impairment to some examiners and only suggest impaired performance to others. A 2 SD score depression is clear evidence of impairment.

Since approximately 15% of intact individuals obtain scores greater than 1 SD below test means, there is concern that too many individuals who are intact with respect to particular functions will be judged impaired when using −1 SD as an impairment criterion. When the criterion is less stringent (e.g., −1 SD rather than −2), more intact performance will be called impaired (i.e., *false positive*) and the more "*hits*" (i.e., impaired performance correctly identified) are to be expected. On the other hand, when criteria become overly strict (e.g., > −2) the possible increase in *misses* occurs such that a truly impaired performance is judged normal (i.e., *false negative*). These errors can be costly to patients with a developing, treatable disease such as some types of brain tumors which will grow and do much mischief if not identified as soon as possible. Should this be a false alarm, the patient is no worse off in the long run but may have paid in unnecessary worry and expensive medical tests. In the case of a possible dementia, this would not be a costly error since there is not successful treatment at the moment and the disorder will progress and have to be managed until the individual dies. However, neuropsychological conclusions will not rest on a single aberrant score. Regardless of the criterion used, the resulting *pattern* of change in performance should make diagnostic sense.

Some neuropsychologists interpret as "probably impaired" any test score 1 or more SD lower than the mean of a normative sample that may or may not take into account appropriate demographics (e.g., Golden, Purisch, and Hammeke, 1991; Heaton, Grant, and Matthews, 1991). This latter group has converted scores from the Halstead-Reitan battery plus other tests into T-scores based on age, education, and sex corrections. In this system a T-score below 40 (> −1 below the mean) is considered likely *to* represent impaired performance. For Heaton, Ryan, and their coworkers (1996), the *pattern* of test scores is also important and must make sense in terms of the patient's history and suspected disorder or disease process. In evaluating test performances, it must be kept in mind that intact individuals are likely to vary in their performance on any battery of cognitive tests and it is not unusual for them to score in the impaired range on one or two tests (Jarvis and Barth, 1994; Taylor and Heaton, 2001).

Concern has been raised that using a criterion for decision making that represents a deviation from the mean of the normative sample rather than change from premorbid level of functioning is likely to result in missing significant changes in very high functioning individuals while suggesting that low functioning individuals have acquired impairments that they do not have.

For instance, a concert pianist might begin to develop slight difficulties in hand functioning in the early stages of Parkinson's disease that were noticeable to him but not to an examiner who uses a criterion for impairment linked to the mean of the distribution of scores for males of his age, education, and sex. In that case another musician might pick up the difference by comparing recordings of an earlier performance with a current performance. Contrast this example with one of several painters who claimed to be brain-damaged after inhaling epoxy paint fumes in a poorly ventilated college locker room. On the basis of his age and education he would be expected to perform at an *average* level. Linking poor performance on many tests to toxic exposure by one psychologist seemed appropriate. However, once his grade school through high school records were obtained, it was found that he had always been functioning at a *borderline* to *retarded* level on group mental ability and achievement tests.

When such evidence of premorbid functioning is available—and often it is not—it far outweighs normative expectations. Robert Heaton (personal communication, 2003 [hjh]) said, "If I had reason to believe that the person was not representative of what appears to be the appropriate normative sample, I would compare the individual with a more appropriate sample [e.g., compare an academically skilled high-school dropout to a higher educational normative sample] and be prepared to defend this decision." This is how competent clinicians tend to decide in the individual case whether to use impairment criteria based on large sample norms or smaller, more demographically fitting norms.

Sensitivity/specificity and diagnostic accuracy

It has become the custom of some investigators in clinical neuropsychology to judge the "goodness" of a test or measure and its efficiency in terms of its diagnostic accuracy, i.e., the percentage of cases it correctly identifies as belonging to either a clinical population or a control group or to either of two clinical populations. This practice is predicated on questionable assumptions, one of which is that the accuracy with which a test makes diagnostic classifications is a major consideration in evaluating its clinical worth. Most tests are not used for this purpose most of the time but rather to provide a description of the individual's strengths and weaknesses, to monitor the status of a disorder or disease, or for treatment and planning. The criterion of diagnostic accuracy becomes important when evaluating screening tests for particular kinds of deficits (e.g., an aphasia screening test), single tests purporting to be sensitive to brain dysfunction, and sometimes other tests and test batteries as well.

The accuracy of diagnostic classification to some degree depends on its sensitivity and specificity. *Sensitivity* refers to the probability of correctly detecting abnormal functioning in an impaired individual (i.e., the "hit rate"). *Specificity* refers to the probability of correctly identifying a normal individual or an individual from another clinical population intact with respect to the test under consideration (i.e., correct rejection of abnormality). Sensitivity/specificity data have been used to validate a criterion for impairment.

The percentage of cases classified accurately by any given test, however, will depend on the base rate of the condition(s) for which the test is sensitive in the population(s) used to evaluate its goodness. It will also depend on the demographics of the population, for instance, level of education (Ostrosky-Solis, Lopez-Arango, and Ardila, 2000). With judicious selection of populations, an investigator can virtually predetermine the outcome. If high diagnostic accuracy rates are desired, then the brain damaged population (e.g., patients with left hemisphere lesions) should consist of subjects who are known to suffer the condition(s) (e.g., communication disorders) measured by the test(s) under consideration (e.g., an aphasia screening test); members of the comparison population (e.g., normal control subjects, neurotic patients) should be chosen on the basis that they are unlikely to have the condition(s) measured by the test. Using a population in which the frequency of the condition measured by the test(s) under consideration is much lower (e.g., patients who have had only one stroke, regardless of site) will necessarily lower the sensitivity rate. However, this lower hit rate should not reflect upon the value of the test. The extent to which sensitivity/specificity rates will differ is shown by the large differences reported in studies using the same test(s) on different kinds of clinical (and control) populations (e.g., Bornstein, 1986a; Mitrushina, Boone, and D'Elia, 1999). Moreover, it will usually be inappropriate to apply sensitivity/specificity data collected on a population with one kind of neurological disorder to patients suspected of having a different condition.

When history, simple observation, or well-established laboratory techniques clearly demonstrate a neurological disorder, neuropsychological tests are not needed to document brain damage (Holden, 2001).

For example, Duffala (1978) used the battery developed by Golden (1979) (see pp. 681–685) to compare 20 "head trauma patients . . . who had injuries resulting from airplane, car, or motor cycle accident, gunshot wound, or severe blow to the head in falling . . . [when] the patients reached an appropriate level of awareness" with "volunteers from a university community or . . . hospital staff." Not surprisingly, she found that this battery "does discriminate between groups of people having brain injury and those without." However, the ability to use a can opener would probably have discriminated as well between these groups.

Since the "sensitivity/specificity diagnostic accuracy rate" standard can be manipulated by the choice of populations studied and the discrimination rate found for one set of populations or one disorder may not apply to others, it is per se virtually meaningless as a measure of a test's effectiveness in identifying brain impaired or intact subjects except under similar conditions with similar populations. A particular test's sensitivity to a specific disorder is, of course, always of interest.

The decision-making procedure (or combination of procedures) that best accomplishes the goal of accurate diagnosis has yet to be agreed upon; and there may be none that will be best in all cases. In the end, decisions are made about individuals. Regardless of how clinicians reach their conclusions, they must always be sensitive to those elements involved in each patient's case that may be unique as well as those similar to cases seen before: qualitative and quantitative data from test performance, behavioral observation, interviews with family members and others as possible, and the history. Disagreements among clinicians are most likely to occur when the symptoms are vague and/or mild; the developmental, academic, medical, psychiatric, psychosocial, and/or occupational histories are complex or not fully available; and the pattern of test performance is not clearly associated with a specific diagnostic entity.

Screening Techniques

Different screening techniques make use of different kinds of behavioral manifestations of brain damage. Some patients suffer only a single highly specific defect or a cluster of related disabilities while, for the most part, cognitive functioning remains intact. Others sustain widespread impairment involving changes in cognitive, self-regulating, and executive functions; attention; and personality. Still others display aberrations characteristic of brain dysfunction (*signs*) with more or less subtle evidence of cognitive or emotional deficits. With such a variety of signs, symptoms, and behavioral alterations, it is no more reasonable to expect accurate detection of every instance of brain disorder with one or a few instruments or lists of signs and symptoms than to expect that a handful of laboratory tests would bring to light all gastrointestinal tract diseases. Yet many clinical and social service settings need some practical means for screening when the population under consideration—such as professional boxers, alcoholics seeking treatment, persons tested as HIV positive, or elderly depressed patients, to give just a few instances—is at more than ordinary risk of a brain disorder.

The accuracy of screening tests varies in a somewhat direct relationship to the narrowness of range or specificity of the behaviors assessed by them (Sox et al., 1988). The specific cognitive defects associated with neurological disorders affect a relatively small proportion of the brain-impaired population as a whole, and virtually no one whose higher brain functions are intact. For instance, *perseveration* (the continuation of a response after it is no longer appropriate, as in writing three or four "e's" in a word such as "deep" or "seen" or in copying a 12-dot line without regard for the number, stopping only when the edge of the page is reached) is so strongly associated with brain damage that the examiner should suspect it on the basis of this defect alone. However, since most patients with brain disorders do not give perseverative responses, it is not a practical criterion for screening purposes. Use of a highly specific sign or symptom such as perseveration as a screening criterion for brain damage results in few persons without brain damage being misidentified as brain

damaged (false positive errors), but such a narrow test will let many persons who are brain damaged slip through the screen (false negative errors) (L. Costa, 1988). In contrast, those defects that affect cognitive functioning generally, such as distractibility, impaired immediate memory, and concrete thinking, are not only very common symptoms of brain damage but tend to accompany a number of emotional disorders as well. As a result, a sensitive screening test that relies on a defect impairing cognitive functioning generally will identify many brain damaged patients correctly with few false negative errors, but a large number of people without brain disorders will also be included as a result of false positive errors of identification.

Limitations in predictive accuracy do not invalidate either tests for specific signs or tests that are sensitive to conditions of general dysfunction. Each kind of test can be used effectively as a screening device as long as its limitations are known and the information it elicits is interpreted accordingly. When testing is primarily for screening purposes, a combination of tests, including some that are sensitive to specific impairment, some to general impairment, and others that tend to draw out diagnostic signs, will make the best diagnostic discriminations.

Signs

The reliance on signs for identifying persons with a brain disorder is based on the assumption that brain disorders have some distinctive behavioral manifestations. In part this assumption reflects early concepts of brain damage as a unitary kind of dysfunction (e.g., Hebb, 1942; Shure and Halstead, 1958), and in part it arises from observations of response characteristics that do distinguish the test performances of many patients with brain disease.

Most pathognomonic signs in neuropsychological assessment are specific aberrant test responses or modes of response. These signs may be either positive, indicating the presence of abnormal function, or negative in that the function is lost or significantly diminished. Some signs are isolated response deviations that, in themselves, may indicate the presence of an organic defect. Rotation in copying a block design or a geometric figure has been considered a sign of brain damage. Specific test failures or test score discrepancies have also been treated as signs of brain dysfunction, as for instance, marked difficulty on a serial subtraction task (Ruesch and Moore, 1943) or a wide spread between the number of digits recalled in the order given and the number recalled in reversed order (D. Wechsler, 1958). The manner in which the patient responds to the task may also be considered a sign indicating brain damage. M. Williams (1979) associated three response characteristics with brain damage:

"stereotyping and perseveration;" "concreteness of behavior," defined by her as "response to all stimuli as if they existed only in the setting in which they are presented;" and "catastrophic reactions" of perplexity, acute anxiety, and despair when the patient is unable to perform the presented task.

Another common sign approach relies on not one but on the sum of different signs, i.e., the total number of different kinds of specific test response aberrations or differentiating test item selections made by the patient. This method has been used with the Rorschach test with some success (Z. Piotrowski, 1937). In practice, a number of behavior changes can serve as signs of brain dysfunction (see Table 6.3). None of them alone is pathognomonic of a specific brain disorder. When a patient presents with more than a few of these changes, the likelihood of a brain disorder runs very high.

Cutting scores

The score that separates the "normal" or "not impaired" from the "abnormal" or "impaired" ends of a continuum of test scores is called a *cutting score*, which marks the *cut-off* point. The use of cutting scores is akin to the sign approach, for their purpose is to separate patients in terms of the presence or absence of the condition under study. A statistically derived cutting score is the score that differentiates brain impaired patients from others with the fewest instances of error on either side. A cutting score may also be derived by simple inspection, in which case it is usually the score just below the poorest score attained by any member of the "normal" comparison group or below the lowest score made by 95% of the "normal" comparison group (see Benton, Sivan, Hamsher, et al., 1994, for examples).

Cutting scores are a prominent feature of most screening tests. However, many of the cutting scores used for neuropsychological diagnosis may be less efficient than the claims made for them (Meehl and Rosen, 1967). This is most likely to be the case when the establishment of a cutting score does not take into account the base rate at which the predicted condition occurs in the sample from which the cutting score was developed (Anastasi and Urbina, 1997; Satz, Fennell, and Reilly, 1970; W.G. Willis, 1984).

TABLE 6.3 Behavior Changes that Are Possible Indicators of a Pathological Brain Process

Functional Class*	Symptoms and Signs	Functional Class*	Symptoms and Signs
Speech and language	Dysarthria	Visuospatial abilities	Diminished or distorted ability for manual skills (e.g., mechanical repairs, sewing)
	Dysfluency		Spatial disorientation
	Marked change in amount of speech output		Impaired spatial judgment
	Paraphasias		Right–left disorientation
	Word finding problems		
Academic skills	Alterations in reading, writing, calculating, and number abilities; e.g., poor reading comprehension, frequent letter or number reversals in writing	Emotional	Diminished emotional control with temper outbursts, antisocial behavior
			Diminished empathy or interest in interpersonal relationships without depression
Thinking	Perseveration of speech or action components		Affective changes without known precipitating factors (e.g., lability, flattening, inappropriateness)
	Simplified or confused mental tracking, reasoning, concept formation		
Motor	Lateralized weakness or clumsiness		Personality changes without known precipitating factors
	Problems with fine motor coordination		
	Tremors		Increased irritability without known precipitating factors
Perception	Diplopia or visual field alterations	Comportment†	Altered appetites and appetitive activities (eating, drinking, play, sex)
	Inattention (usually left-sided, may be perceptual and/or in productions)		Altered grooming habits (overly fastidious, careless)
	Somatosensory alterations (particularly lateralized or confined to one limb)		Hyper- or hypoactivity
			Social inappropriateness

*Many emotionally disturbed persons complain of memory deficits that typically reflect their self-preoccupations, distractibility, or anxiety rather than a dysfunctional brain. Thus memory complaints in themselves are not good indicators of neuropathology.

†These changes are most likely to have neuropsychological relevance in the absence of depression, but they can be mistaken for depression.

Adapted from Howieson and Lezak, 2002; © 2002, American Psychiatric Association Press.

Other problems also tend to vitiate the effectiveness of cutting scores. The criterion groups are often not large enough for optimal cutting scores to be determined (Soper, Cicchetti, et al., 1988). Further, cutting scores developed on one kind of population may not apply to another. R.L. Adams and his coworkers (1982) pointed out the importance of adjusting cutting scores for "age, education, premorbid intelligence, and race–ethnicity" by demonstrating that the likelihood of false positive predictions of brain damage tends to increase directly with age and for nonwhites, and inversely with education and intelligence test scores. Bornstein (1986a) and Bornstein, Paniak, and O'Brien (1987) demonstrated how cutting scores, mostly developed on a small and relatively young normative sample, classified as "impaired" from 57.6% to 100% of normal control subjects in the 60–90 age range.

When the recommended cutting scores are used, these tests generally do identify impaired patients better than chance alone. They all also misdiagnose both intact persons (false positive cases) and persons with known brain impairment (false negative cases) to varying degrees. The nature of the errors of diagnosis depends on where the cutting score is set: if it is set to minimize misidentification of intact persons, then a greater number of organically impaired patients will be called "normal" by the screening. Conversely, if the test-maker's goal is to identify as many patients with brain damage as possible, more intact persons will be included in the brain damaged group. Only rarely does the cutting score provide a distinct separation between two populations, and then only for tests that are so simple that no nonretarded, intact adult could fail. For example, there are few false positive cases screened by the Token Test, which consists of verbal instructions involving basic concepts of size, color, and location.

Single tests for identifying brain disorders

The use of single tests for identifying brain damaged patients—a popular enterprise several decades ago—was based on the assumption that brain damage, like measles perhaps, can be treated as a single entity. Considering the heterogeneity of brain disorders, it is not surprising to find that single tests have high misclassification rates (G. Goldstein and Shelly, 1973; Spreen and Benton, 1965). Most single tests, including many that are not well standardized, can be rich sources of information about the functions, attitudes, and habits they elicit. Yet to look to any single test for decisive information about overall cognitive behavior is not merely foolish but can be dangerous as well, since the absence of positive findings does not rule out the presence of a pathological condition.

Usefulness of screening techniques

In the 1940s and 1950s, when brain damage was still thought by many to have some general manifestation that could be demonstrated by psychological tests, screening techniques were popular, particularly for identifying the brain impaired patients in a psychiatric population. As a result of our better understanding of the multifaceted nature of brain pathology and of the accelerating development and refinement of other kinds of neurodiagnostic techniques, the usefulness of neuropsychological screening has become much more limited. Screening is unnecessary or inappropriate in most cases referred for neuropsychological evaluation: either the presence of neuropathology is obvious or otherwise documented, or diagnosis requires more than a simple screening. Furthermore, the extent to which screening techniques produce false positives and false negatives compromises their reliability for making decisions about individual patients.

However, screening may still be useful with populations in which neurological disorders are more frequent than in the general population (e.g., community dwelling elderly persons: Cahn, Salmon, et al., 1995). The most obvious clinical situations in which neuropsychological screening may be called for are examinations of patients entering a psychiatric inpatient service or at-risk groups such as the elderly or alcoholics when they seek medical care. Dichotomizing screening techniques are also useful in research for evaluating tests or treatments, or for comparing specific populations with respect to the presence or absence of impaired functions.

Once a patient has been identified by screening techniques as possibly having a brain disorder, the problem arises of what to do next, for simple screening at best operates only as an early warning system. These patients still need careful neurological and neuropsychological study to determine whether a brain disorder is present and, if so, to help develop treatment and planning for their care as needed.

Evaluating screening techniques

In neuropsychology as in medicine, limitations in predictive accuracy do not invalidate either tests for specific signs or disabilities or tests that are sensitive to conditions of general dysfunction. We have not thrown away thermometers because most sick people have normal temperatures, nor do we reject the electroencephalogram just because many patients with brain disorders test normal by that method. Thus, in neuropsychology, each kind of test can be used effectively as a screening device as long as its limitations are known and the information it elicits is interpreted accordingly. When testing is primarily for screening purposes, a combination of tests, including some that are sensitive to specific impairment, some to general impairment, and others that tend to draw out diagnostic signs, will make the best diagnostic discriminations.

When evaluating tests for screening purposes, it is important to realize that although neuropsychological tests have proven effective in identifying the presence of brain disorders, they cannot guarantee its absence, i.e., "rule out" brain dysfunction. Not only may cerebral disease occur without behavioral manifestations, but the examiner may also neglect to look for those neuropsychological abnormalities that are present. Inability to prove the negative case in neuropsychological assessment is shared with every other diagnostic tool in medicine and the behavioral sciences. When a neuropsychological examination produces no positive findings, the only tenable conclusion is that the person in question performed *within normal limits* on the tests taken at that time. The neuropsychologist cannot give a "clean bill of health."

Pattern Analysis

The many differences in cognitive performance between diagnostic groups and between individuals within these groups can only be appreciated and put to clinical use when the evaluation is based on test score patterns and item analyses that are taken from tests of many different functions. Neither a narrow range of tests nor interpretation procedures that disregard test and item discrepancies can make available the amount of information generally required for adequate description and analysis of the patient's deficits. Learning what are the relevant variables and how to evaluate them is by far the most difficult part to master of the diagnostic process. A technician or graduate student can be trained over a three month period to give an extensive test battery, to make notes about the qualitative aspects of the patient's performance and behavior, and to score tests reliably. Estimation of premorbid ability, selection of appropriate norms, and conversion of scores to performance levels are not without problems but are still relatively easy to learn. Once test data have been reliably scored and appropriate norms have been chosen to convert scores to standard scores or percentiles, the clinician must determine whether the pattern of performance is typical of individuals with a particular diagnosis. While this may be readily apparent in some cases, it is not in many others. In order to make some sense of the pattern of performance on various tests, the clinician must fully understand the nature of the tests administered, what the various tests have in common and how they differ in terms of input and output modalities, and what cognitive processes are required for successful completion. A thorough understanding of test attributes coupled with thoughtful analysis of why a patient might do poorly on one test but not on another measuring ostensibly similar cognitive processes or even very different ones is necessary to appropriately interpret the data, along with the integration of historical, demographic, and psychosocial data.

The basic element of test score analysis is a significant discrepancy between any two or more scores (Silverstein, 1982). Implicitly or explicitly, all score-based methods of neuropsychological assessment rest on the assumption that one cognitive performance level best represents each person's cognitive abilities generally (see pp. 97–98). Marked quantitative discrepancies in a person's performance—within responses to a test, between scores on different tests, and/or with respect to some expected level of performance—suggest that some abnormal condition is interfering with that person's overall ability to perform at their characteristic level of cognitive functioning. It then becomes the examiner's responsibility to determine the nature of that limitation.

History and observations will help the examiner evaluate the possible contributions that cultural differences or disadvantages, emotional disturbances, developmental anomalies, and so on may make to performance discrepancies. Test score discrepancies may provide the critical information for determining whether the patient is impaired or, in the most usual examinations when diagnosis is not a question, how the impairment affects behavior. Any single discrepant score or response error can usually be disregarded as a chance deviation. A number of errors or test score deviations, however, may form a pattern that can then be analyzed in terms of whether it makes neurological sense, i.e., whether the score discrepancies fit neuroanatomically probable behavior patterns. The possibility that a given pattern of scores reflects the presence of a brain disorder is supported to the extent that the scores conform to a neuropsychologically reasonable discrepancy pattern.

When evaluated in terms of patterns of cognitive strengths and deficits, test scores are compared with one another to determine what factors consistently contribute to high or to low scores. The comparison of two scores is the model for double dissociation, the analytic procedure for localizing lesions by test performances (see p. 113). E.W. Russell (1984) pointed out that by using many tests generating many test scores, "the pattern is essentially one of multiple dissociation between tests" and, as such, is a powerful tool.

A 32-year-old doctoral candidate in the biological sciences sustained a head injury with momentary loss of consciousness just weeks before she was to take her qualifying examinations. She was given a small set of neuropsychological tests two months after the accident to determine the nature of her memory complaints and how she might compensate for them. Besides a few tests of verbal, visuospatial, and conceptual functions, the relatively brief examination consisted mainly of tests of attention and memory as they are often most relevant to mild post-traumatic conditions.

The patient had little problem with attentional or reasoning tests, whether verbal or visual, although some tendency to concrete thinking was observed. Both story recall and sentence repetition were excellent; she recalled all of nine symbol–digit pairs immediately after 3 min spent assigning digits to an associated symbol, and seven of the pairs a half hour later (Symbol Digit Modalities Test); and she recognized an almost normal number of words (12) from a list of 15 she had attempted to learn in five trials (Auditory-Verbal Learning Test). However, this very bright woman, whose speaking skills were consistent with her high academic achievement, could not retrieve several words without phonetic cueing on the Boston Naming Test; and she gave impaired performances when attempting to learn a series of nine digits (Serial Digit Learning), on immediate and delayed recall of the 15-word list, and on visual recall on which she reproduced the configuration of the geometric design she had copied but not the details (Complex Figure Test). Thus she clearly demonstrated the ability for verbal learning at a normal level, and her visual recall indicated that she could at least learn the "big picture." Her successes occurred on all meaningful material and when she had cues; when meaning or cues—hooks she could use to aid retrieval—were absent, she performed at *defective* levels. Analysis of her successes and failures showed a consistent pattern implicating retrieval problems that compromised her otherwise adequate learning ability. This analysis allowed the examiner to reassure her regarding her learning capacity and to recommend techniques for prodding her sluggish retrieval processes.

The question of neuroanatomical or neurophysiological likelihood underlies all analyses of test patterns undertaken for differential diagnosis. As in every other diagnostic effort, the most likely explanation for a behavioral disorder is the one that requires the least number of unlikely events to account for it. Brain dysfunction is suspected when a neurological condition best accounts for the patient's behavioral abnormalities.

Intraindividual variability

Discrepancy, or variability, in the pattern of successes and failures in a test performance is called *scatter*. Variability within a test is *intratest scatter;* variability between the scores of a set of tests is *intertest* scatter (D. Wechsler, 1958).

Intratest scatter. Scatter within a test is said to be present when there are marked deviations from the normal pass–fail pattern. On tests in which the items are presented in order of difficulty, it is usual for the subject to pass almost all items up to the most difficult passed item, with perhaps one or two failures on items close to the last passed item. Rarely do nondefective persons fail very simple items or fail many items of middling difficulty and pass several difficult ones. On tests in which all items are of similar difficulty level, most subjects tend to do all of them correctly, with perhaps one or two errors of carelessness, or they tend to flounder hopelessly with maybe one or two lucky "hits." Variations from these two common patterns deserve the examiner's attention.

Certain brain disorders as well as some emotional disturbances may manifest themselves in intratest scatter patterns. Hovey and Kooi (1955) demonstrated that when taking mental tests, those epileptic patients who suffered paroxysmal brain wave patterns (sudden bursts of activity) were significantly more likely to be randomly nonresponsive or forgetful than were psychiatric, brain damaged, or other epileptic patients. Some patients who have sustained severe head injuries respond to questions that draw on prior knowledge as if they had randomly lost chunks of stored information. For example, moderately to severely injured patients as a group displayed more intratest scatter than a comparable control group, although scatter alone did not reliably differentiate brain injured from control subjects on an individual basis (Mittenberg, Hammeke, and Rao, 1989). Variability, both intertest and over time, characterized responses of patients with frontal lobe dementia (Murtha et al., 2002). E. Strauss, MacDonald, and their colleagues (2002) found a relationship between inconsistency in physical performance and fluctuations on cognitive tests.

Intertest scatter. Probably the most common approach to the psychological evaluation of brain disorders is through comparison of the test score levels obtained by the subject—in other words, through analysis of the intertest score scatter. By this means, the examiner attempts to relate variations between test scores to probable neuropsychological events—or behavioral descriptions in those many cases in which a diagnosis is known. This technique can often clarify a seeming confusion of signs and symptoms of behavioral disorder by giving the examiner a frame of reference for organizing and evaluating the data.

Consistency in the expression of cognitive functions is the key concept of pattern analysis. Damage to cortical tissue in an area serving a specific function changes or abolishes the expression of that function. Once a function is changed or lost, the character of all activities that originally involved that function will change to a greater or lesser degree, depending upon how much the function itself has changed and the extent to which it entered into the activity.

In analyzing test score patterns, the examiner looks for both commonality of dysfunction and evidence of impairment on tests involving functions or skills that are associated neuroanatomically, in their cognitive expression, or with well-described disease entities and neuropathological conditions. First, the examiner estimates a general level of premorbid functioning from the patient's history, qualitative aspects of performance, and test scores, using the examination or historical indicators that reasonably allow the highest estimate (see Chapter 4). This enables the examiner to identify impaired test performances. Following the procedures for dissociation of dysfunction, those functions that contribute to the impaired test performances can be identified. Out of these the examiner notes which if any functions or functional systems are *consistently* associated with lowered test scores, for these are the possible behavioral correlates of brain dysfunction, or represent those areas of function in which the patient can be expected to have the most difficulty. When the pattern of lowered test scores does not appear to be consistently associated with a single pattern of cognitive dysfunction, discrepant scores may well be attributable to psychogenic, developmental, or chance deviations.

Reliable neuropsychological assessment based on impairment patterns requires a fairly broad review of functions. A minor or well-circumscribed cognitive deficit may show up on only one or a very few depressed test scores or may not become evident at all if the test battery samples a narrow range of behaviors. Moreover, most of the behaviors that a psychologist examines are complex. When analyzing behavior in order to identify the deficit(s) contributing to the observed impairments, the psychologist cannot examine a specific function in a vacuum but must look at it in combination with many different functions.

By and large, the use of pattern analysis has been confined to tests in the Wechsler batteries because of their obvious statistical comparability. However, by converting different kinds of test scores into comparable score units, the examiner can compare data from many different tests in a systematic manner, permitting the analysis of patterns formed by the scores of tests from many sources. For example, Heaton, Grant, and Matthews (1991) converted scores from a large number of tests to a single standard score system.

Taking the next step of relating the psychological data to neurological conditions or to behavioral problems that may arise in real life requires more acquaintance with clinical neuropathology and neuro-

logically impaired patients than the scope of this or any other book allows. In describing typical patterns of neuropsychological functioning and some other salient aspects of the major categories of neuropathological disorders, Chapter 7 offers an introduction to neuropathology from a neuropsychologist's perspective.

INTEGRATED INTERPRETATION

Pattern analysis is insufficient to deal with the numerous exceptions to characteristic patterns, with the many rare or idiosyncratically manifested neurological conditions, and with the effects on test performance of the complex interaction between patients' cognitive status, their emotional and social adjustment, and their appreciation of their altered functioning. For the examination to supply answers to many of the diagnostic questions and most of the treatment and planning questions requires integration of all the data—from tests, observations made in the course of the examination, and the history of the problem.

Some conditions do not lend themselves to pattern analysis beyond the use of large and consistent test score discrepancies to implicate brain damage. For example, malignant tumors are unlikely to follow a regular pattern of growth and spread. In order to determine which functions are involved and the extent of their involvement, it is usually necessary to evaluate the qualitative aspects of the patient's performance very carefully for evidence of complex or subtle aberrations that betray damage in some hitherto unsuspected area of the brain. Such painstaking scrutiny may not be as necessary when dealing with a patient whose disease generally follows a well-known and regular course.

Test scores alone do not provide much information about the emotional impact of brain damage on the individual patient's cognitive functioning. However, behavior during the test is likely to reveal a great deal about reactions to the disabilities and how these reactions in turn affect performance efficiency. Emotional reactions of brain damaged patients can affect their cognitive functioning adversely. The most prevalent and most profoundly handicapping of these are anxiety and depression. Euphoria and carelessness, while much less distressing to the patient, can also seriously interfere with expression of a patient's abilities.

Brain impaired patients have other characteristic problems that generally do not depress test scores but must be taken into account in rehabilitation planning. These are motivational and control (executive function) problems that show up in an inability to organize, to react spontaneously, to initiate goal-directed behavior, or to carry out a course of action independently. They are rarely reflected in test scores since almost all tests are well structured and administered by an examiner who plans, initiates, and conducts the examination (see Chapter 16 for tests that elicit these problems). Yet, no matter how well patients do on tests, if they cannot develop or carry out their own course of action, they are incompetent for all practical purposes. Such problems become apparent during careful examination, but they usually must be reported descriptively unless the examiner sets up a test situation that can provide a systematic and scorable means of assessing the patient's capacity for self-direction and planning.

7 | Neuropathology for Neuropsychologists

H. JULIA HANNAY, DIANE B. HOWIESON, DAVID W. LORING,
JILL S. FISCHER, AND MURIEL D. LEZAK

In order to make diagnostic sense out of the behavioral patterns that emerge in neuropsychological assessment, the practitioner must be knowledgeable about the neuropsychological presentation of many kinds of neurological disorders and with their underlying pathology (Houston Conference, 1998). This knowledge gives the examiner a diagnostic frame of reference that helps to identify, sort out, appraise, and put into a diagnostically meaningful context the many bits and pieces of observations, scores, family reports, and medical history that typically make up the material of a case. Furthermore, such a frame of reference should help the examiner know what additional questions need be asked or what further observations or behavioral measurements need be made to arrive at the diagnostic formulation of the patient's problems (Heilman and Valenstein, 2003).

This chapter can only sketch broad and mostly behavioral outlines of such a frame of reference. It cannot substitute for knowledge of neuropathology gained from contact with many patients suffering from many different neuropathological disorders at many different stages in their course and, ideally, in a training setting. However, with its predominantly neuropsychological perspective, this chapter may help to crystallize understandings gained in clinical observations and enhance the clinician's sensitivity to the behavioral aspects of the conditions discussed here.

The major disorders of the nervous system having neuropsychological consequences will be reviewed according to their customary classification by known or suspected etiology or by the system of primary involvement. While this review cannot be comprehensive, it covers the most common neuropathological conditions seen in the usual hospital or clinic practice in this country. The reader may wish to consult R.D. Adams, Victor, and Ropper, *Principles of Neurology* (1997); Asbury et al., *Diseases of the Nervous System* (2002); Lishman, *Organic Psychiatry* (1997); J.N. Walton, *Brain's Diseases of the Nervous System* (1994); and Weisberg's *Essentials of Clinical Neurology* (2002) for more detailed presentations of the medical aspects of these and other less common conditions that have behavioral ramifications.

As in every aspect of neuropsychology, or any other personalized clinical assessment procedure, the kind of information the examiner needs to know will vary from patient to patient. For example, hereditary predisposition is not an issue with infectious disorders or a *hypoxic* (condition of insufficient oxygenation) episode during surgery, but it becomes a very important consideration when a previously unexceptional person begins to exhibit uncontrollable movements and poor judgment coupled with impulsivity. Thus, it is not necessary to ask every candidate for neuropsychological assessment for family history going back a generation or two, although family history is important when the diagnostic possibilities include a hereditary disorder such as Huntington's disease (see pp. 234–241). In certain populations, the incidence of alcohol or drug abuse is so high that every person with complaints suggestive of a cerebral disorder should be carefully questioned about drinking or drug habits; yet for many persons, such questioning becomes clearly unnecessary early in a clinical examination and may even be offensive. Moreover, a number of different kinds of disorders produce similar constellations of symptoms. For example, apathy, affective dulling, and memory impairment occur in Korsakoff's psychosis, with heavy exposure to certain organic solvents, as an aftermath of severe head trauma or herpes encephalitis, and with conditions in which the supply of oxygen to the brain has been severely compromised. Many conditions with similar neuropsychological features can be distinguished by differences in other neuropsychological dimensions. Other conditions are best identified in terms of the patient's history, associated neurological symptoms, and the nature of the onset and course of the disorder.

The presence of one kind of neuropathological disorder does not exclude others, nor does it exclude emotional reactions or psychiatric and personality disorders. With more than one disease process affecting brain function, the behavioral presentation is potentially complex with a confusing symptom picture: e.g., Chui, Victoroff, and their colleagues (1992) offered the diagnostic category of "mixed dementia" for those dementing conditions involving more than one neuropathological entity (see p. 221). Moreover, some conditions may increase the likelihood of other disorders occurring, such as traumatic brain injury, which is a risk factor for Alzheimer's disease (pp. 208–209) and stroke (p. 164), and alcoholism, which increases the likelihood of head injuries from falling off bar stools, motor vehicle accidents, or Saturday night fights.

No single rule of thumb will tell the examiner just what information about any particular patient is needed to make the most effective use of the examination data. Whether the purpose of the examination is diagnosis or delineation of the behavioral expression of a known condition, knowledge about the known or suspected condition(s) provides a frame of reference for the rational conduct of the examination.

TRAUMATIC BRAIN INJURY

> Humpty Dumpty sat on a wall.
> Humpty Dumpty had a great fall.
> And all the king's horses and all the king's men
> Couldn't put Humpty together again.
>
> *Mother Goose*

Traumatic brain injury (*TBI*) can refer generally to injury involving the brain. *Head injury* is still a synonymous term, but in some cases it refers to injury of other head structures such as the face or jaw. Most TBIs are *closed* in that the skull remains intact and the brain is not exposed. *Closed head injuries* (*CHIs*) are referred to as *blunt head injuries* as well. The skull can be fractured and the injury may still be a CHI. *Penetrating head injuries* (*PHIs*), sometimes called *open head injuries*, include all injuries from any source in which the skull and dura are penetrated by missiles or other objects. Not only the nature of the injury but also the pathophysiological processes set in motion by damage to the brain differ in significant ways in CHI and PHI. For some, the term TBI can include other etiologies such as stroke and anoxia. Thus the meaning of TBI continues to be confusing and needs to be clarified in the literature. In this book TBI refers strictly to the effects of CHI and PHI.

TBI is the most common cause of brain damage in children and young adults (Collins, 1990; M.S. Grady and McIntosh, 2002; Thurman et al., 1999). Modern medical techniques for the management of acute brain conditions are saving many accident victims who ten or twenty years ago would have succumbed to the metabolic, hemodynamic, and other complications that follow severe brain trauma (Hsiang and Marshall, 1998; D.F. Kelly, Doberstein and Becker, 1996). As a result, an ever-increasing number of survivors of severe TBI, mostly children and young adults at the time of injury, are rapidly familiarizing us with this relatively new and usually tragic phenomenon of physically fit young people whose brains have been significantly damaged.

Moreover, secondary or delayed injury to the brain from a variety of sources such as hypoxia/ischemia, elevated intracranial pressure (ICP), coagulopathy, and pyrexia may, in fact, be more important than the immediate direct damage to and disruption of brain tissue and neural circuitry (D.I. Graham, 1996; J.D. Miller, Piper and Jones, 1996; D.F. Kelly, Doberstein and Becker, 1996). Better understanding of these conditions has led to the development of specialized clinical monitoring techniques for more serious injuries (J.C. Goodman and Simpson, 1996; J.D. Miller, Piper and Stathan, 1996; Obrist and Marion, 1996; Woodman and Robertson, 1996), investigations into the basic mechanisms underlying these clinical changes, and the search for efficacious pharmacological (Hatton, 2001; Narayan, Michel, et al., 2002) and other interventions such as hypothermia (Clifton and Hayes, 1996) and hypobaric oxygen (Rockswold, 1996). Research findings that seem promising in the laboratory often are not proven to be clearly efficacious in clinical trials in which the same control over a myriad of variables, including genetic and injury characteristics, is not possible (Narayan et al., 2002). (For a detailed description of the series of physiological events that severe TBI is likely to trigger, see Hatton, 2001; McIntosh, Saatman, et al., 1998; J.D. Miller, Piper and Jones, 1996; Novack, Dillon, and Jackson, 1996.)

Prevalence estimates and incidence reports in epidemiological studies vary depending on such decisions as whether to include all grades of severity, to count deaths, to limit the study to hospitalized patients, etc. (Berrol, 1989; R.S. Parker, 2000; Kraus et al., 1996). Incidence of TBI also varies with the study site, as urban centers account for a higher incidence of TBI than rural areas (Gabella et al., 1997; F.B. Rogers et al., 1997). In the United States, the reported incidence of TBI varies across studies but averages about 220 per 100,000 (132 in Maryland to 367 per 100,000 in Chicago) (Kraus et al., 1996). Estimates based on the National Health Interview Survey from 1985–1987 suggested that there are approximately 75,000 deaths, 373,000 hospitalizations, and 1,975,000 medically attended individuals with head injury per year (Kraus et al., 1996; J.T.E. Richardson, 2000). Rates similar to those in the United States in France (281 per 100,000; Cohadon et al., 2002) and higher have been reported in South Africa (316 per 100,000; Nell and Brown, 1991) and South Australia (322 per 100,000; Hillier et al., 1997). Some countries (e.g., England, Japan, Sweden) post half as many fatal injuries as the United States (Kraus et al., 1996; J.T.E. Richardson, 2000); the People's Republic of China's urban TBI rate was one-fourth that of the United States, while the tiny republic of San Marino produced TBIs at an annual rate 16 times that of China (Naugle, 1990).

Even estimates of mortality rates vary greatly (Kraus et al., 1996); mortality rates may change over time for a variety of reasons, including changing admissions and hospital practices and preventive programs (Engberg and Teasdale, 2001). After the initial period of high risk, long-term mortality from TBI is primarily related to the late effects of injury, lack of functional independence, age, and tube feeding (Baguley, Slewa-Younan, et al., 2000; Shavelle et al., 2001; D.J. Strauss et al., 1998).

The peak ages for TBI are in the 15–24 year range with high incidence rates in the first five years and for elderly persons (Hillier et al., 1997; Jager et al., 2000; J.T.E. Richardson, 2000). The most common cause of TBI tends to be falls (Jager et al., 2000; Naugle, 1990) or transportation (Centers for Disease Control, 1997; Kraus et al., 1996; Masson et al., 2001). Falls account for more than half the injuries incurred by infants and young children and by persons in the 64 and older age range. Moving vehicle accidents (MVAs) account for half of all head injuries in the other age groups (Cohadon et al., 2002; Kraus et al., 1996; Masson et al.,2001). Motorcyclists have a higher mortality rate than occupants of motor vehicles, but pedestrians in traffic accidents have the highest rate among these groups (de Sousa et al., 1999; E. Wong et al., 2002).

Helmets have reduced head injuries in sports such as bicycling, hockey, horseback riding, and football although not all helmets reduce craniofacial injuries effectively (S.W. Marshall et al., 2002; P.S. Moss et al., 2002; D.C. Thompson et al., 2003). For instance, motorcycle helmets have noticeably reduced mortality, rate of TBI, severity of injury, length of hospital stay, and acute care costs (Bledsoe et al., 2002; Branas and Knudson, 2001; La Torre, 2003) and increased the likelihood of a favorable outcome (Kraus and Peek, 1995), even for those with severe injuries (P.M. Francis et al., 1991). All helmets are not equal; they need to be designed with each sport in mind (e.g., for motorcycle riding, see Peek-Asa, McArthur and Kraus, 1999; Tsai et al., 1995; Van Camp et al., 1998).

Excepting the over 65 age group in which women outnumber men, men sustain injuries about twice as frequently as women, with this sex differential greatest at the peak trauma years (Cohadon et al., 2002; Naugle, 1990; Jager et al., 2000). Lower socioeconomic status, unemployment, and lower educational levels, too, appear as risk factors, also increasing the likelihood of TBIs that, more frequently than for other groups, are due to falls or assaults (Cohadon et al., 2002; Naugle, 1990). "Typically, TBI occurs in young working class males, who may have had limited educational attainment and who may not have had a stable work history prior to injury" (Ponsford, 1995). Violent TBI specifically (e.g., assault with a blunt or penetrating object, gunshot wound) caused by oneself or another is higher among those who have less than a high school degree (48% vs. 39%), are unemployed (44% vs. 21%), are male (86% vs. 72%), and have a higher blood alcohol level at the time of injury (92.9 vs. 67 mg/dl), as well as among African-Americans (Hanks, Wood, et al., 2003).

In one series of patients, at least 29% had some prior central nervous system condition, including history of alcoholism (18%) and of head injury (8%) among others (J.L. Gale et al., 1983), but higher estimates for heavy drinkers have been reported (Cohadon et al., 2002; Rimel, Giordani, et al., 1981; Bombardier, Rimmele, and Zintel, 2002). While transportation accidents and falls are the leading causes of head trauma, assaults—whether by blows to the head or a penetrating weapon, sports and recreational activities, and the workplace—together account for from about 25% to 40% of reported injuries (Kraus, McArthur, et al., 1996; Naugle, 1990; R.S. Parker, 2001; Templer and Drew, 1992).

The behavioral effects of all brain lesions hinge upon a variety of factors, such as severity, age, site of lesions, and premorbid personality (see Chapter 8). The psychological consequences of head trauma also vary according to how the injury happened, e.g., whether it occurred in a moving vehicle, as a result of a blow to the head, or from a missile furrowing through it. With knowledge of the kind of head injury, its severity, and the site of focal damage, experienced examiners can generally predict the broad outlines of their patients' major behavioral and neuropsychological disabilities and the likely psychosocial prognosis. Of course, only careful examination can demonstrate the individual features of the patient's disabilities, such as whether verbal or visual functions are more depressed, and the extent to which retrieval problems, frontal inertia, or impaired learning ability each contribute to the patient's poor performance on memory tests. Yet, the similarities in the behavioral patterns of many patients, especially those with CHI, tend to outweigh the individual differences.

Severity Classifications and Outcome Prediction

The range of head trauma severity begins with bumps so mild as to leave no behavioral traces: everyone has bruised their head on a protruding shelf or when suddenly jostled by a car or bus, with no lasting ill effects. At the other end of the severity continuum are patients in prolonged coma or a vegetative state (H.S. Levin, Benton, Muizelaar, and Eisenberg, 1996). Neuropsychological assessment is concerned with the patients between these two extremes.

The need to triage patients both for treatment purposes and for outcome prediction has led to the development of a generally accepted classification system based on the presence, degree, and duration of coma, the *Glasgow Coma Scale* (*GCS*) (Jennett and Bond, 1975; Rimel, Giordani, Barth, and Jane, 1982) (see Chapter 18, Table 18.2). Measurement of severity by means of the GCS depends upon the evaluation of both depth and duration of altered consciousness. Coma duration alone is a poor predictor of outcome for the many patients with brief periods of coma (up to 20–30 minutes) (Gronwall, 1989), but it is a good predictor for more severe injuries (B. [A.] Wilson, Vizor, and Bryant, 1991). Although some definitional variations exist between different reporting sites, for all practical purposes the severity of classifications has universal meaning (see Chapter 18, Table 18.3).

Like any other predictor of human behavior, the GCS is not appropriate for many cases (see Chapter 18, pp. 720–721). A single GCS score with no indication of when it was determined and the status of other pertinent variables at the time (e.g., clinical signs, blood alcohol level and level of recreational or prescribed drugs, sedation for agitation, amount and timing of drugs administered earlier or currently, echymosis, intubation, facial injuries, anesthesia for surgery, CT scan results) can lead to an inaccurate assessment of the severity of injury. Indeed, it may take such data including the GCS scores from the first 48–72 hours postinjury to clearly establish the severity of injury in some patients. For instance, a person with a GCS of 15 but abnormalities on the CT scan might perform more like an individual with a moderate TBI on cognitive tests and should perhaps be classified as a complicated mild TBI (D.H. Williams et al., 1990). Persons who enter the TBI trauma system with little or no loss of consciousness but who suffer significant deterioration in mental status, usually within the first 72 hours postinjury from a delayed hematoma (epidural, subdural, or intracerebral), are likely to be misclassified by an early GCS

score (H.A. Young et al., 1984; T.I. Cohen and Gudeman, 1996). A patient who clearly has a severe head injury but recovers fairly rapidly in terms of level of consciousness in the first 24 hours might be misclassified if the *Best Day 1 GCS score* (highest GCS score in first 24 hours) is used as a measure of severity. Moreover, patients with left lateralized PHI are more likely to suffer *loss of consciousness* (*LOC*) than those whose injuries are confined to the right side of the brain; and the duration of coma for those with right-sided lesions tends to be shorter than when lesions are on the left (Salazar, Martin, and Grafman, 1987). As an additional problem in the use and interpretation of the GCS, alcohol intoxication can spuriously lower a GCS score such that the higher the blood alcohol level at time of injury, the more likely it is that the GCS score will improve when reevaluated at least six hours later (Jagger et al., 1984).

Some investigators may rely instead on *posttraumatic amnesia* (*PTA*) to measure the severity of the injury (see Table 7.1; cf. Bigler, 1990a) (M.R. Bond, 1990; W.R. Russell and Nathan, 1946). Not surprisingly, duration of PTA correlates well with GCS ratings (H.S. Levin, Benton, and Grossman, 1982) except for some finer scaling at the extremes. N. Brooks (1989) observed that PTA duration (which begins at time of injury and includes the coma period) typically lasts about four times the length of coma. A number of methods have been devised for standardizing PTA observations (see pp. 719–724).

However, difficulties in defining and therefore determining the duration of PTA have made its usefulness as a measure of severity questionable in some cases (Jennett, 1972; Macartney-Filgate, 1990). For example, while it is generally agreed that PTA does not end when the patient begins to register experience again but only when registration is continuous, deciding when continuous registration returns may be difficult with confused or aphasic patients (Gronwall and Wrightson, 1980). Moreover, many patients with relatively mild head injury are discharged home while still in PTA, leaving it up to the examiner to attempt at some later date to estimate PTA duration from reports by the patient or family members, who often have less than re-

TABLE 7.1 Estimates of Severity of Injury Based on Posttraumatic Amnesia (PTA) Duration

PTA Duration	Severity
<5 minutes	Very mild
5–60 minutes	Mild
1–24 hours	Moderate
1–7 days	Severe
1–4 weeks	Very severe
More than 4 weeks	Extremely severe

liable memories. These considerations have led such knowledgeable clinicians as Jennett (1979) and N. Brooks (1989) to assert that fine-tuned accuracy of estimation is not necessary as judgments of PTA in the larger time frames of hours, days, or weeks will usually suffice for clinical purposes (e.g., Table 7.1). Length of PTA was more accurate than coma duration in predicting cognitive status two years after injury (D.N. Brooks, Aughton, et al., 1980). It is also more predictive than admission GCS of global outcome on the Glasgow Outcome Scale (GOS) at one year postinjury (van der Naalt et al., 1999). Yet failures to discriminate between moderately and severely impaired patients suggest that it may not classify patients with sufficient sensitivity for research (N. Brooks, McKinlay, et al., 1987).

For the patient, PTA can be a psychologically painful issue. When confusion has settled down and continuous registration has returned, patients are likely to become aware that they have no memory or perhaps only a very spotty memory for days—sometimes weeks or months—following their injury. Many are quite uncomfortable about this, sometimes troubled indefinitely by uneasiness about their period of PTA despite being told what happened to them and being reassured as to the propriety of their behavior during that time.

Retrograde amnesia (*RA*), usually involving the minutes, sometimes hours, and more rarely days immediately preceding the accident, frequently accompanies PTA (N. Brooks, 1989; H.S. Levin, High, et al., 1985). Its duration too tends to correlate with severity of injury. Retrograde amnesia, sometimes profound, when reported after minor CHI raises the question of a functional basis (De Renzi, Lucchelli, et al., 1995; Mackenzie, 2000; Papagno, 1998). CT and MRI in the first few weeks were negative in one patient while EEG and SPECT showed marked right temporal dysfunction with parallel dissipation of retrograde amnesia and SPECT findings at three months (Sellal et al., 2002). The anatomical basis of retrograde amnesia in CHI is not entirely clear. Frontal and temporal regions have been implicated as well as the anterior cingulate gyrus (Carlesimo, Sabbadini, Bombardi, et al., 1998; B. Levine, Black, et al., 1998; Markowitsch, Calabrese, et al., 1999). Patients may be less disturbed by their experience of retrograde amnesia than by anterograde amnesia, while their lawyers may find retrograde amnesia difficult to accept.

Some other techniques for evaluating severity have proven fruitful. Auditory and brainstem evoked potentials add to the evaluation of comatose patients during the early postinjury period and to the prediction of outcome (D.C. Anderson et al., 1984; Soustiel et al., 1993). Early serial somatosensory evoked potentials may im-

prove prediction of outcome (Pohlmann-Eden et al., 1997). Visual field defects are strong indicators of severity (Uzzell, Dolinskas and Langfitt, 1988). Anosmia can be a marker of orbitofrontal damage (Varney, Pinkston, and Wu, 2001; Yousem et al., 1999), though other reasons for poor performance on olfactory tests need to be considered (P. Green and Iverson, 2001). Anosmics may have longer hospital stays, longer and deeper coma, more neuropsychological deficits, more abnormal CT/MRI scans, poorer functional outcome (Callahan and Hinkebein, 1999; P.G. Green, Rohling, et al., 2003; Greiffenstein, Baker, and Gola, 2002), and perhaps higher unemployment rates (Varney and Bushnell, 1998), though this has been questioned (Correia et al., 2001; Greiffenstein et al., 2002).

MRI is quite sensitive to traumatic damage even when the injury is not severe, frequently revealing injuries not visualized by CT scanning, especially nonhemorrhagic diffuse axonal injuries and small extra-axial hematomas (Diaz-Marchan et al., 1996; Hankins et al., 1996; Huisman et al., 2003). MRI is also better at visualizing brainstem lesions that are known to predict poorer global and neuropsychological outcome (Firsching et al., 2001; Wedekind et al., 2002). However, MRI studies taken in the acute stages may not predict outcome reliably, whereas later (5 months or more) imaging findings prove highly predictive (J.T.L. Wilson et al., 1988). CT scans are usually done in the early stages of head injury since they detect practically all of the surgically significant lesions, cost less than MRI, are readily available, can even be given in the intensive care setting with a portable unit, visualize blood products and bone fractures and fragments better than MRI, and do not require the specialized life-support equipment and monitoring devices that are not affected by magnetic fields (Diaz-Marchan et al., 1996; Hankins et al., 1996).

A promising development for evaluating the new patient involves blood serum markers of neuronal damage. Such measures are likely to be included in general clinical monitoring of TBI patients and to provide another measure of the severity of damage. Levels of serum S-100B (a marker of glial damage) in the emergency service predict outcome on the Glasgow Outcome Scale at one month postinjury (Townend et al., 2002). Higher median serum S100B protein levels are positively related to mortality, brain death, increased intracranial pressure, and unfavorable outcome, and are sensitive to the presence of mild as well as more severe head injury (Dimopoulou et al., 2003; Savola and Hillbom, 2003; G.J. Shaw et al., 2002). Unlike the GCS score and neuropsychological or behavioral outcome measures, serum levels of S-100B do not seem to be affected by alcohol consumption in head injured or intact individuals (Mussack et al., 2002). Neuron specific endolase (NSE, a neuronal tissue damage marker) also is released after head injury, and its release is related to severity of injury (M. Herrmann, Jost, Kutz, et al., 2000) and outcome (Woertgen et al., 2002). NSE may not be as sensitive to the presence of minor head injury as S-100B (de Kruijk et al., 2001; Mussack et al., 2002). Patterns of S-100B and NSE release may differ in patients with primary cortical contusions, diffuse axonal injury (see pp. 165–167), and signs of cerebral edema indicated by increased ICP without focal mass lesions (M. Herrmann et al., 2000). C-tau, an intracellular protein, is also under investigation as another injury marker since it is elevated with TBI, especially when severe, and appears to predict outcome and the presence of intracranial injuries (G.J. Shaw et al., 2002; Zemlan et al., 2002).

TBI severity generally relates to behavioral and neuropsychological outcomes (Cohadon et al., 2002; H.S. Levin, 1985; J.T.E. Richardson, 2000). The most far-reaching effects of TBI involve personal and social competence, more so than even the well-studied cognitive impairments. Relatively few patients who have sustained severe head injury return to work, and those who do often can hold jobs only in the most supportive settings (Hsiang and Marshall, 1998; N. Rao et al., 1990; Stambrook, Moore, et al., 1990; Vogenthaler et al., 1989), even despite relatively normal scores on tests of cognitive functions (Truelle et al., 1988). Quality of life as reflected in patient and family satisfaction and distress also tends to be increasingly compromised with increased severity of injury (P.S. Klonoff et al., 1986; Lezak and O'Brien, 1990; Peck and Warren, 1989; Ponsford, 1995).

One readily applicable and widely used set of classifications was created for the Glasgow Outcome Scale (Jennett and Bond, 1975; see pp. 725–726). The most severe of the four outcome levels is *Vegetative state*, in which no cortical functioning is apparent. Neuropsychologists are more interested in the next three severity levels which range from *Severe disability* for conscious patients who are more or less dependent on others for accomplishing much of the normal activities of daily living; to *Moderate disability* which includes persons capable of independent living but who are restricted in one or more major activity area by their disabilities; to *Good recovery*[1] for persons who are fully functional socially, although some may have minor residual deficits, whether physical or mental. (See Chapter 18, pp. 726–734, for other outcome measures.)

When discussing severity ratings and outcome prediction, it is as important to note the discrepancies as to document general trends. Exceptions to these general trends occur at all points along the severity continuum. Thus patients whose injuries seem mild, as measured by most accepted methods, may have relatively poor outcomes, both cognitively and socially; and conversely, some others who have been classified as moderately to severely injured have enjoyed surprisingly good outcomes (Newcombe, 1987; Vogenthaler et al., 1989).

Penetrating Head Injuries

Penetrating head injury (PHI) occurs both accidentally and intentionally with everyday objects, tools, weapons, and even plants. For instance, injuries have been reported from such bizarre sources as a ball-point pen (Sharif et al., 2000), a chopstick (Kawamura et al., 1997), a door key (Seex, Koppel, Fitzpatrick, and Pyott, 1997), a TV antenna (Al-Sebeih et al., 2002), a metal doll display stand (Koestler and Keshavarz, 2001), a fishing harpoon (Lopez et al., 2000), and a weed (Nakayama et al., 1995). Some of these objects become embedded in the head and others, including bullets, cause a "through-and-through injury" with both entry and exit wounds. PHI can also result from a tangential injury in which an object glances off the skull and bone fragments are driven into the brain ("Part 2: Prognosis," 2001). Gunshot wounds (GSWs) to the head are, however, the leading cause of PHI and less likely to be associated with multiple trauma than CHI (Aldrich et al., 1992; Peek-Asa et al., 2001; Sosin et al., 1995). The PHI mortality rate is much higher than with CHI, approximately 6.6:1 (Peek-Asa, McArthur, Hovda, and Kraus, 2001) after controlling for initial GCS, gender, age, and presence of multiple trauma. In a prospective study of civilian PHI outcomes, 36% were dead on arrival or died in the emergency center. Of the injuries of survivors admitted for inpatient care, 52% were severe, 7% moderate, and 42% mild. Forty-one percent of these admissions died in the first 48 hours (Zafonte, Wood, et al., 2001a).

Neuropathology

The amount of damage the brain sustains in head injury is determined in large measure by the amount of energy translated to the brain in the course of the damaging event. The kinetic energy transferred from the missile to the brain equals $1/2M(V_{entry} - V_{exit})^2$, where M is the mass of the missile, V_{entry} is the velocity on

---

[1] I (mdl) do not use the term "recovery" when discussing brain injuries. Damage that is severe enough to alter the level of consciousness even momentarily, or to result in even transient impairment of sensory, motor, or cognitive functions, is likely to leave some residual deficits. When the injury is more than mild, the use of the word "recovery," which implies restoration or return to premorbid status (*Webster's Encyclopedic Unabridged Dictionary of the English Language*, 1989), when discussing the patient's prognosis can give the patient and family false hope, delay practical planning, and cause unnecessary anxiety and disappointment (e.g., see Lezak, 1996).

entry, and V_{exit} is the velocity on exit (Trask and Narayan, 1996). Missile velocity on entry is not just a function of muzzle velocity for a bullet but is also determined by how the bullet travels and any deflecting barriers (Trask and Narayan, 1996). Mortality is related to the type of projectile: bullets caused most of the military deaths from injuries in Vietnam (22.7%), relatively few were due to shrapnel (7.6%) (Hammon, 1971; Knightly and Pulliman, 1996). Civilian GSWs more likely come from lower velocity sources at close range with no intervening barriers (though this is changing and mortality rates are high), whereas military GSWs typically come from higher velocity sources but at variable distances and sometimes through barriers such as helmets (Trask and Narayan, 1996). The type of object and the amount of fragmentation, internal ricochet, and indriven debris affect the degree of tissue destruction and the size and configuration of the cavity. Puncture wounds, missile fragments, and low-velocity bullets are most likely to produce "clean" wounds in the sense that significant tissue damage tends to be concentrated in the path of the intruding object (Newcombe, 1969). Since surgical cleansing of the wound (debridement) typically removes damaged tissue along with debris, most of the brain usually remains intact. In most cases, these circumscribed focal lesions produce relatively circumscribed and predictable cognitive losses (with predictability subject, of course, to normal interindividual variations in brain organization). Neuropsychologists who have taken advantage of this "clean" characteristic of penetrating head wounds that received prompt surgical attention have made major contributions to the understanding of functional brain organization (e.g., Luria, 1970; Newcombe, 1969; Newcombe and Russell, 1969; Semmes et al., 1963; Teuber, 1962, 1964).

Extensive scalp wounds may be present with enough blood loss that *hypotension* (abnormally low blood pressure) and *hypovolemia* (abnormally low blood volume) can result (Knightly and Pulliman, 1996; Trask and Narayan, 1996). *Contusions* (bruises) can be widespread with gunshot wounds, especially at entry and contrecoup (see p. 165) sites. Intracranial *hematomas* (swelling filled with blood) develop most often three to eight hours after injury; about 25% of them are in the subfrontal region. They are a relatively common cause of postinjury deterioration. Prevention and treatment of infection are important in surviving PHI since the skull and dura have been breached and brain abcesses can develop. Antibiotics are thus widely used in postoperative management.

Moreover, the penetrating object may also cause damage throughout the brain as a result of shock waves and pressure effects (Reider-Groswasser et al., 2002;

Trask and Narayan, 1996). The extent and severity of diffuse damage to brain tissue depend on such physical qualities as speed, wobble, and malleability of the penetrating object (Salazar, Martin, and Grafman, 1987). Grafman and Salazar (1987) contrasted the relatively restricted area of damage left by a low-velocity (under 1,000 ft/sec) missile that was typical of civilian bullets and older military missiles with the more extensive range of tissue damaged by hemorrhages and apparent *ischemia* (absence of normal blood flow in the affected area) or *edema* (tissue swelling) when the velocity of the penetrating object exceeds 1,000 ft/sec, as in modern weaponry. Of course, low velocity shrapnel fragments also produce evidence of diffuse damage (Reider-Groswasser et al., 2002). The transient physiological conditions (of swelling, bleeding) during the acute stages may leave permanent tissue damage. Some effects of the injury are delayed by many years. It may not be possible to remove all fragments; they usually do not cause complications. Cases of spontaneous migration of fragments occur and produce neurologic deterioration that improves after fragment removal (Zafonte, Watanabe, and Mann, 1998). In one case, a penetrating metal splinter in an 18 year old was associated with a chronic abscess, scar formation, and a malignant glioma 37 years later (Sabel et al., 1999); in another, a brain abscess developed 52 years after a shrapnel injury (Marquardt et al., 2000).

Neuropsychological effects of penetrating injuries

In addition to the behavioral changes and specific cognitive deficits that can usually be traced to the site of the lesion (Grafman, Jonas, et al., 1988), patients with PHI may show some of the impairments of attention and concentration, memory functions, and mental slowing that tend to be associated with diffuse damage. Teuber (1969) noted "subtle but pervasive changes in our patients' capacity to deal with everyday intellectual demands," which he considered to be among the "general effects" of penetrating head wounds. However, in these patients, focal effects are typically more pronounced than diffuse ones (H.H. Kaufman et al., 1985; Newcombe, 1982); and, as one might expect, the larger the lesion, the more general the deficits (Grafman, Jonas, et al., 1988; Teuber, 1962).

Course and outcome

Like other TBI survivors, these patients tend to make relatively rapid gains in the first year or two following injury (A.E. Walker and Jablon, 1961), with further improvement coming very slowly and more likely as a result of learned accommodations and compensations than of return or renewal of function. Cognitive impairments such as language and constructional disorders are among those that may show significant improvement while sensory defects such as visual blind spots and reduced tactile sensitivity persist unchanged indefinitely (Teuber, 1975). Many of the general effects of brain damage, such as distractibility or slowing, tend to improve but may never return to the premorbid level of efficiency. Indeed, Vietnam veterans still had impairments in verbal learning (52%), visual memory (47%), sustained attention (52%), psychological problems (49%), posttraumatic epilepsy (41%), sensory loss (47%), visual field loss (41%), paresis (32%), diminished vision (50%), violence (37%) and difficulties in social interaction (43%–57%) 15 years postinjury, but 56% were working (Schwab et al., 1993). Fifteen years after the Russian invasion of Finland, 89% of the surviving Finnish TBI veterans were working (Hillbom, 1960); and Newcombe (1969) and Teuber (1975) each reported that approximately 85% of their World War II PHI victims were gainfully employed 20 or more years after injury. This large proportion of good outcomes in these older studies may be attributable to low survival rates for the more severely injured soldiers. A small study of Korean War PHI victims also provided "impressive evidence of recovery" such that, despite discrete cognitive impairments in some, most of these men were "working, supporting families, and able to travel alone" approximately 20 years after having been injured (Corkin, Hurt, et al., 1987; see also Dresser et al., 1973). For Vietnam veterans, work status was negatively correlated with posttraumatic epilepsy, paresis, visual field loss, verbal memory loss, psychological problems, and violent behavior (Schwab et al., 1993). Return to work was also related to educational achievement: 84% went back to school and 64% earned degrees (Kraft et al., 1993). The occupational achievement of those returning to work was not related to severity of injury!

Seizure disorders and other sequelae

PHI is associated with a high rate of epilepsy, occurring in up to 80% of patients within the first 24 hours (Yang and Benardo, 2000). Epilepsy may result in serious increase in ICP, worsening ischemic conditions (Trask and Narayan, 1996). Vietnam War veterans had a 53% rate of posttraumatic epilepsy and a 28% rate of persistent epilepsy when seen 15 years postinjury (Salazar, Jabbari, et al., 1985). Yet the seizure patients differed significantly from nonepileptic PHI survivors only on tests involving motor slowing and word list recall (Salazar, Grafman, Jabbari, et al., 1987). Lesions in the left hippocampus were most susceptible to seizure

development, although lesions in other lateralized structures also tended to be epileptogenic (Salazar, Amin, et al., 1987). Larger lesions also characterized the seizure patients (Salazar, Jabbari, et al., 1985). Most of these patients (925) had more than one seizure over an average time of more than seven years, with most seizures initially appearing in the first three years postinjury (G.H. Weiss, Salazar, et al., 1986). More recent examinations of Vietnam veterans indicate that simple partial, complex partial, partial with secondary damage, and generalized seizures are common in this group (Swanson et al., 1995). Posttraumatic epilepsy is also associated with premature death among survivors of penetrating head wounds (Corkin, Sullivan, and Carr, 1984; A.E. Walker and Blumer, 1989), particularly after the age of 50 (G.H. Weiss, et al., 1982).

Cerebrovascular disorders were the most common cause of death in head injured World War I veterans (G.H. Weiss, Caveness, et al., 1982) and occurred frequently among the younger Russo-Finnish War survivors (Hillbom, 1960). Severity in itself did not appear to contribute to a higher death rate except as associated with epilepsy. Corkin and her colleagues (1984) found that for head injured veterans, a lower educational level was also significantly associated with a shortened life expectancy. Achté and his colleagues (1969) reported an increased incidence of psychosis in their war injured population, with severity of injury an important contributing factor. The incidence of psychopathology increased with epilepsy at a similar rate across epilepsy subtypes, though more of the veterans with partial generalized and generalized seizures had inpatient or out-patient psychiatric treatment (Swanson et al., 1995).

Closed Head Injuries

Neuropathology

In *closed head injury* (CHI), brain damage typically occurs in two stages: The *primary injury* is the damage that occurs at the time of impact; the *second injury* consists of the effects of the physiological processes set in motion by the primary injury.

The primary injury. The mechanics of CHI explain many of their common symptom patterns (Bandak, 1995; Gennarelli and Meaney, 1996; Goldsmith, 1966; Nishimoto and Murakami, 1998; D. Pang, 1989; Teasdale and Mathew, 1996). Several kinds of damaging mechanical forces have been identified, such as contact forces and inertial forces (Halliday, 1999). The most obvious of these is *contact force* (force of impact), the predominant cause of brain damage in *static injuries*, in which a relatively still victim receives a blow to the head (Hochswender, 1988). Damage appears to be due to a rapid sequence of events beginning with the inward molding of the skull at the point of impact and compensatory adjacent outbending followed by rebound effects. With sufficient stress, the skull may be fractured, thus dissipating some of the impact energy but complicating the picture with the possibility of infection and additional tissue damage. *Inertial forces* can involve *translational acceleration* in which the head moves in a straight line with the brain's center of gravity or *rotational acceleration* in which the brain rotates around its center of gravity. Movement of the head and neck on impact results in *angular acceleration,* a combination of translational and rotational acceleration.

Cerebral contusions consist of focal damage to brain tissue (*parenchyma*) and vascular structure, are most severe on gyral crests, and may extend into the white matter to a variable degree (D.I. Graham, 1996; Halliday, 1999). When the fine tissue covering the brain (*pia, arachnoid*) is torn, the injury is referred to as a *laceration.* The blow at the point of impact is called the *coup,* and a contusion is likely to appear under the site of impact. *Contrecoup* lesions, in which the brain sustains a contusion in an area opposite the blow, most frequently occur in the frontal and temporal lobes and Sylvian fissure regions (Halliday, 1999). Contrecoup injuries occur in most cases of occipital injury (R.D. Adams, Victor, and Ropper, 1997; Courville, 1942). Frontal blows mainly produce coup lesions. Side blows produce either coup or contrecoup lesions or both (R.D. Adams, et al., 1997; Halliday, 1999); however, A.H. Roberts (1976) reported that 80% of his less seriously injured subjects sustained contrecoup damage as judged by the motorically disabled side. Lateral impacts may produce more injury than frontal or occipital blows (G.A. Ryan et al., 1994; Zhang et al., 2001b). Contrecoup damage results from translational forces and direction of impact to the brain sitting on its flexible stem in a liquid medium (Gurdjian, 1975; Halliday, 1999). The force of the blow may literally bounce the brain off the opposite side of its bony container, bruising brain tissue where it strikes the skull. Coup and contrecoup lesions account for specific and localizable behavioral changes that accompany CHI.

Bruising can also take place at the moment that rapid deceleration begins or within the first few seconds thereafter as a result of the brain being "slammed" against the skull's bony protuberances in response to translational forces and angular acceleration (D. Pang, 1989; D.I. Graham, 1996; Halliday, 1999). These bruises are characteristically most pronounced at the frontal and temporal poles and their undersides, where the cortex normally rests on the rough surface of the base of the skull (Courville, 1942; D.I. Graham, 1996). A direct blow to the head is not necessary for this kind of bruising to occur, only rapid deceleration with energy translation to the brain such as occurs when a vehicle comes to a sudden stop (J.E. Sweeney, 1992). For example, brain damage can result from a whiplash injury (R.W. Evans, 1992, 1996b; R.D. Adams, Victor, and Ropper, 1997; see p. 166, pp. 174–175). With contact or not, under conditions of rapid acceleration or deceleration, single or multiple contusions can occur in deep structures such as the basal ganglia, hypothalamus, brainstem, and corpus callosum. The corpus callosum and brainstem are particularly vulnerable (Gennerelli, Thibault, and Graham, 1998). The degree of corpus callosum injury on MRI may be indicative of clinical severity of diffuse injury and the presence of midbrain injury (Takaoka et al., 2002). Pressure of the medial temporal lobe against the edges of supporting structures or pressure of cerebellar structures onto the *foramen magnum* (opening at the base of the skull where the brainstem becomes spinal cord) at the time of injury produces herniation contusions (D.I. Graham, 1996). Clearly distinguishable focal deficits are much less likely to be seen when there was a great deal of momentum on impact, as occurs in *moving vehicle accidents* (*MVAs*). In such cases damage tends to be widespread so that some deficits associated with damage at the site of impact may be observed as well as deficits that can be attributed only to focal lesions elsewhere in the brain. As a result, victims of trauma occurring with momentum generally present a pattern of multifocal or bilateral damage without clear-cut evidence of lateralization, regardless of the site of impact (Bigler, 1990a; Ponsford, 1995).

Another neuropsychologically important kind of brain damage that occurs in closed head injury results from the combination of translational force and rotational acceleration of the brain within the bony structure of the skull (D. Pang, 1989; Halliday, 1999; R.S. Parker, 2000; Zhang et al., 2001a). The movement of the brain within the skull puts strain on delicate nerve fibers and blood vessels, which can stretch them to the point of shearing (Strich, 1961). Shearing effects, in the form of microscopic lesions that occur throughout the brain (Oppenheimer, 1968; R.S. Parker, 2001), tend to be concentrated in the frontal and temporal lobes (Groswasser, Reider-Groswasser, et al., 1987; Grubb and Coxe, 1978), the interfaces between gray and white matter around the basal ganglia, periventricular zones, corpus callosum (body and splenium), brainstem fiber tracts (dorsolateral), and superior cerebellar peduncles (D. Pang, 1989; Gennarelli, Thibault, and Graham, 1998; Parizel et al., 1998; Halliday, 1999; Leclercq et al., 2001).

When a moving head comes to a fast stop in an accident, the forward-moving energy (in a motor vehicle) or accelerating energy (in a fall) translates into rapid acceleration/deceleration expanding and contracting wave-form movements of the brain matter, usually accompanied by the fast rotational propulsion of the brain within the skull. At the neuronal level, this rapid acceleration and deceleration, along with the rotational forces, results in damage to axons in cerebral and brainstem white matter and, in serious injuries, in the cerebellum (Boström and Helander, 1986; Gennarelli, Thibault, and Graham, 1998; R.S. Parker, 2001). This kind of axonal damage, called *diffuse axonal injury* (*DAI*), appears as torn axons, shearing of axon clusters, retraction balls consisting of sheared back axonal substance (axoplasm), and reactive swelling of strained and damaged axons (J.H. Adams, Graham, and Gennarelli, 1985; D.I. Graham, 1996). Neuronal damage is accompanied by punctate hemorrhages from ruptured blood vessels scattered throughout cerebral white matter and lower structures as well (Boström and Helander, 1986; Parizel et al., 1998). The amount of diffuse damage tends to vary in different parts of the brain since anterior regions are more likely to be involved than posterior ones and deeper structures tend to be more vulnerable than surface areas (J.T.L. Wilson, 1990; D.I. Graham, 1996). Severe DAI without an intracranial mass lesion is present in nearly 50% of severe injuries and 35% of deaths (D.I. Graham, 1996).

The tremendous clinical significance of these microscopic lesions is easily understood if one realizes that myriad microscopic shearing injuries occur simultaneously within a rapidly rotating brain, resulting in myriad axonal and neuronal disruptions within the deep white matter of both cerebral hemispheres, which in essence disconnect the cortex from subcortical structures in widespread regions of the brain. (D. Pang, 1989)

Velocity, duration, acceleration–deceleration rate, and direction of head movement affect severity of DAI (Halliday, 1999). Rotational velocity also appears to play a significant role in producing loss of consciousness (Ommaya and Gennarelli, 1974; R.S. Parker, 2001).

Diffuse axonal injury can occur without any direct impact on the head, as it requires only the condition of rapid acceleration/deceleration such as takes place in *whiplash injuries* due to acceleration/deceleration forces resulting in rapid flexion-extension movement of the neck (Alves and Jane, 1985; R.W. Evans, 1992; Gennarelli, Thibault, et al., 1982; R.S. Parker, 2000; Yarnell and Rossie, 1988; see also pp. 174–175). The possibility of cerebral damage occurring with whiplash is still viewed by some clinicians with skepticism (discussed in R.W. Evans, 1996b).

The effects of these immediate disturbances in neurologic functions created by the mechanical forces of rapid acceleration/deceleration is called *concussion*. Concussion does not require a direct impact to the head; the rapid angular acceleration in itself is sufficient to set these forces in motion (Gennarelli, 1983; R.W. Evans, 1992; Sweeney, 1992). Noting that the concussion syndrome covers a range of symptoms and severity, Gennarelli (1986) suggested that there are two broad categories of concussion: *mild concussion*, without loss of consciousness and characterized by symptoms such as "seeing stars" if the injury was focal and/or a short period of confusion and disorientation with or without amnesia for a brief time before and/or after the event; and *classic concussion*, defined by reversible coma occurring "at the instant of trauma," which may be accompanied by cardiovascular and pulmonary function changes and neurologic abnormalities, including a stiffened body position (*decerebrate posturing*), pupillary changes, and seizure-like activity, all of which dissipate within the first 20–30 minutes after the event. Concussion represents a continuum with varying severity of injury, neuropsychological impairments, and neurobehavioral outcomes (R.C.K. Chan, 2001). When the confusion and disorientation resolve within hours or days, the condition is usually considered a mild TBI (see pp. 168–171), although even seemingly mild injuries can have serious neurobehavioral consequences (R.S. Parker, 2001), including seizure-like symptoms frequently accompanied by chronic cognitive deficits (Verduyn et al., 1992). Indeed, Lovell, Iverson, and coworkers (1999) report mildly decreased performances on tests of information processing and memory acutely after mild TBI that were similar for patients with LOC, no LOC, or uncertain LOC. The neuropsychological sequelae of concussion without LOC do not differ in severity from those occurring when there is a brief comatose period (Leininger, Gramling, et al., 1990; Nemeth, 1991).

In recommending that concussion be defined as "an acceleration/deceleration injury to the head" which is typically but not necessarily accompanied by amnesia, Rutherford (1989) extended this diagnosis to the many cases of minor TBI having behavioral sequelae consistent with this type of brain injury when LOC is questionable. He noted that this definition does not preclude its application to more severely damaged patients. Involvement of brain stem reticular formation structures in the injury may not be necessary for concussion, although postmortem microscopic examination of concussion victims typically shows damage to the corpus callosum, to the rostral (anterior) brainstem, and spread widely throughout the white matter and cortex (Salazar, Martin, and Grafman, 1987; Hankins et al., 1996). Seventy-five percent of a group of mild TBI patients with persistent postconcussional symptoms had a normal MRI or CT scan at the time of injury yet later displayed temporal (75%), frontal (30%), or frontotemporal (40%) abnormalities on PET and SPECT (Umile et al., 2002), indicating that cellular damage not picked up by early neuroimaging continues to have functional and behavioral consequences.

Besides the scattered tiny (*petechial*) hemorrhages seen with diffuse axonal damage and occurring mostly in frontal and temporal lobe white matter, larger blood vessels may be torn on impact. CHI hemorrhages create hematomas within the skull.

Epidural hematomas (EDHs) are formed when the brain's outer, leathery covering, the *dura mater,* is stripped away from the skull by blood from lacerated blood vessels or bleeding from a fracture (Diaz-Marchan et al., 1996). The majority of EDHs occur over the temporoparietal area following a skull fracture that produces arterial damage. EDHs can also occur in frontal, parietal, and posterior areas. Posterior EDH near the brain stem is particularly dangerous since the patient may be conscious until the end stage of development of the blood-filled swelling and minutes from death (J.D. Miller, Piper and Jones, 1996). An EDH can follow contrecoup as well as coup injury (Motohashi et al., 2000; Miyazaki et al., 1995). Most EDHs develop within minutes after the injury but some develop in the first day and even enlarge later on (Diaz-Marchan et al., 1996; T.I. Cohen and Gudeman, 1996).

Subdural hematomas (SDHs) form in the space between the dura and brain, produced most often by torn veins on the brain's surface and the inner side of the dura mater (Diaz-Marchan et al., 1996). They usually appear as a slick of blood that can extend across a hemisphere since their spread is limited only by the dural tissue separating the hemispheres. SDHs may develop within the first 24 hours postinjury (acute SDH), 2–14 days postinjury (subacute SDH), or more than two weeks postinjury (chronic or delayed SDH) (D.I. Graham, 1996). Acute SDHs are often present opposite a skull fracture due to laceration to the brain, especially at the temporal pole (J.D. Miller, Piper, and Jones, 1996; Diaz-Marchan et al., 1996). Chronic SDHs usually develop weeks or months after what seems to be a trivial TBI, might go unnoticed initially (T.I. Cohen and Gudeman, 1996), increasing slowly in size until they have mass effects (D.I. Graham, 1996). They are likely to appear in older individuals who already have some brain atrophy allowing for slow expansion and significant distortion of the brain.

Intracerebral hematomas (ICHs) form within the substance of the brain and may result from a laceration (J.D. Miller, Piper, and Jones, 1996). They usually occur in the frontal and temporal lobes but have been found in the basal ganglia and cerebellum (D.I. Graham, 1996). These hematomas probably result from direct rupture of blood vessels in the brain and are likely to be associated with DAI. *Delayed traumatic intracerebral hematoma (DTICH)* mostly occurs in the first 72 hours postinjury (T.I. Cohen and Gudeman, 1996). These patients ("talk and deteriorate" or "talk and die") are conscious after the injury, may even have an initial GCS of 15, and then deteriorate into a coma. They usually have a mass lesion that needs to be evacuated (D.F. Kelly, Doberstein, and Becker, 1996). A "burst lobe" occurs when an ICH or intracerebellar hematoma joins with an SDH.

When blood flows in between the coverings of the brain, the hematoma it creates acts as a more or less rapidly growing mass. As a hematoma grows, it exerts increasing pressure on surrounding structures. Since the bony cranium does not give way, the air- and liquid-filled spaces surrounding and within the brain are first compressed. The swelling mass then pushes against the softer mass of the brain, deforming and damaging brain tissue pressed against the skull. Ultimately the built-up pressure and swelling may force brain tissue through the base of the cranium (*herniation*) (Diaz-Marchan, et al., 1996; J.D. Miller, Piper, and Jones, 1996; Plum and Posner, 1980). CHIs with hemorrhage tend to be more serious than when damage is due to DAI alone. In one series of 635 fatal CHIs, 75% had skull fractures, 94% had surface contusions (6% mild, 78% moderate, and 10% severe), 29% had DAI, and 60% had intracranial hematomas (10% EDH, 18% SDH, 16% ICH, 23% burst lobe) (D.I. Graham, 1996).

The high velocity of impact in a moving vehicle intensifies shearing, stress, and shock wave effects on brain tissue, thus multiplying the number and severity of small lesions involving nerve fibers and blood vessels throughout the brain. For these reasons, TBIs incurred in MVAs are often treated separately from other head injuries for clinical and research purposes.

The second injury. Secondary damage due to the ensuing physiological processes may be as destructive of brain tissue as the accident's immediate effects, if not more destructive (D. Pang, 1989; R.S. Parker, 2001; J.T.E. Richardson, 2000). Elevated *ICP (intracranial pressure)*, brain swelling/edema, hypoxia/ischemia, pyrexia (fever), and infection are among the complicating processes initiated at the time of injury that lead to secondary damage of the brain (D.I. Graham, 1996; J.D. Miller, Piper, and Jones, 1996) along with a cascade of neurochemical and cellular events (Hatton, 2001; McIntosh et al., 1999; Novack, Johnson, and Greenwood, 1996; Novack, Dillon, and Jackson, 1996). Elevated ICP can result from an increase in cerebral blood volume that produces cerebrovascular congestion; brain *edema*, an increase in tissue water content; and sometimes acute *hydrocephalus* (dilation of the cerebral ventricles) (J.D. Miller, Piper, and Jones, 1996). Brain swelling can be focal or generalized, adjacent to a contusion or diffused throughout one or both hemispheres (D.I. Graham, 1996). Cerebral ischemia results from *cerebral blood flow (CBF)* being insufficient to support the metabolic needs of brain tissue, primarily in the first 24 hours postinjury and especially in the first four (Muizelaar, 1996; Obrist and Marion, 1996). In one study 91% of patients who died due to severe TBI had evidence of cerebral ischemia histologically (D.I. Graham, Adams, and Doyle, 1978). Pyrexia is likely to increase metabolic demands of the brain when CBF is low and associated with brain congestion, edema, and elevated ICP (D.I. Graham, 1996). In most cases, pyrexia is not initially associated with infection.

The most dangerous effects of swelling are on the lower brainstem structures concerned with vital functions, for when compression seriously compromises their activity the patient dies. Moreover, the brainstem is a common site of severe damage. This reflects, at least in part, elevated ICP, which is the most frequent cause of death in CHI (J.H. Adams, Graham, and Gennarelli, 1985; Marmarou, 1985) and tends to be a strong predictor of severe chronic impairment (Uzzell, Dolinskas, and Wiser, 1990). Thus, control of ICP is the most important medical consideration in the acute care of head trauma (J.D. Miller, 1991). The increasing survival rate of patients with such injuries attests to the success of modern medical and surgical techniques for controlling ICP.

As with bruises and tissue damage to other parts of the body, damage to brain tissue, whether from the primary injury or secondary processes, produces swelling as a result of edema. Whereas swelling on the surface of the body—such as the "goose egg" that temporarily bulges out in response to a superficial blow to the head—can expand without putting pressure on body tissue, swelling within the cranium only compounds whatever damage has taken place, whether direct or indirect. Moreover, since edema is one of the normal physiological responses to tissue injury, the development of edema itself further perpetuates and accelerates the edematous process. Like pressure from hematoma, swelling due to edema can produce further direct damage to brain tissue (D. Pang, 1989; J.T.E. Richardson, 2000).

Along with edematous swelling, heightened cerebral blood volume due to loss of normal autoregulatory processes may contribute to increased ICP. This excess of blood in the brain (hyperemia) about the second or third day after severe injury, rather than guaranteeing adequate oxygenation and nourishment when sick and dying brain tissue most need them, tends to cut off normal blood flow. The compression effects of raised ICP can reduce cerebral blood flow generally and create ischemic (bloodless) areas in which no arterial blood gets through to swollen tissues (D.I. Graham, Adams, and Doyle, 1978). Elevated ICP with hyperemia contributes significantly to poorer outcomes in surviving patients (Obrist and Marion, 1996; Uzzell, Obrist,

Dolinskas, and Langfitt, 1986). Hypotension and *hypoxia* (undersupply of oxygen) may contribute to poor outcome (Jeremitsky et al., 2003; Narayan, Wilberger, and Povlishock, 1996; D. Pang, 1989).

Ventricular enlargement, as demonstrated by CT scan, is the most frequent neuroimaging finding in TBI (Bigler, Blatter, et al., 1996). It often occurs in patients with severe closed head injuries (C.A. Meyers, Levin, et al., 1983; see also Bigler, 2001b). This comes from shrinkage of brain substance due to disintegration of severely damaged neuronal tissue, a process that typically is completed within the first six weeks after injury (Bigler, Kurth et al., 1992) but that may continue for months (Haymaker and Adams, 1982). Enlarged ventricles are most likely to occur in patients with prolonged coma following moving vehicle accidents and are associated with poorer outcomes. TBI combined with substance abuse is associated with greater brain atrophy (L.H. Barker et al., 1999; Bigler, Blatter, et al., 1996). Atrophy is also greater with diffuse damage than with localized lesions (Bigler, 2001b). Ventricular dilation is related to poor neuropsychological outcome (C.V. Anderson and Bigler, 1995; S.D. Gale, Johnson, et al., 1999). Reduced corpus callosum size is common with severe CHI, presumably from shear strain and atrophy. This may be a better predictor of long-term cognitive outcome than ventricular enlargement (Verger et al., 2001). Also related to severity are eventual reductions in fornix and hippocampal volume, with associated memory deficits (D.F. Tate and Bigler, 2000). Many other physiological changes take place in the brain, and in other organ systems as well, in response to brain injury (M.S. Grady and McIntosh, 2002). Some are ameliorative; others compound destructive processes. (Full discussions of the body's physiological response to acute brain injury are given in Narayan, Wilberger, and Povlishock, 1996; J.T.E. Richardson, 2000; see also M.S. Grady and McIntosh, 2002, for cellular abnormalities.)

Behavioral alterations associated with common patterns of TBI

Diffuse damage. The diffuse damage that accompanies much TBI consists of minute lesions and lacerations scattered throughout the brain substance that eventually may become the sites of degenerative changes and scar tissue or simply little cavities (Boström and Helander, 1986; Filley, 2001; Strich, 1961). This kind of damage tends to compromise mental speed, attentional functions, cognitive efficiency, and, when severe, high-level concept formation and complex reasoning abilities (Gronwall and Sampson, 1974; R.S. Parker, 2001; van Zomeren and Brouwer, 1994). These problems are typically reflected in patients' complaints of inability to concentrate or perform complex mental operations, confusion and perplexity in thinking, irritability, fatigue, and inability to do things as well as before the accident. The latter complaint is particularly poignant in bright, mildly damaged subjects who may still perform well on standard ability tests but who are aware of a loss of mental power and acuity that will keep them from realizing premorbid goals or repeating premorbid accomplishments.

Problems associated with diffuse damage readily become apparent in an appropriate examination. Slowed thinking and reaction times may result in significantly lowered scores on timed tests despite the capacity to perform the required task accurately. Tasks requiring selective or divided attention tend to be particularly sensitive to diffuse effects (Gronwall, 1977; M. Leclercq and Azouvi, 2002; Stuss, Stethem, Hugenholtz, and Richard, 1989; van Zomeren and Brouwer, 1994). In general, patients with diffuse damage perform relatively poorly on tasks requiring concentration and mental tracking such as oral arithmetic or sequential arithmetic and reasoning problems that must be performed mentally (Gronwall and Wrightson, 1981; Ogden, 1996). Other difficulties experienced by patients with diffuse damage include confusion of items or elements of orally presented questions, feelings of uncertainty about the correctness of their answers, distractibility, and fatigue (Lezak, 1978b, 1988d; Ogden, 1996).

Occasionally, a TBI patient with a strong mathematics background will perform surprisingly well on arithmetic problems, even those involving oral arithmetic with its mental tracking requirements, although many of these patients run into difficulty with problems that require them to juggle several elements mentally. Observations of arithmetically exceptional patients who perform poorly on other tests of mental tracking give the impression that their arithmetic thinking habits are so ingrained that the solutions come to them automatically, before they have time to lose or get confused about the problem's elements. Similar manifestations of other kinds of overlearned behavior can also crop up unexpectedly.

Patients with the mental efficiency problems associated with diffuse damage frequently interpret their experiences of slowed processing and attentional deficits as memory problems, even when learning is affected only mildly, if at all (Howieson and Lezak, 2002b). Thus they complain of "poor memory," but analysis of their performance on memory and attention tests typically implicates reduced auditory span, difficulty doing (or processing) more than one thing (or stimulus) at a time, and verbal retrieval problems. Many are acutely aware that they are mentally inefficient—easily confused, disoriented, overwhelmed, or distracted. These patients may try to compensate for their deficiencies with obsessive-compulsive strategies (Hibbard et al., 2000; Lezak, 1991; McKeon et al., 1984) and tend to avoid stressful (i.e., highly stimulating) situations—such as cocktail parties, the local pub, big family gatherings, and shopping malls—thus becoming somewhat socially withdrawn.

Direct blows to the head. Coup and contrecoup lesions result in discrete impairment of those functions mediated by the cortex at the site of the lesion. Such specific impairment patterns are most likely to appear as the sole or predominant neuropsychological disturbance when the victim has been struck by an object or has struck the head against an object through a sudden move or short fall in which not much momentum was gained.

I (mdl) examined a 28-year-old right-handed man about one year after he was struck by lightning and fell from a work station eight feet above ground, striking the left side of his head. He displayed no language or neurological deficits, and all aspects of response speed, motor control, attention, concentration, and mental tracking were well *above average.* However, he could no longer perform complex mechanical construction work efficiently or safely, nor could he draw a house in perspective. He failed miserably on an employee aptitude test of visuographic functions and had difficulty with block and puzzle construction tasks. His thinking displayed the fragmented quality characteristic of patients with right hemisphere damage, and his wife complained that he had become insensitive to her emotional states as well as socially gauche.

There was no question that this man had localized brain damage. Without further tests, one could not disprove the possibility that he was one of the one-in-a-hundred right-handed persons whose lateral cortical organization was the reverse of normal (see p. 305). However, a more likely explanation was that he was one of the 50% who sustain a localized contrecoup lesion when the traumatic impact is to the side of the head (see Castro-Caldas, Confraria, et al., 1986, for a similar case of contrecoup but with a right-sided coup).

Bruising due to deceleration/acceleration effects. The second pattern of specific impairments that can be associated with localized brain lesions involves the frontal and temporal lobes, those areas most susceptible to the damaging effects of the brain bouncing and twisting within the skull. Thus, problems in the regulation and control of activity, in conceptual and problem-solving behavior, and in various aspects of memory and learning are common among CHI victims (N. Brooks, 1989; Lezak, 1989; R.S. Parker, 2001; Walsh, 1991). The more severe the injury, the more likely it is that the patient will display deficits characteristic of frontal and temporal lobe injuries and the more prominent these deficits will be. Damage involving the frontal and temporal lobes also affects the patient's personality and social adjustment (Blumer and Benson, 1975; Kim, 2002; Lezak and O'Brien, 1990; J.M. Silver et al., 2002; Zhang and Sachdev, 2003). These personality changes, even when subtle, are more likely to impede the patient's return to psychosocial independence than cognitive impairment or physical crippling (Lezak and O'Brien, 1988).

Few persons with TBI exhibit only one pattern of impairment, with the exception of patients with mild injuries. The most severely injured suffer all three. Even many who are moderately damaged will usually have symptoms of focal damage and some temporal and frontal lobe deficits and diffuse impairment as well.

Sensory alterations. An impaired sense of smell (*anosmia*) frequently accompanies bruising of the frontal lobes, as their underside lies on the olfactory nerves (Varney and Menefee, 1993; Yousem et al., 1999). Deficits in smell discrimination may also indicate damage to limbic components of the temporal lobes as these too have connections to the primary olfactory structures (Eslinger, Damasio, and Van Hoesen, 1982; Martzke et al., 1991). Alterations of the sense of smell are directly related to trauma severity and may occur in more than half of patients in contrast to much lower rates of awareness of the deficits (Callahan and Hinkebein, 1999; Costanzo and Zasler, 1992).

Many TBI patients sustain more or less subtle alterations in visual competency (Groswasser, Cohen, and Blankstein, 1990; Padula and Argyris, 1996; R.S. Parker, 2001). These can involve visual acuity, both near and far; visual fields; oculomotor disorders, including fixation difficulties and failure of binocular fusion, which is typically experienced as double vision (*diplopia*) at one or more angle of vision; and aversion to bright lights (*photophobia*) (Gronwall, 1991; J.M. Holmes et al., 1998; London et al., 2003; Suchoff et al., 1999; Weissberg et al., 2000). Prosopagnosia also troubles a few TBI patients (Mattson et al., 2000; Pradat-Diehl et al., 1999).

Dizziness and balance disorders are common problems after head injury that can add to the patient's distress, sense of confusion and disorientation, and cognitive dysfunction (Basford et al., 2003; Furman and Cass, 2003; Grimm et al., 1989). Along with dizziness, hearing defects not infrequently contribute to these patients' cognitive inefficiencies and emotional distress (Lezak, 1989; Jury and Flynn, 2001). Most common of these are ringing or buzzing in the ear (*tinnitus*) (Axelsson, 1995; Coles, 1995) and intolerance of loud/ sudden noises (*hyperacusis*) (Gabriels, 1995).

Closed Head Injury: Nature, Course, and Outcome

Mild traumatic brain injury

Diagnostic criteria. Many different criteria for diagnosing mild TBI have been offered, some relying on PTA, some requiring at least brief LOC (Cohadon et al., 2002, pp. 51–70; Kraus and Nourjah, 1989, pp. 8–10; Ruff and Jurica, 1999; Uzzell, 1999). It is now well recognized that concussion, the characteristic injury of mild TBI, is primarily due to diffuse axonal injury (DAI) in which axons are damaged or destroyed due to acceleration/deceleration forces acting upon the axonal bundles and intracranial blood vessels (Bigler, 1990a, 2001b; Gennarelli, 1986; Y.K. Liu, 1999; Sohlberg and Mateer, 2001; see p. 166). Concussion can also occur without LOC or direct contact with the head, as in whiplash injuries in which the head is jerked with sufficient rapidity and force to cause damage to cerebral and other soft tissue structures (see *Whiplash*, pp. 174–175). Thus, there is increasing acceptance of the diagnostic standard recommended by the American Academy of Physical Medicine and Rehabilitation, which recognizes that concussion can occur without accompanying LOC or PTA (American Congress of Rehabilitation Medicine, 1993) (see Table 7.2). Either translational or rotational forces will be implicated, but many injuries result from a combination of these forces (L. Zhang et al., 2001b).

Neuroimaging in mild TBI. The increasing sensitivity of neuroimaging techniques has raised hopes of resolving questions of the presence or severity of cerebral lesions in persons meeting the diagnostic criteria for mild TBI. Although mild TBI patients with reported LOC are typically scanned by CT in emergency rooms, few display CT abnormalities (Alaoui et al., 1998; Bigler and Snyder, 1995; Kay, 1986), and it is rare for those with no LOC and only brief PTA to show cerebral defects on immediate CT scanning (Bigler, 1999).

TABLE 7.2 Diagnostic Criteria for Concussion

To make the diagnosis of concussion, at least one of the following criteria must be met:

1. any period of loss of consciousness not exceeding 30 mins.; at 30 mins. from onset of loss of consciousness, the patient's Glasgow Coma score must be at least 13
2. any loss of memory for events immediately before or after the accident
3. any alteration in mental state at the time of the accident (e.g., feeling dazed, disoriented, or confused)
4. focal neurological deficits that may or may not be transient
5. posttraumatic amnesia not greater than 24 hrs

From American Congress of Rehabilitation Medicine (1993)

MRI has proven to be more sensitive to the presence of lesions in persons satisfying mild TBI criteria (Bigler, 1999; H.S. Levin, Amparo, et al., 1987; Lewine et al., 1996) but still may not document tissue damage even when history and neuropsychological findings indicate impairment supporting a diagnosis of mild TBI (Bigler and Snyder, 1995). For example, only six of one series of 20 mild TBI patients who had normal CT readings displayed white matter abnormalities on MRI (Mittl et al., 1994). MRI use for scanning mild TBI patients has been limited by cost, length of time required for the examination, problems presented by agitated patients, and technical physical limitations due to magnetic sensitivities (Patterson and Kotrla, 2002; J.T.E. Richardson, 2000). Like lesion patterns for more severe injuries, contusion lesions (i.e., bruises) found by MRI in patients with GCS scores in the 13 to 15 range predominantly involve frontal and temporal regions, and their cognitive deficits tend to reflect impairment in these areas (Bigler, 1999; J.T.L. Wilson, Hadley, et al., 1996). Responding to tendencies to assume normality if neuroimaging by usual procedures is negative, Bigler (2001a) points out that some intracellular damage may not show up on neuroimaging, yet the cell may be dysfunctional due to cytoskeletal abnormalities. Moreover, neuroimaging techniques more sensitive than MRI may reveal lesions when the MRI appears normal. For example, Kant and his colleagues (1997) found that SPECT of 43 mild TBI patients detected cerebral abnormalities in 53% of them, while MRI showed abnormality in only 9%.

Microscopic white matter lesions—due to DAIs, which probably account for much of the cognitive dysfunction associated with concussion—may not be visualized by these imaging techniques. More recent techniques for imaging physiological changes provide some evidence of cerebral dysfunction that does not show up on structural imaging (Bigler, 1999, 2001b; Lewine et al., 1996; A. Jacobs et al., 1996; Sohlberg and Mateer, 2001). For example, Ruff, Crouch and their colleagues (1994) present nine cases with negative CT or MRI who received corroboration of their neuropsychological abnormalities from PET scanning. Yet caution in interpreting data from SPECT or PET studies has been recommended on the basis of the investigational status of these techniques (J.M. Silver et al., 2002; see also p. 16). G.K. Henry and his colleagues (2000) report that quantitative electroencephalography (QEEG) demonstrated abnormal electrophysiological activity in all 32 patients who had sustained whiplash injuries, although 14 had had negative MRI or CT studies. However, most EEG studies of mild TBI patients using standard techniques do not show abnormalities (Schoenhuber and Gentilini, 1989; Wrightson and Gronwall, 1999).

Epidemiology

With less than 20–30 minutes of LOC if any, and PTA measured in hours rather than days, counts or estimates of the percentage of TBIs that can be classified as mild have ranged from 49% to 85%, with most estimates close to the latter figure (T.L. Bennett and Raymond, 1997b; Sherer and Novack, 2003; Wrightson and Gronwall, 1999). Recent incidence figures from the United States (618/100,000) and New Zealand (654/100,000) for TBI patients seen but not hospitalized are comparable (Wrightson and Gronwall, 1999) and consistent with the National Head Injury Foundation (1993) estimate of more than two million persons sustaining mild TBI each year in the United States. Since as many as 25% of mild TBI patients receive medical treatment outside of facilities which keep incidence data (Sosin et al., 1996) and others may never seek treatment, any figure must be regarded as an underestimate (H. Petit et al., 1994). Certain personality traits and behavioral characteristics tend to be predisposing to TBI, such as being a young adult male, impulsive and/or hyperactive, a risk-taker, an alcohol abuser, or having had a learning disability or prior head injury (McAllister and Flashman, 1999). Even among the relatively privileged college student population, mild TBIs have a prevalence rate above 30%, of which more than half are due to sports or other recreational accidents (Laforce and MacLeod, 2001).

Course and duration

Descriptions of the acute condition in mild TBI agree on a triad of neuropsychological dysfunctions—attention deficits, impaired verbal retrieval, and forgetfulness—that usually appear within the first few days after injury (Alves and Jane, 1985; Gasquoine, 1997b; Kay, 1986; Rimel et al., 1981). With extensive examination, more widespread deficits may show up (Reitan and Wolfson, 2000). Other problems, most notably headache, dizziness, irritability, drowziness, sleep disturbance, and fatigability, are also very common early sequelae (Coonley-Hoganson et al., 1984; Gasquoine, 1997b; Ponsford, Willmott et al., 2000) and can exacerbate the effects of the cognitive deficits (Conboy et al., 1986; Dikmen, McLean, and Temkin, 1986). These are the same problems that occur with more severe brain injuries (M.P. Alexander, 1995), compounding and compounded by the additional deficits of severe TBI (see pp. 179–185). These are common problems, acknowledged on a "yes/no" questionnaire by persons who had no acute medical or psychological complaints, but they marked "yes" on fewer items than did mild TBI patients (D.D. Fox et al., 1995; Paniak, Reynolds, et al., 2002); these items did not measure the severity of the problems. Paniak and his coworkers (2002) reported that one month postinjury complaints by mild TBI patients ranged from few to very many such that subjective complaints alone should not be used to identify persons with mild TBI.

When the patient has sustained other injuries, particularly those requiring significant amounts of medication for pain or procedures such as surgery or casting that keep the patient from resuming a full schedule of activities, the cognitive problems may not become disruptive or even evident for days or—in some cases—weeks after the accident. Patients who take a few days away from their normal responsibilities after an accident may not notice mental impairments until returning to work or preparing meals, shopping, and planning for a family. Thus it is not uncommon to find no notes reporting altered mental status in the emergency room record or hospital chart, even when the patient is later observed to suffer from fairly debilitating mental dysfunction.

Many studies report that more than two-thirds of persons sustaining mild TBI will have returned to their premorbid occupations and usual personal activities within the first three to six months after the accident (L.M. Binder, 1997; Gentilini, Nichelli, et al., 1985; P.S. Klonoff and Lamb, 1998; H.S. Levin, Mattis, et al., 1987). This good news was summed up as "neurobehavioral impairment . . . generally resolved during the first 3 months after minor head injury" (H.S. Levin, Mattis, et al., 1987) or "most people recover completely from a mild head injury within a month or two" (Wrightson and Gronwall, 1999).

Yet mild cognitive deficits, primarily associated with slowed processing, persist in many patients meeting the criteria for mild TBI (Gasquoine, 1997b; Ogden and Wolfe, 1998; Stuss, Ely, et al., 1985; Stuss, Stethem, Hugenholtz, et al., 1989). For example, all but one of the 57 mildly injured patients in a three-center study had typical postconcussional complaints immediately following the injury (H.S. Levin, Mattis, et al., 1987). At one month most showed the characteristic evidence of attentional deficits and reduced visuomotor speed. These problems and associated complaints of headache, fatigue, and dizziness diminished significantly in the next two months. However, at three months, almost all of these patients still complained of headaches; and fatigue and dizziness each were reported by 22% of them. These continuing dysfunctions are often subtle and may become evident only with appropriate testing (Gronwall, 1991; Stuss, Stethem, Hugenholtz, and Richard, 1989) or may not become evident at all if an appropriate examination, sensitive to these problems, is not given (Cicerone, 1997).

For example, Gentilini and his colleagues (1985) reported that in their study, "No conclusive evidence was found that mild head injury causes cognitive impairment one month after the trauma." Not surprisingly, their patients and controls had not differed on Digits Forward, one of the most resilient of measures in the neuropsychological armamentarium, nor on four of the other five measures which tend to be relatively insensitive to the processing speed deficits common in mild TBI.

General agreement about the neurobehavioral disorders associated with mild TBI in the acute stage gives way to considerable disagreement regarding their duration (Leininger, Gramling, et al., 1990). The complex of somatic, cognitive, and emotional-reactive symptoms experienced and problems reported acutely may persist for months (the *postconcussional syndrome*) and, in some persons, become chronic (i.e., last longer than a year) (Hartlage et al., 2001; Ogden and Wolfe, 1998; Ruff and Grant, 1999). Estimates of the frequency of chronic postconcussive ailments among persons who have sustained a mild TBI run from a low of 7%–8% (L.M. Binder, 1997) to numbers in the ranges of 10%–15% (M.P. Alexander, 1995; Reitan and Wolfson, 1999), 10%–20% (Ruff and Grant, 1999), 10%–25% (J.T.E. Richardson, 2000), 20%–25% (Hartlage et al., 2001; Malec, 1999), and up to 40% (Alves, Macciocchi, and Barth, 1993). In a British study, only 63% of one group of mildly to moderately injured patients (mean PTA = 3 hrs) claimed few or no residual symptoms at six months (N.S. King et al., 1999). Thornhill and her coworkers (2000) relied on questionnaires filled out by the patients, their family members, or other caregivers for 333 with mild TBI a year after injury and found that only 49% had a "good recovery" (Glasgow Outcome Scale), while 21% continued to be severely disabled.

Other studies, looking at different population groups and at different times postinjury—from three months (Ponsford, Willmott, et al., 2000; Rimel et al., 1981) to three years (Rutherford, 1989)—also found that significant proportions of those diagnosed as having sustained mild TBI had postconcussional symptoms to a troubling degree (Gasquoine, 1997a; Malec, 1999; Ogden and Wolfe, 1998). College students who had sustained mild TBI and seemed "recovered" were abnormally prone to mental inefficiency when physiologically stressed by hypoxic conditions (Ewing et al., 1980) or psychologically stressed by challenging tasks (serial 7s from 500 [!], starting again from 500 after an error, in a very noisy environment) (Hanna-Pladdy, Berry, et al., 2001). W.R. Russell (1974) pointed out that "there is probably no such thing as 'complete recovery' from acceleration concussion of severity sufficient to cause loss of consciousness;" and Ho and Bennett's (1997) response to the question, "Do people recover from mild TBI?" is "Probably not," while reporting on improvements these patients can enjoy from both formal rehabilitation training and developing compensatory strategies on their own. M.P. Alexander (1995) notes that for most "well-recovered" patients, residual symptoms do appear under conditions of stress ("modest alcohol use, sleep deprivation, lengthy travel schedules, or increased workplace demands"), and they may continue indefinitely to experience themselves as having reduced mental efficiency.

Predicting course. The frequently complex interplay between behavioral alterations—cognitive, emotional, executive function—resulting from the brain injury itself, emotional reactions to these alterations, emotional vulnerabilities predating the accident, and social pressures unique for each patient make it virtually impossible in many cases to clarify or partial out the contribution of each of these potentially contributing factors. Recent studies have attempted to identify distinguishing characteristics so that the course for each new patient may be predictable and appropriate treatments instituted early (N.S. King, Crawford et al., 1999; Malec, 1999; see also Ruff and Richards, 2003). So far, most of these efforts have not borne much fruit. Ruff and Jurica (1999) identified severity levels: type I for patients who satisfied mild TBI criteria for the American Congress of Rehabilitation Medicine (p. 170); type III for the more stringent requirements of the American Psychiatric Association (2000), which call for a positive LOC of 5 to 30 min and PTA >12 hrs); and type II, a "bridge" level (positive LOC "with time unknown" or <5 mins and PTA of 60 secs to 12 hrs). All three levels require at least one neurological symptom. A comparison of patient groups at these three levels found no differences between them in quantity of subjective complaints (for physical or emotional symptoms or cognitive problems), nor did these groups differ on any of the 10 tested cognitive dimensions. Similar but short-term findings are reported by Iverson, Lovell, and Smith (2000), who, on comparing patients with brief LOC, equivocal LOC, or no LOC, found no differences on a variety of relatively sensitive cognitive tests one week postinjury (see also Ruff, Crouch, et al., 1994). Yet Hickling and his colleagues' (1998) mild TBI patients who had sustained LOC performed less well on cognitive tests than those who remained conscious during the accident.

N.S. King and his colleagues (1999) reported more success, finding that length of PTA (24 hr maximum), and 7–10 day postinjury measures of life-event problems, emotional distress, processing speed, and mental status were predictive of postconcussion symptom complaints at three months and at six months. However, predictive strength was attenuated after six months: PTA ceased to be predictive but the early measures of life-event problems and emotional distress still correlated—at a lower level—with postconcussion symptom complaints. In the large-scale study by the Thornhill group (2000), the factors predictive of death or disability in mild TBI (defined as GCS 13–15) were age over 40, preexisting physical limitations, and a history of brain illness; yet 35% of the mild TBI subjects without these predisposing factors continued to have moderate to severe disability. In fact, age has probably been the one variable most consistently associated with persisting postconcussion symptoms (Ogden and Wolfe, 1998; see also p. 301). These studies provide further evidence for the generally accepted conclusion that the presence or endurance of postconcussion symptoms as measured by our usual techniques is not clearly related to the early severity measures for mild TBI (presence and duration of LOC, GCS, duration of PTA) (Mateer and D'Arcy, 2000).

The postconcussion syndrome: what is it? Explanations other than severity of the injury have been offered to account for persisting problems and complaints in mild TBI patients. They include residual deficits in brain functioning, psychogenic disorders having their origins in the patients' premorbid personality and attitudes, inclinations—whether or not fully conscious—toward monetary or secondary gains which show up in the neuropsychological examination as poor motivation to perform well; reactions to the cognitive and somatic changes that accompanied the neuropathologic insult, and hypersensitivity to minor alterations in mental efficiency or to somatic problems such as mild headaches or occasional dizziness (Coolidge, Mull, et al., 1998; Gasquoine, 1997b; Malec, 1999; J.T.L. Richardson, 2000). M.P. Alexander (1995) suggests that patients with continuing symptoms were more likely to be under stress at the time of the accident, and that a depressive reaction can maintain or worsen the symptoms. "Functional outcome following mild TBI is determined by the complex interaction of neurological, physical, and psychological factors, the injured individual's premorbid personality and coping style, environmental demands and expectations, and support from others" (Ponsford, Willmott, et al., 2000, p. 577; see also Nemeth, 1996, who illustrates Ponsford's point with case data).

Genetic studies have opened up a new area of investigation. The $\epsilon 4$ allele of the *ApoE* (apolipoprotein E) gene, which has been identified as a risk factor in Alzheimer's disease (see p. 208), also appears to contribute to damage severity in TBI (G.M. Teasdale,

Nicoll, et al., 1997). A six-month outcome study found that although 10 (33%) of the patients with the ε4 allele had a GCS of 13 to 15 (i.e., in the mild TBI range), only one of all the 30 patients with the ε4 allele had a "favorable outcome."

Some workers have implicated premorbid personality or psychiatric disorders as significant contributors to development of the chronic postconcussion syndrome (L.M. Binder, 1997; P.S. Klonoff and Lamb, 1998; Larrabee, 1999; Mayou et al., 1993; see the review by J.T.E. Richardson, 2000). Cohadon and his colleagues (2002) report that of their 27% of mild and moderately injured patients with postconcussional complaints at six months, 68% had histories of antecedant psychosocial problems. Others have not found such relationships between premorbid emotional or personality disturbances and symptom chronicity (Ponsford, 1995; Ponsford, Willmott, et al., 2000; Raskin, Mateer, and Tweeten, 1998). Explanations that are essentially injury-based point out that the cognitive deficits incurred in mild TBI—for the most part due to reduced information processing capacity—are in themselves stress-producing while also putting a strain on cognitive and coping resources and thus creating the potential for continuation, and in some cases, exacerbation of the early postconcussional symptoms (Machulda et al., 1998; J.T.E. Richardson, 2000).

Further complicating efforts to understand the complexities of chronic postconcussional syndromes in individual cases is the role played by hopes for compensation—or reprisal—for injury through the legal system. This has become an issue particularly in the United States, but is also a consideration in other countries which provide monetary relief based on validating complaints of injury (see Cohadon et al., 2002, pp. 345–348). Reports vary greatly on the extent to which expectations for injury compensation contribute to the witting or unwitting exaggeration or persistence of postconcussional symptoms in mildly injured trauma patients (Gasquoine, 1997a,b; J.S. Hayes et al., 1999; Larrabee, 1999). Some workers have reported that the compensation-seeking patients they have studied present more or more enduring symptoms than do patients with similar accident histories and thus conclude that motivation for financial gain is a significant factor for many persons complaining of postconcussional symptoms. However, others have not found noteworthy differences between these groups (Ponsford, Willmott, et al., 2000; Stuss, Ely, et al., 1985). All studies have shown that many—if not most—compensation-seeking patients present symptom patterns similar to those of patients not seeking compensation (J.E. Meyers, Galinsky, and Volbrecht, 1999; Ruff, Wylie, and Tennant, 1993). Moreover, Murrey (2000b) reminds us that

"persons in litigation may actually have a severe cognitive or emotional impairment as a result of the injury which has resulted in their seeking compensation for such injuries" (p. 12).

Whiplash. Debate continues about the validity of complaints after a motor vehicle accident involving rapid acceleration (e.g., halted or slow-moving car rear-ended with force) or rapid deceleration (e.g., sudden stop due to braking or running into an obstacle) but no direct impact (Ferrari, 2001; G.K. Henry, Gross, and Furst, 2001). However, *whiplash injury,* in which the head receives no blow and there may not have been LOC, has been implicated in numerous studies (see, e.g., Bigler, 2001a; G.K. Henry, Gross, et al., 2000; Varney and Varney, 1995; Yarnell and Rossie, 1988). Radanov and Dvorak (1996) documented cognitive deficits in early posttrauma patients whose whiplash injury involved the cervical spine but speculated that pain may be a contributing factor. Kessels, Aleman, and colleagues (2000) performed a meta-analysis of 22 studies comprising a total of 656 "symptomatic" patients examined from a few days to five years after the accident. Compared with healthy controls, the whiplash victims who had symptoms for more than a year were significantly impaired on tests of attention, immediate recall, delayed recall, visuomotor tracking, and cognitive flexibility ($p \leq$ .001), and working memory deficits also appeared ($p \leq$ .05). Abnormal saccadic eye movements have been demonstrated in whiplash cases with persistent cognitive complaints (Furman and Cass, 2003; Mosimann et al., 2000; see also Bigler, 2001a). Comparisons involving persons who were symptomatic in the days following the whiplash injury and those who had also sustained whiplash injuries but did not report symptoms after their accident showed significant differences between test performances on working memory, attention, and visuomotor tracking ($p \leq$ .01) but these two groups did not differ on the recall tests or on cognitive flexibility.

Moreover, six months after the accident, cognitive—primarily attentional—deficits continued to characterize test performances of those patients who had attentional deficits in the first days after the injury (Di Stefano and Radanov, 1996). A two-year follow-up of whiplash patients' psychological status found no differences between those who still complained of pain and those who did not, although the pain patients described themselves as lower on "well-being" and higher on a "nervousness" scale (Radanov, Begré, et al., 1996). This group concluded that "psychological problems are rather a consequence than a cause of somatic symptoms in whiplash."

Explanations for these findings rest on the nature of the mechanical forces generated in rapid impact situations. Under pressure of these forces, hyperextension with possible reactive hyperextension of the head and neck result (Varney and Varney, 1995) along with "induced translational and rotational accelerations" of the brainstem and brain (Liu, 1999). These effects will be muted or aggravated by the angle at which the head and neck are bent—whether front, side, or back, by the flexibility of the neck, by the rigidity of the head rest, by the force itself which can be calculated from the vehicle's speed (Varney and Roberts, 1999b), and by the vulnerability of cervical structures to hyperextension (Froman, 1996). Most residual symptom patterns are similar to those for mild TBI occurring under conditions of rapid acceleration/deceleration and with direct impact to the head. They involve the same kinds of cognitive deficits, somatic complaints, and emotional disturbances as in mild TBI with impact (Kessels, Aleman, et al., 2000). Moreover, as in mild TBI with impact, neurological studies including MRI or CT scanning are most often negative (G.K. Henry, Gross, et al., 2000; Yarnell and Rossie, 1988). However, Henry and his colleagues documented abnormal findings in 11 (of 32) patients who had EEG studies, and one of their patients showed signs of probable brainstem injury; two (of 20 patients) in Yarnell and Rossie's (1988) series had MRI abnormalities, but only three (of 23) showed slowing on EEG.

Posttraumatic stress disorder (PTSD) in mild TBI. As PTSD has been considered to be a more or less severe anxiety reaction to a traumatic event, the relevance of this diagnosis in mild TBI has been questioned on the basis that one cannot have such a reaction with LOC, RA, or PTA in which the patient has amnesia for the traumatic event (Sbordone and Liter, 1995). Pennington (2002) notes that the definition of PTSD requires an "initial exposure to an extreme traumatic stressor" with "reexperiencing" symptoms, a definition that requires some conscious awareness of the event. It follows that patients who cannot remember the event are much less likely to exhibit symptoms of PTSD (Bryant and Harvey, 1995; Warden et al., 1997). Since many mild TBI patients have some recall of the event itself or of circumstances surrounding the event, this would seem to account for reports of PTSD in these patients and general agreement that PTSD and mild TBI do coexist. However, the extent to which PTSD affects mild TBI patients remains an issue with incidence reports varying from one mild TBI patient out of 2,000 (Bontke, 1996), to two satisfying both mild TBI and PTSD criteria out of a series of 312 TBI cases (McMillan, 1996b), to 26% (Bryant and Harvey, 1995) and as many as 33% (moderate and mild TBI combined) (Ohry et al., 1996). Boake (1996a), in a review of study

frequencies of 7% and 11% in mild TBI patients reporting a symptom of PTSD, was surprised to find these percentages so low since many mild TBI patients have at least partial recall of the traumatic event. Findings that rates of PTSD tend to be inverse to TBI severity are consistent and make sense since frequency and density of event amnesia increase with TBI severity (Rattock, 1996; Warden et al., 1997). Moreover, M. Bowman (1997) provides "good evidence of high levels of comorbidity of PTSD with other acute mental disorders, long-standing personality disorders, and substance abuse" in persons presenting PTSD symptoms after exposure to a presumably traumatic event.

Diagnosis of PTSD in mild TBI patients typically relies on patient reports of intrusive memories of the traumatic event and fear and helplessness avoidance responses (Bryant and Harvey, 1999a,b). Ohry and his colleagues (1996), using a standardized inventory to identify patients with PTSD, required the endorsement of a minimum of one intrusion symptom, three avoidance symptoms, and two symptoms of hyperarousal. This diagnosis becomes complicated by the number of symptoms that are identical for PTSD and the chronic postconcussion syndrome. These overlap symptoms include noise sensitivity, fatigue, anxiety, insomnia, poor concentration, poor memory, irritability/anger, and depression (Hickling et al., 1998; N.S. King, 1997; McGrath, 1997). Thus it is not surprising to find that mild TBI patients diagnosed as having PTSD may display more prominent postconcussive symptoms (e.g., problems with concentration, dizziness, fatigue, headaches, and visual disturbances) (Bryant and Harvey, 1999b). Hovland and Raskin (2000) suggest that PTSD can exacerbate cognitive symptoms in mild TBI. In a review of eight studies of PTSD patients with no history of neuropsychological disorder, M.D. Horner and Hamner (2002) noted that a pattern of attention and/or immediate memory impairments emerged, with two studies finding neuroimaging alterations consistent with both emotional complaints and the cognitive data. However, such PTSD-related cognitive effects in TBI patients have been questioned (Hickling et al., 1998; see also M. Bowman, 1997).

Cognitive deficits in mild TBI

During the early stages following mild TBI many patients exhibit moderate to severe communication, perceptual, or conceptual disturbances that, for most patients, ultimately clear up but for others remain as subtle defects that are not always apparent to casual observers (Lezak, 1992; R.S. Parker, 2001; J.T.E. Richardson, 2000; M.T. Sarno, 1980). The uniqueness of each patient's condition was demonstrated in a study of mild and moderate TBI patients that made evident the considerable interindividual variability in kinds of cognitive deficits which grouped data obscures (F.C. Goldstein, Levin, Goldman, et al., 2001). These authors wisely point out that—for mild to moderate injuries—a "patient who was impaired in executive functioning was not necessarily impaired in other areas." This finding of individualized deficit patterns holds true for every other kind of residual cognitive deficit in mild TBI patients. However, by virtue of the nature of many TBIs occuring under conditions of rapid acceleration or deceleration, some cognitive disorders are much more widespread than others.

Attentional deficits. These are the most common of cognitive deficits in mild TBI patients. Slowed reaction times in the acute stage give evidence of slowed mental processing (Hugenholtz et al., 1988; MacFlynn et al., 1984; van Zomeren and Brouwer, 1994). Slowed processing shows up more generally in attentional deficits, including poor concentration, heightened distractibility, difficulty doing more than one thing at a time, and complaints of impaired "short-term memory" (Sohlberg and Mateer, 2001; Spikman, van Zomeren, and Deelman, 1996; Stuss, Ely, et al., 1985; R.L. Wood, 1990). When attentional problems are severe the patient may complain of confusion, inability to think clearly, and disorientation; the latter problem is likely to be compounded by tendencies to underestimate time intervals (C.A. Meyers and Levin, 1992). Most lay persons confuse defective acquisition and recall of new information with "short-term memory." The common complaint of a "memory problem" in mild brain injury is usually the product of attentional (reduced span and distractibility) and verbal retrieval deficits (Howieson and Lezak, 2002; Kay, 1986). Most persons who have had mild head injuries do not have residual learning problems (Dikmen, McLean, and Temkin, 1986; Iverson et al., 2000; Kessels, Aleman, et al., 2000; Ogden and Wolfe, 1998; Ponsford, Willmott, et al., 2000), although exceptions appear in every mild TBI group study.

Verbal retrieval problems. It is not surprising that sluggish verbal retrieval is closely associated with slowed speed of information processing (Bryan and Luszcz, 1996; D.C. Park et al., 1996). After the acute symptoms have subsided, most TBI patients, even some who have sustained severe injuries, tend to show remarkably little deficit on verbal tests that measure overlearned material or behaviors such as culturally common information and reading, writing, and speech (when the damage does not directly involve the language centers). Yet many still have some difficulty recalling words (particularly names of objects, places, persons) readily (Goodglass, 1980; Murdoch, 1990). Verbal retrieval problems (*dysnomia*) show up as slow recall of the desired name, occasional paraphasias (e.g., "shoehorse" for "horseshoe," "wahchi . . . " self-corrected to "walking"), or misnamings, usually giving a semantically related response (e.g., "dice" for "dominoes"). Although verbal retrieval problems are not infrequently misinterpreted as some form of memory or learning disorder (e.g., see J.T.E. Richardson and Snape, 1984; Howieson and Lezak, 2002), they can be readily distinguished using cueing or recognition techniques that enable patients to demonstrate knowledge of the word or name they cannot recall spontaneously.

A 66-year-old lunchroom manager with an eighth grade education sustained significant bodily injuries in a roll-over accident, but her GCS never dropped below 14. Eight months later she was still complaining bitterly of "memory problems" as she felt she had lost her early memories. However, on direct questioning, she told how her schooling began in a two-room schoolhouse but finished in a one-room one; she described her marriage at age 17 by the local preacher and named the city in which she and her first husband had their honeymoon weekend—where they went to the movies. She knew how many siblings she had, where she was in the lineup, and who were her nieces and nephews. She could not give the preacher's name and was distressed that she was unable to recall her nieces' and nephews' names. She also had clear recall of recent trips, the nature and consequences of her mother's recent illness, where she had been living since the accident, and health issues that have developed since the accident.

On testing with the *Memory Assessment Battery*, free recall of stories was *defective*, but on cueing she demonstrated *normal* retention; recall of a word list after six trials was *within normal limits*, it dropped to *defective* after a delay, but when cued she again showed a *normal* retention level. On the *Boston Naming Test* she retrieved 14 words correctly only after phonetic cueing. These findings were consistent with an adequate autobiographic memory lacking only people's names in a woman with a significant verbal retrieval problem.

Sensory/perceptual and motor disorders. Sensory and perceptual problems are frequently reported following mild TBI, particularly in the acute and postacute stages. Thus, symptom reports typically include diplopia, photophobia, dizziness, and—at a low frequency—deafness (T.L. Bennett and Raymond, 1997a; Gasquoine, 1997b; J.D. Miller and Jones, 1990; Sohlberg and Mateer, 1990) and/or tinnitus (Axelsson, 1995; Coles, 1995). Some patients (44%) complained of discomfort in bright light but, on testing, even more displayed a lowered threshold for luminance tolerance (Gronwall, 1991). Headache is a common feature in the acute and postacute stages and may persist after other symptoms have dissipated (Coonley-Hoganson et al., 1984; Ponsford, 1995). It can take the form of most any chronic headache disorder (Speed, 1989). Headaches that do not dissipate with the other acute symptoms require medical attention (Wrightson and Gronwall, 1999). Motor slowing, which will show up on cognitive testing, is probably the most usual change in motor functioning after mild TBI, but some patients may also report coordination problems (Wrightson and Gronwall, 1999).

Common noncognitive sequelae of mild TBI

Emotional distress and fatigue. Many mild TBI patients experience dysphoric emotional alterations in which fatigue may be the chief culprit (Gronwall, 1989; Ponsford, Willmott, et al., 2000; Wrightson and Gronwall, 1999), with both exquisitely acute awareness of deficits and compromised mental efficiency running close seconds to fatigue (Coolidge, Mull et al., 1998; Lezak, 1988d; P.L. Wang and Goltz, 1991). With the slowed processing resulting from many microscopic sites of damage diffusely distributed throughout cerebral white matter and the upper brainstem, activities that were automatic now may be accomplished only with deliberate effort (Stuss, Stethem, Hugenholtz, et al., 1989).

A 53-year-old shopkeeper was only briefly unconscious but quite confused for several days after her car, which had been going about 60 mph (100 kph), spun out of control and into an embankment. Six weeks later she complained of fatigue so severe it allowed her to be active for only two to three hours at a time before she had to stop to rest. Among the many subtle changes she was experiencing was awareness that she no longer could get in or out of her car without thinking about what she had to do and directing each movement consciously.

Activities that are normally automatic but become effortful after the injury, particularly during the first weeks or months, include many that are performed frequently throughout a normal day, such as concentrating, warding off distractions, reading for meaning, doing mental calculations, monitoring ongoing performances, planning the day's activities, attending to two conversations at once, or conversing with background noise, etc. It is little wonder that by late afternoon, if not by noon, many of these patients are exhausted. Making matters worse, as they become fatigued, their efficiency plummets to even lower levels so that activities that were difficult when they were most rested and competent become extremely labored and even more error-prone; e.g., they become more distractible, make more mistakes when speaking, become more clumsy, etc. Further compounding their burdens

is heightened irritability (Gasquoine, 1997a; Machulda et al., 1998; Ponsford, 1995). This is an experience which everyone who has been ill or had surgery should recognize: when one's energy is depleted, patience and frustration tolerance drop and irritability emerges in their stead. Fatigue does not improve anyone's disposition and severe fatigue can make the mildest person scratchy and short-tempered (Boll and Barth, 1983). Galbraith (1985) wisely pointed out that the frustrating experience of mental inefficiency may well contribute to irritability following mild injury. He also noted that it could result from direct damage to the limbic system although no site has been identified.

Abnormal tiredness probably has a more direct effect on a patient's life than any other factor, partly because in itself it limits performance and partly because it increases the effect of the other symptoms, creating a vicious cycle. (Wrightson and Gronwall, 1999, p. 43)

Depression and anxiety. These are common features of mild TBI (T.L. Bennett and Raymond, 1997a; Gasquoine, 1997b; Ponsford, 1995; J.M. Silver et al., 2003). The disorientations and frustrations of headaches, dizziness, abnormal fatigue, and significant changes in mental efficiency experienced in the early days after an accident are likely to engender anxiety in the bewildered and uncomfortable patient (Hovland and Raskin, 2000). When the early symptoms persist, the patient becomes more prone to depression (Cicerone, and Fraser, 1999; Wrightson and Gronwall, 1999). Estimates of depression prevalence range around 35% (Busch and Alpern, 1998). The extent to which depression in mild TBI is reactive to lingering cognitive and somatic disorders, as may be suspected in patients whose depression onset was six or more months after the injury (Fordyce et al., 1983; Varney, Martzke, and Roberts, 1987), and the extent to which it has a neurogenic origin (Busch and Alpern, 1998; Prigatano, 1987; R.J. Roberts, 1999) remain unclear. Contributions from each source probably vary from case to case (M. Rosenthal, Christensen, and Ross, 1998). Premorbid "psychological or social problems" were implicated in one series of patients with continuing emotional disorders (Mayou et al., 1993). However, while depression severity may be associated with functional disability, its contribution to cognitive impairments in mild TBI patients has not been demonstrated (Raskin and Stein, 2000).

Fatigue, anxiety, irritability, and sleep disturbances—symptoms of the postconcussional syndrome—tend to further complicate depression in these patients (Busch and Alpern, 1998; McAllister and Flashman, 1999). Reduced libido is not uncommon following mild TBI (J.D. Miller and Jones, 1990; Wrightson and Gronwall,

1999; Zasler, 1993). Some patients fear they may be going crazy.

Unless specifically forewarned that these problems might occur and that they are natural consequences of an accident that may seem to have been an inconsequential event, patients experiencing the typical postconcussion symptoms, including fatigue and irritability, may become anxious, lose self-confidence, and be bewildered by the puzzling and unpleasant changes in themselves (Conboy et al., 1986; Wittenberg et al., 1996; Wrightson and Gronwall, 1999). Those whose problems with mental inefficiency are relatively severe and enduring are more likely to become distressed. Yet these patients may develop useful compensatory techniques such as working very slowly and double checking themselves to ensure correctness, concerns and traits akin to those of obsessive-compulsive persons (Lezak, 1991; McKeon et al., 1984). Of course, personality predispositions can affect how the patient deals with these symptoms and may contribute to some patients' disablement (Kwentus et al., 1985; Ponsford, Willmott, et al., 2000; Prigatano, 1987; Rutherford et al., 1979).

Moderate traumatic brain injury

Few studies have specifically addressed those levels of damage that are neither mild nor severe, although 8% to 10% of all TBIs fall into this category (Berrol, 1989; Kraus, McArthur, et al., 1996), with one review giving a range of 7% to 28% (S.C. Stein, 1996). The commonly accepted criteria for moderate head trauma are given in Table 7.1, p. 160 (see also Chapter 18, Table 18.3, p. 719). The issue of which GCS score (or combination of GCS scores) is used as a basis for the definition or what clinical events should or should not be present has been raised as well (S.C. Stein, 1996). Some workers include a GCS of 8 or exclude a GCS of 10 for this classification (see Berrol, 1989); some include 13 (S.C. Stein and Ross, 1992). Others only include patients whose GCS never falls below 9 (D.H. Williams et al., 1990) or who have focal deficits, intracranial lesions, or depressed skull fracture with a dural tear (H.S. Levin, Goldstein, High et al., 1988). Although the nature and duration of symptoms vary widely within this group, almost all in one large study continued to suffer significant disturbances at three months postinjury, including the 38% making a "good recovery" on the Glasgow Outcome Scale (Rimel et al., 1982). Headaches, memory problems, and difficulties with everyday living were the most common complaints; and two-thirds of those previously working had not returned to their jobs.

Of course, it is the patient's residual condition that ultimately matters. Here the Glasgow Outcome Scale provides a useful definition of moderate TBI: these are patients who can and, for the most part do, function independently. Many return to work; homemakers resume their usual responsibilities. Yet they tend to differ from intact persons and from what they were in that most exhibit behavioral traces of localized frontal and/or temporal bruising. Frontal damage can be suspected in those who have lost some spontaneity or some initiating capacity; are more impulsive or subject to temper outbursts than before; or whose affective or empathic capacity is muted. Temporal lobe damage makes its appearance as a true learning disorder that often reflects some lateralization of the damage in that the problems may predominantly involve verbal or visual (i.e., nonverbalizable) material; less frequently, as *temporal lobe epilepsy* (*TLE*); or, rarely, in altered affective and drive states associable to damage to limbic structures within the temporal lobes. Most of these patients will have sustained more than one kind of dysfunction; for example, diminished initiative is usually accompanied by affective flattening; a mildly impulsive person may also have a frank learning problem. Planning ability and automatic self-monitoring are also frequently compromised to some extent, not enough to render these patients unemployable but just enough to keep them from being able to rise to supervisory or managerial positions, regardless of their level of skills and cognitive abilities.

Frontal lobe problems, in particular, tend to show up in subtle ways in the moderately impaired person who nonetheless lives independently, works steadily, and maintains family relationships. Patients with diminished initiative and spontaneity typically return to their usual occupations and conduct their routine affairs without difficulty, but they no longer plan for nonroutine activities, including most leisure time activities such as going to a movie, organizing a picnic or a fishing trip, etc. Affective muting often shows up in diminished drives: foods are no longer relished, and sexual activity, while still pleasurable, loses both urgency and importance, so much so in some instances that previously active persons may still respond to another's advances, but it no longer occurs to them to initiate intercourse (R.S. Parker, 2001).

A railroad brakeman in his mid-thirties sustained several hours of LOC after being thrown back on his head when the caboose in which he stood came to an unexpected and abrupt halt. Prior to the injury he had been a devoted family man and churchgoer, spending every Saturday taking his school-age daughters to fairs, movies, shopping malls, etc.; Sundays he ushered at church. His wife described him as having been an affectionate husband and eager sex partner. Two years after the accident he continued in the same job and for all practical purposes was fully competent. Now, however, he spent all his free time at home playing a video game—always the same one, his wife reported. He had ceased interacting with his daughters, dropped all church activities, and was only occasionally responsive when his wife sought intercourse. Affect was dulled but he was not depressed, although a naive examiner could easily interpret his behavior as due to depression. In fact, affectively he was not much of anything—just there.

Severe TBI

I'm alone
I just can't seem to break out
Locked in this cage
Inside my heart I feel full of doubt

I can't seem to free myself
Like I'm stuck in a hole
I'm alone
Can anybody help[1]

Even decades after the injury, severe TBI continues to have significant effects on cognitive, emotional, psychosocial, vocational, and family functioning, as well as independence in living (Hoofien, Gilboa, et al., 2001). Although fewer than 10% of TBI victims are severely injured, this group presents a major and growing social problem because their rehabilitation needs are so great and so costly, because so few return to fully independent living, and because their disabilities create severe financial and emotional burdens for their families (Bigler, 1990a, *passim;* Cohadon et al., 2002; Lezak, 1989; Machamer, Temkin, and Dikmen, 2002; N.V. Marsh, Kersel, et al., 2002). These disabilities tend to be interdependent, may result from a variety of impairments, and are interactive and cumulative in their effects. For example, an instance of poor judgment may have cognitive components, but both impulsivity and loss of appreciation for social context may also contribute. Personality alterations are common; they may be the product of cognitive, emotional, and executive impairments and affect functioning in many domains.

Cognitive and motor defects. This population displays the full range of severity of dysfunction in every aspect of cognition. Excepting the very severely damaged who are most likely to have suffered disruption of cognitive functions generally, each patient's impairment pattern will have at least some unique characteristics as certain functions continue at premorbid or near premorbid levels while others have been more or less

severely affected (D.N. Brooks and Aughton, 1979; Crosson, Greene, et al., 1990; Millis, Rosenthal, Novack, et al., 2001; Newcombe, 1982).

While not universal, *attentional deficits* are very common, particularly among those whose injuries occurred under conditions of rapid deceleration, as in traffic or railroad accidents (Brouwer, Ponds et al., 1989; Stuss, Stethem, Hugenholtz, et al., 1989; van Zomeren and Brouwer, 1990). Distractions can have considerable impact on the ability to work independently and the disruptive effect does not wane quickly (Whyte, Schuster, Polansky, et al., 2000). When severe, attentional deficits can be exceedingly disruptive as these patients can be too distractible or too unable to maintain directed or focused attention that they cannot benefit from retraining (R.L. Wood, 1990). Behavioral slowing, both of mental processing and of response, is characteristic of these patients. Deficits in focused and divided attention may result from slowed information processing but not all attentional deficits can be attributed to this slowness (Bate et al., 2001; Spikman, van Zomeren, and Deelman, 1996). Simple and choice reaction time are commonly impaired with TBI. As the complexity of the task increases or the modality of stimulus presentation is uncertain, the preparatory interval lengthens (Zahn and Mirsky, 1999). Motor complexity (in terms of number of separate movements needed to draw stimuli), however, did not appear to affect response speed while stimulus novelty (letters, familiar and unfamiliar figures) did slow it in these patients, a finding interpreted as implicating slowed information processing (Tromp and Mulder, 1991). Slowed information processing can be a factor in poor executive functioning, but individualizing the pace of presentation of information for each patient can significantly improve processing accuracy (Madigan, DeLuca, Diamond, et al., 2000).

Memory impairments usually consist of problems in the acquisition and retrieval of information; short-term memory is less likely to be affected (Bennett-Levy, 1984b; D.N. Brooks, Hosie, et al., 1986; Lezak, 1979; Zec, Zellers, et al., 2001). Recall tends to be confounded by difficulty discriminating between intrusions, whether purely associative or of similar material presented during the same examination as the target material (Crosson, Novack, et al., 1989; Paniak, Shore, and Rourke, 1989). Spatial learning and memory deficits (Skelton et al., 2000; Shum, Harris, and O'Gorman, 2000) may interfere with way-finding difficulties in everyday life. It is not unusual for recall of verbal or visual information to be impaired with relatively intact recognition (Spikman, Berg, and Deelman, 1995), but recognition memory may be impaired also (Hannay, Levin, and Grossman, 1979). Difficulties in

---

[1]Poem written by a 19-year-old who had been injured at age 5 and was referred for a neuropsychological examination after arrest for a drunken escapade directed by a 16-year-old casual acquaintance.

retrieval of familiar names and learning of new names are common complaints with severe TBI, and impairments are noted on formal testing (Milders, 1998). However, recognition of familiar names is likely to be intact (Milders et al., 1999).

Working memory deficits are often present when these patients attempt two tasks at the same time (S. McDowell et al., 1997; N.W. Park et al., 1999), a task that involves two or more operations at the same time, especially when speeded (e.g., the Paced Auditory Serial Addition Test), or to guide a sequence of actions (Bublak et al., 2000). This is particularly important when TBI patients return to driving, which involves considerable time pressure in carrying out different series of actions as well as making split second decisions (Brouwer, Withaar, et al., 2002). In the extreme case, memory disorders may condemn the patient to awareness of only what is immediately given. Psychomotor skill learning (procedural learning), however, may be preserved despite significant impairment of semantic and event memory (Timmerman and Brouwer, 1999). Not surprisingly, alcoholics—particularly those drunk at the time of injury—are likely to have greater memory impairments than persons with similar injuries but no alcoholic history (N. Brooks, Symington, et al., 1989).

Deficits associated with frontal lobe injury are often the most handicapping as they interfere with the ability to use knowledge and skills fluently, appropriately, or adaptively. When injuries are predominantly frontal, the patient may perform well on time-limited, highly structured examination tasks but still be unable to function independently. One important problem that can occur with both frontal and right cerebral injury is diminished awareness or appreciation of one's deficits (C.C. Allen and Ruff, 1990; Prigatano, 1991b). Without awareness of what has been lost or of the mistakes they make, patients are neither motivated for retraining nor can they monitor their performances properly. The performance of these patients may be significantly compromised, yet they can appear quite untroubled by this, can "talk a good game", and may even continue to announce intentions to return to work, fly airplanes, or enter a profession despite the most obvious cognitive or motor deficits. Moreover, problems in emotional control and social interaction are most likely to be underestimated (Prigatano, Altman, and O'Brien, 1990). Severely damaged patients are also more likely to display reasoning and verbal fluency impairments (D.N. Brooks, Hosie, et al., 1986; D.W. Ellis and Zahn, 1985).

A classic *aphasia* syndrome is relatively rare except with appropriately focal lesions (Sohlberg and Mateer, 1990). It is present in perhaps 2% of surviving severe TBI acute care admissions (Hannay, personal communication, June 26, 2003) with much higher rates, of course, in rehabilitation settings (Gil et al., 1996; Sarno, 1980; Sarno, Buonaguro, and Levita, 1986) and with great variability in their discourse profiles (Hartley and Jensen, 1992; Linscott et al., 1996). Word finding (verbal retrieval) is another common problem, as are misnaming and auditory comprehension (Levin, 1991; Murdoch, 1990). Communication may be compromised due to a lack of logical content and cohesiveness, a lack of clarity, insensitivity to the other's needs and interests, insensitivity to the amount of explanation necessary for another to comprehend the information given, too much or too little information, confabulation and inconsistencies, and impaired *pragmatics* (knowledge and activities of socially appropriate communication) which could include inappropriate cultural and moral content (Linscott, et al., 1996; Sohlberg and Mateer, 1990). Impaired pragmatics also takes in much of the nonverbal aspects of communication, such as gestures, loudness of speech, etc. Conversational discourse may not improve noticeably over time (P. Snow et al., 1998).

A tendency for a *breakdown in linguistic competence* has been associated with severity of damage, supporting observations that trauma patients "talk better than they communicate, while the reverse holds for patients with left hemisphere CVA aphasia" (Wiig et al., 1988). Conversations with TBI patients tend not to be as rewarding, to be more effortful, and to be less appropriate and less interesting (F. Bond and Godfrey, 1997). R.C. Marshall (1989) pointed out how the effects of such cognitive and executive disorders as confusion, disorientation, distractibility, disinhibition, and concrete and rigid thinking can disturb the communication process.

Visuospatial, visuoperceptual, and constructional deficits trouble some of these patients (D.W. Ellis and Zahn, 1985; Newcombe, 1982); but as often as not, the severely damaged patient will have little or no difficulty in one or more of these areas, which may account for the relative paucity of data on these specific dysfunctions. Unfortunately, much of the data on tests involving these functions are imbedded in IQ or other summed scores so that the information is lost to the reader. Of course, such tests in the WIS-A batteries are also timed, introducing the possible effect of reduced information processing speed in these patients (Hoofien, Gilboa, et al., 2001).

Basic motor functions such as primitive reflexes, equilibrium/protective reactions, muscle tone, range of motion, abnormal and voluntary movements, and motor skills involved in sitting, kneeling, standing, and walking may be impaired in the early stages (Swaine and Sullivan, 1996). The profile of motor problems varies across individuals, but significant changes are typically seen in the first few weeks after the injury. Other motor disturbances may be present, perhaps for many years, including decreased manual speed and dexterity, increased reaction time on simple as well as complex reaction time tasks, ataxia, tremors, hemiparesis, hemiplegia, decreased range of motion, spasticity, and contractures (C. Gray et al., 1998; Haaland, Temkin et al., 1994; Hoofien, Gilboa, et al., 2001; Keren et al., 2001). Treatments such as rehabilitation, orthotics, biofeedback, hydrotherapy, hippotherapy (therapeutic horseback riding), medication, nerve blocks, and surgery may be needed at various times to improve motor function.

Executive dysfunction. The most crippling and often the most intractable disorders associated with severe TBI involve capacities for self-determination, self-direction, and self-control and regulation which depend on intact awareness of one's self and surroundings (Crosson, Barco, et al., 1989; Lezak, 1988b; Stuss, 1991b). Self-awareness has important social ramifications: when it is compromised, so are insight and empathy. Reasonably accurate self-awareness is a precondition to accepting the need for rehabilitation and thereby cooperating with it (Ben-Yishay and Diller, 1993; Kay and Silver, 1989; Prigatano, 1991b). It is also a major factor in return to work (Sherer et al., 1998). Making inappropriate, impulsive, unrealistic decisions is common among these patients.

One young man remembered that a business associate of his father's had once said (slapping him on his shoulder) that anytime he wanted a job just to come and see him. Several years later, after his accident, he remembered this comment, found transport several hundred miles to another city, and appeared on the doorstep of this man, saying that he was there for a job. Since the family did not recognize him and he was insistent, somewhat incoherent, and could not properly identify himself, they called the police who checked with regional trauma units and returned him to the original acute care facility. From there he was released to his family.

Executive functions also include aspects of cognition that are not cognitive abilities in themselves but rather concern whether or how they will be expressed (Burgess and Wood, 1990). Thus, the memory disorders of many severely impaired TBI patients will seem more severe than they actually are because the patient may possess the needed information but will not think to use it unless externally prodded or cued (Stuss and Gow, 1992). Self-correcting may follow the same pattern: the patient knows there is an error but does nothing to correct it (Walsh, 1991). Awareness of errors (which must precede their correction) in completing everyday tasks is

lower and affected even more when there is a planning and working memory load (T. Hart et al., 1998). These patients have difficulty dealing with simultaneous competing sources of information in figuring out a sequence of actions, perhaps from processing resource limitations (Cazalis et al., 2001). Automatic, unintended action errors that we all make from time to time (e.g., peeling vegetables and throwing away the vegetables not the peels) occur more frequently in these patients as a result of lapses in sustained attention (I.H. Robertson, Manly, et al., 1997). Severe TBI patients may spontaneously say correctly that the principle on a reasoning task has changed, say how it has changed, but be unable to switch to the new principle, perseverating on the old one in the responses that follow. Perseveration in a response or thought is common. Inflexibility, whether it appears as frank perseveration or as impaired behavioral or conceptual shifting in response to instructions or changing circumstances, can compromise cognitive and social functioning alike (H.S. Levin, Goldstein, et al., 1991).

Often what is needed to perform is available or within these patients' capacity but it does not occur to them to use what is there or to anticipate future needs (Crosson, Barco, et al., 1989). Thus abilities to plan and to recognize and choose alternatives may be impaired. Apathy and disinhibition are discussed below as aspects of emotionality, but from this perspective they become symptoms of dysfunctional ability to control and direct behavior (Truelle, 1987; Walsh, 1991). Apathy has been shown to correlate with reduced executive function, acquisition and memory, psychomotor speed (Andersson and Bergedalen, 2002), and active goal-oriented coping (Finset and Andersson, 2000).

Persons in whom these capacities are compromised cease to be in adequate control of themselves or their destinies: the greater the defect, the more socially dependent and socially dysfunctional they become. It is this order of dysfunction that accounts for the poor outcomes of so many severely damaged patients; why they cannot get or hold jobs, care for their families, or begin new ones; why physically healthy young men stay where they are put, whether it is a rehabilitation center, their family's home, or a street corner; why others get into continual difficulty because of sexual urges clumsily asserted or seemingly senseless aggression (Cohadon et al., 2002; Ponsford, 1995; Varney and Menefee, 1993; R.L. Wood, 1984).

Emotional and psychiatric disorders

Many different kinds of emotional alterations take place as a result of TBI. In severely damaged patients these alterations are predominantly organically based, although reactive disturbances or compensatory changes in attitudes and affective response can have important effects, and premorbid predisposition, too, may enter into this complex equation of why they behave as they do (M.R. Bond, 1984; Lezak, 1989; Prigatano, 1987, 1992; Hibbard, Bogdany, et al., 2000; M. Rosenthal, Christensen, and Ross, 1998).

The emotional changes generally involve either exaggeration or muting of affective experience and response (Prigatano, 1987; J.M. Silver et al., 2002). Both the excitable—affectively florid, impulsive, labile, acting out—and apathetic—emotionally flat, disinterested, noninitiating—patterns of behavioral and emotional alterations have their organic bases primarily in damage to the frontal lobes or underlying structures. Damage to temporal limbic structures will also affect emotionality. Behavioral disturbances associated with temporolimbic lesions may be more episodic, with temper outbursts or sudden alterations of mood that are usually dysphoric in nature. In some patients, both disorders can be seen when a usually emotionally dulled and disinterested patient flares up in rage at some seemingly minor provocation. Interestingly, the focus in reporting about these problems is more frequently on aggressive, acting-out patients rather than on those who are hyporesponsive, although the latter can be as much if not more socially dysfunctional than the former.

Depression and anxiety are particularly common regardless of the severity of injury (Busch and Alpern, 1998; Jorge et al., 1993; M. Rosenthal, Christensen, and Ross, 1998). Anxiety and depression, which trouble many moderately to severely injured patients—particularly after the acute stages—may increase in intensity with time for some (Prigatano, 1992; J.M. Silver et al., 2002; Varney, Martzke, and Roberts, 1987). Hibbard, Uysal, and coworkers (1998) found that major depression was more likely to remit than anxiety. Generalized anxiety disorder for several weeks combined with depression appears to be associated with prolonged depression (Jorge et al., 1993). That anxiety and depression are frequently reactive to patients' appreciation of their physical and cognitive disabilities and social limitations is suggested in a study reporting an inverse relationship between insight into behavioral impairment—which tended to be poorest among patients first examined six months after injury—and emotional distress—which generally worsened with time (Godfrey, Partridge, et al., 1993). This does not rule out the possibility that at least some dysphoric emotional reactions are symptoms of organic alterations in brain functioning (M. Rosenthal, Christensen, and Ross, 1998; Jean-Bay, 2000). Other emotional and psychiatric problems are more common in these patients than in the population at large, such as mania (Shukla et al., 1987), paranoia (Prigatano, 1987), and a schizophrenic-like syndrome that develops after head trauma and is characterized by negative symptoms such as flattened affect, suspiciousness, and social withdrawal rather than the delusions and hallucinations that are the positive symptoms of schizophrenia (M.R. Bond, 1984; J.M. Silver et al., 2002; Zhang and Sachdev, 2003).

Increased rates of personality disorders, including borderline, avoidant, paranoid, obsessive-compulsive, and narcissistic types, have been reported (Hibbard, Bogdany, et al., 2000; Van Reekum et al., 1996). PTSD continues to be a disputed concomitant of TBI, but some evidence suggests that PTSD can occur across the range of injury severity (Feinstein, Hershkop, et al., 2002; Warden et al., 1997). Disinhibited or "impulsive" aggressive behavior with TBI probably results from a loss of frontal inhibition of subcortical limbic structures; verbal confrontations are reported more than actual physical assaults (Grafman, Schwab et al., 1996). Such individuals are more likely to have a history of premorbid aggressive behavior, to be younger, and generally more impulsive, irritable, and antisocial (Greve et al., 2001). Most likely, the relative contributions of psychogenic reactions and organic dysfunction differ among patients and may differ for individual patients at different times.

Social isolation is a common consequence of these emotional alterations, although often not because these head trauma patients generally desire it but rather because they have become boring, difficult, sometimes frankly unpleasant to be with, or because apathy or their cognitive deficiencies keep them from socializing effectively if at all (Fordyce et al., 1983; Lezak and O'Brien, 1990; N.V. Marsh and Knight, 1991). Of course, friends, family, and coworkers frequently do not understand why these patients are no longer "fun to be with" but have become another burden in their lives and withdraw from them. Severe TBI patients may have less opportunity for establishing new contacts and friends after an injury that further isolates them as time goes on (Morton and Wehman, 1995).

Social isolation of the person with TBI is a major determinant of caregiver burden (N.V. Marsh, Kersel, et al., 2002). It is not unusual for adolescent patients with awareness of their situation to comment on the dismal aspects of their future life, perhaps on the fact that they will never go to their prom (high school graduation party), never date or marry and have children, or never work. This is heartbreaking for families, especially parents, just as it is with many other disorders and diseases that are contracted early in life. Parents are not always able to care for a severely injured family member at home and nursing home placement may be the only alternative. This is particularly difficult for the family when a young person with many years of life ahead is involved and nursing home placement may mean further isolation from individuals of their own age. In some cultures TBI may be viewed as a form of madness and the family as well as the patient feel a sense of shame, may not reveal the facts of the injury to others, and withdraw from their social network (Simpson et al., 2000). In our experience, family members are more likely to find the physical deficits acceptable to discuss and deal with than the emotional-personality problems.

Course. Severely injured patients may display a pattern of acute confusional behavior shortly after return to consciousness that can last for days or, rarely, for more than several weeks. The confusional state is typically characterized by motor restlessness, agitation, incomprehension and incoherence, and uncooperativeness, including resistive and even assaultive behavior (Brooke et al., 1992; Eames et al., 1990; Fugate et al., 1997). Reyes and his coworkers (1981) found that agitated or restless behavior on admission to postacute care predicted better outcomes than sluggishness or immobility.

In the next weeks to months both physical status including basic motor functions (Swaine and Sullivan, 1996) and many aspects of cognition improve, some quite rapidly. The more severe the injury, the more pervasive the deficits present one year after the injury (Dikmen, Machamer, Winn, and Temkin, 1995). Perhaps the most frequently impaired cognitive domain with severe TBI is memory and learning (H.S. Levin, 1995; R.L. Tate, Fenelon, et al., 1991) although deficits in information processing speed and executive functions are also very common. Activities, such as new learning which involves the memory system, tend to improve over a longer period of time (K. O'Brien and Lezak, 1981; Vigoroux et al., 1971) but still do not reach normal levels (Paniak, Shore, and Rourke, 1989), even six years after the injury (H.S. Levin, 1995). Those deficits having to do with retrieval rather than registration and learning either are apt to improve as specific verbal or visuospatial functions return to make stored information and response patterns available again. If due to sluggishness in retrieval activity, they may show only minimal improvement and that fairly soon after return of consciousness when the deficits result from extensive frontal or subcortical damage. Activities that have a large attentional component, such as immediate span, tend to improve quickly and reach a plateau within the first six months to a year after injury (Gronwall and Sampson, 1974; Lezak, 1978b).

After the first year improvement may continue but it more likely will come gradually and as a function of new learning and development of compensatory strategies rather than spontaneously as occurs in the first

three to six months or so. For example, a series of severely injured patients showed essentially no change in cognitive functions from year 2 to year 7 (N. Brooks, McKinlay, Symington, et al., 1987). In the course of three examinations taking place over 15 years, aphasic disturbances diminished considerably, concentration problems somewhat, and memory improved very little in 40 severely injured patients (Thomsen, 1984). While the same patients tended to be less childish, a small increase in irritability and restlessness was noted, and there were larger increases in fatigability, "lack of interests," and "sensitivity distress." N. Brooks (1988) did not find any changes in the nature of patient problems as reported by family members from the first to the fifth posttraumatic year. Other than improved physical status, no significant changes were noted from year 1 to year 3 in another group of severely injured patients; and again, no changes appeared from years 3 to 5, although an overall improvement trend in emotional and psychosocial functioning was documented for the entire time span (S.P. Kaplan, 1993).

Despite general agreement in the past that spontaneous improvement levels off no later than some time within the second year after injury, improvements may continue for some individuals many years after the injury (Millis, Rosenthal et al., 2001; Sbordone, Liter, and Pettler-Jennings, 1995). Evidence for test scores that fluctuate both up and down after the first year suggest that more than simple improvement occurs (Kay et al., 1986; Lezak, 1979; Millis et al., 2001). Kay and his coworkers found that these fluctuations are most usual in patients with impaired executive functions and that, rather than reflecting some underlying change in brain function, they merely represent a lack of internal stability and self-regulation. Millis et al. (2001) reported that 22.1% of their patients improved, 15.2% declined, and 62.2% were unchanged. Improvements in verbal fluency, cognitive speed and attention, and problem solving were seen in over 10%, while similar rates of decline were found in cognitive speed and attention, problem solving, and motor coordination in patients whose functioning had declined.

Self-report of severe TBI patients two years after their injury indicates that difficulties continue to plague these individuals in most aspects of daily living to various degrees (Ponsford, Olver, and Curran, 1995). For instance, 40% were still not at their previous level of mobility and 41% still tired more easily. Headaches (36%), dizziness (26%), and visual difficulties (48%) were present also. Most were independent in basic activities of daily living (ADLs) such as feeding (93%), dressing (87%), and personal hygiene (88%) with or without cues to do so; but 30%–40% still could not do light or heavy domestic chores. Full-time employment was only 30% as opposed to 61% preinjury. Only 10% were involved in all previous leisure activities and interests. Sixty percent lived with their family and 61% had never married. Similarly low rates of employment 2–5 years postinjury have been reported (Asikainen et al., 1996). In a study by Masson and colleagues (1996), 58% with severe TBI were working after 5 years. Subjective complaints of memory problems (67%), fatigue (58%), dizziness (26%), pain (48%), depressive temper (41%), anxiety (63%), and irritability (63%) were present. About 25%–50% had problems with washing, dressing, walking, using transport, driving, writing a letter, and dealing with paperwork. Only 41% had made a good recovery, while 15% still had a severe disability. Although the percentage of various difficulties differs somewhat across studies depending on the demographics of the sample (e.g., severity of injury within group, age, and education), it can be said that severe TBI is associated with continuing difficulties in all areas of life for many patients years after the injury.

Thus, in the very long term both good and bad outcomes have been reported for severe TBI patients, although the most usual finding over the years is of no change in cognitive status with persistent complaints of problems—cognitive, school/work, medical, and emotional heading the list—and some continuing social and personality deterioration (N. Brooks, Campsie, et al., 1986; Karol, 1989; Millis, Rosenthal, et al., 2001; Thomsen, 1984, 1989). Gaultieri and Cox (1991) reported significantly increased rates of late-occurring depression and psychotic disorders in addition to a greater likelihood (four to five times that of the general population) of these patients developing dementia. The possibility of further deterioration has been suggested both by findings of delayed neurological deterioration in a small number of children who had mild head injuries (Snoek et al., 1984) and by the identification of prior TBI as a risk factor for Alzheimer's disease (Friedman et al., 1999; Jellinger, Paulus, et al., 2001; G.M. Teasdale, Nicoll, et al., 1997). Age appears to be a major factor in subsequent cognitive decline, the risk being 4.97 times more for each 10 years of age at time of injury (Millis et al., 2001).

Social dysfunction as outcome. The neuropsychological deficits borne by survivors of severe head trauma lead almost inevitably to difficulties in every area of social activity and to the problems encountered by family members, particularly those responsible for their care. Most prominent among areas of concern, and most important for social independence, are work and family.

Severe TBI patients may never return to previous employment levels although some do; others may work at less demanding (and less well paying) jobs than held before injury or in supported or sheltered employment (N. Brooks, McKinley, Symington, et al., 1987; Lezak and O'Brien, 1990; Ponsford, Olver, and Curran, 1995; R.L. Tate, Lulham, et al., 1989). Age at injury seems to be related to employment outcome, those with a severe injury in childhood and early teens (as opposed to late adolescence and early adulthood) having poorer eventual vocational outcome (Asikainen et al., 1996). (Of course, the earlier TBI occurs, the more likely it is to interfere with the normal unfolding of processes developmentally and thus to have greater impact on the cognitive and psychosocial processes.) The problems presented by these patients, and reported by the guidance and rehabilitation people working with them, reflect the full gamut of cognitive, emotional, and executive disorders; but by far the greatest obstacles to vocational reintegration are of an executive nature, i.e., problems of initiating, planning, organizing thoughts and work, self-control, flexibility of thought and response, etc. Attentional and memory problems, impaired reasoning and judgment also contribute to these patients' vocational failures (N. Brooks, McKinlay, Symington, et al., 1987). Appropriate rehabilitation training can increase the employability of a significant number of moderately to severely injured patients (Ben-Yishay, Silver, et al., 1987; Cohadon et al., 2002).

Studies of family adjustment have come to focus on the burden these patients create for their family members (Camplair, Butler, and Lezak, 2003; Florian, Katz, and Labav, 1989; N.V. Marsh, Kersel, et al., 2002). Characteristics most likely to distress family members, reflecting emotional disturbances, are aggression, increased temper and irritability, social withdrawal, and emotional coldness (N. Brooks, 1988; N.V. Marsh et al., 1998, 2002). Other problem behaviors include childishness, emotional lability, and unreasonableness—all qualities that can create tensions, dissension, and stress within the family (Camplair, Kreutzer, and Doherty, 1990; L.C. Peters et al., 1990; Thomsen, 1990). As well as these problems, physical impairments add to family burden at one year after injury (N. Brooks, 1988; Marsh, et al., 1998); but at five years after injury the patients' dependency was experienced as the chief burden on their families (N. Brooks, 1988). Moreover, families with a TBI person tend to become increasingly socially isolated, which can only exacerbate tensions and dissatisfactions (Florian, Katz, and Labav, 1989), and caregiver depression is fairly common (Camplair, Butler, and Lezak, 2003; J.K. Harris et al., 2001).

Physical, cognitive, emotional, and hormonal changes combine to produce sexual difficulties that affect patients and their partners (Crowe and Ponsford, 1999). Loss of libido and hyposexuality occur frequently compared to disinhibition and hypersexuality

(Crowe and Ponsford, 1999; Zasler, 1993). It is possible that cognitive problems interfere with imagery induced sexual arousal independent of the effects of depression (Crowe and Ponsford, 1999; D. Smith and Over, 1987). The issue of sexual relations within a marriage covers a variety of problems, chiefly for spouses whose partners can no longer give or share satisfaction because of altered drives, loss of empathy and patience, clumsiness, tactlessness, or childishness (Camplair, Kreutzer, and Doherty, 1990; Florian, Katz, and Labav, 1989; Zasler, 1993). The most common complaint of male patients and their partners is reduced frequency of sexual relations (Kreuter et al., 1998; R. O'Carroll et al., 1991). Both infrequency of sexual contacts and sexual dissatisfaction were positively related to time since injury—but not to age of patient (R. O'Carroll et al., 1991). Guides for family members and others address many of these problems and more (E.R. Griffith and Lemberg, 1993; Gronwall, Wrightson, and Waddell, 1990). Discussion of sexual changes and problems, a thorough evaluation, and a treatment program that involves, for instance, medical intervention, counseling, behavior modification, or education should be part of any TBI rehabilitation program (Elliott and Biever, 1996; Kreuter et al., 1998; Quintard et al., 2002).

People working with severe TBI patients are consistent in reporting low levels of social interaction with consequent boredom and dissatisfaction (Godfrey, Marsh, and Partridge, 1987; Lezak, 1987b; N.V. Marsh, Knight, and Godfrey, 1990), despite adequate physical mobility and even satisfactory driving behavior (Brouwer, van Zomeren, and van Wolffelaar, 1990). In short, severe TBI significantly reduces the quality of the lives of patients and the people close to them (P.S. Klonoff, Costa, and Snow, 1986; E.A. Peck and Warren, 1989; O'Neill et al., 1998; Steadman-Pare et al., 2001). Yet the emotional status and employment potential of patients who have sustained severe damage bear some relationship to their families' stability and the amount of social support they receive (S.P. Kaplan, 1990, 1991; Sander, Caroselli, et al., 2002; Sander, Sherer, et al., 2003). Of variables relevant within a rehabilitation program for moderately to severely injured patients, appreciation and acceptance of their deficits, emotional and behavioral competence, cognitive functioning, sociability ("involvement with others") and, of course, injury severity are the best predictors of employment success (Cattelani et al., 2002; Ezrachi et al., 1991).

Neuropsychological Assessment of Traumatically Brain Injured Patients

Intensive neuropsychological examinations are not usually undertaken in the acute and postacute stages of TBI since the patient may be in a coma, out of a coma but minimally responsive, delirious, disoriented, unable to understand task instructions, or able to complete only relatively simple tests. Those who assess patients in an intensive care unit and follow them for months and years afterward are likely to stagger the introduction of tests that are predictive of outcome such as the Glasgow Coma Scale, the Glasgow Outcome Scale, the Disability Rating Scale, tests of orientation and PTA, and simple cognitive tests in order to follow improvement and deterioration in the early stages for clinical and research purposes (see Chapter 18, pp. 719–727; Hannay, 2003a,b). For planning rehabilitation of moderately and severely injured patients, neuropsychological assessments are usually introduced once the patient is out of PTA or at specific time points such as three and six months postinjury. Mild TBI patients who are not admitted to hospital usually can participate in an evaluation within days after the injury when required by circumstances (e.g., a high school student wanting to return to school) or for research purposes. However, these ambulatory patients fully capable of self-care may benefit more from early counseling with testing delayed until most of their acute symptoms have stabilized or receded. Patients with a complicated mild TBI (mild TBI plus abnormalities on CT scan) or moderate TBI may be hospitalized in acute care for a week on average (Hannay, 2003a,b; McGarry et al., 2002) and may not be well enough to undergo an extensive evaluation for a while afterward. Severe TBI patients may be hospitalized in acute and postacute care for weeks to months, and some are unable to assist in a complete neuropsychological assessment even at three months postinjury (Hannay, 2003a,b).

Testability has been shown to be predictive of outcome (Boake, Millis, High, et al., 2001; Dikmen, Temkin, Machamer, et al., 1994). Some neuropsychologists use test completion codes that are assigned to each test given to a TBI patient (or indeed to patients with any disorder).

An example of such codes is given in Table 7.3 (Hannay, 2003a,b). This is a code system used for patients admitted to an intensive care unit. Along with reliability codes and impairment codes, these codes can provide a clearer picture of why a patient was not given a test, why a test was not completed, how "good" was the information obtained with the test, and what problems interfered with test performance (e.g., hearing loss interfering with language test performance). Codes such as this can be used for interpreting test findings, writing reports, and analyzing research data since codes come in both written and numeric forms. Codes can be designed for specific clinical situations.

Pastorek et al. (2004) found that test completion codes for relatively simple tests of language compre-

TABLE 7.3 Test Completion Codes

1. Test fully completed

Test not completed because:

2. Patient has acute confusional state, is unable to follow motor commands, or is unable to arouse. This applies to any situation where the test is not fully administered due to arousal problems that are not the result of specific medical complications of traumatic brain injury.

3. Patient has medical complications that make him or her currently untestable (e.g., high fever, respiratory problems, vomiting, etc.).

4. Patient could not complete test because of endotracheal intubation or tracheostomy.

5. Patient refused to complete all or part of a test or was not responsive (not due to 1 or 2).

6. Patient was cooperative and attempted to take test, but testing or part of testing was terminated due to the patient's cognitive, motor, or other limitations not listed elsewhere (e.g., aphasia so does not understand instructions, blindness so only auditory tests given, right-hand paralysis so only left-hand testing completed, understands instructions and completes practice trials but cannot do test).

7. Patient is unable to complete test due to illiteracy.

8. Patient is unable to understand instructions not due to acute confusional state, aphasia, or illiteracy.

9. Test is not applicable at that time (e.g., patient not following commands so cannot administer the GOAT, patient still in the hospital so the CHART is not appropriate to administer).

10. Patient is not available (e.g., in scheduled therapy or medical intervention, no transportation).

11. Examiner is not available (e.g., ill, schedule conflicts).

12. Patient does not give consent.

13. Unknown

GOAT, Galveston Orientation and Amnesia Test; CHART, Craig Handicap Assessment and Reporting Technique.

hension and attention given at one month postinjury were better predictors of outcome at three and six months postinjury than Galveston Orientation and Amnesia Test (GOAT) scores and test scores themselves. It is possible that the results of some studies of TBI patients underestimate their cognitive problems, especially studies of moderate and severe TBI in the first six months postinjury and even later, since untestable patients often are not mentioned or included in the summary data.

As the patient enters acute and postacute rehabilitation, many of the same tests may be administered along with more detailed assessment of functional status. Reintegration into the community leads to further evaluation of disabilities, environmental facilitators, and barriers. In postacute stages, the performance of TBI patients usually improves and eventually levels off, the time taken to do so being quite variable. Then the information from an extensive neuropsychological examination and predictions of the probable long-term neuropsychological status become reasonably reliable. Evaluation of disabilities, environmental facilitators, and barriers at this time and thereafter is particularly useful for clinical and forensic purposes.

Unless direct damage to the left hemisphere has been sustained, most TBI patients have little or no difficulty with verbal tests, excepting subclinical aphasia problems with word naming, language comprehension, and word fluency (Hinchliffe et al., 1998; H.S. Levin, Gary, Eisenberg, et al., 1990; Sarno, Buonaguro, and Levita, 1986). However, about 2% or fewer of surviving severe TBI patients have a residual aphasic disorder (Sarno, et al., 1986), as has been our experience with consecutive admissions to acute care (hjh). TBI patients may also do well on tests that elicit responses primarily mediated by the posterior areas of the cortex, which are less likely to be damaged except when under the point of impact. The latter include tests of constructional abilities and perceptual accuracy that are uncomplicated by memory, organization, or speed requirements. Some memory problems are usually present, but severity varies greatly among patients. These problems tend to be exacerbated by patients' difficulty in identifying what may be relevant among a number of information bits so that their recall is reduced not only by quantity but also by usefulness (Vakil, Arbell, et al., 1992).

Most of the tests used for both general cognitive assessment and examination of brain dysfunction measure abilities likely to withstand TBI. When injuries are very severe, it may be necessary to use tests developed for children in order to elucidate remaining abilities. Unless examination techniques are geared to eliciting impairments that are common to head trauma victims, these often seriously handicapping deficits may not become evident (Lezak, 1989; Newcombe, 1987; Sohlberg and Mateer, 2001; Walsh, 1991). Moreover, many patients can perform on a conventional psychological examination or one of the prepackaged neuropsychological test batteries. Long after the acute stages have passed, many moderately and even severely injured adults may achieve score patterns on Wechsler and Halstead-Reitan batteries that are at least in the *average* ability range (e.g., Dikmen, Machamer, et al., 1990). Yet many of these patients continue to suffer frontal apathy, memory deficits, severely slowed thinking processes, or a mental tracking disability that makes them unable to resume working or, in some instances, to assume any social responsibility at all. Insufficient or inappropriate behavioral examinations of TBI can lead to unjust social and legal decisions concerning employability and competency, can invalidate rehabilitation planning efforts, and can confuse patient and family, not infrequently adding financial distress to their already considerable stress and despair (Nemeth, 1991; Varney and Shepherd, 1991).

In this vein, it should be noted that most patients seeking compensation for their injuries do not present more symptoms or deficits on testing than similar patients who do not have compensation claims (Rimel, Giordani, Barth, et al., 1981; Stuss, Ely, et al., 1985; Suhr, Tranel, et al., 1997), although the opposite has been reported (Paniak, Reynolds, Toller-Lobe, et al., 2002). Claimants may tend to complain more than other patients (McKinlay, Brooks, and Bond, 1983). A negative kind of support for the conclusion that litigation or compensation has little effect on patient behavior was the finding that at three months posttrauma half of a group of mildly injured patients had not returned to work, yet none had compensation claims (R. Diamond et al., 1988). In fact, Shinedling et al. (1990) reported not only no test differences between suing and nonsuing patients but that both groups were deeply involved in denying their trauma-related deficits. Bornstein, Miller, and van Schoor (1988) failed to find any differences in emotional status between patients involved in compensation issues and those who were not, although litigating mild TBI patients have shown higher rates of anxiety, depression, and social dysfunction (Feinstein et al., 2001). Rutherford (1989) suggested that the stress of litigation could affect the duration of symptoms, noting that this would not be apparent at 6 weeks but would become evident some time later. Yet L.M. Binder (1986) noted that "the effect of compensation claims and preinjury pathology is often secondary to organic factors," pointing out that patients with enduring symptoms are the ones most likely to sue.

Moderator Variables Affecting Severity of Traumatic Brain Injury

Age

Advancing age is associated with progressively higher odds of an adverse outcome in terms of mortality and morbidity, especially after age 65 (Gomez et al., 2000; Francel and Jane, 1996; Rothweiler et al., 1998; Susman et al., 2002). These findings cannot be attributed to more severe injuries per se in elderly persons. Susman and coworkers (2002) suggest that intrinsic characteristics of the aging brain, not just the increasing incidence of complications such as hemorrhages, produce a worse outcome after head injury. For instance, changes with advancing age in intracranial compliance, vasoelastic properties, response to mechanical stress, vulnerability to excitotoxic damage, alterations in neurotransmitter metabolism, microvasculature, dendritic spines, and arborization and the blood–brain barrier

probably contribute to the greater morbidity and mortality of older TBI victims (Francel and Jane, 1996).

Throughout most of the adult years age appears to contribute to the severity of cognitive deficits as well (Naugle, 1990; F.C. Goldstein, Levin, Presley, et al., 1994; F.C. Goldstein, Levin, Goldman, et al., 2001). Naming, word fluency, verbal and visual memory, attention, and information processing speed appear to be particularly vulnerable (Finset et al., 1999; F.C. Goldstein et al., 1994, 2001); and elderly patients also experience significantly more depression and anxiety (F.C. Goldstein et al., 2001). Of course, the appropriateness of control groups in such studies is always an issue and can affect the findings (Aharon-Peretz et al., 1997).

The relationship between age and two important predictors of severity—coma duration and PTA—is complex: Gronwall and Wrightson (1974) demonstrated that following concussion more older than younger persons exhibit slowed processing and persistent memory deficits. TBI in elderly persons usually occurs in falls at home rather than in MVAs with resultant higher rates of intracranial hematomas, subarachnoid hemorrhage, epidural and subdural hematomas with increased incidence of elevated ICP, and higher rates of mortality (Francel and Jane, 1996). Pre-existing medical conditions also contribute to the problems (P.T. Munro et al., 2002). Thus the relationship between age and severity of injury is not entirely clear (Kraus, McArthur, et al., 1996). Findings are conflicting with respect to better or worse outcome from mild head injury in the elderly (Kilaru et al., 1996; Rapoport and Feinstein, 2001; Rothweiler et al., 1998; Susman, et al., 2002). Within the narrower category of severe TBI, age seems to make no additional contribution to the severity of cognitive and behavioral deficits (M.B. Glenn et al., 2001; B.A. Wilson, Vizor, and Bryant, 1991). On the contrary, among a group of severely injured patients, outcomes 10 to 15 years later differentiated the younger (15 to 21) from the older (22 to 44) patients in that the younger ones had more behavioral and emotional problems (Thomsen, 1989, 1990). Cost of rehabilitation is higher for older people as it is associated with longer hospital stays and slower rates of functional change (Cifu et al., 1996).

Repeated traumatic brain injuries

Repeated TBIs tend to have a cumulative effect on cognition as a second, even mild, concussion leaves the victim somewhat more compromised than if this had been the sole injury (Gronwall, 1989, 1991; Gronwall and Wrightson, 1975). Moreover, a single traumatic injury to the brain doubles the risk for a future head injury, and two such injuries raises the risk eightfold (Gaultieri and Cox, 1991). Sports injuries, especially from contact sports, have been, unfortunately, a rich source of information about the effects of repeated TBIs and thus can serve as models for the neuropsychological problems associated with repeated head injuries (Boden et al., 1998; Drew and Templer, 1992; Erlanger et al., 1999; Macciocchi et al., 1996; Matser, Kessels, Lezak, et al., 1999).

Data regarding athletes from 114 U.S. high schools during the 1995–1997 academic years show the relative vulnerability to TBIs of participants in high (e.g., football, wrestling, soccer) and low (e.g., baseball, volleyball) contact sports, with the six most serious cases and 598 concussions reported for football (J.W. Powell and Barber-Foss, 1999). In the three academic years from 1997 to 2000, for male college athletes, the concussion rate was highest for football and higher in games than in practice sessions (e.g., 1999–2000 season: games rate = 4.15, practice rate = 0.34) (Covassin et al., 2003). Concussion rates for women athletes were somewhat lower, soccer producing the most concussions in games (e.g., 1999–2000 season games rate = 2.21) with considerably fewer practice injuries. It is interesting to note that football players who had one concussion during a season were at a three times greater risk of having another injury during that season than nonconcussed players (Guskiewicz et al., 2000). The approximately 300,000 sports injuries a year in the United States (Echemendia, Lovell, and Barth, 2003) amount to 18% to 20% of all TBIs (Echemendia and Julian, 2001; McKeever and Schatz, 2003). Impact measurements for hockey, football, and soccer found the highest peak acceleration occurred when heading the ball in soccer (54.7g), with football and hockey peak accelerations trailing at 29.2g and 35g, respectively (Naunheim et al., 2000). In evaluating sports data, the reader must be aware that, for any number of reasons, many athletes underreport injuries (McCrory and Berkovic, 1998) or are unaware that they had a concussion (J.S. Delaney et al., 2001).

Most sports-related injuries—even repeated ones—fall into the category of mild TBI. Young players (age range 14 to 22) examined immediately after receiving a possible concussion showed mild effects in slightly lower scores on the *Standardized Assessment of Concussion (SAC)* (W.B. Barr and McCrea, 2001 [SAC in Appendix, p. 702]). Typically, young and healthy athletes improve rapidly with few if any noticeable cognitive changes within weeks if not days after the injury (J.T. Barth, Alves, et al., 1989). In one study conducted ten days after injury, a comparison between players with one and those with two mild concussions sustained during a college football season did not affect neuropsychological functioning (Macciocchi, Barth, et al., 2001). However, at least six months after their last concussion, youthful athletes (ages 14 to 19) performed as poorly on tests of attention and response speed as did players concussed within the preceding week (Moser and Schatz, 2002). Only attention test scores of young athletes (ages 14–19) who had sustained two or more concussions at least six months earlier showed deficits similar to those with acute concussions (i.e., within the prior week); athletes with a history of one old concussion or none did not display any cognitive deficits (Moser and Schatz, 2002).

Thus, most cognitive test performances of most athletes who have had few concussive injuries will be at or near normal levels, placing them at the "mild" end of what has been called a "dose-related" continuum of deficit. This was seen among professional soccer players as those receiving the lowest "doses" of concussions and *headers* (receiving and batting the ball with their heads) performed tests of cognitive functions at normal levels, with increases in severity of cognitive deficits paralleling increasing incidence of injuries (Matser, Kessels, Jordan, et al., 1998; Matser, Kessels, Lezak, et al., 1999). This dose-related phenomenon showed up in players in "high level" teams who had played within the week of testing, affecting aspects of attention and possibly concept formation (Webbe and Ochs, 2003). Witol and Webbe (2003) found that the current level of heading the ball was less predictive of cognitive impairments than was "lifetime" amount of heading. More soccer players who headed the most (estimated from report: ≥9 times in a game × yrs) had more abnormally low scores on the Complex Figure Test (33%), the Paced Auditory Serial Addition Test (PASAT, 20%), and Trail Making Test-A (14%) than did those whose lifetime heading was "low" (0–4 times in a game × yrs; 21%, 12%, 0%, respectively) (Witol and Webbe, 2003).

A few head injured athletes will suffer a long-lasting postconcussion syndrome, but these have typically sustained a more severe concussion or possibly have a genetic predisposition to trauma vulnerability (see discussions of ApoE4, pp. 173–174 and 208; B.D. Jordan, Relkin, et al., 1997; Erlanger et al., 1999).

Boxing has served as an obvious model for the effects of cumulative blows to the head in that the goal in boxing, of course, is to give one's opponent a sufficiently severe concussion as to render him unconscious (Drew and Templer, 1992; Oates, 1992). Even fighters with no history of having been "knocked out" suffer the effects of years of jabs to the head, as shown by the parkinson-like slowing and motor symptoms and the mental compromise of boxers such as Muhammad Ali (B.D. Jordan, 1987; R.G. Morrison, 1986). The most usual presentation of cumulative damage in boxers is the *punch drunk syndrome,* originally called *dementia pugilistica* but more recently termed *chronic progressive encephalopathy of boxers* (Filley, 1995; Hammerstad and Carter, 1995). Dementing conditions occur in approximately 20% of professional boxers (B.D. Jordan, 2000). This condition is characterized by motor symptoms including, most prominently, clumsiness and incoordination, and *intention tremor* (a chronic fine tremor exacerbated in goal-directed movements) (Lishman, 1997; Martland, 1928; R.G. Morrison, 1986). Impotence has been reported in some of these relatively young men (Boller and Frank, 1982; J. Johnson, 1969). Cognitive deficits in boxers are common, appearing most typically as attentional defects, memory impairment, disorientation, and confusion (Casson, Siegel, et al., 1984; Drew, Templer, Schuyler, et al., 1986; Kaste et al., 1982); and to this list Matser, Kessels, Lezak, and their coworkers (2000) added planning deficits. Neuroradiologic imaging has demonstrated cerebral atrophy in many professional boxers (Casson, Sham, et al., 1982; B.D. Jordan, 1987; B.D. Jordan and Zimmerman, 1990).

The possibility that significant brain damage can result from "well controlled" amateur boxing was questioned by N. Brooks, Kupshik, and their colleagues (1987) who reported none in a group of amateurs averaging five years of boxing. However, the control group's Vocabulary and Raven's Matrices scores were 14 and 24 points, respectively, below that of the boxers, raising doubt about the appropriateness of the group comparisons; and even with their higher ability scores, the boxers' story recall scores fell significantly below those of the control subjects. McLatchie and his coworkers (1987) observed that nine of 15 amateur boxers had some neuropsychological dysfunction; a neuropsychological examination proved to be more sensitive than EEG or CT at uncovering evidence of subtle brain damage. Matser, De Bijl, and Luijtelaar (1992) found a deficit gradient that paralleled the number of matches for 33 amateur boxers with visual recall (Complex Figure) and sustained attention (Trail Making Test-A), showing a significant decline for the 17 boxers who had engaged in more than 30 matches; but an overall pattern of decline was evident for all tests, without exception. Acute effects of boxing were demonstrated by assessments before and immediately after a match, as these 38 amateur boxers displayed pronounced alterations on tests of conceptual reasoning, motor speed, sustained attention, and both verbal and visual recall (Matser, Kessels, Lezak, et al., 2000). On SPECT scans, amateur boxers showed more aberrations in cerebral perfusion than their controls who also outperformed the boxers on tests of divided at-

tention and perceptual recognition; these boxers too showed a dose-related gradient as those who had been in the most matches did less well than those with fewer matches (Kemp et al., 1995). Clinicians working closely with athletes have identified the *second impact syndrome* (*SIS*), a somewhat rare event which is thought to occur when a second TBI is sustained before the physiological reactions to a prior injury have dissipated (Echemendia and Cantu, 2003; Echemendia and Julian, 2001; Erlanger et al., 1999; McRory and Berkovic, 1998). SIS is most likely to be seen in athletes engaged in contact sports as they, more likely than other athletes, tend to receive TBIs in relatively rapid succession. The hallmark of SIS is diffuse swelling of the brain, which may begin within hours of even a mild injury and results from compromised cerebral autoregulation. McRory and Berkovic noted that most reported cases have been of adolescents. Coaches and team physicians are now encouraged to be knowledgeable about the symptoms of concussion and to keep injured players out of the game until they are symptom free (J.T. Barth, Varney et al., 1999; Erlanger et al., 1999). Serial neuropsychological evaluations may provide the best data for determining when it is safe for a concussed player to return to play, although practice effects and player motivation can complicate the evaluation of examination findings (Echemendia and Julian, 2001).

Multiple injuries/polytrauma

Accidents causing head trauma frequently involve trauma to other systems and parts of the body that, in turn, tend to contribute to the severity of the neurobehavioral condition (Macartney-Filgate, 1990; R.S. Parker, 2001), and cognitive deficits contribute to the status of polytrauma patients (Fernandez et al., 2001). The mortality rate does not appear to be increased by polytrauma (Baltas et al., 1998). For example, femur fracture per se in patients with multiple injuries and a CHI does not appear to increase mortality or neurologic disability (Fernandez et al., 2001). However, severely head injured patients who also sustain multiple skeletal injuries are less likely to benefit from rehabilitation than those with only one or no such injury (G. Davidoff et al., 1985; Groswasser, Cohen, and Blankstein, 1990). When sensory disturbances occur in patients whose abilities to concentrate or perform mental operations are already compromised, they can greatly exacerbate the attentional difficulties, add to fatigue, and generally reduce mental functioning, performance efficiency, and capacity to undertake normal social and occupational activities (Sohlberg and Mateer, 1989; Wrightson and Gronwall, 1999). Polytrauma patients improve over time but generally do not return to preinjury levels. Outcome is influenced by age, severity of injury, and previous quality of life (U. Lehmann et al., 1997; Mata et al., 1996; Thiagarajan et al., 1994). Residual impairments and disabilities in ADLs, non-work activities, and work were noted in 80% of individuals with severe multiple trauma, cognitive impairment being related to vocational disability and physical impairment and pain being associated with nonwork disability after three years (Anke et al., 1997).

Preinjury alcohol abuse

It is not surprising to learn that TBI patients with prior histories of alcohol abuse tend to have poorer outcomes as measured by performances on neuropsychological tests (Dikmen, Donovan, et al., 1993). Return to productive activity is related to prior injury and alcohol use (A.K. Wagner et al., 2002). Alcohol appears to have a potentiating effect on head injury severity, neuropathological changes, event-related potentials, and outcome, even when degree of vehicle crush and demographics are taken into account (Baguley, Felmingham, et al., 1997; L.H. Barker, Bigler, Johnson, et al., 1999; R.M. Cunningham et al., 2002; M.P. Kelly, Johnson, et al., 1997; P.S. Tate et al., 1999). The relationship between a history of alcoholism, regardless of its severity, and neuropsychological status after one year is not a simple one: those patients performing least well on tests tend to be poorly educated men whose premorbid lifestyle is more likely to have put them at risk for head injury than are the lifestyles of women or well-educated men.

Uncommon Sources of Traumatic Brain Injury

Although most cases of TBI involve blows to the head or penetration of the skull by missiles or other objects, other sources of TBI include lightning, electrical accidents, and blast injuries. These latter may also have neuropsychological effects as a result of temporary paralysis of brain centers, with consequent cardiac or respiratory malfunction creating a transient hypoxic condition. Some of these accident victims sustain head injuries through falling or being knocked over (e.g., Lezak, 1984a). Other kinds of injury to the brain and associated tissue can also occur in blast or radiation injuries. For a detailed discussion of some less common forms of TBI, see Duff and McCaffrey (2001) and Panse (1970).

Electrical and lightning injuries

Contact with man-made electrical sources results in about 1000 deaths per year, while lightning strikes are associated with 75 to 150 deaths in the United States annually (M.A. Cooper, 1995; Duclos and Sanderson, 1990; Patten, 1992). Lightning causes more deaths in the United States than all other natural disasters but flash floods. Approximately two-thirds of electrical accidents occur at work; the rest happen in the home (Patten, 1992). The number of nonfatal injuries is perhaps five to ten times as high. It has been estimated that 4% to 10% of all admissions to burn hospitals are from electrical injuries (M.M. Brandt et al., 2002; M.A. Cooper, 1995; Tredget et al., 1999).

The effects of electric shock and lightning injuries vary greatly, in part due to the electrical source, points of entry, pathway through the body, as well as associated injuries and victim characteristics. It is thus necessary to have some understanding of the nature of electrical circuits. *Voltage* (potential difference between the inside and outside of a conductor, measured in volts), *amount of current* (movement of charged particles inside a conductor, expressed in amperes), *resistance* (opposition to current flow, measured in ohms), type of current (alternating or direct) as well as exposure duration and path through the body affect the severity of injury (M.A. Cooper, 1995; Rescorl, 1995). These relationships have yet to be clarified with systematic research (Duff and McCaffrey, 2001).

Electrical injuries are often divided into high voltage injuries (greater than 1000 volts) and low voltage injuries (less than 1000 volts), although the division is somewhat arbitrary (M.A. Cooper, 1984; R.C. Lee, 1997). High voltage injuries are usually likely to produce extensive burning and charring of tissues and may even require multiple limb amputation (M.A. Cooper, 1984). However, deaths can occur from low voltages because of "no let-go" mechanical attraction to the source for a long period (R.C. Lee, 1997, see below) while relatively little injury has resulted from some high voltage accidents (Cherington, 1995). M.A. Cooper's 1984 review of electrical injuries is comprehensive.

Household current (generally 1 to 10 milliamps [mA]) is relatively safe under most conditions, whereas higher amperages of 20 to 50 mA can produce respiratory arrest and 50 to 100 mA results in ventricular fibrillation (M.A. Cooper, 1984). Resistance varies with tissue type (Cwinn and Cantrill, 1985). Nerve cells carry electrical impulses and have the least resistance, followed by blood vessels, muscles, skin, tendons, fat, and bone. Electricity usually contacts the body via the skin, with thicker skin—and especially callouses—increasing resistance. Damp or wet skin is a better conductor of electrical current, and sweat can reduce skin resistance from 30,000 to 2500 ohms per cm. When contacting wet skin, even a low amperage household current can cause ventricular fibrillation and sometimes death. Moreover, clean skin has less resistance to current flow than dirty skin, and thin body cross-sections have less resistance than thick ones. For a particular voltage, the injury is therefore likely to be greater in a finger than an arm (M.A. Cooper, 1984).

Once the skin is compromised, current flows primarily internally along nerves, blood vessels, and muscles. Alternating current (AC) is substantially—perhaps three times—more dangerous than the same amperage of direct current (DC) (Bernstein, 1994; Fontanarosa, 1993). Direct current (DC) usually elicits a single, strong skeletal muscle flexion that may push the victim away from the electrical source. Low voltage (1 to 4 mA) AC, such as household current, produces an unpleasant tingling sensation. AC voltages as low as 5 to 20 mA may freeze movement due to repetitive muscle stimulation (*tetany*) such that the victim cannot let go of an object, resulting in dangerously prolonged exposure to internal current flow. Current termination, the sheer weight of the victim's body, or another person pulling the victim away from the current source can release the victim from this frozen state. Continued contact with the current can cause sustained apnea with hypoxemia and respiratory and/or cardiac arrest.

Lightning differs from man-made electrical sources in several ways (M.A. Cooper, 1983; S.R. Craig, 1986). Lightning may involve many millions to a billion volts and from a few to several hundred thousand amperes. Lightning is DC and tends to have a short duration of 1/1000 to 1/100 of a second with a contact temperature of 8,000°C to 30,000°C. In contrast, man-made high voltage sources are usually less than 70,000 volts, less than 1,000 amperes, AC or DC, and involve longer exposure durations.

Risk factors. The risk factors for electric shock and lightning injuries are behavioral, environmental, and geographic—often a combination of these factors in individual cases.

For *electrical injuries,* failure to adhere to electrical safety guidelines is the most common cause of shock. Both low voltage (e.g., contact with defective tools or appliances) and high voltage (e.g., contact with power lines) injuries occur on the job or at home (R.C. Lee, 1997; Mellen et al., 1992). Adolescent male risk-taking behavior, such as climbing utility poles or riding on train roofs, can result in high voltage injuries (Fontanarosa, 1993; Sternick et al., 2000). Children are most likely to put fingers or objects in outlets, to touch live wires, or to suffer electrical burns of the mouth from sucking or chewing on a live wire (Zubair and Besner, 1997), but adults too have such injuries (Shimoyama et al., 1999). High school educated men in their 20s and 30s sustain most (90%) on-the-job electrical injuries and deaths (R.C. Lee, 1997; Mellen et al., 1992).

Lightning can strike in a variety of ways (Cherington, 1995; Cwinn and Cantrill, 1985; M.A. Cooper, 1995). A *direct strike* by a lightning bolt is particularly serious. If the strike is near the head, current may enter by the orifices—ears, eyes nose, and mouth (B.E. Andrews, 1995). A *side flash*, sometimes called a *splash*, occurs when the direct pathway of current, perhaps through a tree, has a higher resistance than a person or another object nearby. It can cause serious injury or death, even to persons indoors, for instance, at a telephone or in the bathtub when a ground current travels along house pipes (B.E. Andrews and Darveniza, 1989). A *ground* or *stride* current occurs when lightning strikes and then travels along the ground to a person. If one foot is closer to the strike point, current may flow up one leg, through the body and out the other leg. M.A. Cooper (2002) describes a fifth mechanism: a *weak upward streamer,* an electric charge that surges up through any object projecting from the ground, induced when the tip of a branch of cloud-to-ground lightning gets within a few hundred meters of the ground. Lightning bolts can strike out of a clear sky (Cherington, Krider, et al., 1997), hence the term "bolt out of the blue." Preceding a storm, this lightning travels nearly horizontally from a lightning head that may be more than 10 km away. Additionally, blunt trauma may occur from the thermoacoustic blast that throws the victim (M.A. Cooper, 1984).

Geographic and climatic variations affect the rate of lightning strikes. For instance, the states of Florida and then Texas had the most lightning-related deaths over an 18-year period in the United States, but Wyoming, followed by New Mexico, Arkansas, Mississippi, and then Florida had the highest rates per capita (M.A. Cooper et al., 2001; Duclos and Sanderson, 1990). Moreover, some natural geographic features such as caves, fissures, faults, metallic ores, and natural radioactivity are likely to be associated with higher strike rates (Patten, 1992). Lightning strikes and related deaths peak in summer, especially the late afternoon (Duclos and Sanderson, 1990), when people are engaged in outdoor recreation or employment (Cherington, 1995, 2001). Lightning-associated deaths occur primarily among males (more than 5:1 male to female ratio), with median age being in the mid twenties (Duclos and Sanderson, 1990). The Lighting Safety Group of the American Meteorological Society's recommendations for reducing the likelihood of a lightning accident are online (http://www.uic.edu/labs/ lightninginjury). Myths about lightning are discussed by Cooper and her colleagues (2001).

Neuroanatomy and pathophysiology. Regardless of its source, the pathway of electrical current through the body is important in determining morbidity and mortality (M.A. Cooper, 1995; Fontanarosa, 1993; Patten, 1992). For instance, the central nervous system (CNS), heart, and internal organs are included in head-to-foot conduction, yet sudden death from ventricular fibrillation is more likely to occur from hand-to-hand, rather than hand-to-foot, current flow. Relatively small currents can have serious and even fatal effects. Alternatively, larger currents passing through the thumb and out other fingers of the hand might have little effect. Presumably, pathways involving the head should lead to higher rates of central nervous system disorders and neuropsychological deficits (Duff and McCaffrey, 2001); however, what pathway has been taken and what systems have been compromised are not always clear.

Central nervous system involvement is common with both electric shock and lightning injuries. It has been estimated that over 70% of all lightning victims have a brief loss of consciousness, and that over 80% have confusion with amnesia and brief periods of paresthesias and paresis (Cherington, Yarnell, and London, 1995; M.A. Cooper, 1980). Cherington and his colleagues (1995) report a wide range of neurologic complications from lightning injuries, such as intracranial and epidural hematomas, cerebral edema, hemorrhage, hemiparesis, infarct that may involve cortical and/or subcortical structures, myelopathy, and concussion. A number of symptoms and syndromes may result, some of which can be delayed in onset. These include hypoxic encephalopathy often from cardiac arrest, ataxia, progressive cerebellar syndrome, Parkinson's disease, polyneuropathy, bulbar palsy, Wilson's disease, spinal atrophy, extrapyramidal syndrome, sagittal sinus occlusion, and autonomic failure. Seizures may be present in the first few days or develop later (M.A. Cooper et al., 2001; Eldad et al., 1992).

A wide variety of neuropathologic findings have been described following electrical and lightning accidents (M. Critchley, 1934; G.S. Davidson and Deck, 1988; M.A. Cooper et al., 2001). Among them are focal petechial hemorrhages throughout the brain—especially in the medulla and the anterior horns of spinal cord gray matter; disintegration of cells in cerebellar structures and the anterior horn; as well as dilation of perivascular spaces, demyelination, coagulation necrosis of gray and white matter, and edema. With a direct hit to the cranium, the entire brain may become swollen and softened. Imaging can elucidate the neuropathology responsible for some symptoms. However, many individuals with cognitive deficits have normal CT/MRI scans (M.A. Cooper et al., 2001), an abnormal EEG being the more frequent finding (Barrash et al., 1996; Hooshmand et al., 1989; van Zomeren, ten Duis, et al., 1998).

Numerous small foci of hyperintensities in the supratentorial white matter, mainly in the immediate subcortical region were apparent on the MRI of a 46-year-old male who was not unconscious but thrown backward violently in a lightning storm (Milton et al., 1996). He had pain in the left arm and paresis in the left leg immediately that resolved while ataxia of gait resolved later and he continued to have mild cognitive difficulties involving abstract reasoning, attention, and concentration.

Cherington, Yarnell, and Hallmark (1993) described three lightning accidents. A spring skier suffered diffuse anoxic brain injury and never regained consciousness. An MRI two days postinjury revealed enlargement of gyri, effacement of sulci, and increased signal intensity in the basal ganglia and cortical gray matter. A mountain camper lost consciousness and complained of numbness and limb stiffness that resolved that day but had residual "red streaks" on his left arm, chest and neck, a perforated eardrum, and finger-to-nose incoordination. Atrophy of the superior cerebellum appeared on MRI. In contrast, a horseback rider also lost consciousness, had amnesia for the event, burns on her forehead, and an exit wound on her right leg with truncal and finger-to-nose ataxia but normal CT and MRI.

In the *peripheral nervous system* (*PNS*) both myelin sheaths and axons can suffer various injuries (M. Critchley, 1934). Mild tingling or numbness may be reported or even a complete loss of sensory or motor function may occur (Mankani et al., 1994). Sensory structures may be injured with findings of perforated eardrums, tinnitus, sensorineural hearing loss, vertigo, loss of vision, cataracts, and inflammation in eye structures (Hawkes and Thorpe, 1992; Ogren and Edmunds, 1995; van Zomeren, ten Duis, et al., 1998). Reports of *autonomic nervous system* symptoms include cardiovascular, temperature, bladder, and erectile dysfunctions (J.A. Cohen, 1995; Fontanarosa, 1993). These symptoms are usually immediate and transient but can be prolonged (Weeramanthri et al., 1991) or delayed (Eldad et al., 1992).

The disease process. Cherington (1995) suggested a four-category classification of the neurologic effects of lightning injury: (1) immediate and transient symptoms, such as loss of consciousness or retrograde amnesia; (2) immediate and prolonged or permanent problems, such as an infarct; (3) delayed sequelae, such as myelopathy or even an intracerebral glioma; and (4) secondary lesions, such as rupture of the tympanic membrane or TBI. This classification could be generalized to electrical injuries and to nonneurologic symptoms as well.

Delayed effects have been noted as long as a decade after the injury. Cherington (1995) suggested several possible explanations for delayed effects: a coincidence, a neurologic condition present from the beginning but not noticed because it was subtle and overshadowed by more pressing medical problems, preexisting but unnoticed symptoms, or structural changes occurring in proteins and other molecules, blood vessel walls, and cellular membranes that are not immediately evident (G.S. Davidson and Deck, 1988; R.C. Lee, 1997). The initiation of a degenerative process is also a possibility (R.C. Lee et al., 1993).

Diagnosis and prediction. Diagnosis of electric shock is generally straightforward as it is based on the history, physical surroundings at the time of the event, entrance and exit wounds, and burns. However, sometimes blunt trauma and falls with absence of burns, blast effects or falling debris, complicate the picture such that a TBI from mechanical forces must be considered (M.A. Cooper, 1984, 1995; Duff and McCaffrey, 2001; see p. 169). Lightning injury may occur when nobody is around, with no reported thunderstorm at the time, and no entrance and exit wounds, burns, or other pathognomonic skin lesions such as "feathering marks" (M.A. Cooper, 1984, 1995). In cases presenting with unconsciousness, paralysis, disorientation, and other cognitive deficits, alternative etiologies must be considered (M.A. Cooper, 1995; Cherington, Kurtzman, et al., 2001).

M.A. Cooper (1980) reported that 30% of lightning victims die and 74% have permanent disabilities. Mortality rates are high for victims with cardiopulmonary arrest (76%), cranial burns (37%), or leg burns (30%). Age, gender, trunk, and arm burns do not appear to contribute significantly to mortality (M.A. Cooper, 1980). Some victims die immediately, usually from arrhythmia (B. Bailey et al., 2001) while others linger for days, weeks, or months before dying of their injuries (e.g., G.S. Davidson and Deck, 1988).

Cognition. Despite many published case studies, research in this area suffers from a variety of problems. These include small sample sizes, little consideration of premorbid factors, incomplete assessments, unspecified test data, little longitudinal data, little or no data on injury severity in terms of electrical characteristics, few body pathway descriptions, treatment of electric shock and lightning strikes as the same condition when that may not be the case, and inappropriate control groups (Duff and McCaffrey, 2001; Primeau et al., 1995).

Some studies report cognitive deficits based on responses to an interview or checklist (A.R. Grossman et al., 1993; Pliskin, Capelli-Schellpfeffer, et al., 1998) but most others involve formal testing (see below). Impairments have been noted in domains indicative of diffuse effects, much like those in TBI (Barrash, Kealey, and Janus, 1996; Duff and McCaffrey, 2001; Primeau et al., 1995).

Mental status alterations are relatively common, particularly occurring as a period of confusion immediately following injury and return to consciousness. Disorientation seems to be reported infrequently (Duff and McCaffrey, 2001), yet it became evident when following a patient whose mental status was examined appropriately (using the GOAT) (Hopewell, 1983).

Sensorimotor status changes include pain, paresthesias and dysesthesias, motor weakness, and incoordination. These are common residual problems for both electric shock and lightning strike victims (Crews et al., 1997; M. Daniel et al., 1984; Primeau et al., 1995).

Complaints of poor *attention/concentration and slower thinking* are common (Pliskin, Capelli-Schellpfeffer, et al., 1998; Primeau et al., 1995). WIS-A Digit Symbol performance is often lower than expected, although WIS-A Arithmetic is usually intact (Barrash et al., 1996; Duff and McCaffrey, 2001; Hopewell, 1983; Varney, Ju, and Shepherd, 1998). Performances on other tests examining attentional functions (e.g., Seashore Rhythm Test, Speech Sounds Perception Test) may also be in the impaired range (M. Daniel et al., 1984; Hopewell, 1983). Van Zomeren, ten Duis, and their coworkers (1998) reported that half of their lightning strike victims scored at *borderline* levels on visual choice reaction time testing with clearly impaired performances on a divided attention task. Information processing speed as measured on the PASAT is sometimes impaired (Crews et al., 1997; van Zomeren, ten Duis et al., 1998).

Memory and learning are often affected. Many victims complain of inability to recall recent events, familiar names, or places, and getting lost in familiar places (M. Daniel et al., 1984). Retrograde amnesia and anterograde amnesia may be present acutely (Van Zomeren, ten Duis, et al., 1998) and improve over time (Hopewell, 1983). Deficits in verbal learning, immediate, and delayed memory are common problems acutely, may continue for months, and may become chronic (Barrash et al., 1996). These deficits have appeared on word list learning tasks (Barrash et al., 1996; Crews et al., 1997) and story recall tests (Crews et al., 1997). Memory for visual information is less likely to be impaired (Barrash et al., 1996; Varney, Ju, and Shepherd, 1998), but visual recall problems have been noted (Crews et al., 1997; Pliskin, Fink, et al., 1999). Some victims had poor tactile recall on the Tactual Performance Test (Crews et al., 1997; M. Daniel et al., 1984).

Verbal functions and academic skills are usually intact, as measured by WIS-A Information, Comprehension, Vocabulary, and Similarities (Barrash et al., 1996; Crews et al., 1997; Duff and McCaffrey, 2001; Varney, Ju, and Shepherd, 1998). In one case, aphasic speech was present two years postelectric arc injury but eventually resolved, although a verbal retrieval deficit remained (Varney et al., 1998). Many electric shock victims complain of verbal retrieval problems (Pliskin, Capelli-Schellpfeffer, et al., 1998), although Barrash and his colleagues (1996) did not find this on verbal fluency testing. The few cases reported in detail suggest considerable variability on academic skill testing. Varney, Ju, and Shepherds' (1998) patient's postinjury reading and spelling scores dropped significantly relative to standardized tests taken in school. In contrast, Crews and his group (1997) studied two patients with intact reading and spelling scores, although one's Arithmetic performance was low.

Perceptual and constructional functions have mostly been measured by WIS-A tests (Block Design, Object Assesmbly, Picture Arrangement, Picture Completion) with patients' performances generally *within normal limits* (Barrash et al., 1996; Crews et al., 1997; Duff and McCaffrey, 2001; Varney, Ju, and Shepherd, 1998). The Complex Figure Test, Benton Visual Retention Test, and Benton's Facial Recognition Test mostly produced similar findings (Barrash et al., 1996; Varney et al., 1998). However, tactile form discrimination tended to be slow and form localization poor in some patients (Crews et al., 1997; M. Daniel et al., 1984).

Executive functions. Few published assessments of these patients have considered executive functioning. The Category Test and Trail Making Test-B have sometimes been associated with impaired performance (Duff and McCaffrey, 2001), but this does not necessarily indicate impaired executive functioning.

Personality and psychosocial behavior. Like many persons who suffer some insult to their brain, victims of electric shock and lightning injury experience changes in their affect and mood (Pliskin, Capelli-Schellpfeffer, et al., 1998; Pliskin, Fink, et al., 1999), but additionally they may develop a post traumatic stress disorder (PTSD) (M. Daniel et al., 1984; A.R. Grossman et al., 1993; Kelley, Pliskin, et al., 1994). Pliskin and his colleagues (1998) found that their patients endorsed increased stress/depression (48%), changes in attitude (41%), and problems with anger/temper (30%), whereas the rates for control subjects were in the 5% to 14% range. These rates are fairly similar to those reported by Janus and Barrash (1996). Depression, emotional lability, increased anxiety and irritability, decreased stress tolerance and self-confidence, indecisiveness, immaturity, irrational violence, low self-esteem, somatic preoccupations, fear of future injury, and nightmares may develop following these injuries (see also Crews, Barth, et al., 1997; Primeau et al., 1995; Varney, Ju, and Shepherd, 1998). Long-term persistence of PTSD-like symptoms has been reported (Lishman, 1997; Pliskin, Fink, et al., 1999).

On personality inventories, elevations on depression are common, with Minnesota Multiphasic Personality Inventory (MMPI) scale elevations on Hs, HY, and sometimes Pt and Sc, as has appeared for brain injured patients in general (see Chapter 19) (Crews et al., 1997; M. Daniel et al., 1984; Pliskin, Capelli-Schellpfeffer, et al., 1998; Primeau et al., 1995). Electric shock victims make significantly poorer psychosocial adjustment than burn patients in vocational functioning, personal and family relationships, social environment, and psychological distress (Pliskin, Fink, et al., 1999).

Treatment. The need for life-saving services acutely has been well-documented (M.A. Cooper et al., 2001). Evaluation and treatment for the wide variety of medical disorders and psychological disorders that occur immediately, after a delay, or are progressive in nature may be necessary and follow protocols developed for these conditions, no matter what their etiology (M.A. Cooper et al., 2001). Treatment may include supportive psychotherapy and rehabilitation (Heilbronner, 1994).

VASCULAR DISORDERS

Knowledge about the structure and dynamics of the cerebrovascular circulation and its relationship to the rest of the circulatory system and its diseases is necessary for understanding the events that characterize the course of cerebrovascular diseases as well as expected patterns of neuropsychological deficits associated with vascular lesions. A technical description of the cerebral circulation and its vicissitudes, however, is beyond the scope of this book. (Readers wishing such a description at a relatively nontechnical level should consult the study course of the American Academy of Neurology, 2002; G.G. Brown, Baird, et al., 1996; Walsh and Darby, 1999; Tatu et al., 2001.)

The considerable variety of disorders affecting cerebral circulation and their many subtypes preclude discussion of all neuropsychological implications of cerebrovascular disease (e.g., see Bogousslavsky and Caplan's *Stroke Syndromes,* 2001; Welch, Caplan, et al., *Primer on Cerebrovascular Diseases,* 1997). Instead, this section deals with those conditions, and the broad outlines of their structural and pathophysiological antecedents, that a neuropsychologist is most likely to see.

Stroke and Related Disorders

The most frequently encountered of the cerebrovascular diseases is the *cerebrovascular accident* (CVA). It was once called *apoplexy* or an *apoplectic attack* and is now commonly referred to as a *stroke.* Unlike myocardial infarction, which is typically announced by pain and shortness of breath, most strokes are painless. Consequently many patients remain at home to see if their symptoms resolve. The term *brain attack,* analogous to *heart attack,* has been introduced to increase the public's awareness of the need for immediate medical attention (Caramata et al., 1994).

Strokes affect approximately 150 persons out of every 100,000 (M.D. Hill and Feasby, 2002; Wolf, Kannel, and McGee, 1986), making it the fifth most common neurological disorder in the United States. Although the incidence of stroke had remained stable for a number of years, it appears to be rising, perhaps because of more sensitive diagnostic techniques (Wolf, 1997; Bogousslavsky, Hommel, and Bassetti, 1998). Stroke is the third most common cause of death after heart disease and cancer (G.G. Brown, Baird, et al., 1996) and is the leading cause of disability in the 60 and over age group (F. McDowell, 1997; Powers, 1990; Wolf, Kannel, and McGee, 1986). The incidence of stroke is actually higher than the patient count, as "silent" strokes—particularly those with no obvious motor or sensory alterations—typically remain undetected until they show up on neuroimaging for some more recent problem or at autopsy (Broderick et al., 1998; Pohjasvaara et al., 1999). The economic burden of stroke in the United States was estimated to be $30 billion in 1993 (Dobkin, 1995; T.N. Taylor et al., 1996) and is undoubtedly considerably more today (Pliskin and Sworowski, 2003).

Risk factors

Risk factors for stroke are well known (J.W. Norris and Hachinski, 2001; Sacco, 2001; Straus et al., 2002). *Atherogenic* processes result in thickening lesions that grow within blood vessel walls; fatty substances are a significant component of these plaque-like lesions (Murros and Toole, 1997; Rajamani and Fisher, 1997; J.N. Walton, 1994). *Hypertension* (high blood pressure), elevated levels of cholesterol and saturated fatty acids, diabetes, and cigarette smoking are all significant contributors to the evolution of *atherosclerosis,* the condition of pathologically thickened arterial walls, which is the source of most strokes. The combination of high estrogen dosage in oral contraceptives and smoking has been associated with a risk of stroke in younger women; recent drug formulations containing reduced estrogen levels may not create as much of a risk for women who smoke (Kittner and Bush, 1997). Kurtzke (1983a) includes hypotension as a risk factor, particularly in elderly persons. Stroke alone increases the risk of dementia by more than a factor of nine (Tatemichi, Desmond, et al., 1992).

Some demographic characteristics are also associated with the incidence of stroke. Generally, the incidence of stroke increases with age, most rapidly from the sixth decade onward; and men are somewhat more stroke-prone than women (J.W. Norris and Hachinsky, 2001). Race may play a role, as both Japanese in Japan and African-Americans have high stroke rates. Japanese in the United States and poor rural Nigerians are less likely to have strokes, yet well-to-do Nigerians have high rates (Hachinsky and Norris, 1985; Wolf et al., 1986). Thus diet and other social factors contribute to the incidence of this disease (G.G. Brown, Baird, et al., 1996; Wolf, 1997). African-Americans with stroke tend to be younger than other stroke patients in the United States. More African-Americans have a greater number of stroke risk factors including hypertension, diabetes mellitus, congestive heart failure, and prior strokes than Caucasian patients (Hassaballa et al., 2001).

Most stroke risk factors can be reduced, typically by making significant lifestyle changes including diet, exercise, smoking cessation, and medical management (C.M. Helgason, 1997; Wolf, 1997). Warning signs of impending stroke, such as *transient ischemic attacks* (*TIAs,* see p. 199), which are often ignored, must be heeded for treatment to be initiated; this requires educating the public.

The pathophysiology of stroke

Medically speaking, a stroke is a "focal neurological disorder of abrupt development due to a pathological process in blood vessels" (J.N. Walton, 1994). The cardinal pathogenic feature of CVAs is the disruption of the supply of nutrients—primarily oxygen and glucose—to the brain as a result of disrupted blood flow (Bogousslavsky, Hommel, and Bassetti, 1998). The inability of nervous tissue of many parts of the brain to survive more than several minutes of oxygen deprivation accounts for the rapidity with which irreversible brain damage takes place. The disruption of normal blood flow, *infarction,* creates an area of damaged or dead tissue, an *infarct.* Most strokes are caused by ischemic infarctions, i.e., infarctions due to tissue starvation resulting from insufficient or absent blood flow rather than from insufficient or absent nutrients in the blood.

In addition to the cells that die in the immediate infarction area, cells surrounding the infarction are at risk. The stroke begins a rapid cascade of neurochemical changes in which brain cells adjacent to the infarct remain viable for several hours (Boysen and Christensen, 2001; K.M.A. Welch et al., 1997, Section II, *passim*) but are subsequently incorporated into the infarction area of irreversible function unless medically treated. This area, called the *ischemic penumbra,* is the target of *thrombolytic* (breakdown of atherosclerotic particles in the bloodstream) therapy to minimize cerebral damage following ischemic stroke (Heiss, 2000). Thrombolytics (aspirin is one) are most likely to be effective during the first three hours following stroke (H.P. Adams et al., 1996). Because "time is brain," it is critical that patients seek medical care as soon as possible so that appropriate evaluation (e.g., CT scanning) and thrombolytic treatment can be instituted within a three-hour window. The primary risk associated with thrombolytic therapy is hemorrhage—a risk well worth taking (H.P. Adams et al., 1996).

Two prominent mechanisms that can account for the tissue starvation of CVAs are obstructions of blood vessels, which create an *ischemic* condition in which blood flow is deficient or absent, and *hemorrhage* (Bogousslavsky, Hommel, and Bassetti, 1998; Yamamoto et al., 2001). Because the symptoms and course of these two major stroke-producing disorders differ, they are considered separately. This separation, however, is an oversimplification, as some kinds of obstructions are hemorrhagic in nature and some hemorrhages give rise to spasmodic constriction of the blood vessels (*vasospasm*) that so severely impedes blood flow as to create focal sites of obstruction.

Obstructive (ischemic) strokes

Cerebral thrombosis. The buildup of fat deposits within the artery walls (called *atherosclerotic* or *arteriosclerotic plaques*) involves fibrous tissue and is susceptible to hemorrhage and ulceration (Ameriso and Sahai, 1997). These deposits are the most common source of obstruction of blood flow to the brain, causing 60% to 70% of all strokes and more than 75% of obstructive strokes (Bogousslavsky, Hommel, and Bassetti, 1998; Powers, 1990). In *thrombotic* strokes, the infarction results from occlusion of a blood vessel by a clump of blood particles and tissue overgrowth, a *thrombus,* that accumulates in arteriosclerotic plaques. These plaques most usually form where blood vessels branch or, less frequently, on traumatic or other lesion sites on the vessel wall. Growth of the thrombus narrows the opening in the blood vessel, thus reducing blood flow, or it closes off the vessel altogether. Thrombotic strokes may occur suddenly with no further increase in symptoms. Often they take as long as half an hour to develop fully. In as many as one-third of cases, thrombotic strokes evolve for hours or even days (Yamamoto et al., 2001). Often (reports range from 50% to 80% of cases) they are preceded by one or more "little strokes," i.e., transient ischemic attacks (TIAs)(see p. 199).

Thrombotic strokes tend to arise from atherosclerotic lesions in the internal carotid or the vertebrobasilar arteries. More than two-thirds of the resultant infarcts in-

volve posterior frontal, temporal, and parietal structures in the region fed by the *middle cerebral artery (MCA)* (Neau and Bogousslavksy, 2001; see Fig. 3.4, p. 44); other infarcts occur in the brainstem, inferior temporal lobe (including the hippocampus), and occipital lobes when the vertebrobasilar system is involved (see Bogousslavsky and Caplan, 2001, Part II, *passim*). About 80% of patients with thrombotic strokes in the territory of the middle cerebral artery enjoy significant spontaneous improvement as swelling and metabolic dysfunction resolve, but close to half continue to be disabled. After three months, relatively little spontaneous improvement can be expected (Bogousslavsky, Hommel, and Bassetti, 1998).

Many methodological issues make outcome literature difficult to interpret. These include how outcome is assessed (e.g., return to work vs. formal outcome scale), severity of motor weakness, association of comorbidities, and whether a consecutive patient series is evaluated vs. only those in formal rehabilitation programs. In addition, expectations for outcome success in patients with prominent language disturbances may differ from those for patients whose deficits are primarily emotional or nonlinguistic.

When the middle cerebral artery is involved, the most obvious cognitive disorders troubling those with right-sided damage will involve visuospatial abilities and gestalt-type concept formation; many with left-sided disease will be more or less aphasic (American Academy of Neurology, 2002). Limb weakness and paralysis as well as somatosensory changes are common in all of these patients. Cognitive deficits involving visual and memory functions tend to occur with strokes due to occlusion of the *posterior cerebral artery (PCA)*, which branches off from the *vertebrobasilar system.* Vertebrobasilar strokes confined to the brainstem or structures below the cerebrum primarily affect aspects of movement, sensation, and consciousness but can also alter cognitive processing.

Cerebral embolism. About 20% to 30% of obstructive strokes are *embolic* (Castillo and Bogousslavsky, 1997). Obstruction in these strokes is caused by an *embolus,* a plug of thrombic material or fatty deposit broken away from blood vessel walls or of foreign matter such as clumps of bacteria or even obstructive gas bubbles. Most emboli are fragments of thrombotic lesions that developed outside the intracranial circulatory system, many in the heart and its blood vessels. Relatively few thrombotic emboli arise from lesions within the major arterial pathways to the brain. Presentation of embolic strokes tends to be abrupt and without the warning precursors of headache or transient ischemic attacks that can accompany other kinds of stroke, although 5% to 6% of embolic strokes begin with fluctuating and evolving symptoms in the first day or two. Symptoms associated with relatively restricted cortical damage are more likely to occur with embolic stroke than with other kinds of stroke. The middle cerebral artery territory is the most common site of embolic strokes although they can occur elsewhere. L.R. Caplan (1980, 2001) introduced the term *top-of-the-basilar syndrome* to refer to visual, oculomotor, and behavioral abnormalities due to emboli that traversed the vertebral arteries but failed to negotiate the hard turn into the posterior circulation and thus occlude posterior cerebral arteries. Memory impairment is common in this syndrome in which the medial thalamus is frequently infarcted.

Variables affecting presentation of obstructive strokes. The effects of ischemic infarctions vary from person to person or from time to time when a person suffers repeated strokes. These variations are due to a host of factors such as individual differences in the anatomical organization of the cerebral circulation, in the capacity to develop and utilize collateral brain circulation, and in cerebral blood pressure and blood flow. Variations in the extent, sites, and severity of arteriosclerotic disease, in the large extracranial arteries that feed the cerebral circulation, in the smaller intracranial and intracerebral vessels, and within the circulatory system of the heart contribute to individual differences in the manifestation of stroke, as do such health variables as heart disease, diabetes, and blood conditions that affect its viscosity or clotting capacity.

Age and sex can play a role in determining the presentation of a stroke (Eslinger and Damasio, 1981; Gates et al., 1986; Sorgato et al., 1990). For example, embolic strokes, usually associated with heart disease, tend to occur at an earlier age than thrombotic strokes. The aphasic women studied by H. Damasio and her colleagues (1989) had more strokes involving anterior regions than the men, whose strokes were more likely to be posterior, with associated differences in the nature of their aphasic disorders. However, conflicting data leave unsettled the question of lateralized sex differences in stroke presentation (Kertesz, 2001).

Cognitive alterations with obstructive strokes. Large artery infarctions tend to produce significant behavioral changes either by direct cortical injury or by disruption of large subcortical areas. Very small artery infarctions may have few behavioral consequences except when they occur cumulatively with more and more little strokes producing an increasing volume of damaged tissue (see pp. 201–202).

Yet with all these variations, certain overall patterns in onset of obstructive strokes and their manifestations tend to stand out. Stroke tends to have one-sided effects. While there is an enormous range of differences between stroke patients with respect to the depth, extent, and site of damaged tissue (e.g., from front to back and crown to base of the brain), most strokes lateralize either to the right or to the left. For this reason many stroke patients have been subjects of neuropsychological research into the lateral organization of the brain and the anatomic correlates of specific cognitive functions (e.g., H. Damasio and Damasio, 1989). The neurobehavioral changes following stroke offer the best examples of both aphasic syndromes and nondominant (hand side, usually right hemisphere) behavioral syndromes (see pp. 70–75, 79–80). As strokes are acute in onset, there is no time for functional compensation (patients with intracranial tumors rarely have classic aphasic syndromes because the tumor grows slowly, allowing for compensation and tissue displacement) (S.W. Anderson, Damasio, and Tranel, 1990). Obstructive stroke syndromes are most prominent acutely and then become less defined over time.

The occurrence of lasting alterations of function in areas of the brain quite distant from the lesion has been suggested by electrophysiological (Gummow et al., 1984) and blood flow (Benke, Kurzthaler, et al., 2002; Chu et al., 2002) studies and by the many patients who experience sensorimotor symptoms in their limbs on the supposedly unaffected side (J.S. Kim, 2001; van Ravensberg et al., 1984). During the acute stages, secondary diffuse effects and *diaschisis* (see p. 288) typically add symptoms of widespread brain pathology as edema and other physiological reactions take place. Sometimes the symptoms improve relatively early in the course of the illness. Such a change for the better is thought to reflect the dislodgement of an embolus and return of more normal blood flow. Swelling and other secondary effects of the stroke can cause more serious bilateral or diffuse damage than the stroke itself and may—as may secondary physiological reactions to trauma—result in death (e.g., see Gewirtz and Steinberg, 1997). Thus, stroke patients frequently display signs of bilateral or diffuse damage during the early stages of their illness. As swelling diminishes and other physiological disturbances return to a more normal state, signs of bilateral or diffuse dysfunction gradually diminish while the severity of the lateralized impairments usually decreases too.

For aphasic stroke patients, speech fluency typically returns by one month if it returns at all; fewer than one-fourth of patients nonfluent at one month regain fluency by six months (Knopman, Selnes, et al., 1983). In contrast, confrontation naming is typically impaired at one month with about one-third of aphasic patients improving to normal or near-normal levels by six months (Knopman, Selnes, et al., 1984). Both site and size of lesion are associated with improvement (see also p. 287). Left-handed aphasic patients too tend to make their greatest gains in the first six months (Borod, Carper, and Naeser, 1990). Sarno and her coworkers (1985) found that their patients made some continuing gains with no sex differences in attained levels of improvement after one to two-and-one-half years.

At one month poststroke, most patients with *hemiplegia* (lateralized paralysis) had perceptual deficits as well, regardless of the side of lesion (Edmans and Lincoln, 1989). These problems affected almost all (97%) of the aphasic patients with hemiplegia and most (81%) of the left hemiplegic patients in this study but fewer than half (47%) of the right hemiplegic patients who did not have aphasia. Although patients in both hemiplegia groups displayed inattention on one or more tests in the Edmans and Lincoln study, those with left hemiplegia had significantly more instances of left-side inattention. (For the many specific visuoperceptual defects that trouble stroke patients, see Barton and Caplan, 2001; for disorders of auditory perception, see R.A. Levine and Häusler, 2001.)

Most patients whose strokes were ischemic in nature have residual defects that are more or less obviously lateralized and display relatively minimal evidence of diffuse damage (American Academy of Neurology, 2002). Thus, with left-sided infarcts, speech and language disorders are common, their specific nature depending on the site and extent of the lesion (Benson, 1988, 1993; D. Caplan, 2003; Goodglass and Kaplan, 1983a; Murdoch, 1990). With lesions on the right, perceptual and visuospatial deficits tend to be among the most prominent (Benton, Sivan, et al., 1994; S. Clarke, 2001). Patients with right-sided damage who have left hemispatial inattention are likely to have lost much of their inattention bias at ten months poststroke but may still display some inattention tendencies (Egelko, Simon, et al., 1989). Their affect comprehension—both visual and auditory—also shows some improvement but is typically compromised (Heilman, Blonder, Bowers, and Crucian, 2000).

For left- and right-sided hemiplegics alike, the largest number of perceptual errors involve aspects of body image. Moreover, their focal deficits typically fit into a pattern of dysfunction associated with areas of the brain that share an artery or network of smaller arterial vessels (e.g., see E. Goldberg, 1989; Babikian et al., 1994; Neau and Bogousslavsky, 2001). Thus, it is unlikely that decreased verbal fluency, suggestive of frontal damage, will occur with alexia without agraphia, a condition that typically implicates an occipital lesion, unless the patient has had two or more successive strokes. In contrast, symptoms that make up

the *angular gyrus syndrome* (Gerstmann's syndrome, see p. 71) occur together because the cortical areas in which these functions are mediated are close together within a common arterial flow pattern (Geschwind and Strub, 1975; Roeltgen, Sevush, and Heilman, 1983).

Emotional disturbances with stroke. Differences in how patients with left or right hemisphere strokes react in the acute stages of their disease have been described in terms of a preponderance of depression and catastrophic reactions with left-sided infarcts, and indifference reactions when the lesion is on the right (Gainotti, 1972, 1989; Heilman, Blonder, Bowers, and Crucian, 2000; R.G. Robinson and Starkstein, 2002). Reports by patients' relatives two weeks after stroke onset indicated that depression was the most prominent emotional change, regardless of lesion side, and that the level of "indifference" (defined in this study as "restricted emotional expression," equated with a psychiatric definition of "apathy," and also including anosognosia) increased greatly in patients with right hemisphere involvement (L.D. Nelson et al., 1993), leading these authors to suggest that left and right hemisphere stroke patients may be experiencing different kinds of depression.

Depression and difficulty in social adjustment affect between one-third and two-thirds of patients (Eslinger, Parkinson, and Shamay, 2002). Moreover, the incidence of depression is likely to increase over time (M. Kauhanen et al., 1999; M.L. Kauhanen et al., 2000a). Posthospitalization development of depression tends to occur more frequently for patients with right-sided lesions; the number of depressed patients with left-sided lesions tends to get smaller after the acute stages (R.G. Robinson and Starkstein, 2002). Cullum and Bigler (1991) found that within the first half-year poststroke (excluding those patients with significantly compromised language functions who are most frequently troubled by depression early in their course, and those unable to fill in a test form) 28% of stroke patients described themselves as clinically depressed; in a similar group who had strokes seven to 24 months earlier, 52% admitted to clinical levels of depressive symptoms. At one year, major depression troubled 26% of stroke survivors in a meta-analysis of five studies (R.G. Robinson and Starkstein, 2002). Two years after stroke, 47% of one large (103) sample were depressed, 27% with symptoms of major depression (R.G. Robinson, Starr et al., 1983). Moreover, one to two years poststroke, severe depression in patients with right-sided damaged was strongly correlated with posterior lesion sites, but depression in patients with left-sided lesions showed no anterior/posterior predilection (R.G. Robinson and Starkstein, 2002). D.W. Desmond and his colleagues

(2003) question these reports of high incidence, suggesting that a history of premorbid depression must be taken into account when examining the relationship between stroke and depression. In this study poststroke depression affected 11.2% of patients; depression occurred more often in women and as severity increased.

Reduction in activities and in socializing are common life style alterations among stroke patients (L.M. Binder, Howieson, and Coull, 1987). Depressed patients in particular are likely to experience restricted activities and social contact. Depression did not predict the quality of social functioning at six months poststroke, but severity of impairment did (R.G. Robinson, Bolduc, et al., 1985). However, four years poststroke, depressive tendencies contributed more to determining the quality of patients' lives than did ability to walk, ability to perform activities of daily living, or memory ability (Niemi et al., 1988). In a more recent report, the most important factors associated with quality of life were depression and marital status (M.L. Kauhanen et al., 2000b).

Transient Ischemic Attacks (TIAs)

These episodes of temporary obstruction of a blood vessel last less than 24 hours by definition, and many last for only minutes, with fully half dissipating within an hour (Bamford, 2001; Hennessy and Britton, 2000; J. Weinberger, 2002). In fact, most stroke specialists consider the standard definition of up to 24 hours to be an unduly long window; its persistence in the literature attests to the power of historical inertia. Two types of TIAs have been identified: those that rarely last more than 45 minutes and leave no evidence of infarction on CT ("most last less than 15 minutes," Tietjen, 1997) and those that last much longer—averaging six hours or so—and show radiological evidence of infarction (Bogousslavsky, Hommel, and Bassetti, 1998). The latter has been termed *cerebral infarction with transient signs* (CITS), referring to its different time course with evidence of brain lesions. It has been suggested, only partly tongue in cheek, that a true TIA should be defined by a transient deficit lasting less than 24 *minutes* rather than less than 24 *hours* (F.T. Nichols, personal communication, October, 2002 [dwl]).

TIAs are characterized by mild stroke-like symptoms that follow the same patterns of presentation—lateralization and clustering of symptoms within defined arterial territories—as do full-blown strokes (Hachinsky and Norris, 1985). Furthermore, like strokes, most TIAs are associated with arteriosclerotic disease and have the same risk factors (Bogousslavsky, Hommel, and Bassetti, 1998). They typically represent reversible ischemia resulting from thrombotic microemboli that pass on before they do much damage. Patients may experience few or many such attacks, relatively frequently or spaced over months or years (Lishman, 1997). Within the first months after a TIA, stroke evolves in approximately 30% of patients (Bogousslavsky, Hommel, and Bassetti, 1998). The risk of stroke following a TIA depends on other clinical factors. For example, TIA patients with more than a 90% stenosis of the ipsilateral internal carotid artery (ICA) have about a 35% chance of stroke in the next two years (Anonymous, 1991), whereas TIA patients with the cardiac disorder, *atrial fibrillation* (extremely rapid heartbeat), have an 8% to 34% chance of a stroke in the next two years (P.A. Scott, 2002).

In stating that TIAs "may resolve completely, leaving no deficit," Powers (1990) reported the common wisdom. However, a closer look at these patients, through the eyes of relatives or a behaviorally oriented clinician (Lishman, 1997; Walsh and Darby, 1999) or with neuropsychological tests (Delaney, Wallace, and Egelko, 1980; G.G. Brown, Baird, et al., 1996), indicates that many patients who have had TIAs suffer mild residual cognitive impairment, the deficits becoming increasingly apparent with repeated attacks. The tests used by Delaney and his coworkers (1980) elicited both problems with slowing and mental tracking suggestive of bilateral or diffuse brain damage and focal deficits indicating that lateralized damage had occurred in those areas in which blood flow is most commonly disrupted by stroke. F.B. Wood and his colleagues (1981) also reported that a substantial number of patients who have had TIAs show some neuropsychological deficits which, in this study, appeared most often on delayed recall tasks.

Treatment of TIA or CITS typically involves chronic antiplatelet coagulation therapy; often aspirin suffices. Anticoagulation therapy may be initiated preventively if a potential embolic source is suspected (e.g., *atrial fibrillation* [abnormal cardiac rhythm]). *Carotid endarterectomy* (surgical removal of atherosclerotic plaques) may be performed when there is significant carotid *stenosis* (arterial narrowing) (Barnett, Meldrum et al., 2002; D.G. Sherman and Lalonde, 1997).

Hemorrhagic strokes

In 10% to 20% of all strokes, hemorrhage is the primary and most significant agent of damage (Bogousslavsky, Hommel, and Bassetti, 1998). Hemorrhagic strokes are associated with a high mortality rate of 35%–52% within the first 30 days (Carhuapoma and Hanley, 2002). Hypertension is the chief risk factor although chronic oral anticoagulants can also increase the likelihood of hemorrhagic stroke if dosages are not well-monitored and controlled. The two most common mechanisms causing arterial rupture are weakening of a vessel wall due to pathological alterations secondary to hypertension which is present in 78 to 88% of cases, and rupture associated with a vascular abnormality such as *aneurysm* (a ballooning weakened arterial wall), *arteriovenus malformation* (*AVM*; see this page), tumor, or deficient coagulation (Qureshi, Tuhrim, et al., 2001; J.N. Walton, 1994). Cocaine, excessive alcohol, and hypertension are additional risk factors for intracerebral hemorrhage (Qureshi, Mohammad, et al., 2001; M.A. Sloan, 1997; van Gijn and Rinkel, 2001). Hypertensive hemorrhagic strokes occur most typically in persons in the 60 to 80 year range: the most commonly affected sites are the putamen, thalamus, and caudate.

The risk of ruptured aneurysm depends more on aneurysm characteristics than patient characteristics. Women and older patients have increased risk of rupture, although patients vary greatly (Rinkel et al., 1998). Symptomatic aneurysms, those larger than 10 mm, and basilar artery aneurysms have a markedly increased likelihood of rupture. The most common site for ruptured aneurysm is subarachnoid (90% of cases); and of these, 41% involve the anterior communicating/anterior cerebral artery, while 34% occur in the middle cerebral artery, each with the potential for profound neuropsychological consequences (Morita et al., 1998).

The manifestations of ruptured aneurysms can be quite dramatic. Early warning symptoms rarely precede these *subarachnoid hemorrhages* (*SAHs*) (van Gijn and Rinkel, 2001; Ogden, 1996). Rather, typically, the patient suffers an extremely painful headache that is often accompanied by nausea and vomiting and followed within the hour by evidence of neurological dysfunction such as stiff neck and focal neurological signs. The patient may or may not lose consciousness depending on the severity of the bleed and the intensity and site of *vasospasm* (contraction of blood vessels in the region of the bleed) which occurs in about 30% of cases and produces ischemia and infarction (Britz and Mayberg, 1997; Mohr, Spetzler, et al., 1986). The condition can be fatal when massive bleeding or extensive vasospasm occurs, with 50% mortality within the first month poststroke (Estol, 2001). Yet, if the bleeding is arrested soon enough, the patient may sustain relatively little brain damage and few cognitive deficits, if any (Ogden, Mee, and Henning, 1993). The in-between cases, in which damage is extensive but not fatal, tend to display serious behavioral impairments attributable to focal damage. For example, patients who have had ruptured aneurysms of the *anterior communicating artery* (*ACA*) are likely to suffer the kind of behavioral disturbances—such as lack of spontaneity, childishness, indifference, and memory retrieval problems—associ-

ated with frontal lobe lesions (Lishman, 1997; Okawa et al., 1980). Cognitive deficits resulting from ruptured aneurysms differ from the impairments of ischemic cerebrovascular accidents in that the damage is likely to be more widespread and does not necessarily follow anatomically well-defined or neuropsychologically common patterns.

Hemorrhages associated with hypertension tend to involve the blood vessels at the base of the cerebral hemispheres so that the damage is usually subcortical (Voelker and Kaufman, 1997). Thus, these strokes mostly affect the thalamus, basal ganglia, and brainstem. These hypertensive cerebral hemorrhages or *intracerebral hemorrhages,* as they are variously called, have a mortality rate of 65% (Kase and Mohr, 1986) to 70% to 80% (Powers, 1990). The condition of surviving patients can be anything from near-vegetative to a relatively good return to independence. Motor system impairments tend to be prominent; residual symptoms and memory disorders may also occur (see Crosson, 1992).

Arteriovenous malformations (*AVMs*) are tangled masses of arteries and veins of congenital origin which grow, usually gradually, much like a tumor (G.G. Brown, Baird, et al., 1996; Hachinski and Norris, 1985; Mohr, Tatemichi, et al., 1986). These are not common, with ruptured and hemorrhaging AVMs comprising about 1% of all strokes. The cognitive effects of nonhemorrhagic AVMs may be relatively mild and not necessarily reflective of lateralized damage (G.G. Brown and Kinderman, 1997). If pronounced, cognitive deficits will show the expected lateralized pattern, but deficits typically associated with damage to the hemisphere contralateral to the AVM may also be present (Mahalick et al., 1991).

Silent strokes

Silent strokes, in which symptoms are not obvious and thus go unremarked, were found in 11% to 15% of subjects in several large studies (Brott et al., 1994; Chodosh et al., 1988; Shinkawa et al., 1995). They may be present in up to 30% of patients with significant internal carotid disease (Furst et al., 2001). Silent strokes are five times as prevalent as symptomatic brain infarcts; their number increases with age and is slightly greater for women (Vermeer et al., 2002). Hypertension, but not other cardiovascular risk factors, appears to be associated with silent infarcts.

For the most part, silent strokes tend to be small, lacunar lesions situated in deep brain structures. Left hemisphere strokes are unlikely to escape notice unless they are small and in deep structures. In the right hemisphere, since symptoms may be less obvious, silent strokes tend to be larger, with a higher percentage involving the cortex. Silent strokes usually become apparent upon CT or MRI scanning of later occurring, obvious strokes or when behavior changes bring the patient to medical attention.

A 62-year-old building inspector was charged with criminal misconduct for issuing hundreds of building permits for plans that did not meet code requirements. He responded with a profound depression, for which he was hospitalized. On neuropsychological examination he was alert, oriented, verbose, illogical but not irrational, and feeling hurt and puzzled by his situation as he thought he had done his work well. While his scores on predominantly verbal tests were generally well above *average,* his performances on construction tests were confused, and both free-hand and copy drawings were confused and distorted. On questioning, he provided a history of a flu-like illness occurring just before he began giving the improper permits. CT scan revealed an old right frontoparietal infarct.

Vascular Dementia

Vascular dementia (*VAD*), broadly conceived, is a decline in cognitive functioning that results from any of a number of vascular etiologies. Yet symptoms necessary to diagnose dementia from vascular disease are a topic of debate with different criteria offered by different authors. For example, some consider that a strategically placed infarct can produce dementia (e.g., left angular gyrus, medial thalamus) (Amar and Wilcock, 1996); others have suggested that a relatively focal constellation of neurobehavioral deficits from a focal lesion constitutes dementia (D.I. Katz et al., 1987); or that diagnosis of dementia requires a decline in memory functioning (Royall and Roman, 2000). Even the term "vascular dementia" lacks agreed-upon diagnostic criteria resulting in significant differences in patient classification (Chui, Mack, et al., 2000).

Given the variety of treatments for cerebrovascular disease, some workers suggest staging by levels of severity beginning with *vascular cognitive impairment* (J.V. Bowler, 2000; Hachinski and Bowler, 1993). This procedure seems to be particularly relevant since memory loss, a prominent feature of Alzheimer's disease and many other dementing conditions, is not necessarily a major symptom of cerebrovascular disease. For example, cardiovascular insufficiency in elderly persons who have not had major cardiovascular disease (e.g., stroke, heart attack) accounted for 28% of the variance on performance of a test of conceptual abstraction and flexibility (the Wisconsin Card Sorting Test) (Dywan et al., 1992).

Multi-infarct Dementia

Multi-infarct dementia (*MID,* also called *arteriosclerotic dementia; arteriosclerotic psychosis*) is an umbrella term for conditions in which widespread cognitive impairment takes place as a result of repeated infarctions, usually at many different sites (Chui, 1989; Chui, Victoroff et al., 1992; Metter and Wilson, 1993; J.S. Meyer, Shirai, and Akiyama, 1997). Although *MID* comes under the broader category of *vascular dementia,* we treat it separately since this is probably the form of vascular dementia most frequently encountered by neuropsychologists.

Chui, Mack, and their colleagues (2000) distinguish two broad categories of this second most common dementing condition: *cortical atherosclerotic dementia* (*CAD*), characterized by repeated infarctions of the large vessels (cerebral arteries) which supply blood to the cerebral cortex, and *subcortical arteriosclerotic dementia* (*SAD*), resulting from infarction and/or ischemia due to blockage or deterioration of the narrower arterioles that feed subcortical structures. MID as a diagnostic category, however, usually refers to subcortical dementias and is used in this way here. MID in turn encompasses a number of conceptually, if not clinically, distinct diagnostic entities (J.S. Meyer, Shirai, and Akiyama, 1997; Peretz and Cummings, 1988). Two— *lacunar strokes* and *Binswanger's disease,* also called *progressive subcortical vascular encephalopathy* (*PSVE*) (Brun et al., 1990)—are generally recognized. In practice, these different conditions tend to be dealt with together as MID. This usage is generally appropriate since the two conditions are similar in many ways and often present together (J.V. Bowler and Hachinsky, 2003; Sultzer and Cummings, 1994; Stuss and Cummings, 1990).

Lacunar strokes occur as small infarcts in deep gray nuclei of the basal ganglia, internal capsule, or pons, with a few appearing in cortical gray matter or in the major cerebral white matter pathways (Cummings and Mahler, 1991; Hommel, 1997; Mohr, Spetzler, et al., 1986). Many lacunar strokes give rise to pure sensory or motor symptoms, and some may be "silent" in that they are discovered only at autopsy (L.M. Binder, Howieson, and Coull, 1987; Stuss and Cummings, 1990). These little strokes are mostly due to occlusion, but occasionally emboli from a nearby lesioned area will plug up the arterioles. Small areas of infarction also have a particular predilection for the white matter around the anterior horns of the lateral ventricles (*periventricular white matter*). All these vulnerable areas are underlying parts of frontal lobe circuitry so it is not surprising that at autopsy most cases with dementia show evidence of softening of frontal white matter (Ishii et al., 1986). Lacunar strokes become a *lacunar state* when an accumulation of lacunae manifest behaviorally in a pattern of motor and cognitive disorders. Not only does dementia result from the amount of brain tissue that is lost but the effects of multiple infarctions may even be synergistic rather than simply cumulative (Wolfe, Babikian, et al., 1994). In about one-third of cases, onset is gradual; the majority of patients experience the *stepwise progressive deterioration* that is one of the hallmarks of MID. These patients typically exhibit signs of frontal system dysfunction, such as deficits in mental shifting, response inhibition, and executive behavior—seen as impaired judgment, apathy, and inertia (Amar and Wilcock, 1996; Ishii et al., 1986; Wolfe, Linn, et al., 1990).

Binswanger's disease differs from the lacunar state in that the onset is slow and insidious (Cummings and Mahler, 1991; Stuss and Cummings, 1990). Moreover, the multiple infarcts are found mostly in periventricular areas and cerebral white matter with accompanying *demyelinization* (loss of the fatty sheath around fast conduction nerve fibers) (Filley, 1995, 2001). CT scan of these patients reveals cortical atrophy with areas of translucency, or white matter hyperintensities (*leukoaraiosis* [LA]) around dilated ventricles. MRI is more sensitive than CT in revealing hyperintensities and "abnormalities" such as small periventricular haloes, although many of these latter phenomena are only age-related. Consequently, Binswanger's disease can be overdiagnosed when based upon radiologic criteria (Nichols and Mohr, 1986). Gait disorders, dysarthria, and incontinence are common problems for these patients. Cognitive and executive dysfunctions typically associated with frontal damage characterize the dementia of Binswanger's disease (Filley, 2001).

Similarities in these two conditions include the common risk factors of hypertension, diabetes, abnormally high fatty content of the blood, and cigarette smoking. Leukoaraiosis, some quite extensive, is seen in large numbers of MID patients (52% in one study [Kobari et al., 1990]). It is strongly associated with risk factors for stroke (Awad, Spetzler, et al., 1987) and with slowed mental processing when stroke risk is high (Junqué et al., 1990) but occurs in only about 20% of the normal aging population and then appears to have no cognitive effects (S.M. Rao, Mittenberg, Bernardin, et al., 1989). The literature gives conflicting reports regarding sex distribution: L.L. Barclay and her colleagues (1985) and Stuss and Cummings (1990) cite studies showing that both sexes are equally affected; but J.V. Bowler and Hachinsky (2003) and Sultzer and Cummings (1994) refer to other studies indicating that slightly more men than women have this disease. Length of survival following diagnosis is shorter than for other dementing conditions.

Communication disorders have a distinctive pattern in which the content and organization of speech remain relatively unaffected but pitch, tone, and melodic qualities are deficient, and rate of production is slow. Most of these patients become dysarthric and may ultimately deteriorate into a kinetic mutism (Cummings and Benson, 1989; A.L. Powell et al., 1988). Writing is affected and auditory span may be diminished.

These patients tend to retain awareness of their disabilities (DeBettignies et al., 1990). Given this awareness it is not surprising to find as many as 60% of MID patients displaying depressive symptoms (Askin-Edgar et al., 2002; Cummings, Miller, et al., 1987). Threatening delusions, such as being robbed or having an unfaithful spouse, are likely to occur in half of these patients at some time in their course.

In some cases the manifestations of MID are sufficiently like those of Alzheimer's disease that it has been mistaken for it (Mesulam, 2000a; J.N. Walton, 1994). It differs from Alzheimer's disease in some important ways (Metter and Wilson, 1993; Walsh and Darby, 1999). Generally symptom onset is acute with fluctuating severity, at times from hour to hour. A history of hypertension along with other risk factors for stroke is almost universal and a stroke history is common (Brinkman, Largen, et al., 1986; Reichman et al., 1993). Focal neurological signs are evident. Significantly better memory test performances distinguished MID patients from those with Alzheimer's disease (J.V. Bowler and Hachinsky, 2003). Relatively better memory test performance plus reduced output, both on verbal descriptions (Cookie Theft Picture) and on unstructured construction tasks (Tinkertoy Test), identified these patients out of a group with dementia of the Alzheimer's type (Mendez and Ashla-Mendez, 1991). Thus MID partakes of some important characteristics of the subcortical dementias. Early in its course, cognitive deficits are likely to predominate while personality deterioration lags behind, although eventually both aspects of behavior may become profoundly disordered. Motor abnormalities, such as gait disturbances and rigidity, which reflect lesions involving subcortical structures, are common but not necessarily predictive of MID (Reichman et al., 1993).

Hypertension

Hypertension, the major precursor of most types of CVA, in itself may alter brain substance and affect cerebral functioning (Johansson, 1997). The major risk factors for hypertension include obesity, excessive use of salt, excessive alcohol intake, lack of exercise, and tobacco use (N.M. Kapla, 2001). Chronic "benign" intracranial hypertension shows evidence of cerebral edema in retinal examinations, but on CT scans cerebral structures generally appear normal (Weisberg, 1985). In one MRI study, twice as many hypertensive persons under age 50 as age-matched normal controls presented high-signal white matter lucencies (R. Schmidt et al., 1991). These hypertensives had poorer performances on tests of verbal and visuospatial learning and memory, visual attention, vigilance, and reaction time, and reported lower activity levels on a mood questionnaire. However, their white matter lesions correlated with age but not with any of the neuropsychological tests or mood scales.

With improved techniques and medications for managing hypertension, an acute condition, *hypertensive encephalopathy*, has become quite rare (Dinsdale, 1986; R.A. Hauser et al., 1988). This potentially fatal condition results from a rapid rise in blood pressure with accompanying headache, seizures, and mental status deterioration along with other symptoms of high intracranial pressure, leaving behind focal high-intensity cerebral white matter lesions, and, in very severe cases, brainstem and cerebellar lesions (Filley, 2001).

Even without documented cerebral changes, hypertension has been associated with mild cognitive impairments which may worsen with the duration and severity of the hypertensive condition (Wilkie, Eisdorfer, and Nowlin, 1976; Swan et al., 1998; Waldstein, Manuck, et al., 1991). Deficits have been reported on a complex concept formation task (the Category Test) (H. Goldman et al., 1974); reduction of blood pressure was related to fewer errors. Other studies also report specific cognitive deficits or tendencies for poorer performance on various tests (Bornstein and Kelly, 1991). For example, P.T. Costa and Shock (1980) observed a tendency for a highly educated group of men with moderately high hypertension to perform less well than controls on a variety of cognitive tasks. A.P. Shapiro and his colleagues (1982) reported psychomotor slowing, reduced sensory–perceptual sensitivity, and impaired time estimation for hypertensive women, with both sexes slowed on a test of complex visuomotor tracking and learning (Digit Symbol) and at normal levels on a test of immediate visual recall (Benton Visual Retention Test). Fifteen months later, effective treatment with antihypertensive medications resulted in improvement trends on the sensory–perceptual and time estimation tests and greater improvement on Digit Symbol than shown by either the untreated or control groups; only performance on the visual recall test deteriorated for both treated and untreated hypertensive groups (R.E. Miller et al., 1984).

Eisdorfer (1977) found that while elderly patients with significant hypertension suffered gradual cognitive deterioration over a ten-year period, those with mild hypertension actually showed some improvement and normotensive subjects did not change appreciably over the years. Wilkie and her coworkers (1976) found that immediate recall of designs (Visual Reproduction) was the only test that hypertensives performed less well, and

then only on six-year follow-up. The Framingham Study Group, reporting on their 2,123 participants in the 55 to 89 age range, found no cognitive changes associated with hypertension (M.E. Farmer, White, et al., 1987); but upon reanalysis of tests taken 12 to 14 years later, hypertension with longer duration was associated with poorer cognitive performance (M.E. Farmer, Kittner, et al., 1990). This finding has been independently observed (Swan et al., 1998). Thus, young hypertensive patients may be more at risk for cognitive impairments than their older counterparts (Waldstein, Jennings, et al., 1996) as the cumulative effects of elevated blood pressure take their toll later in life.

Confusion also exists regarding the cognitive effects of antihypertensive medications as a few studies suggested that medication may contribute to slowed reaction time or memory deficits (M.E. Farmer, White, et al., 1987; Solomon et al., 1983), a few reported improvement (Croog et al., 1986; see also R.E. Miller et al., 1984, noted above), and most registered no significant cognitive changes with medication (e.g., G. Goldstein, Materson et al., 1990; Pérez-Stable et al., 2000). However, drowsiness and listlessness can occur with methyldopa (Aldomet) (Lishman, 1997; Pottash et al., 1981), and β-blockers such as propranolol have been associated with confusion and impaired cognition, especially in elderly persons (Roy-Byrne and Upadhyaya, 2002; M.A. Taylor, 1999). Croog and his colleagues (1986) compared several kinds of antihypertensive medication on quality-of-life measures and found different patterns of effects on such measurement categories as "general well-being," "sexual dysfunction," "work performance," and "life satisfaction," but no differences for "sleep dysfunction" or "social participation." Comparisons of overweight women with and without hypertension showed that more hypertensive women scored in the negative direction than nonhypertensive ones on seven (of eight) measures of well-being (e.g., General Health, Vitality, Social Functioning), and had significantly higher scores on the Beck Depression Inventory as well as self-report measures of fatigue, anxiety, and "vision loss" (Kleinschmidt et al., 2000). Hypertensive women were taking more medications than the nonhypertensives, raising the chicken–egg question of whether medications affected the quality of life of these women, or "perhaps the use of many medications relates to the severity of symptoms and concurrent problems associated with [hypertension]" (p. 324).

Migraine

The second most common neurological disorder, *migraine,* is a headache condition (Kurtzke, 1984) involving 10%–12% of the adult population (M.D. Ferrari and Haan, 2002). The term *migraine* implies a lateralized headache, although only 60% of migraine headaches occur unilaterally (Derman, 1994). *Aura*, frequently associated with migraine, refers to the initial or presaging symptoms which are frequently unpleasant sensations (see Loring, 1999; p. 205 below).

Classification of headaches has always been somewhat ambiguous. Patients can have more than one type of headache, their headaches may change in nature and frequency over their lifetime, and some headaches are not easily classified. In order to standardize the criteria for diagnosis of headaches and to facilitate the comparison of patients in various studies, a hierarchically constructed set of classification and diagnostic criteria was developed (Headache Classification Committee of the International Headache Society, 1988; S. Solomon, 1997). In this classification system, the term *migraine without aura* replaces *common migraine*. *Migraine with aura* refers to *classic migraine*, a disorder with focal neurological symptoms clearly localizable to the cerebral cortex and/or brainstem. Variants of this condition include prolonged aura, familial hemiplegic migraine, basilar migraine, migraine aura without headache, and migraine with acute onset aura (Silberstein et al., 2002). More unusual migraine disorders have been described.

Risk factors

Estimates of prevalence range from 12.9% to 17.6% in women and from 3.4% to 6.1% in men with the ratio of females exceeding males peaking at age 42 (W.F. Stewart, Shechter, and Rasmussen, 1994; Lipton and Stewart, 1997). Migraine rates appear to vary with race: 24.4% for Caucasians, 16.2% for African-Americans, and 9.2% for Asians, perhaps reflecting a genetic component (W. Stewart, Lipton, and Lieberman, 1996). Hereditary factors appear to play a role in susceptibility to migraine, but this has not yet been demonstrated for all cases (Haan et al., 1997). In familial hemiplegic migraine a link to chromosome 19p has been identified (Mathew, 2000).

Comorbidity with mood disorders (depression, anxiety, and panic attacks) (Breslau et al., 1994; W. Stewart, Breslau, and Keck, 1994; Silberstein, 2001) as well as with epilepsy (Lipton, Ottman, et al., 1994; Silberstein, 2001; Welch and Lewis, 1997), stroke, and essential tremor (Silberstein, 2001) has been established. The basis for these associations is not clear (Lipton and Silberstein, 1994; Merikangas and Stevens, 1997; Silberstein, 2001). It may be bidirectional with depression, epilepsy, stroke, and tremor, suggesting one or more common etiologies. Tailoring pharmacologic intervention to migraines and its comorbidities to individual needs has been recommended (Silberstein, 2001). The notion of a migraine personality was introduced by H.G. Wolff (1937) but evidence does not seem to support it (Lishman, 1997). Although some studies report that migraine patients have a relatively high incidence of questionnaire responses associated with "neurotic signs" or "neuroticism" (e.g., Silberstein, Lipton, and Breslau, 1995), this research failed to take into account score inflation resulting from honest reporting of migraine symptoms and their everyday repercussions.

Various triggers have been known to induce migraines. Consumption of foods such as cheese, chocolate, and alcohol—especially red wine and beer—as well as food additives (nitrates, aspartame, and monosodium glutamate) may precipitate a migraine in some individuals (Victor and Ropper, 2001; Peatfield, 1995). Lack of sleep or too much, missing a meal, or stress can precipitate an attack (Lishman, 1997). Some research has indicated that patients are more likely to have migraines on the weekend, perhaps due to habit changes such as consuming less caffeine, getting up later and sleeping longer, or reduced work-related stress (Couturier, Hering, and Steiner, 1992; Couturier, Laman, et al., 1997); but others disagree (T.G. Lee and Solomon, 1996; Torelli et al., 1999). A fall in estrogen levels has been linked to the production of menstruation-related migraines while sustained high levels of estrogen in the second and third trimesters of pregnancy may lead to their reduction (Silberstein, 1992). Migraines may be better, worse, or unchanged with oral contraceptives, menopause, and postmenopausal hormone replacement therapy (MacGregor, 1997). Some drugs (e.g., nitroglycerine, histamine, reserpine, hydralazine, and ronilidene) can be triggers. Even weather changes, high altitudes, and glare lighting have been implicated (Mathew, 2000).

Pathophysiology

The *vascular theory of migraine* (J.R. Graham and Wolff, 1938) proposed that the aura of a migraine is associated with intracranial vasoconstriction and the headache with a sterile inflammatory reaction around the walls of dilated cephalic vessels (Lauritzen, 1994). This theory is supported by the pain's pulsating aspect, occurrence of headaches with other vascular disorders, successful treatment of some headaches with vasoconstrictors, and evidence pointing to the blood vessels as the source of pain. Yet the vascular theory does not explain all aspects of migraine. For instance, in migraine with aura there appears to be a wave of *oligemia* (reduced blood flow) similar to the "spreading cortical depression of Leao," which starts in the posterior part of the brain and spreads to the parietal and temporal lobes at the rate of 2 to 3 mm/min for 30 to 60 minutes and to a varying extent (Lauritzen, 1987; Leao, 1944). This spreading oligemia follows the cortical surface rather than vascular distributions (Lauritzen, 1994). Thus arterial vasospasm does not appear to be responsible for the reduced blood flow (Goadsby, 1997; Olesen et al., 1990).

The *neurogenic theory of migraine* proposes that the headache is generated centrally and involves the serotonergic and adrenergic pain-modulating systems. Several lines of evidence implicate serotonin: its symptomatic relief of headaches, its drop in blood levels during migraine, and the production of migraines by serotonin antagonists. Enhanced serotonin release increases the release of neuropeptides, including substance *P*, which results in a neurogenic inflammation of intracranial blood vessels and migraine pain (Derman, 1994). Pain appears to arise from vasodilation, primarily of the intracranial blood vessels, and from activation of the central trigeminal system as well (Mathew, 2000).

Cerebral atrophy in migraineurs, visualized by CT and MRI, has reported rates of 4% to 58%, but many of these imaging interpretations may have been based on subjective criteria (R.W. Evans, 1996a). Some imaging studies found an incidence of CT or MRI abnormality no higher than in control subjects (deBenedittis et al., 1995; Ziegler et al., 1991). *White matter abnormalities* (WMAs) visualized on MRI range from 12% to 46% of migraine patients, particularly involving the frontal region, while rates of 2% to 14% occur in headache-free controls (R.W. Evans, 1996a; Filley, 2001). WMA rates are relatively high even for migraineurs under age 50 having no other risk factors (Fazekas et al., 1992; Igarashi et al., 1991). Various explanations for the presence of WMAs in migraine patients include increased water content due to demyelination or interstitial edema, multiple microemboli with lacunar infarcts, chronic low-level vascular insufficiency resulting from vascular instability, and release of vasoconstrictive substances such as serotonin (deBenedittis et al., 1995; Igarashi et al., 1991).

Transient global amnesia (*TGA*) is associated with an increased rate of migraine but these disorders differ in age of onset, frequency of symptoms such as nausea and headache, and occurrence of an aura. TGA tends to occur in middle-aged to elderly individuals, usually lasting for a few hours but generally less than 24 hours. Patients typically have total (rare, partial) amnesia for the events during the attack and a period of retrograde amnesia may be present. Complex routine tasks may be carried out during the episode. Whether stressful events and activities are precipitants is unclear. Focal neurologic signs are absent. The suggestion has been made that these are independent conditions involving paroxysmal dysregulation with a similar mechanism (Nichelli and Menabue, 1988; Schmidtke and Ehmsen, 1998).

The migraine condition

Hours and even days before the onset of the headache, migraineurs may experience a prodrome that involves one or more symptoms such as depression, euphoria, irritability, restlessness, fatigue, drowsiness, frequent yawning, mental slowness, sluggishness, increased urination, fluid retention, diarrhea, constipation, food craving, anorexia, stiff neck, a cold feeling, photophobia, phonophobia, and hyperosmia (Victor and Ropper, 2001; Derman, 1994; Silberstein and Lipton, 1994). An aura of neurological symptoms localizable to the cerebral cortex or brainstem occurs around 5 to 30 minutes before the headache in about 20% to 25% of migraine episodes (J.K. Campbell, 1990; Derman, 1994; Silberstein and Lipton, 1994). Homonymous visual auras are most common and include scintillating lights forming a zig-zag pattern (*techopsia*), scotomas due to bright geometric lights or loss of vision, or blurred or cloudy vision (Rossor, 1993). Objects may even change in shape or size (*micropsia* or *macropsia*) or zoom in and out. Unilateral sensory disturbances such as paresthesias and dysesthesias are less common as are motor disturbances that include weakness of one limb or half the body (*monoplegia, hemiplegia*) and language deficits (Derman, 1994; J.S. Saper et al., 1993). Diplopia, vertigo, dysphagia, and ataxia provide evidence of brainstem involvement. Usually the aura lasts less than an hour but it can continue for several days. It is possible to have the aura without a headache.

The more common unilateral pain during the headache phase typically involves one periorbital region—cheek or ear, although any part of the head and neck can be affected (Derman, 1994). Pain is generally associated with nausea, less often with vomiting. Facial pallor, congestion of face and conjunctiva, nasal stuffiness, light-headedness, painful sensations, impaired concentration, memory impairment, scalp tenderness, or any of the prodromal phase symptoms may occur. Orthostatic hypotension and dizziness have been reported (Mathew, 2000). Pain can be more or less severe and frequently has a pulsating quality. It may be aggravated by exercise or simple head movement (Derman, 1994; Silberstein and Lipton, 1994; Lishman, 1997; Rossor, 1993). The headache lasts a few hours to several days. Migraineurs often feel tired, listless, and depressed during the succeeding hours to days though the converse—feeling refreshed and euphoric—sometimes occurs (Derman, 1994).

Migraines can develop at any time but begin most frequently on arising in the morning. Migraines often compromise functioning for hours to days and, in the rare instance, are life threatening (Ferguson and Robinson, 1982). Very occasionally they may be associated with permanent neurological sequelae from ischemic and hemorrhagic stroke (Estol, 2001; Kolb, 1990; Olesen, Friberg, Olesen, et al., 1993).

Migraine does appear to be a risk factor for stroke (Buring et al., 1995; Merikangas et al., 1997: Tzourio et al., 1995) although the relationship between stroke and migraine is not fully understood (Broderick, 1997; Milhaud et al., 2001; K.M.A. Welch, 1994). Concern has been raised about an increased risk for ischemic stroke in women of child-bearing age who have migraine with aura (Donaghy et al., 2002; Milhaud et al., 2001; Tzourio et al., 1995).

Cognition

Findings from neuropsychological studies have been inconsistent. The performance of college students with classic and common migraines was similar to that of nonmigrainous students on the Halstead-Reitan Neuropsychological Battery (HRNB) as well as on memory tests (Burker et al., 1989). Sinforiani and his colleagues (1987) also reported no impairment on any of a set of tests that assessed a wide range of cognitive functions. These patients had normal CT scans, EEG findings, and neurological examination and had not used any prophylactic treatment in the last month. Leijdekkers and coworkers (1990) studied women who had migraine with and without aura, comparing their performances on the Neurobehavioral Evaluation System (NES) to healthy controls and found no group differences on measures of attention, learning and memory, and motor tasks.

In contrast, Hooker and Raskin (1986) found significantly higher Average Impairment Ratings (AIR) on the HRNB in patients with classic and common migraines compared to normal controls. Performance was particularly poor on several tests of motor speed, dexterity, tactile perception, delayed verbal recall, and aphasia screening. On many of the tests, mean scores of the migraine patients were worse than the control group's means, but the large variances—most notably on tests with skewed distributions (e.g., Trail Making Test-B)—obliterated possible group differences (see Lezak and Gray, 1991, for a discussion of this statistical problem). Zeitlin and Oddy (1984) limited their battery to tests thought to be sensitive to mild cognitive deficits. Cognitive deficits appeared on some measures of attention, information processing speed, and recognition memory.

Subject selection seems to be the factor that most clearly distinguishes the studies reporting cognitive deficits from those that do not. In the Hooker and Raskin (1986) and Zeitlin and Oddy (1984) studies, some of the patients were using prophylactic or symptomatic treatments but this did not appear to account for the group differences. Yet these patients were receiving medical attention for their migraines, raising the possibility that they were experiencing more serious migraine-related symptoms and side effects. However, B.D. Bell and his colleagues (1999) recruited mostly patients with common migraines from specialty pain clinics and found that only about 10% of them showed mild cognitive impairment on five or more of 12 test variables. The migraineurs in the three studies that found no differences between them and control subjects were mostly mildly affected individuals (e.g., not seeking medical attention, normal EEG records).

Treatment

Serotonin agonists have proven useful for treating some migraines. Prophylactic pharmacotherapy involving β-adrenergic blocking agents, tricyclic antidepressants, calcium channel blockers, 5-hydroxytryptamine-2 antagonists, nonsteroidal anti-inflammatory medications, antiepileptics, and magnesium replacement are indicated for other migraines (Ferrari and Haan, 2002; Mathew, 2000). A differential diagnosis of migraine from tension-type headaches and cluster headaches needs to be made to provide optimal treatment. Other disorders such as aneurysms, subarachnoid hemorrhage, subdural hematoma, brain tumor, or idiopathic intracranial hypertension need to be ruled out as well (Mathew, 2000).

DEGENERATIVE DISORDERS

Many disease processes involve progressive deterioration of brain tissue and of behavior. Some of these conditions are commonplace, and others are rare. Nerve cell death is central to the manifest neurological and behavioral changes of degenerative neurological diseases. The selective nature in which nerve cell death occurs in these diseases gives them their characteristic symptoms (Agid and Blin, 1987). For the most part their etiology is unknown or only partially comprehended. With their incidence increasing for each year over age 65, degenerative disorders affect a relatively large proportion of elderly persons (Skoog and Blennow, 2001), with recent estimates of three to four million dementia patients in the United States, annual costs of up to 100 billion dollars (DeKosky and Orgogozo, 2001), and future costs estimated in the 150 billion dollar range (Welsh-Bohmer, Attix, and Mason, 2003). Moreover, these estimates may be low because of underreporting in rural areas (Camicioli, Willert, Lear, et al., 2000). An estimated one-third of those affected are severely impaired (i.e., require full-time care) (U.S. Congress, 1987). Since more persons in industrialized countries are living longer, an escalating number of persons with dementia—and burdened caregivers and care facilities—must be anticipated. In the United States, almost half of all Alzheimer patients receive care in a variety of institutions with annual costs for the severely impaired averaging over $35,000 (J. Leon et al., 1998).

Neuropsychological differences between the degenerative disorders typically show up in the early stages before the disease process has become so widespread as to nullify them. By the time these diseases have run much of their course, their victims tend to share many behavioral features. Prominent among these are psychosocial regression; disorders of attention such as inattentiveness, inability to concentrate or track mentally, and distractibility; apathy, with impaired capacity to initiate, plan, or execute complex activities; and the full spectrum of memory disorders. In the long run, most degenerative conditions become neuropsychologically indistinguishable.

Thus, the following descriptions of degenerative disorders pertain to relatively early symptom presentations when distinguishing characteristics are still present. How many months or years it takes from the first appearance of subtle behavioral harbingers of the disorder to full-blown deterioration varies with the condition and with individual differences. As their cognitive functions deteriorate, patients' sense of person, capacity for judgment, and ability to care for themselves will deteriorate too, although some well-ingrained social habits may still be evident. The end point for most persons suffering these conditions is total dependency, loss of general awareness including loss of sense of self, and inability to make self-serving or goal-directed responses. Death typically results from pneumonia or other diseases associated with inactivity and debilitation (Askin-Edgar, White, and Cummings, 2002; Keene et al., 2001; Filley, 1995).

All of the degenerative disorders and many other chronic brain conditions such as stroke can qualify as *dementias* under the broadest interpretations of this variously defined nosological construct (Sungaila and Crockett, 1993; Mesulam, 2000a). A narrower and commonly used definition of dementia as *global cognitive decline* includes several criteria: *global* implies impairment in more than one aspect of cognitive functioning, always including memory dysfunction, and personality alterations may also contribute to the di-

agnosis; and *decline* indicates that this is an acquired condition thereby excluding the mental dullness of retardation. In addition, the patient must be in a clear state of consciousness (awake and alert), thus distinguishing dementia from delirium, stupor, or other states of altered consciousness (American Psychiatric Association, 2000). *Dementia* typically refers to conditions that are both progressive and irreversible (Knopman and Selnes, 2003; Mesulam, 2000a, pp. 444–445; see Rosenstein, 1998, for a summary of the cardinal neurobehavioral features of the major dementing conditions).

CORTICAL DEMENTIAS

Alzheimer's Disease

By far the most common and best known of the dementias is Alzheimer's disease. It is characterized by inexorably progressive degenerative nerve cell changes within the cerebral hemispheres with concomitant progressive global deterioration of intellect and personality. Examination of brain tissue at autopsy shows the accumulation of *amyloid plaques* and *neurofibrillary tangles* (see pp. 209–210). The various brain regions are differentially affected. Early in the course of the disease, cell loss occurs in the hippocampus and adjacent regions of the temporal lobe. The disease process also invades prefrontal and parietal areas. The primary motor and sensory cortical regions are generally spared. The presence of other brain disorders can complicate the clinical picture (Boller and Duyckaerts, 2003).

More than two-thirds of all cases of dementia are attributed to this condition (Skoog and Blennow, 2001; G.W. Small, Rabins, et al., 1997), with estimates ranging up to 80% (Mesulam, 2000a). For the white U.S. population, prevalence has been estimated to be between 1.7 and 1.9 million persons (Hy and Keller, 2000). Because definitive diagnosis has been made only on biopsy or autopsy (Khachaturian, 1985), the clinical diagnosis of Alzheimer's disease is normally qualified as "possible" or "probable" (Bondi, Salmon, and Kaszniak, 1996; McKhann et al., 1984). Recent refinements in neuroimaging and neurochemical profiling have increased the likelihood of making a definitive diagnosis in live patients (Boller and Duyckaerts, 2003). A diagnosis of *dementia of the Alzheimer's type* (*DAT*), acknowledges both its necessarily questionable nature prior to direct examination of brain tissue and that the clinical syndrome may represent more than one pathological process.

Risk factors

Genetic predisposition. In most cases Alzheimer's disease is sporadic. Yet genetic factors contribute to the risk of acquiring Alzheimer's disease (Andreason, 2001; Skoog and Blennow, 2001). Having a first-degree relative (parent or sibling) with the disease doubles an individual's chance of acquiring it compared to cases with no affected first-degree relatives. In identical twins, various studies report concordance ranging from 21% to 67% (Breitner et al., 1995; Gatz et al., 1997; Jarvik, 1988). A small number of patients inherit mutated autosomal dominant genes which are then passed on in their families. So far, three mutations producing familial forms of the disease have been identified: the *presenilin-1 gene* on chromosome 14, the *presenilin-2 gene* on chromosome 1, and the *amyloid precursor protein (APP)* on chromosome 21 (Andreason, 2001).

Moreover, several predisposing genes have been identified. Of these, the best studied is the gene for a protein called *apolipoprotein ε (ApoE)* on chromosome 19. ApoE is a normally occurring protein that helps carry cholesterol and phospholipids throughout the body. The gene has three variants, of which one—the ε4 allele—increases the risk for a variety of disorders including Alzheimer's disease (Corder et al., 1993; Roses and Saunders, 1997). The association of the ε4 allele with development of plaques and tangles may vary with both age and sex (Ghebremedhin et al., 2001).

Most gene studies have examined white populations. African-Americans and Hispanics with the ε4 allele develop Alzheimer's disease at the same rate as whites by age 90 (Tang, Stern, et al., 1998). However, African-Americans and Hispanics lacking the ε4 allele are likely to develop the disease at two to four times the rate of whites who do not have the ε4 allele.

Alzheimer's disease has also been linked with *Down syndrome*, a condition in which mental retardation features prominently, along with skeletal and other developmental anomalies. Both familial early onset (appearing before age 60) Alzheimer's disease and Down syndrome have been localized to chromosome 21 (Andreasen, 2001; Jarvik, 1988; Pirozzolo, Inbody et al., 1989); and almost all Down patients who live more than 30 or 40 years (many die earlier) show both mental and pathological characteristics of Alzheimer's disease (Skoog and Blennow, 2001). Down syndrome occurs significantly more frequently in families with a history of Alzheimer's disease than in those without such a history (Heyman et al., 1983).

Demographic factors. The major risk factor for Alzheimer's disease is age (Bondi, Salmon, and Kaszniak, 1996). Although this disease can appear in people as young as 30, most cases occur after 60. Someone with no family history of Alzheimer's disease has a 15% lifetime risk of getting it (Seshadri et al., 1995),

but this risk varies greatly with age. Approximately 1% of 65-year-olds receive this diagnosis. Its incidence doubles every five years beyond age 65 (D.L. Bachman, Wolf, et al., 1993). As many as 50% of 85-year-olds have Alzheimer's disease. Data on very old people give greatly varying rates of incidence, from almost 50% at age 85 (D.A. Evans et al., 1989) to "a substantial group" of people 100–107 years old "in good cognitive health" (M.H. Silver and Perls, 2000).

Most studies report a higher prevalence in women (Brookmeyer et al., 1998; Gao et al., 1998), although the reverse may be true for African-Americans (Fillenbaum et al., 1998). However, it is likely that this increased prevalence rate merely reflects women's longer life expectancy (Bondi, Salmon, and Kaszniak, 1996). Perhaps genetically based, small differences have appeared among the races. African-Americans and Hispanics may have a slightly higher risk ratio than whites (Tang, Cross, et al., 2001), while whites may have slightly higher risks than Japanese and Chinese people (Jorm and Jolley, 1998). However, racial differences have not always been found (Fillenbaum et al., 1998; Mortimer, 1988b).

Low educational and occupational levels have been associated with an increased risk for developing Alzheimer's disease (Bondi, Salmon, and Kaszniak, 1996; Schmand, Smit, et al., 1997; Y. Stern, Gurland, et al., 1994). One large study found this association only for women (Ott, van Rossum, et al., 1999). For women (men were not studied), even low linguistic ability in early life has been associated with increased risk of the disease (Snowdon et al., 1996). A common explanation of this finding is that people with higher levels of education have more "cognitive reserve" to compensate for the neuropathological changes resulting from the disease and to delay the onset of its clinical presentation (Y. Stern, 2002). The reserve capacity may represent a brain potential present at birth, an acquired factor such as proliferation of synaptic connections related to cognitive stimulation, or ability to use effective compensatory cognitive strategies (Mortimer, 1997; Y. Stern, Gurland, et al., 1994).

Traumatic brain injury. The role of TBI as a risk factor for developing Alzheimer's disease is still somewhat controversial. Many studies have reported a significantly high incidence of TBI history for Alzheimer's patients (e.g., Lye and Shores, 2000; Mortimer, French, et al., 1985; Rocca et al., 1986; Schofield et al., 1997) but not all (A.S. Henderson and Hasegawa, 1992; Mehta et al., 1999). Risk of developing Alzheimer's disease after a severe TBI is greatest for subjects lacking the *ApoE4* allele (Guo et al., 2000; Jellinger, Paulus et al., 2001). In one study of particular interest because of its prospective design, World War II veterans with documented head injuries were assessed for dementia more than 50 years later. Those who had moderate to severe TBIs as young men had higher prevalences of Alzheimer's disease than did veterans without TBI (Plassman et al., 2000).

The cognitive and personality changes that are part of the "punch drunk" syndrome of boxers share many characteristics with the mental alterations of Alzheimer's disease, and the brains of Alzheimer patients and demented boxers show similar pathological changes at autopsy (Mortimer, French, et al., 1985).

Other risk factors. Low levels of estrogen in postmenopausal women may increase the risk of developing Alzheimer's disease. Several epidemiologic studies suggest that women who use estrogen replacement therapy lower their risk of developing the disease (Brinton, 2001; Waring et al., 1999; Yaffe et al., 1998). However, there has been no definitive randomized study of estrogen replacement therapy with long-term follow-up, and data from epidemiological studies may be misleading (V.W. Henderson, 1997). For example, the generally higher educational and socioeconomic levels of women on estrogen replacement therapy could bias study findings. Several randomized, placebo-controlled studies are underway. For example, a relationship between cerebrovascular risk factors and Alzheimer's disease is under investigation (Aguero-Torres and Winblad, 2000; Forette, Seux, et al., 1998).

In some epidemiologic studies smoking appears to have a protective effect (e.g., Fratiglioni and Wang, 2000). A review of epidemiologic studies ruled out this effect and suggested, rather, that smoking may be a modest risk factor but only for persons without the ApoE4 allele (Kukull, 2001; Ott, Slooter, et al., 1998). Yet in another study no effects of smoking appeared (Debanne et al., 2000). Elevated systolic blood pressure ($\geq$160 mm Hg) and high serum cholesterol ($\geq$6.5 mmol/l) in middle-aged persons have also been implicated as risk factors, with increased rate of risk when both blood pressure and cholesterol levels are elevated (Kivipelto et al., 2001).

Neuroanatomy and pathophysiology

The neuropathological hallmark of Alzheimer's disease is the presence of neurofibrillary tangles and senile plaques (W. Samuel et al., 2002; Zubenko, 1997). Neurofibrillary tangles develop when microtubules that transport substances from the nerve cell body to the end of the axon become twisted. The protein that helps maintain the structure of these tubules is *tau*. In Alzheimer's disease tau is altered, allowing twisted tubules to aggregate into tangles. They appear early in the course of the disease in the entorhinal cortex, hippocampus, and other regions of the temporal lobe (Boller and Duyckaerts, 2003; Delacourte et al., 1999; Hyman and Gomez-Isla, 1998). As the disease progresses they show up increasingly in other neocortical areas (with relative sparing of primary sensory and motor cortex) and in specific brainstem nuclei—the nucleus basalis of Meynert (or basal nucleus) in the forebrain, the nucleus raphe dorsalis (raphe nucleus) in the midbrain, and the locus coeruleus at the anterior pontine level (L. Berg and Morris, 1990; Hyman and Gomez-Isla, 1998). Density of neurofibrillary tangles correlates positively with dementia severity (L. Berg, McKeel, et al., 1998; Delacourte et al, 1999). Neurofibrillary tangles also are present in the autopsied brains of elderly nondemented subjects but then are mostly confined to the hippocampal region and rarely occur in the cortex (Crystal, Dickson, et al., 1993; Delacourte et al., 1999). These tangles are many times more numerous in Alzheimer patients than in control subjects (e.g., in one midbrain region 39 times as many were found in Alzheimer patients [Yamamoto and Hirano, 1985]).

Senile (neuritic) plaques are extracellular products by-products of neuronal degeneration. In Alzheimer's disease the *amyloid precursor protein* (*APP*) is clipped at the wrong segment during metabolism, resulting in the production of an undesirable fragment, *beta-amyloid* (β-*amyloid*) (Skoog and Bennow, 2001; Strange, 1992; Zubenko, 1997). These β-amyloid fragments aggregate into plaques which act "like 'brain sludge,' destroying the capacity of neurons to communicate with one another" (Andreasen, 2001, p. 264). Free oxygen radicals have been implicated in β-amyloid production. While commonly seen throughout the cortex of Alzheimer patients, they occur subcortically as well, particularly in the thalamus, hypothalamus, and mammillary bodies (Cummings, 1990; McDuff and Sumi, 1985).

Whether Alzheimer's disease evolves from neurofibrillary tangles and neuritic plaques or whether these are by-products of the disease process is unknown (Andreasen, 2001; Mesulam, 2000a, see pp. 484–485). The autopsied brains of some cognitively intact very elderly persons displayed abundant levels of both these disease markers (Snowdon, 1997). Nevertheless, plaques and tangles in patients younger than 70 are strongly associated with the disease. Current research into treatments for Alzheimer's disease involves drugs that avert the formation of amyloid plaques (Janus et al., 2000) or that may be protective against their formation. Antioxidants such as red wine may have such a protective effect (Orgogozo, Dartigues, et al., 1997). It may also be possible to develop a drug that will keep tau in its normal form, thereby avoiding production of neurofibrillary tangles. The possibility that such drugs could prevent dementia must still be explored (Cutler, Sramek, and Gauthier, 2001).

Neuronal loss is another common feature of Alzheimer's disease (Gomez-Isla, Hollister, et al., 1997). It involves larger neurons in the neocortex, with the greatest loss in the temporal lobes (Strange, 1992) and the brainstem nuclei, particularly the basal nucleus and the locus coeruleus (R.D. Terry and Katzman, 1983; Mann et al., 1984; Yamamoto and Hirano, 1985). Loss of functional synapses in midfrontal and lower (inferior) parietal areas surrounding the temporal lobes correlated highly ($r = .96$) with a global measure of dementia (Mattis Dementia Rating Scale) (R.D. Terry, Masliah, et al., 1991). This patterned loss of cortical function disconnects temporal lobe structures from the rest of the cerebral cortex, thus making an important contribution to the prominent memory disorders in this disease (A.R. Damasio, Van Hoesen, and Hyman, 1990; Geula, 1998; Heun et al., 1997; Juottonen, et al., 1998). This pattern of cortical degeneration also appears to disconnect prefrontal from parietal structures (Braak et al., 2000), which may account for the early compromise of the capacity for divided and shifting attention (Parasuraman and Greenwood, 1998; Parasuraman and Haxby, 1993).

Neuronal loss, especially in the three brainstem areas—the nucleus basalis of Meynert, the raphe nucleus, and the locus coeruleus—appears to be related to reduced production of neurotransmitters by these centers in particular and by other brain structures (Engelborghs and De Deyn, 1997). Neurons in the nucleus basalis of Meynert contain cholinergic enzymes that provide the chief contributions to cholinergic projections to the cerebral cortex and hippocampus. Along with cholinergic depletion, which occurs early in the course of the disease (Cummings, Vinters, et al., 1998), comes loss of cortical nicotinic acetylcholine receptors, which are necessary for effective cortical neurotransmission (Court et al., 2001; Nordberg, 2001). The accompanying degeneration of the cholinergic projection system is a characteristic of Alzheimer's disease that may also play an important role in the memory disorder symptoms (Geula, 1998; Kopelman, 1987c; Van Hoesen, 1990). Abnormalities in the noradrenergic and serotoninergic systems in Alzheimer's disease have been associated with neuronal loss in the locus coeruleus and the raphe nucleus, respectively (Palmer, 1996); and other neurotransmitter systems are also affected (Skoog and Blennow, 2001; W. Samuel et al., 2002).

Loss of neurons typically—ultimately—results in gross anatomic alterations of the brain which appear most obviously as enlarged ventricles and a thinning of the cortical mantle. Neuroimaging techniques show this prominent atrophy pattern (H. Damasio and Damasio, 1989; R.P. Friedland and Luxenberg, 1988; Jack, Petersen, Xu et al., 1999) with pronounced volume reductions in and around the temporal lobes (Heun et al., 1997), and in both the basal ganglia and the thalamus (Jernigan, Salmon, et al., 1991). Temporal lobe volume loss may occur years prior to clinical evidence of dementia (Kaye, Swihart et al., 1997). An inflammatory process may also contribute to the disease manifestations (Akiyama et al., 2000; Fassbender et al., 2000). However, variability in the nature and extent of atrophic changes of both Alzheimer patients and nondemented elderly persons, and the gross pathologic similarities between Alzheimer's disease, other dementing conditions, and mixed dementias preclude reliance on visualization techniques alone for diagnostic discrimination (Ettlin et al., 1989; Skoog and Bennow, 2001). Nevertheless, when coupled with neuropsychological studies, high rates of diagnostic accuracy have been reported (Laakso et al., 2000; P.J. Visser et al., 1999).

Studies of brain metabolism in Alzheimer patients consistently show reduced metabolic activity in both anterior and posterior association areas, occurring most severely in posterior temporal and contiguous parietal and occipital regions (M. Grossman, Payer, et al., 1997; Ibanez et al., 1998; Waldemar et al., 1997). Patients vary considerably both in degree and in anterior/posterior ratio of diminished metabolic activity (Haxby, Grady, et al., 1988). Patterns of reductions in cerebral metabolism correlate with patterns of cognitive deficits (M.S. Albert, Duffy, and McAnulty, 1990; Desgranges et al., 1998; Eustache, Desgranges, et al., 2001). Reduced metabolism in frontal areas is closely associated with dementia severity. Alzheimer patients show a general lowering of cerebral blood flow with some indications that the greatest flow reductions may be in the parietal lobe (Besson et al., 1989; G. Deutsch and Tweedy, 1987; Keilp et al., 1996; Van Hoesen and Damasio, 1987). Nobili and his colleagues (2001) found that measurements of regional cerebral blood flow in a posterior temporal–inferior parietal area were predictive of the disease's evolution. At the cellular level, defective glucose metabolism has been demonstrated (Strange, 1992).

Electrophysiologic studies also reflect the underlying degenerative process (F.H. Duffy, Albert, and McAnulty, 1984; Kurlychek, 1989; A. Stevens and Kircher, 1998). Slowed processing shows up in abnormally long response latencies of evoked and event-related potentials (ERPs) (Goodin and Aminoff, 1986; B.F. O'Donnell, Friedman, et al., 1990; Zappoli, 1988), with slowing increasing as the disease progresses (S.S. Ball et al.,

1989; St. Clair et al., 1988). Slowed brain electrical activity appears on EEG, too (Coburn et al., 1993; Jelic et al., 1998).

Disease process

Course. When the disease progresses slowly, one or more stage will be relatively prolonged; when progression is erratic, the duration of each stage may differ markedly (Rubin, Morris, Grant, and Vendegna, 1989). Estimated from onset, one group of patients had shown symptoms of the disease for an average of 8 years (L.L. Barclay et al., 1985), with duration of about a decade from diagnosis to death (Askin-Edgar, White, and Cummings, 2002). However, the interval between diagnosis and death can be as long as 15 to 20 years (Mesulam, 2000a).

Alzheimer's disease typically begins so insidiously that many families are unaware of a problem until work-related problems pile up or a sudden disruption in routine leaves the patient disoriented, confused, and unable to deal with the unfamiliar situation. Because the early behavioral decline is so gradual and unsuspected and because most basic abilities—e.g., language and sensory and motor functions—usually remain intact in the early stages of the disease, it is difficult to date exactly the onset of the clinical symptoms. Moreover, early evidence of inattentiveness, mild cognitive dulling, social withdrawal, and emotional blunting or agitation are often confused with depression so that it is not uncommon to find an Alzheimer patient who has recently been treated for depression (Kaszniak, Sadeh, and Stern, 1985). Even with hindsight it may be difficult to distinguish the patient's premorbid personality and emotional disturbances from the earliest symptoms and reactions to the evolving experience of personal disintegration (Brun et al., 1990).

The sequence in which cognitive functions first show deterioration generally begins with memory but also with complex mental tracking (e.g., Trail Making Test-B) and verbal fluency (M.S. Albert, Moss, Tanzi, and Jones, 2001). Delayed recall of verbal and visuospatial material often deteriorates quickly to an early floor. Thus immediate recall, category fluency, and confrontation naming may be better for staging dementia severity because they show a steady linear decline (Locascio, Growdon, and Corkin, 1995). Similarly, symbol substitution and construction tests usually decline steadily. As the disease progresses, cognitive impairment becomes broad and severe. Aphasia and apraxia, which may appear in the early stages of the disease, become prominent problems later, along with various agnosias (Chobor and Brown, 1990). Dysfluency, paraphasias and bizarre word combinations, and intrusions are common midstage speech defects. Late in the disease course, many functions can no longer be measured, whether due to patients' inability to cooperate or loss of the functions themselves. In very late stages speech becomes nonfluent, repetitive, and largely noncommunicative, and auditory comprehension is exceedingly limited, with many patients displaying partial or complete mutism (Au et al., 1988). Primitive reflexes appear more frequently in the late stage of the disease (Franssen and Reisberg, 1997; Hogan and Ebly, 1995). In a very general sense, the pattern of functional regression is the inverse of normal developmental stages (Emery, 2000; Reisberg, Ferris, Borenstein, et al., 1990).

When comparing groups, decline appears to take place at a steady rate across functions (e.g., Grady, Haxby, et al., 1988; Storandt, Botwinick, and Danziger, 1986); but examination of individual test protocols shows a great deal of variability between functions as well as between patients (Grady, Haxby, et al., 1988; Marra et al., 2000). After the initial appearance of memory dysfunction, cognitive deterioration may be arrested for as long as nine months to almost three years (Haxby, Raffaele, et al., 1992). Once nonmemory functions begin to decline, mental deterioration proceeds to its inevitable end.

Clinical subtypes. Age-based differences underlie the once generally accepted distinction between *presenile* (onset under age 65) and *senile* (onset at age 65 or later) *dementia.* Although diagnostic codes still make this distinction, there is little reason to believe that someone who develops the disease at age 62 has a different disease from someone who develops it at age 68. However, age at onset does affect the rate of decline (see *Predicting course,* below).

Greater involvement of one hemisphere than the other occurs in approximately 20% to 40% of patients (J.T. Becker, Huff, et al., 1988; A. Martin, Brouwers, Lalonde, et al., 1986; Strite et al., 1997); one study reports a percentage of 77% (N.J. Fisher et al., 1999). Lateralization of deficits tends to appear in typical patterns in which verbal/detail oriented functions or visuospatial/globally (configurationally) oriented functions are coupled, remaining relatively intact or deteriorating together (Delis, Massman, Butters, et al., 1992; Massman, Delis, Filoteo, et al., 1993). Although premorbid abilities and age-related decline might account for some lateralized performances, the presumption is that the disease affects the hemispheres asymmetrically. Asymmetrical lesions have been found at autopsy (Moossy et al., 1989), and greater language impairment or visuospatial deficits tend to correlate with MRI findings (N.C. Fox et al., 1996) or lowered brain metabolism in one hemisphere (Franceschi et al., 1995; R.P.

Friedland et al., 1985; A. Martin, Brouwers, Lalonde, et al., 1986).

Other clinical subtypes have been observed (Mitrushina, Uchiyama, and Satz, 1995). Notable is the *posterior variant* or *visual variant* (Benson, Davis, and Snyder, 1988; Furey-Kurkjian et al., 1996). Early in the course of this subtype prominent visual disturbances occur such as visual agnosia, prosopagnosia, alexia, and Balint's syndrome. Memory may be relatively preserved early on; however, a full dementia syndrome eventually develops (D.N. Levine, Lee, and Fisher, 1993). Unlike typical cases of Alzheimer's disease, neuropathological studies show an occipitoparietal focus (Hof et al., 1993; D.N. Levine, Lee, and Fisher, 1993). These different subtypes—of which a few tend to be recurrent while many others are relatively unique—appears to reflect different pathologic vulnerabilities between or within hemispheres (Joanette, Melançon, et al., 1993; Joanette, Ska, Poissant, 1994).

Diagnosis and prediction

Severity classification. Although "stages" of dementia often refers to its time course (i.e., "early," "middle," "late"), these terms also refer to the severity of the disease, meaning, respectively: "mild," "moderate," and "severe." The *Clinical Dementia Rating (CDR)* scale which is widely used in dementia research, rates severity on a 5-point scale where 0 is no evidence of dementia. Ratings are based on memory and other cognitive abilities; temporal orientation, judgment and problem solving, community activities, and home activities and hobbies. *Questionable dementia* (CDR 0.5) is defined either as mild consistent forgetfulness or slight problems with two or more other cognitive areas. *Mild dementia* (CDR 1) is either moderate difficulty with recent recall that interferes with daily activities or mild forgetfulness with mild to moderate impairment in three or more other cognitive areas, which may also include needing prompting for personal hygiene. *Moderate dementia* (CDR 2) is severe memory loss or moderate memory loss with severe impairment in three or more other cognitive areas, which may also include requiring assistance with personal hygiene or dressing. *Severe dementia* (CDR 3) involves severe memory loss with only memory fragments, orientation to person only, inability to make judgments or solve problems, no independent function inside or outside the home, inability to perform personal care and, often, incontinence.

Diagnostic issues. No single marker or set of markers for reliable positive identification of Alzheimer's disease in living patients has yet been found. Short of autopsy, this is a diagnosis of exclusion, made only af-

TABLE 7.4 Exclusion Criteria for Diagnosis of Alzheimer's Disease

Age-related cognitive decline

Delirium

Depression

Drug abuse

Human immunodeficiency virus

Medical conditions: e.g., hypothyroidism, vitamin B_{12} deficiency, systemic illness

Medication side effects

Other central nervous system degenerative diseases

Vascular disorders: e.g., stroke, multi-infarct dementia

ter ruling out other possible causes of memory disorder or dementia (see Table 7.4). The clinical diagnosis relies on information from a variety of sources, following diagnostic guidelines (Geldmacher and Whitehouse, 1996, 1997; McKhann et al., 1984; Tierney et al., 1988). Such information includes patient and family history, a neurological examination, physiological and neuroradiographic studies, and laboratory assessments to help rule out other—particularly reversible—conditions. With these criteria diagnostic accuracy, as tested by biopsy or autopsy, may run as high as 86% of cases (Tierney et al., 1988; J.C. Morris, McKeel, Fulling, et al., 1988)—100% in one small series (E.M. Martin et al., 1987). Even very mildly impaired early Alzheimer patients can be identified with a high degree of accuracy using informant reports and clinical judgment (J.C. Morris, McKeel, Storandt, et al., 1991). Slowed event related potential (ERP: P300) can occur prior to the appearance of cognitive or behavioral symptoms (Matsumoto, 2002). Yet much of the diagnosis will ultimately rely on the quantitative pattern and qualitative characteristics of cognitive functioning elicited by neuropsychological assessment (e.g., M.S. Albert, Moss, Tanzi, and Jones, 2001). Derrer, Howieson, and their colleagues (2001) found that three memory tests—CERAD Word List Acquisition, WMS-R Logical Memory II (i.e., delayed recall), and Visual Reproduction II—could distinguish patients with mild dementia from age-matched controls with 100% sensitivity and 92% accuracy.

Characteristic cognitive impairment patterns have been determined for most dementing conditions, which aid in identifying the probable Alzheimer patient (Derix, 1994; S. Hart and Semple, 1990; Askin-Edgar, White and Cummings, 2002; see specific disorders below). The most distinguishing cognitive feature of Alzheimer's disease is a relatively severe verbal memory disorder, with other deficits likely in orientation, speeded psychomotor performance, language and speech fluency, and complex reasoning (Howieson, Dame, et al., 1997; D.M. Jacobs, Sano, Dooneief, et al., 1995; Mungas et al., 1998). Constructional deficits are also common. Alzheimer patients typically score highest on tests of overlearned behaviors presented in a familiar format and immediate memory recall. Many perform quite well on WIS-A tests of Information, Vocabulary, many Comprehension and Similarities items, and Digits Forward, some even when they cannot care for themselves. The more the task is unfamiliar, abstract, and speed-dependent and the more it taxes patients' dwindling capacity for attention and learning, the more likely they will do poorly: Block Design, Digit Symbol, and Digits Backward typically vie for the bottom rank among WIS-A test scores.

MRI evidence of hippocampal atrophy can also contribute to a diagnosis of Alzheimer's disease (Jack, Petersen, et al., 1999; Kaye, Swihart, et al., 1997). The combination of memory impairment and hippocampal atrophy is better than either one alone (Laakso et al., 2000; P.J. Visser et al., 1999). PET studies have typically shown reduced glucose metabolism in the inferior parietal, frontal, and lateral temporal cortex and in the posterior cingulate (see p. 210). Similar decreases in perfusion have been seen with SPECT measurements (K.A. Johnson et al., 1998). A meta-analysis of 27 studies examining the diagnosis of Alzheimer's disease found that measures of memory were most sensitive, hippocampus volume on MRI was next and more sensitive than PET or SPECT (P.J. Visser et al., 1999).

Predicting course. No strong predictors of rate of cognitive decline have yet emerged as different studies have provided different findings (R. Gould et al., 2001). Examiners are still missing a "yardstick" that reliably describes the stage of the disease. Many studies have used the Mini-Mental State Examination (MMSE) or the Mattis Dementia Rating Scale to determine disease stage (see Chapter 18). Whether medications will be able to slow the disease course significantly or even halt it remains a question dependent upon continuing pharmacologic research (Bédard, Lévesque, et al., 2003).

Age at onset is a significant predictor in some studies, with early onset associated with faster decline (D. Jacobs, Sano, et al., 1994; Koss, Edland, et al., 1996; Teri, McCurry, et al., 1995; R.S. Wilson, Gilley, et al., 2000b), but not in all studies (Bracco et al., 1994). Higher education has been associated with faster decline (R. Gould et al., 2001; Rasmusson et al., 1996; Teri, McCurry, et al., 1995). No relationship between rate of decline and sex has emerged (B.J. Small, Viitanen, et al., 1997; Teri, McCurry, et al., 1995). Extrapyramidal signs (tremor, rigidity, and bradykinesia) have been associated with a slightly faster course

in some studies (C.M. Clark et al., 1997; Samson et al., 1996; Storandt, Morris, Rubin, et al., 1992) but not all (Rasmusson et al., 1996). Effects of ApoE4 on rate of cognitive decline remain inconclusive (Craft, Teri, et al., 1998; Dal Forno et al., 1996). Nonright-handedness and family history of dementia have been associated with faster decline (Rasmusson et al., 1996). Race showed a slight effect in one study with whites declining faster than African-Americans (Fillenbaum, Peterson, et al., 1998).

Some cognitive variables also have predictive value (Bracco et al., 1994; Faber-Langendoen et al., 1988). Patients with significant language dysfunction deteriorated more rapidly than those with relatively intact language skills. Both syntactic impairment and poor performance on Block Design have been implicated in faster decline (Rasmusson et al., 1996). Studying patients ranging in age from 75 to 95, B.J. Small, Herlitz, and their colleagues (1997) found that higher initial MMSE scores were associated with faster rate of decline but that progression was slower when Digits Forward and Block Design were initially superior; for this group, age, sex, and education had no predictive value.

Cognition

Although Alzheimer's disease affects every area of behavior, the cognitive changes—and particularly the memory deficits—are the most obvious early symptoms and have attracted the most research attention. The overall patterns of cognitive deterioration in Alzheimer's disease are well established. Also well established are the differences among patients: probably no two patients present in the same manner, nor are patterns of deterioration identical as different functions deteriorate at different rates for the individual patient as well as for different patients. Yet the overall course of the disease runs consistently downhill so that at the end all functions are lost and all patients reach a similar stage of behavioral dilapidation.

Sensorimotor status. Visual dysfunction in Alzheimer's disease shows up in reduced contrast sensitivity as well as other changes (Mendola et al., 1995; Gilmore and Whitehouse, 1995); patients may have defects in inferior visual fields (Trick et al., 1995). Visuoperceptual deficits are common (Cogan, 1985; Eslinger and Benton, 1983; Mendez, Martin, et al., 1990). They show up prominently on tests requiring visual discrimination, analysis, spatial judgments, and perceptual organization. Severity increases over time, but the pattern of dysfunction can vary greatly between patients as specific deficits tend to be independent of one another and do not necessarily worsen at similar rates. For example, Della Sala, Kinnear, and their coworkers (2000) found that three of 33 patients displayed impaired color processing. Object recognition, which requires intact inferotemporal cortex, tends to be more impaired than the visuospatial abilities associated with the posterior parietal cortex (Kurylo et al., 1996; see also Fujimori et al., 2000). Auditory acuity appears to be no more of a problem in Alzheimer's disease than in the aging population generally. Tone perception may remain intact (D.A. White and Murphy, 1998).

Olfactory acuity, measured by recognition, is typically impaired early in the disease course (R.L. Doty, Reyes, and Gregor, 1987; Nores et al., 2000; Koss, Weiffenbach, et al., 1988), but pleasantness discrimination is retained (Royet et al., 2001). Olfactory deficits in patients with mild cognitive impairments may predict the eventual development of Alzheimer's disease (Devanand, Michaels-Marston, et al., 2000). On finding neurofibrillary tangles and cell loss in olfactory nuclei, Esiri and Wilcock's (1984) conclusion that "the olfactory sensory pathway is significantly affected in Alzheimer's disease" is consistent with the behavioral data. Reductions in left hippocampal volume are also associated with impaired odor identification in Alzheimer patients (C. Murphy et al., 2003).

Apart from impairments in eye movements and except in the very late stages when all systems are involved, motor system disorders are infrequent, occurring in about 16% of cases (Koller, Wilson, et al., 1984; Mesulam, 2000a). However, patients do poorly on complex motor tasks, better when the tasks are less complex (Kluger, Gianutsos, et al., 1997).

Attention. Attentional deficits are part of the symptom picture of Alzheimer's disease, although all patients may not display such problems, particularly in the early stages (A. Martin, 1990; Parasuraman and Haxby, 1993). Moreover, alertness appears to remain unaffected, at least for mildly to moderately demented patients (McKhann et al., 1984; Nebes and Brady, 1993).

Impairments in nearly all aspects of attention have been reported, including defective focusing and shifting (Freed, Corkin, et al., 1989; Nebes and Brady, 1989; Oken, Kishiyama, et al., 1994) and slowed reaction times (J.K. Foster et al., 1999; Sano, Rosen, et al., 1995). However, simple attention span may remain near normal. For example, many severely impaired patients who still have some verbal skills can correctly repeat five digits forward (e.g., R.S. Wilson and Kaszniak, 1986). Cognitive slowing results in longer reaction times for these patients (J.K. Foster et al., 1999; Sano, Rosen, Stern, et al., 1995). Deficits in dividing and shifting attention may be the earliest indi-

cators of cortical dysfunction, with capacities for arousal and responsive focusing affected only later as the disease progresses (Baddeley, Baddeley, et al., 2001; Nebes, 1992a; Parasuraman and Haxby, 1993; R.J. Perry and Hodges, 1999). These deficits increase in severity with both task complexity and disease progression. The practical implications of these deficits show up in escalating social dependency and deteriorating personal habits (Vitaliano et al., 1984). When talking while walking, patients unable to do more than one thing at a time are at a heightened risk of falling (Camicioli, Howieson, et al., 1997).

Orientation. Temporal orientation and knowledge of current events are often compromised (e.g., Brandt, Folstein, and Folstein, 1988) even early in the course of this disease, although impaired orientation alone is unlikely to be the first symptom (Huff, Becker, et al., 1987). Orientation may remain intact after deterioration of other functions has become evident (Eisdorfer and Cohen, 1980; O'Donnell, Drachman, et al., 1988).

Memory and learning. Early in their course, Alzheimer patients present memory problems. Memory problems—particularly verbal memory deficits—show up on tests several years before the dementia diagnosis is warranted (M.S. Albert, Moss, Tanzi, and Jones, 2001; Bäckman et al., 2001; Bondi, Monsch, Galasko, et al., 1994; Howieson, Dame, et al., 1997; Linn, Wolf, et al., 1995; Masur, Sliwinski, et al., 1994; see Table 7.5, p. 215). Elderly community-dwelling subjects were followed longitudinally: memory functioning of those who subsequently developed Alzheimer's disease was compared with memory findings of those who continued to show no clinical signs of dementia. These studies pave the way for very early treatment of the disease as drugs are now being developed that slow its progression.

The nature of the learning defect has been studied with a variety of techniques, mostly looking at aspects of verbal memory. Almost from disease onset, Alzheimer patients show deficits in acquisition and retention of information. On tests of free recall, whether of meaningful material (sentences, stories) or on rote learning tasks, Alzheimer patients perform very poorly (Brandt, Spencer, et al., 1988; N. Butters, Granholm, et al., 1987; Mitrushina, Drebing et al., 1994; Petersen, Smith, Ivnik, et al., 1994),), displaying the most severe losses on the earliest stimuli presented in a series (*primacy effect*) (Massman, Delis, and Butters, 1993). Learning and/or retrieval processes sustain the most significant impairment in the early stages, with increasingly lower rates of acquisition of new information, whether on rote learning tasks or in remembering ongoing personal experiences or passing events, until the

TABLE 7.5 Memory in Alzheimer's Disease

LEARNING, RECALL, AND RECOGNITION

Learning: flat learning curve across trials

Delayed recall: very poor after even a short delay

Repetitions: often frequent

Intrusions: often frequent

Recognition memory: impaired, indicating storage problems

Positive response bias: false positive errors

ENCODING, STORAGE, AND RETRIEVAL

Encoding and retrieval: impaired, but overshadowed by storage problem

Storage (consolidation): failure to store new information

Rate of forgetting: rapid

AMNESIA

Anterograde: evident early

Retrograde: also early, but difficult to measure

TYPES OF MEMORY

Episodic (verbal and visual): severe early

Semantic: impaired

Implicit (unconscious memory): impaired semantic priming, intact perceptual priming

Procedural relatively intact

Temporal orientation: impaired relatively early and progressive, reflects both anterograde and retrograde amnesia

NEUROPATHOLOGY

Impaired episodic memory: bilateral medial temporal: hippocampus (CA1, entorhinal cortex, subiculum), amygdala, parahippocampal gyrus

Impaired semantic and implicit memory: association cortex

Impaired organization, encoding, and source memory: frontal lobes

Intact procedural memory: relatively intact basal ganglia

Adapted from Zec (1993)

learning capacity is lost (Grafman, Weingartner, Lawlor, et al., 1990; Hodges, 2000). Contributing to this learning deficit is defective encoding, which in turn appears to be due to failure to remember or call up the encoding process, so that impaired learning in Alzheimer's disease appears to be the result of a double impairment in the learning process (J.T. Becker, 1988; Buschke, Sliwinski, et al., 1997; Carlesimo et al., 1998).

The most sensitive measure of the memory deficit is delayed memory. When acquisition scores approach normal levels, this deficit may be seen in low savings scores (Larrabee, Youngjohn, et al., 1993; B.R. Reed, Paller, and Mungas, 1998; Tröster, Butters, Salmon, et al., 1993; Welsh et al., 1994). Rapid forgetting characterizes Alzheimer patients after they demonstrated acquisition on both verbal (e.g., grocery list) and visual-

verbal (e.g., face–name associations) learning trials (Larrabee, Youngjohn, et al., 1993). Once visual stimuli have been learned, some studies showed that rate of forgetting is about that of normal persons although, of course, the Alzheimer patients' initial retention is well below that of normals (Huppert and Kopelman, 1989; Kopelman, 1985); others demonstrated a rapid fall-out over the first two hours, but what is left may be retained for at least two days (R.P. Hart, Kwentus, Taylor, and Harkins, 1987; R.P. Hart, Kwentus, Harkins, and Taylor, 1988). Moreover, some patients in the early stages of the disease show better retention of a set of stimuli at three days than at one day (the *rebound phenomenon*) (Freed, Corkin, et al., 1989).

Retrieval problems show up in several ways: in much lower recall than what is elicited by recognition and priming techniques (Heindel, Salmon, et al., 1989); in impaired performance of verbal fluency tests; and in defective remote memory (R.S. Wilson, Kaszniak, and Fox, 1981). Alzheimer patients' responses may include as many or more intrusions or other kinds of errors as correct answers (Cahn et al., 1997; Gainotti and Marra, 1994; J.H. Kramer, Levin, et al., 1989; Manning et al., 1996), and they do not benefit from repetition (Weingartner, Eckardt, et al., 1993).

Mildly impaired patients may perform normally on recognition tests. However, even when aided by a recognition format, Alzheimer patients beyond the early stage of the disease perform significantly below normal levels on visual as well as verbal tasks (Heindel, Salmon, et al., 1989; Moss, Albert, Butters, and Payne, 1986); they give a large proportion of false positive responses ("false alarms") due to poor discrimination between target items and distractors (Deweer, Pillon, et al., 1993). Cueing has been frequently used to assess the full learning potential of these patients, but many studies found that verbal cueing—whether with learning trials or as an aid to recall—does not help (N. Butters, Albert, Sax, et al., 1983; Herlitz and Viitanen, 1991; Petersen, Smith, Ivnik, et al., 1994). However, strong associational cues at recall can enhance patients' performance (Buschke, Sliwinski, et al., 1997; Granholm and Butters, 1988) and cueing with associated motor acts improves verbal recall (Karlsson et al., 1989). Self-generated cues are more effective than cues provided by the examiner (Lipinska et al., 1994).

Alzheimer patients do not appear to benefit from gist (Nebes, 1992b) or other conceptual relationships (e.g., semantic categories) even when they are built into word lists, again in marked contrast to normal subjects (Herlitz and Viitanen, 1991; Hodges, 2000). Neither do they display the normally seen proactive inhibition when asked to learn several sets of words in the same semantic category (Cushman et al., 1988). High imagery does not improve word retention (Ober, Koss et al., 1985) although familiarity—e.g., of associations in word pairs such as *East–West* (McWalter et al., 1991)—may benefit recall. Memory for the temporal order of events is impaired (Storandt, Kashkie, and Von Dras, 1998).

Studies of testable patients (i.e., mildly to moderately demented) have reported that many but not all have impaired primary memory (holding information for no more than 30 sec) or working memory (J.T. Becker, 1988; Belleville et al., 1996; E.V. Sullivan, Corkin, and Growdon, 1986). The addition of a distractor task to test working memory increases the deficit significantly (R.G. Morris and Kopelman, 1986). Working memory performance correlates with sentence repetition impairment (J.A. Small et al., 2000). Working memory deficits also appear with nonverbal auditory stimuli (D.A. White and Murphy, 1998). These deficits, in turn, compromise learning (secondary memory), which then can proceed only on reduced information.

Older memories tend to be more available than recent ones, thus exhibiting a *temporal gradient* that applies to both publicly available information and personal history (Fama, Sullivan, Shear, et al., 2000b; Fama, Shear, Marsh, et al., 2001; Kopelman, 1989; Nebes, 1992a). As the disease progresses, knowledge of current events and general information is compromised (Brandt, Folstein, and Folstein, 1988; L.E. Norton et al., 1997). Prospective memory—remembering to remember—deteriorates early in the disease (Huppert and Beardsall, 1993) and may be the patient's main complaint. With intensive training, very specific prospective memory responses can be drilled into some Alzheimer patients (C.J. Camp et al., 1996), but this recall is available only for the trained target responses.

Contrasting with the dismal picture of memory and learning in both verbal and visual modalities is evidence that learning ability for simple motor and skill learning tasks is relatively preserved (Bondi and Kaszniak, 1991; Brandt and Rich, 2001; Dick et al., 1995; Eslinger and Damasio, 1986), but it is not for complex tasks (Grafman, Weingartner, Newhouse, et al., 1990). Fortunately, Alzheimer patients may retain skills for pleasurable activities such as playing musical instruments (W.W. Beatty, Winn, et al., 1994). Alzheimer patients are impaired on some implicit memory tests (Brandt, Spencer, et al., 1988) but not others—depending on the type of task, e.g., success with short delays on word-based perceptual tests but failure with long delays (Gabrieli, Vaidya, Stone, et al., 1999; Meiran and Jelicic, 1995). They often show normal perceptual priming (Fleischman et al., 1998; Jelicic et al., 1995; Park et al., 1998). These differential learning patterns reflect anatomical differences between the declarative and pro-

cedural memory systems and demonstrate the selectivity of cerebral degeneration in this disease.

Verbal functions and academic skills. Deterioration in the quality, quantity, and meaningfulness of speech, and in verbal comprehension, characterizes most Alzheimer patients in relatively early stages of the disease and, ultimately, all of them (Bayles, 1988; Bschor et al., 2001; S. Hart, 1988; Hebert et al., 2000). Central to all aspects of this deterioration is a breakdown in semantic relationships and understandings, "a loosening of semantic ties and concept formation that produces a loss of the associated links of words, and the things they represent" (I.M. Thompson, 1988, p. 132). This breakdown appears to follow the sequence of language development in reverse (Emery, 2000).

Semantic disruptions appear in many ways: Word generation, whether to letters, semantic categories (e.g., animals), or situations (e.g., naming things in a supermarket) is greatly reduced even early in the course of the disease and further compromised by many errors such as perseverations and incorrect categories (Bayles, Salmon, et al., 1989; Binetti, Magni, et al., 1995; Salmon, Heindel, and Lange, 1999; see also p. 520). Category fluency appears to be more disrupted than letter fluency (Monsch, Bondi, Butters, et al., 1992; Salmon, Heindel, and Lange, 1999). Their semantic deficits contribute to a virtual inability to use a clustering strategy for word generation (Troyer, Moscovitch, et al., 1998b). Moreover, cueing for subcategories (e.g., "farm animals, pets") does not help them (C. Randolph, Braun, et al., 1993). Fluency tasks are especially difficult for Alzheimer patients because they make demands both on directed generation of ideas and on semantic knowledge (Fama, Sullivan, Shear, et al., 2000a).

Confrontation naming too elicits many fewer responses from Alzheimer patients than from intact persons along with many more errors—usually due either to semantic or to word retrieval failures (Bowles et al., 1987; Gainotti, Daniele, et al., 1989; Hodges, Patterson, et al., 1996; LaBarge et al., 1992; Thompson-Schill et al., 1999), but phonemic errors, as seen in aphasia, are rare (Astell and Harley, 1996; Hodges, Salmon, and Butters, 1991; Huff, Mack, et al., 1988). Perceptual errors may also occur on naming tests, but they are rare until the diseases progresses to the moderate stage (LaBarge et al., 1992). Some studies have found that certain word categories, such as nouns vs. verbs, are especially impaired, although these findings have not been consistent (M. Grossman, Mickanin, et al., 1996; D.J. Williamson et al., 1998). Naming problems may develop somewhat later than the generative problem (Bayles and Tomoeda, 1983). Yet correlations run high between word generation and naming for Alzheimer patients (.79 and .80, respectively) (Huff, Corkin, and Growdon, 1986; A. Martin and Fedio, 1983), suggesting that the same process of semantic deterioration underlies failures on both these tasks.

Even as speech content empties, the basic organizing principles of language—syntax and lexical structure—remain relatively intact: "nouns are placed where nouns should go" and verbs and other types of words are placed where they should go" (Bayles, 1988; K. Lyons et al., 1994). Yet speech may convey little meaning as words lack clear referents (e.g., thing, stuff, it [without an identifiable antecedent]), and statements become irrelevant or redundant (Devlin et al., 1998; Irigaray, 1973; Nicholas, Obler, Albert, and Helm-Estabrooks, 1985).

The other side of this problem is diminished comprehension of both written and spoken language (Bayles, Boone, et al., 1989; Irigaray, 1973; Paque and Warrington, 1995). Reading accuracy diminishes as semantic memory deteriorates (Storandt, Stone, and LaBarge, 1995; Strain et al., 1998). Comprehension deficits increase with grammatic and syntactic complexity (Croot et al., 1999; Grober and Bang, 1995; S. Hart, 1988). Alzheimer patients also have difficulty recognizing emotional tone in speech, a problem closely linked to impaired recognition of emotion-laden facial expressions (Allender and Kaszniak, 1989).

As language functions deteriorate almost all aspects of writing deteriorate as much or more (Appell et al., 1982; J. Horner et al., 1988; Lambert et al., 1996). Many fewer words appear in free writing (Neils et al., 1989) and mechanical aspects of writing typically deteriorate (N.L. Graham, 2000). Not surprisingly, quantity of misspelling is directly related to disease progression (Pestell et al., 2000), with phonologically irregular words most likely misspelled (Rapcsak, Arthur, et al., 1989).

An important aspect of verbal impairment that appears early in the course of the disease is loss of spontaneity so that conversation typically has to be initiated by someone else or something else (Irigaray, 1973; Naugle, Cullum, and Bigler, 1997). In extreme cases, a verbally capable patient may become mute.

A 49-year-old married salesman, father of three, had been variously diagnosed as depressed and paranoid schizophrenic during a six-month period in which he withdrew socially, at one point talking only to the living room radiator. On his third psychiatric hospitalization, he was diagnosed as catatonic as he remained immobile most of the time and mute. Since it is unusual for catatonic schizophrenia to first appear in midlife, someone in the Psychiatry Department suspected aphasia and a neuropsychological consultation was requested. When I [mdl] met him in his room he fixated on the bright yellow button pinned to my white lab coat and slowly began speaking for the first time in weeks, reading the red

printed words over and over, "Thank you for not smoking. Thank you for not smoking," etc. Once he had started talking, it became possible to engage his attention enough for him to answer questions. He was promptly referred for a neurological workup, which resulted in a diagnosis of probable Alzheimer's disease.

Arithmetic skills are often affected early in the disease (Girelli and Delazer, 2001). Performance of patients with mild Alzheimer's disease on oral arithmetic (i.e., WIS-A Arithmetic) correlated highly with sentence repetition ($r = .60$) and digit span (forward $r = .57$, backward $r = .56$). This suggests that the patients had difficulty holding the question in mind long enough to perform the mental calculation (Rosselli, Ardila, Arvizu, et al., 1998). In this study, Arithmetic scores also correlated highly with WMS-R Visual Reproduction ($r = .73$), perhaps because manipulating item elements involves visuospatial memory. As the disease progresses, so do mathematical and number processing impairments (Deloche et al., 1995).

Visuospatial functions, construction, and praxis. Visuospatial competence of Alzheimer patients generally tends to be impaired, as demonstrated by several quite different means: Complex visuoperceptual discriminations become difficult (Kaskie and Storandt, 1995; Nebes, 1992a). Left–right orientation remains relatively intact except when left–right discriminations require mental rotation (Brouwers, Cox, et al., 1984; Flicker, Ferris, Crook, et al., 1988). Unilateral visuospatial inattention is very common among Alzheimer patients, showing up in most as left-sided inattention, but some others display the less common right-sided problem (L. Freedman and Dexter, 1991; see also Mendez et al., 1997). Line orientation judgment tends to be impaired, with severity ranging from almost total failure to overlap with very low performing elderly subjects (Ska, Poissant, and Joanette, 1990).

The constructional disabilities of these patients have been well documented (Zec, 1993). On simple tasks such as clock drawing their performances are generally defective (Cahn-Weiner et al., 1999; Kozora and Cullum, 1994; Rouleau et al., 1996), worsening with disease progression (M. Freedman, Leach, et al., 1994); but a few may achieve scores low in the intact range (T. Sunderland, Hill, et al., 1989). On more difficult copy tasks (e.g., Complex Figure, Mini-Mental State design) most performances are defective (Binetti, Cappa, et al., 1998; Brandt, Folstein, and Folstein, 1988; Brouwers, Cox, Martin, et al., 1984). Block construction, too, is sensitive to this disease (Bozoki et al., 2001; Brandt, Mellits, et al., 1989; Logsdon et al., 1989). In handling constructional material, Alzheimer patients may exhibit the *closing-in phenomenon* when they make their copy of a drawing or construction close to or connected with the model or overlapping into it. The presence of closing-in responses may aid in the differential diagnosis between Alzheimer's dementia and dementing disorders due to vascular disease as the latter patients do not give this response (Gainotti, Parlato, et al., 1992). Patients with visuospatial behavioral symptoms who get lost, wander aimlessly, or can no longer recognize familiar surroundings are also more likely to perform drawing and constructional tasks poorly (V.W. Henderson et al., 1989). Loss of visuospatial information appears in a common inability to use a map (W.W. Beatty and Bernstein, 1989).

Apraxias in Alzheimer patients may show up as impairment in pantomiming (Bayles, Boone, et al., 1989; R.L. Schwartz et al., 2000) and in copying gestural (finger movement) patterns (L. Willis et al., 1998). More commonly, Alzheimer patients have conceptual apraxia in which they make errors of tool–action or tool–object associations (Dumont et al., 2000; R.L. Schwartz et al., 2000). Impairment in the ability to perform everyday activities was correlated with this disturbance of the conceptual system (Dérouesné et al., 2000). Paraphasias and articulatory errors that may be a form of oral apraxia appear as the disease progresses (Obler and Albert, 1980). Dysarthria and jumbling of sounds and words tend to parallel the performance apraxias that eventually interfere with the patient's accomplishment of almost any intentional act, including intentional speech.

Thinking and reasoning. As may be expected, Alzheimer patients display reasoning impairments, some from the earliest stages of the disease. Reasoning about both visual and verbal material is affected (e.g., Cronin-Golomb, Rho, et al., 1987; Grady, Haxby, Horwitz, et al., 1988; Zec, 1993). Semantic knowledge, whether for words or objects, becomes degraded such that concepts lose their distinctiveness and conceptual boundaries blur, resulting in vague and overgeneralized thinking (A. Martin, 1992). Irigaray (1973) further noted that loss of the abstract attitude, appearing in language usage as inability to assume a metalinguistic distance from speech or language, contributes to defective expression as well as comprehension. As reasoning becomes more difficult with progression of the disease, patients may be judged incompetent to participate in decision-making (Marson, Cody et al., 1995; Marson, Ingram et al., 1995).

Executive functions

Aspects of executive functioning critical for social competence and effective behavior are compromised early in the course of this disease. *Self-awareness,* one important component of executive functioning, is typically impaired. Some patients appreciate the extent of their memory and other cognitive problems, and a very few are able to appreciate the impact of their illness on their family and the implications for the future. However, the majority show diminished awareness of their cognitive deficits and inappropriate behaviors early in the course of the disease, with the severity of this problem roughly paralleling the deterioration of memory functions (DeBettignies et al., 1990; Feher, Mahurin, et al., 1991; Vasterling et al., 1997; M.T. Wagner et al., 1997). What is more, insight may appear in a moment of clarity and then disappear just as rapidly.

Perseverations and intrusions in speech and actions represent another aspect of these patients' impaired ability to execute behavior effectively (Irigaray, 1973; Monsch, Bondi, Salmon, et al., 1995; Salmon, Granholm, et al., 1989). Like nonresponsiveness, perseverations are not limited to speech, but it is most common for them to involve semantic material (Lamar et al., 1997). They show up early in written spellings, such as "streeet," "CCCcarl," or "Reagagen;" in the meaningless appearance in writing or speech of words or expressions just recently used (Bayles, Tomoeda, Kaszniak, et al., 1985); in drawings that resemble the last or next-to-the-last thing drawn or in movements or gestures left over from a preceding response or activity. This latter kind of perseverative response (intrusion) has proven useful in differentiating Alzheimer's disease from other dementing processes (Fuld 1983; Fuld, Katzman, et al., 1982). Loewenstein, Wilkie, and their colleagues (1989) identified five kinds of intrusions: *test* intrusions come from distractor tasks; *shift* intrusions reflect difficulties shifting from a previous task; *conceptual* are intrusive responses conceptually similar to previous task items; *confabulatory* consist of a single percept combining two target items; *unrelated* are not from the examination tasks. Intrusions show up on constructional tasks as well (e.g., D. Jacobs, Tröster, et al., 1990).

Executive measures sensitive to mild stage Alzheimer's disease include tests of working memory, set-shifting, and sequencing (M.S. Albert et al., 2001). As the disease progresses, patients have difficulty with more complex tasks involving planning and flexibility of thinking (Brugger, Monsch, Salmon, and Butters, 1996; J.L. Mack and Patterson, 1995).

Personality and psychosocial behavior

Behavioral disturbances, including personality changes and emotional disorders, affect all Alzheimer patients eventually, many of them from the earliest stages of the disease (Gilley, 1993; Mace and Rabins, 1991; Petry et al., 1988; Teri, Borson, et al., 1989). Different traits show different patterns of change—or no change—over time (Marvin et al., 1997). Clinging to caregivers and easily distracted moods are characteristic behaviors of many patients in the early stages of the disease; disinterest and passivity are also prominent behavioral features (Wild, Kaye, and Oken, 1994).

Some very different kinds of behavior problems are among the most common: Bózzola and his coworkers (1992) reported apathy to be by far the most prevalent which, at its mildest, involves passivity, loss of interest and concern, and reduced spontaneity, becoming anergia in which patients are immobilized by their neuropathology. Apathy can be mistaken for depression in these patients (M.L. Levy et al., 1998; D.B. Marin et al., 1997; G.W. Small, Rabins, et al., 1997). Anxiety, depression, psychotic symptoms, sleep disorder, and incontinence are also frequent behavior problems associated with Alzheimer's disease (Cacabelos et al., 1996). Many patients have episodes of hallucinations and visual illusions (G.W. Small, et al., 1997). Poor self-care, including deteriorated hygiene habits and inappropriate dressing, is a common problem that increases in severity with progression of the disease (Haley, Brown, and Levine, 1987; Reisberg, Ferris, Borenstein, et al., 1990; Teri, Larson, and Reifler, 1988).

Other disturbances show up in increased activity as agitation and restlessness, with aimless wandering and bursts of violence and destructiveness presenting serious problems for caregivers (Haley, Brown, and Levine, 1987; Gilley, 1993); but unlike self-care activities, these tend to ease as the patient's capacity for any kind of activity becomes increasingly compromised (Haley and Pardo, 1989). Suspiciousness and paranoia affect the thinking of many of these patients (Rabins, Mace, and Lucas, 1982; Swearer et al., 1988). Negativism, as stubbornness or refusal to cooperate, is frequently reported by caregivers (e.g., C.M. Fisher, 1988). In one large study caregivers rated agitation, dysphoria, irritability, delusions, and apathy as the most disturbing behaviors (Kaufer et al., 1998). These problems are not mutually exclusive. They may appear and disappear at different stages of the disease and are not well predicted by cognitive status (Bózzola et al., 1992; Marvin et al., 1997; Rubin, Morris, Storandt, and Berg, 1987).

Whether more Alzheimer patients suffer from depression than organically intact persons of comparable ages remains unanswered. Some investigators report that 20% to 50% or more of these patients are also depressed (Lazarus et al., 1987; Li et al., 2001; Reifler, 1992; Wragg and Jeste, 1989). Other studies have not found an abnormal amount of depression among Alzheimer patients (Knesevich et al., 1983; Rubin and Kinscherf, 1989; M.F. Weiner et al., 2002). In one study, 4% of dementia (mostly Alzheimer's disease) patients reported suicidal ideation but none had made any

suicide attempts (Draper et al., 1998). By and large, the incidence of depression decreases as severity of dementia increases, but exceptions have been reported (Teri and Wagner, 1992). Depressed patients may be identified better by interviewing their families than by self-report (Mackenzie et al., 1989).

Dementia patients with major depression may constitute a special subset with greater degeneration of subcortical structures than patients who have not been severely depressed (Zubenko, 2000). Such patients are also more likely to have close relatives who have had major depression (Pearlson, Ross, et al., 1990). Thus, both organic and psychological contributions may account for the differences between patients with respect to the presence, timing, and extent of depression. Yet psychiatric problems, particularly in the form of hallucinations and delusions, are not uncommon, troubling from about 20% to as many as 73% of Alzheimer patients (Gormley and Rozwan, 1998; Holroyd, 2000; Teri, Larson, and Reifler, 1988; R.S. Wilson, Gilley, et al., 2000a). The wide differences in these percentages may reflect not only different patient populations and evaluation techniques but also the increasing incidence of emotional and behavioral problems during the early evolution of the disease (Rubin, Morris, and Berg, 1987; Swearer et al., 1988). However, relationships between cognitive deterioration and psychiatric symptoms have not been consistently documented (Wragg and Jeste, 1989). Patients with florid psychotic symptoms appear to deteriorate more rapidly than those without such symptoms (Lopez et al., 1991; R.S. Wilson, Gilley, et al., 2000b).

Whether Alzheimer patients should continue driving is a dilemma. No one wants to restrict the mobility of safe drivers. Yet Alzheimer patients become unsafe drivers at some point during the course of their illness. A review of state motor vehicle records showed no increased rate of crashes or traffic violations of Alzheimer patients compared to age-matched controls, but the Alzheimer patients probably drove fewer miles than did the comparison group (Trobe et al., 1996). Moreover, some reports indicated that more than 80% of those who continue to drive get lost with from about one-third to almost one-half of driving Alzheimer patients involved in accidents (Kaszniak, Keyl, and Albert, 1991). Neuropsychological test scores did not predict future crashes or violations but driving simulators and road tests did (Cox et al., 1998; G.K. Fox et al., 1997; L. Hunt et al., 1993).

Treatment

Current pharmacological treatment of cognitive problems associated with Alzheimer's disease involves use of anticholinesterase inhibitors that enhance cholinergic function (Cummings, et al., 1998). Since cholinergic function declines with Alzheimer's disease, this treatment attempts to restore levels as much as possible. Some patients benefit by becoming able to carry out functions that had been lost before treatment, and some show a slowing in rate of cognitive decline over time compared with nontreated patients (J.C. Morris, Cyrus, et al., 1998; S.L. Rogers et al., 1998). However, not all patients improve. This treatment is symptomatic and does not change the course of the disease. Disease-modifying drugs are under investigation (Cummings et al., 1998); some are in human trials. Patients who are depressed may benefit from antidepressants. Patients with psychotic symptoms—frequently, hallucinations or delusions—may be helped by some typical and some novel antipsychotic agents (Askin-Edgar, White, and Cummings, 2002, see p. 980 for their list). Patients with mild disease and insight may benefit from supportive therapy or a support group. Learning compensation techniques or ways to change the environment to assist the patient is helpful for some patients and their families. However, attempts to increase memory skills are inadvisable because they can create false expectations and lead to unnecessary frustration. When patients lack insight, intervention usually involves family education and counseling.

Frontal Lobe Dementias

Frontotemporal dementias (FTDs) are degenerative diseases of insidious onset and slow progression involving the frontal and temporal lobes with relative sparing of the posterior brain (Askin-Edgar, White, and Cummings, 2002). Their etiology is unknown. They tend to appear between the ages of 40 and 65; the number of women affected is not disproportionately high (Neary and Snowden, 1991). They account for approximately 20% of progressive dementia cases (M. Grossman, 2001). Early studies labeled frontotemporal dementias generally as Pick's disease, although Pick's is now distinguishable as a subtype of frontotemporal dementia (Kaufer and Cummings, 2003; see p. 221).

Frontotemporal dementia and Alzheimer's disease are easily confused because the conditions are similar and, in their later stages, may be indistinguishable. The most characteristic feature of frontotemporal dementia is the profound change in social behavior and personality that occurs, sometimes years in advance of diagnosis (Askin-Edgar, White, and Cummings, 2002). Lack of insight is inevitable (McGlynn and Kaszniak, 1991; Sungaila and Crockett, 1993) and, along with "stereotypic and eating behavior," best differentiated frontotemporal dementia patients from those with Alzheimer's disease (Bozeat et al., 2000). Other common features of the syndrome are alterations in speech and language, extrapyramidal signs (akinesia, rigidity, and tremor), incontinence, and primitive reflexes (Neary, Snowden, Gustafson, et al., 1998).

Risk factors

Approximately 40% to 50% of cases are transmitted by autosomal dominant inheritance (Bird, 1998; Higgins and Mendez, 2000). Most cases have tau pathology, and a small percentage have a mutated tau gene on chromosome 17 (Higgins and Mendez, 2000). The finding of a greater than usual incidence of brain trauma occurring within four years prior to onset of frontotemporal degeneration suggests that TBI may be a contributing factor, but prior TBI is relatively uncommon (12% of one series of 60 patients) and thus may be only a weak causal factor, if at all (Mortimer and Pirozzolo, 1985).

Neuroanatomy and pathophysiology

The parietal and occipital lobes remain unaffected in most cases, with atrophy concentrated in the temporal and frontal neocortex, excepting the posterior one-half to two-thirds of the superior temporal gyrus which is also typically spared. Cortical atrophy can occur asymmetrically. In some cases, a "knife blade" boundary separating frontal and anterior temporal lobes from the nondiseased posterior brain can be seen (Neary and Snowden, 1996). As for subcortical structures, the limbic system and the corpus striatum are affected but much less than the neocortex. The extent of hippocampus and amygdala involvement varies from case to case (Snowden, Neary, Mann, and Benson, 1996, pp. 117–118). The nucleus basalis of Meynert may be reduced in size but not as much as in Alzheimer patients, and a marked cholinergic deficiency would be unusual (Rossor, 1987). The two main cellular findings are prominent microvascular change and/or severe astrocytic gliosis with or without Pick bodies (Neary, Snowden, Gustafson, et al., 1998). In pure frontotemporal cases the tangles and plaques of Alzheimer's disease are absent. Frontal blood flow is significantly reduced as is frontal metabolism but the EEG remains normal (Neary, Snowden, Northen, and Goulding, 1988).

Disease process

Course. These diseases follow a steadily downhill course, but individual rates of decline may differ greatly (Neary and Snowden, 1991). In the initial stages, silliness, socially disinhibited behavior, and poor judgment predominate (Askin-Edgar, White, and Cummings, 2002), although language impairments may herald disease (Chui, 1989; S. Hart and Semple, 1990). Progressive apathy, blunted affect, and cognitive dysfunction characterize the middle stages. In the late stages patients become mute and many display some motor rigidity. The deteriorative process ends as a vegetative state. Duration of these diseases may be anywhere between two and 17 years (Chui, 1989; Neary and Snowden, 1991).

Clinical subtypes. As with all degenerative diseases, the clinical pattern reflects the distribution of disease in the brain (Chui, 1989). Some patients have greater frontal than temporal involvement. In the *disinhibited type,* a frontal atrophy is confined to orbitomedial zones with relative sparing of the dorsolateral cortex. By contrast, patients with the *apathetic type* have disproprotional atrophy of the dorsolateral cortex (Neary and Snowden, 1996). With left frontal and temporal involvement, language impairment is predominant (Edwards-Lee et al., 1997; M. Grossman, Payer, et al., 1998). Patients with predominant right-sided involvement are much more likely to display socially undesirable behavior as an early symptom than those with mostly left-sided disease (Mychack et al., 2001). A rapidly progressing form of frontal lobe dementia develops in some cases of *motor neuron disease* (*amyotrophic lateral sclerosis, ALS*) (Neary, Snowden, Mann, et al., 1990; Askin-Edgar, White, and Cummings, 2002), but relatively few ALS patients have cognitive deficits (Poloni et al., 1986).

Pick's disease, first described over a century ago (Sjögren et al., 1952) is one type of frontotemporal dementia (see p. 220) that is frequently confused with Alzheimer's disease (Mendez, Selwood, et al., 1993). It is estimated that about 20% of patients with frontotemporal dementia have classic Pick's disease with the hallmark intraneuronal inclusions called *Pick bodies* (Higgins and Mendez, 2000). Dysnomia, with both retrieval and confrontation naming impaired, is a regular feature of Pick's disease. Also characteristic of Pick's disease is a Klüver-Bucy-like syndrome, probably associated with amygdala degeneration (Filley and Cullum, 1993; Munoz-Garcia and Ludwin, 1984). Thus these patients tend to become impulsive, hyperoral with indiscriminate eating, and may display compulsive and seemingly meaningless tactile searching. As with other frontotemporal dementias, social dilapidation is a problem.

Diagnosis

The chief diagnostic problem is differentiating frontal lobe degenerations from Alzheimer's disease as many of the verbal defects are similar; and apathy, poor judgment,

and irritability or affective flattening appear in both conditions. Moreover, Alzheimer neuropathology may encroach on the frontal lobes or frontal projection routes producing a mixed diagnostic picture (Sungaila and Crockett, 1993). Using current clinical criteria for differentiating frontotemporal dementia from Alzheimer's disease (Neary, Snowden, Gustafson, et al., 1998), 77% of patients with frontotemporal dementia met the diagnostic criteria for both diseases on confirmed autopsy (Varma et al., 1999). However, in the early stages, silliness and socially inappropriate and even boorish behaviors with relatively intact cognition, including memory, can help distinguish these diseases from other dementing disorders. The end stages for all progressive cortical diseases are similar. A number of behavioral rating scales have been proposed to capture the features that differentiate it from Alzheimer's disease (Kertesz, Nadkarni, et al., 2000; Lebert et al., 1998; Mendez, Perryman, et al., 1998; J.R. Swartz et al., 1997).

Neuroimaging shows degeneration of the frontal and temporal lobes (e.g., Lenzi and Padovani, 1994, pp. 104, 105; Askin-Edgar, White, and Cummings, 2002). Similarly, hypoperfusion signs on SPECT scans are more severe in the anterior frontal or temporal areas than in posterior regions (Elfgren et al., 1993; B.L. Miller et al., 1997). However, imaging may appear normal early in the disease course (C.A. Gregory et al., 1999).

Cognition

Cognitive alterations typically follow personality and behavioral changes, although this is not always the case (Moss, Albert, and Kemper, 1992). Formal assessment is not always possible with these patients, even early in their course, as disinhibited or apathetic behavior may make it difficult to engage their cooperation (Chui, 1989). Frontotemporal dementia patients regularly perform even more poorly on verbal fluency tests than Alzheimer patients (Mathuranath et al., 2000; Pachana, Boone, et al., 1996). Visuospatial orientation and praxis are preserved and arithmetic skills remain relatively intact (Chui, 1989; Askin-Edgar, White, and Cummings, 2002). Speech may be characterized by pressure of speech, stereotypy or echolalia, and perseveration or, alternatively and in later stages, poverty of speech output that progresses to mutism (Neary, Snowden, Gustafson, et al., 1998). These patients are usually oriented.

Executive functions

Executive disorders, abstraction, and reasoning deficits are among the distinctive characteristics of this disease

(Moss, Albert, and Kemper, 1992). In fact, executive impairments are greater than memory deficits—exactly the reverse of the Alzheimer presentation (Mathuranath et al., 2000; Pachana, Boone, et al., 1996; R.J. Perry and Hodges, 2000; Askin-Edgar, White, and Cummings, 2002). Yet these patients can usually maintain routines during the early stages of the disease. With lateralized disease patients exhibit the usual left–right differences with greater impairment on verbal or nonverbal executive tasks, respectively (K.B. Boone, Miller, Lee, et al., 1999).

Personality and psychosocial behavior

Initial symptoms typically appear in "frontal lobish" kinds of personality changes, such as silliness, social disinhibition, poor judgment, and impulsivity, along with apathy or impaired capacity for sustained motivation (M.L. Levy et al., 1996). Compulsive behaviors are common (Mendez, Perryman, et al., 1997), as are stereotyped and utilization behavior, gluttony—particularly in the early stages—food fads, and decline in personal hygiene and grooming (Neary, Snowden, Gustafson, et al., 1998; Sungaila and Crockett, 1993; Askin-Edgar, White, and Cummings, 2002). Hyperorality may occur later in the course, with mouthing of inedible objects (Neary and Snowden, 1991). Affectively these patients tend to be blandly inappropriate (Kertesz, Nadkarni, et al., 2000).

Dementia with Lewy Bodies (DLB)

Another less common form of primary degenerative dementia (Gomez-Tortosa et al., 1998; C. Holmes et al., 1999; McKeith, 2002), *Lewy body dementia (DLB)* was unrecognized before the 1970s. It may account for as many as 20% of patients with dementia (Hansen et al., 1990, McKeith, Perry, et al., 1992). DLB is typically associated with progressive dementia, extrapyramidal signs, visual hallucinations and delusions, and most noteworthy, severe fluctuations in cognitive functioning (McKeith, 2002), although others report less variability (Papka, Rubio, Schiffer, and Cox, 1998). It shares clinical features with both Alzheimer's and Parkinson's disease, and hence is not easily conceptualized as either a cortical or subcortical dementia (see p. 224).

Risk factors and course

Similar to patients with Alzheimer's disease, DLB patients have an elevated ApoE4 allele frequency (C.F. Lippa et al., 1995). DLB is slightly more common in men (M.F. Weiner et al., 1996), with disease onset typically occurring after age 50 (McKeith, 2002). Patients with DLB have a more rapid decline than those with Alzheimer's disease and other degenerative dementias (McKeith, Perry, et al., 1992; Olichney et al., 1998).

Neuroanatomy and pathophysiology

Most DLB patients display neuropathological findings seen in both Parkinson's and Alzheimer's disease (McKeith, 2002; McKeith, Perry, et al., 1992). The defining neuropathological feature is the *Lewy bodies*, protein deposits found throughout the cortex and paralimbic areas and in the substantia nigra, as in Parkinson's disease. In addition, senile plaques are common although neurofibrillary tangles are few (M.F. Weiner, 1999). When Lewy bodies occur with neurofibrillary tangles and amyloid plaques, it is considered a *Lewy body variant* of Alzheimer's disease. Neuronal degeneration is prominent in frontal, anterior cingulate, insular, and temporal areas (McKeith and Burn, 2000).

The EEG is often abnormal, with greater temporal lobe slowing and transient slow wave activity than seen in Alzheimer's disease (Briel et al., 1999). Generalized atrophy may appear on MRI but with less medial temporal lobe atrophy than characterizes Alzheimer's disease (Barber, Ballard, et al., 2000; G.T. Harvey et al., 1999), which may explain why DLB patients typically have less memory impairment in early disease stages than those with Alzheimer's disease. Functional imaging (SPECT) has shown decreased dopaminergic activity (Z. Walker, Costa, Ince, et al., 1999; Z. Walker, Costa, Walker, et al., 2002) and more frequent appearance of occipital hypoperfusion than in Alzheimer's disease (Lobotesis et al., 2001).

Diagnosis and prediction

The pattern of neuropsychological impairment aids in the differential diagnosis of DLB as on cognitive testing these patients usually have prominent visuospatial deficits (Ballard et al., 1999; Lambon Ralph, Powell, et al., 2001) but perform better on memory tests than Alzheimer patients (Ballard et al., 1999; Heyman, Fillenbaum, et al., 1999) and may have deficits associable to frontosubcortical dysfunction (McKeith, 2002). With the expected cognitive and behavioral impairments, the clinical diagnosis of possible DLB is based on the presence of at least two of the following features; just one feature suggests possible DLB: (1) fluctuating levels of cognitive functioning; (2) recurrent visual hallucinations, appearing early in the disease course, that are typically well formed and detailed; (3) spontaneous parkinsonian symptoms.

Cognition

Given the relative recency that DLB has been identified as a distinct clinical entity, published neuropsychological findings are scanty. For example, Gnanalingham and his colleagues (1997) reported that DLB patients failed on a card sorting task, but the literature lacks other studies of functions that may involve frontosubcortical structures.

Sensorimotor findings in DLB patients are entirely consistent with the pathology. Extrapyramidal signs akin to Parkinson symptoms (bradykinesia, rigidity, hypophonic speech, masked facies, stooped posture, and a slow shuffling gait) develop in over 50% of patients. Praxis is often impaired (Z. Walker, Allen, et al., 1997), while sensory function is largely intact (Rockwell et al., 2000).

Fluctuating *attention* is a core feature of the disease. Attention and lucidity may fluctuate for a few minutes or over weeks or months, and transient confusional states occur. Decreased forward and backward digit spans have been reported (Gnanalingham et al., 1997; Hansen et al., 1990). Attentional impairment has also appeared on simple and choice reaction time and computerized vigilance tests (McKeith and Burn, 2000). Early in the disease course, *memory* impairment consists of poor retrieval with relatively preserved acquisition (McKeith, Perry, et al., 1992). The pattern of memory dysfunction in DLB has been attributed not only to better preserved medial temporal lobe structures but also to supported cholinergic neurotransmission (McKeith and Burn, 2000).

Verbal functions follow the Alzheimer pattern of deterioration. Letter and semantic fluency may be decreased, at levels comparable to Alzheimer's disease. Similarly, naming ability may be at Alzheimer levels (Hansen et al., 1990). In contrast, *visuospatial* impairment is an early and prominent feature of DLB. These patients have more difficulty copying designs with blocks than do Alzheimer patients (Hansen et al., 1990). Not only are their clock drawings poor but DLB patients do not improve when allowed to copy a clock drawing, unlike patients with either Parkinson's or Alzheimer's disease (Gnanalingham, et al., 1996, 1997). Patients who are unable to copy the intersecting pentagons on the MMSE are more likely to receive a diagnosis of DLB than of Alzheimer's disease (Ala et al., 2001).

Personality and psychosocial function

Depression may develop in as many as half of DLB patients (McKeith and Burn, 2000). Sleep disturbances are common (Grace et al., 2000). Hallucinations, usually visual, can appear early in the disease course, and their persistence may contribute to a diagnosis of DLB. Patients often have insight into the unreality of the hallucinations. Many patients also have paranoid delusions. The high frequency of these symptoms often leads to an initial psychiatric referral (McKeith and Burn, 2000). Accurate diagnosis is important as inappropriate treatment with neuroleptics can result in severe, nonreversible, motor (extrapyramidal) dysfunction that will exacerbate parkinsonian symptoms (McKeith, 2002; M.A. Taylor, 1999).

Treatment

Patients may show some improvement in both cognitive and behavioral symptoms from cholinesterase inhibitors (Barber, Panikkar, and McKeith, 2001; Maclean et al., 2001; McKeith, Grace, et al., 2000). Patients who respond to cholinesterase inhibitors are more like to have DLB than Alzheimer's disease (McKeith, 2002).

Other Cortical Atrophies

Neurodegenerative disorders sometimes take the form of focal cortical atrophy (S.E. Black, 1996). Two of the more common may be classified as variants of frontotemporal dementia (M.P. Alexander, 2002; Boller and Duyckaerts, 2003). *Primary progressive aphasia* is a gradually progressive aphasia syndrome that occurs without memory impairment or dementia early in the disease. In fact, many patients remain dementia-free for at least two and as long as ten years (Mesulam, 2000a), although almost all progress to a final dementia syndrome. Both fluent and nonfluent types have been described; associated features are acalculia and ideomotor apraxia. The disorder often starts with anomia and proceeds to impaired grammatical structure and language comprehension (Mesulam, 2001). The left temporal lobe is the primary site of degeneration; neuropathological evidence of Pick's disease is frequent (Kertesz and Munoz, 1997; Mesulam, 2001).

Semantic dementia refers to a rare condition in which the meaning of words, objects, and concepts becomes impaired. Contrasting with other dementias, recent memories are better preserved than remote ones (P.J. Nestor, Graham, et al., 2002). Neuroimaging and autopsy show prominent involvement of the lateral temporal lobes, particularly the inferior and middle temporal gyri. The amygdala is affected and hippocampal atrophy may be present (Galton et al., 2001). Word finding difficulties occur (Lambon Ralph, Graham, et al., 1998), but most striking is impaired knowledge of word meaning (Snowden et al., 1996). As traditional language areas are spared, the patient has intact grammar and syntax (Snowden et al., 1996). Unlike anomic patients who know the meaning of a word but cannot retrieve it, these patients, when given a word to define, demonstrate that they do not know the meaning although the word may seem familiar. Less is known about the clinical course and neuropathology because few cases have been reported (Hodges, Patterson, et al., 1992).

SUBCORTICAL DEMENTIAS

Subcortical dementia refers to the behavioral constellation of symptoms associated with diseases of subcortical brain structures (Bondi, Salmon, and Kaszniak, 1996; Cummings, 1990; Derix, 1994). Although the concept of subcortical dementia was originally advanced by M.L. Albert, Feldman, and Willis (1974), awareness of the behavioral effects from differential involvement of cortical and subcortical structures can be traced to the late 19th century. Meynert postulated that certain psychiatric symptoms resulted from a blood flow imbalance between cortical and subcortical structures (discussed in M.A. Turner et al., 2002). *Subcorticale demenz* was used by Von Stockert in 1932 to describe the cognitive impairment of a patient with encephalitis lethargica.

The behavioral changes associated with subcortical dementia include (1) cognitive slowing (*bradyphrenia*) with disturbances of attention and concentration, executive disabilities including impaired concept manipulation and use of strategies, visuospatial abnormalities, and a memory disorder that affects retrieval more than learning; (2) absence of aphasia, apraxia, and agnosia, the classical symptoms of cortical damage; and (3) emotional or psychiatric features of apathy, depression, or personality change (Cummings, 1986; Huber and Shuttleworth, 1990).

Although differences in brain substrate exist, the clinical distinction between cortical and subcortical dementias is largely behavior-based (Bondi, Salmon, and Kaszniak, 1996; Derix, 1994). Cummings (1986) identified the specific cognitive functions affected by *cortical* degeneration—including language abilities, reasoning and problem solving, learning, and praxis—as *instrumental functions*—functions that carry out behavior and are "the most highly evolved of human activities." In *subcortical* dementias, in contrast, cognitive impairments involve the *fundamental functions*—functions that "are crucial to survival and emerge early in phylogenetic and ontogenetic development." These include arousal, attention, processing speed, motivation, and emotionality.

Subcortical dementias arise from many different etiologies, and a partial listing of these includes thalamic stroke or tumors, hypoparathyroidism, acquired immunodeficiency syndrome (AIDS) encephalopathy, and dementia pugilistica (Cummings, 1990; Frederiks, 1985b; M.A. Taylor, 1999). This syndrome complex has also been called *frontal-subcortical dementia* because it involves frontal-subcortical pathways or subcortical structures intimately connected with the frontal lobes (Cummings and Benson, 1990; L.M. Duke and Kaszniak, 2000).

The distinction between "cortical" and "subcortical" dementias is not universally accepted, however (R.G. Brown and Marsden, 1988; Lerner and Whitehouse, 2002; Mayeux, Stern, Rosen, and Benson, 1983; M.A. Turner et al., 2002). Questioning of this dichotomy results from the considerable overlap between the two groups regarding both cognitive deficits and mood alterations. Objections to this distinction further stress the interrelatedness of cortical and subcortical degeneration, the presence of subcortical atrophy in cortical dementias (P.J. Whitehouse, Price, et al. , 1981), and the presence of cortical abnormalities associated with subcortical disease (L.R. Caplan, 1980; Lazzarino et al., 1991; Nicolai and Lazzarino, 1991). "The dense pattern of neuronal interconnections between cortical and subcortical regions suggests that the functional organization of the brain does not respect such conventional anatomical distinctions" (R.G. Brown and Marsden, 1988). Thus, Alzheimer patients and dementia patients with Parkinson's or Huntington's disease can present very similar—often undifferentiable—abnormalities (R.G. Brown and Marsden, 1988; Kuzis et al., 1999; Pillon, Dubois, Lhermitte, and Agid, 1986; Starkstein, Sabe, et al., 1996), while differences between the Parkinson and Huntington groups can be as notable as those between subcortical groups as a whole and Alzheimer patients (Askin-Edgar, White, and Cummings, 2002; Chui, 1989; Derix, 1994).

Although the classification of dementia as either cortical or subcortical may be oversimplified, Alzheimer's disease and each of the major triad of subcortical dementias—Parkinson's disease, Huntington's disease, progressive supranuclear palsy—can often be distinguished by their overall patterns of cognitive deficits (Pillon, Dubois, Lhermitte, and Agid, 1986; Pillon, Dubois, Ploska, and Agid, 1991). Thus, "cortical" vs. "subcortical" categorizations at best represent a continuum of varying degrees of cortical and subcortical pathology, with behavioral distinctions greatest during the earlier stages of disease. However, as a heuristic distinction, this differentiation of dementia types has led to more careful investigations into these disease processes and provides a conceptual framework for organizing and evaluating observations of these patients.

Movement Disorders

The largest group of subcortical dementia patients have movement disorders as their disease involves the *extrapyramidal motor system*. This system consists of physiologically similar but spatially distributed structures including the basal ganglia (caudate, putamen, and globus pallidus), subthalamic nucleus, substantia nigra, and their interconnections to each other and to thalamic nuclei (see Chapter 3, pp. 45–49; Fig. 7.1). In contrast to the pyramidal motor system, which consists of upper and lower motor neurons that guide purposeful and voluntary movement, the extrapyramidal system modulates movement and maintains muscle tone and posture. Movement disorders can be conceptualized as having either excessive abnormal involuntary movements (*dyskinesia*) or halting initiation and slowed execution of directed movement (*akinesia* or *bradykinesia*). The three major neurotransmitters of the basal ganglia are dopamine (DA), acetylcholine (ACh), and γ-aminobutyric acid (GABA). Since DA is an *inhibitory* neurotransmitter, decreased DA levels increase caudate activity, resulting in bradykinesia. In contrast, excess DA levels, which may be associated with L-dopa therapy, (see pp. 233–234) can produce dyskinesia.

ACh is an *excitatory* neurotransmitter that increases caudate activity. One approach to medical management of many movement disorders is to decrease ACh with anticholinergic medication. Because decreased ACh may impair recent memory, however, negative cognitive side effects may be associated with anticholinergic therapy (Nutt, Hammerstad, and Gancher, 1992; Van Spaendonck et al., 1993). GABA is an *inhibitory* neurotransmitter found in the caudate, putamen, and globus pallidus.

Movement disorders share clinical features that are temporarily modifiable. Anxiety, fatigue, and stimu-

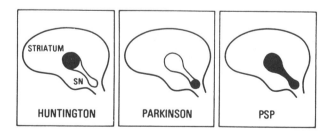

FIGURE 7.1 "The three neurodegenerative diseases classically evoked as subcortical dementia are Huntington's chorea with lesions in the striatum, particularly the caudate nucleus, Parkinson's disease with severe neuronal loss in the substantia nigra, and progressive supranuclear palsy with severe neuronal loss in the striatum and substantia nigra, associated with degeneration of other structures in the basal ganglia, upper brainstem, and cerebellum." (From Agid et al., 1987, reprinted by permission)

lants exacerbate the clinical symptoms, and movements may be decreased temporarily with volition. Involuntary movements, other than tics or *myoclonus* (sudden sharp involuntary jerks), are absent during sleep.

Parkinson's Disease/Parkinsonism (PD)

PD is typically an idiopathic disorder associated with DA depletion in the basal ganglia and its connections from the *substantia nigra,* a small nucleus adjacent to the caudate (see Hurley et al., 2002; Stacy and Jankovic, 1992, for MRI visualization of these structures). Because the symptoms of PD can be also be present with non-idiopathic causes, such as toxic exposure, putamenal hemorrhage, or encephalitis, the term *parkinsonism* is often used to refer to the common features of the disease without reference to etiology.

Parkinson described the cardinal features of PD in his 1817 monograph entitled *Essay on the Shaking Palsy* (Parkinson, 1817). He reported "involuntary tremulous motion, with lessened muscular power, in parts not in action and even when supported; with a propensity to bend the trunk forewards, and to pass from a walking to a running pace: the senses and intellect being uninjured." Parkinson's description fits nicely within the current concept of subcortical dementia. Charcot, who added rigidity as a feature of the disease, named the disorder Parkinson's disease (*la maladie de Parkinson*) (Finger, 1994), which had previously been called *paralysis agitans*.

Parkinsonism's outstanding feature is a movement disorder with a number of component symptoms (M. Freedman, 1990; Nutt, Hammerstad, and Gancher, 1992; Stacy and Jankovic, 1992; Weisberg, 2002). Few patients display all symptoms, particularly early in the course of the disease. Initial complaints are often vague and may include pain and numbness, difficulty with handwriting, and difficulty with repetitive tasks (e.g., brushing teeth). Prominent among the motor symptoms is the "resting tremor," a relatively rapid rhythmical shaking that can affect limbs, jaw, and tongue, which diminishes or disappears during movement and in sleep. Tremor is generally the first sign of PD, seen in approximately 70% of patients (Lieberman, 1995c), and typically begins in a single hand before progressing to the ipsilateral leg and then contralateral limbs. This tremor is also called a "pill rolling" tremor, although Charcot's more vivid metaphor describes the tremors as if the hands were "crumbling bread" (Finger, 2000, p. 186).

The slowed movement of bradykinesia along with the akinesic difficulty initiating movement are the cardinal feature of PD. Bradykinesia may be seen in reduced limb movements such as absence of arm gestures while talking and decreased arm swing while walking. It is also associated with an absence of facial expression (*masked facies*) and decreased spontaneous blink rate. Patients have been known to overcome bradykinesia temporarily under strong emotional arousal such as in an emergency (*kinesia paradoxica*); and when objects—such as keys—are tossed to them as many who cannot readily initiate walking will catch them easily (B.K. Westbrook and McKibben, 1989). Handwriting becomes jerky and decreases in size (*micrographia*). Bradykinesia affects everyday activities, including hygiene, and becomes a very debilitating feature of the disease.

Patients do not typically complain about muscular rigidity as they tend to report it as "weakness" (Nutt, Hammerstad, and Gancher, 1992). Muscular rigidity is common, particularly in the wrists and elbow; examiners describe it as having a "lead pipe" quality, an analogy to the steady resistance associated with attempting to bend a lead pipe. The simultaneous presence of a 4–6/sec. tremor with parkinsonian hypertonia creates the feeling of a "cogwheel" or "ratcheting" resistance when the examiner attempts to move the patient's wrist or arm. Rigidity predominates in the flexor muscles, causing a stooped "simian" appearance (Lieberman, 1995c).

Thus the parkinsonian gait is characterized by a forward stooped posture, narrow base, with decreased arm swing and slow shuffling with little steps (*marche à petits pas*), with difficulty starting to walk and, once started, difficulty stopping. Postural instability may result in frequent tripping and falls. In more advanced stages of PD, motor "freezing" may occur in which the patient appears glued to the ground and unable to take any steps (Ahlskog, 1999; Nutt, Hammerstad, and Gancher, 1992). Autonomic impairment occurs late in the disease.

Estimates of the incidence of dementia in these patients have ranged from 2% to 93%, but most textbooks cite figures of approximately 10%–30% (Mahurin, Feher, et al., 1993). An additional 20% may show signs of cognitive impairment without frank dementia (Lieberman, 1998). The dementia of Parkinson's disease may not be so much a separate condition as the more severe manifestations of a progressive cognitive deterioration affecting almost all Parkinson patients along a continuum ranging from subtle to very severe (Granérus, 1990; E.V. Sullivan, Sagar, Gabrielli, et al., 1989). Some workers, however, have suggested that two types of dementia can occur with this disease, one which generally satisfies the criteria for subcortical dementia, and another which can be more severe and displays neuropathological features of Alzheimer's disease, and affects a higher proportion of Parkinson

patients than the general population (Boller, Mizutani, et al., 1980; Chui and Perlmutter, 1992; Derix, 1994).

Depression is common in PD but, due to reduced movement and expressiveness, some patients may appear depressed who have no affective experience of depression.

Parkinsonism may affect men more than women (S.G. Diamond et al., 1990), although there are also studies indicating no sex difference (Tanner, 1992). The typical age at onset is in the 50s, and it is rarely seen before age 30 years (Martilla, 1987; Rajput et al., 1984). The incidence of PD is approximately 20 per 100,000, with a prevalence of 150–200 per 100,000 in Western countries (Lieberman, 1995c; Malaspina et al., 2002). In the United States, PD has an estimated cost of $27 billion per year (Obeso et al., 2000). Treatment costs alone for L-dopa and related drugs run $1,000 to $6,000+ per year, per patient.

Risk factors

The etiology of Parkinson's disease is unknown. While twin studies have failed to implicate a prominent genetic component (Duvoisin, Eldridge, et al., 1981; Tanner, Ottman, et al., 1999), evidence indicates a greater genetic contribution in patients with earlier onset disease (W.K. Scott et al., 2001; Tanner et al., 1999). A few families show an inheritance pattern, typically appearing as an autosomal dominant with reduced penetrance (N.E. Maher et al., 2002; Mahurin, Feher, et al., 1993; Muenter et al., 1998). Since parkinsonism is a syndrome rather than a disease, it has a number of causative agents, some known or suspected and some unknown (Malaspina et al., 2002). Among known etiologies are viral encephalitis and possibly other postviral conditions; drugs with DA antagonistic properties such as neuroleptics; toxic substances (Hammerstad and Carter, 1995); and rarely, perhaps as a result of better diagnostic criteria, vascular disease (Evatt et al., 2002; Koller, Langston, et al., 1991; Nutt, Hammerstad, and Gancher, 1992). Muhammad Ali, the famous boxer who developed a parkinsonian condition, dramatically illustrates the potential of repeated TBI as a risk factor for this disease (see also Della-Sala and Mazzini, 1990; Erlanger et al., 1999; Jordan, 2000; Mendez, 1995; see also pp. 188–189). However, Parkinson's other celebrity patient—Michael J. Fox—may have contracted the disease from an environmental contaminant. Fox was one of four employees out of approximately 125 TV production workers who has developed Parkinson's disease, giving rise to speculation that this TV crew was exposed to the same environmental toxin.

An environmental etiology was suggested when the disease was first recognized in England at the beginning of the industrial revolution, when toxic industrial byproducts were implicated in the development of Parkinson's disease (Hammerstad and Carter, 1995; Koller, Langston, et al., 1991; Malaspina, 2002; Tanner and Langston, 1990). Tanner (1989) observed that younger patients were more likely to have rural backgrounds, raising the possibility of exposure to toxins in well water or herbicides. A renewed interest in environmental toxins as a cause of PD came from the discovery that MPTP (1-methyl-4-phenyl-1,2,3,6-tetrahydropyridine), a neurotoxin with a predilection for neurons in the substantia nigra, induces parkinsonism (Rajput, 1992). Toxic exposure, postviral conditions, and TBI all fit into a pattern of slow preclinical neuronal degeneration (Koller, Langston, et al., 1991; Strange, 1992; Tanner and Langston, 1990). Despite growing knowledge about this disease, more than 80% of cases are *idiopathic*; i.e., their etiology remains unknown (Lerner and Whitehouse, 2002; Nutt, Hammerstad, and Gancher, 1992).

Epidemiologic studies have consistently implicated smoking as a reverse risk factor, as smokers are half as likely to develop PD as nonsmokers (Fratiglioni and Wang, 2000). A genetic linkage for this phenomenon has been suggested (Checkoway et al., 1998). Benedetti and colleagues (2000) note that fewer patients than control subjects consumed coffee, but they warn against assuming that coffee is protective against PD.

Neuroanatomy and pathophysiology

The pathologic hallmark of Parkinson's disease is loss of melanin-containing DA neurons in the compact zone (*pars compacta*) of the substantia nigra, a pair of small, darkly pigmented bodies that synthesize DA (Agid, Ruberg, et al., 1987; M. Freedman, 1990; Strange, 1992) (see Figs. 3.17 and 7.1, pp. 77, 225). The loss of DA neurons in the substantia nigra is accompanied by reduction of DA in both the caudate and putamen in the basal ganglia. Basal ganglion output goes by way of the thalamus to the neocortex, particularly to prefrontal areas. This DA loss may result in frontal disconnections (D.M. Jacobs, Levy, and Marder, 2003; E.V. Sullivan, Sagar, Gabrieli, et al., 1989; A.E. Taylor et al., 1986a) and appears to be directly related to the presence and severity of motor symptoms (Dubois and Pillon, 1992). When DA levels drop below 30% of normal, the motor and other symptoms of Parkinson's disease become manifest (Agid and Blin, 1987; Koller, Langston, et al., 1991). Cell loss also occurs in other brainstem nuclei such as the locus coeruleus and the nucleus basalis of Meynert, the major cholinergic input to the cerebral cortex (Corkin, Growdon, Desclos, and Rosen, 1989; Granérus, 1990; Lerner and Whitehouse,

2002). The concomitant reduction in nondopaminergic neurotransmitters probably contributes to the symptom picture (S. Hart and Semple, 1990; E.K. Perry et al., 1985; Pillon, Dubois, Cusimano, et al., 1989). Lesions are also often found in other cell populations including the locus coeruleus (noradrenergic source to cortex), the substantia innominata, the hypothalamus, mamillary bodies, the mesencephalic reticular formation, and the dorsal raphe nucleus. Thus, although Parkinson's disease is thought to be a dopamine disease, it involves many systems and many neurotransmitters (Arciniegas and Beresford, 2001). Lewy bodies, a characteristic intracellular marker for this disease, can be found within the remaining neurons in the affected areas (Lerner and Whitehouse, 2002; Nutt, Hammerstad, and Gancher, 1992).

Cortical involvement is suggested by decreased regional cerebral blood flow (rCBF) in numerous cortical regions (Bissessur et al., 1997; Weder et al., 2000). An early study found generally reduced CBF levels but they were not related to the nature or severity of cognitive deficits in Parkinson's disease (Globus et al., 1985). More precisely localized studies have correlated reduced blood flow in frontal and parietal areas with characteristic frontal lobe defects of perseveration and diminished verbal fluency (Goldenberg, Podreka, et al., 1989); in frontal areas and the basal ganglia with motor imagery and execution tasks (M. Samuel et al., 2001); and in the right globus pallidus, with planning and retention of problem solutions (using the Tower of London tasks) (Owen, Doyon, et al., 1998). Abnormally slowed auditory evoked potential patterns differentiate Parkinson's patients from patients with other types of progressive dementia, as well as from healthy control subjects (Goodin, 1992; Kupersmith et al., 1982; B.F. O'Donnell, Squires, et al., 1987), although the degree of slowing is greater in older Parkinson's disease patients compared to age-matched controls than in younger Parkinson's disease patients, who may not differ from controls (Stanzione et al., 1998; Tachibana, Aragane, Kawabata, and Sugita, 1997). Abnormally long evoked potential latencies have been associated with impaired performances on tests of immediate verbal recall and visuoperceptual discrimination (S. Pang et al., 1990).

Disease process

Course. Symptom onset may begin with just one indicator of the disease, usually tremor (Koller, Langston, et al., 1991; McPherson and Cummings, 1996), or other signs of motor impairment, as in fine motor tasks or activities requiring postural change (e.g., getting out of a chair) (Nutt, Hammerstad, and Gancher, 1992). Symptoms may fluctuate before becoming established. They may even appear temporarily during the prodromal stage, typically under stressful conditions, and then recede until years later when the disease becomes obvious.

Since the motor symptoms of Parkinson's disease emerge only after DA levels in the brain are substantially reduced, this can be considered a two-stage disease. Whatever factor is responsible for the degeneration process initiates the prodromal stage, which may begin two or more decades before symptoms become obvious. Degeneration, primarily of substantia nigra cells, then progresses slowly and insidiously until the second stage, when the disease becomes manifest (Granérus, 1990; Langston and Koller, 1991; Wooten, 1990). Progression of the disease in the second stage also tends to be slow, with most patients now surviving ten to 15 years after the first symptoms were noticed (Nutt, Hammerstad, and Gancher, 1992; Peretz and Cummings, 1988). The rate of progression is variable; progression is slower for patients who initially present with tremor (Lieberman, 1995c). In contrast, PD patients who present with postural instability and gait difficultly as their major clinical impairment tend to be older, to be more cognitively impaired, and to have a more rapid disease progression.

Prior to the now almost universal use of dopamine replacement therapy (L-dopa [levodopa] see pp. 233–234), mortality rates were three times that of comparable age and sex groups in the general population. With appropriate medication, this rate approaches normal expectations, with the majority of Parkinson patients surviving beyond age 75 (Granérus, 1990; Rajput et al., 1984). Even with current treatments, PD is slowly and inexorably progressive over several decades (M.M. Hoehn, 1992). Cognitive decline, too, takes place slowly (Corkin, Growdon, et al., 1989; Portin and Rinne, 1980), with different functions deteriorating at different rates (Tweedy et al., 1982). One examination of Parkinson patients over a two year interval showed that reduced cognitive functioning—defined as a loss of at least 4 points on the MMSE—was present in only 22% of 77 patients with idiopathic Parkinson's disease (Bayles, Tomoeda, Wood, et al., 1996). However, most patients in this series who had "normal" MMSE scores during the original assessment declined to the "questionable" range at follow-up. Even in the earliest stages, when cognitive functions generally are intact, mild dysfluency and conceptual rigidity can occur (Lees and Smith, 1983). B.E. Levin, Llabre, and Weiner (1989) also found deficits in focused attention, both verbal and visual immediate recall, and mental flexibility in newly diagnosed patients, a pattern that has been replicated (W.P. Goldman et al., 1998). Cognitive decline is tied to disease duration and

motor symptom severity, but not closely, as other variables also contribute to cognitive changes (Chui, 1989; B.E. Levin, Tomer, and Rey, 1992; Mahurin Feher, et al., 1993). Course may differ for men and women as, with disease progression, men tend to display more severe motor symptoms and women have more L-dopa-associated dyskinesias (K.E. Lyons et al., 1998).

Subtypes. Some differences among patients are predictive of other features of the disease. They appear with sufficient regularity as to permit subtyping, although these classifications are not mutually exclusive.

A *lateralized presentation* of the disease is common, with tremor or stiffness beginning on one side or even just one limb but increasing in severity and gradually spreading so that in the later stages the motor disorder generally involves both sides of the body (Nutt, Hammerstad, and Gancher, 1992; Starkstein, 1992; Wooten, 1990). These variations in disease presentation tend to be reflected cognitively in that many patients with predominantly left-sided motor dysfunction show greater deficits than those with right-sided symptoms on tests with a visuospatial component (F.P. Bowen, 1976; B.E. Levin, Llabre, Reisman et al., 1991; A.E. Taylor, Saint-Cyr, and Lang, 1986), and left visuospatial inattention has been observed in these patients (Starkstein, Leiguarda, et al., 1987; Villardita, Smirni, and Zappala, 1983). Direnfeld and his group (1984) also reported that only patients with left-sided symptoms had significant memory impairments, but both lateralized groups showed visuospatial deficits, which were more severe in patients with lesions on the left. Other workers, however, found no differences between lateralized groups on visuospatial tasks (Hovestadt et al., 1987), complex motor tasks (Horne, 1973), or a battery examining both visuospatial and motor functions (Huber, Freidenberg, et al., 1989). Whether failure to demonstrate lateralization differences results from patient selection and matching procedures, excessive variability within a patient group, or the nature of the tests employed remains an unsettled question. Patients with a right-sided motor disorder are more likely to report depressive symptoms than those whose motor dysfunction is on the left (Starkstein, 1992).

Motor symptom differences may also distinguish two types of Parkinson patient, those in whom tremor is the chief symptom and those who suffer the more disabling problems of bradykinesia and rigidity (Chui, 1989; B.E. Levin, Tomer, and Rey, 1992; Mortimer, Pirozzolo, et al., 1982). When tremor predominates, the course is more likely to be benign (Wooten, 1990). Findings regarding the association of dementia with tremor have been equivocal (Chui, 1989). Dementia and the usual cognitive deficits of Parkinson's disease tend to occur more frequently in patients in whom bradykinesia and rigidity are the prominent motor features.

Early and late onset appear to have quite different clinical implications. Adult patients whose onset is before age 40 or 45 tend to have a slower progression with fewer cognitive disorders, including dementia (Dubois, Pillon, Sternic, et al., 1990; Goetz et al., 1988; Quinn et al., 1987; B.E. Levin, Tomer, and Rey, 1992), with about one-tenth the incidence rate of onset after age 60 (Golbe, 1991). Later-onset patients tend to have a rapid progression of the disease and are more likely to suffer cognitive deficits (Katzen et al., 1998). Rates of dementia increase rapidly when disease onset occurs after age 70 (Mayeux, Stern, Rosenstein, et al., 1988), which may reflect a compounding of normal aging with the cognitive vulnerability of PD.

Diagnosis and prediction

Severity classification. Hoehn and Yahr (1967) developed the first widely used scale for staging of Parkinson's disease, which is based largely on motor impairment and mobility but does not directly address functional status. It is a 5-point scale with unilateral signs and symptoms characterizing stage 1. At stage 5, the patient is wheelchair-bound or bedridden.

The most popular instrument to stage PD is the *Unified Parkinson's Disease Rating Scale (UPDRS)*, which contains three sections: (1) Mentation, Behavior, and Mood; (2) ADL; and (3) Motor function. A total of 199 points are possible, and higher scores represent greater disability. The addition of quality of life and behavioral variables to motor characteristics of the disease has contributed to the UPDRS's success (Calne and Koller, 1998; Fahn et al., 1987).

Diagnosis. Parkinson's disease is diagnosed clinically based upon bradykinesia, rigidity, tremor, and postural instability, although all four symptoms need not be present (Nutt, Hammerstad, and Gancher, 1992). Because there is no diagnostic test specific to Parkinson's disease, the diagnosis of Parkinson's disease may be incorrect in approximately one-fourth of patients when examined at autopsy (A.J. Hughes et al., 1992). Common diagnostic errors include progressive supranuclear palsy (PSP) (see pp. 241–244) and multiple system atrophy. MRI may identify uncommon causes of parkinsonism, such as multiple infarcts. Features not typically associated with Parkinson's disease include early severe dementia, early severe autonomic dysfunction, gaze difficulties (especially downward gaze), and upper motor neuron or cerebellar signs (Arciniegas and Beresford, 2001; Nutt, Hammerstad, and Gancher, 1992).

Prediction. Age, of course, is a significant predictive factor. Neuropsychological test performances may also predict as lower scores of elderly subjects on Picture Completion (WIS-A), Stroop color–word trial, and verbal fluency were associated with later emergence of PD symptoms (Mahieux, Fenelon, et al., 1998). The probability of coexisting dementia has also been predicted by neuropsychological assessment (S.P. Woods and Tröster, 2003). Woods and Tröster found that Parkinson patients who later became demented had poorer performances on digits backward and word list learning and recognition, and they made more perseverative errors on the Wisconsin Card Sorting Test at baseline than Parkinson patients who did not develop dementia by the one-year follow-up.

Sensorimotor status

Sensory complaints may include numbness, coldness, burning, or pain (Koller, 1984b; Nutt, Hammerstad, and Gancher, 1992). Often, these symptoms are restricted to the hemiparkinson side and precede motor symptoms. Some patients have impaired kinesthesia (Jobst et al., 1997). More than 70% of patients had selective olfactory deficits; on pathologic examination, Lewy bodies showed up in every olfactory bulb specimen (Hawkes et al., 1997).

Motor slowing is symptomatic of Parkinson's disease and affects performances on all timed tests. Additionally, beyond just slowness in initiating or carrying out activities, *bradyphrenia* (mental slowing) occurring in excess of motor slowing has been shown to affect the behavior of many PD patients (Agid et al., 1987; Haaland and Harrington, 1990), a phenomenon often associated with depression (D. Rogers, 1992). Bradyphrenia appears to be enhanced by task complexity as Parkinson patients may have normal reaction times but are abnormally slowed on choice reaction time tests (Cummings, 1986). Slowed scanning of items in memory was implicated in one study (R.S. Wilson, Kaszniak, Klawans, and Garron, 1980). However, others have not shown that reaction time slows with greater task complexity (Rafal, Posner, et al., 1984; Mahurin and Pirozzolo, 1993; Poewe et al., 1991; C. Robertson and Empson, 1999; Russ and Seger, 1995).

Cognition

By and large, the cognitive deficits associated with the early stages of PD are similar to, and often indistinguishable from, the cognitive disorders that occur with frontal lobe damage, particularly with involvement of the prefrontal cortex (Bondi, Kaszniak, et al., 1993; Haaland and Harrington, 1990; Mortimer, 1988a; Pillon, Dubois, Ploska, and Agid, 1991; A.E. Taylor, Saint-Cyr, and Lang, 1986). Moreover, Portin and his coworkers (1984) reported that many aspects of cognitive dysfunction in Parkinson patients are associated with cortical atrophy which tends to involve "anterior parts of the convexity." Thus these patients tend to display such characteristics of prefrontal dysfunction as difficulties in switching or maintaining a set, in initiating responses, in serial and temporal ordering, in generating strategies (i.e., executive planning), and in cognitive slowing and diminished productivity. These characteristics of prefrontal dysfunction may account for many of the cognitive deficits manifested in this disease (Dubois, Boller, et al., 1991; M. Freedman, 1990; Pillon, Agid, et Dubois, 1996).

For patients in whom bradykinesia and rigidity are the outstanding motor symptoms, cognitive impairments are most pronounced; when tremor is the most prominent motor disorder they are correspondingly more mild (Chui, 1989; Granérus, 1990) or nonexistent (B.E. Levin, Tomer, and Rey, 1992). Cognitive impairments tend to be greater with increased severity of motor symptoms (Girotti et al., 1988; B.E. Levin et al., 1991; Mortimer, Christensen, and Webster, 1985), especially bradykinesia (Mayeux, Stern, Rosen, and Leventhal, 1981; Mortimer, Pirozzolo, et al., 1982). The pattern of cognitive deficits in parkinsonism has been likened to the pattern of impairment associated with depression (Weingartner, Burns, et al., 1984) and to an exaggeration of the normal mental changes of aging (M.L. Albert, 1978).

Conflicting findings from different studies are not uncommon. They are probably due to variations in cognitive status among these patients, and thus to biases in the groups under study. Moreover, it is important to recognize that many more patients will display one or more kind of cognitive deficit than will meet the criteria of a more globally impaired dementia.

Attention. For attentional capacity as measured by digit span, most studies have found performances to be generally *within normal limits* (R.G. Brown and Marsden, 1988; Huber and Shuttleworth, 1990; Koller, 1984a). Attentional deficits are common in these patients, appearing most usually on complex tasks requiring shifting or sustained attention (Cummings, 1986; Horne, 1973; Huber, Friedenberg, et al., 1989; M.J. Wright et al., 1990) and on mental calculations that require sustained mental tracking (Huber and Shuttleworth, 1990; A.E. Taylor, Saint-Cyr, Lang, and Kenny, 1986). Very short-term memory tested by consonant trigrams was intact with delays up to 15 sec, except when an intervening distractor was introduced (Brown-Peterson technique) making this a test of working memory, for then patients' recall rate dropped below that of normal control subjects (E.V. Sullivan, Sagar, Cooper, and Jordan, 1993). F.L. Bowen (1976) observed that these patients could perform the mental tracking tasks "but were inattentive to their errors." Variability in cognitive status within the Parkinson patient group may account for some contradictory findings as, on many attentional tasks—especially timed ones—Parkinson group means fall considerably below age norms or control scores (Mahurin, Feher, et al., 1993), but relatively large standard deviations reflecting interindividual differences obscure the generally impaired status of the Parkinson patients (see Huber, Shuttleworth, Paulson, et al., 1986; Mayeux, Stern, Sano, et al., 1987; Pillon, Dubois, Lhermitte, and Agid, 1986). Large standard deviations may be expected when bradykinesic and tremorous patients are included in the research sample as bradykinesia correlates significantly with response times but tremor does not (Mahurin, Feher, et al., 1993).

Memory and learning. A fairly consistent pattern of memory and learning impairments has emerged despite some contradictory findings both between and within studies which, in the latter, have been explained by striking variations within the patient group (e.g., see El-Awar et al., 1987; Heindel, Salmon, Shults, et al., 1989). Orientation is typically intact (Cummings, 1986; Huber, Shuttleworth, Paulson, et al., 1986; Pillon, Dubois, Lhermitte, and Agid, 1986).

Short-term recall for word lists or stories is likely to be impaired (R.G. Brown and Marsden, 1988; Massman, Delis, Butters, et al., 1990; A.E. Taylor, Saint-Cyr, and Lang, 1986; Tweedy et al., 1982); delay may enhance short-term recall (Corkin, Growdon, Desclos, and Rosen, 1989), a phenomenon typically found with slowed processing. Recall of unrelated verbal material is typically impaired (R.G. Brown and Marsden, 1988; Mayeux, Stern, Sano, et al., 1987; A.E. Taylor et al., 1986a; Weingartner, Burns, et al., 1984) and often contains an abnormal number of *intrusions* (conceptually or phonetically associated words) (J.H. Kramer, Levin, et al., 1989). With recall aids, these patients will tend to perform *within normal limits*, whether assistance is provided through cueing, as in paired associate learning (Harrington, Haaland, et al., 1990; Koller, 1984a; A.E. Taylor et al., 1986), or in a recognition format (W.W. Beatty, 1992; Flowers, Pearce, and Pearce, 1984; A.E. Taylor et al., 1986a). However, some studies found no improvement with cueing (e.g., Massman et al., 1990; Tweedy et al., 1982). Parkinson patients benefit when given learning strategies, such as categorizing the stimuli, but they are unlikely to initiate strategies (R.G. Brown and Marsden, 1988). Sequencing and other ordering requirements greatly increase the difficulty of the learning task for these patients (Weingartner, Burns, et al., 1984).

When visual memory requires a motor response, Parkinson patients tend to perform poorly (R.G. Brown and Marsden, 1988; Pillon, Dubois, Lhermitte, and Agid, 1986), but intact visual learning is suggested when it is examined by a recognition format (Flowers, Pearce, and Pearce, 1984). Both spatial and pattern recognition have been shown to be deficient but less so with longer delay intervals (W.W. Beatty, 1992), yet spatial learning remains intact (J.A. Cooper and Sagar, 1993). Defective short-term recall has also been reported for visually presented material (E.V. Sullivan and Sagar, 1988). However, unlike verbal working memory, distraction did not impair very short-term recall of 3-item tapping patterns (using the Corsi block board); but when delays were filled with a distracting activity, both patients and control subjects made more errors, patient errors exceeding those of controls after 15 sec delays but not delays of 3 or 9 secs (E.V. Sullivan, Sagar, Cooper, and Jordan, 1993).

Procedural and skill learning is likely to be compromised (Haaland and Harrington, 1990): Harrington, Haaland, and their coworkers (1990) found that degree of impairment related to severity of the disease; Heindel, Salmon, Shults, and their colleagues (1989) reported that procedural learning impairments occurred only in patients with pronounced cognitive deficits; Beatty and Monson (see W.W. Beatty, 1992) found skill learning to be normal for Parkinson patients with or without dementia. Such contradictory findings raises questions of subject selection in a condition with so many symptom variables.

Remote recall, whether semantic or visual, tends to be impaired (W.W. Beatty and Monson, 1989; R.G. Brown and Marsden, 1988; Venneri et al., 1997). Despite the high incidence of depression in PD, depression does not appear to contribute to poor memory performance (Boller, Marcie, et al., 1998).

Verbal functions. Vocabulary, grammar, and syntax remain essentially intact in Parkinson's disease (Bayles, 1988; R.G. Brown and Marsden, 1988; E.V. Sullivan, Sagar, Gabrieli, et al., 1989), although both phrase length and overall output tend to be reduced (Bayles, Tomoeda, Kaszniak, et al., 1985; Cummings and Benson, 1989). However, verbal disturbances, primarily associated with word finding and retrieval, are common (W.W. Beatty, 1992). Thus these patients tend to perform poorly on fluency tasks (R.G. Brown and Marsden, 1988). Whether they generate more words for *semantic* categories (e.g., animals, fruits) than for simple first letter (*phonemic*) associations (Bayles, Trosset, et

al., 1993; Gurd and Ward, 1989) or have greater difficulty generating words to semantic categories (Auriacombe et al., 1993; B.E. Levin, Llabre, and Weiner, 1989; Raskin, Sliwinski, and Borod, 1992) may also depend on the disease characteristics of the patients in these subject groups (Azuma et al., 1997). Subcategory cueing (e.g., jungle animals, farm animals) can bring patient scores up to control subjects' levels (Randolph, Braun, et al., 1993).

Verbal fluency is related to dopamine depletion. On fluency trials both on and off L-dopa, decreased output occurred only when patients were not receiving L-dopa (Gotham et al., 1988). Verbal fluency performances during the earliest, or preclinical, stages of the disease, provide a measure of subsequent dementia risk that exceeds the prognostic value of other cognitive function tests (D.M. Jacobs et al., 1995).

Reports of confrontation naming deficits are almost evenly divided between studies that found them (Bayles, 1988; R.G. Brown and Marsden, 1988; W.P. Goldman et al., 1998) and those that did not (Corkin, Growdon, Desclos, and Rosen, 1989; M. Freedman, 1990; Pillon, Dubois, Lhermitte, and Agid, 1986). Findings linking impaired naming with severity of cognitive deficits suggest that the naming disorder emerges later than other verbal dysfunctions, notably dysfluency (Bayles and Tomoeda, 1983; El-Awar et al., 1987; Gurd and Ward, 1989).

Parkinson patients are particularly distinguished by *hypokinetic dysarthria,* an impairment of the mechanical aspects of speech (Bayles, 1988; Cummings and Benson, 1989; M. Freedman, 1990), which E.M.R. Critchley (1987) attributed to a failure of integration of the "phonation, articulation and language" aspects of speech production. This shows up as dysarthria, loss of melodic intonation which gives a monotonic quality to speech, low volume, and variable output speeds so that words may come out in a rush at one time and very slowly another. Writing problems tend to parallel alterations in speech production. Writing acquires a cramped, jerky appearance and may be greatly reduced in size (*micrographia*) (S. Hart and Semple, 1990; Tetrud, 1991). Not surprisingly, oral reading is slowed (Corkin, Growdon, Desclos, and Rosen, 1989).

Visuospatial functions. Visuospatial impairments have been frequently described in Parkinson patients (R.G. Brown and Marsden, 1988; Cummings and Huber, 1992; McPherson and Cummings, 1996). Deficits have been reported for perceptual judgments requiring matching, integration, and angular orientation; for both drawing to copy and free drawing, with reduced size noted on human figures (Riklan et al., 1962); and for both personal and extrapersonal orientations, except for equivocal findings for left–right orientation (R.G. Brown and Marsden, 1988). These patients have difficulty with WIS-A Block Design and Object Assembly tests (Girotti et al., 1988; Huber, Shuttleworth, and Freidenberg, 1989). Impairments on Block Design are highly correlated with dementia and disease duration (B.E. Levin et al., 1991) as are visuospatial orientation deficits (Raskin, Borod, Wasserstein, et al., 1990). Mortimer, Pirozzolo, and their colleagues (1982) found that good performance on visuospatial tasks was associated with tremor; poor performance with bradykinesia. Cummings and Huber (1992) also noted these visuospatial test differences. They suggest that a general progression of visuospatial deficits takes place, beginning with impaired rod orientation early in the disease course; defective line orientation and failures on Block Design and Picture Arrangement appear in the disease's middle stage; and facial recognition is affected in late-stage Parkinson's disease. Hovestadt and his coworkers (1987) consider the spatial disorientation problem to be supramodal, occurring early and unrelated to duration or severity of the illness, patient's age, medication effects, or verbal skills.

Most studies controlled or accounted for motor disorder before reporting visuospatial deficits (e.g., Boller, Passafiume, et al., 1984; Cummings, 1986). Still the nature of these problems has been questioned by a number of studies that have concluded that visuospatial functions are not unduly impaired in Parkinson patients (B.E. Levin, 1990)—at least in those whose motor problems are not predominantly left-sided. Rather, what appears as a visuospatial disorder may be best understood in terms of executive dysfunctions (see this page). Copy and recall drawings of the Rey-Osterrieth Complex Figure were poorly organized with significant omissions, deficits that implicated executive dysfunctions; but both visuoperceptual and motor defects also contributed to impaired performances, leading to the conclusion that "visual construction impairments in PD are multifactorial in nature" (M. Grossman et al., 1993).

Thinking and reasoning. Test batteries assembled to examine Parkinson patients typically omit tests of reasoning and judgment, but what sparse findings are available indicate that in this area Parkinson patients tend to perform normally—on tests of comprehension of complex ideational material (M.L. Albert, 1978; Haaland, personal communication, 1991; Loranger et al., 1972), on the Cognitive Estimate test (Lees and Smith, 1983), and to have a realistic appreciation of their condition and limitations (R.G. Brown, MacCarthy, et al., 1989; McGlynn and Kaszniak, 1991). Reports on concept formation are contradictory as some studies found impairment on WIS-A Similarities (Huber, Shuttleworth, and Freidenberg, 1989; Pillon,

Dubois, Ploska, and Agid, 1991) but others did not (R.G. Brown, Marsden, et al., 1984; Loranger et al., 1972; Portin and Rinne, 1980). Flowers and Robertson (1985) reported intact abstracting ability.

Executive functions

The attributes of thinking—reasoning, problem solving, judgment, and concept formation—can be distinguished, one from another, and are clearly dissociable from executive functions, yet Parkinson patients consistently fail tests comprising both conceptual and executive functions. Tests which require both concept formation and the ability to shift sets elicit defective performances from most Parkinson patients: e.g., Raven Progressive Matrices (Huber, Shuttleworth, Paulson, et al., 1986; Pillon, Dubois, et al., 1986, 1989), the Wisconsin Card Sorting Test (F.P. Bowen, 1976; Cronin-Golumb, 1990; Lees and Smith, 1983; A.E. Taylor, Saint-Cyr, and Lang, 1986), and the Category Test (C.G. Matthews and Haaland, 1979). These patients typically make errors when they are first required to formulate a strategy; once they have acquired a solution set they perform at near-normal levels (Saint-Cyr and Taylor, 1992). Both the shifting component of any task and maintaining a set are difficult for them (F.P. Bowen, 1976; Cronin-Golumb, 1990; Flowers and Robertson, 1985; Haaland and Harrington, 1990), but problems in set shifting may be predominant (Raskin, Borod, and Tweedy, 1992; M. Richards et al., 1993). Frequently appearing problems in self-monitoring (Girotti et al., 1988) and self-correction have been attributed to difficulties in shifting sets (F.P. Bowen, 1976) or to failure to initiate changes they perceived were needed (Ogden, Growdon, and Corkin, 1990). Parkinson patients consistently have difficulty adapting to novelty regardless of the modality in which it appears (Loranger, 1972; A.E. Taylor and Saint-Cyr, 1992). Response slowing too may contribute to executive deficits (R.G. Brown and Marsden, 1986; Daum and Quinn, 1991; A.E. Taylor, Saint-Cyr, and Lang, 1986). Inability to organize percepts in a planful manner (what Ogden and her colleagues call "forward planning," a problem that shows up as a sequencing deficit when these patients must organize picture stories serially, e.g., WIS-A Picture Arrangement) is another aspect of impaired executive functioning identified in Parkinson patients (Mortimer, 1988a; Ogden, Growdon, and Corkin, 1990; E.V. Sullivan, Sagar, et al., 1989).

Some researchers have postulated that all of these deficits may be due to defective behavioral regulation arising from an impairment of central programming (R.G. Brown and Marsden, 1988; Haaland and Harrington, 1990; Horne, 1973; Stern, Mayeux, and Rosen, 1984). More recently, Harrington and Haaland

(1991b) suggested that visuoperceptual deficits and sluggish shifting may also contribute to these patients' motor regulation disorder. Yet planning on the Tower of London test or the somewhat more demanding Tower of Toronto test proceeds slowly but is likely to remain intact (Goldenberg et al., 1989; Saint-Cyr and Taylor, 1992).

Personality and emotional behavior

Depression is one of the more consistent features of parkinsonism, with most estimates of its occurrence in the 40% to 60% range (Askin-Edgar, White, and Cummings, 2002; Lieberman, 1998), but it has also been reported to be as high as 70% (Bieliauskas and Glantz, 1989). In an extensive review of the literature, Cummings (1992) reported that depression occurs in approximately 40% of PD patients and is distinguishable from other depressive disorders by greater anxiety and less self-punitive ideation. Rates of depression were lower in studies lacking standardized rating or interview protocols. Mean reported scores on the most commonly used instrument, the Beck Depression Inventory (BDI), were high (i.e., in the abnormal direction) in the normal to subclinical ranges. Cummings (1992) observed that depression in Parkinson's disease was initially considered to be a reaction to the patient's chronic and progressive neurologic impairments. However, many studies suggested otherwise as the duration of Parkinson's disease appears unrelated to the presence of depression and item analysis of these patients' responses on the BDI showed greater dysphoria and pessimism, irritability, sadness, and suicidal ideation with little of the guilt, self-blame, feelings of failure, or fear of punishment that characterize classical idiopathic depression. Cummings (1992) further noted that PD patients also have a high frequency of anxiety symptoms with few delusions or hallucinations. Despite frequent suicidal ideation, PD patients have a very low suicide rate (e.g., see Myslobodsky et al., 2001). Cummings (1992) concluded that these subtle differences between depression in PD and idiopathic mood disorders suggest that this may be a disease-specific depression syndrome with distinctive mood profiles, further noting that depression in PD involved mesocortical/prefrontal dysfunction associated with reward, motivation, and stress response systems.

Thus, although depression may seem to be an appropriate response to the crippling symptoms of parkinsonism, it tends to be unrelated to the severity of motor symptoms (S.M. Rao, Huber, and Bornstein, 1992; Mayeux, Stern, Cote, and Williams, 1984), to cognitive impairment when it is not severe (S.M. Rao et al., 1992), or to other patient characteristics such as age or sex, extent of disablement, or medication regimen

(A.E. Taylor, Saint-Cyr, Lang, and Kenny, 1986). It is more likely to develop when cognitive impairments are severe (Mayeux, Stern, et al., 1981, 1983), although only 5% of Parkinson patients were both depressed and demented in a series in which 51% were clinically depressed but without dementia and 11% had dementia but were not depressed (Sano, Stern, et al., 1989). When compared with patients with other equally crippling disorders, most studies have found that more Parkinson patients were depressed (Conn, 1989). Kaszniak, Sadeh, and Stern (1985) point out some of the difficulties in diagnosing depression in bradykinetic patients in whom reduced levels of motor activity, facial impassivity, and slowed responding can make them appear depressed, a problem compounded by the unreliability of self-reports of cognitively impaired patients (see also Arciniegas and Beresford, 2001; Nutt, Hammerstad, and Gancher, 1992).

Depression improves transiently but not significantly when treatment with L-dopa reduces disability (Santamaria and Tolosa, 1992). Parkinson depression has a low remittance rate and tends to be resistant to treatments designed for idiopathic depression, which suggests that rather than being due to serotonin depletion, "depression in PD may be a function of the neurobiology of PD itself" (Arciniega and Beresford, 2001, p. 293). Yet questions about a relationship between depression and serotonin depletion remain unanswered (S.M. Rao, Huber, and Bornstein, 1992) as other workers think serotonin depletion may be part of the disease process (Mayeux, Stern, Cote, and Williams, 1984; Sano et al., 1989). Anxiety and panic attacks may also occur (Askin-Edgar, White, and Cummings, 2002; McPherson and Cummings, 1996), although more frequently during medication "off" periods.

A prodromal personality has been described, characterized by emotional and moral rigidity, introversion, seriousness, and restricted affective expression (Koller, Langston, et al., 1991; Lohr and Wisniewski, 1987). On the one hand, Paulson and Dadmehr (1991) wondered whether these moralistic prodromal tendencies might have led patients-to-be to drink more water and thus increase their exposure to suspected toxic trace elements. On the other hand, these personality characteristics may reflect the first pathological changes due to a disease process that evolves for years, and perhaps decades, before the classical motor symptoms become apparent (Koller, Langston, et al., 1991; Lohr and Wisniewski, 1987).

Treatment

Medical treatment of Parkinson's disease focuses on symptomatic medication and decreasing the rate of disease progression with neuroprotective agents. Perhaps the most important treatment success story in neurology has been the use of L-dopa, begun in 1967, to replace DA depletion due to degeneration of the substantia nigra. Since DA does not cross the blood–brain barrier, the DA precursor L-dopa was employed to replace the diminished DA stores. Although it provides relief from many parkinsonian features, it is also associated with nausea and vomiting due to its effects on the peripheral nervous system. One form of L-dopa is combined with carbidopa which minimizes unwanted side effects. Sinemet, the trade name for the L-dopa/carbidopa combination, means "no vomiting."

Research findings have been equivocal regarding the effect of L-dopa on the cognitive status of many Parkinson patients (Arciniegas and Beresford, 2001), much of them discouraging (Mahurin, Feher, et al., 1993; Pillon, Dubois, Bonnet, et al., 1989). Unfortunately, most of its enhancing effects on motor symptoms begin to diminish after only two or three years, with significant deterioration after eight to ten years of L-dopa therapy (Agid et al., 1987; Askin-Edgar, White, and Cummings, 2002; Gancher, 1992; Portin and Rinne, 1980). Due to reappearance of symptoms following initial success of DA replacement therapy, the timing of L-dopa initiation is a matter of debate. L-dopa therapy is frequently deferred until the disease becomes sufficiently advanced to interfere with daily activities as it may be effective only for five to 20 years.

Thirty percent or more of patients taking L-dopa experience psychiatric side effects, usually as mild psychotic symptoms such as visual hallucinations, paranoid delusions, vivid dreams, confusional states (Askin-Edgar, White, and Cummings, 2002; Conn, 1989; Lohr and Wisniewski, 1987), and *dyskinesias* (involuntary abnormal movements) (Nutt, Hammerstad, and Gancher, 1992; Strange, 1992). L-dopa does not seem to alleviate depression directly but rather the reactive component of depression tends to dissipate as motor symptoms improve (Kaszniak, Sadeh, and Stern, 1985). Although L-dopa may temporarily improve dementia, these patients are very susceptible to its toxic side effects (Mayeux, Stern, Rosenstein, et al., 1988; Peretz and Cummings, 1988).

A complication of L-dopa therapy is the development of response fluctuations and dyskinesias, generally beginning about five years after initiating L-dopa therapy (Hardie et al., 1984; McPherson and Cummings, 1996; Nutt, Hammerstad, and Gancher, 1984). The initial signs of diminished L-dopa efficacy appear as a "wearing off" phenomenon in which motor symptoms fluctuate or increase prior to the next L-dopa dosing. This condition progresses until an "on–off" pattern develops in which the severity of both motor and nonmotor (sensory, autonomic) symptoms fluctuates, generally in relation to time of dosage intake (J.H. Carter et al., 1989; Gancher, 1992; Nutt, Woodward, et al., 1984).

Eventually, motor "freezing" appears during "off" periods and unexpected falling becomes a problem. When "on," patients perform better on cognitive tests, feel more alert and clear-headed, and have faster reaction times than in the "off" condition (R.G. Brown, Marsden, et al., 1984; B.E. Levin, Tomer, and Rey, 1992; Rafal, Posner, et al., 1984). Emotional status may also fluctuate, with elevated mood and less anxiety in the "on" condition and lower mood and increased anxiety when "off" (Richard et al., 2001).

Other medications have been used either alone or in conjunction with L-dopa. Most usually noted are anticholinergic medications used to treat the motor symptoms but which appear to have adverse effects on selective attention and planning (Glatt and Koller, 1992). Selegiline, a monoamine oxidase (MAO) B inhibitor, tends to slow disease progression by reducing the incidence of free radicals (McPherson and Cummings, 1996; Weisberg, 2002) and protecting against L-dopa's "wearing off" tendency (Nutt, Hammerstad, and Gancher, 1992).

Surgical treatments generally include lesioning or placing a deep brain stimulator in regions of either the globus pallidus, subthalamic nucleus, or ventral intermediate thalamic nucleus (Eskandar et al., 2001). Surgery candidates are usually patients whose medical management has become increasingly difficult and who have neither dementia nor evidence of involvement of many brain regions. By and large, these procedures are associated with relatively little cognitive risk (Kubu et al., 2000; Perrine et al., 1998; Soukup et al., 1997), although reduced verbal fluency may occur and some frontal/executive dysfunction has been reported (Askin-Edgar, White, and Cummings, 2002). When successful, along with improvement in motor functions, these patients may enjoy mildly enhanced psychomotor speed and working memory (Pillon, Ardouin, et al., 2000).

Huntington's Disease (HD)

This hereditary condition, first described after studying patients living in Long Island, New York, was originally called *Huntington's chorea* (from the Greek word *choreia*, meaning "dance") because of the prominence in its symptom picture of the involuntary, spasmodic, often tortuous movements that ultimately become profoundly disabling (see Bruyn, 1968). The disease is also manifested both cognitively and in personality disturbances: motor disturbance, cognitive impairment, and psychiatric features together form the symptom triad (Lauterbach et al., 1998). With the possible exception of those persons whose symptoms do not appear until relatively late in life and who, as a group, may not exhibit as severe a degree of cognitive deterioration or emotional disorders as do the others (J.W. Britton et al., 1995; J.B. Martin, 1984), most patients suffer impairment in all three symptom spheres, although each aspect of the disease may differ in time of onset and in severity (S.E. Folstein, 1989; Lohr and Wisniewski, 1987; Schwarcz and Shoulson, 1987). Since most people at risk for this disease are aware of their possible fate, early diagnosis is more common than with other dementias. Thus, estimates of ten to 20 years as the usual duration of the disease are trustworthy. Some patients may live with it as long as 25 to 30 years (Schwarcz and Shoulson, 1987; J.N. Walton, 1994). Estimates of the overall prevalence of Huntington disease run from 5 to 10 per 100,000, although it may be as high as 12 per 100,000 for adults in the 40- to 50-year age range (S.E. Folstein, Brandt, and Folstein, 1990; Tobin, 1990). However, prevalence rates vary greatly both between countries and between regions within countries (S.E. Folstein, 1989; Lerner and Whitehouse, 2002).

Cognitive deficits, typically first interpreted by the patient or observers as memory problems, may be the initial symptoms of this disease (Hahn-Barma et al., 1998; Paulsen, Zhao et al., 2001), or they may not appear until after motor or behavioral changes have become obvious (S.E. Folstein, 1989). Similarly, psychiatric symptoms tend to be independent of cognitive and motor aspects of the disease (Paulsen, Ready et al., 2001). Various estimates of the incidence of dementia have been offered, but they probably reflect the duration of the disease in the sample under study, as all Huntington patients develop dementia unless they die before the disease runs its course (Bayles, 1988; Peretz and Cummings, 1988).

Risk factors

Genetic predisposition. Huntington's disease results from an excessive number of trinucleotide *CAG repeats* (cytosine, adenine, guanine) in the HD gene located on chromosome 4 (Kremer et al., 1994). This autosomal dominant disease has 100% penetrance such that half of all offspring of a carrier parent will acquire the disease if they live long enough (S.E. Folstein, 1989; J.B. Martin, 1984; Schwarcz and Shoulson, 1987; Tobin, 1990). If the pathologic gene is due to a mutation, it cannot be passed to subsequent generations. However, parental sex is related to disease onset and severity, with the infrequent juvenile form more commonly inherited from the father (Lieberman, 1995a). Children who develop HD rarely live until adulthood.

Demographic factors. Disease onset typically occurs between 30 and 40 years, which allows many patients to have children before they know if they are gene carriers, although the range of HD onset is between 2 and 80 years (Lieberman, 1995a). In addition, the age range during which HD most usually becomes evident makes the disease expression especially difficult for family members since these are prime parenting and wage-earning years. HD is less frequently observed in African Americans and rarely in Asians. As would be expected, with an autosomal dominant inheritance pattern, HD affects males and females equally.

Neuroanatomy and pathophysiology

The core anatomic feature of this disease is atrophy of the caudate nucleus and putamen, structures in the corpus striatum (S.E. Folstein, 1989; Schwarcz and Shoulson, 1987; Tobin, 1990; see Fig. 7.1). The atrophy begins along the head of the caudate next to the ventricular wall, producing a distinctive flattening when viewed on CT or MRI (Lieberman, 1995a). The degenerative process may also invade the cerebellum, thalamic nuclei, and other subcortical structures. Decreased basal ganglia volume may predate disease onset (Aylward, Brandt, et al., 1994), although correlations with motor and mental slowing and with decreased verbal memory in the absence of formal disease suggest early disease manifestations that occur prior to being able to identify disease onset (Campodonico et al., 1998). Reports on cortical involvement are inconsistent, as some workers describe cortical changes (M.L. Albert, 1978; Tobin, 1990) but others do not (S.E. Folstein, Brandt, and Folstein, 1990; J.B. Martin, 1984). Loss of cortical neurons has been described on autopsy (Strange, 1992). Frontal lobe MRI volume is correlated with disease severity and general cognitive function but not after accounting for total brain volume, indicating that this association is not specific to the frontal lobes (Aylward, Anderson, et al., 1998). Metabolic alterations visualized by PET scanning indicate reduced metabolism levels in the caudate nucleus and putamen (Berent et al., 1988) and appear to predict disease onset in presymptomatic HD patients (Antonini et al., 1996). Evoked potential patterns resemble those of Parkinson patients; although differences are present, they are not sufficiently specific for diagnostic purposes (Goodin and Aminoff, 1986), but early sensory processes as well as later latency ERP indexes of word recognition and target detection may both be affected (Munte et al., 1997).

Neurological symptoms are essentially limited to the subcortical (extrapyramidal) motor system. As exceptions, olfactory identification becomes impaired early in the course of the disease (Moberg et al., 1987), and tactile perception may be diminished (D.C. Myers, 1983; H.G. Taylor and Hansotia, 1983). Depression is common; suicide rates are much higher than among the general population (S.E. Folstein, Brandt, and Folstein, 1990).

Alterations in the levels of many neurotransmitters accompany the striatal degeneration (S. Hart and Semple, 1990; Strange, 1992). The most prominent and consistent changes occur as reduced levels of the inhibitory neurotransmitter GABA (S.E. Folstein, 1989; J.B. Martin, 1984; Tobin, 1990), with a concomitant increase in excitatory neurotransmitters that, in high concentrations, can have neurotoxic effects (Nutt, 1989; Schwarcz and Shoulson, 1987; Tobin, 1990). These changes are confined to the involved subcortical structures (Cummings, 1986).

Disease process

Course. This is a steadily progressive disorder that typically runs its course in ten to 15 or 20 years (Schwarcz and Shoulson, 1987; Tobin, 1990), but it may last as long as 30 years (J.B. Martin, 1984). In a very few cases, disease onset occurs before age five or as late as 80, but the mean age at onset is in the early 40s, with 25% to 28% late onset (over 50) (J.B. Martin, 1984; Tobin, 1990). Reports of onset age are affected by criteria for diagnosis as some workers date onset from the first associated symptom, which may be cognitive (Hahn-Barma et al., 1998) or psychiatric (Berrios, Wagle et al., 2001), yet others may require motor signs. A higher number of CAG repeats on the HD gene has been associated with earlier disease onset (Duyao et al., 1993), more rapid rate of neuronal loss (Furtado et al., 1996), and more rapid disease progression (Brandt, Bylsma, Gross et al., 1996; Illarioshkin et al., 1994) but not with psychiatric symptoms (Berrios, Wagle, et al., 2001; Lerner and Whitehouse, 2002).

Initial motor signs may be mild restlessness, slowed oculomotor responses, occasional uncontrolled jerks or gestures involving any part of the body (the choreic movements), and manual clumsiness (S.E. Folstein, 1989; Lishman, 1997; Lerner and Whitehouse, 2002). In fact, the chorea is very subtle in the earliest stages of the disease and is often incorporated into voluntary movement, something of which even the patient is unaware and may interpret as signs of restlessness or being uncomfortable. Over time these problems increase in frequency and severity, and other motor abnormalities further impair voluntary motor control. As the disease progresses, chorea is accompanied by dysarthria and dysphagia (Lieberman, 1995a). In the final stages,

akinetic and mute patients are fully dependent. Aspiration pneumonia is the most common cause of death when the disease runs its course (S.E. Folstein, 1989; D.C. Myers, 1983).

In more than half of the cases, psychiatric disturbance or dementia precedes the appearance of obvious motor symptoms (S.E. Folstein, Brandt, and Folstein, 1990; Lieberman, Dziatolowski, et al., 1979; Lohr and Wisniewski, 1987). The rate of progression of each aspect of the disease—motoric, cognitive, and psychiatric—may differ, although in most cases all major features of the disease are present.

Subtypes. Time of onset, rate of progression, and symptom severity tend to differ according to the sex of the affected parent (J.B. Martin, 1984; R.H. Myers, Vonsattel, et al., 1988; Sapienza, 1990). In general, the disease appears earlier in children of Huntington fathers, with a $5^{1}/_{2}$ year difference in average age at onset and thus considerable overlap between offspring of transmitting mothers and fathers. The earlier the onset, the more severe are the symptoms and the faster its progression, with the juvenile form of the disease presenting the most severe motor symptoms and progressing most rapidly although cognition may be relatively preserved (Gomez-Tortosa, del Barrio, Garcia Ruiz, 1998).

Families differ in the incidence of major affective disorder, as it runs abnormally high in some, and very low in others (S.E. Folstein, 1989; S.E. Folstein, Abbott et al., 1983; S.E. Folstein, Franz, et al., 1983). Group differences have also been suggested by findings that African Americans tend to have an earlier onset with fewer psychiatric disturbances (S.E. Folstein, 1989).

Diagnosis and prediction

Severity classification. The *Unified Huntington Disease Rating Scale (UHDRS)* was developed to facilitate disease characterization for research purposes (Anonymous, 1996; Siesling, van Vugt, et al., 1998; see also Siesling, Zwinderman, et al., 1997, for a shortened version). The UHDRS measures four domains of clinical performance and capacity in HD: motor function, cognitive function, behavioral abnormalities, and functional capacity.

Diagnostic issues. The discovery of the HD gene has raised questions about the advisability of genetic testing of persons at risk for developing the disease for fear that positive results may have devastating psychological effects, or that even negative results may produce "survivor guilt" (S. Hersch, Jones, et al., 1994). However, potential carriers' reactions tend to relate to their level of psychological adjustment more than to the test results (Meiser and Dunn, 2000), with no documented long-term emotional distress due to self-knowledge as recently as 1997 (van't Spijker and ten Kroode). Specific ethical and legal issues apply when families seek prenatal testing. Although genetic testing is widely available, it has not become the standard of care. Generally fewer than 5% of eligible individuals have undergone this procedure (S.M. Hersch and Rosas, 2001). Clinical diagnosis typically relies on determination of an otherwise unexplainable and characteristic extrapyramidal movement disorder with appropriate family history.

DNA testing for the number of CAG repeats in the HD gene located on chromosome 4 provides the definitive diagnosis; the trinucleotide protein has been named *huntingtin*. Although slightly different thresholds have been reported, individuals diagnosed with Huntington's disease generally have 36 to 40 or more CAG repeats. Cases of juvenile onset HD typically have more than 60 CAG repeats.

Cognition

Like Parkinson's disease, many of the initial cognitive deficits of Huntington patients are akin to frontal lobe disorders. Studies that have demonstrated relationships between neuropathological characteristics of this disease and cognitive deficits consistently implicate the caudate nucleus in its mental rather than its motor manifestations (Berent et al., 1988; Brandt, Folstein, Wong, et al., 1990; Starkstein, Brandt, et al., 1988). Given the caudate nucleus's intimate connections with the prefrontal cortex, it would appear that atrophy disconnects caudate–prefrontal loops and "frontal-lobish" kinds of alterations emerge in patients with no demonstrable prefrontal lesions (Cummings and Benson, 1990). Cognitive decline has been associated more closely with severity of motor symptoms than duration of the disease (Brandt, Strauss, et al., 1984).

Despite some lack of agreement regarding early symptom appearance (de Boo et al., 1997), cognitive impairment is often the first expression of the disease and may predate motor symptoms by as long as two years (Hahn-Barma et al., 1998; Paulsen, Zhao, et al., 2001). Yet Digit Symbol (WIS-A), optokinetic nystagmus, and rapid alternating movements were most sensitive to decline in another study, illustrating the heterogeneity of early symptom presentation (Kirkwood et al., 1999). Poorer cognitive performance is associated with a larger number of CAG repeats on the HD gene (Jason et al., 1997).

Sensorimotor status. Eye movements become disturbed in several ways (S.E. Folstein, 1989; D.C. My-

ers, 1983): They are generally slowed and have longer latencies in response to stimulation; the approach to targets occurs in short, jerky steps rather than a normal smooth sweep; and visual tracking becomes inefficient because of inability to maintain gaze on a moving target or to repress reflexive responses to unanticipated stimuli (Lasker and Zee, 1997). With these visual problems, it is not surprising that Huntington patients are significantly slowed on visual tracking tasks, such as the Trail Making Test and symbol substitution tasks (Brandt, Folstein, Wong, et al., 1990; Caine, Bamford, et al., 1986). Oepen and his colleagues (1985) described jerkiness on a pencil tracking task, which was most prominent in the left hand; manual operations become increasingly slowed and clumsy as the disease progresses (H.G. Taylor and Hansotia, 1983). Specific defects on a sequential movement task that characterized Huntington patients included difficulty in initiating movements, poor utilization of advance information, and relatively greater deficits in performances by the nonpreferred hand (Bradshaw, Phillips, et al., 1992).

Patients often appear unaware of their involuntary movements, which has been interpreted as reflecting lack of insight associated with decreased cognitive functions or the operation of psychological defense mechanisms (see McGlynn and Kaszniak, 1991). However, Huntington patients may not have the subjective experience of choreic movement, which may or may not be unrelated to degree of cognitive impairment (Snowden, Craufurd, et al., 1998). Huntington patients do have decreased perception of forces and weights, suggesting impaired "effort sensation" similar to that shown by cognitively healthy subjects with weakened muscles who perceive weights as disproportionately heavy (Lafargue and Sirigu, 2002). Slowed mental processing and difficulties in shifting sets may also contribute to performance failures on timed visuomotor tasks (S.E. Folstein, 1989; Huber and Paulson, 1987). Diminished odor identification has also been reported (Bylsma, Moberg, et al., 1997).

Attention. Attention span—usually tested by immediate digit recall—shrinks as the disease progresses: it can be normal in the early stages but inevitably becomes abnormally short (R.G. Brown and Marsden, 1988; N. Butters, Sax, et al., 1978; Caine, Ebert, and Weingartner, 1977). Concentration and mental tracking are impaired at every stage of the disease (Boll, Heaton, and Reitan, 1974; Caine et al., 1977; S.E. Folstein, Brandt, and Folstein, 1990). Difficulties both in maintaining and in shifting attentional sets also characterize Huntington patients (Boll et al., 1974; S.E. Folstein, 1989; Josiassen, Curry, and Mancall, 1983).

Memory and learning. Intensive study of the memory system problems encountered by Huntington patients has found a pattern of specific memory deficits (R.G. Brown and Marsden, 1988; N. Butters, Salmon, Granholm, et al., 1987; Butters, Salmon, Heindel, and Granholm, 1988; Caselli and Yanagihara, 1991; S.E. Folstein, Brandt, and Folstein, 1990). Among the earliest indicators of cognitive decline, these deficits are mild in the beginning stages of the disease, worsening and becoming more inclusive as the disease progresses (M.S. Albert, Butters, and Brandt, 1981; N. Butters, Sax et al., 1978; N. Butters, Wolfe, et al., 1986).

The common features of this pattern include an impaired short-term (working) memory which is extremely vulnerable to interference effects, as demonstrated by the Brown-Petersen procedure (N. Butters and Grady, 1977; Caine, Ebert, and Weingartner, 1977; Meudell et al., 1978), by testing for retention of a few words following several minutes of distractions (S.E. Folstein, Brandt, and Folstein, 1990), and with visual material (Caine, Bamford et al., 1986). Acquisition of new material is slowed (Brandt and Rich, 2001; Delis, Massman, et al., 1991; Massman, Delis, Butters, et al., 1990; Shimamura, Salmon, et al., 1987). This problem is compounded by defective retrieval and thus appears most prominently on recall trials, as semantic cueing or a recognition format tends to aid retrieval (N. Butters, Salmon, Granholm et al., 1987; Granholm and Butters, 1988; Massman, Delis, Butters, et al., 1990). With disease progression patients lose the ability to discriminate between stored and associated material, and a recognition format becomes less helpful in efforts to differentiate learning and retrieval (J.H. Kramer, Delis, Blusewicz, et al., 1988).

Huntington patients display virtually normal priming effects (Brandt and Rich, 2001; Heindel, Salmon, et al., 1989), indicating that some learning does occur, at least while they are still testable. Moreover, like normal subjects, these patients may display both primacy and recency effects, recalling most frequently words at the beginning and end of a list (Caine, Ebert, and Weingartner, 1977; R.S. Wilson, Como, et al., 1987). However, a diminished primacy effect has also been observed (Massman, Delis, Butters, et al., 1990) which may reflect the working memory's sensitivity to interference. Retrieval deficits are more likely due to poor memory search initiation or strategy rather than simply to defective encoding, although coding strategies may be inefficient (Crosson, 1992). Reduced storage capacity may also contribute to the memory disorder.

Unlike normal subjects, Huntington patients are not spontaneously prone to using such learning strategies as rehearsal (N. Butters and Grady, 1977; Weingartner, Caine, and Ebert, 1979a) or encoding with imagery (Caine, Ebert, and Weingartner, 1977; Weingartner, Caine, and Ebert, 1979b). Though they may benefit somewhat from semantic encoding (Massman, Delis, Butters, et al., 1990; R.S. Wilson, Como, et al., 1987), this benefit is not always manifested (Caine et al., 1977; Weingartner, Caine, and Ebert, 1979a). Serial learning is virtually impossible for them (Caine et al., 1977). Story recall is also impaired (N. Butters, Sax, et al., 1978; Caine, Bamford, et al., 1986; Josiassen, Curry, and Mancall, 1983), with some loss of information following a delay (N. Butters, Salmon, Cullum, et al., 1988; Tröster, Jacobs, et al., 1989); but affectively loaded material has an enhancing effect, which is maintained on delayed recall (Granholm, Wolfe, and Butters, 1985). Although these patients tend to be aware of their memory failures they are unlikely to initiate a search for unretrieved material (Brandt, 1985; S.E. Folstein, Brandt, and Folstein, 1990). Thus deficits appear chiefly at input, as defective working memory and encoding; and in spontaneous recall in which reduced retrieval effort and efficiency combine with defective storage to compromise memory abilities, while retention of learned information appears to be fairly stable.

Both visual and verbal remote memory deficits of Huntington patients resemble those of normal subjects in not showing a temporal gradient (M.S. Albert, Butters, and Brandt, 1981; W.W. Beatty, Salmon, et al., 1988). Cueing aids recall significantly in the early stages, but with disease progression, recall levels drop so low that, even with the benefits of cueing, patients recall half of what cued normals recall. Similar to individuals with frontal lobe impairment, HD patients have decreased memory for the source of learned information (Brandt, Bylsma, et al., 1995). However, HD patients do not show a tendency to perseveration despite increased susceptibility to proactive interference during paired-associate learning (Rich et al., 1997).

Visual memory deficits, too, tend to be mild initially and worsen with time (N. Butters, Sax, et al., 1978). Defective visual memory has been reported for designs (N. Butters et al., 1978; Caine, Bamford, et al., 1986), faces (Biber et al., 1981), and other visual stimuli (S.E. Folstein, Brandt, and Folstein, 1990). Exceptions to these findings include one study in which Huntington patients had good recall for designs but made an abnormal number of intrusion errors (D. Jacobs et al., 1990); another showed that patients' recognition memory for pictures following prolonged exposure was at the same level as normal controls after delays of ten minutes, six hours, and one week (Martone et al., 1986). Only a tendency toward impaired spatial memory was documented in one small group of Huntington patients (Boll, Heaton, and Reitan, 1974). Remote visuospatial memory, examined by recall of map locations, was found to be impaired for cities and for regions in which patients lived, yet recall of the gross features of the United States remained intact (W.W. Beatty, 1989b). The various findings—especially of the study by Boll and colleagues—may reflect heterogeneity for disease severity and/or duration in patient group composition. In studies involving designs, recall drawings may have been insufficiently analyzed due to standardization requirements of formal studies.

Motor skill and procedural learning in these patients have consistently proven defective (N. Butters, Salmon, Heindel, and Granholm, 1988; Fedio, Cox, et al., 1979; Heindel, Salmon, Shults, et al., 1989; Paulsen, Butters, et al., 1993). Most studies examining procedural learning deficits show some preserved learning ability on verbal tasks, indicating differential deterioration of the habit-forming and the knowledge acquisition memory systems. Procedural learning, too, is less impaired in the early stages of this disease (N. Butters, Wolfe, Martone, et al., 1985; Saint-Cyr and Taylor, 1992), but generalizing ability is defective, even in minimally impaired patients (Bylsma, Brandt, et al., 1990).

Verbal functions. Language structure—vocabulary, grammar, syntax—tends to be preserved in Huntington disease until the last stages, when the dementia becomes essentially global (Bayles, 1988). However, verbal productions become simplified, shortened, and susceptible to semantic errors (S.E. Folstein, Brandt, and Folstein, 1990; W.P. Gordon and Illes, 1987). Reduced verbal fluency is one of the earliest signs of encroaching cognitive deterioration (Bayles, Tomoeda, et al., 1985; N. Butters, Wolfe, Granholm, and Martone, 1986; Huber and Paulson, 1987), but with category cues these patients can improve their scores, although they are unlikely to get up to control subjects' levels (C. Randolph, Mohr, and Chase, 1993). Suhr and Jones (1998) reported no differences between semantic and category fluency but noted an excessive number of repetition errors. Confrontation naming is less likely to be impaired early in the course of the disease (Bayles and Tomoeda, 1983; R.G. Brown and Marsden, 1988) but becomes impaired as the disease progresses and may show up as an early symptom as well (Caine, Bamford, et al., 1986; W.P. Gordon and Illes, 1987).

The mechanics of speech production suffer significant alterations, with impaired articulation, loss of expressive toning, and reduced control over rate and intensity of delivery (S.E. Folstein, Brandt, and Folstein, 1990; W.P. Gordon and Illes, 1987). With worsening motor or cognitive symptoms, patients ultimately cease talking altogether, due to the same loss of voluntary control over the muscles of speech and breathing that makes eating difficult and swallowing hazardous (S.E. Folstein, 1989).

Visuospatial functions. Almost all studies report impaired visuospatial abilities, including right–left orientation, regardless of whether a motor response is required (R.G. Brown and Marsden, 1988; Caine, Bamford, et al., 1986; Fedio, Cox, et al., 1979). However, Brouwers and his colleagues (1984) found that visuoconstruction and route learning were spared in mildly impaired patients. Apraxia is rarely seen (Derix, 1994; S.E. Folstein, Brandt, and Folstein, 1990).

Administration limitations, imposed by research needs for standardized performances or rigid interpretation of test instructions, may obscure underlying deficits that contribute to low scores on visuoperceptual and construction tests while not permitting residual competencies to come to light.

A 59-year-old law school professor whose mother had died with Huntington disease was referred for neuropsychological assessment when a CT scan revealed reduction in caudate size and enlarged ventricles. His best performance, at a *superior* level, was on the WAIS-R Information test with no other WAIS-R test scores above *average*. Angulation judgment (Judgment of Line Orientation) was of *high average* caliber. However, identification of cut-up pictures (Hooper Visual Organization Test) was very *defective*, primarily because of a persistent tendency to respond to just one of the several pictured pieces in an item rather than conducting the full-scale search required for an integrated response (e.g., he called the truck [item 8] a "dresser," attending only to the rectangle with three parallel double lines that comes from the truck's side; the mouse [item 22] became a "pipe," which is the shape of the tail piece).

His initial approach to copying the Complex Figure was piecemeal: he began without any apparent attempt to scan the whole design (see Fig. 7.2, p. 240). The score for this first copy is difficult to compute but would be no higher than 12 points (of 36). Upon completing the circle and five short lines, he began to look for the next step in the drawing and only then realized that his copy was grossly distorted. He accepted the offer of redrawing the figure and, despite his clumsiness, produced an organized and spatially accurate copy with one intrusion error (see lower drawing of Fig. 7.2) and omission of the left-side cross (see Chapter 14, Fig. 14.2, p. 537, showing the Rey-Osterrieth Complex Figure). Both his immediate and delayed recall drawings preserved the structural outlines of the figure, although most details were lost (see Fig. 7.3, p. 240). It is doubtful that recall would have been even this successful if he had not been given a second copy trial. Thus, while visuospatial abilities remained intact, his performances appeared impaired due to defective scanning and planning. Had this examination followed a research protocol rigidly, this patient's intact visuospatial abilities would not have been adequately documented.

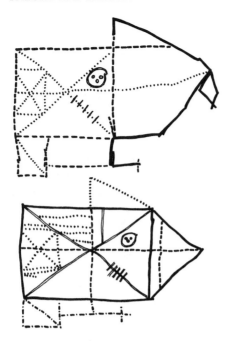

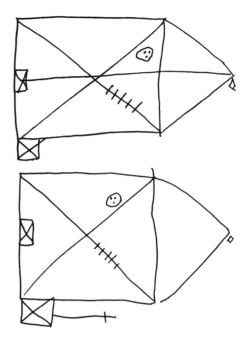

FIGURE 7.2 Tracings of law professor's Complex Figure copies (see text for description of his performance). The colored pens he used to draw the figure were switched in the course of his drawing, permitting this tracing to show the order in which he drew the figures. The drawing sequence for the first (*upper*) figure is indicated by the different lines: ___, _ _ _, ⋯, ═══. The drawing sequence for the second (*lower*) figure was ___, _ _ _, ═══, ⋯, ─·─·─.

FIGURE 7.3 Immediate (*upper*) and delayed (*lower*) recall of the Complex Figure by the law professor with Huntington's disease whose copies of the figure are shown in Figure 7.2.

Thinking and reasoning. Findings on tests of reasoning and concept formation differ a little. Some have indicated near normal retention of conceptual abilities (Similarities [WIS-A]) with a small relative decline in practical reasoning scores (Comprehension [WIS-A]) (Caine, Hunt, et al., 1978; Josiassen, Curry, Roemer, et al., 1982; M.E. Strauss and Brandt, 1985); others found that performances on both of these tests remain within the *average* range, at least in the early stages of the disease (N. Butters, Sax, et al., 1978; Fedio, Cox, et al., 1979), with Similarities (which has a large vocabulary component) holding up better than Comprehension. Calculations are typically affected (Caine, Bamford, et al., 1986; Fedio, Cox, et al., 1979; S.E. Folstein, Brandt, and Folstein, 1990).

Wechsler Intelligence Scale patterns. By and large, the performance pattern of Huntington patients on the WIS is what might be expected: Tests of well-learned material such as Information, Comprehension, Similarities, and Vocabulary hold up best; the more unfamiliar the test material and the greater the role played by reasoning, speed, or manipulation, the lower the scores (S.E. Folstein, Brandt, and Folstein, 1990; Josiassen, Curry, Roemer, et al., 1982; D.C. Myers, 1983). M.E. Strauss and Brandt (1986) reported that lowered

scores on the Digit Symbol, Comprehension, and Arithmetic tests best discriminated Huntington patients from intact subjects, and among WIS-A subtests, Digit Symbol continues to be among the most sensitive to alterations in neuropsychological status from any etiology, including early HD (Kirkwood et al., 1999; Paulsen, Zhao et al., 2001). Small variations in this overall pattern may occur between studies because different stages of the disease are represented in the patient samples and/or because sample sizes tend to be small: e.g., "only 2 of the 9 [Huntington] patient groups [under review] . . . consisted of more than 20 patients, and 3 had only 6" (Lezak, 1988c).

Executive functions

Executive deficiencies are similar to those exhibited by patients with frontal lobe lesions (Blumer and Benson, 1975; R.G. Brown and Marsden, 1988; Caine, Hunt, et al., 1978; S.E. Folstein, Brandt, and Folstein, 1990), including diminished self-generated activity, impaired behavioral regulation, and deficits in planning and organization. Early in the disease these patients are reasonably accurate in reporting their deficits (McGlynn and Kas234niak, 1991), even "acutely aware of their cognitive disabilities" (Caine, Hunt, et al., 1978), although this accuracy tends to diminish as the dementia becomes more severe (Caine and Shoulson, 1983; S.E. Folstein, 1989; McGlynn and Kaszniak, 1991).

Personality and psychosocial behavior

Huntington patients undergo significant personality changes that may precede the appearance of other symptoms, may accompany them, or may occur later in the course of the disease (Cummings, 1986; S.E. Folstein, 1989). Statistics on emotional disorders vary greatly, again probably because of age, severity, and duration differences between patient groups. Bear's (1977) conclusion that the incidence of personality or emotional change approaches 100% "of adequately examined patients" emphasizes the ubiquity of emotional and behavioral disturbances in these patients.

Depression is the most common psychiatric disorder, affecting an estimated 38% to 50% of all Huntington patients at some time, with 20% suffering chronic depression (S.E. Folstein, 1989; S.E. Folstein, Brandt, and Folstein, 1990). Evidence suggesting that it is not simply a reaction to having the disease but very likely an effect of the disease process comes from several sources: depression precedes motor and cognitive symptoms in many cases, and it is much more common in Huntington than in Alzheimer disease (Maricle, 1993). Ventral prefrontal and anterior temporal (paralimbic area) hypometabolism has been implicated in Huntington depression (Mayberg, 2002). A suicide rate around 4% to 5% is far above that for the general population (S.E. Folstein, Brandt, and Folstein, 1990; Lerner and Whitehouse, 2002). Suicide attempts were identified in 27.6% of patients in the National Huntington Disease Research Roster (Farrer, 1986). However, genetic testing confirming HD gene carrier status does not appear to increase suicide risk (Leroi and Michalon, 1998), and mood and coping strategies appear unaffected by diagnosis confirmation (Jankovic, Beach, and Ashizawa, 1995).

Mania or hypomania occurs in about 10% of patients; and anywhere from 4% (S.E. Folstein, Brandt, and Folstein, 1990) to 18% (Lohr and Wisniewski, 1987) may present with schizophrenic-like delusional or hallucinatory symptoms (McHugh and Folstein, 1975). Maricle (1993) points out, however, that the bizarre kinds of hallucinations and delusions that are first rank symptoms of schizophrenia are rare; Huntington patients are more likely to be jealous, suspicious, or obsessional. Obsessive-compulsive tendencies may be expressed by cognitive rigidity, excessive reliance on routines, and perseveration on different topics (Leroi and Michalon, 1998).

Irritability, emotional lability, and anxiety trouble many patients (Caine, Hunt, et al., 1978; Cummings, 1986). Aggressive outbursts are not uncommon, and sexual promiscuity has been reported in the early stages of Huntington's disease and Alzheimer's disease (Dew-hurst et al., 1970; S.E. Folstein, 1989; Maricle, 1993). At least in males, there is an increased crime rate in carriers of the HD gene (P. Jensen, Fenger, Bolwig, and Sorensen, 1998). Irritability and aggression, too, may result from the disease process. Apathy and anergia tend to take over in the later stages of the illness (Cummings, 1986; S.E. Folstein, Brandt, and Folstein, 1990; McHugh and Folstein, 1975) but may also be among the earliest symptoms (Maricle, 1993).

Treatment

Treatment options are limited to palliative care and will differ during different disease stages. Neuroleptic medications are most commonly used to relieve the choreic movements (Lerner and Whitehouse, 2002; Maricle, 1993). While effective for this purpose, they tend to increase rigidity and other parkinson-like symptoms (Schwarcz and Shoulson, 1987). Some newer atypical neuroleptics are often better tolerated. Moreover, dopaminergic drugs that alleviate the Parkinson-like symptoms exacerbate the chorea (Peretz and Cummings, 1988), while antidopaminergics are often effective in treating the movement disorder (Shale and Tanner, 1996). Because patients may be unaware of their chorea, this condition is not always treated. Unfortunately, neither these nor other medications improve the dementia.

Behavioral changes are often of greater disturbance to caretakers than motor or cognitive deficits. In their review of the literature, Leroi and Michalon (1998) observed that most treatment approaches for psychiatric symptoms were anecdotal. Symptoms are managed in much the same way as in mentally deteriorating patients without HD.

Progressive Supranuclear Palsy

PSP, also known as Steele-Richardson-Olszewski syndrome (J.C. Steele, Richardson, and Olszewski, 1964), has received increased attention in the popular press after the comedian/actor/musician Dudley Moore was diagnosed. PSP is classically associated with an inability to look downward on command. Because the eye gaze nuclei in the brainstem are intact, the critical lesion is a level above these nuclei—hence the name *supranuclear*. The triad of disorders that characterize the subcortical dementias—motor dysfunction, cognitive deterioration, and emotional/personality disturbances—comprise the PSP symptom complex (M.L. Albert, Feldman, and Willis, 1974; Duvoisin, 1992; Peretz and Cummings, 1988). PSP is a progressive degenerative disease that erodes subcortical structures and alters cortical—primarily prefrontal—functioning as subcortical–cortical interconnections break down. It can be considered a "Parkinson Plus" syndrome (Lieberman, 1995b).

Onset of this nonfamilial condition is usually in the 60s (Duvoisin, 1992) although it can develop in the 40s. Median survival time is approximately six years from symptom onset (not diagnosis, which is typically delayed for several years following symptom expression) (Litvan, Mangone, et al., 1996). Risk factors are unknown, but there is a suggestion that PSP may be related to an environmental toxin (Golbe, 1996). The prevalence is 1.4 per 100,000 with an estimated incidence of 3 to 4 per million (Golbe, 1996). Men may be more likely to develop the disease (Bower, Maraganore, McDonnell, and Rocca, 1997; Santacruz et al., 1998), although Golbe (1992) found no sex differences.

Neuroanatomy and pathophysiology

The lesion sites in PSP are found from the upper (rostral) brainstem to the basal ganglia (Agid et al., 1987; Jellinger and Bancher, 1992; Lees, 1990; Peretz and Cummings, 1988) and may include thalamic and limbic structures (Jernigan, Salmon, et al., 1991). The degenerative process appears to disconnect ascending pathways from these subcortical structures to the prefrontal cortex, while ascending long tracts from lower structures remain intact. Frontal involvement, due to disconnection from subcortical centers, shows up as hypometabolism (Blin et al., 1990; Burn, Sawle, and Brooks, 1994; N.L. Foster et al., 1992; Garraux et al., 1999). Changes in neurotransmitter levels take place as the degeneration proceeds (Agid et al., 1987; S. Hart and Semple, 1990; Kish et al., 1985; Ruberg, Hirsch, and Javoy-Agid, 1992). Dopamine levels drop drastically and other abnormal neurochemical alterations, both increases and decreases, are present.

The disease process

Course. Initial symptoms vary greatly and become more pronounced as the disease progresses (M.L. Albert, Feldman, and Willis, 1974; Golbe, Davis, et al., 1988; Lees, 1990; Peretz and Cummings, 1988). Postural instability and falling are the most common initial features (Furman and Cass, 2003), often appearing two years or more prior to diagnosis (Santacruz et al., 1998). Although cognitive and behavioral alterations may be the first symptoms, they are rare (Litvan, Mangone, et al., 1996). Difficulty concentrating and word-finding problems are seen in roughly half of PSP patients within 2 years of diagnosis; about half of all patients who survive more than 4 years after diagnosis

complain of failing memory (Santacruz et al., 1998). A small number of patients first display tremor or motor symptoms involving speech, swallowing, or dexterity. The hallmark of the disease—vertical gaze palsy—occurs relatively late. Histologically confirmed cases of PSP without ophthalmoplegia have been reported (Dubas, Gray, and Escourolle, 1983; Santacruz et al., 1998).

About halfway through the disease course most of the other problems emerge and increase in severity. When the disease is full-blown, movement disorders appearing as rigidity, bradykinesia, defective control of mouth and neck muscles with an impassive expression and drooling, plus a variety of oculomotor defects render the patient increasingly dependent. Most patients who live long enough become wheelchair-bound, and many are mute at the end stage. Death often results from respiratory arrest, either secondary to pneumonia or due to degenerative processes involving brainstem respiratory centers.

Diagnosis and prediction

Histologic examination is necessary for a definitive diagnosis which includes an appropriate distribution and density of neurofibrillary tangles and neuropil threads in the basal ganglia and brainstem. PSP is often misdiagnosed clinically as Parkinson's disease by primary neurologists or corticobasal degeneration by movement disorder specialists (Lees, 1990; Litvan, Mangone, et al., 1996). While workers may differ on a few of the specifics, the agreed-upon conditions that are necessary for clinical diagnosis include onset after age 40, postural instability, a progressive course, and the characteristic oculomotor symptoms (Litvan, Agid, Calne, et al., 1996; Litvan, Agid, Jankovic, et al., 1996). PSP tends to be more severe in older patients, who also have a shorter survival time (Santacruz et al., 1998).

Sensorimotor status

PSP patients typically experience visual problems associated with oculomotor defects (D. Kimura, Barnett, and Burkhart, 1981; Lees, 1990; Peretz and Cummings, 1988; Troost, 1992). Most common among these is a gaze defect in the vertical plane such that voluntary downward gaze ultimately becomes impossible. Thus they have difficulty eating or writing. Most patients fall when walking; when they try to compensate by bending the head down, their eyes roll up reflexively. Other oculomotor problems result in blurring or double vision and impaired ability to find or track visual stimuli (Rafal, 1992). They perform extremely slowly and are error-prone on tests calling for visual scanning

(Grafman, Litvan, Gomez, and Chase, 1990; D. Kimura, Barnett, and Burkhart, 1981). Motor impairments show up as slowing and difficulty performing sequential hand movements (Grafman, Litvan, Gomez, and Chase, 1990; Milberg and Albert, 1989). Ideomotor apraxia may be present (Pharr, Litvan, et al., 1999; Pharr, Uttl, et al., 2001).

Cognition

Deficits that tend to accompany prefrontal lesions are prominent. Slowing in all aspects of mental processing and response is pervasive (Au et al., 1988; Dubois, Pillon, Legault, et al., 1988; Grafman, Litvan, Gomez, and Chase, 1990). Lishman (1997), reporting his clinical experience, states that when given an "abnormal amount of time" in which to respond, his patients gave "surprisingly intact" performances: "Memory as such appeared not to be truly impaired, but rather the timing mechanism which enables the memory system to function at normal speed" (p. 667). As with other progressive conditions for which studies are based on small samples of patients at different stages, no fully consistent picture of cognitive disabilities emerges, although many features of cognitive dysfunction in PSP have been identified (E.R. Maher et al., 1985).

Attention. A mean forward digit span of 5.60 ± 1.42 in a sample of 9 patients averaging 65 years indicates that span is *within normal limits* for many if not most of these patients (Milberg and Albert, 1989). Mental tracking problems tend to be mild on relatively simple tasks and increase in severity as tracking tasks become more complex (Grafman, Litvan, Gomez, and Chase, 1990; Pillon, Dubois, Lhermitte, and Agid, 1986). Reaction time and central processing are slowed (Pillon and Dubois, 1992; Grafman, Litvan, and Stark, 1995; R. Johnson, Jr., Litvan, and Grafman, 1991).

Memory and learning. Complaints of forgetfulness are common (M.L. Albert, Feldman, and Willis, 1974; Peretz and Cummings, 1988; Pillon and Dubois, 1992). Memory impairment can occur at every stage of processing except short-term retention without interference (Litvan, Grafman, Gomez, and Chase, 1989; Milberg and Albert, 1989; Pillon, Dubois, Lhermitte, and Agid, 1986). These patients are very susceptible to interference effects (Pillon and Dubois, 1992). Although significantly impaired when compared with an appropriate control group, PSP patients' memory deficits tend not to be as severe as those of Alzheimer patients (Milberg and Albert, 1989; Pillon, Dubois, Lhermitte, and Agid, 1986), near normal verbal and nonverbal memory performances have been reported (M.S. Albert,

Moss, and Milberg, 1989), and within group variations can be very large (E.R. Maher et al., 1985). Implicit learning does take place (Pillon and Dubois, 1992). However, PSP patients display rapid forgetting (Grafman, Litvan, and Stark, 1995).

Verbal functions. Impaired verbal retrieval shows up as word finding problems (Au et al., 1988) and defective performance on fluency tests (Dubois, Pillon, Legault, et al., 1988; Litvan, Grafman, et al., 1989; Pillon, Dubois, Ploska, and Agid, 1991). Confrontation naming tends to be mildly impaired (Cummings, 1986; Milberg and Albert, 1989), although the naming errors often involve an object visually similar to the target object, suggesting that visual misperception is the major source of the naming disorder. As with Huntington and Parkinson patients, the elements of language remain intact. The mechanism of speech production, however, can be affected most prominently by slowing but also by dysarthria and a monotonic delivery (M.L. Albert, Feldman, and Willis, 1974).

Visuospatial functions. Scores on tests requiring analysis and integration of visually presented material tend to be marginal to the *average* range (Picture Completion, see D. Kimura, Barnett, and Burkhart, 1981; Picture Arrangement, see Grafman, Litvan, Gomez, and Chase, 1990), and these patients do poorly on Block Design (Milberg and Albert, 1989; Derix, 1994). These WIS-A tests are all timed, leaving in question how much response slowing contributes to low scores. A finding of impaired cube drawing, however, does implicate a visuospatial deficit (Pillon, Dubois, Lhermitte, and Agid, 1986).

Thinking and reasoning. Clinical observations indicate that PSP patients vary in the degree to which thinking and reasoning are impaired, as some report normal functioning and others describe deficits (M.L. Albert, Feldman, and Willis, 1974; Janati and Appel, 1984). Verbal concept formation as measured by Similarities (WIS-A) has typically been reported to be at an *average* level (excepting a report by Pillon, Dubois, Lhermitte, and Agid, 1986, whose patients performed significantly below the *average* range). When examined by visual tests (Raven's Progressive Matrices, Wisconsin Card Sorting Test), concept formation is consistently impaired (Dubois, Pillon, Legault, et al., 1988; Grafman, Litvan, Gomez, and Chase, 1990; Milberg and Albert, 1989). These patients' ability for mental manipulations, as required by arithmetic story problems, tends to be impaired, although they can perform multiplication adequately (Milberg and Albert, 1989; Pillon et al., 1986).

Executive functions

Executive dysfunction is an important characteristic of this disease. It shows up in both verbal and graphic dysfluency, in impaired sequencing and mental flexibility, and as apathy and behavioral inertia, and difficulty planning and shifting conceptual sets (M.L. Albert, Feldman, and Willis, 1974; Grafman, Litvan, Gomez, and Chase, 1990; Grafman, Litvan, and Stark, 1995; Pillon, Dubois, Ploska, and Agid, 1991). Pillon and Dubois (1992) suggest that many of these patients' abstraction and reasoning failures are essentially due to impaired executive functioning. Significant correlations have been reported between apathy and the Initiation and Perseveration scores from the Mattis Dementia Rating Scale, suggesting a common link to frontal–subcortical abnormalities (Litvan, Mega, et al., 1996).

Personality and psychosocial behavior

Apathy and inertia are the most commonly reported personality features of PSP patients (Aarsland et al., 1999; M.L. Albert, Feldman, and Willis, 1974; Janati and Appel, 1984; Peretz and Cummings, 1988). These problems were identified in 91% of one sample using the Neuropsychiatric Inventory (Litvan, Mega, et al., 1996). Irritability is frequently seen; depression or euphoria may occur in some patients. Dubois, Pillon, Legault, and their colleagues (1988) found a tendency for their patients to report mild depression. Emotional incontinence—either laughing or crying—has also been described in some patients. Disinhibition is present in approximately one-third of PSP patients (Litvan, Mega, et al., 1996).

Treatment

Despite its resemblance to many features of Parkinson's disease, PSP has limited response to dopamanergic or anticholinergic drugs (Kompoliti et al., 1998). The emotional symptoms may be relieved by some antidepressants, but cognitive dysfunction is as yet untreatable (Lees, 1990).

OTHER PROGRESSIVE DISORDERS OF THE CENTRAL NERVOUS SYSTEM IN WHICH NEUROPSYCHOLOGICAL EFFECTS MAY BE PROMINENT

Multiple Sclerosis (MS)

Although typically characterized by relapses and remissions early in its course, MS is grouped with the de-

generative diseases because it often involves more or less progressive accumulation of neurological deficits with persistent cognitive and behavioral dysfunction later in its course. Unlike many other degenerative diseases, however, MS typically strikes during the prime wage-earning years and does not appreciably shorten life span, so it is extremely costly on both individual and societal levels (Whetten-Goldstein et al., 1998). In the United States, an estimated 250,000 to 350,000 persons have physician-diagnosed MS, amounting to a prevalence rate of 0.1% (D.W. Anderson et al., 1992).

MS is distinctive for the often erratic appearance of symptoms that flare up acutely over the course of several days, persist for variable lengths of time, then disappear or at least partially remit for periods of unpredictable length (A.E. Miller, 2001; Noseworthy, Lucchinetti, et al., 2000). Each new attack may involve different areas of brain or spinal cord white matter and consequently may produce very different symptoms. The enormous variability in the physical and cognitive manifestations of MS and in rates of disease progression complicate the determination of "early" and "late" stages. Consequently, MS is more accurately staged with reference to extent of underlying pathology than to symptom duration.

Prominent MS symptoms include weakness, stiffness, or incoordination of an arm or leg; gait disturbance; visual impairments; neurogenic bladder and bowel symptoms (including hesitancy and retention, or urgency and incontinence); sexual dysfunction (affecting all aspects of the sexual response); sensory changes; heat sensitivity; and fatigue, particularly in the afternoon when body temperature rises (A.E. Miller, 2001). Some patients may develop a cerebellar syndrome, including dysarthria characterized by thickened, sluggish sounding speech or by spasmodically paced—"scanning"—speech, *dysphagia* (difficulty swallowing), and tremor. Cognitive impairment—typically involving attentional processes, memory, and executive functions—is common. However, cortical signs (e.g., aphasia and apraxia) are rare, which may explain why neurologists failed for so many years to appreciate the prevalence of cognitive impairment in MS (Fischer, 2001; J.T.E. Richardson, Robinson, and Robinson, 1997).

Diagnosis, course, and prediction
Diagnostic issues. The diagnosis of MS is based on clinical abnormalities observed on neurological examination, supplemented by abnormalities on laboratory studies such as cerebrospinal fluid (CSF) analysis findings indicating immune activation and evoked potential or MRI studies (W.I. McDonald et al., 2001; A.E. Miller, 2001; Noseworthy, Lucchinetti, et al., 2000).

Relapsing forms of MS are considered definite when an individual has had at least two distinct attacks plus neurologic signs confirming involvement of at least two sites in the central nervous system, i.e., evidence of "dissemination in time and space" (C.M. Poser, Paty, et al., 1983). The vast majority of patients who initially have isolated CNS syndromes involving the optic nerve, spinal cord, brain stem, or cerebellum with MRI evidence of additional clinically asymptomatic brain lesions have further clinical attacks (Brex et al., 2002; Optic Neuritis Study Group, 1997). Consequently, now patients with clinically isolated syndromes who have unequivocal MRI evidence of dissemination in time and space can be given a diagnosis of definite MS (Dalton et al., 2002; W.I. McDonald et al., 2001); absent MRI evidence, patients with clinically isolated syndromes receive a diagnosis of possible MS. *Progressive forms* of MS are considered definite if patients have clinical or MRI evidence of disease progression for at least one year and supportive laboratory findings (i.e., abnormal CSF and abnormal MRI or visual evoked potentials), with no other plausible neurologic cause (W.I. McDonald et al., 2001).

Measuring disease severity. Disease severity in MS is traditionally expressed as a score on the Kurtzke *Expanded Disability Status Scale* (*EDSS*; Kurtzke, 1983b), a clinical rating scale derived from the neurologic examination. Walking ability and motor function contribute most strongly to EDSS scores, although brainstem, sensory, bowel and bladder, and visual functions also enter in. The rating of "cerebral" functions is based on clinical judgment rather than formal neuropsychological examination, and it confounds assessment of cognitive function and affective state. The psychometric limitations of the EDSS—ordinal scale of measurement, bimodal score distribution, poor reproducibility, and relative insensitivity to change—are widely acknowledged (Sharrack et al., 1999). Other clinical rating scales for MS have been devised, but they suffer similar psychometric limitations (Rudick, Weinshenker, and Cutter, 2001).

Cognitive function generally correlates weakly with symptom duration and neurologic disability, as assessed by the EDSS (W.W. Beatty, Goodkin, Hertsgaard, and Monson, 1990; S.M. Rao, Leo, Bernardin, and Unverzagt, 1991), excepting perhaps processing speed and working memory (Thornton and Raz, 1997). This should not be surprising. Cerebral atrophy can occur early in an MS course (Rudick, Fisher et al., 1999; Zivadinov, Sepcic, et al., 2001), contributing to the weak relationship between cognitive function and disease duration. Moreover, patients with predominantly spinal cord involvement can have substantial physical disability—resulting in high EDSS scores—but still remain cognitively intact (Lezak, Bourdette, et al., 1989). Consequently, newer quantitative assessments which incorporate measures of sensory, motor, and cognitive function complement severity ratings derived from MS clinical rating scales (Fischer, Rudick, Cutter, et al., 1999; Syndulko, Ke, et al., 1996).

Disease course. MS can follow several distinct courses (Lublin and Reingold, 1996; Vukusic and Confavreux, 2001). In rare cases, it is "clinically silent," with MS plaques showing up on autopsy in individuals who showed no obvious clinical symptoms of the disease during life (J.J. Gilbert and Sadler, 1983). In approximately 80% of patients, MS begins with a clinical attack from which the patient essentially "recovers," followed by clearly defined relapses, with improvement—either full or partial—and clinical stability between attacks: this pattern is termed *relapsing–remitting MS*. Up to 10% of these patients do extremely well, with only infrequent attacks and little observable neurological impairment after 15 years or more (*benign MS*); this subgroup is probably underrepresented in clinic-based studies as patients have no need for follow-up examinations. Most relapsing–remitting patients start deteriorating progressively within 15 years of their initial attack, either with or without occasional relapses (*secondary progressive MS*).

In contrast, about 20% of MS patients have a gradual, nearly continuous progressive course from the time their first symptom appears (A.J. Thompson et al., 2000). Most do not have any clear-cut relapses or remissions (*primary progressive MS*), although some have occasional relapses superimposed on a progressive course (*progressive relapsing MS*). On occasion, MS progresses very rapidly, reducing a patient to helpless dependency or death soon after disease onset (*malignant MS*). However, studies of life expectancy in MS—even those conducted before the availability of disease-modifying medications—indicated a median survival of 35 to 42 years after diagnosis (S. Poser, Kurtzke, et al., 1989), so for most patients, age at death is similar to that for the population at large (Sadovnick, Ebers, et al., 1992).

Although these classifications are based primarily on physical changes appearing on neurological examination, disease course has modest predictive value for cognitive dysfunction. For example, chronic progressive patients (those with primary progressive or secondary progressive MS) generally perform worse on cognitive tests than do patients with relapsing–remitting MS (Fischer, 1988; M. Grossman, Armstrong, et al., 1994; Heaton, Nelson, Thompson, et al., 1985). In addition, secondary progressive MS patients tend to be more impaired than those with a primary progressive course (S.J. Camp et al., 1999; Gaudino et al., 2001), although these differences are much less striking when patients are equated for disease duration and disability (Foong, Rozewicz, Chong, et al., 2000). Relapsing–remitting patients may also have deficits relative to healthy controls, albeit less striking ones than those observed in progressive patients (M. Grossman, Armstrong, et al., 1994; L. Ryan et al., 1996). Relapses may also be associated with fluctuations in cognitive function, particularly attention and processing speed (Foong, Rozewica, Quaghebeur, et al., 1998). However, the relationship between cognitive impairment and disease course is not strong enough to predict the cognitive status of individual MS patients (W.W. Beatty, Goodkin, Hertsgaard, et al., 1990).

Prognosis. Predicting disease course or rate of progression is fraught with inaccuracies, particularly early in the disease (Kantarci and Weinshenker, 2001). Before disease-modifying treatments were available, the common expectation was that half of all MS patients would need assistance to walk within 15 years of clinical onset (Weinshenker et al., 1989). Poor prognosis (i.e., more rapid disability progression) is associated with older age at symptom onset, incomplete recovery from a first attack, a short interval between the first two attacks, frequent relapses over the first five years, a progressive course from disease onset, and early motor, cerebellar, or sphincter symptoms (Kantarci and Weinshenker, 2001; Noseworthy, Lucchinetti et al., 2000). If the initial MS attack consists of optic neuritis, predominantly sensory symptoms, or limited brainstem symptoms, the disease often follows a more favorable course.

Predicting the probability and course of cognitive impairment in an MS patient is also difficult. Early longitudinal studies suggested that, when present, cognitive deficits were reasonably stable—or at least progressed slowly relative to physical impairment—with fewer than 20% of patients deteriorating over three to four year intervals (Bernardin et al., 1993; Jennekens-Schinkel et al., 1990). Amato and his colleagues' (2001) longitudinal study painted a less optimistic picture: 24% of recent onset patients—most of whom had relapsing-remitting disease—worsened within four to five years, and by the ten year follow-up, 42% had deteriorated significantly. Furthermore, nearly all of the cognitively impaired patients in a study of patients with moderate to severe disability and progressive MS deteriorated further over the two to four year follow-up, and nearly one-third of those who were cognitively intact at the initial assessment worsened slightly as well (Kujala, Portin, and Ruutiainen, 1997).

Thus, as with all other MS symptoms, cognitive impairment is often progressive at quite variable rates.

Risk factors

Converging evidence from an extensive body of genetic, epidemiologic, viral, and immunologic studies suggests that MS is the product of multiple factors, none of which is by itself sufficient for the development of MS (Pryse-Phillips and Costello, 2001).

Genetic predisposition. Genetic factors clearly influence susceptibility to MS (Compston and Coles, 2002; Hillert and Masterman, 2001; Noseworhty, Lucchinetti, et al., 2000). Concordance rates in monozygotic twins (approximately 30%) are about six times those for dizygotic twins and other full siblings (2%–5%)—markedly higher than that in the general population. The human leukocyte antigen (HLA) gene complex is considered crucial in determining MS susceptibility, although other candidate genes and chromosomal regions have been implicated as well (Hillert and Masterman, 2001). Some genetic factors (e.g., ApoE 4 allele frequency) may affect rates of disease progression but not susceptibility (Chapman, 2001; Fazekas, Strasser-Fuchs, et al., 2001).

Many chromosome regions containing genes thought to be important in MS also harbor genes that predispose individuals to other autoimmune diseases (K.G. Becker et al., 1998). Autoimmune diseases—but not other diseases types—are more common in first-degree relatives of MS patients than in control subjects, raising the possibility that autoimmunity itself may have a common genetic predisposition (Broadley et al., 2000). MS most likely involves multiple genes and considerable genetic heterogeneity (Hillert and Masterman, 2001; Oksenberg, Baranzini, et al., 2001). However, the lack of perfect concordance in identical twins underscores the importance of nonhereditary factors.

Demographic factors. MS is two to three times more common in women than in men. This gender discrepancy is greatest in patients whose disease initially follows a relapsing–remitting course and virtually nonexistent in patients whose course is progressive from onset (Noseworthy, Lucchinetti, et al., 2000). The average age at MS symptom onset is around 30 (Vukusic and Confavreux, 2001). However, initial symptoms occur before age 16 in nearly 5% of patients (Ghezzi et al., 1997), and after age 50 in close to 10% (Noseworthy, Paty, et al., 1983). Prevalence by race is related to latitude (see below).

Geographic latitude. The prevalence of MS varies greatly around the world, implicating environmental factors. Excepting Japan, temperate zones tend to have higher prevalence rates, with MS becoming less common as one approaches the tropics. For unknown reasons, this north–south gradient has attenuated somewhat over time (Hernán et al., 1999). High prevalence regions (30 or more cases per 100,000) include the northern United States and Canada, northern Europe, eastern Russia, Israel, southeastern Australia, and New Zealand. Regions with medium prevalence rates (5 to 30 cases per 100,000) comprise the southern United States, southern Mediterranean countries, the Ukraine and Russia into Siberia, the remainder of Australia, South Africa, and parts of Latin America. MS remains relatively rare in the rest of Asia, Africa, and northern South America, although the prevalence rate in African Americans—many of whom are of mixed African and Caucasian heritage—is between that of native Africans and Caucasians. Epidemiological studies in the Faro Islands and emigration studies in South Africa, Israel, and England suggest that the risk of developing MS is associated with where one lived before mid-adolescence: by and large, Europeans migrating to areas of relatively low incidence (e.g., Israel, South Africa) after age 15 have the same risk of MS as those remaining in their countries of origin, whereas those migrating before age 15 have the lower risk associated with their new countries (Kurtzke, 2000).

Infection. Several lines of evidence suggest that an infectious agent may initiate—and perhaps maintain—the pathological immune response in MS. On average, MS patients contracted common childhood illnesses at later ages than healthy controls, and they also have elevated levels of serum or CSF antibodies to several viruses (S.D. Cook, 2001). MS exacerbations often seem to be triggered by viral or bacterial infections, even if the infectious agent is not implicated in the development of MS. As yet, however, no infectious agent has been unequivocally linked to MS. Kesselring and Lassman (1997) have suggested that MS probably represents a generalized delayed immune response to multiple infections occurring during a highly vulnerable period for the immune system.

Immunology. While many aspects of the immune response in MS must still be worked out, there is no doubt that the immune system plays a crucial role in this neurologic disease. Many components of the immune system are involved (Compston and Coles, 2002; Oksenberg and Hauser, 1999). For unknown reasons, certain types of immune system cells (T cells), normally located outside the CNS, become activated and are able to penetrate the protective *blood–brain barrier* (*BBB*) to proliferate and stimulate activity in other types of immune

system cells (e.g., B cells, macrophages, and cytokines). Antibodies to components of the myelin sheath are also formed, enter the CNS, and attack myelin directly (Lucchinetti et al., 2000; Noseworthy, Lucchinetti et al., 2000). Additional immune factors and mechanisms may contribute to myelin degradation and predominate during the relapsing and progressive stages of the illness. Neuroimaging studies suggest that active inflammatory lesions are present up to ten times more often than manifest relapses, suggesting that MS is far more active immunologically than is clinically apparent (D.H. Miller, Barkhof, and Nauta, 1993).

Hormonal factors may modify both the complex immune response and the clinical symptoms of this illness. Relapse rates and MS lesion activity typically decline during pregnancy—especially during the third trimester—and then increase in the first three months postpartum, before returning to prepregnancy rates (Confavreux et al., 1998; van Walderveen, Tas, et al., 1994). In addition, MS symptoms often worsen during the premenstrual phase of a woman's cycle (Zordrager and De Keyser, 1998), and MS lesion activity on MRI has been associated with hormone ratios in the luteal phase (Pozzilli, Falaschi, et al., 1999).

Vulnerabilities

Stress. The idea that physical trauma or emotional stress may precipitate MS onset or exacerbations has been around since the late 1800s. Controlled studies have not shown an association between physical trauma and either MS onset or exacerbation (Goodin, Ebers, et al., 1999; Martinelli, 2000). Controlled retrospective studies do suggest a link between psychological stress and MS symptom onset: over 75% of MS patients experienced at least one major negative life event prior to symptom onset compared with slightly over half of those with other chronic illnesses (Warren, Greenhill, and Warren, 1982) and only one-third of healthy adults over comparable time periods (I. Grant, Brown, et al., 1989). Grant and his colleagues found that MS patients were much more likely than healthy persons to have experienced qualitatively extreme events. In a more recent study, events categorized as "moderately stressful"—those that produced conflict and disrupted daily routines but were not considered severe stressors—were prospectively associated with new inflammatory lesions on MRI 8 weeks later (D.C. Mohr, Goodkin, Bacchetti, et al., 2000). Moreover, most patients believe that stress can trigger MS exacerbations (Rabins, Brooks, et al., 1986).

However, other studies do not support a link between stress and MS activation. For example, clinically stable patients and those in exacerbation reported comparable *numbers* of stresses—both major and minor—in the preceding six months (Warren, Warren, and Cockerill, 1991), although other patients in exacerbation reported a *greater number* of "moderately to extremely negative" events in the preceding six months than did clinically stable patients (G.M. Franklin, Nelson, Heaton, et al., 1988). Over a 12-week period the absolute number of major life stressors did not prospectively predict either clinical exacerbations or new inflammatory lesions (on MRI) (D.C. Mohr, Goodkin, Bacchetti, et al., 2000). Furthermore, MS patients and healthy persons displayed similar subjective, physiological, and immunologic responses to simulated stressors (Ackerman et al., 1998).

It may well be that the intensity of a specific stressor and the disruption associated with it are crucial mediating factors in MS. A chronic fluctuating disease like MS undoubtedly increases the proportion of negative to positive stressors, which in turn could affect disease progression (C.E. Schwartz et al., 1999). The relationship between stress and MS exacerbations clearly merits further study (Goodin, Ebers, et al., 1999; Martinelli, 2000).

Heat. In MS heat—whether in the form of hot weather or an overheated room—often worsens existing symptoms and may even precipitate new ones (e.g., blurring of vision). Fever associated with infection and elevated body temperatures with physical exertion or exercise can have the same effect. Fortunately the emergence or worsening of MS symptoms due to elevated body temperature is nearly always transient as symptoms return to baseline when body temperature is reduced (A.E. Miller, 2001).

Fatigue. Over 80% of MS patients cite fatigue as a current symptom, and it is often one of the most disabling (Ford et al., 1998; Krupp, 1997). Patients with significant fatigue cannot actively engage in a task for more than a few hours at a time without it compromising their efficiency or sense of well-being. MS fatigue is relatively independent of disease-related variables such as physical disability and disease duration or course (J.D. Fisk et al., 1994; Ford et al., 1998). It is thought to arise from a combination of impaired nerve conduction, physical deconditioning, depression and anxiety, and cognitive impairment (Krupp, 1997). Central factors such as metabolic abnormalities of the frontal cortex and basal ganglia, increased cortical activation during movement, and immune dysfunction undoubtedly contribute to MS fatigue (Comi, Leocani, et al., 2001).

Although MS patients often report that fatigue affects their cognitive functioning, neuropsychological test performance is not strongly related either to subjective fatigue (as assessed by the 9-item *Fatigue Severity Scale* (*FSS*) (Krupp and Elkins, 2000; R.H. Paul, Beatty, Schneider, et al., 1998b) or to fatigue induced by the testing procedures themselves (R.A. Cohen and Fisher, 1989; S.K. Johnson et al., 1997). However, adverse effects of fatigue have been observed on tasks requiring continuous mental effort over extended intervals (Krupp and Elkins, 2000; Kujala, Portin, Revonsuo, and Ruutiainen, 1995).

Neuroanatomy and pathophysiology

Pathophysiology. The pathological hallmark of MS is the demyelinated plaque, which is characterized by loss of the myelin sheath and proliferation of *astrocytes* (star-shaped connective tissue cells), forming pinkish or grayish scar tissue (*gliosis*) (Compston and Coles, 2002; Noseworthy, Lucchinetti, et al., 2000). Active lesions usually show evidence of both inflammatory cells and *remyelination* ("shadow plaques"). Although all MS lesions from any given patient will have a common structure and immunologic features, the immunologic features of lesions may differ from patient to patient (Lucchinetti, et al., 2000). This raises the possibility that MS is a disease entity that actually comprises several distinct syndromes differing in their etiologies and pathogenic mechanisms.

The early clinical symptoms of MS most likely stem from axonal demyelination, which can slow or even block nerve conduction (Noseworthy, Lucchinetti, et al., 2000). Clinical recovery occurs as edema resolves, sodium channels—essential to the propagation of nerve impulses—become redistributed along demyelinated axons, and remyelination occurs in some axons. After repeated bouts of disease activity, neurologic function is progressively lost due to irreversible axonal injury, scarring, and depletion of the cells from which myelin is formed. Both inflammation and demyelination appear to play a role in axonal degeneration, both within MS plaques and in "normal appearing white matter" outside lesions as a result of *Wallerian degeneration* (loss of axons due to disconnection from their originating cell bodies) (DeStefano et al., 2002; Waxman, 2000), albeit at different disease stages.

Neuroanatomy. Although primarily a disease affecting white matter, MS lesions can nonetheless be found in any part of the CNS, including gray matter in which myelinated axons lie (Kidd, Barkhof, et al., 1999; Noseworthy, Lucchinetti, et al., 2000). Moreover, white matter lesions blocking or compromising subcortical axonal transmission can undercut—and effectively isolate—specific cortical areas (Filley, 2001; Jeffery,

Absher, et al., 2000). Despite the randomness with which MS lesions can appear, certain patterns of lesion location account for the most common symptoms. Specifically, MS has a predilection for the optic nerves, the white matter surrounding the cerebral ventricles (*periventricular region*), the corpus callosum, and the white matter of the brain stem, cerebellum, and spinal cord (Noseworthy, Lucchinetti, et al., 2000).

Neuroimaging. MS lesions appear as hyperintense "bright spots" on conventional T_2-weighted MRI, making MRI one of the most useful diagnostic tools (Fazekas et al., 1999). MRI makes it possible to identify, locate, and study the evolution of both MS lesions and atrophy in the brain and spinal cord (P.M. Matthews and Arnold, 2001; D.H. Miller, Grossman, et al., 1998). However, neurologic disability (as measured by the EDSS) is only modestly correlated with the number or volume of MS lesions appearing on T_2 images—no doubt a function of both the psychometric limitations of the EDSS and the restricted scope of conventional imaging (Barkhof, 1999).

For example, newer T_2 image acquisition procedures—such as fast spin echo (FSE) imaging and fluid-attenuated inversion recovery (FLAIR)—can detect cortical and juxtacortical lesions not apparent on conventional images (Bakshi, Ariyaratana et al., 2001; Moriarty et al., 1999), while MRI procedures such as T_1-weighted imaging with gadolinium are better suited to identifying active inflammatory lesions as well as areas of extensive demyelination and axonal loss—so-called "black holes" (D.H. Miller, Grossman, et al., 1998). Newer quantitative imaging techniques—magnetic transfer imaging (MTI), diffusion-weighted imaging (DWI), and magnetic resonance spectroscopy (MRS)—can detect subtle abnormalities in brain tissue that appear quite normal on T_1 and T_2 images (Filippi and Grossman, 2002; Rovaris, Bozzali, et al., 2001). Subtle abnormalities in brain tissue elicited by these imaging techniques may precede the emergence of enhancing lesions by up to 2 years (Pike et al., 2000).

Not surprisingly, neuropsychological test performance is moderately to strongly related to the overall volume of MS lesions on MRI (S.M. Rao, Leo, Haughton, et al., 1989; Rovaris and Filippi, 2000). Furthermore, patients with the greatest lesion volumes are at heightened risk for further cognitive decline (J.A. Bobholz, personal communication [jsf]). Test performance has also been associated with MRI indicators of brain atrophy, including evidence of periventricular and callosal sites and generalized loss of brain tissue (Fischer, 2001; Zivadinov, De Masi, et al., 2001). Increases in lesion burden and in brain atrophy over one to four year intervals have been associated with deteriorating test performance (Sperling et al., 2001; Zivadinov, Sepcic, et al., 2001).

A purported relationship between executive dysfunction and MS lesion burden in specific brain regions, most notably the frontal lobes (Arnett, Rao, et al., 1994), becomes attenuated when overall lesion burden is taken into account (Foong, Rozewicz, Quaghebeur, et al., 1997). In fact, cognitive impairment in MS is more closely linked to lesions that disrupt cortical–cortical connections than it is to white matter lesions in specific regions (Lazeron, Rombouts, et al., 2000; Moriarty, Blackshaw, et al., 1999). The most robust relationships between neuroanatomic loci on MRI and neuropsychological performance are those between the corpus callosum and several related cognitive functions—complex attention and processing speed, verbal fluency, and interhemispheric transfer (Pelletier et al., 2001; S.M. Rao, Leo, Haughton, et al., 1989). These findings make sense: performance on many cognitive tests is subserved by distributed cognitive networks rather than isolated brain regions, so it is unrealistic to attribute most cognitive abnormalities in MS to focal lesions, particularly when there is widespread disease.

Parameters derived from newer imaging techniques have demonstrated even more striking associations with cognitive function (Rovaris, Filippi, Minicucci, et al., 2000; van Buchem, Grossman, et al., 1998; Zivadinov, De Masi, et al., 20001). Furthermore, MS patients' cognitive function correlates strongly with cerebral glucose metabolism rates on PET (Blinkenberg et al., 2000); their cerebral activation patterns differ from control subjects' on both ERP studies (Pelosi et al., 1997) and functional MRI (fMRI) (Rocca, Falini, Colombo, et al., 2002). Even more intriguing is the observation that differences in cerebral activation patterns are apparent even when MS patients' test performances are superficially similar to those of healthy controls (Filippi and Grossman, 2002), raising the possibility that cognitive and motor circuits can reorganize to compensate for tissue damage.

Cognition

The dissemination of lesions in cerebral white matter plus their affinity for periventricular regions creates some commonalities of cognitive dysfunction in MS (Fischer, 2001; Wishart and Sharpe, 1997). Relatively few MS patients qualify for a diagnosis of dementia as cognitive impairments are often less severe than those seen in neurologic disorders in which dementia is prominent (W.W. Beatty, Goodkin, Monson, and Beatty, 1989; M.A. Butters, Goldstein, et al., 1998).

Moreover, unlike dementing conditions, MS is by its very nature heterogeneous in both its physical and cognitive manifestations. For example, three distinct neuropsychological patterns have been observed in relapsing–remitting patients (Fischer, Jacobs, Cookfair, et al., 1998; L. Ryan et al., 1996). Although many patients—34% to 46% of those studied—appeared to function quite normally from a neuropsychological perspective, nearly one in six were noticeably impaired, with deficits of at least moderate severity in three or more cognitive domains. The most common pattern of impairment in these samples—observed in 37% to 49% of the patients—involved circumscribed deficits in one or two cognitive domains (e.g., attention/processing speed, learning/memory, and/or executive function), in varying combinations. Estimates of the prevalence of cognitive dysfunction—including milder forms of cognitive impairment—hover around 43%–44% on comprehensive neuropsychological assessments (Heaton, Nelson, Thompson, et al., 1985; S.M. Rao, Leo, Bernardin, and Unverzagt, 1991). These figures are much higher than those derived from brief mental status examinations, which are notoriously insensitive to the types of cognitive deficits commonly seen in MS (W.W. Beatty and Goodkin, 1990). *Because of the many different ways in which cognition can be affected in MS patients, neuropsychological examination of these patients requires assessment of a variety of functions.*

Sensorimotor status. Visual disturbances in MS are varied and may include blurred vision, double vision resulting from eye movement incoordination which is usually persistent, total or partial loss of vision due to *optic neuritis* (inflammatory demyelination of the optic nerve, typically of acute onset, unilateral, and transient MS), loss of color perception or blindness in one or both eyes, impaired contrast sensitivity, impaired ability to process individual features of visual stimuli, and eye movement abnormalities (A.E. Miller, 2001; Vleugels et al., 2000). Whitaker and Benveniste (1990) estimated that two-thirds of MS patients would experience at least one of these visual problems at some point in their illness, some transiently and others permanently. Auditory dysfunction is less common but hearing loss—either unilateral or bilateral—does occasionally occur, often in association with brainstem lesions (A.E. Miller, 2001). Examiners must be aware of the possibility of sensory disorders that can affect patients' test performances.

Spontaneous complaints of impaired sense of smell are rare, but up to one-third of all MS patients may have olfactory dysfunction (Doty, Li, et al., 1999). Olfactory deficits are strongly associated with plaque load in inferior frontal and temporal lobes. Deficits in olfaction may alert the examiner to the possibility of defects in cognitive functions subserved by these regions.

At some point in their illness, nearly all MS patients experience sensory alterations—including numbness, tingling or painful sensations, and *Lhermitte's phenomenon* ("electric shock" sensation on neck flexion) (A.E. Miller, 2001). Motor symptoms are also extremely common, with 80 to 90% of MS patients reporting episodic or persistent limb weakness, spasticity, and/or incoordination—usually a combination of these problems. Because MS patients inevitably perform poorly on tests requiring fine sensory discrimination or rapid coordinated motor responses (Heaton, Nelson, Thompson, et al. 1985; van den Burg et al., 1987), test batteries should minimize sensory and motor demands (Benedict, Fischer, et al., 2002; Peyser, Rao, et al., 1990). Alternatively, one can "extract" the motor skill aspects of a task by subtracting the score of a simple visuomotor task from that of its complex form (e.g., Digit Symbol [WAIS-III], Trail Making Test). The examiner should avoid giving tests on which failure is both inevitable and uninterpretable due to sensory or motor confounds while covering a wide range of cognitive functions (see pp. 118–120 for testing which minimizes visual, sensory, and motor demands).

Attention. Many MS patients report feeling mentally "slowed down," noting that they must exert great effort to think quickly or to keep up with the pace of normal conversation. Impaired processing speed is a classical finding in MS (C.J. Archibald and Fisk, 2000; Kail, 1998; Kujala, Portin, Revonsuo, and Ruutiainen, 1994; S.M. Rao, St. Aubin-Faubert, and Leo, 1989). This shows up on well-known tasks such as the PASAT and the oral response format of the Symbol-Digit Modalities Test (SDMT) as well as on tests requiring information transfer between cerebral hemispheres (S.M. Rao, Bernardin, Leo, et al., 1989; Rubens et al., 1985; Wishart, Strauss, et al., 1995), particularly those involving dichotic listening and lexical decision making (Ortiz et al., 2000). MS patients can often perform accurately if stimuli are presented at a sufficiently slow rate as impaired processing speed is a core cognitive deficit (Demaree et al., 1999).

Simple auditory span and visuospatial span are normal in most MS patients (Heaton, Nelson, Thompson, et al., 1985; Minden, Moes, Orav, et al., 1990; S.M. Rao, Leo, Bernardin, and Unverzagt, 1991), although deficits in auditory span—and less commonly, visuospatial span—have been reported (W.W. Beatty, Paul, Blanco, et al., 1995; DeLuca, Barbieri-Berger, and Johnson, 1994; Fischer, 1988). Performance on tests of selective attention varies, depending on task demands and disease factors. Many MS patients will perform normally on self-paced tests with the printed material in front of them (e.g., letter or symbol cancellation tasks) and on tests that have few stimulus or response choices, such as the Brown-Peterson technique (auditory consonant trigrams) and many choice reaction time tasks (W.W. Beatty, Goodkin, Monson, and Beatty, 1989; Kujala, Portin, Revonsuo, and Ruutiainen, 1994; S.M. Rao, Leo, Bernardin, and Unverzagt, 1991). Deficits are often more apparent on tests using auditory verbal stimuli than those using visual stimuli (Foong, Rozewicz, Quaghebeur, et al., 1997; R.H. Paul, Beatty, Schneider, et al., 1998a), although not always (B.J. Diamond et al., 1997). Increased disease activity, whether due to an exacerbation or continuing disease progression, may ultimately compromise a patient's previously adequate attentional resources, leading to performance impairments on even less demanding selective attention tests (I. Grant, McDonald, Trimble, et al. 1984; Grigsby, Ayarbe, et al., 1994).

Regardless of disease status, most MS patients exhibit deficits on tasks with greater stimulus or response complexity—such as supraspan tests, sequence reversal tests, and the Sternberg task—and those requiring inhibition of a previously correct response—including the Stroop interference condition and the PASAT (R.H. Paul, Beatty, Schneider, et al., 1998a; Rao, Leo, Bernardin, and Unverzagt, 1991; Rao, St. Aubin-Faubert, and Leo, 1989; van den Burg et al., 1987). In addition, alternating attention and divided attention are nearly always impaired in MS. Impairments will be immediately apparent on tasks requiring patients to shift attention back and forth from one stimulus to another, such as alphanumeric sequencing and Trails B (Grigsby, Kaye, and Busenbark, 1994; Heaton, Nelson, Thompson, et al., 1985). Performance deficiencies will also be evident when two operations or tasks must be performed simultaneously, the absolute level of impairment increasing with task similarity and the attendant competition for common attentional resources (C.A. Archibald and Fisk, 2000; D'Esposito, Onishi, et al., 1996).

Memory and learning. MS patients often report problems with "short-term memory," meaning that they have difficulty remembering details of recent conversations and events but still recall events from the distant past quite well. In fact, semantic memory is often fairly well preserved in MS, particularly in patients with relapsing disease (W.W. Beatty, Goodkin, Monson, and Beatty, 1989; H. Klonoff, Clark, et al., 1991). However, on occasion deficient recall of remotely learned facts occurs, as on the Information test of the WIS-A (S.M. Rao, Leo, Bernardin, and Unverzagt, 1991), on tests assessing memory for famous people and events (W.W. Beatty, Goodkin, Monson, and Beatty, 1989; R.H. Paul, Blanco, Hames, et al., 1997), and on autobiographical memory measures for personal events (R.H. Paul, Blanco, Hames, et al., 1997).

One classic finding in MS is impaired recall on tests of multitrial learning (W.W. Beatty, Goodkin, Monson, et al., 1988; Minden, Moes, Orav, et al., 1990; S.M. Rao, Hammeke, McQuillen, et al., 1984). Patients often struggle on the first trial to grasp all of the material presented, finding their processing capacity overwhelmed. Typically they do better on subsequent trials, which allows them to learn the list by slow accretion. In fact, MS patients' failure to carry out future actions stems primarily from deficiencies in their initial grasp of information going by them rapidly and only once—as in normal conversational "give and take"—as opposed to failure of prospective memory *per se* (i.e., "remembering to do") (Bravin et al., 2000).

The degree of impairment on verbal and visual learning tests is usually comparable, but we [jsf, mdl] have examined a few patients whose impairment was restricted to the verbal or the visual modality, implying lateralization of cerebral abnormalities. Within the verbal domain, recall of word lists is typically more disrupted than that of prose passages, in which the inherent meaningfulness of the passage provides a kind of "glue" to help the material stick. Impaired memory in MS often takes on a "frontal" quality, with deficits being most pronounced on free recall trials due to inefficiencies in encoding and retrieval while storage is relatively spared. Thus, free recall tends to be poorer than cued recall, which in turn is inferior to recognition (Thornton and Raz, 1997; Wishart and Sharpe, 1997). Many MS patients perform nearly normally on recognition testing, confirming that they have absorbed considerably more material than they are able to dredge up spontaneously.

On the basis of these findings, some investigators have argued that MS preferentially disrupts retrieval while sparing encoding and storage processes (S.M. Rao, Leo, and St. Aubin-Faubert, 1989; S.M. Rao, Grafman, DiGiulio, et al., 1993). However, MS patients as a group are specifically impaired in their ability to activate novel strategies. For example, they are less likely to use semantic clustering (Arnett, Rao, Grafman, et al., 1997) and visual imagery (Canellopoulou and Richardson, 1998). This contributes to deficient encoding on the first trial of multitrial learning tasks and on paired associate learning tasks with weak cue–target associations (Faglioni et al., 2000; Thornton, Raz, and Tucker, 2002). MS patients also tend to be less consistent in recalling items from one learning trial to the next (W.W. Beatty, Wilbanks, Blanco, et al., 1996; Faglioni et al., 2000) and to forget prose material at faster rates than healthy controls (Lokken et al., 1999), again implying ineffective acquisition of new material (J. DeLuca, Barbieri-Berger, and Johnson, 1994; J. DeLuca, Gaudino, et al., 1998).

In contrast, implicit memory—as examined by such priming and perceptual motor skill tasks as pursuit rotor, serial visual reaction time, and mirror-reading—is almost always intact (W.W. Beatty, Goodkin, Monson, and Beatty, 1990; S.M. Rao, Grafman, DiGiulio, et al., 1993).

On examining individual test protocols it becomes clear that MS patients' learning and explicit memory performances are quite heterogeneous. At least three patterns have been observed (W.W. Beatty, Wilbanks, Blanco, et al., 1996; Fischer, 1988; S.M. Rao, Hammeke, McQuillen, et al., 1984). Some patients (24% to 36% of the samples) perform like healthy controls, with essentially intact learning and recall. A more common pattern (43% to 56% of the patients sampled) is that of "inefficient" performance, in which summary scores and learning curves are superficially normal but closer inspection uncovers deficient first trial recall, mildly inconsistent recall across trials, and mildly deficient delayed recall. The remainder (20%–22%) exhibit striking performance deficits, including a flattened learning curve, extremely poor delayed recall, and numerous intrusion errors.

Deficits in processing speed and working memory no doubt contribute significantly to these learning deficits (Gaudino et al., 2001; Thornton, Raz, and Tucker, 2002). Clinical observations suggest that slowed mental processing makes it difficult for many patients to grasp all of a verbal message, particularly when it is long, complex, delivered rapidly, and with competing stimuli—as often occurs in a noisy office or at home when the baby is crying, the TV is blasting, and the patient is trying to perform some household chore (Howiesen and Lezak, 2002). Laboratory studies conducted under quiet and controlled conditions often suggest that such patients recall material reasonably well when permitted to devote all of their attentional resources to learning the material. However, in real life, rapidly passing ambient information that others pick up effortlessly is missed.

Verbal functions and academic skills. Language abilities typically remain intact in MS, except for those dependent on rapid and efficient retrieval. Aphasia syndromes are rare (J.T.E. Richardson, Robinson, and Robinson, 1997). Alexias have also been observed, as have other syndromes usually associated with cortical lesions (Dogulu et al., 1996; Filley, 2001; Jonsdottir et al., 1998). These syndromes typically occur with an acute relapse—occasionally even as the presenting symptom—and most resolve with corticosteroid treatment.

Verbal fluency is often disrupted in MS—whether by reductions in cognitive speed, flexibility, search strategy, and/or access to verbal storage (Friend et al., 1999; S.M. Rao, Leo, and St. Aubin-Faubert, 1989). Clinical experience suggests that phonemic fluency tasks are more sensitive to impairment than are semantic fluency tasks. Deficits in confrontation naming have been reported (Friend et al., 1999; Lethlean and Murdoch, 1994), although generally confrontation naming is better preserved than fluency, particularly in patients with relapsing–remitting disease (W.W. Beatty, Goodkin, Monson, and Beatty, 1989; Fischer, 1988). We [jsf, mdl] have observed that when confrontation naming is impaired in MS, phonemic cuing often facilitates retrieval, implying reasonable preservation of the structure of semantic knowledge.

Subtle language abnormalities do occur in MS, as indicated by testing deficits in comprehension of concept meanings and attributes (Laatu et al., 1999) and in deciphering complex or ambiguous grammatical structures (M. Grossman, Robinson, et al., 1995; Lethlean and Murdoch, 1997). In addition, some MS patients' verbal output often seems "empty," with fewer information units per sentence and fewer complete and grammatically correct sentences (G.L. Wallace and Holmes, 1993). Subtle language difficulties such as these can have devastating effects on interpersonal relationships and on work performance, particularly for patients in verbally demanding professions.

Visuospatial functions and construction. MS patients often complain of problems with "vision". Sensory impairments involving the visual system frequently occur in MS (see p. 250). However, problems that patients attribute to defective "vision" are more often disorders of visual perception, which are surprisingly common in MS (S.M. Rao, Leo, Bernardin, and Unverzagt, 1991; Vleugels et al., 2000). Any aspect of visual perception may be disrupted, including facial perception ("knowing who") (W.W. Beatty, Goodkin, Monson, and Beatty, 1989; J. Ward et al., 1999); visual form perception ("knowing what") (van den Burg, Van Zomeren, and Minderhoud, 1987; Vleugels et al., 2000); and visuospatial perception ("knowing where") (S.M. Rao, Leo, Bernardin, and Unverzagt, 1991). Spatial perception may be affected less often than other aspects of visual perception, particularly for relapsing–remitting patients (J. DeLuca, Gaudino, et al., 1998; D'Esposito, Onishi, et al., 1996).

Test performance on measures of visuospatial abilities and construction must be interpreted cautiously. As Fennell and Smith (1990) astutely noted, these tests draw on numerous abilities, including "visual perception, visuospatial analysis, executive functions, memory, and speed of motor output." Although deficits in motor speed and coordination are well documented in

MS, the impact of poor planning on visuoconstructional task performance is often underappreciated.

Thinking and reasoning. MS patients may perform at normal levels on well-structured tests of verbal reasoning and concept formation (S.J. Camp et al., 1999; J. DeLuca, Johnson, and Nadelson, 1993; Landrø et al., 2000), but deficits in abstract reasoning deficits are likely to show up on less structured tests (W.W. Beatty, Goodkin, Monson, and Beatty, 1989; S.J. Camp et al., 1999; Heaton, Nelson, Thompson, et al., 1985). Impaired problem solving in MS has been attributed to perseverative responses (Beatty, Goodkin, Monson, and Beatty, 1989; Heaton, Nelson, Thompson, et al., 1985; S.M. Rao, Leo, Bernardin, and Unverzagt, 1991). However, studies using tests that disentangle concept formation and concept shifting—such as the California Card Sorting Test—have shown that MS patients shift conceptual frameworks reasonably well when offered several alternatives (W.W. Beatty, Hames, et al., 1995; W.W. Beatty and Monson, 1996). These findings suggest that a deficient ability to generate alternative strategies—rather than perseveration—is at the heart of the conceptual and behavioral inflexibility often exhibited by MS patients.

Executive functions. In addition to their limitations in problem solving, MS patients are often inefficient and error prone on planning and sequencing tasks (Arnett, Rao, Grafman, et al., 1997; W.W. Beatty and Monson, 1994; Foong, Rozewicz, Quaghebeur, et al., 1997). Other aspects of executive functions may be disrupted as well, including temporal ordering (W.W. Beatty and Monson, 1991), monitoring internal and external stimuli (Grafman, Rao, Bernardin, and Leo, 1991; Landrø et al., 2000), cognitive estimation (Foong, Rozewicz, Quaghebeur et al., 1997), and self-regulation (Benedict, Priore, et al., 2001; Grigsby, Kravcisin, et al., 1993). Deficiencies in executive functions are often more apparent to family members and friends than they are to the affected individual. Persons close to the patient may erroneously attribute these behaviors to personality features, such as "stubbornness" or "disorganization." Helping friends and family members to understand the neurologic basis for these deficits and to develop strategies for managing them may ease household tensions considerably (Benedict, Shapiro, et al., 2000).

As noted earlier, impairments in conceptual reasoning and executive functions may contribute to MS patients' deficiencies on tests of other cognitive abilities, such as memory and visuoconstruction. Performance on measures of executive functions is moderately to strongly correlated with overall recall (Troyer et al., 1996), spontaneous use of systematic learning strategies

(Arnett, Rao, Grafman, et al., 1997), and how readily patients learn to apply imagery-based mnemonic techniques (Canellopoulou and Richardson, 1998). Often poor performance on visuoconstructional tasks can be traced to impaired planning and organizational abilities as well (see Fennell and Smith, 1990, for a case example).

The following case illustrates several important features of MS-related cognitive dysfunction.

A 39-year-old woman was seen for neuropsychological assessment to evaluate complaints of subtle difficulties with concentration, word retrieval, and memory that affected her work as a customer service manager, a job she had held for close to ten years. Some 15 years prior to the evaluation, she had an acute onset of right-sided numbness and weakness, gait disturbance, eyelid droop, and dysarthria, although her neurologic work-up at the time was negative and no diagnosis was established. Most of her symptoms resolved, but she was left with diminished right-sided sensation and persistent fatigue and then later developed right-sided pain, bladder dysfunction, and major depression. She was diagnosed with MS shortly before the neuropsychological evaluation, at which time she had an EDSS of 3.5. Despite her cognitive complaints, this patient performed in the *average* to *high average* range in most domains of cognitive function (verbal, visuospatial, calculation ability, attention/processing speed, learning/memory, and planning). This was consistent with her history of completing two years of college. The only exception was her reduced problem-solving flexibility, in the *low average* range (18% perseverative errors on the Wisconsin Card Sorting Test).

The patient was coached on compensatory strategies to apply at work and at home and referred for psychological counseling and reassessment of her antidepressant medication. Her depression was successfully treated and her MS symptoms remained clinically stable, but she continued to have difficulty performing her job and took a medical leave six months after the evaluation. When reassessed 18 months later, she had clearly deteriorated neuropsychologically: her problem-solving abilities had slipped into the *defective* range (29% perseverative errors and only 3 categories achieved on the Wisconsin Card Sorting Test), attention/processing speed had worsened (PASAT-3" Total of 31/60 vs. her previous 45/60), and learning was also *defective* (California Verbal Learning Test ΣTrials 1–5 = 47, −2.1 SD).

As in this case, memory is not always impaired in MS. Patients often interpret their cognitive difficulties as "memory problems" when functions other than memory—in this case problem solving—are compromised. This case also demonstrates that even circumscribed cognitive deficits can have a potentially devastating impact on daily functioning, and that cognitive impairment can progress in a patient who appears to be clinically stable in other respects.

Similar disparities between patients' cognitive complaints and their objective performance are common

(Fischer, 1989; Landrø et al., 2000; R. Taylor, 1990). Some patients—particularly those who are emotionally distressed—greatly underestimate their objective performance, whereas others—patients with deficits in concept formation and self-monitoring and those with severe memory deficits—often overestimate their abilities. Consequently, all cognitive functions commonly impaired in MS—attention and processing speed, learning and memory, visuospatial abilities, and executive functions—must be examined, not just those that the patient says are impaired.

The case example also illustrates how fatigue can affect a patient's daily functioning. Ideally MS patients should be tested in the morning to minimize the effects of late day fatigue, and in a quiet environment with a relatively cool ambient temperature to accommodate the heat sensitivity that troubles so many MS patients. Tasks requiring continuous cognitive effort should be intermingled with less attention-demanding tasks, and ample opportunities for breaks should be provided. Lengthy batteries may need to be administered in two or three separate testing sessions.

Psychosocial consequences of cognitive impairment in multiple sclerosis

Cognitive impairment can have far-reaching consequences for MS patients and their families. For example, it affects the employability of many MS patients (Amato et al., 2001; Beatty, Blanco, et al., 1995; S.M. Rao, Leo, Ellington, et al., 1991). In a study contrasting MS patients with prominent spinal cord disease and minimal cognitive dysfunction with others who had primarily cerebral involvement, only one of the 14 "cerebral MS" patients remained employed compared with over half of the 11 "spinal MS" group, who remained employed despite a longer disease duration and greater physical disability (Wild, Lezak, et al., 1991). Cognitively impaired MS patients also have poorer driving skills, with a greater risk of motor vehicle accidents (Schultheis et al., 2001).

Cognitive impairment can also constrain independence within the community and at home (Amato et al., 2001; Higginson et al., 2000) and limit a patient's ability to benefit from rehabilitation programs (Langdon and Thompson, 1999). Cognitively impaired MS patients partake of fewer social activities than their cognitively intact counterparts and require more assistance in performing complex household tasks such as cooking and, in extreme cases, even basic self-care activities (S.M. Rao, Leo, Ellington, et al., 1991). They often need help making decisions and managing their finances, yet patients with no obvious physical disabilities or lacking appreciation of their cognitive limitations may thwart efforts to assist them. Not surprisingly, cognitive impairment is a significant source of caregiver strain (Chipchase and Lincoln, 2001; R.G. Knight, Devereux, and Godfrey, 1997). In the study comparing "cerebral" and "spinal" MS patients, those with predominantly cerebral involvement had fewer stable marriages—although more marriages per capita—than those with spinal disease (Wild, Lezak, et al., 1991).

Disorders of mood, affect, and behavior

Disturbances of affect and behavior—euphoria, affective instability, and pathological laughing and crying—are not uncommon in MS (Feinstein, 1999; Minden and Schiffer, 1990). *Euphoria*—unusual cheerfulness and optimism about the future that is inconsistent with a patient's clinical condition—was widely discussed in early writings on MS (Finger, 1998); more recent surveys suggest that true euphoria is rare and typically associated with advanced disease and extensive frontal white matter involvement (Feinstein, 1999). Much more common than euphoria is *affective instability*—abrupt shifts in mood and behavior. In a recent survey, up to 40% of MS patients were described by family members as "agitated" and/or "irritable" (Diaz-Olavarrieta et al., 1999). These patients often do not monitor their behavior effectively either in social situations or on neuropsychological testing (e.g., making more errors than control subjects on reasoning tests) (Benedict, Priore, et al., 2001). Diaz-Olavarrieta and colleagues found that 13% of patients in their sample were frankly disinhibited and impulsive. "Sudden mood changes" and "partner upsetting other people" are among the behaviors that caregivers report as most burdensome.

Feinstein and colleagues (1997) observed that nearly 10% of patients in their series developed *pathological laughing and crying* (PLC), a socially disabling condition in which outward affective expression becomes disconnected from internal emotional experience (see also, pseudobulbar state, p. 37). Patients with PLC suddenly lose emotional control, either laughing or crying uncontrollably—or sometimes both—in the absence of an apparent triggering stimulus or corresponding mood state. These patients, many of whom have progressive disease, often have cognitive deficits as well, particularly on tasks requiring rapid mental activity (e.g., Stroop, Controlled Oral Word Association Test) (Feinstein, O'Connor, and Feinstein, 1999). Prefrontal/anterior cingulate circuits have been implicated, as have cerebropontocerebellar pathways (Parvizi et al., 2001).

Mood disturbances, such as major depression and bipolar disorder, are also very common in MS (Cummings and Mega, 2003; Schiffer and Babigian, 1984). Feinstein's (2002) study confirms that patients with severe major depression, particularly those who live alone and who also abuse alcohol, are at heightened risk for suicide. In structured psychiatric interviews, 34% to 54% of MS clinic patients give a history consistent with major depression (Joffe et al., 1987; Sadovnick et al., 1996), a rate up to three times that for healthy adults (Blazer et al., 1994). Bipolar disorder—with a lifetime prevalence of 13%–16%—is 10 to 15 times more common in MS patients than in the general population (Joffe et al., 1987). At any given point in time, approximately one in six MS patients meets criteria for current major depression, with prevalence rates reaching 40% among newly diagnosed patients (M.J.L. Sullivan et al., 1995).

Often the cardinal symptoms of uncomplicated major depression—such as apathy and social withdrawal—are less pronounced in MS, whereas symptoms such as irritability—and to a lesser extent, worry and discouragement—are more prominent (Minden, Orav, and Reich, 1987; Ron and Logsdail, 1989). Depressed mood in MS patients has been associated with poorer quality of life (J.L. Wang et al., 2000) and poorer performance on selected neuropsychological measures—specifically, processing speed and working memory (Arnett, Higginson, Voss, et al., 1999a,b) and planning efficiency (Arnett, Higginson, and Randolph, 2001). Assessment of depression can be complicated by fatigue, sleep disturbance, and concentration difficulties. Careful queries about a patient's fatigue, sleep, and concentration difficulties—including diurnal variations, heat sensitivity, and responsiveness to mental and physical activity—can help the clinician discern the extent to which MS itself may be contributing to these symptoms.

Clinically significant anxiety—with or without depression—is also fairly common, as reported by 25% of MS patients (mostly women) (Feinstein, O'Connor, et al., 1999). Combined anxiety and depression in MS patients is associated with increased somatic complaints, suicidal thoughts and plans, and greater social dysfunction. So-called "subsyndromal" distress (i.e., personally disruptive emotional symptoms that do not fulfill criteria for a major depression or anxiety disorder) is present in nearly half of all MS patients (Feinstein and Feinstein, 2001).

Although one might assume that depression is a not an inappropriate reaction to what can be a very devastating disease of young adulthood, it is only weakly related to disease severity as measured by the EDSS (Huber, Rammohan, et al., 1993; Joffe et al., 1987; Patten and Metz, 1997). Many patients with substantial physical disability function effectively using such adaptive coping strategies as positive reappraisal and social support seeking. Depression is reportedly more common in "cerebral" than in "spinal" MS (Schiffer, Caine, et al., 1983). Correlations between depression and cerebral atrophy and axonal loss are modest (Bakshi, Czarnecki, et al., 2000; Zorzon et al., 2002), and efforts to link depression with MS lesion load (on T_2 MRI) have been disappointing (Ron and Logsdail, 1989; Sabatini, Pozzilli, et al., 1996).

As it turns out, psychological factors—such as life stresses and coping strategies (Aikens et al., 1997; Gilchrist and Creed, 1994), and cognitive appraisal (Pakenham, 1999; Shnek et al., 1995)—are much stronger predictors of mood than disease variables. Most patients do become more distressed during clinical relapses (Dalos et al., 1983; Kroencke et al., 2001) or bouts of CNS inflammation (Fassbender et al., 1998; Feinstein, Ron, and Thompson, 1993). At these times psychological and immunologic factors clearly interact (Foley et al., 1992; Mohr, Goodkin, Islar, et al., 2001).

Treatment

Medications. The treatment of MS was revolutionized in the mid 1990s when beneficial effects of disease modifying medications were demonstrated in large-scale clinical trials with relapsing–remitting MS patients (M. Freedman, Blumhardt, et al., 2002; Goodin, Frohman, et al., 2002). These injectable medications (β-interferons and glatiramer acetate) suppress immune activation, although their mechanisms of action vary (see Comi, Filippi, and Wolinsky, 2001; IFNB Multiple Sclerosis Study Group, 1993; L.D. Jacobs, Cookfair, et al., 1996; K.P. Johnson et al., 1995; Li and Paty, 1999). Each medication has an immediate impact on disease activity, reducing clinical relapse rates and impeding new lesion formation. In addition, some have been shown to retard clinical disease progression as defined by the EDSS (L.D. Jacobs, Cookfair, et al., 1996; K.P. Johnson et al., 1995) or to attenuate cerebral lesion accumulation (Li and Paty, 1999). The results of recent clinical medication trials led to revision of the diagnostic criteria for MS (W.I. McDonald et al., 2001) and to the recommendation that patients be treated at the first sign of clinical disease (Goodin, Frohman, et al., 2002). High dose corticosteroids hasten the recovery of function after an MS exacerbation and are considered standard treatment for acute attacks of MS although they may have a transient adverse effect on memory performance (Foong, Rozewicz, Quaghebeur et al., 1998).

Clinical trials of disease modifying medications for MS typically assess so-called "clinical" outcomes—EDSS or quantitative measures of function—or MRI studies. Neuropsychological effects of disease modifying medications for MS have been less well studied (Fischer, 2002). While some medications showed neither beneficial nor adverse neuropsychological effects (Kappos et al., 2004; Weinstein et al., 1999), beneficial effects were observed on composite cognitive measures in a two-year trial of interferon-β1a for relapsing–remitting MS (Fischer, Priore, Jacobs, et al., 2000): attention and memory showed the most striking improvements. J.A. Cohen and colleagues (2002) also reported a beneficial trend on the PASAT, the only measure of cognitive function administered, in a trial of interferon-β1a for secondary progressive MS. In another clinical trial for progressive MS, in which a comprehensive neuropsychological battery was used, the PASAT also proved to be the mea-sure most sensitive to treatment effects (Goodkin and Fischer, 1996).

Cholinesterase inhibitors—developed as a treatment for dementia—may also improve cognitive function in MS patients (Fischer, 2002; Y.M. Greene et al., 2000; Leo and Rao, 1988). They clearly merit further investigation in MS. Medications for fatigue, including psychostimulants, may also be of neuropsychological benefit in MS. Amantadine had a modest beneficial effect on selective attention in two small studies of MS patients being treated for fatigue (R.A. Cohen and Fisher, 1989; Geisler et al., 1996), although not in a third trial (Sailer et al., 2000).

Psychological treatments. Cognitive rehabilitation may also benefit some MS patients (Fischer, 2002). Both process-specific and general beneficial effects on attention were maintained over a nine week follow-up period by MS patients with documented attentional impairments who had 18 weeks of computerized process-specific attention training (Plohmann et al., 1998). A six week cognitive rehabilitation program combining restorative and compensatory techniques improved visual perception, with a trend for better visuospatial memory (but not attention), in a group of cognitively impaired inpatients who then maintained gains over a six month follow-up period (Jønsson et al., 1993). Recent fMRI studies documenting alterations in cortical activation associated with simple hand movements in MS patients raise the intriguing possibility that compensatory cerebral reorganization may underlie the relatively lasting benefits of cognitive rehabilitation (Reddy et al., 2000; Rocca et al., 2002).

Nonspecific supportive counseling can prevent worsening of depression (D.C. Mohr and Goodkin, 1999), but a major depressive episode generally does not fully resolve without specific treatments. Clinical experience suggests that depressed MS patients respond well to methods developed for treating patients with primary depressive disorders [jsf]. A handful of treatment outcome studies confirm the effectiveness of both cognitive behavior therapy (Larcombe and Wilson, 1984; D.C. Mohr, Boudewyn, et al., 2001) and antidepressant medication (D.C. Mohr and Goodkin, 1999; Schiffer and Wineman, 1990). Antidepressant medications are often remarkably effective for pathological laughing and crying as well (Dark et al., 1996; Schiffer, Herndon, and Rudick, 1985). Finally, "neuropsychological compensatory training"—a combination of education, social skills training (including empathic listening), and cognitive behavioral techniques (self-monitoring, problem-solving, self-control)—can help modify the affective instability and behavioral disturbances associated with MS (Benedict, Shapiro, et al., 2000).

Normal Pressure Hydrocephalus (NPH)

This often reversible condition involving mental deterioration has also been called *occult hydrocephalus* (Pincus and Tucker, 2003) or *communicating hydrocephalus* (Hurley et al., 1999). It is not a primary degenerative disorder, such as the dementias. Rather, it results from impaired reabsorption or obstruction of the flow of *cerebral spinal fluid* (CSF), most usually by scarring from old trauma or subarachnoid hemorrhage but also from other sources of hemorrhage or tumor (R.D. Adams, 1980; Filley, 2001; Geocadin and Williams, 2002). Sometimes the source of the obstruction cannot be identified. It is primarily a disease of older adults.

The neuropathology involves ventricular enlargement with associated white matter damage (Filley, 2001; Geocadin and Williams, 2002). As the volume of CSF increases, pressure builds up within the ventricles, which gradually enlarge by eroding adjacent tissue and by stretching to accommodate the pressure: outward pressure on the surrounding white matter also stretches and compresses blood vessels producing ischemic damage, and pushes the cortex against the skull. As the ventricles enlarge to accommodate the steady, usually slow, fluid increase within them, CSF pressure returns to normal. The onset of this condition can be very slow and insidious.

If left to run its course, NPH produces a classic symptom triad of slowly progressive gait disturbance, urinary incontinence, and cognitive impairment typified by confusion, disorientation, and memory problems, with progressive mental debilitation. The shuffling, apractic gait, which somewhat resembles that of Parkinson patients, eventually interferes with ambulation. Although their enlarged ventricles readily show up on neuroimaging, a casual or naive observer can easily misdiagnose the steadily deteriorating mental and physical condition of these patients as, in the later stages, it resembles primary dementias such as Alzheimer's disease (Pincus and Tucker, 2003). Hippocampal and temporal lobe atrophy differentiates Alzheimer's disease from NPH on neuroimaging studies (A.E. George et al., 1995; W.G. Bradley, 2001). It is estimated that up to 6% of patients evaluated for dementia may in fact have NPH (Hurley et al., 1999). Because the deteriorating process may be reversed by a relatively simple surgical procedure involving placement of a ventricular shunt for CFS drainage, correct diagnosis is of the utmost importance (Geocadin and Williams, 2002).

Gait disturbances, incontinence, and memory impairment are also features of Alzheimer's disease, as well as of normal pressure hydrocephalus; and some NPH patients—particularly those with the greatest cognitive impairment—may have concomitant Alzheimer's disease pathology (i.e., neuritic plaques) (Golomb et al., 2000; Tedeschi et al., 1995). However, the usual order of appearance of these symptoms can help the examiner distinguish between the two conditions (R.D. Adams, 1980; Pincus and Tucker, 2003; Stambrook, Gill, et al., 1993). Incontinence and a clumsy, wide-based gait are commonly but not necessarily among the earliest symptoms of normal pressure hydrocephalus (Geocadin and Williams, 2002). Cognitives changes are often subtle at first but when apparent involve disorientation, confusion, apathy, decreased attention span, both mental and motor slowing, and impaired new learning with relatively good preservation of many cognitive functions, judgment, and self-awareness until late in the disease course. Poor performance on tests of immediate recall, short-term memory, and learning in the early stages may reflect confusion and impaired attention rather than a primary registration or learning disability. Thus the common sequence of events in NPH runs counter to the course of Alzheimer's disease in which memory deficits are among the earliest symptoms, and incontinence and loss of walking ability herald the terminal stages (Iddon et al., 1999).

Similarity between this pattern of deficits and behavioral alterations frequently associated with frontal lobe disease is not surprising as enlargement of the lateral ventricles can damage frontal tissue (Filley, 2001; Stambrook, Gill, et al., 1993). Learning and recall of both visual and verbal material is typically compromised, although recall of both recent and remote events (episodic memory) is likely to remain intact. Executive dysfunction, slowed processing, and perseveration occur early in the disease process (Lerner and Whitehouse, 2002).

Reports of success rates for ventricular shunt range from 20% to 80% with symptomatic relief lasting up to four years in some cases (Hurley et al., 1999). Improvement in patients' cognitive functioning indicates that they were relatively intact (Ogden, 1986) as surgery is most likely to be successful in patients with secondary NPH (i.e., having an identifiable origin), symptom duration less than six months, onset of gait disturbance before cognitive deterioration, no cerebrovascular disease, and a positive CSF tap test (i.e., giving temporary relief) (Boon et al., 2000; Geldmacher and Whitehouse, 1997; Hurley et al., 1999). Shunt failures have been documented (Lerner and Whitehouse, 2002).

Since patients with normal pressure hydrocephalus retain self-awareness and are appreciative of their socially handicapping impairments until they become severely confused, they may be quite appropriately depressed, but diagnosis of depression can be confused by frontal symptoms of apathy or abulia (Filley, 2001). Although frank psychoses are rare (Nagaratnam et al., 1994), patients may have other mood disturbances, anxiety, and aggressive outbursts, which often improve with successful shunting (Askin-Edgar, White, and Cummings, 2002; Rice and Gendelman, 1973). Physical symptoms are more likely to improve or resolve after ventricular shunting than are cognitive deficits (Geocadin and Williams, 2002; Iddon et al., 1999).

TOXIC CONDITIONS

The list of substances that can be deleterious to brain tissue is virtually endless (e.g., Hartman, 1995; Spencer and Schaumburg, 2000). It includes substances that are poisonous in any form or amount, as well as the substances of abuse and drugs that may promote central nervous system efficiency at one dose level but interfere with it at another. There is not space in this chapter to review the many kinds of neurotoxic substances, the variety of pathological processes they can produce, or their multitudinous effects.

The examiner must keep in mind the possibility of a toxic reaction with every patient. With the exception of patients with an alcohol-related condition, relatively few people seen for neuropsychological assessment have disorders that are primarily due to toxicity. Not infrequently, however, the effects of medications or street drugs, of industrial and other chemicals, or of alcoholism will complicate the presentation of another kind of neurological disorder. The examiner needs to remain alert to this possibility, particularly with patients inclined toward the use of street drugs and alcohol, and those prone to self-medication or likely to be careless about a medical regimen.

Problems of medicinal drug toxicity are addressed in the section on medication effects in Chapter 8 (pp. 317–

319). This section reviews the salient neuropsychological features of the most commonly occurring toxic brain injuries—alcohol abuse and other, representative, neurotoxic substances.

Alcohol-Related Disorders

First: the benefits of alcohol consumption in moderation

Before entering into this review of the many and varied neurocognitive disorders associated with alcohol abuse, the reader should also learn of the benefits of a reasonable alcohol intake.

Several studies have shown that a modest level of alcohol consumption (see below, *Social drinking*) may lower the risk of dementia (Orgogozo, Dartiques, et al., 1997; Ruitenberg et al., 2002; Zuccala et al., 2001). Moreover, protective effects of moderate alcohol intake have been described for cardiovascular and cerebrovascular disease (Klatsky, 1994; Renaud et al., 1993; Thun et al., 1997). Some studies found that red wine afforded the greatest protection (Criqui and Ringel, 1994; Korsten and Wilson, 1999; Orgogozo, Dartiques, et al., 1997; Reinke and McCay, 1996); this has been attributed to its high level of polyphenic antioxidants (Sun et al., 2002). Others indicate that any kind of alcoholic beverage taken in moderation is beneficial (Hennekens, 1996; Klatsky et al., 1997; Mukamal et al., 2003).

Alcohol abuse and brain–behavior effects

Different kinds of brain changes have been associated with alcohol-related behavioral disturbances (Filley, 2001; Jernigan, Butters, et al., 1991; S.B. Rourke and Løberg, 1996). Alcohol (ethanol) acts as a central nervous system depressant and has effects like those of some tranquilizing and hypnotic drugs. The metabolism of alcohol and its metabolites initiates chains of biochemical and physiological events involving many other organ systems of the body. Thus, "the characteristic action of alcohol . . . may reflect not only the intrinsic properties of the drug, but also the whole constellation of secondary events that are determined by the amounts, routes and frequencies with which [it is] customarily used" (Kalant, 1975).

Several distinctive patterns of behavioral alterations and neuropsychological deficits can occur with alcohol abuse. They can overlap in a single person or a particular clinical group and may simply represent stages of neurotoxicity along a continuum of neurobehavioral deterioration (C. Ryan and Butters, 1980a). Yet they can differ greatly in their behavioral presentations, their

etiologies (in terms of such risk factors as duration and quantity of alcohol consumption, premorbid nutritional status, and length of abstinence), and underlying neuropathology.

Social drinking

Alcohol intake in moderation is typically defined as one to two normal portions (shot of liquor, highball, glass of wine, small mug of beer) which provides 0.75 to 1.5 fluid ounces (21 to 42 milliliters) in a day; definitions of heavy or high intake begin at four to five drinks a day (Arciniegas and Beresford, 2001). Annual intake reported by self-described social drinkers tends to run from around 4 to 11 or 12 liters (MacVane et al., 1982; E.S. Parker and Noble, 1977). Some studies of social drinkers have shown a relationship between the amounts and frequency of consumption and mild cognitive impairments appearing mostly in slightly reduced short-term verbal recall, subtle deficits in concept formation and mental flexibility, and a mild perseverative tendency (I. Grant, 1987; MacVane et al., 1982; E.S. Parker and Noble, 1977). However, other studies of social drinkers have not found that that quantity of consumption (or even a little more: Schinka, Vanderploeg, et al., 2002a,b) affects performances on many different kinds of neuropsychological tests (I. Grant, 1987; Parsons, 1986; S.B. Rourke and Løberg, 1996). R.G. Knight and Longmore (1994) noted that the evidence of neuropsychological impairment in social drinkers "remains inconclusive, inconsistent, and open to a variety of explanations" (p. 219). One series of studies suggested that small amounts of alcohol taken immediately after a learning session improve memory consolidation (E.S. Parker et al., 1980, 1981), although learning attempted shortly after ingestion tends to be compromised (B.M. Jones and Jones, 1977), except when retrieval is also attempted in an intoxicated state (Weingartner, Adefris, et al., 1976).

Chronic alcoholism

Definitions of alcoholism abound: most rely upon alcohol-related psychosocial maladaptations (e.g., American Psychiatric Association, 2000) or on the quantity and frequency of drinking (S.B. Rourke and Løberg, 1996). Identifying who is an alcoholic, however, is not as straightforward as might be expected. These people typically come to professional attention when they are seeking relief from the problem or help for a medically related one, or as a result of misbehavior while under alcohol's influence. In one report, a physician recognized the problem in fewer than half of a group of chronic alcoholics; alcoholics are more likely to be identified if they present with a medical condition (R.D. Moore et al., 1989). Moreover, women with alcohol problems are even less readily recognized (Amodei et al., 1996). Most studies of alcoholics rely on patient reports of how much and how often they drink within a given time period for diagnosis or for measuring the severity of the drinking problem, recognizing that self-reports of alcoholics are often unreliable.

Risk factors. Besides the obvious risks of drinking too much too often, many other risk factors may contribute to cognitive dysfunction in alcoholics (K.M. Adams and Grant, 1986). This multifactorial aspect of chronic alcoholism accounts for the range and variety of presentations of cognitive disorders and a literature replete with contradictory findings (R.E. Meyer, 2001; S.B. Rourke and Løberg, 1996; Tarter and Alterman, 1984). *Aging* has been considered a risk factor (Carlen, Wilkinson, et al., 1981; Freund, 1982; I. Grant, 1987) but is confounded with duration and intensity of drinking and longer exposure to *medical risk factors* such as TBI (N. Brooks, Symington, et al., 1989; I. Grant, Adams, and Reed, 1984; Naugle, 1990) and alcohol-related diseases (I. Grant, 1987; Korsten and Wilson, 1999; J.R. Taylor and Combs-Orne, 1985). *Race* may play a role as one study found African-American alcoholics were more seizure-prone than their white counterparts (Tarter, Goldstein, et al., 1983). *Sex differences* have also been considered to be a possible factor since women generally drink less (York and Welte, 1994) and metabolize alcohol differently (Lieber, 2000). However, no consistent pattern of differential sex response has been documented (E.V. Sullivan, Fama, et al., 2002). A *family history* of alcoholism weighs heavily as a risk factor, even when the children have been raised in a nonalcoholic environment, suggesting some genetic vulnerability (I. Grant, 1987; S.B. Rourke and Løberg, 1996; M.A. Taylor, 1999). *Diet* plays a role as well, both in the deleterious effects of malnutrition on cognitive functioning and in the development of neuropathogenic deficiency diseases (Brust, 2000b; I. Grant, 1987; Lishman, 1997).

Neuroanatomy and pathophysiology. Alcohol is a neurotoxin in itself Filley, 2001; Brust, 2000b). Its metabolism proceeds through several different routes, which may account for alcohol's many different effects on the central nervous system and on other organ tissues (Brust, 2000b, M.A. Taylor, 1999). Cognitive deficits have been correlated with both white and gray matter abnormalities (Brust, 1993). Cerebral atrophy is a common finding among dedicated alcoholics compared to age-matched controls (Jernigan, Butters, et al., 1991; Ron, 1983). It has been associated with the toxic

effects of alcohol, especially cerebral white matter (Brust, 2000b; Filley and Kleinschmidt-DeMasters, 2001). White matter atrophy is more prominent than gray matter changes (de la Monte, 1988; G.B. Jensen and Pakkenberg, 1993) and is identifiable with specialized MRI techniques (e.g., diffusion tensor imaging) (Pfefferbaum et al., 2000). It is generally related to age. The degree of cortical atrophy is not a reliable predictor of cognitive dysfunction (W. Acker, Ron, et al., 1984; I. Grant, 1987; Lishman, 1997).

Along with overall brain shrinkage marked by enlarged ventricles and widened spaces between cortical folds, gray matter in the dorsolateral frontal and parietal regions may be especially affected (Jernigan, Butters, et al., 1991; Lishman, 1997; D.A. Wilkinson and Carlen, 1981). Chronic heavy alcohol ingestion reduces the elaboration of dendrites in the brain, mostly in the hippocampus and cerebellum (Korsten and Wilson, 1999; Lishman, 1997). Subcortical atrophy is frequently observed at autopsy or by scanning and may involve the cerebellum, the caudate nucleus, and limbic system structures (Jernigan, Butters, et al., 1991; Ron, 1983). Ethanol may disturb hippocampal function directly and by disrupting critical hippocampal afferents (A.M. White et al., 2000). All measures of regional cerebral blood flow (rCBF) are relatively reduced, mostly in frontal and parietal regions (Berglund et al., 1987; S.B. Rourke and Løberg, 1996). Strokes may complicate the chronic alcoholic's neuropathologic and neuropsychologic presentation (M.A. Sloan, 1997).

Abnormal EEG findings are common in chronic alcoholics (Brewer and Perrett, 1971; S.B. Rourke and Løberg. 1996). Lukas and his colleagues (1986) reported that normal subjects given measured doses of alcohol exhibited heightened parietal lobe α wave activity, which was associated with subjective feelings of euphoria, while increased θ activity paralleled the rising blood alcohol level. Studies of visual evoked potentials in alcoholics have found abnormalities suggestive of frontal and parietal involvement (D.A. Wilkinson and Carlen, 1981), with particular slowing noted in right hemisphere regions (Kostandov et al., 1982). The P3 event related potential amplitude may also be decreased (Enoch et al., 2001; J.M. Nichols and Martin, 1996; Oscar-Berman, 1987), especially when there is a family history of alcoholism (S.B. Rourke and Løberg, 1996).

Although probably contributing in some cases to the acquisition of an addiction to alcohol (Lukas et al., 1986), the transient euphoria that alcohol can generate does not account for the desperate need for alcohol experienced by truly addicted persons. Rather, sudden withdrawal can trigger serious and potentially life-threatening problems in long-term very heavy drinkers (Ballenger and Post, 1989; Brust, 2000b; Lishman, 1997; M.A. Taylor, 1999). Initial withdrawal symptoms include nausea, tremulousness, and insomnia, but can progress to seizures and *delirium tremens* (*DTs*), an acute disorder in which the most prominent symptoms are tremulousness, visual and other sensory hallucinations, and profound confusion and agitation that can lead to death from exhaustion. Alcohol-precipitated seizures are not uncommon among seizure-prone persons such as those who have had a TBI or who have focal lesions from some other cause (A. Hopkins, 1981; Lechtenberg, 1999). Seizures and transient amnesic episodes ("blackouts") also occur in chronic alcoholics of long standing, usually during a heavy bout of drinking or soon after (Brust, 1993; J.N. Walton, 1994).

Cognitive functions. Chronic alcohol abuse affects some specific aspects of cognition and executive functioning including complex visuospatial abilities and psychomotor speed, while many well-established abilities and skills such as arithmetic and language—abilities examined within well-structured and familiar formats—and attention remain relatively unimpaired (Parsons, Butters, and Nathan, 1987; C. Ryan and Butters, 1986; S.B. Rourke and Løberg, 1996; Tarter, 1976). The severity of the specific deficits associated with chronic alcoholism has been related to intake quantity (De Renzi, Faglioni, Nichelli, and Pignattari, 1984) and duration of the drinking problem (Parsons and Farr, 1981; C. Ryan and Butters, 1986; J.J. Ryan and Lewis, 1988) in some studies but not in others (K.M. Adams and Grant, 1984; I. Grant, 1987) as well as to age (Carlen, Wilkinson, et al., 1981; Parsons and Farr, 1981; C. Ryan and Butters, 1986). Pishkin and his colleagues (1985) found that age at which drinking began was a strong predictor of conceptual level and efficiency and may account for positive correlations between age or duration and cognitive dysfunction reported in other studies. Binge drinkers appear to be less prone to alcohol-related cognitive deficits than those with a heavy daily alcohol intake (Sanchez-Craig, 1980). In noting the conflicting data between studies of variables that might be associated with cognitive dysfunction, C. Ryan and Butters (1986) called attention to "the myriad demographic and alcoholism-related factors which interact to produce the pattern of cognitive impairment found in the alcoholic individual." Consumption variables alone can explain relatively little of alcoholics' neuropsychological test performances (S.B. Rourke and Løberg, 1996).

Similarities in the cognitive alterations that occur with aging and that are exhibited by many alcoholics prompted the hypothesis that alcoholism accelerates aging of the brain (Blusewicz et al., 1977; Graff-Radford, Heaton, et al., 1982). These similarities involve impairments of executive functions such as mental flexibility and problem-solving skills and of short-term memory and learning (Craik, 1977; C. Ryan and Butters, 1980b). However, careful comparisons also expose significant differences between elderly persons and chronic alcoholics in both psychometric deficit patterns and qualitative aspects of test performance, which suggest that the processes underlying the cognitive deficiencies in these two groups are not the same (I. Grant, Adams, and Reed, 1984; J.H. Kramer, Blusewicz, and Preston, 1989; Oscar-Berman and Weinstein, 1985; M.D. Shelton et al., 1984).

Sensorimotor status appears to be vulnerable in chronic alcoholism. Mergler, Blain, and their colleagues (1988) found impaired color vision in all the heavy drinkers (more than 25 ounces [751 grams] per week) they examined, and increasing incidence of the impairment with increased consumption (see also Brust, 2000b). The efficiency of visual search and scanning tends to be impaired (Kapur and Butters, 1977; C. Ryan and Butters, 1986). Glosser and her colleagues (1977) suspected that visual scanning problems may contribute to alcoholics' relatively slowed performances on symbol substitution tasks. Tendencies to response slowing have been documented on many different kinds of tests (e.g., S.W. Glenn and Parsons, 1990; Parsons and Farr, 1981; S.B. Rourke and Løberg, 1996). In some serious drinkers, manual slowing may be exacerbated by peripheral neuropathies experienced as numbness or paresthesias of the hands or feet (Brust, 2000b; Lishman, 1997; J.N. Walton, 1994). Peripheral neuropathies in alcoholics are always associated with vitamin deficiencies but the contribution of alcohol toxicity is unknown (L.H. Van den Burg et al., 1998).

Memory deficits are common but far from universal. Chronic alcoholics tend to sustain subtle but consistent short-term memory and learning deficits that become more evident as task difficulty increases (e.g., by increasing the number of items to be learned or inserting distractor tasks between learning and recall trials) (C. Ryan and Butters, 1982, 1986). These deficits appear to be the product of a reliance on superficial encoding strategies which limit discriminability between stimuli and access to effective associations. For example, intrusions (recall errors, often associations to target stimuli; e.g., "teacher" offered in recall of a word list including "parent" and "school") appear in greater number than is normal and tend to persist throughout successive trials (J.H. Kramer, Blusewicz, and Preston, 1989; Weingartner, Faillace, and Markley, 1971). Normal rates of forgetting further implicate encoding rather than retrieval (J.T. Becker, Butters, et al., 1983; Nixon et al., 1987).

Many studies indicate that chronic alcoholics, particularly those with lower intake histories, perform normally on verbal learning tests but may do poorly on visual and spatial learning assessments (Bowden, 1988; De Renzi, Faglioni, Nichelli, and Pignattari, 1984; Kapur and Butters, 1977; C. Ryan and Butters, 1986; M.D. Shelton et al., 1984). Both verbal and visual memory deficits have also appeared concurrently (Nixon et al., 1987), with visual impairments probably more susceptible to duration of alcoholism than verbal ones (J.J. Ryan and Lewis, 1988). However, serious memory and learning deficits are not a regular feature of chronic alcoholism. Remote memory is particularly resistant to deterioration in alcoholics (M.S. Albert, Butters, and Brandt, 1980). Alcoholics tend to underestimate their memory impairments or deny them altogether (J.J. Ryan and Lewis, 1988). Moreover, when complaints of cognitive dysfunction are elicited, they are more likely to reflect emotional distress than accurate self-perceptions (Errico et al., 1990).

Visuospatial functions remain essentially intact, although chronic alcoholics may perform relatively poorly on tests requiring visuospatial organization (Parsons and Farr, 1981; C. Ryan and Butters, 1986). Here too exceptions can occur, as Bowden (1988) found with young alcoholics whose Block Design performances were unimpaired. Perceptuomotor problems associated with chronic alcoholism may appear at first to implicate functions associated with the right hemisphere. However, analysis of the visuospatial failures of chronic alcoholics suggests that they involve slowed visual organization and integration (Akshoomoff et al., 1989). Furthermore, alcoholics show no consistent performance decrement on perceptuomotor tasks or motor coordination tasks that require little or no synthesizing, organizing, or orienting activity (Oscar-Berman and Weinstein, 1985; Tarter, 1976). No neuropathological data support a hypothesis of right hemisphere susceptibility to the depredations of alcohol (S.B. Rourke and Løberg, 1996; C. Ryan and Butters, 1982).

Deficits in *adaptive or executive behavior* are frequently observed, appearing on tasks involving functions associated with frontal lobe activity (I. Grant, 1987; S.B. Rourke and Løberg, 1996; C. Ryan and Butters, 1986; Talland, 1965a). Thus, difficulties in maintaining a cognitive set, impersistence, decreased flexibility in thinking, defective visual searching behavior, simplistic problem-solving strategies, deficient motor inhibition, perseveration, loss of spatial and temporal orientation, and impaired ability to organize perceptuomotor responses and synthesize spatial elements characterize the test behavior of chronic alcoholics. Al-

coholics' abilities to make abstractions and to generalize from particulars may remain intact, but these abilities are vulnerable to the ravages of excessive alcohol use (S.B. Rourke and Løberg, 1996). The performance defects listed here also contribute to alcoholics' failures on tests involving abstractions (C. Ryan and Butters, 1982).

Abstinence effects. There has been much interest in the extent to which cognitive deficits associated with alcohol consumption are ameliorated by abstinence. During the detoxification period, usually the first two weeks after cessation of drinking, most alcoholics will exhibit a variety of neuropsychological deficits involving just about every cognitive function that has been subject to testing, including the ordinarily stable verbal skills (M.S. Goldman, 1982; C. Ryan and Butters, 1986). Thus, most newly abstinent alcoholics show remarkable "improvements" when test scores obtained weeks or months later are compared with performance levels obtained during the acute withdrawal stage. Measurements of improvement of function are only valid when compared with baseline scores obtained after the acute condition has dissipated. The greatest amount of return of function takes place in the first week of abstinence (C. Ryan and Butters, 1986). Rate of return slows down rapidly thereafter, leveling off at three to six weeks. Reports of continuing improvement are inconsistent (C. Ryan, Di Dario, et al., 1980; Tarter, 1976; Unkenstein and Bowden, 1991) but there is some reason to be cautiously optimistic (M.S. Goldman, 1983; I. Grant, Adams, and Reed, 1984; Guthrie and Elliott, 1980; see p. 262). For social drinkers performing generally *within normal limits* on neuropsychological tests, two weeks of abstinence made no difference in test scores (Parsons, 1986).

Memory tends to improve first but less than completely in the initial weeks of abstinence (M.S. Goldman, 1982, 1983; Parsons and Farr, 1981). Both recently detoxified and abstinent (for 18 months or longer) alcoholics in their late 30s performed *within normal limits* on a variety of neuropsychological tests (I. Grant, Adams, and Reed, 1979). However, the group that had been detoxified for only three weeks when first tested did not exhibit the practice effects displayed by the other group on retest one year later (K.M. Adams, Grant, and Reed, 1980). This learning failure suggests the presence of subtle learning deficits at three weeks of abstinence that usual test procedures do not detect. Improvements in short-term memory approaching normal levels were observed in alcoholics abstinent for five or more years (C. Ryan and Butters, 1982). Some studies reported complete return of impaired perceptuomotor skills following prolonged sobriety (R.H. Farmer, 1973; Tarter and Jones, 1971); but despite improvement with prolonged abstinence, performance on tests involving these skills may remain depressed (Parsons, 1977). Response speed and attention measured in symbol substitution tasks, for example, may also improve over a year or more of abstinence (C. Ryan and Butters, 1982). Whether impaired functions continue to improve with prolonged abstinence is questionable. For example, five or more years of abstinence resulted in no improvements for 30 previously alcoholic men on a paired-associated learning test used to measure long-term memory (Brandt, Butters, et al., 1983).

Age may be a significant variable in determining the reversibility of alcohol-related deficits. On a variety of speed-dependent perceptual and motor tasks, younger subjects (under 35 to 40) generally returned to normal performance levels within three months after they stopped drinking, while older ones improved but remained relatively impaired (M.S. Goldman, 1982). Other reports confirm that neuropsychological functions, primarily memory and executive abilities, are less likely to improve or will improve more slowly in older abstinent patients (Munro, Saxton, and Butters, 2000; S.B. Rourke and Grant, 1999).

Reports that the CT scans of some chronic alcoholics with cerebral atrophy show evidence of reduced atrophy following abstinence suggest a parallel between the structural status of the brain and the cognitive functioning of these patients (Carlen, Penn, et al., 1986; S.B. Rourke and Løbert, 1996; Lishman, 1997; Ron, 1983), a parallel that is maintained along the age continuum (Trabert et al., 1995). Since alcohol toxins act preferentially on white matter, improvements may be due to remyelination of nerve fibers (Filley, 2001).

Alcoholic dementia

A condition of significant mental and personality deterioration occurring after years of alcohol abuse, *alcoholic dementia* features widespread cognitive deterioration without the profound amnesia of Korsakoff's syndrome (Lishman, 1997; S.B. Rourke and Løberg, 1996; C. Ryan and Butters, 1986). These patients sustain extensive cerebral atrophy which involves white matter to a disproportionate degree (Filley, 2001). Along with memory deficits, they display poor performances on tests of cognitive abilities and behavioral dysfunctions typically associated with frontal lobe pathology. Alcoholic dementia may represent the end stage of a dementing process associated with alcohol-induced atrophy (S.B. Rourke and Løberg, 1996; M.A. Taylor, 1999). Some patients diagnosed as having alcoholic dementia display some of the symptoms typi-

cal of Korsakoff's syndrome (Brust, 2000b; Lishman, 1997) and vice versa, which suggests that these patients have sustained more than one kind of alcohol-related brain injury. Cortical changes similar to those present in frontotemporal dementia have also been described (Brun and Andersson, 2001).

Korsakoff's syndrome

The most striking neuropsychological deficit associated with alcoholism is the gross memory impairment of *Korsakoff's syndrome*. This alcohol-related disorder is sometimes referred to as *Wernicke-Korsakoff syndrome* as, in acute and untreated patients, the initial symptoms are, typically, massive confusion and disordered eye and limb movements (*Wernicke's encephalopathy*) (American Academy of Neurology, 2002; Arciniegas and Beresford, 2001; Brust, 2000b; O'Connor and Verfaillie, 2002; S.B. Rourke and Løberg, 1996). This condition of nutritional depletion—especially thiamine—typically affects alcoholics with a long drinking history. It may be brought on by a particularly heavy bout with alcohol (usually two weeks or more) during which the patient eats little if any food. Alcohol interferes with gastrointestinal transport of vitamin B (thiamine) and chronic liver disease compromises thiamine metabolism (Brust, 1993; Reuler et al., 1985). When the alcoholic's diet is insufficient to meet the body's needs, those regions of the brain that are most thiamine dependent will suffer impaired neuronal function which, if not treated, can lead to cell death—and to the anatomical lesions associated with this brain disease (N. Butters, 1985; Joyce, 1987; Lishman, 1997). A genetic defect in thiamine metabolism with heightened vulnerability to thiamine deficiency when dietary intake is insufficient has been identified in some Korsakoff patients (Blass and Gibson, 1977; Reuler et al., 1985). If treated promptly in the acute stage with thiamine, both Wernicke's and Korsakoff's syndromes may be ameliorated (Arciniegas and Beresford, 2001; Brust, 2000b; Victor et al., 1971). Deficiency of another vitamin, nicotinic acid, has been associated with a confusional disorder that occurs in alcoholic patients (Brust, 2000b; Lishman, 1997).

Neuroanatomy and neuropathology. Hemorrhagic lesions in specific thalamic nuclei and in the mammillary bodies, usually with lesions occurring in other structures of the limbic system, have been implicated in Korsakoff's syndrome (Brust, 1993; S.B. Rourke and Løberg, 1996; Victor et al., 1971). Neuronal depletion also appears in two of the three known sources of input to the cholinergic system, the nucleus basalis of Meynert and another basal forebrain nucleus (N. Butters and Stuss, 1989; Joyce, 1987; Salmon and Butters, 1987). Other neurotransmitter deficiencies have also been noted (Joyce, 1987; McEntee et al., 1984; D.A. Wilkinson and Carlen, 1981). MRI scans show significant loss of gray matter in orbitofrontal and mesiotemporal cortex and in the thalamus and other diencephalic structures, along with enlarged ventricles (Jernigan, Schafer, et al., 1991). Neuronal loss in the medial anterior thalamic nuclei is thought to be the primary source of the recent memory impairment (Harding et al., 2000; P.J. Visser et al., 1999). Olfactory deficits further implicate limbic system dysfunction (N. Butters and Cermak, 1976; Hulshoff Pol et al., 2002; B.P. Jones, Moskowitz, et al., 1975).

Cognitive functions. Most early studies of Korsakoff's syndrome concentrated on the memory deficits with relatively little attention paid to other functions. Perhaps that was because Korsakoff patients' scores on the usual tests of cognitive functions (e.g., Wechsler Intelligence Scales) are virtually identical with those of chronic alcoholics (Kapur and Butters, 1977; C. Ryan and Butters, 1986). Thus, their performances hold up on well-structured, untimed tests of familiar, usually overlearned material such as vocabulary and arithmetic, while their scores on the other tests decline only to the extent that speed and visuoperceptual and spatial organization are involved. However, Korsakoff patients take an abnormally long time (85 msec compared to 25 msec for normal subjects) to identify visually presented material due to their greatly slowed visual processing capacities (Oscar-Berman, 1980). Auditory processing, too, is significantly slowed in Korsakoff patients (N. Butters, Cermak, Jones, and Glosser, 1975; S.R. Parkinson, 1979).

On clinical examinations of *attention,* many Korsakoff patients perform quite well on Digit Span, Subtracting Serial Sevens, and other tasks involving simple components of attention (N. Butters and Cermak, 1976; Kopelman, 1985), although they are unlikely to resume interrupted activities (Talland, 1965a). They fail on more complex aspects of attention such as shifting and dividing (Oscar-Berman, 1980, 1984) and working memory (O'Connor and Verfaillie, 2002).

The *memory* impairment in Korsakoff's syndrome involves declarative memory and includes both antegrade and retrograde deficits (N. Butters, and Stuss, 1989; O'Connor and Verfaillie, 2002; Parkin, 1991; S.B. Rourke and Løberg, 1996). Their functional relationship in Korsakoff's syndrome is suggested by their inconsistent and then relatively mild and not necessarily paired appearance in chronic alcoholism, indicating that the Korsakoff memory deficit is not simply a more severe presentation of the memory impairment of chronic alcoholism; and by their inevitable togetherness in Korsakoff's syndrome. In an ingenious series of studies, N. Butters and his coworkers (N. Butters, 1984a; N. Butters and Brandt, 1985; N. Butters and Cermak, 1980; C. Ryan and Butters, 1986; Salmon and Butters, 1987) implicated defective encoding of new information as the common component of the Korsakoff memory disorder. Defective encoding results in the patient's retaining access to much of the immediate experience of the past two or three minutes, with little or no ability to utilize whatever might have been stored in recent memory (i.e., since the onset of the condition), and a tendency toward inconsistent and poorly organized retrieval of remote memory with retrograde amnesia occurring on a steep temporal gradient. It is as though letters and papers were slipped randomly into a set of files: the information would be there but not readily retrievable, and whatever is pulled out is probably not what was sought.

The anterograde deficits are the most readily apparent since, for all practical purposes, patients with a full-blown Korsakoff's syndrome live in a time zone of about three to five minutes, having little or no ready access to events or learning drills in which they participated prior to the space allowed by their short-term memory. These learning deficits are not modality specific but extend to all kinds of material (N. Butters, 1985; Huppert and Piercy, 1976; O'Connor and Verfaillie, 2002). What little learning ability they do manifest on recall is extremely vulnerable to proactive inhibition (N. Butters and Cermak, 1976; Leng and Parkin, 1989), although they benefit from long rehearsal times (N. Butters, 1984a; Meudell et al., 1978). Moreover, they show little if any learning curve on repeated recall trials (Talland, 1965a). Given the analogy to a disorganized filing system, it is not surprising that Korsakoff patients have difficulty both learning and recalling information in temporal sequence (Shimamura, Janowsky, and Squire, 1990). They also display tendencies to perseverate errors or responses from one set of stimuli to the next (N. Butters, 1985; N. Butters, Albert, Sax, et al., 1983; Meudell et al., 1978) and to make intrusion errors in both verbal and visual modalities (N. Butters, Granholm, et al., 1987; D. Jacobs, Tröster, et al., 1990).

Short-term recall does not differ greatly from that of normal subjects, even with interference procedures (N. Butters and Grady, 1977; Kopelman, 1985, 1986), although contradictory findings have been reported (Leng and Parkin, 1989). Moreover, when given a recognition format rather than a recall format, they do demonstrate some learning, particularly if given long exposure times; they benefit only inconsistently from contextual information and not at all from verbal mediators (N. Butters, 1984; Huppert and Piercy, 1976; Martone, Butters, and Trauner, 1986). Yet when given a strategy for remembering (e.g., judging the likability of faces) their recognition scores improved (Biber, Butters, et al., 1981). Their almost normal recall of stories with sexual content (D.A. Davidoff, Butters, et al., 1984; Granholm, Wolfe, and Butters, 1985) and improved recall with visual imagery (Leng and Parkin, 1988) also indicate that these patients have some learning potential (see also N. Butters and Stuss, 1989; Parkin, 1982). When new information is acquired (albeit slowly), Korsakoff patients show normal forgetting rates, further implicating a retrieval problem rather than a storage problem (Huppert and Piercy, 1976; Kopelman, 1985).

The retrograde defect shows up as difficulty in recalling either past personal or public information (M.S. Albert, Butters, and Levin, 1979; N. Butters and Albert, 1982; R.A. McCarthy and Warrington, 1990). This difficulty follows a steep temporal gradient with poorest recall of the most recent events and recall improving as the time of memory acquisition is more removed from the date of onset of the Korsakoff condition (N. Butters and Cermak, 1986; Kopelman, 1989). As with new learning, these patients perform significantly better with a recognition format, again demonstrating that retrieval is a significant part of the Korsakoff memory problem (Kopelman, 1989). As N. Butters and Cermak (1986) have shown, this deficit occurs with material learned and available to the patient premorbidly, while the patient's memory was still reasonably intact. These observations thus cast doubt on faulty encoding (e.g., Parkin, 1991) as an explanation of impaired retrieval of long-stored information in this condition.

One interesting aspect of their memory disorder is a breakdown in the capacity to appreciate or use time relationships to guide or evaluate their responses. Korsakoff patients tend to be oblivious to chronology in their recall of remote events so that they report impossible sequences unquestioningly and without guile, such as going into service before going to high school, or watching television before World War II. When they attempt to answer questions about events, it is as though they respond with the first association that comes to mind no matter how loosely or inappropriately it might be linked to the questions (Lhermitte and Signoret, 1972). Korsakoff patients are also prone to confabulation, particularly in the early stages of their disorder (N. Butters, 1984; De Renzi, 2000; Kopelman, 1987a). For example, they tend to produce unconsidered, frequently inconsistent, foolish, and sometimes quite exotic confabulations in response to questions for which they feel they ought to know the answer, such

as "What were you doing last night?" or "How did you get to this place?" The greater presence of confabulation during the initial stages of the disease may be related to orbital and medial frontal hypometabolism which normalizes over time (Benson, Djenderedjian, et al., 1996).

Implicit memory (examined, e.g., by response times or primed recall) remains relatively intact. It is only when active (conscious, directed) retrieval is required that Korsakoff patients fail to exhibit what they may have learned (Graf et al., 1984; Nissen, Willingham, and Hartman, 1989; Shimamura, Salmon, et al., 1987). Skill learning is intact (Martone, Butters, et al., 1984).

Conceptual and regulatory (executive) impairments, such as premature responding, diminished ability to profit from mistakes (i.e., change unrewarding response patterns), and diminished ability to perceive and use cues, have been described in these patients (Oscar-Berman, 1980, 1984). They also do poorly on tests requiring hypothesis generation and testing as well as problem solving (N. Butters, 1985; Laine and Butters, 1982).

Emotional and psychosocial behavior. Behavioral defects specifically and consistently associated with the Korsakoff syndrome are disorientation for time and place; apathy characterized by a virtually total loss of initiative, insight, and interest; and a striking lack of curiosity about past, present, or future. Patients are emotionally bland but with a capacity for momentary irritability, anger, or pleasure that quickly dissipates when the stimulating condition is removed or the discussion topic is changed. Thus they are at the mercy of whatever or whoever is in their immediate environment. Despite their many residual abilities and skills, unlike the chronic alcoholic whose memory functions remain relatively intact, the memory defects and inertia of the Korsakoff syndrome render the severely impaired patient utterly dependent.

The relationship between Korsakoff's syndrome and chronic alcoholism. It has been suggested that Korsakoff's syndrome represents the extreme end stage of the organic alterations in chronic alcoholism. However, Korsakoff's syndrome differs from chronic alcoholism in a number of important respects: Since most Korsakoff patients have a history of chronic alcoholism, they also are likely to have acquired the kind of cerebral atrophy typically associated with heavy alcoholic intake over the years, and some chronic alcoholics will also have mild diencephalic involvement. Only Korsakoff patients, however, will have sustained significant lesions in structures throughout the diencephalon along with depressed neurotransmitter levels. Unlike the gradual deterioration associated with chronic alcoholism, Korsakoff's syndrome has a sudden onset, usually appearing as a residual of *Wernicke's encephalopathy* (a condition due to thiamine deficiency in which involuntary rapid eye movements [*nystagmus*], gaze paresis, ataxia, confusion, and amnesia are prominent symptoms) (Heindel, Salmon, and Butters, 1991; Lishman, 1997). Korsakoff patients exhibit marked personality alterations with the cardinal features of extreme passivity and emotional blandness, and thus are unlike chronic alcoholics who, for the most part, do not lose their individuality or capacity to generate self-serving or goal-directed activity. Chronic alcoholics are further distinguished by the absence of confabulation and—not least—by the relative mildness and scattered incidence of their memory deficits.

Another difference is in improvement potential. Korsakoff patients require thiamine replacement early in their course to make any gains but, while the Wernicke features of the condition improve with thiamine (e.g., visual and gait disturbances), the Korsakoff condition is more likely to last (Brust, 2000b). Again unlike alcoholics, many Korsakoff patients do not regain enough capacity to maintain social independence, and the nature of the condition precludes effective cognitive remediation: patients who do not have self-directed access to new information cannot make behavioral changes. For Korsakoff patients, further neurologic deterioration is unlikely since most of them end up in custodial care.

Street Drugs

The effects of any one of the many illicit substances taken by drug users are compounded and often obscured by background variables, such as histories of head trauma and poor school performance, and by the polydrug habits of most street drug users. Thus knowledge about any single drug often comes from studies of one or a few persons who came to medical attention and then includes all the biases that can distort the findings of such limited studies. Despite these research problems, characteristic and enduring neuropsychological effects have been identified for a few street drugs (D.E. Hartman, 1995).

Marijuana (cannabis)

Marijuana's acute effects include hallucinatory and reactive emotional states, some pleasant, some unpleasant and even terrifying; time disorientation; and recent—transient—memory loss (Brust, 2000a; Lishman, 1997; Solowij, 1998). The intensity of these effects, including both visual and auditory hallucinations, in-

creases as the dose gets higher; very high doses can result in psychotic states (Brust, 1993; Colbach and Crowe, 1970). Yet the most apt generalization that can be made about studies of the long-term neurological and neuropsychological effects of marijuana use is that the findings are equivocal (A.S. Carlin and O'Malley, 1996; Parsons and Farr, 1981).

Long-term effects on cognitive abilities. A comparison of test scores of college student marijuana users and nonusers on the Wechsler Intelligence Scale and the Halstead Battery taken a year apart showed no difference on any measure (Culver and King, 1974). This finding was supported by a Danish study of several groups of polydrug users, all of whom used marijuana, in which the same set of tests plus learning and reaction time tests showed no differences between the users and control groups (P. Bruhn and Maage, 1975). Similar studies have come up with similarly negative results (Brust, 1993; Satz, Fletcher, and Sutker, 1976; J. Schaeffer et al., 1981). I. Grant, Adams, Carlin, and their coworkers (1978a,b) concluded, on the basis of a large-scale collaborative study of polydrug abuse, that marijuana "is not neurotoxic, at least in the short run (i.e., approximately 10 years of regular use)." However, they qualified this conclusion by noting that their subjects "were not, in general, heavy hallucinogen consumers." In a review of studies on cognition in marijuana users, A.S. Carlin and O'Malley (1996) suggest that absence of conclusive findings may reflect the insensitivity of the instruments used in many studies.

Long-term effects on personality. Some studies point to personality changes in heavy users of marijuana or hashish (Brust, 1993; A.S. Carlin and O'Malley, 1996; Lishman, 1997). The most commonly described characteristics are affective blunting, mental and physical sluggishness, apathy, restlessness, some mental confusion, and poor recent memory.

For example, Sharma (1975) found that Nepalese who used cannabis at least three times a day for more than two years show diminished motivation, poor work records and social relationships, reduced libido, and inefficiency; these problems resolved with abstinence. However, these findings have been subject to debate as many studies have found no significant long-term deficits (A.S. Carlin and O'Malley, 1996; Hannerz and Hindmarsh, 1983; Lishman, 1997; J. Schaeffer et al., 1981).

Acute effects. Laboratory studies of behavior during marijuana use also tend to be equivocal. In a very detailed review, L.L. Miller (1976) found that for each study that demonstrated a marijuana-related change on one or another test of cognitive functions, at least one and usually more did not. Yet, Miller's data suggest a deficit pattern. While studies using Digit Span were too equivocal to allow any conclusions to be drawn, scores on symbol substitution tests showed a possible dose-related tendency toward response slowing on this task. On simple tracking tasks, no deficits were found, but a study using a complex tracking task did elicit evidence of impairment following marijuana inhalation. Memory test data are the most conclusive, generally showing reduced memory efficiency during marijuana usage (Brust, 2000a). This deficiency appears to be associated with storage but not retrieval (C.F. Darley et al., 1973) and may be due more to impaired attention, loss of ability to discriminate between old and new learning, or insufficient rehearsal than to a storage defect per se. Slowed visual processing during marijuana use has also been demonstrated (Braff et al., 1981). This may have contributed to poor driving performance in a study combining alcohol and marijuana at low levels, although neither drug alone affected driving (Sutton, 1983). Time perception, which under normal conditions tends to be underestimated (i.e., one thinks less time has passed than actually has), may be underestimated even more when marijuana is used. However, this effect, observed in the laboratory within 30 minutes of administration of the drug, tended to dissipate within the subsequent 40 minutes (Dornbush and Kokkevi, 1976), and no effect on time sense was obtained in one study of young adult males (Heishman et al., 1997). R.J. Mathew and colleagues (1998) found cerebellar blood flow differences in healthy volunteers, with time sense altered only for those with decreased flow.

Cocaine

This potent central nervous system stimulant is highly addictive both through the euphoric "rush" experience obtained by inhaling freebase smoke and through nasal inhalation of the powder form. The effect is less rapid and sharp when the drug is taken intravenously because increasingly greater amounts of the drug are required to reexperience the early highs (Ballenger and Post, 1989; Brust, 1993; J.R. Taylor and Jentsch, 2001; Washton and Stone, 1984). Other positive aspects of cocaine intoxication include increased alertness and arousal levels, increased sense of well-being and confidence, and motor activation much like the stimulating qualities of amphetamines. At the neurotransmission level, cocaine increases dopamine in reward circuits (Dackis and O'Brien, 2002), contributing to a vicious cycle of craving and ever higher thresholds for a euphoric reaction to the drug. In the early stages of use

it acts as an aphrodisiac, heightening libido and sexual response (Lukas and Renshaw, 1998), but in the long run cocaine can reduce libido and cause impotence. Psychiatric reactions include agitation, paranoia, delusions and hallucinations, panic attacks, and self- or other-directed violence (M.A. Taylor, 1999). "There is significant evidence that repeated stimulant exposure disrupts the functional integrity of the brain's reward centres" (Dackis and O'Brien, 2002, p. 435).

Seizures occurring within 90 minutes of ingestion affect a small percentage of habitual cocaine users; when taken in the purified form of "crack," newcomers to the drug may also have a seizure reaction (Berliner, 2000; Brust, 1993; Mody et al., 1988; Pascual-Leone et al., 1990). Cocaine users with prior seizure histories are more likely than others to have a seizure reaction. Acute hypertension and other symptoms of central nervous system overstimulation can lead to strokes, which are more often hemorrhagic than infarcts (Brust, 1993; D.C. Klonoff et al., 1989; S.R. Levine et al., 1987), or to death from respiratory or cardiac failure or acutely elevated body temperature (Washton and Stone, 1984). Chronic users who have cocaine-associated seizures tend to show brain atrophy on CT scans with evidence of white matter lesions (*leukoencephalopathy*) (Berliner, 2000; Filley and Kleinschmidt-DeMasters, 2001). Cerebral functional neuroimaging (fMRI) shows abnormal metabolism and hypoperfusion, both when using cocaine and in chronic users even after sustained abstinence (Strickland, Miller, et al., 1998). These neuroimaging abnormalities were consistent with findings of slowed mental processing, memory impairments, and reduced mental flexibility.

Unlike many other addicting drugs, withdrawal is neither potentially life-threatening nor physically agonizing; but transient depression, irritability, listlessness, restlessness, confusion, sleep disturbances, and abnormal movements can occur (M.A. Taylor, 1999). Cognitive problems may develop with long-term use of the drug, especially memory and concentration deficits and impaired executive functioning (Rosselli, Ardila, Lubansky, et al., 2001; Washton and Stone, 1984). The memory problem appears to be due mostly to reduced retrieval efficiency but a mild storage deficit is also suggested (Mittenberg and Motta, 1993). Many chronic users, when abstinent, become dysphoric (Berliner, 2000). Both the amount of cocaine use and length of abstinence contribute to response patterns.

Opiates

Opiate addiction, usually to heroin in Europe and North America, creates a familiar picture of mental and physical sluggishness and personal neglect which can worsen with continuing use of the drug (J.N. Walton, 1994) and is paralleled by EEG slowing (Brust, 2000c). Cognitive effects are generally less debilitating even in persons who had long-term addictions (A.S. Carlin and O'Malley, 1996; S. Fields and Fullerton, 1975; Parsons and Farr, 1981).

A few studies have suggested that long-term opiate users sustain permanent impairments that show up in lowered scores on tests involving visuospatial and visuomotor activities (A.S. Carlin and O'Malley, 1996; I. Grant, Adams, Carlin, et al., 1978a). One study of 72 opiate users reported poorest performances on tests requiring integration of different kinds of functions, with an overall pattern of dysfunction suggestive of diffuse impairment (Rounsaville, Novelly, and Kleber, 1981). In this study, a review of risk factors for the approximately four-fifths who had cognitive deficits (53% severe, 26% mild) found significant relationships between neuropsychological impairments and poor school performance, childhood hyperactivity, cocaine use (≥24%), and greater alcohol use (≥40%) than the nonimpaired opiate addicts. Yet, no relationships between test performance and levels or duration of opiate use showed up, nor were there performance differences between the opiate users and matched controls (Rounsaville, Jones, et al., 1982). Long-term opiate users in another study had lowered scores on tests involving visuospatial and visuomotor activities (I. Grant, Adams, Carlin, et al., 1978a). However, this study's subjects were "polydrug" users which, along with demographic disadvantages, makes it difficult to arrive at any cause-and-effect conjectures (A.S. Carlin and O'Malley, 1996). Pau and his colleagues (2002) reported that attention, mental flexibility, and abstract reasoning appeared unaffected in 30 abstinent addicts who used heroin for an average of 4 and 8 months, although impulsivity appeared on the Porteus Mazes. These findings were not inconsistent with others indicating that in abstinent persons prolonged use of opiates alone does not seem to affect cognitive functioning (Brust, 2000c; S. Fields and Fullerton, 1975; Lishman, 1997; Parsons and Farr, 1981).

Other street drugs

MPTP (1-methyl-4-phenyl-1,2,3,6-tetrahydropyridine) is among the better-known of these. When administered intravenously a very few (of thousands of users) developed a parkinson-like syndrome (Di Monte and Langston, 2000). Like Parkinson patients, these patients have a compromised dopaminergic system with neuropathologic alterations in the substantia nigra. Mental changes also follow the Parkinson pattern of poor performances on tests of perceptuomotor and executive/conceptual functions, although these patients are not demented (Y. Stern, Tetrud, et al., 1990).

Methamphetamine intake, whether oral, by inhalation, or intraveous, can result in strokes, some due to spastic occlusion of intracranial arteries producing a characteristic "beading" effect that shows up on arteriograms (Rothrock et al., 1988). Hemorrhagic stroke also occurs (Heller et al., 2000). Other cardiopulmonary and neurologic findings can have neuropsychological consequences: e.g., cerebral edema, hematoma of the corpus callosum. Cognitive alterations are associated with damage to whatever areas of the brain are involved. However, even heavy amphetamine use, in itself, does not appear to lead to cognitive impairment (I. Grant, Adams, Carlin, et al., 1978a,b), although frontal dysfunction has been reported. Characteristically paranoidal psychotic episodes with vivid hallucinations, both auditory and visual, and vulnerability to psychotic relapses have occurred in long-term heavy users (M.A. Taylor, 1999; Heller et al., 2000; Lishman, 1997).

PCP (phencyclidine) can be smoked, sniffed, or swallowed. Acutely, users may become confused, disoriented, excited, and display psychotic symptoms which, in some 20% of hospitalized users, may last for several weeks (Javitt, 2000). Users have been described as showing more general cognitive impairment than nonusers (A.S. Carlin and O'Malley, 1996); but the historical confounds of high rates of TBI, seizures, childhood chronic otitis media, and attention and learning disorders together with the questionable nature of substances sold as PCP make these studies difficult to interpret. Among the physiological disturbances associated with PCP, hypertension is most common and, in rare cases, has been fatal (Javitt, 2000).

Polydrug abuse

When examined within the first several weeks of abstinence, from about two-fifths to one-half of polydrug abusers show impairment on neuropsychological tests, these impairments found almost exclusively in subjects using central nervous system depressants (sedatives, hypnotics and opiates) (A.S. Carlin and O'Malley, 1996; I. Grant, Adams, Carlin, et al., 1978a; I. Grant, Reed, et al., 1979). Some studies reported a pattern of performance slowing and impaired memory, both verbal and visual, with verbal concept formation remaining intact (McCaffrey, Krahula, et al., 1988; J.A. Sweeney et al., 1989). A large collaborative study found both visuoperceptual and verbal/academic deficiencies in a newly detoxified group of polydrug users, many of whom also used alcohol (I. Grant et al., 1978a, 1979). Unfortunately, except for the memory trials on the Tactual Performance Test, this Halstead-Reitan battery-based study did not examine memory functions. When retested three months later, at least two-fifths of the subjects were urine positive for drugs, and their neuropsychological status generally remained unchanged (I. Grant, Adams, Carlin, et al., 1978b). Risk of cognitive impairment was also linked with increasing age, poor education, and medical and developmental problems.

Social Drugs

Caffeine

Both caffeine and nicotine have stimulant/arousal properties (Koelega, 1993). Caffeine tends to increase motor activity and rate of speech and reduces reaction times (Judd et al., 1987), these effects being more pronounced in children than in adults (Rapoport et al., 1981). It also increases fine motor unsteadiness when taken by persons who normally use little or no coffee but has no negative effects on those who consume coffee regularly (B.H. Jacobson and Thurman-Lacey, 1992). These arousal effects have been documented in EEG and evoked response studies (Curatolo and Robertson, 1983; Tharion, et al., 1993). Tharion and his colleagues also found that with caffeine, subjects were better able to maintain their focus of attention to a visual vigilance task.

Nicotine

The immediate arousal effects of nicotine have shown up on EEG (O'Shanick and Zasler, 1990). Its impact on cognitive functions, however, remains unclear as some studies have shown improvements in memory and on complex tasks (Elgerot, 1976; Peeke and Peeke, 1984) and others have found poorer performances on learning tasks (Houston, 1978) and on speeded, vigilance, and problem solving tests (G.G. Brown, Baird, and Shatz, 1986). A recent study found no substantial effects from long-term smoking (10 to 20 years) on a range of cognitive tests (Schinka, Vanderploeg, et al., 2002a,b). Brust's (2000d) observation that, "Human smokers experience increased alertness followed by relaxation" (p. 861) suggests an explanation for these contradictory data.

Some idea of the complexity of the neuropsychological effects of nicotine can be obtained from recent studies involving smokers, nonsmokers, and Alzheimer patients. Smokers show faster reaction times after smoking a cigarette than when tested without a pretest cigarette, suggesting that information processing speed increases with smoking (Pritchard et al., 1992). However, when smokers who inhale deeply were compared with those who do not, the latter—"light inhalers"—had faster reaction times to nontarget items on the Continuous Performance Test. Further, after smoking a cigarette, light inhalers performed mental tracking tasks (serial addition and subtraction of 3s) faster than before smoking; but deep inhalers, whose performance rate after smoking did not change appreciably, instead showed a pattern of EEG change that was similar to that of persons taking anti-anxiety medication (Pritchard, 1991). Unlike deep inhalers, nonsmokers improved steadily with practice and without benefit of nicotine, ultimately exceeding the highest scores made by light smokers whose response rate increased after smoking but not from practice alone.

A series of studies examined the reported memory enhancement property of nicotine (Rusted and Warburton, 1992; Warburton, Rusted, and Fowler, 1992; Warburton, Rusted, and Muller, 1992). These workers found that nicotine facilitates memory retention following learning trials but not the amount of initial learning. They attributed this phenomenon to increased availability of attentional resources. When given to Alzheimer patients, nicotine did not increase the amount of material learned but patients showed a dose-related reduction in intrusion errors (Newhouse et al., 1993). Temporary improvements with nicotine usage in Alzheimer patients have also been documented (Fant et al., 1999). Some epidemiologic studies of Alzheimer's and Parkinson's disease suggest that nicotine may be protective (see pp. 209, 227).

Withdrawal symptoms begin a day or two after cessation of smoking and may continue for several days thereafter, creating a mental miasma of drowsiness, confusion, and impaired concentration exacerbated by low frustration tolerance and irritability (Brust, 1993; O'Shanick and Zasler, 1990). Indirect effects of smoking on mentation show up in habitual smokers who develop chronic obstructive pulmonary disease (COPD) with resultant insufficient oxygenation and compromised brain function (see p. 282). It has been suspected of speeding up the evolution of AIDS in HIV+ persons (Fant et al., 1999). While not directly associated with functional impairment, nicotine is the most lethal of the addictive drugs as its usual methods of delivery create the most serious health hazards.

Environmental and Industrial Neurotoxins

More than 850 substances, some common, some rare, have been identified as having known or potential neurotoxic effects (Anger, 1990). Most fall into three major categories: solvents and fuels, pesticides, and metals (B. Weiss, 1983; R.F. White, Feldman, and Proctor, 1992). In addition to the drugs discussed above, many medications and commonly used substances can have neurotoxic effects, especially when taken in excessive amounts (Schaumburg, 2000b), e.g., water (Schaumburg, 2000d) and inhalation of nitric oxide from whipped cream dispensers (Scelsa, 2000).

In evaluating exposed persons, it is important to take the nature of the exposure into account (Morrow, Stein, et al., 2001; Morrow, Steinhauer, et al., 1997): high-level acute exposure is typically a one-time event occurring, for example, as an accidental release of toxic substances; long-term chronic exposure to lower levels of toxins may not have observable effects with a single exposure, but cumulative effects may result in neurotoxic disorders. Symptoms may differ greatly with differences in the amount and duration of exposure (Arezzo and Schaumburg, 1989; R.F. White, Feldman, and Proctor, 1992). Moreover, some neurotoxic effects may take time to evolve, first appearing even decades after exposure (Calne et al., 1986; Ogden, 1996) or exacerbating preexisting nervous system dysfunction (Arezzo and Schaumberg, 1989). Comprehensive reviews of environmental toxins and their neuropsychological effects are provided by D.E. Hartman (1995) and Spencer and Schaumburg (2000).

In order to compare patients and patient groups for severity of work-related exposure, an *estimated exposure index (EEI)* has been proposed (Morrow, Kamis, and Hodgson, 1993). This index takes into account *duration of exposure* measured in years, months, and days; *intensity of exposure* as either "background exposure" with no direct physical contact or "intense exposure" involving direct contact with the toxic substance by inhalation, skin absorption, or both, or "intermediate when the substance was in the work area but direct contact was avoided;" *frequency of exposure* measured as either less than 5%, between 5% and 30, or greater than 30% per job; and history of peak exposure graded as "no," "yes without hospitalization," or "yes with hospitalization." The EEI is calculated as intensity × frequency × peak + duration.

Solvents and fuels

The symptoms of neurotoxicity from solvent exposure, often in the form of fumes in the environment, are so nonspecific that they can be mistaken for everything from the common cold to neurasthenia or other emotional disturbances. Moreover, they are so varied and vague that a casual observer may easily misinterpret them.

A pattern of widespread behavioral disturbances reflects the acute sensitivity of the central nervous system to toxic substances and the especial predilection of solvents for fat-rich neuronal tissue (Anger, 1990;

Schaumburg, 2000c; Spencer, 2000a), i.e., white matter (Filley, 2001). Most clinical and laboratory findings point to a depression of brain function in solvent toxicity (Morrow, Muldoon, and Sandstrom, 2001). Abnormal EEGs and, in some studies, brain atrophy have been documented in solvent-exposed persons (Arlien-Søborg et al., 1979; Eskelinen et al., 1986; Juntunen et al., 1980). Long-term exposure can lead to lowered cerebral blood flow, particularly in frontotemporal areas (Hagstadius et al., 1989; Risberg and Hagstadius, 1983). While citing evidence of the neurotoxic effects of high-level exposure, Grasso (1988) notes that questions still remain regarding the toxicity of low-level exposure. For example, more recent studies of workers with very low-level exposure have demonstrated only mild deficits on attentional tasks requiring mental shifting and/or response speed, with no memory or distress symptoms (Schaumburg and Spencer, 2000). However, low-level exposure to agents used in cosmetic nail studios and beauty salons has been associated with reports of mild cognitive inefficiencies (LoSasso et al., 2001).

Acute exposure. During and immediately following acute solvent exposure, many persons complain of headache, dizziness, undue fatigue, nausea, and mental confusion (Furman and Cass, 2003; Spencer and Schaumburg, 2000; R.F. White, Feldman, and Travers, 1990). Some will have respiratory symptoms or skin irritation. We have had patients report an acute flushing that subsides only after a few hours away from the exposure site (dwl, mdl). A transient euphoric reaction to high-intensity intake of toluene, a constituent of such common items as glues, paints, marking pens, and thinners, has led to sniffing for pleasure. Laboratory studies of the cognitive effects of short-term exposures have identified tests of attention and monitoring as sensitive to this type of exposure, but many of the most sensitive clinical tests have not been used in laboratory research (Anger, 1992). Severity of dysfunction tends to be positively associated with the duration and intensity of exposure.

Chronic exposure. Most chronic solvent toxicity occurs in the workplace as a result of long-term exposure to fumes from such substances as paints, glues, and cleaning fluids (e.g., toluene, perchlorethylene, solvent mixtures) (R.M. Bowler, Mergler, Huel, et al., 1991; Spencer and Schaumburg, 2000); to petroleum fuels (Knave et al., 1978); to lubricating and degreasing agents (Grandjean et al., 1955); or to materials used in the manufacture of plastics (e.g., styrene) (Eskenazi and Maizlish, 1988; O'Donoghue, 2000). Long-term inhalant abusers (e.g., glue sniffers) have incurred such long-term neurological and neuropsychological disasters as cognitive impairments ranging in severity from mild deficits to full-blown dementia; disordered gait, balance, and coordination along with spasticity and oculomotor defects in some patients; and white matter atrophy (*toxic leucoencephalopathy*) (Filley and Kleinschmidt-DeMasters, 2001; N.L. Rosenberg et al., 1988; Schaumburg, 2000c). Possibly reversible damage to the liver and renal system has also been reported in glue-sniffing adolescents (Schaumburg, 2000c).

Among subjective complaints, fatigue, memory and concentration problems, emotional lability and depression, sleep disturbances, and both sensory and motor symptoms involving the extremities are most prominent (R.M. Bowler, Mergler, Rauch, et al., 1991; Eskelinen et al., 1986; Morrow, Muldoon, and Sandstrom, 2001). Morrow, Stein, and their colleagues (2001) found that 50% of subjects reporting prior exposure to workplace solvents met psychiatric criteria for depression. The similarity of these complaints to those of neurotic or depressed patients, coupled with the absence of distinctive neurological symptoms, can mislead a naive examiner into discounting the patient's complaints if supporting neuropsychological findings are not available.

Sensory and motor changes include impaired visual acuity (Härkönen et al., 1978; Mergler, Frenette, et al., 1991) and color vision (R.M. Bowler, Lezak, et al., 2001; Mergler and Blain, 1987; Bowler, Mergler, Huel, et al., 1991); vestibular disorders (Furman and Cass, 2003; Morrow, Furman et al., 1988); altered smell sense with hypersensitivity to common environmental odors which, interestingly, has been related to a supramodal learning and recall deficit (C.M. Ryan, Morrow, and Hodgson, 1988); reduced manual dexterity (R.M. Bowler, Mergler, et al., 1991); and numbness and/or weakness of the extremities (E.L. Baker, Letz, et al., 1988). Peripheral nerve conduction velocities were slowed in more than half of one group of patients with long-term exposure (Flodin et al., 1984). Slowed latencies of event-related potentials were documented in all of a small group of persons with organic solvent exposure that occurred two years or more before testing (Morrow, Steinhauer, and Hodgson, 1992; see also Morrow, Steinhauer, and Condray, 1996). Sensory and motor symptoms tend to reflect both peripheral and central neuronal involvement (Cone et al., 1990; Schaumburg and Spencer, 2000; J.R. Williams et al., 1987).

The most prominent *cognitive deficits* involve many aspects of attention, memory, and response slowing (Anger, 1990, 1992; R.M. Bowler, Lezak, et al., 2001; R.M. Bowler, Mergler, Huel, et al., 1991; Morrow, Stein et al., 2001). Morrow, Robin, and their colleagues (1992) documented specific deficits in both forward and reversed digit span, acquisition of new information, and a variation of the Brown-Peterson distractor technique. Their findings suggested that the amount of material these patients are capable of processing is reduced. Abnormal slowing on the Trail Making Test characterized the performance of many—but not all—workers with severe chronic toxic encephalopathy due to solvent exposure (Nilson et al., 1999). Slowing was most pronounced on the Trail Making Test-B and increased with age. It is noteworthy that similar deficit patterns occur with other conditions in which brain damage is known or presumed to be diffuse, such as mild TBI and multiple sclerosis. Reasoning and problem solving abilities may also be compromised (Linz et al., 1986).

Executive disorders show up as reduced spontaneity, impaired planning ability, and situation dependency, for example (Hagstadius et al., 1989; Hawkins, 1990; Lezak, 1984b). Frontal dysfunction has been described using PET during performance of working memory tasks in subjects with solvent exposure (Haut et al., 2000).

Emotional disturbances often present as somatic preoccupations, depressive tendencies, or anxiety with social withdrawal (R.M. Bowler, Lezak, et al., 2001; R.M. Bowler, Mergler, Rauch, et al., 1991; R.M. Bowler, Rauch, et al., 1989; Linz et al., 1986) and can persist two years or more after removal from exposure (R.M. Bowler, Mergler, Rauch, and Bowler, 1992; Morrow, Muldoon, and Sandstrom, 2001). These essentially dysphoric reactions appear to occur without significant changes in personality or interpersonal interactions (Morrow, Kamis, and Hodgson, 1993). The absence of a relationship between emotional distress and cognitive dysfunction suggests that distress is not necessarily reactive to mental ability deficits, nor that distress contributes significantly to poor test performance (R.M. Bowler, Lezak, et al., 2001; Morrow, Ryan, Hodgson, and Robin, 1990; Morrow, Stein, et al., 2001). However, dysphoric emotional states and cognitive impairments tend to occur together (Ogden, 1993). Alterations in adaptive capacity (e.g., sleep disturbance, lethargy) are frequently reported (Anger, 1990; E.L. Baker, Letz, et al., 1988; Filley and Kleinschmidt-DeMasters, 2001).

Differences between the effects of particular solvents and how patients have been affected are the result of interactions between many variables, including duration and intensity of exposure, age, physical and even emotional status of the patient at the time of exposure (Morrow, Ryan, Hodgson, and Robin, 1991), the different kinds of neurotoxins to which a person has been exposed, and the metabolic alterations induced by specific toxic substances (E.L. Baker, Letz et al., 1988; Oscarsson, 1980; Schaumburg, 2000b). Relatively low but enduring exposures can result in slight—often subtle—but demonstrable neuropsychological deficits (Bleecker, Bolla, Agnew, et al., 1991). Both recency of exposure and exposure to a single, sudden high dose have been related to symptom severity (Morrow, Ryan, Hodgson, and Robin, 1990; Morrow, Steinhauer, Condray and Hodgson, 1997). Overall intensity of exposure, rather than duration, may be a key factor in determining symptom severity (E.L. Baker, Letz, et al.,,, 1988; Morrow, Ryan, Hodgson, and Robin, 1990, 1991; Risberg and Hagstadius, 1983). After two or more years of no further exposure, some patients have fewer complaints of subjective distress, particularly with problems of fatigue, headache, and dizziness (Orbaek and Lindgren, 1988). However, patients with brain atrophy visualized by CT scan showed no cognitive improvement during a two-year period with no further exposure to industrial solvents, nor did their symptoms progress (P. Bruhn, Arlien-Søborg, et al., 1981).

The possibility that *long-term solvent exposure* may ultimately produce an Alzheimer-like dementia has been suggested by reports of such syndromes in chronically exposed painters (Arlien-Søborg et al., 1979; Calne et al., 1986; Morrow, Muldoon, and Sandstrom, 2001). Freed and Kandel (1988) found that 37% of a large sample of probable Alzheimer patients had a minimum of two years of occupational exposure, significantly more than the 12% in the control group with similar occupational histories. However, some studies have questioned the association of solvent exposure with a dementing disorder. One found no differences in occupational exposure to presumed neurotoxins when comparing British men who died in the 1970s with and without death certificate diagnoses of "presenile dementia" (O'Flynn et al., 1987). Weaknesses in the early Danish studies, such as inadequate or nonexistent control groups and insufficient data regarding the nature and length of exposure, have been pointed out (Errebo-Knudsen and Olsen, 1986). Studies of workers in industrial settings in which exposure levels had been maintained at relatively low levels for years do not report the cognitive deficits or emotional distress found among less protected workers, although several heavily exposed patients had shown symptoms of toxic encephalopathy (Triebig, 1989; Triebig et al., 1988). Even in the absence of a frank dementia, solvent exposure may contribute to poorer cognitive functioning by interacting with the normal aging process (Nilson et al., 2002).

Pesticides

Most pesticides have neurotoxic effects that, in high doses and/or long exposures, produce a deficit pattern which appears to be similar to the core pattern of solvent toxicity, although fewer formal studies of pesticide neurotoxicity have been reported (Anger, 1990; A.A. Frank et al., 2000; Kurlychek, 1987; B. Weiss, 1983). On acute exposure, patients experience many symptoms associated with central nervous system involvement, such as headaches, blurred vision, anxiety, restlessness, apathy, depression, mental slowing and confusion, slurred speech, and ataxia (Eskanazi and Maizlish, 1988). Coma, convulsions, and death due to respiratory failure can occur with very severe exposure.

Chronically exposed persons are subject to motor system symptoms (H.A. Peters et al., 1982). These patients frequently complain of irritability, anxiety, confusion, and depression. Attention, memory, and response speed are most often mentioned as impaired. Reidy and his colleagues (1992) found impaired short-term visuospatial memory in addition to mental speed and manual dexterity deficits in a group of workers. Gardeners and farmers exposed to pesticides may be at increased risk for mild cognitive impairment (Bosma et al., 2000). Sleep disturbances trouble patients after both acute and chronic exposure. Reports of improvement or symptom stability vary greatly and may depend on the methods of assessment as much or more than the type of pesticide or the duration of exposure.

Metals

The two metals best known for their toxicity potential are lead—the mental dulling of children exposed to lead paint and leaded gas fumes, and Clare Booth Luce's unhappy encounter with lead paint in her Italian villa decades ago, were headline stories—and mercury—made famous by Lewis Carroll's Mad Hatter (hatmakers in the late 19th century used mercury to process felt) and by headline stories on several large-scale illness epidemics traceable to organic mercury that entered the food chain after being dumped into heavily fished waters.

Lead. Lead neurotoxicity can compromise virtually the whole gamut of cognitive functions: attention, memory and learning, visual and verbal abilities, both motor and processing speed, and coordination (Anger, 1990; Gross and Nagy, 1992; R.F. White, Feldman, and Travers, 1990). Lead-exposed workers frequently report fatigue as a problem, along with headache, restlessness, irritability, and poor emotional control (Eskenazi and Maizlish, 1988; H. Hanninen, 1982; Pasternak et al., 1989). Development of toxicity symptoms requires weeks or longer of exposure; they do not occur acutely (Cory-Schlecta and Schaumburg, 2000). Serious effects on infants and children (R.G. Feldman and

White, 1992; B. Weiss, 1983) continue to depress cognitive functioning into adulthood (R.F. White, Diamond et al., 1993).

H. Hänninen (1982) reported specific deficits on visual tasks, both construction and memory. Visuospatial and executive function impairments are often the most prominent effects (A. Barth et al., 2002). In one series of lead-exposed workers, cognitive abilities progressively declined over an average of 16 years after past occupational exposure (B.S. Schwartz et al., 2000). Bolla-Wilson and her colleagues (1988) found that higher lead levels in blood were associated with poorer performances on tests of both verbal and visual learning, word usage, and construction. Yet some studies reported no or few abnormal cognitive findings (Braun and Daigneault, 1991; Pasternak et al., 1989; C.M. Ryan, Morrow, Parkinson, and Bromet, 1987), which may be due to moderate or low exposure or current blood levels.

Lead toxicity also can affect motor functions, showing up as a wrist- or foot-drop and reduced motor speed and strength (Morrow, Muldoon, and Sandstrom, 2001; Pasternak et al., 1989; B. Weiss, 1983). High exposure levels have been shown to have adverse effects on the central nervous system as well as kidneys, the reproductive system, and blood content (Morrow, Muldoon, and Sandstrom, 2001).

Organic lead, used in leaded gasoline, for example, is highly toxic. As such it is an important contributor to the neurobehavioral disorders of chronic gasoline sniffers, including pronounced memory impairment (Lishman, 1997; Schaumburg, 2000a).

Mercury. Mercury toxicity can have many different central nervous system effects, consistent with autopsy findings of encephalopathy, particularly involving the cerebellum, the basal ganglia, the primary visual cortex in the occipital lobe, and spinal cord degeneration (R.G. Feldman, 1982; Verity and Sarafian, 2000). When acute intoxication does not result in death due to respiratory, gastrointestinal, and/or renal dysfunction, such problems as motor slowing and clumsiness, paresthesias, tremor, visual and hearing defects, agitation, and mental dulling may evolve in as few as two days after exposure or as long as six weeks and persist indefinitely (Maghazaji, 1974; B. Weiss, 1983). Even one exposure, if the dose is high enough, can result in serious sensory and motor dysfunction, cognitive deficits, and even death (Verity and Sarafian, 2000).

Deficits due to chronic low-level exposure become evident on tests of visuomotor coordination and construction; these patients also have attentional, memory, and reasoning problems (H. Hänninen, 1982; R.F. White, Feldman, and Travers, 1990). Mercury levels in urine have been associated with short-term memory deficits (P. Smith et al., 1983). With the very low level of exposure incurred by dentists when working with amalgam, those with highest (but still low) exposures made, on the average, a few more drawing errors and reported a few more emotional disturbances than low-exposure dentists, although cognitive functions remained intact (the status of memory and attention was not reported in these studies) (I.M. Shapiro et al., 1982; Uzzell, 1988). Uzzell and Oler (1986) found that dental technicians, too, report a pattern of emotional distress that has been associated with cognitive inefficiencies and display a short-term memory deficit. Patients with a history of relatively severe exposure suffer a chronically depressed mood with apathy and social withdrawal (Maghazaji, 1974), but depression, shyness, irritability, nervousness, and fatigue also trouble patients with chronic mild exposures (L.S. Gross and Nagy, 1992). Very mild tremor, motor slowing, and reaction times may improve in time (J.M. Miller et al., 1975). EEG abnormalities tend to be associated with age at time of exposure and the severity of intoxication: children sustain the greatest brain damage with the most pronounced cognitive and neurological deficits, which are not likely to improve (Brenner and Snyder, 1980).

Other metals. The list of metals with known toxic effects is long and research on most is scanty (Anger, 1990; R.M. Bowler and Cone, 1999, *passim*; Spencer and Schaumburg, 2000). Of these, aluminum and manganese are of particular neuropsychological interest.

Aluminum's previously conjectured role in the etiology of dementia (A.S. Schwartz, Frey et al., 1988) has not been supported, but it is definitely implicated in *dialysis dementia,* a condition that had affected fewer than 1% of kidney dialysis patients (L.S. Gross and Nagy, 1992; Spencer, 2000a). The incidence of dialysis dementia has significantly decreased following the removal of aluminum from the dialysate and purification of the water used in dialysis (G.B. Young and Bolton, 2002). It is more likely to be a problem when dialysis is conducted at home with a water supply containing high concentrations of aluminum (A.M. Davison et al., 1982).

Onset of dialysis dementia is typically marked by stuttering and inarticulate or dysfluent speech (J. Barron et al., 1980). Concentration and memory problems can qualify the condition as a dementia. Personality changes can include just about everything from agitation to depression and apathy to paranoia (G.B. Young and Bolton, 2002). Motor problems show up in uncontrolled jerking (myoclonus) and difficulty swallowing. EEG abnormalities typically implicate both frontal areas and the diencephalic reticular activating system and, if identified early in their evolution, may be reversed with a prompt response to the problem.

Manganese is used in the manufacture of many products, particularly metal alloys. It is an essential trace element for normal metabolism (Chu et al., 2000). Chronic poisoning, typically seen among miners and metal workers, evolves slowly and may take years to reach a fully established stage characterized by both mental and motor disorders (J.B. Sass et al., 2002). Severity of symptoms increases with prolongation of exposure. Once established, the motor and mental symptoms of *manganism* tend to progress, even with no further exposure.

Initially workers complain about drowsiness, dizziness, sleep disturbances with nightmares, emotional lability, and apathy (Chu et al., 2000; Hua and Huang, 1991; Q. Huang, et al., 1990). Clumsiness, abnormal gait and posture, trembling, and numb hands typically occur later in exposure. A Parkinson-like movement disorder with rigidity and bradykinesia may be associated with impaired visuoperceptual accuracy, visual learning, construction, and slowed response and processing times in exposed workers (Hua and Huang, 1991); these problems have appeared at lower levels with environmental airborne exposures (Mergler, Baldwin, et al., 1999). Some may have neither motor symptoms nor cognitive deficits except for mild slowing. Decreased cortical metabolism was widespread in four exposed workers with mild parkinsonism who did not have abnormal neuropsychological examinations or subcortical metabolic changes (Wolters et al., 1989). Other workers presenting with the Parkinson motor syndrome have had problems only on tests of facial recognition and construction (C.-C. Huang et al., 1989). A large group of manganese workers, not separated with respect to motor symptoms, displayed slowed response speed, impaired dexterity and eye–hand coordination, and deficits in verbal short-term memory and learning, with education levels also contributing to poor performances on the verbal and speeded tests but not to dexterity or coordination problems (Q. Huang et al., 1990).

Formaldehyde

Because it is so widely used in buildings, furnishing materials, and household products, formaldehyde in vapor or derivative form is often present in home environments (Schenker et al., 1982). Laboratory animals exposed steadily for three months to somewhat higher than normally encountered air levels of formaldehyde incurred brain lesions, particularly involving the parietal cortex (Fel'man and Bonashevskaya, 1971). Both

acutely and chronically, persons exposed to formaldehyde have complaints implicating the central nervous system, such as headache, dizziness, irritability, memory problems, and sleep disturbances (Consensus Workshop on Formaldehyde, 1984; Olsen and Dossing, 1982). Impairments on tests of attention and short-term memory have been reported for exposed workers (B. Bach, 1987; Kilburn et al., 1987), and reduced vigilance was observed in nine of 14 persons living in homes insulated with formaldehyde foam (Schenker et al., 1982).

My experience with a number of persons complaining of memory problems associated with formaldehyde exposure is that many of them displayed attentional deficits which interfered with effective communication and normal information storage and were interpreted by them as "memory" problems [mdl]. However, using the Halstead-Reitan battery and the Wechsler Memory Scale to examine a small series of persons exposed to low levels of formaldehyde fumes in their homes, Cripe and Dodrill (1988) reported no notable differences between them and matched control subjects.

INFECTIOUS PROCESSES

Many of the infectious diseases that have long-lasting mental effects, such as measles encephalitis and tuberculous meningitis, can be severely crippling, if not fatal (Gelb, 1990; Lishman, 1997). Others, such as general paresis (neurosyphilis) and certain fungal infections, may have a fairly long course that leaves the patient's mental capacities progressively impaired, with very specific deficits that are peculiar to the disease or that relate to a focal lesion. Some idea of how many infectious diseases can have direct effects on brain functioning is given by Lishman (1997), who lists 24 varieties of encephalitis and notes several other conditions suspected of having a viral etiology. Three among these are of current neuropsychological interest: the *human immunodeficiency virus* (*HIV*) because of its clinical importance, and *herpes simplex* because of the theoretically interesting nature of its effects on brain function.

HIV Infection and AIDS

HIV attacks and progressively destroys the immune system, and it has a morbid predilection for the brain (Fernandez et al., 2002; Kaemingk and Kaszniak, 1989; M.D. Kelly et al., 1996; Lishman, 1997). The usual infection agent for the *acquired immunodeficiency syndrome* (*AIDS*) is HIV-1. HIV-2 has also been associated with AIDS, particularly in western and central Africa (I. Grant and Martin, 1994). The range of central nervous system disorders associated with HIV is broad, but generally they involve either the direct effects of the virus on the nervous system or indirect effects from opportunistic illnesses and infections or from complications from HIV treatment (Fernandez et al., 2002).

Course

HIV+. In its early stages before breakdown of the immune system becomes evident, this disease is quite benign (Sidtis and Price, 1990). The potential patient may continue in apparent good health for years, with few if any of the mental changes that eventually trouble most patients before the disease runs its ultimate course (Janssen et al., 1989; Selnes, Miller, et al., 1990). Estimates vary on the percentage of patients whose initial symptoms involve the central nervous system (10%: R.M. Levy, 1988; 20%: Clifford, 2002) or are neuropsychological (10% to 30% of cases: A.C. Collier et al., 1987). Some studies have reported some slight but significantly depressed test performances in medically asymptomatic patients (M.D. Kelly et al., 1996; S. Perry et al., 1989; Y. Stern, Marder, et al., 1991), which may reflect population differences between studies or different sets of tests (e.g., word fluency tests seem to be particularly sensitive to early changes). Some of these "prepatients" may have positive EEG findings and auditory (Kaemingk and Kaszniak, 1989) or visual (Ollo et al., 1991) evoked potential slowing before other neurological symptoms appear (Fernandez et al., 2002).

AIDS. AIDS is defined by the presence of an active disease state associated with immunological compromise, such as a wasting disease with fever and diarrhea, a condition of neurological deterioration, or an opportunistic infection or malignancy (A.C. Collier et al., 1987; Faulstich, 1987). As HIV infection evolves into AIDS, the incidence and virulence of brain damage increase greatly: a positive relationship between the status of the immune system, disease severity, and cognitive functioning has been consistently documented (Lishman, 1997; Saykin et al., 1988; Skoraszewski et al., 1991). Cerebral changes usually show up on MRI scanning as brain atrophy and in multiple small diffuse or larger bilateral subcortical (mostly white matter but also deep gray matter) lesions, and occasionally in a single focal lesion (Fernandez et al., 2002; Filley, 2001; I. Grant, Atkinson, et al., 1987; J.G. Jarvik et al., 1988). Many patients have EEG abnormalities, particularly as the disease progresses (Kaemingk and Kaszniak, 1989). From 75% to 90% of all patients will have some CNS involvement by the time they die (A.C. Collier et al., 1987; R.M. Levy and Bredesen, 1988a) due to opportunistic infections, HIV, or both. Most untreated patients die within two to three years after AIDS onset, but some patients live five years or longer (Faulstich, 1987).

Neuropsychopathology

Prodromal. The very earliest stages of this disease are notable for the absence of symptoms in most HIV infected persons; diagnosis is made on blood serum in the laboratory. Most—an estimated 70% (M.D. Kelly et al., 1996)—HIV carriers without obvious health problems show no evidence of cognitive dysfunction regardless of their immune system status or duration of HIV infection (Goethe et al., 1989; E.N. Miller, Selnes, et al., 1990). For most HIV[+] persons, this prodromal stage lasts from two to ten years (Selnes, Miller, et al., 1990) with some infected persons remaining symptom-free for 20 years (Lishman, 1997). However a subgroup of HIV[+] patients does show subtle memory and verbal fluency deficits before developing immunosuppression-related illnesses (S. Perry et al., 1989; Skoraszewski et al., 1991). One large study of seropositive HIV subjects, for example, found that one-third had relatively small but widespread performance decrements when compared to the other seropositive subjects, whose performance levels were generally comparable to healthy subjects in their age groups (Van Gorp, Hinkin, et al., 1993; see also M.D. Kelly et al., 1996).

In time the prepatient may experience mild episodes of mental inefficiency or confusion. The early symptom pattern, before opportunistic diseases appear or the virus becomes active within brain substance, includes the common indicators of diffuse damage—attentional and memory deficits, and slowed processing and responses. Deficits may also show up on naming and fluency tests, conceptual problem solving, motor sequencing, and self-monitoring, without aphasia, apraxia, or agnosia. This cluster of symptoms thus presents a pattern typically seen with subcortical disorders and white matter disease (Filley, 2001; M.D. Kelly et al., 1996; Kent et al., 1994; Van Gorp, Mitrushina, Cummings, et al., 1989). Some patients may have more or less transient localized problems with verbal or visuospatial abilities, for example, or clumsiness or paresthesias in one limb or on one side.

The earliest symptoms can be difficult to identify or evaluate as the patient may also be run down physically, have frequent respiratory or other infections, take medications or drugs that affect alertness or processing speed, and be often—not inappropriately—depressed, somatically preoccupied, or anxious (Hestad et al., 1993; R.M. Levy and Bredesen, 1988b; Sidtis and Price, 1990; Skoraszewski et al., 1991), all conditions that can affect mental efficiency by compromising otherwise intact cognitive functioning or by worsening organically based dysfunction. It is not surprising to learn that persons at risk and those with HIV infection but with no or just the earliest physical symptoms acknowledge higher stress levels than AIDS patients (Faulstich, 1987; Tross and Hirsch, 1988; see also Lishman's [1997] discussion of the "worried well"). Depression appears to affect the neuropsychological test performances of HIV$^+$ patients little if at all (I. Grant, Olshen, et al., 1993; Hinkin et al., 1992).

AIDS dementia complex. This progressive condition has other names, such as *HIV-associated encephalopathy, AIDS encephalopathy,* or *HIV-associated dementia (HAD)* (A.C. Collier et al., 1987; Diesing et al., 2002). They all refer to an evolving dementia due to direct HIV infection of the brain which, in its final stages, typically involves rapid deterioration of cerebral functioning (Fernandez et al., 2002; Lishman, 1997; Sharief and Swash, 1998). The dementing process may begin insidiously with very subtle symptoms, such as depression or complaints of concentration and memory problems and of mental sluggishness. Before evolving into a full-blown dementia, concentration and memory deficits and slowed mental processing are the most usual cognitive impairments. Most patients develop motor disorders, with weakness, tremor, incoordination, and gait disturbances prominent among them. Patients may exhibit emotional disturbances, such as irritability, depression, apathy, agitation, and blunted affect; hallucinations, delusions, and paranoidal thinking—and more extremely, psychotic mania or delirium—have also been reported. Occasionally emotional and personality changes show up before cognitive dysfunction becomes apparent. Mental disorders can develop into full-blown dementia in just a few days from the appearance of the first symptom or take as long as two months, sometimes longer (Tross and Hirsch, 1988).

In late stage AIDS dementia, patients' mental dilapidation shows up in confusion, disinhibition, and prominent motor disorders. Mutism, incontinence, seizures, and coma are among the catastrophic problems heralding death. Cerebral atrophy appears on radiographic scans: autopsy findings reveal cortical sparing with diffuse lesions in white matter and subcortical structures which have substantiated the subcortical dementia nature of this condition (Filley, 2001; Van Gorp, Mitrushina, Cummings, et al., 1989).

Treatment. HIV antiretroviral therapy and protease inhibitors, together termed *highly active antiviral therapy (HAART)*, have significantly increased life expectancy and quality of life while decreasing neurologic complications. Prior to its introduction, more than 60% of AIDS patients became demented. Now, mostly in developed countries, probably fewer than 10% of HIV$^+$ patients will develop dementia (Clifford, 2002). In the United States, this treatment has resulted in 75% fewer deaths from AIDS or AIDS-related diseases between 1994 and 1997 (Palella et al., 1998).

Some patients with AIDS dementia will have more than one kind of brain disease (R.M. Levy and Bredesen, 1988a,b), and some with two or more other brain disorders may appear to have AIDS dementia. Thus even when the patient has deteriorated to the point of dementia, a diagnostic effort may identify other treatable conditions. The treatment of AIDS dementia itself continues to evolve (Fernandez et al., 2002; Lishman, 1997). Some centers may delay initiation of treatment due to long-term toxicity, expense, and inevitable evolution of virus resistance over time (Clifford, 2002). Yet AIDS treatment has significantly improved quality of life for affected patients.

Herpes Simplex Encephalitis

This infectious condition is of special neuropsychological interest. Relatively few people contract this disease, and of these, relatively few survive the acute stage without treatment (Lishman, 1997; Victor and Ropper, 2001). Of those who do survive, reports of a return to normal function range from 3% (Kennedy and Chaudhuri, 2002) to one-third (Snowden, 2002), depending upon whether treatment is initiated before damage is irreparable (Sharief and Swash, 1998). However, many of those who survive have lost much medial temporal and orbital brain tissue, usually including the hippocampal memory registration region, the amygdala with its centers for control of primitive drives, and that area of the frontal lobes involved in the kind of response inhibition necessary for goal-directed activity and appropriate social behavior. In calling attention to the selective affinity of this virus for limbic system gray matter, A.R. Damasio and Van Hoesen (1985) suggested that distinctive neurochemical and neuroimmunological properties of this specialized cerebral subsystem may account for its being the only site of this virulent infection. Alternatively, the predilection for the temporal lobe may stem from the virus's entry by means of the olfactory pathway, allowing the disease to travel along the base of the brain to the inferior temporal lobes (R.T. Johnson, 1998). Another hypothesis suggests that the virus spreads from the trigeminal ganglia to the temporal and frontal cortices (L.E. Davis and Johnson, 1979). Risk factors are unknown: 80% to 90% of adults carry herpes simplex antibodies. The disease can occur at any age in any season.

Due to the significant involvement of the temporal lobes bilaterally, these patients typically display an exceedingly dense memory defect with profound anterograde amnesia, considerable retrograde amnesia, and severe social dilapidation (O'Connor, Verfaillie, and Cermak, 1995; Lhermitte and Signoret, 1972; Sharief and Swash, 1998). Their hippocampal lesions compromise new learning, in contrast to Korsakoff patients with thalamic and mammillary body lesions who demonstrate some new learning but have difficulty with retrieval. Many of these patients become perseverative in their recall of old information or activities.

A 35-year-old real estate broker with severe memory impairment wandered aimlessly in the hospital corridor, stopping in front of every man wearing a tie to say, "What a nice tie! That's a very attractive tie you're wearing." He repeated himself virtually verbatim, day after day, and many times the same day to interns and residents working on that ward. He ate everything he could get, regardless of when or how much he had last eaten and with no recall of having eaten.

The profound behavioral changes that accompany the viral invasion of limbic structures resemble the *Klüver-Bucy syndrome* displayed by monkeys with bilateral temporal lobectomies and are probably most directly associated with damage to the amygdala (Greenwood et al., 1983; Lishman, 1997; Tranel, 2002). The Klüver-Bucy-like behavior may show up as uncontrolled eating (*bulimia*); hyperorality, including licking, lip-smacking, and oral searching; loss of fear, social responsivity, and social and personal inhibitions; and affective blunting and incapacity for discriminating or meaningful relationships. Impaired ability to make discriminations is one of the important elements in the disordered behavior of persons who have survived herpes encephalitis.

Lyme Disease

Lyme disease is a tick-borne infection caused by the bacterium *Borrelia burgdorferi* and is named after Lyme, Connecticut, where the disease was first described. Although more than 15,000 cases are reported in the United States each year, this is likely a low estimate due to underreporting (Orloski, Campbell, et al., 1998). Lyme disease is more prevalent in the northeastern and mid-Atlantic states, in regions where the small hard-bodied Ixodid ticks are abundant. Its highest concentrations are in Connecticut (67.9/100,000) and Rhode Island (44.8/100.000) (Orloski, Hayes, et al., 2000). It occurs most usually during late spring and summer when ticks and people are most active outdoors.

After the tick bite, spirochetes spread to other areas by cutaneous, lymphatic, and blood-borne routes. The incubation period before symptoms appear is generally one to two weeks, with the development of a single "bull's-eye" rash (*erythema migrans* [*EM*]) usually the first symptom. This is followed by nonspecific flu-like symptoms such as fever, malaise, fatigue, headache, and joint and muscle aches. The disease may spread to other organ systems in up to 20% of patients approximately one month after initial infection (Pachner et al., 1989). Neurologic disorders, such as aseptic meningitis, facial nerve palsy, motor and sensory nerve inflammation, and encephalitis, may occur in 15 to 20% of patients (Garcia-Monco and Benach, 1995). Neuropsychologists may see patients who have developed Lyme encephalopathy since their conditions usually involve cognitive impairments, sleep disturbance, fatigue, and personality changes, which—along with arthritis and other musculoskeletal illnesses—may become chronic (Fallon, Nields, et al., 1992). Cardiac abnormalities are uncommon, occurring in approximately 8% of patients (Nagi et al., 1996).

Lyme disease is rarely, if ever, fatal. On MRI, Lyme patients with encephalomyelitis have white matter lesions that are similar to MS lesions in appearance, although patients with mild encephalopathy often have normal MRIs or relatively small white matter lesions (Filley, 2001; Morgen et al., 2001). SPECT scanning has revealed multifocal areas of hypoperfusion in both the cortex and the subcortical white matter in patients with Lyme encephalopathy, suggesting functional or mild structural abnormality not visible on conventional MRI (Fallon, Das, et al., 1997; Logigian et al., 1999). Treatment typically includes antibiotic therapy for 3–4 weeks, which is most effective if initiated early. Later, in cases with evident neurologic dysfunction, the disease may be treated with intravenous antibiotics.

The pattern of neuropsychological performance includes memory impairment (Westervelt and McCaffrey, 2002). Some investigators report reduced word generation (Benke, Gasse, et al., 1995; Gaudino, Coyle, and Krupp, 1997) whereas others have not observed this (R.F. Kaplan et al., 1999; Svetina et al., 1999). Inconsistency in neuropsychological study findings may be due, in part, to relatively small sample sizes as well as heterogeneity in study group composition (Westervelt and McCaffrey, 2002).

Chronic Fatigue Syndrome (CFS)

This somewhat controversial diagnosis requires complaints of severe chronic fatigue lasting at least six months with other etiologies excluded; thus it is a diagnosis of exclusion. A large portion of the controversy, however, stems from the tendency of some health care providers to give this diagnosis when no other explanation for fatigue can be found, even when the patient's fatigue falls within expected levels of variation (Wessely, 2001). The diagnosis of CFS is typically given to patients who become greatly fatigued with minor physical or mental exertion, but this severe fatigue pattern must not have been a life-long condition. In addition, CFS fatigue is not relieved with bed rest. Somatic complaints are common, including sore throat, tender or swollen lymph nodes, muscle pain, multijoint pain without swelling or redness, and headaches. This cluster of symptoms, with memory deficits, contributes to a clinical diagnosis (Fukuda et al., 1994).

CFS is diagnosed up to four times more often in women than in men (Reyes et al., 1997). Prevalence estimates are difficult to obtain, but the Reyes study of four U.S. cities reports an incidence of 4.0 to 8.7 per 100,000. The etiology of CFS is probably multifactorial. Although there has been speculation about a link between viruses such as Epstein-Barr and CFS, these patients do not have active infection. Because fatigue is common after viral infection, at least come cases of CFS may represent a postinfectious syndrome (Jain and DeLisa, 1998). Reduced activity of the hypothalamic–pituitary–adrenal axis has been implicated (Cleare et al., 2001).

Cognitive impairment often involves poor concentration, impaired learning, and word finding difficulty (Barrows, 1995). In their summary of neuropsychological deficits in CFS, Michiels and Cluydts (2001) report that slowed processing speed and impaired working memory and learning are the most prominent and most consistent. Others report that cognitive deficits are relatively subtle and involve complex information processing speed or efficiency (Jain and DeLisa, 1998). The literature is inconsistent, in part due to the heterogeneity of diagnosis and group composition; and when deficits are present, they generally tend to be subtle (Tiersky et al., 1997). Although depression is common in CFS and can be considered a possible explanation for mild neuropsychological impairment, CFS patients without psychiatric illness may even perform more poorly than psychiatrically troubled CFS patients (J. DeLuca, Johnson, et al., 1997). Subjective memory complaints are usually greater than what is observed in formal neuropsychological examinations (Tiersky et al., 1997).

BRAIN TUMORS

One of every four cancer patients will develop tumors that invade or impinge on brain tissue (*intracranial neoplasms*) at some point in their illness (Victor and Ropper, 2001). In any given year, 46 of every 100,000 adults in the United States will develop a brain tumor, which amounts to approximately 115,000 new U.S. cases, mostly metastisized from lung cancer (C.A. Meyers and Cantor, 2003). In adults, secondary intracranial neoplams outnumber primary brain tumors by a factor of 2:1, with the reverse being true in children (see Packer, 1999, for a review of pediatric brain tumors).

Primary Brain Tumors

Gliomas

Tumors that arise from the glial cells forming the connective tissue of the brain—*gliomas*—are the most common primary brain tumors in adults, accounting for nearly half of all brain tumors in adults (DeAngelis, 2001; Victor and Ropper, 2001). They are slightly more common in men than in women (1.6:1). Gliomas can be further subdivided into *astrocytomas*, *oligodendroglial* tumors, and *mixed gliomas*. Brain tumors are graded according to the most malignant area identified within them, ranging from highly malignant (grade 3 or 4) to relatively benign (grade 1 or 2) (Kleihues and Cavenee, 2000; Laterra and Brem, 2002, Victor and Ropper, 2001).

Malignant astrocytic tumors—*glioblastoma multiforme* and *anaplastic astrocytoma*—are the most common glial tumors in adults (DeAngelis, 2001; Laterra and Brem, 2002). Glioblastomas—which constitute 80% of the malignant gliomas—usually present in the sixth or seventh decade of life, while anaplastic astrocytomas appear slightly earlier (fourth or fifth decade). These rapidly growing malignancies infiltrate the brain's tissue—typically the white matter—making clean surgical removal all but impossible. On MRI they are easily identified by their irregular ring-like gadolinium enhancement, surrounding edema, and mass effect. Treatment of malignant astrocytomas is essentially palliative, consisting of surgical removal (*resection*) of as much of the tumor as possible, followed by focused cranial radiation (DeAngelis, 2001; Laperriere et al., 2002). Adding chemotherapy prolongs survival time, albeit modestly (Glioma Meta-Analysis Trialists Group, 2002). Even with aggressive treatment, median survival time for glioblastoma patients is only one year from diagnosis and for patients with anaplastic astrocytomas, two to four years after diagnosis (DeAngelis, 2002; Laterra and Brem, 2002; Victor and Ropper, 2001).

Lower grade astrocytomas generally occur in young adults in their twenties or thirties (DeAngelis, 2001). Like malignant gliomas, these tumors are infiltrative, although they grow much more slowly. Patients are often neurologically intact until they have a focal or generalized seizure. On MRI, low grade astrocytomas appear as diffuse nonenhancing masses without surrounding edema or mass effect; on positron emission tomography (PET), they are hypometabolic (hypermetabolic areas would suggest a more malignant process).

Treatment of low grade astrocytomas is the subject of some debate, particularly in patients who are essentially free of symptoms and whose seizures are well controlled with anticonvulsant medication (Bampoe and Bernstein, 1999; DeAngelis, 2001; Recht et al., 2000). Complete surgical removal of a low grade astrocytoma is ideal but may not be possible because these tumors frequently impinge on crucial brain regions or are too large to be completely excised. Chemotherapy is of limited benefit. Postsurgical radiation therapy is often recommended (DeAngelis, 2001)—specifically low dose radiation therapy, which is as efficacious as higher doses but produces fewer side effects (Karim et al., 1996). Sadly most of these tumors ultimately evolve into malignant gliomas. Median survival time for patients with low grade astrocytomas is approximately five years, but with considerable variability (DeAngelis, 2001). Poorer prognosis is associated with ages over 40, specific tumor characteristics (histology, larger size, and whether it crosses the midline), and the presence of neurological deficits prior to surgery (Pignatti et al., 2002).

Originally thought to be rare, oligodendrogliomas, which originate from the oligodendrocytes or their precursors, may constitute up to 20% of all glial neoplasms (Fortin et al., 1999). They are about twice as common in men as in women and occur most often in young adults in their twenties or thirties (Victor and Ropper, 2001). Most arise from the deep white matter underlying the frontal or temporal lobes. Oligodendrogliomas are often low grade and may be difficult to distinguish pathologically from low-grade astrocytomas. However, oligodendrogliomas have been associated with specific genetic alterations (Bigner et al., 1999), which has important treatment implications (J.S. Smith et al., 2000). A seizure is often the first sign that something is awry; headache or hemiparesis (most often progressive, although onset is typically acute if there has been a hemorrhage) may also be presenting signs.

As with low grade astrocytomas, treatment may be deferred unless disabling symptoms are present or progression is evident on clinical evaluation or imaging studies. Unlike astrocytomas, oligodendrogliomas are unusually sensitive to chemotherapy, making both chemotherapy and focal radiation therapy viable treatments (J.D. Olson et al., 2000; J.R. Perry et al., 1999). Highly malignant oligodendrogliomas necessitate immediate and aggressive treatment: surgical resection, if feasible, followed by chemotherapy and/or radiation

therapy. Fortunately, 75% of patients with malignant oligodendrogliomas respond to chemotherapy, and nearly half of these can function at premorbid levels or at least have sustained remissions with meaningful clinical improvement (K. Peterson et al., 1996).

Meningiomas

Meningiomas are technically not brain tumors as they arise from the cells forming the external membranes covering the brain (the meninges). They are the next most common primary intracranial tumor in adults, constituting approximately 15%–20% of intracranial neoplasms (DeAngelis, 2001). Meningiomas grow between the brain and the skull, at times penetrating the skull itself and producing characteristic changes in its bony structure. Unlike gliomas, meningiomas are more common in women than in men (2:1). Most are benign (Victor and Ropper, 2001), although radiation-induced meningiomas can be malignant (Bondy and Ligon, 1996). Meningiomas usually occur over the cerebral convexities or at the base of the skull, and they tend to grow relatively slowly, causing symptoms by compressing adjacent neural structures (e.g., cranial neuropathies, headache, progressive hemiparesis). Symptomatic meningiomas are found most often in patients in their sixth and seventh decades, although 75% of them are so small that they are discovered only incidentally on autopsy (DeAngelis, 2001).

Because meningiomas are often self-contained and do not invade the brain itself, many can be completely removed by surgery, particularly if they do not involve the skull base (DeAngelis, 2001; Victor and Ropper, 2001). However, up to 20% will recur within ten years. Patients with inoperable or malignant meningiomas may undergo radiation therapy, but chemotherapy is generally not helpful.

CNS lymphoma

Primary central nervous system *lymphoma* used to be quite rare (≤1% of primary brain tumors). Its incidence in the United States has tripled over the last two decades, partly due to the heightened frequency of CNS lymphoma in immunosuppressed populations (including AIDS patients) (Schabet, 1999). Primary CNS lymphomas can occur in persons with intact immune systems, though typically not until the sixth and seventh decades (DeAngelis, 2001). Lesions associated with primary CNS lymphoma may be single or multifocal and they often cluster around the ventricles. Consequently these patients may initially present with behavioral and cognitive changes typically associated with subcortical involvement or with focal cerebral signs (e.g., hemiparesis, aphasia, or visual field defects) instead of headaches or seizures (DeAngelis, 2001; Victor and Ropper, 2001).

Treatment of CNS lymphoma consists of cranial irradiation and corticosteroids which produce transient improvement but, unfortunately, these tumors almost always recur: median survival time is only 12 to 18 months, and even less in immunocompromised patients (D.R. Nelson et al., 1992). In patients with intact immune systems, high-dose methotrexate regimens coupled with radiation therapy can extend median survival to four years or more. Many patients who undergo these combined chemotherapy–radiation regimens—particularly those over age 60—experience delayed neurotoxic effects (Abrey et al., 1998).

Secondary (Metastatic) Brain Tumors

Metastatic intracranial neoplasms are secondary carcinomas originating in solid tumors elsewhere in the body that are transported into the CNS and settle in brain tissue—the skull and dura or, less commonly, the meninges (Patchell, 2002). (These are distinct from the less common *paraneoplastic disorders*—neurologic syndromes associated with carcinoma that stem not from direct invasion or compression of the nervous system, but rather from indirect mechanisms that are incompletely understood [Dropcho, 2002].) The most common source of cerebral metastases is the lung, followed by the breast, melanoma, gastrointestinal tract, and kidney (Patchell, 2002; Victor and Ropper, 2001).

Cerebral metastases are multiple in at least 50% of cases, are generally solid (but occasionally ring-like), and are typically accompanied by edema (Patchell, 2002; Victor and Ropper, 2001). These tumors tend to grow faster and thus show effects sooner than the tumor of origin (Patchell, 2002). Patients with cerebral mestastases often present with symptoms similar to those of glioblastoma multiforme: headache, seizures, focal cerebral signs, or cognitive and behavioral alterations that progress over weeks to months (Victor and Ropper, 2001). Metastases to the skull and dura typically arise from breast or prostate tumors or multiple myelomas. They are often asymptomatic, particularly if located on the skull convexity, but can be symptomatic when skull base metastases involve the cranial nerves or pituitary. Treatment of secondary intracranial carcinomas may involve corticosteroids (to relieve edema), surgery (if there is a single accessible metastasis and primary tumor growth has been controlled), whole-brain irradiation, and/or chemotherapy (particularly if the primary tumor is sensitive to chemotherapy). Whole brain irradiation is the most widely used treatment although, even with radiation therapy, me-

dian survival time is a meager four to six months (van den Bent, 2001).

CNS Symptoms Arising from Brain Tumors

Brain tumors can compromise brain function in one or more of four distinct ways: (1) by producing generalized symptoms associated with increased ICP—such as headache (which occurs in about half of all patients and is typically diffuse and most pronounced on wakening) and occasionally nausea, vomiting, and sixth nerve palsy (paralysis of lateral eye movements); (2) by inducing seizures, which are typically focal or secondarily generalized; (3) by producing focal symptoms—such as hemiparesis and aphasia—that reflect progressive invasion or displacement of brain tissue and can suggest tumor location; and (4) by secreting hormones or altering endocrine patterns involving a variety of body functions (DeAngelis, 2001).

To some extent, tumors act as localized lesions, affecting behavior in much the same way that other kinds of discrete brain lesions do (S.W. Anderson, Damasio, and Tranel, 1990; Scheibel et al., 1996). For example, memory is often compromised—particularly with frontal tumors and those in the region of the third ventricle, in or near the thalamus (T.R.P. Price, Goetz, and Lovell, 2002). Many primary brain tumors either are located in the frontal lobes or involve brain regions with rich connections to the frontal lobes, so executive dysfunction—impairments in conceptual flexibility, planning and organization, and the like—is nearly universal (C.A. Meyers, Weitzner, et al., 1998; T.R.P. Price, Goetz, and Lovell, 2002). Brain tumors often interfere with dopaminergic pathways in the frontal–brainstem reticular system, so deficits in processing speed and working memory are also common (C.A. Meyers, Weitzner, et al., 1998).

However, lesion site may not be of primary importance in determining the nature of associated neuropsychological symptoms because the neuropsychological effects of a tumor depend not only on its location but also on its rate of growth (Gleason and Meyers, 2002; Hom and Reitan, 1984). Fast-growing tumors tend to put pressure on surrounding structures, thereby disrupting function, whereas the gradual displacement of brain tissue by lower grade tumors may allow for shifts in position and reorganization of structures with minimal behavioral repercussions until the tumor has become quite large (C.A. Meyers, 2000b). By increasing intracranial pressure and contributing to displacement of brain structures, edema often exacerbates neurologic symptoms and adds diffuse effects to the focal symptom picture. The degree to which edema may contribute to the severity of symptoms is probably best appreciated when one sees the often dramatic effects of corticosteroids, which can rapidly shrink edema-swollen tissues. Severely confused patients with serious impairments in all aspects of brain function may in relatively short order return to an alert and responsive state with control over many of the functions that seemed lost even hours before.

Neurobehavioral changes in cancer patients can occur as cognitive deficits, mood disturbances, behavioral alterations, diminished adaptive capacities (e.g., somnolence, apathy, loss of spontaneity), and any combination thereof. These changes are characteristic of patients with high-grade glioma (Dropcho, 2002; M. Klein et al., 2001) but are also seen surprisingly often in patients with systemic cancers (e.g., small-cell lung carcinoma) and no evidence of brain metastases (C.A. Meyers, Byrne, and Komaki, 1995). Neurobehavioral changes tend to be subtle at first, insidious in their development, and may fluctuate in severity, particularly early on. A patient's neurobehavioral status may actually signal the extent to which carcinoma has infiltrated the CNS: neuropsychological function independently predicts survival in patients with recurrent high-grade gliomas, over and above what can be gleaned from knowing tumor histology and number of recurrences (C.A. Meyers, Hess, et al., 2000; R. Thomas et al., 1995).

Mood disorders, psychotic symptoms, and personality changes (ranging from disinhibition to apathy) associated with intracranial neoplasms may be difficult to disentangle from primary psychiatric disorders. These neuropsychiatric symptoms are often associated with disruption of cortical interconnections with limbic structures (Weitzner, 1999). Fatigue is also a significant problem for cancer patients—in some cases being a direct function of the tumor but more often being associated with cognitive or mood disturbances or stemming from cancer treatments (Valentine and Meyers, 2001). Emotional distress and fatigue often contribute more to subjective complaints of impaired cognitive function in cancer patients than does objective neuropsychological impairment (Cull et al., 1996), as is often the case in patients with nonneurologic disorders (van Dam et al., 1998).

CNS Symptoms Arising from Cancer Treatment

Compounding the direct effects of a brain tumor on CNS function are the adverse effects associated with many cancer treatments (*iatrogenic effects*) (Anderson-Hanley et al., 2003).

Radiation therapy

Consistent evidence from multiple studies suggests that 25%–30% of patients undergoing either therapeutic or prophylactic radiation therapy develop radiation-associated encephalopathy (J.R. Crossen et al., 1994). Whole brain irradiation can produce not only acute effects (i.e., transient confusion and worsening neurological function during radiation therapy, presumably due to edema), but also "early delayed effects" consisting of a diminution of cognitive and functional status within the first weeks and months after treatment— usually attributed to transient cerebral demyelination— as well as "late delayed effects" associated with severe demyelination and necrosis, i.e., a progressive subcortical dementia developing months to years after treatment (Filley, 2001).

Cerebral atrophy is common in patients treated with radiation therapy, as are a variety of white matter changes (T.J. Postma et al., 2002; Vigliani, Duyckaerts et al., 1999) and neuropsychological deficits (Cheung et al., 2000; M.S. Hua, Chen, et al., 1998). Total radiation dose is the strongest factor determining the magnitude of white matter changes as well as neuropsychological effects (Corn et al., 1994; C.A. Meyers, Geara, et al., 2000). Specific cognitive functions (e.g., retrieval from verbal memory) may be particularly vulnerable to adverse radiation therapy effects (C.L. Armstrong, Corn, et al., 2000; C.L. Armstrong, Stern, and Corn, 2001), as are certain patient populations (e.g., young children, elderly persons, patients with vascular risk factors, and patients receiving concomitant chemotherapy). With revisions in radiation therapy methods and elimination of confounding factors, the delayed effects of cranial irradiation may be more transient and more circumscribed than initial studies suggested (Vigliani, Sichez, et al., 1996).

Chemotherapy

Many of the current chemotherapy treatments for intracranial neoplasms as well as other forms of cancer, including those without evidence of CNS metastases, are toxic to the central nervous system, inducing white matter changes akin to those produced by radiation therapy (Ahles et al., 2002; Olin, 2001). Cognitive deficits have been observed with standard dose as well as high dose systemic regimens, even after completion of chemotherapy. Many different cognitive functions may be impaired, including information processing speed, memory, executive function, spatial abilities, and simple attention span (Anderson-Hanley et al., 2002). Not all patients are equally affected, suggesting that as yet unidentified factors related to the individual or to the treatment may predispose certain patients to develop neuropsychological sequelae.

Methotrexate was the first anticancer medication to produce documented neurobehavioral changes, although numerous cytotoxic (e.g., bischloroethylnitrosourea, cisplatin), immunosuppressive (e.g., cyclosporine, FK-506), and antimicrobial (e.g., amphotericin B) medications—and combinations—have subsequently been observed to have these effects (Schagen et al., 1999; Troy et al., 2000; van Dam et al., 1998). Metastatic cancer patients treated with biological response modifiers, or *cytokines*—interferon-α, tumor necrosis factor-α, interleukin-2, alone or in combination—may be especially vulnerable. Adverse effects of cytokines appear to be less a function of the dose administered in any one treatment than a function of either the route of administration—intrathecal or intraventricular administration being associated with the greatest risk—or treatment duration (total cumulative dose) (Capuron et al., 2001; C.A. Meyers, 1999). Mood disturbances are also common in patients undergoing cytokine treatment—particularly those treated with interferon-α, which exerts diverse effects on the neuroendocrine system, neurotransmitters, and other cytokine pathways (Licinio et al., 1998; Valentine, Meyers, et al., 1998). Finally, opioids—commonly used to control the pain associated with advanced cancer—may produce or intensify preexisting neurobehavioral changes including psychomotor slowing, mood alterations and, in extreme cases, hallucinations or delirium (Clemons et al., 1996; P. Sjøgren et al., 2000).

Psychostimulants may benefit patients whose cognitive function is compromised, regardless of whether these deficits stem from the brain tumor itself, radiation or chemotherapy treatments designed to eradicate the tumor, or opioid treatments for cancer pain (C.A. Meyers, Weitzner, et al., 1998; Rozans et al., 2002). Attentional rehabilitation has also shown benefits in survivors of childhood cancer (R.W. Butler and Copeland, 2002).

OXYGEN DEPRIVATION

When oxygen deprivation is sufficiently severe and lasts long enough, it produces mental changes. *Anoxia* refers to a complete absence of available oxygen; in *hypoxic* conditions oxygen availability is reduced; in *anoxemia* the blood supply lacks oxygen. Anoxia and anoxemia occur as a result of acute oxygen-depriving conditions, which may be fatal if they last longer than 5 to 10 minutes. Hypoxia is distinct from ischemia. The latter refers to reduced blood flow that affects the delivery of glucose and other substances in addition to oxygen and the removal of metabolic by-products, while during hypoxia cerebral blood flow continues and only oxygen level is altered. (Miyamoto and Auer, 2000). Hypoxia without ischemia can be relatively benign (Simon,

1999). When hypoxia is severe it can result in brain damage acutely, but lower levels of oxygen deprivation are also associated with brain damage if the hypoxic episodes continue or frequently recur (Gibson et al., 1981).

The brain is more oxygen dependent than many other tissues. The hippocampus, basal ganglia, and cerebral cortex are particularly vulnerable to oxygen deprivation (D. Caine and Watson, 2000). PET studies (DeVolder et al., 1990) and CT scanning (Tippin et al., 1984) have also demonstrated both cortical damage and subcortical lesions in the cerebellum in very severely impaired patients.

Acute Oxygen Deprivation

Medical emergencies

Almost all persons surviving five or more minutes of complete oxygen deprivation or 15 minutes of "substantial" hypoxia sustain permanent brain damage (J.N. Walton, 1994). Patients who do not become permanently comatose typically incur impaired learning ability with normal retrieval of information stored prior to the event (Barat et al., 1989; Cummings, Tomiyasu, et al., 1984; Filley, 2001). Involvement of other cognitive functions varies greatly, as many persons remain intact but others present evidence of cortical damage such as anomia or apraxia (e.g., see Parkin et al., 1987). A review of 67 individual case reports found that 54% had memory disturbance, 46% had personality and behavioral changes, and 31% had visuospatial or visual recognition problems (D. Caine and Watson, 2000).

Cardiac failure and respiratory failure are probably the most usual conditions leading to acute oxygen deprivation (Barat et al., 1989; DeVolder et al., 1990; Volpe and Hirst, 1983). Anesthesia, near-drowning accidents, and failed hanging are other causes of acute oxygen deprivation. These conditions are more likely to cause brain injury than cases of pure hypoxia because they involve reduced blood flow (Miyamoto and Auer, 2000).

Social competency can be compromised, as was the case with two professional men examined after anesthesia accidents (mdl). Both sustained memory problems, but their social crippling resulted more from reduced spontaneity, impaired planning ability, diminished self-control, and deterioration in grooming and social habits than their memory disorders.

Hypoxia at high altitudes

Acute transient effects of oxygen deprivation in high altitude environments have been studied in airplane pilots who ascend rapidly and mountaineers whose ascent is gradual. Headache, nausea, and vomiting may accompany increasing mental dulling, diminished alertness with loss of normal self-protective responses, and affective disturbances such as euphoria or irritability (K.M. Adams, Sawyer, and Kvale, 1980; Lishman, 1997). Transient deficits on a symbol substitution task and in motor speed appeared when, for brief periods, normal subjects were exposed to oxygen levels comparable to those at 3,000–5,000 meters above sea level; vigilance, verbal fluency, and immediate memory remained intact (D.T.R. Berry, McConnell, et al., 1989). In a study of Mount Everest climbers, the time needed to comprehend simple spoken sentences increased by 50% as they ascended (P. Lieberman et al., 1995).

Chronic impairments in short-term memory, mental flexibility, and concentration showed up in five of eight world-class high mountain (above 8,500 meters without oxygen) climbers; the three most impaired had abnormal EEG findings involving frontal and temporal areas (Regard, Oelz, et al., 1989). Other studies found similar effects in climbers at high altitudes who, acutely, sustained reduced verbal and visual memory performances, motor slowing (finger tapping), and mild verbal expressive deficits (Hornbein et al., 1989; Sarnquist et al., 1986; Townes et al., 1984). On follow-up examinations 11 months later, delayed (30 min) verbal recall improved significantly, as did verbal fluency, but rate of verbal learning remained slowed, as did motor speed. Insufficient brain oxygenation, decreased CBF, and—in experienced mountaineers with high hematocrit levels—increased blood viscosity appeared to contribute to the neuropsychological deficits.

Chronic Oxygen Deprivation

The most usual medical condition underlying chronic hypoxia is *chronic obstructive pulmonary disease (COPD)* (Lishman, 1997; J.N. Walton, 1994), also called *chronic airflow obstruction* (CAO) (Prigatano and Levin, 1988). As a group, patients with COPD tend to show small but wide-ranging impairments which afflict even mildly hypoxic patients and increase with heightened severity of their hypoxic condition (I. Grant, Heaton, McSweeny, et al., 1982; I. Grant, Prigatano, et al., 1987; Prigatano, Parsons, et al., 1983). Most likely to be affected are complex attention, speed of information processing, and memory (Stuss, Peterkin, Guzman, et al., 1997). Prolonged oxygen therapy may partially ameliorate these patients' cognitive deficits or at least halt the progression of cognitive deterioration in those who are more severely hypoxic (Heaton, Grant, McSweeny, et al., 1983; Kozora et al., 1999). Regardless of the degree of their hypoxia, these patients

report a diminished quality of life with a relatively great amount of emotional distress showing up particularly as depression and somatic preoccupations (Kales et al., 1985; McSweeny, Grant, et al., 1985; Prigatano, Wright, and Levin, 1984).

Chronic hypoxia can also occur in *sleep apnea*, in which breathing frequently stops for ten or more seconds at a time and more than ten times an hour during sleep (R.O Hopkins and Bigler, 2001). Sleep apnea typically occurs in overweight people and in men (4%–12% in the general population) more than in women (2%–5%). These patients too may have cognitive deficits, which one study reported were associated with their degree of hypoxia and showed up particularly on visual memory and speeded tasks (D.T.R. Berry, Webb, et al., 1986). Impaired short-term memory and/or long-term memory and/or visuospatial performances were found in approximately three-fourths of a group of 50 persons suffering from sleep apnea (Kales et al., 1985). Bédard and his coworkers (1993) identified impairments in planning and organizing abilities and in manual dexterity as those least likely to resolve with treatment. These patients also have sleep fragmentation due to apneic events throughout the night that disrupt sleep. An investigation of the role of sleep in sleep apnea patients concluded that cognitive dysfunction could be attributed to sleep disturbance (Verstraeten et al., 1996). Sleepiness, depression, and general malaise are problems for many sleep apnea suffers. Treatment with continuous positive airway pressure helps ameliorate cognitive deficits (Valencia-Flores et al., 1996).

Carbon Monoxide Poisoning

In carbon monoxide (CO) poisoning, oxygen deprivation occurs as CO supplants oxygen in the bloodstream. Oxygen will always lose in the race for binding sites in hemoglobin as CO's affinity for these sites is about 250 times greater (Ginsberg, 1985). Brain damage appears to be centered in the globus pallidus area of the basal ganglia, but it may also involve the cerebral cortex, hippocampus, cerebellum, and fornix (Crystal and Ginsberg, 2000; Kesler et al., 2001; see also C.R. Reynolds, Hopkins, and Bigler, 1999). Decreased metabolic activity primarily involving frontal lobe structures but also temporal lobe areas has been reported (Pinkston et al., 2000). Recent imaging studies have also indicated that some demyelinization can also occur which, in mild cases, can be asymptomatic (Filley, 2001). Dunham and Johnstone (1999) note the variability in symptom expression, even among persons with similar exposure levels.

Acute CO poisoning effects begin with disorientation, headache, a racing heartbeat, dizziness, fainting, and somnolence, and if sufficiently severe, the patient deteriorates into coma and death. Mild residual problems affecting cognition are common and may include impaired attention, processing speed, memory, and executive functions (Gale, Hopkins, et al., 1999). Patients may also suffer apathy, fatigue, and emotional lability with lowered frustration threshold (Lishman, 1997). Severe chronic effects may include symptoms of both cortical and subcortical involvement, including apraxias, agnosias, cortical blindness, dementia, paralysis, Parkinson-like movement disorders, and incontinence. An estimated 40%–50% of these patients will have continuing verbal memory problems (Kesler et al., 2001), and some may undergo personality deterioration characterized by lability, irritability, and impulsivity (D.L. Jackson and Menges, 1980; Olson, 1984). Verbal memory impairments were associated with fornix atrophy (Kesler et al., 2001). In a study of patients six months after CO poisoning, cognitive impairments correlated with unconsciousness for greater than five minutes but not with periventricular white matter hyperintensities (R.B. Parkinson et al., 2002).

A fairly unique feature of CO poisoning is the delayed appearance of significant cerebral white matter damage—with personality alterations, mental deterioration, incontinence, a gait disorder, and mutism with frontal release signs and the masked facies seen in parkinsonism—in coma patients who had seemed to recover (Choi, 1983; Crystal and Ginsberg, 2000). Such relapses may occur four days or as much as six weeks after return to seemingly normal functioning; they are relatively rare (Crystal and Ginsberg, 2000, report 3% of cases; C.R. Norris and his colleagues, 1982, estimated 10% to 30% following acute CO exposure). The majority of these patients will improve, some to near-normal functioning within a year after the initial relapse (Crystal and Ginsberg, 2000). However, Bryer and his colleagues (1988) noted that patients who appear to have "totally recovered" may actually have sustained permanent subtle neuropsychological deficits. In line with this hypothesis, comparison of neuroimaging (quantitative MRI) done six months after exposure with baseline imaging studies for a large series of CO exposed subjects found generalized atrophy of the corpus callosum with from 7% to 43% of subjects performing at lower levels on one or more cognitive test (S.S. Porter et al., 2002).

METABOLIC AND ENDOCRINE DISORDERS

Metabolic disorders of the brain are secondary to pathological changes that occur elsewhere in the body. Many of the cerebral concomitants show up as transient confusion, delirium, or disordered consciousness during acute conditions of metabolic dysfunction (Godwin-Austen and Bendall, 1990; Victor and Ropper, 2001). Mental disturbances are usually global in nature, with particular involvement of attentional and memory functions and often reasoning and judgment. Psychiatric disturbances are a more common feature of endocrine disorders than are neuropsychological impairments (Boswell et al., 2002).

Diabetes Mellitus (DM)

Children and adults with diabetes are at increased risk for cognitive impairment. Young and middle-aged adults with insulin dependent diabetes are at risk for impairments in working memory and psychomotor slowing, while older adults are likely to have verbal learning and aspects of memory affected as well (Knopman, Boland, et al., 2001; M. Kovacs et al., 1994; C.M. Ryan and Geckle, 2000b). Having observed more repetitions on a verbal fluency task, Perlmuter, Hakami, and their colleagues (1984) reported that poorer scores on a learning test were due to impaired retrieval rather than deficient learning ability. Others have noted impaired letter fluency (Wahlin et al., 2002). U'Ren and his colleagues (1990) specifically examined response speed of older adults (ages 65 to 75) on several tests and found that only on the one requiring mental shifting (Perceptual Speed) did the diabetics perform less well than a control group, suggesting that the mental flexibility component may have been the significant variable here.

In adult studies deficits appeared mostly on attentional and short-term memory and learning tests. Diabetic women who were at least 65 years old performed more poorly than older women without the disease on a short battery including Digit Symbol, Trail Making Part B, and a modified Mini-Mental Status Examination (Gregg et al., 2000). The diabetic women had a greater rate of decline when tested again at least three years later. Women with diabetes for at least 15 years had a three-fold increase in baseline cognitive impairment. Recent reviews suggest that verbal memory and complex information processing are the areas typically affected in DM (Stewart and Liolitsa, 1999; Strachan et al., 1997).

The critical variable contributing to the cognitive dysfunction in diabetes appears to be impaired control of glucose levels in the blood (Holmes, 1986; C.M. Ryan and Geckle, 2000a). When hypoglycemic, diabetics displayed notable slowing on complex reaction time tests (C.S. Holmes, Koepke, and Thompson, 1986), reduced verbal fluency and naming ability (C.S. Holmes, Koepke, Thompson, et al., 1984), and slowed visuomotor tracking and shifting (Hoffman et al., 1989); but when hyperglycemic, test performances showed only a nonsignificant impairment trend or were not impaired (Draelos et al., 1995; Hoffman et al., 1989; C.S. Holmes, Koepke, and Thompson, 1986). Sommerfield and his colleagues (2003) found that all memory systems were impaired during acute hypoglycemia, with working and delayed memory particularly vulnerable. However, in young adults, recurrent severe hypoglycemic episodes were not associated with persistent cognitive dysfunction (S.C. Ferguson et al., 2003). Chronic hyperglycemia, at least for adults, appears to be the critical risk factor for cognitive dysfunction (C.M. Ryan, Williams, et al., 1993; C.M. Ryan, 1997). Complicating the neuropsychological status of diabetics are other frequently associated neuropathogenic conditions such as hypertension and cerebrovascular disease (Bornstein and Kelly, 1991; Godwin-Austen and Bendall, 1990; Lishman, 1997), age-associated brain changes (C.M. Ryan and Geckle, 2000a), and such psychological factors as depression and questionable motivation to perform well in patients with a chronic disease (Perlmuter, Goldfinger, et al., 1990; Von Dras and Lichty, 1990).

In addition to cognitive impairments, diabetic patients are at increased risk for dementia (Leibson et al., 1997; Ott et al., 1999). In a large prospective population-based study, persons with diabetes were roughly twice as likely to develop dementia than their healthy peers (Ott et al., 1999). Their rate of having a stroke is two to three times greater than the rate for nondiabetic persons (F.W. Whitehouse, 1997).

Hypothyroidism (Myxedema)

Cognitive deterioration is a fairly consistent feature of pronounced thyroid insufficiency, or *hypothyroidism* (*myxedema*) (Beckwith, 2001; Godwin-Austen and Bendall, 1990). The onset and development of the cognitive impairments in this condition are usually subtle and insidious. The patient gains weight, becomes sluggish and lethargic, and suffers concentration and memory disturbances (G.M. Abrams and Jay, 2002; Lishman, 1997). Cognitive disorders occur in 46% of cases (Boswell et al., 2002). Specific visuospatial impairments were documented in adolescents who were hypothyroid at birth and during very early infancy, although visual recognition was intact (Leneman et al., 2001). Low thyroid functioning, but still within the normal range, has been associated with cognitive impairment in older adults (Prinz, Scanlan, et al., 1999; Volpato et al., 2002). Psychiatric disturbances, such as hallucinations, paranoid ideation, or delirium, can occur when hypothyroidism is severe (G.M. Abrams and Jay, 2002). This condition is reversible with thyroid replacement therapy (Baldini et al., 1997; Boswell et al., 2002).

Liver Disease

Among the many sources for liver disease are infection, alcohol and other toxic agents, and a variety of idiopathic and inherited metabolic disorders (Tarter and Van Thiel, 2001). Abnormalities on electrophysiological studies (EEG, ERP) are common. As would be expected in a condition which increases the level of toxic blood substances and affects basic metabolic functions, many patients display attentional disorders and response slowing with conceptual and memory abilities generally preserved. Many of these patients have especial difficulty with tasks calling upon visuospatial abilities.

Uremia

The neuropsychological effects of uremic poisoning, which occurs with kidney failure, are quite typical of the mental changes associated with metabolic disorders. A progressive development of lethargy, apathy, and cognitive dysfunction with accompanying loss of sense of well-being takes place as the uremic condition develops (Lishman, 1997; Pliskin et al., 2001). While untreated renal patients often show general cognitive dulling, pronounced deficits may appear on tests of attention, psychomotor speed, immediate recall—both visual and verbal—and construction. However, since the construction tests are timed, without further information it is not possible to determine whether the lower scores were due simply to slowing or to visuospatial or conceptual components of the task. Depression, emotional withdrawal, and negativism are common problems with these patients (Lishman, 1997; Pliskin et al., 2001). Episodes of compromised consciousness, delirium, or hallucinations occur in about one-third of patients; about one-third have seizures. When the disease is out of control, problems associated with acute hypertension may further disrupt mental functioning.

Treatment with chronic hemodialysis appears to improve cognitive status as patients receiving dialysis function better cognitively than undialyzed patients. Yet even with dialysis, uremia patients continue to display memory and learning problems and reduced mental flexibility (Pliskin et al., 2001). However, interpretation of neuropsychological studies is complicated by the associated high incidence of hypertension and atherosclerosis in these patients. Aluminum toxicity, while still affecting some dialysis patients, is no longer as common a problem as it once was (see pp. 272–273).

NUTRITIONAL DEFICIENCIES

The contributions of malnutrition to mental deficiencies in children are now well known (Grantham-McGregor and Ani, 2001; D.K. Katzman et al., 2001; von Schenck et al., 1997; Wasantwisut, 1997; Winick, 1976). In adults the best known of the disorders of nutritional deficiency is Korsakoff's psychosis and the related vitamin B_1 deficiency disease, beriberi (Lishman, 1997; Victor and Ropper, 2001; J.N. Walton, 1994; see also p. 262). The importance of other B vitamins for the health of the nervous system is increasingly appreciated (Goebels and Soyka, 2000; Selhub et al., 2000). For example, low levels of B_{12} were associated with reduced speed of information processing (i.e., on a coding task), in elderly (ages to 85) nondemented persons (Jelicic, Jonker, and Deeg, 2001). Many conditions of mental deterioration have been attributed to dietary deficiency (Chafetz, 1990; Essman, 1987; Lester and Fishbein, 1988; Lishman, 1997).

Folic acid—or *folate*—deficiency, provides a good example of insufficient intake of a specific nutritional component. It can result in a progressive condition of mental deterioration with concomitant cerebral atrophy (M.I. Botez, Botez, et al., 1979; M.I. Botez, Botez, and Maag, 1984). This condition, most usually appearing in elderly and incapacitated persons with poor dietary habits or opportunities, gives rise to a variety of neurological and neuropsychological symptoms, including sensory and reflex abnormalities, depressed mood, and impairments on memory, abstract reasoning, and construction tests specifically (Lishman, 1997). Folate deficiency is often accompanied by other nutritional problems. It has beeen implicated in general depression of cognitive functions which, when severe, presents as dementia (Lishman, 1997). Significant improvements on neuropsychological testing have been observed with folate replacement therapy (M.I. Botez, Botez and Maag, 1984). This crippling disorder is unnecessary as it can be avoided with a moderate intake of lettuce or other greens. Low levels of folic acid have also been implicated as a risk factor for cardiovascular disease and stroke; increasing folic acid intake has been directly related to reduced stroke incidence (Wolf, 1997).

How general malnutrition may affect the functioning of the mature or almost mature central nervous system is demonstrated in adolescent and young adult women with *anorexia nervosa*, whose self-inflicted starvation regimen was sufficiently severe to bring them to psychiatric attention. Reports on these young people's neuropsychological status suggest that they may show a variety of mild impairments. In one study, nine of 20 young women performed poorly on two or more tests of cognitive functions, with slowed reaction times, reduced short-term memory, and retrieval deficits being the most prominent problems (Hamsher, Halmi, and Benton, 1981). The incidence of specific deficits diminished over the subsequent year when two-thirds of the group either maintained or gained weight, although many of them still had lower scores on digit span (the combined score) and almost the same number continued to show reaction time slowing. Another group's abnormally low performances on complex speed-dependent attention tests, Block Design, and a problem-solving task improved after three months during which group members made "substantial" weight gains, although more than half of these young women were still impaired on one to two (of eight) measures (Szmukler et al., 1992). Anorexic women were significantly impaired in every area of neuropsychological functioning except on vigilance tasks—on which a trend toward impairment appeared—compared to women with prior starvation habits who maintained normal weight for at least six months and performed poorly only on speed-dependent attentional tasks or tests of concept formation and conceptual shifting (B.P. Jones et al., 1991). The question remains of whether, with adequate nutrition after a period of relative starvation, cognition returns fully to normal levels or equally across all neuropsychological domains (D.K. Katzman et al., 2001).

Malnutrition can also occur toward the end of life among elderly people whose intake of nutrients falls below recommended dietary standards (J.S. Goodwin et al., 1983). Disease-free, fully independent, and financially comfortable adults ages 60+ whose blood levels of vitamin C, riboflavin, vitamin B_{12}, and folic acid were below recommended levels generally had the poorest performances on the Category Test and the Wechsler Memory Scale, thus reflecting problems similar to those found in anorexic young people. Greater understanding of the relationship between nutrition and cognitive functioning can insure adequate dietary intake of the nutrients needed to maximize quality of life in our increasingly older society (Riedel and Jorissen, 1998).

8 | Neurobehavioral Variables and Diagnostic Issues

DIANE B. HOWIESON, DAVID W. LORING, AND H. JULIA HANNAY

Like all other psychological phenomena, behavioral changes that follow brain injury are determined by multiple factors. Size, location, kind, and duration of a lesion certainly contribute significantly to the altered behavior pattern. Other important predisposing variables are the individual's premorbid abilities and experiences. Age at the onset of the neuropathologic disorder, the pattern of cerebral dominance, cultural and historical background, life situation, and psychological makeup also affect how patients respond to the physical insult and to its social and psychological repercussions. Moreover, life changes experienced by brain impaired patients are dynamic, reflecting the continually evolving interactions between behavioral deficits and residual competencies, patients' appreciation of their strengths and weaknesses, and family, social, and economic support or pressure.

LESION CHARACTERISTICS

Focusing on the Hole rather than the Doughnut.
A. Smith, 1979

Diffuse and Focal Effects

The concepts of "diffuse" and "focal" brain injury are more clear-cut than their manifestations. Diffuse brain diseases do not affect all brain structures equally, and it is rare to find a focal injury in which some diffuse repercussions do not take place either temporarily or ultimately (Bigler, 1990a; Ferro, 2001; Teuber, 1969; see also Diaschisis, p. 288).

Diffuse brain injury typically results from a widespread condition such as infection, anoxia, hypertension, intoxication (including alcohol intoxication, drug overdose, and drug reactions), certain degenerative, metabolic, and nutritional diseases, and it occurs in most closed-head injuries, particularly those sustained under conditions of rapid acceleration or deceleration as in falls or moving vehicle accidents. The behavioral expression of diffuse brain dysfunction usually includes memory, attention, and concentration disabilities; impaired higher level and complex reasoning resulting in conceptual concretism and inflexibility; and general response slowing (Hsiang and Marshall, 1998; A.J. Thompson, 1998; Wrightson and Gronwall, 1999; see also pp. 168–169; 270). Emotional flattening or lability may also be present. These symptoms tend to be most severe immediately after an injury or the early stages of a sudden onset disease, or they may first appear as subtle and transient problems that increase in duration and severity as a progressive condition worsens.

Trauma, space-displacing lesions (e.g., tumors, blood vessel malformations), localized infections, and cerebrovascular accidents cause most focal brain injuries. Some systemic conditions, too, such as a severe thiamine deficiency, may devastate discrete brain structures and result in a predominantly focal symptom picture. Occasionally, focal signs of brain damage accompany an acute exacerbation of a systemic disorder, such as diabetes mellitus, confusing the diagnostic picture until the underlying disorder is brought under control and the organic symptoms subside. Symptoms of diffuse damage almost always accompany focal lesions of sudden onset. Initially, cloudy consciousness, confusion, and generally slowed and inconsistent responsiveness may obscure focal residual effects so that clear-cut evidence of the focal lesion may not appear until later. However, the first sign of a progressive localized lesion such as a slow-growing tumor may be some slight, specific behavioral impairment that becomes more pronounced and inclusive. Ultimately, diffuse behavioral effects resulting from increased intracranial pressure and circulatory changes may obliterate the specific defects due to local tissue damage.

Focal lesions can often be distinguished by lateralizing signs since most discrete lesions involve only or mostly one hemisphere. Even when the lesion extends to both hemispheres, the damage is apt to be asymmetrical, resulting in a predominance of one lateralized symptom pattern. In general, when one function or several related specific functions are significantly impaired while other functions remain intact and alertness, response rate, either verbal or nonverbal learning ability, and orientation are relatively unaffected, the examiner can safely conclude that the cerebral insult is focal.

Site and Size of Focal Lesions

From a neuropathological perspective, the site of the lesion should determine many characteristics of the attendant behavioral alterations (Filley, 1995; Heilman and Valenstein, 2003, *passim;* Mesulam, 2000b). Yet the expression of these changes—their severity, intransigence, burdensomeness—depends upon so many other variables that predicting much more than the broad outlines of the behavioral symptoms from knowledge of the lesion's location is virtually impossible (S.W. Anderson, Damasio, and Tranel, 1990; E. Goldberg, 1995; Markowitsch, 1984, 1988; A. Smith, 1980). In discussing Hughlings Jackson's tenet stated a century ago that localizing a lesion and localizing a function cannot be considered identical operations, Vallar (1991) pointed out that, "localizing a given mental function in a specific area of the brain is simply nonsense" (p. 344). Certain areas of the brain may be critical for specific cognitive functions, but brain regions are not isolated (Fuster, 2003; E. Goldberg, 2001). They work together as fully interconnected, distributed neural networks. Functional neuroimaging has made this point clear. Complex mental functions such as memory (K.L. Hoffman and McNaughton, 2002; Markowitsch, 2000) and appreciating the moral of a story (Nichelli et al., 1995) involve brain regions distributed over wide areas. Lesions in one area may disrupt the network and produce impairment similar to lesions of another area within the network. Each territory contributes to some aspect of cognitive processing. For example, like lesions of the inferotemporal cortex and the medial temporal lobe, lesions of the prefrontal cortex have been associated with impairment on face recognition memory (Rapcsak, Nielsen, et al., 2001). Rapcsak and his colleagues suggested that the role of the prefrontal cortex was to enhance the efficiency and accuracy of the temporal lobe memory system.

In ordinary clinical practice relatively few patients with primary focal lesions have damage confined to the identified area. Stroke patients may have had other small or transient and therefore unrecognized cerebral vascular accidents and, at least in the first few weeks after the stroke, depression of neural functioning may affect some areas of the brain other than the site of the defined lesion. Yet, in these patients, lesion site is more likely to predict the nature of the accompanying neuropsychological deficits than is its size (volume) (Powers, 1990; Turkheimer et al., 1990). For example, small subcortical lesions can produce major effects. A wide array of cognitive deficits have been associated with small thalamic infarcts (Kalashnikova et al., 1999) and with small lesions in the internal capsule (Madureira et al., 1999). Naeser, Alexander, and their colleagues (1982) considered the complexity of the site versus size question in observing that "site . . . was most important in determining language behavior" while lesion size "may be a factor in the severity of articulatory impairment." In contrast, Kertesz (2001) notes that language comprehension of stroke patients is not closely related to lesion size. Both the size of the lesion and its site contribute to severity of dysfunction and its improvement in stroke patients (Altieri et al., 2001; Kertesz and Gold, 2003; Naeser, Helm-Estabrooks, et al., 1987). Based on CT measures of mostly stroke patients, Turkheimer and colleagues (1990) concluded that the severity of deficit may be best estimated for a specific function by taking into account jointly both size and hemisphere side of lesion, as the importance of lesion size differs between the hemispheres and the importance of hemispheric contributions differs with the task.

With the exception of some missile or puncture wounds, TBIs are rarely "clean," for damage is generally widespread. Here the size of the lesion may be an important determinant of residual functional capacity (Grafman, Jonas, Martin, et al., 1988; Salazar, Grafman, Jabbari, et al., 1987). Tumors do not respect the brain's midline or any other of the landmarks or boundaries we use to organize our knowledge about the brain, and they can be erratic in their destruction of nervous tissue (S.W. Anderson, Damasio, and Tranel, 1990). In most cases, information about where in the brain a discrete lesion is located must be viewed as only a partial description that identifies the primary site of damage. Patterns of behavior or neuropsychological test performances often may not meet textbook expectations for a lesion in the designated area.

Depth of Lesion

Subcortical damage associated with a cortical lesion compounds the symptom picture with the added effects of disrupted pathways or damaged lower integration centers (Kumral, 2001; H.S. Levin, Williams, et al., 1988; Filley, 2001). The depth and extent to which a cortical lesion involves subcortical tissue will alter the behavioral correlates of similar cortical lesions. Depth of lesion has been clearly related to the severity of impairment of verbal skills (Ferro, 2001; Naeser, Palumbo, et al., 1989; Newcombe, 1969). The varieties of *anosognosia* (impaired awareness of one's own disability or disabled body parts, associated with right parietal lobe damage) illustrate the differences in the behavioral correlates of similarly situated cortical lesions with different amounts of subcortical involvement. Gerstmann (1942) reported three forms of this problem and their subcortical correlates: (1) Anosognosia with neglect of the paralyzed side, in which patients essentially ignore the fact of paralysis although they may have some vague awareness that they are disabled, is associated with lesions of the right optic region of the thalamus. (2) Anosognosia with amnesia for or lack of recognition of the affected limbs or side occurs with lesions penetrating only to the transmission fibers from the thalamus to the parietal cortex. (3) Anosognosia with such "positive" psychological symptoms as confabulation or delusions (in contrast to the unelaborated denial of illness or nonrecognition of body parts of the other two forms of this condition) is more likely to occur with lesions limited to the parietal cortex.

Distance Effects

Diaschisis

Diaschisis refers to depression of activity that takes place in areas of the brain outside the immediate site of damage, usually in association with acute focal brain lesions (E.M.R. Critchley, 1987; Niimura et al., 1999; Ferro, 2001). Von Monakow ([1914], 1969) originally conceived of diaschisis as a form of shock to the nervous system due to disruptions in the neural network connecting the area damaged by the lesion with functionally related areas that may be situated at some distance from the lesion itself, including the opposite hemisphere. Some investigators have extended the concept of diaschisis to include acute depression of neuronal activity in areas outside the immediate site of damage resulting from physiological reactions such as edema (Kertesz and Gold, 2003; E.W. Russell, 1981). However, the concept of diaschisis applies more appropriately to the depression of relatively discrete or circumscribed clusters of related functions (Cohadon et al., 2002; C.J. Price, Warburton, et al., 2001; A. Smith, 1984) than to the global dampening of cerebral activity associated with the often radical physiological alterations that take place following an acute injury to the brain. Diaschisis has typically been viewed as a transient phenomenon that, as it dissipates, allows the depressed functions to improve spontaneously. It may also account for the appearance of permanent changes in functions that are not directly associated with the lesion site (Gummow et al., 1984; A. Smith, 1984).

Depressed functioning in cerebral areas that have not been structurally damaged can be seen most clearly in stroke patients who exhibit deficits associated with the noninfarcted hemisphere (L. M. Binder, Howieson, and Coull, 1987; Chukwudelunzu et al., 2001). Reduced blood flow and electroencephalographic abnormalities in the noninfarcted hemisphere have been documented, particularly within the first few weeks poststroke (Derdeyn and Powers, 1997; Kertesz, 2001). Normalization of the noninfarcted hemisphere typically occurs in young patients but elderly stroke victims are likely to experience persisting diaschisis effects (Gummow et al., 1984).

Disconnection syndromes

The chronic condition of diaschisis is similar to disconnection syndromes in that both show up as depression or loss of a function primarily served by an area of the brain that is intact and at some distance from the lesion. Both phenomena thus involve disrupted neural transmission through subcortical white matter. However, the similarity ends here. Cortical lesions that may or may not extend to white matter give rise to diaschisis, while *disconnection syndromes* result from damage to white matter that cuts cortical pathways, disconnecting one or another cortical area from the communication network of the brain (Filley, 1995, 2001; Geschwind, 1965; Mesulam, 2000b). These disconnection problems can simulate the effects of a cortical lesion or produce an atypical symptom pattern (e.g., Naeser, Palumbo, et al., 1989; Vuilleumier, 2001; Zaidel, Iacoboni, et al., 2003). Even a small subcortical lesion can result in significant behavioral changes if it interrupts a critical pathway running to or from the cortex or between two cortical areas. Thus, cortical involvement is not necessary for a cortical area to be rendered nonfunctional.

Geschwind (1972) analyzed a case in which a patient with normal visual acuity suddenly could no longer read, although he was able to copy written words. Postmortem examination revealed that an occluded artery prevented blood flow to the left visual cortex and the interhemispheric visual pathways, injuring both structures and rendering the patient blind in his right visual field. His left visual field and right visual cortex continued to register words that he could copy. However, the right visual cortex was disconnected form the left hemisphere so that this verbal information was no longer transmitted to the left hemisphere for the symbol processing necessary for verbal comprehension and therefore he could not read.

The most dramatic disconnection syndromes are those that occur when interhemispheric connections are severed, whether by surgery or as a result of disease or developmental anomaly (Bogen, 1969a,b; Sergent, 1987;

Sperry, 1974, 1982; E. Zaidel, Iacoboni, et al., 2003). For example, under laboratory conditions that restrict stimulation to one hemisphere, information received by the right hemisphere does not transfer across the usual white matter pathway to the left hemisphere that controls the activity of the right hand. Thus, the right hand does not react to the stimulus or it may react to other stimuli directed to the left hemisphere while the left hand responds appropriately.

Disrupted systems

Given the profuse and elaborate interconnections between cerebral components and the complexity of most ordinary human behaviors, it is not surprising that damage in a given area would have secondary adverse effects on the activity of distant but normally interacting areas, such as those in a homologous position contralateral to the lesion. In citing instances of this phenomenon, Sergent (1988b) explained that "an intact hemisphere in a damaged brain cannot operate as it does in an intact brain."

Nature of the Lesion

Type of damage

Differences in the nature of the lesion also affect the symptom picture. Where there has been a clean loss of cortical tissue, as a result of surgery or missile wounds, those functions specifically mediated by the lost tissue can no longer be performed. When white matter has also been removed, some disconnection effects may occur. In short, when the lesion involves tissue removal with little or no diseased tissue remaining, repercussions on other, anatomically unrelated functions tend to be minimal and the potential for rehabilitation runs high (Newcombe, 1969; Teuber, 1969).

Dead or diseased brain tissue, which alters the neurochemical and electrical status of the brain, can produce more extensive and severe behavioral changes than a clean surgical or missile wound that removes tissue. Thus, the functional impairments associated with diseased or damaged tissue, as in strokes or closed-head injuries, tend to result in behavioral distortions involving other functions, to have high-level cognitive repercussions, and to affect personality. Studies of patients with a resected epileptogenic temporal lobe point to the cognitive benefits of removing diseased tissue. These patients may show both impairment of those modality-specific memory functions typically associated with the ablated area, and memory improvements in the other modality, most usually when the nondominant anterior temporal lobe is removed (Chelune,

Naugle, et al., 1991; Loring and Meador, 2003b; P. Martin et al., 2002). In most cases, evidence for improved verbal memory after partial resection of the right temporal lobe is weak at best (T.M. Lee et al., 2002). Many of these patients perform better on visuospatial tasks, regardless of the side of resection, with some patients showing more general improvement. Moreover, improvement on tests of verbal comprehension and fluency has even been reported following anterior resection of the speech dominant temporal lobe (Hermann and Wyler, 1988). Hécaen (1964) found that fully two-thirds of his frontal lobe tumor patients presented with confused states and dementia, whereas patients who had had extensive surgical loss of prefrontal tissue were apt to be properly oriented and to suffer little or no impairment of reasoning, memory, or learned skills.

The presence of diseased or dead brain tissue can also affect the circulation and metabolism of surrounding tissue both immediately and long after the cerebral insult has occurred, with continuing psychological dysfunction of the surrounding areas (Finger, LeVere, et al., 1988; Hillbom, 1960; D.G. Stein, 2000). This may include such secondary effects of tissue damage as build-up of scar tissue, microscopic blood vessel changes, or cell changes due to lack of oxygen following interference with the blood supply, which often complicate the symptom picture. Yet some lesions, such as slow-growing tumors, can become quite large without significant cognitive repercussions (S.W. Anderson, Damasio, and Tranel, 1990).

Severity

There is little question that the severity of damage plays an important role in determining the behavioral correlates of a brain lesion. Yet no single measure of severity applies to all the kinds of damage that can interfere with normal brain functioning. Even neuroimaging, which usually provides reliable information about the extent of a lesion, does not reliably detect some kinds of damage such as the very early degenerative changes of many dementing processes, and some recent as well as old traumatic lesions. Duration of coma is a good index of the severity of a stroke or traumatic injury but much less useful for assessing the severity of a toxic or hypoxic episode in which loss of consciousness does not occur with predictable regularity. Extent of motor or sensory involvement certainly reflects the dimensions of some lesions, so that when large portions of the body are paralyzed or sensory deficits are multiple or widespread, an extensive lesion with important behavioral ramifications should be suspected. However, injury or disease can involve large areas of frontal or posterior association cortex or limbic structures and yet have only minimal or subtle motor or sensory effects.

In many cases, to evaluate the severity of a brain disorder one should rely on a number of different kinds of measures, including the behavioral measures obtained in neuropsychological assessment. The latter are often quite sensitive to subtle alterations in the brain's activity or to changes in areas of the brain that do not involve consciousness, or motor or sensory behavior directly.

Momentum

Dynamic aspects of the lesion contribute to behavioral changes too. As a general rule, regardless of the cause of damage, the more rapid the onset of the condition, the more severe and widespread will its effects be (Finger, LeVere, et al., 1988; Hom and Reitan, 1984; A. Smith, 1984). This phenomenon has been observed in comparisons of the behavioral effects of damage from rapidly evolving cerebrovascular accidents with the behavioral effects of tumors in comparable areas, for stroke patients usually have many more and more pronounced symptoms than tumor patients with similar kinds of cerebral involvement (S.W. Anderson, Damasio, and Tranel, 1990). Rapid-onset conditions such as stroke or TBI tend to set into motion such alterations in brain function as release of cytotoxic compounds, reduced cerebral circulation, depressed metabolism, diaschisis, and apoptosis (Cohadon et al., 2002; J.M. Silver et al., 2002; K.M.A. Welch et al., 1997, Section II: Pathogenesis and Pathology, *passim*). The effect of the rapidity with which a lesion evolves shows up when comparing behavioral deficits of tumors developing at different rates. Self-contained, slow-growing tumors that only gradually alter the spatial relationships between the brain's structural elements but do not affect its physiological activity or anatomical connections tend to remain "silent;" i.e., they do not give rise to symptoms until they become large enough to exert pressure on or otherwise damage surrounding structures (Feinberg, Mazlin, and Waldman, 1989). A fast-growing tumor is more likely to be accompanied by swelling of the surrounding tissues, resulting in a greater amount of behavioral dysfunction with more diffuse effects than a slow-growing tumor (Hom and Reitan, 1984).

TIME

Brain disease is a dynamic phenomenon, even when the lesions are static and nonprogressive. Regular trends in patterns of improvement or deterioration depend on the nature of the cerebral insult, the age of the patient,

and the function under study. The length of time following symptom or disease onset must be taken into account in any evaluation of neuropsychological examination data.

Nonprogressive Brain Disorders

In this category can be found all brain disorders that have time-limited direct action on the brain. TBI, ruptured aneurysms, anoxia, successfully treated infectious or toxic/metabolic conditions, and nutritional deficiencies are the usual sources of "nonprogressive" brain injury. Conceptually, strokes fall under this heading since each stroke is a finite event with a fairly predictable course and outcome. Once a patient has suffered a stroke, however, the likelihood of reoccurrence is high, particularly when vascular risk factors are not controlled (e.g., hypertension, diabetes, smoking, cardiac arrhythmias) (Bogousslavsky, Hommel, and Bassetti, 1998; Mead and Warlow, 2002). Therefore, in some patients, cerebrovascular disease behaves like a progressive brain condition in which the ongoing deterioration is irregularly slowed by periods of partial improvement (Powers, 1990; Babikian et al., 1994), and in fact, the concept of "multi-infarct dementia" describes cognitive impairment resulting from repeated infarctions, usually at different sites (see pp. 201–202).

Psychological characteristics of acute brain conditions

With nonprogressive or single-event brain disorders, the recency of the insult may be the most critical factor determining the patient's cognitive status. Patients tend to make the most rapid gains in the first weeks and months following medical stabilization (Bode and Heinemann, 2002; Jorgensen et al., 1999). When patients with serious injuries associated with a prolonged coma regain consciousness, and usually for several weeks to several months thereafter, they are often confused, unable to track the sequence of time or events, emotionally unstable, unpredictably variable in their alertness and responsiveness, behaviorally regressed, and likely to display profound cognitive deficits. In less severely affected patients, symptoms of acute disorganization recede rapidly and noticeable improvement takes place from day to day during the first few weeks or months until the rate of improvement levels off. Yet some patients with less severe injuries experience confusion to some degree for days, weeks, and sometimes months following a TBI or stroke. This confusion is often accompanied by disorientation, difficulty in concentration, poor memory and recall for recent experiences, fatigability, irritability, and labile affect. Structural imaging such as CT or MRI does not fully indicate the areas in which functional impairment is likely to occur due to a variety of factors, such as edema (Betz, 1997; Bigler, 1990a; Kreiter et al., 2002) and diaschisis.

Apart from variations in specific functional defects arising from personal and lesion differences, the most common behavioral characteristics of an acute brain lesion in conscious patients are impaired retention, concentration, and attention; emotional lability; and fatigability. The disruption of memory formation can be so severe that months later these patients recall little or nothing of the acute stage of their condition, although they appeared to be fully conscious at the time (posttraumatic amnesia). So much of a patient's behavioral reintegration usually takes place the first month or two following brain injury that psychological test data obtained during this time, although related to eventual long-term outcome (Boake et al., 2001; Jeffery and Good, 1995), may apply for only an extremely short time, during which they reflect the patient's transient abilities (Hier, Mondlock, and Caplan, 1983b; Ruff, Levin, et al., 1989).

Psychological characteristics of chronic brain conditions

Even after the acute stages have passed and a brain lesion has become "static," a patient's condition rarely remains fixed. Cognitive functions, particularly those involving memory, attention, and concentration, and specific disabilities associated with the site of the lesion generally continue to improve markedly during the first six months or year. Spontaneous improvements that continue beyond a year are generally slight (Geschwind, 1985; Kertesz and Gold, 2003; H.S. Levin, 1995; Newcombe and Artiola i Fortuny, 1979). However, full recovery is rare (Gronwall, 1989; Jorgensen et al., 1999; D.E. Levy, 1988; Yeates et al., 2002; see footnote p. 162). The status of cognitive functions at six months for stroke, or a year following moderate to severe TBI, is unlikely to change greatly for most patients, although improvement for patients with more severe TBI may extend beyond a year (Millis, Rosenthal, et al., 2001). Cognitive rehabilitation, by retraining or use of compensatory aids, may further improve cognitive status (Sohlberg and Mateer, 2001; B.A. Wilson, 1998).

Both the rate and nature of improvement are almost always uneven. Improvement does not follow a smooth course but tends to proceed by inclines and plateaus, and different functions improve at different rates (A. Basso, 1989; Kertesz and Gold, 2003). Old memories and well-learned skills generally return most quickly (*Ribot's law*); recent memory, ability for abstract thinking, mental flexibility, and adaptability are more likely

to return more slowly. Of course, these general tendencies vary greatly depending upon the site and extent of the lesion and the patient's premorbid abilities.

Brain injured patients' test scores are likely to fluctuate considerably, over time and between functions, particularly during the first few years after injury (D.N. Brooks, 1987; Lezak, 1979; A. Smith, 1984). Therefore, predicting a patient's ultimate ability to perform specific functions or activities can be very chancy for at least a year after the event. Unless the patient's handicaps are so severe as to be permanently and totally disabling, it is unwise for binding decisions or judgments to be made concerning legal, financial, or vocational status until several years have passed.

Some functions that appear to be intact in acute and early stages may deteriorate over the succeeding months and years (Dikmen and Reitan, 1976; A. Smith, 1984). Findings from studies of traumatically injured patients (Anttinen, 1960; M.R. Bond, 1984; Daghighian, 1973; Hillbom, 1960) and of patients who underwent brain surgery for psychiatric disorders (Geschwind, 1974; E.C. Johnstone et al., 1976; A. Smith and Kinder, 1959) suggest that for both these conditions, following an initial improvement and a plateau period of several years or more, some mental deterioration may take place. Behavioral deterioration generally involves the highest levels of cognitive activity having to do with mental flexibility, efficiency of learning and recall, and reasoning and judgment about abstract issues or complex social problems. Prior brain injury may also increase vulnerability to such degenerative disorders as Alzheimer's disease (Mortimer and Pirozzolo, 1985) and parkinsonism (e.g., Muhammad Ali, the once world champion boxer; see Jordan, 1987, 2000).

Repeated brain trauma, such as that associated with boxing, is a known risk factor for the development of dementia (see pp. 188–189, 208–209). However, the risk of developing dementia following a single TBI is less well established. Several large longitudinal studies indicate no relationship (Launer et al., 1999; Mehta, Ott, et al., 1999) but others suggest some increased risk (Mortimer and Pirozzolo, 1985; Nemetz et al., 1999; Schofield et al., 1997).

Patients with neurological disorders who have been invalids and patients institutionalized over long periods of time tend to perform with a sameness characterized chiefly by poor memory and attention span, apathy, concrete thinking, and generally regressive behavior. Such behavioral deterioration can obscure the pronounced test performance discrepancies between differentially affected functions that are characteristic of acute, reversible, or progressive brain conditions.

Few symptoms distinguish the behavior of persons suffering chronic brain injury of adult onset with sufficient regularity to be considered characteristic. The most common complaints are of temper outbursts, fatigue, and poor memory (N. Brooks, Campsie, et al., 1986; Jorge and Robinson, 2002; Lezak, 1978a,b, 1988a; J.M. Silver et al., 2002). Rest and a paced activity schedule are the patient's best antidotes to debilitating fatigue. Patients who read and write and are capable of self-discipline can aid failing memory with notebooks (e.g., see Sohlberg and Mateer, 2001; B.A. Wilson, 1986) or with the use of a paging system (J.J. Evans et al., 1998; B.A. Wilson, Emslie, et al., 2001).

However, the reality of memory complaints is not always apparent, even on careful examination. When this occurs, the complaints may reflect the patient's feelings of impairment more than an objective deficit. Care must be taken to distinguish true memory defects from attention or concentration problems, for patients may easily interpret the effects of distractibility as a memory problem (Howieson and Lezak, 2002b). A common chronic problem is an abiding sense of unsureness about mental experiences (*perplexity*) (Lezak, 1978b). Patients express this problem indirectly with hesitancies and statements of self-doubt or bewilderment; they rarely understand that it is as much a natural consequence of brain injury as fatigue. Reassurance that guesses and solutions that come to mind first are generally correct, and advice to treat the sense of unsureness as an annoying symptom rather than a signal that must be heeded, may relieve the patient's distress.

Another difficulty is poor self-awareness, which can limit vocational options (Sherer et al., 1998) and interfere with rehabilitation efforts (Cohadon et al., 2002; Prigatano, 1991b; Trexler et al., 2000). For example, severely impaired TBI patients report fewer behavioral problems and more somatic complaints than do family members (Santos et al., 1998) and may describe themselves as less impaired or disturbed than those with mild TBI (Greiffenstein, Baker, Donders, and Miller, 2002).

Depression troubles most adults who were not rendered grossly defective by their injuries. It is usually first experienced within the year following the onset of brain injury but can remain high for decades (Holsinger et al., 2002). The severity and duration of the depressive reaction vary greatly among patients, depending on a host of factors both intrinsic and extrinsic to their brain condition (J.M. Silver et al., 2002; R.G. Robinson and Starkstein, 2002; see pp. 329–330). Patients whose permanent disabilities are considerable and who have experienced no depression have either lost some capacity for self-appreciation and reality testing, or are denying their problems. In both cases, rehabilitation prospects are significantly reduced, for patients must have a fairly realistic understanding of their strengths

and limitations to cooperate with and benefit from any rehabilitation program. For some patients, the depression resolves or becomes muted with time (e.g., Lezak, 1987b) and, in others, may be successfully treated with pharmacotherapy (Jorge and Robinson, 2002; M. Rosenthal, Christensen, and Ross, 1998; Roy-Byrne and Upadhyaya, 2002).

Heightened irritability is another common complaint of both patients and their families (N. Brooks, 1988; Galbraith, 1985; Niemi et al., 1988; van der Naalt et al., 1999). Delayed onset irritability may, in part, reflect poor social functioning and greater impairment in activities of daily living (S.H. Kim et al., 1999). A greatly—and permanently—decreased tolerance for alcohol should also be anticipated following brain injury of any consequence (Zasler, 1991). Unfortunately, persons who drink postinjury are unlikely to be "light" or social drinkers (Kolakowsky-Hayner et al., 2002).

Predicting outcome

Outcome can be evaluated on a number of dimensions (A. Hopkins, 1998; Sohlberg and Mateer, 2001). Self-report and the presence and severity of sensory and motor symptoms are most often used in clinical practice. This custom can create serious problems for the many brain injured patients whose motor or sensory status and ability to respond appropriately to such simple questions as, "How are you feeling today?" far exceed their judgment, reasoning abilities, self-understanding, and capacity to care for themselves or others (e.g., Prigatano 1991b). Neuropsychological data and evaluations of the status of particular impaired functions, such as speech, also serve as outcome measures. Social outcome criteria tend to vary with the age of the population. The usual criterion of good outcome for younger adults, and therefore for most TBI patients, is return to gainful employment. For older people, usually stroke patients, the social outcome is more likely to be judged in terms of degree of independence, self-care, and whether the patient could return home rather than to a care facility.

Variables influencing outcome. Regardless of the nature of the lesion, its severity is by far the most important variable in determining the patient's ultimate level of improvement. Etiology plays some role since traumatically injured patients tend to enjoy more return of impaired functions such as arm or leg movements or speech than do stroke patients (A. Basso, 1989; Kertesz and Gold, 2003). Of course, trauma patients are generally younger than stroke patients and less likely to have preexisting brain disease or conditions that may work against the healing process. Among stroke patients, those whose strokes are due to infarction, whether thrombotic or embolic, have longer survival times than patients with hemorrhagic strokes (Abu-Zeid et al., 1978; Bogousslavsky, Hommel, and Bassetti, 1998; Lishman, 1997); but it is unclear whether hemorrhagic strokes or infarcts have a better prognosis for the surviving patients (A. Basso, 1989; Hier et al., 1983b).

Age may affect outcome at the age extremes but appears to have little influence within the young to middle-aged adult range (see pp. 294–296). *Premorbid competence,* both cognitive and emotional/social, may contribute to outcome and may be related to *cognitive reserve* (see p. 315). *General physical status* may be associated with outcome for stroke patients (J.F. Lehmann et al., 1975; R.C. Marshall, Tompkins, and Phillips, 1982). For example, perceptual problems—especially unilateral visuospatial inattention—have been identified as important in contributing to post-stroke dependency (Edmans, Towle, and Lincoln, 1991; Kertesz and Gold, 2003). Nutrition, both pre- and post-morbid, is another physical status variable that can significantly affect a patient's potential for improvement (Finger, LeVere, et al., 1988; Wolf, 1997; B. Young et al., 1991). Yet physical impairments may be far outweighed by emotional and personality disturbances in determining the quality of the psychosocial adjustment following TBI (Lezak, 1987b). A positive mood along with high levels of consciousness and normal speech are early predictors of good outcome for stroke patients (Henley et al., 1985). *Early stroke rehabilitation* has also been associated with higher levels of improvement (R.C. Marshall et al., 1982); but as the healthier patients are the more likely candidates for early entry into a rehabilitation program, the salutary effects of early rehabilitation become questionable (M.V. Johnston and Keister, 1984).

Family support contributes to good outcomes for both trauma and stroke patients (Camplair, Butler, and Lezak, 2003; J.F. Lehmann et al., 1975). On reviewing outcomes of 41 epilepsy patients following temporal lobectomy, Rausch found that poor family support was the most important predictor of a poor outcome (personal communication, November, 1992, mdl). For example, married stroke patients have better outcomes (Henley et al., 1985) and tend to outlive single ones (Abu-Zeid et al., 1978). Yet, the extent to which family and friends continue their involvement with the patient may, in turn, be related to the severity of the patient's behavior and self-care problems. Thus, at least in some instances, the presence of family support and social stimulation may depend on how well the patient is doing rather than serve as an independent predictor of outcome success (Drummond, 1988; M.G. Livingston and Brooks, 1988).

Side of lesion can be relevant to outcome, as right hemisphere stroke patients may have poorer outcomes than those with left-sided injury (Pimental and Kingsbury, 1989), but this is not a universal finding (Sundet et al., 1988; D.T. Wade et al., 1984). However, expectations for aphasic patients may differ from those for patients with visuospatial disorders. Denes and colleagues (1982) suggested that lower improvement rates among patients with right cerebral lesions are due to unilateral spatial agnosia, not indifference reaction; but Gialanella and Mattioli (1992) reported that anosognosia contributes more to poor motor and functional outcomes in these patients than either personal or extrapersonal inattention. Moreover, among patients with right hemisphere damage, those who show the inattention phenomenon tend to be more impaired and improve less than the ones who are not troubled by it (D.C. Campbell and Oxbury, 1976).

With left hemisphere strokes, significantly greater improvement takes place in right-handed aphasic patients whose brains developed atypical asymmetry such that, contrary to the usual pattern, their left frontal lobe is wider than the right and these relative proportions are reversed for the occipital lobe (Pieniadz et al., 1983; Schenkman et al., 1983). These patients—atypical both for their cerebral structure proportions and their greater improvements, particularly in verbal comprehension—might be benefiting from some relatively well-developed posterior right hemisphere language capabilities. This possibility is also suggested by both evoked potential (EP) and PET studies which document more right hemisphere activation during the performance of language tasks by aphasic patients than by patients with right hemisphere damage or normal controls (Papanicolaou, Moore, Deutsch, et al., 1988; Leff et al., 2002). Moreover, aphasia in left-handed and ambidextrous stroke patients is more likely to be mild or transient than in right-handers, suggesting that they benefit from bilateral cortical involvement of language (A. Basso, 1989; Gloning and Quaterner, 1966).

Mechanisms of improvement

Explanations of how improvement occurs after brain injury are either based on behavioral constructs or refer to the neurologic substrates of behavior (Pöppel and von Steinbüchel, 1992). Compensatory techniques and alternative behavioral strategies enable patients to substitute different and newly organized behaviors to accomplish activities and skills that can no longer be performed as originally developed or acquired (Almli and Finger, 1988; Grafman, Lalonde, et al., 1989; D.G. Stein, 2000; B.A. Wilson, 2000). These compensatory and substitute techniques often evolve quite unconsciously and become very useful for many brain injured patients. They are the major focus of rehabilitation programs for a wide range of impaired functions.

Among functional/neurological explanations of how brain injured patients improve are phenomena that do not imply alterations in the neural substrate but, rather, reflect receding *diaschisis effects* (Almli and Finger, 1988; Kertesz, 2001; Rothi and Horner, 1983; Seitz et al., 1999). Of the many neurologically based theories involving neuronal reorganization or alteration, increasing participation by homologous regions of the contralateral hemisphere has received significant support. For certain functions, most notably receptive language, areas in the intact hemisphere homologous to the lesioned areas appear to be able to take over at least some of the functions that were rendered defective (G. Deutsch and Mountz, 2001; Feinberg et al., 1989; Mimura et al., 1998; Rothi and Horner, 1983; see p. 57).

Progressive Brain Diseases

In progressive brain disease, behavioral deterioration tends to follow an often bumpy but fairly predictable downhill course for particular sets of functions that may deteriorate at varying rates, depending on the disease. When the diagnosis is known, the question is not so much *what* will happen, but *when* will it happen. Past observations provide some rules of thumb to guide clinicians in their predictions. The clinical rule of thumb for predicting the rate of mental decline holds that conditions that are progressing rapidly are likely to continue to worsen at a rapid rate whereas slow progressions tend to remain slow.

Patients with newly diagnosed progressive brain disease may benefit from an early baseline assessment of their psychological status with one or two reexaminations at two- to four- or six-month intervals. Such a longitudinal study can give a rough basis for forecasting the rate at which mental deterioration is likely to take place, to aid the patient and the family in planning for ongoing care. Further repeat assessments may document improvements—or slowed progression—with pharmacotherapy.

Predicting the course of the behavioral effects of a brain tumor differs from making predictions about other progressively deteriorating diseases. Biopsy, performed in the course of surgery, takes much of the guesswork out of estimating the rate of progression, for different kinds of brain tumors grow at fairly predictable rates. The severity of the behavioral disorder, too, bears some relationship to the type of tumor. On the one hand, extensive edema and elevated intracranial pressure, for instance, are more likely to accompany fast-growing astrocytomas and glioblastomas

than other tumorous growths and thus involve more of the surrounding and distant tissue. On the other hand, the *direction* of growth is not as predictable so that the neurologist cannot forewarn patients or their families about *what* behavioral changes they can expect as the disease runs its course, short of terminal apathy, stupor, and coma.

SUBJECT VARIABLES

Age

For thousands of years the average human life expectancy was 32–45 years (Angel, 1975). According to the Federal Interagency Forum on Aging-Related Statistics (2000), at the beginning of the 20th century the life expectancy at birth in the United States was about 48 years compared to 79 years for women and 74 years for men by 1997. The figure of four million Americans aged 85 and above in 2000 is expected to grow to almost 18 million by the year 2050 based on projections by the U.S. Bureau of the Census (Schneider, 1999). It is fitting that neuropsychological studies of this age group have become more frequent in the past decade in response to this aging revolution. Reflecting this trend, the 1997 versions of the Wechsler batteries were expanded to include normative data for persons up to age 89 years compared to only 74 years in previous versions.

A variety of factors have been identified that contribute to cognitive status with advanced age. In some studies individuals with higher education or higher intelligence show less age-related decline and less susceptibility to dementia (see p. 315). An active lifestyle in a favorable environment seems to preserve cognitive health (Schaie, 1994). Emotional status, and the habits and interests of decades may also contribute to older persons' considerable interindividual variability on measures of neuropsychological relevance (Neugarten, 1990; Schaie, 1995). Conditions that can affect cognition, such as infections, chronic systemic illness, medication side effects, and sensory loss (Lindenberger and Baltes, 1994; Tranel, Benton, and Olson, 1997), are all more common in elderly people. Genetics appears to play a substantial role, perhaps more so than in younger individuals. In studies of elderly twin pairs, estimates of heritability were greater than 60% for general cognitive ability (McClearn al., 1997; Plomin et al., 1994) and varied from 40% to 56% for learning and memory. Aging effects can be different for men and women, depending on the variable. For example, age-specific brain changes are greater in men than women for sulcal cerebrospinal fluid volume and Sylvian fissure cerebrospinal fluid volume, and the parieto-occipital region area as reported in a study of 330 elders aged 66 to 96 years (Coffey, Lucke, et al., 1998).

Brain changes with age

With advancing age every organ system undergoes alterations to some degree. The dynamic effects of aging on the brain are well documented. All measures of brain size register little or no change from the early adult years until the 40s to 50s. The brain's volume is at its peak around the early 20s and then declines very gradually over many decades (E.A. Mueller et al., 1998). Some structures are affected more than others. Cortical atrophy first shows up in the 40s, with increasingly widened sulci, narrowed gyri, and thinning of the cortical mantle. Ventricular size follows a similar pattern of slow change with increasing dilatation beginning in the 40s for men but not until the 50s for women (Kaye, DeCarli, et al., 1992). Studies have shown modest age-related changes in a number of specific brain regions, particularly the temporal lobe, hippocampus, and basilar–subcortical region (see E.A. Mueller et al., 1998 for a review).

Different kinds of alterations at the cellular level may account for the overall changes in brain size. At least some shrinkage in brain tissue appears to be due to neuronal loss, which occurs unevenly in both cortical and subcortical structures (Haug et al., 1983). The hippocampus and anterior dorsal frontal lobe, including the frontal poles, are the areas most susceptible to neuronal loss. For example, for every decade after the mid-40s, the hippocampus loses approximately 5% of its cells (M.J. Ball, 1977). Other areas lose fewer neurons or, as is the case for the occipital lobes, virtually none. In fact, neuronal loss in the cortex is either not significant or not as extensive as earlier reports (M.S. Alberts, 1998; R.D. Terry, DeTeresa, and Hansen, 1987; Wickelgren, 1996). Among subcortical structures some, such as the thalamus, basal ganglia, locus coeruleus, and Purkinje cells in the cerebellum, are particularly vulnerable to neuronal loss while other nuclei and pathways remain intact for the full life span (Filley, 1995; Kemper, 1994). With advanced age, the size of pyramidal neurons in the neocortex and hippocampus, and their dentritic arborization reduce and the number of neocortical synapses decreases (Katzman, 1997). White matter loss may also account for significant amounts of brain shrinkage (Meier-Ruge et al., 1992; Salat et al., 1999). White matter hyperintensities are more common in elderly persons than young adults (M.S. Albert, 1998). White matter tract integrity deteriorates with advancing age (O'Sullivan et al., 2001), which may contribute to subtle cognitive deficits (K.B.

Boone, Miller, et al., 1992; Skoog et al., 1996; Ylikoski et al., 1993). However, others have not found a significant correlation between white matter hyperintensities and cognitive impairment (R. Schmidt et al., 1999; Wahlund et al., 1996). In a review, Gunning-Dixon and Raz (2000) concluded that white matter abnormalities correlate with poorer performance on tasks of processing speed, memory, and executive functions but not on other cognitive abilities or fine motor performance.

Other brain changes seen in nondemented elderly persons include the presence of senile plaques and neurofibrillary tangles, abnormalities associated with Alzheimer's disease (Gomez-Isla and Hyman, 2003). The presence of these neuropathological features in both normal aged brains and Alzheimer's disease would seem to blur the distinction between normal and a disease state, except for findings of significant neuronal loss in Alzheimer's disease. Undoubtedly, some brains of "normals" come from aging individuals who have early, undetected dementia. However, many studies support a distinction between normal aging and Alzheimer's disease based on the distribution and extent of neuropathological features (M.J. Ball and Murdoch, 1997; Hof et al., 1996).

Recently identified cellular mechanisms that could underlie the brain changes associated with aging include the following: *apoptosis* (gene-directed cell death); cumulative biological errors in DNA replication, protein synthesis, or protein structure; and free radical production (Drachman, 1997). During metabolism and energy production, oxygen may be generated with an unpaired electron. Evidence suggests that oxidative stress caused by these extra electrons, or *free radicals,* plays significant roles in various neurodegenerative disorders (D.G. Morgan and Gordon, 1996). Mitochondrial DNA is particularly susceptible to oxidative stress, and there is evidence of age-dependent damage. This may contribute to the delayed onset and age dependence of neurodegenerative diseases (Beal, 1995).

Most measures of physiological brain function also reflect the aging process. Cerebral blood flow tends to show a progressive decline through the early adult years, which varies in intensity in different parts of the brain (Krausz et al., 1998; Hagstadius and Risberg, 1989; J.S. Meyer et al., 1994). Blood flow is reduced in various parts of the brain with the greatest diminution in flow often involving prefrontal and temporal lobe areas. Patterns of regional cerebral blood flow tend to become more widespread in older than in younger persons (Esposito et al., 1999; Grady, Maisog, et al., 1994). This pattern suggests that the ability to focus neural activity may be impaired in older subjects or that older adults recruit larger brain regions to support task performance as a form of compensation for increasing inefficiencies (Madden et al., 1999). Brain metabolism, measured by glucose or oxygen utilization, tends to diminish, but considerable variation has been reported (M.S. Albert and McKhann, 2002; J.S. Meyer et al., 1994; Petit-Taboue et al., 1998). Additionally, age does not appear to have a significant effect on *cerebral acetylcholinesterase activity*, an important indicator of the functioning central cholinergic system that is affected in Alzheimer's disease (Kuhl et al., 1999; Namba et al., 1999).

Changes in brain wave frequencies have been consistently reported. Older individuals show fewer waves in the α frequency than do younger persons (Oken and Kaye, 1992; F.H. Duffy, Albert, McAnulty, and Garvey, 1984). Half of a group of subjects in the 85 to 98 year age range showed intermittent temporal slowing which was associated with the appearance of white matter hyperintensities on MRI, but not with either blood pressure levels or cognitive functioning (Oken and Kaye, 1992). Other electrophysiological changes appeared in evoked potential studies as transmission velocities become slower with age, particularly beginning around the late 40s, and latencies increase (W.J. Evans and Starr, 1994; Oken and Kaye, 1992; Prinz, Dustman, and Emmerson, 1990).

Normal cognitive aging

Despite proliferating research, disagreements on the nature of cognitive changes in the aged are far from settled, with some studies reporting more extensive age-related cognitive loss than others. Divergent findings among studies may be due to different methodological approaches (La Rue and Markee, 1995). For ease and efficiency, most studies use a cross-sectional design comparing different age groups. However, cross-sectional designs potentially confound aging effects and cohort differences in culture, environment, medical status, education, and experience (Hertzog, 1996). For example, educational experiences cannot be equated in persons of much different ages who may have had the same number of years of education. Imagine comparing a young group with an elderly group on a computerized test. The young group would be expected to feel at ease with the computer format, while the elderly group might have a number of individuals with no computer experience. In the Seattle Longitudinal Aging Study, which was designed so that cohort and age effects could be compared, cohort effects were stronger than age effects on cognitive measures (J.D. Williams and Klug, 1996).

Longitudinal research eliminates cohort differences by examining the same persons over time. However, two main limitations are inherent in this approach. Bias associated with selective attrition may be introduced in which participants completing the project are generally higher functioning and thus not representative of the original group (Ruoppila and Suutama, 1997; Siegler et al., 1982). Research programs are more likely to retain persons with good health, financial security, high social status, and wide-ranging interests. Additionally, repeated examinations of the same individuals in longitudinal studies can produce practice effects that favor subsequent examinations and mask potential decline (R. Frank et al., 1996; Mitrushina and Satz, 1991; Storandt, 1990). The difficulty in eliminating practice effects is compounded by the limited availability of alternate forms of many neuropsychological tests that have been constructed for equivalent level of difficulty. By and large, longitudinal studies show less age-related decline in cognition than cross-sectional studies (J.D. Williams and Klug, 1996).

Another problem in interpreting aging research involves the "normality" of some elderly volunteers who may appear to be healthy and intact but have early or subtle brain disease, which cannot be identified in many instances without extensive and expensive examination procedures. Thus the typical "normal" control group of elderly persons probably includes at least a few subjects with some brain disorder or as yet undiagnosed dementia. Moreover, even among healthy older subjects, many will obtain scores suggestive of impairment on some tests (B.W. Palmer, Boone, Lesser, and Wohl, 1998).

The pattern of cognitive aging. Large individual differences in aging patterns have been observed, especially on memory tests (Sinnett and Holen, 1999); any attempt to draw conclusions is limited by this underlying variability (Schaie, 1995; R.S. Wilson, Beckett, et al., 2002). Historically, researchers have relied on the concepts of *crystallized* and *fluid* intelligence to distinguish those abilities that hold up with advancing age from the ones that decline (Baltes and Graf, 1996; J.L. Horn and Donaldson, 1976). Thus, over-learned, well-practiced, and familiar skills, ability, and knowledge are "crystallized," continuing to be fully operative and even showing gains into the 60s, then remaining stable until at least the mid-70s (Sinnett and Holen, 1999); while activities requiring "fluid" intelligence, which involves reasoning and problem solving for which familiar solutions are not available, follow the typical pattern of relative slow decline through the middle years until the late 50s or early 60s, when decline proceeds at an increasingly rapid pace (A.S. Kaufman and Horn, 1996). A review of mean scores for various age groups from the normative data of the WAIS III battery shows the least age effect on measures of over-learned skills: Vocabulary, Information, Comprehension, and Arithmetic (Wechsler, 1997a). The greatest age effects are on Picture Arrangement, Matrix Reasoning, Digit Symbol, and Object Assembly. Except for Digit Symbol, which has a significant speed component, these measures could be described as "fluid" intelligence measures.

Other workers propose that slowing—psychomotor slowing, slowed cognitive processing—can account for much if not all of the measured changes in performances that decline with age (Fisk and Warr, 1996; Klein, 1997; Van Gorp, Satz, and Mitrushina, 1990). Many measures of "fluid" intelligence are timed tasks, raising the possibility that response speed has an important confounding effect. Still others suggest that a visuospatial component (Koss, Haxby, et al., 1991) or frontal lobe dysfunction (Mittenberg, Seidenberg, et al., 1989) might explain much of what influences these changes. The common pattern of cognitive functioning in elderly persons has been likened to that seen in (presumably early) subcortical dementia (Van Gorp and Mahler, 1990).

Yet cognitive decline in elderly persons affects only some functions. Verbal abilities are usually well retained (Schum and Sivan, 1997), although word fluency may be reduced (Bäckman and Nilsson, 1996). Overall, many persons 85 years of age and older perform less well than younger persons in cross-sectional comparisons on tests of visual perception, constructional tasks, and memory, at least for visuospatial material (Howieson, Holm, al., 1993; Koss, Haxby, et al., 1991). Nevertheless, the decline in test performance does not translate into impairment in daily activities (Corey-Bloom et al., 1996). For example, with aging, scores on tests involving communication decline; yet studies of elderly people in natural situations have found no differences between younger and older persons in communication for the great majority of cases (Ska, Montellier, et Nespoulous, 1991).

Longitudinal studies generally show fewer age changes. A large study of a representative sample living near Copenhagen stratified by geographical location, age, and sex found that cognitive functions were relatively stable over an 11-year interval for adults up to age 70 (Laursen, 1997). The major change with aging was slower processing speed. Over time, performance tended to decline slightly on measures of nonverbal learning and memory, retention of verbal material, psychomotor speed, visuospatial processing speed, and concentration; however, most of the changes were without practical significance. A similar, ten-year longitudinal study beginning with 65- to 79-year-old subjects reported minimal if any compromise in "language, in-

tellect, perception, and decision making" among those participants who maintained good health (Tranel, Benton, and Olson, 1997). Similar findings were obtained for an 84- to 93-year-old group over a four-year interval (Hickman et al., 2000). These oldest old had minimal decline on most tests and did not show a greater rate of cognitive decline compared to subjects 15 years younger. In recent years, much normative data on cognitive test performance of elderly subjects have become available (Ganguli et al., 1991; Ivnik, Malec, Smith et al., 1996; Richardson and Marottoli, 1996).

Sensory and motor changes with aging. The sensory and motor aspects of aging are familiar: sensory modalities decline in sensitivity and acuity, response times are increasingly slowed, and fine motor movements seem somewhat clumsy (Swihart and Pirozzolo, 1988). Visual acuity, *stereopsis* (binocular vision), and oculomotor functions first show losses in the 40s to 50s, so that most persons age 60 and older experience several kinds of visual compromise (Fozard, 1990; Matjucha and Katz, 1994). Decline in hearing parallels that of vision (Fozard, 1990; E. Wallace et al., 1994). Mild to moderate hearing impairment is associated with lower performance on auditory administration of verbal memory tests (van Boxtel et al., 2000); presumably other auditorily administered cognitive test performances would be affected as well. Odor sensitivity, too, follows a similar pattern of decline with peak sensitivity in the 20s to 40s and first gradual then rapid loss (R.L. Doty, 1990). Disequilibrium (*presbyastasis*) occurs as a result of degeneration of vestibular system structures in normally aging persons (Furman and Cass, 2003).

Slowing in all aspects of behavior characterizes older persons (Salthouse, 1991b; Swihart and Pirozzolo, 1988; Van Gorp and Mahler, 1990). Beginning at age 30 simple reaction time follows a regular pattern of relatively gradual incremental slowing so that by age 60 it may have dropped by no more than 20% of what it was in the 20s and probably by less than that (Nebes and Brady, 1992; R.T. Wilkinson and Allison, 1989).

Diminished dexterity and coordination tend to compromise fine motor skills (Swihart and Pirozzolo, 1988). Balance problems (Kaye, Oken, et al., 1994) decreased vibratory sense in the lower extremities. Gait and posture defects (J.C. Morris and McManus, 1991) likely contribute to the tendency for many elderly persons to fall (Furman and Cass, 2003). Motor strength begins to diminish a little around the 40s with accelerated losses thereafter (Bornstein, 1985; 1986c; Spirduso and MacRae, 1990).

Attentional functions in aging. Although closely allied with and reflecting processing speed, the effects of age on attentional efficiency vary with the complexity of the task or situation. Thus simple span tends to remain essentially intact into the 80s (Benton, Eslinger, and Damasio, 1981; Craik, 1991). Participants from the WAIS-III normative sample over 80 years of age had a respectable mean digit span of nearly 6 forward although digits reversed was 4 (J.J. Ryan, Lopez, and Paolo, 1996). Individuals with higher education and higher occupational status performed better than those with less education who worked as laborers. Simple stimulus detection is unaffected by age (P.M. Greenwood, Parasuraman, and Haxby, 1993). However, elderly persons respond more slowly or make more errors when divided attention is called for, as on choice reaction time tests or dual task formats (P. Greenwood and Parasuraman, 1991; A.A. Hartley, 2001) and are slow to shift attention when given an invalid cue (P.M. Greenwood and Parasuraman, 1994). Elderly people have difficulty adjusting the size of attentional focus (P.M. Greenwood, Parasuraman, and Alexander, 1997; Oken, Kishiyama, et al., 1999). Deficits in sustained and selective attention and in increased distractibility also accompany normal aging (Filley and Cullum, 1994; Klein, Ponds, et al., 1997).

Memory functions in aging. As in most other areas of cognitive activity, different aspects of memory and learning differ in how they hold up with advancing age (Balota et al., 2000; Parkin, Walter, and Hunkin, 1995; Rybash, 1996). When older persons complain of memory problems, most frequently they are referring to sluggish word-finding, particularly proper names. Although this may be related to other memory problems, it can be dissociated from them (see *Verbal abilities in older persons,* below).

Interpretation of differences between age groups on memory tests is not always straightforward. Many memory tasks lend themselves to different retention and recall strategies. Thus response characteristics such as diminished self-monitoring (Nyberg et al., 1997), reduced flexibility (Dobbs and Rule, 1989; Parkin, Walter, and Hunkin, 1995), and poor use of strategies (M.S. Albert, 1994; Brebion et al., 1997; Daigneault and Braun, 1993) may contribute to the performance decline of elderly persons.

Short-term—or primary—memory as measured by brief retention of simple span shows only a slight age effect. Short-term memory becomes vulnerable to aging when the task requires mental manipulation of the material, as when reversing a string of digits (Craik, 1991; J.J. Ryan, Lopez, and Paolo, 1996) or when mentally organizing the stimuli or trying to remember the material while engaging in another activity—i.e., working memory (Baddeley, 1986; Brebion et al., 1997;

Hultsch et al., 1992). For example, the Letter–Number Sequencing test (Wechsler, 1997a) measures the ability to reorder sets of numbers and letters and is sensitive to an age effect. Unfortunately, auditory discrimination problems in the elderly also contribute to poor performance on this task due to identical vowel sounds of the stimulus items, such as "b," "c," "d." Age differences also show up on a self-ordered pointing task in which subjects are asked to make unique responses on each trial in a series; success requires them to keep in mind their earlier responses (Daigneault and Braun, 1993; Shimamura and Jurica, 1994; R. West et al., 1998). Yet elderly subjects can place a random series of words in alphabetical order as well as controls (Belleville et al., 1996). Differences between studies are likely related to differences in task demands which are not well understood. Reduced storage capacity (R.L. Babcock and Salthouse, 1990), and reduced ability to ignore irrelevant information (Hasher and Zacks, 1988), have been proposed (see also N.D. Anderson and Craik, 2000). Slowed processing speed as a significant contributor to benign memory problems in older persons has been implicated in a number of studies (Bryan and Luszcz, 1996; B.J. Diamond, De Luca, et al., 2000; Luszcz and Bryan, 1999; D.C. Park et al., 1996; Salthouse, 1991a). The Diamond group found no modality-specific differences in processing speed for either younger and faster subjects ($M_{age} = 26$) or the older ones ($M_{age} = 77$).

Many clinical studies using standard neuropsychological tests have shown small declines in verbal memory with age, with larger changes in memory for visuospatial material (Howieson, Holm, et al., 1993; Koss, Haxby, et al., 1991) or faces (Diesfeldt and Vink, 1989), although an incidental learning paradigm produced contrary findings (Janowsky, Carper, and Kaye, 1996). The primary deficit appears to be in the efficiency of acquiring new information with retention over time relatively well retained (Haaland, Price, and LaRue, 2003; Petersen, Smith, Kokmen, et al., 1992; Trahan, 1992; Youngjohn and Crook, 1993a). For example, recognition memory is relatively well retained with advanced age (Whiting and Smith, 1997). Tombaugh and Hubley (2001) found that increasing age was associated with faster rates of forgetting for short delay intervals (20 minutes and one day) but not over longer intervals (greater than one day). Some longitudinal studies suggest that the rate of memory decline over time is not more precipitous in the very old compared to those under 70 (Hickman et al., 2000; Zelinski and Burnight, 1997), yet Giambra and colleagues (1995) found increased vulnerability to decline in their very old subjects. The type of material to be retained probably is a factor as visual memory may show sharper declines in later years than verbal memory (Arenberg, 1978; Haaland, Linn, et al., 1983). Other age-related declines occur in source memory (Craik, Morris, et al., 1990; Erngrund et al., 1996; Schacter, Kasniak, Kihlstrom and Valdiserri, 1991), in memory for temporal order (Fabiani and Friedman, 1997; Parkin et al., 1995), and in prospective memory (Mäntyla and Nilsson, 1997; Maylor, 1998), although findings have varied (Craik, 1991; Einstein and McDaniel, 1990; R.L. West, 1986). While the data are not perfectly consistent, implicit memory appears to be relatively preserved with aging, particularly for perceptual priming tasks (see Rybash, 1996 for a review). Procedural memory and skill learning also are relatively intact in the elderly (Vakil and Agmon-Ashkenazi, 1997).

Memory complaints by elderly persons are unreliable predictors of significant cognitive deficits. Many older people with age-appropriate memory performances complain of poor memory, comparing their ability now to when they were young. Yet many persons in the early stages of dementia do not appreciate that their memory is failing. The perception of memory problems can be affected by sex, education, depression, and overall cognitive ability (B. Johansson, Allen-Burge, and Zarit, 1997).

Several standards have been proposed for classifying memory impairment in the elderly. For example, the diagnosis of *Age-Associated Memory Impairment* (*AAMI*) requires at least one score of at least one standard deviation (SD) below the young adult mean on the Benton Visual Retention Test, the verbal memory tests of the Wechsler Memory Scale, or other appropriate memory tests plus Scaled Scores of 9 or higher on Wechsler Intelligence Scale tests and scores of 24 or higher on the Mini-Mental State Exam (Crook, Bartus, et al., 1986; Larrabee, McEntee, et al., 1992). Elderly persons who satisfy the AAMI criteria show little or no change on a wide variety of memory tests, suggesting that this is a benign condition (Hanninen and Soininen, 1997; Nielsen et al., 1998; Youngjohn and Crook, 1993b). Blackford and LaRue (1989) proposed two other diagnostic standards for describing decline in the elderly: one for *age-consistent memory impairment* (*ACMI*), specified when 75% or more of the memory test scores fall within the ±1 *SD* range of the test mean for the subject's age, and one for *late-life forgetfulness* (*LLF*), identified when 50% or more of memory test performances fall within 1 or 2 *SD* below the tests' age means. These diagnostic concepts were compared in a study of 202 individuals between the ages of 60 and 64 and in good health. The prevalence rates were 13.5% for AAMI, 6.5% for ACMI, and 1.5% for LLF (Schroder et al., 1998), reflecting the increasing leniency of these diagnoses. In the Schroder study, complaints of cognitive deficits were significantly correlated with higher scores on depression and neuroticism scales but not with neuropsychological measures.

Verbal abilities of older persons. Most verbal abilities resist the regressive effects of aging (Bayles, Tomoeda, and Boone, 1985; Obler and Albert, 1985; Schum and Sivan, 1997). Thus vocabulary and verbal reasoning scores remain relatively stable throughout the life span of the normal, healthy individual and may even increase a little. However, reports differ depending upon whether comparisons between age groups are done on a cross-sectional or a longitudinal basis (Huff, 1990).

Two areas that have received much attention are age effects on verbal fluency and confrontation naming. Findings in verbal fluency studies can be confusing as advanced age may be associated with no decline (Mittenberg, Seidenberg, et al., 1989; Parkin and Java, 1999), little decline (Salthouse, Fristoe, and Rhee, 1996), or significant decline (Huff, 1990; Hultsch et al., 1992). Tombough, Kozak, and Rees (1999) found that age played a greater role in animal naming (23.4% of the variance) than in phonemic fluency (FAS [see pp. 518–519, 520–521], 11% of the variance). These differences may account for some of the seemingly contradictory findings of other studies.

Conflicting findings also have appeared in confrontation naming studies in which subjects are asked to name on sight real or pictured objects. Huff (1990) noted that fluency tends to decline more with advancing age than confrontation naming. He attributed this difference to the degree to which the task is more or less automatic or effortful: confrontation naming provides a cue that may trigger a habitual association, while naming tasks measuring fluency require the subject to perform a word search. Response speed is also more important in the fluency task. Some samples show little, if any, decline in performance on confrontation naming tasks (Goulet et al., 1994; Hickman et al., 2000); but in a Hong Kong study using a test "blueprinted" on the Boston Naming Test, subjects in a 60- to 80-year-old group were both slower and less accurate than a younger comparison group (Tsang and Lee, 2003). It is noteworthy that persons over 70 years frequently complain of word finding difficulties. In conversation and normal social interactions, the verbal retrieval problem becomes embarrassing for many older people who cannot dredge up a familiar name quickly or who block on a word or thought in mid conversation (M. Critchley, 1984).

Visuospatial functions, praxis, and construction in aging. Although object and shape recognition remain relatively intact throughout the life span, visuoperceptual judgment, for both spatial and nonspatial stimuli, declines—not greatly but rather steadily—from at least age 65 on into the 90s (Eslinger and Benton, 1983; Howieson, Holm, et al., 1993; Koss, Haxby, et al., 1991; Schaie, 1994). Basic perceptual analysis appears intact, whereas perceptual integration and reasoning show age-related declines, particularly on tasks requiring substantial problem solving (Libon, Glosser, et al., 1994). In evaluating performances on the most commonly used constructional tests—Block Design and Object Assembly—the time factor is closely associated with aging (Van Gorp, Satz, and Mitrushina, 1990; Wechsler, 1981, 1997a). Nevertheless, when scores are determined without regard to time, small age effects often still persist (Libon, Glosser, et al., 1994; Ogden, 1990). Elderly people tend to be less accurate than younger ones in copying an elaborate geometric design (the Complex Figure) (Ska and Nespoulous, 1988a), but they use good strategies (Janowsky and Thomas-Thrapp, 1993). When copying simpler designs, their productions are as accurate as those of younger subjects, suffering somewhat only from compromised graphomotor control (Ska, Desilets, and Nespoulous, 1986). On free drawing tasks, whether the subject matter be as complex as a person or a bicycle or as simple as a pipe or a star, older subjects' drawings tend to be simplified and less well articulated than those done by younger persons (Ska, Desilets, and Nespoulous, 1986; Ska and Nespoulous, 1987, 1988a; Swihart and Pirozzolo, 1988).

Reasoning, concept formation, and mental flexibility. Reasoning about familiar material holds up well with aging (Bayles, Tomoeda, and Boone, 1985). Arithmetic problem solving, for example, changes little with age (Compton et al., 2000; A.S. Kaufman, Reynolds, and McLean, 1989; Wechsler, 1981, 1997a). In contrast, when reasoning is brought to solving unfamiliar or structurally complex problems and to those requiring the subject to distinguish relevant from irrelevant or redundant elements, older persons tend to fare increasingly less well with advancing age (Arenberg, 1982; Cronin-Golomb, 1990; Hayslip and Sterns, 1979).

Concept formation and abstraction, too, suffer with aging, as older persons tend to think in more concrete terms than the young and the mental flexibility needed to make new abstractions and to form new conceptual links diminishes with age, with an increasingly steep decline after age 70 (M.S. Albert, Wolfe, and Lafleche, 1990; Arenberg, 1982; Cronin-Golomb, 1990; Isingrini and Vazou, 1997). Advanced age is associated with impairment on tests requiring concept formation and mental flexibility such as the Category Test (Heaton,

Grant, and Matthews, 1991), the Wisconsin Card Sorting Test (WCST) (Isingrini and Vazou, 1997; Parkin and Java, 1999; Salthouse, Fristoe, and Rhee, 1996) the Tower of Hanoi task (Brennan et al., 1997), Trail Making Test Part B (Arbuthnott and Frank, 2000; Keys and White, 2000), and Matrix Reasoning (Wechsler, 1997a). Yet in healthy older persons, problems with concept formation and mental flexibility may not become pronounced—or even noticeable—until the 80s (Haaland, Vranes, et al., 1987). Generally, age has been shown to be associated with slowness on the conflict condition of the Stroop Test, which requires inhibiting a stronger response tendency to produce a less potent response (Rush et al., 1990; Wecker et al., 2000). However, an age effect has not always been found on this test (K.B. Boone, Miller, et al., 1990; Verhaeghen and De Meersman, 1998).

Studies designed to compare older persons to patients with frontal lesions have come up with equivocal findings. Elderly persons, like patients with frontal lesions, tend to use less efficient memory strategies on list learning tasks than younger adults (Stuss, Craik, Sayer et al., 1996). In an analysis of the relationship between prefrontal cortex volume and performance on cognitive tasks, perseverations on the WCST were predicted by age and age-related changes in prefrontal cortex volume (Raz et al., 1998). However, older subjects did not resemble patients with frontal lesions on a spatial association memory task (Salmoni et al., 1996).

Health and cognitive aging

The cognitive effects of systemic diseases that commonly occur with aging—e.g., hypertension, diabetes, cerebrovascular pathology—are well known (see Chapter 7). Nutritional habits and metabolism may change in the elderly, resulting in undernutrition for such cognitively important substances as vitamins B_{12} and B_6 and folate (I.H. Rosenberg and Miller, 1992). Although health status must be taken into account when examining older persons, health problems alone are unlikely to account for most age-related declines in cognitive functioning (Salthouse, 1991b). Even healthy elderly volunteers show age-related decline on some cognitive tests.

Research also shows the positive side of health status and, better yet, that regular aerobic exercise may slow the rate of cognitive decline and even reverse it (Dustman, Emmerson, and Shearer, 1990; Spirduso and MacRae, 1990). When sedentary individuals in the 55- to 75-year age range were compared with similar groups who either participated in an aerobics program or did strength and flexibility training, those in the aerobics program made significant gains on a set of cognitive tests while the other groups differed little from pre- to posttesting. Improvements with exercise have shown up in cognitive speed and efficiency (Dustman, Ruhling, et al., 1984) and executive control processes (A.F. Kramer et al., 1999). Another study found that fitness in both young and middle-aged (50 to 62) men was associated with higher scores on tests of visual as well as cognitive functioning (Dustman, Emmerson, Ruhling, et al., 1990). It was suggested that the increase in cerebral blood flow with exercise provides for better oxygenation of the brain. Even playing video games may be good mental exercise for older persons, as it can speed up reaction time (Dustman, Emmerson, Steinhaus, et al., 1992).

Age at onset

Studies of adult patients who have suffered head trauma or stroke demonstrate how age and severity are likely to interact with advancing age, enhancing the impact of severity of damage. When severity is not taken into account, age alone does not appear to make much difference in outcome for patients within the young to middle age adult range. Older adults show less improvement one year after TBI than younger ones, have a greater number of complications including subdural hematomas, and are less likely to survive a severe injury (Cohadon et al., 2002; Rothweiler et al., 1998). In progressive deteriorating conditions, the normal mental changes of advancing years, such as reduced learning efficiency, can compound mental impairments due to the disease process. However, degenerative diseases differ in their effects, as early onset is associated with a more virulent form of some conditions (e.g., Huntington's disease) and later onset is predictive of greater severity in others (e.g., Parkinson's disease).

Brain disease and aging

Cerebrovascular and degenerative diseases of the brain increase sharply with advancing age, creating an ever-growing social burden (U.S. Congress, 1987). Moreover, the magnitude of this problem is expected to increase as more and more individuals live into their ninth and tenth decades. The social burden of the problem is further compounded in that, with advancing age, patients presenting with dementia symptoms are more apt to be suffering from an irreversible disease than from any treatable condition. With advancing age, elderly people generally have fewer social resources, such as family availability and income. Thus, when they require care, it is increasingly likely to be given in a nursing home or institution, where unfamiliar surroundings and lack of stimulation and personalized care contribute to

the severity of their symptoms. Unfortunately, the option of care in a well-managed foster home or assisted living facility is available only for some, a problem which is worsening in the United States.

Sex Differences

Sex-related patterns of brain structure and function

Sex-related variations in anatomical structures and functional characteristics of the brain are still controversial. When sex differences are found, and they often are not, they tend to indicate that lateral asymmetry is not as pronounced in women as in men and—as with all bimodal curves—there is considerable overlap (J. Levy and Heller, 1992; Hiscock, Inch, Jacek, et al., 1994; Hiscock, Israelian, et al., 1995; Hiscock, Inch, Hawryluk, et al., 1999). Both cortical and subcortical differences in some anatomic structures occur with normal sexual differentiation (Witelson, 1991).

Asymmetry in cortical temporal and parietal areas tends to be greater in right-handed men than in women generally, and the region of the corpus callosum that connects the functionally asymmetric temporoparietal regions (posterior body and isthmus) is smaller in men than in women (Witelson, 1989, 1991). Men are more likely to have a larger left versus right planum temporale (the posterior superior temporal gyrus), with essentially symmetric regions in women (Witelson, 1991; see Aboitiz et al., 1992; Kulynych et al., 1994, regarding measurement issues that can affect the findings). Increased fissurization of the anterior cingulate gyrus in the left hemisphere of men has been reported (Yucel et al., 2001). Heschl's gyri may be larger bilaterally in women (Rademacher et al., 2001) while the putamen and globus pallidus may be larger in men (Giedd et al., 1996). Sex-related asymmetries have been found in regions possibly involved in sexual differentiation, such as the hypothalamus (Chung et al., 2002; Swaab and Fliers, 1985).

Brain size is generally the same for infants of both sexes until age two or three, at which time the male brain begins to grow faster until adult brain weight is reached, at about 5 to 6 years (Witelson, 1991). Interestingly, girls and boys do not differ in height until about 8 years (Dekaban and Sadowsky, 1978), so body size per se is not the determinant of brain size. Female fetuses appear to have a thicker corpus callosum at each gestational age (16–36 weeks) (Achiron et al., 2001). The consistently smaller brains of adult women primarily involve the cerebral hemispheres and sometimes the cerebellum (Beaton, 1997; Nopoulos et al., 2000; Witelson, 1991). An overall larger corpus callosum has been reported for women (Witelson, 1989) but no difference between men and women has also been reported (Oka et al., 1999). When brain size is taken into account, callosum findings vary (S.C. Johnson, Farnworth, et al., 1994; H. Steinmetz et al., 1995; Parashos et al., 1995), but the corpus callosum in females still tends to be larger. The corpus callosum in men tends to shrink with advancing age between ages 25 to 68 and perhaps later; but no such change occurs in women, suggesting that brain aging may take place earlier in men than in women (Witelson, 1989). Brain differences between men and women have been reported at the microscopic level. Greater neuronal density has been reported in language areas in men (Witelson, Glezer, and Kigar, 1995) and larger *neuropil* (interlacing of dendrites and axonal branches) volumes in women (Rabinowicz et al., 2002).

Physiological activity in the brain tends to support these anatomical implications. Blood flow values appear to run higher in the right frontal lobe of men but not women, although on the average, overall cerebral blood flow in women is 11% higher than in men (Rodriguez et al., 1988). However, sex-related regional CBF (rCBF) findings seem to vary from study to study, methodology, and task (or cognitive state) (Esposito, Van Horn, et al., 1996; Frost et al., 1999; Kastrup et al., 1999). Notably, CBF decreases with advancing age in women but not men (Pagani et al., 2002). More marked lateralization in EEG patterns in men has been reported (Flor-Henry, Koles, and Reddon, 1987; L.J. Harris, 1978), a difference not always observed (Galin, Ornstein, et al., 1982). In a magnetic field evoked potential study of vowel processing, women showed greater N100m responses over the left hemisphere (Obleser et al., 2001). Siegel and colleagues (1996) found greater right than left asymmetry of cortical glucose metabolism in women but not men with Alzheimer's disease, suggesting that Alzheimer's disease has a greater effect on the left hemisphere of men.

Hormonal influences appear to be intimately involved with sexual differentiation during the course of development (Bradshaw, 1989; Burstein et al., 1980; Witelson and Swallow, 1988). Another line of research has looked at cognitive changes in women in the course of their normal hormonal fluctuations (H.W. Gordon and Lee, 1993); while suggestive, these findings are not always robust. On visuoperceptual tasks, left field superiority is typically highest during the menstrual phase when female hormone levels are lowest, and then diminishes to the point of no left field advantage or even a shift to right field superiority in the premenstrual phase (Hampson, 1990; Heister et al., 1989). Heister and her colleagues proposed that this variability may account for some of the conflicting findings on male–

female differences in cerebral lateralization. In complementary studies, healthy young males given a one-time injection of female hormones showed reduced practice effects on a spatial orientation test, but their verbal fluency increased significantly when the female hormone blood levels were high (H.W. Gordon, Corbin, and Lee, 1986). A single injection of testosterone blocked practice effects of verbal ability in older males but did not affect verbal or spatial memory (O.T. Wolf et al., 2000). Changes over the menstrual cycle have been reported for verbal and music dichotic listening (G. Sanders and Wenmoth, 1998), language (G. Fernandez et al., 2003), and olfactory acuity asymmetries (Purdon, Klein, and Flor-Henry, 2001); in working memory (Janowsky, Chavez, and Orwoll, 2000; A. Postma et al., 1999), arithmetic (Kasamatsu et al., 2002), implicit memory (Maki et al., 2002), and spatial ability and fine motor skills (Hampson, 1990). Cognitive processing seems to be, to some degree, plastic and altered by gonadal steroids (Y.R. Smith and Zubieta, 2001).

Unilateral brain disease effects may also offer clues to sex differences in brain organization. On the one hand, some studies show that with left hemisphere lesions, men's verbal test scores typically decline relative to their visuospatial performances; but with lesions on the right the opposite pattern appears (L.J. Harris, 1978; Inglis, Ruckman, et al., 1982; McGlone, 1976). Women, on the other hand, may not show these effects with the same degree of regularity, as 20% of women patients in a large-scale study did not have speech strictly lateralized to the left, although many more men (71.8%) than women (46%) had compromised visuospatial functions with right-sided lesions (Bryden, Hécaen, and DeAgostini, 1983; see also Blanton and Gouvier, 1987). These findings have been interpreted as reflecting the lesser degree of right hemisphere visuospatial superiority that women have relative to the left hemisphere: when right hemisphere functioning is compromised, not as much visuospatial competence is lost by women as by men (J. Levy and Heller, 1992). However, with lateralized brain lesions, women appear to have a distinct right hemisphere superiority for recognizing facial expressions, which contrasts with the male right hemisphere visuospatial advantage; women's ability to discriminate melodic patterns or environmental sounds with the left ear is also superior to that of men. Other studies have not found these effects (Bryden, 1988; A. Smith, 1983; W.G. Snow and Sheese, 1985). Studying aphasic patients, H. Damasio, Tranel, and her colleagues (1989) reported a greater incidence of comprehension problems among men and expressive deficits in women, but the men tended to have posterior lesions and the women's strokes were more anterior, which may explain these findings. In another study of aphasic patients, more verbiage, but also more neologisms, differentiated men's speech from women's; these differences were ascribed to psychosocial characteristics (Dressler et al., 1990). A possible sex difference in the location of language regions in the brain was suggested by the sites of infarcts producing aphasia in men and women (Hier, Yoon, et al., 1994).

Improvement following stroke may vary with sex differences as left hemisphere lesioned women have shown greater improvements in some aspects of aphasia than men (A. Basso, Capitani, and Moraschini, 1982; Pizzamiglio, Mammucari, and Razanno, 1985). Regardless of side of lesion, women may develop a greater degree of independence following stroke than their male counterparts (Sundet et al., 1988) and survive longer (Chambers et al., 1987). However, one study found better functional outcome in men after stroke (Wyller et al., 1997). Other studies (of right- and left-lesioned patients, respectively) offered no evidence of improvement differences between the sexes (Hier, Mondlock, and Caplan, 1983b; Sarno, Buonaguro, and Levita, 1985). Relatively few studies of outcome from TBI have included sex as a variable, but a meta-analysis suggests that men do better than women even though clinical opinion tends to be the opposite (Farace and Alves, 2000).

Cognitive differences between the sexes

The nature–nurture issue remains unsettled in questions of sex differences in cognitive abilities. Differences in brain anatomy have been demonstrated, but so too have the effects of education and socialization (Geary, 1989; L.J. Harris, 1978; Nash, 1979). Moreover, while some general trends in male or female superiority have been documented, few performance differences between the sexes have remained unquestioned or unequivocal. Thus, the issue of sex differences in cognitive functioning is far from simple and far from settled.

Laterality studies of cognitive performances report fairly consistent trends of men showing more pronounced lateralization effects than women (Coney, 2002; Hannay, 1976; B.W. Johnson et al., 2002; Witelson, 1976). These trends may be rather weak (Bryden, 1988) and do not appear universally (e.g., Mc-Keever, 1986). Laterality research also has demonstrated female superiority on verbal tasks and a male advantage on predominantly nonverbal visuospatial tasks (Coltheart, Hull, and Slater, 1975; Schaie, 1994). The finding of sex-related differences on laterality tasks has been controversial with many explanations (H. Hiscock, Inch, Jacek, et al., 1994). An exhaustive survey of auditory, visual, tactile, and dual-task studies pub-

lished in six well-known journals tends to support the hypothesis of greater lateralization of function in males, especially since the findings seem to be independent of stimulus-task variables and impressively consistent (H. Hiscock et al., 1994, 1995, 1999).

Clinical data based on the Wechsler Intelligence Scales suggest that men perform better on two academically influenced tests, Arithmetic and Information, while women tend to achieve higher scores on symbol substitution (A.S. Kaufman, McLean, and Reynolds, 1991; W.G. Snow and Weinstock, 1990). However, on two well-standardized American batteries on which boys have performed best on spatial visualization, mechanical aptitude, and high school mathematics tests, and girls did better on grammar, spelling, and perceptual speed, the differences between the sexes has declined greatly from 1947 to 1980 with the single exception of high school mathematics with no differences on arithmetic or either verbal or figural reasoning (Feingold, 1988). In Germany, sex differences on tests of visuospatial abilities decreased from 1978 to 1987 (Stumpf and Klieme, 1989). Sex differences were small on Israeli military mental ability tests (Flynn, 1998a).

Perceptual speed and accuracy. On tests of psychomotor speed and accuracy using visual stimuli, women tend to outperform men (Majeres, 1988, 1990; S.L. Schmidt et al., 2000) but this is not always the case (Klinteberg et al., 1987; M. Peters, 1997; Roig and Placakis, 1992). This advantage appeared to be pronounced among children on the Symbol Digit Modalities Test, but on these kinds of tests the differences between adults as measured by speed, while still present to some degree, are not large enough to warrant separate test norms (Heaton, Taylor, and Manly, 2003; A.S. Kaufman, McLean, and Reynolds, 1988; A. Smith, 1982). Contradictory findings on tactile discrimination are simply confusing, as each study offers conclusions based on very disparate results (H. Cohen and Levy, 1986; Genetta-Wadley and Swirsky-Sacchetti, 1990; Tremblay et al., 2002; Witelson, 1976).

Verbal functions. Left lateralized processing for speech is present in both sexes from early childhood, but this left-cerebral specialization appears to become greater in males during later childhood, when tested by laboratory techniques (D.P. Gordon, 1983). Yet, on many different kinds of verbal skill tests, no significant differences between the sexes emerged when data were combined from 165 studies on subjects ranging in age from 2 to 64 (Hyde and Linn, 1988). More of these studies (27%) showed females performing better than males, with 7% favoring males, yet 66% of them produced no significant differences. Of these 165 studies, the greatest (although small) female advantages appeared on tests of general verbal ability, making words out of letters (anagrams), and the quality of speech production. The extent to which culture and ethnicity might contribute to disparate results is suggested by a study that found American Caucasian girls outperformed boys on all of a three-part naming task (a version of the Stroop test), but boys and girls of three different Asian ethnic subgroups did equally well (P.H. Wolff et al., 1983). When the inclusion of a memory or learning component makes the verbal task more difficult, women consistently perform better than men (Bleecker, Bolla-Wilson, Agnew, and Meyers, 1988; Ivison, 1977; J.H. Kramer, Delis, and Daniel, 1988; Rabbitt et al., 1995). A sex difference may not be present on all verbal memory tasks (Herlitz, Nilsson, and Backman, 1997). Women often demonstrate better word fluency (Acevedo et al., 2000; T. Lee et al., 2002), although it may depend on the type of category (Capitani, Laiacona, and Barbarotto, 1999).

Visuospatial functions. Males tend to fare better on many visuospatial tests, but considerable overlap in the score distributions of the two sexes will be found on any given task in which there is a male advantage (Witelson and Swallow, 1988). Differences are not prominent until the seventh grade, when girls' performances become poorer (Karnovsky, 1974). Moreover, research findings are not unequivocal (P.J. Caplan et al., 1985; Filskov and Catanese, 1986). A male advantage shows up particularly on tests of spatial orientation (W.W. Beatty and Tröster, 1987; Hiscock, 1986; McKeever, 1986; Stumpf and Klieme, 1989), object location memory (Postma, Izendoorn, and De Haan, 1998), in learning spatial placement by touch (Heaton, Ryan, et al., 1996)—although this finding is not always duplicated (Dodrill, 1979)—and on mental rotation and spatial perceptual tasks (such as estimating water levels) (Gladue and Bailey, 1995). Findings are mixed for tests requiring visuospatial analysis and synthesis (e.g., Embedded Figures Test, Block Design) (A.S. Kaufman, McLean, and Reynolds, 1988; A.S. Kaufman, Kaufman-Packer, et al., 1991; R.S. Lewis and Harris, 1990). Memory assessment may heighten sex differences on visuospatial tasks (Ivison, 1977; Orsini, Chiacchio, et al., 1986). Men's advantage in visuospatial processing may be more evident when tasks involve active processing (e.g., mentally following a task) rather than passive processing (e.g., recalling previously memorized spatial positions) (Vecchi and Girelli, 1998). Experience with spatial activities (e.g., exploring a neighborhood vs. jump rope) may be related to the sex difference (Corballis, 1991; Siegel-Hinson, 2000).

Mathematical abilities. Differences in mathematical performances of adolescents and adults almost always favor males over females (Benbow, 1988; Feingold, 1988; A.S. Kaufman, Kaufman-Packer, et al., 1991). In grade school, however, girls average slightly higher scores than boys in computation skills with no differences in problem solving ability (Hyde, Fennema, and Lamon, 1990). Performance differences favoring boys begin to appear around the seventh grade, even before high school when spatially based mathematics become important and fewer girls take advanced mathematics courses (Benbow and Stanley, 1982). Twenty years later, both males and females in the Benbow and Stanley study were high achievers but males were more likely to receive degrees at all levels in mathematics and the inorganic sciences and females, in life sciences and the humanities (Benbow, Lubinski et al., 2000). Males may be more likely to match strategies to problem characteristics when advanced mathematical problem solving is required (Gallagher et al., 2000). Patrick (1998) found that for females only, mathematical problem solving was related to mental rotation ability. From their meta-analysis of studies which included mathematics test data on more than 3 million subjects, Hyde and her colleagues (1990) concluded that the size of sex differences has diminished over the years and is now quite small. Many models have been offered to account for these differences, from purely psychosocial to purely biological, with many mixed models in between; but the questions remain intriguingly resistant to easy explanations.

Sex and handedness interactions

Compounding much of the data on sex differences in cognitive abilities is the effect of handedness, as left-handed males tend to perform more like right-handed females in showing some superiority on tests of verbal skills and sequential processing, while left-handed females and right-handed males appear to have an advantage on visuospatial tasks (H.W. Gordon and Kravetz, 1991; R.S. Lewis and Harris, 1990) and nonverbal auditory stimuli (Piazza, 1980). Having left-handed family members (*familial sinistrality*) may enhance the effects of sex and handedness on visuospatial orientation (Healey et al., 1982). Notable exceptions include left-handed females whose language dominance appears to be in the right hemisphere, as they tend to perform least well on spatial rotations (L.J. Harris, 1978), and the varying and complex effects of having left-handed family members (Carter-Saltzman, 1979; McKeever, 1986; Tinkcom et al., 1983). The relationship between hemispheric organization and handedness may differ between men and women (Eviatar et al., 1997).

Further complicating the issue of sexual differences are findings suggesting that homosexual men as a group tend to have performance patterns more like women, but almost half of the group under study were nonright-handers (McCormick and Witelson, 1991). A study by Lippa (2003) with almost 2,000 subjects suggests that homosexual men and women have much higher rates of nonright-handedness than heterosexuals. Left-handedness was associated with more female-typical occupational preferences, self-ascribed femininity and nonmasculinity in male homosexuals and a tendency for male-typical occupational pursuits along with nonfeminine and masculine preferences in female homosexuals.

Caveat

When taking an examinee's sex or gender preference into account in evaluating neuropsychological test performances, it is perhaps most important to keep in mind that group differences rarely amount to as much as one-half of a standard deviation (e.g., Ivison, 1977; A.S. Kaufman, McLean, and Reynolds, 1988; Mitrushina, Boone, and D'Elia, 1999, *passim*): *overlap in the distribution of scores for men and women is much greater than the distance between them.* Interpretation of individual test performances in the context of general knowledge about cognitive differences between the sexes must be done with caution.

Lateral Asymmetry

Asymmetrical cerebral lateralization and unilateral hand preference are not exclusively human but characterize our ancestral line. Some research suggests that monkeys and apes tend to use their right hands for fine manipulation (R.D. Morris, Hopkins, and Bolser-Gilmore, 1993), while the left serves a more supportive function or engages in large visually guided movements, such as reaching (MacNeilage, 1987). Some workers found fairly equal right- and left-hand preferences in fewer than half of observed primates, the others having mixed preference (Annett, 2002). However, skulls of our hominoid ancestors present a pattern of differential lateralized brain size similar to that of humans today, and their tool-making remnants display a right preference (Corballis, 1991). Evidence that humans evolved as asymmetrically lateralized further appears in Neolithic carvings that show traces of right-handed tool use (Spenneman, 1984), and the right hand preference for holding tools or weapons as shown in

statues and paintings dating as far back as 3000 B.C.E. (Coren and Porac, 1977). In most cases handedness is genetically determined (Annett, 2002), although early trauma or even prenatal events may affect adult hand preference. A left-hand preference after an early left hemisphere lesion is called *pathological left-handedness* (Corballis, 1991; Satz, Orsini, Saslow, and Henry, 1985).

Hand preference and cerebral organization

Right-handers. Studies of adults generally estimate that 90% to 95% are right-handed (Annett, 2002; Fennell, 1986). These figures tend to vary with age as the incidence of right-handedness increases from 70% or less in early childhood to 86% to 90% in childhood and the teen years (Briggs and Nebes, 1975), and to go as high as 97% to 99% in middle aged and older persons (Annett, 2002). While the very high percentages for older persons may be explained in part by the practice of forcible repression of left-handedness, it is also likely that some born left-handers simply learn to accommodate to the many dextral biases in the environment (S.J. Ellis et al., 1988). Estimated handedness percentages may also vary according to the stringency with which hand preference is defined and how it is measured or otherwise determined (Annett, 2002). Some variations across races and ethnic groups have been documented (Fennell, 1986) but are far from universal (e.g., Maehara et al., 1988). By small percentages fewer males are right-hand dominant than females throughout the life span (Annett, 2002). Right-handers tend to be consistent, using the right hand for almost all one-handed acts (M. Peters, 1990). The less frequent exceptions in which they use the left hand are more likely to occur with relatively simple hand or arm movements requiring little modification once the act begins (e.g., pointing, screwing in a light bulb) (Healey, Liederman, and Geschwind, 1986).

Studies of right-handers have found left hemisphere language representation in the 95%–99% range (Borod, Carper, Naeser, and Goodglass, 1985; J. Levy and Gur, 1980). Roughly 95% of right-handed subjects have left cerebral language dominance as determined by Wada testing (Branch, Milner, and Rasmussen, 1964; Loring, Meador, Lee, et al., 1990), fMRI (J.A. Springer et al., 1999), or functional transcranial Doppler (Knecht, Drager, et al., 2000).

Left-handers. Left-handers (or technically more accurate, *nondextrals*) can be distinguished in terms of the strength of the left-hand tendency (i.e., whether it occurs in every instance a right-hander would use the right hand, or just some), and the variability of this tendency (whether different hands are used for the same activity at different times) (Annett, 2002; M. Peters, 1990; M. Peters and Servos, 1989). Familial sinistrality also contributes to the left-handed typology (Corballis, 1991). Nondextrals can be grouped either as strong left-handers with no family history of left-handedness or as weak left-handers with familial sinistrality or as very infrequently occurring strong left-handers with familial sinistrality. In addition, *ambiguous-handed* persons who are inconsistent in their use of hands constitute another small group of neuropsychologically normal persons (Satz, Nelson, and Green, 1989), although ambiguous-handedness is more likely to appear among persons with severe developmental disabilities presumably due to early trauma (Soper and Satz, 1984).

The majority (70%–80%) of nondextral patients are left cerebral language dominant, a finding that has been obtained with Wada testing (Branch et al., 1964; Loring, Meador, Lee, et al., 1990), fMRI (Szaflarski et al., 2002), or functional transcranial Doppler (Knecht, Drager, et al., 2000). However, the incidence of right cerebral dominance has been more difficult to estimate, in part due to criteria issues regarding what constitutes right hemisphere language (P.J. Snyder, Novelly, and Harris, 1990) and the tendency to treat language laterality as a discrete rather than a continuous variable (Loring, Meador, Lee, et al., 1990). Consequently, language lateralization is often simply characterized as typical or atypical, although most patients who are not left language dominant by Wada testing display bilateral rather the right language dominance (Risse, Gates, and Fangman, 1997).

Handedness is often used as a marker to indicate increased likelihood of atypical cerebral language representation. Only recently, with the development of noninvasive techniques to determine language representation, has the relationship between handedness and language representation been studied. The incidence of right hemisphere language dominance determined by functional transcranial Doppler increased linearly with the degree of left-handedness, from 4% in strong right-handers to 15% in ambidextrous individuals and 27% in strong left-handers (Knecht, Drager, et al., 2000). Thus, the relationship between left-handedness and right cerebral dominance is not an artifact of pathology (i.e., pathologic left-handedness) but reflects a natural relationship.

In an fMRI study of nondextrals, 78% were left language dominant, 14% had bilateral language, and 8% displayed right dominance (Szaflarski et al., 2002). Language laterality was related not only to the strength of hand preference as reported by Knecht, Drager, et al. (2000), but of particular importance, also to family history of left-handedness. Subjects were more than two-and-one-half times as likely to have atypical language representation (right or bilateral) with a history of familial left-handedness than those with no left-handed relatives (35% vs. 13%). The link between both personal handedness and family handedness history to language laterality suggests a common genetic feature, and this undoubtedly will be the focus of future, larger scale studies. Even though most nonright-handed persons are left cerebral language dominant, they are more likely to have atypical language representation, particularly in the context of a left-handed family history.

In approximately one-quarter to one-third of nondextrals, aphasic disorders are associated with right-sided lesions (Borod, Carper, Naeser, and Goodglass, 1985), and about one-half of these (reports from different studies range in the neighborhood of 13% to 16%) appear to have bilateral language representation (Blumstein, 1981). These latter are the familial left-handers who usually have only a moderate degree of left-hand preference, showing some ambidexterity (i.e., while fairly consistent in their hand preferences for specific activities, they use different hands depending upon the activity). Aphasia patterns in left-handers with unilateral lesions also indicate that for a few of them, speech comprehension may be processed by one hemisphere—usually the left, while expressive ability is a function of the other hemisphere (Naeser and Borod, 1986). Strongly biased familial left-handers are apt to resemble nonfamilial strongly left-handed people more than other familial left-handers in having predominantly left hemisphere representation of language. Moreover, right-handers with left-handers in the family tend to show more and faster improvement from aphasia due to left hemisphere lesions than do other right-handers, suggesting that they too may have some bilateral cerebral representation for language functions (Carter-Saltzman, 1979; Thiery et al., 1982).

Neuroanatomic correlates of handedness. The thickness of the mid and anterior regions of the corpus callosum and the size of the callosal area tend to vary with handedness (Witelson and Kigar, 1987; Witelson, 1989). Thus, persons classified in Witelson's series of subjects as having a nonconsistent right hand preference have more callosal substance than those with a consistent right hand preference. However, this relationship holds only for men: callosal size does not differ for women, regardless of hand preference (Witelson and Goldsmith, 1991). Studies of brain lateralization and handedness using radiographic visualization suggest a somewhat decreased tendency to lateral asymmetry among left-handers, although nonfamilial left-handers showed asymmetry patterns like those of right-handers (Witelson, 1980). A correlation also exists between planum temporale asymmetry and handedness, although the strength of this relationship depends on how the planum temporale borders are defined (Zetzsche et al., 2001).

Handedness and cognitive functions

In determining patterns of cognitive functioning, in addition to sex and handedness, familial sinistrality may play a role (McKeever, 1990), although its relevance has been questioned (Orsini, Satz, et al., 1985). A tendency for right-handers to perform better than left-handers on visuospatial tasks has been consistently observed (Bradshaw, 1989; Cerone and McKeever, 1999; J. Levy, 1972). These group differences in visuospatial abilities may be due to the greater likelihood that left-handers, like women, have visuospatial functions mediated in a more diffuse manner by both hemispheres than localized on the right, as is most typical for male right-handers. Levy wisely cautioned that these data represent overall group tendencies and cannot be indiscriminately applied to individuals.

A higher proportion of nondextrals than right-handers are represented at the extremes of cognitive competency. At the lower end are persons whose left-handedness resulted from early brain injury (Coren and Searleman, 1990; O'Boyle and Benbow, 1990; Soper and Satz, 1984). At the other end can be found higher percentages of skilled mathematicians (Benbow, 1988; F. Gaillard, Converso, and Amar, 1987; Witelson, 1980) along with professional athletes, architects, lawyers, and chess players (O'Boyle and Benbow, 1990; Schachter and Ransil, 1996). However, the mathematical advantage appears to be a male prerogative. More left-handers generally enjoy artistic (graphic) talents, and a higher proportion of right-handers are proficient in music (B.D. Smith et al., 1989). Smith and his colleagues noted that, while significant, these tendencies—observed among college psychology students—are relatively weak.

Determining cerebral lateralization

Identification of the language dominant hemisphere or whether language is represented in either hemisphere can be an important issue in neuropsychological assessment. When the side of a lateralized lesion is known, the pattern of test performance will generally provide the needed information. However, most brain injury does not come in neatly lateralized packages or express itself in a theoretically ideal pattern of lateralization. The need to identify the language dominant hemisphere is most critical when neurosurgical intervention is planned. It can also be useful in developing individualized assessment protocols, in interpreting assessment findings, and in making a rehabilitation plan.

Observational methods. In the clinic, the easiest and perhaps the surest way to identify right-handed subjects is to observe which hand is used for writing or drawing. This method alone correctly identified the side for language dominance determined by Wada testing in 89.5% of patients (all of the seven men, 10 of the 12 women) (E. Strauss and Wada, 1987). However, this simple approach to the question of handedness does not identify persons with a left-sided or mixed (ambilateral) preference who, by training or as a result of illness or injury, learned to write with the right hand.

Handedness and footedness are highly correlated in right-handed persons, but about 60% of left-handers are right-footed (J.P. Chapman et al., 1987; Searleman, 1980). Thus the side and strength of foot preference may be an even more reliable predictor of the direction and extent of lateral asymmetry in cortical organization, probably because it is less subject to cultural pressure. However, foot preference for kicking may reflect compensatory behavior, not dominance. Freides (1978) recommended that when investigating footedness, the examiner inquire into the subject's preference for hopping or standing on one foot rather than kicking since children with lateralized dysfunction often learn to stand on the stronger leg and kick with the weaker one.

J. Levy (1972; with Reid, 1976) hypothesized that hand position in writing may reflect cerebral lateralization. She reported that both right- and left-handers using a normal hand position tended to have language representation on the hemisphere side opposite the writing hand while subjects holding their writing instrument in an inverted position (i.e., "hooked") were more likely to have language represented in the hemisphere on the same side as the writing hand. This looked like an easy solution to a difficult problem. Unfortunately, research—including Wada testing—has not supported it (E. Strauss, Wada, and Kosaka, 1984; Weber and Bradshaw, 1981, 1987). Yet, R. Gregory and Paul (1980) reported that male left-handed "inverters" tended overall to perform a little less well on neuropsychological test batteries (WAIS, Halstead-Reitan Battery [HRB]) than left- or right-handers who wrote in the usual position. They suggested that these performance differences reflected "the inefficiency of bilateral organization of cerebral functions."

Laboratory methods. While far from a routine procedure, the surest method of identifying the pattern of cerebral organization is the Wada test. Although direct cortical stimulation methods map language representation, they are performed only unilaterally, thereby precluding any conclusion about bilateral language. Data from Wada studies have served as standards for measuring the effectiveness of noninvasive laboratory techniques such as dichotic listening tests or examination of visual half-field performances. These techniques tend to produce results in the expected direction, yet many findings have proven equivocal or contradictory, particularly with nonright-handed subjects, who are the ones who most need to have their lateralization patterns identified correctly (Bryden, 1988; Segalowitz, 1986). Moreover, conclusions drawn from these techniques do not always agree with Wada test findings (Hugdahl et al., 1997).

A variety of functional imaging procedures have been used to identify cerebral language lateralization. Of these, the most widely studied is fMRI, which has produced good correlations with Wada language data (J.R. Binder et al., 1996), although their concordance is not perfect (W.D. Gaillard et al., 2002; Westerveld, Stoddard, et al., 1999). Other noninvasive procedures for identifying language representation include functional transcranial Doppler (Knecht, Deppe, et al., 1998) and magnetic source imaging (Breier, Simos, et al., 1999).

Behavioral techniques. In the clinic, congruent handedness and footedness probably gives the best indication of the pattern of cerebral lateralization, short of a formal laboratory study (E. Strauss and Wada, 1983). However, when they are not congruent other methods of ascertaining the lateralization of language functions can be used. Eye preference does not help to clarify lateral preference in left-handed persons, as many have a right or mixed eye preference regardless of their strength of handedness (Annett, 2002). Nevertheless, eye preference may give some indication of visual field superiority for nonverbal stimuli (E. Strauss and Goldsmith, 1987).

A number of behavioral techniques have been devised to help ascertain both lateral preference and its strength (as measured by the consistency of side of choice). Many clinicians use an informal set of tasks or questions having to do with a variety of one-sided activities. For example, D. Kimura and Vanderwolf (1970) asked their subjects to show how they "write, brush teeth, comb hair, hammer a nail, cut bread, use a key, strike a match, and hold a tennis or badminton racquet." Subjects were classified as right- or left-handed if they met at least six of these criteria on one hand. M. Peters (1990) found that a variety of manual tasks sorted out consistent from inconsistent (ambidextrous) left-hand writers. The inconsistent ones have more strength in the right hand as measured by a

hand dynamometer (Grip Strength Test) and throw with the right, but they use their left hands for tasks requiring dexterity and speed (Purdue Pegboard, finger tapping). On the *Hand Preference Test* (Spreen and Strauss, 1998), subjects show how they would perform the following six manual tasks: writing, throwing a ball to a target, holding a tennis racquet, hammering a nail, striking a match, and using a toothbrush. If all six acts are not performed with the same hand the subject is classified as "mixed-handed." Not all one-handed tasks can be used to evaluate lateral preference. For tasks that do not require skill (e.g., "Pick up piece of paper," "Pet cat or dog") and those that require strength (e.g., "Pick up briefcase"), strongly lateralized people are likely to use either hand (Obrzut, Dalby, et al., 1992).

On retaking the *Lateral Dominance Examination* after five years, 92 to 100% of normal control subjects showed the same preference on all seven hand preference items (e.g., throw a ball, use a scissors), all three eye preference items (e.g., look through a telescope), plus the football kick item; but only 81% used the same foot to "squash a bug" (Dodrill and Thoreson, 1993). The high level of lateral preference stability found with this very typical set of preference tasks can be easily generalized to other such assessments of lateral preference.

Two tests requiring fine motor coordination and speed appeared at about the same time. The *Target Test* requires subjects to mark the center of each target, first with the preferred hand and then with the nonpreferred one (Borod, Koff, and Caron, 1984; this article contains detailed administration and scoring instructions) (see Fig. 8.1, p. 309). It is individually administered, first as a speed test, then for accuracy. Instructions for the speed trial emphasize the need to work fast. For the accuracy trials, speed is controlled by requiring the subject to tap in time to a metronome. Expected left and right hand differences appeared, with speed predicting hand preferences slightly better than accuracy. On the accuracy test, however, familial left-handers showed a left hand advantage while nonfamilial left-handers' advantage was in the right hand.

Another dotting test was developed for group administration (Tapley and Bryden, 1985) (see Fig. 8.2, p. 309). Subjects are instructed to "make a dot in each circle following the pattern as quickly as you can," with additional emphasis on getting dots in the circles without touching an edge. Four 20 sec trials are given, with the first and fourth trials performed by the preferred hand. The score is the number of correctly dotted circles made by the right hand minus the number made by the left, divided by the total number, $(R - L)/(R + L)$, so that scores favoring the right hand are positive and those favoring the left are negative. This method generated a bimodal curve with virtually no

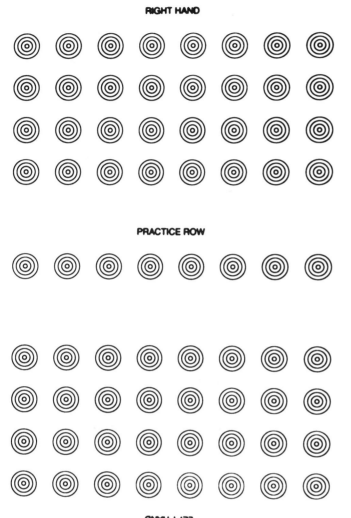

FIGURE 8.1 The target matrix for measuring manual speed and accuracy. (Courtesy of Joan Borod)

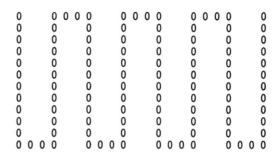

FIGURE 8.2 Tapley and Bryden's (1985) dotting task for measuring manual speed. Four reproductions of this pattern appear in a 2 × 2 array on a sheet with instructions on the upper left and lower right patterns to "Use the hand you write with" and, on the other two, to "Use the hand you *don't* write with" (p. 216).

overlap between right- and left-handers, but it did not distinguish between familial and nonfamilial lefties.

Annett (2002) relies on "the peg moving task" to ascertain side and strength of handedness. The subject moves ten dowel pegs in one row of holes on a board to a parallel row of holes, first with the right hand going from right to left, then with the left going from left to right. The score for each hand is the average time for five completed trials. Relative response speed determines the nature of handedness.

Questionnaires and inventories. Formal questionnaires typically ask about choice of side in performing a variety of one- and two-hand activities and other acts such as choice of foot for kicking or for dressing first. They may vary in length from as many as 55 items or more to as few as 10 (see Table 8.1). Many inquire into

only hand activities and some are simply variants of others with one or two items added or removed (e.g., Briggs and Nebes, 1975; B. Milner, 1975; see Fig. 8.2). Some inventories inquire into other kinds of preferences as well. A 13-item inventory was developed which has only four hand items (throwing, drawing, erasing, card dealing), but three each for foot (kick a ball, pick up pebble with toes, step onto chair), eye (peek through keyhole, look into bottle, sight rifle), and ear (listen through a door, listen for heartbeat, put on single earphone) (Coren, Porac, and Duncan, 1979).

Findings generated by different questionnaires of different lengths and composition on very different populations (e.g., African children, Hawaiian adults, Israeli teenagers, etc.) differ in the percent of left-handers identified, ranging from as few as 0.4% of 4,143 Taiwanese children and adults to 11.8% of 5,147 Canadian and American adults (Salmaso and Longoni, 1985). These investigators also found that the addition of one eye preference and one foot preference item to the *Edinburgh Handedness Inventory* (Oldfield, 1971; see also S.M. Williams, 1991) increased the number of right-handers showing variability in their laterality preferences.

Another important difference between preference inventories is whether items are dichotomized or offer a range of responses that better reflect the natural distribution of laterality preferences (i.e., strong, weak, or none) for any given activity. With either method the items that most clearly discriminate right- and left-handers are those inquiring into the hand for writing, drawing, and throwing (Raczkowski et al., 1974; Salmaso and Longoni, 1984; Steenhuis and Bryden, 1989). More complex two-handed activities, such as using a broom to sweep or opening a box lid, did not discriminate well.

A revision of Annett's (2002, p. 29) hand preference questionnaire, developed in the late 1960s, takes into account the fact that, for many left-handed and am-

TABLE 8.1 Some Lateral Preference Inventories and Their Item Characteristics

Name and Reference	Body Parts*	Number of Items	Response Choices per Item†
Edinburgh Handedness Inventory: S.M. Williams, 1991	H-1, H-B	10	5 (L or R strong or weak or NO)
Edinburgh Handedness Inventory (variant): Salmaso & Longoni, 1985	H-1, H-B, F, EY	22	3 (L, R, either)
Handedness inventory: Briggs & Nebes, 1975‡	H-1, H-B, EY	13	5 (L or R always or usually or NO)
Hand preference inventory: Healey et al., 1986	H-1 (54 items) + direction of axe swing	55	5 (L or R always or preferred or NO)
Handedness questionnaire: Raczkowski et al., 1974	H-1	23	3 (L, R, both)
Self-report inventory: Coren, Porac, & Duncan, 1979	H-1, F, EA, EY	13	3 (L, R, both)
Waterloo Handedness Questionnaire: Steenhuis & Bryden, 1989	H-1	60	5 (L or R always or usually or either)

*H-1, one hand act; H-B, both hands act; F, foot; EA, ear; EY, eye.
†NO, no preference; L, left; R, right.
‡See Figure 8.3.

bidextrous persons, lateral preference is not easily dichotomized (Briggs and Nebes, 1975; see Fig. 8.3). The five-point scale measuring strength of laterality for each item was added to make this inventory more sensitive to ambidexterity than Annett's questionnaire. A handedness score can be obtained by assigning two points to "always" responses, one point to "usually," and none to "no preference." Scoring left preferences as negative and right preferences as positive gives a range of scores from −24 for the most left-handed to +24 for the most right-handed. The authors arbitrarily called persons receiving scores of +9 and above right-handed, those with scores between −9 and +8 were called mixed-handed, and scores from −9 to −24 indicated left-handedness. Using this method, 14% of a large (n = 1,599) group of students were designated nonright-handers, a figure in accord with the literature. Factor analysis of the items in this inventory identified three distinct factors (power, skills, and rhythm), as well as distinctive factor structures for two different student populations (Loo and Schneider, 1979).

Although the incidence of right hemisphere or mixed cerebral lateralization is low in right-handed people, test behavior must be evaluated with these possibilities in mind. The first hint that there has been an unexpected switch is often the examiner's bewilderment when a hemiplegic patient displays the "wrong" set of behavioral symptoms. Since left-handed patients generally are less likely to conform to the common lateralization pattern, their behavior should be routinely scrutinized for evidence of an irregular lateralization pattern. When deviations from the normal left–right or-

ganization of the brain appear, a very thorough study of all functional systems is necessary to delineate the nature of the patient's cognitive disabilities fully, for in these exceptional cases no systematic relationships between functions can be taken for granted.

PATIENT CHARACTERISTICS: RACE, CULTURE, AND ETHNICITY

Race, culture, and *ethnicity* tend to be used almost interchangeably as terms for categorizing individuals with respect to background, perhaps because they are somewhat interrelated and there is some conceptual confusion concerning their meaning (Betancourt and Lopez, 1993; Okazaki and Sue, 1995; Rohner, 1984). It is thus unlikely that one set of definitions for these terms would be acceptable to everyone (but see American Psychological Association, 2003, for definitions to be used with practice guidelines). Regardless of which term is used to group individuals, researchers rarely clarify their use of the term and the assumptions that were made about the characteristics of their samples in this regard.

Race generally suggests that distinctive biological groups have obvious physical characteristics (e.g., skin color, facial features, and hair texture) that differentiate one group from another. It is often implied that behavioral characteristics, such as mental abilities and personality differences, are inherited along with the physical differences (S.J. Gould, 1981; Okazaki and Sue, 1995; Schaefer, 1998). Human history makes this

Name_____   Sex_____   Age_____

Indicate hand preference	Always left	Usually left	No preference	Usually right	Always right
1. To write a letter legibly					
2. To throw a ball to hit a target					
3. To play a game requiring the use of a racquet					
4. At the top of a broom to sweep dust from the floor					
5. At the top of a shovel to move sand					
6. To hold a match when striking it					
7. To hold scissors to cut paper					
8. To hold thread to guide through the eye of a needle					
9. To deal playing cards					
10 To hammer a nail into wood					
11. To hold a toothbrush while cleaning teeth					
12. To unscrew the lid of a jar					

Are either of your parents left-handed? If yes, which? _____
How many siblings of each sex do you have? Male _____ Female _____
How many of each sex are left-handed? Male _____ Female _____
Which eye do you use when using only one (e.g., telescope, keyhole)? _____
Have you ever suffered any severe head trauma? _____

FIGURE 8.3 *The handedness inventory.* (Modified from Annett, 1967. Source: Briggs and Nebes, 1975)

position untenable. Given the migrations, explorations, and invasions of peoples over the ages, there are no genetically isolated distinct groups (Kristof, 2003; Schaefer, 1998; Schwartz, 2001). Individuals belonging to any designated racial group may have ancestors who originated in different world regions. In actuality, within-group variations in physical and behavioral characteristics are tremendous, much more so than variations between groups (Zuckerman, 1990). Thus designation of race is to some degree arbitrary. Sometimes a legal–cultural definition (e.g., degree of "blood") identifies individuals as belonging to a particular racial group, but such definitions vary by community and country. In clinical practice and psychological research, individuals usually self-identify as belonging to a particular racial group spontaneously or in response to categories given by the examiner. These "racial" categories may mix racial, ethnic, and cultural groups, as is the case with the labels *black, white,*

Latino, Asian, and *American Indian.* Latinos, for instance, can belong to any of these categories or any combination of them (Betancourt and Lopez, 1993). Others disagree, citing research indicating that racial categorizations are associated with some genetic differentiation and susceptibility to disease (Risch et al., 2002). Finally, race is not in itself an explanatory variable since it is often confounded with culture, language, educational attainment, environmental, and socioeconomic factors (Betancourt and Lopez, 1993; Olmedo, 1981).

It cannot be assumed that differences between designated racial groups in cognition, personality, or other aspects of human behavior have a genetic, i.e., biologically determined, basis (S.J. Gould, 1981). Nowhere has this issue been more hotly contested and still not resolved than with respect to the measurement of cognitive abilities (Fraser, 1995; Herrnstein and Murray, 1994; Mackintosh, 1998). Much attention has been given to the higher performance of Americans of only European ancestry when compared to Americans of African—and mostly also European—ancestry on some cognitive tests (e.g., A.S. Kaufman, McLean, and Reynolds, 1988), but African Americans have also been and continue to be more socioeconomically disadvantaged (Amante et al., 1977). Yet, for years other such group comparisons have been made with the results favoring various groups, for instance, Chinese and Japanese over persons of European ancestry (e.g., R. Lynn, 1991; B.J. Stone, 1992). Furthermore, factor analytic studies demonstrate congruent factor structures indicating that the underlying abilities are identical for white and black groups (A.S. Kaufman, McLean, and Reynolds, 1991; Faulstich, McAnulty, et al., 1987).

Much of this discussion has focused on the degree to which variations in cognitive abilities are inherited or the result of environmental influences. Such factors as socioeconomic level, prenatal and perinatal complications, nutrition and health, family size, birth order, and education have been shown to be correlated with cognitive performance (Broman and Fletcher, 1999, *passim*; C.A. Nelson, 2000, *passim*). Cognitive differences between groups that tend to be demonstrated repeatedly, regardless of their origin, should be of concern to clinicians. These differences raise the possibility of an increased rate of misdiagnoses of impairment, particularly in neurological disorders such as dementia, when a single set of norms is applied to all groups (Gladsjo, Schuman, et al., 1999).

Culture typically refers to learned experiences that form a way of life shared by a group of people (Rohner, 1984). Culture is transmitted in social interactions that communicate social norms, roles, beliefs, and values and by socially created aspects of the environment such as architecture, art, and tools (Betancourt and Lopez, 1993). The evaluation of patients' reponses in a neuropsychological examination must take into account the contributions of their social and cultural experiences and attitudes to test performance and to their feelings about and understanding of their condition (Anastasi and Urbina, 1997; Greenfield, 1997). For example, persons growing up under conditions of physical or cultural/social deprivation, without adequate medical care, nutrition, environmental stimulation, or other benefits of modern society are more prone to developmental and other childhood disorders that can affect brain function (C.A. Nelson, 2000, *passim*; R. Rao and Georgieff, 2000; Rosenzweig, 1999). These conditions may make them less resilient to brain damage incurred in adulthood (Jennett, Teasdale, and Knill-Jones, 1975).

When characteristics of cultural background or socioeconomic status are overlooked, test score interpretations are subject both to confusion of culturally determined ignorance or underdeveloped skills with brain dysfunction, giving rise to false positive errors, and to missing evidence of deficit on overlearned or overpractised behaviors resulting in false negative errors (Pérez-Arce, 1999). Poorly learned or insufficiently practiced skills can produce a test profile with a lot of scatter which may be misinterpreted as evidence of organic disease. Members of some subcultures that stress intellectual development at the expense of manual activities may be so clumsy and perplexed when doing tasks involving hand skills as to exhibit a large discrepancy between verbal and visuoconstructional test scores (Backman, 1972). On the one hand, a bright but shy farmhand may fail dismally on any task that requires speaking or writing. On the other hand, the test performance of a patient whose cognitive development was lopsided and who sustained brain injury involving her strongest abilities may show so little intertest variability as to appear, on casual observation, to be cognitively intact.

In urging clinicians to be sensitive to differences in cultural values and behavior, Pankratz and Kofoed (1988) gave us the example of the "geezer," a self-made, independent-minded, poorly educated but proud traditionalist who distrusts doctors of all kinds and their "ologies" so as to make him a reluctant, suspicious, and frequently uncooperative patient. In a similar vein, I. Shepard and Leathem (1999) found that the Maori in New Zealand would be more satisfied with their experience of a neuropsychological examination when given the choice of incorporating elements of the Maori culture such as family involvement, the opportunity for sharing background, and a blessing. It was also important for the staff to be aware of the Maori health model which involves a balance between spiritual, family, cognition, and physical elements. Unless treated with an appreciation of their values, ways of looking at things, and special concerns, the clinician risks compromising the care of such patients and perhaps losing them as patients altogether despite their medical or psychological needs.

Ethnicity generally refers to groups that have a common nationality, religion, language, or culture and has been confounded with *race* (Betancourt and Lopez, 1993; Okazaki and Sue, 1995). Ethnicity, like race and culture, is not an explanatory variable in itself. Without a valid demonstration that relevant cultural variables do differ between identified groups (e.g., Americans of Polish descent, Americans of German descent), ethnic differences cannot be used as an explanatory variable in research and must be used only with great caution in the individual case.

The Uses of Race/Ethnicity/Culture Designations

The mapping of the human genome and the DNA microarray are moving medical diagnosis and treatment of a variety of disorders into a new era. It may be possible eventually to identify the genes and their variants that influence (but do not completely determine) the risk of a disease or the response to a particular pharmacological intervention (Risch et al., 2002). It may be possible to determine an individual's genetic risk for many diseases and treatment responses with a *DNA microarray* (*DNA array, gene chip*) consisting of a "lawn of . . . DNA molecules (probes) that are tethered to a wafer no bigger than a thumbprint" (Friend and Stoughton, 2002). When arrays are designed to detect various genetic disorders, precise sources of infections, and the most appropriate drug treatment—and if DNA technology is cheap enough—the practice of medicine will be revolutionized.

In the meantime, we do not know the genetic makeup of each individual, diagnosis is far from perfect, and treatment is often by "trial-and error." Within these present limitations, racial designation may have some usefulness. If a particular disease is more frequent in a particular racial/ethnic/cultural group, then it raises the possibility of some genetic basis (e.g., sickle cell disease in persons of African descent [Sekul and Adams, 1997]). Alternatively, the increased frequency could be a result of environmental variables associated with living in a particular region or socioeconomic level or of ethnic/culturally related variables (e.g., the high mortality rate among Russian men). In any case, it can be argued that self-designation of racial and/or ethnic groups can be useful in identifying a genetic basis for disease risk and treatment response as well as the role of environmental and other variables (Risch et al., 2002).

The Language of Assessment

Bilingualism

Individuals who say that they speak two or more languages vary greatly in the relative knowledge of the languages they speak—from those who are truly bilingual to others with native knowledge of one language and barely passable comprehension and/or conversational facility with the other language. Those who spent their early years in one culture using one language and then, as adults, moved to another culture and adopted its language are likely to have different linguistic capabilities than those who spoke both languages from birth. Test instructions and concepts may be understood better when given in one as opposed to the other language and different test scores may result. Moreover, comfortably bilingual people may respond differently to the same questions depending upon the language in which they are presented (Hong et al., 2000). Even different symptoms may become prominent depending on the language of the examination (Marcos et al., 1973; Sabin, 1975). When the examination is not conducted in the patient's dominant language, inaccu-

rate diagnostic decisions may be made on the basis of the apparent symptoms rather than actual cognitive impairments. Experience working in a multicultural acute care setting has shown that just asking which is the patient's primary language or which language is preferred for testing is not an adequate way of deciding which language should be used [hjh]. If a patient's English appears to be adequate and the patient maintains that this is so when English is really a second language, the clinician who is not bilingual is likely to conduct the examination in English without further questioning.

Lydia Artiola i Fortuny, a bilingual neuropsychologist goes through a series of steps to decide on the language she will use (personal communication, hjh). Careful educational history-taking asks exactly how many years patients have been educated in their country of origin and in the country of residence. (Exceptions are foreign residents in a country for many years who attended a school using the language of their country of origin.) An informal interview includes a broad range of everyday topics discussed in both languages so that native competence in each language can be assessed. Formal language testing conducted in both languages includes Verbal Fluency (Letter and Semantic), the Boston Naming Test, WIS-A Vocabulary, the Token Test, and the Peabody Picture Vocabulary Test. The final decision about language dominance is based on the number of tests in which the individual excels in one vs. the other language and the information gained in the interview regarding educational and residence history. The interviewer must be bilingual and have native competence in each language. Ideally, the neuropsychologist is bilingual or can compare notes with a bilingual technician or colleague.

Regional linguistic variations

Linguistic subgroups (e.g., Mexican, Puerto Rican, Cuban Hispanics) and regional differences in any language can create problems for test administration, scoring, and interpretation. The clinician needs to be sensitive to the nuances of the languages spoken when moving from one region of a country to another or seeing patients from various linguistic groups and subgroups.

For instance, the words "pin" and "pen" when pronounced aloud are frequently pronounced the same way by Texans. As "pin" appears in Form 2 of a commonly used Selective Reminding Test format, this can become a problem for both administration and scoring as well as subsequent interpretation. If the examiner says "pin," and the patient appears to say "pen," the examiner must quickly decide whether this was an accurate response: Did the patient correctly perceive the word "pin" but has a Texas pronunciation that sounds like "pen"? If this is the case, "pin" was correctly recalled and should not be given on the next trial. Did the patient misperceive the word as pronounced by the examiner or remember it incorrectly? If either of these is the case, this response should be scored as an intrusion and the word "pin" repeated on the next trial. The clinician's decision will affect the final scores.

Test translation and development

Most people in the west (Europe and North America) live in countries with a dominant culture and language as well as a particular tradition for conducting clinical examinations, developing psychological tests, treating patients, and designing research. Moreover, Western culture and cultural biases about various population groups determine, in part, interpretations of symptoms and, sometimes, even the diagnoses and the treatments (Betancourt and Lopez, 1993; Garb, 1997; Marcos et al., 1973). The Western tradition of standardized testing, its psychometric and administration aspects, and many tests developed in Western countries have been exported to other cultures, sometimes in an indiscriminate manner that invites errors of interpretation on the part of the clinician and researcher (Ardila, 1995; Artiola i Fortuny and Mullaney, 1997; Olmedo, 1981; Rogler, 1999). Whether due to cultural insensitivity or naiveté, the consequences can be harmful.

When tests are translated literally, many problems can occur (Olmedo, 1981; Artiola i Fortuny and Mullaney, 1997). Item, construct, or method bias can compromise test validity (Van de Vijver and Hambleton, 1996). Poor wording, inappropriate item content, and inaccurate translation may introduce item bias. Translated items may sample different domains and have substantially different meanings and psychometric properties. Test developers need to be wary of items subject to regional variations in language, which can occur at phonological, lexical, syntactic, and semantic levels (Artiola i Fortuny and Mullaney, 1997). Method bias can enter a test protocol in many ways: by an unfamiliar stimulus and response format, in test instructions and administration, in the testing situation and its physical conditions, in patient variables such as motivation, in examiners' characteristics, and in the kind of communication taking place between examiner and patient. A multicultural, multilingual team is necessary for cross-cultural test development. Since cross-cultural differences may be evident in the conceptualization of a construct and the behaviors associated with it, an adaptation or an entirely new test may have to be developed to measure a construct.

In a Chinese medical school in 1986, a psychiatry resident was puzzled about the preponderance of "schizophrenic" patients she was seeing. Questioning disclosed that this diagnosis was arising from MMPI "testing" in which most Chinese patients received high scores on the Sc scale. This inventory had been translated quite literally from English.

The norms—developed on Minnesota citizens in the 1930s—were applied unquestioningly to Chinese patients, most of whom had survived the Cultural Revolution in which arbitrary attacks and deprivations were commonplace, and beliefs in interested spirits abounded. In 1986, many Sc items would be marked in the "abnormal" direction by persons who had lived through these ten years of fear, abuse, and hostile displacements of themselves and their families, who were anxiety-ridden or depressed, and who felt in touch with local spirits, but were not schizophrenic [mdl].

Ethical concerns in training and practice

In the United States, professional psychology training programs at all levels are expected to provide knowledge and experiences concerning cultural and individual diversity as it relates to psychological phenomena and professional practice (American Psychological Association, 2003). Practicing psychologists should be aware of ethical issues in test development, assessment, diagnosis, and intervention as they pertain to cultural and individual diversity (American Psychological Association, 2002; T.M. Wong et al., 2000). They should have a meaningful appreciation of the consequences that insensitivity to these issues can have for patients (Artiola i Fortuny and Mullaney, 1998; LaCalle, 1987). Several principles and standards from the American Psychological Association's *Ethical Principles of Psychologists* and *Code of Conduct* (2002) concern competence, integrity, professional and scientific responsibility, and nondiscriminating respect for people's rights and dignity and for human differences.

While these standards do not address language competence specifically they include it by implication (Artiola i Fortuny and Mullaney, 1998; LaCalle, 1987). Thus, when not fluent in the patient's language, ethical practice should lead the neuropsychologist to refer the patient to a colleague who is fluent in the patient's language or to collaborate with a bilingual clinician—not necessarily a clinical neuropsychologist—if at all possible. When the patient speaks an uncommon language, the use of an interpreter may be necessary, but caution should always be exercised in drawing conclusions from the findings.

PATIENT CHARACTERISTICS: PSYCHOSOCIAL VARIABLES

> It is not only the kind of injury that matters, but the kind of head.
>
> *Symonds, 1937*

Demographic, experiential, and some specific developmental and physical status variables (e.g., childhood nutrition, medications, seizure disorders) can significantly affect responses to a neuropsychological examination. Although these variables are dealt with singly in this book, they can and do attenuate, exacerbate, or simply complicate their mutually interactive effects on cognitive functioning and emotional status. No simple formula can be devised for teasing out their presence or the degree of their contribution to an individual patient's behavior. Rather, the clinician must be aware of what variables may be relevant in the individual case and sensitive to how they can affect examination behavior.

Premorbid Mental Ability

Nowhere is the fallacy of a nature–nurture dichotomy more out of place than in considering mental abilities: Brain size, as measured by MRI, correlates modestly (r = "approximately" .35) but consistently with summed scores from test sets (Bigler, 1995). Thus brain size contributes to premorbid ability level which, in turn, is closely tied to academic achievement and academic exposure (see *Education* and *Illiteracy*, below). No single variable in this complex stands alone; when considered conceptually, each is a product of its interaction with all the many inherent characteristics and environmental experiences and exposures that go into human development (e.g., see Huttenlocher, 2002; Pennington, 2002). Brain injury or disease, in reducing the amount and connectivity of brain tissue, also diminishes mental abilities and psychosocial competencies. The intimacy of these interactions shows up clearly in findings that the level of premorbid mental ability determines—to some extent—not only the amount of cognitive loss following injury (Bigler, 1995; Grafman, Lalonde, et al., 1989) but also the risk of dementia and the rate at which it evolves.

The cognitive reserve hypothesis

On reviewing consistent findings of a significant relationship between estimated or known premorbid ability and level of cognitive impairment with brain injury or disease, Satz (1993) proposed a "threshold theory," which postulates that the amount of *brain reserve capacity* (BRC) represents structural or physiological brain advantages (such as size, redundancy of interconnections) or disadvantages. BRC advantages will show up in higher educational levels, higher scores on mental ability tests both pre- and postmorbidly, and better functioning after brain injury or disease. Level of education, brain size, and academic achievement have all been found to be positively related to later and slower onset of Alzheimer's disease (Y. Stern, 2002). Bigler (1995) demonstrated that test scores and

brain volume were positively correlated in TBI patients. A greater learning capacity is one mechanism for greater cognitive enhancement in already bright people—the more you can learn, the more you learn or, to quote Rapport, Brines, and their colleagues (1997) on demonstrating that brighter subjects show greater practice effects than those with lower test scores: "The rich get richer."

Education

The effects of education on neuropsychological functioning are potent and pervasive (e.g., Heaton, Grant, and Matthews, 1991; Heaton, Ryan, et al., 1996; Ivnik, Malec, Smith, et al., 1996; Malec, Ivnik, Smith, et al., 1992a; Mitrushina, Boone, D'Elia, 1999, *passim*). While education effects have been amply demonstrated for verbal tests, they also show up on just about every other kind of test involving cognitive abilities, including some that would seem to be relatively unaffected by schooling (e.g., Benton Visual Retention Test [Coman et al., 1999]; Digit Span [Karakas et al., 2002]; spatial memory [Capitani, Barbarotto, and Laiacona, 1996]; a cancellation task [Le Carret et al., 2003]; and even copying simple line drawings with sticks [Matute et al., 2000]). Le Carret and his collaborators (2003) found that education was associated with greater control over processing and with conceptualization ability, capacities inherent in substantial cognitive reserve. Their potency becomes obvious when one subject group has had significantly less education than comparison groups or the population on which the test had been developed.

This was the case for a sample of rural Nicaraguan males, of whom 74% had at most three years of schooling (Anger, 1992; Anger, Cassito, Liang, 1993). When compared with groups of men from nine other countries (e.g., People's Republic of China, Hungary), all of whom had a minimum of eight years of education, the Nicaruagans consistently performed at levels significantly below any others, even on tests that would seem relatively invulnerable to education effects such as digit span, Digit Symbol, and a test of visuomotor coordination. Only on a dexterity test did the Nicaraguans' performances approach those of the other groups.

Education can so greatly influence test performances that poorly educated but cognitively intact persons may get lower scores than mildly impaired but better educated patients, or they may perform within a range of "impairment" based on samples of healthy persons whose educational levels approximate that of the general population of the country in which the test was developed.

For example, using the recommendation that scores below cut-offs in the mid to high 20s indicate impaired cognitive functioning on the Mini-Mental State Examination (MMSE), most of a group of healthy rural-dwelling adults with less than seven years of education would seem to be cognitively impaired (Marcopulos, McLain, and Giuliano, 1997). Moreover, most of this study's subjects in the 55 to 74 age range who had less than five years of school made scores lower than a group of older ($M_{\text{age}} = 76.4$) diagnosed dementia patients averaging 11 years of education (Mast et al., 2001).

On finding that some poorly educated persons—particularly those with eight or fewer school years—may be misclassified as demented on the basis of test scores alone, Y. Stern, Andrews, and their colleagues (1992) recommended that behavioral data, such as activities of daily living, also be taken into account. Illiteracy, the extreme condition of educational deprivation, demonstrates the importance of education to brain development and cognitive competence (see below).

However, brain injury can attenuate education effects (Zillmer, Waechtler, et al., 1992), or education may have positive effects for only some patients. For soldiers with bullet wounds to the brain, education was associated with higher posttrauma test scores only for those whose general ability level fell below the group mean, a phenomenon that may reflect "motivation" and persistence in learning "that enabled these less bright men to become academic achievers" (Grafman, Jonas, et al., 1988).

Many people in the United States now have the General Education Degree (GED) certificate rather than a high school diploma. When evaluation of their test performances requires an educational level, the examiner may want to follow the practice of Prof. Charles Matthews who simply gave them the 12 years of credit to which their passed examination entitles them. When taking years of education into account, it may sometimes be necessary to pay attention to the quality of that education as well as the years, as similar grade levels may have quite different knowledge and skill implications as attested by the generally higher achievement levels of children in suburban schools compared with those from inner city or small rural schools [hjh]. This point was clearly demonstrated in lower reading levels and test-wiseness of elderly African-Americans compared with whites matched for age and education, as school quality for many African-Americans differed greatly from that of their white peers when these subjects were young (Manly, Jacobs, Touradji, et al., 2002).

Illiteracy

Illiteracy can affect the development of cognitive abilities, processing strategies, processing pathways, and functional brain organization (Castro-Caldas, Peter-

sson, et al., 1998; Ostrosky-Solis, Ardila, and Rosselli, 1999; Reis and Castro-Caldas, 1997). Illiterate persons tend to give poorer performances in many cognitive domains (Manly, Jacobs, Touradji, 2002; Ostrosky-Solis, et al., 1999; Salmon, Jin, et al., 1995). For instance, real objects may be named correctly by persons with no formal schooling while they are likely to make noticeably more errors naming photographs and especially line drawings (Lecours, Mehler, et al., 1987; Reis, Guerreiro, and Castro-Caldas, 1994). Illiterate individuals may have had little exposure to two-dimensional representations and the more abstract representation of a line drawing. They may not be competent in using a pen or pencil and thus have difficulty making the simple drawings that can be found in screening instruments such as the MMSE (Katzman, Zhang, et al., 1988). To give another example, a lack of knowledge of the grapheme–phoneme correspondence acquired through reading can result in poorer phonological processing in an adult and have consequences for functional organization of the brain. Illiterate individuals are apt to have difficulty repeating pseudowords, memorizing phonologically as opposed to semantically related word pairs in a paired associate learning task, and generating words beginning with a particular phoneme in a verbal fluency task (Reis and Castro-Caldas, 1997). Repetition of real words has been shown to activate similar brain regions in illiterate and literate individuals, while pseudowords do not (Castro-Caldas et al., 1998).

Normative data infrequently include individuals with very low levels of education or illiterate individuals (Artiola i Fortuny, Romo, et al., 1999; Ivnik, Malec, Smith, et al., 1992a–c). Individuals with less than ten years of education often are treated as a homogeneous group (Gladsjo, Schuman, et al., 1999; Mitrushina, Boone, and D'Elia, 1999, pp. 38–40, 69, 82, 137, 196, 197, and *passim*). Since the effects of education may be negatively accelerated (i.e., be greater as the educational level goes down), the impact on test performances is likely to be magnified at the lower end of the educational continuum (Ostrosky-Solis, Ardila, et al., 1998). Failure to develop appropriate test norms for individuals who are illiterate or have a very low level of education can lead to an overestimation of mental disorders such as dementia (LeCours, Mehler, et al., 1987; Katzman, Zhang, et al., 1988). This problem is likely to be particularly evident among some ethnic/cultural groups, older individuals, and those from rural settings who have had less opportunity for educational attainment or exposure to the culture at large (Artiola i Fortuny, Romo, et al., 1999; Marcopulos, McLain, and Giuliano, 1997). For this reason, functional measures should be included when giving a comprehensive neuropsychological examination for dementia to persons with little or no schooling (Loewenstein, Rubert, et al., 1995; Salmon, Jin, et al., 1995).

Premorbid Personality and Social Adjustment

The premorbid personal and social adjustment of brain impaired patients also can have an effect, not only on the quality of their ultimate adjustment but also on the amount of gain they make when benefiting from good work habits and high levels of expectation for themselves (Newcombe, 1982). Premorbid personality can contribute both directly and indirectly to the kind of adjustment a patient makes following brain injury (Lezak, 1989; Lishman, 1973; Tate, 1998).

Direct effects are fairly obvious since premorbid personality characteristics may not be so much changed as exaggerated by brain injury (M.R. Bond, 1984; J.M. Silver et al., 2002). Impulsivity, anger outbursts, or other forms of acting out and disinhibited behavior can be symptomatic of significant frontal lobe damage in a premorbidly benign and well-socialized person. However, when these disruptive behavioral traits have been present premorbidly—as is so often the case among the young, poorly educated males who comprise a large proportion of the moderately to severely damaged TBI population—they can contribute to some of the severe behavioral disturbances found among this group of brain damaged persons (M.R. Bond, 1984; Grafman, Lalonde, et al., 1989; Prigatano, 1987). However, Tate (1998) found that TBI severity was the overriding outcome predictor for both poorly socialized and adequately socialized patients. Tendencies to dependent behavior, hypochondriasis, passivity, perfectionism, irresponsibility, etc., can be major obstacles to patients whose rehabilitation depends on active relearning of old skills and reintegration of old habit patterns while they cope with a host of unrelenting and often humiliating frustrations.

The indirect effects of premorbid adjustment may not become apparent until the handicapped patient needs emotional support and acceptance in a protective but not institutional living situation (S.P. Kaplan, 1990). Patients who have conducted their lives in an emotionally stable and mature manner are also those most likely to be supported through critical personal and social transitions by steadfast, emotionally stable, and mature family and friends. In contrast, patients with marked premorbid personality disorders or asocial tendencies are more apt to lack a social support system when they need it most. Many of this latter group have been social isolates, and others are quickly rejected by immature or recently acquired spouses, alienated children, and opportunistic or irresponsible friends who want nothing of a dependent patient who can no longer cater to their needs. The importance of a stable home environment to rehabilitation often becomes inescapable when determining whether a patient can return to the community or must be placed in a nursing home or institution.

Medication

In the outpatient setting, many patients take medications, whether for a behavioral or mood disturbance, tension, anxiety, sleep disturbance, or neurological or other medical disorder. Others may be treating themselves with nonprescription cold or headache remedies or an over-the-counter (OTC) analgesic. The effects of medications on different aspects of behavior can significantly alter assessment findings and may even constitute the reason for the emotional or cognitive changes that have brought the patient to neuropsychological attention. Not only may medications in themselves complicate a patient's neuropsychological status, but some combinations or incorrect dosages of drugs can further complicate the complications (Andrewes, Schweitzer, et al., 1990; Bjorkman et al., 2002). In the treatment of epilepsy, where physicians have long been sensitive to cognitive side effects of antiepileptic drugs (AEDs), the goal is always to use multiple medications only as a last resort and to use the lowest efficacious dosage (Meador, 2002). This is the ideal goal for every other kind of medical disorder but is not always realized.

A 56-year-old sawmill worker with a ninth grade education was referred to an urban medical center with complaints of visual disturbances, dizziness, and mental confusion. A review of his recent medical history quickly identified the problem as he had been under the care of several physicians. The first treated the man's recently established seizure disorder with phenytoin (Dilantin), which made him feel sluggish. He went to a second physician with complaints of sluggishness and his seizure history but neglected to report that he was already on an anticonvulsant, so phenytoin was again prescribed and the patient now took both prescriptions. The story repeated itself once again so that by the time his problem was identified he had been taking three times the normal dose for some weeks. Neurological and neuropsychological examinations found pronounced nystagmus and impaired visual scanning, cerebellar dysfunction, and an attentional disorder (digits forward/backward = 4/4; WAIS Arithmetic = 8, WAIS Comprehension = 13 probably is a good indicator of premorbid functioning), and some visuospatial compromise (WAIS Block Design = 8 [age-corrected], see Fig. 8.4, p. 318). Off all medications, he made gains in visual, cerebellar, and cognitive functioning but never enough to return to his potentially dangerous job.

Delirium occurs in 7% of inpatients examined by neurologists (H. Moses and Kaden, 1986). Although

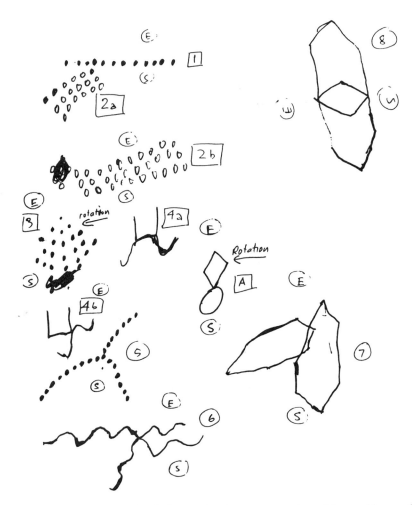

FIGURE 8.4 Copies of the Bender-Gestalt designs drawn on one page by a 56-year-old sawmill worker with phenytoin toxicity.

the causes of such a severe mental status disorder in this group are often multiple, medication effects alone may be responsible in as many as 17% of these patients. Unfortunately, although these cases of delirium are often considered to be "reversible dementia," they are in fact better conceptualized as "treatable" since patients rarely completely return to baseline (Larson et al., 1984).

The effect of medications on cognitive functioning is a broad and complex issue involving many different classes of drugs and numerous medical and psychiatric disorders. Although many medications can be associated with cognitive impairment, the drugs with the highest incidence of cognitive side effects are anticholinergics, benzodiazepines, narcotics, neuroleptics, antiepileptic drugs, and sedative-hypnotics (Meador, 1998a,b; R.A. Stein and Strickland, 1998). Even nonprescription (in the United States) antihistamines may produce significant cognitive effects (G.G. Kay and Quig, 2001; R.A. Stein and Strickland, 1998). Nevertheless, medications differ within each drug class, and newer agents are likely to have fewer cognitive side effects. The reader needing information on specific drug effects or on medications used for particular medical or psychiatric conditions should consult the current volume of the American Medical Association's *Drug Evaluations Annual*, Blain and Lane (1991) in D.M. Davies *Textbook of Adverse Drug Reactions*, the *Compendium of Drug Therapy*, the *Physicians' Desk Reference (PDR), Goodman and Gilman's The Pharmacological Basis of Therapeutics* (Hardman et al., 2001), or similar medication reviews. Commonly prescribed medications for psychiatric and some neurologic disorders are reviewed in P.F. Smith and Darlington's (1996) *Clinical Psychopharmacology* and Stahl's (2002) *Essential Psychopharmacology of Antipsychotics and*

Mood Stabilizers. This latter book goes into some detail describing how these medications work at the intracellular and neurotransmitter levels. A sampling of neuropsychologically relevant drug effects appears in the sections on hypertension (pp. 202–203), Parkinson's disease (pp. 233–234), tumors (pp. 280–281), and epilepsy (pp. 322–323); these should give some sense of the variety and clinical presentations of adverse medication reactions.

Examiners should also be aware that it often takes patients several weeks to adjust to a new drug, and they experience changes in mental efficiency in the interim. Geriatric patients are particularly susceptible to drug reactions that can affect—usually negatively—some aspect(s) of cognitive functioning, alertness, or general activity level (Godwin-Austen and Bendall, 1990). Factors associated with the increased risk of cognitive impairment associated with medication use in elderly persons include imbalances in neurotransmitter systems such as acetylcholine, age-related changes in pharmacodynamics and pharmacokinetics, and high levels of concomitant medication use (S.L. Gray et al., 1999). Elderly people are often on multiple medications (on average seven different drugs according to one report [Bjorkman et al., 2002]), which by itself is a significant risk factor. Complicating matters, patients are often poor historians about what drugs they are taking, their doses, or their dosing intervals (Chung and Bartfield, 2002).

The anticholinergic action of some drugs used in Parkinson's disease or for depression can interfere with memory and, in otherwise mentally intact elderly persons, create the impression of cognitive dilapidation or greatly exacerbate existing dementia (Pondal et al., 1996; R.L. Taylor, 1990; Vollhardt et al., 1992). Brain injury may also increase susceptibility to adverse cognitive reactions to various medications (Cope, 1988; O'Shanick and Zasler, 1990). Brain injury certainly makes drug effects less predictable than for neurologically intact persons (Eames et al., 1990). In many instances, the treating physician must weigh the desired goal of medication—such as the amelioration of anxiety or depression, seizure control, or behavioral calming—against one or another kind of cognitive compromise. Monitoring the neuropsychological status of patients who might benefit from medications known to affect cognition can provide for an informed weighing of these alternatives.

Epilepsy

Etiology and diagnostic classifications

Epilepsy is not a single disease or condition but reflects an episodic disturbance of behavior or perception arising from hyperexcitability and hypersynchronous discharge of nerve cells in the brain that can be associated with a variety of etiologies. Thus, the different syndromes associated with epilepsy are often collectively referred to as "epilepsies" to reflect this heterogeneity. The underlying causes are many and relate to scarring or brain injury from birth trauma, TBI, tumor, the consequences of infection or illness (e.g., complex febrile seizures), metabolic disorder, CVA, progressive brain disease, or a host of other conditions, including genetic factors.

Epilepsy is among the most prevalent of the chronic neurological disorders, affecting approximately 1% of the population or over two million Americans (Hauser and Hesdorffer, 1990), with 30% of incidence cases younger than 18 at diagnosis (G.L. Holmes and Engel, 2001). The annual total cost for the 2.3 million Americans with epilepsy is approximately $12.5 billion. Indirect costs due to the psychosocial morbidity of epilepsy account for 85% of this total with direct costs concentrated among patients with intractable epilepsies (Begley et al., 2000). The public health implications of epilepsy are substantial and have been documented through targeted initiatives and conferences sponsored by the National Institute of Neurological Disorders and Stroke (2002), the Centers for Disease Control and Prevention (1997), and the Agency for Healthcare Research and Quality (2001).

Seizures can arise from any condition that heightens the excitability of brain tissue and may be associated with high fever, drug use, drug withdrawal, and metabolic disorders. Epilepsy, in contrast, requires the presence of at least two unprovoked seizures (i.e., occurring in the absence of acute systemic illness or brain insult). Unfortunately, the diagnosis of epilepsy continues to carry with it a large psychosocial burden, and consequently, the term *seizure disorder* is often used to soften social stigma.

Epilepsies are generally classified along two dimensions—whether they are focal or generalized, and whether their etiology is known, suspected, or unknown (International League against Epilepsy, 1989; Tran et al., 1998). Seizures that have a localized area of onset are called *partial* or *focal,* and seizures that appear to involve large regions of both hemispheres simultaneously are referred to as *generalized.* Etiology is characterized as idiopathic, cryptogenic, or symptomatic. *Idiopathic* epilepsies have no known etiology and usually are not associated with any other neurologic disorders, and consequently, neuropsychological deficits are generally absent (Perrine, Gershengorm, and Brown, 1991). Etiologies of *cryptogenic* epilepsy are also unknown, but neurologic and neuropsychological functions are usually not normal. Seizures from a known etiology are called *symptomatic.* In clinical practice, however, a syndrome diagnosis is often given (e.g., temporal lobe epilepsy, Landau-Kleffner syndrome, juvenile myoclonic epilepsy), which also more narrowly characterizes individual patients as to prognosis and treatment options (Wyllie and Lüders, 1997). A newer classification system has attempted to combine EEG, etiology, and syndrome approaches (Hamer and Lüders, 2001).

Partial seizures arise from a specific focal area of the brain, may be *simple* without any alteration of consciousness, and may involve only one mode of expression (motor, somatosensory, autonomic, or psychic). *Complex partial seizures*, by definition, involve altered consciousness. In addition, it is not uncommon for a partial seizure to progress. For example, a seizure may be preceded by an aura (simple partial seizure) and then develop into a complex partial seizure. This may subsequently progress to involve the entire brain, a process called *secondary generalization* (e.g., secondary generalized tonic-clonic seizure). The most common site for complex partial seizures to originate is the temporal lobes followed by the frontal lobes. In practice, however, it is sometimes difficult to distinguish frontal lobe from temporal lobe seizures due to the direct projections between these areas.

Primary generalized seizures involve all or large portions of both hemispheres from seizure onset. They may be *nonconvulsive*, appearing as *absence* spells (*petit mal attacks*) in which consciousness is briefly lost while eyes blink or roll up, or *convulsive*, which involves major motor manifestations (*generalized tonic-clonic seizures*, or *grand mal seizures*). Note that the term *absence* is reserved for nonconvulsive primary generalized seizures and is not used when loss of awareness occurs with complex partial seizures. The distinction between focal and generalized seizures has practical implications since different seizure types often respond to different anticonvulsant medications (*antiepileptic drugs: AEDs*).

Specific EEG patterns are associated with many epilepsy syndromes and assist in formal diagnosis (e.g., 3 Hz spike and wave complexes in absence seizures; see Klass and Westmoreland, 2002), although some seizure patients may at times have normal EEG recordings. EEG monitoring is also important for determining if a patient's spells may be psychogenic or due to a nonneurologic conditions such as fainting (*syncope*). EEG characteristics are important in evaluations of a patient's candidacy for epilepsy surgery (Cascino, 2002).

Risk factors and vulnerabilities

Genetic predisposition. Epilepsy may run in families, appearing either in conjunction with an inheritable condition which makes the patient seizure-prone or simply as an inherited predisposition to seizures. It is interesting that different seizure types can occur in family members who have epilepsy (Berkovic et al., 1998; Choeiri et al., 2001; Ottman et al., 1998). Genetic factors appear to be more important in the generalized epilepsies but also play a role in some partial epilepsies (Berkovic et al., 1998). Studies of twins have shown a higher concordance rate among monozygotic twins compared to dizygotic twins. However, the mode of inheritance is complex and varies with seizure types and epilepsy syndromes. Evidence is accumulating that pathogenesis of many forms of epilepsy reflects a channel pathology at the microphysiologic level, with K^+, Na^+, or Ca^{2+} channels being affected in different types of epilepsies (Kaneko et al., 2002).

Posttraumatic epilepsy. The risk of developing epilepsy following penetrating head wounds is high. A notably lower incidence of epilepsy among World War II survivors of missile wounds to the brain (25% to 30%) was seen than among Vietnam War survivors (53%) (Newcombe, 1969; Salazar, Jabbari, and Vance, 1985; A.E. Walker and Jablon, 1961). This may reflect a lower survival rate for the severely injured patients, as TBI in itself increases the risk of developing epilepsy, and severity contributes significantly to that risk (Jennett, 1990).

Brain contusion, subdural hematoma, skull fracture, loss of consciousness or amnesia for more than one day, and an age of at least 65 years increased the risk of developing posttraumatic seizures in a civilian TBI patient study (Annegers, Hauser, et al., 1998). In general, the presence of any focal lesion, such as intracerebral hemorrhage and hematomas, increases the likelihood of posttraumatic epilepsy (D'Alessandro et al., 1988; Jennett, 1990). A slight seizure risk for patients following mild TBI does persist after five years (Annegers, Hauser, et al., 1998). In contrast, severe TBI is associated with a much higher posttraumatic seizure risk that is much more longstanding; the first unprovoked seizure may occur more than 10 years after the injury. Although a seizure in the first week after a penetrating head injury is not necessarily predictive of eventual posttraumatic epilepsy, 25% of TBI patients who have a seizure in the first week will have seizures later. However, only 3% of patients who do not have an early seizure will develop late-onset seizures. The cognitive impairment seen in posttraumatic seizure patients probably reflects the effects of the brain injuries that give rise to seizures, rather than effects of the seizures (Haltiner et al., 1996; Pincus and Tucker, 2003).

Other symptomatic epilepsies. Any other kind of insult to the brain also increases susceptibility to seizures (A. Hopkins, 1981; Lishman, 1997). Approximately

10% of all stroke patients experience seizures (Bladin and Norris, 1997; T.S. Olsen, 2001; Silverman et al., 2002), with roughly half of these occurring during the first day and the other half peaking between 6 and 12 months post-CVA event. Seizures occur three times more often following hemorrhagic stroke than ischemic stroke and are usually associated with cortical involvement. Few stroke patients (3%–4%) develop epilepsy; those with late-onset seizures are at greater risk (Bladin, Alexandrov, et al., 2000). Epilepsy can also occur with CNS infections, brain tumors, and degenerative dementia (Annegers, 1996).

Precipitating conditions. Although most seizures happen without apparent provocation, some conditions and stimuli are associated with increasing seizure likelihood. The disinhibiting effects of alcohol can provoke a seizure, as can the physiological alterations that occur with alcohol withdrawal during the "hangover" period and alcohol interactions with medications (Kreutzer, Doherty et al., 1990). Alcohol withdrawal seizures usually develop after prolonged alcohol abuse; the alcoholic patient suddenly stops drinking and generalized convulsions typically occur 48–72 hours later. Physical debilitation, whether from illness, lack of sleep, or physical exhaustion increases the likelihood of seizures. In some women with epilepsy, seizure frequency varies with the menstrual cycle (i.e., *catamenial epilepsy*) (Tauboll et al., 1991). This phenomenon appears to be related to the ratio of estrogen to progesterone. Emotional stress, too, has been implicated as a provocative factor, and seizures may be also be affected by voluntary and spontaneous changes in behavior and thinking (Fenwick and Brown, 1989). *Reflex epilepsy* refers to epilepsies characterized by a specific mode of seizure precipitation, the most common of which is photosensitivity although other precipitants have been reported, such as hearing the voice of a specific female TV celebrity (Mary Hart!) (Ramani, 1991) or even eating (Ahuja et al., 1988). Video games and watching television may also trigger seizures (Badinand-Hubert et al., 1998; Ricci et al., 1998).

Cognitive functioning

Behavior and cognition in epilepsy patients can be affected by multiple factors, including: seizure etiology, type, frequency, duration, and severity; cerebral lesions acquired prior to seizure onset; age at seizure onset; ictal and interictal physiological dysfunction due to the seizures; structural cerebral damage due to repetitive or prolonged seizures; hereditary factors; psychosocial conditions; and antiepileptic drug effects (Lennox, 1942; Lesser et al., 1986; Loring and Meador, 2001;

Meador, 2001). Overall, patients with epilepsy tend to have impaired cognition compared to matched control subjects (D.B. Smith et al., 1986).

Seizure etiology is a principal factor affecting cognitive abilities (Perrine et al., 1991). Patients with seizures due to progressive cerebral degeneration typically have generalized cognitive impairment, patients with mental retardation have an increased incidence of epilepsy, and patients with seizures due to a focal brain lesion may exhibit a specific neuropsychological pattern of deficits. In contrast, patients with idiopathic epilepsy are more likely to have normal mental abilities (Perrine et al., 1991). Similarly, seizure type is strongly associated with cognitive performance (Huttenlocher and Hapke, 1990). Patients with *juvenile myoclonic epilepsy* (*JME*) showing classic 3 Hz spike and wave absence usually have normal cognitive abilities interictally; children with infantile spasms have generally depressed neuropsychological profiles. Earlier seizure onset age is associated with greater cognitive impairment (Hermann, Seidenberg, and Bell, 2002). Patients with mental retardation are more likely to have refractory epilepsy (Dodrill, 1992; Huttenlocher and Hapke, 1990).

Focal seizures and cognitive dysfunction. Focal seizures originate from one side of the brain, although seizure activity may subsequently spread to other brain areas. In some cases, patients with focal seizure onset display a pattern of test performance like that of patients with nonepileptogenic lesions in similar locations. Thus, seizure onset from the left hemisphere may be associated with impaired verbal functions, including verbal memory deficits and some compromise in abstract reasoning. Patients with right hemisphere seizure onset are more likely to display visuoperceptual, visual memory, and constructional disabilities. However, the magnitude of the deficits is often less than with comparable nonepileptic lesions. Atypical cerebral language reorganization resulting from early seizure onset may affect the lateralizing and localizing patterns on neuropsychological tests (Gleissner et al., 2002; Loring, Strauss, et al., 1999; Seidenberg, Hermann, et al., 1997; E. Strauss, Satz, and Wada, 1990). In addition, many AEDs depress neuropsychological test performance, particularly for those measures that are timed or have a prominent motor component (Dodrill and Temkin, 1989; Meador, 1998a,b). The magnitude of lateralized behavioral deficits may be more pronounced when testing occurs during the immediate postictal period (Andrewes, Puce, and Bladin, 1990; Meador and Moser, 2000; Privitera et al., 1991).

Memory. Memory and learning disorders are common among epilepsy patients (Helmstaedter and Kurthen, 2001; Milner, 1975; P.J. Thompson and Trimble, 1996). They become most pronounced with temporal lobe epilepsy (TLE), reflecting the degree of medial temporal lobe pathology (Helmstaedter, Grunwald, et al., 1997; Rausch and Babb, 1993; Trenerry, Westerveld, and Meador, 1995). Material specific memory deficits occur primarily for verbal memory in association with left TLE (Barr, Chelune, et al., 1997; Hermann, Seidenberg, Schoenfeld, and Davies, 1997; T.M. Lee et al., 2002; Rausch and Babb, 1993). As with other neuropsychological functions, there is a risk to memory with some AEDs which increases with multiple medications (*polypharmacy*) (Meador, Gilliam, et al., 2001).

Personality and emotional behavior

Although the psychosocial behavior and emotional status of many persons with seizure disorders do not differ from normal, behavior and personality disorders are much more common among seizure patients, with estimates of psychiatric comorbidity ranging from 29% to 50% (Lishman, 1997; Tucker, 2002; Trimble, 1983, 1989). All behavioral disorders seem to appear with greater frequency among seizure patients than in the general population. For example, seizure patients are more likely to suffer affective disorders, particularly depression; and they have a higher rate of suicide attempts (Pincus and Tucker, 2003; D.C. Taylor, 1989; see Blumer and Altschuler, 1997, for a comprehensive review). The incidence of psychosis and psychiatric hospitalization is elevated (P.J. McKenna et al., 1985; Pincus and Tucker, 2003; J.R. Stevens, 1991; Trimble, 1983). Psychiatric symptoms and other behavioral disorders tend to increase with indices of severity such as seizure frequency (Csernansky et al., 1990; Pincus and Tucker, 2003) and a pattern of seizures of multiple types (Hermann and Whitman, 1986; R.J. Roberts, Paulsen et al., 1988). Persons whose epilepsy is associated with known brain injury (symptomatic epilepsy) are more prone to emotional and behavioral disturbances than those with idiopathic seizures (Hermann and Whitman, 1986).

The generally high rates of psychiatric comorbidity among epilepsy patients reflect more than just the underlying brain dysfunction (Hermann and Whitman, 1992; Tucker, 2002; Whitman and Herman, 1986, *passim*). By virtue of having a condition that may be due to brain injury—often incurred early in life—that places restrictions on many activities, limits employment opportunities, and frequently is associated with social stigma, persons with epilepsy tend to have lower levels of education and socioeconomic status, poorer work histories, and fewer social supports than healthy persons (Dodrill, 1986; Zielinski, 1986). Moreover, sources of distress often experienced by epilepsy patients include fear of seizures, concerns about activity restrictions (e.g., driving) and their consequences, and emotional reactions to social stigma, all of which can contribute to emotional disturbances and diminished quality of life (Whitman and Hermann, 1986, *passim*). However, these social and intrapersonal variables cannot account for the much greater number of emotional and psychosocial disorders among persons with temporal lobe epilepsy than any other seizure group (Lishman, 1997; P.J. McKenna et al., 1985; Trimble, 1989).

Temporal lobe epilepsy. A relationship between personality and temporal lobe epilepsy was described by Waxman and Geschwind (1975) in which some patients displayed excessive verbal output, circumstantial thinking, stickiness or viscosity in thinking and social interactions, hypergraphia, altered sexuality (usually hyposexuality), and intensified mental life (obsessional cognitive and spiritual/religious ideation) (see also p. 76). However, whether this syndrome is a distinctive personality disorder continues to be a controversial issue (Benson, 1991; Blumer, 1999; Devinsky and Najjar, 1999). Selection bias may be one factor contributing to the reported relationship between epilepsy and psychopathology (Hermann and Whitman, 1992).

Depression is reported more frequently in patients with temporal lobe epilepsy and left-sided foci, although not all studies support this finding (Harden, 2002). When depression occurs in TLE, it may involve more "negative" than "positive" depression symptoms (Getz et al., 2002). Generally, depression can be treated with antidepressant medications. In cases of psychotic depression, ECT can be considered (Harden, 2002).

Aggression in epilepsy. One concern that has received much attention over the years is the possible relationship between epilepsy and aggression or criminal behavior. What has often been described as violence or aggression may appear in postictal confusion or postictal psychosis (Kanemoto et al., 1999). Although postictal psychotic aggression is usually not severe, when it is driven by prominent delusions and hallucinations, it can result in self-destructive acts or serious violence (Fenwick, 1989). Interictally, epilepsy patients display episodes of aggressiveness that are no more common than in other populations with comparable neurologic disease (Pincus and Tucker, 2003). Planned, directed aggression related to seizures is distinctly unusual in epilepsy patients (Treiman, 1986, 1991).

Antiepileptic drug effects

AEDs are designed to reduce neuronal irritability. In addition to their effects on abnormal brain activity, however, AEDs decrease normal neuronal excitability, which may affect cognitive function. Fortunately, the cognitive side effects of AED monotherapy are generally not pronounced when anticonvulsant blood levels are maintained within the standard therapeutic range (Meador, 2001). Cognitive side effects may be partially offset in patients with frequent seizures simply by virtue of their therapeutic effects on seizure control. The risk of significant cognitive side effects increases, however, with increasing drug dosages (anticonvulsant blood levels) and when multiple AEDs are necessary to obtain seizure relief (Meador, Gilliam, et al., 2001; see Fig. 8.4).

The neuropsychological functions most likely to be adversely affected by AEDs are psychomotor speed, vigilance, memory, and mood (P.J. Thompson and Trimble, 1996). Interpretation of much of the older literature on cognitive side effects is difficult due to the many design confounds such as nonrandom assignment to treatment conditions and nonequivalence of drug doses (Dodrill and Troupin, 1991). For the older anticonvulsant medications, the most pronounced effects show up with barbiturates and benzodiazepines, but smaller and less consistent problems have been associated with carbamazepine, phenytoin, and valproate (Meador, 1998a, 2001). The cognitive profiles of the newer AEDs continue to be established. Generally, patients taking these newer medications have more favorable cognitive profiles than those on older AEDs (Aldenkamp et al., 2000; Dodrill, Arnett, et al., 1998; Loring and Meador, 2001; Meador, Loring, Ray, et al., 2001). Topiramate (Topamax) is an exception as it has been associated with impaired verbal fluency.

Prognosis

Is epilepsy progressive? A continuing controversy in epilepsy is whether poorly controlled seizures contribute to progressive cognitive decline. The debate is due, in part, to confounding variables that are difficult to control (A.J. Cole, 2000). Since there are often abnormalities that extend far beyond the seizure focus, it is certainly possible that poorly controlled seizures may have significant cumulative brain effects (Hermann, Seidenberg, and Bell, 2002). In a 10-year follow-up study of patients with poorly controlled seizures, no consistent changes were observed with comprehensive neuropsychological testing although subtle "very mild" losses were noted on several neuropsychological measures, including Digit Symbol, Visual Reproduction, Tactual Performance Test time, Seashore Rhythm Test, and Trail Making Part B (M.D. Holmes, et al., 1998). The decline in memory in patients with chronic epilepsy, and in particular visual memory, has been attributed to the interaction of seizure control, seizure

severity, cognitive reserve capacity, and test–retest interval (Helmstaedter, 2002).

Others have attributed at least a portion of progressive memory change in epilepsy to the interaction of preexisting disease with the aging process (Helmstaedter and Elger, 1999). There is an absence of strong human data supporting the theory that "seizures beget seizures" (A.T. Berg and Shinnar, 1997). However, both case reports and patient series have documented MRI changes in hippocampal volumes over a period as short as four years in patients with poorly controlled seizures (Briellmann et al., 2002; Hermann, Seidenberg, and Bell, 2002; T.J. O'Brien et al., 1999; Theodore and Gaillard, 2002). Some authors believe that, even in the absence of overall deterioration, epilepsy "refractoriness" is related to cumulative effects resulting from the many negative neural events associated with a seizure and, hence, aggressive intervention to interrupt this process is warranted (Kwan and Brodie, 2002). Definitive understanding must await longitudinal studies controlling for the many potentially relevant confounds (Sutula and Pitkänen, 2002).

Effects of surgical treatment. Surgery is often an effective treatment option for selected patients whose seizures cannot be satisfactorily controlled with medication (Pincus and Tucker, 2003; Wiebe, Blume, et al., 2001). As it is rare for a person who has failed two different AEDs to become seizure-free with a third medication (Kwan and Brodie, 2000), these patients may become candidates for surgery.

Patients undergoing anterior temporal lobectomy can be selected who have little risk of significant cognitive morbidity (e.g, loss of speech, severe memory disorder) with a high degree of confidence. In general selection factors include early age at seizure onset, evidence of hippocampal atrophy on MRI, and patterns of neuropsychological and Wada test findings that are compatible with the seizure onset laterality. The risk factors associated with increased likelihood of cognitive change are now more widely appreciated than originally understood (e.g., Milner, 1958).

Surgery removes or decreases the burden of seizures for many patients, but the practical outcome depends on other factors as well (Awad and Chelune, 1993; Loring and Meador, 2003b). The side of the lesion affects the cognitive outcome. Although right temporal lobectomy can be associated with visual memory impairments (Gleissner et al., 1998; R.C. Martin, Hugg, et al., 1999), it often leaves few, if any, clinically apparent deficits (Barr, Chelune, et al., 1997; T.M. Lee et al., 2002). Left temporal lobectomy is robustly associated with declines in verbal memory and confrontation naming (Hermann, Wyler, Somes, and Clement, 1994;

T.M. Lee et al., 2002), although Chelune, Naugle, and their colleagues (1993) note that when base rates are factored into outcome data, patients with right temporal lobectomies also do a little less well on verbal memory tests after surgery. The largest postoperative declines in verbal memory tended to appear in patients who, preoperatively, have more normal verbal memory test performances (Chelune, Naugle, Luders, and Awad, 1991). These patients lose the most functional tissue in the resection (Chelune, 1995). This has been demonstrated by MRI (Trenerry, Jack, et al., 1993), formal pathology (Hermann, Wyler, Somes, et al., 1992; Rausch and Babb, 1993), and Wada memory testing (Loring, Meador, Lee, et al., 1995). The best predictors of postoperative psychosocial outcome following anterior temporal lobectomy are the patient's preoperative psychosocial adjustment, and whether they become seizure-free (Hermann, Wyler, and Somes, 1992). Although short-term data (two to five year follow-ups) indicate that 60% to 80% of surgery patients have a significant, if not complete reduction in seizures, data for long-term prognoses are as yet insufficient (Tran et al., 1998).

Nonepileptic spells/pseudoseizures

Psychogenic spells resembling seizures have been recognized since the 18th century (Trimble, 1986). They have been called *pseudoseizures, hysterical pseudoseizures, pseudoepileptic seizures, hysteroepileptic psychogenic seizures,* and most recently, *nonepileptic seizures (NES)* (J.R. Gates, 2000). This latter name reflects the current viewpoint that these spells are evidence of psychiatric disease which can seriously affect a patient's functioning. Calling these symptoms "seizures" can mislead patients since the spells are not true seizures and can also mislead health care professionals because there are many types of nonepileptic seizures (e.g., associated with hypoglycemia) that are genuine seizures but are not epilepsy. To avoid this confusion, we will use the term *nonepileptic spells*.

Nonepileptic spells are paroxysmal spells that may superficially resemble seizures. The diagnosis of nonepileptic spells implies a psychological origin: most often they occur with anxiety disorder, depression, schizophrenia, conversion disorder, factitious disorder, and malingering. However, seizures and nonepileptic spells coexist in 10% to 20% of cases, complicating the diagnostic problem (Benbadis et al., 2001; Pincus and Tucker, 2003). No single cognitive or personality pattern characterizes persons who have nonepileptic spells as they are a very heterogeneous group, differing among themselves in mental abilities, emotional functioning, demographic backgrounds, and neurological

status (Lesser, 1996; Sackellares et al., 1985; Vanderzant et al., 1986). Many have a history of a traumatic event and depression (Barry and Sanborn, 2001), including sexual or physical abuse (Harden, 1997; Pincus and Tucker, 2003). Approximately 75% are women (Lesser, 1996). New onset nonepileptic spells following TBI have been reported (L.E. Westbrook et al., 1998).

Nonepileptic spells mimic just about every type of genuine seizure pattern and can display almost every associated symptom or problem including urinary incontinence, reports of *auras* (premonitory sensations common in true epilepsy), and even—though rarely—self-injury such as tongue biting (Groppel et al., 2000; Selwa et al., 2000). However, nonepileptic spells may be identified by a number of characteristics not seen with seizures including a longer duration than most true seizures (Rechlin et al., 1997), the ability of patients to recall their "spells" since seizures are rarely remembered, and clear consciousness during the event (W.L. Bell, 1998). In addition, many patients having nonepileptic spells display bizarre or purposeful movements such as kicking, slapping, and striking out; pelvic thrusting is not uncommon. These too are patterns not typical of seizures. Complicating the diagnostic picture are complex partial seizures with frontal foci as these can generate bizarre behaviors such as pelvic thrusting, masturbatory activity, and kicking or other aggressive acts (Barry and Sanborn, 2001). However, patients who have nonepileptic spells perform at or near normal levels on neuropsychological testing, which may be helpful in differentiating them from patients with epilepsy (J.A. Walker, 2000). A normal EEG recorded during the spell without evidence of epileptiform activity is the "gold standard" for diagnosis (Pincus and Tucker, 2003).

PROBLEMS OF DIFFERENTIAL DIAGNOSIS

Many referrals to neuropsychologists raise questions of differential diagnosis. The most common ones, the ones in which differential diagnosis is the central issue, have to do with the possibility that brain disease may underlie an emotional or personality disturbance, or that behavioral dilapidation or cognitive complaints may have a psychological rather than a neurological basis. The distinction between neurological disorders and some psychiatric disorders is now largely historical. Brain abnormalities occur in many psychiatric disorders, while for others abnormalities are suspected but as yet not clearly identified. Psychiatric symptoms accompany, and may even be prominent in many neurological diseases. Here the focus is on conditions in which psychiatric and neurological conditions, using traditional distinctions, often require an understanding of both for correct diagnosis. A review of the neuropsychology of psychiatric disorders is beyond the scope of this book. Useful resources for this information are I. Grant and Adams' (1996) *Neuropsychological Assessment of Neuropsychiatric Disorders*, B.S. Fogel, Schiffer, and Rao's (1996) *Neuropsychiatry*, and Yudofsky and Hales' (2002) *The American Psychiatric Publishing Textbook of Neuropsychiatry and Clinical Neurosciences*.

Often, questions of differential diagnosis are asked as "either–or" problems, even when lip service is given to the likelihood of interaction between the effects of a brain lesion and the patient's emotional predisposition or advanced years. In perplexing cases of differential diagnosis, a precise determination may not be possible unless an ongoing disease process eventually submerges the functional aspects of the patient's confusing behavior or unless "hard" neurological signs are evident. Before the era of neuroimaging, patients with frontal lobe tumors were often misdiagnosed as having psychiatric illnesses (Ron, 1989). Today's misdiagnoses may occur with diseases such as frontotemporal dementia (without aphasia) (C.A. Gregory and Hodges, 1996) or with multiple sclerosis as early manifestations are easily misinterpreted (Johannsen et al., 1996; Skegg, 1993). Large test batteries that serve as multiple successive sieves tend to reduce but still do not eliminate neuropsychodiagnostic errors.

Pankratz and Glaudin (1980) applied the two kinds of classification errors to problems in diagnosing these patients. *Type I errors* (false positive) involve the diagnosis of a physical disease when a patient's condition represents a functional solution to psychosocial stress. *Type II errors* (false negative) are diagnoses of functional disorders when a patient's complaints have a neurological basis. The subtle behavioral expression of many brain diseases, particularly in their early stages, and the not uncommon sameness or overlap of symptoms of organic brain diseases and functional disturbances make both kinds of errors common (Godwin-Austen and Bendall, 1990; Howieson and Lezak, 2002; M.J. Martin, 1983; Strub and Wise, 1997). When the findings of a neuropsychological examination leave the examiner in doubt about a differential diagnosis, repeated examinations may bring out performance inconsistencies in persons with functional disturbances (Kapur, 1988a) or—if spaced at 6 to 12 month intervals—may reveal progressive deterioration (A. Smith, 1980).

Emotional Disturbances and Personality Disorders

Patients who complain of headaches, dizziness, "blackout" spells, memory loss, mental slowing, peculiar sensations, or weakness and clumsiness usually find their way to a neurologist. These complaints can be very difficult to diagnose and treat: symptoms are often subjective and wax or wane with stress or attention; with regular events such as going to work, arriving home, or family visits; or unpredictably. The patient's complaints may follow a head injury or a bout with an illness as mild as a cold or as severe as a heart attack, or they may simply occur spontaneously. When there are objective neurological findings, they may be unrelated to the patient's complaints or, if related, insufficient to account for the level of distress or incapacitation. Sometimes treatment—medication, counseling, physical therapy, rest, activity, or a change in the patient's routine or living situation—will relieve the problem permanently. Sometimes relief lasts only temporarily, and the patient returns for help again and again, each time getting a new drug or a different regimen that may provide respite for a while. The temptation is great to write off as neurotic, inadequate, or dependent personalities patients who present these kinds of diagnostic problems or who do not respond to treatment (J.M. Goodwin et al., 1979; E.A. Klonoff and Landrine, 1997; Pincus and Tucker, 2003) or—if there is a pending law suit or disability claim—as compensation seekers (Alves and Jane, 1985; R.S. Parker, 2000).

However, many serious and sometimes treatable neurological diseases first present with vague, often transient symptoms that can worsen with stress and temporarily diminish or even disappear altogether with symptomatic or psychological treatment (Pincus and Tucker, 2003). The first symptoms of multiple sclerosis and early vascular dementia, for instance, are often transient, lasting hours or days, and may appear as reports of dizziness, weakness, ill-defined peculiar sensations, and fatigue. Diagnostically confusing complaints can herald a tumor and persist for months or even years before clear diagnostic signs emerge. Vague complaints are also common to postconcussion patients. TBI survivors tend to show significantly elevated profiles on the popular Minnesota Multiphasic Personality Inventory (MMPI) suggestive of emotional disturbances involving anxiety, depression, health concerns, and attentional problems (Cripe, 1997; Dikmen and Reitan, 1974; Fordyce et al., 1983; see p. 749). These patients may be diagnosed as emotionally disturbed when they are simply reporting common postconcussion symptoms (Cripe, 2002; Lezak, 1992).

Early diagnosis of neurological disease can be complicated by the fact that these are the same complaints expressed by many persons for whom functional disorders serve as a life-style or a neurotic reaction to stress. Particularly when patients' symptoms and their reactions to them appear to be typically neurotic or suggestive of a character disorder may their neurological complaints be discounted.

A 34-year-old high school teacher originally sought help for seizures that began without apparent reason. Each of several neurologists, upon finding no evidence of organic disease, referred him for psychiatric evaluation and treatment. Since his wife, a somewhat older woman, continued to press for a neurological answer to his seizures, by the end of the first year following seizure onset he had been seen by several neurologists, several psychiatrists, and at least one other psychologist besides myself.

The patient's passive-dependent relationship with his wife, the tendency to have seizures in the classroom—which ultimately gained him a medical retirement and relief from the admitted tension of teaching—and his history as an only child raised by a mother and grandmother who were teachers led to agreement among the psychiatrists that he had a hysterical seizure disorder. Personality and cognitive test data supported this diagnosis. When his seizures dissipated during a course of electroconvulsive therapy, all of the clinicians were relieved to learn that their diagnostic impressions were validated in such a striking manner. After several symptom-free months, however, his psychiatrist observed a slight facial asymmetry suggesting weakness or loss of innervation of the muscles around the left side of his mouth and nose. He immediately referred the patient for neurological study again. An abnormal EEG was followed by radiographic studies in which a small right frontotemporal lesion showed up that, on surgery, proved to be an inoperable tumor. The patient died about a year and a half later. [mdl]

Complaints of headache, dizziness, fatigue, and weakness can be accurate reports of physiological states or the patient's interpretation of anxiety or an underlying depression (Pincus and Tucker, 2003). The presence of anxiety symptoms or depression in the absence of "hard" findings is not in itself evidence that the patient's condition is functional, for the depressive reaction may be reflecting the patient's awareness or experience of as yet subtle mental or physical symptoms of early neurological disease (Askin-Edgar, White, and Cummings, 2002; Lishman, 1997; Reifler, Larson, and Hanley, 1982). Memory complaints are common symptoms of depression and may be particularly prominent among the complaints of elderly depressed patients.

Neuropsychological decisions about the etiology of these symptom pictures rely on criteria for both functional and neurologic disorders. An inappropriate—usually bland or indifferent—reaction to the complaints, symbolic meaningfulness of the symptoms, secondary gains, perpetuation of a dependent or irresponsible life-style, a close association between a stressful event and the appearance of the patient's problem, and an unlikely or inconsistently manifested pattern of cognitive impairment suggest psychogenic contributions to the patient's problems, regardless of the pa-

tient's neurological status. Occasionally, a happily unconcerned patient will maintain frankly bizarre and medically unlikely symptoms with such good will that their psychogenic origin is indisputable.

Consideration of a brain disorder in the differential diagnostic process is no different than any other diagnostic questions. A behavioral aberration indicative of a brain disorder that appears on neuropsychological examination as a single sign, such as rotation on a visuoconstructional task or perseverative writing, or a few low scores on tests involving the similar or associated functions should prompt the examiner to look for a pattern of cognitive impairment that makes neuroanatomical or neuropsychological sense. Evidence of lateralized impairment lends strong support to the possibility of neurological involvement.

It is unusual to see patients in whom behavioral manifestations of brain disease are uncomplicated by emotional reactions to their mental changes and consequent personal and social disruptions. As a rule, only the most simplistic or severely impaired persons will present clear-cut symptoms of brain damage without some emotional contribution to the symptom picture. Several varieties of emotional disturbances and their organic contributions illustrate many of the problems of separating organic manifestations from purely psychopathological phenomena.

Conversion disorders (conversion hysteria)

With complaints of various weaknesses and sensory disorders, these patients' unconcerned attitude of *la belle indifference*—which leads the list of hysteria's "classical signs"—may be the first clue to a conversion hysteria.[1]

A 37-year-old woman arrived for an evaluation in an elaborate, motorized wheelchair. She developed shoulder weakness of unknown etiology ten years earlier that progressed to leg weakness. She lived in a nursing home where, for over a year, she claimed to be even too weak to stand. Attendants bathed, dressed, transferred, and turned her. She said that she had a muscle weakness disorder despite normal findings on multiple medical tests including nerve conduction and EMG studies. Neurological examiners repeatedly noted *give-away weakness* (poor effort on strength testing) indicating that she was actively preserving a disability status. She expressed contentment with her situation and vehemently denied current emotional problems. Past history included an abusive and un-

---

[1]The other six signs are: 2. anomalous sensory complaints; 3. changing patterns of sensory loss; 4. sensory and motor findings changing with suggestions; 5. hemianaesthesia that splits the midline exactly; 6. unilateral loss of vibratory sense with sequential bilateral stimulation of forehead or sternum; and 7. "lapses" into normal exertion on motor testing of a supposedly weakened limb (the "giveaway" sign).

happy childhood, teenage anorexia with suicide attempts and self-mutilating behaviors prior to development of her "weakness." Tragically, this woman had not received care for her very evident emotional disorder for a number of years.

These kinds of chronic conversion disorders are difficult to treat. One approach that has been successful in some cases of functional motor disorder is *strategic-behavioral intervention* (Teasell and Shapiro, 1994) which places patients in a double bind by telling them that recovery would prove the disorder was neurological but failure to recover would confirm a psychiatric etiology.

In studies of patients originally diagnosed as having a conversion reaction, however, as many as half of them had significant medical problems, usually involving the CNS (Ron, 1996; R.L. Taylor, 1990). Moene and colleagues (2000) urge caution in diagnosing hysteria in adults older than 35 years, in cases where symptoms last a long time, and in cases where a neurological disorder had been suspected.

Medical folklore has held that only women can suffer a conversion hysteria (*hysteria* means "uterus" in Greek), which was originally thought to result from a displacement of that organ). However, men as well as women present this problem (Walsh and Darby, 1999). Occasionally this thinking still leads to misdiagnosis in a male patient with a conversion reaction. Cheerfully unrealistic attitudes about visual or motor defects or debilitating mental changes may also mislead the examiner into making an erroneous functional diagnosis when the inappropriate behaviors mask an appropriate underlying depressive reaction from the patient himself as well as others or reflect impaired self-perceptions due to brain damage (e.g., see Prigatano, 1991b; Schachter, 1991). Far from being pathognomonic for hysteria, at least one and, in one case, all seven of the classical signs of hysteria appeared in a series of patients with acute structural CNS damage (mostly from stroke) (R. Gould et al., 1986).

Psychogenic memory disorders

Schachter and Kihlstrom (1989) distinguished pathological from nonpathological functional amnesias. In the latter category fall commonplace losses of memory experienced by everyone, such as forgetting one's dreams and much of the events of childhood—particularly early childhood. Pathological psychogenic amnesias can take a number of forms, some of which mimic neuropathologically based memory disorders (Kopelman, 1987a; Kopelman, Christensen, et al., 1994; Mace and Trimble, 1991).

Dissociative amnesia is an inability to recall important personal information, such as a stressful event or a series of gaps in one's life experiences that is too ex-

tensive to be explained by ordinary forgetfulness (Y. Stern and Sackeim, 2002). While these may be purely psychogenic responses to emotional stress; when relatively brief they are often not dissimilar to alcoholic "blackouts" (p. 260). Situational amnesias can occur for specific traumatic events and are reversible, which distinguishes them from the irreversible retrograde amnesia for time preceding a concussion with loss of consciousness. Patients in a *dissociative fugue* have a loss of self-knowledge, including identity and history, without awareness of this loss; upon return to their normal state these patients typically have no recall of the fugue.

Nowhere does the problem of differentiating organic amnesia from functional amnesia become more acute or more complicated than when a criminal suspect pleads loss of memory for the critical event (Kopelman, 1987a,b; Schacter, 1986a). The alleged perpetrators have frequently been under the influence of alcohol at the time the crime was committed, in some instances they sustain head injury in the course of the criminal activity or shortly thereafter, and a few have impaired memory due to a preexisting neurological disorder, all conditions predisposing to a genuine inability to recall the relevant events. Emotional shock reactions, acting out in a fugue state, and other—rare—psychogenic memory disorders may also leave the defendant without access to recall of the crime. Since the self-serving effects of memory impairment are obvious to all but the dullest criminal defendants, the temptation to simulate a memory disorder is great, and the task of clarifying the nature of the suspect's memory complaints can be difficult.

Psychotic Disturbances

A neurological disorder can also complicate or imitate severe functional behavioral disturbances (Lishman, 1997; Skuster et al., 1992; Strub and Wise, 1997; Weinberger, 1984). The primary symptoms may involve marked mood or character change, confusion or disorientation, disordered thinking, delusions, hallucinations, bizarre ideation, ideas of reference or persecution, or any other of the thought and behavior disturbances typically associated with schizophrenia or the affective psychoses. The neuropsychological identification of a neurologic component in a severe behavior disturbance relies on the same criteria used to determine whether neurotic complaints have a neurological etiology. Here, too, a pattern of cognitive dysfunction selectively involving predominantly lateralized abilities and skills makes a strong case for a brain disorder, as does a pattern of memory impairment in which recent memory is more severely affected than remote memory, or a pattern of lowered scores on tests involving attention functions and new learning relative to scores on tests of knowledge and skill. The inconsistent or erratic expression of cognitive defects suggests a psychiatric disturbance (G. Goldstein and Watson, 1989). Organic behavioral disturbances are not likely to have symbolic meaning (Malamud, 1975).

Identifying those psychotic conditions that have a neuropathologic component is often more difficult than distinguishing emotional disturbances or character disorders from symptoms of brain damage because some psychiatric disorders are as likely to disrupt attention, mental tracking, and memory as are some neurological conditions (D.A. King and Caine, 1996; R.S. Goldman, Axelrod, and Taylor, 1996; Seidman, 1983). Psychiatric disorders may also disrupt perceptual, thinking, and response patterns as severely as neurological conditions (Pincus and Tucker, 2003). Therefore, a single test sign or markedly lower score cannot identify the brain injured patient in a psychotic population. Before concluding that a psychotically disturbed patient is neurologically impaired, the examiner will require a clear-cut pattern of lateralized dysfunction or neurological memory impairment, a number of signs, or a cluster of considerably lowered test scores that make neurological or neuropsychological sense.

Neuropsychological differentiation of organic and functional disorders tends to be easier when the condition is acute and to become increasingly difficult with chronicity, for institutionalization can have a behaviorally leveling effect on brain injured and functional patients alike. In this situation one must be wary of a "chicken and egg" effect, as those psychotic patients without demonstrable brain disease who are retained in institutions for any considerable length of time are also those most severely disturbed and probably most likely to have some neurological basis to their disorder. In some cases, the history is useful in differentiating the neurological from the psychogenically disturbed patients. Neurological conditions are more apt to develop during or following physical stress such as an illness, intoxication, TBI, or some forms of severe malnutrition. Emotional or situational stress more often precedes functionally disturbed behavior disorders. Unfortunately for diagnosticians, stress does not always come neatly packaged: an illness that is sufficiently severe to precipitate an organic psychosis or a TBI incurred in a family feud or a traffic accident is also emotionally upsetting.

Schizophrenia

The mechanisms underlying the brain's malfunction in schizophrenia have eluded scientists for decades. Even with the latest structural and functional neuroimaging, many questions remain unanswered. What is known is that schizophrenic patients' symptoms of hallucinations and delusions improve with drugs that block dopamine neurotransmission. The high incidence of premorbid neurological disorders (such as head injury, perinatal complications, childhood illnesses) suggests that in many cases the schizophrenic disorder may not be so much a disease entity but a mode of response to earlier cerebral insults (Pennington, 2002; Pincus and Tucker, 2003). A high familial incidence implicates a hereditary factor in some cases (Pincus and Tucker, 2003). Considerable heterogeneity among patients leads to descriptions of various subtypes (R.S. Goldman, Axelrod and Taylor, 1996; G. Goldstein, Allen, and Seaton, 1998; Heinrichs, 1993; S.K. Hill et al., 2001). This disorder usually begins in late adolescence or early adulthood. It does not have a long-term course of progressive deterioration in most cases (Rund, 1998). Rather, behavioral deterioration typically continues for several years and then plateaus for decades with many instances of improvement documented for these patients in their sixth decade and later (Tamminga, Thaker, and Medoff, 2002).

Structural and functional neuroimaging shows a variety of subtle abnormalities, particularly in the hippocampus, entorhinal and cingulate cortices, and other limbic areas (Pincus and Tucker, 2003; Tamminga, Thaker, and Medoff, 2002). Decreased cortical gray matter has been reported (E.V. Sullivan, Lim, et al., 1998). Several lines of evidence suggest that frontal lobe dysfunction is a core feature of schizophrenia (Weinberger et al., 1991). One theory holds that schizophrenia results from aberrations in the neural circuitry that links the prefrontal cortex with the thalamus, cerebellum, and—perhaps—basal ganglia (Andreasen, Paradiso, and O'Leary, 1998). Functional imaging studies report hypometabolism of the frontal lobes in schizophrenics with so-called negative symptoms (Tamminga, Thaker, Buchanan, et al., 1992). These patients are notable for their flat affect, behavioral passivity, and indifference. They tend to have a history of childhood cognitive and social dysfunction preceding the gradual evolution of the full-blown schizophrenic condition and are more likely to have structural brain anomalies (Andreason, 2001; Pennington, 2002).

As a group, schizophrenics perform below expectation on a wide range of cognitive tests, particularly those associated with frontal lobe regulation: attention, strategy use, and problem-solving (Jeste et al., 1996; R.S. Goldman, Axelrod, and Taylor, 1996). The memory impairment of schizophrenics resembles that of patients with subcortical pathology (Paulsen, Heaton, Sadek, et al., 1995). Cognitive performance may be affected, at least in part, by poor motivation or inefficient use of strategies so that individual's response levels can vary considerably from one test session to the next (Heinrichs, 1993). Moreover, some persons diagnosed as schizophrenic have neither the neurological stigmata nor significant neuropsychological deficits, which raises further questions about the etiology and nature of brain involvement in this condition and the accuracy of diagnosis (Heinrichs, 1993; Pincus and Tucker, 2003). For example, in one study employing a control group, 27% of the schizophrenic patients were blindly rated as "normal" based on their neuropsychological performance (Palmer, Heaton, et al., 1997).

Neurological disorders with psychotic features

The behavioral symptoms of some neurological conditions are easily misinterpreted. Unlike many postcentral lesions that announce themselves with distinctive lateralized behavioral changes or highly specific and identifiable cognitive defects, the behavioral effects of frontal lobe tumors may be practically indistinguishable from those of progressive character disorders or behavioral disturbances. Hécaen (1964) found that 67% of patients with frontal lobe tumors exhibited confused states and dementia and that almost 40% had mood and character disturbances. Their confusion tends to be relatively mild and is often limited to time disorientation; the dementia, too, is not severe and may appear as general slowing and apathy, which can be easily confused with chronic depression. Euphoria, irritability, and indifference resulting in unrealistically optimistic or socially crude behavior may give the appearance of a psychiatric disturbance, particularly when compounded by mild confusion or dullness. Degenerative brain diseases can produce psychiatric symptoms including psychosis (Lishman, 1997; Pincus and Tucker, 2003; see also pp. 219, 223, 241). Some patients with dementia, usually of moderate severity, will become delusional, often believing that someone has stolen something from them or that their spouse is unfaithful. Hallucinations, usually visual, may occur in Alzheimer's and Parkinson's diseases and may be an early symptom of Lewy body dementia. Marked personality changes with loss of social graces are characteristic of patients with frontotemporal dementia, including Pick's disease. Absence of an earlier psychiatric history, the insidious onset of symptoms, and an accompanying memory impairment usually distinguish these dementia patients from psychiatric patients. Diseases of the basal ganglia often produce psychiatric symptoms with depression being common in Parkinson's and Huntington's diseases (Sano, Marder, and Dooneief, 1996), but psychotic episodes can also occur

in Parkinson's disease, sometimes triggered by drug treatment. The movement disorder associated with these latter diseases helps differentiate them from purely psychiatric disorders.

Another difficult to diagnose group are psychiatric patients with suspected temporal lobe lesions. These patients tend to be erratically and irrationally disruptive or to exhibit marked personality changes or wide mood swings (Blumer, 1975; Heilman, Blonder, Bowers, and Valenstein, 2003; Pincus and Tucker, 2003). Schizophrenic-like symptoms can appear in patients with temporal lobe seizure disorders (Pincus and Tucker, 2003; Tucker, 2002) or temporal lobe tumors (T.R.P. Price et al., 2002). Severe temper or destructive outbursts, or hallucinations and bizarre ideation may punctuate periods of rational and adequately controlled behavior, sometimes unpredictably and sometimes in response to stress. Positive neuropsychological test results may provide clues to the nature of the disturbance when EEG or neurological studies do not. Memory for auditory and visual, symbolic and nonsymbolic material should be reviewed as well as complex visual pattern perception and logical—propositional—reasoning.

Patients with right hemisphere disease may also display behavioral and emotional abnormalities of psychiatric proportions, including paranoidal ideation, hallucinations, and agitation (Cutting, 1990; B.H. Price and Mesulam, 1985; Schomer et al., 2000). When the lesion is restricted to the parietal lobe so that motor functions are unaffected, a bright, highly verbal, and distressed patient can appear to be cognitively and neurologically intact unless visuospatial abilities are appropriately tested or the examiner is alert to the subtle verbalistic illogic that often characterizes the thinking of these patients.

Other brain diseases that can produce psychiatric symptoms include strokes, tumors of other regions, and infections (e.g., AIDS, neurosyphillis). Psychiatric symptoms can also accompany a variety of non-neurological illnesses including thyroid and parathyroid disease, pituitary disease, and metabolic and toxic conditions (Skuster et al., 1992; Tarter, Butters, and Beers, 2001, *passim*).

Depression

Depression can complicate the clinical presentation of a brain disorder (Jorge and Robinson, 2002; Sano, Marder, and Dooneief, 1996; Sweet, 1983) or the effects of aging. Even in neurologically intact young persons, depression may interfere with the normal expression of cognitive abilities (Mayberg et al., 2002; Walsh and Darby, 1999). For example, slowed mental processing and mild attentional deficits characterize many of these patients (Brand and Jolles, 1987; D.A. King and Caine, 1996; H. Christensen et al., 1997; Massman, Delis, Butters, et al., 1992).

Most cognitive studies of depressed patients have focused on memory functions. Impairments in recall and in learning for both verbal and visuospatial material have been demonstrated (Brand and Jolles, 1987; Otto et al., 1994; P.M. Richards and Ruff, 1989). Most studies have found that recognition memory is also affected by depression (D.B. Burt et al., 1995; Veiel, 1997a). Contrary to previous assumptions that memory dysfunction in depression results from insufficient or poorly sustained effort (e.g., Weingartner, 1986), recent reviews have concluded that impaired memory performance by depressed patients is not due to effort demands or poor motivation (H. Christensen et al., 1997; Kindermann and Brown, 1997). For example, patients have as much difficulty on WIS-A tests requiring less effort, such as Vocabulary, as on effortful ones, such as Block Design.

Some studies have not demonstrated significant memory impairments in depressed patients (Niederehe, 1986) or have elicited impairments for some abilities (e.g., verbal fluency) and not others in some groups but not others (D.A. King and Caine, 1996). Others have reported slowed speed of responding and diminished visuospatial abilities and mental flexibility (Veiel, 1997a). Inconsistent findings may be due to differences in severity between patient groups (H. Christensen et al., 1997), length of depressive illness (Denicoff et al., 1999), and medications (Crews et al., 1999). Crews and his associates found no difference on a variety of cognitive tests of concentration and executive functions between moderately depressed, unmedicated outpatient women compared to matched control subjects which, they suggested, might be due to the relatively short duration and less severe condition of their subjects compared to patients in studies finding a positive effect. While hospitalized medical patients showed deficits on tests of speed, recognition memory, and abstraction, those who were depressed performed as well as those who were not, indicating that deficits for these patients were not due to depression (Cole and Zarit, 1984). M.R. Basso and Bornstein (1999) reported that young patients with recurrent depression had deficits on a word list learning task while young patients hospitalized for a single episode of depression performed as well as control subjects.

Another possible resolution of the contradictory findings is suggested by the data reported by Massman and his colleagues (1992), as about half of their depressed patients performed no differently from control subjects: if all of their patients had been lumped together in the statistical analysis, rather than treated as discrete sub-

groups of depressed patients, it is likely that these interesting findings would have been obscured. B.W. Palmer, Boone, and their colleagues (1996) observed that depressed outpatients with vegetative symptoms had a variety of cognitive deficits while those with only psychological symptoms performed as well as control subjects. Poor cognitive performance by patients with bipolar disorder, during periods of well-being, was associated with hippocampal asymmetry (right > left), suggesting that variations in limbic structure or function may be an important variable (Ali et al., 2000). Some studies have reported that emotionally neutral or negative stimuli are better remembered by depressed patients than positive material, which suggests that a response bias favoring negative contents could account for some of the differences reported about the memory functioning of depressed persons (D.B. Burt et al., 1995; H. Christensen et al., 1997; Niederehe, 1986).

Depression in older persons

The most common problem complicating differential diagnosis of behavioral disturbances in older persons is depression, which can mimic or exacerbate symptoms of progressive dementing conditions (Jenike, 1994). While the incidence of depression is only a little higher among persons aged 65 and over than in the younger population (Blazer, 1982; Marcopulos, 1989), it may be the most frequently occurring emotional disorder among the elderly (Hassinger et al., 1989; L.W. Thompson et al., 1987). In elderly persons who have not been chronically depressed, it is often preceded by stressful events, particularly of loss—of loved ones, status, meaningful activity. In these cases the condition takes on more of the character of a reactive depression than a major depressive disorder (Alexopoulos, Young, et al., 1989; Blazer, 1982). Chronic physical illness greatly increases the likelihood of depression in elderly persons as a number of physical disorders and medications can produce depression-like symptoms (Kaszniak and Allender, 1985; MacKinnon and DePaulo, 2002). Enlarged ventricles and decreased brain density have been associated with late-onset depression (Alexopoulos, Young, et al., 1989); among elderly psychiatric inpatients, depression has been associated with cortical infarctions and leukoencephalopathy (white matter lacunae) (Filley, 2001; Zubenko et al., 1990). The "vascular depression" hypothesis is supported by the comorbidity of depression with vascular disease and vascular risk factors (Alexopoulos, Meyers, et al., 1997; Filley, 1995) and the presence on imaging of hyperintensities in white matter, particularly in deep white matter (Nebes, Vora, et al., 2001). Studies of memory functions in elderly depressives are similar to those of younger depressed persons in producing contradictory findings (Bieliauskas and Lamberty, 1995; Lamberty and Bieliauskas, 1993; L.W. Thompson et al., 1987). Some studies have not found depressed elderly persons' memory performances to differ significantly from those of normal subjects (K.A. Boone, Lesser, Miller, et al., 1995; Niederehe, 1986); others have documented deficits (Kaszniak, 1987; Kaszniak, Sadeh, and Stern, 1985). Depressed older psychiatric inpatients performed worse than controls on most learning and recall measures of the California Verbal Learning Test, except for retention (D.A. King, Cox, et al., 1998). Also, as in younger depressives, attention and concentration may be somewhat impaired (Larrabee and Levin, 1986) and responses may be abnormally slowed (K.A. Boone, Lesser, Miller, et al., 1995; Comijs, Jonker, et al., 2001; R.P. Hart and Kwentus, 1987). One distinguishing feature of older depressed persons is that they tend to complain a lot about poor memory, even when testing shows that memory is *within normal limits* for their age (Comijs, Deeg, et al., 2002; Kaszniak, 1987; J.M. Williams, Little, et al., 1987). Deficits on language tasks, particularly on the more complex test items, show up among elderly patients with long histories of major depression (Emery and Breslau, 1989; Speedie et al., 1990). However, depressed elderly patients did not differ from their normal controls in either accuracy or quality (richness, aptness) of vocabulary test responses (Houlihan et al., 1985).

Differentiating dementia and depression

> Demented patients often appear to be depressed. Depressed patients can also appear demented.
> *Pincus and Tucker, 2003, p. 160*

Probably the knottiest problem of differential diagnosis is that of separating depressed dementia patients who, early in the course of the disease, do not yet show the characteristic symptoms of dementia, from psychiatrically depressed patients in the depths of their depression when they may display a pattern of dysfunctional behavior that appears similar to dementia. Depressive reactions may be the first overt sign of something wrong in a person who is experiencing the very earliest subjective symptoms of a dementing process (Devanand, Sano, Tang, et al., 1996; Geerlings et al., 2000; Yaffe, Blackwell, et al., 1999). Those aspects of the clinical presentation of both an early dementing process and depression that are most likely to contribute to misdiagnosis are depressed mood or agitation; a history of psychiatric disturbance; psychomotor retardation; impaired immediate memory and learning abilities; defective attention, concentration, and track-

ing; impaired orientation; an overall shoddy quality to cognitive products; and listlessness with loss of interest in one's surroundings and, often, in self-care (Lishman, 1997; Strub and Wise, 1997; C.E. Wells, 1979).

Nonetheless, functionally depressed patients and those with neurological disease may differ in a number of ways. Elderly depressed patients often somatize their distress, some becoming quite hypochondriacal (Hassinger et al., 1989; Kaszniak, Sadeh, and Stern, 1985), while demented patients are less likely to experience the vegetative features of depression (Hoch and Reynolds, 1990). The structure and content of speech remains essentially intact in depression but deteriorates in dementia of the Alzheimer type. The severity of memory impairment is much greater in Alzheimer patients, and this is an important distinguishing feature (H. Christensen et al., 1997; desRosiers, Hodges, and Berrios, 1995; R.P. Hart, Kwentus, Taylor, and Harkins, 1987; P.J. Visser, Verhey, et al., 2000). Intact incidental learning in depressed patients will be reflected in fairly appropriate temporal orientation, in contrast to demented patients who are less likely to know the day of the week, the date, and time of day (R.D. Jones et al., 1992). Inconsistency tends to distinguish the orientation disorder of depressives from the more predictable disorientation of dementia patients. The presence of aphasias, apraxias, or agnosias clearly distinguishes an organic dementia from the pseudodementia of depression (Golper and Binder, 1981; Lishman, 1997). Quite early in the course of their illness, many dementia patients show relatively severe impairment on both copy and recall trials of drawing tests and on constructional tasks (R.D. Jones et al., 1992), making inappropriate responses or fragments of responses that may be distorted by perseverations, despite their obvious efforts to do as asked. In contrast, the performance of depressed patients on drawing and construction tasks may be careless, shabby, or incomplete due to apathy, low energy level, and poor motivation but, if given enough time and encouragement, they may make a recognizable and often fully adequate response. Lamberty and Bieliauskas (1993) point out that while depressed elderly patients' performances on neuropsychological tests tend to run below those of age-matched controls, these patients' test scores, on the whole, will be higher than those of dementing patients.

Moreover, depressed patients are more likely to be keenly aware of their impaired cognition, making much of it; in fact, their complaints of poor memory in particular may far exceed measured impairment and they can often report just where and when the memory lapse occurred (Reifler, 1982). Dementia patients, in contrast, are typically less aware of the extent of their cognitive deficits, particularly after the earliest stages (McGlynn and Kaszniak, 1991), and may even report improvement as they lose the capacity for critical self-awareness, although striking exceptions can occur. A tendency to give "don't know" answers may distinguish depressives who are poorly motivated from demented patients who respond uncritically with erroneous answers (Kaszniak, Sadeh, and Stern, 1985; Lishman, 1997); but this has not been a consistent finding (R.C. Young et al., 1985).

Historical information can greatly help to differentiate dementia patients who are depressed from depressed patients who appear to be demented (Godwin-Austen and Bendall, 1990; Lishman, 1997; C.E. Wells, 1979). The cognitive deterioration of a dementing process typically has a slow and insidious onset, while cognitive impairments accompanying depressive reactions are more likely to evolve over several weeks' time. The context in which the dysfunctional symptoms appear can be extremely important in the differential diagnosis, as depressive reactions are more likely to be associated with an identifiable precipitating event or, as so often happens to the elderly, a series of precipitating events, usually losses. However, precipitating events, such as divorce or loss of a job or a business, may also figure in depressive reactions of dementia patients early in their course. In the latter cases, hindsight usually shows that what looked like a precipitating event was actually a harbinger of the disease, occurring as a result of early symptoms of ineptitude and social dilapidation. Most often, the disturbed behavior of elderly psychiatric patients has a mixed etiology in which emotional reactions to significant losses—of loved ones, of ego-satisfying activities, or of physical and cognitive competence—interact with the behavioral effects of physiological and anatomical brain changes to produce a complex picture of behavioral dilapidation. Many of the physical disorders to which elderly persons are prone may create disturbances in mental functioning that mimic the symptoms of degenerative brain disease (Godwin-Austen and Bendall, 1990; Hassinger et al., 1989; Lishman, 1997). Since these conditions are often reversible with proper treatment, the differential diagnosis can be extremely important. Although enumerating distinguishing characteristics may make the task of diagnosing these patients seem reasonably simple, in practice, it is sometimes impossible to formulate a diagnosis when the patient first comes to professional attention. In such cases, only time and repeated examinations will ultimately clarify the picture.

Effects of electroconvulsive therapy (ECT) for depression

Complaints of poor memory are common among persons who have undergone ECT for depression (J.

Rosenberg and Pettinati, 1984). Memory problems trouble patients most often during the course of the treatments and shortly thereafter (Abrams 1988; Calev et al., 1993; Y. Stern and Sakeim, 2002). These problems include impaired learning ability and defective retrieval as well as apparent loss of memories: memories of events immediately preceding the treatments are most likely to be permanently lost; recent personal memories are more vulnerable than older ones (Cahill and Frith, 1995). Patients receiving bilateral ECT are more likely to have persisting memory complaints (Squire, Wetzel, and Slater, 1979) and to exhibit memory deficits at least shortly after treatment, which are also more likely to be more severe than those whose treatments were unilateral (typically applied to the right side of the head) (Sackeim, Prudic, et al., 2000; Shimamura and Squire, 1987). Return to normal memory function has been reported for patients who have had fewer than 20 treatments although some of these patients continue to voice memory complaints. In the last several decades it has become relatively rare for the number of treatments to exceed 20—more usually, reports indicate a course of six to 12 treatments (e.g., Sackeim, Prudic, et al., 2000).

Pincus and Tucker (2003) among others report that in the long run ECT's effects on memory and other aspects of cognition are benign. However, some patients continue to have memory deficits; vulnerability to subtle but persistent impairments shows up especially in patients who already have cognitive impairments (Y. Stern and Sackeim, 2002). When the mental efficiency of elderly depressed patients who had undergone ECT when younger was compared with that of other elderly depressed patients with no history of ECT, those with an ECT history took significantly longer to complete the Trail Making Test-B (Pettinati and Bonner, 1984).

Transcranial magnetic stimulation is a rapidly developing, noninvasive tool for treating medication-resistant major depression (Triggs et al., 1999). It appears to pose no cognitive danger (Y. Stern and Sackeim, 2002). Whether it will replace ECT will depend on further study of the durability of its antidepressant effect (T. Burt et al., 2002).

Depression with brain disease

Depression may be a prominent feature of a number of neurological disorders, including Parkinson's disease, Huntington's disease, AIDS dementia, and stroke (Mayberg, Keightley, et al., 2002; Mesulam, 2000c; R.G. Robinson and Travella, 1996). Clinically significant depression affects about one-quarter to two-fifths of patients with primary progressive dementia at some time during their course (Lazarus et al., 1987; Mayberg, Keightley, et al., 2002; Pincus and Tucker, 2003; Reifler, 1986). Depression tends to add to cognitive compromise, particularly affecting memory functions. Many of these patients respond to medication for their depression with some cognitive improvement although, of course, the underlying dementia will be unaffected (Hoch and Reynolds, 1990; Reifler, 1986). Discriminating between depressed and nondepressed dementia patients can be well-nigh impossible. Reifler and his colleagues (1982) observed that a past history of psychiatric disorder may increase the likelihood of depression in a dementia patient, and they suggest that when in doubt the clinician should begin a "carefully monitored empirical trial" of an antidepressant medication.

It can also be important to identify treatable depression in patients with other brain diseases whose poor insight or impaired capacity to communicate may prevent them from seeking help on their own. E D. Ross and Rush (1981) suggest a number of clues to the presence of depression in these patients. Among these are an unexpectedly low rate of improvement from the neurological insult or unexpected deterioration in a condition that had been stable or improving, uncooperativeness in rehabilitation and other "management" problems, or "pathological laughing and crying in patients who do not have pseudobulbar palsy." Ross and Rush recommended that the family as well as the patient be interviewed regarding the presence of vegetative indicators of depression. They also noted that the monotonic voice and reduced emotional responsiveness of patients with right hemisphere lesions may deceive the observer who, in these cases, must listen to what the patients say rather than how they say it.

Malingering

Malingering is a special problem in neuropsychological assessment because so many neurological conditions present few "hard" findings and so often defy documentation by clinical laboratory techniques, particularly in their early stages. The problem is complicated by the compensation and retirement policies of companies and agencies which can make poor health worth some effort. Yet White and Proctor (1992) note that it "is much less common than might be expected given the amount of attention it receives in the literature" (p. 146).

A critical determinant in differentiating malingering from other pseudoneurologic disorders is the extent to which the patient is aware of the nature of the dysfunctional behavior (Walsh and Darby, 1999). Yet self-awareness of an assumed disability may not be an all-or-none experience for the complainant. Depth psychology has demonstrated that the continuum of self-awareness with full self-awareness, at one end and complete self-deception at the other, contains every possible gradation of self-awareness in between its extremes. Thus sometimes an effort to identify malingering will involve determining whether and to what extent the patient's problems are symptomatic of a psychogenic disturbance rather than deliberate pretense (Lishman, 1997). Here the history and a review of the patient's current psychosocial circumstances may provide the most useful information. Moreover, malingering itself often serves as an unwitting effort to work out disturbing life problems or emotional obstacles and thus may, in itself, be symptomatic of a psychological disorder (Pankratz and Erickson, 1990). This common aspect of malingering adds further to difficulties in discriminating between a clearly invidious attempt to gain some not entitled advantage and a psychogenic disorder.

Some specific performance characteristics may alert the examiner to the possibility that the patient is malingering. When a disability would be advantageous, complaints and expressions of distress that appear to exceed by far what the injury or illness would be expected to cause signal the possibility of malingering. Inconsistency in performance levels or between a patient's report of disability and performance levels, unrelated to any fluctuating physiological conditions, is perhaps the most usual indicator of malingering, or at least a pseudoneurologic condition. Research has shown that it is easier to fake successfully on sensory and motor tests than on tests of higher level cognitive abilities (Cullum, Heaton, and Grant, 1991). Suggestions about how difficult a task is may bring out failure on tests that most persons with neurological disorders perform well.

As poor memory is a common complaint in malingering, the evaluation of its validity has received special attention (Brandt, 1988; Kapur, 1988a). Some approaches to the problem have looked at discrepancies within the examination. For example, an abnormally short digit span in the absence of any other speech or language disorder or a much better performance on a difficult memory test compared to a usually easier task should raise the examiner's suspicions of malingering. Attitudes toward memory aids distinguished study subjects who simulated forgetting from those who had actually forgotten the target material as the former were much less likely to agree that cueing could aid recall of the target material than were subjects who had actually forgotten it (Schacter, 1986b). The case below illustrates a number of these rules of thumb for identifying a pseudoneurotic complaint.

A 45-year-old college graduate claimed that severe memory impairment and some hearing loss resulted from an anoxic episode brought on by a beating by a business competitor. He initiated a lawsuit requesting $1,000,000 for damages and expenses. He had not worked since being injured but, by report, had become an excellent cook and volunteered on the telephone at a community service center. My technician, Jeanne Harris, and I [mdl] saw this man four years after the event and three years after an initial neuropsychological examination, in which slowing and an erratic performance pattern that made no neuropsychological sense were reported (e.g., recall of only 4 digits forward but an Associate Learning [WMS] score of 12 was *within normal limits* for his age; only one error on the Seashore Rhythm Test while failing 14 of the 60 items on the Speech Sounds Perception Test). He had been reexamined recently but the data were not available.

Ms. Harris saw him first and made the following notes: "When asked to tell his age, P replied, 'In my 40's. I was born (he gave the correct date).' Again I asked his age: '45 or 46? Do you know which?' 'I'm not sure what year it is.' (I asked him what year he thought it might be). 'I think it's (correct year).' Later when asked to date his Complex Figure drawing he was unable to recall the date. He looked at his watch and wrote '7th' (the correct day of the month)." Continuing Ms. Harris' notes: "When asked, for example, what is the population of the U.S., he didn't hesitate at all before saying '200 million.' While doing Picture Completion he asked only one time, 'something wrong with it?' and I repeated, 'What is missing?' Otherwise he remembered for each picture what he was supposed to do but he gave seven 'don't knows' and one erroneous response for a score low in the *average* range. When asked to rhyme alphabet letters with 'tree,' he immediately understood the instructions and gave no repetitions even though he said letters out of sequence. Suddenly, during the Picture Arrangement test, he commented, 'I've seen these recently,' yet when asked for a delayed recall of the Complex Figure he said he could not remember having seen a drawing."

On this occasion he repeated only three digits forward correctly and only two reversed. When given the date and day of the week, on immediate recall he said only "Friday." He was exceedingly slow to respond on many tests (e.g., scores of 28 on both trials of the Symbol Digit Modalities Test), yet he produced 44 words in the three 1-minute trials of the Controlled Oral Word Association Test with only two repetitions.

There was little question in my mind that most if not all the "deficits" paraded by this man were functional in nature.

The fact that the past four years of his life had been given over to these symptoms with the resulting diminished quality and very dead-end nature of his life further suggested psychogenic contributions to his complaints. In explaining to his lawyer that a good case for cognitive impairment could not be made on the basis of this examination, I recommended counseling for the patient and his very supportive and overly protective wife.

While it is often possible to differentiate between organically based impairment and functional neuropsychological complaints, efforts to differentiate between simulated and psychogenic dysfunction typically remain unsuccessful (Puente and Gillespie, 1991; Schacter, 1986c). Moreover, even when the patient's behavior or the history strongly suggest some deliberate simulation, brain damage may also be contributing to the symptom picture. Nowhere does this become clearer than in studies of Munchausen patients. These are persons who deliberately fake their histories and medical records, and may even go so far as to injure themselves to simulate illness in a pattern of behavior that can continue for years, with the apparent goal of being a patient (Pankratz, 1988, 1998). A number of them, on neuropsychological examination, were found to have significant cognitive deficits reflecting well-defined syndromes of cerebral dysfunction (Pankratz and Lezak, 1987).

Generally, but not always, a thorough neuropsychological examination performed in conjunction with careful neurological studies will bring out performance discrepancies that are inconsistent with normal neuropsychological expectations. If inpatient facilities are available, close observation by trained staff for several days will often answer questions about malingering. There are a number of special techniques for testing the performance inconsistencies characteristic of malingerers (e.g., see pp. 760–761, 768). When malingering is suspected, the imaginative examiner may also be able to improvise tests and situations that will reveal deliberate efforts to withhold or mar a potentially good performance.

II | A COMPENDIUM OF TESTS AND ASSESSMENT TECHNIQUES

The apparent precision of numerical scores fosters an overdependence on test scores that must be resisted.
Bert F. Green, Jr., American Psychologist, 1978

I N the final 12 chapters of this book, most adult tests of cognitive functions and emotional status, and of behavioral observations in common use plus some relatively uncommon examination techniques are reviewed. These are tests and assessment techniques that are particularly well-suited for *clinical* neuropsychological examinations.

An effort has been made to classify the tests according to the major functional activities they elicit, and for many of them this was possible. Many others, though, call upon several functions so that their assignment to a particular chapter was somewhat arbitrary. Moreover, some tests will provide more information about one or another function, depending upon the patient (Dodrill, 1997). The most obvious example is the Wechsler oral Arithmetic test which reflects an approximate level of arithmetic achievement for many people, but for those with significant attentional disorders it provides much more information about their attentional problems than their arithmetic prowess.

In the following discussion, any mention of a test will refer only to individual tests, not batteries (such as the Wechsler Intelligence Scales) or even those test sets, such as Digits Forward and Digits Backward, that custom has led some to think of as a single test. This consideration of individual tests comes from demonstrations of the significant intertest variability in patient performances, the strong association of different patterns of test performance with different kinds of brain pathology, the demographic and other factors which contribute to the normal range of intraindividual test score variations, and the specificity of the brain-behavior relationships underlying many cognitive functions (e.g., see Grant and Adams, 1996, *passim;* Mesulam, 2000b; Naugle, Cullum, and Bigler, 1997).

This knowledge of intraindividual variations in test performances does not support the popular concept of "intelligence" as a global—or near-global—phenomenon which can be summed up in a single score (Ardila, 1999a). Nor does it support summing scores on any two or more tests that measure functions differing in any way, whether it be in their nature, such as combining the scores for Wechsler's Block Design test which involves abstract visual analysis and visuospatial response with Wechsler's Matrix Reasoning test which engages conceptual analysis and abstraction with minimal visuospatial demands and no motor requirements (Wechsler, 1981; The Psychological Corporation, 1997); or in their complexity, as Digits Backwards is a more complex activity than Digits Forward (Lezak, 1979; F.W. Black, 1986).

Not all of these tests are well-standardized, and thus they do not satisfy all of the criteria recommended by the American Psychological Association (1999). Those which have been insufficiently or questionably standardized were included because their clinical value seems to outweigh their statistical weaknesses. In many instances standardized tests are not appropriate, due to the patient's limitations, the rarity in normative populations of the condition being assessed (e.g., visuospatial inattention, perseveration), or the experimental nature of the examination. We recommend that clinicians try out those that appear to meet their—and their patients'—clinical needs. It is hoped that clinicians in situations where new techniques can be tested will do so and publish their findings.

Space, time, and energy set a limit to the number of tests we reviewed. Selection favored tests that are in relatively common use, represent a subclass of similar tests, illustrate a particularly interesting assessment method, or uniquely demonstrate some significant aspect of behavior. Criteria of availability and ease of administration eliminated those tests that require bulky, complicated, expensive equipment or material that cannot be easily obtained or reproduced by the individual clinician. These criteria cut out all tests that require a fixed laboratory installation as well as all those demanding special technical knowledge from the examiner.

Most of the testing materials can be ordered from test publishers (see listing with addresses, p. 785) or they are easily assembled by the examiner; a few must be ordered from the author or an unusual source for which information is provided in footnotes. Some instruments, such as the Trail Making Test, are in the public domain. These tests are identified wherever possible so that the user can decide whether to copy test forms or purchase them from a test purveyor. The Science Directorate of the American Psychological Association (1995) offers *A Guide for Locating and Using Both Published and Unpublished Tests*.[1] Psychophysiological tests of specific sensory or motor functions, such as tests of visual and auditory acuity or of one- and two-point tactile discrimination are also part of the standard neurological examination. Because they are well-described elsewhere, this book will not deal with them systematically. With few exceptions, the tests considered here are essentially psychological.

Use of computers in neuropsychological assessment, whether for administering tests, scoring and compiling data, or formula-based "interpretation," continues to proliferate. A comprehensive and critical review of this field is beyond the scope of this book. A number of tests that are hand administered, scored, etc. also have computer programs for administration, scoring, etc.; this is noted for most of the tests that we know about. However, as it is not possible to keep up with the pace of computerization, we recommend that readers refer to the test catalogue to learn whether computerized software is available for the test of interest. Computerization of neuropsychological assessment requires a book of its own—preferably in a loose-leaf binding to keep pace with its growth.

[1]Copies may be ordered from Science Directorate, American Psychological Association, 750 First Street, NE, Washington, DC 20002-4242; (202) 336-6000.

9 | **Orientation and Attention**

ORIENTATION

Orientation, the awareness of self in relation to one's surroundings, requires consistent and reliable integration of attention, perception, and memory. Impairment of particular perceptual or memory functions can lead to specific defects of orientation; more than mild or transient problems of attention or retention are likely to result in global impairment of orientation. Its dependence on the integrity and integration of so many different mental activities makes orientation exceedingly vulnerable to the effects of brain dysfunction.

Orientation defects are among the most frequent symptoms of brain disease. Of these, impaired awareness for time and place is the most common, accompanying brain disorders in which attention or retention is significantly affected. It is not difficult to understand the fragility of orientation for time and place, since each depends on both continuity of awareness and the translation of immediate experience into memories of sufficient duration to maintain awareness of one's ongoing history. Moreover, disorientation can result from a confusion of memory traces from different events or different temporal contexts that sometimes results in confabulations (Schnider et al., 1996). Thus, impaired orientation for time and place typically occurs with widespread cortical involvement (e.g., in Alzheimer-type dementia, acute brain syndromes, or bilateral cerebral lesions), lesions in the limbic system (e.g., Korsakoff's psychosis), or damage to the reticular activating system of the brain stem (e.g., disturbances of consciousness). Lesions involving the orbitofrontal cortex, basal forebrain, or limbic system are common in confabulators (Schnider, 2000). However, when cognitive impairments or deficits in attention are relatively mild, orientation can still be intact. Thus, while impaired orientation, in itself, is strongly suggestive of cerebral dysfunction, good orientation is not evidence of cognitive or attentional competence (Varney and Shepherd, 1991).

Inquiry into the subject's orientation for time, place, and basic personal data such as name, age, and marital status is part of all formalized mental status examinations (pp. 698–699) and most memory test batteries (e.g., General Information section of the Randt Memory Scales; Orientation section of The Rivermead Behavioural Memory Test; Orientation test of the Wechsler Memory Scales). Time orientation is usually covered by three or four items (e.g., day of week, date, month, year) and orientation for place by at least two (name of place where examination is being given, city it is in). In these formats, orientation items fit into scoring schemes such that, typically, if two or more of the five or seven time/place orientation items are failed, the score for that section of the test or battery falls into the *defective* range.

Tests of specific facets of orientation are not ordinarily included in the formal neuropsychological examination. However, their use is indicated when lapses on an informal mental status examination call for a more thorough evaluation of the patient's orientation or when scores are needed for documenting the course of a condition or for research. For these purposes, a number of little tests and examination techniques are available.

Time, place, and person orientation can be quite naturally examined by asking the subject to provide the examination identification data requested on most standardized test forms. For example, relevant identification data for the Wechsler Intelligence Scales include subject name, address, age, marital status, and date of birth, place of testing, and date tested. Inpatients can be asked the reason for their hospitalization to assess their understanding of their situation. By the time subjects have answered questions on these items or—even better, when possible—filled these items out themselves, the examiner should have a good idea of how well they know who and where they are and when. Although patients with compromised consciousness or dementia usually respond unquestioningly, alert patients who are guarded or sensitive about their mental competence may feel insulted by the simplicity of these "who, where, when" questions. Asking time, place, and person questions in the context of filling out a test form comes across to the subject as an integral part of the proceedings and is thus less likely to arouse negative reactions.

In a patient population, orientation status was related to memory impairment and age but was independent of education and simple attention as measured by digit span (Sweet, Suchy, et al., 1999). However, even normal, healthy older persons may have mild orientation difficulty, especially when experiencing the routine sameness of hospital days.

Awareness Interview (S.W. Anderson and Tranel, 1989)

This structured interview format consists of questions relevant to patient orientation for person, place, and time, plus items dealing with patients' appreciation of deficits in motor functioning, thinking, memory, speech and language, and visuoperceptual functions. An additional question asks how patients evaluate their test performances. This interview not only provides a graded scoring schedule for evaluation of overall severity of awareness problems but also gives examiners useful wording for the questions they must ask in evaluating patient orientation and awareness. Although the 3-point ratings for each item are subjective, the authors reported a high ($r = .92$) interrater reliability coefficient. High awareness scores correlate with patient abilities to successfully function in daily activities such as telephone use, money management, and cooking (LaBuda and Lichtenberg, 1999).

Time

To test for time orientation, the examiner asks for the date (day, month, year, and day of the week) and the time of day. Sense of temporal continuity should also be assessed, since the patient may be able to remember the number and name of the present day and yet not have a functional sense of time, particularly if in a rehabilitation unit or similarly well-structured setting (J.W. Brown, 1990). Likewise, some patients will have a generally accurate awareness of the passage of time but be unable to remember the specifics of the date. Poor performances on time orientation items have been demonstrated with control subjects with less than eight years of schooling (J.C. Anthony et al., 1982). Questions concerning *duration* will assess the patient's appreciation of temporal continuity. The examiner may ask such questions as "How long have you been in this place?"[1] "How long is it since you last worked?" "How long since you last saw me?" "What was your last meal (i.e., breakfast, lunch, or dinner)?"[2] How long ago did you have it?" Time disorientation occurs more commonly in patients with impaired memory who are older, have limited education, and perform digits reversed poorly (Sweet, Suchy, et al., 1999).

Temporal Orientation Test (Benton, Sivan, Hamsher, et al., 1994)

This is a scoring technique in which negative numerical values are assigned to errors in any one of the five basic time orientation elements: day, month, year, day of week, and present clock time. It has a system of differentially weighted scores for each of the five elements. Errors in naming or numbering days and errors in clock time are given one point for each day difference between the correct and the erroneously stated day and for each 30 minutes between clock time and stated time. Errors in naming months are given 5 points for each month of difference between the present and the named month. Errors in numbering years receive 10 points for each year of difference between the present and the named year. The total error score is subtracted from 100 to obtain the test score. Scores from the original study in which 60 patients with brain disease were compared with 110 control patients are given in Table 9.1. For more comprehensive and recent test data, see the 1994 manual or the manual for the *Iowa Screening Battery for Mental Decline* (Eslinger, Damasio, and Benton, 1984). However, elaborate normative tables are not necessary here: suffice it to say that any loss of score points greater than 5 indicates significant temporal disorientation as only 4% of one study's elderly (ages 60–88) control subjects received an error score greater than 2 (Eslinger, Damasio, Benton, and Van Allen, 1985).

Neuropsychological findings. Both control subjects (hospitalized patients without cerebral disease) and brain damaged patients most commonly erred by missing the number of the day of the month by one or two. For both groups, the second most common error was misestimating clock time by more than 30 minutes. The brain damaged group miscalled the day of the week with much greater frequency than the control patients. Patients with undifferentiated bilateral cerebral disease performed most poorly of all. Applying this test to frontal lobe patients, Benton (1968) found that it discriminated between bilaterally and unilaterally brain injured patients, for none of the frontal lobe patients with unilateral lesions gave defective performances but 57% of those with bilateral lesions did. For many patients with a history of alcoholism, failure on this test predicted poor performances on several tests of short-term

---

[1]It is important not to give away answers before the questions are asked. The examiner who is testing for *time* orientation before *place* must be careful not to ask, "How long have you been in the *hospital?*" or "When did you arrive in *Portland?*"

[2]Some mental status examinations for recent memory include questions about the foods served at a recent meal. Without checking with the family or dietitian, one cannot know whether the patient had chicken for dinner or is reporting an old memory of what people usually eat in the evening. The menu problem is most apparent with breakfast as the variety is usually limited making it impossible to tell whether the patient's memory is old or new when "toast, cereal, eggs, and coffee" are given as breakfast items.

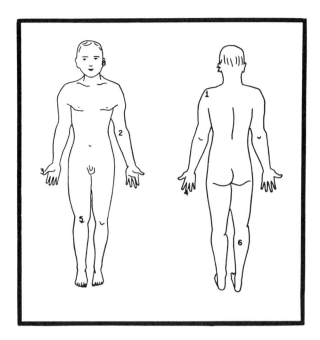

FIGURE 9.1 One of the five diagrams of the Personal Orientation Test (Semmes et al., 1963).

A comparison of left and right hemisphere damaged patients' performances on this task indicated that the left hemisphere patients have greatest difficulty following verbal directions, whereas patients with right hemisphere lesions are more likely to ignore the left side of their body or objects presented to their left (i.e., left hemi-inattention) (Raghaven 1961). Parkinson patients tend to have difficulty with this test (Raskin, Borod, and Tweedy, 1992). Using part 5 of this test, which is mostly nonverbal, F.P. Bowen (1976) showed that Parkinson patients suffered some defects in body orientation. Those whose symptoms were predominantly left-sided or bilateral made many more errors than patients with predominantly right-sided symptoms.

Finger Agnosia

Impaired finger recognition is associated with different kinds of deficits. When the impairment involves only one hand it may be due to a sensory deficit resulting from brain damage contralateral to the affected hand (Denburg and Tranel, 2003). The bilateral disorder will typically be a *finger agnosia,* a specific manifestation of autotopagnosia, and be most evident on examination of the middle three fingers (Frederiks, 1985a). A variety of techniques designed to elicit finger agnosia have demonstrated that it can occur with lesions on either side of the brain (Denburg and Tranel, 2003), but most lesions associated with finger agnosia involve the left angular gyrus (Mesulam, 2000b). The problem shows up in impaired finger recognition, identification, differentiation, naming, and orientation, whether they be the patient's fingers or someone else's, and regardless of which hand. Finger agnosia is one of the four disorders that make up Gerstmann's syndrome (see p. 71).

As the stimulus in both the following tests is tactile, it becomes important to distinguish between a sensory deficit due to impaired somatosensory processing and the perceptual/conceptual problem of somatic disorientation. The Boston Diagnostic Aphasia Examination supplementary section includes items for examining finger identification. When the problem is associated with compromised speech functions and involves the hand ipsilateral to the lesion—for which sensation should be relatively intact—as well as the contralateral one, then it probably reflects a finger agnosia. Other tests of the hands' sensory competence can help distinguish between a sensory deficit and the agnosic condition.

Finger Localization (Benton, Sivan, Hamsher, et al., 1994)

This technique for examining finger agnosia has three parts: Part A requires subjects to identify their fingers when touched one at a time at the tip by the examiner. Part B differs from Part A only in shielding the hand from the subject's sight using a curtained box in which the hand is placed (see Fig. 9.2, p. 342). In Part C two fingers are touched at a time. Ten trials are given each hand for each of the three conditions. Benton and his colleagues (1994) provide outline drawings for each hand with the fingers numbered so that speech-impaired patients can respond by pointing or saying a number (see Fig. 9.3, p. 342).

Of 104 control subjects, 60% made two or fewer errors with fewer than three errors on average. There were no differences between sexes or between hands. Both patients with right and with left unilateral hemisphere disease made errors, but a higher proportion of aphasic patients were impaired than any other group, and most of the patients with right-sided lesions who performed poorly were also "mentally deteriorated." Both control subjects and brain damaged patients made a larger proportion of errors on Part C than the other two parts. Seven to nine errors is considered a *borderline performance,* 10 to 12 errors is *moderately defective,* and performances with 13 or more errors are *defective.* The test manual also provides normative data for children.

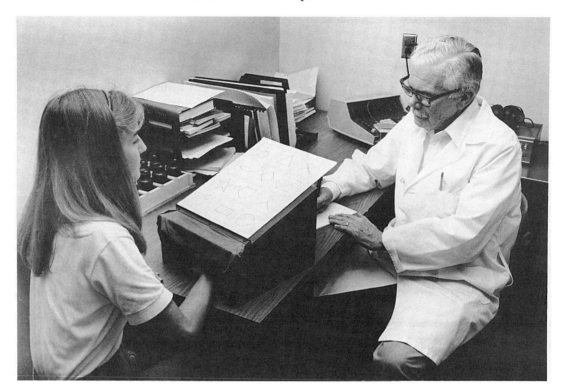

FIGURE 9.2 Curtained box used by Benton to shield stimuli from the subject's sight when testing finger locationation and other tactile capacities (e.g., see p. 341). (Photograph courtesy of Arthur L. Benton)

Tactile Finger Recognition (Reitan and Wolfson, 1993; called Tactile Finger Localization by Boll, 1974)

In this test the examiner assigns a number to each finger. When subjects' eyes are closed and hands extended, the examiner touches the fingers of each hand in a predetermined order, and subjects report the number of the finger they think was touched. Patients with right-sided lesions made more both contralateral and ipsilateral errors than patients with left hemisphere damage (Boll, 1974). This test is part of the Halstead-Reitan Battery.

Directional (Right–Left) Orientation

As the examination of body orientation almost necessarily involves right–left directions, so the examination of right–left orientation usually refers to body parts (e.g., Strub and Black, 2000). Healthy normal adults make virtually no mistakes on right–left discriminations involving their own body parts or those of others (Benton, Sivan, Hamsher, et al., 1994; T.J. Snyder, 1991; see Right–Left Orientation Test, below), although women tend to respond more slowly than men and report more susceptibility to right–left confusion. When verbal communication is sufficiently intact, gross testing of direction sense can be accomplished with a few commands, such as "Place your right hand on your left knee," "Touch your left cheek with your left thumb," or "Touch my left hand with your right hand." Standardized formats such as in the Boston Diagnostic Aphasia Examination supplementary section (which includes items exploring right–left orientation to body parts) or the following tests are useful for determining

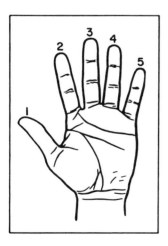
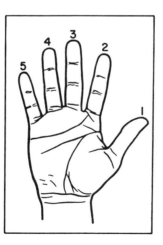

FIGURE 9.3 Outline drawings of the right and left hands with fingers numbered for identification. (© Oxford University Press. Reproduced by permission)

the extent and severity of a suspected problem when a detailed documentation of deficits is required, or in research.

Right–left Orientation Test (RLOT) (Benton, Sivan, Hamsher et al., 1994)

This 20-item test challenges the subject to deal with combinations of right and left side with body parts (hand, knee, eye, ear) and with the subject's own body or the examiner's (or a front view model of a person). Excepting items 13 to 16, the side of the responding hand and the indicated body part are specified to randomize and balance right and left commands and combinations. Items 1 to 4 each ask the subject to show a hand, eye, or ear; items 5 to 12 give instructions to touch a body part with a hand; then items 13 to 16 request the subject to point to a body part of the examiner; the last four items have the subject put a hand on the body part of the examiner or of a model that is at least 15" (38 cm) in height. The A and B forms of this test are identical except that "right" and "left" commands are reversed. Two other forms of this test (R, L) are available for examining hemiplegic patients. The maximum number of errors in the normal range is 3, with no more than one error on the first 12 items involving the subject's own body. No sex differences have shown up on this test (T.J. Snyder, 1991). On a small patient sample, aphasics gave the largest number of impaired performances (75%), while 35% of patients with right-sided lesions made all their errors on the "other person" items, in which right and left must be reversed conceptually (Benton, Sivan, Hamsher, et al., 1994).

Standardized Road-Map Test of Direction Sense (Money, 1976)

This easily administered test provides developmental norms for a quick paper-and-pencil assessment of right–left orientation (D. Alexander, 1976; Fig. 9.4). The examiner traces a dotted pathway with a pencil, asking the subject to tell the direction taken at each turn, right or left. The test is preceded by a demonstration trial on an abbreviated pathway in a corner of the map. Although norms for ages above 18 are not available, a cutoff point of ten errors (out of 32 choice points) is recommended for evaluating performances, regardless of age. Since it is unlikely that persons who make fewer than 10 errors are guessing, their sense of direction is probably reasonably well-developed and intact.

Test characteristics. Women tend to make more errors than men, but their average is well under 10

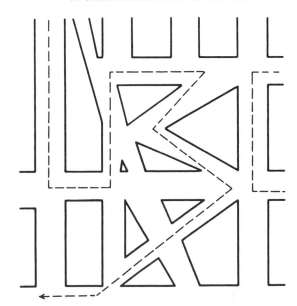

FIGURE 9.4 A section of *The Standardized Road-Map Test of Direction Sense* (© J. Money. Courtesy of the author)

(Brouwers et al., 1984; W.W. Beatty and Troster, 1987); both age and dementia may exaggerate this difference. Young and elderly control groups performed equally well, making on the average fewer than two errors on the unrotated turns; but subjects age 62 and older had significantly more errors than younger ones when judging the direction of rotated turns, and more errors than for unrotated turns (Flicker, Ferris, Crook, et al., 1988). Still, the older subjects' average score for both kinds of turns combined did not exceed 10. Almost all brain injured patients who are capable of following simple instructions pass this test, so that failure is a clear sign of impaired right–left orientation. It may also result from inability to shift right–left orientation, which will show up particularly at those choice points involving a conceptual reorientation of 90° to 180° (e.g., see Vingerhoets, Lannoo, and Bauwens, 1996).

Neuropsychological findings. N. Butters, Soeldner, and Fedio (1972) examined the performances of four groups of patients with localized lesions (right parietal and temporal, left frontal and temporal). The left frontal group averaged 11.9 errors, more than twice as many as the right parietal patients who were next highest with a mean error score of 5.5. The authors suggested that the failures of the left frontal patients reflect the test's conceptual demands for making mental spatial rotations. Without left parietal and right frontal groups, this study did not address the question of whether the right–left confusion that some patients with left hemisphere damage experience may have contributed as much or more than conceptual disabilities to the left frontal patients' poor performances. A more recent study showed that parietal injuries affect Road-Map orientation much more than do frontal injuries (Vingerhoets, Lannoo, and Bauwens, 1996). Although not statistically significant, a tendency for patients with left parietal injuries to have greater error scores (6.0 ± 7.7) than those with right parietal lesions (4.5 ± 3.4) suggests that impaired coordinate orientation was a relevant factor in left-lesioned patients' performances.

Patients with early probable Alzheimer's disease made an average number of errors that is still less than ten although somewhat higher than the average for elderly controls (Brouwers et al., 1984; Flicker, Ferris, Crook, et al., 1988). They tended to show a differential between unrotated and rotated turns similar to that of elderly control subjects. Moderately impaired Alzheimer patients have difficulty on this task even when the paper is rotated so that all intersections are aligned with the participant (Rainville et al., 2002). Their impairment may be based on visuoperceptual difficulties specific for this disease (H.L. O'Brien et al., 2001). The average performance for patients with advanced dementia is at chance levels for both kinds of turns. This test was instructive in bringing out differences between Alzheimer and Huntington patients, as the Huntington patients' near-normal unrotated performances indicate that simple right–left orientation was intact while their much lower scores on rotated turns implicate a conceptual problem (Brouwers et al., 1984).

Space

Spatial disorientation refers to a variety of defects that in some way interfere with the ability to relate to the position, direction, or movement of objects or points in space. Different kinds of spatial disorientation do not arise from a single defect but are associated with damage to different areas of the brain and involve different functions (Farah, 2003; McCarthy and Warrington, 1990; Schachter and Nadel, 1991). As in every other kind of defective performance, an understanding of the disorientated behavior requires careful analysis of its components to determine the extent to which the problem is one of verbal labeling, inattention, visual scanning, visual agnosia, or a true spatial disorientation. Thus, comprehensive testing for spatial disorientation requires a number of different tests.

Spatial orientation is one of the components of visual perception. For this reason, some tests of visuospatial orientation are presented in Chapter 10, such as Judgment of Line Orientation, which measures the accuracy of angular orientation, and line bisection tests, which involve distance estimation and are susceptible to left visuospatial inattention.

Distance estimations

Both spatial disorientation (Benton, 1969b) and visual scanning defects (Diller, Ben Yishay, Gerstman, et al., 1974) can contribute to impaired distance judgment. Benton divided problems of distance estimation into those involving local space, i.e., "within grasping distance," and those involving points in the space "beyond arm's reach." He noted a tendency for patients with disordered spatial orientation to confuse retinal size with actual size, ignoring the effects of distance.

In examining distance estimation, Hécaen and Angelergues (1963) gave their patients a number of informal tasks. They asked for both relative (nearer, farther) and absolute (in numerical scale) estimations of distances between people in a room, between the patient and objects located in different parts of the room, and for rough comparisons between the relative estimates. Patients also had to indicate when two moving objects were equidistant from them. These distance estimation tasks were among other tests for visuospatial deficits. Although some visuospatial deficits accompanied lesions in the left posterior cortex, more than five times as many such deficits occurred in association with right posterior—particularly occipital—lesions.

Mental transformations in space

Abilities to conceptualize such spatial transformations as rotations, inversions, and three-dimensional forms of two-dimensional stimuli are sensitive to various kinds of brain disorders (e.g., Boller, Passafiume, and Keefe, 1984; N. Butters and Barton, 1970; Royer and Holland, 1975). Examination methods are mostly paper-and-pencil tests that require the subject to indicate which of several rotated figures matches the stimulus figure, to discriminate right from left hands, or to mark a test figure so that it will be identical with the stimulus figure. Luria (1966, p. 371) showed samples of the last two kinds of items in the "parallelogram test" and the "hands test." These items and others have been taken from paper-and-pencil intelligence and aptitude tests (e.g., the *California Tests of Mental Maturity* [E.T. Sullivan et al., 1963]; the *Primary Mental Abilities Tests* [L.L. Thurstone and Thurstone, 1962], among others). For example, the multiple-choice *Cognition of Figural Systems* subtest of the *Structure of Intellect Learning Abilities Test (SOI-LA)* has one section requiring the subject to identify figures rotated 90° and another section calling for 180° rotation (Meeker and Meeker, 1985; see also Sohlberg and Mateer, 1989).

Performance deficits on tests requiring mental rotations have been associated with parietal lobe lesions;

neuroimaging studies support clinical findings that mental rotation requires bilateral parietal involvement with greatest contributions from the right (Farah, 2003). Studies involving conceptual transformations from two to three dimensions have consistently demonstrated the importance of the right hemisphere to these operations (Nebes, 1978). These tests were not designed for diagnostic discriminations; but rather, they are of value in gaining information about visuospatial orientation for planning, treatment, and research purposes.

Mental Re-orientation (Ratcliff, 1979)

This spatial orientation test, devised for neuropsychological studies, has also been called the *Left–Right Reorientation Test* (see Fig. 9.5). The "Little Men" figures can be presented by slide projection or on cards. Each of the four positions is shown eight times; in half the cases the black disc is on the figure's right, in half on the left. The subject's task is to state whether the black disc is on the figure's right or left side. Before and after the test, the subjects were given 12 trials of a simple right–left discrimination task (indicating whether a black circle was right or left of a white one) that did not involve reorientation in order to evaluate accuracy of simple right–left discrimination. When given to healthy college students, the sexes did not differ with respect to accuracy, but women had longer response latencies than men, with male left-handers having the shortest latencies, female left-handers the longest (T.J. Snyder, 1991). Not surprisingly, these subjects made fewer errors to the upright figures, regardless of whether forward or backward, than to the in-verted figures. This test proved to be more sensitive to left–right confusion than the Right-Left Orientation Test (T.J. Snyder, personal communication, 1990). Comparing small patient samples (e.g., only 11 in the "nonposterior" group), Ratcliff (1979) found that those with right posterior lesions made more errors ($p < .05$) than any other group.

The *Puppet Test,* a variation of the Mental Reorientation task, examines spatial reorientations on visuoperceptual and visuomotor tasks (Boller, Passafiume, and Keefe, 1984). The visuoperceptual format displays 12 multiple-choice items; for each the subject must match a Little Man, each oriented differently, to one of four differently oriented alternatives. The visuomotor format presents pairs of variously oriented Little Men, only one with a black disc; the task here is to blacken the disc on the same side of the other figure as the sample figure's black disc. Despite the motor response required by this test's visuomotor format, factor analysis indicated that both parts of the test have a significant visuoperceptual component, while the motor response part has a relatively low loading on a factor strongly associated with drawing and other motor response tests.

Space Thinking (Flags) (L.L. Thurstone and Jeffrey, 1984)

This 21-item multiple-choice test of spatial orientation was developed for use in industry but is readily applicable to neuropsychological questions. Each item displays a rectangular geometric design, the "flag," with six other designs which may differ in their spatial rotation, mirror the target design, or both (see Fig. 9.6). The subject's task is to indicate whether the flag shows the same or the opposite side of the flag as the target. Norms are available for a 5-minute time limit. For different items, from 0 to 4 responses may be correct.

Spatial dyscalculias

Difficulty in calculating arithmetic problems in which the relative position of the numbers is a critical element of the problem, as in carrying numbers or long division, tends to occur with posterior lesions, particularly involving the right hemisphere (A. Basso, Burgio, and Caporali, 2000; Denburg and Tranel, 2003). This shows up in distinctive errors of misplacement of numbers relative to one another, confusion of columns or rows of numbers, and neglect of one or more numbers, although the patient understands the operations and appreciates the meaning and value of the mathematical symbols.

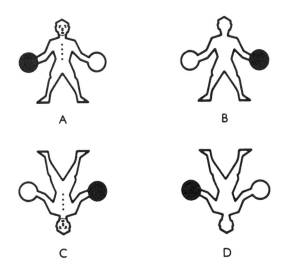

FIGURE 9.5 "Little Men" figures of the Mental Re-orientation Test.

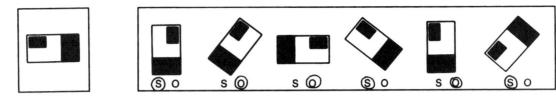

FIGURE 9.6 *Space Thinking* (*Flags*) example, marked correctly for *same* (S) or *opposite* (O) positions relative to the model on the left of the figure. (Courtesy of Pearson Reid London House, Inc.)

Tests for spatial dyscalculia are easily improvised (e.g., see Macaruso et al., 1992; Strub and Black, 2000). When making up arithmetic problems to bring out a spatial dyscalculia, the examiner should include several relatively simple addition, subtraction, multiplication, and long division problems using two- to four-digit numbers that require carrying for their solution, written out in fairly large numbers. The examiner can also dictate a variety of computation problems to see how the patient sets them up. Items involving multiplication and division are particularly challenging for patients with this disorder. With unlined letter-size sheets of paper, the patient does not have ready-made lines for visual guidance. A large sheet of paper gives the patient a greater opportunity to demonstrate spatial organization and planning than do smaller ones on which abnormally small writing or unusual use of space (e.g., crowding along one edge) may be less apparent.

Some items of the Arithmetic subtest of the Wide Range Achievement Test–Revised (WRAT-3) (Wilkinson, 1993) will elicit spatial dyscalculia. However, writing space is limited so that subjects may work out their calculations on various parts of the problem sheets, making it difficult for the examiner to see how an erroneous answer was computed. A useful set of problems that are graduated in difficulty, but none too hard for the average 11- or 12-year-old, are shown in Figure 15.12, p. 609. On this untimed test patients are instructed to work out the problems on the sheet as sufficient space is provided for each problem. Most of the problems require spatial organization and are thus sensitive to spatial dyscalculia.

Topographical orientation

Defective memory for familiar routes or for the location of objects and places in space involves an impaired ability for *revisualization*, the retrieval of established visuospatial knowledge (Benton, 1969b; Farah, 2003). Testing for this defect can be difficult, for it typically involves disorientation around home or neighborhood, sometimes in spite of the patient's ability to verbalize the street directions or descriptions of the floor plan of the home.

When alert patients or their families complain that they get lost easily or seem bewildered in familiar surroundings, topographical memory can be tested by asking first for descriptions of familiar floor plans (e.g., house or ward) and routes (nearest grocery store or gas station from home), and then having them draw the floor plan or a map, showing how to get from home to store or station, or a map of the downtown or other section of a familiar city. The catch here is that the locale must be familiar to both patient and examiner to be properly evaluated. One way of getting around this problem is to find the patient's spouse or a friend who can draw a correct plan for comparison (e.g., see Fig. 9.7a,b, p. 347).

A reasonably accurate performance of these kinds of tasks is well within the capacity of most of the adult population. Thus, a single blatant error, such as an east–west reversal, a gross distortion, or a logically impossible element on a diagram or map, should raise the suspicion of impairment. More than one error may be due to defective visuospatial orientation but does not necessarily indicate impaired topographical memory. Visuographic disabilities, unilateral spatial inattention, a global memory disorder, or a confusional state may also interfere with performance on tests of visuospatial orientation. Evaluation of the source of failure should take into account the nature of the patient's errors on this task and the presence of visuographic, perceptual, or memory problems on other tasks.

Topographical Localization (Lezak, no date)

Topographical memory can be further tested by requesting the patient to locate prominent cities on a map of the country. An outline map of the United States of convenient size can be easily made by tracing the Area Code map in the telephone directory onto letter-size paper. When using this technique, I [mdl] first ask the patient to write in the compass directions on this piece of paper. I then ask the patient to show on the map where a number of places are located by writing in a number assigned to each of them. For example, "Write 1 to show where the Atlantic Ocean is; 2 for Florida;

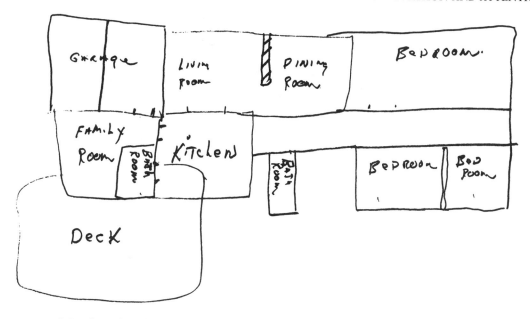

FIGURE 9.7a Floor plan of his home drawn by a 55-year-old mechanic injured in a traffic accident who complained of difficulty finding his way around his hometown.

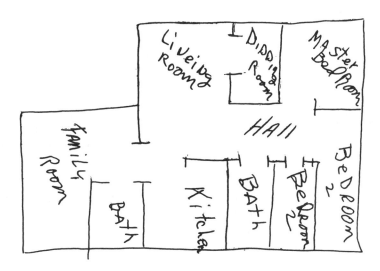

FIGURE 9.7b Floor plan of their home drawn by the mechanic's spouse.

3 for Portland; 4 for Los Angeles; 5 for Texas; 6 for Chicago; 7 for Mexico; 8 for New York; 9 for the Pacific Ocean; 10 for the Rocky Mountains, and 11 for your birthplace" (see Fig. 9.8, p. 348). The places named will be different in different locales as appropriate for different patients. To insure this test's sensitivity to visuospatial inattention, at least as many of the places named should be in the west as in the east.

For clinical purposes, scoring is not necessary as disorientation is usually readily apparent. It is important, however, to distinguish between disorientation and ig-

norance when a patient misses more than one or two items. Committing a few errors, particularly if they are not all eastward displacements of western locales, probably reflects ignorance. Many errors usually reflect disorientation. Most patients mark the points of the compass correctly. However, a scoring system that gives one point for each correct compass direction and one point for each of the 11 named locales (including the patient's place of birth) discriminated better than chance ($p < .05$) between performances made by 45 head injury patients in the second year posttrauma or

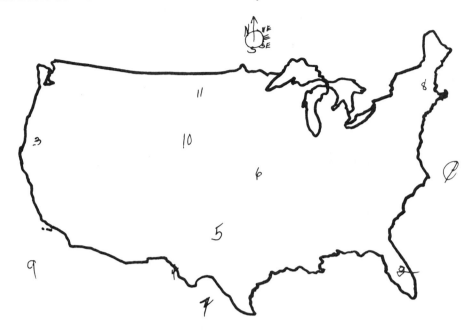

FIGURE 9.8 Topographical Localization responses by a 50-year-old engineer who had been hemiparetic for 14 years since suffering a ruptured aneurysm of the right anterior communicating artery. Although only two of his respones are notably displaced (4 and 6), he betrayed left visuospatial inattention in an overelaborated set of compass points from which the West was omitted.

later ($M = 12.40 \pm 3.07$) and 27 normal control subjects ($M = 14.26 \pm 1.26$).[1] In contrast, none of an older (age range 42–76) group of six patients with right CVAs achieved scores above 11 ($M = 7.83 \pm 2.79$).

Fargo Map Test (FMT-S)[2]
(W.W. Beatty, 1988, 1989a)

This test of geographic knowledge takes into account not only familiarity with the major features of the United States but also the regions with which the subject, by history, should have familiarity. It tests a variety of functions, particularly recent and remote spatial memory and visuospatial orientation. The materials consist of two kinds of maps, an outline map of the United States and 17 regional outline maps, including two of states (New York, Florida), one for New England, with the rest covering from two- to four-state regions (e.g., California, Nevada; Nebraska, Iowa, Kansas, Missouri); and lists of numbered target geographic features (e.g., Atlantic Ocean, Canada) and

cities. After recording all of the places in which subjects have lived for a year or more and their age when residing in each place, subjects locate from 12 to 16 designated target items on each map. A near-correct location receives a score of 1; a less precise approximation earns .5, and of course 0 is scored for a complete failure. Only targets within correctly identified maps count in the scoring. Percent correct can be calculated for each regional map to make regional comparisons with respect to the subject's dates of residence.

Test characteristics. Normative studies indicated that test scores increased directly with education and age—even past age 70 for men, although women's accuracy declined a little after 70 (W.W. Beatty, 1988, 1989a). Men tend to outperform women but not in every comparison (W.W. Beatty and Troster, 1987). The standard form takes about an hour to complete. A shortened revised version (*FMT-R*) provides outline maps on which numbered dots correspond to gross geographic features and cities, with answer sheets for writing in the number associated with printed place names (W.W. Beatty, 1988). This procedure is less difficult for those who lack fine motor control than the standard requirement of positioning the code number on the outline map.

Neuropsychological findings. Parkinson patients whose mental status is intact performed normally ex-

---

[1]The control subjects and 41 of the patients had been given neuropsychological examinations as part of a Veterans Administration funded research project on the long-term cognitive consequences of nonprogressive brain damage. All of the control subjects were in the 19–49 year age range; the patients were in that age range when injured. Two were in their 50s when tested.

[2]To obtain copies of the Fargo Map Test, contact W.W. Beatty, Ph.D., Dept. of Psychiatry and Behavioral Sciences, University of Oklahoma Health Sciences Center, POB 26901, Oklahoma City, OK 73190.

cept for excessive errors in locating cities, but deteriorated patients were impaired on all test sections requiring geographic localization (W.W. Beatty and Monson, 1989). Huntington patients did poorly for both where they lived earlier and their present region (W.W. Beatty, 1989b). Mildly and moderately demented Alzheimer patients achieved higher scores for their early region of residence than for their current one (W.W. Beatty, personal communication, 1992); these patients were only moderately impaired for knowledge of gross geographical features but severely impaired in locating cities with any precision.

Route finding

The inability to find one's way around familiar places or to learn new routes is not uncommon in brain impaired patients. The problem can be so severe that it may take days before an alert and ambulatory patient can learn the way to the nurses' station. It often dissipates as the acute stage of the illness passes, but some confusion about locations and slowness in learning new routes may remain.

The *Rivermead Behavioural Memory Test* (B.A. Wilson, Clare, et al., 1999) includes a test of learning and recalling a route. A more challenging technique shows a videotape of an unfamiliar neighborhood; later the examiner asks the subject about routes through the neighborhood and the location and relationship of landmarks. Compared to control subjects, patients with either right or left temporal lobe lesions were less accurate in their topographical orientation (Maguire et al., 1996). The only difference between these patient groups was the inaccuracy of the right-side lesion group in judging the proximity of landmarks.

ATTENTION, CONCENTRATION, AND TRACKING

> There are no tests of attention . . . one can only assess a certain aspect of human behavior with special interest for its attentional component.
> *van Zomeren and Brouwer, 1992*

Although attention, concentration, and tracking can be differentiated theoretically, in practice they are difficult to separate. Purely attentional defects appear as distractibility or impaired ability for focused behavior, regardless of the patient's intention. Intact attention is a necessary precondition of both concentration and mental tracking activities. Concentration problems may be due to a simple attentional disturbance, or to inability to maintain a purposeful attentional focus or, as is often the case, to both problems. At the next level of complexity, conceptual tracking can be prevented or interrupted by attention or concentration problems and also by diminished ability to maintain focused attention on one's mental contents while solving problems or following a sequence of ideas.

Clarifying the nature of an attention problem depends on observations of the patient's general behavior as well as performance on tests involving concentration and tracking, for only by comparing these various observations can the examiner begin to distinguish the simpler global defects of attention from the more discrete, task-specific problems of concentration and tracking. Further, impaired attention is not always a global disability but may involve one receptive or expressive modality more than others.

Reaction Time

As slowed processing speed often underlies attentional deficits (see pp. 35, 176), reaction time tests can serve as relatively direct means of measuring processing speed and understanding the nature of the associated attentional deficits (Godefroy et al., 2002; Posner, 1978; Shum, McFarland, and Bain, 1994). Simple reaction time is frequently slowed with brain disease or injury, and slowing increases disproportionately with increases in the complexity of the task, whether it be the addition of choices requiring discrimination of stimuli (J.K. Foster et al., 1999; Gronwall, 1987; Ponsford and Kinsella, 1992; van Zomeren, Brouwer, and Deelman, 1984) or introduction of a distractor (van Zomeren and Brouwer, 1987; van Zomeren, Brouwer, and Deelman, 1984). This slowing is particularly apparent in patients with severe TBI (Spikman, van Zomeren, and Deelman, 1996; Spikman, Deelman, and van Zomeren, 2000) and in many multiple sclerosis patients (Kail, 1998). What additionally may distinguish TBI patients from control subjects is inconsistency in levels or individual performances (Stuss, Stethem, Hugenholtz, et al., 1989). Simple reaction time slowing in itself distinguishes dementing patients from matched elderly control subjects, but differences between the healthy and dementing groups become much larger when stimulus choices (e.g., red or green light) and/or response choices (e.g., right or left hand) are introduced (Ferris, Crook, Sathananthan, and Gershon, 1976). Depressed patients too tend to have slowed reaction times on simple as well as complex formats (Cornell et al., 1984), although depression did not add to slowing in one group of cognitively impaired elderly patients (Bieliauskas and Lamberty, 1995). Should reaction time apparatus be unavailable, slowed processing can also be inferred from sluggish performances on other speeded attention tasks (van Zomeren and Brouwer, 1992).

Vigilance

Successful performance of any test of attention, concentration, or tracking requires sustained, focused attention. Vigilance tests examine the ability to sustain and focus attention in itself. These tests typically involve the sequential presentation of stimuli (such as strings of letters or numbers) over a period of time with instructions for the patient to indicate in some way (tap, raise hand) when a given number or letter (the target stimulus) is perceived. Thus, lists of 60 or more items can be read, played on a tape, or presented in a visual display at a rate of one per sec (Strub and Black, 2000). The simplest form of the task presents only one target item but two or more can be used. More complex variations of the vigilance task require the subject to respond only when the target item is preceded by a specified item (e.g., to tap B only when it follows D). Strub and Black's *"A" Random Letter Test* (p. 42) contains one run of three As and two runs of two embedded among other alphabet letters randomly sequenced; the triplet and pairs additionally sample the patient's ability to stop an ongoing activity. These vigilance tasks are performed easily by persons whose capacity for sustained attention is intact, and they are unaffected by age, at least well into the 80s (M.S. Albert, Duffy, and Naeser, 1987). Thus, even one or two lapses on these tests may reflect an attention problem. Tests for assessing unilateral spatial inattention, such as letter or line cancellation, are discussed in Chapter 10, pp. 378–383. In addition to the tests reviewed in this section, the Speech Sounds Perception Test and/or the Seashore Rhythm Test may be useful for examining a known or suspected concentration or tracking problem.

Continuous Performance Test (CPT) (1)
(Rosvold et al., 1956)

Computerized vigilance tests usually present stimuli briefly and provide reaction times as well as accuracy data. Letters of the alphabet in random order appear briefly in the center of the screen. In the simple condition, subjects are asked to respond to every X and, in the more difficult version, X only if it follows A. Although the CPT is intended to measure sustained attention, failure can occur for a variety of reasons, including impulsivity or dyscontrol, anxiety, and environmental noise (Ballard, 1996; Halperin et al., 1991). Total error scores mask the differences between errors of omission and commission and should be avoided as these two types of errors have different interpretations (Halperin et al., 1991).

Continuous Performance Test (CPT) (2)
(Conners, 1992)

In this format the subject indicates every time a letter other than X appears on the screen, which allows for measures of commission as well as omission. Because the test takes 14 min., it also measures ability to sustain attention—or waning attention—over a relatively long period for such a monotonous task. A newer version, the *CPT-II* (Conners, 2000), has a larger normative sample and includes data from adults with brain disorders as well as people with attention deficit disorders (ADD, ADHD). Adults with ADHD have a higher rate of commission errors than control subjects, which suggests that they have trouble inhibiting responses (Barkley, 1997; Epstein et al., 2001). They also make omission errors and have high reaction time variability (A.J. Walker et al., 2000). Patients with temporal lobe epilepsy are less able to sustain attention throughout the test (Fleck et al., 2002).

Continuous Performance Test of Attention (CPTA)
(Cicerone, 1997)

An auditory CPT presents a series of letters read at the rate of one per sec on an audiotape. Subjects are asked to tap their finger each time they hear a target letter. Task difficulty is heightened by increasing the complexity of the target. In the first three conditions the targeted letters increase from one to two to five specified letters. In the fourth condition subjects are asked to respond only when they hear **A** immediately following **L**. In the last condition, letters and numbers are intermingled randomly; targets are one letter and one number. Responses are scored for omission and commission errors. An average 13 months post mild TBI, patients made significantly more errors than control subjects on this task.

Short-term Storage Capacity

The dissociation between processing speed, as measured by speed-dependent and mental tracking tests, and short-term capacity reflects the basic dimensions of attention: how fast the attentional system operates and how much it can process at once. Of course speed and quantity are related: the faster a system can process information the more will be processed within a given time. Yet, since this relationship is far from perfect (Shum, McFarland, and Bain, 1990), these two dimensions can—and should—be examined separately insofar as possible. Attentional capacity is measured by span tests which expose the subject to increasingly larger (or smaller, in some formats) amounts of information with instructions to indicate how much of the stimulus was immediately taken in by repeating what was seen or heard or indicating what was grasped in some other kind of immediate response. Depending upon the theoretical bias of the examiner, or the battery in which the test is embedded, these tests have been considered measures of attentional capacity or of short-term memory. While they require short-term memory, performances on these tests are more strongly associated with attention than memory and are covered in this chapter (Howieson and Lezak, 2002). Tests requiring immediate recall of more information than can be grasped at once (e.g., supraspan, story recall) or which interpose an activity or other stimulus between administration and response (e.g., Consonant Trigrams) are presented in Chapter 11, Memory I: Tests.

Digit Span

The *Digit Span* test in the Wechsler batteries (the intelligence and memory scales) is the format in most common use for measuring span of immediate verbal recall. In these batteries it comprises two different tests, *Digits Forward* and *Digits Backward,* each of which involves different mental activities and are affected differently by brain damage (see Banken, 1985; E. Kaplan, Fein, et al., 1991). Both tests consist of seven pairs of random number sequences that the examiner reads aloud at the rate of one per sec, and both thus involve auditory attention. Additionally, both depend on a short-term retention capacity (Shum, McFarland, and Bain, 1990). Here much of the similarity between the two tests ends.

A note on confounded data

In combining the two digit span tasks to obtain one score, which is the score that enters into most statistical analyses of the Wechsler tests, these two tests are treated as if they measured the same behavior or very highly correlated behaviors. The latter assumption holds for most normal control subjects into their 70s (E. Kaplan, Fein, et al., 1991) and 80s (Storandt, Botwinick, and Danziger, 1986). Differences between these two tests become most evident in studies of brain damaged patients in which forward and reverse digit spans are dissociated in some patient groups (F.W. Black, 1986; Lezak, 1979; E.V. Sullivan, Sagar, et al., 1989) but not in others (F.W. Black and Strub, 1978).

For example, of 52 patients (age range 18-63) with TBI of mild to moderate severity, 24 could reverse no more than four digits, yet 41 had digit forward spans ranging from 6 to 9, in the *average* or better range (clinical record review, mdl). This difference, significant at the .05 level ($\chi^2 = 3.938$), clearly demonstrates that these two tests each measure something different. Yet with so many of these patients unable to recall more than four digits in reverse, only seven of the 52 received WIS-R Digit Span scaled scores below 8, the lowest score in the *average* ability range. The difference between the number of patients receiving *below average* scores on Digits Reversed and the number with *average* or better scores when Digits Forward and Digits Reversed were combined for the scaled score was significant ($\chi^2 = 5.797$, $p < .02$), further demonstrating how combining scores from these two tests obscure the data that each test generates.

The risk of losing information by dealing with these two tests as if they were one and combining their scores becomes obvious when one considers what the Wechsler Adult Intelligence Scale scaled score, based on the combined raw scores, might mean.

To obtain a scaled score of 10, the *average* scaled score, young adults need to achieve a raw score of 11 which, in the majority of cases, will be based on a Digits Forward score of 6 and a Digits Backward score of 5. However, they can get this *average* rating based on a Digits Forward score of 7 and a Digits Backward score of 4 with a three-point difference between the scores, a difference that occurs more often in brain damaged groups than in intact populations. The same scaled score of 10 may also be based on a Digits Forward score of 8 and a Digits Backward score of 3. A disparity between scores of this magnitude is almost never seen in normal, intact subjects. Moreover, a Digits Backward score of 3 in a young adult, in itself is indicative of brain dysfunction in a compliant, attentive, subject.

The problem of obscuring meaningful data is further compounded in all recent revisions of Wechsler's tests, WAIS-III and WMS-III. In order "to increase the variability of scores," two trials are given of each item (i.e., at each span length) and the subject receives one raw score point for each correct trial. Thus, information about the length of span is confounded with information about the reliability of span performance.

A person in the 18- to 34-year-old range who passes only one of the two trials on each pair of Digits Forward items containing four to six digits and Digits Backward items of three to five digits in length would receive a total raw score of 10, which would be classified at the level of a scaled score of 6, just above the *borderline* level. Yet, for neuropsychological purposes, this subject has demonstrated an *average* span for both digit span forward and the reversed digit span. That this subject is more prone to error than most people whose span for digits of the same length is interesting information. However, neither the subject's *average* capacity nor proneness to error is evident in the final score. Rather, the final score can easily be misinterpreted by anyone who does not know that both the subject's forward and reversed span of recall were *within normal limits* (i.e., 6 and 5).

For neuropsychological purposes, none of the Wechsler scoring systems is useful. Digit span forward and digit span reversed are meaningful pieces of information that require no further elaboration for interpretation. The examiner seeking to place the subject's performance into a statistically meaningful context will find the cumulative percentiles for the longest digit spans (forward and reversed data are presented separately) in the manual for the *WAIS-R as a Neuropsychological Instrument* (*WAIS-RNI*) (E. Kaplan, Fein, et al., 1991). The examiner who is interested in assessing the *reliability* of a patient's attention span should give at least three trials at each span length (J.R. Shelton and her coworkers [1992] recommend "at least 10"), but should not confound data about the consistency of response with data concerning its length.

Forward Span: Digits, Verbal

All WIS-A and Wechsler Memory Scale (WMS) batteries use the same digit sequences, except that the original two WMS batteries began with the four-digit sequence. Table 9.2 provides four other lists, drawn from a table of random numbers, for repeat examinations. These are most likely to be useful when examinations are frequently repeated, as may be required in drug studies; or for patients whose problems are due to attentional and not learning deficits and who fail after only two or three trials but learn one or more of these short sequences, particularly if retested several times. These sequences can be used with any kind of number-based span test.

For digit span recall, the subject's task is to repeat each sequence exactly as it is given. When a sequence is repeated correctly, the examiner reads the next longer number sequence, continuing until the subject fails a pair of sequences or repeats the highest (9 digits in WIS-A batteries, 8 in WMS) sequence correctly. Occasionally a patient's failure will appear to be due to distraction, poor cooperation, inattentiveness, etc., such that a third trial at the twice-failed sequence seems appropriate to the examiner whose interest is in finding out span length. The other occasion for giving a third trial arises when the patient recalls more digits reversed than forward and the examiner can assume that the patient is capable of doing at least as well on the much less difficult Digits Forward as on Digits Backward. This infrequently occurring disparity probably reflects the patient's lack of effort on a simple task. Almost invariably, such a patient will pass a third trial and occasionally will pass one or two of the longer sequences. When giving the third digit series, the easiest method is to take the requisite number of digits out of one of the nine forward or eight backward sequences that are unlikely to be used. Another administration variant has been introduced by Edith Kaplan and her colleagues (see Milberg, Hebben, and Kaplan, 1996) who give the next longer series of digits when failure on both trials results from mixing up the sequence of the correct digits. They then score for both the longest correct span and the longest span of correct but out-of-sequence digits.

Although examiners are instructed to begin with the three-digit sequence in the WAIS-R and WMS-R, and two digits in the WAIS-III and WMS-R, this is a waste of time and can try the patience of most alert and responsive patients. Beginning with four digits loses no data in most cases. Subjects who have tracked well in conversation and already have performed adequately on the Sequential Operations Series (see p. 362) may

TABLE 9.2 Randomized Digit Lists for Span Tests

Forward Span		Reversed Span	
3-6-5	4-8-5	2-9	5-1
2-4-9	2-6-8	9-4	3-7
3-1-7-4	5-7-2-4	8-7-2	9-1-8
4-6-2-9	7-6-2-9	5-8-1	6-2-9
1-8-5-2-4	4-7-1-5-9	7-8-6-4	9-7-1-3
8-7-1-9-5	2-8-3-6-9	8-4-1-7	3-9-8-6
2-4-7-3-9-1	8-3-7-1-4-2	8-2-5-9-4	5-9-6-8-1
1-9-5-7-4-3	7-8-4-9-3-6	5-8-6-3-9	2-1-8-9-3
5-6-3-9-2-1-8	8-2-1-9-3-7-4	9-2-4-8-7-1	9-5-7-4-3-8
6-4-3-2-8-5	2-9-5-4-9-6-8	3-7-4-9-1-6	1-9-3-7-4-2
2-7-5-8-6-4-9-3	3-1-7-9-4-2-5-8	8-7-5-2-6-3-9	6-9-4-2-7-3-1
9-4-3-7-6-2-5-8	7-2-8-1-9-6-5-3	4-8-1-2-5-9-7	5-8-4-2-1-9-6

begin with five digits. If they fail at the four- or five-digit level it is easy to drop down to a lower one. For most clinical purposes, subjects who recall seven digits correctly have demonstrated performance well *within normal limits;* whether they can recall 8 or 9 digits is usually irrelevant for the examination issues, and the test can be discontinued at this point without losing important clinical information. Of course, when following a research protocol, such clinical liberties cannot be taken.

Test characteristics. The WIS-A manuals provide a method to convert raw scores into standard scores that can be juggled into separate standard score estimates for each of the two Digit Span tests. However, because Digit Span has a relatively restricted range (89% of a large normative sample had spans within the 5 to 8 digit range [E. Kaplan, Fein, et al., 1991]) and does not correlate very highly with other measures of cognitive prowess, it makes more sense to deal with the data in raw score form than to convert them. Taking into account that the normal range for Digits Forward is 6 ± 1 (G.A. Miller, 1956; Spitz, 1972), and that education appears to have a decided effect on this task (Ardila and Rosselli, 1989; A.S. Kaufman, McLean, and Reynolds, 1988), it is easy to remember that spans of 6 or better are well *within normal limits,* a span of 5 may be *marginal to normal limits,* a span of 4 is definitely *borderline,* and 3 is *defective.* Age tends to affect forward span only minimally beyond ages 65 or 70 as reported in most studies (Craik, 1990; Jarvik, 1988); even healthy subjects in the 84–100 age range achieved a forward span mean of 5.7 ± 1.0, range 4–8 (Howieson, Holm, et al., 1993; see also Hickman et al., 2000).

What Digits Forward measures is more closely related to the efficiency of attention (i.e., freedom from distractibility) than to what is commonly thought of as memory (A.S. Kaufman, McLean, and Reynolds, 1991; P.C. Fowler, Richards, et al., 1987; Spitz, 1972). Anxiety tends to reduce the number of digits recalled (J.H. Mueller, 1979; Pyke and Agnew, 1963), but it may be difficult to identify this effect in the individual case. For example, one study of 144 students (half tested as high anxiety; half, as low anxiety) reported a Digits Forward mean score of 7.15 for the high-anxiety students and 7.54 for the low-anxiety students, a difference indicating a large overlap between the two groups (J.H. Mueller and Overcast, 1976). Stress-induced lowering of the Digits Forward score has been shown to dissipate with practice (Pyke and Agnew, 1963). When it appears likely that a stress reaction is interfering with a subject's Digit Span performance, the examiner can repeat the test later. If the scores remain low even when the task is familiar and

the patient is presumably more at ease, then the poor performance is probably due to something other than stress. Practice effects are negligible (McCaffrey, Duff, and Westervelt, 2000a), with test–retest reliability coefficients ranging from .66 to .89 depending on interval length and subjects' ages (Matarazzo and Herman, 1984; W.G. Snow, Tierney, et al., 1989).

Neuropsychological findings. Digit repetition is resistant to the effects of many brain disorders. It tends to be more vulnerable to left hemisphere involvement than to either right hemisphere or diffuse damage (Hom and Reitan, 1984; Risse et al., 1984; Weinberg et al., 1972). Since it appears to be primarily a measure of attention, it is not surprising to find that, in the first months following head trauma or psychosurgery, the Digits Forward span of some patients is likely to fall *below normal limits,* but it is also likely to show returns to normal levels during the subsequent years (Lezak, 1979; Uzzell, Langfit, and Dolinskas, 1987). However, repeated blows to the head appear to impair span, as the number of concussions in soccer players was inversely correlated with Digits Forward performance (Matser, Kessels, Lezak, et al., 1999). It tends to be reduced in individuals with long-term exposure to industrial solvents (Morrow, Robin, et al., 1992). Although among the tests least sensitive to dementia, once past the early, mild stage, forward span becomes noticeably reduced in length (Kaszniak, Garron, and Fox, 1979; Storandt, Botwinick, and Danziger, 1986). In previously healthy persons, shrinkage of both forward and reversed span was likely to herald death within several years (B. Johansson and Berg, 1989).

If systematic studies of digit span error types associated with different kinds of neuropsychological conditions have been conducted, they must be rare and unreported. However, clinical experience does provide some suggestive error patterns. For example, patients with conditions associated with diffuse damage who have mental tracking difficulties (e.g., mild TBI, many multiple sclerosis patients) are apt to repeat the correct digits but mix up the order, usually among the middle digits. More severely impaired TBI patients with significant frontal lobe involvement may substitute bits of overlearned sequence strings (e.g., 3-5-6-7 instead of 3-5-9) or perseverate from the previous series. With severe brain injury, span tends to be reduced (Ruff, Evans, and Marshall, 1986). When moderately demented patients fail they are likely to repeat no more than their limit (e.g., 4-8-2-9 or 4-8-9-5 instead of 4-8-2-9-5). The WAIS-RNI record form contains a section for recording Digit Span errors in detail, and possible interpretations are discussed in the manual (E. Kaplan, Fein, et al., 1991).

Point Digit Span (A. Smith, 1975)

Along with the standard administration of forward and reversed digit span, Aaron Smith (1975) also had his subjects point out the digit series on a numbered card. The "point" administration parallels the digit span tests in all respects except that the response modality does not require speech, so that the verbal span of patients who are speech impaired can be tested. It has been used with aphasic patients for both auditory and visual digit presentations (Risse et al., 1984). When given with Digit Span to the speaking patient, marked performance differences favoring the "point" administration suggest a problem in speech production. A "point" performance much below the performance on the standard presentation suggests problems in integrating visual and verbal processes (A. Smith, personal communication, 1975 [mdl]). J.R. Shelton and her colleagues (1992) advised that this technique always be used with patients whose ability for expressive speech is compromised.

Point Digit Span requires a large (approximately 30 cm × 30 cm) white cardboard card on which the numbers 1 through 9 appear sequentially in a 3 × 3 arrangement in big (approximately 6 cm high) black print. The subject is instructed to point out the number sequence read by the examiner, or the reverse sequence for Digits Backward. The procedure is identical with that of Digit Span; i.e., presentation begins with three digits (two for Digits Backward), and increases one digit following each success. As with the Digit Span tests, the examiner may begin with longer sequences than those prescribed in the WIS-A. The test is usually discontinued after two failures at the same level. To keep language-handicapped patients from developing a spatial strategy that would then obscure their verbal attention span, J.R. Shelton and her colleagues (1992) gave them a response sheet with a different layout of numbers for each succeeding set of numbers of a given length.

Letter span

Normal letter span (6.7 in the 20s, 6.5 in the 50s) is virtually identical with digit span except beyond age 60 when some relative loss has been documented (5.5 in the 60s, 5.4 in the 70s) (Botwinick and Storandt, 1974). McCarthy and Warrington (1990) suggested that letter span is likely to be a little smaller than digit span as random letters are less susceptible to "chunking" into "higher order units" than digits (e.g., 3-2-6-8 converts readily into "thirty-two sixty-eight").

Every localization group in Newcombe's (1969) study of missile wound patients had lower average scores on a simple letter span task, analogous to Digits Forward, than on the digit version of the task, as did the control subjects and two groups of head trauma patients studied by Ruff, Evans, and Marshall (1986). With a mean age of 28, these control subjects' average letter span was 6.3 ± 1.3. On Letter Span, with the single exception of the left frontal group, the left hemisphere damaged groups also obtained lower average scores than the right hemisphere groups. The mean score range for the left hemisphere groups was from 5.00 (temporal or temporoparietal, and mixed) to 5.75 (frontal); for the right hemisphere patients, group mean scores ranged from 5.50 (frontal and mixed) to 6.00 (temporal or temporoparietal). The overlap of scores of the different patient groups was too great to permit inferences about localization of the lesion in any individual case.

Forward Span: Visual

Since the first appearance of a test for immediate recall of visually presented sequences, several variations on this concept have been developed. Not only is it useful for immediate visual span but the format can be adapted for examining visuospatial learning as well (see pp. 466–467).

Knox Cube Test (KCT)

This is one of the tests in the *Arthur Point Scale of Performance* battery (Arthur, 1947). The four blocks of the Knox Cube Test are affixed in a row on a strip of wood. The examiner taps the cubes in prearranged sequences of increasing length and complexity, and the subject must try to imitate the tapping pattern exactly. Administration time runs from two to five minutes.

Test characteristics. Correlational studies supported the clinical impression that this test measures immediate visuospatial attention span with the addition of a "strong" sequencing component (Bornstein, 1983a; see also Shum, McFarland, and Bain, 1990). The ease of administration and simplicity of the required response recommend this task for memory testing of patients with speech and motor disabilities and low stamina, and elderly or psychiatric patients (Inglis, 1957). Edith Kaplan has pointed out that the straight alignment of four blocks allows the patient to use a numerical system to aid recall so that there may be both verbal and nonverbal contributions to responses. Mean scores of a large general hospital population of middle-aged and elderly men tested twice on four different administrations of this test correlated significantly ($p < .01$) with the WAIS Digit Span, Arithmetic, Block Design, and Picture Arrangement tests, but less highly with Vocabulary (Sterne, 1966). Bornstein and Suga (1988) reported a significant ($p < .01$) education effect. Having demonstrated improved performance on the Knox Cube Test immediately following electroconvulsive shock therapy to the right hemisphere, Horan and his colleagues (1980) concluded that this test examines the sequential, time-dependent functions of the left hemisphere.

Corsi Block-tapping Test

B. Milner (1971) described the Block-tapping task devised by P. Corsi for testing memory impairment of patients who had undergone temporal lobe resection. It consists of nine black $1^{1}/_{2}$-inch cubes fastened in a random order to a black board (see Fig. 9.9). Each time the examiner taps the blocks in a prearranged sequence, the patient must attempt to copy this tapping pattern.

Test characteristics. Using the Corsi format, block span tends to run about one block lower than digit span (E.V. Sullivan, Sagar, Gabrieli, et al., 1989; Ruff, Evans, and Marshall, 1986), although Canavan and his colleagues (1989) found more than a two-point disparity for healthy young control subjects. Smirni and coworkers (1983) observed that, due to the layout of the blocks on the Corsi board, different sequences vary in length and spatial configuration. This will be true of the WAIS-RNI version too (see below). Beyond the 3-block items which almost all healthy young adults repeated correctly, the sequences with the shortest distances between blocks were most likely to be failed. When the length of the paths was equal, success was associated with the sequence pattern.

Education contributed significantly to performance levels in an Italian study in which more than one-third of the subjects had less than a sixth grade education (Orsini, Chiacchio, et al., 1986). Men tended to achieve slightly (in the general range of one-third of a point) but significantly ($p < .001$) higher scores than women, although this discrepancy became smaller with more years of schooling and was virtually nonexistent for persons with more than 12 years of education. Age effects did not appear in this study until after 60 when they became increasingly pronounced. In another study, despite the subjects' wide age range (20–75), no age effects appeared, but these subjects averaged 13+ years of schooling and it is unlikely that any had less than an eighth grade education (Mittenberg, Seidenberg, et al., 1989).

Neuropsychological findings. DeRenzi, Faglioni, and Previdi (1977) found that stroke patients with visual field defects had a shorter immediate recall span on Corsi's test than patients without such a defect, regardless of hemisphere side of lesion. In another study, patients with right hemisphere lesions performed more poorly than those with lesions on the left (Kessels et al., 2001). Although their score range was wide (2 to 8), right temporal lobectomy patients' average score equaled that of the control group (5.0), while those with left temporal lobectomies had a much smaller range (4 to 6) and a slightly but not significantly higher average score (5.6) (Canavan et al., 1989). Patients with frontal lobe lesions performed least well ($M = 4.4$). With only one to three moves to copy, Alzheimer patients achieved relatively normal scores (E.V. Sullivan, Corkin, and Growdon, 1986); but following the standard procedure of increasing the number of blocks in a sequence after each successful trial, mildly and moderately impaired Alzheimer patients' scores were lower ($M = 4.4$) compared to control subjects ($M = 5.5$), and severely impaired patients had an average span of only 2.5 (Corkin, 1982). Severe anterograde amnesia did not appear to affect this visuospatial attention task. Patients

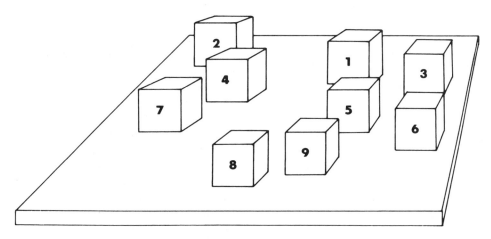

FIGURE 9.9 Corsi's Block-tapping board. (From Milner, 1971)

with moderately severe TBI lagged behind normal subjects about 0.5 point (6.4 to 5.8), and those with severe head injuries performed on the average another half-point lower (*M* = 5.3) (Ruff, Evans, and Marshall, 1986).

Corsi variants. Three variations on the Corsi theme are found in the WMS-R, WMS-III, and WAIS-RNI. For a comprehensive discussion of many other variations, see Berch et al. (1998). The difficulty level of a particular variant depends on many factors, including the length of the spatial path and the number of crisscrosses (Orsini, Pasquadibisceglie, et al., 2001). The Wechsler variants most like the original Corsi format are the WAIS-RNI and WMS-III *Spatial Span,* which use ten cubes on a board attached in an irregular arrangement. Separate WMS-III norms are available for total span (i.e., counting both trials at each level) forward and total span backward. The WAIS-RNI version too requires two administrations at each level but registers only the longest span. E. Kaplan, Fein, and their coworkers (1991) observed that block span will normally be one to two points below digit span. If it is much lower than the longest digit span, right hemisphere dysfunction is implicated; and when the block span exceeds the digit span, left hemisphere dysfunction may be suspected. These workers also noted the usefulness of the block array in eliciting evidence of lateralized dysfunction.

The WMS-R *Visual Memory Span* provides two cards on each of which are printed eight squares in a nonlinear pattern—red squares for forward span and green for reversed span. The administration procedure is the same as for Digit Span, requiring two trials at each level regardless of whether the first was passed. It thus also confounds span length with response consistency, producing a score that is uninterpretable except at the extremes of the continuum.

Finding herself without a Corsi board when this test seemed to have clinical utility, but in an office with a blackboard, a Veterans' Administration Hospital Psychology Service intern (Jeanne Taylor) marked up nine X's in random fashion with chalk and was able to examine her patient's visuospatial span this way. Lacking any of these materials, an examiner can gain some sense of a patient's visuospatial span by drawing X's or circles on a piece of paper. The chief advantage of having either a block board or the WMS-R cards is that number cues (on the block side facing the examiner or diagramed in the WMS-R manual) enable the examiner to keep track of the patient's performance more easily.

Still another variant is the *Dot Location* task (D.L. Roth and Crosson, 1985), which consists of a pattern of dots on a sheet of paper. Following the Corsi administration format, the examiner points to two or more dots (up to nine), but instead of repeating the examiner's movements, the subject must draw the dots on a blank sheet of paper in the correct order and general location (within a 4 cm radius of the original dot position). This test proved to be the most sensitive to the presence of brain damage when compared with other span formats (digit and word span, Corsi blocks).

Sentence repetition

Unlike many span tests, this technique for assessing auditory span has a naturalistic quality that can be directly related to the patient's everyday functioning. Patients with intact language skills but an abnormally short sentence span are like persons with a reading knowledge of a second language but little conversational experience trying to understand native speakers who always seem to be talking too fast. Foreign language beginners tend to grasp only fragments of what they hear, often losing critical elements of speech that go by them too quickly to be fully accessed. The difference between patients with a reduced sentence span and the foreign language novice is that, because it is their native tongue, patients frequently do not realize how much they are missing. Their experience, typically, is that the people around them have become argumentative and disagreeable to them. Family members perceive these patients as not paying attention because of disinterest or self-absorption, or as having a memory disorder when this is not the case. These problems of mishearing verbal instructions or getting only part of telephone messages can seriously affect work as well as disrupt family interactions.

The number of data bits grasped in a meaningful sentence is normally considerably greater than digit or word span (McCarthy and Warrington, 1990), with only small decrements occurring after age 65 and appearing more prominently in men's than women's performances. Repeatability of sentences by normal subjects depends on their length, complexity, and meaningfulness, and the speed at which they are spoken (Butterworth et al., 1990; J.R. Shelton et al., 1992). The importance of meaningfulness to length of span becomes evident in studies of patients whose span for unrelated items may be very short but whose recall of sentences is relatively well preserved (R.C. Martin, 1990; McCarthy and Warrington, 1990). Comparing sentence span with word or digit span, the examiner can determine the extent to which meaning contributes to the patient's span of auditory-verbal attention. Goodglass and Kaplan (1983a) and Goodglass, Kaplan, and Barresi (2000) also acknowledged the role that familiarity can play in the rapidity and efficiency with which a sentence is grasped by providing two lists of phrases and sentences in a sentence repetition test, *Repeating Phrases*. The "high probability" set contains commonplace words and expressions (such as, "I drove home from work"), which contrast with "low probability" sentences composed of less frequently used words and phrases (e.g., "The spy fled to Greece").

Some mental status examinations include one or two sentences for repetition (e.g., Mini-Mental State Examination [MMSE], Neurobehavioral Cognitive Status Examination). Godwin-Austen and Bendall (1990) recommended inclusion of a sentence for repetition when examining older persons, suggesting the "Babcock" sentence: "One thing a nation must have to be rich and great is a large secure supply of wood." The *Memory for Sentences* test in the 1986 revision of the Stanford-Binet scales contains sentences appropriate for the range of difficulty levels from two years to late adolescence (Thorndike et al., 1986).

Administration of sentence repetition tests typically proceeds from easy items to the most difficult, or until the subject has made four or five failures (e.g., Benton and Hamsher, 1989; Spreen and Strauss, 1998; Thorndike et al., 1986). When the test is given this way, the patient who is having difficulty on this task will experience repeated failures until the criterion for stopping has been reached. John A. Walker (personal communication, 1985 [mdl]) suggested that skipping around between shorter and longer items in a quasi-random manner will avoid unnecessary unpleasantness for the patient, as successes will be intermixed with failures. Moreover, when giving this test to persons whose language abilities are intact, it is not necessary to begin with the easiest items. For example, on the original version of Sentence Repetition (Table 9.3), a good place to start with nonaphasic patients is item 7, both because it is getting close to the length where many attentionally impaired patients begin to fail, and because missing the pronoun shift may indicate confusion about the instructions. This pronoun error suggests that the subject may not have understood the requirement of repeating the sentence *exactly*, and instructions must be given again carefully before proceeding further. Some Americans whose normal speech has a grammar base that differs from the usual English forms (e.g., "black English," some rural dialects) will not be able to respond appropriately because they "hear" what is said in their vernacular. Persons with strong dialects should not be given this test.

Neuropsychological findings. As on other highly verbal tasks, failure on sentence span tests has long been associated with lesions of the left hemisphere.

TABLE 9.3 Sentence Repetition: Form I

1. Take this home
2. Where is the child?
3. The car will not run.
4. Why are they not living here?
5. The band played and the crowd cheered.
6. Where are you going to work next summer?
7. He sold his house and they moved to the farm.
8. Work in the garden until you have picked all the beans.
9. The artist painted many of the beautiful scenes in this valley.
10. This doctor does not travel to all the towns in the country.
11. He should be able to tell us exactly when she will be performing here.
12. Why do the members of that group never write to their representatives for aid?
13. Many men and women were not able to get to work because of the severe snow storm.
14. The members of the committee have agreed to hold their meeting on the first Tuesday of each month.

Failures may occur at the level of auditory comprehension or articulation of words, or because of a dissociation between auditory input and speech output (Goodglass and Kaplan, 1983a). The attentional aspects of this span test show up in the difficulty patients with attentional deficits have in accurately recalling sentences containing as many as 18 or 20 syllables. Patients with conditions in which damage tends to be diffusely distributed, such as TBI and multiple sclerosis—which are also conditions in which attentional deficits are prominent—are most likely to perform *below normal limits* on this task. Alzheimer patients have reduced sentence repetition span, particularly when the sentences are complex (J.A. Small et al., 2000).

Sentence Repetition (1) (Benton and Hamsher, 1989)

This subtest of the Multilingual Aphasia Examination (MAE) can do double duty. The 14 sentences in Form I graduate in length from three syllables to 24 syllables (Table 9.3). They thus provide a measure of span for meaningful verbal material ranging from abnormally short to the expected normal adult length of 24 syllables. In addition, seven different linguistic constructions are represented among each of the two sets of sentences, Forms I and II (e.g., positive declaration, negative interrogation, etc.). This allows examiners to test for the patients' sensitivity to syntactical variations in what they hear. This feature appears useful for registering mild or subtle linguistic deficits of patients whose communication abilities may seem intact when they take the usual tests in a neuropsychological examination. A scoring

TABLE 9.4 Sentence Repetition (MAE):
Demographic Adjustments for
Raw Scores

Add	Education	Age
0	≥ 12	≤ 59
1	≥ 12	≥ 60
2	= 9-11	≤ 59
3	= 9-11	≥ 60
3	= 6-8	≤ 59
4	= 6-8	≥ 60

From Benton, Hamsher and Siran (1994)

system gives one point for each sentence repeated correctly and provides an adjustment formula for additional points to be added to the raw score of persons in the age groups 25 to 29 and 60 to 64 who have had 15 years or less of schooling (see Table 9.4). Scores of 11 to 13 are in the *average* range (%iles 25–75, approximately); scores between 9 and 10 are considered *borderline* to *low average;* below 9 performances are *defective.* Scores of 14 or higher were obtained by 35% of the control group. Developmental norms offer age-equivalent values that can be meaningful in interpreting impaired performances to lay persons (Carmichael and MacDonald, 1984); e.g., recall no better than sentence 8 is at the level of an eight-year-old child.

Sentence Repetition (2) (Spreen and Strauss, 1998)

The overall format of this test is similar to Benton and Hamsher's Sentence Repetition test, but the 22 sentences in each of the two forms (A and B) are unique to this version (printed in Spreen and Strauss, 1998, p. 368). The first item is a one-word statement (e.g., "Look") with graduated lengths up to the last 26-syllable item. Although the sentences can be read, the recommended administration is by audiotape. Both adult and developmental norms are provided by Spreen and Strauss.

Silly Sentences (1) (Botwinick and Storandt, 1974)

The contribution of meaning to retention was examined by means of a set of long silly sentences developed as a parallel task to paragraph recall:

1. The Declaration of Independence/sang/overnight/while/the cereal/jumped/by the river./
2. Two dates/ate/the bed/under the car/seeing/pink flowers/forever./
3. They slept/in the fire/to avoid the draft./It was cold there/and their sweaters kept them/cool./
4. I eat pink mice./They are delicious/but their green fur/gives me heartburn./

Each of these silly sentences is read to the subject and is immediately followed by a recall trial. Correct recall of each unit—marked by slashes—merits one point so that the total possible score is 24. The average recall of subjects by decades was 21.9 for the 20s, 20.7 for the 30s, 20.6 for the 40s, 20.0 for the 50s, 19.0 for the 60s, and 15.6 for the 70s. A comparison of these data with scores obtained for paragraph recall indicated that meaningfulness of material played an increasingly greater role in recall in the later decades.

Silly Sentences (2) (Baddeley, Emslie, and Nimmo-Smith, 1993)

Speed of comprehension is the central feature of this test. The subject reads 100 short sentences, half of which are sensible, and indicates whether each is sensible or silly. The score is the total number of correct responses completed within two min. An alternate form is available for retesting. Test–retest reliability using the alternate form is high (*r* = .78). However, a practice effect was observed with scores 11 points higher on a second administration one to two weeks later (Hinton-Bayre et al., 1997). These authors found this test to be more sensitive to the effects of concussion 24 to 48 hours after injury in rugby players than either the WAIS-R Digit Symbol or Symbol Digit Modalities Test.

Mental Tracking: Tests of Working Memory

Working memory tests require people to hold information in mind while performing a mental operation. Thus tests which require the subject to keep track of ongoing mental activity typically involve at least very short-term memory of what was just done or heard while performing another operation. For instance, the WIS Arithmetic test questions must be held in mind while the subject performs the mental operations. A good example of this process is the paper clip item on the WAIS-III, which requires that the long, convoluted problem be held in mind in order to recall the number of green paper clips while mentally adding all (red, yellow, and green) paper clips. Many examinees require that this item be re-read and some require a visual assist. Working memory is a favorite paradigm for functional imaging studies; the left dorsolateral prefrontal cortex is activated for verbal working memory tests and the right dorsolateral prefrontal cortex for spatial versions (Cabeza and Nyberg, 2000; Dolan et al., 1997; Henson, 2001).

The simplest test of mental tracking is digit span reversed, also known as *Digits Backward* (WIS-A, WMS), which tests how many bits of information a person can attend to at once and repeat in reverse order. Tests of mental tracking may involve some perceptual tracking or more complex mental operations, and many of them also involve some form of scanning. The role of visual scanning in conceptual tracking has become apparent in studies demonstrating the scanning eye movements that accompany the performance of such conceptual tracking tasks as digit span reversed or spelling a long word or name in reverse (Weinberg, Diller, et al., 1972).

A general attentional deficit has also been implicated in these problems (I.H. Robertson, 1990). Tracking tasks can be complicated by requiring the subject to track two or more stimuli or associated ideas simultaneously, alternatively, or sequentially on double or multiple tracking tests involving divided and/or shifting attention. The capacity for double or multiple tracking is one most likely to break down first with many brain disorders. Occasionally, loss of this capacity may be the only documentable mental change following TBI or a brain disease. The disturbance appears as difficulty in keeping two or more lines of thought going, as in a cocktail party conversation, in solving two- or three-number addition or multiplication problems mentally, or in remembering one thing while doing another, and thus can be very burdensome for the patient.

Reversing serial order: digits

The *Digits Backward* number sequences of the Wechsler Intelligence and Memory Scales are two to eight digits long and two to seven digits long, respectively. On hearing them, the subject's task is to repeat them in an exactly reversed order. Although Wechsler's instructions suffice for most subjects, when dealing with patients who are known or suspected to have brain impairment, some variants may help to elicit maximum performance on this test without violating the standardization.

Patients whose thinking is concrete or who become easily confused may comprehend the standard instructions for Digits Backward with difficulty if at all. Typically, these patients do not appreciate the transposition pattern of "backward" but only understand that the last number need be repeated first. To reduce the likelihood of this misconception, the digits backward task can be introduced using the wording in the Wechsler manuals, giving as the first example the two-digit number sequence, which even very impaired patients can do with relative ease. Everyone who seems likely to have difficulty on this task but recalls two digits reversed on either the first or second trial then receives the following instructions: "Good! [or some other expression of approval], Now I am going to say some more numbers, and once again, when I stop I want you

to say them backwards. For example, if I say 1-2-3, what would you say?" Most patients can reverse this three-number sequence because of its inherently familiar pattern. If the subject fails this example, it is given again verbally with the admonition, "Remember, when I stop, I want you to say the numbers backwards—the last number first and the first one last, just as if you were reading them backwards." The examiner may point in the air from the patient's left to right when saying each number, and then point in the reverse direction as the patient repeats the reversed numbers so as to add a visual and directional reinforcement to the concept "backwards." If the patient still is unable to grasp the idea, the examiner can write each number down while saying "1-2-3" the third time. The examiner needs to write the numbers in a large hand on a separate sheet of paper or at the top of the Record Form so that they face the subject and run from the subject's left to right, i.e., Ɛ-Ƨ-Ɩ. Then the examiner points to each number as the patient says or reads it. No further effort is made to explain the test. As soon as the subject reverses the 1-2-3 set correctly or has received all of the above explanations, the examiner continues with as much more of Digits Backward as the patient can do. The WAIS-III manual gives the cumulative percentages of differences between the longest Digits Forward and Digits Backward spans for each age group.

Test characteristics. The normal raw score difference between digits forward and digits reversed tends to range a little above 1.0 (E. Kaplan, Fein, et al., 1991), with a spread of reported differences running as low as .59 (J.H. Mueller and Overcast, 1976) and as high as 2.00 (Black and Strub, 1978). The examiner who chooses to evaluate the Digits Backward performance on the basis of the raw score should consider raw scores of 4 to 5 as *within normal limits;* 3 as *borderline defective* or *defective,* depending on the patient's educational background (Botwinick and Storandt, 1974; Weinberg, Diller, et al., 1972); and 2 to be *defective* for everyone. The Digits Backward span typically decreases about one point during the seventh decade. However, as age groups 60 and over are increasingly likely to be better educated than the groups examined in the reported studies, these classifications may be appropriate at least to age 70. Howieson and her colleagues (1993) reported that for 34 subjects in the 84–100 age range, digit span reversed did not differ greatly from normal expectations ($M = 4.5 \pm 1.0$, range 3-6). Thus some but not all older subjects get lower scores than younger ones (Canavan et al., 1989; Kaszniak, Garron, and Fox, 1979).

The reversed digit span requirement of storing a few data bits briefly while juggling them around mentally is an effortful activity that calls upon the working memory, as distinct from the more passive span of apprehension measured by Digits Forward (Banken, 1985; F.W. Black, 1986). The task involves mental double-tracking in that both the memory and the reversing operations must proceed simultaneously. Many people report that they perform this task by making a mental image of the numbers and "reading" them backward. Impairment is found in patients with unilateral spatial inattention or with attentional bias to the right-side of space, supporting the role of mental imagery in performing this task (Rapport, Webster, and Dutra, 1994). Factor analysis indicated that both visual and verbal processes contribute to the reversed digit span performance (Larrabee and Kane, 1986).

Neuropsychological findings. Like other tests involving mental tracking, digit span reversed is sensitive to many different brain disorders. By and large, patients with left hemisphere damage (F.W. Black, 1986; Newcombe, 1969; Weinberg, Diller, et al., 1972) and patients with visual field defects have shorter reversed spans than those without such defects. Yet following temporal lobectomy neither right- nor left-lesioned patients performed much differently than control subjects (Canavan et al., 1989). In general, the more severe the lesion the fewer reversed digits can be recalled (Leininger, Gramling, et al., 1990; Uzzell, Langfitt, and Dolinskas, 1987). This test is very vulnerable to the kind of diffuse damage that occurs with solvent exposure (Morrow, Robin, et al., 1992) and in many dementing processes. Patients with frontal lesions may also have difficulty (Leskela et al., 1999). Frontal lobe lesions, such as those produced by psychosurgical procedures, may lower reversed span (Canavan et al., 1989; Scherer et al., 1955), but not necessarily (Stuss, Kaplan, et al., 1981).

Reversing serial order: spelling and common sequences

The sensitivity of digit span reversed to brain dysfunction also is seen in other tasks requiring reversals in the serial order of letters or numbers (M.B. Bender, 1979). Bender used a variety of reversal tasks to assess normal children, adults, and several groups of older persons (over age 60); adult patients with a dementing disease or diffuse encephalopathy, or with aphasia; and dyslexic children. In addition to counting forward and backward (mostly to establish a set for reversing serial order on subsequent tasks), subjects were given the following reversing tasks. Spelling two- (I-T), three- (C-A-T), four- (H-A-N-D), and five- (W-O-R-L-D) letter words backward was the first. Any word of the designated length in which each letter appears only once can

be substituted as needed (e.g., H-O-U-S-E, Q-U-I-C-K). Bender also compared letter reversing with serial word reversing; for example, days of the week, months of the year. Reading words forward and backward and vertically printed words from top to bottom and bottom to top were examined next.

Approximately one in ten normal adults and older subjects over age 60 made reversed spelling errors. The older the subject group, the greater the incidence of errors, up to an error rate of 38% for a group of normal adults aged 75 to 88. The percentage of patients with diffuse encephalopathy making reverse spelling errors was less (78%) than the percentage of aphasic patients failing this task (90%). Aphasic patients also had more difficulty than others reading in reverse or from bottom to top, although many who failed these tasks could read satisfactorily in the left–right or top to bottom directions. Bender (1979) suggested that the ability to reverse letter, number, and word strings is characteristic of normal thinking and language processes. It is vulnerable to many different kinds of cerebral disorders because defects in reversal ability can result from (a) reading disability; (b) memory disorder; (c) aphasia; (d) the mental rigidity that may accompany aging; (e) perseverative tendencies; (f) a specific disability for learning to reverse symbolic material; or (g) "latent" alexia that shows up on the unfamiliar reversing task.

Jenkyn and his coworkers (1985) asked their subjects to spell *world* forward as well as backwards. When misspelled, the reversal of the misspelling becomes the correct backwards response. In their normative group the incidence of failure increased from 6% at ages 50–54 to 21% in the 80+ age range.

Mental Control (Wechsler Memory Scales) (Wechsler, 1945, 1987, 1997b)

This section of the original Wechsler Memory Scale and its revisions (WMS-R) has little to do with memory. Its attentional character has been consistently attested by factor analytic studies (e.g., Bornstein and Chelune, 1989; D.L. Roth, Conboy, et al., 1990). This three-item test of mental tracking requires the subject to (1) count backwards from 20 in 30 sec; (2) repeat the alphabet in 30 sec[1]; and (3) count from 1 to 40 by 3's in 45 sec. Only items completed within the time limits are scored on a 3-point scale on which no errors earns 2 points, reduced to 1 point if there is one error, with no credit for two or more errors. Item scores are summed, making this a 7-point scale (WMS-R) on which 0 indicates failure on all three items and 6 is a perfect score; each

---

[1]Examiners should be aware that the Spanish alphabet has two additional letter units.

WMS item is credited one more point for responses completed within 10 sec, resulting in a 10-point scale for the original version of this test.

The WMS-III has expanded items to include counting from 1 to 20, saying the days of the week and the months of the year forward and backward, and counting by 6's while alternating with the days of the week beginning, "0—Sunday–6—Monday, etc." For patients unable to recite the alphabet and who appear to be too dilapidated to succeed on even the simplest sequencing task, it is unnecessary to give the more difficult items. Recitation of the alphabet indicates whether the subject recalls it sufficiently to do alphabet-based tasks such as Trail Making and provides some evidence of whether old over-learned sequences are intact.

Test characteristics. There appear to be virtually no age effects for either the WMS-R version of Mental Control (Ivnik, Malec, et al., 1992c; Wechsler, 1987) or the WMS version (Storandt, Botwinick, and Danziger, 1986). Hulicka (1966) reported that the lowest Mental Control mean scores she obtained were made by the 60 to 69 and 70 to 79 age groups, while 80- to 89-year-olds achieved higher scores ($n = 25$, $M = 6.92$) than 30- to 39-year-olds ($n = 53$, $M = 6.75$), a finding that may reflect selective processes allowing some persons to reach their 80s sufficiently intact to participate in a study such as this one. A moderate age effect is seen with the WMS-III version. Average scores for 21- to 29-year-olds range from 21 to 29 while for 80- to 84-year-olds scores were in the 15 to 22 range with practically no overlap. Education effects have been documented for the WMS version of Mental Control, with a 1.4-point differential between persons with less than 12 years of schooling (5.6) and those with more than 15 years (7.0) (Ivnik, Smith, et al., 1991).

Neuropsychological findings. Performance on this test reflects the progressive deterioration of Alzheimer's disease (Storandt, Botwinick, and Danziger, 1986). However, it did not discriminate either between depressed patients and normal controls or between depressed patients and mildly to moderately demented Alzheimer patients, although the latter group's Mental Control scores were significantly lower than those of control subjects (R.P. Hart, Kwentus, Taylor, and Hamer, 1988). It also did

TABLE 9.5 Consistency of Serial Addition (Wechsler Memory Scale–Revised Scoring) and Sequential Operations Series Performances for 67 Patients

Serial Addition	NUMBER OF SEQUENTIAL OPERATION SERIES ITEMS FAILED			
	0	*1*	*2*	*3*
Pass	28	15	6	6
Fail	3	3	3	3

not discriminate between multiple sclerosis patients and normal subjects (Fischer, 1988) despite the prominence of attentional problems in MS.

In reviewing examinations by others who routinely gave the WMS or WMS-R in its entirety and relied on Mental Control data for evaluating mental tracking, I [mdl] came across a number of patients who had failed one or more items in the more difficult *Sequential Operations Series* (*SOS*) that I generally give but succeeded on Mental Control items (see above and Tables 9.5 and 9.6). As all but very dilapidated persons can count from 20 to one in reverse, and—excepting the few, usually with limited educational backgrounds, who placed U after Q in the alphabet—almost every adult raised in a Western culture can recite the alphabet, these two items are not sensitive techniques for measuring mental tracking or any other attentional activity.

To investigate the sensitivity of the sequential addition task, my colleagues (Katherine Wild, Julia Wong-Ngan) and I [mdl] administered it, along with the more difficult tasks comprising SOS (alphabet reversed, subtracting 3's from 50, 7's from 100) to 67 subjects. This group of adult patients mostly came from the MS clinic or for evaluation of postconcussion complaints, but it also includes a few referred for a dementia workup or with other conditions. Of this group, only three who failed serial addition succeeded on the SOS tasks, while 27 who failed one or more of the SOS tasks passed the serial addition task (see Table 9.5, see Table 9.6 for pass/fail criteria). A χ^2 comparison of failures on the serial addition task and the three SOS tasks was significant ($p < .05$), as was a comparison of the number of perfect performances on each of these tests ($p < .001$).[1]

---

[1]These data were analyzed by Gary Ford.

TABLE 9.6 Performances on Serial Addition and the Sequential Operation Series for 67 Patients

	Serial Addition (1 → 40)	*Subtracting Serial 3's* (50 → 14)	*Subtracting Serial 7's* (100 → 16)	*Alphabet Reversed* (R → A)
Criteria for failure (in errors)	≥2	≥2	≥4	≥4
n perfect performances	41	39	15	27
n satisfactory performances	14	14	31	16
n failures	12	14	21	24

Sequential Operations Series (SOS)

Typically I begin an examination with these little tasks, often introducing them as "brain teasers" [mdl]. They can be scored for errors, time, or—as in the WMS serial attention test—for both. Time to completion is one way of measuring the subject's ease of responding (e.g., Shum, McFarland, and Bain, 1990). I count the number of 5 sec intervals between responses. Most persons who can do these tasks pause for 5 sec or more only once or twice in a sequence, if at all. More than three such pauses suggest difficulty with the task. While these tasks examine the ability to maintain an activity and retain an item while performing another kind of mental operation (complex mental tracking), they also require continuous self-monitoring. Most failures will result from subjects' inability to keep track of where they are in a sequence or, less often, what they are supposed to do (e.g., "Subtract threes or fours?"). Occasionally failure occurs for subjects who demonstrate adequate concentration and tracking abilities but who neglect to monitor errors of carelessness. Close attention to the subject's responses, including self-corrections, expressions of confusion, etc., will help the examiner understand the nature of the failure.

Alphabet Reversed. Following a correct alphabet recitation at the beginning of the examination, I [mdl] ask for the alphabet reversed beginning with the letter R. **R** was chosen both to shorten the task to 16 items and because it is within the "**Q-R-S-T**" sequence that often appears in rhythmic recitations of the alphabet, thus forcing subjects to break up an habituated sequence. This is a not infrequent problem for patients with impaired mental flexibility or perseverative tendencies who understand the instructions but, having difficulty wresting themselves free from an ingrained "**Q-R-S**" habit, will begin with "**R-S**" several times before being able to say "**R-Q**." Approximately two-thirds of the sample patient group performed similarly on the serial subtraction and the alphabet reversed tasks (32 passed and 12 failed both). Alphabet Reversed was the only successful performance for 14 patients, while nine who failed it passed both subtraction tasks. M.A. Williams, LaMarche, and their colleagues (1996) had patients repeat the entire alphabet backwards: cardiac transplant candidates were slower than control subjects but did not make more errors. Comparing this task to other tests of attention in a larger group with brain disorders, these authors found that alphabet backwards was most related to performance on the PASAT and Serial 7s and least to tests of attention involving visuomotor responses.

Serial Subtractions. There is little statistical data on Subtracting Serial Sevens (SS7) for it is not generally used by psychologists except for the truncated version in the Mini-Mental State Examination. It is part of the mental status examination given by psychiatrists, neurologists, and other medical examiners (e.g., Strub and Black, 2000). Subjects are first instructed to "Take seven from 100." When they have done this, they are told, "Now take seven from 93 and continue subtracting sevens until you can't go any further." Some workers ask for serial subtraction by 13's, a task which should probably be reserved only for bright subjects as it can be very frustrating (Shum, McFarland, and Bain, 1990). Whether SS13 adds information not elicited on SS7 is questionable. Occasionally a patient will have recited SS7 so many times that much, if not all, of the number sequence will have been committed to memory. When a well-oriented patient has been given many mental status examinations, particularly during the previous weeks or months, the examiner should start the test at 101 or 102 instead of 100.

Many patients who are unable to perform SS7 can handle serial threes (SS3): "Take three from 50 . . . " (see Table 9.6). When the patient's attention abilities seem questionable, SS3 can be given first in order to accustom subjects to serial subtraction and to see whether they can perform the task at all. When SS3 is failed (3 or more errors), SS7 should not be given; even two SS3 errors should give the examiner pause. Patients who cannot perform the simpler serial subtraction task can be asked to count from 20 backward or say the months of the year backward, both very simple mental tracking tasks. A. Smith (1967) gave SS7 to 132 employed adults, most of them with college or professional educations, and found that only 99 performed the task with two errors or less. He thus showed that this test's usefulness in discriminating between normal and brain injured populations does not rest simply on the presence or absence of errors. He also demonstrated that grossly impaired performances are rarely seen in the normal population—only three (2%) of Smith's subjects were unable to complete the task and only six made more than five errors. The women in Smith's study were more error-prone than the men, particularly women over 45 who had not attended or completed college. J.C. Anthony and his colleagues (1982) found that, even on the 5-item MMSE version of this test, control subjects with less than eight years of schooling performed poorly. Patients with serious cardiac disease made few errors but their completion time was 58% longer than that of matched controls (M.A. Williams, LaMarche, et al., 1996). Very defective recitations of SS7 are fairly common among brain injured patients (Luria, 1966).

Other mental tracking tests

In a Chinese version of the WMS, since alphabet tasks are not usable, subjects are asked to count backwards from 100 to 0. This task is more sensitive than the 20 to 1 counting task, as persons with impaired mental tracking tend to slip decades (e.g., . . . 63-62-61-60-69, etc.) or simply get lost among all the numbers. These problems are more likely to show up after the first 20 or 30 numbers. This task can be given to persons with very limited education and those who cannot recite the alphabet correctly.

Alpha Span (Craik, 1990)

Subjects listen to increasingly longer lists of common, unrelated words and recall them in alphabetical order. Two trials are presented at each length (from two to eight). The test ends when both trials are failed. Age accounted for 6.3% of the variance in a large sample of 50- to 90-year-old participants (Lamar et al., 2002). Correlations were strongest with Digits Forward and Backward and category fluency (r = .34, .30, .27, respectively), very weak (r = .16) with letter fluency, and unrelated to Trail Making Test performances.

Alphanumeric Sequencing (Grigsby, Kaye, and Busenbark, 1994)

The patient alternates between counting and reciting the alphabet aloud beginning with "1-A-2-B . . . " continuing through L. Scores are obtained for time and errors. Chronic progressive MS patients performed worse than control subjects on both measures, while patients with the relapsing-remitting form of MS performed poorly only on time to completion (Grigsby, Ayarbe, et al., 1994).

Using essentially the same format, Ricker and Axelrod (1994) administered an oral version of the Trail Making Test to three groups of adults, two younger and one elderly. The comparability of oral and written performances, as assessed by oral-to-written ratios, was consistent across age groups. This task can be used for patients who are unable to perform visuographic tasks. This test differs from the Trail Making Test in that visual scanning is not required but demand is greater on working memory because visual cues are lacking.

Letter–Number Sequencing (WAIS-III, WMS-III) (Wechsler, 1997a,b)

Many elderly persons and patients with brain disorders have an immediate memory span as long as that of younger, intact adults. Thus digit span, as traditionally administered, frequently does not distinguish brain impaired or aged persons from normal, young ones, nor does it elicit the immediate recall problems characteristic of many persons with brain disorders. Because of these limitations, longer and more complex span for-

mats have been devised in the hope that they will have greater sensitivity to attentional deficits.

In this test subjects hear lists of randomized numbers and letters (in alternating order) of increasing lengths (from two to eight units). Subjects are asked to repeat numbers and letters from the lowest in each series, and numbers always first. For example, on hearing "6-F-2-B," the subject should respond, "2-6-B-F." This requires subjects to keep the items in mind long enough to rearrange their order. The span is increased until the subject fails all three items of one length. This test is not recommended for persons with impaired hearing who may have difficulty discriminating the rhyming letters, such as C, V, and Z. It may even be difficult for them to differentiate A from 8. Normative data show a moderate age effect. Scores obtained by healthy young adults correlate with performance on WIS-III Digits Forward and Backward, Arithmetic, Symbol Search, and on visual spatial learning (Crowe, 2000).

Neuropsychological findings. Alzheimer patients have difficulty on this test (Earnst et al., 2001). For age and education matched HIV$^+$ and HIV$^-$ subjects, no differences were observed on the standard condition (E.M. Martin, Sullivan, et al., 2001). When asked simply to repeat the letter–number sequences as heard, many in the HIV$^+$ group repeated more of the long sequences than did the HIV$^-$ group. However, when ability to reorder the sequences was corrected for repetition length, the HIV$^-$ subjects outperformed the HIV$^+$ ones. Performance is also related to TBI severity as mild TBI patients did not differ from control subjects but those with moderate injury performed more poorly (Donders, Tulsky, and Zhu, 2001). However, these authors note that more variance was accounted for by level of education (r = .13) than by injury severity. *They urge caution in interpreting scores.*

N-Back Task

Used primarily for research, this task asks the subject to report when a stimulus item presented serially is the same as an item "n" steps back from the item at hand. For the 2-back condition, if the sequence were 8-7-1-8-6-3-6, the subject would say "yes" following the second 6. Working memory is required to keep previous items in mind while attending to the current item. Imaging studies have consistently shown prefrontal cortex involvement (e.g., C.S. Carter et al., 1998; D'Esposito, Ballard, et al., 1998), making this technique attractive for research purposes. An age effect showed up in comparisons of 68-year-olds to 20-year-olds (See and Ryan, 1995) and of persons over 70 years to 30-year-olds (Salat et al., 2002). The Salat team found that both groups made increasingly more errors when the demands expanded from 1-back to 3-back; the difference between age groups was present for all conditions. Although mild TBI patients did not differ from control subjects, functional MRI showed that the TBI group had higher activation during the high demand condition than the control group; they may have been working harder to achieve this performance level (McAllister, Saykin, et al., 1999).

Paced Auditory Serial Addition Test (PASAT)[1]
(Gronwall, 1977; Gronwall and Sampson, 1974)

This sensitive test simply requires that the patient add 60 pairs of randomized digits so that each is added to the digit immediately preceding it. For example, if the examiner reads the numbers "2-8-6-1-9," the subject's correct responses, beginning as soon as the examiner says "8," are "10-14-7-10." The digits are presented at four rates of speed, each differing by 0.4 sec and ranging from one every 1.2 sec to one every 2.4 sec. Precise control over the rate at which digits are read requires a taped presentation. The tape begins with a brief repetition task that is followed by a ten-digit practice series presented at the 2.4-sec rate. Sixty-one digits are given at each rate (see Brittain et al. [1991] or Spreen and Strauss [1998] for detailed instructions). The performance can be evaluated in terms of the percentage of correct responses or the mean score for all trials.

This task is difficult. Normal middle age adults achieved 72% correct responses at the slowest rate but only 45% at the fastest (J.D. Fisk and Archibald, 2001). Comprehensive adult norms are available (Mitrushina, Boone, and D'Elia, 1999) and include most normative studies (e.g., D.D. Roman et al., 1991; Spreen and Strauss, 1998). P.J. Snyder and Cappelleri (2001) noted that on faster trials many patients will skip every third item to make the task more manageable. They suggest scoring the total number of times that two correct responses are given in a row, which they refer to as "dyads."

A shorter form of this test, the *Paced Auditory Serial Addition Test-Revised* (*PASAT-R*) contains only 26 digits in each trial, making a total of 100 possible responses for all four trials (H.S. Levin, 1983). Presentation rates run 0.4 sec. slower for each trial than in the original version.

Test characteristics. Not surprisingly, performance levels on this speed-dependent test decline with age (Brittain et al., 1991; Spikman, Deelman, and van Zomeren, 2000), a decline that Roman and her colleagues (1991) found to be most prominent after age 50. The Brittain group observed that on average men perform a trifle better than women, but while statistically significant, this trifle is of "minimal practical significance." Other studies have not found sex differences (D.D. Roman et al., 1991; Wiens, Fuller, and Crossen, 1997). Education effects have been reported (Stuss, Stethem, and Poirier, 1987) although Wiens and his colleagues found intelligence test scores but not education to be significantly related to PASAT performance. A factor analytic study showed that the PASAT had more in common with other tests of attention and information processing than with tests of memory, visuoconstruction, or verbal knowledge (Larrabee and Curtiss, 1995). Modest correlations with mental ability measures other than attention (which includes WIS-A Arithmetic) have been reported, leading to the recommendation that the PASAT may only be suitable for high functioning subjects who are not mathematically impaired (E.M.S. Sherman, Strauss, and Spellacy, 1997). Practice effects have been reported, ranging from modest and stopping at the second administration (Gronwall, 1977) to continuing significant gains leveling off only between the fourth and fifth administration (Feinstein, Brown, and Ron, 1994; Stuss, Stethem, Hugenholtz, and Richard, 1989). In her examinations of dysarthric patients, Jeanne Harris (personal communication, 1992 [mdl]) observed that it is impossible to differentiate between attentional deficits and motor speech slowing, a problem which Spreen and Strauss (1998) recommend should deter PASAT use with dysarthric patients.

Neuropsychological findings. Postconcussion patients consistently perform well below control group averages immediately after injury or return to consciousness (Gronwall and Sampson, 1974; Stuss, Stethem, Hugenholtz, and Richard, 1989). For most postconcussion patients, scores return to normal within 30 to 60 days; yet others continue to lag behind the performance level of their control group (Leininger, Gramling, et al., 1990). With severe head injuries, performance levels are significantly reduced from the outset and remain low (Ponsford and Kinsella, 1992; Stuss, Stethem, Hugenholtz, and Richard, 1989). Based on an evaluation of how the PASAT performance was associated with performances on memory and attention tasks, Gronwall and Wrightson (1981) concluded that the PASAT is very sensitive to deficits in information processing ability. Ponsford and Kinsella (1992) interpreted their findings as reflecting abnormally slowed information processing. Roman and her colleagues (1991) pointed out that patients whose head injuries are most likely to have produced diffuse damage are

---

[1]This tape can be ordered from the Neuropsychology Laboratory, University of Victoria, P.O. Box 1700, Victoria, B.C. V8W 2Y2, Canada.

also those most likely to perform the PASAT poorly. By using the PASAT performance as an indicator of the efficiency of information processing following concussion, the examiner may be able to determine when a patient can return to a normal level of social and vocational activity without experiencing undue stress, or when a modified activity schedule would be best (Gronwall, 1977). Sohlberg and Mateer (1989) reported use of this test to measure treatment outcome in traumatically brain injured patients with attentional disorders. This test is also sensitive to cognitive slowing associated with multiple sclerosis (S.M. Rao and National Multiple Sclerosis Society, 1990). A strong inverse correlation has been reported between amount of white matter disease associated with MS and correct responses (Hohol et al., 1997). This correlation improves when correct dyads are scored instead of total correct responses (Fisk and Archibald, 2001; P.J. Snyder, Cappelleri, et al., 2001).

Unfortunately, people experience this sensitive test as very stressful: most persons—whether cognitively intact or impaired—feel under great pressure and that they are failing even when doing well (see also Spreen and Strauss, 1998; Stuss, Stethem, Hugenholtz, and Richard, 1989). Holdwick and Wingenfeld (1999) documented sad or anxious mood states after taking the PASAT, even in healthy college students who had described themselves as happy before taking this test. Since attentional deficits can be elicited in less painful ways, it is frequently not necessary to give the PASAT. However, it can be useful for those patients whose subtle attentional deficits need to be made obvious to the most hidebound skeptics for some purpose very much in the patient's interest. When circumstances necessitates its use, patients can be prepared beforehand by letting them know that it can be an unpleasant procedure and that they may feel that they are failing when they are not.

Stroop Tests (Stroop, 1935; A.R. Jensen and Rohwer, 1966)

This technique has been applied to the study of a host of psychological functions since it was first developed in the late nineteenth century and then, late in the twentieth, it metamorphosed into a popular neuropsychological assessment method. Stroop tests are based on findings that it takes longer to call out the color names of colored patches than to read words and even longer to name the color of the ink in which a color name is printed when the print ink is a color different than the color name (Dyer, 1973; A.R. Jensen and Rohwer, 1966). This latter phenomenon—a markedly slowed naming response when a color name is printed in ink

of a different color—has received a variety of interpretations. Some workers have attributed the slowing to a response conflict, some to failure of response inhibition, and some to a failure of selective attention (see Dyer, 1973; Zajano and Gorman, 1986). Patients who become slowed or hesitant on this part of the Stroop task tend to have difficulty concentrating, including difficulty in warding off distractions. The activity required by this test has been described as requiring the selective processing of "only one visual feature while continuously blocking out the processing of others" (Shum, McFarland, and Bain, 1990). The conflicting shape of the word serves as a prepotent stimulus and thus a distractor when combined with a stimulus (the different color) that has a less habituated response. Thus, it is as a measure of concentration effectiveness that this technique appears to make its greatest contribution to neuropsychological assessment.

Stroop formats. Formats can differ in many ways, some enhancing the Stroop technique's usefulness more than others. (1) The number of trials generally runs from 2 to 4. Some formats use only two trials: one in which reading focuses on color words printed in ink of different colors, and the other requiring naming of the printed colors (e.g., Dodrill, 1978b; Trenerry et al., 1989); some use three, adding one with words printed in black ink (e.g., Golden, 1978) or color dots for simple color naming (e.g., Spreen and Strauss, 1998); some use four, including both a black ink and a simple color-naming trial along with the first two (e.g., N.B. Cohn et al., 1984; Stroop, 1935). In order to increase the test's complexity, Bohnen and colleagues (1992) added a fourth trial to color naming, word reading, and the color–word interference trial by printing a rectangle around 20 color names randomly placed within a 10 line 10 column format and requiring the subject to read these words while naming the colors of the 90 other color names. (2) The number of items in a trial may vary from as few as 17 (N.B. Cohn et al., 1984) or 20 (Koss, Ober et al., 1984) to as many as 176 (Dodrill, 1978b). Two commercially available Stroop formats contain 100 (Golden, 1978) and 112 (Trenerry et al., 1989). (3) The number of colors may be three (e.g., Daigneault et al., 1992; Stuss, 1991a), four (e.g., Dodrill, 1978b; Spreen and Strauss, 1998), or five (Obler and Albert, 1985; Stroop, 1935). (4) Presentation of the stimuli also varies greatly: the 17 items in the format used by N.B. Cohn and her colleagues are arranged vertically but most formats present the stimuli in orderly rows and columns. Koss, Ober, and their coworkers (1984) used a slide projector to display their 20-item trials. The *Press Test* (Baehr and Corsini, 1980) is a paper-and-pencil form of the Stroop Test that was modified for group administration but is suitable for clinical use as well. (5) A random switching condition in which subjects read the color word of some items and name the ink color of other words—designated by being enclosed in boxes—is part of the *California Stroop Test* (Delis, Kaplan, and Kramer, 2001). (6) Scoring may be by time, error, both, or the number of items read or named within a specified time limit (Golden, 1978). Some other names for commercially available Stroop formats are *Modified Stroop Test* (Spreen and Strauss, 1998); *Stroop Color and Word Test* (Golden, 1978); *The Stroop Neuropsychological Screening Test* (*SNST*) (Trenerry et al., 1989). Norms appropriate for response in sign language have been developed for the Stroop Color and Word Test (A.B. Wolff et al., 1989).

I [mdl] prefer the Dodrill format for a number of reasons, not least of which is that two trials are sufficient for eliciting the Stroop phenomenon of slowing on the color–word interference trial. Of perhaps greatest importance is that it is the longest of formats in current use and, as such, may well be the most sensitive. My experience has been that even patients with significant problems in maintaining focused attention and warding off distractions begin the color–word interference trial with a relatively good rate of speed, but they slow down as they proceed, doing much more poorly on the latter half or quarter of the test.

For example, one TBI patient, a high school educated 35-year-old woman whose reading vocabulary is at the 80th percentile, named 50 color words with no errors in the first minute of Trial II (the interference trial), 41 in the second minute with three errors, 27 in the third minute with no errors, 25 in the fourth minute with three errors, and in the last minute (total time was 301 sec) she named 32 color words, again with three errors. Had the number of items been 100 or less, or the time limited to one minute or even two, this impressive slowing effect would not have appeared and her overall performance would not have been judged to be significantly impaired.

An additional virtue of the Dodrill format is that it is quite inexpensive and the scoring sheets may be copied (see p. 367). Moreover, T.L. Sacks and his colleagues (1991) have developed five equivalent forms. Norms are available for this format as well as those that have been published (Mitrushina, Boone, and D'Elia, 1999).

Test characteristics. The Stroop technique has satisfactory reliability (Franzen, Tishelman, Sharp, and Friedman, 1987; Spreen and Strauss, 1998). Reports of practice effects vary from study to study with some studies showing virtually none but others showing considerable gains on a second administration (McCaf-frey, Duff, and Westervelt, 2000b), or even a third one, but not on subsequent ones (Connor et al., 1988; T.L. Sacks et al., 1991). However, Franzen and his group (1987) found practice effects only for the second administration of the word reading trial. A slight reduction in response speed (about 10%) can be expected on the second half of the 176-item (Dodrill format) color–word interference trial but not on the word reading trial, a change in rate ascribed to fatigue (T.L. Sacks et al., 1991). An anxiety arousing testing situation resulted in lowered scores on all three trials of the Stroop Color and Word Test, affecting men more than women (N.J. Martin and Franzen, 1989); and anxiety in TBI patients contributed somewhat to their slower performances but did not fully account for their slowing (Batchelor et al., 1995). A.R. Jensen and Rohwer (1966) reported that in laboratory studies of the Stroop technique women consistently performed better on simple color naming than men, yet N.J. Martin and Franzen (1989) found that, without anxiety-arousing stimuli, men tended to respond a little faster than women on all three trials. However, no male–female differences were found in a large normative study (Ivnik, Malec, Smith, et al., 1996). Slowing with advanced age has been consistently documented (Boone, Miller, et al., 1990; Spreen and Strauss, 1998; Wecker et al., 2000). Age effects may appear most prominently on the color–word interference trial (N.B. Cohn et al., 1984; Daigneault et al., 1992), barely showing up on other trials, if at all.

Neuropsychological findings. Nehemkis and Lewinsohn (1972) found that left hemisphere patients took approximately twice as long as control subjects to perform each trial, but the interference effect was similar for both right and left hemisphere lesioned patients. The Stroop technique is quite sensitive to the effects of closed head injury as even patients with ostensible "good recovery" continue to perform abnormally slowly five months or more after the injury (Stuss, Ely, et al., 1985). However, two to five years following moderate to severe brain injury, patients performed as well as control subjects (Spikman, Deelman, and van Zomeren, 2000). Impaired performance (three trials: reading names, naming colors, and the interference trial) by patients with severe TBI was closely associated with failures on the other attentional tasks and interpreted as reflecting a slowed rate of information processing (Ponsford and Kinsella, 1992). The added requirement of having subjects read some of the color–word items as words while naming the colors of most of these items made this test more sensitive to the subtle attentional deficits of mild head injury patients (Bohnen et al., 1992). Perret (1974) reported slowed performance by patients with left frontal lobe lesions on both Stroop and word fluency tests, with the Stroop test—particularly the color–word interference trials—eliciting the slowing effects most prominently. In contrast, one study reported that right but not left frontal lesions impaired performance (Vendrell et al., 1995). Consistent with the importance of frontal lobe functions, another study found that only bilateral superior medial frontal damage was associated with both increased errors and slowed response times for the interference trial, and that posterior lesions were not associated with any impairment (Stuss, Floden, et al., 2001). Frontal leukotomy patients did not differ from controls on any (of three) Stroop trials (Stuss, 1991a).

Pronounced slowing on the interference trial characterized the performances of mildly and moderately demented patients (Bondi, Serody, et al., 2002; L.M. Fisher et al., 1990; Koss, Ober, et al., 1984), but response slowing in later stage patients tends to be so generalized that the Stroop effect (i.e., interference effect) diminishes. On a happier note, aerobic exercise programs maintained for four months by previously sedentary persons in the 55–70 age range resulted in significantly ($p < .001$) faster performances, even on the very abbreviated 17-item format (Dustman, Ruhling, et al., 1984).

Cautions. This test is unpleasant to take, particularly for patients with concentration problems. I [mdl] therefore always give it last and introduce it by explaining that the patient may find some of it difficult to do but the information it provides is often helpful for understanding the patient's condition. If the patient's attentional problems are sufficiently severe that they have shown up prominently elsewhere in the examination, I may not give the Stroop at all and spare the patient—and myself—the pain.

Visual competence is important. Color blindness may preclude use of this test. Patients whose vision is so hazy that the shape of the words is somewhat degraded will have a decided advantage on the color–word interference task as the interference effect will be diminished (Dyer, 1973).

Stroop Test (Dodrill's Format).[1] This format consists of only one sheet containing 176 (11 across, 16 lines down) color names (red, orange, green, blue) randomly printed in these colors. In Part I of this test, the subject reads the printed word name. Part II requires the subject to report the color in which each word is printed. The times taken to complete the readings are recorded halfway through and at the end, on a sheet the examiner uses for recording the subject's responses. The Part I side of the examiner's record sheet shows the correct word names, the other side has printed in correct order the color names for Part II. This device greatly facilitates the recording of this task since many patients move along quite rapidly, particularly on Part I. Dodrill evaluates the performance on the basis of the total time for Part I, the total time for Part II, and the difference between the total time for Parts I and II (Part II minus Part I) (see Table 9.7). The time at which the subject is halfway through each part, when compared with the total time, indicates whether task familiarity and practice or difficulty in maintaining a set or attention changes the performance rate. A more precise way of documenting response rate changes is to make a slash mark following the color name at the end of each minute. Some patients who have great difficulty doing the interference trial would take longer than five minutes, but Dodrill stops them at ten; I [mdl] stop at five minutes: enough is enough. Dodrill discontinues Part I at five minutes but this would be rare as in well over 200 examinations I have never had a patient take more than three minutes on Part I.

[1]This format may be ordered for $20 a set from Carl Dodrill, Ph.D., 4488 West Mercer Way, Mercer Island, WA 98040. When sending the Stroop material, Dr. Dodrill includes norms based on 100 control subjects, 727 epileptic patients, plus one set from 140 patients in a private neurology practice and one from 160 patients in a "Psychiatric/Neurologic" group. Mean ages for these groups range from 27.66 ± 10.5 to 32.23 ± 13.2; limiting their use with older patients (Dodrill, 1999, unpublished).

TABLE 9.7 Time to Completion (sec)* on Dodrill's Modification of the Stroop Test for Normal Subjects and Three Clinical Groups

	Normal Control (n = 100)	Epileptic (n = 727)	Psychiatric/Neurological (n = 160)	Private Neurological (n = 140)
Part I (300 ″ max)				
Mean ± SD	88 ± 20	117 ± 46	105 ± 47	120 ± 60
Part II (600 ″ max)				
Mean ± SD	230 ± 71	301 ± 114	266 ± 97	284 ± 121
Part II − I				
Mean ± SD	141 ± 55	176 ± 69	160 ± 64	158 ± 67

*Rounded to nearest whole number
From Dodrill (1999)

Complex Attention Tests

Visuographic tasks

Persons unused to handling pencils and doing fine handwork under time pressure are at a disadvantage on these tests. The great importance that motor speed plays in the scoring, particularly below age 35, renders them of doubtful validity for many low-skilled manual workers and for anyone whose motor responses tend to be slow. They are particularly difficult for elderly subjects whose vision or visuomotor coordination is impaired or who have difficulty comprehending the instructions (Savage et al., 1973). Storandt's (1976) report that half of the total score value of Digit Symbol is contributed by copying speed alone is supported by Le Fever's (1985) finding that copying speed accounts for 72% of its variance. Thus the examiner needs to be sensitive to motor and manual agility problems when deciding to give these tests. However, I [mdl] do give one and sometimes both of the symbol substitution tests to patients suspected of having visual perception or visual orientation problems whose defects might show up as rotations, simplifications, or other distortions under the stress of this task. For example, I typically give a symbol substitution test to patients with known or suspected right hemisphere damage, particularly if it is right frontal, since these patients are most likely to make orientation errors, usually reversals.

Digit Symbol (Wechsler, 1944, 1955, 1981),
Digit Symbol-Coding (Wechsler, 1997a)

This symbol substitution task is printed in the WIS test booklet. It consists of rows containing small blank squares, each paired with a randomly assigned number from one to nine (see Fig. 9.10). Above these rows is a printed key that pairs each number with a different nonsense symbol. Following a practice trial on the first ten (WAIS) or seven (WAIS-R or WAIS-III) squares, the subject must fill in the blank spaces with the symbol that is paired to the number above the blank space for 90 sec or 120 sec for the WAIS-III. The score is the number of squares filled in correctly. Subjects are encouraged to perform the task as quickly and accurately as possible.

To make this test more interpretable when it is given to older persons or others who appear to be motorically slowed, Edith Kaplan, Fein, and their colleagues (1991; Milberg, Hebben, and Kaplan, 1996) have developed the Symbol Copy test in which the subject simply copies the symbol above each empty square into that square, thus bypassing the visual search and shifting and the memory components of this test. In this manner, the Digit Symbol performance can be com-

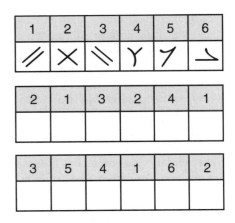

FIGURE 9.10 The symbol-substitution format of the WIS Digit Symbol Test.

pared with a somewhat purer visuomotor task to allow evaluation of its more cognitive aspects. Dr. Kaplan and her colleagues also recommended that the examiner note how far the subject has gone at 30 sec and 60 sec as rate changes, particularly at the beginning or toward the end of the trial, may indicate such performance problems as sluggishness in developing a set when beginning a new task or very low fatigue or boredom thresholds.

A variety of format alternatives are described in the literature, such as symbol sets in which the symbols are more or less familiar (e.g., arrow, diamond, or lambda) (Glosser, Butters, and Kaplan, 1977) or sets with fewer symbol pairs (Salthouse, 1978; Teng, Wimer, et al., 1989). Most have been developed with specific research questions in mind. Their clinical usefulness is limited without adequate norms, although they may be applicable to specific cases. Variations on Digit Symbol are provided by the Repeatable Cognitive-Perceptual-Motor Battery in formats in which the symbols are quite similar to the Wechsler format. Comprehensive norms are available in Mitrushina, Boone, and D'Elia (1999) and Heaton, Grant, and Matthews (1991).

Test characteristics. For most adults, Digit Symbol is a test of psychomotor performance that is relatively unaffected by intellectual prowess, memory, or learning (Erber et al., 1981; Glosser, Butters, and Kaplan, 1977). Comparing Digit Symbol with Digit Symbol Copy, the copy component accounted for 52% of the variance for a group of older persons (Joy et al., 2000), and 48% of the variance of performance by a group of veterans with a mean age of 52 years (Kreiner and Ryan, 2001). These findings are consistent with Storandt's earlier report (1976) that half of the total score value of Digit Symbol is contributed by copy speed alone. Motor persistence, sustained attention, response speed, and visuomotor coordination play important roles in a normal person's performance; but visual acuity does not (Schear and Sato, 1989). Learning the paired combinations does not appear to be an important factor (Joy et al., 2000; Kreiner and Ryan, 2001) although incidental memory is another component of this test (see pp. 472–473 for assessment procedures and evaluation). Perceptual organization components show up on this test (A.S. Kaufman, McLean, and Reynolds, 1991; Zillmer, Waechtler, et al., 1992), but a selective attention factor was most prominent for seizure patients (P.C. Fowler, Richards, et al., 1987). The natural response slowing that comes with age seems to be the most important variable contributing to the age differential on this test.

Test–retest reliability tends to run high, with correlation coefficients in the .82 to .88 range (Matarazzo and Herman, 1984; Wechsler, 1981). The level of test-retest reliability varies with different clinical populations, being very unstable for schizophrenics ($r = .38$) but at the normal adult level for patients with cerebrovascular disorders (G. Goldstein and Watson, 1989). Reliability was near normal levels for people with mild TBI ($r = .74$) (Hinton-Bayre et al., 1997). Reports of practice effect sizes have varied, probably because they are modest (McCaffrey, Duff, and Westervelt, 2000a), but a small sample of younger (average age in the 30s) control subjects showed a 7% gain on retest following a 15-month interval (R.E. Miller et al., 1984). A change in scaled scores of less than one point was seen in young volunteers retested nearly one year later (Dikmen, Heaton, et al., 1999). Moreover no practice effects appeared when this test was given four times with intervals of one week to three months (McCaffrey, Ortega, and Haase, 1993).

Age effects are prominent (Jarvik, 1988; A.S. Kaufman, Reynolds, and McLean, 1989; Wielgos and Cunningham, 1999), showing up as early as the 30s (Wechsler, 1997a) with raw scores dropping sharply after the age of 60 (Ivnik, Malec, Smith, et al., 1992b). Women outperformed men in the U.S. (A.S. Kaufman, McLean, and Reynolds, 1988) and Canada (W.G. Snow and Weinstock, 1990), but not in France (Mazaux, Dartiques, et al., 1995). Estes (1974) pointed out that skill in encoding the symbol verbally also appears to contribute to success on this test, and may account for the (almost) consistently observed feminine superiority on symbol substitution tasks. Storandt (1976) found no relationship between cognitive ability as measured by WAIS Vocabulary scores and Digit Symbol performances although Digit Symbol and the WAIS-R Vocabulary test were found to be related ($r = .50$). Education contributed significantly to performances by elderly volunteers (Mazaux et al., 1995) and seizure patients (Kupke and Lewis, 1989). However, Digit Symbol correlations with other WAIS-R tests ranged from .44 to .21 (Wechsler, 1981), suggesting that mental ability does not contribute greatly to success on this test.

Neuropsychological findings. This test is consistently more sensitive to brain damage than other WIS-A tests in that its score is most likely to be depressed even when damage is minimal, and to be among the most depressed when other tests are affected as well. Because Digit Symbol tends to be affected regardless of the locus of the lesion, it is of little use for predicting the laterality of a lesion except for patients with hemi-inattention or a lateralized visual field cut, who may omit items or make more errors on the side of the test form opposite the side of the lesion (Egelko, Gordon, et al., 1988; E. Kaplan, Fein, et al., 1991; Zillmer, Waechtler, et al., 1992). Aphasics typically earn greatly lowered scores due to exceedingly slow but relatively error-free performances (Tissot et al., 1963).

Digit Symbol's nonspecific sensitivity to brain dysfunction should not be surprising since it can be affected by so many different performance components. Failures on this test may be the result of different factors or their interplay, including a sore shoulder, stiff fingers, or a carpal tunnel syndrome. High levels of arousal can result in performance decrements (S.F. Crowe et al., 2001).

This test is extremely sensitive to dementia, being one of the first tests to decline with little overlap with control subjects' scores; and declining rapidly with disease progression (Storandt, Botwinick, and Danziger, 1986; Larrabee, Largen, and Levin, 1985). L. Berg, Danziger, and their colleagues (1984) found Digit Symbol to be a good predictor of the rate at which dementia progresses. It is also one of the few WIS-A tests on which Huntington patients performed poorly before the disease became manifest (M.E. Strauss and Brandt, 1986). Lower scores distinguish patients with rapidly growing tumors from those whose tumors are slow-growing (Hom and Reitan, 1984). Digit Symbol performance is correlated with coma duration in head trauma patients (Correll et al., 1993; B. Wilson, Vizor, and Bryant, 1991) and tends to run below the other WIS-A performances in these patients (Crosson, Greene, et al., 1990). It is likely to be the lowest WIS-A score for chronic alcoholics (W.R. Miller and Saucedo, 1983). Not surprisingly, elderly depressed patients do Digit Symbol slowly, making its use in the differential diagnosis of depression versus dementia questionable, except when a test of incidental learning of the digit–symbol pairs follows the Digit Symbol test (pp. 472–473) (R.P. Hart, Kwentus, Wade, and Hamer, 1987).

Digit Symbol proved to be an effective measure of cognitive improvement in medically treated hypertensives (R.E. Miller et al., 1984). Again, the good news is that for previously sedentary elderly persons Digit Symbol scores improved significantly (an average of 6 raw score points) after aerobic training of three hours a week for four months (Dustman, Ruhling et al., 1984).

Symbol Digit Modalities Test (SDMT)
(A. Smith, 1982)

This test preserves the substitution format of Wechsler's Digit Symbol test, but reverses the presentation of the material so that the symbols are printed for the numbers to be written in (see Fig. 9.11). This not only enables the patient to respond with the more familiar act of number writing but also allows a spoken response trial. Both written and oral administrations of the SDMT should be given whenever possible to permit comparisons between the two response modalities. When, in accordance with the instructions, the written administration is given first the examiner can use the same sheet to record the patient's answers on the oral administration by writing them under the answer spaces. Neither order of presentation nor recency of the first administration appears to affect performance (A. Smith, personal communication). As with WAIS and WAIS-R Digit Symbol, 90 sec are allowed for each trial; but there are 110 items, not 100. The written form of this substitution test also lends itself to group administration for rapid screening of many of the verbal and visual functions necessary for reading (A. Smith, 1975).

Test characteristics. The SDMT primarily assesses complex scanning and visual tracking (Shum, McFarland, and Bain, 1990) with the added advantage of providing a comparison between visuomotor and oral responses. Manual speed and agility contribute significantly to SDMT performance, but visual acuity is not an important factor (Schear and Sato, 1989). A signif-

TABLE 9.8 Symbol Digit Modalities Test Norms for Ages 18 to 74

Age Group	Mean Education	Mean Written Administration	Mean Oral Administration
18–24 (n = 69)	12.7	55.2 (± 7.5)	62.7 (± 9.1)
25–34 (n = 72)	13.5	53.6 (± 6.6)	61.2 (± 7.8)
35–44 (n = 76)	12.1	51.1 (± 8.1)	59.7 (± 9.7)
45–54 (n = 75)	11.7	46.8 (± 8.4)	54.5 (± 9.1)
55–64 (n = 67)	11.3	41.5 (± 8.6)	48.4 (± 9.1)
65–74 (n = 61)	10.7	37.4 (± 11.4)	46.2 (± 12.8)

Based on studies by Carmen C. Centofanti.

icant performance decrement in one response modality relative to the other naturally points to a dysfunction of that modality. In a comparison of symbol-substitution test formats that differed in familiarity of the symbols and whether a digit or symbol response was required, all subjects—normal controls as well as brain impaired patients—performed both the familiar and unfamiliar digit response tests more slowly than those calling for symbol responses (e.g., Digit Symbol) (N. Butters and Cermak, 1976; Glosser, Butters, and Kaplan, 1977). This phenomenon was attributed, at least in part, to absence of an orderly sequence in the symbol stimulus array. Test–retest reliability was .74 in young athletes tested one to two weeks apart (Hinton-Bayre et al., 1997).

The adult normative population was composed of 420 persons ranging in age from 18 to 74 (see Table 9.8). When applied to 100 patients with "confirmed and chronic" brain lesions, these norms correctly identified 86% of the patient group and 92% of the normal population, using a cut-off of ≥1.5 standard deviations below the age norm (A. Smith, 1982). Smith considered scores below this cut-off to be "indicative" and those between 1.0 and 1.5 SDs below the age norm to be "suggestive" of cerebral dysfunction. A cut-off greater than −1 SD gives a somewhat high (9% to 15%) rate of false-positive cases (Rees, 1979). More complete norms are available in the test manual—

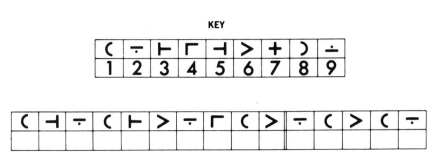

FIGURE 9.11 The Symbol Digit Modalities Test (SDMT). (By Aaron Smith, Ph.D. © 1982 by Western Psychological Services. Reprinted by permission.)

which includes child norms, and in the compilation by Mitrushina, Boone, and D'Elia (1999). Education- and age-corrected norms for people older than 75 have been developed (E.D. Richardson and Marottoli, 1996). Small gains on both the written and oral formats showed up on retesting after an interval of approximately one month with correlation coefficients of .80 and .76, respectively (A. Smith, 1982); with a year-long interval, a reliability coefficient correlation was .78 (W.G. Snow, Tierney, et al., 1988). A small sample (24) of control subjects made a 7% gain on retest after a 15-month interval (R.E. Miller et al., 1984). The trend for small gains shows up on most but not all retest studies (McCaffrey, Duff, and Westervelt, 2000b).

The oral format can be particularly useful with patients whose attentional disorders tend to disrupt ongoing activities, as these patients are apt to skip or repeat items or lines (since no pencil marks guide them) unless they figure out that they can keep track of their place with their finger. These tracking failures provide telling evidence of the kinds of problems these patients encounter when trying to perform their everyday activities. Another virtue of the SDMT format is the three pairs of mirrored figures, which bring out problems of inattentiveness to details or inappreciation of orientation changes.

The norms in Table 9.8 show how early and how rapidly response slowing occurs. Even in an educationally privileged sample ($M = 14.12$ years), men's scores dropped approximately 10% in the fourth decade on both forms of the test, although women's performances remained virtually unchanged during these years (Yeudall, Fromm, et al., 1986). While the female advantage has been documented consistently (A. Smith, 1982; Yeudall, Fromm, et al., 1986), it shrinks when handedness is taken into account, as non-right-handed men do almost as well on the oral format as non-right-handed women who, in turn, do less well than their right-handed counterparts (Polubinski and Melamed, 1986). Educational levels are positively associated with higher scores (E.D. Richardson and Marottoli, 1996; Selnes, Jacobson, et al., 1991; A. Smith, 1982).

Neuropsychological findings. Pfeffer and his colleagues (1981) found the SDMT to be the "best discriminator" of dementia and depression out of a set of eight tests, which included the Trail Making Test plus tests of immediate and short-term memory, reasoning, and motor speed. The average performance of severely injured TBI patients was more than ten points lower than that of controls on the written format, and almost 20 points lower on the oral format, with little overlap between the groups (Ponsford and Kinsella, 1992). MS

patients who reported memory problems performed worse on the SDMT than those who did not (Randolph, Arnett, and Higginson, 2001), while the report of memory problems had a weaker association with their performances on memory tests, such as story recall and the California Verbal Learning Test. These comparisons led the authors to suggest that the memory complaints of MS patients represent cognitive domains other than memory (e.g., see Howieson and Lezak, 2002). SDMT scores also correlated significantly with neuroradiologic evidence of caudate atrophy in Huntington patients (Starkstein, Brandt, et al., 1988).

Comparability of Digit Symbol and Symbol Digit Modalities Test

Although these tests tend to be as highly correlated with one another as each is on retesting (.78 for workers exposed to neurotoxins, .73 for their controls [Bowler, Sudia et al., 1992]; .91 for neurology clinic outpatients [Morgan, 1992]), SDMT raw scores run consistently lower than those of Digit Symbol. Both tests can be used to examine incidental learning by having subjects fill in the bottom line (or a blank line on a fresh test form) without seeing the key (see pp. 472–473). Symbol Digit Modalities Test, which allows a comparison of auditory and graphic response speed on a symbol substitution task, and is sensitive to tendencies toward spatial rotation or disorientation, may provide more information than Digit Symbol. When a symbol substitution test is given to patients with pronounced motor disability or motor slowing who will obviously perform poorly on these highly time-dependent tests, their low scores add no new information although qualitative response features may prove informative, and the incidental memory trials always add useful data.

Trail Making Test (TMT)

This test, originally part of the *Army Individual Test Battery* (1944), has enjoyed wide use as an easily administered test of scanning and visuomotor tracking, divided attention, and cognitive flexibility. Developed by U.S. Army psychologists, it is in the public domain and can be reproduced without permission. It is given in two parts, A and B (see Fig. 9.12, p. 372). The subject must first draw lines to connect consecutively numbered circles on one work sheet (Part A) and then connect the same number of consecutively numbered and lettered circles on another worksheet by alternating between the two sequences (Part B). The subject is urged to connect the circles "as fast as you can" without lifting the pencil from the paper.

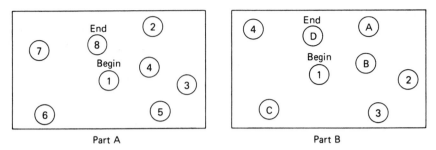

FIGURE 9.12 Practice samples of the Trail Making Test.

Three alternate forms of Part B are offered in the Repeatable Cognitive-Perceptual-Motor Battery (see p. 676). Their comparability to the original format appears to be satisfactory. The *California Trail Making Test* contains five conditions, one of which is similar to the original Part B (see pp. 637–638). One new visual search condition has subjects locate those numbers and letters that have curved parts (e.g., **3, D**). Two conditions involve sequencing only numbers or letters where both appear on the page, and one condition involves motor speed in tracing an existing line.

Some administration and scoring procedures for the original version have changed over the years. Originally, the examiner removed the work sheet after three uncorrected errors. Each trial received a score on a 10-point scale, depending on the amount of time taken to complete it. Armitage (1946) changed this procedure, allowing the patient to finish regardless of the number of errors but accounting for the errors by giving a score of zero to performances in which errors were left uncorrected. Reitan (1958) made further changes, requiring the examiner to point out errors as they occur so that the patient could always complete the test without errors and to base scoring on time alone. Spreen and Strauss (1998) provide very detailed administration instructions. It is unnecessary and probably unkind to allow a trial to continue beyond five or even four minutes.

The scoring method introduced by Reitan is the one in most common use today. However, the price for a simplified scoring system may have been paid in diminished reliability, for the measured amount of time includes the examiner's reaction time (in noticing errors) and speed in pointing them out, and the speed with which the patient comprehends and makes the correction. This method penalizes for errors indirectly but does not control for differences in response times and correction styles that can conceivably result in significant biases in the time scores obtained with different examiners (see W.G. Snow, 1987b). A difference score (B − A) essentially removes the speed element from the test evaluation. This score correlates highly with scores on other mental ability tests (e.g., WIS-A) and with severity of cognitive impairment (Corrigan and Hinkeldey, 1987). Mitrushina, Boone, and D'Elia (1999) report test norms for adults, as do Heaton, Grant, and Matthews (1991). Stuss, Stethem, and Poirier (1987) offer a compilation of adult norms; and norms for older adults have also been developed (Ivnik, Malec, Smith, et al., 1996; E.D. Richardson and Marottoli, 1996).

Test characteristics. This test of complex visual scanning has a motor component such that motor speed and agility make a strong contribution to success (Schear and Sato, 1989; Shum, McFarland, and Bain, 1990). Like most other tests involving motor speed and attention, the Trail Making Test is highly vulnerable to the effects of brain injury (Armitage, 1946; Spreen and Benton, 1965). When the number of seconds taken to complete Part A is relatively much less than that taken to complete Part B, the patient probably has difficulties in complex—double or multiple—conceptual tracking. Korrte and colleagues (2002) found that performance on Part B is sensitive to cognitive inflexibility to a modest degree as Part B scores correlated more highly with the Wisconsin Card Sorting Test perseverative errors than with digit span, letter fluency, or memory test scores. However, Part B also correlates very highly with Part A, which argues against cognitive flexibility being the primary determinant. Many patients with mild brain dysfunction will not have difficulty on this test (Nilson et al., 1999).

In general, reported reliability coefficients vary considerably, with most above .60 but several in the .90s and more in the .80s (Spreen and Strauss, 1998). A low reliability coefficient ($r = .36$) comes from schizophrenic patients on Part A; a very high one ($r = .94$), also on Part A, was generated by a group of neuropsychiatric patients with "vascular disorder" (G. Goldstein and Watson, 1989). With few exceptions, some improvement is typically registered for both TMT parts on retesting (Dikmen, Heaton, et al., 1999; McCaffrey, Duff, and Westervelt, 2000b); yet only improvement on

Part A is likely to reach statistical significance because group variances for Part B tend to be very large (e.g., Leininger, Gramling, et al., 1990). As an exception, no practice effect was observed in one study when the second administration occurred one year later (M.R. Basso, Bornstein, and Lang, 1999). With four successive examinations spaced a week to three months apart, Part B showed significant practice effects, although the gains made in the third testing were lost three months later on the fourth examination (McCaffrey, Ortega, and Haase, 1993). The distribution of scores on this test has a positive skew such that use of cut-off scores may be more appropriate than standard scores (Soukup, Ingram, Grady, and Schiess, 1998).

Normative data vary markedly according to characteristics of the normative samples (Mitrushina, Boone, and D'Elia, 1999; Soukup, Ingram, Grady, and Schiess, 1998). Mitrushina and her colleagues recommend care in selecting the most appropriate data set for clinical comparisons. For example, performance times increase significantly with each succeeding decade (Ernst, Warner, et al., 1987; Stuss, Stethem, and Poirier, 1987). In healthy volunteers the age effect is large on component skills (visual search, sequencing, and motor speed) and not dependent on the switching component (Salthouse, Toth, et al., 2000; Wecker et al., 2000). Education, too, plays a significant role in this test (Bornstein, 1985; Ernst, 1987), these effects showing up more strongly on Part B than Part A (Stuss, Stethem, Hugenholtz, and Richard, 1989). Bornstein and Suga (1988) documented the biggest differences between subjects with a tenth grade education or less and those with 11 years or more of formal education. Women may perform somewhat slower than men on Part B (Bornstein, 1985), particularly older women (Ernst, 1987).

Interpretations of TMT performances have typically rested on the assumption that the circled arrangement of symbols on the two test forms calls upon response patterns of equivalent difficulty. To the contrary, Fossum and his coworkers (1992) showed that the spatial arrangements on Part B are more difficult; i.e., response times become slower on Part B even when the symbols are the same as those of Part A as the Part B pathway is 56 cm longer and has more visually interfering stimuli than Part A (Gaudino et al., 1995).

Neuropsychological findings. Both Parts A and B are very sensitive to the progressive cognitive decline in dementia (Greenlief et al., 1985), so much so that Storandt, Botwinick, and their colleagues found that Part A alone contributes significantly to differentiating demented patients from control subjects (1984) and that it documents progressive deterioration, even in the early stages of the disease (Botwinick, Storandt, et al.,

1988). The elderly persons who perform poorly on Part B are likely to have problems with complex activities of daily living (Bell-McGinty et al., 2002). Both parts of this test are highly correlated ($r_A = .72$, $r_B = .80$) with caudate atrophy in patients with Huntington's disease (Starkstein, Brandt, et al., 1988).

TMT performances by patients with mild TBI are slower than those of control subjects, and slowing increases with severity of damage (Leininger, Gramling, et al., 1990). However, the large variances on TMT-B keep apparent group differences from reaching statistical significance (e.g., 16+ sec on Part B between mild and more severely concussed patients in the Leininger study; the same difference between mildly injured patients and control subjects in Stuss, Stethem, Hugenholtz, and Richard, 1989). Two to five years following moderate to severe TBI, patients were slower on Trails B than control subjects, although differences between these groups did not show up on the PASAT or the original Stroop format (Spikman, Deelman, and van Zomeren, 2000). Both Parts A and B contributed significantly to prediction of degree of independence achieved in their living situations for a group of moderately to severely injured head trauma patients (M.B. Acker and Davis, 1989).

The kinds of errors made can provide useful information. Among TBI patients, both errors of impulsivity (e.g., most typical is a jump from 12 to 13 on Part B, omitting L in an otherwise correct performance), and perseverative errors may occur such that the patient has difficulty shifting from number to letter (Lezak, 1989). McCaffrey, Krahula, and Heimberg (1989) found some of both kinds of errors made by polydrug users 7 days after detoxification, but few of these patients continued to make these errors after another drug-free week to ten days. Errors are not uncommon among normal control subjects. One study found that 12% and 35% of healthy subjects made at least one error on Parts A and B, respectively (Ruffolo, Guilmette, and Willis, 2000). However, in another study all participants who made more than one error had frontal lesions when compared to patients with posterior lesions and control subjects (Stuss, Bisschop, et al., 2001). Electrophysiological measures that appear to be "associated with frontothalamic functioning"—early stages of the Contingent Negative Variation (CNV)—correlated significantly with both TMT-A and -B, lending support to hypotheses linking the TMT to frontal activation (Segalowitz, Unsal, and Dywan, 1992). However, the importance of frontal lesions to impaired TMT performances has been questioned by findings of no significant differences in failure rates between patients with frontal lesions and those whose lesions were retrorolandic (Reitan and Wolfson, 1995a).

Emotionally disturbed patients, as suggested by elevated scores on the Minnesota Multiphasic Personality Inventory (MMPI), tend to perform more poorly than persons whose emotional status scores are not elevated (Gass and Daniel, 1990). No differences on TMT scores appeared between hospitalized schizophrenic and depressed patients, although the performances of patients with and without brain damage were clearly distinguishable (Crockett, Tallman, et al., 1988). On TMT-B depression has a slowing effect which interacts with the slowing of aging such that elderly depressed patients require a disproportionately greater amount of time to complete the test than emotionally stable elderly subjects or depressed younger ones (D.A. King et al., 1993).

The TMT's clinical value does not rest on what it may contribute to diagnostic decisions. Visual scanning and tracking problems that show up on this test can give the examiner a good idea of how effectively the patient responds to a visual array of any complexity, follows a sequence mentally, deals with more than one stimulus or thought at a time (Eson et al., 1978), or is flexible in shifting the course of an ongoing activity (Pontius and Yudowitz, 1980). When patients have difficulty performing this task, careful observation of how they get off the track and the kinds of mistakes they make can provide insight into the nature of their neuropsychological disabilities.

Color Trails (Maj et al., 1993)

Because the TMT format requires good familiarity with the English alphabet, this sensitive test cannot be given to persons whose written language is not based on this alphabet. In order to capitalize on the value of the TMT format as a neuropsychological test, this version uses color to make a nonalphabetical parallel form of the test for use in cross-cultural World Health Organization studies. In Color Trails-1 subjects are given a page with scattered circles numbered from one to 25, with even-numbered circles colored yellow and odd-numbered ones colored pink. The task is the same as TMT-A, requiring the subject to draw a line following the number sequence. Color Trails-2 also presents the subject with a page containing 25 circles, but on this sheet each color set is numbered: to 13 for the yellow odd numbers, to 12 for the pink even ones. The task is to follow the number series with a pencil but to alternate between the two colors as well (**1Y-1P-2Y**, etc.). Correlations with the two forms of the TMT are .41 and .50 for Color Trails 1 and 2, respectively. TMT-B and Color Trails-2 correlated better ($r = .72$) when the participants were older and had higher levels of education. This format discriminated HIV$^+$ and HIV$^+$ subjects well ($p < .001$). Normative data are available for Latinos (Pontón, Gonzalez, et al., 2000) and Chinese (T.M. Lee and Chan, 2000).

Everyday attention

Most everyday activities are dependent on intact attentional mechanisms for directing attention, dividing attention when necessary, and sustaining attention until an activity is complete. Many so-called memory problems are actually problems with attention (Howieson and Lezak, 2002), including the familiar complaint of being unable to recall the name of a recently introduced person—or, worse yet, the name of someone known well.

Test of Everyday Memory (TEA) (I.H. Robertson, Ward, Ridgeway, and Nimmo-Smith, 1994, 1996)

Attention is assessed with activities that are meaningful to patients, such as searching maps, looking through telephone directories, and listening to lottery number broadcasts. The eight tasks measure selective attention, sustained attention, attentional switching, and divided attention. Normative data are presented for 154 adults (J.R. Crawford, Sommerville, and Robertson, 1997). In a study of patients with severe TBI, the Map test of the TEA and a modified Stroop test distinguished the patients from control subjects better than did the Symbol Digits Modalities Test or the PASAT (Bate et al., 2001)

10 | Perception

The tests considered in this chapter are essentially perceptual, requiring little or no physical manipulation of the test material. Most of them test other functions as well, such as attention, spatial orientation, or memory, for the complexities of brain function make such overlap both inevitable and desirable. Only by testing each function in different modalities, in combination with different functions, and under different conditions can the examiner gain an understanding of which functions are impaired and how that impairment is manifested.

VISUAL PERCEPTION

Many aspects of visual perception may be impaired by brain disease. Typically brain impairment involving one visual function will affect a cluster of functions (Zihl, 1989); infrequently the visuoperceptual disorder will be confined to a single or small-set dysfunction (Riddoch and Humphreys, 2001). These latter instances of defective visuoperception provide the substance for theorizing on the nature of visuoperception. Some of the stimulus dimensions that highlight different aspects of visual perception are the degree to which the stimulus is structured, the amount of old or new memory or of verbalization involved in the task, the spatial element, and the presence of interference.

Visual functions can be broadly divided along the lines of verbal/symbolic and configural stimuli. When using visually presented material in the examination of lateralized disorders, however, the examiner cannot categorically assume that the right brain is doing most of the processing when the stimuli are pictures, or that the right brain is not engaged in distinguishing the shapes of words or numbers. Visual symbolic stimuli have spatial dimensions and other visual characteristics that lend themselves to processing as configurations, and most of what we see, including pictorial or design material, can be labeled. Materials for testing visuoperceptual functions do not conform to a strict verbal/configurational dichotomy any more than do the visual stimuli of the real world. Moreover, impairment of basic visual functions (e.g., acuity, oculomotor skills) is likely to result in poor performances on the more complex visuoperceptual tasks (Cate and Richards, 2000). These authors recommend screening for visual competency when evaluating responses to visuoperceptual tests.

The theoretical separation of attentional from perceptual functions reflects more how we conceptualize complex mental phenomena than how they work. The arbitrariness of this division of receptive activities is never more obvious than when considering the inattention phenomenon. It is dealt with in this chapter because *imperception*—conscious unawareness of stimuli—is its most striking aspect, but a good case could be made for placing this topic under *Attentional Functions*.

Visual Inattention

The *visual inattention* phenomenon (also called "visual neglect" or "visual extinction") usually involves absence of awareness of visual stimuli in the left field of vision, reflecting its common association with right hemisphere lesions. Visual inattention is more likely to occur with posterior lesions (usually parietal lobe) than with anterior lesions when the damage is on the right, but it may result from frontal lobe lesions as well (Heilman, Watson, and Valenstein, 2003). The presence of homonymous hemianopsia increases the likelihood of visual inattention, but these conditions are not necessarily linked (Halligan, Cockburn, and Wilson, 1991; Mesulam, 2000a). Visual inattention is more apt to be apparent during the acute stages of a sudden-onset condition such as stroke or trauma, when patients may be inattentive to people on their neglected side, even when directly addressed, or eat only food on the side of the plate ipsilateral to the lesion and complain that they are being served inadequate portions (N.V. Marsh and Kersel, 1993; Samuelsson et al., 1996). Long after the acute stages of the condition and blatant signs of inattention have passed, when these patients' range of visual awareness seems intact on casual observation, careful testing may elicit evidence that some subtle inattention to visual stimuli remains (e.g., see Fig. 10.1, p. 376).

Close observation of the patient when walking (bumping into walls, furniture on one side), talking (addressing persons only on one side), or handling an array of objects (as when eating) may disclose inattention deficits. The inattention phenomenon may also show up on tests designed for other purposes, such as

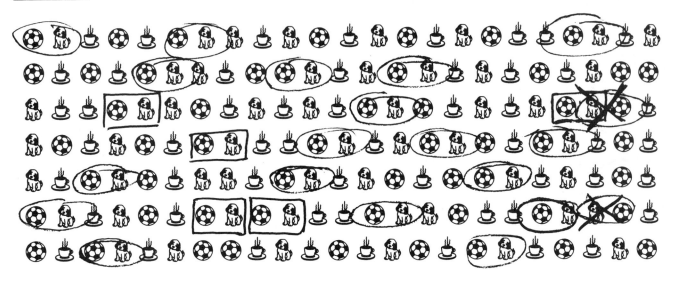

FIGURE 10.1 This sample from the *Pair Cancellation* test (Woodcock-Johnson III Tests of Cognitive Abilities; Woodcock, McGrew, and Mather, 2001c) shows how scanning cancellation tests with horizontally aligned stimuli can elicit subtle unilateral inattention—usually on the left. These top seven (of 21) lines contain four of the eight left-sided omissions (enclosed in rectangles), one of the three right-sided omissions, and two right-sided errors (X'd) made by the 55-year-old dermatologist who had sustained a blow to the left side of his head in a skiing accident (see p. 87). (© Riverside Press. Reprinted with permission)

a page of arithmetic problems (Egelko, Gordon, et al., 1988; see Figs. 3.16, 4.1, pp. 72, 87), or tests in which the stimuli or answers are presented in a horizontal array (see Fig. 10.1).

Testing for unilateral inattention

Different tests for inattention appear to have different levels of sensitivity as indicated by the number of patients in a sample who fail one or more of them, as the nature of the inattention phenomenon varies among patients (e.g., see L. Bachman et al., 1993; Ferber and Karnath, 2001; Halligan, Cockburn, and Wilson, 1991). J. Binder and his colleagues (1992), studying the effects of right hemisphere stroke, reported that cancellation tasks are much more likely to elicit evidence of inattention in patients with anterior or subcortical lesions than line bisection tasks, while the bisection tasks tend to be specifically sensitive to posterior lesions. Thus, the careful examiner will not rely on just one test of inattention if the patient's behavior suggests an inattention problem or the lesion site makes one likely.

On finding that patients were more likely to make errors when fatigued by a task, Fleet and Heilman (1986) recommended that inattention tasks such as letter cancellation tests be given in a long series to increase the likelihood of eliciting evidence of inatten-

tion. Meaninglessness and discontinuity of stimuli may also increase a task's sensitivity to inattention (Kartsounis and Warrington, 1989). Distracting stimuli on the side of space ipsilateral to the lesion (in the intact visual field) also enhance the inattention phenomenon (e.g., bilateral simultaneous stimulation; Kinsella, Packer, et al., 1995; Mesulam, 2000a; Strub and Black, 2000). Where patients begin cancellation tests for unilateral inattention also has diagnostic value (Mesulam, 2000a). On several of these tests, 94% of right-lesioned patients began at least one on the right side of the page, about half of patients with right-sided stroke began on the right (Samuelsson et al., 1996; see also Chatterjee, 2003), although normally people in most Western cultures work from left to right (e.g., Rousseaux et al., 2001; Samuelsson, et al., 1996, 2002).

In showing visual material to brain impaired patients, the examiner must always be alert to the possibility that the patient suffers visuospatial inattention and may not be aware of stimuli that appear on one side (usually the left) of the examination material. For tests in which response choices are laid out in a horizontal format (e.g., 3 × 2 or 4 × 2, as in the Test of Facial Recognition or WAIS-III Matrix Reasoning), the examiner may wish to realign the material so that all response choices are set in a column that can be presented to the patient's midline (or right side, if left-sided inattention is pronounced). Alternatively, when visuospatial inattention is obvious or suspected, tests with horizontal formats must be shown to the patient's right side.

Line Bisection Tests

The technique of examining for unilateral inattention by asking a patient to bisect a line has been used for decades (Diller, Ben-Yishay, et al., 1974). The examiner draws the line for the patient or asks the patient to copy an already drawn horizontal line. The patient is then instructed to divide the line by placing an "X" at the center point. The score is the length by which the patient's estimated center deviates from the actual center. When Diller's technique is used, a second score can be obtained for the deviation in length of the patient's copied line from that of the examiner's line. Numerical norms are not available for this technique.

Line bisection characteristics. Examinations of this technique with normal subjects have shown that they tend to mark horizontal lines to the left of center, typically deviating one to two mms, or about 1.6% (Bradshaw, Nettleton et al., 1985; Scarisbrick et al., 1987), but not always (Butter, Mark, and Heilman, 1988). Left-handed performances exacerbate this effect as left-handed subjects show the left-sided deviation more than right-handed ones (Rousseaux et al., 2001; Scarisbrick et al., 1987). The length of the line also affects line bisection accuracy for both normal subjects and patients with lateralized lesions: Short lines are less likely to elicit a deviation from center than long ones,

and the longer the line the greater the deviation (Butter, Mark, and Heilman, 1988). Most patients with right-sided lesions give greater deviations to the right, and most left-lesioned patients move the "bisection" further left with increases in line length (Pasquier et al., 1989). Noticeable errors are most often made by patients with visual field defects who tend to underestimate the side of the line opposite to the defective field, although the reverse error appears occasionally (Benton, 1969b). However, many patients with visuospatial inattention do not err consistently (Ferber and Karnath, 2001, see p. 378). Thus, a single trial is often insufficient to demonstrate the defect. The importance of having an adequate sampling of bisection behavior was demonstrated by N.V. Marsh and Kersel (1993) who, using only four lines, reported that this technique was among the least sensitive in their battery.

Line Bisection Test (LB)[1] (Schenkenberg, Bradford, and Ajax, 1980)

In a multiple-trial version of this technique, the subject is shown a set of 20 lines of different sizes arranged so that six are centered to the left of the midline of a typewriter-paper size page (21.5 x 28 cm), six to the right of midline, six in the center. A top and bottom line, to be used for instructions, is also centered on the page (see Fig. 10.2). Since only the middle 18 lines are scored, 180° rotation of the page produces an alternate

[1]This test is in the public domain. The figure may be copied and enlarged.

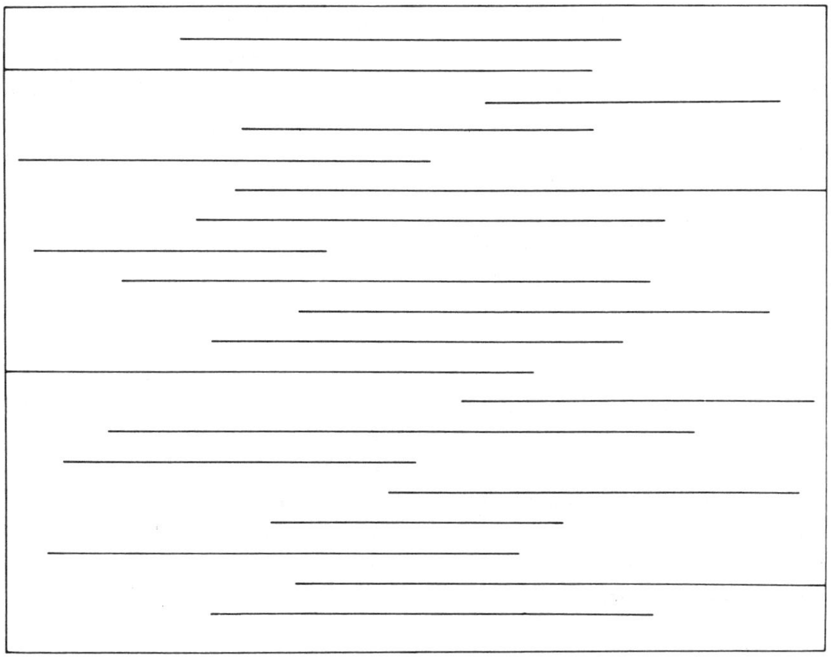

FIGURE 10.2 The Line Bisection test. (Schenkenberg et al., 1980)

form of the test. Instructions ask the patient to "Cut each line in half by placing a small pencil mark through each line as close to its center as possible," to take care to keep the nondrawing hand off the table, and to make only one mark on a line without skipping any lines. All capable patients take one trial with each hand, with randomized orientation of the page on first presentation and 180° rotation of the page on the second trial. Two scores are obtained. One gives the number and position of unmarked lines (e.g., 4R, 1C, 2L). The other is a Percent Deviation score for left-, right-, and center-centered lines derived by the formula:

$$\text{Percent Deviation} = \frac{\text{Measured Left Half} - \text{True Half}}{\text{True Half}} \times 100$$

Percent Deviation scores are positive for marks placed right of center and negative for left-of-center marks. Average Percent Deviation scores can be computed for each of the three sets of differently centered lines or for all lines. For a six-line modification of this test, Ferro, Kertesz, and Black (1987) recorded the score in millimeter deviations from the line centers. With control subjects making an average 2.9 mm deviation to the left, a right deviation cutting score of 15.3 mm indicated left hemispatial inattention. Test–retest correlations run in the .84 to .93 range for the 20-line format (Schenkenberg, Bradford, and Ajax, 1980).

Neuropsychological findings. Schenkenberg and his colleagues found that 15 of 20 patients with right hemisphere lesions omitted an average of 6.6 lines, while only 10 of the 60 subjects in the left-side lesioned, diffusely damaged, and control groups omitted any lines; these 10 omitted an average of only 1.4 lines each. Patients with right hemisphere lesions tended to miss lines, mostly the shorter ones on the left and center of the page, regardless of hand used. Only one control subject overlooked one line. When patients with right hemisphere damage used their right hands, their cutting marks tended to deviate to the right on both left- and center-centered lines, but not on right-centered lines. The other groups displayed no consistent deviation tendencies when using the right hand. A tendency to deviate to the left was generally manifested on left-hand trials, regardless of the site or presence of a brain lesion. Examining right-sided stroke patients, Kinsella, Packer, and their colleagues (1995) found that this test distinguished between those having demonstrated inattention in occupational therapy and those without apparent inattention. The identified inattention group performed significantly differently than the other stroke patients or control subjects,

deviating most on left-sided lines, least on lines on the right of the paper. Using a cut-off criterion of 14% relative displace of the bisection, Ferber and Karnath (2001) reported that 60% of their well-documented inattention patients were identified by the line bisection technique.

Using a similar format with 12 horizontal lines, Egelko, Gordon, and their colleagues (1988) reported correlations between this test and damage site as shown on CT scan for temporal ($r = -.59$), parietal ($r = -.37$), and occipital ($r = -.42$) lobes of right brain lesioned patients. On the six-line version of this test, 10 of 14 patients with lesions limited to right-sided subcortical structures exhibited the right-directional deviation with most of their failures due to their not fully exploring the left side of the lines rather than inattention per se (Ferro, Kertesz, and Black, 1987).

How the test is presented may affect its sensitivity. Rather than varying line length and center as in Figure 10.2, Halligan, Cockburn, and Wilson (1991) used only three same-length lines placed in step-wise fashion on the page. This format identified 65% of right hemisphere–damaged patients with evidence of unilateral inattention along with 75% (3 of 4) patients whose lesions were on the left.

Cancellation tasks for testing visual inattention

These are dual-purpose tests: when given to elicit unilateral inattention they may be untimed or response speed may be secondary as the examiner looks for the location and number of omissions and errors. When timed, these tests require visual selectivity at fast speed with a repetitive motor response. However, the motor response is typically so minimal that it hardly qualifies them as tests of visuomotor functions. These techniques assess the capacity for sustained attention, accuracy of visual scanning, and activation and inhibition of responses. When timed, lowered scores on these tasks can reflect the general response slowing and inattentiveness of diffuse damage or acute brain conditions; disregarding timing brings out the more specific defects of response shifting and motor smoothness or of unilateral inattention.

One common format for these tests consists of rows of stimuli with targets randomly interspersed among a larger number of foils (e.g., Figs. 10.1, 10.5). Another format scatters the stimuli in a seemingly random manner. Stimuli may be short lines, letters, numbers, other symbols, or even little pictures (e.g., Figs. 10.3, 10.4, 10.6). The patient is instructed to cross out all designated targets. Performance is typically scored for omissions and errors, and may be scored for time to completion; or, if there is a time limit, scoring is for errors and number of targets crossed out within the allotted time. Several similar tasks can be presented on the same page. The task can be made more difficult by decreasing the space between target characters or the number of foils between targets (Diller, Ben Yishay, et al., 1974). Talland (1965a) made the task more complex by using gaps in the line as spatial cues (e.g., "cross out every [specified letter] that is preceded by a gap") or by designating two targets instead of one (e.g., Fig. 10.5).

Test of Visual Neglect (M.L. Albert, 1973), also called Line Crossing (B. (A.) Wilson, Cockburn, and Halligan, 1987a)

In this technique for eliciting visual inattention, patients are asked to cross out lines scattered in a seemingly random manner over a sheet of paper. Albert's version consists of a sheet of paper (20×26 cm) with 40 lines, each 2.5 cm long, drawn out at various angles and arranged so that 18 lines are widely dispersed on each side of a central column of four lines, nine in each upper and lower quadrant (see Fig. 10.3).

M.L. Albert (personal communication, January, 1993 [mdl]) advises:

I administer the test in two different ways, depending on whether or not I have an actual copy of the test on hand. If I don't, I start with a blank sheet of paper, and draw all the lines on it, free hand, in approximately the correct position. If I am starting with a copy of the test, I present it to the patient or subject and overdraw each line once. My purpose is to assure myself that I have drawn all the lines in front of the subject. I usually start by saying, "I'm going to draw a whole bunch of lines on this paper, and I want you to watch me while I do it." (Or, "Take a look at all of the lines on this paper," at which point I overdraw each line). Then I say, "I'd like you to cross out all of the lines on this paper, like this," at which point I draw a line through one of the lines in the middle of the page, and hand the pencil to the subject.

Neuropsychological findings. Different criteria for abnormality produce somewhat different and even puzzling findings. One or no omissions was the criterion for normality; only one of 40 control subjects made a right field omission and none omitted lines on the left (Vanier et al., 1990). With the inattention criterion of ≥ 2 omissions on the three left or three right columns, unilateral inattention was identified in seven of the 40 patients. Using a fairly strict criterion of six omissions, 24 of 41 right-lesioned patients were classified as having left-sided inattention, but 22 crossed out all the lines, leading to the conclusion that for patients with right-sided lesions, the distribution of inattention is bimodal (Plourde et al., 1993).

This test compares favorably with other commonly used tests for visuospatial inattention (Halligan, Cockburn, and Wilson, 1991); although N.V. Marsh and

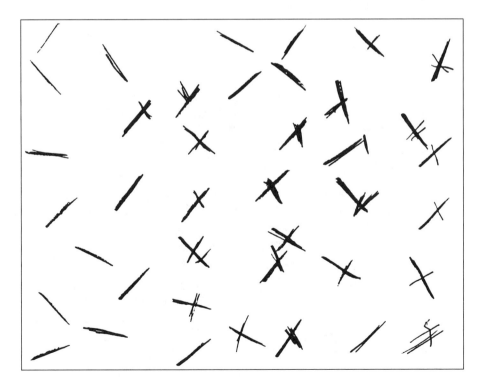

FIGURE 10.3 Performance of patient with left visuospatial inattention on the Test of Visual Neglect. (Courtesy of Martin L. Albert)

Kersel (1993) reported that it identified only 23% of patients who had displayed inattention on at least one of four tests. A few patients with left-sided lesions may also display unilateral inattention on this test but those whose lesions involve the right hemisphere tend to leave many more lines uncrossed (M.L. Albert, 1973; Halligan, Cockburn, and Wilson, 1991; Plourde et al., 1993). Halligan and Marshall (1989) noted that this test also documents the two-dimensional aspect of inattention as patients with inattention may differ not only in neglecting to cross out lines on the left or right side of the page but are likely to omit responses in a quadrant, reflecting a vertical dimension to this phenomenon.

Bells Test (Test des cloches) (Gauthier et al., 1989)[1]

In this test, rather than angled lines, 315 little silhouetted objects are distributed in a pseudo-random manner on the page with 35 bells scattered among them (see Fig. 10.4). Despite their random appearance, the objects are actually arranged in seven columns with five bells to a column. As the subject circles bells, with the admonition to do so "without losing time," the examiner notes by number on a diagramed page the order in which the subject finds the bells. This enables the examiner to document the subject's scanning strategy—or lack thereof.

For the original sample of a small control group and patients with left- or right-sided strokes, no sex or age

[1]This test can be ordered from Ortho Édition, 76, rue Jean Jaurès, 62330 Isbergues, France (Tel: [33]-3-61-94-94, Fax: [33] 3-21-61-94-95).

TABLE 10.1 The Bells Test: Omissions by Age and Education

AGE (YEARS)			
20–34 (n = 163)	35–49 (n = 156)	50–64 (n = 140)	65–79 (n = 117)
1.50 ± 1.79	2.15 ± 2.18	2.24 ± 2.34	2.54 ± 2.24

EDUCATION (YEARS)		
≤8 (n = 189)	9–12 (n = 172)	≥13 (n = 215)
2.55 ± 2.24	2.13 ± 2.20	1.59 ± 1.95

Adapted from Rousseaux et al. (2001)

differences showed up (Gauthier et al., 1989). Half of the control group made no omissions; the other half made up to three, leading to the recommendation that any more than three omissions on one or another side of the page indicates a lateralized attention deficit. Two-week test–retest reliability was .69. A normative study of commonly used tests of inattention involved 450+ healthy subjects from three areas in northeast, north central, and northwest France (Rousseaux et al., 2001). Scoring for omissions, sex did not influence Bells Test performances. Age and education effects were small (see Table 10.1). Most subjects began the task on the left. Errors were virtually nonexistent. Both number of omissions and time to completion increased with age (from ≤ 142 sec for age group 20–34 to ≥ 253 sec for ages 65–80). In comparisons with M.L. Albert's Test of Visual Neglect, this test identified a higher number of stroke patients with visual inattention (22/40 vs.

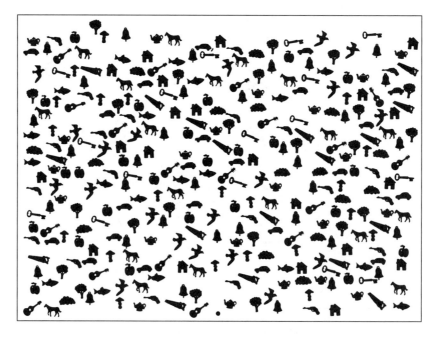

FIGURE 10.4 The Bells Test (reduced size). (Courtesy of Louise Gauthier and Yves Joanette)

7/40, Vanier et al., 1990; 33/35 vs. 22/31, Ferber and Karnath, 2001).

The Balloons Test (Edgeworth, Robertson, and McMillan, 1998)

This test consists of two pages each with 202 circles of the same size scattered in a random appearing fashion. On the first page (subtest A) to be administered, 22 have a short line extending down, much like a balloon with a short string. All but 22 circles have the balloon-like line on the second page (subtest B). For each page the task is the same: to cross out as many balloons as possible in a 3-min time limit. The first task is easy, relying on the "pop-out" phenomenon in which a few different objects are easily detected. The second page requires effortful search. When a patient makes more errors on subtest B than subtest A, the authors suggest that the better A performance demonstrates that visual fields are intact so that B omissions may be interpreted as due to inattention. This test, based on perceptual theory, is simple to administer. It certainly appears to be a promising addition to inattention assessment.

Letter cancellation tests and variants

Diller, Ben Yishay, and their colleagues (1974) constructed nine different cancellation tests; two forms for each of four stimulus categories (digits, letters, easy three-letter words, and geometric figures) plus one form using pictures. For the two-form sets, the first form has one target, the second two (see Fig. 10.5). The basic format consists of six 52-character rows in which the target character is randomly interspersed approximately 18 times in each row. The median omission for 13 control subjects was 1 for both letter and digit cancellation; median time taken was 100 sec on Letters, 90 sec on Digits. For just the letter cancellation task, normal performance limits have been defined as 0 to 2 omissions in 120 sec (Y. Ben Yishay, personal communication, 1990).

Stroke patients with right-sided lesions were not much slower than the control subjects but had many more omissions (*Mdn* Letters = 34; *Mdn* Digits = 24),

always on the left side of the page, and no errors. Patients with lesions on the left made few errors but took up to twice as long (*Mdn* Letters time = 200 sec; *Mdn* Digits time = 160 sec). Performance deficits appeared to be associated with "spatial neglect" problems with right-sided strokes, and slowed information processing when strokes involved the left hemisphere.

The *Behavioural Inattention Test* includes a shorter letter cancellation task (Halligan, Cockburn, and Wilson, 1991; B. (A.) Wilson, Cockburn, and Halligan, 1987a). Upper case letters are printed in five lines of 34 items each, of which 40% are targets (E, R), distributed equally on either side of the array. The average number of omissions for 50 control subjects was 2 ± 2.0 (range = 33–40), 26 patients with strokes on the left made an average 5.2 ± 8.1 omissions; 54 patients with right-sided strokes averaged 9.2 ± 9.8 omissions. Using a cut-off score of 8 for patients with documented unilateral inattention, inattention was identified in all left-lesioned stroke patients with this format and 77% of those with right-sided lesions.

Cancel H consists of three letter cancellation forms used to document normal response patterns over the life span (Uttl and Pilkenton-Taylor, 2001). The first, a practice form, consists of 60 upper case letters, 20 to a line, with 13 targets (always H) and 47 foils. The "Trial 1 and Trial 2" forms contain 180 letters each arranged in three rows with 12 H's in each row spaced so that 3 H's went into each of four line sections of equal length. Subjects were 351 healthy adults, ages 18 to 91, divided into seven decades: 20–29 to 80–91 plus an 18–19 age group. No surprises were reported for this study. The youngest group worked the fastest (*M* = 36.36 sec for Trials 1 and 2); the oldest group was slowest (*M* = 52.74 sec for these trials). Time increments climbed steadily. The difference between age groups for the number of omissions was negligible; more than two omissions was relatively rare for any but the two oldest age groups. Neither sex, age, nor education was related to cancellation efficiency, but significant correlations were found with tests involving visual search and visuomotor skills. Though relatively rare, more omissions occurred on the rows' right side.

```
B E I F H E H F E G I C H E I C B D A C H F B E D A C D A F C I H C F E B A F E A C F C H B D C F G H E

C A H E F A C D C F E H B F C A D E H A E I E G D E G H B C A G C I E H C I E F H I C D B C G F D E B A

E B C A F C B E H F A E F E G C H G D E H B A E G D A C H E B A E D G C D A F C B I F E A D C B E A C G


C D G A C H E F B C A F E A B F C H D E F C G A C B E D C F A H E H E F D I C H B I E B C A H C D E F B

A C B C G B I E H A C A F C I C A B E G F B E F A E A B G C G F A C D B E B C H F E A D H C A I E F E G

E D H B C A D G E A D F E B E I G A C G E D A C H G E D C A B A E F B C H D A C G B E H C D F E H A I E
```

FIGURE 10.5 Letter Cancellation task: "Cancel C's and E's" (reduced size) (Diller, Ben-Yishay, et al., 1974)

Star Cancellation (Halligan, Cockburn, and Wilson, 1991; B. [A.] Wilson, Cockburn, and Halligan, 1987a)

This untimed test was designed to increase cancellation task sensitivity to inattention by increasing its difficulty. Within this apparent jumble of words, letters, and stars are 56 small stars which comprise the target stimuli (see Fig. 10.6). The page is actually arranged in columns to facilitate scoring the number of cancelled small stars. The examiner demonstrates the task by cancelling two of the small stars, leaving a total possible score of 54. The test is available in two versions, A and B. Normal control subjects rarely miss a star: mean score of misses for 50 subjects was 0.28, with two missed at most so that three or more missed stars constitutes failure. A sample for copying and a scoring template are included in the Behavioural Inattention Test kit (B. [A.] Wilson, Cockburn, and Halligan, 1987a). This test correlates well with other tests of inattention ($r = .65$; [with drawing a clock face, a person, a butterfly] to $r = .80$ [with copying a star, a cube, a daisy, and three geometric shapes]). It identified all of a group of 30 patients (26 left, 4 right) with inattention (H. Marshall and Wade, 1989), 33 of 35 stroke patients with documented inattention (Ferber and Karnath, 2001), and was reported to be the most sensitive of a set of four tests (N.V. Marsh and Kersel, 1993).

Two and Seven Test[1] (Ruff, Evans, and Light, 1986; Ruff, Niemann, Allen, et al., 1992)

This test was developed to assess differences between automatic (obvious distractors) and controlled (less obvi-

[1]This test can be ordered from Neuropsychological Resources, 909 Hyde St., Suite 620, San Francisco, CA 94109-4839.

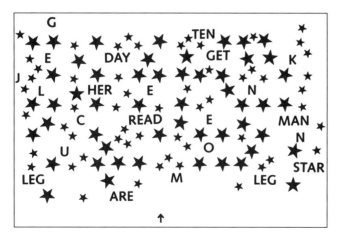

FIGURE 10.6 Star Cancellation test (reduced size). (Courtesy of Barbara A. Wilson)

ous distractors) visual search. The "automatic" condition consists of lines of randomly mixed capital letters with the digits 2 and 7 randomly intermixed; "controlled" search is presumably called upon by a format in which 2's and 7's are randomly mixed into lines of also randomly mixed digits. The test consists of 20 3-line blocks of alternating "automatic" or "controlled" search conditions. Each line of 50 characters contains ten 2's and 7's. Time allowed is five min. Scores are obtained both for correct cancellations and for omitted items up to the last item completed within the time limit.

Test characteristics. Test–retest reliability was in the .84 to .97 range although an average 10-point practice effect appeared. The average score for the "automatic" condition was 147, and that for "controlled" search was 131; this difference was significant ($p \le .001$). No sex differences appeared on normative studies. Slowing increased linearly with age on both conditions; the relationship between speed and education was also linear up to 15 years, when education effects leveled off.

Neuropsychological findings. On medication trials, patients with AIDS and AIDS-related complex (ARC) showed relatively large differences between medication and placebo performances (F.A. Schmitt, Bigley, et al., 1988). As on other cancellation tasks, a small group (14) of patients with right-sided lesions were faster than patients with left hemisphere involvement but slower than normal subjects (Ruff, Niemann, et al., 1992). Anterior lesions on the right were associated with poorer accuracy than left anterior lesions, but no laterality differences in accuracy scores showed up for patients with posterior lesions. Anticipated differences between the two search conditions showed up most prominently in the right frontal group.

Visual Search and Attention Test (Trenerry, Crosson, DeBoe, and Leber, 1990)

Still another cancellation test consists of four 60 sec trials: one is a straightforward letter cancellation format; the second displays typewriter symbols (e.g., [,], <, >, %); the third and fourth are composed of letters and typewriter symbols, respectively, with color serving as an additional distractor as the characters are randomly printed in red, green, or blue. Each line is 40 characters long with 10 targets to a line and 10 lines to a trial. Performance is evaluated for left and right sides separately to facilitate evaluation of hemi-inattention, and for a total score.

Test characteristics. A pronounced age effect was shown by a normative sample covering the age groups from 18 to 19 years and then each decade through age 60+: the youngest group's mean total score of 166.93 ± 21.88 was the highest, with scores steadily diminishing to the 60+ age group's low mean of 98.98 ± 25.23. Normative tables for the six age groups provide scores for the left and right halves of each worksheet along with the total scores. Education did not contribute to score differences. In validation studies involving the control subjects and patients with various kinds of brain damage, discriminant function analysis generated 13% to 14% false positive and 12% to 22% false negative classifications, which both supports a claim that this test is sensitive to brain damage and suggests the need for caution about using it for screening purposes.

Picture description tasks for testing visual inattention

Symmetrically organized pictures can elicit "one-sided" response biases indicative of unilateral visual inattention. I [mdl] use two pictures taken from travel advertisements: One has a columned gazebo in its center with seven lawn bowlers pictured along the horizontal expanse of foreground; the other is a square composed of four distinctly different scenes, one in each quadrant. I ask patients to count the people and the columns on the first card and to tell me everything they see on the second one. Each of these pictures has successfully brought out the inattention phenomenon when it was not apparent on casual observation.

Picture Scanning (B. [A.] Wilson, Cockburn, and Halligan, 1987a)

This test, part of the Behavioural Inattention Test, consists of three large color photographs of common views: a plate with food on it; a bathroom sink with toiletries set around it; and the window wall (of an infirmary?) flanked by a steel locker and wheelchair on the left, a walker and privacy screen on the right. The subject is instructed to "look at the picture carefully" and then both name and point out the "major items" in the pictures. The test is scored for omissions. Fifty intact subjects averaged 0.62 ± 0.75 omissions, with three omissions at most. Of stroke patients with inattention, 65% of those with right-sided lesions failed this task but only one of four whose lesions were on the left (Halligan, Cockburn, and Wilson, 1991).

Reading tasks for testing visual inattention

Two kinds of word recognition problems can trouble nonaphasic patients. Both aphasic and nonaphasic patients with visual field defects, regardless of which hemisphere is damaged, tend to ignore the part of a printed line or even a long printed word that falls outside the range of their vision when the eye is fixated for reading. This can occur despite the senselessness of the partial sentences they read. Patients with left hemisphere lesions may ignore the right side of the line or page, and those with right hemisphere lesions will not see what is on the left. This condition shows up readily on oral reading tasks in which sentences are several inches long. Newspapers are unsatisfactory for demonstrating this problem because the column is too narrow. To test for this phenomenon, Battersby and his colleagues (1956) developed a set of ten cards on which were printed ten familiar four-word phrases (e.g., GOOD HUMOR ICE CREAM, NEWS PAPER HEAD LINE) in letters 1 inch high and 1/16 inch in line thickness. Omission or distortion of words on only one side was considered evidence of a unilateral visual defect.

Two reading tests are part of the Behavioural Inattention Test battery, each appearing in two versions (B. [A.] Wilson, Cockburn, and Halligan, 1987a). One test, *Menu Reading*, is on a large card containing two columns of five food items each, printed in large letters on either side of a centerfold. A number of these items consist of two words (e.g., fried haddock, jam tart). The other test, *Article Reading*, is presented in three columns in print a little larger than newspaper copy. Both articles deal with political economy—one Britain's, the other about Gorbachev's plans for the Soviet Union. Control subjects had no problems with either task. Menu Reading proved to be more sensitive to errors of inattention than Article Reading, respectively identifying 65% and 38% of patients with inattention (Halligan, Cockburn, and Wilson, 1991).

Indented Paragraph Reading Test (IPRT) (B. Caplan, 1987)

The Indented Paragraph is just that (see Fig. 10.7, p. 384). As can be seen on this example of the errors made by the 45-year-old pediatrician described on pp. 73–74, this test is effective in eliciting inattention errors as well as tendencies to misread. The subject reads the text aloud. Caplan recommends that the examiner record "the first word read on each line" and omissions, as well as the time taken to complete the reading. The examiner can follow the subject's reading on another test sheet, noting errors of commission as well as those of omission (e.g., Fig. 10.7). For clinical purposes, when a subject has completed half of the paragraph without errors, the test can be discontinued, as little more information will be gained. By the same token, if many errors are made on the first 14 or 15 lines, these should be sufficient to warrant discontinuing what—in these

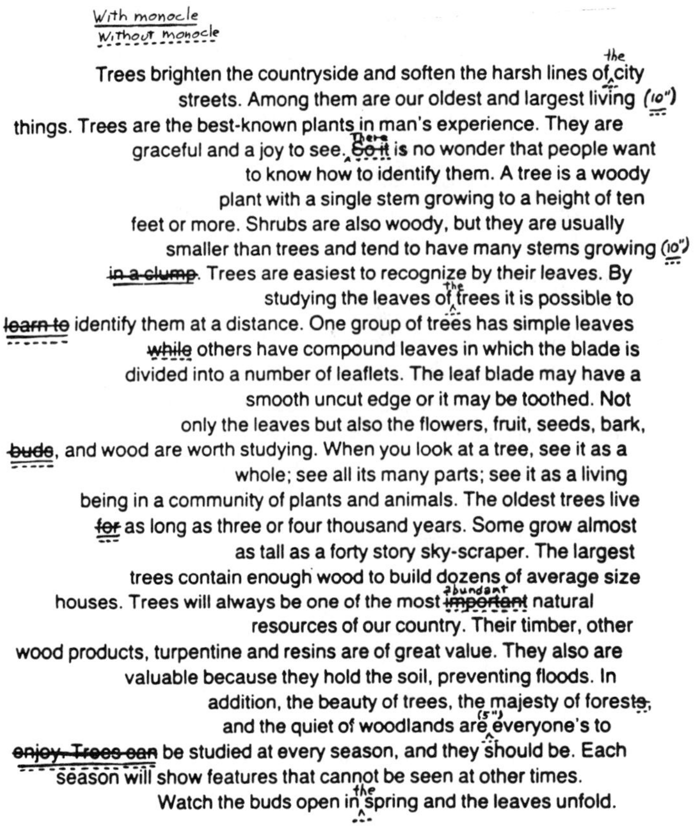

With monocle
Without monocle

Trees brighten the countryside and soften the harsh lines of city
streets. Among them are our oldest and largest living (10")
things. Trees are the best-known plants in man's experience. They are
graceful and a joy to see. So it is no wonder that people want
to know how to identify them. A tree is a woody
plant with a single stem growing to a height of ten
feet or more. Shrubs are also woody, but they are usually
smaller than trees and tend to have many stems growing (10")
in a clump. Trees are easiest to recognize by their leaves. By
studying the leaves of trees it is possible to
learn to identify them at a distance. One group of trees has simple leaves
while others have compound leaves in which the blade is
divided into a number of leaflets. The leaf blade may have a
smooth uncut edge or it may be toothed. Not
only the leaves but also the flowers, fruit, seeds, bark,
buds, and wood are worth studying. When you look at a tree, see it as a
whole; see all its many parts; see it as a living
being in a community of plants and animals. The oldest trees live
for as long as three or four thousand years. Some grow almost
as tall as a forty story sky-scraper. The largest
trees contain enough wood to build dozens of average size
houses. Trees will always be one of the most important natural
resources of our country. Their timber, other
wood products, turpentine and resins are of great value. They also are
valuable because they hold the soil, preventing floods. In
addition, the beauty of trees, the majesty of forests,
and the quiet of woodlands are everyone's to (5")
enjoy. Trees can be studied at every season, and they should be. Each
season will show features that cannot be seen at other times.
Watch the buds open in spring and the leaves unfold.

FIGURE 10.7 Indented Paragraph Reading Test with errors made by the 45-year-old traumatically injured pediatrician described on pp. 73–74. Errors made in each of two trials (with a small range magnifying monocle and without it) are marked.

cases—can be a painful task for patient and examiner alike. Of course, for research purposes, a standardized administration is necessary. The patient can be asked to describe what was read as an informal test of reading comprehension (and occasionally of short-term memory). Caplan defines mild neglect as one to nine omissions on the left side of the page; ten or more omissions earn a classification of moderate to severe neglect.

Neuropsychological findings. In the original study, most (78.3%) patients with left-sided damage read this passage without error, but barely half (53.5%) with lesions on the right read it perfectly. This test elicited the inattention phenomenon in patients in each lateralization group who had given no signs of such a problem on other tests. Of a sample of patients with right hemisphere disease similar to Caplan's original group, 20% scored in the mild inattention category while 50% met the criteria for moderate to severe inattention (L. Bachman et al., 1993). Although only 36% of this patient group had more than a high school education and 8% had at most five years of schooling, educational level was not associated with left-sided omissions. In a com-

parison of reading errors made by right hemisphere stroke patients on paragraphs with straight margins, doubly indented margins, and the Indented Paragraph, the doubly indented paragraph elicited the most errors ($M = 15.21 \pm 34$), fewer appeared on the Indented Paragraph ($M = 12.50 \pm 25$), and even fewer on the straight-sided paragraph, but these differences were not significant (Towle and Lincoln, 1991). Correlations with the Star Cancellation and Article Reading tests were .37 and .49, respectively. Towle and Lincoln pointed out that the different tests identified somewhat different clusters of patients, again illustrating the need for more than one kind of assessment for visuospatial hemiinattention.

Writing techniques for examining inattention

Left unilateral visual inattention for words, a defect that interferes with the reading accuracy and pleasure of many patients with right brain damage, may be clearly shown by having the patient copy sentences or phrases. Names and addresses make good copying material for this purpose since missing words or numbers

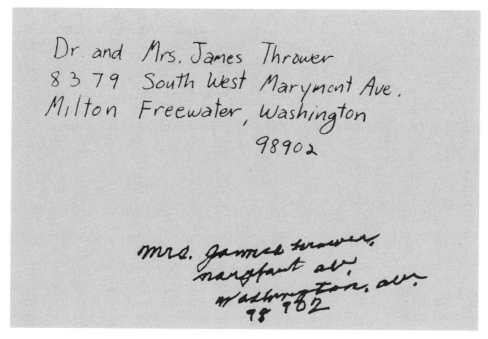

FIGURE 10.8 This attempt to copy an address was made by a 66-year-old retired paper mill worker two years after he had suffered a right frontal CVA. His writing not only illustrates left visuospatial inattention but also the tendency to add "bumps" (e.g., the m in "James") and impaired visual tracking (e.g., "Ave" is repeated on the line below the street address line)—all problems that can interfere with the reading and writing of patients with right hemisphere lesions.

are less apparent than a word or two omitted from the left-hand side of a meaningful line of print. When set up in a standard address format, patients' efforts to copy model addresses readily reveal inattention defects (see Fig. 10.8). The Behavioural Inattention Test contains two little copying tasks in the *Address/Sentence test* (B.[A.] Wilson, Cockburn, and Halligan, 1987a). One consists of a four-line address similar in the number and placement of elements to the one shown in Figure 10.8. The second task is a three-line sentence, such as might be in a newspaper article but presented in type a little larger than ordinary print. The top left-hand word in each is "The," on the left at the bottom is "St.," words that could readily be omitted without compromising the meaning of the sentence. Of a group of right brain damaged patients with inattention, 65% failed this test (Halligan, Cockburn, and Wilson, 1991).

Drawing and copying tests for inattention

Both free drawing and drawing to copy can elicit the inattention phenomenon (e.g., see Figs. 3.13 and 3.15a, pp. 67, 69). Thus most batteries designed to elicit inattention will contain one or both of these techniques. For example, Strub and Black (2000) ask their patients to copy five items (a diamond, a cross, a cube, a three-dimensional pipe, and a triangle within a triangle) and to draw free hand a clock with numbers and hands (time not specified), a daisy in a flower pot, and a house in perspective showing two sides and a roof. The Behavioural Inattention Test (B. [A.] Wilson, Cockburn, and Halligan, 1987a) has both *Representational drawing* (a "clock face with numbers," a man or woman, a butterfly) and *Figure and shape copying* (a star, a cube, a daisy) tasks. The characteristic common to these stimuli is their bilateral nature: many are bilaterally symmetrical (e.g., see Fig. 10.9, p. 386); in the others, left- and right-sided details are equally important.

The bilateral asymmetry of the Complex Figure proved effective in eliciting evidence of left visuospatial inattention (Rapport, Farchione, Dutra, et al., 1996) (see Fig. 14.2, p. 537). The side of errors and omissions on copies of the Complex Figure clearly distinguished right-lesioned stroke patients with ($n = 36$) and without ($n = 32$) already identified unilateral inattention: the former made an average of 3.31 ± 1.33 omissions from the left of the figure; the latter's left omission average was 0.72 ± 0.68. Similar data distinguished patients with left-sided strokes (right-sided omission $M = 0.45 \pm 0.89$) and control subjects who rarely omitted a design element. Of the 36 patients with left visuospatial inattention, 35 gave evidence of this problem when copying the Complex Figure.

Drawings tend to be somewhat less sensitive in eliciting inattention than cancellation tasks generally. In an evaluation of the Behavioural Inattention Test, fig-

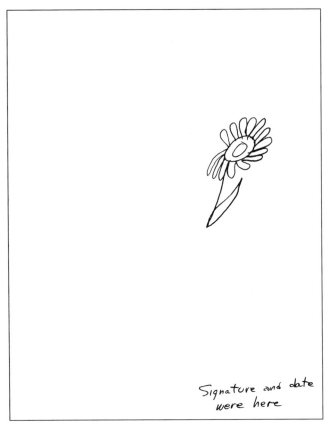

FIGURE 10.9 Flower drawn by patient with left visuospatial neglect. Note placement of flower on the page.

ure and shape copying were much more sensitive than drawing specified objects (eliciting inattention errors for 96% and 42%, respectively, of patients with right-sided strokes) (Halligan, Cockburn, and Wilson, 1991).

Inattention in spatial representation

Unilateral visuospatial inattention is a spatial as well as a visual phenomenon. This can be demonstrated in tests of spatial representation in which the visual component has been eliminated. Left-sided spatial inattention was elicited by requesting the subject to describe a familiar locale (Bisiach and Luzzatti, 1978). Patients were asked to name the prominent features of a scene from two specific viewing points directly opposite one another. Their left-sided inattention appeared as either absence or scant mention of features on the left, in marked contrast to detailed descriptions of structures to the right of each given perspective.

Behavioural Inattention Test (BIT) (B. [A.] Wilson, Cockburn, and Halligan, 1987a)

This test battery was developed to provide a more naturalistic examination of tendencies to hemi-inattention, whether right or left. It consists of two sections, the "conventional subtests" and the "behavioural subtests." The six "conventional" subtests have been described above (Line crossing, Star cancellation, Figure and shape copying, Line bisection, Representational drawing, Letter cancellation). Picture scanning, Menu reading, Article reading, and Address and sentence copying are four of the nine "behavioural subtests." The others are *Telephone dialing* (which uses a disconnected telephone on which the patient must dial three numbers presented in large print on separate cards); *Telling and setting the time* (includes reading numbers pictured on a digital clock; reading a large clock face, and setting time with the movable hands of the face); *Coin sorting* (requires identification of six denominations of coins laid out in three rows in front of the subject); and *Map navigation* (presents a grid of paths with a different letter at each choice point: the examiner calls out letter pairs which the subject must trace by finger, e.g., from A to B).

Test characteristics. Available reliability studies involve very small groups of patients (as few as six, up to 10), but they indicate satisfactory ($r = .75$ for parallel forms of the set of conventional tests) to excellent reliabilities ($r = .97$ for test–retest of the set of behavioral tests) (Halligan, Cockburn, and B. Wilson, 1991). The two sets of tests correlated highly with each other ($r = .79$) and each correlated well (rs of .65, .67) with occupational therapists' reports and an assessment of activities of daily living (ADLs). All of 14 control subjects passed all of the behavioral tests except Map navigation (failed by three) and Picture scanning and Digital time (each failed by one) (B. [A.] Wilson, Cockburn, and Halligan, 1987b). Map navigation was the most sensitive of these tests (eliciting inattention from 14 of 28 patients with lateralized damage), with Coin sorting running a close second (11 patients displayed inattention). This battery identified inattention in 18 of 41 right hemisphere stroke patients (Samuelsson et al., 2002).

Visual Scanning

The visual scanning defects that often accompany brain lesions can seriously compromise such important activities as reading, writing, performing paper-and-pencil calculations, and telling time (Diller, Ben Yishay, et al., 1974), and they are also associated with accident-prone behavior (Diller and Weinberg, 1970). Tests for inattention and cancellation tasks will often disclose scanning problems as will other perceptual tests requiring scanning.

Counting dots

This very simple method for examining visual scanning can be constructed to meet the occasion. The subject is asked to count aloud the number of dots—20 or more—widely scattered over a piece of paper, but with an equal number in each quadrant. Errors may be due to visual inattention to one side, to difficulty in maintaining an orderly approach to the task, or to problems in tracking numbers and dots consecutively. McCarthy and Warrington (1990, p. 85) noted that this technique can make poor scanning strategies evident, as some patients count the same dot more than once thus overestimating the number while others miss or neglect dots and report too few.

Visual Scanning Test (Samuelsson, Hjelmquist, Jensen, and Blomstrand, 2002)

Samuelsson and his coworkers used the Behavioural Inattention Test with acute and postacute stage right hemisphere stroke patients to identify those exhibiting unilateral inattention (*n* = 18) and those who did not (*n* = 23). Thirty-two letters and numbers appear scattered on a standard European size paper (approximately 29.5 × 21 cm), but are actually arranged in 8 rows × 4 lines providing 32 "cells" for tracking subject responses. Subjects read the letters and numbers while the examiner tracks the path of target selection on a separate graphed page.

Most of the demographically matched control subjects (29/34) followed a single search strategy (24 by row, 5 by column); all but three of them began at top left; 29 missed no target and no one missed more than one. Patients giving no evidence of inattention differed little from control subjects, but omitted more targets, shifted strategies a bit more, and a few subjects read the same target more than once. Inattention patients showed direction shifts—which were not made by either control subjects or noninattention patients, and more strategy shifts, with a median of 8.7% repeated targets (interquartile range = 23.8%), this latter kind of error being the most important correlate of inattention. A follow-up study six to seven months later found only six (of 36) patients still manifesting unilateral inattention and even their search patterns had become less erratic.

Visual Search (R.F. Lewis and Rennick, 1979)

This test is part of both the computer-assisted and manual forms of the Repeatable-Cognitive-Perceptual-Motor Battery. More recently it was included in the National Institute of Mental Health Core Neuropsy-

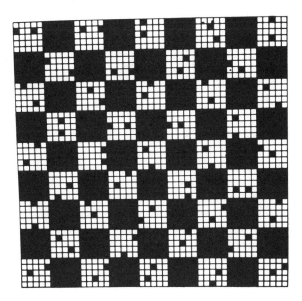

FIGURE 10.10 One of the Visual Search stimulus figures.

chological Battery and in this battery's abbreviated version (N. Butters, Grant, et al., 1990). The test booklet contains four versions of the 9 × 9 checkerboard pattern stimulus figure (see Fig. 10.10). The subject's task is to indicate in which of the outlying grids is the position of the two little black squares like that of eight center test grids. The test is scored for time and errors. For 30 healthy adults (M_{age} = 37.6 ± 11.8, M_{educ} = 15.5 ± 2.7), mean total time was 116.8 ± 36.9 sec., with 1.09 ± 1.4 average errors (McCaffrey, Westervelt, and Haase, 2001). Over five trials given over $1^1/_2$ years, scores remained essentially flat.

In the original format of 16 stimulus figures projected on a screen, brain impaired patients were much slower than normal control subjects and considerably slower than neurologically intact psychiatric patients (G. Goldstein, Welch, et al., 1973). Error scores did not discriminate between these groups. Time scores also proved useful in evaluating the effects of medication changes in epileptic patients (R.F. Lewis, Rennick, Clifford, et al., 1976, cited in Kelland and Lewis, 1994).

In my experience the evaluation standards (provided with the test material) may be too generous [mdl]. A comprehensive normative study would be welcomed.

Color Perception

Tests of color perception serve a dual purpose in neuropsychological assessment. They can identify persons with congenitally defective color vision, or "color blindness," whose performance on tasks requiring accurate color recognition might otherwise be misinterpreted. Knowledge that the patient's color vision is defective will affect the evaluation of responses to such colored material as the color cards of the Rorschach technique, and should militate against use of color-dependent tests such as Stroop tests. Color perception tests can also be used to test for color agnosia and related defects. Evaluation of color recognition (usually measured by color association tasks such as Coloring of Pictures or Wrongly Colored Pictures, discussed below) is important in examining aphasic patients since many of them have pronounced color recognition deficits (Denburg and Tranel, 2003; Vuilleumier, 2001). A small proportion of patients with lesions on the right and of nonaphasic patients with left-sided lesions also have color recognition problems. Color perception itself can be attentuated by some toxic exposures (Mergler, Bowler, and Cone, 1990; Spencer, 2000b). Rarely, brain disease will destroy the ability to see colors (*achromatopsia*) (Bauer and Demery, 2003; Farah, 2003).

Testing for accuracy of color perception

In neuropsychological assessment, the *Dvorine* (1953) and the *Ishihara* (1983) screening tests for the two most common types of color blindness are satisfactory. The *H-R-R Pseudoisochromatic Plates* (Hardy et al., 1957) screen for two rare forms of color blindness, which would not be correctly identified by the Ishihara or Dvorine tests, as well as for the two common types (Hsia and Graham, 1965). The stimulus materials of all three of these tests are cards printed with different colored dots, which form recognizable figures against a ground of contrasting dots.

Farnsworth's Dichotomous Test for Color Blindness (D-15), Lanthony's Desaturated 15 Hue Test (D15-d)[1]

These tests each consist of 16 color caps, all of similar brightness but a little different in hue, together representing a continuous color range. The Lanthony set colors are desaturated (i.e., very pale pastels) and sensitive to even mild forms of defective color vision. In each test set, 15 color caps are spread out randomly in front of the subject, whose task initially is to find the color cap with the hue closest to that of a cap fixed to one end of a horizontal tray. Then, one by one, the subject must try to line up the 15 movable caps in a consistent color continuum, always seeking the hue closest to the one just matched. A scoring form permits discrimination of three kinds of impaired color vision. This tech-

nique has identified color vision impairments associated with toxic solvent exposure (Mergler, Bowler, and Cone, 1990) and with alcoholism (Mergler, Blain, et al., 1988). A scoring table is now available for the desaturated test which can be used when conducting field studies (e.g., of toxic exposures) (Geller, 2001).

Neitz Test of Color Vision (J. Neitz, Summerfelt, and Neitz, 2001)

This paper-and-pencil color perception test is suitable for both individual and group testing of both blue–yellow and red–green discrimination deficiencies. The subject sees a sheet with nine grayish circles, each filled with rows and columns of small, mostly grayish dots, but some dots are in muted colors forming a geometric figure (square, circle, etc.; and one large circle has randomly placed colored dots) within the circle that can only be discerned by color competent viewers. Eight of the nine circles have other dots making patterns not normally viewed but seen by persons with color blindness. The type of errors made help to discriminate between the two most common color vision defects. Responses are checked in one of five small circles below each large one: in each array of response circles one contains the outline of each of the four geometric figures and one is empty. The correct response is the circle containing the normally discerned pattern in the large stimulus circle. Error patterns indicate the kind of color blindness a person has. Three parallel versions each test for the same kinds of color defect but the circle patterns are placed differently.

This test was developed for children but can be easily used with adults. In a validity study, failures were compared with genotypes: none of the subjects with an identified gene type for color blindness passed this test; 94% of normal adult males did pass it. In one published study, the authors (M. Neitz and Neitz, 2001) reported on color testing of 5,129 boys. Comparisons with conventional tests of color vision found good agreement.

Color-to-Figure Matching Test (Della Sala, Kinnear, Spinnler, and Stangalino, 2000)

Questioning whether Alzheimer patients had impaired color vision (*dyschromatopsia*), Della Sala and his colleagues showed nine black on white line drawings of common objects which "are not linked with a unique prototypical color" (e.g., an artichoke, a rabbit, a priest [!]) along with 30 colored pencils including many shades of some colors (e.g., five of red, four of green, but just one for black and for white). Correctness of

---

[1]This test may be ordered from Luneau Ophtalmologie, B.P. 252, 28005 Chartres Cedex, France (e-mail: luneau.export©free.fr).

color choices was defined by 33 control subject responses to this test: any color selected for a drawing by 11 or more of them was considered "correct;" colors which six or fewer control subjects had selected for a drawing were "wrong;" colors selected for a drawing by 7 to 10 of the control subjects were classified as "doubtful." Each color choice was scored on a 3-point scale (2–0); with eight drawings (the first, cherries, is a practice trial), the maximum score is 16. Alzheimer patients' average score was 13.18 ± 2.66. Color choice failures correlated significantly ($r = .59$) with disease severity. A designated cut-off score clearly distinguished mildly impaired patients who performed well on this test from moderately impaired patients who made most of the errors.

Discriminating between color agnosia and color anomia

The problem of distinguishing color agnosia, in which colors are seen but have lost their object context (Farah, 2003; see Bauer and Demery, 2003, for a somewhat different definition) from an anomic disorder involving use of color *words* was ingeniously addressed in two tasks devised by A.R. Damasio, McKee, and Damasio (1979). *Coloring of Pictures* requires the subject to choose a crayon from a multicolored set and fill in simple line drawings of familiar objects that have strong color associations (e.g., banana—yellow; frog—green). In *Wrongly Colored Pictures*, the examiner shows the subject a line drawing that has been inappropriately colored (e.g., a green dog, a purple elephant), and asks what the picture represents.

In a refinement of these techniques which investigates the correctness of color associations, Varney (1982) developed a set of 24 line drawings of familiar objects (e.g., banana, ear of corn). Each drawing is accompanied by samples of four different colors, of which only one is appropriate for the item. This format requires only a pointing response. Just four of 100 normal subjects failed to identify at least 20 colors correctly. In contrast, 30% of the 50 aphasic patients failed this standard. It is of interest that all of the aphasic patients who failed the color association test also failed a reading comprehension task, while none who succeeded on the reading task failed the color association test.

Three kinds of color tests together may help to distinguish a color agnosia from an anomia for colors (Beauvois and Saillant, 1985). In the purely verbal "colour name sorting" test, the examiner names a color (e.g., blush, scarlet) and the subject must identify the general color category to which it belongs (brown, red, or yellow). A second verbal task asks for a color name for a purely verbal concept (e.g., "what colour name would you give for being jealous?" " . . . to royal blood?"). Visual tasks include the Color Sorting Test and a test of "pointing out the correctly coloured object." These latter two tests require little if any verbal processing. A third test category, "visuo-verbal tests," asks for "colour naming on visual confrontation;" "pointing out a colour upon spoken request" asks the subject to "show me the colour of a banana" for example; and conversely, the subject is asked to "give the colour name of an object" drawn without color.

Goodglass, Kaplan, and Barresi (2000) include some color items in the Boston Diagnostic Aphasia Examination. *Word Discrimination* asks the subject to point to six colors named by the examiner. The *Visual Confrontation Naming* section asks the subject to name these six colors. In *Written Confrontation Naming*, two colors are shown for their names to be written. Performance on these three tasks may help the examiner sort out the presence and nature of a problem with colors, or at least alert the examiner that a problem with colors needs further investigation.

Although these tests can aid in differentiating an agnosic from an anomic condition, examiners must remain alert to the possibility that the agnosia or the anomia involves much more than colors. Moreover, problems with object recognition or other naming disorders may have contributed to erroneous responses (see also Coslett and Saffran, 1992; De Renzi and Spinnler, 1967).

Visual Recognition

Interest in visual recognition has grown with the rapid expansion of knowledge of the different roles played by the hemispheres and with more precise understanding of the different functional systems. When brain dysfunction is suspected or has been identified grossly, the examination of different aspects of visual recognition may lead to a clearer definition of the patient's condition.

Angulation

The perception of angular relationships tends to be a predominantly right hemisphere function except when the angles readily lend themselves to verbal description (e.g., horizontal, vertical, diagonal) so that they can be mediated by the left hemisphere as well as the right. Thus inaccurate perception of angulation is more likely to accompany right hemisphere damage than damage to the left hemisphere (Benton, Hannay, and Varney, 1975; McCarthy and Warrington, 1990).

Judgment of Line Orientation (JLO)[1] (Benton, Hannay, and Varney, 1975; Benton, Sivan, Hamsher, et al., 1994, test manual)

This test examines the ability to estimate angular relationships between line segments by visually matching angled line pairs to 11 numbered radii forming a semicircle (see Fig. 10.11). The test consists of 30 items, each showing a different pair of angled lines to be matched to the display cards. Its two forms, H and V, present the same items but in different order. A five-item practice set precedes the test proper. The score is the number of items on which judgments for both lines are correct; thus, the score range is 0–30. Scores ≥23 are in the *average* or better ranges (e.g., 29–30 = *superior*). Score corrections are provided for both age and sex (see Table 10.2).

Test characteristics. Internal consistency is high (.90) (Qualls et al., 2000). After one year a retest correlation for elderly control subjects was .59 (B.E. Levin, Llabre, Reisman, et al., 1991). For control subjects and patients in a stable course, practice effects were inconsequential (McCaffery, Duff, and Westervelt, 2000b), and nil for Parkinson patients and controls after 20 min (Alegret et al., 2001). Normative data show that only 5.5% of 137 normal subjects obtained scores below 19 while only two of that group scored below 17 (Benton,

[1]The test material is sold by the Medical Sales Department, Oxford University Press, 198 Madison Ave., New York, NY 10016.

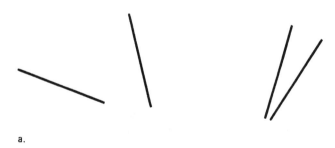

a.

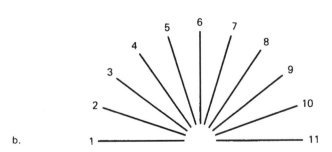

b.

FIGURE 10.11 Judgment of Line Orientation (Benton, Sivan, Hamsher, et al., 1994). Examples of double-line stimuli (*a*) to be matched to the multiple-choice card below (*b*).

TABLE 10.2 Judgment of Line Orientation: Score Corrections

Add	
0	Men under age 65
1	Men between ages 65 and 74
2	Women under age 65
3	Men over age 65, women between ages 65 and 74
4	Women over age 75

Adapted from Benton, Sivan, Hamsher, et al. (1994)

Sivan, Hamsher, et al., 1994). Scores between 17 and 20 represent mild to moderate defects in judging line orientation; scores below 17 indicate a severe defect.

Women's scores tend to run about two points below those of men, a finding virtually identical to that of an Italian study cited in the manual; male superiority also appeared for college students in a group-administered variation of this test (Collaer and Nelson, 2002). Performance declines with age, most noticeably after 65 (Eslinger and Benton, 1983; Mittenberg, Seidenberg, et al., 1989), but in one study this decline did not reach statistical significance (Ska, Poissant, and Joanette, 1990). A group of well-educated elderly people scored well within the normal range until after age 75 (Benton, Eslinger, and Damasio, 1981). JLO performances by over 750 persons ages 55 to 97 generated small correlations with age ($r = -.25$), with sex ($r = -.24$), with education ($r = .21$), and thus required virtually no changes in standard score conversions from ages 56 to 77 (Ivnik, Malec, Smith, et al., 1996). The mean raw score range for this large sample remained at 21–22 from age 56 to 80, dropping to 20–21 for the 81 to 83 age group, and to 19–21 for ages 84 to 97.

Neuropsychological findings. While performing an rCBF using a shortened version of this test, cerebral blood flow in temporo-occipital areas increased bilaterally, with the greatest increases on the right (Hannay, Falgout, et al., 1987). Most patients with left hemisphere damage performed in the *normal* range, as shown when 50 left- and 50 right-lesioned patients were compared with the normative subjects (age-corrected scores): 41 with left-sided lesions performed at *average* or better levels, only one scored below 17; of the patients with right-sided lesions, 21 achieved an *average* or better score and 18 made scores in the *severely defective* range (Benton, Sivan, Hamsher, et al., 1994). Patients with visual field defects showed a slightly greater tendency to failure than those with intact fields. Aphasia in left-hemisphere lesioned patients increases somewhat their likelihood of failure. Most failures were made by patients with posterior or mixed anterior–posterior lesions (see also A.R. Damasio and Anderson, 2003).

Dementia patients frequently fail this test (Eslinger and Benton, 1983; Ska, Poissant, and Joanette, 1990), many receiving scores much below the 18-point cutoff. However, 51.6% of patients with probable Alzheimer's disease overlapped a control group of similar age, and 60.7% of Parkinson patients also overlapped the control group, although the means of both groups were lower (Finton et al., 1998). An analysis of error types in this study did not differentiate these groups with the exception of Parkinson patients' greater incidence of misjudgment of both lines with their spatial relationship maintained. The failures of 16% of a group of Parkinson patients were not associated with general cognitive ability, or with disease severity (Hovestadt et al., 1987), nor were failures associated with PD duration (B.E. Levin, Llabre, et al., 1991). Alegret and his colleagues (2001) concluded that the nature of errors made by Parkinson patients—disproportionately involving intraquadrant dissimilar lines and horizontal lines—demonstrated a visuospatial disorder in this disease.

Short forms. Randomized JLO items comprise two 15-item forms; scores were doubled to make them comparable to the 30-item JLO (Qualls et al., 2000). Using protocols from rehabilitation patients (mostly stroke, some TBI, and a few other neuropathological disorders), these forms had good internal consistency and one form correlated very well (.94) with full score data. However, on testing a different group of stroke patients, scores did not discriminate well between right- and left-lesioned patients. Ten percent of these patients produced scores in the normal range, leading the authors to recommend these forms for visuospatial screening and use of the original JLO when visuospatial impairment is an issue.

Unusual views of pictured objects

Warrington and Taylor (1973; see also McCarthy and Warrington, 1990) examined the relative accuracy with which patients with right or left hemisphere lesions could identify familiar objects under distorting conditions. In the first condition, involving 20 enlarged drawings of small objects such as a safety pin, both patients and control subjects recognized objects drawn in their usual size. The patients made significantly more errors than the control subjects in recognizing the enlarged objects, with only a negligible score difference between the right and left brain lesioned groups. The second condition presented photographs of 20 familiar objects taken from a conventional and an unconventional view. For example, a bucket was shown in a side view (the conventional view) and straight down from above (the unconventional view). This condition resulted in a clear-cut separation of patients with right brain damage, who did poorly on this task, from the left damaged group or the control subjects. In addition, patients with right posterior lesions made the most errors by far.

Riddoch and Humphreys (2001) developed a set of object pictures taken from unusual angles (e.g., a corkscrew: from the side of the handle, facing the handle from the tip of the greatly foreshortened screw). On showing these pictures to patients with right hemisphere lesions, they found a "double dissocation" as one patient failed to recognize only objects reduced to their minimal features (side view of corkscrew) while other patients' recognition impairment was restricted to objects with a foreshortened main axis (view from tip of corkscrew). They note that for the most part these patients had adequate recognition for objects seen in familiar perspectives, and offer some theories to account for these phenomena. Turnbull and his colleagues (1997) suggest that both dorsal (involving the parietal lobes) and ventral (involving the temporal lobe) pathways contribute to unusual view deficits: the temporal lobes are necessary for object recognition; the parietal lobes provide for the spatial conceptualization necessary to identify objects from strange perspectives.

Perceptual Speed (Identical Forms)
(L.L. Thurstone and Jeffrey, 1987)

This is a timed paper-and-pencil picture matching task in which both visuoperceptual accuracy and speed in making perceptual judgments contribute to the performance (Fig. 10.12, p. 392). Each of the 140 items displays a target figure—an abstract design of an object such as a clock, a bird, or a shoe or a geometric design—with five similar designs, of which one is identical to the target. A five min time limit insures that virtually no one can complete the test, although most of the items are neither tricky nor difficult. Norms were developed for personnel selection in industry, but this easy to administer test is well-suited to neuropsychological applications.

Test characteristics. Norms are given for jobs in industry and government organizations. Thurstone and Jeffrey (1987) obtained split-half reliability coefficients ranging from .92 to .98 based on a 60-item format. Correlations with nine discrete clerical test scores ranged from .32 (Error Location) to .52 (Alphabetizing). Like its name, this test has had highest or second highest loadings on a Perceptual Speed factor in numerous studies (reported in test manual).

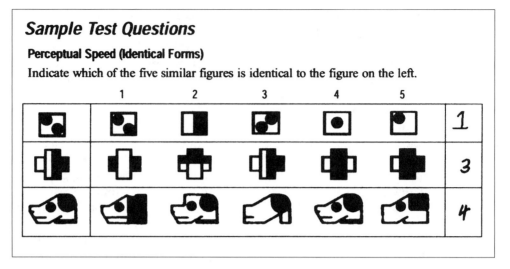

FIGURE 10.12 Perceptual Speed. (© 1984 by L.L. Thurstone, Ph.D. All rights reserved.) This sample test question may not be duplicated in any manner without written permission from the publisher. (Courtesy of Pearson Reid London House, Inc.)

Face recognition

Warrington and James's (1967b) demonstration that there is no regular relationship between inability to recognize familiar faces (*prosopagnosia*) and impaired recognition of unfamiliar faces has led to a separation of facial recognition tests into those that involve a memory component and those that do not (see also Chatterjee and Farah, 2001; McCarthy and Warrington, 1990). Tests of familiar faces call on stored information and ease of retrieval. Typically, these tests require the subject to name or otherwise identify pictures of well-known persons (Warrington and James, 1967b). Two kinds of errors were noted in the earlier studies: Left hemisphere damaged patients identified but had difficulty naming the persons, whereas defective recognition characterized the right hemisphere damaged patients' errors. A third error pattern appears among patients with frontal lesions who lack a search strategy (Rapcsak, Nielsen, et al., 2001). Facial recognition deficits tend to occur with spatial agnosias and dyslexias, and with dysgraphias that involve spatial disturbance (Tzavaras et al., 1970).

Recognition tests of unfamiliar faces involving memory have appeared in several formats. Photos can be presented for matching either one at a time or in sets of two or more. When the initial presentation consists of more than one picture, this adds a memory span component, which further complicates the face recognition problem. The second set of photos to be recognized can be presented one at a time or grouped, and presentation may be immediate or delayed. By having to match unfamiliar faces following a delay, patients with brain damage involving the right temporal lobe demonstrated significant performance decrements, again linking memory for configural material with the right temporal lobe (Warrington and James, 1967b).

Test of Facial Recognition[1] (Benton, Sivan, Hamsher, et al., 1994)

This test was developed to examine the ability to recognize faces without involving a memory component. The patient matches identical front views, front with side views, and front views taken under different lighting conditions (see Fig. 10.13). The original test has 22 stimulus cards and calls for 54 separate matches. Six items involve only single responses (i.e., only one of six pictures on the stimulus card is of the same person as the sample), and 16 items call for three matches to the sample photograph. It may take from 10 to 20 minutes to administer, depending on the patient's response rate and cautiousness in making choices.

In order to reduce administration time, a short form of this test was developed that is half as long as the original (H.S. Levin, Hamsher, and Benton, 1975). The 16-item version calls for only 27 matches based on six one-response and seven three-response items. Correlations between scores obtained on the long and short forms range from .88 to .93, reflecting a practical equivalence between the two forms. Instructions, age and education corrections (see Table 10.3, p. 393), and norms for both forms are included in the test manual.

[1]This test material is sold by the Medical Sales Department, Oxford University Press, 198 Madison Ave., New York, NY, 10016.

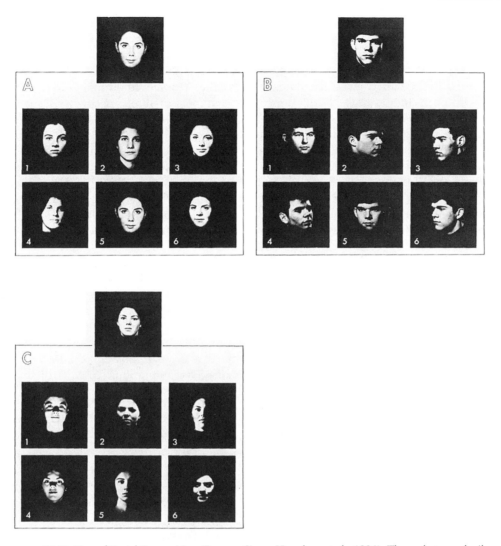

FIGURE 10.13 Test of Facial Recognition (Benton, Sivan, Hamsher, et al., 1994). These photographs illustrate the three parts of the test. *A:* Matching of identical front-views. *B:* Matching of front-view with three-quarter views. *C:* Matching of front-view under different lighting conditions.

Test characteristics. One-year retesting of elderly control subjects gave a reliability correlation of .60 (B.E. Levin, Llabre, Reisman, et al., 1991). Practice effects appear to be mostly negligible (McCaffrey, Duff, and Westervelt, 2000b). A 1.9-point difference between

TABLE 10.3 Facial Recognition Score Corrections

Add	
0	Everyone ages 16 to 54
1	Ages 55 to 64, 12+ years' education
2	Ages 65 to 74, 12+ years' education
3	Ages 55 to 64, 6–12 years' education
4	Ages 65 to 74, 6–12 years' education

Adapted from Benton, Sivan, Hamsher, et al. (1994)

older (55–74) subjects who had completed high school and those who had not was significant ($p < .01$), but the difference in the two education groups at younger ages was smaller and insignificant (Benton, Sivan, Hamsher, et al., 1994). Older age is negatively related to success on this test (Eslinger and Benton, 1983; Mittenberg, Seidenberg, et al., 1989). Even well-educated intact subjects show a significantly large failure rate (10%), beginning in the early 70s and increasing (to 14%) after age 75 (Benton, Eslinger, and Damasio, 1981). No sex differences have been reported.

Neuropsychological findings. Normal subjects who are weakly left-handed may do less well on facial recognition tests than right-handed or strongly left-handed normal control subjects (J.G. Gilbert, 1973). This tendency has been related to the relatively decreased lateralization of functions hypothesized as characterizing the brain organization of weakly left-handed persons. A comparison of patients with lateralized brain lesions found that 80% of the 33 with right-sided damage made scores below the median of the left-sided lesioned patients (Wasserstein, Barr, et al., 2003). Patients with right posterior lesions have the highest failure rate on this test (Benton, Sivan, Hamsher, et al., 1994). Patients with right parietal lesions perform more poorly than those with right temporal lesions on the facial recognition task reflecting this task's substantial visuospatial processing component (Warrington and James, 1967b). Wasserstein, Zappulla, and their colleagues (1984) found, for example, that their three patients with right medial–temporal lesions performed in the 85th to the 97th percentile range. However, following temporal lobe resection for intractable epilepsy, patients' ($n =$ 158) Facial Recognition scores dropped a small but significant amount regardless of resection side, although their Judgment of Line Orientation performances remained at the preoperative level (Hermann, Seidenberg, Wyler, and Haltiner, 1993). That the task may have a linguistic component is suggested by findings that aphasic patients with defective language comprehension fail on this test at rates a little lower than those with right parietal damage (Benton, Sivan, Hamsher, et al., 1994). Many more patients with posterior lesions had defective performances than did patients with anterior lesions. Patients with left hemisphere lesions who were not aphasic or who were aphasic but did not have comprehension defects made as few errors as healthy subjects. Visual field defects do not necessarily affect facial recognition scores although they are significantly correlated ($r = .49$, $p < .001$) with failure on this test (Egelko et al., 1988).

The group of dementing patients that had an 80% failure rate on Judgment of Line Orientation performed much better on this test with only a 58% failure rate (Eslinger and Benton, 1983). However, many more (39%) of a group of Parkinson patients failed on this test than on JLO (Hovestadt et al., 1987). This test correlated with the duration of Parkinson's disease and, as may be expected, was sensitive to the dementia that may accompany Parkinson disease (B.E. Levin, Llabre, Reisman, et al., 1991). It also elicited deficits in mildly impaired Parkinson patients (B.E. Levin, Llabre, and Weiner, 1989).

Recognition of the facial expression of emotion

Assessment procedures. A variety of photograph sets for examining facial expressions are available (e.g., Ekman and Friesen, 1975 [facial photos showing anger,

disgust, fear, happiness, sadness, surprise, neutral]; Izard, 1971). Some are included in batteries designed to examine various aspects of emotion perception. Borod, Tabert, and their colleagues (2000) list several of these. Some emotional test batteries require more equipment than pictures or cards, such as the *New York Emotion Battery* (*NYEB*), which presents photos of facial expressions on slides using a timed slide projector with exposure times ranging from 5 sec (a matching task) to 20 sec (an identification task) (Borod, Welkowitz, and Obler, 1992). Others have devised their own photo sets. H.D. Ellis (1992) observed that this diversity of stimuli makes it difficult to compare study findings.

Moreover, test formats differ considerably as well. For example, A.W. Young and his colleagues (1996) showed six of the seven emotions depicted in the Ekman and Freisen set in four conditions that paired: same person same expression, same person different expression, different person same expression, and both person and expression different. This technique permitted the examiners to distinguish affect discrimination from facial discrimination. To test for expression recognition, individual photos were shown with emotional names to be selected; for expression matching, target photos were shown with a set of five containing one expression like the target plus four foils. Another group of investigators used all seven emotions in the Eckman and Freisen set: emotion recognition was tested by showing the photographs each with a list of seven emotion adjectives to be selected (Hornak et al., 1996). These subjects had been previously tested with Warrington's Recognition Memory for Faces to ensure their competency in facial recognition. Using the basic emotions photographed by Eckman and Friesen, A. Young, Perrett, and their colleagues (2002) have developed a computerized package that provides both the original Eckman and Freisen stimuli and the capacity to "computer-morph" both emotions onto faces to provide a range of intensity of expression.

Neuropsychological findings. The right hemisphere makes both the earliest and most rapid responses to faces associated with affective states (Pizzagalli et al., 1999; E. Strauss and Moscowitsch, 1981). Thus it is not surprising that when patients with unilateral brain lesions are tested for accuracy in identifying facial affect, those with damage on the right are much more likely to perform poorly than those with left-sided lesions (Borod, Bloom, et al., 2002; see also Heilman, Blonder, Bowers, and Valenstein, 2003). However, this difference may hold only when the task requires identification of emotion (i.e., which of several printed choices does a face photo express?) and not discrimination of expressions (i.e., do paired face photos exhibit the same emotion or different emotions?) (Borod, Cicero, Obler, et al., 1998). Patients with lateralized lesions show a differential sensitivity to different kinds of emotional expressions: patients with right brain damage recognized happy emotional expressions to about the same degree as did patients with left brain disease (83% accuracy vs. 79%), but they were significantly impaired in recognition of negative (38% accuracy to 76% for left brain damage) or neutral expressions (42% accuracy vs. 93%) (Borod, Koff, Lorch, and Nicholas, 1985; see also Borod, Welkowitz, Alpert, et al., 1990). Interestingly, patients with left-sided lesions were more accurate in identifying neutral expressions than were control subjects (93% to 81%). Etcoff's (1986) patients with right hemisphere lesions attempted to analyze the faces they were shown by rather unsystematic efforts at matching features, and, for the most part, they failed. Again, patients with brain lesions on the left side performed much like controls. In using a more complex experimental design that required recall as well as identification of emotional expression, Prigatano and Pribram (1982) found that patients with right posterior lesions were relatively more impaired than those with anterior lesions or than left hemisphere damaged patients.

Frontal leucotomy patients exhibited overall an even greater degree of emotional incomprehension than the right hemisphere damaged group (Cicone et al., 1980). Patients with ventral lesions of the frontal lobe also do poorly identifying facial expressions (Rolls, 1999). Although deficits in recognizing emotional expressions of faces or in voices did not necessarily go together, these deficits were strongly associated with severity of such behavior problems as disinhibition.

Figure and design recognition

Accuracy of recognition of meaningless designs is usually tested by having the patient draw them from models or from memory (e.g., Bender-Gestalt, Complex Figure Test). When design reproductions contain the essential elements of the original from which they are copied and preserve their interrelationships reasonably well, perceptual accuracy with this kind of material has been adequately demonstrated. A few responses to the WIS-A Picture Completion test or a similar task will show whether the subject can recognize meaningful pictures. At lower levels of functioning, picture tests can assess recognition of meaningful pictures (e.g., Peabody Picture Vocabulary Test, Boston Naming Test, or Picture Vocabulary items from Verbal Comprehension of the Woodcock-Johnson Battery-III Tests of Cognitive Abilities). The first 12 items of both forms of Raven's

Progressive Matrices test simple recognition of designs. For patients with verbal comprehension problems, children's tests may be useful. When patients' graphic reproductions are inaccurate, markedly distorted or simplified, or have glaring omissions or additions, or when patients are unable to respond correctly to drawings or pictures, there is further need to study perceptual accuracy.

Visual Form Discrimination[1] (Benton, Sivan, Hamsher, et al., 1994)

This is a multiple-choice test of visual recognition. Each of the 16 items consists of a target set of stimuli and four stimulus sets below the target, one of which is a correct match (see Fig. 10.14). The other three sets contain small variations of displacement, rotation, or distortion. No age, sex, or education effects were found for the control subjects (Benton et al., 1994). An internal consistency coefficient (*alpha*) of .66 was thought to be reduced by the similarity of the sample (acute TBI) (Malina et al., 2001). With a cut-off of 28 specificity was 84% although sensitivity was only 59% for the TBI patients.

Based on a 3-point scoring system (2 = fully correct, 1 = a peripheral error response, 0 = all other errors), 68% of the control subjects achieved scores of 30 or

[1]The test material is sold by the Medical Sales Department, Oxford University Press, 198 Madison Ave., New York, NY 10016.

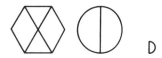

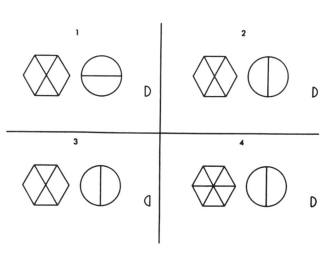

FIGURE 10.14 An item of the Visual Form Discrimination test. (© Oxford University Press. Reprinted by permission)

more, 95% had scores ≥26, and none scored below 23. In contrast, half of a "brain diseased" group (*n* = 58) made scores of 22 or less. Left anterior, right parietal, and bilateral-diffuse lesions were associated with the highest percentages of impaired performances. With a simple right/wrong scoring system, recently diagnosed Alzheimer patients failed, on average, ten of the 16 items, with most errors involving the small, peripheral figures (Mendez, Mendez, et al., 1990). However, only 32% of the acute TBI sample scored below the cut-off of 26 set by Benton and his colleagues (Malina et al., 2001). For both control subjects and these TBI patients, scores were markedly skewed such that the median and interquartile range describe these populations better than parametric statistics.

The multiple-choice format easily converts to a memory test. Following an immediate recall procedure, B. Caplan and Caffery (1996) showed the target designs for 10 sec to 51 control subjects of wide ranging ages (*M* = 36, range 21–79) and education levels (*M* = 14.9, range 7–20). Using the 3-point scoring system (2, 1, 0), a cut-off at 2 *SD* is 21.2. Number correct correlated positively with education (*r* = .33), negatively with age (*r* = −.43). Acknowledging the limitations of this "normative" sample, the authors called for more normative and clinical data for this procedure.

Visual Organization

Tests requiring the subject to make sense out of ambiguous, incomplete, fragmented, or otherwise distorted visual stimuli call for perceptual organizing activity beyond that of simple perceptual recognition. Although the perceptual system tends to hold up well in the presence of brain disorders for most ordinary purposes, any additional challenge may be beyond its organizing capacity. For this reason, tests of perceptual organization were among the earliest psychological instruments to be used for evaluating neuropsychological status. Roughly speaking, there are three broad categories of visual organization tests: those requiring the subject to fill in missing elements; tests presenting problems in reorganizing jumbled elements of a percept; and test stimuli lacking inherent organization onto which the subject must impose structure.

Tests involving incomplete visual stimuli

Of all tests of visual organization, those in which the subject fills in a missing part, such as Wechsler's Picture Completion, are least vulnerable to the effects of brain damage, probably because their content is usually so well structured and readily identifiable. Thus, although technically they qualify as tests of perceptual organization, they are not especially sensitive to problems of perceptual organization except when the perceptual disorder is relatively severe.

Gestalt Completion Tests

Several sets of incomplete pictures have been used to examine the perceptual closure capacity (e.g., see Fig. 10.15). Poor performance on gestalt completion tests has generally been associated with right brain damage (McCarthy and Warrington, 1990; Newcombe and Russell, 1969), yet correlations between four such tests were relatively low (.35 to .60), although each correlated highly (.70 to .90) with a total score when given to college students (Wasserstein, Zappulla, Rosen, et al., 1987). These included the *Street Completion Test* (Street, 1931), unpublished Street items (see Thurstone, 1949), Mooney's *Closure Faces Test* (not available for clinical use), and the *Gestalt Completion Test* (Ekstrom et al., 1976). Wasserstein and her colleagues suggested that differences in performances on these various closure tasks were due to variations in such stimulus characteristics as whether lines were straight or curved, perspective or content information cues, verbalizable features, or subjective contour illusions. Thus these tests cannot be used interchangeably. The several meanings of the concept of "closure" could account for low intercorrelations of tests purporting to measure a "closure" function (Wasserstein, 2002). Moreover, when Closure Faces was included in factor analyses with non-facial closure measures (including one set of subjective contour illusions) plus the Test of Facial Discimination, two factors emerged, a *closure* factor and a *facial discrimination* factor: Closure Faces was related to both of them (Wasserstein, Barr, et al., 2003). This held for separate analyses for left- and right-brain injured subjects. The facial discrimination factor was positively related to education; the closure factor was negatively related to age.

Test characteristics. Age contributed significantly to performance differences on all four tests for normal subjects (*r* = −.49 to −.73) and patients with left hemisphere damage (*r* = −.42 to −.78) but generally less to the scores of patients with right-sided lesions (*r* = .09 to −.45) (Wasserstein, Zappulla, Rosen, et al., 1987). Small sex differences favoring males showed up on Street Completion and Closure Faces Test performances of the control subjects, and a larger male advantage appeared on the unpublished Street items and Closure Faces for left brain damaged patients but not those with right brain damage. These authors note that performance on closure tests appears to be independent of performance on facial recognition tests, sug-

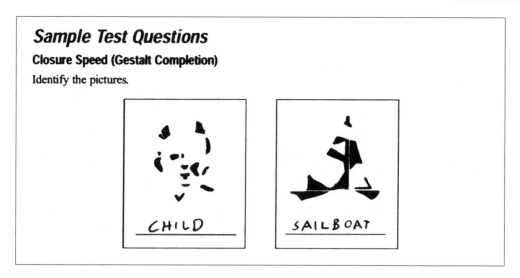

FIGURE 10.15 Closure Speed (Gestalt Completion) (© 1984 by L.L. Thurstone, Ph.D. All rights reserved.) This sample test question may not be duplicated in any manner without written permission from the publisher. (Courtesy of Pearson Reid London House, Inc.)

gesting that two different perceptual processes having different anatomical correlates underlie the two different tests.

Neuropsychological findings. Analysis of the performances of unilaterally brain lesioned patients indicates a relationship between performance on the gestalt completion tests and the perception of subjective *contour illusions* (i.e., visual illusions in which brightness or color gradients are seen when not present [Tovée, 1996]) (Wasserstein, Zappulla, Rosen, et al., 1987). For example, most people will see Figure 10.16 as a solid white triangle overlying an inverted triangular frame and three black circles, although no solid triangle is physically present. Performances on the gestalt completion tests and on a subjective contours task by patients with right hemisphere damage demonstrated lower levels of relationship than did performances by

patients with left-sided lesions. This latter group appeared to use a common solution mechanism for solving both gestalt completion and subjective contour problems. Patients with left brain damage consistently made higher scores than those with right-sided lesions on all four of the gestalt completion tests, and had scores close to the control subjects' scores on two tests (actually having a higher mean than the control subjects on one of the two). Performances on the subjective contour tests clearly differentiated right and left hemisphere–damaged groups.

Closure Speed (Gestalt Completion) (L.L. Thurstone and Jeffrey, 1983)

This "figural" test presents 24 degraded pictures of objects or animals to be identified within three minutes. Space is provided for the subject to write in each item name (see Fig. 10.15). The test manual provides norms derived from groups of workers at different technical and professional levels. E.W. Russell, Hendrickson, and Van Eaton (1988) used this paper-and-pencil test to study occipital lobe functions. Some patients dictated their answers. Mean score for 55 male control subjects was 11.23. The average score for patients with left-sided anterior/lateral (i.e., temporal and parietal) lesions was barely higher than for those with occipital lesions (8.58 ± 5.33 to 7.75 ± 4.53); but with lesions on the right, the anterior patients outperformed those with occipital lesions significantly (7.00 ± 5.02 to 2.92 ± 2.23). The ease of administration and accessibility of materials recommends this test for both clinical and research work.

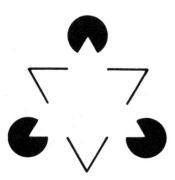

FIGURE 10.16 Example of the subjective contour effet. (From E.L. Brown and Deffenbacher, 1979. © Oxford University Press)

Gollin Figures (Gollin, 1960)

Another test that uses incomplete drawings to assess perceptual functions consists of 20 picture series of five line drawings of familiar objects (e.g., duck, tricycle, umbrella) ranging in completeness from a barely suggestive sketch (Set I) to a complete drawing of the figure (Set V). The score is the sum of all the set numbers at which each picture is correctly identified. Warrington and James (1967a) and Warrington and Rabin (1970) used Gollin's original procedure, but Warrington and Taylor (1973) included only three rather than five items in each picture series. Another shortened format used only three sets of figures, one three-item set for practice and two containing the original five-item series, to be used as alternate versions of the test (J.L. Mack, Patterson, et al., 1993). These workers found that a 30-sec exposure afforded sufficient response time for each stimulus picture. Age effects appeared when younger age (M = 34.8) and older (M = 69) healthy, well-educated subjects were compared (M.B. Patterson et al., 1999). The younger group identified pictures at a greater level of fragmentation and were faster than the older subjects. However, these two measures were not correlated: fragmentation level appears to relate to perceptual accuracy, reaction time to the cognitive slowing associated with aging. A factor analysis of elderly subjects' and Alzheimer patients' performances on a set of tests assessing visual, verbal, and memory functions demonstrated a significant visuoperceptual component for the Gollin test (J.L. Mack, Patterson, et al., 1993).

Neuropsychological findings. The Gollin figures did not discriminate between right and left hemisphere lesioned groups in the Warrington and Rabin study, patients with right parietal lesions showing only a trend toward poor performance. However, this test was more sensitive to right brain lesions than other perceptual tests used in the Warrington and James or Warrington and Taylor studies, successfully discriminating between patients with right- and left-sided lesions and implicating the right posterior (particularly parietal) lobe in the perception of incomplete contours. With just one picture series, Gollin scores differentiated Alzheimer patients from elderly control subjects (J.L. Mack, Patterson, et al., 1993). An investigation into the nature of TBI patients' difficulties with this test found that they failed to recognize the fragmented drawings and displayed inconsistent search strategies with some tendency to perseverate responses from one drawing to the next (Rahmani et al., 1990). Control subjects were faster than depressed patients in identifying the pictured object, but the difference did not reach significance (Grafman, Weingartner, Newhouse, et al., 1990). Both these groups recognized the degraded pictures much sooner than Alzheimer patients.

Visual Object and Space Perception Battery (Warrington and James, 1991)

Experimental techniques for exploring visual perception have been incorporated into this nine-test battery. As normative data and cutting scores are provided for each little test, these tests can be used individually or the battery can be given as a whole. Factor analysis of test data from a large sample of healthy older (50 to 84 years) adults supported the distinction between space and object perception (Rapport, Millis, and Bonello, 1998).

The first test, *Shape Detection Screening,* only checks whether the patient's vision is sufficiently intact to permit further examination. Half of its 20 cards display an all-over pattern with an embedded and degraded X, the other half have just the all-over pattern; the subject must find the cards with the X. It is rare that any items are failed by patients with right hemisphere disease, and rarer still for intact persons to fail.

Object perception tests. The next four tests present views of letters, animals, or objects that have been rendered incomplete in various ways. Rotated silhouettes (tests 2 to 4) has the effect of obscuring recognizable features of an object to a greater or lesser degree (Warrington and James, 1986). 1. *Incomplete Letters* shows 20 large alphabet letters, one to a card, which have been randomly degraded so that only 30% of the original shape remains. 2. *Silhouettes* are blackened shapes of 15 objects and 15 animals as they appear at angular rotations affording a range of difficulty beginning with an item identified correctly by only 36% of the controls and ending with highly recognizable stimuli (100% recognition by control subjects) (see Fig. 10.17, p. 399). 3. *Object Decision* presents the subject with 20 cards each printed with four black shapes of which one is a silhouette of a real object, thus giving only minimal clues to the object's identity (see Fig. 10.18, p. 399). 4. *Progressive Silhouettes,* presents only two items—both elongated objects—to be identified, first at a virtually unrecognizable 90° rotation from the familiar lateral view, then sequential rotation of the other nine silhouettes gradually approaches the familiar lateral view (the tenth silhouette). The score is the number of silhouettes seen before correct identification of the object.

Age contributed to control subject performances on these four tests, requiring a 1-point difference in cutoff scores between persons under 50 and 50+. As pre-

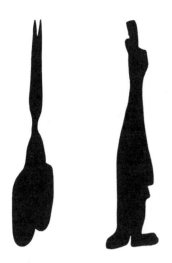

FIGURE 10.17 Two items from the Silhouettes subtest of the Visual Object and Space Perception Test. (© 1991, Elizabeth Warrington and Merle James. Reproduced by permission)

dicted, the average scores for each of these four tests discriminated patients with right and left hemisphere lesions, the latter group performing at levels within the average score range of the control subjects. Failure rate for patients with right hemisphere disease was from 25.7% to 34.5%; patients whose lesions were on the left failed at rates from 3.8% to 12%.

Space perception tests. The last four tests examine different aspects of space perception. 5. *Dot Counting* presents ten arrays of five to nine dots each, randomly arranged on separate cards. The cut-off for failure is 8 correct, as few normal subjects made any errors. 6.

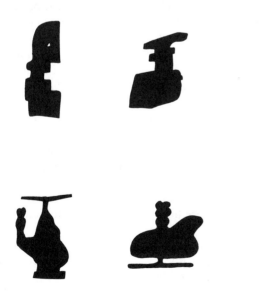

FIGURE 10.18 Multiple-choice item from the Object Decision subtest of the Visual Object and Space Perception Test (© 1991, Elizabeth Warrington and Merle James. Reproduced by permission)

Each of the 20 items of *Position Discrimination* presents a card with two identical horizontally positioned squares, one containing a black dot in the center, the other with a black dot slightly off-centered—to the left on half of the items, to the right on the other half. The subject must decide which square contains the centered dot. This too was very easy for intact subjects, resulting in a cut-off score of 18. 7. *Number Location* also presents two squares each on ten stimulus cards, this time one square is above the other with the numbers from 1 to 9 randomly spaced within the top square. The bottom square contains a dot in the location of one of the numbers which the subject must identify. 8. *Cube Analysis* is a ten-item block counting task (see Fig. 15.11, p. 607 for a similar task). A cut-off score of 6 reflects the greater difficulty of this task relative to the others in the space perception set.

Age was not associated with performance on any of these four tests. On all of them, more patients with right hemisphere disease failed (from 27.0% to 35.1%) than patients whose damage was on the left (from 9.3% to 18.7%), although the left-damaged patients consistently failed in greater numbers than normal expectations would warrant.

Tests involving fragmented visual stimuli

Perceptual puzzles requiring conceptual reorganization of disarranged pieces test the same perceptual functions as does Object Assembly. The visual content can be either meaningful or meaningless (e.g., Minnesota Paper Formboard [Likert and Quasha, 1970]).

Hooper Visual Organization Test (HVOT), (Hooper, 1983)

The HVOT was developed to identify mental hospital patients with "organic brain conditions". It consists of 30 pictures of more or less readily recognizable, cut-up objects (see Fig. 10.19, p. 400). The subject's task is to tell each object's name if the test is individually administered, or to write the object's name in spaces provided in the test booklet. The finding that, on the individual administration, a cut-off of 5 consecutive errors changed the rating of only 1% of a large subject sample, allows for early discontinuation of a poor performance (Wetzel and Murphy, 1991).

Test characteristics. On three administrations repeated after 6 months and again after 12 months, mean HVOT scores did not shift to any appreciable degree, and a coefficient of concordance (W) of .86 indicated that test–retest reliability is high (Lezak, 1982c). A one-year retest reliability coefficient for elderly controls was

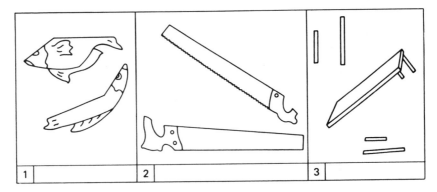

FIGURE 10.19 Easy items of the Hooper Visual Organization Test. (By H. Elston Hooper. © 1958 by Western Psychological Services. Reprinted by permission)

.68 (B.E. Levin, Llabre, Reisman, et al., 1991). This test does not correlate significantly with sex or education, at least for ages below 70, but it has a modest correlation with mental ability. Reports on aging effects are contradictory. Whelihan and Lesher (1985) found a significant drop in the performance of "old-old" (ages 76 to 92) intact subjects compared to a "young-old" (ages 60 to 70) group. Montgomery and Costa's (1983) finding of a median score of 23.7 for a large sample of older persons (ages 65 to 85) suggests that some score drop with advanced age can be expected. E.D. Richardson and Martolli's (1996) age × education data for mostly white men and women show little loss between the <12 years' schooling groups ages 76 to 80 and 81 to 91, as the younger group's mean score (17.90) already fell within the "high probability of impairment" range; but with education level ≥12, the older group scored an average 2 points below the younger one. Merten and Beal (2000) found that item order does not correspond to ranking for item difficulty and raised questions about both the nature of items and scoring standards. Two multiple regression studies including WAIS-R and naming tests found that a perceptual integration/organization factor accounted for 44% (Ricker and Axelrod, 1995) and 45% (Greve, Lindberg, et al., 2000) of HVOT variance, together lending strong support to its validity as a test of perceptual integration/organization. Moreover, the 11% or 15% (respectively) contribution of confrontation naming to HVOT variance indicates that naming ability plays only a minor role (see *Multiple-choice HVOT,* below). Still, Spreen and Strauss (1998) advise that, "Since the test requires naming, results in even mildly aphasic patients may be questionable" (pp. 509–510).

Cognitively intact persons generally fail no more than six HVOT items. Persons who make 7 to 11 failures comprise a "borderline" group that includes emotionally disturbed or psychotic patients as well as those with mild to moderate brain disorders. Persons with scores in this range have a low to moderate likelihood of brain impairment. More than 11 failures usually indicates brain pathology. When this many errors result from a psychiatric rather than a neuropathologic condition, qualitative aspects of the responses will generally betray the etiology. Many brain injured persons perform well on the HVOT (Wetzel and Murphy, 1991). However, a low score on this test usually indicates the presence of brain damage, as false positive performances are rare.

Neuropsychological findings. The frequency of low scores on this test does not differ on the basis of side of lesion or presence of diffuse/medial injury (J.L. Boyd, 1981; P.L. Wang, 1977; Wetzel and Murphy, 1991). However, lesion laterality may be distinguished by the *nature* of the errors as patients with right-sided lesions are more likely to give fragmented or part responses (see paragraph below for examples), those with lesions on the left will make more naming errors (Nadler, Grace, et al., 1996). Brain tumors and stroke tend to be associated with much lower scores than does TBI (J.L. Boyd, 1981). Relatively few in one sample of Alzheimer patients performed *within normal limits;* their average score (11 ± 5.34) was greater than 4 SD below that of control subjects (25 ± 3.03) (Mendez, Mendez, et al., 1990). The HVOT proved to be very sensitive to both dementia and disease duration in Parkinson patients (B.E. Levin, Llabre, Reisman, et al., 1991). Sohlberg and Mateer (1989) recommend it for examining temporal lobe dysfunction. However, it has only little predictive value for rehabilitation outcome (Greve, Lindberg, et al., 2000).

Several of the HVOT items are particularly effective in eliciting the kind of perceptual fragmentation that tends to be associated with lesions of the right frontal lobe, although all patients with right frontal lesions do not make this kind of error. Patients who exhibit this phenomenon will often be able to identify most of the items correctly, thus demonstrating both perceptual accuracy and understanding of the instructions. Yet, on one or more of the three items that contain one piece most clearly resembling an object in itself, patients who have a tendency to view their world in a fragmented manner will interpret that one piece without attending to any of the others in the item (see also Lezak, 1989). For example, the top piece of item 1 may be called a "duck" or a "flying goose" (see Fig. 10.19, also see pp. 564–565 for a discussion of the relationship of the HVOT and constructional tasks). Item 21 becomes "a desert island" when only the center piece is taken into account, and the tail of the "mouse" of item 22 turns into "a pipe." When fragmentation is more severe, the mesh of item 12 may be called "a tennis net," item 14 becomes "a pencil," and item 30 "a plumber's helper" or "plunger."

A multiple-choice HVOT. To reduce the problem of object naming for anomic patients—and to make manifest the HVOT visual integration component—a multiple-choice format (*MC-HVOT*) was developed in which four possible responses are listed vertically in large print under each item (Schultheis, Caplan, et al., 2000). For example, response alternatives for item 1 are "fish, tomato, boomerang, globe." On a small sample of both TBI and stroke patients whose Boston Naming Test scores fell below the 10th percentile, MC-HVOT showed notable improvements for both patients with lesions on the right (M_{gain} = 8 points) and on the left (M_{gain} = 10.9 points), gains which permitted a better understanding of these patients' visual integration capacities.

Tests involving ambiguous visual stimuli

Some tests that use ambiguous stimuli were developed as personality tests and not as tests of cognitive functioning. They were applied to neuropsychological problems as examiners became familiar with the kinds of responses made by different patient groups.

Rorschach technique

This projective technique exemplifies how ambiguous stimuli, originally used for personality assessment, can provide information about a patient's perceptual abilities. When handling Rorschach responses as data about personality (e.g., behavioral predispositions), the examiner looks at many different aspects of the test performance, such as productivity, response style, and the affective quality of the subject's associations. In neuropsychological assessment, Rorschach protocols can be evaluated for a variety of qualitative and quan-

titative response characteristics that tend to be associated with brain disease (see pp. 740–742). Although perceptual accuracy enters into both personality evaluations and diagnostic discriminations, it can also be treated in its own right, apart from these broader applications of the test.

Evaluation of the perceptual component of a Rorschach response can focus on four aspects of perceptual activity. The first is the accuracy of the percept. Since the inkblots are ambiguous and composed by chance, no *a priori* "meaning" inheres in the stimulus material. Nevertheless, certain areas of the blots tend to form natural gestalts and to elicit similar associations from normal, intact adults. The test for perceptual accuracy, or "good form," is whether a given response conforms in content and in the patient's delineation of a blot area to common ways of looking at and interpreting the blot. A reliable method of determining whether a given response reflects a normal organization of the stimulus uses a frequency count, differentiating "good form" (F+) from "poor form" (F−) responses on a strictly statistical basis (S.J. Beck, 1981; S.J. Beck et al., 1961; Exner, 1986). Beck (1961) lists usual and rare responses to all the commonly used parts of the Rorschach inkblots so that the examiner need only compare the patient's responses with the listed responses to determine which are good and which are poor form. Of the hundreds of good form responses, 21 are given with such frequency that they are called "popular" (P) responses. They are thought to reflect the subject's ability not merely to organize percepts appropriately but also to do so in a socially customary manner. The percentage of good form responses (F+%) and the incidence of popular responses thus can be used as measures of perceptual accuracy.

That these response variables do reflect the intactness of the perceptual system can be inferred from the consistent tendency for brain damaged patients to produce lower F+% and P scores than normal control or neurotic subjects (Aita, Reitan, and Ruth, 1947; D.W. Ellis and Zahn, 1985; Z. Piotrowski, 1937). In normal Rorschach protocols, 75 to 95% of unelaborated form responses are of good quality, with bright persons achieving the higher F+% scores (S.J. Beck, 1981). Brain damaged patients tend to produce less than 70% good form responses (e.g., DeMol, 1975/1976; C. Meyers et al., 1982). Their poor form responses reflect the kind of perceptual problems that are apt to accompany brain injury, such as difficulties in synthesizing discrete elements into a coherent whole, in breaking down a perceptual whole into its component parts, in clarifying figure–ground relationships, and in identifying relevant and irrelevant detail (G. Baker, 1956). Patients' verbatim associations will often shed light on the nature of their perceptual disabilities. Their behavior too may betray the perceptual problems, for only brain damaged patients attempt to clarify visual confusion by covering parts of the blot with the hand.

A second aspect of perceptual organization that may be reflected in Rorschach responses is the ability to process and integrate multiple stimuli. Some brain disorders reduce the capacity for handling a large perceptual input at once, resulting in a narrowed perceptual field and simplified percepts. This shows up in relatively barren, unelaborated responses in which one characteristic of the blot alone dictates the content of the response, for the patient ignores or does not attempt to incorporate other elements of the blot into the percept. The reduced capacity for handling multiple stimuli also appears as difficulty in integrating discrete parts of the blot into a larger, organized percept or in separating associations to discrete blot elements that happen to be contiguous. Thus, the patient may correctly interpret several isolated elements of card X as varieties of sea animals without ever forming the organizing concept, "underwater scene." Or, on card III, the side figures may be appropriately identified as "men in tuxedos" and the central red figure as a "bow tie," but the inability to separate these physically contiguous and conceptually akin percepts may produce a response combining the men and the bow tie into a single forced percept such as, "they're wearing tuxedos and that is the bow tie." Sometimes mere contiguity will result in the same kind of over-inclusive response so that the blue "crab" on card X may be appropriately identified, but the contiguous "shellfish" becomes the crab's "shellfish claw." These latter two responses are examples of confabulation on the Rorschach.

Moreover, the number of form responses that also take into account color (FC) is likely to be one per record for brain damaged patients, whereas normal subjects typically produce more than one FC response (D.W. Ellis and Zahn, 1985; Lynn et al., 1945). Some patients simply name colors (Cn), whereas normal subjects do not give this kind of response (DeMol, 1975/1976). There may be relatively few responses involving texture and shading (FT, FY) (D.W. Ellis and Zahn, 1985), and those introducing movement into the percept (M or FM) are apt to be minimal (Dörken and Kral, 1952; Z. Piotrowski, 1937).

A third aspect of perception is its reliability. Many brain impaired patients feel that they cannot trust their perceptions. Uncertainty—the Rorschach term for expressions of doubt and confusion is *perplexity*—about one's interpretations of the inkblots is relatively common among brain damaged patients but rare for other patient groups or normal subjects (G. Baker, 1956, Z.

Piotrowski, 1937). Lastly, brain damaged patients tend to have slower reaction times (i.e., ≥ 1 min) on the Rorschach than do normal persons (Goldfried et al., 1971; C. Meyers et al., 1982).

Visual Interference

Tasks involving visual interference are essentially visual recognition tasks complicated by distracting embellishments. The stimulus material contains the complete percept but extraneous lines or designs encompass or mask it so that the percept is less readily recognizable. Visual interference tasks differ from tests of visual organization in that the latter call on synthesizing activities, whereas visual interference tests require the subject to analyze the figure–ground relationship in order to distinguish the figure from the interfering elements. Sohlberg and Mateer (1989) included these kinds of tests in their examination of temporal lobe disorders.

Figure–ground tests

Hidden Figures (L.L. Thurstone, 1944), Closure Flexibility (Concealed Figures) (L.L. Thurstone and Jeffrey, 1982)

Thurstone proposed a 34-item version of Gottschaldt's (1928) *Hidden Figures Test* that has been used in many studies of abilities of patients with brain damage (see Fig. 10.20, p. 403). The Hidden Figures task requires the subject to identify the hidden figure by marking the outline of the simple figure embedded in the more complex one. At the most difficult levels, the subject has to determine which of the two intricate designs contains the simpler figure. Spreen and Benton (see Spreen and Strauss, 1998) developed a 16-item test, the *Embedded Figures Test*. Closure Flexibility is a 49-item multiple-choice version of this task with two correct solutions for each item. In Thurstone's study of normal perception, successful performance on this task was strongly associated with "the ability to form a perceptual closure against some distraction . . . [and] the ability to hold a closure against distraction" (L.L. Thurstone, 1944, p. 101).

Test characteristics. The normative sample of 3,073 comes from three levels of managerial hierarchies for four occupational categories (Line, Professional, Sales, and Technical). Scores can be evaluated either by a centile scale or a normalized standard score scale providing comparisons with these 12 occupational groupings. The manual cites studies conducted by Thurstone and his students who found significant correlations ($r = .59$, .63) with inductive reasoning. Factor analytic studies

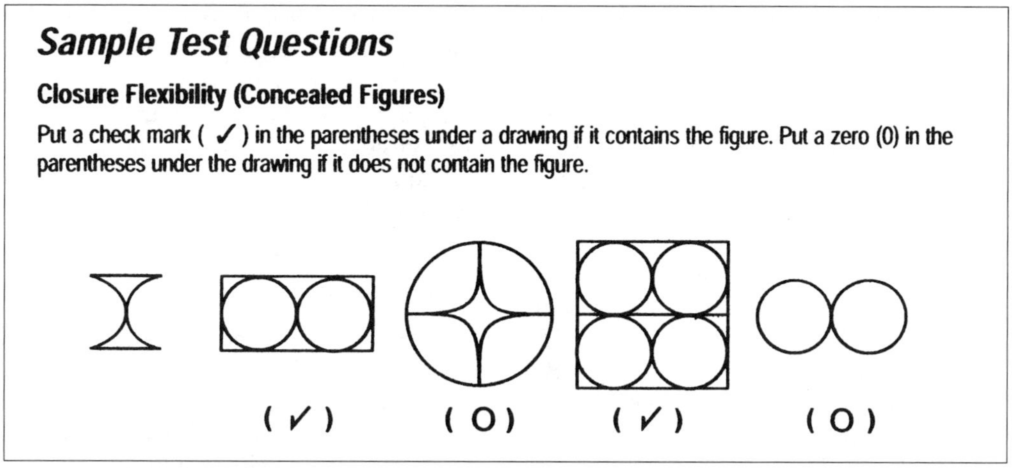

FIGURE 10.20 Closure Flexibility (Concealed Figures). (© 1984 by L.L. Thurstone, Ph.D. All rights reserved.) This sample test question may not be duplicated in any manner without written permission from the publisher. (Courtesy of Pearson Reid London House, Inc.)

have shown significant associations with both analytic reasoning and a space factor.

Neuropsychological findings. Teuber, Battersby, and Bender (1960) found that all groups with brain injuries due to missile wounds performed more poorly on the Hidden Figures Test than did normal subjects. Moreover, the degree of impairment of test performance has been related to the size of the lesion regardless of side (Corkin, 1979). Patients who had had surgery involving the frontal cortex (Teuber, Battersby, and Bender, 1951) and aphasic patients made significantly lower scores than other brain injured patients. Patients whose aphasia resulted from other kinds of brain lesions, mostly vascular, also did poorest among patients studied for the effects of lateralized lesions (Russo and Vignolo, 1967). Interestingly, nonaphasic patients with left-sided lesions performed within the control group range. The scores of patients with right sided lesions were midway between the two groups with left hemisphere damage. The presence of visual field defects did not affect these performances. Talland (1965a) reported that patients with Korsakoff's psychosis performed very poorly on this test, attributing their almost total failure to problems in perceptual shifting and focusing.

Overlapping Figures Test

This little test was originally devised by Poppelreuter ([1917] 1990) to study the psychological effects of head injuries incurred during World War I (see Fig. 10.21). Its popularity is reflected in the number of formats that have been devised. For most formats subjects are asked to name as many of the figures as they can.

Ghent (1956) employed nine similar figures, each with four overlapping line-drawn objects, to examine the development of perceptual functions in children. Luria (1966) used several versions of an overlapping or "*superimposed figures*" test to examine the phenomenon of simultaneous agnosia. In her systematization of Luria's examination methods, A.-L. Christensen (1979) included three Pöppelreuter-type figures as part of "the investigation of higher visual functions." An expanded version of this test that included ten stimulus figures with a total of 40 objects presented in such categories as "clothing" or "animals" was developed by Masure and Tzavaras (1976) under the name of *Ghent's Test* (i.e., *le test de Ghent*). Total time to completion was recorded and subjects indicated their responses on a multiple-choice form. Gainotti, D'Erme, and their colleagues (1986, 1989) devised an *Overlapping Figures* test, consisting of five overlapping line drawings on each of six cards with a multiple-choice presentation of target figures and foils; both test figures and responses are vertically aligned. The most

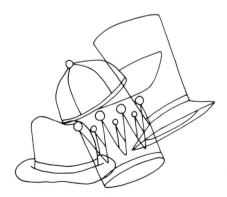

FIGURE 10.21 Example of a Poppelreuter-type overlapping figure.

complex of the overlapping figure tests, the *15-objects test*, contains two figures, each an overlapping drawing of 15 different items (Pillon, Dubois, Bonnet, et al., 1989). This format was scored for both response time and erroneous identifications. A more recently developed format contains three sets of overlapping figures, each set presenting a different number and category of figures (3 simple geometric figures; 4 man-made objects; 5 fruits) (Mori et al., 2000). Subjects name items in the first two categories; fruits is a matching task. In all but the Mori sets, Overlapping Figures, and the 15-objects test, the figures are composed of items in the same category (e.g., fruits, clothes) and some examiners also ask subjects to identify the general category of items (e.g., Rahmani et al., 1990).

Neuropsychological findings. Both Luria and A.-L. Christensen described several ways in which a patient can fail this test. Both pointed out the difference between the inability to perceive more than one object at a time or to shift gaze that may accompany a posterior lesion and passivity or inertia of gaze, perseverated responses, or confused responses, which are more likely to be associated with an anterior lesion. Christensen also noted that a perceptual bias to the right may indicate left visuospatial inattention. On a multiple-choice format, right-lesioned patients performed significantly more poorly than control subjects and patients with left-sided damage, who also did less well than the controls (De Renzi and Spinnler, 1966; Gainotti, D'Erme, et al., 1986, 1989). Patients with posterior lesions performed more poorly than the anterior group and those with left posterior lesions were by far the slowest.

Responding to the three different figure categories with a maximum score of 12, patients with probable Alzheimer's disease made significantly more correct identifications (10.6 ± 1.8) than did patients with Lewy body dementia (LBD) (8.1 ± 2.6) (Mori et al., 2000), and LBD patients who did not have visual hallucinations outperformed those who did (10.2 ± 1.5 vs. 7.4 ± 2.5); unfortunately, control data were not provided. Alzheimer patients' difficulty on this task was attributed to impaired analysis of figure–ground relationships (Mendez, Mendez, et al., 1990). Parkinson patients responded much slower than the controls and made more errors on the most complex format of this test (Pillon, Dubois, Bonnet, et al., 1989). Performances on this test correlated significantly with verbal and memory test scores. A simpler version with only three or four overlapping figures also proved sensitive to mental deterioration in Parkinson patients and was significantly related to disease duration (B.E. Levin, Llabre, Reisman, et al., 1991). Rahmani and his colleagues (1990) listed the kinds of errors made by TBI patients: misidentification; objects not perceived as related to one another; perseveration of a concept from one card to another; only part of an item is noted and then misidentified; only the most prominent items are noted; idiosyncratic relationships are drawn about the items in the figure.

Picture search

Hidden Pictures of the *Snijders-Oomen Nonverbal Intelligence Test (SON-R 5¹/₂-17; rev. ed.)* (Tellegen et al., 1998) involves visual search and recognition of parts of objects or of objects at unusual angles. It has much in common with children's playbook puzzles that ask for a count of objects (e.g., kites) hidden in drawings, in unlikely places as well as likely ones. In this test, line drawings of four different scenes contain 7 or 8 items in whole or part view. Following two trial scenes on which the examiner can provide explanations and examples, the subject is allowed 1¹/₂ min to search each scene. The 17-year-old norms of the SON-R 5¹/₂-17 provide an adequate standard for evaluating most adult performances.

AUDITORY PERCEPTION

As is the case with vision, the verbal and nonverbal components of auditory perception appear to be functionally distinct (Bauer and Demery, 2003; McGlone and Young, 1986; I. Peretz, 2001). Also as with vision, many techniques are available for examining the verbal auditory functions. Unlike visual perception, however, psychologists have paid less systematic attention to nonverbal auditory functions. Thus, the examination of nonverbal aspects of auditory perception is limited to a few techniques. The most common sources of defective auditory comprehension are deficiencies in auditory acuity resulting from conduction and/or sensorineural hearing losses, and deficits in auditory processing associated with cortical damage (Ceranic and Luxon, 2002).

Auditory Acuity

Many patients whose hearing is impaired are aware of their problem. Unfortunately, some individuals with mild to moderate deficits are embarrassed and do not report them to the examiner, or they may try to hide their disability even at the cost of a poor performance on the tests. When hearing loss is mild, however, or involves very specific defects of sound discrimination without affecting loudness, the patient may not appreciate the problem. Occasionally a patient incurs a reduction in hearing sensitivity as a result of brain injury, in which case hearing on the ear opposite the side of the lesion is likely to be the more impaired. More common is diminished auditory acuity with aging (E. Wallace et al., 1994). When such a hearing loss is slight, and particularly when it is recent or when aphasic defects also contribute to speech comprehension problems, the patient may be unaware of it.

Frequently, patients who do not report their hearing problem betray it in their behavior. Persons whose hearing is better on one side tend to favor that side by turning the head or placing themselves so that the better ear is closer to the examiner. Mild to moderately hard of hearing persons may display erratic speech comprehension as the examiner's voice becomes louder or softer, or not hear well if the examiner turns away when speaking to them. The examiner who suspects that the patient has a hearing loss can test for it crudely by speaking softly and noting whether the patient's level of comprehension drops. When the patient appears to have a hearing loss, the examiner should insist that the patient see an audiologist for a thorough audiological examination. An audiological assessment is of particular importance when a tumor is suspected, for an early sign of some forms of brain tumor is decreased auditory acuity. It is also important for brain impaired patients with other sensory or cognitive defects to be aware of hearing problems so that they can learn to compensate for them and, when indicated, get the benefits of a hearing aid or, for some conditions, surgical remediation.

Auditory Discrimination

Some patients have difficulty discriminating sounds even when thresholds for sound perception remain within the normal hearing range and no aphasic disability is present (Ceranic and Luxon, 2002; R.A. Levine and Häusler, 2001). Auditory discrimination can be tested by having the patient repeat words and phrases spoken by the examiner, or by asking the patient to tell whether two spoken words are the same or different, using pairs of different words, such as "cap" and "cat" or "vie" and "thy," interspersed with identical word pairs. Auditory discrimination is evaluated routinely in audiometric examinations. When the problem is suspected, referral to an audiologist is indicated.

Phoneme Discrimination (Benton, Sivan, Hamsher, et al., 1994)

Rather than real words, this 30-item tape-recorded task uses half identical, half similar pairs of nonsense words (e.g., "ur–ur," "pedzap–pelzap") as stimuli. The word list may be read by the examiner, as explicit pronunciation instructions are given in the manual. Since by chance alone subjects can get 15 items correct, only scores above 15 are considered (scores that fall much below 15 may indicate a motivation problem). Using a cut-off score of 22 (the lowest score made by normal subjects), auditory discrimination problems were found in 24 of 100 aphasic patients, and all but two of the 24 had defective oral comprehension.

Wepman's Auditory Discrimination Test (Wepman and Reynolds, 1987)

Wepman formalized the technique of testing auditory discrimination by using single syllable word pairs, some identical, some differing only by a phoneme coming from the same phoneme category. Thirteen word pairs differ in their initial consonant, thirteen in their final consonant, and four differ in the middle vowel sound. The test comes in two equivalent forms.

Although this test was originally devised to identify auditory discrimination problems in young school children, and the present norms were developed on samples of four- to eight-year-olds, norms for the 8–0 to 8–11 age range are adequate for adults since auditory discrimination is generally fully developed by this age. Alternate form reliabilities of .92 are reported, based on child studies. Test–retest reliabilities in the .88 to .91 range have been obtained on child samples. W.G. Snow, Tierney, and their colleagues (1988) found a test–retest correlation of .68 for 100 normal elderly persons.

Sound Blending and Incomplete Words (W-J III) (Mather and Woodcock, 2001)

The Woodcock-Johnson III *Tests of Cognitive Abilities* contain two tests of auditory–verbal perception, both administered by audio recording. Sound Blending examines the ability to synthesize language sounds by presenting familiar words (e.g., "bunny," "picnic") slowly with syllables separated in time; the subject's task is to identify the word. Age norms are available to >26 which are appropriate for most adults with intact hearing. Incomplete Words is also described as a test of "auditory processing," in which the subject hears words lacking one or more phonemes; again the task is to identify the word. Age norms for this test go to >33 years. While factor and cluster analyses associate Sound Blending with a "general intellectual ability" factor plus "phonemic awareness," Incomplete Words is associated only with "phonemic awareness." Reliability coefficients for adults are in the .90 to .93 range.

Speech Sounds Perception Test (SSPT)
(Reitan and Wolfson, 1993)

This test is in the Halstead-Reitan Battery. Sixty sets of nonsense syllables each beginning and ending with different consonants but based on the vowel sound "ee" comprise the items, which are administered by tape recording. Subjects note what they think they heard on a four-choice form laid out in six 10-item sections (called "series") labeled A to F.

The appropriateness of the examination format has been questioned. Reddon, Schopflocher, et al. (1989) point out that for 58 of the 60 test items the correct response is always the second or third response of the four listed horizontally in each item, with the first response choice containing the correct prefix and the last containing the correct suffix. A 14-year-old girl of just *average* mental ability figured this pattern out early in the course of taking the test (Bolter et al., 1984), leading to the suggestion that patients who make few errors should be queried about strategy upon completing the test. However, for 56 patients with diffuse brain injuries, the type of error (prefix, suffix, or both) identified these patients at the same rate as the error score (Charter, Dutra, and Lopez, 1997). Items differ in the degree to which correct choices are phonetically similar or identical to common words, and these items tend to be identified with relatively greater frequency than those that sound less familiar (Bornstein, Weizel, and Grant, 1984). Patients with hearing impairments, particularly those with high-frequency loss, which is common among elderly persons, are likely to perform poorly on this test (Schear, Skenes, and Larsen, 1988). For example, Ernst (1988) found that a group of 85 intact elderly persons achieved a mean score of 7.8 [failures]; when evaluated by Halstead's (1947) recommended cut-off score of 7 [failures], 37% of them failed the test.

Test characteristics. Test–retest correlations rarely run below .60 and most are well above it (G. Goldstein and Watson, 1989). Retesting control subjects show essentially no practice effects, not even a trend (McCaffrey, Duff, and Westervelt, 2000b). Not surprisingly, given the issue of impaired auditory acuity, accuracy diminishes with age; age accounts for about 10% of the variance; education contributes about 17% (Heaton, Ryan, et al., 1996). No sex differences have been reported (Filskov and Catanese, 1986; Heaton, Ryan, et al., 1996). An item analysis found that 19 of the items were more sensitive than the others, and sufficiently sensitive to discriminate between patients and control subjects (Charter and Dobbs, 1998).

Neuropsychological findings. This test is sensitive to brain damage generally, and to left brain damage in particular. Patients with left-hemisphere damage made the most errors when compared with those whose lesions were in the right hemisphere or were bilateral (Bornstein and Leason, 1984; Hom and Reitan, 1990). These latter patient groups also differed in patterns of failure, as those with left-sided lesions made the highest percentage of suffix errors and relatively fewer prefix errors than those with right-sided or bilateral lesions. Bornstein and Leason suggested that patients making more than 70% suffix errors and fewer than 29% prefix errors are likely to have left-sided damage. The SSPT is also sensitive to attentional deficits: Hom and Reitan (1990) categorize this rapidly paced test as one of "Attention and Concentration", a conclusion that my clinical experience supports (mdl). The examiner must be wary of concluding that a patient has left hemisphere damage on the basis of a high error score on this test alone as it may test the subject's capacity to attend to a boring task.

Short form alternatives. Most errors occur on the first two sections, Series A and B, with fewest on D and E (Bornstein, 1982; Crockett, Clark et al., 1982). When scored for just the 30 items in the first three 10-item series (A, B, and C), 96% and 90% of two patient groups achieved similar scores on both this and the full 60-item format (Bornstein, 1982). Crocket, Clark, and their colleagues found an error difference of 2.13 between the half test and the full test. Since the first three (A, B, C) series elicit the most errors, Charter and Dobbs (1998) recommend a cut-off of 5. This form, *SSPT-30*, has a lower reliability than the full test leading Charter and Dobbs to recommend using the 60-item test whenever possible.

Alternatively, Charter (2000) tested a short form consisting of just the last 30 items (*SSPT-DEF*) for use when the original short form is invalid. Based on statistical analyses, Charter concluded that this can be a satisfactory substitute for SSPT-30, but that the original test is always preferable, when possible.

Aphasia

It is always important to look for evidence of aphasia in patients displaying right-sided weakness or complaining of sensory changes on the right half of the body (see pp. 70–71, 75, 77). Aphasia must also be considered whenever the patient's difficulty in speaking or comprehending speech appears to be clearly unrelated to hearing loss, attention or concentration defects, a foreign language background, or a thought disorder associated with a psychiatric condition. The patient's performance on tests involving verbal functions should help the examiner determine whether a more thorough study of the patient's language functions is indicated.

Auditory Inattention

Some patients with lateralized lesions involving the temporal lobe or central auditory pathways tend to ignore auditory signals entering the ear opposite the side of the lesions, much as other brain damaged patients exhibit unilateral visual inattention on the side contralateral to the lesion (Heilman, 2002). Auditory inattention can be tested without special equipment by an examiner standing behind the patient so that stimulation can be delivered to each ear simultaneously. The examiner then makes soft sounds at each ear separately and simultaneously, randomly varying single and simultaneous presentations of the stimuli. Production of a soft rustling sound by rubbing the thumb and first two fingers together is probably the method of choice (e.g., G. Goldstein, 1974) as, with practice, the examiner can produce sounds of equal intensity with both hands.

Auditory–Verbal Perception

Every thorough neuropsychological examination provides some opportunity to evaluate auditory perception of verbal material. When presenting problems of judgment and reasoning, learning, and memory orally, the examiner has an opportunity to make an informal estimate of the patient's auditory acuity, comprehension, and processing capacity. Significant defects in the perception and comprehension of speech are readily apparent during the course of administering most psychological tests. For example, a patient must have a fairly intact capacity for auditory–verbal perception in order to give even a minimal performance on the WIS-A. If just a few tasks with simple instructions requiring only motor responses or one- or two-word answers are given subtle problems of auditory processing may be missed. These include difficulty in processing or retaining lengthy messages although responses to single words or short phrases may be accurate, inability to handle spoken numbers without a concomitant impairment in handling other forms of speech, or inability to process messages at high levels in the auditory system when the ability to repeat them accurately is intact (D.L. Bachman and Albert, 1988). In the absence of a hearing defect, any impairment in the recognition or processing of speech usually indicates a lesion involving the left or speech-dominant hemisphere.

When impairment in auditory processing is suspected, the examiner can couple an auditorily presented test with a similar task presented visually. This kind of paired testing enables the examiner to compare the functioning of the two perceptual systems under similar conditions. A consistent tendency for the patient to perform better under one of the two stimulus conditions should alert the examiner to the possibility of neurological impairment of the less efficient perceptual system. Test pairs can be readily found or developed for most verbal tests at most levels of difficulty. For example, both paper-and-pencil and orally administered personal history, information, arithmetic reasoning, and proverbs questions can be given. Comprehension, sentence building, vocabulary items, and many memory and orientation tasks also lend themselves well to this kind of dual treatment.

Testing for Auditory Comprehension

Most aphasia tests contain a set of items for examining verbal comprehension. The section, *Complex Ideational Material,* of the *Boston Diagnostic Aphasia Examination* (Goodglass, Kaplan, and Barresi, 2000) begins with eight paired questions requiring "yes" or "no" answers. These are followed by four little stories of increasing complexity, each accompanied by four questions, again calling for a "yes" or "no" response.

Putney Auditory Comprehension Screening Test (PACST) (Beaumont, Marjoribanks, Flury, and Lintern, 2002)

This is a 60-item set of a mix of half true, half false statements testing auditory comprehension. The two practice questions are exemplars: "Can babies look after themselves?" "Do surgeons operate on people?" Like the practice questions, the vocabulary consists of words and names in common usage. All questions can be answered with "yes" or "no." Seven different topics are represented in the questions (e.g., "Comparatives," "General Knowledge"). Sentence lengths range from three to eight words. Most sentences are syntactically simple in active tense; a few use passive tense and/or a coordinating or subordinating clause. Impairment is defined as a score ≤ 56.

The test was validated on 112 neurology service inpatients (age range, 18–90), most of whom took it three times at monthly intervals. Most patients could respond verbally; others used signals or buzzers. No sex differences showed up but performances were positively correlated with education and socioeconomic status and—surprisingly—with lower age, a finding the authors attribute to the relatively greater severity of disability among younger patients. Satisfactory reliability was demonstrated. Validity was tested by correlations of the PACST scores with ward manager and speech therapist evaluations (r = .52, .83 respectively).

Although this kind of evaluation is more often needed with neurologically impaired inpatients than outpatients, it may clarify some communication problems of speaking patients quickly and effectively. The authors observe that the PACST is likely to be most useful with nonverbal patients with severe physical disabilities, such as those with "*locked-in syndrome*" (in which motor control may be limited to eye movements) or advanced multiple sclerosis.

Nonverbal Auditory Reception

So much of a person's behavior is organized around verbal signals that nonverbal auditory functions are often overlooked. However, the recognition, discrimination, and comprehension of nonsymbolic sound patterns, such as music, tapping patterns, and the meaningful noises of sirens, dog barks, and thunderclaps are subject to impairment much as is the perception of language sounds (Kolb and Wishaw, 1996; I. Peretz, 2001). Defects of nonverbal auditory perception tend to be associated with both aphasia and bilateral temporal lobe lesions (D.L. Bachman and Albert, 1988) and, more rarely, with right hemisphere damage alone (Hécaen and Albert, 1978).

Most tests for nonverbal auditory perception use sound recordings. H.W. Gordon (1990) included taped sequences of four to seven familiar nonverbal sounds (e.g., rooster crowing, telephone ringing) in a battery designed to differentiate right and left hemisphere dysfunction. Subjects are asked to recognize the sounds and then write the names of the sounds in the order in which they were heard. Although developed for lateralization studies on sex, age, and psychiatric disorders, this technique has clinical potential.

Seashore Rhythm Test (Reitan and Wolfson, 1993; Seashore et al., 1960)

This test is the one used most widely for nonverbal auditory perception since Halstead (1947) incorporated it into his test battery. This subtest of Seashore's *Test of Musical Talent* requires the subject to discriminate between like and unlike pairs of musical beats. Normal control subjects average between 3 and 5 errors (Bornstein, 1985b; Reitan and Wolfson, 1989); the original cut-off was set between 5 and 6 errors (Halstead, 1947).

Test characteristics. For groups with average ages in the middle 50s or lower, age does not appear to affect ability to do this test (Bornstein, 1985; Reitan and Wolfson, 1989). In the 65- to 75 year age range, one-third of a normal group had scores in the "impaired" range (Ernst, 1988). Similar findings were reported for normal subjects in the 55- to 70 year range (Bornstein, Paniak, and O'Brien, 1987). In a large sample, education contributed to approximately 15% of the variance (Heaton, Ryan, et al., 1996). No sex differences were reported. Musical education, however, can make a significant difference as many cognitively impaired patients with musical backgrounds achieve scores in the normal range; thus Karzmark (2001) recommends that normal scores of patient with musical training be interpreted with caution.

Test–retest differences are small (McCaffrey, Duff, and Westervelt, 2000b). Internal reliabilities (split–half and odd–even) of .77 and .62 have been reported (Bornstein, 1983b). However, Charter and Webster (1997), reporting a reliability coefficient of .78 (n = 617), found that many of the items were too easy to be very discriminating. They also reported that this test is sensitive to fatigue and/or reduced concentration as the last items were passed at a lower rate than the initial ones. "From a purely psychometric standpoint, Seashore Rhythm test is *not* [sic] an example of a good test" (Charter and Webster, 1997, p. 167).

Neuropsychological findings. Although originally purported to be sensitive to right hemisphere dysfunction, most studies indicate no differences in performance levels between patients with right-sided lesions and those with lesions on the left (Hom and Reitan, 1990; Reitan and Wolfson, 1989), even for patients with lesions confined to the temporal lobes (Boone and Rausch, 1989). Rather, this test is most useful as a measure of attention and concentration, as brain impaired patients generally perform significantly below the levels of normal control subjects; patients with bilateral and diffuse lesions tend to make even more errors than those with lateralized lesions (Reitan and Wolfson, 1989). Thus, not surprisingly, the number of errors made correlates positively with a measure of severity of TBI. Categorization of this test as one that is most sensitive to attention and concentration deficits (Hom and Reitan, 1990) accords with our clinical experience [hjh, mdl].

Testing for amusia

Defective perception of music or of its components (e.g., rhythm, pitch, timbre, melody, harmonics) is usually associated with temporal lobe disease, and is more likely to occur with right-sided involvement than with left (see I. Peretz, 2001, who notes the importance of differentiating recognition of melody, primarily reduced with right temporal lesions, and rhythm recognition which may be affected by lesions on either hemisphere side).

Tests for this aspect of auditory perception can be easily improvised. The examiner can whistle or hum several simple and generally familiar melodies such as "America" ("God Save the Queen"), "Silent Night," or "Frère Jacques." Pitch discrimination can be tested with a pitch pipe, asking the patient to report which of two sounds is higher or whether two sounds are the same or different. Recognition for rhythm patterns can be evaluated by requiring the patient either to discriminate similar and different sets of rhythmic taps or to mimic patterns tapped out by the examiner with a pencil on the table top. Zatorre (1989) prepared 3- and 6-note melodies, presenting them in pairs that were either the same or differed in the tone or rhythmic value or both of one note. Patients with right temporal lobectomies performed significantly below normal levels on this task. Zatorre (1984) reviewed a variety of other techniques for examining melody discrimination, including use of bird songs and dichotic listening. In evaluating patient responses, the effects of musical training must be considered (Botez et Botez, 1996).

Formalized batteries may be used for systematic examination of musical functions. Benton (1977a) outlined a seven-part battery developed by Dorgeuille that contains four sections for assessing receptive functions: II Rhythmic expression (reproduction of tapped rhythm patterns); IV Discrimination of sounds (comparing two tones for highest pitch); V Identification of familiar melodies; and VI Identification of types of music (e.g., whether dance, military, or church). Wertheim and Botez (1961) developed a comprehensive examination for studying amusic phenomena in musically trained patients with cerebral disorders that, in its review of perceptual aspects of musicianship, tests for: A. Tonal, Melodic, and Harmony Elements; B. Rhythmic Element; C. Agogical (tempo-related) and Dynamic Elements; and D. Lexic Element (testing for ability to read musical notation). Each of these sections contains a number of subsections for examining discrete aspects of musical dysfunction. While providing for a comprehensive review of residual musical capacities in musicians who have sustained brain damage, this battery is too technical for general use.

Recognition of emotional tone in speech

That nonverbal aspects of speech may be as important to communication as its verbal content becomes evident when listening to the often flat or misplaced intonations of patients with right hemisphere damage. The emotionally toned techniques described here may bring to light another dimension of the deficits that are likely to accompany left visuospatial neglect, which can debase the quality of these patients' social adjustment, and can lead to an underestimation of their affective capacity when their problem is one of perceptual discrimination rather than emotional dulling.

Using four sentences with emotionally neutral content (e.g., "He tossed the bread to the pigeons."), Daniel M. Tucker and his coworkers (1977) examined whether the capacity to identify or discriminate the emotional toning of speech was impaired with lateralized cerebral damage. Tape recordings were made of each sentence read with a happy, sad, angry, or indifferent intonation, making a total of 16 sentences presented in random order on a recognition task. These sentences were paired for a discrimination task, in which the subject was asked to indicate which of the pair expressed a specified one of the four moods. Although their patient sample was small those whose damage involved right-sided brain structures (i.e., had left visuospatial inattention) were much less able to appreciate the emotional qualities of the sentences than the conduction aphasics who comprised the left-lesioned group with no overlap of scores on either task. In a similar study using four neutral sentences and three emotional tones, patients with right hemisphere disease performed below normal levels on both test tasks (Borod, Welkowitz, et al., 1990). Several other tests of emotional perception and batteries which include such tests are reviewed by Borod, Tabert, et al. (2000). Regardless of format or test length, patients with right brain lesions consistently performed poorly. Following are two sample formats.

In the *Emotional Perception Test* (*EPT*), recordings of three sentences are each read in five different emotional tones: happy, angry, frightened, sad, and neutral (P. Green, Flaro, and Allen, 1999). One sentence is neutral, the second is a request, the third voices a complaint. An equivalent test (three "sentences," each heard in the five emotional modes) uses nonsense sentences to separate tone from content. Scoring forms can be used for clinical examinations or group administrations, the latter consisting of half the original items. Normal subjects' accuracy did not differ significantly whether heard by the right ear, the left, or both, nor did subjects differ on the two test sets. Errors increased significantly after age 50 and even more so for a 70- to 90-year-old group. Women outperformed men on all measures. The manual reports no studies on neurologically impaired patients.

The *Prosodic perception* task in the New York Emotion Battery (Borod, Welkowitz, and Obler, 1992) uses four neutral sentences, each spoken in one of eight emotional tones. The *discrimination* part of this test presents these sentences in 56 pairs for the subject to decide whether the intoned emotion is the same or different. For the *identification* subtest, subjects must choose which of eight emotional words printed on a card describe the tone of each of 24 spoken sentences (Borod, Cicero, et al., 1998). The mean scores for control subjects and patients with left-sided lesions were identical; patients with right-sided lesions made more errors ($p = .035$).

TACTILE PERCEPTION

Investigations into defects of touch perception have employed many different kinds of techniques to elicit or measure the different ways in which tactile perception can be disturbed. Most of the techniques present simple recognition or discrimination problems. A few involve more complex behavior.

Tactile Sensation

Before examining complex or conceptually meaningful tactile-perceptual functions, the integrity of the somatosensory system in the area of neuropsychological interest—usually the hands—should be evaluated. Some commonly used procedures involve asking patients to indicate whether they feel the sharp or the dull end of a pin, pressure from one or two points (applied simultaneously and close together), or pressure from a graded set of plastic hairs, the Von Frey hairs, which have enjoyed wide use in the examination of sensitivity to touch (A.-L. Christensen, 1979; Luria, 1966; Varney, 1986). The patient's eyes should be closed or the hand being tested kept out of sight when sensory functions are tested.

Tactile Inattention

The tactile inattention phenomenon, sometimes called "tactile extinction" or "tactile suppression," most often occurs with right hemisphere—particularly right parietal—damage. Although it frequently accompanies visual or auditory inattention, it can occur by itself. Testing for tactile inattention typically involves a procedure used in neurological examinations in which points on some part of the body (usually face or hands) on each side are touched first singly and then simultaneously (*double simultaneous stimulation*) (Strub and Black, 2000). This is the method, in standardized format, that is used in the Sensory-Perceptual Examination of the Halstead-Reitan battery (e.g., Reitan and Wolfson, 1993). Patients experiencing left hemi-inattention

will report only a right-sided touch on simultaneous stimulation, although when just one side is touched they may have no difficulty reporting it correctly.

Face–Hand Test (FHT) (Kahn and Miller, 1978; Zarit, Miller, and Kahn, 1978)

An examination for tactile inattention that involves two bilateral stimulation points on each trial—the method of double simultaneous stimulation—has been formalized as a brief 10- or 20-trial test administered first with the subject's eyes closed. Upon each stimulation trial, the subject must indicate the point of touch (see Table 10.4). Should subjects make errors with their eyes closed, the test is readministered with their eyes open. Interestingly, under the eyes-open condition, only 10% to 20% of patients who had made errors with their eyes closed improved on their original performances (Kahn, Goldfarb, et al., 1960-61). The original format had 10 touch trials, but this was expanded to 16 trials (Zarit, Miller, and Kahn, 1978). Subjects who do not have an inattention problem and elderly persons who are not demented may make one or two errors on the first four trials but typically make no further errors once they have grasped the idea of the task. Impaired patients show no such improvement. Four or more errors indicates impairment (e.g., Eastwood et al., 1983).

Neuropsychological findings. This technique demonstrates the presence of tactile inattention. Not all errors, though, are errors of inattention. Errors on trials 2 and 6 suggest that the patient has either a sensory impairment or difficulty following instructions. Displacement errors, in which the patient reports that the stimulus was felt on another part of the body, tend to occur with diffuse deteriorating conditions (M. Fink et al., 1952). Beyond middle age, errors on this test tend to increase with advancing years (Kahn and Miller,

TABLE 10.4 The Face-Hand Test

Trial			
1.	Right cheek	and	left cheek
2.	Left cheek	and	left hand
3.	Right cheek	and	right hand
4.	Left cheek	and	right hand
5.	Right hand	and	left hand
6.	Right cheek	and	right hand
7.	Right hand	and	left hand
8.	Left cheek	and	right hand
9.	Right cheek	and	left hand
10.	Left cheek	and	left hand

Adapted from Kahn and Miller (1978)

1978). This test is a sensitive indicator of dementia progression; many mildly demented patients make some errors on this test, but with advancing deterioration they tend to fail more than half of the items on the expanded test format (L. Berg, Danziger, et al., 1984; Eastwood et al., 1983). In contrast, with repeated testing, elderly control subjects improved from an average of almost one error on initial testing to virtually none on a third examination (G. Berg, Edwards, et al., 1987).

Quality Extinction Test (QET) (A.S. Schwartz, Marchok, and Flynn, 1977)

Dissatisfaction with the number of patients with parietal lobe damage who did not display the tactile extinction phenomenon on the usual testing procedures led to the development of a test that requires more complex discriminations. In this test, after becoming familiarized by sight and touch with an assortment of different surface textures (e.g., wire mesh, sandpaper, velvet), blindfolded subjects are required to identify these materials when they are brushed against their hands. On some trials, each hand receives the same material; on the other trials, different material is brushed against each hand. This method elicited the inattention phenomenon when it did not show up with usual testing procedures. Tactile inattention is strongly associated with spontaneous visual inattention but when visual or auditory inattention shows up only on testing, tactile inattention is less likely to be found (A.S. Schwartz, Marchok, and Kreinick, 1988).

Tactile Recognition and Discrimination Tests

Stereognosis (recognition of objects by touch)

Object recognition (testing for astereognosis) is commonly performed in neurological examinations (Strub and Black, 2000; L.A. Weisberg, Garcia, and Strub, 1996). Patients are asked to close their eyes and to recognize by touch such common objects as a coin, a paper clip, a pencil, or a key. Each hand is examined separately. Size discrimination is easily tested with coins. The examiner can use bits of cloth, wire screening, sandpaper, etc., for texture discrimination (Varney, 1986). Intact adults are able to perform tactile recognition and discrimination tests with virtually complete accuracy: a single erroneous response or even evidence of hesitancy suggests that this function may be impaired (Fromm-Auch and Yeudall, 1983). Somesthetic defects are generally associated with lesions of the contralateral hemisphere, although bilateral deficits can occur with right hemisphere lesions (Bauer and Demery, 2003; Benton, Sivan, Hamsher, et al., 1994; Caselli, 1991).

Luria (1966) used four procedures to satisfy reasonable doubts about whether a patient's inability to identify an object placed in the palm results from astereognosis or some other problem. Patients who do not identify the object on passive contact with the hand are encouraged to feel the object and move it around in the hand. Should they not be able to name the object, they are given an opportunity to pick out one like it from other objects set before them. Should they still not recognize it, Luria put the object in the other hand, noting that, "if the patient now recognizes the object without difficulty, when he could not do so before, it may be concluded that astereognosis is present." Of course, as soon as the patient accurately identifies the object, the remaining procedural steps become unnecessary.

Wooden letters and formboard shapes were the stimuli in a study of lateralized tactile discrimination (Pandey et al., 2000). Following a somewhat complex testing protocol, these workers showed differential hemispheric success: patients with right-sided lesions needed fewer trials to recognize letters; those with lesions on the left recognized forms in fewer trials. The almost universal availability of letter and geometrically shaped blocks recommends them for testing tactile perception.

Some workers (e.g., Benton, Sivan, Hamsher, et al., 1994 [see also Fig. 9.2, p. 342, which shows how the Tactile Form Perception test is administered]; Reitan and Wolfson, 1993, 2002) have standardized procedures for examining stereognosis and developed scoring systems for them.

For example, using their scoring system to evaluate the *Tactile Form Recognition Test*—which Reitan and Wolfson (2002) say may take as long as 15 min, these authors compared a group of 50 (diagnosticaly not defined) "brain-damaged persons" with a demographically similar group without apparent neurological disease for ability to identify the shape of four flat plastic pieces (cross, square, triangle, and circle). They found not only a highly significant difference between the two groups' mean scores, but reported that their cut-off score (scoring procedures were not provided in this article) identified 82% of patients, 84% of control subjects.

The refinements of scoring are necessary for many research purposes. However, the extra testing they entail adds little to a clinical examination that gives the patient three or four trials with different objects (or textures) for each hand that has sensation sufficiently intact to warrant the testing.

Skin writing

The technique of tracing letters or numbers on the palms of the subject's hands is also used in neurological examinations. A. Rey (1964) formalized the skin-

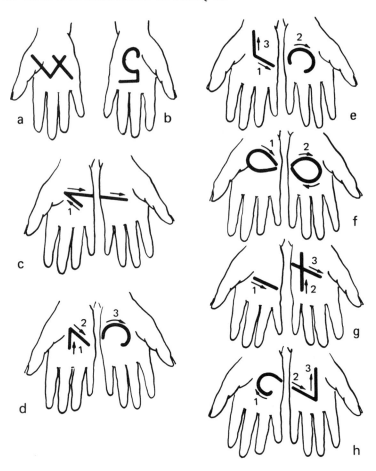

FIGURE 10.22 Rey's skin-writing procedures. (Courtesy of Presses Universitaires de France)

writing procedure into a series of five subtests in which the examiner writes, one by one in six trials for each series (1) the figures 5 1 8 2 4 3 on the dominant palm (see Fig. 10.22a); (2) V E S H R O on the dominant palm; (3) 3 4 2 8 1 5 on the nondominant palm (Fig. 10.22b); (4) 1 3 5 8 4 2 in large figures extending to both sides of the two palms held 1 cm apart (Fig. 10.22c–h); and (5) 2 5 4 1 3 8 on the fleshy part of the inside dominant forearm. Each subtest score represents the number of errors. Rey provided data on four different adult groups: manual and unskilled workers (M), skilled technicians and clerks (T), people with the baccalaureate degree (B), and persons between the ages of 68 and 83 (A) (see Table 10.5). In the absence of a

TABLE 10.5 Skin-Writing Test Errors Made by Four Adult Groups

Group		Right-Hand Numbers	Right-Hand Letters	Left-Hand Numbers	Both-Hands Numbers	Forearm Numbers
M	Mdn	0	1	0	2	1
$n = 51$	CS*	2	3	2	5	3
T	Mdn	0	1	0	1	0
$n = 25$	CS	2	3	1	3	3
B	Mdn	0	1	0	0	0
$n = 55$	CS	1	2	1	2	2
A	Mdn	1	2	1	2	2
$n = 14$	CS	3	4	3	6	3

*CS, cutting score.
Adapted from Rey (1964)

sensory deficit or an aphasic condition, when the patient displays an error differential between the two hands, a contralateral cortical lesion is suspected; defective performance regardless of side implicates a tactile perceptual disability.

Skin-writing tests are useful for lateralizing the site of damage when there are no obvious signs such as hemiparesis or aphasia. The two tests presented here can also provide some indication of the severity of a tactile-perceptual defect. Moreover, in finding that toe writing responses can be indicative of severity of TBI, P. Richards and Persinger (1992) hypothesized that this is due to "the particular vulnerability of the medial hemispheric surfaces to the consequences of shear and compressional forces." They followed the same procedures used in Fingertip Number-Writing Perception (below).

Fingertip Number-Writing Perception (G. Goldstein, 1974; Reitan and Wolfson, 1993)

As part of his modification of Halstead's original test battery, Reitan added these formalized neurological procedures in which the examiner writes with a pencil each of the numbers 3, 4, 5, 6 in a prescribed order on each of the fingertips of each hand, making a total of 20 trials for each hand. Normal subjects are more accurate in identifying stimulation applied to their left-hand fingers than those on the right, and the three middle fingers are more sensitive than the other two (Harley and Grafman, 1983). On this symbol identification task, stroke patients with right hemisphere disease made many fewer errors than those whose damage was on the left, but each group performed best with the hand ipsilateral to the lesion (G.G. Brown, Spicer, et al., 1989).

OLFACTION

Diminished olfactory sensitivity accompanies a number of neurological disorders (R.L. Doty and Bromley, 2002; Jones-Gotman and Zatorre, 1988; Mesholam et al., 1998) and has proven useful in discriminating neurodegenerative disorders from depression in elderly persons (McCaffrey, Duff, and Solomon, 2000; G.S. Solomon et al., 1998), or in predicting cognitive decline (Graves et al., 1999) or possible advent of Parkinson's disease (Berendse et al., 2001). Thus olfaction testing should be considered when preparing an assessment battery. Informal olfaction testing is frequently performed by neurologists using a few common odors (coffee, peppermint, vanilla, vinegar, etc.) (e.g., American Academy of Neurology, 2002; Bannister, 1992; Weisberg et al., 1996). This technique will

suffice for most clinical work. In some cases, patient reports alone may provide the necessary information: Varney (1988) found that TBI patients who reported olfactory dysfunction were less likely to be employed. However, almost all of a group of Alzheimer patients were unaware of their olfactory deficits (R.L. Doty, Reyes, and Gregor, 1987).

For the more precise odor detection needed for research, the *University of Pennsylvania Smell Identification Test (UPSIT)*[1] is probably the most widely used olfaction assessment technique (R.L. Doty, 1992). The 40 odors in this test include different kinds, both pleasant and unpleasant. They are encapsulated in plastic microtubules positioned in strips, each odor on a page in one of four 10-page booklets. When scratched, the strip releases an odor. For each odor four alternative answers are presented on the page. Additionally, odor detection is assessed in a forced-choice paradigm in which a relatively faint odor is presented with an odorless substance. The odor stimulus is gradually increased to a level at which the subject can make four correct choices; and then it is gradually reduced as a check on the subject's threshold response.

Norms are available for the identification and detection tests of the UPSIT. Women tend to identify odors better than men, even across cultures which show differences, as Korean Americans outperformed African and white American groups, with native Japanese doing least well on this set of comparisons (R.L. Doty, Applebaum, et al., 1985). The sex difference did not hold up when memory for odors was tested (Moberg et al., 1987). Age effects are significant for normal control subjects, with the greatest losses occurring in the seventh decade (R.L. Doty, 1990; R.L. Doty and Bromley, 2002). A smoking habit does not seem to affect olfaction sensitivity for some subjects (R.L. Doty, Applebaum, et al, 1985; Moberg et al., 1987).

Other olfactory testing techniques include presentation of odors discretely to each nostril. This allows testing of lateralized sensitivity and showed that the right nostril tends to be more sensitive among normal control subjects, regardless of sex or apparent hemispheric biases (Zatorre and Jones-Gotman, 1990, 1991). To test olfactory memory, Moberg and his colleagues (1987) developed a 30-item set of odors. Five minutes after smelling a set of 10 target odors, one by one, subjects were exposed to 20 odors, including the original 10 plus five similar and five dissimilar foils. Both Huntington and Alzheimer patients were significantly deficient in odor recall when compared with normal control subjects.

---

[1]This test, under its trademark name *Smell Identification Test,* can be ordered from Sensonics Inc., Haddon Heights, NJ 08035.

11 | Memory I: Tests

Memory is the capacity to retain information and utilize it for adaptive purposes (Fuster, 1995). Efficient memory requires the intact functioning of many brain regions, including some that are especially susceptible to injury or disease. Moreover, many common neurological and psychiatric conditions produce a decline in that efficiency. One in three individuals aged 75 and above without dementia complains about memory deficits (Riedel-Heller et al., 1999). Moreover, memory complaints in outpatient settings may be the most frequent reason for neuropsychological referral. Thus memory assessment is often the central issue in a neuropsychological examination.

The use of the same word—memory—to identify some very different mental activities can create confusion. Patients as well as some clinicians lump many kinds of cognitive dysfunction under the umbrella of "memory impairment." In contrast, some patients whose learning ability is impaired claim a good memory because early recollections seem so vivid and easy to retrieve. Many older adults report memory problems when referring to an inability to retrieve common words or proper names consistently. This word finding difficulty—*dysnomia*—can occur along with efficient retrieval of episodic memories and, conversely, patients who have problems recalling episodic memories are not necessarily dysnomic. Deficits in processes outside the memory system can affect memory performance: these include attention and concentration, information processing speed, organization, strategy, effort, and self-monitoring (Ganor-Stern et al., 1998; Howieson and Lezak, 2002). Maintaining terminological distinctions between the different aspects of memory and the other functions necessary for efficient memory will help the clinician keep their differences in mind when evaluating patients and conceptualizing findings and theory.

Because memory impairments can take a variety of forms, no one assessment technique demonstrates the problem for all patients. Knowledge about presenting complaints, the nature of the brain injury or the neuropsychological syndrome, and the differing etiologies of memory disorders should guide the selection of memory tests. In every examination the examiner's choice of memory tests should depend upon clinical judgment about which tests are most suitable for answering the question under study for *this patient*. Therefore this chapter presents the tests in most common use plus a few of particular interest because of their potential research or clinical value, or because the format merits further exploration. Most tests of short-term and working memory are discussed in Chapter 9, pp. 351–358 because of their kinship to attentional processes (Cowey and Green, 1996; Howieson and Lezak, 2002). At least as many more memory tests show up in the literature as are described here.

EXAMINING MEMORY

For most adults it is useful to begin the examination of attention before proceeding with memory tests because of its fundamental role in memory performance. If someone performs poorly on simple attentional tasks such as span of immediate verbal retention (e.g., Digit Span Forward) or simple mental tracking (e.g., counting backwards by 3s or 7s), it may not be possible to get a valid measure of retention. For some patients, it may be necessary to delay the examination until a different time or under different circumstances in order to get a valid memory assessment.

A comprehensive memory evaluation should include (1) orientation to time and place; (2) prose recall to examine learning and retention of meaningful information which resembles what one hears in conversation, such as Wechsler's Logical Memory stories or other stories developed to test verbal recall; (3) rote learning ability which gives a learning curve and is tested with both free and recognition trials, such as the Auditory Verbal Learning Test or the California Verbal Learning Test; (4) visuospatial memory such as the Complex Figure, followed by a recognition trial when available; (5) remote memory, such as fund of information; and (6) personal—autobiographical—memory. All tests designed to measure learning should include one or more trials following a delay period filled with other tasks to prevent rehearsal, and both free recall and recognition or cued recall should be examined following the delay. When tests calling upon a motor response are not appropriate or produce equivocal findings, visual recognition tests can be substituted. A unilateral lesion may affect recall of verbal and nonverbal material differentially with left hemisphere lesions more likely to compromise verbal memory and right hemisphere lesions particularly disrupting visuospatial recall (Abrahams et al., 1997; Loring, Lee, Martin, and Meador, 1988; Milner, 1958; Sass et al., 1995). Thus, inclusion of both verbal and visuospatial tests is necessary for the assessment of memory problems specific to the type of material being learned.

When assessing memory the examiner should also compare aspects of cognition that are not heavily dependent on memory with the memory performance. The examiner can usually integrate the memory tests into the rest of the examination so as to create a varied testing format, to avoid stressing those memory-impaired patients who may be concerned about their deficits, and to use nonmemory tests as interference activities when testing delayed recall. Much mental status information can be obtained quite naturalistically during the introductory interview. For example, rather than simply noting the patient's report of years of schooling and letting it go at that, the examiner can ask for dates of school attendance and associated information such as dates of first employment or entry into service and how long after finishing school these events took place. Although the examiner will frequently be unable to verify this information, internal inconsistencies or vagueness are usually evidence of confusion about remote personal memory or difficulty retrieving it.

Three memory testing procedures must be part of every aspect of memory assessment if a full understanding of the patient's strengths and weaknesses is to be gained. (1) Immediate recall trials are insufficient tests of learning, retention, or the efficiency of the memory system. To examine learning (i.e., whether material has been stored in more than temporary form), a delay trial is necessary. In addition, a few patients who process information slowly will recall more on a delay trial than initially, thus demonstrating very concretely their slowed ability to digest and integrate new information. Freed, Corkin, and their coworkers (1989) call this late improvement *rebound* when it follows diminished performance on an early delay trial. (2) Interference during the delay period will prevent continuous rehearsal. Absence of some intervening activity between exposure to the stimulus and the subject's response leaves in question whether recall following delay was of learned material or simply of material held in continually rehearsed temporary storage. (3) When the subjects' recall is *below normal limits,* it is not possible to know whether reduced retrieval is due to a learning impairment or a retrieval problem. In these situations,

some means of assessing learning that bypasses simple recall must be undertaken to decide this critical issue. The most direct of these, and often the simplest, is to test learning by recognition. Other techniques include use of cues, comparing recall of meaningful material with recall of meaningless material (as meaning can serve as an internal cue), or the method of *savings* (in which the patient is given the same test at a later time to see whether the material is learned more quickly the second time, i.e., as a measure of forgetting; see p. 478).

The examiner needs to take special care to recognize when a poor performance on memory tests occurs because of impairment from other possible sources of reduced functioning. Elderly persons frequently have vision or hearing problems that adversely affect proper registration of the stimulus. Patients with frontal lobe or certain kinds of subcortical damage may lack the spontaneity or drive to reproduce all that they remember. When the patient exhibits diminished initiation or persistence, the examiner should press for additional responses. With story material, for example, it may be possible to encourage a complete recall by asking such questions as, "How did it begin?" or "What was the story about?" or "What happened next?" and so on. When the task involves reproduction of configural material, the patient can be encouraged with, "That's fine; keep going," or by being asked, "What more do you remember?" Depressed patients also may lack the drive to give their best performance on memory tests and may benefit from supportive prompting.

Memory tests, perhaps more than most cognitive tests, are influenced by practice effects (see pp. 116–117; McCaffrey, Duff, and Westervelt, 2000b). Many patients are examined repeatedly to measure their course over time or to examine the validity of data in forensic cases. In these cases it is desirable to have alternate test forms of equivalent difficulty for reassessment purposes. Using different but equivalent forms of verbal memory tests can reduce if not eliminate significant practice effects. A small practice gain is more likely to occur on visuospatial memory tests even when different forms are used due to "learning to learn" the even less familiar visuospatial procedures (Benedict and Zgaljardic, 1998). There has been a paucity of memory tests with multiple equivalent forms although more and more they are being developed.

VERBAL MEMORY

While many verbal memory tests are available, only a few have reliable norms based on careful standardization. Even with many tests available, the examiner may occasionally find that none quite suits the needs of a particular patient or research question, and will devise a new one. Verbal memory tests are presented here by content in order of increasing complexity. Not every kind of test is represented under every content heading, but taken altogether, the major techniques for examining verbal memory functions are reviewed.

Verbal Automatisms

Material learned by rote in early childhood and frequently used throughout life is normally recalled so unthinkingly, effortlessly, and accurately that the response is known as an *automatism*. Examples of automatisms are the alphabet, number series from 1 to 20 or 100 by 10's, days of the week and months of the year, a patriotic slogan or a long-practiced prayer. Automatisms are among the least perishable of the learned verbal habits. Loss or deterioration of these well-ingrained responses in nonaphasic patients may reflect attentional disturbances or fluctuations of consciousness in acute conditions. It occurs in nonacute conditions only when there is severe, usually diffuse, cerebral damage, such as in advanced dementia. To test for automatisms, the examiner simply asks the subject to repeat the alphabet, the days of the week, etc. More than one error usually indicates brain dysfunction.

Letters and Digits

Brown-Peterson Technique (L.R. Peterson and Peterson, 1959; L.R. Peterson, 1966; Baddeley, 1986)

To study short-term retention, a popular method has been this distractor technique which is also called the *Peterson task* (e.g., Baddeley, 1986), the *Peterson and Peterson procedure* (e.g., H.S. Levin, 1986), and other variations on the Peterson name, or it may be referred to as *Auditory Consonant Trigrams* (*ACT*) (Mitrushina, Boone, and D'Elia, 1999; Spreen and Strauss, 1998, use the acronym CCC). The purpose of the distractor task is to prevent rehearsal of material being held for short-term retention testing. The Brown-Peterson technique is included in this chapter because it assesses short-term memory and, unlike many working memory tests (covered on pp. 358–364), it does not require manipulating information held in memory. Rather, the task is to recall the information as presented.

Upon hearing (or seeing) three consonants presented at the rate of one-per-second, the subject is required to count backward from a given number until signaled to stop counting, and then to report or identify the stimulus item. The examiner tells the subject the two- or three-digit number from which to begin counting immediately after saying or showing the test item. For ex-

TABLE 11.1 Example of Consonant Trigrams Format*

Stimulus	Starting Number	Delay (sec)	Responses
QLX	—	0	
SZB	—	0	
HJT	—	0	
GPW	—	0	
DLH	—	0	
XCP	194	18	
NDJ	75	9	
FXB	28	3	
JCN	180	9	
BGQ	167	18	
KMC	20	3	
RXT	188	18	
KFN	82	9	
MBW	47	3	
TDH	141	9	
LRP	51	3	
ZWS	117	18	
PHQ	89	9	
XGD	158	18	
CZQ	91	3	

Number correct
0″ Delay _____
3″ Delay _____
9″ Delay _____
18″ Delay _____
   Total
*Courtesy of Edith Kaplan.

ample, the examiner says, "V J R 186" when the subject begins counting—"185, 184," etc.—until stopped at the end of a predesignated number of seconds and is expected to recall the item (see Table 11.1 for a consonant trigram stimulus format). With this technique, normal subjects have perfect recall with no distraction delay: they recall about 80% of the letters correctly with a distraction duration of 3 sec, approximately 70% to 80% correct recall with 9 sec delays (Stuss, Stethem, and Poirier, 1987). Longer durations produced a wider range of normal performances: from 50% to 80% with delays of 18 sec, and around 67% when the delay is as long as 36 sec. Giving five trials of three consonants each for a total of 15 possible correct responses at each delay interval, Stuss and his colleagues report standard deviations typically within the 1.6 to 2.8 range for the 9 sec delay, increasing to 2.1 to 3.6 for the 36 sec delay for various age groups (see also N. Butters, Sax, et al., 1978; Mitrushina, Boone, and D'Elia, 1999, report on two versions of the test).

This technique has also been administered with visual stimuli. In the sequential format the consonants are printed individually on cards and shown one at a time in sets of three; in the simultaneous format all three consonants appear together on each stimulus card (Edith Kaplan, personal communication [mdl]).

Test characteristics. Differences in sex, age—from late teens up to 69 years—or education levels (high school completion or less vs. more than high school) were not statistically significant (Stuss, Stethem, and Poirier, 1987). Nevertheless, women showed a tendency for better recall than men, persons with more than a high school education had slightly higher scores on average, and older subject groups did a little less well than younger ones. Education effects penalized those with fewer years of schooling regardless of age (Bherer et al., 2001). Small but significant practice effects do occur (Stuss, Stethem, and Poirier, 1987). Stuss noted that,

The Brown-Peterson is an interesting test. My concern is that it is very sensitive but not necessarily very specific. I think it is a wonderful working memory test, and one has to be very careful about interpreting [failure] as "poor test motivation." However, the test is very multifactorial and people can fail for various reaons. I am therefore cautious in its interpretation. (personal communication, Dec., 1996 [mdl]).

Neuropsychological findings. The Brown-Peterson technique is useful for documenting very short-term memory deficits (i.e., rapid decay of memory trace) in a variety of conditions. One of the early uses of the Brown-Peterson task in a patient population was Baddeley and Warrington's (1970) study of amnesic patients in which they reported no difference between Korsakoff patients and controls. Subsequent investigators, however, found severe impairments in Korsakoff patients (N. Butters and Cermak, 1980). Leng and Parkin (1989) noted that the performance deficits of Korsakoff patients were associated with their frontal lobe dysfunction rather than the severity of their memory problems, and also that patients with temporal pathology did better than those with Korsakoff's syndrome. Further implicating the sensitivity of this technique to frontal lobe dysfunction is Kapur's (1988b) finding that patients with bifrontal tumor, but not those with a tumor in the region of the third ventricle, recalled significantly fewer items than control subjects. B. Milner (1970, 1972) found that patients with right temporal lobectomies performed as well as normal controls on this test, but the amount recalled by those with left temporal excisions diminished as the amount of hippocampus loss increased. Again temporal lobe epilepsy patients with a left hemisphere focus performed less well than patients with a right hemisphere focus on a task recalling a single word after interference, but in this study both patient groups scored lower than controls (Giovagnoli and Avanzini, 1996). However, a visual presentation of word triads resulted in equally impaired recall by right and left temporal lobe seizure patients (Delaney, Prevey, and Mattson, 1982).

Data on multiple sclerosis patients are mixed: in one set of studies, they tended to differ very little from control subjects (Rao, Leo, Bernardin, and Unverzagt, 1991; Rao, Leo, and St. Aubin-Faubert, 1989); in others, MS patients exhibited deficits (I. Grant, McDonald, Trimble, et al., 1984; Grigsby, Ayarbe, et al., 1994). The distraction effect is much greater for Alzheimer patients than for normal subjects in their age range (E.V. Sullivan, Corkin, and Growdon, 1986), and it distinguishes both Huntington (N. Butters, Sax et al., 1978; D.C. Myers, 1983) and Parkinson patients (Graceffa et al., 1999) from controls. Schizophrenics show a rapid decline in recall on this task and produce an unusual number of intrusion errors (Fleming et al., 1995). Stuss, Ely, and their colleagues (1985) report that this test was the most sensitive to mild head injury in a battery of commonly used tests.

Occasionally consonant trigrams offers bonus information about a patient's susceptibility to attentional disorders. When counting backwards, the patient may skip or repeat a decade, or drop numbers out of sequence without being aware of the error(s). This occurrence suggests mental tracking and/or self-monitoring problems which should be further explored.

A 30-year-old native English speaker of Polynesian stock incurred an episode of cerebral hypoxia during a surgical procedure. She had dropped out of high school to work as a cashier in a fast food outlet. In the neuropsychological examination she obtained only *low average* to *average* scores on verbal skill and academic tests—excepting for a *high average* verbal fluency production. Yet on tests of visuoperception and construction she achieved scores in the *high average* and even *superior* (Block Design SS = 14) ability ranges and performed *within normal limits* on both the Category Test and Raven's Matrices. Chief complaints (of her family) involved executive disorders: passivity, anergia, impaired organizing ability, and disinhibited shopping. Together these problems have rendered her socially dependent.

On Consonant Trigrams this cooperative patient recalled 9/15 letters after the 3 sec delay trials, 5/15 after the 9 sec delay, and 2/15 after 18 sec, demonstrating a significant working memory problem. In addition she had difficulty keeping track of what she was doing when counting backwards: of the 15 items, she made no errors on only six; on others she skipped decades ("51-40-49-48 . . . ok"), she counted forward ("82-83-84 . . . I'm going upwards") but was usually not aware of errors, and she tended to skip numbers ("81-79-78 . . . " "156-154-153 . . ."), thus also displaying a severe mental tracking disability made worse by defective self-monitoring.

Variants of the Brown-Peterson technique. This paradigm has been adapted to specific research or clinical questions in a number of ways. The mode of presentation may be written—usually the stimuli are presented on cards—as well as oral. The stimuli may be words instead of consonants, and the number of stimuli—whether words or consonants—may be as few as 1 (e.g., see Leng and Parkin, 1989; E.V. Sullivan, Corkin, and Growdon, 1986). While the distracting subtraction task is usually by 3's, some studies have used 2's. Of three different distracting conditions in one study, two called for subtraction (by 2's, by 7's), and one simply required rapid repetition of "the" during the different time intervals (Kopelman and Corn, 1988). "The" repetition produced minimum interference compared with subtraction distractors, while subtraction by 2s or by 7s was equally effective. In another study, of three conditions using 10, 20, and 30 sec intervals between presentation of three consonants and request for response, one "distractor" involved repeating the syllable "bla," one required simple addition, with no distractor in the third; recall was almost perfect with no distractor and a little less than perfect in the "bla bla" condition, but dropped significantly with addition—particularly for subjects with ≤12 years' education (Bherer et al., 2001). In yet another variant, subjects had to recall eight triads of women's given names after counting backwards for 20 sec (Kapur, 1988b). Using three stimuli at a time—whether words or consonants—and subtraction by 3s for the usual duration ranges resulted in similar findings across studies (D.C. Myers, 1983), suggesting that the paradigm is more important than the contents in eliciting the Brown-Peterson phenomenon. Using recall of three monosyllabic words, Eustache and his colleagues (1995) observed an age effect for subjects ranging from 20 to 69 years.

Increasing the Tested Span

Many elderly subjects and patients with brain disorders have an immediate memory span as long as that of younger, intact adults. Thus, simple span tests, as traditionally administered, frequently do not elicit the immediate recall deficits of many persons with reduced memory capacity. To enhance sensitivity to these problems, longer and more complex span formats have been devised.

Supraspan

A variety of techniques for examining recall of strings of eight or more random numbers have demonstrated the sensitivity of the supraspan task to age, educational level, brain impairment, and anticholinergic medication (Crook, Ferris, et al., 1980; H.S. Levin, 1986). When given strings of numbers or lists to learn that are longer than normal span (i.e., span under *stimulus overload* conditions), the excess items serve as interference stimuli so that what is immediately recalled upon hearing the list represents partly what span can grasp, and partly what is retained (learned) despite interference. Problems in identifying and scoring the supraspan (e.g., it may begin at 7, 8, 9, or 10 in the normal population; should partial spans be counted?) resulted in some complex scoring systems that are unsuited to clinical use.

In normal subjects, supraspan recall will be at or a little below the level of simple span (e.g., see S.M. Rao, Leo, and St. Aubin-Faubert, 1989; pp. 421, 426 for initial recall of word list learning tasks) but will be two or more items shorter than simple span in many brain disorders. Digit span—forward or reversed—did not discriminate multiple sclerosis patients from normal subjects in the Rao, Leo, and St. Aubin-Faubert study, yet when given just one digit more than their maximum forward span, patients averaged two and one-half recalled digits fewer than the controls (2.95 vs. 5.46, respectively). Patients with right temporal lobe resections had impaired performances on a verbal supraspan learning task despite achieving intact verbal memory scores on the Wechsler Memory Scale (WMS) (Rausch and Ary, 1990).

Telephone Test (Crook, Ferris, et al., 1980; Zappalá et al., 1989)

To make the span test practically meaningful, 7- or 10-digit strings have been presented in a visual format, as if they were telephone numbers to be recalled. It is interesting to note that the longer the string, the shorter the amount of recall (see Table 11.2).

Serial Digit Learning (or Digit Sequence Learning) (Benton, Sivan, Hamsher, et al., 1994)

Subjects with less than a twelfth grade education hear a string of eight digits to learn (form D8); subjects with 12 or more years of schooling learn a nine-digit span (form K9). The digit string is repeated either until the subject has recalled it correctly for two consecutive trials or through all 12 trials. The maximum score of 24 is based on a scoring system in which each correct trial earns two points, one omission or misplacement drops

TABLE 11.2 Telephone Test Scores for Two Age Groups

	AGE (YEARS)	
Digit String	*≤50*	*>50*
Seven	5.93 ± .20	4.79 ± .29
Ten	4.24 ± .28	2.93 ± .26

From Zappalá et al. (1989)

the score to 1 point, and 2 points are added for each trial to 12 that did not have to be given. Defective performance is defined by a score of 7 or less for high school graduates (form K9), and 6 points or less for those at lower education levels. Age becomes a relevant variable after 65 years, which makes this test more sensitive to the mental changes of aging than simple digit span (Benton, Eslinger, and Damasio, 1981). Education contributes positively to performance on this test, but sex does not affect recall efficiency (Benton, Sivan, Hamsher, et al., 1994). Factor analysis suggests that performance is more closely a function of attention and information processing than learning (Larrabee and Curtiss, 1995).

Neuropsychological findings. Although intragroup variability for right and for left temporal lobe seizure patients was so great that the difference between their respective mean scores of 12.7 ± 7.2 and 8.3 ± 8.5 did not reach significance (Loring, Lee, Martin, and Meador, 1988), a χ^2 comparison of the number of failures in each group was significant ($p < .045$; see Lezak and Gray, 1991). However, even the large intragroup variability did not obscure pre–post left temporal lobectomy changes as documented on this test, with this group's average score dropping from an initial 13 to 5 after surgery (G.P. Lee, Loring, and Thompson, 1989). Patients with right temporal lobectomies showed, on the average, only a 2-point drop from their presurgery scores. This test is sensitive to more than verbal memory deficits, as patients with bilateral damage tend to perform less well on it than those with strictly lateralized dysfunction (Benton, Eslinger, and Damasio, 1981; Benton, Sivan, Hamsher, et al., 1994). Patients with lead toxicity also perform below expectation on this test (Stewart et al., 1999).

Tombaugh and Schmidt (1992) present a similar 12-trial format but use a sequence two digits longer than the subject's longest span and require three correct trials before discontinuing early. The rationale for this procedure is that adjusting the supraspan length on the basis of each individual's forward digit span equates the level of difficulty for everyone. They include a delayed recall trial with as many as six additional learning trials should the initial delayed recall be failed. Normative data for adults 20–79 years show a significant age effect. Scores of 70- to 80-year-old persons run 25% lower than scores for normal subjects under 40 (Tombaugh, Grandmaison, and Schmidt, 1995).

Words

The use of words, whether singly in word lists or combined into phrases, sentences, or lengthier passages, introduces a number of dimensions into the memory task that can affect test performances differentially, depending upon the patient's age, nature of impairment, mental capacity, etc. These dimensions include familiar–unfamiliar, concrete–abstract, low–high imagery, low–high association level, ease of categorization, low–high emotional charge, and structural dimensions such as rhyming or other phonetically similar qualities (e.g., see Baddeley, 1976; Mayes, 1988). The amount of organization inherent in the material also affects ease of retention. This is obvious to anyone who has found it easier to learn words than nonsense syllables or sentences than word strings. When using words for testing memory—and particularly when making up alternate word lists, sentences, etc.—the examiner must be alert to the potential effects that these dimensions can have on the comparability of items, for instance, or when interpreting differences between groups on the same task.

When developing material for testing memory and learning functions, the examiner may find Toglia and Battig's *Handbook of Semantic Word Norms* (1978) a useful reference. These authors give ratings for 2,854 English words (and some "nonwords") along the seven dimensions of concreteness, imagery, categorizability, meaningfulness, familiarity, number of attributes or features, and pleasantness, thus enabling the examiner to develop equatable or deliberately biased word lists on a rational, tested basis. A "meaningfulness" list of 319 five-letter (alternating consonant with vowel, e.g., "vapor," "money," "sinew") words and word-like constructs (i.e., *paralogs*) was developed by Locascio and Ley (1972). Paivio and his colleagues (1968) graded 925 nouns for concreteness, imagery, and meaningfulness. Palermo and Jenkins's *Word Association Norms* (1964) provides a great deal of data on word frequencies and their relatedness. An exhaustive reference for frequency of 86,741 English words is available (J.B. Carroll, Davies, and Richman, 1971).

Brief word learning tests

When circumstances require that memory be assessed quickly, such as at the hospital bedside, a short word learning task provides useful information. Probably the word-learning test familiar to most clinicians comes from the mental status examination used by medical practitioners, especially psychiatrists and neurologists, to evaluate their patients' mental conditions. In the course of the evaluation interview the patient is given three or four unrelated, common words (some examiners use a name or date, an address, and a flower name or florist's order, such as "two dozen yellow roses") to repeat, with instructions to remember these items for recall later. The patient must demonstrate accurate immediate repetition of all the words or phrases so that there is no question about their having been registered.

For some patients, this may require several repetitions. Once assured that the patient has registered the words, the examiner continues to question the patient about other issues—work history, family background—or may give other brief items of the examination for approximately 5 min. The patient is then asked to recall the words. The widely used Mini-Mental State Examination (MMSE) tests memory with recall of three words after a few minutes with an intervening task (M.F. Folstein et al., 1975; see pp. 706–709). Strub and Black (2000) give *Four Unrelated Words* with recall after delays of 5, 10, and 30 mins and provide norms for five decades from the 40s to 80s.

Most persons under age 60 have no difficulty recalling all three or four words or phrases after 5 or 10 mins (Strub and Black, 2000). Thus, correct recall of two out of three or even three out of four raises the question of a retention deficit in middle-aged and younger persons (Beardsall and Huppert, 1991). Most data sugggest that approximately 50% of adults, including those over 85 years, can recall all three words and another 30%–40% can recall two of the words (Bleeker, Bolla-Wilson, Kawas, and Agnew, 1988; Heeren, Lagaay, von Beek et al., 1990). In another study approximately 25% of healthy adults aged 50 and older (up to 95) recalled all three words and 40% recalled two of the three words (Cullum, Thompson, and Smernoff, 1993). All studies agree that recall of only one of three words at any age usually indicates that verbal learning is impaired. Using a cut-off of less than two words, this memory test had an 82% accuracy rate in distinguishing patients with mild dementia from controls (Derrer et al., 2001). Stuss, Binns, and their collaborators (2000) report that when TBI patients could recall "three little words" predicted return of continuous memory.

A three-item stimulus (table, red, 23 Broadway) has been used as a brief memory assessment with 2,000 presumably intact persons in the 50 to 93 age range (Jenkyn et al., 1985). With a criterion of failure of one or more errors, failed performances were made by 14% to 19% of subjects between the ages of 50 and 64, by 24% to 28% of those in the age range 65 and 79, and by 55% of persons over age 80. Unfortunately, how many persons made only one error is not reported. Yet it is evident that the one error = failure criterion may be too stringent for older persons. Again using only three words, 28 healthy subjects 75 years and older recalled an average of 2.0 ± 1.0 words (Beardsall and Huppert, 1991). The relative crudity of the three-word format has led some clinicians to favor one with four words (Petersen, 1991; Strub and Black, 2000). Godwin-Austen and Bendall (1990) use a 7-word address.

Among the many variants to the basic three- or four-word format is one in which the examiner identifies their categories when naming the words (e.g., "Detroit, a city; yellow, a color; lily, a flower; apple, a fruit."). On the first recall trial, the examiner asks for the words. Should the patient omit any, the examiner can then see whether cuing by category will aid the patient's recall. When cuing improves recall, a retrieval rather than a storage problem is implicated. Upon satisfying himself that the patient could recall several words after a short time span, Luria (1973b) used two three-word lists, giving the patient "Series 2" after the patient had learned the three common words in "Series 1." When the second series had been learned, Luria then asked for recall of Series 1 as a test of the patient's capacity to maintain the organization and time relationships of subsets of learned material.

C. Ryan and Butters (1982) used four words in a version of the Brown-Peterson technique. Following the one-per-second reading of four unrelated words (e.g., anchor, cherry, jacket, and pond), patients were given a three-digit number with instructions to count backward from that number by threes for 15 or 30 seconds, at which time they were instructed to recall the words. This technique was quite sensitive in eliciting an age gradient for normal subjects that was paralleled, at significantly lower levels, by alcoholics at the three tested age levels. Since the four (or three) words differ on each subsequent trial, this format is effective in bringing out perseverative tendencies (N. Butters, 1985).

In still another variation, two three-word sets (rose, ball, key; brown, tulip, honesty) were given for immediate recall, each word set administered at a different time during the examination (Cullum, Thompson, and Smernoff, 1993). Subjects were not told that they would be asked to recall the words later. Although the words are repeated up to three times as needed to retain for immediate recall, and the delayed recall trial comes only two to three minutes later, fewer than 30% of subjects age 50+ recalled all three of the first set of words, while one-third of them recalled one or none; only 10% recalled all three of the second set, with 60% recalling none. The expected age gradient appeared, with subjects in the 80- to 95-year age range remembering the fewest words; education was not associated with recall prowess. As the lower word frequency for "tulip" and "honesty" may account for the very great differences in rate of recall between the two word lists, the authors caution that word difficulty be considered when giving word learning tests.

Strub and Black (2000) use four words that can be cued in several ways and ask for recall at 10 and 30 min as well as 5 min. Should any words be missed on spontaneous recall, the examiner provides different cues, such as the initial phoneme of the abstract word, the category of the color, a familiar characteristic of the flower, etc. When cueing fails, they recommend a recognition technique (e.g., "Was the flower a rose, tulip, daisy, or petunia?") to help determine whether the patient's problem is one of storage or retrieval. The additional 10 and 30 sec recalls elicited a rebound effect in which recall improved with delay for each of their five age groups (e.g., recall at 5 and 10 secs for subjects in their 60s was 2.0 and 3.0 words, respectively; for the 80s it was 2.1 and 2.7 words); 30 sec recalls for all but the 40s group were even higher than 10 sec recall (e.g., 3.5 for the 60s group). Moreover, both stage I and II Alzheimer patients showed the rebound effect at 10 sec with a slight drop at 30 sec that was still higher than the 5 sec recall (e.g., stage I: 1.6, 1.9, 1.8 at 5, 10, and 30 secs).

Benson Bedside Memory Test (D. Frank Benson, personal communication [dbh])

Frank Benson used eight words in an informal examination of memory (see Table 11.3). The eight words are read to the patient and with recall after each of four trials. Free recall is obtained after a 5 to 10 min delay followed by a category-cued recall for any omissions, followed by multiple choice prompting if necessary. Although this task takes only minutes it is sensitive to delayed recall impairment. Most adults can acquire 7 or 8 of the words during the four presentations and should be able to recall approximately 6 freely and the remainder with cues.

Word Span and Supraspan

The number of words normal subjects recall immediately remains relatively stable through the early and middle adult years. Five age groups (20s to 60s) comprising a total of 200 men, were tested with familiar one-syllable words in lists ranging in length from four

TABLE 11.3 Benson Bedside
Memory Test

Words	Category Cue
Cabbage	Vegetable
Table	Furniture
Dog	Animal
Baseball	Sport
Chevrolet	Automobile make
Rose	Flower
Belt	Article of clothing
Blue	Color

to 13 words (Talland, 1965b). Beyond five-word lists, average recall scores hovered around 5.0. The five age groups did not differ on recall of lists of four to seven words. The two oldest groups showed a very slight but statistically significant tendency to do a little less well than the youngest groups on the 9- and 11-word lists, and the three oldest groups did less well on the 13-word list. The greatest difference between the oldest and youngest groups was on the 9-word list on which the 20–29 age group averaged 5.6 words and the 60–69 age group averaged 5.0 words. A significant drop with aging in number of words recalled was also documented by Delbecq-Derouesné and Beauvois (1989). Recall data from 12 lists of 15 words each for five age ranges (20–25 to > 65) indicated that subjects in the 55–65 age range and older retrieved significantly fewer words, recalling many fewer from the beginning and middle of the lists than did three younger age groups. When tested first with a two-word list and adding a word with each successful repetition while maintaining the original word order, the word span of a group of control subjects again averaged 5.0 (E. Miller, 1973). Control subjects learned word lists of one, two, and three words longer than their word span in two, four, and more than ten trials, respectively.

Word list learning tests provide a ready-made opportunity to examine supraspan. Rather than use random words, some examiners test supraspan with shopping lists to enhance the task's appearance of practical relevance (Delis, Kramer, Kaplan, and Ober, 1987, 2000; Flicker, Ferris, and Reisberg, 1991; Teng, Wimer, et al., 1989). Of those tests with unrelated words in most common use, the Selective Reminding procedure usually presents a 12-word list and the Auditory-Verbal Learning Test (AVLT) list contains 15 words. Based on tests from 301 adults, Trahan, Goethe, and Larrabee (1989) found that on first hearing a 12-word list, the average recall of younger adults (18–41) was approximately six, recall dropped to an average of five words for persons age 54–65, persons 66–77 years old recalled between four and five words, and the average for a 78+ group was four words. On the basis of these data, Trahan and his colleagues recommended that recall of fewer than four words be considered impaired up to age 54; and that for ages 54 and older, the impaired classification begin with recalls of two or less. Slightly higher spans have been reported for Trial I of the AVLT in samples of healthy, well-educated subjects (Ivnik, Malec, Smith, et al., 1992a). M. Schmidt (1996) computed metanorms for nine adult age groups divided by sex.

On supraspan learning tasks, it appears that both short-term retention and learning capacities of intact subjects are engaged (S.C. Brown and Craik, 2000; see also Vallar and Papagno, 2000, for a discussion of the many systems contributing to supraspan recall). Many brain impaired patients do as well as normal subjects on the initial trial but have less learned carry-over on subsequent trials (e.g., Lezak, 1979). Short-term retention in patients whose learning ability is defective also shows up in a far better recall of the words at the end of the list than those at the beginning (the *recency effect*), as the presentation of new words in excess of the patient's immediate memory span interferes with retention of the words first heard. Normal subjects, on the other hand, tend to show a *primacy* as well as a recency effect, consistently having better recall for the words at the beginning of the list than for most of the other words. Moreover, when the full list is repeated for each learning trial, subjects whose memory system is intact are much more likely to develop an orderly recall pattern that does not vary much from trial to trial except as new words are added. By trial IV or V, many subjects with good learning capacity repeat the list in almost the same order as it is given.

On word list tests in which unrelated words are presented in the same order on each learning trial, the subject's learning strategy can be examined for efficiency. On the initial hearing most normal individuals show a primacy and recency effect in which they recall most easily the first and last few words from the list but they tend to switch strategies after the second or later trials and begin their recall with the words they had not yet said, thereby minimizing proactive interference effects. In addition to these strategies, many subjects make semantic associations between the words and recall subgroups of words in the same order from trial to trial (e.g., on the AVLT, school-bell; on the California Verbal Learning Test [CVLT], recognition of one or more of the predefined categories). A review of the order in which patients recall words over the five trials will show whether they are following this normal pattern. Patients who fail to show this or any other pattern may have approached the task passively, may be unable to develop a strategy, or may not appreciate that a strategy is possible. Asking the patient at the conclusion whether any particular technique was used for learning the words often clarifies whether strategies were developed intentionally.

Impairment in the ability to put time tags on learned material is assessed by the subject's accuracy in distinguishing each of the two lists on the short-term and delayed recall trials and on the recognition trial of the AVLT or CVLT, or by the presence of intrusions from previously administered tests. For example, items from the Boston Naming Test when seen earlier might appear among the recalled words. For confused patients, even words from the instructions, such as "remember,"

may be produced. Intrusions of words not in any test shows a tendency for interference from internal associations and, sometimes, disinhibition.

A few times in the course of the series of learning trials most persons will repeat on the same trial a word already given on that trial. This kind of repetition is not "perseveration." Rather, most patients who repeat an abnormal number of words on word list learning tests have attentional problems such that they have difficulty keeping track of what they have already said while searching their memory for other words; in short, they cannot do two things at once: monitor their performances and engage in a memory search. *Perseveration* refers to mental stickiness or "stuck in set" phenomena that are more likely to occur with specific patterns of cognitive dysfunction such as those associated with significant frontal lobe damage, some aphasic disorders, etc. *Repetition* must not be confused with *perseveration*.

Auditory–Verbal Learning Test (AVLT)
(A. Rey, 1964; M. Schmidt, 1996)

In 1916 Edouard Claparède developed a one-trial word list learning test composed of 15 words which were later used by André Rey to form the AVLT (Boake, 2000). This easily administered test affords an analysis of learning and retention using a five-trial presentation of a 15-word list (list A), a single presentation of an interference list (List B), two postinterference recall trials—one immediate, one delayed—and recognition of the target words presented with distractors. By this means the examiner easily obtains measures that are crucial for understanding the kind and severity of a patient's memory deficits: immediate word span under overload conditions (trial I), final acquisition level (trial V), total acquisition (ΣI–V), amount learned in five trials (trial V − trial I), proactive interference (trial I − trial B), retroactive interference (trial V − trial VI), delayed recall (trial VII), recognition, number of repetitions, and number and types of intrusions. Retention should be examined after an extended delay, from 20 to 45 minutes—most usually, around 30. In some instances the examiner may wish to determine retention after longer periods, such as one hour or the next day. The original French words and their order were translated without change to English. Other language versions include Flemish (Lannoo and Vingerhoets, 1997), German (H. Mueller et al., 1997), Hebrew (Vakil and Blachstein, 1993), and Spanish (Miranda and Valencia, 1997).

For trial I, the examiner reads a list (A^1) of 15 words (see Table 11.4) at the rate of one per second after giving the following instructions:

TABLE 11.4 Rey Auditory-Verbal Learning Test Word Lists

List A[1]	B[1]	AC[2]	BC[2]	A/JG[3]	B/JG[3]	C
Drum	Desk	Doll	Dish	Violin	Orange	Book
Curtain	Ranger	Mirror	Jester	Tree	Armchair	Flower
Bell	Bird	Nail	Hill	Scarf	Toad	Train
Coffee	Shoe	Sailor	Coat	Ham	Cork	Rug
School	Stove	Heart	Tool	Suitcase	Bus	Meadow
Parent	Mountain	Desert	Forest	Cousin	Chin	Harp
Moon	Glasses	Face	Water	Earth	Beach	Salt
Garden	Towel	Letter	Ladder	Knife	Soap	Finger
Hat	Cloud	Bed	Girl	Stair	Hotel	Apple
Farmer	Boat	Machine	Foot	Dog	Donkey	Chimney
Nose	Lamb	Milk	Shield	Banana	Spider	Button
Turkey	Gun	Helmet	Pie	Radio	Bathroom	Log
Color	Pencil	Music	Insect	Hunter	Casserole	Key
House	Church	Horse	Ball	Bucket	Soldier	Rattle
River	Fish	Road	Car	Field	Lock	Gold

[1]Taken from E.M. Taylor, *Psychological Appraisal of Children with Cerebral Defects.* © 1959 by Harvard University Press.

[2]Developed by Crawford, Stewart, and Moore (1989). © Swets and Zeitlinger.

[3]Developed by Jones-Gotman, Sziklas, and Majdan (personal communication, March 1993).

I am going to read a list of words. Listen carefully, for when I stop you are to tell me as many words as you can remember. It doesn't matter in what order you repeat them.

On first hearing the long list some patients may be distracted by fear of failure, so it is desirable to include in the instruction:

There are so many words that you won't remember them all the first time. Just try to remember as many as you can.

The examiner writes down the words recalled in the order in which they are recalled, thus keeping track of the pattern of recall, noting whether the patient has associated two or three words, proceeded in an orderly manner, or demonstrated hit-or-miss recall. *Examiners should not confine themselves to a structured response form* but rather take down responses on a sheet of paper large enough to allow for many repetitions and intrusions as well as for high-level—and therefore very wordy—performances. Use of record sheets in which words from the list are checked or numbered in order of recall from trial to trial delays the inexperienced examiner as some patients recall the words so fast that finding the words to check is difficult. Moreover, preformed record sheets do not allow the examiner to keep track of where intrusions or repetitions occur in the course of the subject's verbalizations on any one trial. It is usually possible to keep up with fast responders by simply recording the word's initial first two or three letters when more than one word on the list begins with the same letter (e.g., CUrtain, COFfee, COLor). Should patients ask whether they have already said a word, the examiner informs them, but does not volunteer that a word has been repeated as this tends to distract some patients and interfere with their performance. It also may alert some patients to monitor their responses—a good idea that may not have occurred to them without external advice.

When patients indicate that they can recall no more words, the examiner rereads the list, following a second set of instructions:

Now I'm going to read the same list again, and once again when I stop I want you to tell me as many words as you can remember, *including words you said the first time.* It doesn't matter in what order you say them. Just say as many words as you can remember, whether or not you said them before.

This set of instructions must emphasize inclusion of previously said words, for otherwise some patients will assume it is an elimination test.

The list is reread for trials III, IV, and V, using trial II instructions each time. The examiner may praise patients as they recall more words. Patients may be told the number of words recalled, particularly if they are able to use the information for reassurance or as a challenge. On completion of each ten-word trial of a similar word learning test, Luria (1966) asked his patients to estimate how many words they would recall on the next trial. In this way, along with measuring verbal learning, one can also obtain information about the accuracy of patients' self-perceptions, appropriateness of their goal setting, and their ability to apply data about themselves. This added procedure requires very little time or effort for the amount of information it may afford, and it does not seem to interfere with the learning or recall process. On completion of trial V, the examiner tells the patient:

Now I'm going to read a second list of words. This time, again, you are to tell me as many words of this second list as you can remember. Again, the order in which you say the words does not matter. Just try to tell me as many words as you can.

The examiner then reads the second word list (B^1), and writes down the words in the order in which the patient says them. Following the B-list trial, the examiner asks the patient to recall as many words from the first list as possible (trial VI). Also without forewarning, the 20- to 45-minute delayed recall trial (VII) measures how well the patient recalls what was once learned. Normally few if any, words recalled on trial VI are lost after this short a delay (e.g., Mitrushina, Boone, and D'Elia, 2000; M. Schmidt, 1996).

The score for each trial is the number of words correctly recalled. A total score, the sum of trials I through V, can also be calculated. Words that are repeated can be marked R; RC when patients repeat themselves and then self-correct; or RQ if they question whether they have repeated themselves but remain unsure. Subjects who want to make sure they did not omit saying a word they remembered may repeat a few words after recalling a suitable number for that trial. However, lengthy repetitions, particularly when the subject can recall relatively few words, most likely reflect a problem in self-monitoring and tracking, along with a learning defect.

Words offered that are not on the list are errors and marked E. Frequently an error made early in the test will reappear on subsequent trials, often in the same position relative to one or several other words. Intrusions from list A into the recall of list B or from B into recall trial VI are errors that can be marked A or B.

See Table 11.5 for an example of scored errors. The 28-year-old ranch hand and packer who gave this set of responses had sustained a right frontotemporal contusion requiring surgical reduction of swelling just two years before the examination. Since the accident he had been unable to work because of poor judgment, disorientation, and personality deterioration.

This method of marking errors enables the examiner to evaluate the quality of the performance at a glance. Patients who make intrusion errors tend to have difficulty in maintaining the distinction between information coming from the outside and their own associations; those who give a List A response on Trial B, or a List B response on later trials tend to confuse data obtained at different times. Some, such as the patient whose performance is given in Table 11.5, have difficulty maintaining both kinds of distinctions, which suggests a serious breakdown in self-monitoring functions.

TABLE 11.5 Sample AVLT Record Illustrating Error Scoring

I	II	III	IV	V	B	VI
Hat 1	Drum 1	River 1	Drum 1	River 1	Desk 1	Drum 1
Garden 2	Curtain 2	House 2	Curtain 2	House 2	Ranger 2	Curtain 2
Moon 3	Bell 3	Turkey 3	Hat 3	School 3	Glasses 3	Bell 3
Turkey 4	House 4	Farmer 4	School 4	Bell 4	Bell A	Parent 4
Hose EA	River 5	Water EC	Parent 5	Farmer 5	Pet EA	School 5
	Hose EA	Color 5	Farmer 6	Drum 6	Fish 4	Moon 6
	Drum R	Drum 6	Color 7	Curtain 7	Glasses R	Teacher EA
	Bell R	Curtain 7	Nose 8	Bell R	Mountain 5	Turkey 7
	Curtain R	Garden 8	Turkey 9	School R	Cloud 6	Coffee 8
	Drum R	Hat 9	Color R	Parent 8	Bell AR	Color 9
		Hose EA	School R	Coffee 9		
		Garden R	Nose R	School R		
		Turkey R	Drum R	Parent R		
		Farmer R	Turkey R	Color 10		
		School 10	Farmer R	Moon 11		
		Parent 11				
4	5	11	9	11	6	9
1 EA	1 EA	1 EA	6 R	4 R	2 A (1 R)	1 EA
	4 R	1 EC			1 EC	
		3R			2 R	

A recognition trial should be given to all patients except those who recall 14 or more words on trial VII and have made no errors (confabulations, list confusions, associations, or other intrusions), for the likelihood of recognition errors by these latter subjects is slim. In testing recognition, the examiner asks the patient to identify as many words as possible from the first list when shown (or read if the patient has a vision or literacy problem) a list of 50 words containing all the items from both the A and B lists as well as words that are semantically associated (S) or phonemically similar (P) to words on lists A or B; or the alternate word sets (see Table 11.6). The instruction is given as the patient is handed the recognition sheet and a pencil:

I am going to show you a page with words on it. Circle the words from the first list I read to you. Some of the words you see here are from the first list and some are from the second list I read to you only once. Some of these words were not on either list. Just circle the ones from the first list, the list I read five times.

Some subjects circle relatively few words and need encouraging. It is possible to keep two scores by giving them a different colored pencil after they said they were finished, telling them:

TABLE 11.6 Word Lists for Testing AVLT Recognition, Lists A–B

Bell (A)*	Home (SA)	Towel (B)	Boat (B)	Glasses (B)
Window (SA)	Fish (B)	Curtain (A)	Hot (PA)	Stocking (SB)
Hat (A)	Moon (A)	Flower (SA)	Parent (A)	Shoe (B)
Barn (SA)	Tree (PA)	Color (A)	Water (SA)	Teacher (SA)
Ranger (B)	Balloon (PA)	Desk (B)	Farmer (A)	Stove (B)
Nose (A)	Bird (B)	Gun (B)	Rose (SPA)	Nest (SPB)
Weather (SB)	Mountain (B)	Crayon (SA)	Cloud (B)	Children (SA)
School (A)	Coffee (A)	Church (B)	House (A)	Drum (A)
Hand (PA)	Mouse (PA)	Turkey (A)	Stranger (PB)	Toffee (PA)
Pencil (B)	River (A)	Fountain (PB)	Garden (A)	Lamb (B)

Recognition Lists AC-BC[1]

Nail (A)	Envelope (SA)	Ladder (B)	Foot (B)	Water (B)
Sand (SA)	Car (B)	Mirror (A)	Bread (PA)	Joker (SB)
Bed (A)	Face (A)	Screw (SA)	Desert (A)	Coat (B)
Pony (SA)	Toad (PA)	Music (A)	Street (SA)	Captain (SA)
Jester (B)	Silk (PA)	Dish (B)	Machine (A)	Tool (B)
Milk (A)	Hill (B)	Pie (B)	Head (SPA)	Fly (SPB)
Plate (SB)	Forest (B)	Wood (SB)	Girl (B)	Song (SA)
Heart (A)	Sailor (A)	Ball (B)	Horse (A)	Doll (A)
Jail (PA)	Dart (PA)	Helmet (A)	Soot (PB)	Stall (PA)
Insect (B)	Road (A)	Stool (PB)	Letter (A)	Shield (B)

Recognition Lists A/JB-B/JB

Rock (PB)	Star (SA)	Soap (B)	Television (SA)	Violin (A)
Corn (PB)	Peel (SA)	Frog (SB)	Hotel (B)	Beach (B)
Pear (SA)	Lock (B)	Dog (A)	Piano (SA)	Radio (A)
Tree (A)	Banana (A)	Orange (B)	Spider (B)	Bus (B)
Cork (B)	Toad (B)	Cousin (A)	Bucket (A)	Doctor
Bread	Uncle (SA)	Bathroom (B)	Soldier (B)	Chest
Sofa (SB)	Earth (A)	Gloves (SA)	Scarf (A)	Knife (A)
Stair (A)	Hospital (SB)	Field (A)	Wife (SA)	Donkey (B)
Ham (A)	Grass (SA)	Armchair (B)	Train (SB)	Hunter (A)
Casserole (B)	Lunchbox (SA)	Blanket (PA)	Suitcase (A)	Chin (B)

*(A) Words from List A; (B) words from list B; (S) word with a semantic association to a word on list A or B as indicated; (P) word phonemically similar to a word on list A or B, (SP) words both semantically and phonemically similar to a word on the indicated list.
[1]Reprinted with permission (Crawford, Steward, and Moore, 1989).

There were 15 words on that list. See if you can find the rest of them even if you have to guess.

This technique allows the examiner to distinguish between those patients who do not recognize the additional words and make many errors from those who are overly cautious and use a high confidence threshold in their responding.

Others—often patients whose judgment appears to be compromised in other ways as well—check 20 or even 25 of the words, indicating that they neither appreciated the list's length nor maintained discrimination between list A, list B, and various kinds of associations to the target words. These patients can be instructed that the list contained only 15 words and asked to review the recognition sheet, marking with an X only those they are sure were on the list. Without this procedure the accuracy of their recall and ability to sort out what comes to mind cannot be ascertained.

The recognition procedure measures how much was learned, regardless of the efficiency of spontaneous retrieval. Comparison of the recognition and delayed recall scores provides a measure of the efficiency of spontaneous retrieval. Recognition scores below 13 are relatively rare among intact persons under age 59 (Mitrushina, Boone, and D'Elia, 2000; M. Schmidt, 1996), and scores under 12 are infrequent among 55- to 69-year-olds (Ivnik, Malec, Smith, et al., 1992a; Mitrushina, Boone, and D'Elia, 1999). Further, the recognition score examines the patient's capacity to discriminate when or with what other information a datum was learned. This technique may elicit evidence of disordered recall like that which troubles patients with impaired frontal lobe functions who can learn readily enough but cannot keep track of what they have learned or make order out of it. If the patient's problem is simply difficulty in retaining new information, then recognition will be little better than recall on trial VII.

The third word list (C) is available should either the A- or B-list presentations be spoiled by interruptions, improper administration, or confusion or premature response on the patient's part. List C is really an emergency list as words from it are not represented on the AB recognition sheet, thus reducing the recognition format's sensitivity to intrusion and confusion tendencies. Evidence that list C is easier than list B suggests that scores one point higher might be expected for list C trial B and for list A trials VI and VII when using list C as a distractor (Fuller et al., 1997). However, list C was found to be comparable to list A, with individual measures correlating in the .60 to .77 range, and all but three mean differences (favoring list A and appearing on trials IV, V, and VI) no greater than one word (J.J. Ryan, Geisser, et al., 1986). When list C was compared with list A as an alternate learning list in a large study of young gay and bisexual men who were HIV seronegative, it was mostly equivalent although it was slightly more difficult to learn (Uchiyama et al., 1995). Another study found essentially no difference between lists A and C for trials I, III, V, VI, VII, and the recognition trial (Delaney, Prevey, et al., 1988).

As is typical of memory tests practice effects can be pronounced (see pp. 116–117; McCaffrey, Duff, and Westervelt, 2000b). For example, significant improvement on almost all measures appeared on retesting after almost one month, with many increases exceeding one word and an almost three-word difference appearing on trial I (Crawford, Stewart, and Moore, 1989). Thus, the same lists should not be given twice in succession. Ideally, the examiner will have alternate lists with the recognition trial sheet available. Alternate forms are *parallel forms* if they produce results equivalent to the original versions. Crawford, Stewart, and Moore (1989) and Majdan and her colleagues (1996) have developed parallel lists (see Table 11.4) with appropriate sets of words for recognition testing (see Table 11.6). M. Schmidt (1996) provides other parallel forms in English and in German plus three of the four lists Rey (1964) said he had "borrowed [*emprutées*]" from Claparède.

However, it is not always possible to know in advance that the patient had been given the AVLT in a recent examination by someone else. When the parallel list material is not at hand for a second examination, the examiner can reverse the A and B lists, giving the B list five times and using the A list as interference. This manipulation reduces practice effects for all trials except the interference trial, as some patients will show remarkably good recall of the A list even after a year or more.

Normative data. Most young adults (ages 20–39) recall six or seven words on trial I and achieve 12 or 13 words by the fifth trial. The change in number of words recalled from trials I to V shows the rate of learning—the learning curve—or reflects little or no learning if the number of words recalled on later trials is not much more than given on trial I. In general, approximately 1.5 words are lost from trial V to trial VI, i.e., following the interference trial list (B); although after age 64 the spread between trials V and VI gradually increases from almost 2.0 (ages 65–69) to 3 (ages 75–79, 80+) (Sinnett and Holen, 1999). Little if any loss occurs between trials VI and VII, the delayed recall trial. Usually no more than one error shows up on the recognition trial (Mitrushina, Boone, and D'Elia, 1999; M. Schmidt, 1996). Marked variations from this general pattern will likely reflect some dysfunction of the memory system.

Michael Schmidt's (1996) metanorms are reliable for most purposes as several normative studies with relatively large samples have contributed to them. M.E. Harris and his colleagues (2002) have updated their recognition trial accuracy norms. A study of 1,818 homosexual men provides norms for this demographic group as part of a multicenter study of HIV (Uchiyama et al., 1995). M. Schmidt (1996) summarized the AVLT literature through 1995. Extensive reviews of normative data also appear in other sources (Mitrushina, Boone, and D'Elia, 1999; Spreen and Strauss, 1998).

Test characteristics. Word list learning is among the most sensitive verbal memory test formats because of the relative freedom from associative context compared with, for example, prose material. In offering an explanation for the effectiveness of every AVLT learning measure (each trial, Σ trials I–V, *learning* [high score − trial I], in distinguishing normal control subjects from a group of patients with "medically confirmed neuropathologies," J.B. Powell and his colleagues (1991) suggested that these scores "reflect the combined functioning of a wider cross section of neurobehavioral mechanisms, including arousal, motivation, attention/concentration, auditory perception, verbal comprehension, immediate verbal memory span, short-term verbal memory storage and retrieval, and progressive learning abilities" (p. 248). This study found that each of these AVLT scores discriminated between these groups better than each of the Halstead-Reitan measures, the Stroop (Dodrill format), and either Logical Memory or Visual Reproduction (WMS).

It is not surprising that age effects show up on word list tests. Using a Hebrew version of the AVLT, Vakil and Blachstein (1997) found modest changes below the age of 60 compared to increasingly reduced recall after 60. In this study the measures most affected by age were trial V and total acquisition score (ΣI–V), list B, and the first delayed recall (trial VI). Minimal age effects were found for the forgetting rate. This task becomes challenging for persons over 70 years. They typically recall five words on trial I, achieve 10 words by trial V, lose two or three words between trials V and VI, and make two or three errors on the recognition task (M. Schmidt, 1996). Healthy elderly subjects, in comparison with younger ones, show greater forgetting of words at the end of the list during delayed recall (Carlesimo et al., 1997). This suggests that older subjects rely much more on short-lived memory processes—i.e., the immediate recall of the last words on the list—than do younger people.

Sex too plays a role, as women's means on many of the AVLT measures tend to run higher than men's means, from as little as .1 (on a recognition trial) to more than 2.0 words (on recall items) (Bleecker, Bolla-Wilson, Agnew, and Meyers, 1988; Geffen, Moar, et al., 1990). Instances in which men's mean scores are the same or better than women's scores are relatively rare (e.g., R.M. Savage and Gouvier, 1992). Education, verbal facility as measured by vocabulary (WAIS-R), and general mental ability also contribute significantly to performances on this test (Bolla-Wilson and Bleecker, 1986; Ripich et al., 1997; Selnes, Jacobson, et al., 1991; Uchiyama et al., 1995; Wiens et al., 1988).

This test has high test-retest reliability. Using alternate forms with a retest interval of one month, correlations ranged from .61 to .86 for trials I–V and from .51 to .72 for delayed recall and recognition (Delaney, Prevey, Cramer, et al., 1992). Test–retest reliability correlation coefficients after one year ranged from .38 (for trial B) to .70 (for trial V) (W.G. Snow, Tierney, Zorzitto, et al., 1988). Factor analytic studies show that the learning measures of the AVLT (V, VI, recognition) correlate significantly—mostly in the .50 to .65 range—with other learning measures (Macartney-Filgate and Vriezen, 1988; J.J. Ryan, Rosenberg, and Mittenberg, 1984). The supraspan measure, trial I, probably reflects its large attentional component in negligible (.17 to −.13) correlations with the learning measures (Macartney-Filgate and Vriezen, 1988). An evaluation of the comparability of the AVLT with the CVLT produced correlations of .32 for trial I, .33 for trial V, .47 for total words recalled, and .37 for short delay recall (Crossen and Wiens, 1994). A factor analysis of scores made by 146 normal volunteers for Trials I, V, B, VI, VII, Recognition, and a temporal order measure produced three basic factors: retrieval, storage, and acquisition (short-term memory) (Vakil and Blachstein, 1993). The first factor included performance on temporal order and trials VII, B, and V; the second factor included only the Recognition score; and trials I and B entered into the third factor.

Neuropsychological findings. Ordinarily, the immediate memory span for digits and the number of words recalled on trial I will be within one or two points of each other, providing supporting evidence regarding the length of span. Larger differences usually favor the digit span and seem to occur in patients with intact immediate memory and concentration who become confused by too much stimulation (stimulus overload). These patients tend to have difficulty with complexity of any kind, doing better with simplified, highly structured tasks. When the difference favors the more difficult word list retention task, the lower digit span score is usually due to inattentiveness, lack of motivation, or anxiety at the time Digit Span was given.

Slowness in shifting from one task to another can show up in a low score on trial I. When this occurs in a person whose immediate verbal memory span is *within normal limits,* recall B will be two or three words longer than that of trial I, usually *within normal limits.* In these cases trial II recall will show a much greater rate of acquisition than what ordinarily characterizes the performance of persons whose initial recall is abnormally low; occasionally a large jump in score will not take place until trial III. When this phenomenon is suspected, the examiner should review the pattern of the patient's performance on other tests in which slowness in establishing a response set might show up, such as Block Design (e.g., a patient who gets one point at most on each of the first two standard administration designs [i.e., 5 and 6], and does designs 7, 8, and 9 accurately and, often, faster than the first two; or a verbal fluency performance in which the patient's productivity increases with each trial, even though the difficulty of the naming task may also have increased). In those cases in which recall of list B is much lower (by two or three words) than immediate recall on trial I, what was just learned has probably interfered with the acquisition of new material; i.e., there is a *proactive interference* effect. When proactive interference is very pronounced, intrusion words from list A may show up in the list B recall too.

Most patients with brain disorders show a learning curve over the five trials. The appearance of a curve, even at a low level—e.g., from three or four words on trial I to eight or nine on V—demonstrates some ability to learn if some of the gain is maintained on the delayed recall trial, VII. Such patients may be capable of benefiting from psychotherapy or personal counseling and may profit from rehabilitation training and even formal schooling since they can learn, although at a slower rate than normal. Occasionally a once-bright but now severely memory impaired patient will have a large immediate memory span, recalling eight or nine words on trial I, but no more than nine or ten on V and very few on VI. Such a performance demonstrates the necessity of evaluating the scores for each trial in the context of other trials.

This test has proven useful in delineating memory system deficits in a variety of disorders. Some TBI patients will have a reduced recall for each measure but demonstrate a learning curve and some loss on delayed recall but a near normal performance on the recognition trial, indicating a significant verbal retrieval problem (Bigler, Rosa, et al., 1989; Peck and Mitchell, 1990). These patients tend to make a few intrusion errors. The AVLT has been effective in predicting psychosocial outcome after TBI (S.R. Ross et al., 1997).

With localized lesions, the AVLT elicits the expected memory system defects: Frontal lobe patients perform consistently less well than control subjects on recall trials but, given a recognition format for each trial, they show a normal learning curve (Janowsky, Shimamura, Kritchevsky, and Squire, 1989). Patients with left anterior temporal lobectomies show impaired delayed recall of words from the list (Majdan et al., 1996). Degree of left hippocampal atrophy measured by MRI in patients with temporal lobe epilepsy has been associated with severity of total recall and delayed recall deficits on this test (Kilpatrick et al., 1997). Before anterior temporal lobectomy, patients with left temporal lesions differed from those with lesions on the right only in lower scores on recall trials (VI and VII) and recognition; but after surgery they differed greatly on all AVLT measures (Ivnik, Sharbrough, and Laws, 1988). Miceli and his colleagues (1981) also found that patients with right hemisphere lesions did significantly better than those with lesions involving the left hemisphere, even though these latter patients were not aphasic. Korsakoff patients showed minimal improvement on the five learning trials, but when provided a recognition format for each trial they demonstrated learning that progressed much slower than normal and never quite reached the trial V normal level of virtually perfect recognition (Janowsky, Shimamura, Kritchersky, and Squire, 1989; Squire and Shimamura, 1986). These latter authors note that the usual recall format of the AVLT discriminates effectively between different kinds of amnesic patients.

Degenerative diseases have differing AVLT patterns. Low recall on almost all measures except for rate of forgetting, has been reported for multiple sclerosis patients compared to controls (Bravin et al., 2000). Patients with advanced Huntington's disease have, on the average, a greatly reduced immediate recall (fewer than four words), show a small learning increment, and drop down to trial I levels on delayed recall; a recognition format demonstrates somewhat more learning, and they are very susceptible to identifying a word as having been on the learning list when it was not (a false positive error) (N. Butters, Wolfe, et al., 1985, 1986). Patients with early Alzheimer type dementia have a very low recall for trial I and get to about six words by trial V (Bigler, Rosa et al., 1989; Mitrushina, Satz, and Van Gorp, 1989). They have particular difficulty recalling words after a delay with distraction (Woodard, Dunlosky, and Salthouse, 1999). While they recognize about two more words than they can recall, their performances are characterized by many more intrusions than any other diagnostic group (Bigler, Rosa, et al., 1989). Patients with mild cognitive deficits who are at risk for subsequent development of dementia have impaired performance (Petersen, Smith, Waring, et al., 1999; Tierney et al., 1996).

AVLT variants. Patients obviously incapable of learning even 10 of the 15 words experience the standard administration as embarrassing, drudgery, or both. Others may be easily overwhelmed by a lot of stimuli, or too prone to fatigue or restlessness to maintain performance efficiency with a 15-word format. Yet these patients often need a full-scale memory assessment. They can be given only the first 10 words, using the standard procedures. Although a 10-word ceiling is too low for most persons—controls and patients alike—it elicits discriminable performances from patients who, if given 15 words, would simply be unable to perform at their best. Minden, Moes, and their colleagues (1990) used this method to examine multiple sclerosis patients who, by virtue of impaired learning and retrieval functions, easy fatigability, and susceptibility to being overwhelmed and confused due to a reduced processing capacity, may perform better on a 10-word list. The 35 normal control subjects recalled 6 ± 1.4 words on trial I, 9.1 ± 1.2 on trial V, 5.1 ± 1.2 on list B, 7.6 ± 2.3 on trial VI, 7.1 ± 2.9 on trial VII, and then recognized 9.4 ± 1.0 of the words. MS patients were impaired on all measures relative to the controls.

In order to minimize cultural bias in the original AVLT word list for World Health Organization (WHO) research on HIV-1 infection (e.g., there are no turkeys and few curtains in Zaire), two new word lists were constructed from five common categories: body parts, animals, tools, household objects, and vehicles—all presumed "to have universal familiarity" (WHO/UCLA-AVLT) (Maj et al., 1993). List lengths and administration format remain the same. A comparison between subjects in Zaire and Germany indicated low intercultural variability with this new form. When given along with the original word list to persons in a Western country, correlations were in the .47 to .55 range.

Another administration variation ensures that the patient has attended to the words on the list. Using a list of ten words taken from AVLT lists B and C, Knopman and Ryberg (1989) required patients to read each word aloud, shown individually on index cards, and follow each word with a sentence they make up using that word. Dementia patients were able to accomplish this task. This was repeated for a second learning trial. Recall followed an interposed task five minutes after the second learning trial. This technique discriminated 55 normal subjects (M recall = 6.0 ± 1.8) from 28

Alzheimer patients (M recall = 0.8 ± 1.0), with no overlaps between the two groups. Correlations with a retest of the normal subjects six months later gave a coefficient of .75.

Vakil, Blachstein, and Hoofien (1991) also use this task to examine incidental recall of temporal order by giving subjects the A list, on which the order differs from the administration sequence, and asking them to rewrite the list in its original form. By giving two sets of administration instructions—one for intentional recall in which subjects are told that they should remember the word order, the other for incidental recall in which the need to remember the word order is not mentioned—Vakil and his colleagues demonstrated that much of temporal order judgment comes automatically. Correlations with other AVLT scores indicate a relationship between the incidental recall of temporal order and retention but not acquisition (Vakil and Blachstein, 1993).

California Verbal Learning Test (CVLT) (Delis, Kramer, Kaplan, and Ober, 1987); California Verbal Learning Test–Second Edition (CVLT-II) (Delis, Kramer, Kaplan, and Ober, 2000)

This word list task is designed to assess the use of semantic associations as a strategy for learning words. Each of the 16 words in each CVLT list belongs to one of four categories of "shopping list" items: for example, List A—"Monday's" list—contains four names of fruits, of herbs and spices, of articles of clothing, and of tools; List B—the "Tuesday" interference list—also contains names of fruits and of herbs and spices plus four kinds of fish and four kitchen utensils. The CVLT-II categories—no more shopping lists—for List A are vegetables, animals, ways of traveling, and furniture, with vegetables and animals in List B along with musical instruments and parts of buildings. The CVLT-II includes an alternate form and a short form (CVLT-IISF). The words are read at a rate slightly slower than one per second.

Category items are presented in a randomized order with instructions to recall the words in any order, thereby assessing the subject's spontaneous use of semantic associations. While examination of the use of strategies offers an advantage, it creates disadvantages as well. CVLT performance is a measure of the interaction between verbal memory and conceptual ability, so scores cannot be evaluated as exemplars of the patient's learning ability *per se* because of the possible confounding effects of concept apprehension and conceptual organization (Delis, 1989). However, when it is important to assess whether and how well a patient uses learning strategies based on concept formation, this test offers an advantage.

The procedure is identical for the two CVLT editions and similar to the AVLT. Following five trials with List A, the interference List B is read to the subject. Two "short delay" recalls of List A are obtained. The first of the two recall trials is "free" recall in which the request for the subject to "tell me all" remembered items from List A is identical to the AVLT free recall procedure. Immediately following the free recall trial the examiner asks the subject to recall items in each of the categories (fruits, then herbs and spices, etc.). For subjects who used semantic clustering during the learning phase, cueing at delayed recall offers little additional benefit. However, subjects who failed to make the semantic associations during the learning trials often benefit from this cueing. The enhanced recall due to cueing at the short delay also should carry over to the free recall requested 20 minutes later. This "long delay" trial measures recall of List A under the same two conditions, "free" and "cued." In one study, category cueing following short delay free recall failed to facilitate long delay recall in college students. The students receiving standard cueing instructions recalled the same number of words as students receiving no cueing during short delay recall even though the cued students used more semantic clustering in their delayed free recall than did those who received no cueing (P.K. Shear et al., 2000). The failure to find performance enhancement associated with cueing might have been due to a near ceiling effect as these students recalled an average of over 14 of the 16 words on trial 5.

The recognition trial format also differs from that of the AVLT in its oral presentation of just 44 items (48 on CVLT-II): of course all items of List A are included, but only eight from List B, two from each of the two overlapping categories and two from each of the two new categories. On the CVLT, four nonlist items each come from one of the four List A categories (e.g., tools: hammer; spices and herbs: pepper), eight items bear a phonetic resemblance to List A items (e.g., grapes: tapes, parsley, pastry); and the remaining eight are simply items one might find in a very large supermarket (e.g., film, clock). In my experience [mdl], these latter items have never elicited false positive errors.

Practice effects, which tend to be particularly prominent on memory tests (McCaffrey, Cousins, Westervelt, et al., 1995), led to the development by Delis, Kramer, and their coworkers (1983, 1987) of an alternate form of the CVLT that is parallel to the original in every respect (Delis, McKee, et al., 1991). Sixteen of the 19 scores (Principal CVLT Variables, see below) generated by this test were significantly correlated, half of these equal to or greater than $r = .67$.

Responding to the problems inherent in the original CVLT, Delis and his coworkers developed the CVLT-II. It is intended to replace the first test and not simply serve as an alternate form. Differences in the normative samples between tests preclude the interchangeability of standard score equivalents of raw scores between versions. The major changes are that the CVLT-II uses different categories of items that have higher familiarity than on the original form and the normative sample is much larger. An optional forced-choice recognition measure is obtained approximately 10 to 15 minutes after the yes/no recognition. Because forced-choice with completely unrelated items is easier than yes/no recognition, this measure was added to detect motivation lapses. Revisions have been made in calculating certain scores; repetitions are now called "repetitions," not "perseverations" and a new clustering score has been added.

A comparison of the CVLT and CVLT-II in a sample of 62 healthy adults tested approximately seven days apart on the two tests showed good equivalency in Total Trials 1–5 recall and Long-Delay Free Recall (Delis, Kaplan, Kramer, and Ober, 2000). Data for Short-Delay Recall and the cued recalls were not given. The CVLT and AVLT were compared in 60 normal adults and were found to provide similar information although scores were slightly higher on the CVLT (Crossen and Wiens, 1994). Raw scores for learning and short delay retention were nearly identical across tests for a TBI group given both in spite of the design differences in the tests (Stallings et al., 1995). German (Hildebrandt et al., 1998) and Korean (Kim and Kang, 1999) versions of the CVLT have been validated.

CVLT scores. In addition to the acquisition scores for trials 1, 5, and B, and retention of List A following free and cued trials for short and long delays, and *Recognition Hits,* other scores include: *List A Total Recall,* which is the sum of trials 1 through 5; *Learning Slope,* which quantifies the rate of learning; *Recall Consistency* on the learning trials; plus scores that reflect learning strategies (i.e., *Semantic Cluster Ratio, Serial-order Cluster Ratio,* and scores for primacy, recency tendencies); plus still more scores for comparing Trials I and B, free and cued recall, and recall and recognition and scores for such other response characteristics as repetitions (given the misnomer, *Perseverations,* see p. 422), *False Positives,* and *Intrusions* (for free and for cued recall trials). Together, not counting Number Correct scores for trials 2, 3, and 4, these total at least 19 different CVLT scores (27 on the research edition of the alternate CVLT form).

The CVLT-II changes the ways in which semantic and serial clustering scores are calculated, and a new subjective clustering score has been added. *Intrusions* and *repetitions* are scored and subtyped according to noncategory or category characteristics, and further into synonym/subordinate intrusions and across-list intrusions. Both *proactive* (intrusions from List A into List B recall) and *retroactive* (from List B into delayed recall and recognition trials) interference can be documented. Also included are scores for evaluating signal detection efficiency and response biases.

Many of the 27 CVLT scores (42 CVLT-II scores) with normative data are highly intercorrelated such that the most useful data are obtained from the List A trial 5, List A Σ1–5, semantic clustering, free and cued recall (both short and long delays), intrusions (both free and cued recall), and recognition hits and false positives (Elwood, 1995). All but semantic clustering is easily scored by hand, and in most cases the examiner knows whether or not the subject has used semantic clustering based on the obtained recall pattern without using a complex computational formula. A guide for calculating all of the supplementary scores by hand is included in the test manual. The publisher markets a computer scoring system which is helpful for complex calculations of such scores as Recognition Discriminabilty (CVLT-II) and Learning Slope, although the neuropsychological import of these scores remains in question.

Normative data. The CVLT manual provides normative data for 273 males and females in seven age groups covering 17 to 80 years. These data have been criticized for poor standardization and inflated norms (Elwood, 1995). Norms demographically corrected for age, education, ethnicity (Caucasians and African Americans), and sex are available (M.A. Norman et al., 2000). Norms for elderly males and females have been compiled by Paolo, Tröster, and Ryan (1997a). The CVLT-II has an improved normative sample of 1,087 adults in seven age groups ranging from 16 to 89 years and stratified according to the U.S. census by age, sex, ethnicity, educational level, and region of the country. Because age and sex account for significant differences between individuals, norms are provided for males and females within each age group.

Test characteristics. Age-associated CVLT performance decrements are seen, particularly at age 65 and beyond (Paolo, Tröster, and Ryan, 1997a; Pope, 1987). Significant age × Total Trials 1–5 correlations of −.61 for the original test and −.65 for the alternate form reflect the important contribution of age to recall (Delis, McKee, et al., 1991). For example, the learning curve is a little flatter for older persons. However, at least into the 60s, immediate span (trial 1) and recognition

remain essentially unchanged, with relatively few false positive errors (J.H. Kramer, Blusewicz, and Preston, 1989). A trend toward fewer clusters with advancing age has been reported (Pope, 1987). Interestingly, while the number of intrusions increased with advancing age, false positive errors on the recognition trial continue to be small (around 1.1 ± 2.2) into the 75 to 91 age range (Pope, 1987). Education correlations are positive and significant, but lower than those for age (.36 and .39 for original and alternate test forms, respectively) (Delis, McKee, et al., 1991).

In the sample used to produce demographically corrected norms, Caucasians outperformed African Americans and women were superior to men (M.A. Norman et al., 2000). It is unknown if the ethnicity effect would have been significant if the African Americans had been as well-educated as the Caucasians. Many studies show that women tend to outperform men on learning and recall measures of this test (Paolo, Tröster, and Ryan, 1997a; Ragland et al., 2000; Reite et al., 1993; Wiens, Tindall, and Crossen, 1994) although no sex differences showed up for the recognition trial or for error types (J.H. Kramer, Delis, and Daniel, 1988). Women use a semantic clustering strategy more often than men (Berenbaum et al., 1997; J.H. Kramer, Delis, and Daniel, 1988). Personal experience [dbh] suggests that men are less likely than women to make a distinction between the categories of fruit and herbs/spices, instead treating them all as "edibles." Some men are unfamiliar with spices such as paprika, further contributing to a breakdown in use of categories on the original CVLT. Based on a study of elderly men twin pairs, CVLT measures of learning and recall have a large genetic component (56% of total variance), whereas the genetic component is not significant on learning strategy or recognition memory (Swan et al., 1999).

Reliability studies undertaken by the test's authors give split-half (odd–even item, odd–even learning trials, 2 × 2 categories) reliability correlation coefficients of .77 to .86 (Delis, Kramer, Fridlund, and Kaplan, 1990). In older adults tested slightly over a year later, the stability coefficient for acquisition and long-delay free recall was .76 (Paolo, Tröster, and Ryan, 1997b). CVLT-II reliability correlations are also high (Delis, Kaplan, Kramer, and Ober, 2000). Split-half reliability correlations of scores from Total Trials 1–5 range from .87 to .89, and alternate form reliability ranges from .72 to .79 for various measures. Test–retest (21 days later) reliability was .82 for Total Trials, although it was much lower for some of the many variables, most notably Total Learning Slope (.27) and Total Repetitions (.30).

Factor analyses have consistently shown a large general verbal learning factor with small effects of response discrimination, learning strategy, proactive interference, and serial position (Delis, Freeland, et al., 1988; Millis, 1995; Schear and Craft, 1989; Vanderploeg, Schinka, and Retzlaff, 1994). An alternative four-factor model (attention span, learning efficiency, delayed recall, and inaccurate recall) has also been described (Wiegner and Donders, 1999). Together these studies demonstrate how different are various aspects of verbal memory, thus supporting the conceptual framework of this test. Attention plays a significant role in performance (Rapport, Axelrod, et al., 1997; Vanderploeg, Schinka, and Retzlaff, 1994). WAIS-R Vocabulary alone accounted for up to 13% of the variance (P.A. Keenan, Ricker, Lindamer, et al., 1996). Correlations with other memory tests are reported to be "modest" (Schear and Craft, 1989).

Neuropsychological findings. Clinical studies using the CVLT-II are few in number at the time of this writing. The CVLT-II performance of a small group of patients with circumscribed frontal lobe lesions was compared to that of control subjects (Baldo, Delis, et al., 2002). The frontal patients had a depressed learning curve, an increased tendency to make intrusions, reduced semantic cluster, and impaired yes/no recognition performance because of a tendency to endorse semantically related distractors and words from the interference list. Both groups slightly benefited from cueing and both recalled slightly more words in the Long-Delay Free Recall than in the Short-Delay Free Recall. The interpretation of these findings supported the theory that the frontal lobes play an important role in strategic memory processes and source memory. Using a 12-item version of the CVLT (three categories, four items each), Ricker, Müller, and their coworkers (2001) looked for cerebral blood flow changes by PET scanning during recall and recognition trials, and found differences between small samples of normal control subjects and of patients with severe traumatic injuries. Changes occurred predominantly in frontoparietal regions for both groups. On free recall, controls showed significant blood flow increases in the left middle frontal gyrus, left medial cerebellum, and left angular/ supramarginal gyrus whereas the patients showed only increase in the left angular supramarginal gyrus. On recognition testing, both groups had increased blood flow in the middle frontal gyri bilaterally, with the TBI patients experiencing a greater increase than control subjects.

Performance patterns generated by the CVLT effectively discriminate many—but not all—patient groups. The CVLT has been used to examine the interaction between memory and the frontal executive impairments associated with TBI (Deshpande et al., 1996; Haut and Shutty, 1992; Kibby et al., 1998; Novack et al., 1995). Crosson, Novack, and their colleagues (1989) describe three different memory problem patterns among TBI patients—consolidation deficits, impaired encoding, and retrieval deficiencies—which show up primarily in their *number correct* and *error* scores on the recognition trial. Deshpande and her colleagues (1996) elicited five learning subtypes using cluster analysis: "Active, Disorganized, and Passive" and two similar to a "Deficient subgroup." For example, the Active group were least impaired, the Disorganized group the most impaired, unable to profit from repetitions.

The interpretation of recognition–recall discrepancies as retrieval deficits has been challenged (Cicchetti, 1997; M.C. Wilde et al., 1995, 1997) and defended (Veiel, 1997a,b). Briefly, the argument is that recognition is easier than free recall for patients with retrieval deficits as it puts less demand on retrieval. Wilde and his colleagues (1995) tested this assumption by comparing TBI patients who had recognition–recall discrepancies with those who did not. Two predictions about patients with these discrepancies were not supported: that they would have better cued recall than free recall, and that they would have less consistent recall as measured by the Consistency Index. One prediction, that patients with recognition–recall discrepancies would show fewer intrusions during both free and cued recall, was supported. Wilde and his colleagues concluded that this study gave little support for the retrieval interpretation while Veiel accepted the partial support.

The CVLT performances of patients with left temporal lobe seizures differ from those of patients with seizures associated with right temporal lobe dysfunction and from normal control subjects on a number of variables including fewer words learned and fewer total number of words recalled, less semantic clustering, and poorer retrieval, although their recognition level was similar to that of the other two groups (B.P. Hermann, Wyler, Richey, and Rea, 1987). Mean scores also showed that patients with left temporal lobe involvement had a greater loss from trial V to short-term delayed recall and more false positive errors, but intragroup variability was so large that these differences did not reach significance. Most of the CVLT variables did not discriminate between patients with right temporal lobe involvement and normal subjects. Left anterior temporal lobectomy seizure patients have greater deficits after surgery than patients with comparable surgeries in the right hemisphere (K.G. Davies et al., 1998a,b). Using a German language version of the CVLT, Hildebrandt and his colleagues (1998) found that patients with strokes involving both the left prefrontal cortex and left temporal lobe were impaired in encoding and recall compared to a group with right posterior lesions. Performance of the left temporal lobe groups was significantly worse than that of the left prefrontal group for final learning level, short-term cued recall, and learning slope. Reliance on a serial clustering strategy was a distinguishing characteristic of patients with left mediotemporal lesions. Recognition performance was relatively intact in all the stroke groups. B.J. Diamond and his colleagues (1997) observed that patients with anterior communicating artery aneurysm were defective in both acquisition and retention of information, in scanty use of semantic cluster, and in making an abnormally large number of intrusion and false positive errors.

The CVLT readily elicits the memory problems of Alzheimer patients, even those with very mild disease (Bayley et al., 2000; Bondi, Monsch, Galasko, et al., 1994). Alzheimer patients recall fewer words from the beginning of the list than controls (Bayley et al., 2000); their greatest difficulty is with free recall on long delay (Massman, Delis, and Butters, 1993; Zakzanis, 1998). Learning and retention deficits in Alzheimer patients are associable to atrophy of the mesial temporal lobe and thalamus (Libon, Bogdanoff, et al., 1998; Stout et al., 1999). Many Parkinson patients do not spontaneously use semantic strategies as well as do controls (Knoke et al., 1998; van Spaendonck et al., 1996b). Because of the many variants of this disease, not all Parkinson patients will be impaired on the CVLT (Filoteo et al., 1997). Multiple sclerosis patients show a diminished acquisition rate, tend to use serial rather than semantic clustering, and recall fewer words than controls after delay (B.J. Diamond et al., 1997). However, their percentage savings score and recognition discrimination are unimpaired. Patients with HIV associated dementia perform poorly on acquisition but show relatively good retention over time (D.A. White et al., 1997). Using 14 CVLT scores, Murji and colleagues (2003) identified four subtypes in their 154 HIV patient subgroups, based on different loadings of four factors: Attention Span, Learning Efficiency, Delayed Recall, and Inaccurate Recall. The subtypes—Normal, Atypical, Subsyndromal, and Frontal–striatal—varied with respect to scores on a depression inventory and on tests of cognitive functioning. Interestingly, the poorest performers (Frontal–striatal) had less education than those in the other groups: the effects of a cognitive reserve were offered as one possibility to account for this; certainly others can be conjectured.

Each of the major degenerative diseases affects the CVLT variables somewhat differently, permitting a number of group-by-group discriminations and potentially aiding differential diagnosis in the individual case (Delis, Massman, et al., 1991; J.H. Kramer, Levin, et al., 1989). For example, more than 35% of the responses made by a group of Alzheimer patients were intrusions, compared with less than 10% for high functioning Huntington and Parkinson patients. Alzheimer patients forgot almost 80% of trial 5 recall following delay, high functioning Parkinson patients' loss was almost 30%, and delay allowed high functioning Huntington patients to improve their recall a little. "Perseveration" (i.e., repetitions, which may or may not have been true perseverations) also helped to differentiate these three groups, as high-level Huntington patients repeated themselves eight times on the average during the learning trials while Alzheimer patients made an average of about three repetitions and high level Parkinson patients averaged only one. Both Alzheimer and Huntington patients displayed very poor recall of the words at the beginning of the list, but Huntington patients recognized these words while Alzheimer patients gave no evidence of having learned them (Massman, Delis, and Butters, 1993). Compared to Alzheimer patients, patients with ischemic vascular dementia show superior recognition discriminability as their performance pattern is more similar to patients with subcortical dementia (i.e., Parkinson's disease, Huntington's disease) (Libon, Bogdanoff, et al., 1998). Patterns of deficits in Huntington patients also have been reported in asymptomatic Huntington gene carriers (Hahn-Barma et al., 1998).

Alcoholic patients differ from normal controls on most variables of this test, but their level of semantic clustering is similar and their learning curves have similar slopes although consistently lower than those of normal subjects (J.H. Kramer, Blusewicz, and Preston, 1989). Alcoholics are also relatively susceptible to interference effects. Korsakoff patients produced a profile similar to that of Alzheimer patients, making this test a poor discriminator of these two conditions, particularly in the early stages of Alzheimer's disease (Delis, Massman, et al., 1991). The CVLT may aid discrimination between early Alzheimer's disease and depression, as depressed patients show about the same score increase on the recognition trial relative to recall as normal subjects, but Alzheimer patients' recognition score is only a little better than their recall if at all (Massman, Delis, Butters, et al., 1992). Schizophrenic patients do not organize their recall by semantic categories (Kareken et al., 1996).

CVLT short forms. Shorter versions have been developed for severely impaired patients; being briefer they will be less stressful for both failing patients and concerned examiners. On a 9-word list composed of three 3-word categories, dementia patients of mild to moderate severity perform worse than controls (Libon,

Mattson, et al., 1996). Vascular dementia patients were superior to Alzheimer patients on delayed recall measures and made fewer intrusions and false positive recognition responses. Woodard, Goldstein and their coworkers (1999) found moderate correlations with the WMS-R Logical Memory and Visual Memory as well as with nonmemory tests, suggesting that dementia patients' low memory test scores may indicate general cognitive deterioration. A six-word version containing three exemplars of two categories is useful for demonstrating the learning and recall impairment of patients with moderate Alzheimer's disease (Kaltreider et al., 1999).

The CVLT-II manual also gives a short version of the test. The CVLT-IISF has nine words in three categories, uses only one list instead of two, and gives only four learning trials. It calls for delayed recall at two intervals—30 secs (filled with counting backward as a distraction) and 10 mins, followed by a yes/no recognition trial. As with the standard version, a forced-choice recognition trial is optional.

CERAD Word List Memory (W.G. Rosen, Mohs, and Davis, 1984)

The Consortium to Establish a Registry for Alzheimer's Disease (CERAD) (J.C. Morris, Heyman, et al., 1989; J.C. Morris, Edland, et al., 1993) includes a list of ten unrelated words for examining memory, a procedure incorporated in the Alzheimer's Disease Assessment Scale (ADAS) (W.G. Rosen, Mohs, and Davis, 1984). The short list is a suitable length for the very elderly and for Alzheimer patients who are likely to become distressed by longer lists. Its brevity is also useful for patients who are difficult to manage (Lamberty, Kennedy, and Flashman, 1995) and also would be appropriate for severely amnesic patients for whom longer word lists would be too taxing. The procedure has the advantage that the patient reads the words printed in large letters on cards, bypassing the hearing problems common to this age group and assuring registration of each word. The words are shown at a rate of one every 2 secs and presented in a different order on each of the three learning trials. Recall follows each trial. After a 3 to 5 min delay retention is tested by free recall and a recognition trial in which ten unrelated distractor words are intermixed with the target words. An alternate list of words of equal difficulty is available for repeat testing.

Age and education norms have been developed for Caucasian Americans (Ganguli et al., 1991; Welsh, Butters, Mohs, et al., 1994; Welsh-Bohmer et al., 2000) and African Americans (Unverzagt, Hall, Torke, et al., 1996). A significant age effect is reflected in the norms

(Howieson, Holm, Kaye, et al., 1993; Unverzagt, Hall, Torke, et al., 1996; Welsh, Butters, Mohs, et al., 1994). In a sample of Caucasian Americans, women outperformed men and education affected final acquisition level but not delayed free recall (Welsh, Butters, Mohs, et al., 1994); yet no sex differences were reported in a more recent sample (Welsh-Bohmer et al., 2000). For African Americans, education contributed to acquisition, recall, and recognition scores; the only score on which women were superior was acquisition (Unverzagt, Hall, Torke, et al., 1996).

Correlations of CERAD and CVLT performances of probable Alzheimer patients on comparable variables were mostly at the $p < .001$ level (e.g., Total Words, $r = .65$; Last Trial Recall, $r = .48$; Recognition Hits, $r = .40$). However, lower correlations (e.g., False Positives, $r = .22$; Forgetting Rate Percent, $r = .15$) indicate that while, for the most part, these two tests measure similar aspects of verbal learning in this patient group, differences in CERAD and CVLT scores are sufficiently great that conclusions drawn from one of these tests cannot be automatically assumed for the other (Kaltreider et al., 2000).

The acquisition and free recall measures are sensitive to memory loss associated with early stage dementia (Greene et al., 1996; Howieson, Dame, Camicioli, et al., 1997; Welsh, Butters, Hughes, et al., 1992). Performance declines progressively with increasing severity of dementia (Welsh, Butters, Hughes, et al., 1991). K. Welsh and her colleagues (1991) observed that the delayed recall measure was the most useful in detecting Alzheimer's disease while others have suggested that the total acquisition score identifies Alzheimer patients best (Derrer et al., 2001). Impaired word recognition becomes evident with progression of dementia. Test sensitivity and scores were approximately the same for African American and Caucasian Alzheimer patients when differences between groups in age, education, and disease severity were statistically corrected (Welsh, Fillenbaum, Wilkinson et al., 1995).

Hopkins Verbal Learning Test (HVLT) (Brandt, 1991), Hopkins Verbal Learning Test-Revised (HVLT-R) (R.H.B. Benedict, Schretlen, et al., 1998)

In its original form this is a word list learning task in which 12 words, four in each of three semantic categories, are presented for three learning trials. This is followed by a 24-word recognition list containing all 12 target words plus six semantically related foils and six unrelated ones (Brandt, 1991). The words on each of six 12-word lists differ for each list. The six lists and the recognition format for each are given in Brandt (1991). The 1998 revision includes a 20 to 25 minute delayed recall trial that is forewarned plus the subsequent yes/no 24-word recognition trial. Scores include one for each learning trial, a total acquisition score, a learning measure, delayed free recall, percent retention, and delayed recognition. Recognition scores are calculated for true positives, false positives, a discrimination index (true positives − false positives), and a measure of the recognition trial response bias, *Br* (the sum of "yes" responses).

Test characteristics. Stability coefficients over nine months using different forms were moderate for total recall ($r = .50$) in healthy older adults (Rasmusson et al., 1995). The six alternate forms are equivalent for the recall trials but recognition scores differ slightly (R.H.B. Benedict, Schretlen, et al., 1998).

In many ways this is a short version of a CVLT-type task, as indicated by a relatively high correlation ($r = .74$) for total learning for the two tests (Lacritz and Cullum, 1998). Validity studies demonstrated the comparability of HVLT-R recall and recognition measures to memory measures from other tests, particularly verbal memory tests (Lacritz, Cullum, al., 2001; A.M. Shapiro et al., 1999). Unimpaired adults achieve ceiling scores easily (Lacritz and Cullum, 1998). Normative data from unimpaired young adults on the HVLT-R produced a mean recall of 11 out of 12 words on the last learning trial, and the delayed recall mean was 10.6. Healthy, well-educated older adults (mean age, 70.7 ± 9.3) approach ceiling on the last learning trial. By contrast, mean performance of the normative group ages 70–88 did not approach ceiling. In a larger study of older adults, women performed better than men and there was a significant effect of age but not education (Vanderploeg, Schinka, Jones, et al., 2000). These authors provide normative data for Form A for ages 60 to 84 with adjustments for sex.

Neuropsychological findings. Patients with Alzheimer's disease and those with vascular dementia show a learning deficit on the HVLT (A. Barr et al., 1992; Frank and Bryne, 2000; Hogervorst et al., 2002; A.M. Shapiro et al., 1999). Comparing Huntington and Alzheimer patients on recognition trial scores, Brandt, Corwin, and Krafft (1992) found Alzheimer patients more likely to say "yes" to semantically related foils than the Huntington patients, and unlike control subjects who had made no false positive errors on unrelated foils, both kinds of dementia patients said "yes" to some of them. The HVLT has been useful in predicting which males will have a postconcussive syndrome after minor head injury (Bazarian et al., 1999). Of those with scores of 25 or greater on the summed learning trials, 92% did not have a postconcussive syn-

drome one month after injury. This relationship did not hold for females with minor head injury. In young adults the delayed recall and recognition measures proved sensitive to the effects of a relatively low blood alcohol level (0.07 mg/dl) compared to the drug-free state (Acheson et al., 1998).

Interference Learning Test (M.M. Schmidt and Coolidge, 1999)

This verbal learning task is uniquely designed to evaluate the effect of interference on learning a list of words. The ideal patient for this test would seem to be a high functioning adult who has performed adequately on a more standard word list learning task despite complaints of everyday memory problems in settings with more distractions than occur in a quiet testing room. The initial list, given in four trials, consists of 20 target words intermixed with 24 distractors, each exposed for three secs. The subject is instructed to read each word from a card but remember only the words printed on white cards and ignore those on blue cards. The target words consist of four nouns from each of three categories and eight abstract nouns. The to-be-ignored distractor words include 20 concrete nouns, some from target categories, and four abstract nouns, making them suitable for taxing source memory and inviting intrusion errors. Sixteen target words and no distractors make up a second list which is presented twice. Four words come from each of two categories, one the same as the original list and one different, and eight abstract nouns.

Recall of List 1 is obtained after two trials with List 2 (short delay) and after 30 mins (long delay). The delayed free recall is followed by a category cued recall trial and a yes/no recognition trial. The recognition words include the 20 target words from List 1, five to-be-ignored words, three words from List 2, and 14 words either from List 1 categories or unrelated to any lists. Finally, recall of the to-be-ignored words is tested with yes/no recognition. This test yields measures of learning under conditions of interference, source memory, intrusion errors, and organizational strategies. Computer scoring is available.

The normative sample consisted of 393 mostly Caucasian participants in the 16 to 93 age range ($M = 35.7$) with an average education of 14.2 years. Although the age group sizes are not given, older individuals appear to be underrepresented. Normalized *T*-scores were derived from a regression equation taking into account age and "premorbid IQ." A subsample of 20- to 29-year-olds gave no more intrusions on this test than on the AVLT or the CVLT despite efforts to produce interference with the to-be-ignored words.

Supporting the hypothesis that multiple sclerosis patients are particularly sensitive to the disruptive effects of interference during learning, a group of 30 MS patients had poorer overall recall when the distractor words were included (List 1 recall compared to List 2 recall) and made more intrusion errors than controls (Coolidge, Middleton, and Griego, 1996). In samples of patients with a variety of brain disorders, only the MS group made significantly more source errors than the control group (M.M. Schmidt and Coolidge, 1999). Clinical usefulness will determine whether the extra time needed to administer this complex task compared to the AVLT or CVLT is time well spent.

Selective Reminding (SR) (Buschke and Fuld, 1974)

The differentiation of retention, storage, and retrieval may also be accomplished with the selective reminding procedure. As this is a procedure, not a specific test, it has been given in many different ways. Subjects usually hear (or may be shown one by one on cards [Masur, Fuld et al., 1989]) a list of words for immediate recall. On all subsequent trials, subjects are only told those words they omitted on the previous trial. The procedure typically continues until the subject recalls all words on two successive trials or to the twelfth trial, although the original procedure called for repeated trials until all the words were recalled at one time. Those subjects who recall all words before the twelfth trial must reach a standard recall criterion (complete recall on three consecutive trials) before given a delayed recall trial. Not all subjects reach this criterion in 12 trials. Considerable variation can exist between subjects on the number of times each word must be presented (i.e., was not recalled in the previous trial). Some examiners give both a cued and a four-choice recognition trial after the last or twelfth trial (H.S. Levin, 1986; Spreen and Strauss, 1998) (see Table 11.7, p. 437). Most examiners ask for a free recall after 30 minutes (e.g., Hannay and Levin, 1985; Spreen and Strauss, 1998) or one hour (Ruff, Light, and Quayhagen, 1989).

The original version called for ten items, all of the same category (animals, clothing) to be read at a 2-per-sec rate (Buschke and Fuld, 1974); 12 items is the most common list length today. Erickson and Scott (1977) pointed out that such category-restricted lists lent themselves to successful guessing. Most examiners now use lists of unrelated words. A set of four comparable 12-word lists developed by Hannay and Levin (1985) is in most common use. Loring and Papanicolaou (1987) noted that different examiners have reported findings on different lists of different composition and length, making it difficult to draw generalizations from the literature. For example, McLean, Temkin, and their colleagues (1983) used a 10-item list giving a maximum of ten trials; Gentilini and his coworkers (1989) also gave ten trials but with a 15-item list; and Masur and his colleagues (1989, 1990), using the usual 12-item list, gave a maximum of six trials. See p. 437 for lists.

SR scores. Unique to selective reminding procedures is a measure of those words consistently recalled from trial to trial without further reminding: *Consistent long-term retrieval (CLTR).* (Masur and his colleagues [1990] further restricted the definition of this score as "the number of items the subject is able to recall on at least the last three trials without reminding.") Ten other scores can be obtained (Hannay and Levin, 1985; Spreen and Strauss, 1998) although some workers compute fewer (e.g., Ruff, Light, and Quayhagen, 1989). The full score roster for the learning trials includes, along with CLTR: *Sum recall (ΣR); Long-term retrieval (LTR)* or *Long-term storage (LTS),* the number of words recalled on two or more consecutive trials (i.e., without intervening reminding); in *Short-term recall (STR)* are words recalled only after reminding; *Random long-term retrieval (RLTR)* refers to words in LTS that do not reappear consistently but require further reminding; *Reminders* is the sum of reminders given in the course of the procedure; *Intrusions* are words not on the list. Three additional scores are given for the number of words recalled on cueing, by means of the multiple choice procedure, and on the delayed free recall trial. Additionally, Spreen and Strauss (1998) recommend noting the number of words recalled on the first trial (i.e., the supraspan).

Test characteristics. The test format provides numerous intercorrelated scores (Burkart and Heun, 2000; Loring and Papanicolaou, 1987; Spreen and Strauss, 1998) that are assumed to represent short-term recall, long-term recall and storage, and retrieval. Only words recalled on two consecutive trials are assumed to be in long-term storage. In support of this assumption, Beatty, Krull, and colleagues (1996) found that words retrieved from CLTR on the last acquisition trial were more likely to be recalled after delay than were words not consistently retrieved. An inadequate recall of words from long-term storage is assumed to represent a retrieval failure. However, other interpretations are possible. Loring and Papanicolaou (1987) pointed out that RLTR may represent weak encoding of words rather than a retrieval failure. Low CLTR scores of multiple sclerosis patients was interpreted as representing difficulties in the acquisition/encoding of information (J. DeLuca, Gaudino, Diamond, et al., 1998). Given the popularity of this test, the lack of comparisons

TABLE 11.7 Multiple-Choice and Cued-Recall Items for Forms 1–4 of SRT

Form 1

1. bowl	dish	bell	view
2. love	poison	conform	passion
3. dawn	sunrise	bet	down
4. pasteboard	verdict	judgement	fudge
5. grand	grant	give	jazz
6. see	sting	fold	bee
7. pain	plane	pulled	jet
8. county	state	tasted	counter
9. voice	select	choice	cheese
10. flower	seed	herd	seek
11. date	sheep	wool	would
12. mill	queen	food	meal

Form 2

1. shine	glow	chime	cast
2. dispute	disappear	contour	disagree
3. fat	oil	trail	fit
4. stopwatch	affluent	wealthy	worthy
5. trunk	drunk	stoned	blunt
6. fin	peg	wake	pin
7. glass	grass	plan	lawn
8. moon	beam	spark	noon
9. propose	ready	prepare	husband
10. award	prize	pot	size
11. bark	bird	duck	luck
12. leap	ranch	blade	leaf

Form 3

1. throw	toss	through	plate
2. flower	lilt	intent	lily
3. film	movie	slave	kiln
4. waver	cautious	discreet	distinct
5. soft	loft	attic	tack
6. beet	meat	clue	beef
7. stream	street	speed	road
8. helmet	armor	bacon	velvet
9. smoke	serpent	snake	pool
10. hoed	dug	hay	dog
11. blank	bundle	pack	puck
12. ton	shirt	foil	tin

Form 4

1. egg	shell	beg	source
2. airline	runner	darling	runway
3. fort	castle	sink	fork
4. boldness	dentist	toothache	headache
5. blown	drown	float	rib
6. body	infant	middle	baby
7. larva	lava	echo	rock
8. damp	moist	hook	stamp
9. purse	clean	pure	bare
10. ballot	vote	dish	note
11. chain	peal	strip	slip
12. trust	rise	fact	truth

Cued Recall Words

Form 1		Form 2		Form 3		Form 4	
BO	PL	SH	GR	TH	ST	—	LA
PA	COU	DI	MO	LI	HE	RU	DA
DA	CH	FA	PRE	FI	SN	FO	PU
JUD	SE	WEA	PR	DI	DU	TO	VO
GR	WO	DR	DU	LO	PA	DR	ST
—	ME	—	LE	BE	—	BA	TR

From Spreen and Strauss (1998).

of the selective reminding procedure with other word learning tasks with full reminding procedures in the same individuals is disappointing. Such comparisons would indicate whether the unique measures of this procedure, including CLTR, identify memory problems better than scores from the less complicated rote learning procedures.

Up to age 70, women tend to outperform men, with age of lesser importance and education contributing only little and that mostly below the college level (Ruff, Light, and Quayhagen, 1989). The Ruff group present normative data for LTS and CLTR for men and women separately, each data set stratified by age (four ranges from 16–24 to 55–70) and education (three levels, ≤12, 13–15, ≥16). They attributed at least some of the women's advantage to their greater use of a clustering strategy (e.g., by their temporal relationships—primacy or recency effects, or conceptually, e.g., *plane* and *bee* both fly). When the age range includes subjects over 70, age becomes an important variable, with sex effects of smaller but still significant consequence (Larrabee, Trahan, et al., 1988). Larrabee and his colleagues published norms for seven age groups from 18–29 to 80–91 which include all 11 of the usual scores. They provided correction values to bring men's scores up to women's levels (reproduced in full in Spreen and Strauss, 1998). See Table 11.8 for these age × sex norms for the three most used scores, CLTR, ΣR, and LTS.

Versions of this test using both six and 12 trials have been compared for sensitivity. Because 12 trials can be tedious, the shorter version would be preferable if it were shown to be as sensitive as the longer version. Norms have been reported for all scores generated on a six-trial version for cognitively intact 56 adults, ages 18 to 58 (Ehrenreich, 1995). Revised normative data for a six-trial administration have also been extracted from Larrabee and colleagues' 1988 data (Larrabee, Trahan, and Levin, 2000). As with other comparisons between six- and 12-trial versions (Drane et al., 1998; R.L. Smith et al., 1995), the correlations for various measures were high, ranging from .81 to .95 with the

notable exception of a lower correlation (.51) for RLTR. The authors point out that the correlations are likely to be inflated because scores on the 12-trial version are based, in part, on cumulative scores at trial 6.

Reliability has been examined by test–retest procedures using the different forms. Test–retest reliability has correlations in the .41 to .62 range using seven of the learning measures for all four forms (Hannay and Levin, 1985), and higher—.73 and .66—for ΣR and CLTR using only Forms I and II (Ruff, Light, and Quayhagen, 1989). Hannay and Levin (1985) reported that Form I is more difficult than Forms II, III, and IV, which were comparable (see also Larrabee, Trahan, et al., 1988). However, equivalency among the four forms has also been documented (Westerveld et al., 1994). A substantial practice effect for most of the scores appeared with four administrations using different forms of the test regardless of the order of the forms (Hannay and Levin, 1985). Correlational studies with other memory tests consistently bring out this procedure's significant verbal memory component (Larrabee and Levin, 1986; Macartney-Filgate and Vriesen, 1988).

Neuropsychological findings. Typically, studies report only one or a few scores, mostly CLTR, often with ΣR or LTS. SR measures of storage and retrieval have not only distinguished severely head injured patients from normal control subjects, as expected (H.S. Levin, Mattis, et al., 1987; Paniak et al., 1989), but have effectively documented impairment in mildly injured patients (McLean, Temkin, et al., 1983). Differences in learning efficiency show up between patients whose head injuries differ in their severity (H.S. Levin, Grossman, Rose, and Teasdale, 1979): on long-term storage, only the seriously damaged group did not continue to show improvement across all 12 trials, but leveled off (with an average recall of approximately six words) at the sixth trial. The mildly impaired group achieved near-perfect scores on the last two trials, and the moderately impaired group maintained about a one-word-per-trial lag behind them throughout, showing a much

TABLE 11.8 Norms for the Most Used SR Scores for Age Groups with 30 or More Subjects

	AGE (YEARS)			
	18–29	*40–49*	*60–69*	*70–79*
Education (years)	12.88 ± 1.7	14.71 ± 2.7	13.40 ± 3.6	13.46 ± 3.8
M/F	23/28	19/12	33/17	38/21
Scores				
CLTR	115.12 ± 19.7	107.10 ± 26.6	88.92 ± 35.8	69.68 ± 36.0
ΣR	128.18 ± 9.2	125.03 ± 12.0	114.82 ± 15.8	105.27 ± 16.7
LTS	125.00 ± 10.5	122.45 ± 15.6	107.00 ± 21.8	95.54 ± 24.9

From Larrabee, Trahan, Curtiss, and Levin (1988). Reprinted with permission.

less consistent retrieval pattern than the mildly impaired group. ΣR and CLTR also were sensitive to continuing improvements in moderately to severely injured patients over a two-year span (Dikmen, Machamer, et al., 1990). Paniak and his colleagues (1989) observed that CLTR in itself did not adequately account for a tendency of severely head injured patients to have an abnormally high rate of random recall which these authors attribute to inefficient learning but, rather, may reflect erratic retrieval mechanisms.

Lateralized temporal lobe dysfunction, whether identified on the basis of seizure site or due to anterior lobectomy, is readily discriminated by significantly depressed CLTR and LTS scores when the damage is on the left (Drane et al., 1998; Giovagnoli and Avanzini, 1996; G.P. Lee, Loring, and Thompson, 1989). However, neither CLRT nor LTS differentiated those patients whose left temporal lobectomies did not include the hippocampus from those with larger resections that did (Loring, Lee, Meador, et al., 1991). More impairment is associated with left than right frontal lesions for total words recalled, although impairment is evident with both lesion sites (Vilkki, Servo, and Surmaaho, 1998).

The selective reminding format has been used successfully to elicit memory impairment in patients with very mild Alzheimer's disease or with mild cognitive impairment that does not yet meet criteria for a dementia diagnosis (Devanand et al., 1997; Petersen, Smith, Waring, et al., 1999). Masur and his colleagues (1989) found that LTR and CLTR were the scores that best distinguished patients with early Alzheimer's disease from normal controls. They also report (1990) that SR scores—ΣR and the delayed recall score—were particularly sensitive predictors of which apparently normal elderly persons might develop Alzheimer's disease within two years of the initial examination, predicting well above baseline rates (37% and 40%, respectively) for these two scores. Prediction rates of most other SR scores were comparable, except STR (i.e., supraspan), which is generally relatively insensitive to very early dementia. In a more recent study the Buschke research group caution that using age- and education-corrected scores reduces the sensitivity for detecting dementia by as much as 28% compared to uncorrected scores (Sliwinski et al., 1997). They recommend using memory scores without age corrections for detecting mild dementia. Patients with dementia alone or combined with Parkinson's disease or stroke achieved scores significantly below those of nondemented Parkinson or stroke patients (Stern, Andrews et al., 1992). Multiple sclerosis patients performed significantly below normal control subjects on CLTR but not on delayed recognition (DeLuca et al., 1998; S.M. Rao, Leo, and St. Aubin-Faubert, 1987). However, considerable variability exists among MS patients. Beatty and his colleagues found that 25% of these patients performed normally while the remainder showed varying degrees of impairment with the SR procedure (Beatty, Wilbanks, et al., 1996).

SR variants. One variant of the SR procedure is *Free and Cued Selective Reminding (FCSR)* (Buschke, 1984; Grober, Merling, et al., 1997). The FCSR uses category cues at both acquisition and retrieval in an attempt to ensure semantic encoding and enhance recall. The subject is asked to search a card containing line drawings of four objects and to identify the one that belongs to a category named by the examiner. Each of the 16 items to be learned appears on one of four of these cards. After each item on the card is correctly identified, the card is removed and immediate recall of the four items is tested by cueing with the category prompt. The subject is corrected for any errors. Additional items are presented four at a time in the same manner. After the study phase, four recall trials are obtained in which free recall is followed by cued recall for items not spontaneously reported. Missed items are presented again with their cues. Elderly subjects recall twice as many words from long-term memory in FCSR than in SR (Grober, Merling, et al., 1997). Normative data for the elderly have been reported from the MOANS project (Ivnik, Smith, Lucas, et al., 1997) and the Einstein Aging Project (Grober, Lipton, Katz, and Sliwinski, 1998). The latter group found that age, education, and sex influenced performance but race did not. Free recall impairment on the FCSR predicted the development of dementia as much as five years in advance of the diagnosis (Grober, Lipton, Hall, and Crystal, 2000). However, the usefulness of this test is limited by ceiling effects because category cueing makes recall much easier for most adults, including well-functioning elderly.

The *Double Memory Test (DMT)* was designed to be a more difficult version of the FCSR by increasing the items per category cue from one to four and increasing the list length to 64 items (Buschke, Sliwinski, et al., 1995). Two lists are used, one in which category cues are presented during acquisition as well as retrieval, the other in which category cues are presented only during retrieval. Both patients with dementia and controls benefit when category cues are presented during acquisition compared to cueing only during retrieval. The benefit in the dementia patients is inversely related to the severity of the dementia (Buschke, Sliwinski, et al., 1997).

Tuokko and her colleagues (with Crockett, 1989; with Gallie and Crockett, 1990) offered a pictorial form of the test that documented memory deterioration in elderly patients. Two Spanish versions of the SR have been developed (Campo et al., 2000).

Word List (Wechsler, 1997)

An optional verbal memory test that comes with the Wechsler Memory Scale-III models the AVLT procedure but is shorter. The examiner reads the list of 12 unrelated words in the same order for each of four trials at the rate of one word per $1^1/_2$ secs and instructs the patient to recall them in any order. A short delayed recall of the original list follows a one-trial interference list. The patient is told to expect another recall 30 min later. Recognition is obtained with a yes/no format in which the subject identifies the target words from an equal number of foils, also semantically unrelated. The manual provides normative data for eight measures: List A trial 1 recall, total recall, learning slope, the difference between trial 4 recall and short delay recall, long delay recall, recognition, and the percent of trial 4 recall retained in the long delay recall condition. Also, norms for a "contrast" measure of recall of the first trials of both lists are available.

A floor effect with a pronounced distribution skew for long delay recall begins with a relatively young age group. It is unlikely that this score distribution justifies conversion to scaled scores (see p. 145). For example, the mean number of words recalled in the long delay condition by the 55–65 year-old group is 3.5 and a recall of only one word is the lower limit of the *average* range. No obvious reason explains the low performance by the normative group. Although the word frequency of the items is slightly lower than for some word lists, it appears comparable on such important variables as concreteness, imagery, meaningfulness, and pleasantness. Other word lists do not use exactly the same procedure, making direct comparisons impossible. However, a similar age group (55–59 years) given five trials in which to learn the 15 AVLT words, an interference trial, and tested 30 mins later with no warning gave an average recall of 10.4 words with the lower limit of the *average* range at 8.3 words (Ivnik, Malec, Tangalos, et al., 1990). Given ten words (CERAD), three trials, and no interference list, a 50–69 year-old group with low education (9.1 years) recalled an average of 7.0 words with 5.8 words at the lower limit of the *average* range (Welsh, Butters, Mohs, et al., 1994). The relatively lower education of the older groups in the WMS-III normative population may contribute to the seemingly large age effect. For the elderly, the acquisition and recognition scores appear to provide better measures of memory impairment than does recall following long delay.

Paired associate word learning tests

The format of paired associate tests consists of word pairs that are read to the subject with one or more re-

call trials in which the first of the pair is presented for the subject to give the associated word. Thus it is a word-learning test with built-in cueing.

Associate Learning (PAL) (Wechsler, 1945);
Verbal Paired Associates (VePA)
(Wechsler, 1987, 1997)

This is perhaps the most familiar of the paired word learning tests. The original Wechsler format consists of ten word pairs, six forming "easy" associations (e.g., baby-cries) and the other four "hard" word pairs that are not readily associated (e.g., cabbage-pen) (Wechsler, 1945). The PAL list is read three times, with a memory trial following each reading. Total score is one-half the sum of all correct associations to the easy pairs plus the sum of all correct associations to the hard pairs, made within five secs after the stimulus word is read. Thus, the highest possible score is 21. The word pairs are randomized in each of the three learning trials to prevent positional learning. In its original format this was a test of cued new learning with no procedure in place for measuring retention. Some workers have added a 30-min delayed recall (e.g., Spreen and Strauss, 1998; Stuss, Ely, et al., 1985). A fourth-trial variation on the standard administration of the Associate Learning task reverses the order of word pair presentation by telling the patient, "I'm going to give you the second word and you give me the first" (Milberg, Hebben, and Kaplan, 1996). In this way, the examiner can determine whether the word associations were truly learned, or whether the patient's correct responses represent strings of passively learned phonetic associations. WMS-II provides an alternate form of the PAL (C.P. Stone et al., 1946) which tends to be significantly more difficult than Form I. Suspected dementia patients scored one-and-one-half points higher on Form I with a correlation between Forms I and II of .73 (Margolis et al., 1985). These studies found correlations between PAL Forms I and II of .61 and .73, respectively.

Verbal Paired Associates (VePA-R) in the 1987 revised edition of the Wechsler Memory Scale (WMS-R) contains just eight pairs, four of the original easy pairs and four hard pairs. Scoring is based on the first three trials, although subjects who have not learned all the pairs by the third trial get up to three more trials. Approximately one-half hour later a single recall trial is given. Scoring differs from the original format in that, while correct recall of easy and hard pairs is still counted separately, easy and hard pairs alike receive the same one-point value for each correct response.

On both forms—WMS and WMS-R—the score is evaluated only for the total sum. The WMS doubled value for the hard pairs gives more weight to the presumed new learning they require making them more vulnerable to many kinds of brain damage than easy pairs, which depend to a large extent on old learned associations (R.S. Wilson, Bacon, et al., 1982). The relative weight contributed by the easy associates increases with age (DesRosiers and Ivison, 1986).

The weight differential was demonstrated in a comparison of mildly injured TBI patients, patients whose injuries were severe, and normal subjects on the WMS version of paired associates, for the difference between the average recall of severely injured patients and control subjects for easy pairs was only 3.6 words, but for the hard pairs it was 4.9 (Uzzell, Langfitt, and Dolinskas, 1987). It also showed up when performances of multiple sclerosis patients were compared with those of control subjects as here easy words did not distinguish the groups on any of the three trials, but the hard word score differed significantly for the two groups on all trials (Minden, Moes, et al., 1990). However, these studies, in which easy and hard pairs were evaluated separately, are thoughtful exceptions to the WMS manuals' norms based on the combined scores. Of course the juxtaposition of hard and easy pairs in one test has the practical result of testing two different activities (i.e., recall of well-learned verbal associations and retention of new, unfamiliar verbal material), but the combined score obscures the status of each.

In *Verbal Paired Associations-III* (1997), all items are "hard," thus doing away with the relative insensitivity of the easy items. Administration and scoring are based on four trials with eight pairs. Following a delayed recall approximately 30 mins later, a recognition trial includes the previously presented word pairs intermixed with pairs of new words. This latter task, for which no norms are provided, appears to be too easy for most patients. Rather, the score from this recognition test is combined with the Logical Memory II recognition score in the normative tables which precludes comparison of this score with the normative sample!

In including only hard pairs, the test publishers eliminated one of the virtues of the earlier pair sets, as easy pairs provide opportunities for memory impaired patients to have some experience of success on otherwise consistently frustrating and even humiliating failures in a memory examination. When examining a psychologically frail elder, I [mdl] still use the word pair set from the WMS-R. Moreover, a subject's failure to make these easy associations can no longer alert the clinician to possible poor motivation.

Clinical experience [dwl, mdl] suggests that the delayed recall format lacks useful sensitivity. Although a paired associate recognition trial is given immediately after the delayed free recall, there are no item pairs in which the first word is incorrectly paired with the second word of a different word pair or a new, nonlist word. Thus the patient need only recognize either of the two words since they always appear as the correct target pair, defeating the purpose of testing acquired *word associations*.

Test characteristics. By inspection, small but consistent age decrements show up for this test (see Mitrushina, Boone, and D'Elia, 1999; Spreen and Strauss, 1998; Wechsler, 1987, p. 52). Within age ranges above 60, some studies found that age contributes little to score differences on the WMS version of this test (J.S. Bak and Greene, 1981; Ivnik, Smith, et al., 1991), while pronounced score declines for elderly subjects have been documented too (Kaszniak, Garron, and Fox, 1979; Margolis and Scialfa, 1984; Zagar et al., 1984). It may be suspected that when scores from the oldest age groups are similar to those in young–old groups, differences in the demographic composition of these age groups contribute to their performance similarities as education and income tend to be positively correlated with health and longevity. McCarty, Siegler, and Logue (1982), avoiding the demographic factors involved in longevity, retested their subjects over a decade or more and found that only the hard-pairs score decreased significantly. The more difficult VePA-III version shows a steady decline with age; subjects over 75 years generally recall no more than three or four of the pairs.

Despite the preponderant evidence for sex effects on word learning tests, evaluations for sex biases with appropriate norms or correction scores are not given in the WMS-R or WMS-III manuals. Commingling of scores from the story recall task, Logical Memory, on which men perform equally well if not better than women and Verbal Paired Associates for most test evaluation purposes possibly masks sex differences. One study considering sex differences on this test in the WMS version found that women performed better only on the hard associates, which makes sense in light of the sex differences that appear on other tests of rote verbal learning. In two other WMS studies, women tended to average about 1 point higher than the men at each age level until the 60s, when they had an approximately two-point lead (Ivison, 1977). However, sex differences have not always shown up on the WMS version (Trahan, 1985). Young women outperformed young men on the VePA-III first trial recall, total recall, and percent retention but not delayed recall (M.R. Basso et al., 2000). Education effects have been reported for both easy and hard pairs on the WMS version (Ivnik, Smith, et al., 1991).

Normative data from a number of studies have been compiled for the WMS forms of Verbal Paired Associates (Mitrushina, Boone, and D'Elia, 1999; see also Spreen and Strauss, 1998). The manuals give normative data for ages 16–74 for the VePA-R and 16–89 for the VePA-III. Unfortunately, for the WMS-R, only extrapolated data are provided for age groups 18–19, 25–34, and 45–54 as these groups were not included in the standardization (see p. 483).

A short-term (7 to 10 days) test–retest reliability correlation of .53 and a significant 1.33 point gain in mean score were documented for hypertensive patients (McCaffrey, Ortega, et al., 1992). This correlation is in line with a test–retest (after one year) reliability correlation of .63 obtained by W.G. Snow, Tierney, and their colleagues (1988). Three-week retesting of subjects from a broad age range (17–82) produced a relatively high reliability coefficient (.72) with an average 1.31 score gain ($p < .05$) (Youngjohn, Larrabee, and Crook, 1992). On retesting with the WMS-R, only small gains accrued on the learning trials for all three standardization groups (ages 20–24, 55–64, 70–74), with virtually no gains on delayed recall (Wechsler, 1987; see also McCaffrey, Duff, and Westervelt, 2000b for more test–retest data). Stability coefficients were highest on the VePA compared to all other WMS-III tests; retesting 2 to 12 weeks later resulted in a 1 to $1^{1}/_{2}$ point gain (The Psychological Corporation, 1997).

Examination of the construct validity of this test generally demonstrates a significant verbal learning component (Bornstein and Chelune, 1989; Larrabee and Levin, 1986) or a general learning factor that is relatively independent of verbal skills (Chelune, Ferguson, and Moehle, 1986; Larrabee, Kane, et al., 1985), depending on the mix of tests being studied. When easy and hard pairs are analyzed separately, the association of hard pairs with other verbal learning measures becomes evident (Macartney-Filgate and Vriezen, 1988).

Neuropsychological findings. Jones-Gotman (1991b) pointed out that this test falls short of the ideal for a verbal memory test as the words lend themselves readily to visual imagery, thus allowing the enterprising subject to use a dual encoding strategy. Yet, despite this potential drawback, both earlier versions of the test are sensitive to the effects of lateralized lesions: with patient groups of mixed etiologies, both learning and delayed recall means of patients with left-sided lesions were significantly below those made by patients whose dysfunction was on the right side (WMS-R: Chelune and Bornstein, 1988; WMS: Saling et al., 1993; Vakil, Hoofien, and Blachstein, 1992). These findings are supported by studies of patients who had temporal lobectomies for seizure control, as those with left-sided excisions not only performed at significantly lower levels than those whose surgery involved the right temporal lobe (WMS-R: L.H. Goldstein et al., 1988), but they also performed below their already depressed presurgery scores on this test (WMS: Ivnik, Sharbrough, and

Laws, 1988). In a study of patients with temporal lobe epilepsy, poor VePA delayed recall of the left temporal group was the only WMS-III test that statistically distinguished patients with left and right foci (N. Wilde et al., 2001). Slightly but significantly and fairly consistently lower scores on delayed recall of the WMS version distinguished patients who had apparently "recovered" from mild head injuries from normal control subjects (Stuss, Ely, et al., 1985).

Paired-associate learning has proven useful not only in eliciting the learning deficits of Alzheimer type dementia (Bondi, Salmon, and Kaszniak, 1986) but also in documenting the progress of deterioration, even in the early stages (Kaszniak, Poon, and Riege, 1986; Storandt, Botwinick, and Danziger, 1986). However, of a group of seven patients with memory complaints associated with neurological disorders, of whom four had Alzheimer diagnoses, only one performed WMS paired associates at a level below that of the 12-person control group (Lussier et al., 1989). N. Butters, Salmon, Cullum, and their coworkers (1988) found that by calculating a *savings score* (delayed recall ÷ last immediate recall [whether trial 3 or higher] × 100) they could demonstrate retention levels by both young and old control subjects that were significantly better than those of patients with Huntington's disease or amnesia due to head injury or Korsakoff's psychosis. This differential did not show up for Alzheimer patients who, it may be presumed, had such low immediate recall scores that they could not lose much and still make any response at all. Moreover, the savings differential was smaller than for other WMS-R tests (Logical Memory and Visual Reproduction). Unfortunately these workers did not evaluate patients' learning and retention performances per se on this test as they used the WMS-R manuals' recommended combined VePA and Logical Memory score.

The paired associate format is useful in showing memory impairment in patients with basal ganglia disease. Although newly diagnosed Parkinson patients were impaired on the PAL, they showed a good savings score at a 1-hour delay (J.A. Cooper, Sagar, Jordan, et al., 1991). Memory for the hard pairs of the PAL distinguished presymptomatic gene carriers for Huntington's disease from noncarriers (Hahn-Barma et al., 1998). The VePA-R differentiated relatively young patients with Parkinson's disease from matched controls even though the groups were indistinguishable on the Logical Memory WMS-R test (Camicioli, Grossmann, et al., 2001). Squire and Shimamura (1986) found that the PAL discriminated very well between a group of amnesics of mixed etiology and persons with mildly depressed memory functioning due to either depression or chronic alcoholism. It also proved to be sensitive in documenting the more subtle differences between depressed patients and normal control subjects. TBI patients can be taught to improve their performance on this test using mental imagery instructions (Twum and Parente, 1994).

Paired associate learning variants. The paired associate learning format lends itself to a seemingly unlimited number of modifications—in length, difficulty level, number of trials, scoring methods, etc. (e.g., Delbecq-Dérouesné and Beauvois, 1989; Morrow, Robin, et al., 1992; see also H.S. Levin, 1986). Some examples are given here.

In an early study, Inglis (1959) randomized the order of administering just three word pairs (cabbage–pen, knife–chimney, sponge–trumpet), giving them until the subject reached a criterion of three consecutive correct responses for all three pairs or until 30 trials, dropping out word pairs once the criterion was reached. The score was the number of times a word pair had to be repeated. Not surprisingly, a control group's mean score of 13 ± 6.6 was significantly lower than that for elderly psychiatric patients (59 ± 25).

The first ten word pairs of Wechsler's Similarities test given to TBI patients were used to test incidental learning by asking for a free recall of the pairs, and then giving a cued recall trial using the first word of each pair as the cue (Vilkki, Holst, Öhman, et al., 1990). Both free and cued recall correlated significantly with duration of coma (−.48 free recall, −.43 cued recall) and ventricular enlargement (−.33, −.32 for free and cued recall, respectively). This technique was also highly sensitive to the presence of diffuse damage and to the left-lateralized damage after surgical repair of subarachnoid hemorrhage due to a ruptured aneurysm (Vilkki, Holst, Öhman, et al., 1989). A year after surgery, free recall, but not cued recall, discriminated between patients functioning normally and those with obvious neuropsychological deficits.

Rich and her colleagues (1997) examined the interference effect of using a different set of second words during a second learning task, following an AB–AC paradigm. Huntington patients were slow to learn the initial pairs relative to controls and were disproportionately impaired in learning the new associations. However, they did not recall more B words during the AC portion of the test and, therefore, did not show increased suceptibility to proactive interference as was hypothesized.

Choosing among word-learning tests [mdl]

Many word list tasks are available today. The examiner's selection should depend on what test characteristics are most relevant to the examination questions, the patient's condition and demographic status, and the ease of administration and scoring.

For verbal learning per se, my preference for the AVLT rests on a number of test variables: Unlike the SR procedure, all subjects are exposed to the same number of stimuli, and since they are given in the same order, position effects (primacy, recency) become evident as well as other strategies the subject might use. The addition of both immediate and delayed recall trials and a recognition trial allows the examiner to see both the effects of interference and those of delay on recall; the recognition trial, of course, is the best measure of how much the subject has actually learned and the extent of recall efficiency. Both administration and scoring are much simpler than those of the SR, requiring no arithmetic operations, and the data are immediately available. In fact, I score as I give the test. Moreover, little seems to be gained (but much time lost) by the elaborate SR scoring procedures. Moreover, as Loring and Papanicolaou (1987) note, a number of SR measures "have typically . . . high correlations in both clinical and control samples (i.e., total recall, LTS, LTR, CLTR), suggesting that these measures are assessing similar constructs." These authors further note that the seeming parcellation into "long-term storage" and "retrieval" makes an arbitrary distinction between these terms, basing LTS on Buschke's definition requiring two consecutive trials and overlooking the possibility that erratic recall of a word may reflect tenuous storage rather than a retrieval problem. In fact, this test does not measure retrieval as understood in the usual sense of the efficiency of delayed recall compared with recognition tested immediately following delayed recall (e.g., see Delis, 1989; Loring and Papanicolaou, 1987).

In comparing the SR procedure with the AVLT and CVLT list learning administration (standard procedure), using 20 words for ten trials and college undergraduates as subjects, MacLeod (1985) discovered that with the SR procedure these subjects required only 30 to 40 item exposures to reach the 20-word criterion, compared to more than 100 single-item exposures for the standard procedure. However, criterion was reached one full trial sooner for an animal list by means of the standard procedure compared to the SR procedure, and the standard procedure also led to criterion an average of one-half trial sooner than the SR procedure on a random word list. In recommending the SR procedure as "faster to administer . . . because fewer items need be presented on each study trial," MacLeod did not reckon with the learning problems of neurologically impaired patients who may require many more word repetitions during 12 (often discouraging, certainly boring) trials in which half or more of the words must be repeated each time. MacLeod's work indicates that, overall, the SR and the standard procedure are about equally effective in measuring learning competency, at least in bright young people.

When examining the incidental use of concept formation (compared with the structured format of Similarities, e.g.), the subject's use of strategy in learning, and/or whether cueing helps (e.g., when focusing on a patient's potential to benefit from remediation training), the CVLT provides valuable information as it documents the benefits of prepackaged concepts for learning. However, because of the CVLT's built-in conceptual confounds, the AVLT is a better test for verbal rote memory in itself. The CVLT may also be used for a second examination to avoid practice effects on the AVLT, although CVLT produces slightly higher scores (Crossen and Weins, 1994).

Verbal Paired Associates (WMS-R) are particularly useful when the patient appears incapable of learning more than a very few words on a list test (administration of story recall early in the examination gives a general idea of the patient's level of verbal learning). With VePA, verbal learning can be examined by means of the hard pairs while the easy ones give the patient some success opportunities so that the test is not experienced as too defeating. Moreover, the built-in cues also help to determine whether the patient can benefit from cueing strategies for remediation. Although the WMS version with its greater weighting on hard pairs appears to work a little better as a measure of verbal learning, the availability of normative data, particularly for the delayed recall trial, facilitates WMS-R interpretation.

Story Recall

In many ways story recall tests most resemble everyday memory demands for the meaningful discourse found in conversation, radio and television, and written material. They provide a measure of both the amount of information that is retained when the material exceeds immediate memory span, and the contribution of meaning to retention and recall. Prior experience may prompt the story listener to attend to the setting, characters, actions, and outcome of a story. The comparison of a patient's memory span on a story recall test with a word list task will tell how much the inherent organization and meaningfulness of the prose material can facilitate memory or, conversely, how much syntactic processing or overload of data can compromise functioning.

Story recall administration presents a number of problems because not all examiners present the test material in exactly the same way. Ideally, the stories are enunciated carefully in a natural speech pattern with a slight pause between sentences for clarity. Presentation rates that are too fast hinder recall in intact persons (Shum, Murray, and Eadie, 1997), an effect likely to be greatest in the elderly and patients whose brain disorder has slowed their processing of information. Also, asking patients "Anything else?" at the end of recall allows them an opportunity to provide information out of order that might have come to mind during or after the recall process. Some patients will spontaneously provide this additional recall while others will not [dbh].

Scoring issues. Scoring story recall presents a number of problems since few people repeat the test material exactly. This leaves the examiner with the problem of deciding how much alterations differ from the text to require loss of score points. Common alterations include a variety of substitutions (of synonyms, of similar concepts, of less precise language, of different numbers or proper names); omissions (large and small; irrelevant to the story, relevant, or crucial); additions and elaborations (ranging from inconsequential ones to those that distort or alter the story or are frankly bizarre); and shifts in the story's sequence (that may or may not alter its meaning).

Rapaport and his colleagues (1968) addressed questions of how to judge these alterations by scoring as correct all segments of the story in which "the change does not alter the general meaning of the story or its details." Without a more elaborate scoring scheme, this rule is probably the most reasonable one that can be followed in a clinical setting. Talland and Ekdahl (1959) made a welcome distinction between verbatim and content (semantic) recall of paragraphs. They divided meaningful verbal material into separate scoring units for verbatim recall and for content ideas, which are credited as correctly recalled if the subject substitutes synonyms or suitable phrases for the exact wording (see p. 449). Several scoring methods have been devised for the Logical Memory (LM) test that take minor alterations and/or gist into account (see p. 445). These may be generally applicable to tests of story recall. Unless scoring rules for alterations are specified or a method for scoring slight alterations is used, the examiner will inevitably have to make scoring decisions without concise, objective standards. In most cases, the likelihood that a score for a story recall test may vary a few points (depending on who does the scoring and how the scorer feels that day) is not of great consequence. The sophisticated psychological examiner knows that there is a margin of error for any given score. However, alterations in some patients' responses may make large segments unscorable as verbatim recall, although the patient demonstrated a quite richly detailed recall of the story. Other patients may reproduce much material verbatim, but in such a disconnected manner, or so linked or elaborated with bizarre, confabulated, or perseverated introjections that a fairly high verbatim recall score belies their inability to reproduce newly heard verbal material accurately.

Logical Memory (LM-O, LM-R) (Wechsler, 1945, 1987, 1997)

Free recall immediately following auditory presentation characterizes most story memory tests. The original Wechsler Memory Scale version, Logical Memory (LM-O) employs this format. The examiner reads two stories, stopping after each reading for an immediate free recall. The LM manuals do not specify the speed of presentation of the stories, which may vary considerably across examiners (Shum, Murray, and Eadie, 1997). The format for the WMS-R Logical Memory test (LM-R) differs in a number of ways from the WMS-O. Most important for the usefulness of the test is the addition of a 30-minute delayed recall of the stories. The Anna Thompson story has remained the first story in all versions with only minor variations in each subsequent edition. The second story was changed for the 1987 revision. In WMS-III, not only is another new paragraph paired with the venerable Anna Thompson (the WMS-R Robert Miller story was considered too likely to evoke an emotional reaction in some people and thus bias recall), but it is given in two learning trials which increases the likelihood of retention over a 30-minute delay. The second reading may aid patients who are so overwhelmed by the amount of information contained in the story that they lose track of what they are hearing. Repeating the first story rather than the second may have better addressed the problem of anxious patients "freezing" at the beginning of the test (Cannon, 1999). Delayed recall may be prompted with a set of cues provided for each story. Two alternate paragraphs of equivalent difficulty to LM-R have been developed for use when repeat testing is required (J. Morris et al., 1997).

Scoring. Scoring of the stories requires the examiner's judgment. Score differences due to variability both in subjective criteria and in scoring methods produced a variegated set of LM-O average performances by normal young and middle-aged subjects (Loring and Papanicolaou, 1987; see also Mitrushina, Boone, and D'Elia, 1999). Scoring guidelines introduced with the LM-R improved interrater reliability with coefficients above .95 (K. Sullivan, 1996; Wechsler, 1987). The manuals for both LM-R and LM-III provide a general rule—based on "item(s) correctly repeated," for scoring each of the 25 items of a story and examples of both satisfactory and failed responses. However, the size, complexity, and scoring criteria of individual items differ considerably: several items consist of just one name with no variations credited, other one-name items allow several variations; some words have to be precisely included (e.g., cafeteria), while others may be indicated by similar expressions (e.g., "cops" is an acceptable substitute for "police"); some words can be scored as correct even if they occur in an incorrect context (e.g., South). These scoring anomalies suggest that two persons with similar recall abilities may earn quite different scores if one hit on the items calling for a single word response and the other recalled the same amount of material or even more but did not give many of the specified person and place names. For these reasons—and to capture distortions or confabulations—recall should be recorded verbatim. Unfortunately the WMS record forms do not leave space for recording subjects' responses on them.

A detailed scoring system proposed for LM-O is designed to bring out qualitative response differences that classify response segments (single ideas) according to whether they are essential propositions (e.g., that a robbery took place), detail propositions (e.g., the protagonist's name was Anna Thompson), or self-generated propositions (i.e., intrusions) (Webster et al., 1992). These authors also developed a cued recall format for the Anna Thompson story which contains 12 questions, each open-ended and followed by a choice of three answers. A recognition task consisting of multiple-choice questions developed for LM-R showed a ceiling effect for well-educated subjects (Fastenau, 1996b). A thematic scoring option has also been added for both LM-III stories, designed to indicate the number of main ideas recalled.

The score for the additional learning provided by the second presentation of Story B is referred to as a "learning slope;" the manual provides comparison data from the normative sample. In some cases this score may be critical in the interpretation of overall performance.

An 85-year-old man without memory complaints in a study of healthy aging recalled seven elements each from LM-III A and the first administration of Story B. Following the second presentation of Story B his recall doubled, showing the advantage of giving a second trial, perhaps because of age-related slow information processing. His benefit from the second trial held through the delay interval. He retained ten elements of Story B while recalling only four from Story A. However, following WMS-III scoring rules, combining his delayed recall score of Story A with that of Story B (Σ = 21) placed him only in the *average* range for his age thus failing to show his *above average* ability to retain well-learned information over time.

TABLE 11.9 WMS-III Logical Memory Recognition Scores as a Function of Age or LM-II Scores in an Elderly Sample

| Age (years) | Sample (n) | LM-II (mean) | RECOGNITION SCORES | | |
			Recognition (mean)	Range	25th Percentile
70–79	26	31.6 ± 8.3	27.1 ± 2.3	21–30	25
80–89	70	27.3 ± 7.0	25.7 ± 2.7	16–30	24
90–99	30	21.2 ± 8.8	23.1 ± 3.2	16–29	20
LM-II Range					
All	7	0–9	19.1 ± 2.6	16–23	16
All	16	10–19	23.1 ± 2.4	18–26	21
All	56	20–29	24.9 ± 2.5	18–30	23
All	47	30–39	27.4 ± 2.5	24–39	26
All	6	40–45	29.9 ± 0.9	28–30	28

From the Oregon Brain Aging Study.

A formula is provided for calculating percent retention of the LM-III stories over the delay interval. The manual gives no normative story content data for the LM-III yes/no recognition test which follows the 30-minute delayed recall of both stories. Rather, the recognition score from this test is added to the Verbal Paired Associates recognition score to produce a composite recognition score, again leaving interpretation of the data to the examiner's imagination. To correct this deficiency, at least for a group of healthy, well-educated ($M = 14.7$ years) subjects in a longitudinal study of aging (Hickman et al., 2000), recognition scores are given in Table 11.9. This sample (61 men, 71 women) had a mean age of 84.8. No sex effect appeared on the delayed recall (LM-II) or the Recognition trial. Recognition scores ranged from chance (16) to perfect in a negatively skewed distribution. They correlated with age ($r = -.46$), but the correlation with LM-II scores ($r = .73$) was stronger.

Test characteristics. Immediate recall of both earlier LM versions remains fairly stable through middle age and then progressively declines (Mitrushina, Boone, and D'Elia, 1999; Sinnett and Holen, 1999; Wechsler, 1987). The LM-III immediate recall shows a slow, steady decline between the ages of 55 and 89 years with the oldest age group (85–89 years) recalling about half of the recall of the youngest normative group (Wechsler, 1997b). Delayed recall data vary for LM, perhaps in part because of administration and test differences. Delayed recall on LM-R may begin its decline as early as the 20s, level off until the 50s, and then continue to shrink (Wechsler, 1987). However, the omission of data for years 18–19, 25–34, and 45–54 makes this a tenuous generalization. Norms have been developed for LM-R for older age groups (Ivnik, Malec, Smith, et al.,

1992c; Lichtenberg and Christensen, 1992; Marcopulos, McLain, and Giuliano, 1997; E.D. Richardson and Marottoli, 1996). Delayed recall on LM-III begins to decline fairly steadily from about age 45. Age decline on LM-III delayed recall is largely explained by poorer immediate recall (Haaland, Price, and LaRue, 2003). A steady decline in recall of thematic units also occurs with age. The relatively lower education of the older groups in the WMS-III normative population makes these norms questionable when evaluating the performances of better educated older persons.

Sex effects are not prominent. Overall, women have the advantage. They outperformed men on immediate recall of LM-R (Ragland et al., 2000). Ivison (1986) found slightly higher scores by women on "Anna Thompson," slightly higher scores by men on the second LM-O story, perhaps reflecting the stories' different content. Women with greater temporal lobe cerebral blood flow performed better on immediate and delayed recall of the LM-R than those with lower blood flow, but this correlation was not found in males (Ragland et al., 2000). Education, often used as the most convenient measure of intellectual ability, makes a significant contribution to performance on LM (Abikoff et al., 1987; Compton et al., 1997; E.D. Richardson and Marottoli, 1996; Ylikoski et al., 1998), as does socioeconomic status (Sinnett and Holen, 1999).

Correlations between LM-R stories A and B for different age groups were in the .68 to .80 range for immediate recall and .68 to .85 for the delay trial (Wechsler, 1987). The WMS manual does not give any information about the relationship between the two LM stories. For LM-R the test manual reports that subjects in the 20–24 year age group made the greatest gains when retested within four to six weeks: +7.4 on immediate recall of the two stories, +9.4 on delayed recall (out of a possible 50 points) (Wechsler, 1987; see also McCaffrey, Duff, and Westervelt, 2000b, for other control group gains). Two raters scoring LM-R blindly achieved almost perfect agreement (Woloszyn et al., 1993). The retest gain on LM-III over 2 to 12 week intervals was reported to be about 2 points for immediate and delayed recall when the age groups were combined (The Psychological Corporation, 1997). Practice effects can be observed with lengthy retest intervals, even up to a year (Hickman et al., 2000; Theisen et al., 1998).

Correlational studies consistently demonstrate a relationship between the immediate recall trial of this test and other learning tests (Kear-Colwell, 1973; Macartney-Filgate and Vriezen, 1988), and an even stronger association of delayed recall with other learning tests (Bornstein and Chelune, 1989; Woodard, Goldstein, et al., 1999). This latter group described LM-R as the "purest" measure of episodic memory compared to a word list learning task and a visuospatial memory task because of its relatively low association with nonmemory measures. Both immediate and delayed trials have larger associations with verbal tests (e.g., WIS Information, Vocabulary) than does the associate learning format, probably reflecting the verbal organization and syntax required both for repeating the stories and giving answers to these two WIS tests (Larrabee, Kane, et al., 1985).

Neuropsychological findings. Because of its age and popularity, a wealth of clinical studies have used LM. Thus LM data exist for almost all known brain disorders. This review covers LM patterns for the most commonly seen or neuropsychologically relevant conditions.

A delayed LM-O recall distinguished a group of mild TBI patients with apparent "good recovery" from control subjects whose average recall score was $2\frac{1}{2}$ units greater than that of the patients (Stuss, Ely, et al., 1985). In another study, TBI patients recalled less of the Anna Thompson story than controls, particularly losing details in the middle portion of the story while showing relatively well-preserved primacy and recency effects (S. Hall and Bornstein, 1991). Soccer (European football) concussions in long-term adult players are associated with impaired LM-R performance (Matser, Kessels, Lezak, et al., 1999). LM-R was more accurate than a word list learning task and a paired associate learning task in differentiating patients with mild head injuries from matched controls (Guilmette and Rasile, 1995). However, not all studies have found LM to be sensitive to mild TBI. Brooker's (1997) review identifies other WMS-R tests as more sensitive to the effects of mild TBI and mild dementia in group comparisons, apparently because of LM's large within-group vari-

ability. For example, the LM-O version of this test did not distinguish moderately injured from severely injured head trauma patients prior to entrance into a rehabilitation program, although the moderately injured group's average score (5.85) was barely *marginal to normal limits*, while that of the severely damaged group was *defective* (4.25) (Trexler and Zappala, 1988). Yet, significant improvement in the first year after head injury was registered by LM-O, which also distinguished the head injured patients from their controls even after showing improvement at two years posttrauma (Dikmen, Machamer, et al., 1990); moreover, the LM-R score contributed to the prediction of improvement and level of social integration of TBI patients six months after discharge from acute rehabilitation (Hanks, Rapport, et al., 1999).

A "percent forgetting" score reflecting the difference between immediate and delayed recall showed that right temporal lobectomy patients were more likely than those with temporal excisions on the left to have improved verbal memory, and less likely to perform worse than preoperatively (Ivnik, Sharbrough, and Laws, 1988). Delaney, Rosen, and their colleagues (1980) found that only delayed recall differentiated right from left temporal lobectomy patients. Similar findings showed the expected right–left differential in recall score levels for patients with seizure foci who subsequently had temporal lobectomies, but a "percent retained" score was the only one that correlated significantly with neuronal loss in the excised tissue (Sass et al., 1992). The volume of the left hippocampus significantly predicted LM-R immediate, delayed, and percent retention scores in seizure patients who had not undergone surgery (R.C. Martin, Hugg, Roth, et al., 1999). Groups of patients with lateralized lesions of mixed etiologies also performed differently on LM-R, of course with the patients whose damage was on the right outperforming the left lesioned group (Chelune and Bornstein, 1988; P.M. Moore and Baker, 1996). Patients with carotid artery disease performed significantly better than Alzheimer patients but significantly worse than control subjects on LM; no differences showed up between the two groups with lateralized carotid involvement (Kelly, Kaszniak, and Garron, 1986). A scoring system that distinguishes between "Essential," "Detail," and "Self-generated" propositions brought out response differences between patients with lateralized lesions and normal control subjects (Webster et al., 1992). For example, normal control subjects gave more essential and detail propositions than did the patients, patients with left-sided lesions tended to make fewer responses in all categories, and patients with lesions in the right hemisphere gave more intrusion responses.

Like other learning tests, LM has been useful as an aid both in identifying dementia and in tracking its progression (Storandt, Botwinick, and Danziger, 1986; R.S. Wilson and Kaszniak, 1986). Scores below those of controls have been found in patients before the appearance of clinical evidence of Alzheimer's disease (Howieson, Dame, et al., 1997; Rubin, Storandt, Miller, et al., 1998) or in asymptomatic Huntington's disease gene carriers (Hahn-Barma et al., 1998). Characteristically, Alzheimer patients have poor recall after the delay interval. The Savings Score developed by Nelson Butters, Salmon, Cullum, and their coworkers (1988; Tröster, Butters, Salmon et al., 1993) (see p. 442) shows that Alzheimer patients have more pronounced forgetting over the delay interval than Huntington patients). This test is also sensitive to the memory and learning deficits of multiple sclerosis (Minden, Moes, et al., 1990). MS patients show the usual pattern of recalling main elements compared to nonessential details but recall less than controls (Lokken et al., 1999).

Babcock Story Recall Format (Babcock, 1930; Babcock and Levy, 1940)

Like Logical Memory in the Wechsler tests, the modified format uses a pair of stories of similar length and difficulty.[1] After initial reading and recall of the first story, the first story is reread and one or two tests are interpolated for approximately 10 min when a recall is requested. Immediate thereafter, a second story is read and its administration follows the Babcock format of immediate recall upon first hearing, then rereading, and another approximately 10 min interference period, and then delayed recall of the second story. One set of data on normal subjects found an approximately 4-point gain on second recall of 21-item stories (Rapaport et al., 1968). Freides, Engen, and their colleagues (1996) used the double reading format on two 29-unit stories and the original Babcock-Levy[1] story divided into 22 units; recall after the second reading immediately followed a drawing recall trial so that delay was only from 80 to 120 sec. College students' average unit gain was from 5 (story 1 [Babcock-Levy], first reading $M = 12.8 \pm 3.5$) to 6.6 (story 2, first reading $M = 16.5 \pm 5$). Given only the Babcock-Levy story, elderly subjects (in 60s, 70s, 80s) on average made 5 unit gains from first reading: $M = 10.5 \pm 3.4$ (60s), $M = 9.0 \pm 3.3$ (70s), $M = 8.0 \pm 3.6$ (80s) (see p. 449 for second story and Table 11.10).

It is noteworthy that LM-III now includes the Babcock format for the second of its two stories.

When using story pairs, the decision about which story recall format to use, one without rereading after the first recall or Babcock's, depends on whether the examiner is more interested in testing for proactive interference or learning. The stories in each of these tests can be adapted to either format. The Babcock format may be more likely to elicit interference effects because it was read twice and the second story is introduced immediately after the delayed recall of the first. The two readings in the Babcock format seem to make more neuropsychological sense than a single reading of a story, as patients with a limited auditory span, or whose grasp of information as it goes by them is restricted by slow processing, will register only a small portion of the story on first hearing it. Immediate recall provides an appropriate opportunity for documenting these problems which then can be distinguished from defective learning by rereading the story. Delayed recall will then give a clearer picture of learning capacity. By the same token, patients whose delayed recall drops significantly even with a second reading leave little doubt about the fragility of their recall capacity. Of special interest are intrusions of content or ideas from the first to the second paragraph and wide disparities in amount of recall.

Story Sets

Story recall elicits the most information about a subject's ability to handle meaningful verbal information when two stories are given in tandem. Since neuropsychological examinations are often repeated, sometimes within weeks or even days, the best way to deal with practice effects is to have multiple story sets available.

Each of the four forms of the Rivermead Behavioural Memory Test (B. [A.] Wilson, Cockburn, and Baddeley, 1985) contains a 21-unit (from 54 to 65 words in each) story suitable for tandem presentations. The authors acknowledge the local nature of some place names and colloquialisms in the stories, advising examiners to substitute more familiar ones as needed (e.g., I substitute "Beaverton," a Portland suburb, for "Brighton" [mdl]).

P. Green and Kramar (1983)[2] developed the *CogniSyst Story Recall Test,* a series of stories at five levels of difficulty (from 22 words, 10 items to 56 words, 25 items) with six stories in each set.

Two/ semi-trailer trucks/ lay on their sides/ after a tornado/ blew/ a dozen trucks/ off the highway/ in West Springfield./ One person/ was killed/ and 418 others/ were injured/ in the

---

[1]December 6./ Last week/ a river overflowed/ in a small town/ ten miles/ from Albany./ Water/ covered the streets/ and entered the houses./ Fourteen persons/ were drowned/ and 600 persons/ caught cold/ because of the dampness/ and cold weather./ In saving/ a boy/ who was caught under a bridge,/ a man/ cut his hands.

[2]The complete test sets and norms can be ordered from Wm. Paul Green, Ph.D., 17107-107 Ave., #201, Edmonton, Alberta, T5S 1G3, Canada. (e-mail: paulgreen@shaw.ca)

TABLE 11.10 Expected Scores for Immediate and Delayed Recall Trials of the Babcock Story Recall Test

Mental Ability Level*	Sample (n)	IMMEDIATE RECALL			DELAYED RECALL		
		Q_1	Median	Q_3	Q_1	Median	Q_3
Average	27	12	13	14	13	15	16
High average	41	12	14.5	17	16	17	19
Superior	45	13	15	18	15	17	19

*For statistical definitions of these levels, see Chapter 6.
Adapted from Rapaport et al. (1968).

Wednesday storm/ which hit an airport/ and a nearby residential area./ The governor/ will ask/ the President/ to declare/ the town/ a major disaster area.

Cowboy Story

Because it has been included in many mental status examinations since it first appeared in 1919, this is the paragraph best known to medical practitioners. Talland (1965a; with Ekdahl, 1959) used it to make a welcome distinction between verbatim and content recall of paragraph. He divided it into 27 memory units for quantitative verbatim recall and identified 24 content ideas (italicized words or phrases), which are credited as correctly recalled if the subject substitutes synonyms or suitable phrases for the exact wording.

A cowboy/ from Arizona/ went to San Francisco/ with his dog,/ which he left/ at a friend's/ while he purchased/ a new suit of clothes./ Dressed finely,/ he went back/ to the dog,/ whistled to him,/ called him by name/ and patted him./ But the dog would have nothing to do with him,/ in his new hat/ and coat,/ but gave a mournful/ howl./ Coaxing was of no effect/; so the cowboy went away/ and donned his old garments,/ whereupon the dog/ immediately/ showed his wild joy/ on seeing his master/ as he thought he ought to be./ (Talland, 1965a).

On immediate recall testing, a 22-subject control group gave an average of 8.32 of the 27 verbatim memory units; their average content recall score was 9.56. Healthy subjects in three age groups (M_{ages} = 43.5, 55.9, and 67.5) read this story aloud (Fastenau, Denburg, and Abeles, 1996). The youngest group recalled 15.1 units immediately and lost an average of less than one unit after a 20-minute delay. The oldest group recalled less, 13.5 units, but retained this level of recall over delay. Age accounted for about 10% of the variance in these data.

Story Memory Test (Heaton, Grant, and Matthews, 1991)

This story recall test is unique in its multiple presentations and normative data that includes a 4-hour delay.

The 29-item story authored by Ralph Reitan is presented for up to five trials or until the subject has obtained at least 15 points, whichever comes first. The procedure is advantageous for patients with slow information processing or attentional deficits who may not have sufficient exposure when material is presented only once. A tape recording of the story presents items at the rate of one scorable unit per second. Patients with attentional or hearing problems might benefit from a "live" presentation. Recall units are scored so that partially correct information receives partial credit. The *Learning* score is the number of points recalled on the last learning trial divided by the number of trials taken to reach criterion. The *Memory* score is a percent of loss over time: percentage of the difference between the amounts recalled on the last learning trial and on the 4-hour recall. Age- and education-corrected norms are presented in the manual.

African Americans do not perform as well as Caucasians on this test, which has been attributed in part to differences in dialect (Manly, Miller, Heaton, et al., 1998). In this study the use of Black English affected the Learning score because different word usage by African Americans resulted in loss of points. Memory was not affected by the use of Black English because it is scored as a percent loss. A factor analysis of immediate memory (trial 1) showed loading with CVLT trial 1 while the Learning score loaded with CVLT learning (trials 1–5); verbal fluency contributed to both of these scores (DiPino, Kabat, and Kane, 2000). Delayed recall loaded positively with CVLT delayed recall and negatively with digits backward and Judgment of Line Orientation.

Stories in memory batteries

Memory batteries frequently include story recall tests. The *Memory Assessment Scales* (J.M. Williams, 1991; see pp. 488–490) contains a short story that is read once to the patient. Immediate and delayed recalls are obtained, although only responses to nine questions about the stories are scored. This story would be useful for severely impaired patients who might fail other memory tests as the cueing provided by questions about the stories facilitates recall. The *Denman Neuropsychology Memory Scale* (Denman, 1984, 1987; see pp. 490–491), on the other hand, offers a 42-item story, which is longer than most tests in order to avoid the ceiling effects that can occur with shorter stories. The *Learning and Memory Battery* (*LAMB*) (Tombaugh and Schmidt, 1992; see pp. 493–494) contains a 31-item paragraph of information about a person which is read twice with free and cued recall trials following each reading. Delayed recall takes place after 20 minutes and includes free and cued recall as well as multiple-choice questions regarding missed material. The *Randt Memory Test* (Randt and Brown, 1986; Randt, Brown, and Osborne, 1980; see pp. 487–488) contains five 25-word, 20-item stories, which could be used in pairs. All five stories follow an identical formula in identical sequence: date (3 items), place (2 items), catastrophe (3 items), locale (4 items), consequence that includes three numbers (8 items). Erickson and Howieson (1986) suggested that they read more like a list than a story. Since the strict similarity of the items could lead to confusion for even the most efficient learner, these stories should be used together—or even a day apart—only with caution.

VISUAL MEMORY

Tests of visual memory often call for a visuomotor response, typically drawing. This, of course, can complicate the interpretation of defective performance since failure may arise from constructional disability, impaired visual or spatial memory, or an interaction between these or other factors. Even on recognition tasks without a constructional response, perceptual impairments such as hemispatial inattention are potential performance confounds. Therefore, the quality of a patient's responses when compared to other neuropsychological measures should enable the examiner to estimate the relative contributions of perception, constructional or visuomotor skill, and memory to the final product.

To minimize verbal mediation, visual memory test stimuli often use abstract designs or nonsense figures, although some visual memory tests (e.g., Continuous Recognition Memory Test; WMS-III Family Pictures) contain both visual and verbal elements and do not strive to assess material-specific memory function. Even attempts to create a hypothetically "pure" nonverbal visual memory test by using complex or unfamiliar stimuli cannot fully eliminate verbal associations—which are thought to contribute to the poorer lateralizing ability of most visual memory tests compared to their verbal counterparts (Barr et al., 1997; Feher and Martin, 1992).

The measurement of learning (rate, efficiency, retention) requires material of sufficient difficulty that only very exceptional persons would be able to grasp and retain it with one or two exposures, and there must be enough learning trials to permit emergence of a learning curve. A number of visual learning tests meet these requirements—some do not. Several more or less follow André Rey's AVLT paradigm.

Facial recognition is another form of visual memory. The Recognition Memory for Faces portion of the Recognition Memory Test (Warrington, 1984) and the Wechsler Memory Scale-III Faces test (Wechsler, 1997b) use this format. The Warrington test is discussed in Chapter 12 and the WMS-III Faces is discussed below.

Visual Recognition Memory

Recognition testing is important for evaluating visual memory when free recall is impaired. It also overcomes the output limitations of patients who cannot adequately draw due to hemiparesis or some other physical limitation. Most newer visual memory test formats include a recognition component. In this section, only visual memory tests that solely rely on recognition testing will be discussed.

Recurring Figures Test (D. Kimura, 1963)[1]

This test is important, in part, because it established the recurring stimulus paradigm for visual memory assessment. The material consists of 160 cards containing either geometric or irregular nonsense figures which are each shown for 3 sec in eight trial blocks. The trial sets are not apparent to the subject as the stimuli are continuously presented. Eight of the first 20 designs repeat in each subsequent trial block. The subject indicates which designs were seen previously. Because the targets are "new" during the first trial block, correct recognition of all targets yields a score of 56. False positive responses are subtracted from the total to correct for guessing. Normative information is based upon corrected recognition performance.

Test characteristics. Performance appears unaffected by age (Rixecker and Hartje, 1980): Kimura's control subjects, all in their 20s, had an average corrected score

[1]The test material may be ordered from D.K. Consultants, Department of Psychology, University of Western Ontario, London, Ontario, Canada, N6A 3K7.

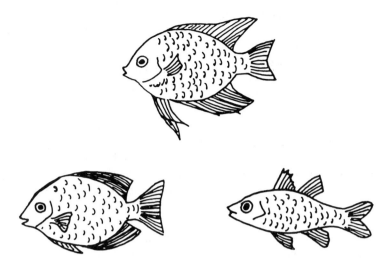

FIGURE 11.1 One of the eight target figures (top) of the Continuous Recognition Memory Test and two foils. (Courtesy of H. Julia Hannay)

of 38.9 which is similar to the performance of an independent sample of healthy young subjects ($M = 37.5$) (Aguirre et al., 1985) and other, older, groups in their 30s ($M = 40.9$) and 40s ($M = 36.6$) (Nielsen, Knudsen, and Daugbjerg, 1989). One exception ($M = 28.5$) was reported for control subjects of whom most were in their forties (Newcombe, 1969). For subjects in the 20 to 65 year age range, performance was unaffected by age but education differences were found (Rixecker and Hartje, 1980). A reliability coefficient of .94 was reported.

Neuropsychological findings. Kimura (1963) found no difference between right and left temporal lobectomy patients. Right temporal lobe patients made more false positive errors, however, producing a significant left vs. right group difference for education corrected scores. Both groups remembered geometric better than nonsense figures but left temporal patients recognized a greater proportion of nonsense figures.

Corrected scores differentiated TBI patients from healthy control subjects, although no difference in number of false positive errors was observed (D.N. Brooks, 1974). Patients with histories of alcoholism obtained an average score of 32.7, in sharp contrast to the *defective* scores ($M = 11.3$) made by six Korsakoff patients (Squire and Shimamura, 1986). Noting some extreme instances of intragroup variability (range = 5 to 24 for Korsakoff patients, which overlaps the control subjects' range of 20 to 40), Squire and Shimamura suggested that, "this test may fail to detect amnesia in some cases because it does not incorporate a long delay, and because the critical items are repeated several times" (p. 873). This criticism can be applied to all re-

curring recognition tests that do not incorporate a delayed recall component.

Continuous Recognition Memory Test (CRMT) (Hannay and Levin, no date; Hannay, Levin, and Grossman, 1979)[1]

This test consists of 120 line drawings of various flora (e.g., mushrooms, flowers, a cauliflower, a potato) and fauna (e.g., fish, seashells, dogs) organized into six blocks of 20 drawings each (see Fig. 11.1). The first set of blocks introduces the eight target drawings plus 12 foils. Each of the subsequent blocks contains all eight target figures plus eight similar ones (in each of the eight categories from which target figures are drawn), plus four drawings from other-than-target categories (e.g., vegetables). The subject sees each drawing for 3 sec and, similar to Kimura's Recurring Figures, indicates whether the drawing is "old," i.e., previously seen, or "new." The original format of the test includes a set of drawings with each target figure on top of a page and repeated again with the similar foils randomized below to test perceptual accuracy. This format can be readily turned into a recognition trial simply by covering the target figures on top of each page with a 3 × 5 card and asking the subject to point out the drawing which is exactly like the one seen before, "six different times."

This test extends Kimura's scoring system to include signal detection techniques. Scores are obtained for *Hits*

---

[1]This test may be ordered from H.J. Hannay, 4046 Grenoch Lane, Houston, TX 77025.

(correct recognition of recurring targets), *False Alarms* (incorrectly calling a new, nonrecurring figure "old"), and *Misses* (failure to recognize a target stimulus). The *Correct Responses* score is calculated from the formula Hits + (60 − False Alarms). A d' score can also be calculated as a measure of perceptual discrimination. Impairment levels have been determined for each of these scores: Correct Responses < 87; Hits < 36; False Alarms > 16; Misses > 4 (Hannay, Levin, and Grossman, 1979). Although this test appears similar to the Continuous Visual Memory Test described below, they cannot be used interchangeably.

The application of signal detection methods to recognition memory testing is not universally accepted (J.T.E. Richardson, 1994). Drake and Hannay (1992) explained that signal detection analysis is justifiable for evaluating scores when it meets the necessary assumptions of signal detection theory (i.e., a constant sensory input [signal and noise], random presence of signal that occurs with a fixed signal strength, with signal and noise at times being indistinguishable).

Test characteristics. For 66 TBI patients, neither age nor education was associated with scores on this test (Hannay, Levin, and Grossman, 1979). However, both age and education effects, but not sex differences, were observed in a large (n = 299) sample of healthy subjects in the 10 to 89 year age range (Trahan, Larrabee, and Levin, 1986). Hits and False Alarms tap into different aspects of memory performance, with Hits associated with learning and memory, and False Alarms reflecting attention to visual detail (Fuchs et al., 1999).

Larrabee and Curtiss (1995) modified this test by including a 30 min delayed recognition trial. Unlike the Visual Reproduction test of the Wechsler Memory Scale, spatial ability did not contribute to CRMT performance. Somewhat surprisingly, the relationship to the Wechsler Memory Scale "general memory factor" was similar for both immediate acquisition and delayed recognition.

Neuropsychological findings. While this test did not discriminate between healthy subjects and patients with mild TBI, Correct Response did identify from 67% to 85% of moderately and severely injured patients from a broad age range (Hannay, Levin, and Grossman, 1979). Relatively fewer brain injured adolescents with moderate (29.4%) to severe (41.5%) injuries performed at *defective* levels (Hannay and Levin, 1989). Correct Response scores of patients with brain injury, mostly due to trauma, tended to be negatively associated with ventricular enlargement (H.S. Levin, Meyers, et al., 1981). Adolescents with left hemisphere contusions or hematoma or with diffuse damage performed at a

somewhat lower level than those with identifiable right-sided or bilateral lesions (Hannay and Levin, 1989).

Continuous Visual Memory Test (CVMT) (Trahan and Larrabee, 1988)

With the Hannay and Levin CRMT format as a model, this test differs only in the abstract nature of the stimulus designs and in such details as number of items (112), number of target figures (7), number of times each target figure appears (7), and exposure time (2 sec). Scoring follows the CRMT procedures. Besides a trial for perceptual accuracy, the CVMT includes a recognition trial after a 30-minute delay. Normative data are available for ages 18 to 70+ (Trahan and Larrabee, 1988; Trahan, Larrabee, and Quintana, 1990). Cut-off scores for *Total* (score), a d' score (the perceptual discrimination measure calculated from z-scores for *Hits* and *False Alarms* listed in the record form), and *Delay* have been calculated for four age groups, 18–29, 30–49, 50–60, and 70+, and are presented with the normative data in the test booklet. However, several studies in independent samples suggest that the recommended cut-off scores tend to misclassify some healthy elderly subjects as impaired (S. Hall, Pinkston, et al., 1996; Paolo, Tröster, and Ryan, 1998a).

Test characteristics. Performance levels go down slowly but steadily from age 30 on, mostly due to an increase in false alarms (Trahan, Larrabee, and Quintana, 1990). Because of these age declines, the suggested cut-off scores for younger subjects are inappropriate for elderly application (S. Hall, Pinkston, et al., 1996). A comparison between subjects with 12 or fewer years of education and those with 16 or more years found no differences between groups (Trahan and Larrabee, 1988). Interitem reliability correlations go from .80 to .98 (for both recurring and nonrecurring items) (Trahan and Larrabee, 1988). Trahan and Larrabee (1988) reported a strong association between Total score and the WMS-R Visual Reproduction test's delay trial while finding no association between Delay and Block Design. These and other congruent data indicate that Delay is a measure of visual memory "relatively independent of visual–spatial ability" (Trahan and Larrabee, 1988). In their factor analytic studies, d' was associated with "a general cognitive factor" but no memory factors. The delayed recognition score has been reported to be the best measure of visual memory in some factor analytic studies (Larrabee, Trahan, and Curtiss, 1992) but not in others (Larrabee and Curtiss, 1995). However, like the Continuous Recognition Memory Test, spatial ability contributes little when compared to Wechsler's Visual Reproduction test (Larrabee and Curtis, 1995).

Test–retest stability coefficients in 12 healthy subjects reported in the manual are .85 for Total score, .80 for d', and .76 for Delayed Recognition, although somewhat lower scores have been reported for larger samples (.53 to .66) (Trahan, Larrabee, Fritzsche, and Curtiss, 1996). As with other memory tests, stability coefficients after a one year retest delay were substantially lower (.44 to .49) in one healthy elderly sample (Paolo, Tröster, and Ryan, 1998b). Based upon these test–retest reliability data, an 11-point difference in Total score between assessments reflects a significant change ($p = .10$) that exceeds the standard error of the difference score and is not likely due to chance (Paolo, Tröster, and Ryan, et al., 1998b). An alternative form of the CVMT is available for repeat testing (Trahan, Larrabee, Fritzsche, and Curtiss, 1996).

Neuropsychological findings. The average scores for both right- and left-lateralized stroke patient groups were significantly lower than those for control subjects on all measured variables (Trahan, Larrabee, and Quintana, 1990). However, while 50% of patients with right-sided lesions failed on Total and 63% performed in the impaired range on Delay, of the patients with left-sided strokes only 20% and 23% failed on these measures, respectively. In a sample of patients with lateralized temporal lobe epilepsy, the CVMT did not discriminate seizure onset laterality, although overall cognitive functional and visuoperceptual processing were related to CVMT scores (Snitz et al., 1996). Almost all (92%) of a small group of Alzheimer patients had difficulty discriminating targets from false alarms. However, only about half had Total or Delay scores below the acceptable level (Trahan and Larrabee, 1988).

WMS-III Faces (Wechsler, 1997b)

Memory for faces has a rich tradition in memory assessment (Warrington, 1984), and in particular, for assessing memory functions associated with the non-dominant hemisphere (B. Milner, 1968). This test of facial recognition memory is similar to Warrington's Recognition Memory subtest. A series of 24 faces is shown at the rate of one every 2 sec. Memory is assessed with a recognition format in which the target face pictures are shown one-by-one interspersed among 24 foils. The subject's task is to indicate which faces had been previously seen. Delayed recognition is tested with the 24 target faces mixed in with 24 new foils. Three scores can be obtained: *Recognition Total* ("yes" for targets, "no" for foils) on the immediate and on the delay trials, and *percent recalled*. Scores are converted

to standard scores ($M = 10 \pm 3$) for each age group (see p. 142). As with many other WMS-III tests, the percent recalled score can be compared to normative tables as a supplemental score.

Test characteristics. The following data come from the Psychological Corporation's (1997) statistical analyses of this test. Performance for both the immediate and delayed components is fairly stable through young adulthood. It begins to decline in middle age and decreases more rapidly in the 70s and beyond. Percent recall shows little age effect as the average recall (i.e., with scaled score = 10) in the oldest age group (85–89 years) corresponds to a retention of 92 to 94%. The average reliability coefficient was .74 for both the immediate and delayed conditions. The test–retest stability coefficient over a short period of 2 to 12 weeks is .67 for immediate and .62 for delayed recognition. The stability for percent retention ranged from 81% to 89% for the two groups.

Although men may outperform women on visuospatial tests such as Judgment of Line Orientation, this difference is not seen on the WMS-III Faces test (M.R. Basso, Harrington, et al., 2000). Faces scores do not correlate as well with the WMS-III "general visual memory factor" or with other visual memory tests as do other measures of visual memory (Millis, Malina, et al., 1999). This low correlation may simply reflect a different aspect of visual memory assessed by Faces than the other tests.

A yes/no recognition format with no built-in control for guessing or response bias lends itself to guessing. This creates a problem when the accuracy of "normal" recognition does not differ much from 50%, i.e., chance. For example, for the oldest age group (85–89 years), a score of 24 (half right) on either the immediate or delayed condition results in a scaled score of 7 (16th–24th percentile range)! Moreover, a score of 34 might be obtained either by correctly recognizing all 24 target faces and correctly saying "no" to 10 foils (making 14 false positive errors), or 10 correct recognitions (14 false negative errors) while correctly saying "no" to all 24 foils. Yet the inferences from these two patterns should be very different despite identical scores.

Clinical findings. Schizophrenia patients tend to perform poorly on tests of memory for faces, including the WMS-III Faces test (Conklin et al., 2002). In addition, first-degree relatives of these patients perform poorly on WMS-III Faces.

Family Pictures (Wechsler, 1997b)

This new test in the Wechsler Memory Scale-III is designed to measure "complex, meaningful, visually presented information," which the test developers consider a "visual analogue to the Logical Memory subtest" (Wechsler, 1997b, p. 15). Like the Continuous Visual Recognition Memory test, many aspects of Family Pictures are easily verbalized.

The test is introduced by showing a "family portrait"—colored drawings of six family members (mother, father, grandfather, grandmother, son, and daughter) and their dog. Subjects then see individual pictures for 10 sec that contain four family members appearing in different situations performing everyday tasks. Subjects are simply instructed to remember as much about each scene as possible for recall after the picture is removed. Recall is scored for reports of which of the characters were in the scene, where they were located in the picture using a 2 × 2 grid, and what each character was doing. A 30-minute delayed recall is also obtained.

Test characteristics. This test can present some scoring problems. Scoring is "character based," meaning that unless the correct person is identified, points for what was going on in the picture and in which quadrant cannot be earned. This can create a problem for some older patients who, based upon their age, may refer to the "father" as "son" and the "son" as "grandson." Further, in a least one picture (i.e., yard scene), the distinction between "father" and "son" is not as clear as in others; even when the subject correctly identifies the activity and place, misclassification of the son results in a score of 0 (it could be argued that in these cases a perfect score of 4 should be awarded since the person confusion is not due to memory failure). The examiner can usually avoid this problem by taking a little extra time during the initial identification of each family member.

Other concerns about the test have surfaced. For example, patients often confuse the picnic with the yard scene on delayed recall, making the scores difficult to interpret (e.g., describing the activities for the yard scene when prompted with "tell me everything about the picnic scene" receives no memory credit). Also, very indistinct actions are portrayed for the characters in the meal scene, and their intended actions are often missed: patients may simply report that everyone is eating, which gets credit for only one of the four persons at the table. This scene has the potential for an additional scoring problem as "looking" is listed as an example of both a 0-point and 1-point action response for two separate characters. Moreover, a verbal memory impairment (i.e., forgetting the picture titles) may also be a source of low scores.

The three components of Family Pictures (who, what, and where) are summed into a single score. Given the

potential neuropsychological differences associated with a ventral "what" stream that processes object information and a dorsal "where" stream involved with spatial processing (Mishkin, Ungerleider, and Macko, 1983), it is unfortunate that normative data for each discrete component were not provided. Thus, one cannot easily tell what this test is measuring in the individual case.

Visual Recall: Design Reproduction

A number of abbreviated tests of memory for designs call for a 5- or 10-sec exposure followed immediately, or after a brief delay, by a drawing trial in which subjects attempt to depict what they remember. Probably the most popular designs are the two Memory for Designs I tasks at age levels IX and XI from the Stanford-Binet (Terman and Merrill, 1973; see Fig. 11.2, p. 455). These appear in slightly modified form in the Wechsler Memory Scale-III and in other test sets as well (e.g., Gainotti and Tiacci, 1970). Both the Stanford-Binet and the Wechsler Memory Scale administrations call for a 10-sec exposure followed by an immediate response. A third Binet design, composed of embedded diamonds, appears at age level XII (see Fig. 11.2).

Memory tests requiring reproduction of a design have been used to assess right hemisphere damage. McFie (1960) found a significant number of impaired Binet design reproductions associated with right hemisphere lesions regardless of their specific site within the hemisphere, although this disability was not associated with left hemisphere patients. More recently, extrahippocampal volumes in the right medial temporal lobe, but not the hippocampus, have been associated with Visual Reproduction performance (Kohler et al., 1998; R. Martin et al., 1999).

Visual Reproduction (Wechsler, 1945, 1987, 1997b)

This was originally developed as an immediate recall test, but many examiners added a delayed trial to the original version (VR-O) (e.g., E.W. Russell, 1988). Each of the three VR-O cards with printed designs is shown for five seconds (the third card of each form of the test has a double design; form I contains the IX- and XI-year level designs of the Binet pictures shown in Fig. 11.2). The other two form I designs are from the Babcock-Levy test battery (1940). Following each exposure, subjects draw what they remember of the design. The maximum score is 14. Scoring discrepancies can be quite large and mostly arise from differences of opinion about the degree of accuracy required, with

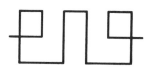 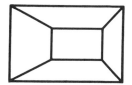

IX- and XI-year level

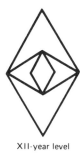

XII-year level

FIGURE 11.2 Memory for Designs models (Terman and Merrill, 1973. Courtesy of Houghton Mifflin Co.)

questions of proportions concerning card B drawings in particular (M. Mitchell, 1987).

Delayed recall trials have been given anywhere from 20 min to an hour later; most examiners ask for a 30-min recall. The procedures described by Trahan, Quintana, and their colleagues (1988) are typical in requesting recall after 30 min of testing during which other drawing tasks are not given ("to limit interference"). Using the same scoring criteria as those for the first trial, these workers offer normative data for four age groups from 18–19 to 70+ (for more normative data for both immediate and delay trials, see also Mitrushina, Boone, and D'Elia 1999; Spreen and Strauss, 1998).

The first formal revision of this test (VR-R) included both immediate and 30-min delay trials (Wechsler, 1987). It consists of four items, of which three contain a single figure (design A is the same on both forms of VR, B is new involving circles within circles, C is VR-O card B) and on the fourth item card, D, are two designs, one containing three and the other two geometric elements. Examples accompany very detailed scoring guidelines with new criteria for the designs retained from the original version. The maximum score is 41 points with the same scoring criteria applied to both the immediate and delayed trials.

Further modifications were introduced in the second revision (VR-III) (Wechsler, 1997b). A simple design was added to lower the floor of the test, one of the cards from VR-R was deleted, and one of the cards from the original scale that was not included in VR-R resurfaced in slightly modified form. As with VR-R, a

30-minute delayed recall is obtained. The newest version contains a 48-item recognition test and a seven-item discrimination test to identify differences in recall and recognition capacities. In addition, a copy task can be given to examine the potential role of motor difficulty. Scoring for the VR-III has been modified so that partial credit may be earned; the manual provides good examples of 0-, 1-, and 2-point responses. The maximum score is 104 points with scaled score conversions for the different age groups (see p. 484).

A scheme for scoring intrusion errors for the VR-O and VR-R was devised to document these often very interesting abnormal response distortions (D. Jacobs, Salmon, et al., 1990; D. Jacobs, Tröster, et al., 1990). Fewer intrusion errors appeared on VR-R performances compared to VR-O, which these authors suggest may be due to the introduction of circular figures along with the rectilinear ones of VR-O.

Test characteristics. All versions of this test display steep age gradients (Wechsler, 1987; see also Mitrushina, Boone, and D'Elia, 1999; Spreen and Strauss, 1998). The score drop-off is particularly sharp in the later years: for example, on VR-R, average performances in the 30–35 point range at ages 56–66 drop to a 20–28 point range at ages 77–87 (Ivnik, Malec, Smith, et al., 1992); on the VR-III, average performances in the 43–51 point range at ages 55–64 are in the 28–34 point range at ages 70–79 (Wechsler, 1997b).

In a large-scale Australian standardization, women obtained an average score that was almost 1 point lower than that of the men (Ivison, 1977), a pattern that has been seen in other studies (Reite et al., 1993). Findings of a sex difference in VR age-related decline are inconsistent (Barrett-Connor and Kritz-Silverstein, 1999; Suutama et al., 2002). Neither the WMS-R nor the WMS-III manual reports on sex effects for VR (Wechsler, 1987, 1997b).

For a sample of subjects with educational backgrounds ranging from 0 to >12 years, education effects were prominent on both immediate and delayed recall trials ($p < .0001$) (Ardila and Rosselli, 1989). Education was also a significant variable in a study of older persons, ages 60 to 94, whose average education levels were in the $10^1/_2$ to $13^1/_2$ year range but within-group variability was large (SDs ranged from 4.78 to 6.71; Ivnik, Malec, Smith, et al., 1992c). However, no significant education effects were found on this test for any of four, mostly younger, patient groups, with education levels averaging from $11^1/_2$ to $13^1/_2$ years although the range of scores within groups was narrower (SDs from 2.34 to 3.61; Trahan, Quintana, et al., 1988). Together these studies suggest that educationally deprived persons may do poorly on this test—and perhaps any other unfamiliar task requiring paper and pencil—but beyond the level of a basic educational foundation, education effects may be small.

As with most memory tests, practise effects occur (McCaffrey, Duff, and Westervelt, 2000b). A group of older subjects (M age = 69.3) gained almost 2 points on retesting a year later, losing most of this gain on the next year's retesting (Kaszniak, Wilson, Fox, and Stebbins, 1986). Moreover, with only a 7 to 10 day difference between test and retest, hypertensive patients gained 1 point on immediate recall and 1.62 points on delayed recall; chronic smokers made even greater gains of 1.49 and 2.90 on immediate and delay trials, respectively, with all gains statistically significant (McCaffrey, Ortega, et al., 1992). When tested over multiple sessions, the practice effect for VR-R was less than that for other WMS-R tests (Reite et al., 1993). However, for both immediate and delayed recall trials, gains made on retesting were so small as to be practically inconsequential. Further, on immediate recall of VR-O no practice effects showed up at one year for a youthful group of TBI patients (Dikmen, Machamer, et al., 1990), which probably reflects the patients' diminished learning capacities.

An interscorer reliability coefficient of .97 was reported for VR-R, with scoring differences of 4 points or less and an average difference between two scores of 1.50 (Wechsler, 1987). Woloszyn and his colleagues (1993) report interscorer reliability coefficients of similar magnitude. Internal consistency estimates for VR-R (six age groups) ranged from .46 to .71 on im-

mediate recall and from .38 to .59 on delayed recall (Wechsler, 1987).

For the individual components scored according to VR-R criteria, Card A (flags) is a better measure of visual memory, whereas Card B (boxes) is associated more with conceptual reasoning ability (M.A. Williams et al., 1998). VR correlates significantly with tests involving predominantly visuospatial problem solving and visual memory; the association with other visual memory tests is stronger for the delay trial (Larrabee, Kane, and Schuck, 1983; Leonberger et al., 1991; Trahan, Quintana, et al., 1988). Chelune, Bornstein, and Prifitera (1990) called attention to the consistency with which a visual construction component emerges most prominently when other tests are included in the factor analysis. That Visual Reproduction is often affected by constructional skill has been demonstrated by both factor analysis (Larrabee and Curtiss, 1995) and clinical group comparisons (Gfeller, Meldrum, and Jacobi, 1995).

Neuropsychological findings. On immediate recall, neither version discriminated between patients with right- and left-sided lesions (Chelune and Bornstein, 1988; Delaney, Wallace, and Egelko, 1980), although in one study of patients with lesions confined to the temporal lobes, those with left-sided damage performed significantly better (Jones-Gotman, 1991a). On delayed recall, patients with right temporal lesions obtained significantly lower scores on VR-O than those with lesions on the left or healthy control subjects (Delaney, Rosen, et al., 1980), but VR-R showed only a nonsignificant trend favoring patients with left hemisphere damage (Chelune and Bornstein, 1988). In a large multicenter study of over 500 patients with lateralized temporal lobe epilepsy, there was no effect of seizure onset laterality for the immediate or delayed VR-R conditions, nor for the percentage retention over 30 minutes (Barr, Chelune, et al., 1997).

The relative simplicity of the designs encourages verbal encoding and may account for the general absence of pronounced differences between performances by patients with right-sided or left-sided lesions (see also Jones-Gotman, 1991a). The stimuli were revised in the most recent version to minimize verbalization further. Certainly, this test cannot be used to aid in lesion lateralization. VR-O is sensitive to the effects of TBI, correlating significantly with ventricular enlargement (Cullum and Bigler, 1986). It even distinguished a group of patients with mild TBI from control subjects by virtue of an average 1.3 point difference that was significant (Stuss, Ely et al., 1985). While registering improvement over the first year postinjury, VR-O stabilized at that point, with no further change when these TBI patients were examined at the second postinjury year (Dikmen, Machamer, et al., 1990).

Like other memory tests, VR is very sensitive to cognitive deterioration associated with dementia (Kaszniak, Fox, et al., 1978; Laakso et al., 2000). A correlation between delayed VR-R and right hemisphere parahippocampal gyrus volume has been reported in patients with probable Alzheimer's disease (Kohler et al., 1998). D. Jacobs, Tröster et al., 1990) found that the number of intrusions from previously seen stimuli distinguished Alzheimer and Huntington patients from TBI patients who, like control subjects, made very few intrusion errors; Alzheimer patients had the most intrusions of all. In one study, VR-O surpassed the diagnostic accuracy of MRI hippocampal volume measurements (Laakso et al., 2000). "Wineglass" confabulation has been described in some alcoholic patients in which patients rotated the design on VR-R Card D to become a "bowl and stem" (L.W. Welch, Nimmerrichter, et al., 1997). It is interesting to note these patients' reports of drawing the designs as originally presented, i.e., not rotated.

Multiple sclerosis patients tend to do poorly on both immediate and delay trials (Minden, Moes, et al., 1990), although those treated with high doses of interferon beta-1b demonstrated improved VR-O performance at 2–4 years following treatment initiation (Pliskin, Hamer, et al., 1996). Solvent-exposed workers with subclinical symptoms did not give abnormal performances on VR-O (Bleecker, Bolla, et al., 1990), although meta-analysis suggests that VR is sensitive to lead exposure effects (Seeber et al., 2002).

Complex Figure Test: Recall Administration (CFT)
(A. Rey, 1941; Osterrieth, 1944;
Corwin and Bylsma, 1993b)

Recall of the Complex Figure typically follows the copy trial immediately, on delay, or both. The Rey-Osterrieth (or "Rey-O," see Fig. 14.2, p. 537) is the most commonly used figure, although other figures designed to be comparable have been developed for repeated assessments (e.g., Taylor figure, see Fig. 14.3, p. 538; Medical College of Georgia [MCG] figures, see Fig. 14.5, pp. 539–540; Emory figures, see Freides, Engen, et al., 1996). Because Taylor figure scores tend to run higher than R-O scores, Hubley and Tremblay (2002) modified the Taylor Figure by decreasing the number of distinctive features (e.g., star, circle in square), including additional lines to increase the complexity of the visual array and modifying the placement of other figure features (see Fig. 14.4, p. 538). A different complex figure was developed for the Repeatable Brief Assessment of Neuropsychological Status (RBANS, see pages 696–697).

In most administrations, subjects are not forewarned when given the copy instructions that they will be asked to reproduce the figure from memory. Because the four MCG figures were designed for drug trials with repeated assessments over relatively short periods of time, subjects are informed that memory will be tested upon completion of the copy trial so the task demands remain fairly constant across testing sessions.

Perhaps because of its popularity, many variations in CFT administration and scoring have been reported; precise scoring criteria are a more recent development. Even among the formal scoring systems, the criteria range from relatively liberal (Loring, Martin, et al., 1990) to strict (Jones-Gotman, personal communication, 1992 [mdl]; J.E. Meyers and Meyers, 1995b). This variability may be due to Rey's omission of scoring criteria in the original test description.

Recall trials follow either a single delay or two delays, the later delay assessing retention. The timing of the recall trials differs among examiners. The "immediate" recall trial has been given in as brief a delay as 30 sec (Loring, Martin, et al., 1990), but following Osterrieth's (1944) convention, some examiners test after a three-min (short) delay (e.g., see Table 11.11) (see also D.T.R. Berry, Allen, and Schmitt, 1991; Delbecq-Dérouesné and Beauvois, 1989). A longer delayed recall, from 30 min (D.N. Brooks, 1972; Corwin and Bylsma, 1993a; Spreen and Strauss, 1998) to 45 min or an hour (Ogden, Growdon, and Corkin, 1990; L.B. Taylor, 1979) has been obtained with or without the early recall (Spreen and Strauss, 1998). Within the limits of an hour, the length of delay appears to be of little consequence (D.T.R. Berry and Carpenter, 1992; Freides and Avery, 1991). As with the copy trial, the examiner may record how subjects go about drawing the figure, either by giving them different colored pencils to track their progress as suggested by Rey (Corwin and Bylsma, 1993b), or by having the examiner note the sequence of their drawings (Milberg, Hebben, and Kaplan, 1996). Although there are advantages and disadvantages to each of these procedures, switching pencils does not appear to distract subjects and may actually be associated with improved memory performance compared to the "flowchart" method (Ruffolo, Javorsky, et al., 2001).

Standardized systems call for scoring the number of elements correctly produced (see pp. 541–543). Adding to them are a number of systems for evaluating and scoring qualitative features of the drawings. Problems in knowing which of the various published norms to use are raised by differences in test administration and scoring, and by poor reliabilities for individual item scoring (Tupler et al., 1995). In addition, simple clerical scoring errors may further confound score validity (Charter, Walden, and Padilla, 2000).

Most studies have found the Rey figure to be harder to recall than the Taylor which typically elicits scores several points higher than the Rey (D.T.R. Berry, Allen, and Schmitt, 1991; Kuehn and Snow, 1992; Loring and Meador, 2003a; Tombaugh and Hubley, 1991). Comprehensive norms are given in Mitrushina, Boone, and D'Elia (1999) and J.E. Meyers and Meyers (1995). Spreen and Strauss (1998) provide a set of age-graded norms for the copy and 30 min recall trials. For the 16- to 30-year sample the 30 min delay norms are roughly comparable to Osterrieth's (1944) findings for 3-minute delayed recall, as were 30 min delay performances of young college students (Loring, Martin, et al., 1990; see Table 11.11). For all older age levels, the Spreen and Strauss 30 min delay scores run 2 or more points lower than Osterrieth's median score of 22, as do J.E. Meyers and Meyers'. In addition to reporting data for the 3-min recall for three subject groups (ages 45–59, 60–69, and 70–83), K.B. Boone, Lesser, and their coworkers (1993) computed a percent retention score ([recall score − copy score] × 100) for their subjects. Normative data for copy, immediate, and delayed recall are available for 211 subjects, as well as recognition and matching trials (Fastenau, Denberg, and Hufford, 1999). These norms are presented in a user-friendly table that transforms the values into the commonly used standard scores ($M = 10 \pm 3$). The MCG figures produce scores that are more comparable to the Taylor than the Rey figure. Despite some variability among the MCG figures (Loring and Meador, 2003a), they generally provide comparable results (Ingram, Soukup, and Ingram, 1997).

Immediate and delayed memory performances are usually similar. Most studies found that few performances using either the Rey or Taylor showed more than a 1- or 2-point difference between immediate and delayed recall trials (e.g., D.T.R. Berry Allen, and Schmidt, 1991; Heinrichs and Bury, 1991; Shorr et al., 1992; see Mitrushina, Boone, and D'Elia, 1999, for these and many more norm sets).

In a comparison of immediate and delayed recall scores of 40 unselected cases (27 men, age range 18–67), 30 (75%) had score differences no greater than 2 points, although four (10%) had 5-point differences. The average difference between immediate and delayed recall was .425. One-third (13) of the delay scores were higher than the immediate scores. Score distributions of ten Taylor figure protocols did not differ from that of the Rey-O. Half the cases were TBI; the others had such various diagnoses as seizure disorder, Huntington's disease, multiple sclerosis, HIV+, toxic encephalopathy, and cerebral vascular disease. Neither age nor diagnosis appeared to contribute to the higher delay scores.

It is important to note, however, that a short-term recall preceding a delayed recall trial may result in a higher delay score than if a delay trial only is given (Loring, Martin, et al., 1990; see Table 11.11). Freides and Avery (1991) reported a 4- to 5-point score increase from immediate to delay for undergraduate students, probably showing this large an increase because they gave no copy trial.

Since the presence or absence of an immediate recall trial will affect performance, this must be kept in mind when choosing a norm set. Alternative scoring systems (e.g., see pp. 461, 490) further complicate efforts to integrate findings from so many different sources. Additionally, Bennett-Levy (1984a) noted that some examiners tend to score recall trials less strictly than the copy trial, based on the rationale that subjects often do not exercise the same degree of care as when copying so that small lapses in precision probably do not represent lapses in memory. He therefore scored both strictly (following the Montreal Neurological Institute standards) and with more lax criteria. He found that although the correlation between these two scoring methods was high (.94), scoring differences amounted to an average of more than 4 points.

TABLE 11.11 Percentiles for Adult Accuracy Scores on Memory Trials of the Complex Figure Test (Rey-O)

	PERCENTILE										
	≤5	10	20	30	40	50	60	70	80	90	99+
Osterrieth*	—	15	17	19	21	22	24	26	27	28	31
Loring†	15	21	24	26	28	29	29.5	30.5	32	33	36
Loring‡	16	22.5	25	28	29	30.5	31	32	33	35	36
Loring§	13.5	16	19.5	20	21	23	24.5	26	28	30.5	32

*$n = 60$.
†$n = 49$, 30 sec recall.
‡$n = 49$, 30 min recall following 30 sec trial.
§$n = 38$, 30 min recall with no prior recall trial.
From Loring, Martin, et al. (1990)

The role of strategy. How the test-taker goes about copying the complex figure will bear a significant relationship to figure recall (Bennett-Levy, 1984a; Heinrichs and Bury, 1991; Shorr et al., 1992). By and large, persons who approach the copying task conceptually, dealing first with the overall configuration of the design and then—only secondarily—with the details, recall the figure much better than subjects who copy the details one by one, even if they do so in a systematic manner (such as going from top to bottom or left to right). The organizational strategy or lack thereof employed during the copy trial is often a strong predictor of subsequent recall (L.K. Dawson and Grant, 2000; Deckersbach et al., 2000; P.D. Newman and Krikorian, 2001), particularly for subjects at lower mental ability levels (Fujii et al., 2000). This difference may be due to the need to recall many more items when they are processed in individual pieces rather than combined into conceptually meaningful units (e.g., see Ogden, Growden, and Corkin, 1990). Somewhat surprisingly, the orientation of the figure during copy (0°, 90°, 180°, or 270°) is not related to recall success (Ferraro et al., 2002). Thus, the CFT may still be a useful test of visual memory when a fixed stimulus position is not possible, such as in bedside assessment.

Applying Osterrieth's system to scoring copying strategies (pp. 544–545), Ska and Nespoulous (1988a) found that until age 74 the usual relationship between strategy and recall level held but that their 75+ group showed a marked decline in both copy ($M = 30.8 \pm 4.1$) and recall ($M = 13.3 \pm 5.4$), although overall, the older subjects' strategic approaches did not differ significantly from those of the younger groups. Moreover, from 41% to 50% of their younger groups of healthy subjects used Osterrieth's level IV, additive details approach (as did six of the ten persons in the 75+ group).

A "perceptual cluster ratio" devised by Shorr and her coworkers (1992, see p. 546) demonstrated this phenomenon. This score correlated significantly with both the copy score (.55) and an "encoding score" (obtained by dividing the immediate recall score by the copy score) (.55) at a much higher level than the correlation between the usual copy score and the encoding score (.35). In regression analyses, the "strategy total" score calculated by Bennett-Levy (1984a, see p. 546) proved to be the first "of the major determinants of copy scores" (sharing this honor with copy time and age)

and the first of three "best predictors of later recall" (along with copy score and age).

In an investigation of the role of verbalization versus visualization strategy and the verbalizability of the Rey-O and Taylor figures, those college students who generally tend to use visual strategies recalled both figures better than those who rely on verbal strategies (M.B. Casey et al., 1991). The visualizers were at a greater advantage on the Rey-O figure, but no differences between these two strategy groups obtained for the Taylor figure.

Test characteristics. Significant age effects on recall trials show up consistently (Delbecq-Dérouesné and Beauvois, 1989; Fastenau, Denburg, and Hufford, 1999; Spreen and Strauss, 1998). Spreen and Strauss' data based only on the 30 min delayed recall suggest that decline begins in the 30s, continuing fairly steadily until the 70s when a larger drop in scores appears. On three-minute short-term recall, however, a tendency to an average decrease in scores was first shown by a 41–55 age group, but it did not become pronounced until around age 60, with marked decline continuing into the 65+ ages (Delbecq-Dérouesné and Beauvois, 1989). For relatively well-educated subjects (averaging $14\frac{1}{2}$ years of schooling), on 3 min delay recall scores did not decrease notably until after age 69 (K.B. Boone, Lesser, et al., 1993). The ubiquitousness of the late age decline is seen on the Medical College of Georgia figures (see Table 11.12).

Some studies have reported that men tend to recall the figures better than women (Bennett-Levy, 1984a; M.B. Casey et al., 1991; Rosselli and Ardila, 1991). However Freides and Avery's (1991) college students showed no sex differences, nor did the large sample of 211 subjects across different ages (Fastenau, Denburg, and Hufford, 1999). No sex differences were found for recall of the MCG figures (Ingram et al., 1997).

A "cultural level" score derived from education levels contributed significantly ($p < .05$) to recall of the Rey figure (Delbecq-Dérouesné and Beauvois, 1989). Rosselli and Ardila (1991) reported a significant correlation between recall scores and education (.37, $p < .001$), but the inclusion of persons with less than six years of schooling in a sample also containing about equal numbers of persons with more than 12 years of schooling probably exaggerates the contribution of education,

TABLE 11.12 Medical College of Georgia Complex Figure (MCGCF) Data for Two Older Age Groups

Age	N	Copy	Short Delay	Long Delay
55–64	48	35.7 ± .61	30.3 ± 3.8	29.6 ± 4.1
65–75	29	35.6 ± .87	26.9 ± 7.1	26.4 ± 7.2

at least for application to populations with a generally higher average educational level.

Interscorer reliability is good ($r = .91$ to $.98$) (D.T.R. Berry, Allen, and Schmitt, 1991; Loring, Martin, et al., 1990; Shorr et al., 1992). Test–retest reliabilities using alternate forms (CF-RO, CF-T) were in the .60 to .76 range (D.T.R. Berry, Allen, and Schmitt, 1991). The Rey-O figure is a little more difficult to remember than the Taylor figure (M.B. Casey et al., 1991; Duley et al., 1993; Kuehn and Snow, 1992; Tombaugh and Hubley, 1991) or the MCG figures (Meador, Loring, Allen, et al., 1991) such that CFT-RO scores run a little lower than CFT-T scores. Both immediate and delayed recall trials have a strong visual memory component (Baser and Ruff, 1987; Loring, Lee, Martin, and Meador, 1988) and an almost as strong visuospatial component (D.T.R. Berry, Allen, and Schmitt, 1991).

Neuropsychological findings. Performance on the two recall trials helps the examiner sort out different aspects of the constructional and memory disabilities that might contribute to defective recall of the complex figure. Patients whose defective copy is based more on slow organization of complex data than on disordered visuospatial abilities (more likely with left-sided lesions) may improve their performances on the immediate recall trial (Osterrieth, 1944), and improve further with a second, later trial. These patients tend to show preserved recall of the overall structure of the figure with simplification and loss of details. Patients with right-sided lesions who have difficulty copying the figures display even greater problems with recall (L.B. Taylor, 1979). As a result of the distortions made by patients with right temporal lesions and of loss of details by those whose lesions involve the left temporal lobe, these two groups could not be discriminated on the basis of delayed recall scores alone, although a qualitative error score did differentiate them (Loring, Lee, and Meador, 1988; Piguet et al., 1994). The Loring group cautioned against relying on just one material-specific memory test when attempting to make such an identification. Although both figural and spatial features of the CFT are affected by right medial temporal impairment, the effect is greater for the spatial components, which may be less verbalizable than figural features (Breier, Plenger, et al., 1996).

In addition to scoring in the "traditional" manner (i.e., following Osterrieth's 1944 guidelines), a system for scoring qualitative errors was developed for distinguishing performances by patients with right or left temporal lobe damage (Loring, Lee, and Meador, 1988; Piguet et al., 1994; see Table 14.5, p. 544). These qualitative errors are most likely to occur in recall drawings of patients with right-sided temporal lobe lesions, but they may be applicable to drawings by patients whose right-sided dysfunction is not confined to the temporal lobe, and to TBI patients and those with frontal damage as well.

Patients with right hemisphere damage also tend to lose many of the elements of the design, making increasingly impoverished reproductions of the original figure as they go from the immediate to the delayed recall trial. Those right hemisphere damaged patients who have visuospatial problems or who are subject to perceptual fragmentation will also increasingly distort and confuse the configurational elements of the design.

This showed up in the three trials—copy (a), immediate recall (b), and (approximately) 40 min delayed recall (c)—drawn by a 50-year-old graduate civil engineer 12 years after suffering a ruptured aneurysm of the right anterior communicating artery, which resulted in left hemiparesis, significant behavioral deterioration, and pronounced impairment of arithmetic and complex reasoning abilities along with other cognitive deficits (see Fig. 11.3, p. 461).

CFT recall is sensitive to mild neuropsychological impairment in a variety of clinical populations. Alcoholic patients perform more poorly on recall than controls (L.K. Dawson and Grant, 2000; E.V. Sullivan, Mathalon, et al., 1992), and recall of the CFT continues to be impaired for a longer period following abstinence in older alcoholics than in younger patients (Munro, Saxton, and Butters, 2000). The magnitude of severe postoperative pain was found to be inversely related to CFT recall (Heyer et al., 2000), although the independent contribution of analgesia (i.e., morphine) is difficult to determine since patients experiencing greater pain receive more aggressive pain treatment.

Traumatically brain injured patients also tend to have difficulty on CFT recall trials. Patients with mild TBI showed significant deficits on 3 min recall trials within the first 21 months postinjury (Leininger, Gramling, et al., 1990). Two to five years posttrauma, moderately injured patients (PTA < 3 weeks) achieved significantly higher delayed recall scores than those whose injuries were severe (Bennett-Levy, 1984b). D.N. Brooks' (1972) TBI patients did as well as control subjects on immediate recall but gave impaired performances after a 30 min delay.

Following generally piecemeal copy trials, Parkinson patients had very poor recall scores ($M = 7.55$) (Ogden, Growdon, and Corkin, 1990), as might be expected from other studies, demonstrating the inefficiency of a fragmented copy approach for memory storage. Even after being asked to remember the design before beginning the copy trial, Huntington patients recalled significantly fewer elements than did either control subjects or persons at risk for the disease (whose

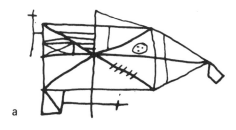

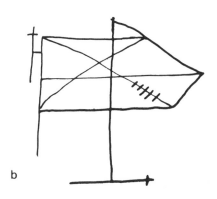

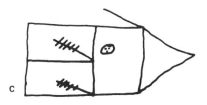

FIGURE 11.3 Complex Figure Test performance of a 50-year-old hemiparetic engineer with severe right frontal damage of 14 years' duration (see text; Chapter 9, Fig. 9.8). (*a*) Copy trial. (*b*) Three-minute recall with no intervening activities. (*c*) Recall after approximately 40 minutes of intervening activities, including other drawing tasks. This series illustrates the degradation of the percept over time when there is a pronounced visual memory disorder.

average scores on both copy and recall trials exceeded those of the control group by a nonsignificant bit) (Fedio, Cox, et al., 1979).

Patients with gliomas who survived at least 4 years after diagnosis differed in CFT recall according to their treatment (Gregor et al., 1996). Patients receiving whole brain irradiation and surgery displayed poorer CFT recall than those with focused irradiation and surgery. Children with acute lymphoblastic leukemia who were treated with intrathecal methotrexate therapy or whole brain irradiation performed more poorly on CFT recall (Lesnik et al., 1998; Waber, Shapiro, et al., 2001).

Complex figure modifications

Several modifications to the Complex Figure test have been developed to overcome limitations in the procedure as originally presented. Patterning their procedure after the Babcock-Levy story recall (see pages xx-xx), Freides and Avery (1991) had subjects study the Taylor figure for 60 sec, recall it, and then gave a second presentation of the figure for additional study with recall following a 20 min delay. Using their two new figures, they decreased exposure time to 30 sec to avoid ceiling effects (Freides, Engen, et al., 1996). Expected age declines appeared. The authors cite Erickson and Scott (1977) in support of using repeated learning trials:

> Basing one's inferences about learning and memory capabilities on immediate recall or recognition of material that has been presented one time seems a poor way of assessing memory. (p. 1144)

Tombaugh, Faulkner, and Hubley (1992) also used the Taylor figure in a learning paradigm with four learning trials, a 30 sec exposure on each trial, and a 2 min limit to recall time. Delayed recall is requested 15 min later, followed by a copy trial that lasts for only 4 min. This technique was sensitive to age differences over a 20- to 79-year range, with prominent score decrements beginning in the 50s for all the memory and learning measures. An apparently faster rate of learning for older subjects simply reflected the very much lower scores made by them on the first trial; even by the fourth learning trial, subjects over 50 never caught up with the younger ones and retained less. In providing a learning curve, this method adds potentially important information not obtainable by standard administration of either Verbal Reproduction or the CFT. It is a somewhat lengthy and possibly tedious procedure for which they developed a 69-point scoring system that greatly increases scoring time and effort; Freides, Engen, et al. (1996) report no psychometric benefit using Tombaugh's system in comparison to traditional scoring methods. In deciding whether to use this technique, the clinician must weigh its potential benefits against the suspected drawbacks of time (for administration and scoring), patient discontent, and examiner impatience with all that scoring.

Complex Figure Test recognition formats. J.E. Meyers and Meyers (1995) devised a recognition trial. Fastenau (1996a; with Denburg, and Hufford, 1999) supplemented the CFT by adding a recognition and a matching trial following delayed free recall (Extended Complex Figure Test, see below). Important differences distinguish these two recognition formats.

J.E. Meyers and Meyers' *Complex Figure Recognition Trial* (1995) presents 12 items for the figure along with 12 foils. The items are copies of internal details from the Rey-O and Taylor figures, both small (e.g., R-O: circle with dots, Taylor: wavy line) and large (the structure of each figure). The subject is asked to encircle each figure that belongs to the "whole design" just drawn. Norms were compiled from performances by 208 intact subjects in the 14 to 60 age range; their average age of 26.55 ± 8.62 attests to the relative youth of this group. Neither age nor education contributed significantly to these scores. This technique distinguished brain injured patients, psychiatric patients, and healthy subjects effectively. Brain injured patients identified more CFT parts than they recalled after either a 3 min or a 30 min delay, although healthy control subjects' recall exceeded recognition (J.E. Meyers and Lange, 1994).

In the *Extended Complex Figure Test* (ECFT) (Fastenau, Denburg, and Hufford, 1999; Fastenau, 2003), for each of 30 items, five stimulus figures are presented vertically, decreasing the effect of bias due to response preference associated with visual field or inattention defects. Each target contains one of the original 18 elements from the figure with four distractor elements. In addition to assessing recognition of the different elements, elements recalled are evaluated in different sets to provide a *global score* (the large rectangle, diagonal cross, and horizontal and vertical midlines), a *detail score* (the cross at the far left of the figure, diamond at the far right, circle with three dots, and five horizontal lines), and *left* and *right element scores*. The detail score was divided so that right- and left-sided elements could be considered separately. The foils for these details also have distractor elements in either the left or right portion of the figure. Normative data on 211 healthy subject ranging from 30 to 85 years of age are presented as scaled scores. The mean age of this group (62.9 years) is older than that of the J.E. Meyers and Meyers (1995) sample indicating its appropriateness for a larger range of patents. Sex effects on the supplemental recognition and matching trials are negligible. "This test adds a little more time but it will have significant yield for some patients" (Fastenau, personal communication, April 2003 [mdl]).

Benton Visual Retention Test (BVRT) (Sivan, 1992)

This widely used visual recall test is often called by its originator's name alone, "the Benton." It owes its popularity to a number of virtues. It has three forms that are roughly equivalent; some studies demonstrate no differences in their difficulty level and other studies indicate that Form D may be a little more difficult than Forms C or E (Benton, 1974; Riddell, 1962), or that Form C is a bit easier than the other two forms (Sivan,

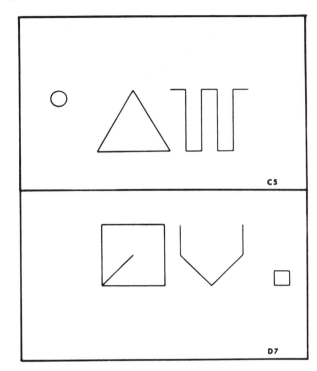

FIGURE 11.4 Two representative items of the Benton Visual Retention Test. (© A.L. Benton. Courtesy of the author)

1992). Its norms include both age and estimated original mental ability.

The three-figure design format is sensitive to unilateral spatial neglect (see Fig. 11.4). All but two of each ten-card series have more than one figure in the horizontal plane; most have three figures, two large and one small, with the small figure always to one side or the other. Besides its sensitivity to visual inattention problems, the three-figure format provides a limited measure of immediate span of recall since some patients cannot keep in mind the third or both of the other figures while drawing a first or second one, even though they may be able to do a simple one-figure memory task easily. Further, spatial organization problems may show up in the handling of size and placement relationships of the three figures.

Both the number of *correct* designs and the number of *errors* are scored. The complex but easily learned scoring system helps the examiner identify error patterns. The manuals furnish adult norms for two administration procedures, Administrations A and C. Administration A allows a 10 sec exposure to each card with immediate recall by drawing (see Table 11.13, p. 463 for adult norms; norms for children ages 8 through 14 can be found in the manuals and in Spreen and Strauss, 1998). Administration B, like A, is also a simple recall test but follows a five-second exposure. Administration B Number Correct norms run about an

TABLE 11.13 BVRT Norms for Administration A: Adults Expected Number Correct Scores, by Estimated Premorbid IQ and Age*

	EXPECTED NUMBER CORRECT SCORE, BY AGE		
Estimated Premorbid IQ	15–44	45–54	55–64
100 and above	9	8	7
95–109	8	7	6
80–94	7	6	5
70–79	6	5	4
69 and below	≤5	≤4	≤3

BVRT Norms for Administration A: Adults Expected Error Scores

	EXPECTED ERROR SCORE, BY AGE			
Estimated Premorbid IQ	15–39	40–54	55–59	60–64
110 and above	1	2	3	4
105–109	2	3	4	5
95–104	3	4	5	6
90–94	4	5	6	7
80–89	5	6	7	8
70–79	6	7	8	9
69 and below	≥7	≥8	≥9	≥10

*These data are identical to those given in Sivan's 1992 test manual except for slight differences in age range: The three new age ranges for Number Correct scores at 15–49, 50–59, and 60–69; for Error scores they are 15–44, 45–59, 60–64, and 65–69.

average of 1 point below those reported for Administration A. Administration C is a copying test in which the subject is encouraged to draw the designs as accurately as possible. On Administration D, which requires the subject to delay responding for 15 sec after a 10 sec exposure, the average Number Correct score may be lower than that for Administration A by 0.1 to 0.4 points (Sivan, 1992); however, intersubject variations can be great as some patients improve with delay while others' scores drop.

Mitrushina, Boone, and D'Elia (1999) have compiled a comprehensive collection of norms for this test. Spreen and Strauss (1998) present a data set of error norms organized by sex, seven age levels (from 10–19 to 80–89), and two levels of education (with or without college degree) that may be useful in evaluating performances of educationally advantaged subjects. Also focusing on better educated subjects, Youngjohn, Larrabee, and Crook (1993) give norms for five age groups (18–39, each of the next three decades, and 70+) and three levels of education (12–14, 15–17, and 18+). Extensive norms based on 156 healthy volunteers between 61 and 97 years of age, in addition to 625 subjects with memory concerns and 196 patients with mixed etiology are presented by Coman et al. (1999).

The examiner should give the patient a fresh sheet of paper, approximately the size of the card for each design. The test publisher sells a response booklet, but half sheets of letter-size paper work well. To avoid the

problem of a patient "jumping the gun" on the memory administrations—and particularly on Administration D—the pad of paper may be removed after completion of each drawing and not returned until it is time for the patient to draw the next design.

When the copy administration is given first, the examiner is able to determine the quality of the patient's drawings per se and also familiarize the subject with the three-figure format. Well-oriented, alert patients generally do not require the practice provided by administration C, so it need not be given if there is another copying task in the battery. Patients who have difficulty following instructions and lack "test-wiseness" should be given at least the first three or four designs of a series for copy practice.

Six types of errors are recognized for scoring purposes: *omissions, distortions, perseverations, rotations, misplacements* (in the position of one figure relative to the others), and errors in *size*. Thus, there can be, and not infrequently are, more than one error to a card.

Interpretation of performance is straightforward. Taking the subject's age and "estimated premorbid" ability into account, the examiner can enter the normative tables for Administration A and quickly determine whether the Number Correct or the Error score falls into the impairment categories. On Administration B, the normal tendency for persons in the age range 16–60 is to reproduce correctly one design less than under the 10-second exposure condition of Administration A. The examiner who wishes to evaluate Administration B performances need only add 1 point and use the A norms. Only Error Score norms with no age or mental ability corrections are available for Administration C. The Number Correct Scores of Administration D for healthy control subjects are, on the average, 0.4 point below Administration A scores.

Tabulation of errors by type allows the examiner to determine the nature of the patient's problems on this test. Impaired immediate recall or an attention defect appears mostly as simplification, simple substitution, or omission of the last one or two design elements of a card. Healthy subjects exhibit these tendencies too; the difference is in the frequency with which they occur. The first two designs of each series consist of only one figure so simple and easily named that it is rare for even patients with a significantly impaired immediate memory capacity to forget them. Unilateral spatial neglect shows up as a consistent omission of the figure on the side opposite the lesion. Visuospatial and constructional disabilities appear as defects in the execution or organization of the drawings. Rotations with preserved gestalts suggest a problem with spatial orientation, perhaps linked to deficient appreciation of figure–ground relationships. Consistent design distortions may indicate a perceptual disorder.

Perseverations should alert the examiner to look for perseveration on other kinds of tasks. Widespread perseveration suggests a monitoring or activity control problem; perseveration limited to this test is more likely evidence of a specific visuoperceptual or immediate memory impairment. Simplification of designs, including disregard of size and placement, may be associated with overall behavioral regression in patients with bilateral or diffuse damage.

When given with Administration A, Administration D (10 sec exposure, 15 sec delay) sometimes provides interesting information about the patient's memory processes that is not obtainable elsewhere. Occasionally, the 15-second delay elicits a gross memory impairment when memory defects were not pronounced on Administration A. A few brain injured patients do better on Administration D than on A, apparently profiting from the 15 sec delay to consolidate memory traces that would dissipate if they began drawing immediately. For example, patients with left lateralized lesions achieved better scores on delayed than on immediate recall trials (Vakil, Blachstein, et al., 1989). Patients who improve their performance when they have the quiet delay period may be suffering attention and concentration problems rather than memory problems per se, or they may need more than an ordinary amount of time to consolidate new information due to slowed processing.

Test characteristics. Aging effects show up in decreasing Number Correct scores, at least from age 45 or 50 (Benton, 1974; Sivan, 1992), although the decrements in succeeding decades tend to stay below 1.00 until the mid-seventies. Although Benton's (1974) young adult age group extended to age 44 and Sivan (1992) further extended it to age 49, other normative data for Administration A suggest that decline in memory efficiency (at least in increasing errors) may begin as early as in the 30s, with a greater number of errors in each succeeding decade (Arenberg, 1978; Coman et al., 1999; Spreen and Strauss, 1998). This gain in the average number of errors never exceeds 1.40 (between the 60s and 70s) until the 80+ years, when average increases in error number from 1.70 to more than 5 have been found (e.g., 7.4 ± 3.7 for 122 subjects with a mean age of 72.2 ± 9.0 [Robiinson-Whelen, 1992]). For over 1,000 subjects in the 18 to 70+ age range with 12 to 18+ years of schooling, age and education together accounted for approximately 12% of the variance for both number correct and number of errors (Youngjohn, Larrabee, and Crook, 1993). With testing repeated after intervals of less than a year, Error scores vary negligibly at any age (McCaffrey, Duff, and Westervelt, 2000b). With retest intervals of seven or more years, only control subjects over age 60 tended to make more errors, a tendency that increased with advancing age. By and large, Number Correct scores do not vary greatly for control subjects regardless of age when the time interval does not exceed eight to ten years, except for subjects in the very older age ranges.

With respect to error types, older healthy subjects (ages 65 to 89) made mostly distortion errors (45%) with many fewer rotation errors (18%) and omissions (14%), the next two most frequent error types (Eslinger, Pepin, and Benton, 1988). These amount to about three distortion errors and 1.2 rotation and omission errors on the average (La Rue, D'Elia, et al., 1986). The authors noted that distortion and rotation errors involve "either a partially or completely correct reproduction of the stimulus form . . . suggesting at least a partially intact memory capacity." Younger subjects (ages 18 to 30) too make mostly distortion errors, with misplacements and rotations following in frequency (Randall et al., 1988). Mental ability, as measured by the Satz-Mogel short form of the WAIS-R, contributed significantly to both Number Correct and Error scores for persons achieving scores in the *borderline* and *mentally retarded* ranges; but no differences showed up in BVRT performances for all other ability categories (from *low average* to *superior*) which, Randall and her colleagues suggest may be due to a ceiling effect.

Swan, Morrison, and Eslinger (1990) obtained interrater reliability coefficients of .96 for Number Correct and .97 for Error scores, although Randall and her colleagues (1988) found interrater reliability coefficients of only .85 and .93, respectively. The BVRT was stable and had a high reliability on one set of repeated administrations (Lezak, 1982c). Three administrations given to healthy control subjects 6 and 12 months apart produced no significant differences between either Number Correct or Error score means. Coefficients of concordance (W) between scores obtained for each administration were .74 for Number Correct and .77 for Error. In one factor analytic study, the highest loading (.55) was on a visuospatial factor with only secondary loadings (.45, .42) on memory and concentration factors, respectively (Larrabee, Kane, Schuck, and Francis, 1985). Number Correct and Error scores are highly correlated (e.g., −.86: Vakil, Blachstein, et al., 1989; Benton, 1974). Although the wider range of Error scores would seem to permit them to make more sensitive discriminations, for at least some conditions, either set of scores appears to be useful for this purpose (Vakil, Blachstein, et al., 1989; but see also column 2, this page).

Neuropsychological findings. When deciding whether to give the BVRT or some other visually presented memory test, it is important to recognize that many of the designs can be conceptualized verbally (e.g., for C5 in Fig. 11.4, "small circle up, triangle, and a squared-off 'W'"). Thus, this test is sensitive to left brain injury as well as right. Taken with the findings of factor analysis and with reports that the BVRT has higher correlations with tests of design copying ability than with memory tests (e.g., A.B. Silverstein, 1962), these data suggest that the constructional component may well outweigh the memory component measured by this test. Vakil, Blachstein, et al., (1989) found that scores achieved by patients with right hemisphere disease fell from Administration C (immediate recall) to the 15-sec delay series, which was opposite the pattern of improvement shown by patients with left-sided dysfunction. TBI patients made significantly more errors (M = 5.0 ± 5.0) than matched control subjects (M = 2.0 ± 4.0) (H.S. Levin, Gary, et al., 1990).

Since this test involves so many different capacities— visuomotor response, visuospatial perception, visual and verbal conceptualization, immediate memory span—it is not surprising that it is quite sensitive to the presence of a brain disorder. For example, in a group of healthy elderly subjects living at home independently, BVRT performance was related to the presence of MRI signal abnormalities (Kasahara et al., 1995). It identified cognitive impairment several years after a bout of viral meningitis in patients without evidence of residual brain abnormality (Sittinger et al., 2002).

The BVRT is sensitive to cognitive decline in early Alzheimer's disease (Storandt, Botwinick, and Danzinger, 1986). The Number Correct score emerged as the best single discriminator of dementia patients from healthy controls in a small (seven contributing test scores) examination battery (Eslinger, Damasio, Benton, and Van Allen, 1985), and was among the more sensitive predictors of deterioration in a larger test battery (L. Berg, Danziger, et al., 1984). However, Number Correct did not discriminate between elderly depressed and dementia patients in another study, but the Error score did (La Rue, D'Elia, et al., 1986). BVRT performance may be a preclinical predictor of subsequent dementia both in patients with (G.W. Small, La Rue, et al., 1995) and without (Dartigues et al., 1997; Fabrigoule et al., 1998) memory complaints. Number Correct was not sensitive to the effects of solvent exposure (Bleeker, Bolla, et al., 1990).

The number of omissions may differentiate depressed from dementia patients (La Rue, D'Elia, et al., 1986). Thus both the Number Correct and Error test scores are useful for making diagnostic discriminations, as is the pattern of errors. However, like other single tests, the BVRT must not be used alone as it does not identify brain impaired patients with enough reliability for individual diagnostic decisions.

The BVRT can serve several purposes. When perseveration or visuospatial inattention is suspected or when there is a need to record these problems in the patient's own hand, the BVRT may be the instrument of choice. It can be particularly useful for documenting these problems in patients who monitor their performances and are thus apt to catch inattention or perseveration errors when they see them. The 15-minute delay administration can be given following Administration A to patients who either seem overwhelmed by too many stimuli or are slow to process information, to see whether they can use the brief interlude to sort out and consolidate the material. This test may also be used to measure the immediate retention span of language-impaired patients. However, it is not a test of visuospatial learning and should neither be confused with one nor used as one.

Visual Learning

The measurement of learning (rate, efficiency, retention) requires material of sufficient difficulty that only very exceptional persons would be able to grasp and retain it with one or two exposures, and there must be enough learning trials to permit emergence of a learning curve. A number of visual learning tests meet these requirements—some do not. Several more or less follow André Rey's AVLT paradigm.

Biber Figure Learning Test (BFLT)[1] *(Glosser, Goodglass, and Biber, 1989)*

This test consists of ten test items each composed of two geometric figures (e.g., two truncated rectangles back to back, a triangle with an inside triangle rotated 180°) and 30 distractors (three for each target figure, of which one differs in orientation, one in shape, and one in being quite different from the target). Following exposure to all ten items, shown one by one for two seconds, the subject is asked to draw them from memory for five learning and recall trials. An immediate recognition trial follows the free recall trials, then a 20-minute delay period ends with Delayed Free Recall and Delayed Recognition. A final two trials involve Immediate Reproduction of each design after a 3 sec exposure, and then a Copy trial for all designs just drawn "with any error."

For four age groups from 40–49 through to 70–79, a significant age effect appeared on free recall but not on recognition trials. Test–retest reliabilities were in the .79 to .91 range, with a year-and-one-half wait between tests. Correlations of the various BFLT scores with visual reasoning, construction, and other visual memory tests were in the .46 to .71 range; the highest correlation was with Wechsler's Paired Associate Learning test. Free recall on learning trials did not differentiate patients with right hemisphere disease from those whose lesions were on the left, and both groups performed significantly below the level of healthy subjects. Although delayed recall for both patient groups was also below that of the healthy subjects, the right hemisphere group had a retention score (Delayed Recall divided by Trial 5) proportionally like that of the healthy subjects and significantly higher than the retention score made by the left hemisphere patients. However, on recognition trials the relationship between the two lateralized lesion groups was reversed in that patients with left hemisphere involvement performed like the control subjects but the right brain injury group recognized significantly fewer designs. The lower retention score made by left brain injury subjects and the high correlation with a verbal learning test together implicate a significant verbal learning component for this test.

A 15-item format—the *Biber Figure Learning Test–Extended (BFLT-E)*—is patterned after the AVLT (Glosser, Cole, et al., 2002). It includes two parallel versions for repeat assessment. After five trials in which the original 15 designs are shown at a rate of one every 3 sec, each trial followed by a drawn recall, a second set of designs is presented also followed by an immediate recall trial. Then, without additional exposure, patients are asked to draw the original 15 items. After 20 to 30 min, delayed recall and recognition memory are tested, the latter with a 45-item, yes/no procedure displaying the original 15 items, seven items from the distractor set, and 23 foils.

With this longer version of the test, significant left vs. right temporal lobe epilepsy focus differences showed up on Learning trial 5, a score for learning across trials, immediate and delayed memory, as well as recognition measures (Glosser, Cole, et al., 2002); poorer performances were associated with right seizure-onset patients. For discriminating lateralized seizure onset, the BFLT-E was superior to traditional memory measures (Rey Auditory Verbal Learning Test and Wechsler Memory Scale-Revised) which failed to identify to group differences.

Visual Spatial Learning Test (VSLT)[2] *(Malec, Ivnik, and Hinkeldey, 1991)*

These authors sought a visuospatial learning task suitable for patients with movement disorders. The test consists of a 6 × 4 grid and seven different nonsense designs that are (truly) difficult to verbalize. After seeing the designs placed on squares on the grid, subjects are given an empty 6 × 4 grid and 15 designs with the task of selecting the target seven and placing them as they were when seen on the grid. Five learning trials are followed by a 30 min delayed recall trial. Performance is scored for recognition learning of the designs, recall of the target positions on the grid, and recall of designs in their proper places on the grid.

The usual age gradient appeared for both learning and delay trials. Highest correlates of VSLT scores were with Visual Reproduction scores (in the .29 to .46 range), but the VSLT also had correlations with some verbal memory tests that fell within this range. Before temporal lobectomies, both right and left temporal lobe seizure patients performed at similar levels on all VSLT measures. After surgery these two groups tended to diverge, with right-resected patients performing less well (see also Ivnik, 1991). Nevertheless, a factor analytic study failed to demonstrate the VSLT as a measure of nonverbal memory distinct from verbal memory (G.E. Smith, Malec, and Ivnik, 1992).

Normative data are available for elderly patients ranging from 56 to 97 years of age (Malec, Ivnik, Smith, et al., 1992). The VSLT is a good discriminator of de-

---

[1]Dr. Glosser provides her fax (215-349-5579) and e-mail (glosser©mail.med.upenn.edu) addresses.

[2]This material may be requested from James F. Malec, Ph.D., PM & R-1D-SMH, Mayo Medical Center, Rochester, MN 55905. (e-mail: malec.james©mayo.edu)

mentia patients from intact elderly persons, reportedly classifying 78.9% of healthy subjects and 87.9% of dementia patients correctly (Malec et al., 1992).

Diagnosticum für Zerebralschäde–Revision (Diagnostic workup for cerebral disease–Revised) (Helmstaedter, Pohl, Hufnagel, and Elger, 1991)

This visual memory test asks the patient to learn nine simple geometric designs, all of which can be produced by connecting five separate lines. The designs are individually presented to the subject at the rate of one design every 2 sec for the patient to recall by using 5 wooden sticks of equal length to reconstruct the designs. A maximum of six trials are given but testing is stopped when the patient reproduces all items. Performance feedback is not given.

In reports about this test several different measures have been scored. The primary measures include a learning score summing performance over trials, total number of rotations (at least 30°) or mirror inversions, failures (false positive reproductions), and a 30 min delayed recognition with drawings of the target figures interspersed with 12 foils.

Sex differences have been reported, with men displaying an advantage (Helmstaedter, Kurthen, and Elger, 1999). This test has predictive value for everyday memory performance in healthy controls in that performances was directly related to subjects' ability to recall specifics of the assessment examination when questioned one week later (Helmstaedter, Hauff, and Elger, 1998).

Neuropsychological findings. Patients with right temporal lobe epilepsy and epilepsy patients with bitemporal EEG abnormalities performed significantly poorer on immediate recall and learning compared to either healthy controls or patients with left temporal lobe seizures (Helmstaedter et al., 1991). Patients with right temporal lobe epilepsy had a greater number of rotated or mirrored responses. In a subsequent study in which hippocampal sclerosis was identified by MRI, patients with right TLE with hippocampal sclerosis performed more poorly on learning, recognition, rotations, and failures than those without MRI evidence of sclerosis; the latter did not differ from healthy controls (Gleissner, Helmstaedter, and Elger, 1998). These findings suggest that the right–left differences reported in the early 1991 study resulted from the inclusion of large numbers of right TLE patients in whom hippocampal atrophy or sclerosis was present. This test also appears to be sensitive to "crowding," in which language shifts from the left to the right hemisphere following an early left hemisphere lesion (Helmstaedter, Kurthen, Linke, and Elger, 1994).

Heaton Figure Memory Test (Heaton, Grant, and Matthews, 1991)

This test uses the Visual Reproduction stimuli from the original Wechsler Memory Scale but introduces several important changes. Each card is shown for 10 seconds, although the patient does not reproduce the designs until all three cards (four designs) have been presented. The three cards are again shown up to a maximum of five trials or until a criterion of 15 points is reached. Thus, this format incorporates a learning component in which acquisition rate can be examined. In addition, a four hour delay trial is obtained.

In a mixed patient sample, factor analysis has generally linked the initial trial with immediate visual memory (DiPino et al., 2000). Although a distinct visual memory factor was not extracted, overall performance was related to the California Verbal Learning Test, supporting its use as a memory measure. In elderly patients with age-associated memory impairment, immediate recall was correlated with left amygdala volume while delayed recall correlated with both right and left amygdala volume (Soininen et al., 1994). No correlation with hippocampal volume emerged in this study.

Ruff Light Trail Learning Test (RULIT) (Ruff, Light, and Parker, 1996)

This nonverbal learning task asks the subject to learn a specific pathway or trail through circles spread over a piece of paper; the circles are interconnected by lines (see Fig. 11.5, p. 468), and the "start" and "end" circles are labeled as such. Subjects are told that they will be learning a 15-step path that is not the shortest route between the start and end circles. Subjects are not told how to choose the correct response from the different alternatives but must find it by trial and error. On moving their finger from one circle to the next, subjects are informed whether they are correct or not; if incorrect, they go back to the last correct circle and make a different choice. A trial is completed when the end point is reached following the correct path, regardless of the number of digressions made on the way. The task is discontinued after two consecutive trials in which the 15-step sequence is correctly traced, up to a maximum of 10 trials. Performance can be evaluated across learning trials and for "step errors," errors that are repeated at the same circle. Factor analysis of a group of healthy subjects suggests that the RULIT assesses visual learning/

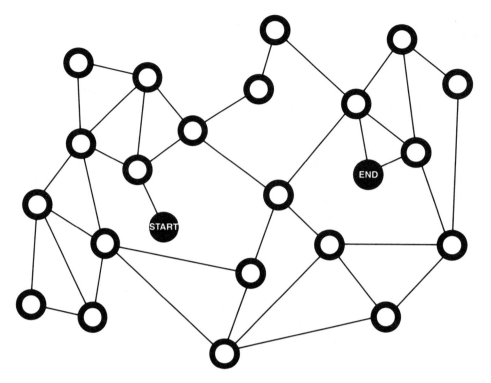

FIGURE 11.5 Ruff-Light Trail Learning Test (RULIT) (reduced size). Reproduced by special permission of the publisher, Psychological Assessment Resources, Inc., from the Ruff-Light Trail Learning Test by Ronald M. Ruff, Ph.D., and C. Christopher Allen, Ph.D. © 1999 PAR, Inc. Further reproduction is prohibited without permission of PAR, Inc.

memory and is distinct from its verbal counterpart, the Selective Reminding Test (C.C. Allen and Ruff, 1999).

Shum Visual Learning Test (SVLT)[1]
(Shum, O'Gorman, and Eadie, 1999)

This test uses Chinese characters as stimuli since they are not easily verbalized (by non-Chinese, that is!). The format is similar to the Rey AVLT: five learning trials, a second character set designed to measure interference, then a recognition trial for the original stimulus set. The addition of the second set is a slight modification of the test from its original presentation (Eadie and Shum, 1995), and the new stimulus set is included to measure interference effects in retention.

The ten target stimuli are displayed one-by-one for 2 sec each on each of the first five learning trials. Retention is tested by means of a recognition format, with the ten stimuli interspersed with ten distractors. These foils were created by modifying the target stimuli through adding, deleting, or relocating a stroke from

the Chinese character. The same set of distractors is used for each recognition memory trial. Subjects are giving up to 5 sec to respond. After the fifth learning trial, the second stimulus set is presented and recognition memory is tested with a new distractor set; this is followed by a recognition trial of the original stimulus set. After a 20-min delay, recognition of the first set is again tested.

Normative data are available for three major indices: *learning* (difference between the first and fifth trials), *retention after interference* (difference between trials 5 and 7), and *delayed retention* following a 20-min delay (difference between trials 7 and 8). Unlike most clinical memory measures, however, performance criteria are reported using a nonparametric measure of recognition memory based on signal detection theory which incorporates hit rate and false alarms for descriptive purposes. Correct responses for individual trials, the sum of correct responses for the five learning trials, and the number of false positives can be scored and evaluated.

Neuropsychological findings. TBI patients with severe injuries performed more poorly than healthy controls both during the first year after injury and later (D.H. Shum, Harris, and O'Gorman, 2000) although

[1]Dr. Shum can be reached at School of Applied Psychology, Griffith University, Nathan, Queensland, Australia 4111. (e-mail: d.shum@mailbox.gv.edu.au)

no group effect for time after injury appeared. In addition to poorer learning scores, TBI patients made more false positive recognition errors. No effect of TBI compared to healthy controls was present on the Retention after Interference or Delayed-Retention trial, an unexpected finding.

Hidden Objects

Testing the patient's immediate memory and learning for spatial orientation and span of immediate memory by asking for recall of where and what objects have been hidden is an examination technique in the Terman and Merrill (1973) Stanford-Binet tests and in mental status examinations (e.g., Strub and Black, 2000). Strub and Black hide four common objects, such as a pen, keys, watch, or glasses, in the examining room while the patient observes, naming each object as it is hidden. The patient's task is to find or point out each hiding place after at least ten minutes of interpolated activity. Adults with unimpaired visual learning remember all four objects and hiding places. Barbizet and Duizabo (1980) also used familiar objects (e.g., pen, button, cork) in their version of the hidden objects test: The examiner gives the patient five objects to name and place in a box, which is then hidden from view. After 15 min, the examiner asks the patient which objects had been hidden, where, and to describe them. Recall is tested again at one and 24 hours. Barbizet and Duizabo pointed out that the technique of asking for immediate recall and then delayed recall at two subsequent times helps to differentiate among conditions in which memory disorders occur. They demonstrated this by describing a jovial *grand alcoolique,* who found a bottle of wine that had been hidden behind him 3 minutes earlier but after 10 minutes more recalled neither the hiding place nor what had been hidden.

TACTILE MEMORY

Tactual Performance Test (TPT)

Like the Knox Cubes, the material for this test came from the Arthur (1947) battery of tests (*Seguin Formboard,* see Fig. 11.6). Although originally administered as a visuospatial task, Halstead (1947) converted it into a tactile memory test by blindfolding subjects and adding a drawing recall trial. Halstead incorporated this version of the test into his battery which has continued to be used for neuropsychological testing (Reitan and Wolfson, 1993). Halstead's administration requires three trials, the first two with the preferred and nonpreferred hands, respectively, and the third with both hands. The score for each trial is the time to completion, which Halstead recorded to the nearest tenth of a minute. Their sum is the *Total Time* score.

Differences in administration time were reported by Snow (1987b) who noted that Reitan (1979) suggested ending a trial after 15 minutes for patients who are "getting discouraged and . . . making very slow progress" unless they are close to a correct performance; but other workers discontinue at 10 minutes routinely or at the examiner's discretion.

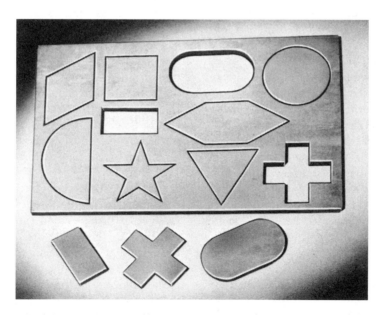

FIGURE 11.6 One of the several available versions of the Sequin-Goddard Formboard used in the Tactual Performance Test. (Courtesy of the Stoelting Co.)

On completion of the formboard trials it is concealed, the examiner removes the blindfold, and instructs the subject to draw the board from memory indicating the shapes and their placement relative to one another. Thus two measures of incidental memory are obtained (Hom and Reitan, 1990): the *Memory* score is the number of shapes reproduced with reasonable accuracy; the *Location* score is the total number of blocks placed in proper relationship to the other blocks and the board. Scoring of Memory and Location is at the examiner's discretion.

Cutting scores, developed by Halstead on a limited and skewed subject sample (see p. 671) were retained by Reitan to indicate "organic" impairment. They are now superseded by adequate normative data (Mitrushina, Boone, and D'Elia, 1999; Heaton, Grant, and Matthews, 1986, 1991; Spreen and Strauss, 1998).

Test characteristics. Age contributes significantly to TPT performances, so much so that when using Halstead's cutting scores for older persons, many will fall into the impaired range (Ernst, 1987; L.L. Thompson and Parsons, 1985). For example, Heaton, Ryan, et al., (1986) found that 30% and 58% of their healthy subjects in the 40-59-year age range had Total Time and Location scores (respectively) in Halstead's *defective* range; by ages 60+, 77% and 91% "failed" on their Total Time and Location scores.

Whether sex makes a difference has not yet been satisfactorily determined differences have shown up on one or more of the three scores (Ernst, 1987; Heaton, Ryan, et al., 1996; L.L. Thompson and Parsons, 1985) but not always (Filskov and Catanese, 1986). Where differences appear, men tend to perform better than women on Total Time while women make higher scores on one or both of the recall drawing measures. A small education contribution showed up for all three scores on the large-scale normative study by Heaton and his colleagues (1996) but Ernst (1987) examined a group of elderly Australians and found none. Bernard (1989) reported that, using the Halstead cut-off scores, 36% of a relatively poorly educated group of healthy young men had Location scores in the impaired range, and 18% were classified as "impaired" on their Total Time scores.

Reviewing reliability studies, L.L. Thompson and Parsons (1985) concluded that with between-test delays of three months to one year, test–retest reliability was generally adequate, and best (.68–.93) for Time (see also Spreen and Strauss, 1998). On three week retesting the reliability correlation for Time was .69, for Memory it was .80, and .77 for Location (Bornstein, Baker, and Douglass, 1987). With few exceptions, performances improve for control subjects after as

much as a two-year interval between tests (McCaffrey, Duff, and Westervelt, 2000b). Some score gains on each of the TPT measures have also been documented for a variety of patient samples. However, E.W. Russell (1985) found the Location score to be particularly unreliable. Moreover, Snow (1987b) noted a report (P.W. Martin and R.L. Green, cited in Snow) that scoring for Memory produced agreements in 71% to 76.3% of cases, but for Location the agreement between judges dropped to 56.7% and 63.8%, with some judge pairs agreeing as little as 36% on Memory and 29% on Location, which puts the reliability of these measures on somewhat shaky ground.

Internal consistency coefficients of the Memory score ranged from .64 for a group of healthy subjects to .74 for a group of patients with diffuse injuries (Charter and Dutra, 2000). Internal consistency coefficients for Location were higher, ranging from .77 (the healthy subjects) to .82 (the patient group). As observed by Charter and Dutra, these scores fall into the border zone of the "unacceptable/fair" and "fair/good" classifications describing strength of internal consistency according to Cicchetti's 1994 guidelines. The rhombus is the most difficult block to remember and the circle is the easiest (Charter and Dutra, 2001). Using discrimination indexes which vary from −1.00 to +1.00 depending upon how well performance by an individual block discriminates between groups, three blocks for Memory (diamond, oval, and rhombus) and one block for Location (oval) were considered unacceptable (discrimination values ≤.3) (Charter and Dutra, 2001).

L.L. Thompson and Parsons (1985) remarked on the relatively high level of intercorrelations between the three TPT measures, especially between Memory and Location (.56 to .71), with TPT Time correlating in the .32 to .72 range with Memory, in the .26 to .62 range for Location. Out of one large group of tests, all TPT measures loaded on the same factor with the most commonly scored five measures showing a very narrow range of correlations (.50 to .69) (P.C. Fowler, Richards, et al., 1987). This further supports the impression that these different trials are essentially measuring much the same thing.

Neuropsychological findings. Although there appears to be little doubt that markedly slowed or defective performances on the formboard test or the recall trial are generally associated with brain damage, the nature of the defect remains in dispute. Most investigators have found a right–left hemisphere differential favoring performance by patients with left hemisphere lesions (Heilbronner and Parsons, 1989; Teuber and Weinstein, 1954; L.L. Thompson and Parsons, 1985). Halstead (1947) considered this test to be particularly sensitive to frontal lobe lesions; yet Teuber and Weinstein's posterior brain injured patients performed least well, and their anterior brain injured patients made the best scores of their three brain injured subgroups (1954; Teuber, 1964; see also L.L. Thompson and Parsons, 1985). Teuber (1964) noted that their findings are "not unreasonable, in view of the known symptomatology of parietal and temporal lesions. What is difficult to understand is that this formboard task should have been considered a test of frontal pathology at all" (p. 421).

The difference between the time taken on the preferred hand and that on the nonpreferred hand trials may provide a clue as to the side of the lesion. Normally, as learning takes place, trial II takes a little less time than trial I even though it is performed with the nonpreferred hand, and trial III takes the least amount of time. When this pattern is reversed in right-handed subjects (i.e., Trial II with the left hand takes longer than Trial I, the right-handed trial) depressed functioning of the right hemisphere may be suspected (L.L. Thompson and Heaton, 1991).

Like other tests calling upon a complex of neuropsychological functions for optimum performance, TPT scores are typically lower for brain damaged populations than for intact persons (e.g., Spreen and Strauss, 1998; L.L. Thompson and Parsons, 1985). A fairly consistent pattern of dysfunction on this test has emerged in studies of chronic alcoholics (Fabian, Jenkins, and Parsons, 1981; W.R. Miller and Saucedo, 1983; Parsons and Farr, 1981). When administered in the Halstead-Reitan format, right-handed alcoholics showed the most slowing on the nonpreferred hand trial, significant slowing on the preferred hand trial, impaired performance with both hands, and an abnormally low Location score with a normal or near normal Memory score. This pattern was essentially the same for both male and female alcoholics, although women (both alcoholics and controls) tended to outperform men on the Memory score but do relatively poorer than their male counterparts on the Location task (Fabian et al., 1981).

Shortcomings of the TPT. Probably because of its inclusion in the popular Halstead-Reitan Battery—and perhaps because this battery is so often administered by a technician rather than by the clinician responsible for deciding which tests to give—the TPT continues to enjoy wide usage despite several important drawbacks. The chief clinical drawback is the enormous discomfort experienced by many patients when blindfolded, which, when added to their frustration in performing a trial that may take as many as ten or even more minutes for some to complete, creates a degree of psycho-

logical distress that does not warrant use of an instrument that may give very little new information in return. The other major problems are the amount of time consumed in giving this test to older and brain injured patients, and the equivocal and often redundant nature of the data obtained. It is most appropriately used with visually compromised persons [mdl].

TPT variants. De Renzi (1968) used a six-figure rather than the ten-figure formboard in his studies. The smaller board may reduce time about one-third, making this test feasible for ordinary clinical use (C. Clark and Klonoff, 1988). Certainly the reduction in number of forms does not seem to have reduced the discriminating power of this technique (see De Renzi, 1968; also, E.W. Russell, 1985, Spreen and Strauss, 1998). Rather, Clark and Klonoff found that both Memory and Location scores are higher with the six-hole board, improving the discrimination potential of these scores. They also found that the six-hole formboard showed good reliability over two years and four testing sessions, with essentially no gain from session to session. Further, construct validity was comparable to that of the ten-hole board. In comparing the six and ten hole formboards, E.W. Russell (1985) concluded that the six hole board was actually more sensitive to performances by severely impaired patients because the ten hole board was so difficult for them that their very large time scores registered neither differences in severity of dysfunction nor lateralization deficits. Russell suspected that the larger number of blocks contributes to disrupted performances of very impaired patients by confusing them.

Teuber and Weinstein (1954) administered this test somewhat differently than Halstead and Reitan. They gave only two trials to blindfolded subjects, one with the board in the usual position and one with the board rotated 180°. Like Halstead and Reitan, they followed the formboard task with a drawing recall, but scored only for memory, not for location. Performances of their frontal lobe injured patients were consistently superior to those of patients whose injuries involved other cortical areas (Teuber, 1964). The frontal lobe patients also recalled more forms on the drawing trial than any other group, and the occipital lobe patients recalled the fewest.

Tactile Pattern Recognition (B. Milner, 1971)

Four pieces of wire, each twisted into a distinctly different nonsense shape (see Fig. 11.7, p. 472), comprise the material for a tactile test of immediate memory. Subjects never see the wire figures. After several training trials on matching the figures with no time delay,

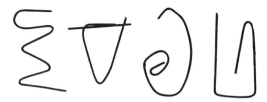

FIGURE 11.7 Tactile nonsense figures (Milner, 1971. © 1971, Pergamon Press. Reprinted by permission)

matching follows an increasing delay length up to two minutes. During 30 sec delay trials, a distractor task of copying matchstick patterns was introduced (B. Milner and Taylor, 1972).

Six out of seven commissurotomized patients performed best with their left hand, indicating that complex perceptual learning can take place without words and that it is mediated by the right hemisphere. B. Milner and Taylor (1972) found little difference between patients with unilateral surgical lesions and intact interhemispheric connections, and control subjects on this task. Both groups performed rapidly and virtually without errors except for a single error made by each of two left temporal lobectomy patients using their right hands. These findings suggest that, even after delay with an intervening distractor task, this test may be too easy for patients whose lesions are as localized and circumscribed as temporal lobectomy patients.

INCIDENTAL LEARNING

The virtue of testing for incidental learning is that this technique looks at learning as it occurs naturally in the course of events. The WIS-A provides an opportunity for assessing incidental learning. E. Kaplan, Fein, and their colleagues (1991) devised a technique for using the WAIS-R Digit Symbol (see pp. 368–369) to measure incidental learning in addition to obtaining a score on a standardized coding performance. They note which square the patient filled in at 90 seconds (the time allotted for the test) but allow the patient to continue until the end of the next-to-the-last row. They then fold the test sheet under so that only the unmarked last row shows and request subjects to fill in from memory as many of the symbols as can be recalled. After this, subjects are asked to write out as many of the symbols as they can remember. A recall of six of the nine symbol pairs is at the low end of the range of normal recall. Patients who cannot place seven or more correctly are encouraged to write as many of the symbols as they can recall in the margin below. Significant age and education effects were seen. As a guideline, the authors state that 80% of healthy older adults will correctly match at least three symbols with digits; scores below three should be noted but only scores of zero may be regarded as definitely abnormal. The exception is participants in their 80s with no more than a high school education, who recalled an average of two associations. Over 85% of adults over 50 years of age will produce at least six correct symbols, and any score below five may be treated as abnormal except for the group noted above. Age and education norms are provided for 177 adults ranging in age from 50 to 90 using the Kaplan procedure for administering the WAIS-R (Joy et al., 2000). Age-related decline was found on a shortened version of this task with 131 South African adults of Anglo-Saxon origin ranging in age from 20 to 89 (Shuttleworth-Jordan and Bode, 1995). Participants completed 42 coding pairs rather than the 68 pairs used in the Kaplan version. Age-related decline was greatest in participants 70 years and older.

The WAIS-III changed the name of this test to Digit Symbol-Coding, increased the time to completion to two minutes, and included a procedure for assessing incidental learning similar to the one proposed by E. Kaplan and her colleagues (Wechsler, 1997a). The Administration and Scoring Manual does not provide normative data for this test, but the Technical Manual (The Psychological Corporation, 1997) provides cumulative percentages of participants performing at different levels up to the 50th percentile.

With 110 items in 7½ rows, the Symbol Digit Modalities Test (SDMT) (A. Smith, 1982; see pp. 370–371) has both more items and several more rows than Digit Symbol. Its length usually allows for both immediate and delayed recall trials to be examined on the same test form, as few patients get as far as the next-to-last row. Thus, in most cases, immediately upon completion of the test proper the examiner can fold the last two rows back and ask the subject to fill in only the now top row from memory, marking it at the left with a big **X**. Folding this row back makes it possible to give the delayed trial on the last row. In addition to the examination of both incidental learning and retention, impaired self-regulation may show up in a patient who continues the immediate recall trial on the bottom line, despite specific instructions to fill in only the line marked with an **X**. Impaired self-regulation may also become evident when patients pair up two different symbols with the same number, or write in different numbers for two of the same symbols. Since incidental recall on SDMT is based on two 90 sec trials, the cutoff score between 5 and 6 recommended for Digit Symbol may be a little generous. However, in clinical practice it is usefully discriminating. Most patients recall as many or almost as many digit–symbol pairs correctly on delayed recall as they had recalled immediately. Patients with significant retention problems recall fewer—sometimes only one or even none—on delayed recall. A few patients will improve from immediate recall to delayed recall. A close inspection of their test performances typically provides other indications that theirs is a slowed processing problem.

A procedure for examining incidental memory using WIS-A Similarities (Vilkki, Holst, Ohman, et al., 1992) gives a nice example of such an examination and how it can be incorporated into the usual test proceedings. Upon completing Similarities, subjects were asked for both free recall and cued recall of test items, the latter trial presented as a paired associates test. When given to patients who had undergone surgical repair of a subarachnoid hemorrhage a year earlier, free recall but not cued recall discriminated between patients functioning normally and patients with obvious neuropsychological deficits.

A 15-item version of the Boston Naming Test has also been used for incidental recall of the items (Bryan and Luszcz, 2000). Because the task was used to assess incidental learning rather than confrontation naming only, correct names were given for incorrect or unnamed items. On this task, age accounted for only 8% of the variance and speed. Performance was predicted by scores on verbal knowledge, speed, and retrieval on other tasks.

A female superiority has been observed for verbal memory on incidental learning tasks too (McGivern et al., 1998). For example, using pictorial material with varying degrees of verbalizable stimuli (e.g., complex scenes vs. easily labeled stimuli), Chipman and Kimura (1998) found that women performed better than men when the stimuli were verbalizable. Incidental learning is not often examined in patients with brain disorders. For Parkinson patients the findings are mixed. Ivory and colleagues (1999) reported that patients with Parkinson's disease without dementia were impaired in learning verbal material under incidental learning conditions; but another study found that incidental learning of Parkinson patients without dementia equalled that of control subjects, while only Parkinson patients with dementia were impaired (Azuma et al., 2000).

PROSPECTIVE MEMORY

Remembering to execute an action planned for the future requires a mechanism for signaling when the appropriate time has arrived and recall of the nature of the intent. Signals may be either time or event based (Einstein and McDaniel, 1990). An alarm clock may serve as a signal for a *time-based intention,* while remembering to tell a friend something at the next encounter would be an *event-based intention.* Most people depend on prospective recall of numerous tasks in their daily activities. Investigators are beginning to explore ways to examine prospective memory systematically (see Brandimonte et al., 1996). The Rivermead Behavioral Memory Test (RBMT) contains several tasks designed to measure prospective memory (Wilson, Cockburn, and Baddeley, 1985; see pp. 491–493). The *Cambridge Behaviour Prospective Memory Test* (Groot et al., 2002) has four time-based items such as, "In 20 minutes please ask me for a copy of the newspaper;" and four event-based prospective memory tasks, one of which is, "When the alarm rings, please put this briefcase under the desk."

Many studies of prospective memory have looked at the influence of age, prompted by knowledge of age-related decline on tests of episodic memory and the frequent complaints of elderly persons that they forget to carry out actions or go to a room and cannot recall what they intended to do while there. Findings of an age-related decline in prospective memory have been mixed, dependent on the demographic characteristics of the subjects and the type of prospective memory studied. Einstein and McDaniel (1990) instructed subjects to press a response key every time a designated word appeared in a word list task. Performance was examined under both external-aid and no-aid conditions. No age effect was found for well-educated younger and older subjects (mean age 69 years) on this prospective memory task, although the younger group outperformed the elderly on the more traditional tasks of free recall and recognition of word lists. Using a memory aid facilitated prospective memory at similar levels for both groups. While no age differences were found on an event-based task, such as the one above, age differences were found with a time-based task in which subjects were instructed to perform an action every 10 minutes (Einstein, McDaniel, et al., 1995). Studying subjects with more varied educational attainment, occupational status, and verbal ability, K.E. Cherry and LeCompte (1999) found a significant age-related decline in older adults (mean age 70 years) with lower ability level but not for higher ability older adults. Studying prospective memory in subjects up to 92 years of age, Bisiacchi (1996) found age effects only for subjects over 70 years. Other data suggest that age-related decline in prospective memory occurs when conditions of learning and recalling are sufficiently complex (Einstein, Smith, et al., 1997).

The roles of "hippocampal" memory and "frontal" functioning in prospective memory were examined in elderly (64 to 85 years) adults who showed differential performances on these functions (McDaniel et al., 1999). Hippocampal function was assessed with traditional memory tests and the Wisconsin Card Sorting Test, Controlled Oral Word Association Tests, WAIS-R Arithmetic, and WMS-R Mental Control and Digits Backward were used to evaluate frontal competence. The prospective memory task involved pressing a response key every time a target word appeared in a multiple-choice test of general knowledge. The subjects with the best performance on "frontal" tasks responded significantly more often to the target words than those who did poorest on these tasks. The "hippocampal" memory factor did not produce a significant effect. The authors concluded that the results were in line with theoretical speculation that prefrontal systems subserve significant processes in prospective memory.

A few studies have examined prospective memory in patients with brain disorders. Cockburn (1996a) asked patients with mixed brain disorders and controls to indicate when a task duration reached five minutes (time-based intention) and to change color pens when numbers on a cancellation task changed from two-digit to three-digit and to initial the last page of the test booklet (event-based intentions). Subjects also did other memory tasks and tests of executive function. Control subjects generally performed better than patients, particularly on the time-based task. No relationship was found between performance on executive and memory measures and success on the time-based prospective task. Patients who had poorer prose recall were more likely to fail event-based tasks.

Prospective memory is impaired in many severely injured TBI patients (Kinsella, Murtagh, et al., 1996). For a group of patients with brain injury, mostly TBI, the total perspective memory score for both time-based and event-based tasks correlated significantly with scores on traditional episodic memory tests and executive function tests (Groot et al., 2002). No significant correlations were found for attention, speed of processing, or years of education. Event-based tasks were easier than time-based tasks for patients and control subjects. Note-taking improved performance. In a study comparing patients with focal lesions in various sites, P.W. Burgess, Veitch, and their colleagues (2000) found that patients with lesions of medial regions in the left hemisphere had problems in prospective memory as measured by ability to follow self-generated plans for completion of multiple tasks. All six patients with severe memory impairment from herpes encephalitis failed prospective memory tasks, both time-based and event-based, even though the patients showed variable performance on traditional verbal memory tests (Sgaramella et al., 2000). Huppert and Beardsall (1993), using the Rivermead Behavioural Memory Test, found that impairment in event-based prospective memory was more prominent than impairment in learning and recall of words and objects in patients with very mild dementia.

REMOTE MEMORY

The need to assess very long-term memory arises particularly when retrograde amnesia is present and the examiner wants to know how far back it extends. Thus, testing for the integrity of remote memory usually concerns persons with brain conditions that result in retrograde amnesia, such as Korsakoff's disease, temporal or frontal lobe pathology, and those with memory problems incurred in special circumstances, such as treatment with electroconvulsive therapy (ECT). Usually, the retrograde amnesia shows a temporal gradient in which it is most severe for the period preceding the precipitating event. Several strategies for measuring retrograde amnesia involve recall or recognition of information that is commonly held. Unfortunately, in using test items that range from recent to remote topics, an instrument developed to assess gradients of long-term memory must be constantly updated or it will soon become obsolete. This precludes the development of a well-standardized test of remote memory because of the impossibility of going through elaborate standardization procedures every few years. Bahrick and Karis (1982) described methods for assessing remote memory (what they call "long-term ecological memory") and discussed some of the attendant methodological problems.

The interpretation of data from remote memory studies has been questioned since some of the material may have been relearned years after the event (when presented in an article, a book, or a television program, e.g.) (M.G. O'Connor et al., 2000; Sanders, 1972). Sanders also wondered how even-handed this examination technique was since the amount of interest in events such as the death of a prime minister of another country or in personalities such as politicians or movie stars varies so greatly from person to person. McCarthy and Warrington (1990) point out that various items of current salient information will acquire differing retention values as decades pass. Scores on a test of familiarity with television program titles, for example, were positively related to the amount of time the subjects watched television (Harvey and Crovitz, 1979). These tests also presuppose a degree of nationwide cultural homogeneity that one may no longer be able to count on, not just in the United States but in most sizable English-speaking countries and perhaps in some continental European countries too.

Recall of Public Events and Famous Persons

News events tests

A variety of remote memory tests have been based on information from well-known news events. Recall and recognition of public events were investigated in Great Britain by Warrington and Silberstein (1970), who examined the usefulness of both a recall and a multiple-choice questionnaire for assessing memory of events that had occurred in the previous year. Subjects took this test three times at six-month intervals. This technique showed that both age and the passage of a year's time affected recall and recognition of once-known information, and that recall was much more sensitive to age and time effects than was recognition. This method was then extended over longer periods with the development of a multiple-choice *Events Questionnaire* using events for the four preceding decades selected to give even coverage over the 40-year span (McCarthy and Warrington, 1990). A companion test of "well-known" faces covering the previous (approximately) 25 years was also developed in both free recall and multiple-choice versions. With long time periods, both recognition and recall techniques registered significant decrements for age and the passage of time.

Hodges and Ward (1989) used the *Famous Events Test*, consisting of 50 famous events from the 1930s to the 1970s randomly interspersed with 50 made-up events. The subject must identify the true event and, if correct, tell the decade in which it occurred. Patients with transient global amnesia could adequately identify true events but were deficient in dating those in the two decades prior to the amnesic episode. Squire, Haist, and Shimamura (1989) developed a later updated (Reed and Squire, 1998) *Public Events Test* composed of 145 events reported in the news from the 1940s through the 1990s that asks first for free recall and then provides a four-choice format. Patients with the most extensive temporal lobe damage showed the greatest memory loss for facts and events in the most recent decades preceding their brain injury. Kopelman (1989) developed a now updated *News Events Test* (Kopelman, Stanhope, and Kingsley, 1999). Memory for events familiar to British subjects is tested by asking them to identify what was happening in 40 pictures from each decade from the 1960s to the 1990s. Partial credit is given for incomplete identification. Patients with temporal lobe lesions (mostly herpes encephalitis), frontal lobe lesions, and Korsakoff's syndrome performed poorly, showing temporal gradients such that items from the 1960s were recalled better than items from the 1970s and 1980s. The *Dead-or-Alive* memory test (Kapur, 1989) asks subjects to indicate whether a famous personality from the past is dead or alive, whether the cause of death was natural, and what the year of death was, expressed in five-year bands. The items consist of 30 famous people who have died and 10 who are still living. This test demonstrated the remote memory deficits of a patient with severe TBI (Kapur, Scholey, Moore, et al., 1996).

The *Transient News Events Test* (M.G. O'Connor et al., 2000) tests recall of remote events that had time-limited media exposure. Selected news items had had extensive popular appeal but discontinued coverage. Amounts and durations of news coverage were obtained from *New York Times*' records; to be considered, an item had to radically decrease in frequency of mention over a three-year period. The resulting 40 items cover the years from 1952 through 1992. Free recall is scored for both correct and partially correct answers. Recognition probing is used for any items that the subject does not recall. No age-related decline was observed for the 20 to 80 year-old range. All ages demonstrated a recency effect in that events from the recent past were recalled better than remote ones. Younger subjects were unable to tell about events that predated their birth, as expected. Men had superior recall for the remote time periods compared to women, but no other sex differences were observed.

Famous people tests

As part of a series of studies of memory disorder in Korsakoff's disease, several tests involving recall or recognition of famous people were developed (M.S. Albert, Butters, and Levin, 1979; M.S. Albert, Butters, and Brandt, 1980). The *Famous Faces Test* consists of black and white photographs of people who achieved fame in each of six decades (1920s to 1970s) and, in the free recall portion, subjects are asked to name the person shown in the photograph. *Facial Recognition Test* is a multiple-choice recognition of the sample people. Twenty-nine photographs, taken when the subjects were young, were paired with photographs of these same people who were still famous when they were old (e.g., Charlie Chaplin) and presented in randomized order to make up the *Old–Young Test*. In addition, two questionnaires about famous people from these decades were constructed, one testing recall, the other, recognition. Patients with Korsakoff's disease averaged almost 60 years of age and 12 years of education. Control subjects were matched on these variables. This latter group did not show a gradient of loss of information with the passage of time. On most analyses of the data from these tests, the patients showed a marked gradient, from low scores for recent material to scores approaching normal for material from early decades. When this set of tests was given to patients recently diagnosed with Huntington's disease and to advanced Huntington patients, no temporal gradient was found for either of the patient groups, as both sets of patients performed poorly on material from all decades (M.S. Albert, Butters, and Brandt, 1981). However, both patients with Alzheimer's disease and control subjects recognized photographs of familiar faces taken when the person was old more readily than those taken earlier (R.S. Wilson, Kaszniak, and Fox, 1981).

The Famous Faces Test was updated to study remote memory in Alzheimer patients (Hodges, Salmon, and Butters, 1993). The new version has photographs of 85 people who were famous from the 1940s through the 1990s. Both semantic and phonemic prompting cues are given along with a four-choice recognition format. Alzheimer patients were significantly impaired in all test conditions, displaying a temporal gradient for recognition, identification and naming with phonemic cues, but impairments for spontaneous naming or naming with semantic cues did not vary with decades. Thus, they appeared to have lost stored knowledge about the person and not simply a naming deficit. Patients with dorsolateral frontal lobe lesions were impaired on free recall of famous faces but less impaired when given multiple-choice recognition alternatives (Mangels et al., 1996). Unlike Alzheimer patients, they appeared to have knowledge of the person but were unsuccessful in retrieving the information in the free recall condition.

Presidents Test[1] (Hamsher and Roberts, 1985)

While this test requires updating every four to eight years, barring unfortunate circumstances, the update involves only the addition of the photo of the new president and discarding that of the last of the six which had been serving as items in this test. Four different administrations examine: (1) *Verbal Naming* (VN), which asks for free recall of the current president and his five immediate predecessors; (2) *Verbal Sequencing* (VS), in which six cards with the presidents' names are handed to subjects in a "fixed, quasi-random" order with instructions to arrange them chronologically; (3) *Photo Naming* (PN), which shows the presidents' pictures in the same order as the VS cards for the subject to name; and (4) *Photo Sequencing* (PS), which asks for a chronological sequencing of the photos. The naming tests each have a maximum score of 6. The sequencing tasks are scored by rank order correlation (Spearman's

rho) between the correct sequence and the one given by the subject.

Test characteristics. For VN scores, an age effect was found only for subjects with 12 or fewer years of schooling. For PN and PS, only educational differences showed up, while neither age nor education affected VS performances. Score corrections are provided for VN and PN but not PS because of the great variability within the lower education group. VN, PN, and VS each have one cutting score, but two were determined for PS for ≥ 13 and ≤ 12 years of education. In one factor analytic study this test loaded on a remote memory factor which, interestingly, also included a significant weighting (.42) for Digit Symbol (Larrabee and Levin, 1986).

Neuropsychological findings. No control subjects failed more than two tests, and only 8% failed one or two although only 33% of brain damaged patients succeeded on all four tasks (Hamsher and Roberts, 1985). A comparison of patients with lateralized damage found that significantly more with right-sided lesions failed the sequencing tasks than those with left-sided involvement (R.J. Roberts, Hamsher, et al., 1990). Patients with bilateral/diffuse damage or dementia are likely to have memory failures, but few with lateralized lesions fail the memory parts of the test. A significant relationship was found between general cognitive deterioration and number of task failures.

Black and white photographs of the seven most recent U.S. presidents before George Bush and seven other well-known figures, e.g., Neil Armstrong, were used for testing recognition memory of the presidents and for obtaining temporal order of their terms (Storandt, Kaskie, and Von Dras, 1998). Both healthy older persons and patients with mild dementia of the Alzheimer type correctly recognized the presidents and both groups produced U-shaped patterns of errors in temporal ordering, although the dementia group produced more overall errors.

Fama, Sullivan, Shear, et al. (2000b) made the task more difficult by asking patients to write down all the presidential candidates since 1920 and to identify their party affiliation and the years they ran for office. They were then asked to: select from six choices which candidates ran against each other in a particular election and choose the year that the election occurred; sequence the names written on cards of presidential candidates within a single political party from 1920 to 1988; and, identify photographs of presidential candidates from the elections of 1920-1980, giving the candidate's name, party affiliation, and year(s) of the election. Con-

---

[1]This test can be obtained from Kerry de S. Hamsher, Ph.D., Neuropsychology Clinic, 1218 W. Kilbourn Ave., #415, Milwaukee, WI, 53233–1325.

trol subjects had correct free recall of approximately 65% of the elected candidates since 1920 and less than 25% of the defeated candidates. Parkinson patients without dementia performed as well as controls, while Alzheimer patients were severely impaired. A similar pattern was seen on free recall photo naming. Although the Alzheimer patients performed better on recognition tasks compared to free recall, they were impaired compared to Parkinson patients and control subjects except for recognition of names of elected candidates.

Autobiographic Memory

Another aspect of remote memory is the ability to recall one's own history. Rarely, retrograde amnesia involves autobiographical events and even more rarely affects autobiographical mempory more than knowledge of public events and people (J.J. Evans et al., 1996), although some amnesic patients have greater loss of personal memory than general information (Kopelman, 2002). The virtue of examining autobiographic recall is that all people have had full exposure to their history, making it a rich and culture-fair examination resource. It taps a different aspect of memory, and may be useful for patient counseling (B.A. Wilson, 1993). The drawback, of course, is the difficulty of verifying someone else's personal names, dates, and events. I can tell you that Miss Donovan was my first grade teacher [mdl], but how can you check up on me? Only the exceptional case, such as the prominent scientist who had written an autobiography just two years before succumbing to Korsakoff's psychosis, provides a reliable history for the examination of remote memory (N. Butters and Cermak, 1986). For the rest, the examiner can only test the validity of a patient's self-report by interdata comparisons (e.g., do dates and events make chronological sense?), clinical judgment of the clarity and integrity of the patient's responses and, where possible, by reports of others.

The Crovitz Test (Crovitz and Schiffman, 1974)

This test or its modification (Sagar, Cohen, et al., 1988) has been used to examine the efficiency of autobiographic recall from specific time periods. Subjects are asked to describe from any time period personal experiences of a unique episode associated with each of ten common nouns (e.g., car, bird), and estimate the date of occurrence. Four minutes is allowed for each noun, and if necessary, prompts or cues are offered after two minutes. Responses are scored according to the specificity in time and place of the recalled memory and the richness of details. Recollection of memories from var-

ious ages is noted. In a restrained time condition subjects are asked to recall memories from particular ages, such as "before the age of 17" (N.E. Kroll, Markowitsch, et al., 1997). Healthy subjects tend to produce memories from all decades, most from the previous decade (Hodges and Oxbury, 1990). Patients tested during transient global amnesia episodes showed impaired uncued recall and a virtual absence of recent memories (Hodges and Ward, 1989). Six months after resolution of an episode of transient global amnesia, patients' recall of autobiographical memories was impaired in both cued and uncued conditions. Patients with severe TBI produced very few memories from before the onset of their injuries (N.E. Kroll, Markowitsch, et al., 1997).

Autobiographical Memory Interview (AMI) (Kopelman, Wilson, and Baddeley, 1989, 1990)

This questionnaire was developed to standardize the collection of autobiographical data and to provide a range of time spans and item types. It contains two sections: an *Autobiographical Incidents Schedule* and a *Personal Semantic Memory Schedule*. Each schedule asks three questions from each of three time blocks: Childhood (e.g., preschool, primary school), Early Adult Life (e.g., first job, courtship, marriage in 20s), and Recent Events (e.g., a recent visitor, an event in place where interviewed). Patients who cannot respond to a question are given prompts (e.g., for childhood block, first memory? involving brother or sister? etc.). Responses are graded on a 0–3 scale which takes into account the clarity and specificity of the response so that the maximum score for each time block is 9. The Personal Semantic Memory Schedule has four parts, inquiring into Background Information, Childhood, Early Adult Life, and Recent Information. Here the three questions in each part concern the specifics of names, dates, and places. Background Information was allocated a maximum of 23 points, each other section has a maximum score of 21 points. Questionnaire scores were examined in a correlational study with other remote memory tests, producing coefficients in the .27–.76 range, with most .40 or above. Interrater reliability coefficients were satisfactory ($r = .85$). While full confidence in patients' veracity cannot be achieved, this technique appears to satisfy practical requirements as a test of remote memory.

Neuropsychological findings. Amnesic patients performed significantly below control subjects on all variables, with the greatest difference between these groups occurring on recent memory as the controls made almost perfect scores here while amnesics' recent recall (both semantic and event) was poorest (Kopelman, Wilson, and Baddeley, 1989). Examples provided by the authors show how patients' confusion or acuity tends to relate to their performance on the AMI. Patients with some conditions show impairment with a temporal gradient: for Korsakoff patients it is steep with relative sparing of earliest memories (Kopelman, Stanhope, and Kingsley, 1999); of two herpes encephalitis patients, the one with the more extensive temporal lobe lesion did show a temporal gradient on the AMI, but remote memories of the other were relatively spared, as were the temporal lobes (J.M. Reed and Squire, 1998). When multiple sclerosis is severe, overall performance is poor with a slight temporal gradient (Kenealy et al., 2002). Eslinger (1998a) studied the effect of focal temporal lobe lesions in eight patients. Four with bilateral lesions had more severe retrograde memory deficits on the AMI than one patient with unilateral lesions; the other three with unilateral lesions were entirely normal on this inventory. In Eslinger's study a patient with a bilateral prefrontal lesion also showed striking defects in autobiographical memory, except for childhood personal–semantic memories.

FORGETTING

Forgetting involves memory decay over time. Inability to retrieve information either by free recall or recognition suggests that forgetting has occurred. Most techniques for measuring learning can be used to examine forgetting by adding recall or recognition trials spaced over time. Examining Korsakoff patients, Talland (1965a) used a delayed recall format—for example, with recall trials of hours, days, and up to a week to establish forgetting curves for many different kinds of material.

The *savings* method provides an indirect means of measuring the amount of material retained after it has been learned (H.S. Levin, 1986). This method involves teaching the patient the same material on two or more occasions, which are usually separated by days or weeks, but the second learning trial may come as soon as 30 min after the first. The number of trials the patient takes to reach criterion is counted each time. Reductions in the number of trials needed for criterion learning (the "savings") at a later session are interpreted as indicating retention from the previous set of learning trials. Warrington and Weiskrantz (1968) demonstrated some retention in severely amnesic patients over one- and four-week intervals by using the savings method with both verbal and nonverbal material. No other method they used gave evidence that

these patients had retained any material from their initial exposure to the tests. In another application of the savings technique, both postacute brain damaged patients and control subjects were given Logical Memory and Verbal Paired Associate Learning (WMS-R) 24 hours apart and then compared for savings on the second administration (B. Caplan, Reidy, et al., 1990). Their savings scores "produced the sharpest differentiation" between the two groups.

The score devised by D.N. Brooks (1972) to document the relative amount of information lost between the various trials of the Complex Figure Test can be applied to other tests as well:

$$\frac{\text{CFT-I} - \text{CFT-D}}{\text{CFT-I}} \times 100$$

Brooks demonstrated this by also using his "% Forgetting" score to compare performances on immediate and delayed trials of the Logical Memory and Associate Learning subtests of the Wechsler Memory Scale. Tröster, Butters, Salmon, and their colleagues (1993) devised another formula for calculating savings:

$$\% \text{ savings} = \frac{\text{Delayed recall}}{\text{Immediate recall}} \times 100$$

Using this technique for Logical Memory and Visual Reproduction (WMS-R), these authors demonstrated that for both memory tasks older normal subjects had a somewhat higher rate of forgetting than younger ones; Huntington patients' rate of forgetting was higher than elderly subjects', and Alzheimer patients' rate of forgetting greatly exceeded that of the Huntington patients. The WMS-III uses this formula for calculating the "% Retention" for delayed recall measures.

These formulas work well for patients whose recall scores are not at the extremes of the distribution. Patients who have very little immediate recall may achieve a good savings score based on equally scanty delayed recall.

On WMS-III, for example, a 45-year-old patient whose Logical Memory I (immediate recall) raw score is 9 and LM-II (delayed recall) is 7 will have a good % Retention Score of 78, even though the delayed recall score is only *borderline defective* for this age. Another patient of the same age whose LM-I raw score is 65 and LM-II is 40 will have *superior* performances on both recall trials, but the % Retention Score will be 62.

Therefore, forgetting scores should never be interpreted in isolation from initial learning levels.

When the effects of acquisition differences were controlled, rates of forgetting verbal material over a 20-min interval were similar for ages 20–79 (Tombaugh and Hubley, 2001). These authors found that when the retest interval was increased to one day, more forgetting occurred with increasing age. No further differential decline appeared for delays up to 62 days. Age-associated differences were greatest on a word list task, which provides limited opportunity for encoding, and least on paragraph and word pairs in which the format provides a more associative structure. The standardization sample from the WMS-III shows that forgetting rates are similar for ages 16 to 89 on Logical Memory and Visual Reproduction (Haaland, Price, and La Rue, 2003). Age-related decline on these tests was mostly due to poor immediate recall. Nonverbal forgetting may have a steeper age-related decline. For example, older subjects exhibited faster rates of forgetting than younger ones when tested for recognition of magazine photographs one day and one week after initial viewing (Huppert and Kopelman, 1989).

Some patients with degenerative disorders, such as Huntington's disease, have normal retention but forgetting is accelerated in Alzheimer's disease (Massman, Delis, and Butters, 1993). Reports of forgetting rates in other memory disorders are inconsistent and probably relate to the length of delay intervals and the method of study. By extending exposure to the material to be learned and with a 10 min delay, Huppert and Piercy (1979) found normal rates of forgetting for Korsakoff and Alzheimer patients. Patients who have undergone electroconvulsive shock treatments have accelerated forgetting (P. Lewis and Kopelman, 1998; Squire, 1981), and TBI patients have accelerated forgetting during posttraumatic amnesia (H.S. Levin, High, and Eisenberg, 1988). Rapid rates of forgetting new information can continue for months and years following moderate to severe TBI (Vanderploeg, Crowell, and Curtiss, 2001).

12 | Memory II: Batteries, Paired Memory Tests, and Questionnaires

MEMORY BATTERIES

To provide thorough coverage of the varieties of memory abilities, batteries of memory tests are often used. By and large, the older batteries have only haphazard norms, and each has limitations in its scope and emphases such that none provides a suitably well-rounded and generally applicable means of examining memory functions (see Erickson and Scott, 1977). A well-standardized battery that could provide an overall review of memory functions taking into account modality (or material) differences and major aspects of the memory system without requiring much more than an hour would be most welcome. The ideal memory battery would be more extensive than intensive. When a review of memory systems indicates likely areas of impairment, the examiner can undertake a more detailed assessment of deficits.

Even a general review is often not needed, however, for the problem areas requiring careful study are apparent from observation or history. Moreover, a comprehensive memory assessment need not be conducted within the framework of a battery any more than any other aspect of cognitive assessment. Many interesting memory assessment techniques examine different aspects of memory problems with varying degrees of suitability for different patients. Of course, using tests from different sources does not enjoy the advantages of identical scoring systems with intertest equivalencies. Nevertheless, increased statistical refinements of most newer tests provide reasonable comparability across test scores, whether they are expressed in standard deviation or percentile units, or as raw scores accompanied by their statistical descriptions. Thus, many neuropsychologists pick and choose memory tests based upon the appropriateness for the individual patient and the limitations and opportunities of the particular examination situations.

The primary advantage of most batteries is that they include a variety of memory tasks, with the most recently developed ones likely to have good age-graded norms. The chief drawbacks are three: (1) Battery instructions for the examiner typically assume that the entire battery will be given at one time, so that one memory test immediately follows another. Patients with impaired memory thus have to give one deficient performance after another without respite from a succession of failures. Instructions usually fail to remind the examiner that the individual tests comprising the battery can be reorganized or resequenced for an examination format in which memory tests are thoughtfully interspersed with tests of other functions that are more likely to be preserved. Patients who can experience some successes along with their failures are thus somewhat more protected from experiencing the examination as depressing, if not devastating to their self-esteem and anxious hopes for a normal life. Naive and inexperienced examiners, however, may not appreciate this problem as they conscientiously follow the battery makers' administration directions. (2) Having completely given one of the larger batteries, some examiners may imagine that they have given an adequately comprehensive examination without realizing that not all important aspects of the patient's memory problems have necessarily been addressed. (3) Additionally, not all tests in a battery will be relevant for a particular patient or issue; some tests are either redundant or not particularly relevant for anything, including the patient's memory problems. Bundling tests into a formal battery increases the likelihood that unnecessary tests are given.

Wechsler Memory Scale (WMS-O, WMS-R, WMS-III) (Wechsler, 1945; Stone et al., 1946; Wechsler and Stone, 1974, Wechsler, 1997b)

The *Wechsler Memory Scale* (WMS), and its revisions, is likely the most widely used and most recognizable memory battery (M. Butler, Retzlaff, and Vanderploeg, 1991). First published in 1945, the most recent WMS edition was released in 1997. The original 1945 version (WMS-O) is rarely used now and will not be discussed here. Interested readers may refer to previous editions of *Neuropsychological Assessment* for information about the original scale.

The *Wechsler Memory Scale-Revised* (WMS-R) and

Wechsler Memory Scale-III both continue to be popular choices for memory assessment. There are, however, important differences between the two versions of the test as well as from the WMS-O, and each will be discussed separately.

Wechsler Memory Scale-Revised (WMS-R) (Wechsler, 1987)

The original WMS was criticized for many reasons, and the WMS-R represents a major effort to correct its most glaring defects: (1) the unitary Memory Quotient (MQ) score; (2) the scanty assessment of visual/nonverbal memory; (3) the absence of delayed recall measures; (4) the inadequate norming procedures and normative sample. In each of these respects, the WMS-R is an improvement over the original, but in each, it falls short. Unlike the WMS-O, the WMS-R has only one form—a serious limitation since retesting is so often required in clinical neuropsychology and memory and learning tests are particularly susceptible to practice effects (e.g., see McCaffery, Duff, and Westervelt, 2000b, *passim*). Fortunately, for patients who are assessed on more than one occasion, independent tables providing information about reliable changes that incorporate practice effects and measurement error can be consulted (Sawrie, Chelune, et al., 1996).

The WMS-R contains nine tests, six of which originated in the WMS: *Information and Orientation (I/O)*, which appeared as separate tests in the WMS, were combined into a single scale. *Mental Control* and *Digit Span* remain unchanged. Alterations in *Logical Memory (LM)*, *Associate Learning* (now called *Verbal Paired Associates [VePA]*), and *Visual Reproduction (VR)* are described in Chapter 11. Two tests added to the battery in an effort to provide a more balanced assessment of visual relative to verbal memory are *Figural Memory* and *Visual Paired Associates (Visual PA)*. Delayed recall of Logical Memory (LM II), Visual Reproduction (VR II), Verbal and Visual Paired Associates contribute four more scores, for a total of 13.

Information and Orientation questions ask for age, date of birth, identification of current and recent public officials ("Who is president of the United States? Who was president before him?"), and tests orientation to time and place. *Mental Control* assesses automatic speech (alphabet recitation) and simple conceptual tracking. *Figural Memory* is an immediate recognition test of abstract designs. *Logical Memory I and II* test immediate and 30 minute delayed recall of short verbal stories. *Visual Paired Associates* pairs abstract line drawings with colors with a color pointing response required; immediate and delayed conditions are tested. *Verbal Paired Associates* tests verbal associative ability for words and contains both immediate and delayed conditions. *Visual Reproduction I and II* assesses immediate and delayed recall for a visual drawing task. *Digit Span* measures forward span, beginning with 3 and up to 8 digits and backward span from 2 up to 7 digits. Unlike the original WMS, both trials of each span length are administered until failure on both trials of a span length is obtained (see note on giving two trials, pp. 351–352). *Visual Memory Span* is a nonverbal analog of Digit Span which measures the ability to reproduce the spatial pattern of tapping sequences on an array of blocks beginning with 2 and going up to 8 blocks plus the ability to reverse the spatial block tapping sequence from 2 up to 7 blocks (see Chapter 9, Fig. 9.9, p. 355, for a model). As with Digit Span, both trials of a span length are given until the length is reached at which both are failed.

Battery characteristics

1. Trading in the MQ for indices. The WMS-R no longer includes a "memory quotient," or MQ, having been replaced by five indices (*Verbal Memory, Visual Memory, General Memory, Attention and Concentration,* and *Delayed Memory*).

Verbal Memory is the sum of (Logical Memory I × 2) + Verbal PA I; Logical Memory I can contribute more than twice the number of score points as Verbal PA-I by virtue of its greater score potential and the doubled weighting. *Visual Memory* is computed from scores on Figural Memory, Visual PA-I, and Visual Reproduction I. Visual Reproduction I also has a greater score potential and thus contributes more to this index than the other tests. *General Memory* is a compound of both Verbal and Visual memory indices. *Attention and Concentration* is computed from Digit Span, Visual Memory Span, and Figural Memory scores; Digit Span and Visual Memory Span each have double the weighting of the Figural Memory score and more than double the score potential making the Figural Memory contribution quite negligible. Finally, *Delayed Recall* sums delayed recall on 4 tasks (Logical Memory II, Visual Reproduction II, Verbal Paired Associates II, Visual Paired Associates II); here too Logical Memory II and Visual Reproduction II have much greater score ranges and thus the potential of far outweighing performances on the two paired associates tasks. Weighted raw score index sums are converted to individual "Indexes" by means of age-graded normative tables. No rationale for the differential weightings of the tests is given.

These procedures certainly are an improvement over the single summary MQ. A review of the composition of the indices, however, raises some important questions.

2. Disconnections between Index names and contributing factors. The Attention/Concentration Index appears to be appropriately named since it separates out much of the attentional tests in this battery, which, in the previous edition, were simply lumped into the MQ. Although each of the other indices appears from the titles of the component tests to bear a meaningful relationship to its given name, neither the indices nor the contributing tests are always discriminated by factor analyses (Bornstein and Chelune, 1989; Bowden et al., 1997; Elwood, 1991; Hunkin et al., 2000; Moore and Baker, 1997). Moreover, factor analytic studies based on individual test scores that result in a 3-factor solution invariably have an attention/concentration factor, and may have separate factors for immediate memory and delayed recall (D.B. Burton et al., 1993; D.L. Roth, Conboy, et al., 1990, using scores made by TBI patients), or verbal and nonverbal (i.e., predominantly visual) factors with loadings varying somewhat according to sample age and education (Bornstein and Chelune, 1989, for WMS-R performances of persons referred for neuropsychological assessment). Factor analysis solutions appear to vary widely according to population types and what other test data have been included.

The absence of any clear and consistently meaningful factor pattern supports the impression gained from just reviewing the tests and how they fit into the index scheme: Intercorrelations between these measures tend to be low, mostly below .31, indicating that they are mostly measuring different functions; but the pattern of intercorrelations varies considerably with different age groups, raising questions as to just what is being measured. In one report, TBI patients performed more poorly than control subjects on all WMS-R indices, yet did not differ across all component tests when examined individually (Wilhelm and Johnstone, 1995). Thus, it appears that the indices are not to be literally interpreted as measures of the constructs that they purportedly assess (Chelune, Bornstein, and Prifitera, 1990). For example, General Memory, which is based only on immediate learning (Paired Associates I) and immediate recall (Logical Memory I, Visual Reproduction I) is not only a composite score including both poorly delineated visual components and heavily weighted verbal ones, but the contributions of learning (as opposed to immediate recall) are small, and delayed recall is not included although it is a more sensitive measure of what is generally considered to be "memory" than is immediate recall (Loring, 1989). Moreover, reliabilities for discrepancy scores between indices run from .00 to .89, and can vary considerably at different ages (Charter, 2002).

It seems one could anticipate that Verbal and Visual Memory indices would be sensitive to lesion laterality, particularly if the lesions are due to temporal lobectomies, although many epilepsy surgery centers have failed to find the comparison of these two measures to reliably discriminate lesion laterality (Barr, 1997; Kneebone et al., 1997; Loring, Lee, Martin, and Meador, 1989; P.M. Moore and Baker, 1996). Part of this failure, however, may be due to the intrinsic difficulty in assessing right temporal lobe memory function (Barr, Chelune, Hermann, et al., 1997); there is some evidence that the Verbal Memory scores are affected by left temporal lobe lesions (Chelune, Naugle, Lüders, et al., 1993; P.M. Moore and Baker, 1996).

3. Lengthened administration time. The additional tests needed to calculate factor scores significantly lengthened the administration time for the entire battery. Because potential time constraints may limit testing for certain assessments, the WMS-R manual states that a short form can be given by eliminating the delayed recall components. We wonder how widespread this practice is, however, since a major criticism of the original WMS was the absence of a delayed memory component (E.W. Russell, 1975).

An alternative method for reducing test administration time uses immediate and delayed recall of the three tests that appeared in the original scale (Logical Memory, Verbal PA, and Visual Reproduction) to predict the General and Delay Memory summary scores (Woodard and Axelrod, 1995). Favorable findings with this method appear in several validation studies (Axelrod, Putnam, et al., 1996; Hoffman, Scott, et al., 1997; van den Broek et al., 1998). This short form has the advantage of examining delayed recall, which is sacrificed if using the short-form procedure advocated by the test publisher. By eliminating marginally relevant tests administration time was reduced by approximately 50%. The omission of Verbal and Visual Memory indices appears to be of little concern since they have not been effective in documenting lateralized material-specific memory deficits.

4. Enhanced nonverbal representation? Superficially, it would appear that the addition of Figural Memory and Visual PA would remedy the predominantly verbal bias of the WMS. Unfortunately, it has not. Figural Memory is more an attentional task than anything else; Visual PA is quite verbalizible (see Chapter 11; Chelune, Bornstein, and Prifitera, 1990; Loring, 1989) and does not cluster with other measures of nonverbal memory (Wong and Gilpin, 1993). It is of interest that the new nonverbal tests developed for the WMS-R were removed in the subsequent WMS-III edition.

5. *Addition of delayed recall measures.* While the WMS-R has remedied the lack of delayed recall trials in the original WMS, by encouraging the confusion of visual and verbal measures in the Delayed Recall Index (DRI), much of the potential gain has been vitiated for those who attempt to interpret WMS-R performances based solely on index performances. The problem of interpreting—or, more likely, misinterpreting—the Delayed Recall Index is further compounded by the inexplicable—or at least as yet unexplained—score weightings and relative contributions of the four different measures that enter into it. Weightings given to tests in the Delayed Recall Index differ from those in the General Memory Index, although these are the same four tests for both indices (Loring, 1989). The maximum possible scores for the two paired associates tests also differ considerably for their immediate and delayed administrations, adding to the difficulty in comparing the General Memory Index with the Delayed Recall Index. A little prompting for the delayed recall of LM-R is encouraged but not for VR-R, which introduces still another bias into the composite Delayed Recall Index.

Moreover, appropriate recognition testing was not included by test publishers so that the relationship between storage and retrieval must remain obscure for all persons whose delayed recall performances are appreciably lower than their immediate recall. Several authors, fortunately, have developed recognition formats for the Logical Memory and Visual Reproduction which partially offset this important omission (Fastenau, 1996b; Gass, 1995).

6. *Samples and norms.* The manual gives normative data for nine age groups from 16–17 to 70–74. However, for age groups 18–19, 25–34, and 45–54 the data are extrapolated as only six age groups were actually tested. Although the extrapolations are based on assumptions of linear decline for all Index Scores, Attention/Concentration Index in particular may show a different decline pattern which can produce erroneously large discrepancies between this and other "Indexes" for persons in the 45–54 age range (see Loring, 1989). However, Attention/Concentration tends to run lower than General Memory for normal control subjects generally, and is even lower for younger than older ones! (Tröster, Jacobs, et al., 1989). In this same study, younger control subjects tended to have lower Delayed Memory scores relative to General Memory, much like the pattern for Huntington patients. Fischer (1988) found that the manual's norms ran somewhat lower than scores made by community control subjects, resulting in a much more benign estimation of memory deficits in multiple sclerosis patients than when they were compared with local controls. Her reported discrepancies

between the number of patients whose scores on DRI were at levels below -1 SD of the manual's norms (1/3) and of the local norms (68.9%) suggest that even the norms based on normative testing may not have general applicability.

For a test battery produced as a commercial enterprise, the WMS-R sample sizes (50 to 55) for each of the six examined age groups are somewhat small. Sensitivity to age effects was studied by the savings method developed by Cullum, Butters, and their colleagues (1990; see also p. 478). Comparisons of young-old (50 to 70) and old-old (75 to 95) subjects found that vulnerability to forgetting increased greatly with age on both immediate and delayed trials of Visual Reproduction; the elderly subjects' rate of forgetting was also higher on both trials of Logical Memory, Verbal PA, and on the delayed trial of Visual PA. No other WMS-R test showed differences between these two groups. Sex comparisons were made for both index and individual test scores with the finding that no differences appeared. All five indices showed education effects leading the manual to recommend that education be taken into account when interpreting these scores. The restriction of the normative sample to age 74 or less is regarded as a major deficiency by workers who are dealing with an increasingly older population (Ivnik, Malec, Smith, et al., 1992c; Loring, Lee, and Meador, 1989; Tröster, Jacobs, et al., 1989). Alternate norms from the Mayo Clinic derived from 441 cognitively healthy persons ranging from 56-94 years (i.e., MOANS) are available (Ivnik, Malec, Smith, et al., 1992c).

Neuropsychological findings. Despite their deficiencies, the "Indexes" do reflect some disease-associated patterns of memory impairment (N. Butters, Salmon, Cullum, et al., 1988). With memory deterioration, scores on other indices, particularly Delayed Recall, will fall below Attention/Concentration scores (Tröster, Jacobs, et al., 1989). Tröster and his group reported that patients in the early stages of Huntington disease differ from the early Alzheimer pattern in having better DRI scores. However, index scores did not differentiate early and middle stage patients for either of these conditions. A savings score comparing delayed recall as a function of immediate recall appears particularly sensitive to the memory impairment of Alzheimer patients compared with Huntington patients (Tröster, Butters, et al., 1993). In a separate report, however, the WMS-R failed to reliably differentiate these two patient groups (E. Mohr, Walker, et al., 1996).

The restriction of index scales to a low end standard score of 50 appears to create a "floor" effect which does not allow for discrimination of memory deficits in patients with more advanced disease, or in patients with severe memory disorders generally (Leng and Parkin, 1990). In a study comparing patients with frontal lobe lesions to Korsakoff patients, Attention/Concentration tended to run considerably lower than the memory indices for frontal patients, with Delayed Recall holding up quite well (Janowsky, Shimamura, Kritchevsky, and Squire, 1989). The Korsakoff patients performed *within normal limits* on Attention/Concentration but very poorly on all other indexes, achieving an average score of 56.0 on Delayed Memory. Moderately to severely injured TBI patients averaged one standard deviation below the mean on Attention/Concentration as their best index score, with their Delayed Recall average falling more than three standard deviations below the mean (Crossen and Wiens, 1988). These workers found that PASAT scores were a much more sensitive indicator of their patients' attentional deficits than Attention/Concentration, on which about half the patients had *borderline* or *within normal limits* scores. Fischer (1988) reported that three distinctive groups of multiple sclerosis patients were identified by the pattern of their index scores: One group performed at near-normal levels with only Delayed Recall scores dropping just under one standard deviation below the mean (without a recognition trial, the reason for this lowered score remains unknown, but it could well represent a retrieval rather than a learning problem); for a second group all index scores were higher than one standard deviation above the mean, except for a near-average Attention/Concentration (103.82); the third group's average index scores were all in the impaired range.

Patients with temporal lobe epilepsy perform more poorly on all the memory indices and lower on most of the individual subtests. As noted above, most indices did not provide useful lateralization information. However, in temporal lobe epilepsy patients with bilateral hippocampal atrophy on MRI, WMS-III Logical Memory retention scores provided meaningful lateralization information (Sawrie, Martin, et al., 2001).

Wechsler Memory Scale-III (Wechsler, 1997b)

This revision represents the latest attempt to present a balanced approach to memory assessment. The WMS-III contains an even larger number of tests than the WMS-R, further lengthening the battery, but classifies many of them as "optional." The core battery consists of six tests, three of which appeared in the WMS-R, to calculate the various memory indices. Five tests are optional, four of which appeared in a slightly different form in the previous edition. These tests do not contribute to any of the summary memory indices. As with the WMS-R, parallel forms are lacking although a table

containing the confidence intervals for test–retest measurement error reproduced in the technical manual can provide some guidance in interpreting change scores from follow-up testing (Iverson, 2001).

The WMS-R tests included—with slight alterations—as core battery tests are *Logical Memory, Verbal Paired Associates,* and *Spatial Span.* The new WMS-III core battery tests are *Letter-Number Sequencing, Faces,* and *Family Pictures* (Letter–Number Sequencing is discussed in Chapter 9, Faces and Family Pictures are reviewed in Chapter 11). *Visual Paired Associates* and *Figural Memory,* which were developed for the WMS-R, have been dropped from the battery. *Information and Orientation, Mental Control, Digit Span,* and *Visual Reproduction* are now classified as optional tests along with a newly developed verbal task that is appropriately named *Word Lists.* Most tests contain separate immediate and delayed recall components, acknowledging the importance of assessing the ability to retain information for approximately 30 minutes.

The WMS-III battery no longer characterizes performance on Logical Memory and Verbal Paired Associates as "verbal", instead using the label "auditory." This corresponds to "visual," which has historically been applied to visually presented verbalizable memory tests such as Visual Reproduction. Although accurate, it does fundamentally change the focus of the test from one that purportedly measured material-specific memory, which has the implication of more precise clinical/anatomical correlations, to modality-specific memory, which refers only to the sensory modality of material presentation.

The normative age range of the WMS-III has been considerably extended, with the highest age bracket now 85–89 years. This is a significant improvement over the WMS-R's upper limit of 70–74 years, and is comparable to the oldest age range in the MOANS normative sample (Ivnik, Malec, Smith, et al., 1992c; G.E. Smith, Wong, Ivnik, and Malec, 1997). Similarly improved is the size of the normative sample (1,250 vs. 300 in WMS-R). Raw scores convert to standard scores for which M = 10, S.D. = 3.

The decision to classify some of the tests as "core" and others as "optional" does create some unintended consequences since this classification implies that the optional tests should be given "in addition" to the core battery rather than explicitly allowing the examiner the flexibility to choose tests that might be more appropriate for a given referral question.

Battery characteristics. The core WMS-III tests generate eight primary "memory indices" (Auditory Immediate, Visual Immediate, Immediate Memory, Auditory Delayed, Visual Delayed, Auditory Recognition Delayed, General Memory, and Working Memory). In the WMS-R, the General Memory Index was computed from performance on the immediate recall portions of different tests. The General Memory Index of the WMS-III, in contrast, is based solely on the delayed recall performances of the core "memory" tests (Logical Memory II, Faces II, Verbal PA II, Family Pictures II). Thus, the two measures are not comparable. Separate Immediate and Delayed "Indexes" now exist for both the Auditory and Visual tests.

Working Memory Index is the new name for what was *Attention/Concentration* in the WMS-R. It is the popular term for active processing of information in the short term, although all the tests in this index do not fully qualify as tests of working memory (see pp. 25, 358–359). *Working Memory* is equally weighted for auditory and visual stimuli. The auditory task is *Letter-Number Sequencing,* also a WAIS-III test (see p. 363). The visual task is *Spatial Span,* which now uses 3-dimensional, rather than 2-dimensional stimuli. Thus, in contrast to the WAIS-III, which also boasts a *Working Memory Index* but is based only upon auditory processing (i.e., Arithmetic, Digit Span, and Letter–Number Sequencing), the WMS-III index includes attention tests in both auditory and visual modalities.

Verbal memory tests and the Auditory Indexes have changed in several ways from previous formats. Not only is a new paragraph again paired with the venerable Anna Thompson (the WMS-R Robert Miller story was considered too likely to evoke an emotional reaction and thus bias recall in some people), but there is also a slight change in the administration of the new story (see p. 445). Upon immediate recall of story two, it is read again following the Babcock procedure (see p. 445), although unlike the Babcock, memory is tested following the second presentation and again after a delay. This has the advantage of minimizing the effects of brief attentional lapses during stimulus presentation. This leads to improved learning, with the ultimate goal of examining retention over a 30-minute delay. A thematic scoring option has also been added for both stories. Recognition is tested in a two-choice format after delayed free recall for the stories.

Verbal Paired Associates contains only words that are not readily associated (i.e., so-called "hard" items from previous versions of the test, see pp. 440–441). Although the rationale to no longer include "easy" items may be justifiable from a psychometric perspective, there is also an important downside. For example, patients with significant memory impairment will no longer have the easy items as a "face saving" condition in which they are able to "succeed" on some memory tasks. Similarly, a subject's failure to make these easy associations can no longer be used to alert the clinician to possible poor task motivation by the patient. Although a paired associate recognition trial is given immediately after the delayed free recall, there are no incorrect answers in which the first word is incorrectly paired with the second word of a different word pair or is paired with a new, nonlist word. Thus, patients need only recognize either of the two words since they always appear as the correct target pair, making this an extremely easy task with a very low ceiling that all but the most severely impaired patients perform very well. This recognition format does not provide for a recall trial.

Word Lists is a word learning task patterned after the common format exemplified in the Auditory Verbal Learning Test (pp. 422–424). It contains 12 words that have no semantic association presented over 4 trials, followed by a single trial of a second, interference, list. Then, without further additional presentation, recall of the first list is requested. Two delayed trials follow: free recall, and yes/no recognition in which the examiner reads the 12 words interspersed among 12 foils.

Computation of the main auditory memory indices (immediate and delayed) relies on Logical Memory and Verbal Paired Associates scores. Since Word List learning is an optional test, it does not contribute to the Auditory Index, and further, cannot be formally substituted to calculate the Auditory Memory Index—a puzzling omission.

In addition to the indices, the WMS-III provides for the computation of four "Auditory Process Composites" derived from immediate and delayed performances on Logical Memory and Verbal Paired Associates. *Single-Trial Learning* is the score for recall after the first hearing of the material, *Learning Slope* measures performance improvements over trials, *Retention* is a measure of the ability retain material over the delay interval, and *Retrieval* documents differences between free recall and recognition scores.

Less verbalizible memory tests and the Visual Memory Indexes now include two completely new tests, *Faces* and *Family Pictures,* as the only tests in the core battery. Neither new test requires drawing so that the core memory battery could be given to patients unable to use their dominant hand.

Faces, which has both immediate and delayed components, is a recognition task in which 24 faces are first shown one at a time for approximately 2 seconds each. Immediate and delayed recognition are tested using a yes/no format in which the targets are interspersed with an equal number of foils.

Family Pictures is designed to measure "complex, meaningful, visually presented information" and is considered a "visual analogue to the Logical Memory subtest" (Wechsler, 1997b, p. 15). Four pictures are each shown to the subject for 10 seconds. Memory is tested using free recall for the four persons from a family of seven (i.e., mother, father, grandmother, grandfather, son, daughter, dog), what they were doing in the picture, and their location in a 2 × 2 grid. Immediate and delayed recall are obtained.

It is surprising that the highly verbalizible Family Pictures was included as part of the Visual Memory Index, particularly at the expense of Visual Reproduction. This latter test has been part of the scale since its inception and has an extremely rich research literature, yet was marginalized as an "optional" test. Moreover, as the manual states, "Family Pictures is . . . new not only to the *Wechsler Memory Scale* but also to clinical practice and research" (Wechsler, 1997b, p. 15). Thus, neither formal nor informal experience with this type of measure can help guide performance interpretation, at the level of either the individual test or the summary index, to which Family Pictures contributes.

Visual Reproduction, in contrast, is immediately recognizable to users of previous WMS versions, although it includes two new design cards which extend the range of the test upward and downward. In addition to a delayed recall condition, yes/no recognition is tested. Also, scores for copy and discrimination trials are available. As with Word Lists, performance on the Visual Reproduction cannot be substituted for the core memory tests when calculating the summary score.

The contribution of the new visual memory tests to the Immediate Memory and Delayed Memory scores appears less than that of either Logical Memory or Verbal PA. Either summary score can be adequately predicted using the two verbal tests with either one of the two core visual tests (Faces and Family Pictures) (Axelrod and Woodard, 2000). Given the absence of a strong relationship of the Visual Memory Index to lateralized right hemisphere memory dysfunction, omitting one of the visual tasks appears a reasonable procedure for reducing memory assessment time. For example, Family Pictures can take up to 25% of test administration time needed to calculate the primary memory indices (Axelrod, 2001). Further, both these individual tests and the Visual Memory Indexes, are among the least reliable measures included in the WMS-III (Tulsky, Zhu, and Ledbetter, 1997).

Auditory Recognition Index is based on performance of the recognition portions of Logical Memory and Verbal PA. No Visual Recognition Index is calculated, presumably because Faces II already is a recognition measure and because Family Pictures does not lend itself to a recognition assessment format. Unfortunately, separate recognition score norms are not provided by the test publisher for the verbal memory tests individually since the two test scores combine to form a single recognition score. In addition, the recognition scores suffer from a low ceiling effect in healthy populations. This,

along with relatively spared recognition in all but more severely memory impaired patients, limits the clinical utility of this index for many patient evaluations. Many patients obtain perfect scores on Verbal PA. The recognition portion for Logical Memory appears more difficult yet some Logical Memory recognition items can be correctly answered at a better than chance level even without hearing the story, and others may be answered incorrectly at a better than chance level (Killgore and DellaPietra, 2000a,b). A general indication of Logical Memory recognition performance alone can be obtained by adding 24 points (presuming perfect Verbal PA recognition) to the Logical Memory recognition score and applying the Auditory Recognition norms.

Other optional WMS-III tests are *Information and Orientation, Mental Control,* and *Digit Span*. The first two tests were only slightly modified from the WMS-R. Digit Span contains easier and harder sequences, which makes it identical to the WAIS-III test.

Discrepancy Scores appear in multiple tables in the manual that provide information about how likely are differences between different summary scores at different levels of statistical significance. Some of these are potentially helpful, the difference between the intelligence quotient and memory quotient being of interest for relatively isolated memory disorders such as Korsakoff's syndrome (e.g., N. Butters and Cermak, 1976).

Unfortunately, reliance solely on the information presented in the WAIS-III/WMS-III Technical Manual (The Psychological Corporation, 1997) can lead to erroneous conclusions since the manual does not provide tables stratified for general level of intellectual function. A higher General Memory Index score is common in the standardization sample for subjects with lower general mental ability scores, while subjects with higher mental ability levels are likely to have lower relative memory indices (Hawkins and Tulsky, 2001). This demonstrates the relative independence of functions measured by the WIS-A and memory abilities, an independence related at least in part to the differences in how many of the cognitive functions measured by WIS-A are normally distributed differently than most memory abilities.

Statistical properties. For the most part, summary score reliability coefficients are good. Excluding Auditory Recognition Delay (.74), reliability coefficients range from .82 to .93. Individual test reliabilities are somewhat lower, with the lowest reliabilities associated with Faces I and II (both .74). The only test with very high reliability is Verbal Paired Associates I (.93).

Neuropsychological findings. Despite the many improvements over its predecessors, a variety of criterion validity studies have offered only limited support. In one multicenter study, both immediate and delayed Auditory-Visual Memory score discrepancies were related to seizure onset laterality, with a stronger effect present in comparisons of the Delayed Memory Indexes (Wilde et al., 2001). Interestingly, the expected pattern appeared in both left and right temporal lobe groups, with lower Auditory Memory scores occurring in left temporal lobectomy candidates and lower Visual Memory scores present in right temporal lobectomy candidates. Unfortunately, the index discrepancies were not sufficiently robust for individual patient application.

Not surprisingly, several WMS-III measures appear more sensitive to the effects of mild TBI than WAIS-III summary measures (Immediate and Delayed Auditory Indexes, Immediate Memory, Visual Delayed Index, and General Memory) (D.C. Fisher, et al., 2000). Although even greater memory impairment was associated with moderate to severe TBI for most WMS-III measures, no group effect was present for the Auditory Recognition Delayed Index, calling into question the clinical usefulness of this scale. It should be noted that this index has the lowest reliability coefficient (.74) of any WMS-III summary measures.

The Camden Memory Tests (Warrington, 1996a)

Five tests of different aspects of memory and learning are included in this battery. All are first shown at a one per 3 sec rate with the recognition trial following immediately. All tests had the expected age gradients. The tests can be purchased individually (the manual comes with each) or as a battery with some savings.

(1) The *Pictorial Memory Test* (CPRMT) consists of 30 color photos of a wide variety of distinctive subjects (e.g., a pig, a pile of books, two women taking tea outside flower-decorated pub windows). The recognition trial presents 30 pages each containing three photos, one target, and two foils (e.g., telphone booth, outdoor market are foils for the pig). This test was made to be very easy (none of 104 subjects in the normative pool under age 40 failed more than two items, 77% had a perfect score) to identify both patients too impaired to proceed to the other tests and subjects performing below their capacity. In evaluting failed performances, it must be noted that 12.8% and 25% of patients with left- and right-lateralized lesions, respectively, had "significant deficit" scores.

(2) The *Topographic Recognition Memory Test* (CTRMT) substitutes for Face Recognition by presenting 30 more colored photos, detailed pictures of a variety of places (e.g., three cars [red, blue, white] in a gas station; two elderly people buying produce in a market from a young woman). Unlike the CPRMT, the two foils that go with each picture on the recognition trial are quite similar to the target (e.g., gas station at two different angles: one with only the red car, one with the red and a bit of the blue one). That these photos are more or less verbalizable becomes apparent in the larger disparity in "significant deficit" scores between left (10%) and right (29.1%) lesioned patients.

(3) The word pairs in the three 8-item sets of the *Paired Associate Learning Test* (CPALT) are supposed to be moderately related, but associations may be too easy for many subjects (e.g., water–bath, window–curtain). The subject is asked to read aloud the word pairs which are in large print. Immediate recall after each pair exposure is the initial format; in the second format, all eight pairs are shown before association to the initial word is requested. With 3 points given for each correct trial, trial 2 clearly distinguishes the laterally lesioned groups (left $M = 17.1 \pm 8.4$; right $M = 22.3 \pm 2.5$; $p < .002$).

(4 & 5) Included in this battery are two briefer forms of the Warrington Recognition Memory Test (WRMT, pp. 495–497): *Short Recognition Memory Test for Words* (CSRMT-W) and *Short Recognition Memory Test for Faces* (CSRMT-F). These tests have 25 items each and the same administration format as the longer form. For patients with diffuse brain damage, a greater proportion of mildly impaired patients were recognized as having a deficit (% *Deficit Score*) on Faces by the WRMT (67% vs. 40%), more of the severely impaired patients scored as impaired on the long form for Words (70% vs. 61%). Both tests showed greater sensitivity for moderately impaired patients. Normal subjects under 40 rarely missed more than two words (1.9%), but 13% made 5 or more errors on Faces.

Randt Memory Test (Randt and Brown, 1986)

This set of tests was "specifically designed for . . . longitudinal studies" of patients with mild to moderate impairment of storage and retrieval functions. Randt and his coworkers anticipated that this instrument may be useful in investigating drug effects, particularly memory-enhancing drugs (Davies et al., 1990; Parnetti et al., 1996; Salvioli and Neri, 1994), although it has also been successfully used to examine cognitive side effects of different anxiolytics (Barbee et al., 1991) as well as to characterize the memory effects of ECT (Ng et al., 2000; Zervas and Jandorf, 1993).

Although this easy to administer test contains seven subtests (referred to as "modules"), it is brief, taking approximately 20 min. It has a set order of presentation in which acquisition and retrieval from storage are differentiated by separating immediate recall and recall following fixed tasks (a subsequent subtest serves as the distractor task for each one of the four subtests that have delayed-recall trials). An interesting feature is the use of telephone interviews to obtain 24-hour recall data.

This memory test has five different forms for repeated examinations. The first and last modules (General Information and Incidental Learning) are identical in all forms. For patients with at least some ability to recall new experiences, Incidental Learning, which asks for recall of the names of the subtests, cannot remain a test of "incidental learning" for more than one or two repeated administrations. Each form of the other five modules has been equated based on such relevant characteristics as word length, frequency, and imagery levels. Thus, each form appears to be quite similar. The middle five modules test recall of five words using the selective reminding technique, of digits forward and backward, of word pairs, and of a paragraph, and also include a module testing recognition and name recall of 7 out of 15 line drawings of common objects. Scores between subtests are not comparable. In addition to subtest acquisition scores and the two recognition (following interference within the testing session, 24 hours later) scores for the Five Items, Paired Words, Short Story, and Picture Recognition subtests, summation scores for Total Acquisition and Total score plus a Memory Index (or Memory Quotient, which is an overall summation score) are calculated. Conversion to standard scores allows the examiner to make subtest comparisons and draw a memory profile.

Battery characteristics. Reliability studies have been done with community and medical inpatient volunteers. Fioravanti and coworkers (1985) had their subjects take all five forms in the same testing session; Randt and Brown (1986) gave two tests 10 to 14 days apart, and Franzen, Tishelman, et al. (1989) gave the test to college students. Of the subtests, Five Items had the lowest between-forms reliability coefficient (.55 for Acquisition: Fioravanti et al., 1985) and Digit Span the highest at .90 (Randt and Brown, 1986) with most coefficients above .70. Both of these studies reported correlations of .82 and above for the three summary scores. However, test-retest correlations for the summary scores between forms A and B after one- and two-week intervals ranged from .32 to .64, but the mean level of scores on these forms was essentially equivalent (Franzen, Tishelman, et al., 1989). Significant practice effects showed up for Incidental Learning, acquisition of Paired-Words and Short Story, and recall of Five Items, Paired-Words, and Short Story (see also McCaffrey, Duff, and Westervelt, 2000b).

Excepting General Information, at least one trial of each subtest module has demonstrated sensitivity to the effects of aging (D.P. Osborne et al., 1982) or to the memory impairments of a group of patients with memory complaints of one or more years' duration. However, this highly verbal test cannot qualify for general use in neuropsychological assessment since it necessarily penalizes patients with language disorders and would probably be relatively insensitive to memory impairments involving nonverbal (e.g., configural, spatial) material. Moreover, Erickson and Howieson (1986) note that some of the subtests are so easy that ceiling effects can be expected, particularly with younger subjects who may have memory problems. Thus, its usefulness in evaluating memory dysfunction appears to be limited to conditions associated with aging and diffuse brain diseases.

Memory Assessment Scales (MAS) (J.M. Williams, 1991)

This set of memory tests was developed to be a "comprehensive, well-designed, standardized memory assessment battery" that would fulfill the most usual clinical assessment needs in a manner suitable for various kinds of clinical situations and demands. It was originally called the *Vermont Memory Scale (VMS)* (Little et al., 1986). It addresses three kinds of memory functions: attentional functions and short-term memory; learning and immediate (as distinguished from short-term) memory; and memory following a delay. These functions are examined in both verbal and (purportedly) nonverbal modalities; and one test involves the integration of verbal (names) and nonverbal (faces) material.

Two tests contribute to *Short-term Memory,* the summary score for attentional functions. *Verbal Span* is composed of Numbers Forward, which is the longest span in a two- to nine-digit series with two trials for each length; and Numbers Backward, which presents span lengths from two to nine and scores in like manner. In Visual Span the subject sees a card on which is printed a randomized array of stars. The examiner touches the stars following a predetermined pattern that the subject must copy. The test begins with two stars and continues until both trials of the same length are failed or the subject recalls the longest sequence of nine.

Verbal learning is examined by two tests that have immediate and delayed recall trials but the summary score, *Verbal Memory,* is based only on the immediate recall trials. *List Learning* consists of 12 words equally divided among four categories (countries, colors, birds, and cities), which are read to the subject in six learning trials or until 12 words are recalled in a single trial. This test generates six learning or recall scores: *List Acquisition* is the total number recalled including a score of 12 for each trial that did not have to be given; *List Recall*, which is a free recall following interference (the immediate trial of Prose Recall); *Cued* (by categories) *List Recall*, which follows the free List Recall trial; a *Delayed List Recall*, also followed by a Cued List Recall; and finally a *List Recognition* trial, in which each item is paired with a similar foil. Intrusions and clustering in the two free recall trials are also scored. Prose Memory presents a 60-word story about a robbery for immediate free recall followed by nine questions asking for specific details. Only responses to the questions receive scores. Free recall and the same nine questions constitute the delayed recall trial.

The *Visual Memory* summary score is based on two tests with only the immediate trials contributing to it: Immediate Visual Recognition presents more or less simple geometric designs for 5 sec followed by a 15-sec visual distraction task, after which the subject must identify a newly presented design as same or different, or pick which of five designs is the one seen in the learning trial. In Delayed Visual Recognition, the subject must try to identify the original ten target figures from an array of 20. Visual Reproduction has two trials in each of which the subject sees a design for 10 sec that must be drawn after a 15 sec interference by a visual distraction task. The MAS does not include a separate summary scale for delayed memory, so the user measures retention on an individual test basis.

In *Names and Faces,* the subject sees a set of ten named faces for two learning trials, each followed by a recall trial. A delayed trial is given about 15 minutes later. Although this latter trial is labeled a "recall" trial, it is actually a multiple-choice name recognition test.

The data sheet provides a test profile for all immediate and delayed test scores and two other sets of scores: Evaluated as Verbal Process Scores are Intrusions, Clustering, Cued List Recall, and List Recognition scores. In addition to the three summary scores for different aspects of memory, a *Global Memory Scale* score can be calculated by adding together the Verbal and Visual Memory summary scores.

Raw scores can be converted into scaled scores on a 19-point scale in which 10 is the mean and 3 the standard deviation. The normative sample was divided into six age groups from 18–29 to 70+. The fewest subjects (71) are in the 30–39 age group; the 60–69 age group has the most (190). Means and standard deviations for each test score, including intrusions and clustering scores, are given for the six age groups and for four age groups (18–49 to 70+) by education (<11, 12, ≥13). Scoring examples are provided.

Battery characteristics. Reliability (generalizability) coefficients for subtests and summary scales averaged

from .85 to .91 based on a sample of 20 subjects ages 20 to 89. Test–retest reliabilities of .62 to .88 have been reported for the subscales (Little et al., 1986). Interrater coefficients for the drawings were in the .95–.97 range. Detailed factor analytic studies generated two factors for the normal sample: one was associated with a Verbal Comprehension and Perceptual Organization factor of the WAIS-R; the other was an Attention/Concentration factor. When using test performances by neurologically impaired patients, three factors emerged: one associated with nonverbal memory and reasoning, the second a short-term memory and concentration factor, and the third a verbal memory factor.

Neuropsychological findings. Patients with lateralized lesions differed in the expected directions on the Verbal Memory and Visual Memory summary scores. TBI patients had their least difficulty on the Short-term Memory component. Dementia patients scored below all other groups on all subtests except Visual Memory, on which patients with right-sided lesions had a slightly lower average score. However, all patient groups performed significantly *below normal* expectations. A study of how depression affects memory functions in middle-aged and older subjects found that on only the acquisition and free recall trials of List Learning did the depressed group make scores significantly lower than the nondepressed subjects (J.M. Williams et al., 1987). The Prose Memory scores, based on responses to questions, did not differentiate these groups, although the content-based Logical Memory scores did.

This is a carefully developed battery with a number of interesting features, such as the Verbal Process scoring for list learning, the visual interference trial format, and the Name–Face learning test, which may have considerable practical significance. It loses something in not scoring story recall per se, nor delayed design recall. Another problem is that the designs appear to be verbalizable despite the manual's references to them as "nonverbal" tests. It also appears that the standard score conversion system may put at least some of these memory measures into a kind of Procrustean bed in which scores are pulled, pushed, or otherwise manipulated (e.g., pooling scores that measure somewhat different functions) to fit a parametric conception of memory that is not in accord with the way in which many memory functions distribute in normal populations.

Compared to the WMS-R, a sample of mixed neurologic patients tended to obtain lower scores on the Verbal, Visual, and General Memory measures of the MAS (4 to 5 points) (Golden, White, et al., 1999). However, comparisons between comparable scales from the two tests elicited considerable variability and correlations between the scales were modest (Verbal

Memory $r = .57$, Visual Memory $r = .54$, General Memory $r = .52$). Almost two-thirds of the patients had higher WMS-R than MAS scores. Lower MAS scores were also reported in an independent study, although the low correlations between comparable MAS and WMS-R scales led to the suggestion that the tests are measuring different constructs and are not comparable (Hilsabeck et al., 1996). Again, lower scores were associated with the MAS compared to the WMS-R scales that purportedly measure similar constructs.

The utility of the material-specific memory indices is not clear. In one sample of patients who were evaluated prior to temporal lobectomy, no differences were observed between left seizure onset and right seizure onset patients for the Global Memory or Verbal Memory indices, although there was a mild group effect for Visual Memory ($p < .04$) (Loring, Hermann, Lee, et al., 2000). Although a Verbal–Visual Memory difference index is not part of the scale, this measure separated the groups at a high level of significance ($p < .004$). When applied on an individual basis, though, over one-third of the patients (19/54) had a 14-point discrepancy or greater between indices in the unexpected direction, which is the level the manual suggests were classified incorrectly. Using a simple difference score evaluation, these scores would have incorrectly predicted lesion laterality in a mixed neurologic sample in 22/51 patients.

Denman Neuropsychology Memory Scale (Denman, 1984, 1987)

Denman's goal in developing this test battery has been to create "a useful set of measures of selected memory functions (for) clinical settings" (personal communication, December, 1985 [mdl]). The battery includes eight tests, of which four are classified as "Verbal" and four as "Non-Verbal." Only one form of this test is available.

In the Verbal section, *Story Recall* is based on a single 42-item story, of which the gist is similar to the WMS Anna Thompson stories with several identical words and phrases. It was made almost twice as long as most other stories in general use to avoid a ceiling effect, which Denman had found with shorter stories, and the paragraph has been used as a verbal memory measure (J.L. Ross et al., 2000). *Paired Associate Learning* contains 14 word pairs, of which five are conceptually related (easy) and the rest are unrelated (hard). However, no use is made of the easy–hard pair difference. The longer than usual word pair list also reflects Denman's concerns about ceiling effects. *Remote Verbal Information* contains 30 questions about popular culture, newsworthy events and persons, and general knowledge. The *Memory for Digits* format and administration are identical to that of the Wechsler Adult Intelligence Scale-Revised in that both trials at each length are given until the subject fails both, thus generating confounded data, which is further confounded by summing "forward" and "backward" scores to get the score for this test. Both Story Recall and Paired Associate Learning have delayed recall trials for a total of six scores contributing additively to a "Verbal Memory Score."

Four tests come under the "Non-Verbal Memory" heading. In *Figure Recall*, the Rey-Osterrieth complex figure is administered in the usual manner with a copy trial and two recall trials—immediate and delayed. The 24 three-point scoring categories make scoring a rather unwieldy process and generates scores that cannot be compared with most of the complex figure data in the literature. *Musical Tones and Melodies* is a tonal matching task with a format like that of the Seashore Rhythm Test. *Memory for Human Faces* contains one card with 16 facial photos printed in a 4×4 array, which is shown to the subject for just 45 sec. Following a 90-sec distractor task, another card is presented with 48 photos on it, including the original 16 to be identified. Denman explained the relatively large number of target faces as due to the need to avoid a ceiling effect; and the larger number of foils was chosen to avoid the "chance factor" that can result from having only 16 or even 32 foils. The fourth "Non-verbal" test poses 30 questions about visual details of familiar objects, signs, symbols, and sights, such as the poison symbol. The two complex figure trials bring the number of "Non-Verbal Memory" scores to 5.

Raw scores are converted to scaled scores with a range of 1 to 19 by means of age-graded conversion tables. The 1984 standardization was based on 250 subjects with as few as 20 people in the 60–69 age range and only one age group containing more than 40 people (48 at ages 30–39). The appropriateness of these scaled scores comes into question as six out of the seven age ranges (from 10–14 to 60–69) mostly have less than twice as many subjects as scores. By almost doubling the population for the 1987 restandardization to 462, four of the age groups now contain more than two-and-one-half as many subjects as scores; but increasing the number of age groups to 11 (from 10–12 to 80–89) stretches these subject samples to an unacceptably thin extent as four of them still have fewer than 38 subjects to provide norms for a 19-point scale. Since it is not possible to derive parametric data on this refined a scale from such small numbers, one can only suspect that many of the recommended raw score to scaled score conversions are extrapolations from scanty data. Moreover, 65% of subjects over the age of 25 had 13 or more years of education, and more than half of these had completed 16 or more years. Without further information about education effects, these norms must be considered unsuitable for persons with much less schooling. Memory quotients can be derived for the three score totals: Verbal, Non-Verbal, and Full-Scale.

Battery characteristics. In a brochure describing this test, Denman reported internal consistency and interscorer reliability correlations in the .98 to .99 range for the 1984 standardization; .97 for the more recent one. Reliability estimates "derived from commonalities obtained through a factor analysis" were mostly >.87, but three (Digit Span, Musical Tones and Melodies, and Memory for Faces) were unacceptably low (.43, .47, and .25, respectively).

Factor analytic studies have not produced consistent patterns. A factor analysis of the 1984 standardization data found that both the Remote Verbal and Remote Non-Verbal tests load heavily (.81, .78, respectively) on the same factor suggesting that these measures of semantic memory are not clearly differentiable (Larrabee and Curtiss, 1985). For subjects aged 39 and younger, Memory for Digits and Immediate Story Recall loaded together on a second factor, which suggests that they share immediate memory span and attention/concentration components. With the addition of delayed recall scores to the analysis, Tonal Memory tended to be associated with Figure Recall. Paired Associates was most closely associated with Story Recall on immediate trials but the delayed trial of Paired Associates loaded most highly on the same factor as delayed Figure Recall and Tonal Memory, while delayed Story Recall had a factor all to itself. Memory for Human Faces did not load on any factors in this study, leaving questions about what this test may be measuring. A factor analysis that included Memory for Human Faces with some of Wechsler's ability and memory tests found its highest loadings on a general memory factor (J.J. Ryan, Geisser, and Dalton, 1988). For the 1987 standardization, a five-factor solution is reported (Denman, 1987) with both trials of Paired Associates loading on one factor, both trials of Figure Recall on a second, both trials of Story Recall on a third, and two remote recall tests load at somewhat lower levels than the other tests on a fourth; Musical Tones and Melodies, Digit Span, and delayed Face Recall (at a much lower level than its factor-mates) were associated on the fifth factor.

Rivermead Behavioural Memory Test (RBMT, RBMT-11) (B.A. Wilson, Cockburn, and Baddeley, 1985, 2003)

This test was developed to provide measures that could be directly related to the practical effects of impaired memory and for monitoring change with treatment for memory disorders. It was also designed to have face validity so that nonpsychologists could readily understand its findings.

In keeping with its title as a "behavioural" memory test, the RBMT includes mostly practically relevant tasks such as *Remembering a name* associated with a photograph; *Remembering a hidden belonging,* in which the examiner hides from sight some object belonging to the patient (e.g., a comb, a key) while the patient looks on, instructing the patient to remember where it is hidden and to ask for it when the examiner gives a specific cue (such as "We have now finished this test"); *Remembering an appointment* and asking about it on hearing the ring of a timer set for 20 minutes; *Remembering a newspaper article* (story recall) both upon hearing it read and 20 minutes later; *Face recognition* in which five photos seen a few minutes earlier must be identified out of a group of ten; *Remembering a new route,* both immediately and after a 10-minute delay, that the examiner traces between fixed points in the examination room; *Delivering a message* during the route-recall task according to instructions given prior to setting out on the route; *Orientation* for time and place; and knowing the *Date,* which is treated separately from the Orientation questions—as in the pilot study, its correlation with Orientation was low. Only *Picture recognition*—in which ten pictures are shown the subject who, a little later, is asked to identify them when they are mixed in with ten foils—does not directly reflect an everyday activity, although it does measure visual recognition at an easy level.

The test comes in four parallel forms that differ for every subtest except Orientation and Date (e.g., recommended places to hide the object for each form A to D are A—in a desk drawer, B—in a cupboard, C—in a filing cabinet, D—in a briefcase or bag). The original stories have a British character; four similar stories are available for American subjects.

Subtest means for raw scores and their standard deviations are provided for persons in the adult age range (16–69) (B. [A.] Wilson, Cockburn, Baddeley, and Hiorns, 1989). Each test may also be scored on a 2- (0, 1) or 3-point scale (0 to 2) based on the score distribution of the standardization sample. Scores of 2 indicate *normal* functioning; *borderline* performances are scored 1; and 0, of course, measures performances that with few exceptions were at levels at or below the lowest 5% of the standardization population. A *Total Memory Score* is the sum of the test scores that make up a test profile. In addition, screening scores for each test except Delivering a Message are given according to pass/fail criteria for normal functioning in that area: these scores can be combined into a Total Screening Score.

The revision (RBMT-II) preserves essentially the same format as its predecessor. Two sets of adult norms are available, for ages 16–64 and 65–96. The authors state that this revision can also be used with children in the 11–15 age range. The tests themselves differ from the original in that the five faces for "Face recognition" include persons from other than European stock; and instructions for "Remembering a new route" have been clarified to facilitate scoring. Picture stimuli are now presented in booklets rather than on separate cards. This version does not seem to be so different from the original that data gained from one set cannot be compared with data acquired with the other.

Test characteristics. Neither age nor sex differences contributed to the scores for the standardization group (B. (A.) Wilson, Cockburn, Baddeley, and Hiorns, 1989). About 10% of the variance appeared to be associated with mental ability (as measured by either Raven's Matrices or the National Adult Reading Test).

Additional norms for subjects in the 70–94 age range have been developed (Cockburn and Smith, 1989). Although performances within this 25-year range were not separate by age grouping, the older group's mean scores were lower than those of the 16–69-year-old standardization group, and correlation of the Total Profile Score with age was −.44 for the elderly subjects. The total age range for the RBMT-II is 16–96; the authors indicate that this format can be used with children as young as 11. Age affected story recall most profoundly but did not contribute to scores for remembering the first name, picture memory, face memory, route recall, and orientation. Education contributed a little to story recall for the older age group.

Interscorer agreement was reported to be 100% (B.[A.] Wilson, Cockburn, Baddeley, and Hiorns, 1989). Parallel form reliability was measured by correlating performances on B, C, or D with A. For the Screening Score, B and C correlations were .84 and .80, but D correlated at .67. However, Profile Score correlations were in the .83 to .88 range, suggesting that this score may be a more sensitive measure of memory abilities. A slight practice effect appeared, essentially due to improved scores on Remembering a Hidden Belonging.

Both the Profile and the Screening Score Totals correlated highly (−.75 and −.71, respectively) with recorded memory errors of brain injured patients (B.[A.] Wilson, Cockburn, Baddeley, and Hiorns, 1989). Both score totals also correlated significantly with these patients' performances on a variety of memory and learning tests. This finding is similar to that of Malec, Zweber, and DePompolo (1990), who reported that the RBMT scores of a group of brain-injured patients correlated in the .39 to .68 range with other memory tests, but in a lower range (.09 to .47) for nonmemory tests. RBMT scores correlated −.47 with the Activities and Social Behavior Scale of the Portland Adaptability Inventory (Lezak and O'Brien, 1988, 1990).

Neuropsychological findings. The memory problems of moderately to severely injured TBI patients are brought out by this test. Geffen, Encel, and Forrester (1991) found that length of coma was significantly associated with lower RBMT scores. Compared with control subjects under age 50 who passed all of the RBMT items, TBI patients passed on average only 47% of the items (Baddeley, Harris, et al., 1987). When compared with stroke patients, TBI patients tend to do more poorly on remembering names, the appointment, pictures, and the story on both immediate and delayed trials, and are not as well oriented; on no items did the stroke patients' average scores fall below those of the trauma patients (B.[A.] Wilson, Cockburn, Baddeley, and Hiorns, 1989). Perceptual impairment contributed significantly to failures on "Orientation" and "Date," both "Remembering a new route" trials, and "Face recognition" (Cockburn, Wilson, et al., 1990b), but language impairment (dysphasia) affects performances only on the language-loaded tasks of recalling a name, orientation for time and place, and story recall (Cockburn, Wilson, et al., 1990a). However, when comparing stroke patients with lateralized brain injury, only the relatively lower scores on name recall and delayed story recall distinguished those whose damage was on the left. The three subtests given dementia patients—"Remembering a newspaper article" (immediate and delayed recall), "Remembering a new route" (immediate and delayed recall), and "Remembering a name"—were very sensitive to gradations of dementia, including distinguishing "minimal dementia" from a "low-scoring normal" group (Beardsall and Huppert, 1991). Of these, name recall was one of the two most discriminating tasks (recalling six photos of familiar objects was the other). "Remembering a hidden belonging," in itself, is useful in identifying patients with impaired prospective memory; invariably, persons who fail this test have sustained frontal lobe damage [mdl].

This is essentially an atheoretic test; its development was shaped by clinical experience with memory impaired patients. It does have practical value, but with only a two or three point scoring range, it lacks sensitivity at both the high and low ends of memory functioning (Leng and Parkin, 1990). Most outpatients with memory complaints—patients with mild TBI or still employed and recently retired multiple sclerosis patients—perform at perfect or near-perfect levels making this test useless for identifying subtle or small memory deficits. However, for patients with middle-range memory disorders—too severe to be fully independent but not so severe as to require custodial care—this test can be discriminating. Moreover, although it does not provide for small gradations of severe impairment, failure on most of the tests in this battery is unequivocal evidence of a socially crippling memory disorder. Thus, the RBMT has been a useful instrument in the characterization of memory impairment in disorders ranging from basal forebrain amnesia (Goldenberg, Schuri, et. al., 1999), Parkinson's disease (Benke, Hohenstein, et al., 2000), cardiac failure (N.R. Grubb et al., 2000), TBI (B. Levine, Black, et al., 2001), MS (Cutajar et al., 2000), normal aging (Ostrosky-Solis, Jaime, and Ardila, 1998), liver failure (Jalan et al., 1995), methylenedioxy-*n*-methylamphetamine (MDMA, "ecstasy") (Morgan, 1999), stroke (Sunderland, Stewart, and Sluman, 1996), Alzheimer's disease and dementia (Glass, 1998; Huppert and Beardsall, 1993; Kotler-Cope and Camp, 1995) to limbic encephalitis (T.H. Bak et al., 2001).

The Rivermead Behavioural Memory Test (RBMT-E)
(B.A. Wilson, Baddeley, Cockburn, and Tate, 1998)

The test has been modified for patients with more subtle memory problems. The RBMT-E is sensitive to memory disorders in patients who score in the "normal" range on the RBMT (de Wall, Wilson, and Baddeley, 1994; Wills et al., 2000). The RBMT-E increases the level of difficulty by doubling the amount of material to be remembered and by combining material from Forms A and B, and Forms C and D of the original test to produce two parallel versions of the new extended test which avoids the ceiling and floor effects associated with the original scale. Raw scores are converted to 5-point "profile" scores differentially: some differ by age levels, some differ by mental ability levels, and some are converted without regard to these variables. The five profile score classifications go from 0-Impaired to 4-Exceptionally good memory; a profile score of 2 indicates "average" performance. The authors note that because tasks are similar to real-life activities, this battery has not only ecological validity but face validity which may make it more acceptable to some subjects.

Learning and Memory Battery (LAMB)
(Tombaugh and Schmidt, 1992)

In this effort to develop a memory battery "within an information processing framework," seven tests are offered: *Paragraph* lists 31 items about a person (e.g., age, color of house, activities), which is read twice with free and cued recall trials following each reading. Delayed recall trials on this and the next two word-learning tests take place after 20 minutes and include both free and cued recall and multiple-choice recognition. *Word List* contains 15 words, each from a different category. Administration follows the selective reminding procedure, with the difference that following each free recall trial a cued trial is given for missed words. This continues for five acquisition trials or until the subject recalls all words in two consecutive trials. *Word Pairs* consists of three easy (antonyms) and 11 difficult (unrelated) word pairs given in four acquisition trials using the selective reminding procedure. Nothing is made of easy–difficult differences. *Digit Span* scores are the longest number of digits recorded in the forward and backward series. *Supraspan* is a 12-trial task testing learning of a span two digits longer than Digit Span forward. *Simple Figures* presents four simple geometric (and readily verbalizable) figures for 15 sec in three acquisition trials with a 20 min delayed recall trial, which is followed by a copy trial. The authors included this apparently quite easy task to assess persons unable to learn the *Complex Figure*. This complex figure format uses the Taylor figure, gives four acquisition trials exposing the figure for 30 seconds each time, and like Simple Figures, gives the copy trial after the delay trial. In keeping almost perfectly with cognitive science principles, the only summed score is for the two digit span tests, but that comes after the individual span scores, each with its own set of norms. Only a single form of the test is available.

Each subtest yields three scores. The *initial trial* score is a measure of attention; *total trial* measures acquisition; *retention* measures consolidation. Unlike other batteries, composite scores are not generated, which encourages the examiner to choose those memory tests thought to be the most appropriate for clinical evaluation. A "brief LAMB" has been suggested, consisting of the Paragraph, Word List, and Complex Figure subtests for higher-functioning individuals and Paragraph, Word List, and Simple Figure subtests for individuals who are more impaired.

Battery characteristics. Norms for raw scores are derived from a sample of 480 subjects and given in eight age groupings from 20–29 to 75–79 (Tombaugh and Schmidt, 1992). Trial-by-trial norms for just the three verbal tests, Paragraph (also called *Passage* in this report), Word List, and Word Pairs, are given for the six decades between ages 20 and 79, for a slightly smaller subject sample (J.P. Schmidt, et al., 1992). The expected age effects appear for the different tests. Digit Span, for example, shows a nice differential between the slight decline of Digits forward and the steeper Digits backward slide. Sex contributions, while significant for a number of the many scores, were of little or no practical consequence, producing at most a correlation of .18 on Word Pairs. Education's highest correlations were .37 with Paragraphs and .29 with Word Pairs (J.P. Schmidt et al., 1992). WAIS-R Vocabulary scores also correlated significantly with Paragraphs but at the much lower— almost negligible—level of .18, which was also its highest correlation. Block Design scores correlated at .36 and .37 with the two figure learning tasks. A factor analysis resulted in a three-factor solution: verbal memory, visual memory, and general intelligence.

This battery represents an ambitious undertaking and a lot of work. The most interesting and clinically valuable contribution of this battery may be the acquisition format developed for the two visual learning tests. Because norms are available for every trial for every test, these—or any other of this battery's tests—can be used apart from the battery. The relatively long lists of items in the three list-learning tasks may well provide for finer gradations of deficits than tests with fewer items, and their thoughtfully selected foils for the multiple-choice recognition trials is a potentially useful addition.

Unfortunately, neither the apparent attempt to be appropriately inclusive nor the conceptual structure claimed for it may compensate for its flaws as a clinical instrument. The administration is organized so that all word-based tests succeed one another; the two number-based tests are cheek by jowl, as are the two drawing tests. Such close proximity is very useful when the examiner wants to draw out suspected tendencies to perseveration, proactive inhibition, or inability to keep recently received stimuli sorted out, but it can confound interpretations when the goal is simply to document memory and learning. Of course, this administrative procedure may also be unnecessarily stressful for both memory-impaired and language-impaired patients, who will experience a string of defeats unrelieved by any chance of success.

When given as a whole, many of the battery's findings will very likely be redundant: it is difficult to imagine that in the individual case, whether memory impaired or memory intact, much distinguishing data will emerge from the Paragraph, Word List, or Word Pair tests; each is a form of cued list learning (see Erickson and Howieson [1986] for lists in "story" form). For example, correlations between these three tests run in the .56 to .66 range (J.P. Schmidt et al., 1992). The cued trials before both the second and the delayed recall trials of these tests can serve a rehearsal function and certainly focus more attention on the stimulus material than do most other memory test formats, making it difficult to compare learning on the LAMB word list tests with data coming from more commonly used formats. Additionally, the selective reminding procedure further confounds the data such that after the initial free recall trial it will be impossible to know what or how much cueing and/or stimulus repetition contributes to performances. The lack of a story recall test to assess the role of meaning in learning and retention reduces this battery's usefulness for evaluating rehabilitation potential or contributing to rehabilitation planning. Although the cueing trials may be informative on this score, with each word on Word List coming from a different category, this test will not provide information about subjects' spontaneous use of categories for organizing their learning.

There is no doubt that the tests in this battery will examine memory efficiently and will distinguish memory problems as well as those in most other batteries. However, many clinically relevant questions about memory and learning can probably be answered with fewer tests more appropriately administered.

PAIRED MEMORY TESTS

Each test set in this category consists of two tests, one verbal and one presumably nonverbalizable, with the stated or implied purpose of examining material-specific memory disorders. Two test sets—E.W. Russell's (1988) and Warrington's (1984)—have been evaluated for their efficacy as verbal–nonverbal test sets and found wanting in some respects. Hubley and Tombaugh's (2002) test is too new for systematic evaluation.

Russell's Version of the Wechsler Memory Scale (RWMS) (E.W. Russell, 1988)

Dissatisfaction with the many weaknesses of the Wechsler Memory Scale prompted Russell to devise a memory testing procedure using *Logical Memory* (LM) and *Visual Reproduction* (VR), the two tests that he identified as measures of immediate recall which together provide a balanced assessment of verbal (Russell calls it "semantic") and configural (i.e., "figural") memory. Administration of each test follows the same procedures: Each test is first given as originally directed by Wechsler and then in a second recall trial one-half hour later, during time which the subject takes "quite different" tests. This method produces two sets of three scores for each test. One is the *short-term memory* score used in the original WMS; a second, calculated by the same criteria as the first, is the *long-term memory* score for the delayed recall trial; the third score is a computation of *Percent Retained*, that is,

$$\left(\frac{\text{Delayed Recall}}{\text{Immediate Recall}} \right) \times 100.$$

On the delay trials, the examiner is instructed to prompt the subject who denies any recall for either the stories or the designs. For stories, Russell suggests questions such as, "Do you remember a story about a washerwoman?" He also suggests verbal cueing for the "figural" subtest—e.g., "Do you remember a design that looks like flags?"

Test set characteristics. Despite the well-documented decline of Logical Memory and Visual Reproduction scores with aging, Percent Retained scores are unaffected as both immediate and delayed recall tend to decline at the same rate (Haaland, Linn, et al., 1983). Education and mental ability, too, do not contribute to the Percent Retained score (Ivnik, Smith, Tangalos, et al., 1991). Reliability (measured by correlating the scores for the two LM stories and by correlating scores on two pairs of the four designs) was .83 or higher for all scores except "figural percent retained" (E.W. Russell, 1975). When examining reliability between both WMS forms, Percent Retained correlation coefficients were very low (.40 for LM, .42 for Visual Reproduction) (McCarty, Logue, et al., 1980). As is typical for memory tests, significant practice effects appeared over the course of four administrations of the two tests in this set when given at one week to three month intervals (McCaffrey, Ortega, and Haase, 1993). These effects were cumulative for LM but occurred predominantly on the first retest of Visual Reproduction and the gain was then maintained in the subsequent two examinations. A set of "scale scores," which range from 0 for best performance to 5 for most defective, was developed so that scores from the semantic and figural tests could be compared (E.W. Russell, 1975). Impairment ratings generated by these scaled scores yield unacceptably high proportions of false positive classifications (Crosson, Hughes, et al., 1984), a problem that was addressed with a new set of Scale Scores (E.W. Russell, 1988). This renormed version of the RWMS provides corrections to be added or subtracted to all raw scores for six age groups (20–39 to 80+) and three education levels (<12, 12, and >12).

Neuropsychological findings. Comparisons between semantic/verbal and figural scores distinguished between left and right lateralized lesions (E.W. Russell, 1975). Percent Retained also proved effective in discriminating between a group of dementia patients and normal aging (55- to 85 years) control subjects matched for age, sex, and education (Logue and Wyrick, 1979).

Russell (1975) was quick to identify the critical drawback to using the percent retained method of comparing immediate and delayed recall scores (see p. 478 for a discussion of this problem). For example, subjects who recall only one item on immediate recall get a score of 100% if just one item is recalled later; if they recall no items they receive a 0% score, but their item loss has been just one. This problem showed up in a group of dementia patients, of whom almost half (12 of 25) had immediate semantic recall scores of 2 or less so that, "Small changes in absolute amount of [delayed] recall . . . tended to produce spuriously high Percent Retained scores" (Brinkman, Largen, et al., 1983). Consequently, Percent Retained scores for demented patients had a bimodal distribution with standard deviations consistently larger than means. In short, the Percent Retained score, in itself, can tell nothing about the subject's performance. When reported with the immediate and delayed recall scores it becomes superfluous: the relationship of delayed to immediate recall should be obvious.

Recognition Memory Test (RMT) (Warrington, 1984)

This is actually a set of two tests, parallel in form but providing verbal (words) and relatively nonverbalizable (faces) stimuli for assessing material-specific memory deficits for adults in the 18–70 age range. Both tests contain 50 target memory items followed by a recognition trial pairing the targets with 50 distractors. The recognition format allows memory assessment without the potentially confounding effects associated with poor copying ability. All items in the *Recognition Memory for Words (RMW)* test are one-syllable high frequency words. The target words are printed in letters 1 cm high, each on a different page of the test booklet; for the recognition trial, subjects see a large card with each target word listed and paired to the left or right of a foil. *Recognition Memory for Faces (RMF)* also contains 50 stimulus items and 50 distractors. All faces are male, although clothing below the neck is included in the picture. The recognition trial pairs each target face with a photo of a man of similar age and with similar hairline, again with randomized right–left positions.

For both tests, the order of stimulus presentation for recognition differs from the order on the learning trial. Stimulus items are shown at a one-per-three-second rate. Engagement of subjects' attention is assured by requiring them to indicate whether each target item seems pleasant or unpleasant ("yes" or "no"). The direction of these judgments does not appear to affect recognition scores (Delbecq-Dérouesné and Beauvois, 1989).

Retention is assessed immediately after the learning trial by asking the subject which item of each word or face pair had been seen earlier. Raw scores can be converted to percentile scores for three age groups (18–39, 40–54, 55–70) or to "normalized" scores (i.e., standardized scaled scores with a 3 to 18 score range) for the three age groups. A coarse-grained percentile score conversion (for percentiles 75, 50, 25, 10, and 5) is provided for evaluating differences between RMW and RMF scores (the *discrepancy score*).

Test characteristics. In Warrington's (1984) standardization studies, age contributed significantly to both RMW ($r = -.35$) and RMF ($r = -.13$) scores, but only the RMW correlation is practically meaningful. However, a smaller group of subjects in five age ranges (20–25 to 65–86) displayed a significant score reduction with aging on RMF which became particularly prominent for the oldest group (Delbecq-Dérouesné and Beauvois, 1989). The older persons in this latter study, the finer age gradations, or perhaps both conditions may account for this study's finding of important age differences on RMF when Warrington did not. Among Dutch subjects 69 years and older, neither sex nor education correlated significantly with RMW or RMF (Diesfeldt, 1990). Warrington found that both RMW and RMF correlate positively with WIS Vocabulary (.38, .26, respectively) and Raven's Matrices (.45, .33, respectively), indicating that mental ability levels must be considered in interpreting RMT scores (Leng and Parkin, 1990). On RMW, 47% of normal control subjects in the 18–39 age range made no more than three errors, and 45% in the 40–54 age group made four errors or fewer, reflecting ceiling effects (Leng and Parkin, 1990). RMF scores are less bunched at the top. With combined age group scores, the word–face discrepancy was equally distributed, although inspection of the data suggests that many more of the below 40 group in particular recognized somewhat fewer faces than words (Warrington, 1984). No reliability data are given in the manual, although a Cronbach's *alpha* of .86 for RMW and .77 for RMF was reported in a TBI sample (Malina et al., 1998). RMW and RMF were not highly correlated either for dementia patients (.40) or an age-matched group of control subjects (.29), indicating that each of these tests is measuring something(s) different (Diesfeldt, 1990).

Neuropsychological findings. In a study of the effects of lesion lateralization, patients with right-sided lesions performed in the impaired range only on RMF, as expected, but patients with left-sided brain injury performed poorly on both tests, although better on RMF than those with right-sided damage (Warrington, 1984), a finding that has been replicated with a larger sample (Sweet, Demakis, et al., 2000). Since clothing is present in the face pictures in the WMT, but is typically excluded in other tests of memory for faces that have reported lateralized memory impairment, it has been suggested that some patients may use the additional nonfacial material to help remember particular faces (Kapur, 1987).

Warrington (1984) cautioned that interpretation of RMW or RMF performance biases must take into account the status of patients' verbal and visuoperceptual functions. When used with TBI patients, neither test correlated with Glasgow Coma Scale scores and only RMW had a significant correlation ($-.46$) with PTA (M.P. Kelly, Johnson, and Govern, 1996). For this TBI group, both tests had significant correlations with both immediate and delayed trials of the WMS Logical Memory and Visual Reproduction tests, although all RMW correlations ran higher than those for RMF except for RMF's highest correlation (.47) with Visual Reproduction delayed. By and large, these patients performed more poorly on RMF than on RMW. These data suggest that RMT floor effects limit discriminations at low levels of functioning.

Examination of the sensitivity of the RMT to diffuse damage compared somewhat older patient groups to the oldest normative group and found both tests to be highly discriminating (Warrington, 1984). However, in comparing patients with cerebral atrophy, only RMF distinguished patients with mild ventricular atrophy from those with moderate ventricular atrophy; patients with mild or moderate atrophy of the sulci did not differ significantly on either test. When comparisons were made between demented patients and intact subjects of their own age on a Dutch version of this test, both RMW and RMF again differentiated these groups significantly and the discrepancy scores did not (Diesfeldt, 1990). Moreover, for subjects below age 80, RMW scores were 81% effective and RMF was 100% effective in differentiating the dementia and intact groups; but only 59% of the 80 and older groups were differentiated on RMW scores, with RMF scores differentiating these groups somewhat better (76%). Diesfeldt interpreted the relatively high correlations of RMF scores with Raven's Coloured Progressive Matrices for both demented and control subjects ($r = .45, .48$, respectively) as demonstrating the important role that visuoperceptual discrimination plays in this test.

A one-day delay trial enhanced identification of memory impairment in several small groups of patients with amnesic conditions of different etiologies (Squire and Shimamura, 1986). Although RMW did differentiate between patient groups, this did not occur with RMF because of considerable within-group variability. These authors point out that some Korsakoff patients performed well on one test but not the other, indicating that variables other than lesion laterality may contribute to test score discrepancies.

Warrington's (1984) data suggested that this test pairing may be one of the few to discriminate visual memory deficits associated with right-sided lesions. However, the RMT has not been shown to identify material-specific memory deficits with consistency for patients with left-sided lesions, who tend to do poorly on face recognition as well as on word recognition; nor does it, in itself, provide the means for differentiating memory problems from aphasia or visuoperceptual disorders. That Korsakoff patients too may produce intertest discrepancies only adds to RMT limitations in identifying material-specific memory deficits.

Since the RMT is relatively easy to administer and does not take long, Leng and Parkin (1990) suggested that it may perform its best service as a screening device. They also deemed it suitable for measuring mild memory disorders. However, Mayes and Warburg (1992) considered it a poor choice for screening since it is limited to just two tasks that take a disproportionately long time. It is certainly appropriate for patients with motor disorders. It is possible that the addition of a delayed-recall trial would increase its sensitivity and perhaps its specificity as well. Unfortunately, with data on reliability as yet unavailable, practice effects have not been addressed, an omission that is all the more glaring as there is no alternate RMT form.

Memory Test for Older Adults (MTOA) (Hubley and Tombaugh, 2002)

The MTOA consists of paired memory tests (*Word List, Geometric Figure*) explicitly designed for persons 55 years and older. It comes in two forms, the longer one (MTOA:L) is intended for diagnostic use when the question is whether memory is impaired. The shorter form (MTOA:S) contains less difficult stimuli to be used when memory impairment is no longer in doubt. The materials were designed "so that the average older adult can experience the same level of mastery that younger adults experience on many of today's commonly used memory tests." Both forms of the MTOA contain multiple learning trials for both the Word List and Geometric Figure components.

The short and long forms employ the same overall format. The MTOA:L Word List presents 15 words over five trials. In contrast to most verbal memory tests, category cueing is offered for each word not recalled on each trial. This procedure allows patients greater success, minimizing performance anxiety and frustration. Approximately 10 min after the final trial, memory is tested again for both free and cued recall. Recognition memory testing has the patient circle the 15 correct words interspersed among 30 foils. MTOA:S uses a 10-word list, three learning trials, and recognition with 20 foils.

The visual memory test, Geometric Figures, consists of either a 13-component (26 point) design for MTOA:L or a 9-component (18 point) design for MTOA:S. In each of three learning trials, the Geometric Figure is shown for either 30 sec (MTOA:L) or 15 sec (MTOA:S). The subject draws the figure following each presentation. Approximately 10 min after the final trials, delayed recall is tested, followed by a copy trial. The scoring manual contains many examples of 0-, 1-, and 2-point responses for each scoring component.

Normative data are available for ages 55–84, divided into three age ranges. The normative sample for the MTOA:L is 187 subjects, and 213 for the MTOA:S. Performances are reported in cumulative percentage scores empirically derived from frequency counts in the normative data. Interscorer reliabilities for Geometric Figures, which involves some subjectivity, are in the upper .90s for all recall reproductions.

MEMORY QUESTIONNAIRES

Questionnaires that document patients' self-perceptions can be used to characterize the nature of a patient's memory problems or—when compared with test responses or observers' reports—as measures of the accuracy of the patient's self-perceptions. This latter function can contribute significantly to differentiating the often exaggerated memory complaints of depressives from the often underplayed memory deficits of dementia, and it can help evaluate self-awareness in TBI patients and others who may not appreciate their deficits. Questionnaires may also be used when counseling the families of patients whose lack of appreciation of their memory deficits can create very practical problems for both themselves and their families. Memory questionnaires should not be used as proxies for memory assessment, however, as memory self-reports correlate poorly with objective memory scores (A. Barker et al., 1995; Feher, Larrabee, et al., 1994; Helmstaedter, Hauff, and Elger, 1998; Krupp, Sliwinski, et al., 1994; Lannoo et al., 1998; McGlone, 1994; Vermeulen et al., 1993).

Memory questionnaires differ on a number of dimensions: Their length will vary depending on the degree to which memory problems are detailed and differentiated. Responses may be given simply as "yes" or "no" or on a range of choices on scales of severity and/or frequency of a problem. Questionnaires may be presented under the guise of a general or everyday inventory (e.g., *A General Self-Assessment Questionnaire*, Schachter, 1991) or—in most instances—with "memory" in the title. Many memory questionnaires have been developed and new ones continue to appear. Most of them probably accomplish what their authors hoped for them, but with more or less ease of administration, scoring, interpretation, and reliability. These questionnaires are typically made up with a specific population in mind (older people, TBI patients), but are usually applicable to other person/patient categories as well.

The usefulness of memory questionnaires to predict memory impairment has been called into question. In comparisons of questionnaire responses and interviews of TBI patients and their relatives, responses on the *Everyday Memory Questionnaire (EMQ)* were unrelated to the severity of their injuries while relatives' reports did accord with severity classifications (A. Sunderland, Harris, and Gleave, 1984). Using interviews, retesting both community living elderly subjects and their relatives, and also giving subjects a small battery of both verbal and visual learning and recognition tests to examine the reliability and validity of the 1984 questionnaire, A. Sunderland, Watts, and their collaborators (1986) found that correlations between subjects' questionnaire responses and the reliability measures were moderate at best (highest correlation coefficients were for test–retest [.57 for subjects, .51 for relatives]). Validity measures were, by and large, nil excepting for low correlations with story recall.

Others report only weak to moderate relationships between patient reports and memory test performance as well. Bennett-Levy and Powell (1980) found the highest correlations (.37–.41) between self-report items on the *Subjective Memory Questionnaire (SMQ)* and formal test items with the same content (i.e., face–name recall). Only 28% of the items of another self-rating scale, the *Memory Problem Questionnaire,* correlated significantly with clinical memory tests, and those items mostly concerned general memory ratings and ratings on memory problems in reading (Little et al., 1986).

A review of all memory questionnaires is not feasible here. Rather, a number of them will be briefly presented to provide examples of their range, depth, and effectiveness (see also Hickox and Sunderland, 1992).

Memory Functioning Questionnaire (MFQ)
(Gilewski, Zelinski, and Schaie, 1990)

This quite complex questionnaire was devised for examining memory complaints of older people. Its 64 items come in seven sections, each to be rated on a 7-point scale (in which 1 always represents the worst condition), which refers to frequency in some sections and quality (very bad to very good) or "seriousness" in others. It begins with a general rating about the presence of memory problems, from "major problems" to "no problems." *Frequency of forgetting,* the first section (18 items) asks how often common memory problems occur (e.g., remembering faces, keeping up corre-

spondence); two items (taking a test, losing the thread of thought in public speaking) are omitted when this questionnaire is used in dementia studies. The second and third sections (5 items each) have to do with the frequency of poor reading recall. Section four (4 items) asks about quality of recall of "things that occurred" anywhere from "last month" to "between 6 and 10 years ago." The fifth section repeats each of the 18 items of the first, asking for a rating of seriousness of the memory problem. The sixth section, *Retrospective Function,* asks for comparisons of current memory with five time frames from "1 year ago" to "when you were 18." The last section, *Mnemonics Usage,* gives a list of eight compensatory techniques to be graded for frequency of usage.

The 92-item *Memory Questionnaire (MQ)* (Zelinski, Gilewski, and Thompson, 1980) was the parent item source for the MFQ. Following factor analysis, items were selected that loaded on one of four factors: General Frequency of Forgetting, Seriousness of Forgetting, Retrospective Functioning, and Mnemonics Usage. Each MFQ item score comes under one of these headings following a "unit-weighted" procedure that takes indicated severity of each problem into account.

Age effects were related to Frequency of Forgetting and Retrospective Functioning; good health was associated with better scores on General Frequency of Forgetting and Seriousness of Forgetting; Mnemonics Usage was reported more often by persons with more education (Gilewski et al., 1990). Using elderly subjects (in the sixth to the ninth decade), this questionnaire correlated significantly with both memory tests and records of memory failures kept by the subjects (Zelinski, Gilewski, and Thompson, 1980).

This format effectively distinguished depressed middle-aged persons from a nondepressed group as the depressed patients had higher scores in almost every content area with more than half of these scores significantly different (J.M. Williams, Little, et al., 1987). Apart from the scoring problem, while this questionnaire may be used with intact adults, its complexity may make it unreliable for assessment of more than quite mildly impaired persons.

Inventory of Memory Experiences (IME)
(Herrmann and Neisser, 1978)

Recall of both remote and recent personal experiences is examined by this inventory. Forty-eight questions (Part F, frequency) have to do with how often one forgets personal day-to-day events and details. Examples of items in this section are, "How often are you unable to find something that you put down only a few minutes before?" or "When you want to remember an experience, a joke, or a story, how often do you find that you can't do so?" Part R (remote) consists of 24 questions of remote memory such as, "Do you remember any toys you had as a young child?" and "Do you remember the first time you earned any money yourself?" Each of these questions is accompanied by a follow-up question that asks, "How well do you remember . . . ?" All 72 questions are answered on a 7-point scale that ranges from "not at all" to "perfectly."

Data on this inventory come from a study using college students. Eight factors emerged when the scores for Part F were factor analyzed: (1) rote memory (e.g., telephone numbers); (2) absent-mindedness; (3) names; (4) people; (5) conversations (e.g., forgetting jokes, conversations); (6) errands (e.g., forgetting lists of chores); (7) retrieval (i.e., inability to account for a sense that something is familiar); and (8) places (i.e., forgetting the location of something). The college students' greatest problems were with rote memory and names, while they remembered people and conversations best. On Part R, women recalled memories from early childhood a little better than men. Response patterns having to do with other aspects of long-term memory were not well differentiated. The advantages of being able to use the same format for making comparisons between recall of recent and of remote memories should make this an attractive instrument for neuropsychological investigators. Herrmann (1982) reviews similar questionnaires.

Subjective Memory Questionnaire (SMQ) (Bennett-Levy and Powell, 1980; Bennett-Levy, Polkey, and Powell, 1980)

This shortened and somewhat simplified variation on the Inventory of Memory Experiences consists of only 43 questions on which subjects rate themselves on a 5-point scale. Most questions call for an evaluation of how good is memory or learning for specific material (e.g., "Learning new skills;" "Shopping lists"), and seven require judgment of the frequency of a problem (e.g., "Set off to do something, then find you can't remember what"). The questionnaire generally covers an appropriate range of everyday memory activities (Hickox and Sunderland, 1992).

No overall differences were found between three age groups (16–24, 25–34, 35–65), but age effects were found on seven questions by McMillan (1984) and on four by Bennett-Levy and Powell (1980), with only better recall by older subjects of the "Shoe sizes of others" showing an age difference. More items were answered differently by men or women, for a total of nine in Bennett-Levy and Powell's study and of 13 in McMillan's, but no overall sex differences appeared in either study. For the questionnaire as a whole, McMillan (1984) reported a test–retest reliability coefficient of .89 after 50 days.

This questionnaire differentiated moderate (PTA < 3 weeks) from severe (PTA > 3 weeks) TBI patients: the latter patients tended to report more favorably about their memory prowess than did cognitively intact control subjects (Bennett-Levy, 1984b). Comparisons of self-ratings by TBI patients living at home with those of their relatives found that the patient group's average score was higher (indicating better memory) than that given by their relatives, but still significantly lower than the control subjects' self-ratings which, by contrast, were a little lower than what their relatives reported (A.F. Schwartz and McMillan, 1989). Patient self-ratings correlated significantly with their Rivermead Behavioural Memory Test scores. Temporal lobe patients, too, reported significantly more memory problems than control subjects on this questionnaire, with differences between right and left temporal lobe patients showing up on only three items (Bennett-Levy, Polkey, and Powell, 1980). Their overall levels of memory problems brought to light some unexpected interactions between age at time of surgery, time since surgery, sex, and side of excision.

Memory Assessment Clinics Self-rating Scale (MAC-S) (Crook and Larrabee, 1990, 1992)

This 49-item questionnaire addresses the *Ability* to remember and the *Frequency of Occurrence* of memory problems in two separate scales containing 21 and 24 items, respectively, plus four Global Rating items involving comparisons with others, comparisons to previous best memory, speed of recall, and degree of concern about memory. Each Ability scale item is rated on a 5-point scale of *very poor* to *very good*; the 5-point Frequency of Occurrence scale ranges from *very often* to *very rarely* for each item. Factor analytic studies of an original pool of 102 items identified five Ability factors: Remote Personal Memory, Numeric Recall, Everyday Task-Oriented Memory, Word Recall/Semantic Memory, and Spatial Topographic Memory; and five Frequency of Occurrence factors: Word and Fact Recall/Semantic Memory, Attention/Concentration, Everyday Task-oriented Memory, General Forgetfulness, and Facial Recognition (Winterling et al., 1986). Score allocation is based on the factor on which each item had loaded to a significant degree (Crook and Larrabee, 1992). The four Global Rating items are treated separately. More than 1,000 subjects contributed the data for norms for five age ranges (from 18–39 to 70+), which provide means and standard deviations for the five Ability and five Frequency scores each based on item raw scores, for the Total score for each of these scales, and for the Global items (Crook and Larrabee, 1992). Both subject and relative forms are available.

Statistically significant but practically inconsequential age and sex effects showed up on several factors for each scale, with women tending to report fewer problems than men (Crook and Larrabee, 1992). WAIS Vocabulary and education level had some significant factor correlations on each scale. With three-week intervals, test–retest reliabilities for four testing sessions ranged from .82 to .94 for the factor and scale Totals. Self-reports of depressive symptoms by some of the intact, community-dwelling normative population made small (6.5 to 8.9%) but significant contributions to Global score variances (Crook and Larrabee, 1990).

Memory Questionnaire (Mateer, Sohlberg, and Crinean, 1987)

Mateer and her colleagues developed a 30-item scale in which each item is associated with one of four "factor-driven memory" classes, or scales: Attention/prospective memory (15 items: e.g., "I can't remember when I last took my medicine"); Retrograde memory (7 items: e.g., "I can't remember old TV shows"); Anterograde memory (3 items: e.g., "I can't remember what I had for breakfast"); Biographic/overload memory (3 items: e.g., "I lose my way around my old neighborhood or my family's house"); plus two items of currently relevant memory (therapists' and doctors' names, recall of current news). Subjects respond on a 5-point frequency scale from "Never" to "Always."

Comparisons between two groups of TBI patients, with and without coma history, and control subjects found that all groups reported the most problems with attention/prospective memory and least with historic, overlearned information. TBI patients in rehabilitation reported more memory problems in all four memory categories than did control subjects. Control subjects' ratings tended to be consistent with memory test performances but patients' self-ratings were not. Although patients with and without a coma history had similar complaints regarding anterograde memory, noncoma patients reported more memory problems on the other three scales. The authors interpreted this finding as possibly reflecting the considerable distress and critical self-appraisal frequently associated with mild TBI.

Everyday Memory Questionnaire (EMQ) (A. Sunderland, Harris, and Gleave, 1984)

While this questionnaire has even fewer (27) items than those described above, each item must be rated on a 9-point scale, ranging from "Not in the last three months" to "More than once a day." Items are divided into three classes: six "floor" items concern memory problems that typically trouble only very impaired persons (e.g., "Forgetting important details about your-self, e.g., your birthdate or where you live"); six additional items were added to the original list when reported by two or more of the original study patients or their relatives (e.g., "Forgetting where things are normally kept or looking for them in the wrong place"), and discriminator items, which had characterized severely head injured patients but not control subjects. Positively skewed total scores were "normalised by taking their square roots," which then became the vehicle for this study's reporting and research.

Mild and severe TBI patients' scores did not differ appreciably on this questionnaire, although relatives' response totals did differentiate patient groups at a low but significant level. Again, severely head injured patients gave fairly benign self-reports. Another group of TBI patients and their relatives showed a similar response pattern in that self-reports on the EMQ did not discriminate patients from controls but relatives reports did, possibly due to the EMQ's very large variances as, using raw scores, self-report score standard deviations were fully half as large as the means for both patient and control groups (A.F. Schwartz and McMillan, 1989). However, on a somewhat simplified version of this test (as "not at all in the last month" set the longest duration end of the frequency range thus shrinking response choices from nine to seven), stroke patients one month post-onset reported significantly more memory problems than control subjects, and their relatives reported even more than the patients (Tinson and Lincoln, 1987). Six months later this questionnaire registered patient reports of more memory problems, but relatives reported fewer.

Memory Symptom Test (Kapur and Pearson, 1983)

Based on spontaneous memory complaints of 100 patients with different kinds of brain injury, this memory quiz asks patients to compare their current memory in ten areas of common memory complaints with what it was before it was impaired: (1) knowing the day of the week; (2) knowing the month; (3) remembering names of people known for some time; (4) remembering names of people met recently; (5) recognizing faces of persons known for some time; (6) remembering having met someone once before; (7) remembering something told by someone; (8) remembering where something was put; (9) remembering how to get to a familiar place; (10) remembering something recently read. Responses are registered on a 3-point scale: unimpaired, slightly impaired, and very much impaired. When given to a small group of head trauma patients and to a relative or spouse, the other person tended to report more problems than did the patient but patient and observer reports were highly correlated (p < .005). However, neither patient nor observer reports correlated significantly with any of four memory tests.

13 | **Verbal Functions and Language Skills**

The most prominent disorders of verbal functions are the aphasias and associated difficulties in verbal production such as *dysarthria* (defective articulation) and apraxias of speech. Other aspects of verbal functions that are usually affected when there is an aphasic disorder, such as fluency and reading and writing abilities, may be impaired without aphasia being present. Assessment of the latter functions will therefore be discussed separately from aphasia testing.

APHASIA

Aphasic disorders can be mistakenly diagnosed when the problem actually results from a global confusional state, a dysarthric condition, or elective mutism. The reverse can also occur when mild deficits in language comprehension and production are attributed to generalized cognitive impairment or to a memory or attentional disorder. Defective auditory comprehension, in particular, whether due to a hearing disorder or to impaired language comprehension, can result in unresponsive or socially inappropriate behavior that is mistaken for negativism, dementia, or a psychiatric condition. In fact, aphasia occurs as part of the behavioral picture in many brain disorders (Mendez and Cummings, 2002) so that often the question is not whether the patient has aphasia, but rather how (much) the aphasia contributes to the patient's behavioral deficits. Questions concerning the presence of aphasia can usually be answered by careful observation in the course of an informal but systematic review of the patient's capacity to perceive, comprehend, remember, and respond with both spoken and written material, or by using an aphasia screening test. A review of language and speech functions that will indicate whether communication problems are present will include examination of the following aspects of verbal behavior:

1. *Spontaneous speech.*
2. *Repetition* of words, phrases, sentences. "Methodist Episcopal" and similar tongue-twisters elicit disorders of articulation and sound sequencing. "No ifs, ands, or buts" tests for the integrity of connections between the center for expressive speech (Broca's area) and the receptive speech center (Wernicke's area).
3. *Speech comprehension.* a. Give the subject simple commands (e.g., "Show me your chin." "Put your left hand on your right ear."). b. Ask "yes-no" questions (e.g., "Is a ball square?"). c. Ask the subject to point to specific objects.

The wife of a patient diagnosed as a global aphasic (expression and comprehension severely defective in all modalities) insisted that her husband understood what she told him and that he communicated appropriate responses to her by gestures. I examined him in front of her, asking him—in the tone of voice she used when anticipating a "yes" response—"Is your name John?" "Is your name Bill?" etc. Only when she saw him eagerly nod assent to each question could she begin to appreciate the severity of his comprehension deficit [mdl].

An inpatient with new onset global aphasia nodded enthusiastically and said "yes" to all questions, causing his physicians to believe that he had consented to a surgical procedure because they had not asked him a question in which "no" was the appropriate answer [dbh].

4. *Naming.* The examiner points to various objects and their parts asking, "What is this?" (e.g., glasses, frame, nose piece, lens; thus asking for object names in the general order of their frequency of occurrence in normal conversation). Ease and accuracy of naming in other categories, such as colors, letters, numbers, and actions, should also be examined (Goodglass, 1980; Strub and Black, 2000).
5. *Reading.* To examine for accuracy, have the subject read aloud. For comprehension, have the subject follow written directions (e.g., "Tap three times on the table"), explain a passage just read.
6. *Writing.* Have the subject copy, write to dictation, and compose a sentence or two.

When evaluating speech, Goodglass (1986) pointed out the importance of attending to such aspects as the ease and quantity of production (*fluency*), articulatory error, speech rhythms and intonation (*prosody*), grammar and syntax, and the presence of misspoken words (paraphasias). Although lapses in some of these aspects of speech are almost always associated with aphasia, others—such as articulatory disorders—may occur as speech problems unrelated to aphasia. The examiner should also be aware that familiar and, particularly, personally relevant stimuli will elicit the patient's best responses (Van Lancker and Nicklay, 1992). Thus, a patient examined only on standardized tests may actually communicate better at home and with friends than test scores suggest, particularly when patients augment their communication at home with gestures.

Formal aphasia testing should be undertaken when aphasia is known to be present or is strongly suspected. It may be done for any of the following purposes:

(1) diagnosis of presence and type of aphasic syndrome, leading to inferences concerning cerebral localization; (2) measurement of the level of performance over a wide range, for both initial determination and detection of change over time; (3) comprehensive assessment of the assets and liabilities of the patient in all language areas as a guide to therapy. (Goodglass and Kaplan, 1983a, p. 1)

The purpose of the examination should determine the kind of examination (screening, symptom focused, or comprehensive?) and the kinds of tests required (Mazaux, Boisson, et Daverat, 1989; Spreen and Risser, 1991).

Aphasia tests differ from other verbal tests in that they focus on disorders of symbol formulation and associated apraxias and agnosias. They are usually designed to elicit samples of behavior in each communication modality—listening, speaking, reading, writing, and gesturing. The examination of the central "linguistic processing of verbal symbols" is their common denominator (Wepman and Jones, 1967). Aphasia tests also differ in that many involve tasks that most adults would complete with few, if any, errors.

Aphasia Tests and Batteries

The most widely used aphasia tests are actually test batteries comprising numerous tests of many discrete verbal functions. Their product may be a score or index for diagnostic purposes or an orderly description of the patient's communication disabilities. Most aphasia tests involve lengthy, precise, and well-controlled procedures. They are best administered by persons, such as speech pathologists, who have more than a passing acquaintance with aphasiology and are trained in the specialized techniques of aphasia examinations.

Aphasia test batteries always include a wide range of tasks so that the nature and severity of the language problem and associated deficits may be determined. Because aphasia tests concern disordered language functions in themselves and not their cognitive ramifi-

cations, test items typically present very simple and concrete tasks most children in the lower grades can pass. Common aphasia test questions ask the patient (1) to name simple objects ("What is this?" asks the examiner, pointing to a cup, a pen, or the picture of a boy or a clock); (2) to recognize simple spoken words ("Put the spoon in the cup"); (3) to act on serial commands; (4) to repeat words and phrases; (5) to recognize simple printed letters, numbers, words, primary level arithmetic problems, and common symbols; (6) to give verbal and gestural answers to simple printed questions; and (7) to print or write letters, words, numbers, etc. In addition, some aphasia tests and examination protocols ask the patient to tell a story or draw. Some examine articulatory disorders and apraxias as well (Goodglass, 1986; Stringer, 1996).

Aphasia test batteries differ primarily in their terminology, internal organization, the number of modality combinations they test, and the levels of difficulty and complexity to which the examination is carried. The tests discussed here are both representative of the different kinds of aphasia tests and among the best known. Some clinicians devise their own batteries, taking parts from other tests and adding their own. Detailed reviews of many batteries and tests for aphasia can be found in A.G. Davis, *A Survey of Adult Aphasia* (1993); Spreen and Risser, *Assessment of Aphasia* (2003); and Spreen and Strauss, *A Compendium of Neuropsychological Tests* (1998).

Boston Diagnostic Aphasia Examination (BDAE-2) (Goodglass and Kaplan, 1983a,b), Boston Diagnostic Aphasia Examination (BDAE-3) (Goodglass, Kaplan, and Barresi, 2000)

This test battery was devised to examine the "components of language" that would aid in diagnosis and treatment and in the advancement of knowledge about the neuroanatomic correlates of aphasia. It provides for a systematic assessment of communication and communication-related functions in 12 areas defined by factor analysis, with a total of 34 subtests. Time is the price paid for such thorough coverage, for a complete examination takes from one to four hours. As a result many examiners use portions of this test selectively, often in combination with other neuropsychological tests. The BDAE-3 has a new short form that takes only an hour or less. A number of "supplementary language tests" are also provided, to enable discrimination of such aspects of psycholinguistic behavior as grammar and syntax and to examine for disconnection syndromes (see below). The extended version of the BDAE-3 contains instructions for examining the praxis problems which may accompany aphasia.

Evaluation of the patient is based on three kinds of observations. The score for the *Aphasia Severity Rating Scale* has a 6-point range for the 1983 BDAE and a 5-point range for the BDAE-3, based on examiner ratings of patient responses to a semistructured interview and free conversation. Subtests are scored for number correct and converted into percentiles derived from a normative study of aphasic patients, many presenting with relatively selective deficits but, unlike the original 1972 standardization, also including the most severely impaired. These scores are registered on the *Subtest Summary Profile* sheet, permitting the examiner to see at a glance the patient's deficit pattern. In addition, this battery yields a "Rating Scale Profile" for qualitative speech characteristics that, the authors point out, "are not satisfactorily measured by objective scores" but can be judged on seven 7-point scales, each referring to a particular feature of speech production. For some of these scales requiring examiner judgment, relatively low interrater reliability coefficients have been reported (Kertesz, 1989). However, interrater agreement correlations typically run above .75, and percent agreement measures also indicate generally satisfactory agreement levels (A.G. Davis, 1993). Based on his review of BDAE research, Davis suggested that BDAE scores predict performance on other aphasia tests better than patient functioning in "natural circumstances." Data from a 1980 (Borod, Goodglass, and Kaplan) normative study of the BDAE and the supplementary spatial-quantitative tests (see below) contributed to the 1983 norms. The 1999 standardization sample includes 85 adults with aphasia and 15 normal elderly persons. Subjects with low education have lower scores (Borod, Goodglass, and Kaplan, 1980; Pineda, et al., 2000).

Supplementing the verbal BDAE as part of the comprehensive examination for aphasics is a Spatial Quantitative Battery (called the Parietal Lobe Battery [PLB]) (Goodglass and Kaplan, 1983a). This set of tests includes constructional and drawing tasks, finger identification, directional orientation, arithmetic, and clock drawing tasks. While sensitive to parietal lobe lesions, patients with both frontal and parietal damage are most likely to be impaired on this battery (Borod, Carper, Goodglass, and Naeser, 1984).

The range and sensitivity of the "Boston" battery makes it an excellent tool for the description of aphasic disorders and for treatment planning. However, an examiner must be experienced to use it diagnostically. Normative data for the individual tests allow examiners to give them separately as needed, which may account for some of this battery's popularity. Of course, not least of its advantages are the attractiveness and evident face validity of many of the subtests (e.g., the

Cookie Theft picture; a sentence repetition format that distinguishes between phrases with high or low probability of occurrence in natural speech).

Two translations of this battery are available. Rosselli, Ardila and their coworkers (1990) provide norms for a Spanish language version (Goodglass and Kaplan, 1986). A French version developed by Mazaux and Orgogozo (1985) has retained the *z*-score profiling of the BDAE first edition.

Communication Abilities in Daily Living, 2nd ed. (CADL-2) (Holland, Frattali, and Fromm, 1999)

The disparity between scores that patients obtain on the usual formal tests of language competency and their communicative competency in real life led to the development of an instrument that might reduce this disparity by presenting patients with language tasks in familiar, practical contexts. The original CADL (Holland, 1980) examined how patients might handle daily life activities by engaging them in role-playing in a series of simulated situations such as "the doctor's office," encouraging the examiner to carry out a dual role as examiner/play-acting participant with such props as a toy stethoscope.

The CADL-2 revision eliminated items that require role playing and most props. This reduced the number of items from the original 68 to 50 but retained the focus on naturalistic everyday communications (e.g., with a telephone, with real money). The number of communication categories was reduced from ten to seven in the CADL-2: (1) reading, writing, and using numbers; (2) communication sequences; (3) social interactions; (4) response to misinformation or proverbs; (5) nonverbal communication; (6) contextual communication; (7) recognition of humor, metaphor. Examination informality is encouraged.

A series of evaluations of CADL performances of 130 aphasic patients demonstrated that this test was sensitive to aphasia, age, and institutionalization (unspecified) but not sex or social background (Holland, 1980). The CADL differentiated patients with the major types of aphasia on the single dimension of severity of communicative disability based on the summation score. The ten category scores also identified aphasia subtypes. The CADL-2 normative sample includes 175 adults with communication disorders, primarily from stroke or TBI. Test-retest reliability for CADL-2 was .85, and interrater reliability for stanine scores was .99.

Because responses need not be vocalized to earn credits, this test tends to be more sensitive to the communication strengths of many speech-impaired (e.g., Broca's aphasia) patients than are traditional testing instruments. Spreen and Risser (2003) recommend the

CADL to provide the descriptive information about functional communication that is lacking in all the larger, comprehensive, batteries: "it allows an estimate of the patient's communication ability rather than . . . accuracy of language" (Spreen and Strauss, 1998). Yet, A.G. Davis (1993) warned, CADL findings cannot be interpreted as representing naturalistic behavior as it "is still a test" and, as such, "does not provide for observing natural interactions."

Functional Communication Profile (FCP) (M.T. Sarno, 1969)

This is a 45-item inventory that takes 20 to 40 minutes to administer. It permits serial scaled ratings of a patient's practical language behavior elicited "in an informal setting," as distinguished from language on more formal testing instruments since "improvement as measured by higher (formal) test scores does not always reflect improvement" in the patient's day-to-day activities (J.E. Sarno et al., 1971). Like battery type aphasia tests, the Functional Communication Profile also requires an experienced clinician to apply it reliably and sensitively. Evaluation proceeds in five different performance areas: "Movement," "Speaking," "Understanding," "Reading," and "Other," not exclusively verbal, adaptive behaviors. The test has no sex bias (M.T. Sarno, Buonagura, and Levita, 1985). Scoring is on a 9-point scale, and ratings are assigned on the basis of the examiner's estimate of the patient's premorbid ability in that area. Scores are recorded on a histogram. Sarno (1969) recommended color coding to differentiate the initial evaluation from subsequent reevaluations for easy visual review. She also offered a rather loose method of converting the item grades into percentages that may be too subjective for research purposes or for comparisons with clinical evaluations made by different examiners. However, this test is of practical value in predicting functional communication (Spreen and Risser, 2003) and for documenting post-stroke improvement (M.T. Sarno, 1976).

Multilingual Aphasia Examination (MAE) (Benton and Hamsher, 1989; Benton, Hamsher, and Sivan, 1994)

A seven-part battery was developed from its parent battery, the Neurosensory Center Comprehensive Examination of Aphasia (see below), to provide for a systematic, graded examination of receptive, expressive, and immediate memory components of speech and language functions. The Token Test and Controlled Oral Word Association are variations of tests in general use; others, for instance the three forms of the Spelling test

(Oral, Written, and Block—using large metal or plastic letters), were developed for this battery. Most of the tests have two or three forms, thus reducing practice effects on repeated administrations. For each test, age and education effects are dealt with by means of a *Correction Score*, which, when added to the raw score gives an *Adjusted Score*. Percentile conversions for each adjusted score and their corresponding classification have been worked out so that scores on each test are psychometrically comparable. This means of scoring and evaluating subtest performances has the additional virtue of allowing each test to be used separately as, for instance, when an examiner wishes to study verbal fluency or verbal memory in a patient who is not aphasic and for whom administration of many of the other subtests would be a waste of time. A Spanish version of this test (MAE-S) is available (G.J. Rey and Benton, 1991). Most of these tests are both age and education sensitive; the effects of age and education have been reported for many of them (Ivnik, Malec, Smith, et al., 1996; Mitrushina, Boone, and D'Elia, 1999; Ruff, Light, and Parker, 1996).

Neurosensory Center Comprehensive Examination for Aphasia (NCCEA)[1] (Spreen and Benton, 1977; Spreen and Strauss, 1991)

This battery consists of 24 short subtests, 20 involving different aspects of language performance, and four "control" tests of visual and tactile functions. Most of the subtests normally take less than five minutes to administer. The control tests are given only when the patient performs poorly on a test involving visual or tactile stimuli. A variety of materials are used in the tests, including common objects, sound tapes, printed cards, a screened box for tactile recognition, and the Token Test "tokens." An interesting innovation enables patients whose writing hand is paralyzed to demonstrate "graphic" behavior by giving them "Scrabble" letters for forming words. All of the materials can be easily purchased, or they can be constructed by following instructions in the manual. Age and education corrected scores for each subtest are entered on three profile sheets, one providing norms for the performance of intact but poorly educated adults, a second with norms based on the performance of aphasic patients, and the third giving performance data on nonaphasic brain damaged patients. The first two profiles taken together enable the examiner to identify patients whose performance differs significantly from that of normal

---

[1]This battery may be obtained from the University of Victoria Neuropsychology Laboratory, P.O. Box 1700, Victoria, British Columbia, V8W 3P4, Canada.

adults, while providing for score discriminations within the aphasic score range so that small amounts of change can be registered.

This test has proven sensitivity, particularly for moderately and severely aphasic patients (Spreen and Risser, 2003) and also for distinguishing kinds and degrees of speech and language impairments after head injury (Sarno, 1980). It suffers from a low ceiling which diminishes its usefulness for examining well-educated patients with mild impairments (Spreen and Risser, 2003), and it omits assessment of spontaneous speech.

Porch Index of Communicative Ability (PICA) (Porch, 1983)

The PICA was developed as a highly standardized, statistically reliable instrument for measuring a limited sample of language functions. This battery contains 18 ten-item subtests, four of them verbal, eight gestural, and six graphic. The same ten common items (cigarette, comb, fork, key, knife, matches, pencil, pen, quarter, toothbrush) are used for each subtest with the exception of the simplest graphic subtest in which the patient is asked to copy geometric forms. Spontaneous conversation is not addressed. The examiner scores each of the patient's responses according to a 16-point multidimensional scoring system (Porch, 1971). Each point in the system describes performance. For example, a score of **1** indicates no response; a score of **15** indicates a response that was judged to be accurate, responsive, prompt, complete, and efficient. Qualified PICA testers undergo a 40-hour training period after which they administer ten practice tests. This training leads to high interscorer reliability correlation coefficients. Its validity as a measure of language and communication ability has been demonstrated (Spreen and Risser, 2003).

By virtue of its tight format and reliable scoring system, the PICA provides a sensitive measure of small changes in patient performance. This sensitivity can aid the speech pathologist in monitoring treatment effects so long as the patient's deficits are not so mild that they escape notice because of the test's low ceiling. Its statistically sophisticated construction and reliability make it a useful research instrument as well (McNeil, 1979). A.D. Martin (1977) called into question a number of aspects of the PICA, such as the assumption that the scaling intervals are equal, which can lead a score-minded examiner to misinterpret the examination, particularly with respect to the patient's capacity for functional communication. Auditory comprehension is not adequately examined by these procedures (Kertesz, 1989; Spreen and Risser, 2003). Thus, while some

aphasia syndromes may be indicated by PICA findings, the data it generates are too limited for making diagnostic classifications or inferences about underlying structural damage (A.G. Davis, 1993).

Western Aphasia Battery (WAB) (Kertesz, 1979, 1982)

This battery grew out of efforts to develop an instrument from the Boston Diagnostic Aphasia Examination that would generate diagnostic classifications and be suitable for both treatment and research purposes. Thus, many of the items were taken from the Boston examination. The Western Aphasia Battery consists of four oral language subtests—*spontaneous speech, auditory comprehension, repetition,* and *naming*—that yield five scores based on either a rating scale (for Fluency and Information content of speech) or conversion of summed item-correct scores to a scale of 10. Each score thus can be charted on a ten-point scale; together, the five scores, when scaled, give *a profile of performance.* An *Aphasia Quotient (AQ)* can be calculated by multiplying each of the five scaled scores by 2 and summing them. Normal (i.e., perfect) performance is set at 100. The AQ gives a measure of discrepancy from normal language performance, but like any summed score in neuropsychology, it tells nothing of the nature of the problem. The profile of performance and the AQ can be used together to determine the patient's diagnostic subtype according to pattern descriptions for eight aphasia subtypes. In addition, tests of reading, writing, arithmetic, gestural praxis (i.e., examining for apraxia of gesture), construction, and Raven's Progressive Matrices are included to provide a comprehensive survey of communication abilities and related functions. Scores on the latter tests can be combined into a *Performance Quotient (PQ)*; the AQ and PQ together give a summary *Cortical Quotient (CQ)* score for diagnostic and research purposes. The language portions of the test take about one and one-half hours, and less time with more impaired or particularly fluent patients. Reliability and validity evaluations meet reasonable criteria. Its statistical structure is satisfactory (Spreen and Risser, 2003).

Only the two scores obtained by ratings should present standardization problems. However, the other items leave little room for taking the qualitative aspects of performance into account and thus may provide a restricted picture of the patient's functioning which may account for some of the reported disparities between diagnostic decisions made by clinicians or generated by other aphasia tests and diagnostic classifications based on WAB data (e.g., see A.G. Davis, 1993). Another drawback is that the classification system does not address the many patients whose symptoms are of a "mixed" nature (i.e., have components of more than one of the eight types delineated in this classification system) (Spreen and Risser, 2003).

The WAB has been used to evaluate the language abilities of patients with a variety of neurological diseases. Patients with right hemisphere strokes performed as well as control subjects on all five scales while those with strokes on the left were significantly impaired (K.L. Bryan and Hale, 2001). Early language impairment in patients with primary progressive aphasia was detected on items involving fluency and naming, while comprehension and nonverbal cognition were retained (Karbe et al., 1993). Lower fluency, repetition, and naming scores distinguished left hemisphere stroke patients from patients with mild Alzheimer's disease; however, those with right hemisphere strokes could not be distinguished on any AQ measures (J. Horner, Dawson, et al., 1992). Patients with vascular dementia performed worse than Alzheimer patients on the writing scale while the latter scored lower on the repetition scale (Kertesz and Clydesdale, 1994).

Aphasia Screening

Aphasia screening tests do not replace the careful examination of language functions afforded by the test batteries. Rather, they are best used as supplements to a neuropsychological test battery. They signal the presence of an aphasic disorder and may even call attention to its specific characteristics, but they do not enable the examiner to make either a reliable diagnosis or the fine discriminations required for understanding the manifestations of an aphasic disorder. These tests do not require technical knowledge of speech pathology for satisfactory administration or determination of whether a significant aphasic disorder is present. However, excepting the Token Test which can elicit subtle deficits, conversations with the patient coupled with a mental status examination should, in most cases, make an aphasia screening test unnecessary. "All we need is a concept of what needs to be assessed, a few common objects, a pen, and some paper" (A.G. Davis, 1993, p. 215). Davis considers screening tests to be useful to the extent that "a standardized administration maximizes consistency in diagnosis, supports a diagnosis, and facilitates convenient measurement of progress" (p. 215).

Aphasia Screening Test (Halstead and Wepman, 1959)

This test was created by Wepman, not Halstead; Wepman was a member of Halstead's department at the

time the article describing it was published. This is the most widely used of all aphasia tests since it or one of its variants has been incorporated into many formally organized neuropsychological test batteries. As originally devised, the Aphasia Screening Test has 51 items which cover all the elements of aphasic disabilities as well as the most common associated communication problems. It is a fairly brief test, rarely taking longer than 30 minutes to complete. There are no rigid scoring standards, but rather, the emphasis is on determining the nature of the linguistic problem once its presence has been established. Erroneous responses are coded into a diagnostic profile intended to provide a description of the pattern of the patient's language disabilities. Obviously, the more areas of involvement and the more a single area is involved, the more severe the disability. However, no provisions are made to grade test performance on the basis of severity, nor information provided for classifying patients, nor are guidelines given for clinical application.

Wepman (personal communication, 1975 [mdl]) rejected this test about 30 years after he had developed it, as he found that it contributed more confusion than clarity to both diagnosis and description of aphasic disorders. Aphasia and related conditions require more than an item or two to be identified and understood within the totality of the patient's communication abilities.

Reitan included it in the Halstead-Reitan Battery along with tests developed by Halstead and others. Reitan pared down the original test to 32 items but still handled the data descriptively, in much the same manner as originally intended (Jarvis and Barth, 1994; Reitan and Wolfson, 1993). A second revision of the Aphasia Screening Test appeared in E.W. Russell, Neuringer, and Goldstein's (1970) modification of Reitan's modification of Halstead's battery. This version, called the Aphasia Test, contains 37 items. It is essentially the same as Reitan's modification except that four easy arithmetic problems and the task of naming a key were added. E.W. Russell and his colleagues established a simple error-counting scoring system for use with their computerized diagnostic classification system, which converts to a 6-point rating scale. Other scoring systems have been developed typically based on a number correct (or error) score in which each item is evaluated on a "right" or "wrong" basis (W.G. Snow, 1987b).

In his item-by-item comparisons of responses made by 50 patients with lateralized lesions, W.G. Snow (1987a) found that only one item—copying the drawing of a key—discriminated the two groups: significantly more patients with right hemisphere disease made errors on this item than those with left-sided lesions. By and large, patients with left-sided damage did worse on verbal items; those with damage on the right had poorer performances on naming the triangle, on drawing, and on reading "7 SIX 2." More than half of a group of normal elderly (ages 65–75) subjects failed one or more of the repetition items, at least one drawing item was failed by a similar number, and more than one-third of this group failed at least one item classified as measuring language comprehension (Ernst, 1988). Additionally, significant correlations between this test and both mental ability and education have been recorded (Spreen and Risser, 1991). Thus, if one goes by score alone, this test cannot qualify for aphasia screening. Moreover, the manner in which it is presented to examiners allows naive ones to ascribe very serious neuropsychological deficits to a single error, such as reporting "acalculia" on the basis of a patient's inability to multiply 27×3 mentally (usually reflecting an attention disorder!) or interpreting the careless drawing of a key as "constructional apraxia." Ridiculous as it seems, I [mdl] have seen such crude and potentially harmful interpretations many times when reviewing examination protocols and reports. Probably the best way of handling this test is Wepman's: *junk it altogether.*

A very shortened version of Wepman's Aphasia Screening Test consists of four tasks (Heimburger and Reitan, 1961):

1. Copy a square, Greek cross, and triangle without lifting the pencil from the paper.
2. Name each copied figure.
3. Spell each name.
4. Repeat: "He shouted the warning"; then explain and write it.

This little test may aid in discriminating between patients with left and right hemisphere lesions, for many of the former can copy the designs but cannot write, while the latter have little trouble writing but many cannot reproduce the designs.

Token Test (Boller and Vignolo, 1966; De Renzi and Vignolo, 1962)

The Token Test is extremely simple to administer, to score and, for almost every nonaphasic person who has completed the fourth grade, to perform with few if any errors. Yet it is remarkably sensitive to the disrupted linguistic processes that are central to the aphasic disability, even when much of the patient's communication behavior has remained intact. Scores on the Token Test correlate highly both with scores on tests of auditory comprehension (Morley et al., 1979) and with language production test scores (Gutbrod et al., 1985). The Token Test performance also involves immediate

memory span for verbal sequences and capacity to use syntax (Lesser, 1976). It can identify those brain damaged patients whose other disabilities may be masking a concomitant aphasic disorder, or whose symbolic processing problems are relatively subtle and not readily recognizable. However, it contributes little to the elucidation of severe aphasic conditions since these patients will fail most items quite indiscriminately (Wertz, 1979).

Twenty "tokens" cut from heavy construction paper or thin sheets of plastic or wood make up the test material. They come in two shapes (circles and squares[1]), two sizes (big and little), and five colors. The tokens are laid out horizontally in four parallel rows of large circles, large squares, small circles, and small squares, with colors in random order (e.g., see De Renzi and Faglioni, 1978). The only requirement this test makes of the patient is the ability to comprehend the token names and the verbs and prepositions in the instructions. The diagnosis of those few patients whose language disabilities are so severe as to prevent them from cooperating on this task is not likely to depend on formal testing; almost all other brain injured patients can respond to the simple instructions. The test consists of a series of oral commands, 62 altogether, given in five sections of increasing complexity (Table 13.1).

Examiners must guard against unwittingly slowing their rate of speech delivery as slowed presentation of instructions (*stretched speech* produced by slowing an instruction tape) significantly reduced the number of errors made by aphasic patients without affecting the performance of patients with right hemisphere lesions (Poeck and Pietron, 1981). However, even with slowed instructions, aphasic patients still make many more errors than do patients with right-sided lesions.

Items failed on a first command should be repeated and, if performed successfully the second time, scored separately from the first response. When the second, but not the first, administration of an item is passed, only the second performance is counted, under the assumption that many initial errors will result from such nonspecific variables as inattention and disinterest. Each correct response earns 1 point on the 62-point scale. The examiner should note whether the patient distinguishes between the Part 5 "touch" and "pick up" directions.

Boller and Vignolo (1966) developed a slightly modified version of De Renzi and Vignolo's (1962) original Token Test format. Their cut-off scores correctly classified 100% of the control patients, 90% of patients with right-hemisphere lesions, and 91% of apha-

---

[1]When originally published, instructions called for rectangles. Squares have been universally substituted to reduce the number of syllables the patient must process.

TABLE 13.1 The Token Test

PART I

(Large squares and large circles only are on the table)

1. Touch the red circle
2. Touch the green square
3. Touch the red square
4. Touch the yellow circle
5. Touch the blue circle (2)*
6. Touch the green circle (3)
7. Touch the yellow square (1)
8. Touch the white circle
9. Touch the blue square
10. Touch the white square (4)

PART II

(Large and small squares and circles are on the table)

1. Touch the small yellow circle (1)
2. Touch the large green circle
3. Touch the large yellow circle
4. Touch the large blue square (3)
5. Touch the small green circle (4)
6. Touch the large red circle
7. Touch the large white square (2)
8. Touch the small blue circle
9. Touch the small green square
10. Touch the large blue circle

PART III

(Large squares and large circles only)

1. Touch the yellow circle and the red square
2. Touch the green square and the blue circle (3)
3. Touch the blue square and the yellow square
4. Touch the white square and the red square
5. Touch the white circle and the blue circle (4)
6. Touch the blue square and the white square (2)
7. Touch the blue square and the white circle
8. Touch the green square and the blue circle
9. Touch the red circle and the yellow square (1)
10. Touch the red square and the white circle

PART IV

(Large and small squares and circles)

1. Touch the small yellow circle and the large green square (2)
2. Touch the small blue square and the small green circle
3. Touch the large white square and the large red circle (1)
4. Touch the large blue square and the large red square (3)
5. Touch the small blue square and the small yellow circle
6. Touch the small blue circle and the small red circle
7. Touch the large blue square and the large green square
8. Touch the large blue circle and the large green circle

TABLE 13.1 (continued)

9. Touch the small red square and the small yellow circle
10. Touch the small white square and the large red square (4)

PART V

(Large squares and large circles only)

1. Put the red circle on the green square (1)
2. Put the white square behind the yellow circle
3. Touch the blue circle with the red square (2)
4. Touch—with the blue circle—the red square
5. Touch the blue circle and the red square (3)
6. Pick up the blue circle or the red square (4)
7. Put the green square away from the yellow square (5)
8. Put the white circle before the blue square
9. If there is a black circle, pick up the red square (6)

N.B. There is no black circle.

10. Pick up the squares, except the yellow one
11. Touch the white circle without using your right hand
12. When I touch the green circle, you take the white square.

N.B. Wait a few seconds before touching the green circle.

13. Put the green square beside the red circle (7)
14. Touch the squares, slowly, and the circles, quickly (8)
15. Put the red circle between the yellow square and the green square (9)
16. Except for the green one, touch the circles (10)
17. Pick up the red circle—no!—the white square (11)
18. Instead of the white square, take the yellow circle (12)
19. Together with the yellow circle, take the blue circle (13)
20. After picking up the green square, touch the white circle
21. Put the blue circle under the white square
22. Before touching the yellow circle, pick up the red square

*A second number at the end of an item indicates that the item is identical or structurally similar to the item of the number in De Renzi and Faglioni's "short version" (see p. 510). To preserve the complexity of the items in Part 5 of the short version, item 3 of the original Part IV should read, "Touch the large white square and the *small* red circle."

From Boller and Vignolo (1966)

sic patients, for an overall 88% correctly classified (see Table 13.2, p. 509).

Part V alone, which consists of items involving relational concepts, identified only one fewer patient as "latent aphasic" than did the whole 62-item test of Boller and Vignolo. This finding suggests that Part V could be used without the other 40 questions to identify those patients with left hemisphere lesions misclassified as nonaphasic because their difficulties in symbol formulation are too subtle to impair communication for most ordinary purposes. Doubling the number of items increased the power of Part II to discriminate between patients with right hemisphere lesions and aphasics to 92.5% (R. Cohen, Gutbrod, et al., 1987).

TABLE 13.2 A Summary of Scores Obtained by the Four Experimental Groups on The Token Test

| | | BRAIN DAMAGED PATIENTS | | |
| | | RIGHT | LEFT | |
Partial Scores	Control Patients (n = 31)	(n = 30)	Nonaphasic (n = 26)	Aphasic (n = 34)
Part I				
10	31	30	26	30
9 & lower				4
Part II				
10	31	29	25	23
9 & lower		1	1	11
Part III				
10	29	28	25	13
9	2	2	1	10
8 & lower				11
Part IV				
10	29	25	21	5
9	2	3	3	4
8 & lower		2	2	25
Part V				
20 and above	28	22	14	3
18 & 19	3	7	5	2
17 & lower		1	7	29
Total score				
60 & above	26	21	14	2
58–59	5	6	4	1
57 & lower		3	8	31

Adapted from Boller and Vignolo (1966)

Test characteristics. Age effects have been documented (De Renzi and Faglioni, 1978; Ivnik, Malec, Smith, et al., 1996; Spreen and Strauss, 1998). Although De Renzi and Faglioni (1978) reported education effects, Spreen and Strauss (1998) suggest that age corrections are unnecessary for persons with greater than eight years of education. Correlations with general mental ability (as measured by Raven's Matrices) become apparent only with brain impaired patients (Coupar, 1976). Men and women perform similarly (M.T. Sarno, Buonaguro, and Levita, 1985). Test-retest reliability was high with correlation coefficients between .92 and .96 when measured on aphasic patients (Spreen and Strauss, 1998); with intact elderly persons who make very few errors, the reliability coefficient was only .50 after a year's interval (W.G. Snow, Tierney, Zorzitto, et al., 1988). Practice effects measured on patients with no intervention and no degenerative disease are virtually nil (McCaffrey, Duff, and Westervelt, 2000b). Validation of its sensitivity to aphasia comes from a variety of sources (Spreen and Risser, 2003).

Neuropsychological findings. Despite the simplicity of the called-for response—or perhaps because of its simplicity—this direction-following task can give the observant examiner insight into the nature of the patient's comprehension or performance deficits. Patients whose failures on this test are mostly due to defective auditory comprehension tend to confuse colors or shapes and to carry out fewer than the required instructions. They may begin to perseverate as the instructions become more complex. A few nonaphasic patients may also perseverate on this task because of conceptual inflexibility or an impaired capacity to execute a series of commands.

For example, although he could repeat the instructions correctly, a 68-year-old retired laborer suffering multi-infarct dementia was unable to perform the two-command items because he persisted in placing his fingers on the designated to-kens simultaneously despite numerous attempts to lead him into making a serial response.

This clinical observation was extended by a study of a group of dementia patients who performed consider-ably *below normal limits* on a 13-item form of this test (Swihart, Panisset, et al., 1989). These patients did best on the first simple command, "Put the red circle on the green square," with high failure levels (56% and 57%) on the two following items because of tenden-cies to perseverate the action "Put on" when these sub-sequent item instructions asked for "Touch." This study found the Token Test to be quite sensitive to de-mentia severity: it correlated more highly with the Mini-Mental State Examination ($r = .73$) than with an auditory comprehension measure ($r = .49$), indicating that failures were due more to general cognitive deficits than to specific auditory deficits.

When patients have difficulty on this task, the prob-lem is usually so obvious that, for clinical purposes, the examiner may not find it necessary to begin at the be-ginning of the test and administer every item. To save time, the examiner can start at the highest level at which success seems likely and move to the next higher level if the patient easily succeeds on three or four items. When a score is needed, as for research purposes or when preparing a report that may enter into litigation proceedings, the examiner may wish to use one of the several short forms.

Token Test variants. Spreen and Benton developed a 39-item modification of De Renzi and Vignolo's long form, which is incorporated in the Neurosensory Cen-ter Comprehensive Examination for Aphasia (repro-duced in Spreen and Strauss, 1998). From this, Spel-lacy and Spreen (1969) constructed a 16-item short form that uses the same 20 tokens as both the original and the modified long forms and includes many of the relational items of Part V. A 22-item Token Test is part of Benton, Hamsher, and Sivan's Multilingual Aphasia Examination battery. The first ten items contain rep-resentative samples from sections I to IV of the origi-nal test; the last 11 items involve the more complex re-lational concepts found in the original section V. A 16-item short form identified 85% of the aphasic and 76% of the nonaphasic brain damaged patients, screen-ing as well as Part V of the 62-item long form but not quite as well as the entire long form. These data sug-gest that, for screening, either Part V or a short form of the Token Test will usually be adequate. Patients who achieve a borderline score on one of these shorter forms of the test should be given the entire test to clar-ify the equivocal findings. Age-corrected norms have been developed for the MAE version (Ivnik, Malec, Smith, et al., 1996).

TABLE 13.3 Adjusted Scores and Grading Scheme for the "Short Version" of the Token Test

CONVERSION OF RAW SCORES TO ADJUSTED SCORES		SEVERITY GRADES FOR ADJUSTED SCORES	
For Years of Education	*Change Raw Scores By*	*Score*	*Grade*
3–6	+1	25–28	Mild
10–12	−1	17–27	Moderate
13–16	−2	9–16	Severe
17+	−3	8 or less	Very severe

Adapted from De Renzi and Faglioni (1978)

A "Short Version" of the Token Test (De Renzi and Faglioni, 1978). This 36-item short version takes half the time of the original test and is therefore less likely to be fatiguing. It differs from others in the inclusion of a sixth section, Part 1, to lower the test's range of difficulty. The new Part 1 contains seven items requir-ing comprehension of only one element (aside from the command, "touch"); e.g., "1. Touch a circle"; "3. Touch a yellow token"; "7. Touch a white one." To keep the total number of items down, Part 6 has only 13 items (taken from the original Part 5), and each of the other parts, from 2 through 5, contains four items (see the double-numbered items of Table 13.1 and its footnote). On the first five parts, should the patient fail or not respond for five seconds, the examiner returns misplaced tokens to their original positions and repeats the command. Success on the second try earns half a credit. The authors recommend that the earned score be adjusted for education (see Table 13.3). The adjusted score that best differentiated their control subjects from aphasic patients was 29, with only 5% of the control subjects scoring lower and 7% of the patients scoring higher. A scheme for grading auditory comprehension based on the adjusted scores (see Table 13.3) is offered for making practical clinical discriminations. De Renzi and Faglioni reported that scores below 17 did distin-guish patients with global aphasia from the higher-scoring ones with Broca's aphasia.

VERBAL EXPRESSION

. . . sudden fits of inadvertency will surprise vigilance, slight avocations will seduce attention and casual eclipses will darken learning; and that the writer shall often in vain trace his memory at the moment of need, for that which yesterday he knew with intuitive readi-ness, and which will come uncalled into his thoughts tomorrow.

Samuel Johnson

Tests of confrontation naming provide information about the ease and accuracy of word retrieval and may also give some indication of vocabulary level. Individually administered tests of word knowledge typically give the examiner more information about the patient's verbal abilities than just an estimate of vocabulary level. Responses to open-ended vocabulary questions, for example, can be evaluated for conceptual level and complexity of verbalization. Descriptions of activities and story telling can demonstrate how expressive deficits interfere with effective communication and may bring out subtle deficits that have not shown up on less demanding tasks.

Naming

Confrontation naming, the ability to pull out the correct word at will, is usually called *dysnomia* when impaired. The left temporal lobe is essential for this task in most right-handers (Hamberger et al., 2001). Lesions of the posterior superior temporal and inferior parietal regions are associated with semantic paraphasic errors, while lesions of the insula and putamen contribute to phonologic paraphasic errors (Knopman, Selnes, Niccum, and Rubens, 1984). Repetitive transcranial magnetic stimulation over the temporal lobe can facilitate picture naming (Mottaghy et al., 1999). The speech-dominant hippocampus also is a significant component of the overall neuroanatomical network of visual confrontation naming (Sawrie, Martin, et al., 2000). Dysnomia is usually a significant problem for aphasic patients. In its milder form, dysnomia can be a frustrating, often embarrassing problem that may accompany a number of conditions—after a concussion or with multiple sclerosis, for example.

Two months after being stunned with a momentary loss of consciousness when her car was struck from behind, a very bright doctoral candidate in medical sociology described her naming problem as "speech hesitant at times—I'm trying to explain something and I have a concept and can't attach a word to it. I know there's something I want to say but I can't find the words that go along with it."

In neurological examinations, confrontation naming is typically conducted with body parts and objects beginning with the most frequently used terms (e.g., *hand, pen*) and then asking for the name of the parts, thus going from the most frequently used name to names less often called upon in natural speech (e.g., *wrist* or *joint, cap* or *clip*) (e.g., Strub and Black, 2000). In formal aphasia and neuropsychological assessment, pictures are the most usual stimulus for testing naming facility. The examination of patients with known or suspected aphasia may also include tactile, gestural, and nonverbal sound stimuli to evaluate the naming process in response to the major receptive channels (Rothi, Raymer, et al., 1991).

Kremin (1988), noting that most confrontation naming tasks assess only nouns, recommended asking for verbs and prepositions to delineate the nature of the naming deficit for more accurate diagnosis. Identifying activities, shown in line drawings, with the appropriate verb appears to be a slightly easier task for intact adults than naming objects (M. Nicholas, Obler, Albert, and Goodglass, 1985). A little loss of retrieval efficiency for older adults in the 70s was documented on this task. The Boston Diagnostic Aphasia Examination has a number of activity pictures for just this purpose. Picture sets containing only very common objects are unlikely to prove discriminating when examining suspected or early dementia patients (Bayles and Tomoeda, 1983; Kaszniak, Wilson, et al., 1986).

For picture naming, Snodgrass and Vanderwart's 1980 set of 260 pictures has norms for "name agreement, image agreement, familiarity, and visual complexity." A.W. Ellis and his colleagues (1992) provided a list of 60 picture items taken from the Snodgrass and Vanderwart collection, arranged both according to frequency of occurrence in English and in sets of three. Each word in a set contains the same number of syllables but differs according to its frequency (high, medium, low), thus enabling the examiners to make up naming tasks suitable for particular patients or research questions. The vulnerability of object names to retrieval failure is related to the age of acquisition of the names, with later acquisition (usually less commonly used words) associated with more errors (B.D. Bell, Davies, Hermann, and Walters, 2000; Hodgson and Ellis, 1998).

Boston Naming Test (BNT) (E.F. Kaplan, Goodglass, and Weintraub, 1983; Goodglass and Kaplan, 2001)

This test consists of 60 large ink drawings of items ranging in familiarity from such common ones as "tree" and "pencil" at the beginning of the test to "sphinx" and "trellis" near its end. Adults begin with item 30 and proceed forward unless they make a mistake in the first eight items, at which point reverse testing is continued until eight consecutively correct responses are obtained. The test is discontinued after eight consecutive failures. When giving this test to patients with dementia or suspected dementia, K. Wild (personal communication, 1992 [mdl]) recommends the following instructions: "I'm going to show you some pictures and your job is to tell me the common name for them. If you can't think of the name and it's something you know you can tell me something you know about it." She advises that semantic cueing be conservative to assess for perceptual errors. When patients are unable to name a drawing, the examiner gives a semantic cue; if still unable to give a correct name, a phonetic cue is provided (e.g., for *pelican,* "it's a bird," "pe"). The examiner notes how often cues are needed and which ones are successful. The cueing procedure lacks clinical utility when studying some nonaphasic patients: the effect of phonemic cueing was similar for patients with Alzheimer's disease, temporal lobe epilepsy, and normal control subjects (Randolph, Lansing, et al., 1999).

An item review of responses from 1383 adults ranging from 17 to 97 years from diverse parts of the United States showed that alternative responses, some of which are accepted synonyms, were common for four items (see Table 13.4) (D. Goldstein et al., 2000). The frequency with which these alternative responses were given varied according to age, education, race, and geographic region. For example, 16% of African Americans called the "harmonica" a "harp." Accepting these substitutions as correct resulted in small but significantly improved scores for 175 individuals. No practice effect was observed at one-year retest intervals (Mitrushina and Satz, 1995b; see also McCaffrey, Duff, and Westervelt, 2000b).

The number of recent studies offering normative data attests to the test's popularity: Heaton, Avitable, et al., 1999 (full adult age range); Ivnik, Malec, Smith, et al., 1996 (age range 56–95+); T.P. Ross et al., 1995 (age range 70–80+); Tombaugh and Hubley, 1997 (full adult age range); L.W. Welch et al., 1996 (age range 60–93). Mitrushina, Boone, and D'Elia (1999) present a comprehensive compilation of 19 norm sets, most for late middle-age to elderly persons.

The revised edition has a 15-item short version as well as the standard 60-item picture set. A new multiple-choice format for recognition testing can be used when items are missed. The examiner reads four printed choices for the patient to select the one that matches the drawing. Nine error types are coded. Since the same picture set is used in the 2001 edition, the examiner need only find the set of norms most suitable (by demographic characteristics) for the patient at hand.

Test characteristics. No appreciable score decline appears to occur until the late 70s when the drop is slight, although standard deviations increase steadily from the

60s on, indicating greater variability in the normal older population (T.P. Ross et al., 1995; Van Gorp, Satz, et al., 1986; L.W. Welch et al., 1996). More than just the score changes, though, Obler and Albert (1985) described qualitatively different response features that increase in frequency with aging, such as comments about the test or an item, circumlocutions describing the picture without naming it, and responses to dotted line drawings which provide context to the target stimulus (e.g., a boy portrayed by dotted lines on solid line stilts). These changes are not obvious until the 70s; 30-year-olds and 50-year-olds do not differ in scores or qualitative responses on the BNT (M.S. Albert, Heller, and Milberg, 1988). However, older people are less likely to make phonologically similar errors than young adults. While educational level is a contributing variable, particularly for older persons, sex is a weak variable, producing mixed results (Randolph, Lansing, et al., 1999; Spreen and Strauss, 1998; L.W. Welch et al., 1996). High correlations with verbal ability tests have also been reported (e.g., $r = .83$ with the Gates-MacGinitie Reading Test [Form K 7–9] [Hawkins et al., 1993]; $r = .65$ with WAIS-R Vocabulary [Killgore and Adams, 1999]). Hawkins and his coworkers found that normal control subjects whose reading vocabulary was at a twelfth-grade level or lower performed *below normal limits* when evaluated by the meager 1983 edition norms (five age levels for 84 adults, range 18 to 59 years).

Neuropsychological findings. This test effectively elicits naming impairments in aphasic patients (Margolin, Pate, et al., 1990). Aphasic patients make significantly more perseveration errors than do patients with right hemisphere damage, with a greater tendency for those with posterior lesions to perseverate than those with lesions confined to the frontal lobes (Sandson and Albert, 1987). Although this test was designed for the evaluation of naming deficits, Edith Kaplan recommends using it with patients with right hemisphere damage, too. She notes that, particularly for patients with right frontal damage, some of the drawings elicit responses reflecting perceptual fragmentation (e.g., the mouthpiece of a harmonica may be reinterpreted as the line of windows on a bus!).

The BNT is also widely used in dementia assessment as a sensitive indicator of both the presence and the degree of deterioration. Alzheimer patients have both lexical retrieval deficits and semantic deficits (Laine, Vuorinen, and Rinne, 1997). They tend to name a superordinate category instead of the target word (e.g., "boat" instead of "canoe") (Lukatela et al., 1998). An analysis of error types shows that mildly impaired Alzheimer patients are likely to make significantly

TABLE 13.4 The Most Frequent Alternative Responses to Boston Naming Test Items

Test Item	Alternative Responses
Mask	False face, Face
Pretzel	Snake, Worm
Harmonica	Harp, Mouth organ
Stilts	Tom(my) walkers, Walking sticks, Sticks

Adapted from D. Goldstein et al. (2000)

lower scores than age-matched controls as they have difficulty inhibiting visually or phonologically incorrect responses (Chosak Reiter, 2000). However, unlike stroke patients, in dementia patients PET scanning did not demonstrate any regular association between poor performance on the BNT and lateralized metabolic dysfunction (Parks, Duara, et al., 1987). Patients with vascular dementia also have naming difficulties (Chosak Reiter, 2000); Laine et al., 1997; Lukatela et al., 1998).

Not surprisingly, naming deficits occur in patients with left hippocampal damage (K.G. Davies et al., 1998a). The BNT is effective in identifying word-finding problems in multiple sclerosis patients (Lezak, Whitham, and Bourdette, 1990) and following mild head trauma (Lezak, 1991). These latter groups of patients, who are more likely to have difficulty giving the correct word due to problems with retrieval rather than loss of stored information, often benefit greatly from cueing. The number of words recalled on phonemic cueing can provide a useful indicator of the degree to which verbal retrieval problems interfere with everyday conversation. Randolph, Lansing, and their colleagues (1999) report that phonemic cueing increased correct responses by an average of 4.2 responses for normal control subjects in the 50–83+ age range. Tombaugh and Hubley (1997; also in Mitrushina, Boone, and D'Elia, 1999) offer a comprehensive stratified table which gives averages for spontaneous responses (SR) alone and with stimulus cues (SR + SC), and with phonemic cues (SR + SC + PC). Subtracting (SR + SC) from (SR + SC + PC) gives the amount of expected gain from phonetic cueing for normal control subjects (see Table 13.5). When patients in the younger age group with adequate educational backgrounds give two or three or more correct responses with phonemic cueing, a retrieval problem should be suspected.

Short versions ranging from 15 to 30 items have been used with reasonable clinical sensitivity (Fastenau, Denburg, and Mauer, 1998; N.J. Fisher et al., 1999). When used as part of the CERAD (Consortium to Establish a Registry for Alzheimer's Disease) battery, only the same 15 words—representing the full range of difficulty—are given at a time, thus allowing for brief repeated examinations (J.C. Morris, Heyman, et al., 1989). Even this short form is sensitive to the presence and severity of dementia (Lansing et al., 1999; Larrain and Cimino, 1998; W.J. Mack et al., 1992). A Korean version of a 60-item naming test has been developed (Kim and Na, 1999).

Visual Naming Test (Benton, Hamsher, and Sivan, 1994)

This 30-item confrontation naming test is in the Multilingual Aphasia Examination. The normative adult sample consisted of 360 individuals ranging in age from 16 to 69. Schum and Sivan (1997) extended the norms for well-educated elders (ages 70 to 90) who show very little change in score with advanced age. Urban African-American normative data run below those for whites (R.J. Roberts and Hamsher, 1984). In an educationally diverse sample of 100 men, education accounted for 13% of the variance (Axelrod, Ricker, and Cherry, 1994). This test has a strong ($r = .86$) concurrent validity with the Boston Naming Test (Axelrod et al., 1994). A Spanish version contains translations of most of the original items with substitution of more culturally familiar items where appropriate (E.F. Kaplan, Goodglass, and Weintraub, 1986; G.J. Rey, Feldman, Hernandez, et al., 2001).

Graded Naming Test (GNT) (McKenna and Warrington, 1980)

This 30-item test was designed so that early items would be correctly named by most adults and the final ones would be so difficult that many normal people would fail them. As such, education would be expected to influence performances. The 100 people of *average* intelligence in the standardization sample with an age range from 18 to 77 had a mean score of 20.4 ± 4.1 (Warrington, 1997). Normative data for an older sample (ages 70 to 90) have been reported for New Zealanders (J.A. Harvey and Siegert, 1999). A mean score of

TABLE 13.5 Normal Boston Naming Test Score Gain with Phonemic Cueing

Score (percentiles)	AGE			
	25–69		70–88	
Education	9–12 (n = 78)	13–21 (n = 70)	9–12 (n = 45)	13–21 (n = 26)
90	+1	0	+1	+1
75	+2	+1	+1	+2
50	+3	+2	+3	+2
25	+3	+3	+5	+5
10	+5	+5	+7	+8

Data calculated from Tombaugh and Hubley (1997)

14 for patients with mild Alzheimer's disease was significantly below the performance of demographically matched control subjects (S.A. Thompson et al., 2002).

Other naming tests

The tests described above involve object naming. Proper name retrieval has also been studied. Many older people report difficulty in quick recall of names of familiar persons. Arguably, this is a more difficult task as proper names have an arbitrary link with their reference. A few studies have compared the retrieval of proper names with object names. A 71– to 84-year-old group had no more difficulty in recalling names of people compared to object names than a younger (53 to 63) age group (Maylor, 1997). Relative to normal subjects, mild Alzheimer patients had more difficulty naming famous people based on information than on pictures (Semenza, Borgo, et al., 2000). Rarely, patients with focal lesions have a selective impairment for proper names (Lucchelli and De Renzi, 1992).

Other forms of category-specific naming difficulties have been reported. Warrington and Shallice (1984) studied four patients who showed a specific disability for naming living things and foods compared to inanimate objects. A naming test consisting of 60 items belonging to one of six categories (fruits, vegetables, animals, furniture, vehicles, and tools) was used to study the naming deficit in seven survivors of herpes simplex encephalitis (Barbarotto et al., 1996) and a patient anomic for objects but not names of familiar people (F. Lyons et al., 2002). Four of the seven herpes patients were significantly more impaired on the animal category. The *Category Specific Names Test* (McKenna, 1998) has four categories (animals, fruits/vegetables, man-made objects requiring an action [such as a wallet], and man-made objects not associated with a specific action [e.g., a barometer]) with normative data for 400 adults.

The *Action Naming Test* (Obler and Albert, 1979) was designed to study verb naming. Its 55 line drawings of actions range from common (e.g., *running*) to less common (e.g., *knighting*). Normal subjects (age range from 30s to 70s) correctly named more than 90% of the items (Ramsay et al., 1999). Elderly participants named significantly fewer items than younger ones. In a comparison of object and action naming in older adults, 14 items from both the Boston Naming Test and the Action Naming Test were matched for level of difficulty (Mackay et al., 2002). Similar age-related declines in naming showed up on each task. Alzheimer patients have difficulty with both action and object naming but less for naming actions when items from both categories are matched for word frequency (D.J.

Williamson et al., 1998). Based on a study of patients who had anterior temporal lobectomies for seizure control, L.H. Lu and colleagues (2002) postulated that the left temporal lobe is important for activating nouns and verbs that had human action attributes, such as "tools" or "dialing." The *Object and Action Naming Battery* assesses naming of 162 objects and 100 actions (Druks and Masterson, 1999).

Vocabulary

Vocabulary level has long been recognized as an excellent guide to the general mental ability of intact, well-socialized persons. Vocabulary tests have proven equally valuable in demonstrating the effects of dominant hemisphere disease. This dual function has placed vocabulary tests among the most widely used of all mental ability tests, whether alone or as part of test batteries.

Vocabulary (Wechsler, 1955, 1981, 1997a)

The individually administered vocabulary test in most common use throughout the world consists of 40 words (following the 1955 WAIS format) and some of its translations (e.g., Chinese), 35 in the WAIS-R and other translations (e.g., Czech), and 33 in its 1997 reincarnation. The words are listed in order of difficulty. The examiner reads the question, "What does ____ mean?" The easiest word on the list is "bed," but the administration usually begins with the fourth word, "winter," which practically all adults can define. The test continues until the subject fails five (WAIS, WAIS-R) or six (WAIS-III) words consecutively or until the list is exhausted. The most difficult word on the WAIS-R and WAIS-III is "tirade," item 36 of the WAIS. One or two points are given for each acceptable definition, depending on its accuracy, precision, and aptness. Thus, the score reflects both the extent of recall vocabulary and the effectiveness of speaking vocabulary.

Vocabulary normally takes 15 to 20 minutes to administer, and about five minutes to score, which makes it the most time-consuming of the WIS tests by far (L.C. Ward et al., 1987). In clinical practice, particularly with easily fatigued brain impaired patients, the high time cost of administering Vocabulary rarely compensates for the information gain it affords. Vocabulary is often omitted from assessments using WIS-A tests because the information it adds is redundant when the other verbal tests have been given. Even with reduced item formats (e.g., WAIS-III), Vocabulary takes longer than any other of the verbal tests to administer and score. A vocabulary test can be included in a paper-and-pencil battery or a picture vocabulary test substituted for patients unable to read or write (see pp. 516–517).

Test characteristics.[1] Vocabulary score performances tend to peak in the middle adult years, rising from the early 20s as more knowledge is acquired and beginning a slow decline in the sixth to seventh decades for all forms (Wechsler, 1955, 1981, 1997a). Using an identical testing format (Stanford-Binet, Form L-M), Storck and Looft (1973) noted that synonyms are the most common form of response among normal adults, but their frequency tends to decrease a little in the sixth or seventh decade. Definitions in terms of descriptions, use, or demonstrations are relatively uncommon, except among children, and explanations—although also not commonly given—tend to increase in frequency gradually throughout the adult years.

However, education affects Vocabulary scores to a much greater extent than age (Malec, Ivnik, Smith, et al., 1992a), particularly for older persons who tend to have had less schooling (A.S. Kaufman, Reynolds, and McLean, 1989). Older subjects are the only ones for whom urban/rural differences show up, favoring urban dwellers (A.S. Kaufman, McLean, and Reynolds, 1988). At least into the early 70s, educational differences may account for most, if not all, later age differences on the WAIS-R standardization (A.S. Kaufman, Kaufman-Packer, et al., 1991). Sex differences are negligible (A.S. Kaufman, Kaufman-Packer, et al., 1991; A.S. Kaufman, McLean, and Reynolds, 1991; W.G. Snow and Weinstock, 1990). African-Americans consistently perform below whites (A.S. Kaufman, McLean, and Reynolds, 1988), but how this may be related to educational differences was not examined. Early socialization experiences tend to influence vocabulary development even more than schooling, so that the Vocabulary score is more likely than WIS-A Information or Arithmetic to reflect the patient's socioeconomic and cultural origins and less likely to have been affected by academic motivation or achievement (Anastasi, 1988; P.E. Vernon, 1979; see also J. Huttenlocher et al., 1991).

A large amount of interscorer disagreement ultimately shows up in the summary scores to which Vocabulary contributes (Verbal Scale IQ, Full Scale IQ) (J.J. Ryan, Prifitera, and Powers, 1983). As one of the three open-ended tests in the "verbal" set of WIS tests, Vocabulary scoring differences may contribute significantly to the (60% to 68%) interscorer disagreements; even though item disagreements may be small, they can add up. However, practice effects are minimal (Mc-

[1]Most of the following data come from WAIS-R studies; WAIS and WAIS-III studies are identified as such.

Caffrey, Cousins, et al., 1995; McCaffrey, Duff, and Westervelt, 2000a). Vocabulary has one of the highest test–retest reliability correlations (Iverson, 2001): for most patient samples, they are in the .78 to .84 range (J.J. Ryan, Georgemiller, et al., 1985), excepting a very low (.38) correlation for schizophrenics, which tells more about the patients than the test (G. Goldstein and Watson, 1989). For normal elderly subjects, retesting after a year produced a reliability coefficient of .71 (W.G. Snow, Tierney, Zorzitto, et al., 1989). Split-half correlations for different age groups for both forms of this test are in the .92 to .96 range (J.J. Ryan, Arb, et al., 2000; Wechsler, 1955, 1981; Zhu et al., 2001). Probably without exception, factor analytic studies locate Vocabulary on a Verbal factor, reflecting its invariably high intercorrelations with the three other distinctively verbal tests in the WIS battery—Information, Comprehension, and Similarities (The Psychological Corporation, 1997; L.C. Ward, Ryan, and Axelrod, 2000). As WAIS Vocabulary and Information tests correlated at virtually identical levels with a variety of both verbal and nonverbal tests, indicating that they measure essentially the same abilities, Feingold (1982) suggested that either can be used as a best single ability measure (except, of course, with speech- and language-impaired patients) and that when used together, one of them is redundant.

Neuropsychological findings. When brain injury is diffuse or bilateral, Vocabulary tends to be among the least affected of the WIS battery tests (McFie, 1975; Zillmer, Waechtler, et al., 1992). Thus it also holds up relatively well in early dementia (Melvold et al., 1994; E.V. Sullivan, Sagar, et al., 1989) but, like all else, will eventually decline (R.G. Morris and Kopelman, 1992). The quality of responses given by Alzheimer patients deteriorates with an increased frequency of inferior explanations and generally less precision than responses made by older persons whether depressed or not (Houlihan et al., 1985). Like all other highly verbal tests, Vocabulary is relatively sensitive to lesions in the left hemisphere (Parsons, Vega, and Burn, 1969). Among the WIS battery verbal tests, however, Vocabulary is generally not one of those most depressed by left hemisphere damage (McFie, 1975; Zillmer, Waechtler, et al., 1992). Patients with right hemisphere damage may tend to give verbosely elaborated and not infrequently circumstantial definitions.

A Vocabulary variant. The Wechsler Adult Intelligence Scale-Revised as a Neuropsychological Instrument (WAIS-R NI) provides a multiple-choice list for the 35 Vocabulary words, each with five alternatives, which the subject reads, giving a verbal response

(E. Kaplan, Fein, et al., 1991). Among each set of choices are one 2-point definition, a 1-point definition, and three 0-point definitions, including one that is phonetically similar to the test item word. This format is particularly helpful for patients with word retrieval problems who can recognize but not bring up spontaneously the correct definition.

Paper-and-pencil vocabulary tests

Single paper-and-pencil vocabulary tests are rarely used. Most of the time, the assessment of vocabulary takes place as part of an academic aptitude test battery, a reading test battery, or one of the multiple test guidance batteries. One single vocabulary test that has been used in numerous neuropsychological studies is the 80-word Mill Hill Vocabulary Scale (Raven, 1982). This multiple-choice test takes relatively little time to administer and is easily scored. Mill Hill raw scores convert to percentiles and a standard score (expressed as a "deviation IQ" score [Raven et al., 1976]) for age levels from 20 to 65. This well-standardized test has proven sensitivity to left hemisphere disease (L.D. Costa and Vaughan, 1962) and to dementia (R.G. Morris and Kopelman, 1992). Performance on the Mill Hill was only slightly (5 IQ score points) but significantly diminished in a group of TBI patients mostly tested within six months of injury (D.N. Brooks and Aughten, 1979). No Mill Hill score differences were found between groups of elderly patients with and without diffuse brain disease (Irving, 1971).

The *Gates-MacGinitie Reading Tests* (GMG) are well-suited for clinical evaluations of vocabulary level as they have both a vocabulary and a reading comprehension test presented in a four-choice format (see p. 523). The most recent edition expands the number of formats by including one for adults in addition to the senior high school norms which are applicable for many adult patients.

For research purposes, the *Verbal Comprehension* test of the *Employee Aptitude Survey* (EAS) (Ruch et al., 1963) provides a quick, simple means for assessing vocabulary. The four-choice format contains 30 words ranging in difficulty level from "keen" to "prolix," thus sampling a more mature vocabulary range than similar tests. L.M. Binder, Tanabe, et al., 1982 found that scores remained stable during treatment for cerebrovascular disorders, although some other measures showed improvement with middle cerebral artery bypass. I [mdl] included it in a study on mental efficiency with type II diabetes mellitus under the assumption that, as a vocabulary test, it would be relatively unaffected by disease severity: comparisons were made between one group whose members had newly identified

diabetes, another of diagnosed and treated diabetics, and a healthy control group (U'Ren et al., 1990). However, contrary to expectations, scores on this test did reflect diabetes severity ($p < .001$), which suggested that selecting definitions for these mostly abstract words involves a significant amount of conceptual prowess, at least for persons within the 67–77 year age range.

Nonverbal response vocabulary tests

Vocabulary tests in which patients signal that they recognize a spoken or printed word by pointing to one of a set of pictures permit evaluation of the recognition vocabulary of many verbally handicapped patients. These tests are generally simple to administer. They are most often used for quick screening and for estimating the general ability level of intact persons when time or circumstances do not allow a more complete examination. Slight differences in the design and in standardization populations of the picture vocabulary tests in most common use affect their appropriateness for different patients to some extent.

Peabody Picture Vocabulary Test (PPVT-III)
(L.M. Dunn and Dunn, 1997)

This easily administered vocabulary test has been standardized for ages 2½ to 90+. It consists of 204 picture plates, each with four pictures, one plate for each word in the two reasonably equivalent test forms with the words arranged in order of difficulty. The subject points to or gives the number of the picture most like the stimulus word, which is spoken by the examiner or shown on a printed card. The simplest words are given only to young children and obviously retarded or impaired adults. The PPVT items span both very low levels of mental ability and levels considerably above average adult ability. Care should be taken to enter the word list at the level most suitable for the subject so that both basal (the highest six consecutive passes) and ceiling (six failures out of eight) scores can be obtained with minimal effort. Points for passed items are simply counted and entered into tables giving a standard score equivalent, percentile rank, stanine, and an age equivalent score. A Spanish version is available from the PPVT publisher.

The standardization for the current revision of the PPVT is based on a sample of 2,725 subjects drawn from different regions and occupational groups according to representation in the 1994 U.S. Census. Split-half and alternate form reliabilities were .94 (L.M. Dunn and Dunn, 1997). A study of adults found correlations of the PPVT-R (L.M. Dunn and Markwardt,

1981) with the WAIS-R VIQ score of .82 and .78 for Forms L and M respectively, with much lower correlations with the PIQ score (.46, .38) (Stevenson, 1986). Correlational studies between the original 1965 version of the PPVT and a number of other cognitive tests plus education found WAIS-R Vocabulary to be the only important contributor to PPVT variance (J.K. Maxwell and Wise, 1984). This research appears to reflect the essentially verbal nature of this test. Stevenson (1986) also found that PPVT-R mean scores ran consistently lower than did WAIS-R summation scores. The next edition, PPVT-III, underestimated the *superior* WIS-A scores in one study of college students (N.L. Bell et al., 2001).

Since administration begins at a level near that anticipated for a subject, this test goes quickly and, as such, may be a useful instrument for estimating mental ability levels generally. Although PPVT scores are often interpreted as representing premorbid intelligence, patients with lesions of the left hemisphere may have difficulty with this test (A. Smith, 1997). For severely impaired patients, particularly when their ability to communicate has been compromised, this test may give the examiner the best access to the patient's residual vocabulary and fund of information. In addition, the simplicity of the pictures makes it eminently suitable for those brain damaged patients who have so much difficulty sorting out the elements in a complex stimulus that they are unable to respond to the intended problem.

Quick Test (Ammons and Ammons, 1962)[1]

Although billed as an intelligence test from which IQ scores can be derived, this 50-item test primarily examines vocabulary (Swartz, 1985)—but vocabulary used in situational contexts. The subject is shown a card with four pictures: one, for example, depicting a traffic policeman with a whistle to his mouth guarding children on the way to school. As the examiner reads words from the list the subject points to the appropriate picture (e.g., "belt," "pedestrian," and "imperative" go with the policeman picture). Words are scaled in difficulty from "easy," ages six through 18+, to "hard." Its three forms are roughly equivalent. Based on data from ten studies, median correlations with the WAIS VIQ, Information, and Vocabulary tests were .82, .82 and .83 (Feingold, 1982). This test may underestimate the mental ability of the brightest subjects but is quite accurate for persons in the *average* ability ranges (Traub and Spruill, 1982). M.B. Acker and

Davis (1989) found that scores on this test contributed significantly to predictions of outcome for TBI patients almost four years later as measured by both degree of independence and level of community activity. Taken together, these studies recommend the Quick Test for rapid screening of verbal ability.

Discourse

Story telling

Pictures are good stimuli for eliciting usual speech patterns. The *Cookie Theft* picture from the Boston Diagnostic Aphasia Examination (Goodglass and Kaplan, 1983b) is excellent for sampling propositional speech since the simple line drawing depicts familiar characters (e.g., mother, mischievous boy) engaged in familiar activities (washing dishes) in a familiar setting (a kitchen). Patients' stories about this picture can help differentiate the types of language impairment of different aphasic groups (Ardila and Rosselli, 1993). Alzheimer patients have difficulty in describing the central meaning of stories and tend to focus on less important details (S.B. Chapman et al., 1995).

Describing activities

Open-ended questions about patients' activities or skills also elicit samples of their normal speech. I [mdl] have asked patients to describe their work (e.g., "Tell me how you operate a drill press"), a behavior day ("Beginning with when you get up, tell me what you do all day"), or their plans (see *Script Generation* [pp. 620–621] for a formalized procedure to elicit patients' descriptions of familiar activities). While these questions may enable the examiner to learn about the patient's abilities to plan and carry out activities, they do not allow for much comparison between patients (e.g., How do you compare a farmer's description of his work with that of a sawmill worker who pulls logs off of a conveyor belt all day?). Moreover, the patient's work may be so routine or work plans so ill-formulated that the question does not elicit many words. De Renzi and Ferrari (1978) solved the problem of comparability for their Italian population by asking men to describe how they shave and women how to cook spaghetti. "Tell me how to make scrambled eggs" is a counterpart of the spaghetti question that most Americans can answer. L.L. Hartley and Jensen (1991) instructed their patients to explain how to buy groceries in an American supermarket. I [mdl] ask patients what they like to cook and then have them tell me how to make it, or I may ask men to describe how to change a tire. Borod, Rorie, and their colleagues (2000) asked patients to recollect

---

[1]This test can be obtained from Psychological Test Specialists, Box 9229, Missoula, MT 59807.

emotional and nonemotional experiences. Interestingly, emotional content enhanced discourse of left hemisphere lesioned patients and suppressed performance when the lesion was on the right.

Verbal Fluency

Following brain injury, many patients experience changes in the speed and ease of verbal production. Greatly reduced verbal productivity accompanies most aphasic disabilities, but it does not necessarily signify the presence of aphasia. Impaired verbal fluency is also associated with frontal lobe damage (R.W. Butler, Rorsman, et al., 1993; Janowsky, Shimamura, Kritchevsky, and Squire, 1989), particularly the left frontal lobe anterior to Broca's area (Baldo, Shimamura, Delis et al., 2001; B. Milner, 1975; Tucha et al., 1999). Stuss, Alexander, and their coworkers (1998) found that patients with left dorsolateral and/or striatal lesions were the most significantly impaired on a letter fluency task. Lesions restricted to the inferior medial area of the frontal lobes did not produce impairment. However, patients with superior medial frontal lesions of either left or right hemisphere had moderate impairment. Fluency also diminished with left parietal lesions. Patients with left frontal lesions perform poorly on verb generation tasks as well (Thompson-Schill et al., 1998). In keeping with these clinical data, the frontal lobes show increased activation on imaging studies during fluency tasks (Brannen et al., 2001; Warkentin and Passant, 1993).

Reductions in fluency may occur in patients with diffuse brain injury. In TBI patients, reduced verbal fluency is associated with both measures of severity (coma and PTA duration) and computed tomography suggesting that diffuse axonal injury is a major contributor to the cognitive inflexibility reflected in their poor fluency performances (Vilkki, Holst, Öhman, et al., 1992).

A fluency problem can show up in speech, reading, and writing; generally, it will affect all three activities (Perret, 1974; L.B. Taylor, 1979) and both free and responsive speech (Feyereisen et al., 1986). However, with aging, writing fluency tends to slow down much earlier than speech fluency, which healthy persons maintain well into the 70s (Benton and Sivan, 1984). Problems in word generation are prominent among the verbal dysfunctions of dementia.

Fluency of speech

Fluency of speech is typically measured by the quantity of words produced, usually within a restricted category or in response to a stimulus, and usually within a time limit. Almost any test format that provides the opportunity for unrestricted speech will test its fluency. Fluency has been measured by rate of speech production as well as word counts of spoken responses to pictures, to directed questions, or to questions stimulating free conversation (Feyereisen et al., 1986; L.L. Hartley and Jensen, 1991).

As Estes (1974) suggested, word fluency tests provide an excellent means of finding out whether and how well subjects organize their thinking. He pointed out that successful performance on these tests depends in part on the subject's ability to "organize output in terms of clusters of meaningfully related words." He also noted that word-naming tests indirectly involve short-term memory in keeping track of what words have already been said. Fluency tests requiring word generation according to an initial letter give the greatest scope to subjects seeking a strategy for guiding the search for words and are most difficult for subjects who cannot develop strategies of their own. Examples of effective strategies are use of the same initial consonant (e.g., content, contain, contend, etc.), variations on a word (shoe, shoelace, shoemaker), or variations on a theme (sew, stitch, seam). Fluency tests calling for items in a category (e.g., animals, what you find in a grocery store) provide the structure lacking in those asking for words by initial letter. However, even within categories, subjects to whom strategy-making comes naturally will often develop subcategories for organizing their recall. For example, the category "animals" can be addressed in terms of domestic animals, farm animals, wild animals, or birds, fish, mammals, etc.

Laine (1988) defined two kinds of conceptual clustering appearing as two or more successive words with similar features: *phonological clusters* share the same initial sound group for letter associates (*salute, salvage* for *S*) or the same initial sound for animals (*baboon, beaver*); and *semantic clusters* in which meanings are either associated (soldier, salute) or shared (salt, sugar). When a cluster is exhausted, the subject must efficiently switch to a new one (Troyer, Moscovitch, and Winocur, 1997).

Age (particularly for persons over 70), sex, and education have been found to influence performance on these tests (Benton, Hamsher, and Sivan, et al., 1994), with women's performances holding up increasingly better than men's after age 55. Some studies have found no age differences on letter fluency tasks (D. Hughes and Bryan, 2002) but positive age effects appear on semantic fluency, e.g., "animals" (Troyer, 2000). In Troyer's study, advancing age was associated with slightly larger cluster sizes and fewer category switches. In evaluating fluency performances, premorbid ability levels need also be taken into account (Crawford,

Moore, and Cameron, 1992), and especially educational and vocational accomplishments.

Controlled Oral Word Association (COWA) (Benton and Hamsher, 1989; Spreen and Strauss, 1998)

Benton and his group have systematically studied the oral production of spoken words beginning with a designated letter. The associative value of each letter of the alphabet, except *X* and *Z*, was determined in a normative study using normal control subjects (Borkowski et al., 1967; see Table 13.6). Control subjects of low ability tended to perform a little less well than brighter brain impaired patients. These findings highlight the necessity of taking the patient's premorbid verbal skill level into account when evaluating verbal fluency (Crawford, Moore, and Cameron, 1992).

The Controlled Oral Word Association test (first called the *Verbal Associative Fluency Test* and then the *Controlled Word Association Test*) consists of three word-naming trials. The set of letters that were first employed, F-A-S, has been used so extensively that this test is sometimes labelled "F-A-S." The version developed as part of Benton and Hamsher's (1989) Multilingual Aphasia Examination provides norms for two sets of letters, C-F-L and P-R-W. These letters were selected on the basis of the frequency of English words beginning with these letters. In each set, words beginning with the first letter of these two sets have a relatively high frequency, the second letter has a somewhat lower frequency, and the third letter has a still lower frequency. In keeping with the goal of developing a multilingual battery for the examination of aphasia, Benton and Hamsher also give the frequency rank for letters in French, German, Italian, and Spanish. For example, in French the letters P-F-L have values comparable to C-F-L. The COWA is one of three tests in the *Iowa Screening Battery for Mental Decline* (Eslinger, Damasio, and Benton, 1984; see p. 691). The FAS version is part of the Neurosensory Center Comprehensive Examination for Aphasia.

To give the test, the examiner asks subjects to say as many words as they can think of that begin with the given letter of the alphabet, excluding proper nouns, numbers, and the same word with a different suffix.

TABLE 13.6 Verbal Associative Frequencies for the 14 Easiest Letters

	WORDS/MINUTE		
	9–10	*11–12*	*>12*
Letters	A C D G	B F L M	P
	H W	R S T	

From Borkowski et al. (1967)

TABLE 13.7 Controlled Oral Word Association Test: Adjustment Formula for Males (M) and Females (F)

Education (Years Completed)	AGE (YEARS)					
	25–54		*55–59*		*60–64*	
	M	F	M	F	M	F
<9	9	8	11	10	14	12
9–11	6	5	7	7	9	9
12–15	4	3	5	4	7	6
≥16	—	—	1	1	3	3

Adapted from Benton, Hamsher, and Sivan (1994)

The Multilingual Aphasia Battery version also provides for a practice trial using the very high frequency letter "S." The practice trial ends when the subject has volunteered two appropriate "S" words. This method allows the examiner to determine whether the subject comprehends the task before attempting a scored trial. (The practice trial I [mdl] give lasts one minute to provide a genuine "warm-up"). The score, which is the sum of all acceptable words produced in the three one-minute trials, is adjusted for age, sex, and education (see Table 13.7). The adjusted scores can then be converted to percentiles (see Table 13.8). In addition, the examiner counts both errors (i.e., rule violations such as nonwords, proper nouns) and repetitions (noting whether they are repetitions, true perseverations, or variations on the just previously given word, e.g., "look," "looking," the latter word being a rule violation). Repeated words that count as repetitions do not occur successively but are evidence of an impaired ability to generate words and keep track of earlier responses simultaneously. A greater number of words is usually produced early compared to later in the trial. Fernaeus and Almkvist (1998) suggest scoring the first and second halves of each one-minute trial separately. Although this pattern holds for Parkinson patients, the COWA performance that best distinguished them from

TABLE 13.8 Controlled Oral Word Association Test: Summary Table

Adjusted Scores	Percentile Range	Classification
53+	96+	Superior
45–52	77–89	High normal
31–44	25–75	Normal
25–30	11–22	Low normal
23–24	5–8	Borderline
17–22	1–3	Defective
10–16	<1	Severe defect
0–9	<1	Nil–Trace

Adapted from Benton, Hamser, and Sivan (1976)

control subjects was fewer words produced in the first 15 sec (Fama, Sullivan, Shear, et al., 1998).

Spreen and Strauss (1998) give means and standard deviations for different age and educational groups. Tombaugh, Kozak, and Rees (1999) report means and standard deviations for large normal samples ranging from 20 to 89 years with percentiles stratified by age and education. Norms are also available stratfied for education and sex (Ruff, Light, Parker, and Levin, 1996); for age, education, and ethnicity (African American and Caucasian: Gladsjo, Schuman, et al., 1999); and for age and ethnicity (African American, Hispanic, and Caucasian: Johnson-Selfridge et al., 1998). Sumerall and his colleagues (1997) provide data about qualitative errors in an elderly sample (70–95) without neurologic or psychiatric disease: perseverations (23% repeated the same word within 30 sec., 28% repeated the same word after 30 sec, and 40% repeated a word stem with a different ending), breaking set (4.3% gave words in which the first letter differed from the one required), and *proper noun* (13% gave one or more). Only subjects ages 81–95 and with fewer than 15 years' education broke set. Age did not affect productivity. (See Mitrushina, Boone, and D'Elia [1999] for a compilation of earlier norm sets.) Metanorms based on data from 32 studies with a total of 17,625 scores provide a "Summary of aggregate statistics for FAS Totals" giving means and standard deviations by sex, for four age groups (<40, 40–59, 60–79, 80–95) and for two education levels (0–12, >12) (Loonstra et al., 2001). Since variability at lower educational levels tends to be wide (e.g., Loonstra and her colleagues found the SD for 0–12 years = 13.09, for >12 = 12.37), the performances of persons with less education, particularly levels below high school, must be interpreted with caution.

Test characteristics. While mean scores for less educated older subjects slowly slide from a 50–54 year high (which at 41.52 does not differ from younger groups nor from their better educated age peers), means remain about the same for those with 13+ years of schooling until the 75+ years when the mean drops by an apparently nonsignificant amount (Spreen and Strauss, 1998). The performances of men and women do not differ (Ruff, Light, Parker, and Levin, 1996; Sarno, Buonaguro, and Levita, 1985; Zec, Andrise, et al., 1990).

On retesting elderly persons after one year, only the letter *A* (of the FAS set) had a reliability coefficient below .70 or .71, which were the reliability levels for the other letters and the total score, respectively (W.G. Snow, Tierney, Zorzitto, et al., 1988). COWA performance had a moderate correlation with WIS-A Digit Span (.45) and Vocabulary (.41), but practically inconsequential correlations with memory (.17 to .22)

and figural fluency (.24) (Ruff, Light, Parker, and Levin, 1997). Comparing the first and second halves of the one-minute productions, initial responses related to Digit Span and memory free recall, while later responses were related to WIS-A Information, Similarities, and Vocabulary (Fernaeus and Almkvist, 1998). These researchers concluded that initial responses depended on rapid access of words from semantic memory with very little effort, while late productions depended on strategies for effortful searching of semantic memory.

Neuropsychological findings. Word fluency as measured by FAS, COWA, and similar techniques calling for generation of word lists has proven to be a sensitive indicator of brain dysfunction. Frontal lesions, regardless of side, tend to depress fluency scores, with left frontal lesions resulting in lower word production than right frontal ones (Miceli et al., 1981; Perret, 1974; Ramier et Hécaen, 1970). Benton (1968) found that not only did patients with left frontal lesions produce on the average almost one-third fewer FAS words than patients with right frontal lesions, but those with bilateral lesions tended to have even lower verbal productivity. Patients with left dorsolateral and superior medial frontal lobe lesions switched categories less frequently but produced normal cluster sizes (Troyer, Moscovitch, Winocur, et al., 1998a). Although both left and right temporal lobe partial resections for seizure control produced declines in COWA performance in the days following surgery, one year later performance exceeded preoperative levels for both groups (Loring, Meador, and Lee, 1994). Left temporal lobe epilepsy (N'Kaoua et al., 2001), multiple sclerosis (Matotek et al., 2001), and mild TBI (Raskin and Rearick, 1996) are often associated with deficits on letter fluency tests. Reduced capacity to generate words has been associated with every dementing process, although the underlying defect tends to vary (Tröster, Fields, et al., 1998; Troyer, Moscovitch, Winocur, et al., 1998b). In some conditions mental inflexibility seems to make an important contribution to the naming disorder (e.g., in some patients with Parkinson's disease); in others, semantic processing and recall abilities are impaired (e.g., Alzheimer's disease). Lexical–phonological functions are compromised in left hemisphere stroke patients. Performances on this test did not differentiate elderly depressed patients from those with diagnosed dementia (R.P. Hart, Kwentus, Taylor, and Hamer, 1988).

Category fluency

Category fluency is less difficult than letter fluency for adults. Whereas elderly control subjects generate about 12 to 16 words/min for letter fluency, animal fluency averages for control subjects range from 20.95 (50 to 59 age range) to 18.96 (70 to 79 age range) (e.g., see Mitrushina, Boone, and D'Elia, 1999). Even control subjects in their 80s produced more animals than FAS words (Koroza and Cullum, 1995). Category fluency declines with age (Fama, Sullivan, Shear, et al., 1998). Using the categories of animals, fruits, and vegetables, normative data stratified by language, age, sex, and education are available for well-educated elder (Lucas et al., 1998a) and for English and Spanish speakers living in the United States (Acevedo et al., 2000). In a study of four ethnic groups, Hispanics and African Americans named the fewest animals, Chinese and Vietnamese the most (Kempler et al., 1998). The authors suggested that variations in word lengths among languages contributed to these findings.

Patients with frontal lobe lesions have reduced letter and category fluency, which is consistent with the theory that they have deficent retrieval strategies (Baldo and Shimamura, 1998). Alzheimer patients have more difficulty with category fluency than letter fluency (Fama, Sullivan, Shear, et al., 1998), an impairment usually attributed to a breakdown in semantic knowledge about categories (Monsch, Bondi, Butters, et al., 1994). Using optimal cut-off scores, category fluency was superior (100% sensitivity, 90.9% specificity) to letter fluency (81.8% sensitivity, 84.1% specificity) in correctly differentiating Alzheimer patients from control subjects. Parkinson patients also have more difficulty with category than letter fluency compared to control subjects (Fama, Sullivan, Shear, et al., 1998). Monsch and her colleagues (1994), finding that Huntington patients were equally impaired on both types of tasks, suggested that their failures were due to reduced general initiation and/or retrieval capacities. However, another study reported that Huntington patients were relatively more impaired on categories (Baldo and Shimamura, 1998).

When both animal and letter naming tasks were used to compare dementia and depression effects on verbal fluency, depressed patients' better animal naming scores distinguished the two patient groups, although even on this easier task the depressed patients' output was inferior to that of the control subjects (R.P. Hart, Kwentus, Taylor, and Hamer, 1988). Compared to control subjects, category production of right brain damaged patients may be a little lower than their letter production and they tend to produce fewer clusters, perhaps due to reduced ability to develop semantic strategies (Joanette et al., 1990).

Other categories have been used to study verbal fluency. Examining the nature of the naming deficits of Parkinson, Huntington, and Alzheimer patients, Randolph, Braun, and their colleagues (1993) used "name things found in a supermarket" along with subcategory cues (e.g., "fruits and vegetables," "things people drink"); the subcategory cueing aided the Parkinson and Huntington patients substantially, but not those with Alzheimer's disease. In addition to the more usual fruit and vegetable naming task, Fuld (1980) asked her elderly subjects to name happy and sad events and found that, contrary to the usual pattern, depressed subjects named more sad than happy events. Other categories that have been used to examine fluency are "types of transportation" and "parts of a car" (Weingartner, Burns, et al., 1984). Studying the effect of set on the verbal productions of patients with Korsakoff's psychosis, Talland (1965a) asked his subjects to "name as many different things as you can that one is likely to see in the street." A 17 person control group (WAIS Vocabulary $M = 10$) averaged 15.7 street sights.

Action fluency

Subjects are instructed to "tell me as many different things as you can think of that people do. I don't want you to use the same word with different endings, like 'eat,' 'eating,' 'eaten.' Also, just give me single words, such as 'eat' or 'smell,' rather than a sentence. Can you give me an example of something that people do?" (Piatt et al., 1999). Parkinson patients were compared with elderly subjects on three fluency tasks: animal naming, FAS, and verb generation. Parkinson patients without dementia and control subjects generated more verbs than FAS words, but patients with dementia had disproportionate difficulty with action fluency. Yet others have reported impaired action fluency in Parkinson patients without dementia (Peran et al., 2003).

Writing fluency

Thurstone Word Fluency Test (TWFT) (L.L. Thurstone and Thurstone, 1962). A written test for word fluency first appeared in the *Thurstones' Primary Mental Abilities* tests (1938, 1962). Subjects must write as many words beginning with the letter S as they can in five minutes, and then write as many four-letter words beginning with C as they can in four minutes. The average 18-year-old can produce 65 words within the nine-minute total writing time. Adult norms are available (Heaton, Grant, and Matthews, 1991). B. Milner (1964, 1975) found that the performance of patients with left frontal lobectomies was significantly impaired on this test relative to that of patients with left temporal lobectomies whose frontal lobes remained intact, and to that of patients whose surgery was confined to the right hemisphere. She observed that this task is more discriminating than object naming fluency tests because the writing task, particularly for C words, is harder. This pattern of relative impairments (frontal output < nonfrontal, left < right hemisphere, left frontal < right frontal) showed up among patients with brain damage due to many different etiologies (Pendleton, Heaton, Lehman, and Hulihan, 1982). Those patients with diffuse damage (trauma and degenerative diseases) performed much like the frontal patients. In a validity study, patients with many kinds of brain injuries performed below control subjects' levels, but the test did not discriminate anterior from posterior lesions, left from right hemisphere lesions, or focal from diffuse lesions; test–retest reliability was high (M.J. Cohen and Stanczak, 2000).

Quantity of writing content

Clinical observations that many patients with right hemisphere damage tend to be verbose led to speculation that these patients may use more words when writing than do other persons (Lezak and Newman, 1979). The number of words used to answer personal and WAIS-type questions, complete the stems of a sentence completion test, and write interpretations to proverbs and a story to Thematic Apperception Test (TAT) card 13MF was counted for 29 patients who had predominantly right hemisphere damage, 15 whose damage was predominantly in the left hemisphere, 25 with bilateral or diffuse damage, and also for 41 control subjects hospitalized for medical or surgical care. On a number of these items, proportionately more patients with predominantly right hemisphere damage gave very wordy responses than patients with other types of brain damage or the control patients. This phenomenon appeared most clearly on the open-ended questions of the sentence-completion test and a personal history questionnaire, neither of which required much conceptual prowess or writing skill. On proverb interpretations and the TAT story, education level played the greatest role in determining response length except for the tendency of the left brain damaged group to give the shortest responses to proverbs.

Quality of writing

At the suggestion of David Spaulding, I [dbh] often ask dementia patients to write "Help keep America clean" on an unlined sheet of paper. This brief writing-to-dictation task gives an opportunity to observe spelling, use of capitalization, and orthographic skills as well as planning in the use of space on the page. More complex tasks offer an opportunity to examine grammar, syntax, and organization of thought processes. Croisile, Ska, and their associates (1996b) compared moderately demented Alzheimer patients' oral and written descriptives of the BDAE Cookie Theft picture, scoring for total number of words and their subtypes (nouns,

adjectives, etc.), lexical errors, syntactic complexity, grammatical errors, amount of information, implausible details, and irrelevant comments. Oral descriptions were longer than written ones for both patients and control subjects. Oral descriptions proved to be more sensitive to word-finding difficulty in Alzheimer patients, while written descriptions showed a greater reduction in number of functor words and more implausible details. In addition, Alzheimer patients made more spelling errors.

Speed of writing

Talland (1965a) measured writing speed in two ways: speed of copying a 12-word sentence printed in one-inch type and speed of writing dictated sentences. On the copying task, his 16 control subjects averaged 33.9 seconds for completion, taking less time ($p < .05$) than patients with Korsakoff's psychosis. No significant score differences distinguished control subjects from patients in their speed of writing a single 12-word sentence. However, when writing a 97-word story, read to them at the rate of one to two seconds per word, the control subjects averaged 71.1 words within the three-minute time limit, whereas the patient group's average was 53.1 ($p < .02$). When writing speed has been slowed by a brain disorder, the slowing may become more evident as the length of the task increases. Moreover, the amount of time it took to write the word "television" with the nonpreferred hand differentiated neurologically normal and abnormal schizophrenic patients better than 30 other measures, mostly taken from the standard Halstead-Reitan Battery (G. Goldstein and Halperin, 1977). These investigators acknowledged being at a loss to explain this finding and wondered whether the task's sensitivity might be a function of its midrange level of complexity. Writing times in the range of 6.6 and 5.7 seconds were reported for the schizophrenic patients without neurological disease studied by Goldstein and Halperin and for medicated epileptics (R. Lewis and Kupke, 1992), respectively. Nondominant hand times tend to run just about twice as long as times for the dominant hand, suggesting that pronounced deviations from this pattern may reflect unilateral brain damage.

The Repeatable Cognitive-Perceptual-Motor Battery includes a test of writing speed, *Sentence Writing Time,* which requires subjects to write "The large dog runs fast" (Kelland and Lewis, 1994; R. Lewis, Kelland, and Kupke, 1990). They report a mean writing time of 7.4 ± 1.4 sec for 40 persons (20 of each sex) in the 18–to 30 year range. Writing time ranges for older age groups ran from 7.8 ± 1.3 for 33 subjects 45–59 years old to 11.0 ± 3.3 for 38 subjects age 70 and over. Administration of diazepam to healthy volunteers did not affect their writing time as measured by this test.

VERBAL ACADEMIC SKILLS

With the exception of aphasia tests, surprisingly few neuropsychological batteries contain tests of learned verbal skills such as reading, writing, spelling, and arithmetic. Yet impairment in these commonplace activities can have profound repercussions on a patient's vocational competence and ultimate adjustment. It can also provide clues to the nature of the underlying organic condition.

Reading

Reading may be examined for a number of reasons: to obtain a general appraisal of reading ability in patients without a distinctive impairment of reading skills; to evaluate comprehension of verbal material; for diagnostic purposes, particularly with patients who are aphasic or have significant left hemisphere involvement; or for fine-grained descriptions of very specific deficits for research or treatment purposes. Diagnosis and fine-grained descriptions require specialized knowledge that is usually available from speech pathologists or reading specialists who are also well acquainted with the appropriate test instruments. Cognitive neuropsychologists studying reading aberrations frequently devise their own examination techniques, designed for the specific problem or patient under study (e.g., see Baddeley, Logie, and Nimmo-Smith, 1985; Coslett, 2003; McCarthy and Warrington, 1990; Rapp et al., 2001).

Examiners are cautioned about evaluating reading ability on the basis of the multiple-choice questions for the reading passages in the Boston Diagnostic Aphasia Examination or the Western Aphasia Battery (L.E. Nicholas et al., 1986). Both control subjects and aphasic patients answered considerably more than half the items correctly (far beyond 25% correct by chance) without reading the passages, simply on the basis of inherent meaningfulness. TBI patients earned almost as high scores without reading the BDAE and WAB passages as after reading them (Rand et al., 1990). The paragraph in the Minnesota Test for Differential Diagnosis of Aphasia is so difficult that normal control subjects answered only 80% of the sentences correctly (L.E. Nicholas et al., 1986).

Gates-MacGinitie Reading Tests (GMRT), 4th ed. (MacGinitie, MacGinitie, Maria, and Dreyer, 2000)

These are academic skill tests that lend themselves to neuropsychological assessment. Although these paper-and-pencil multiple-choice tests come in separate forms for each year from Pre-Reading to sixth grade, three will be appropriate for most adults: grade 7/9, grade 10/12, and AR (Adult Reading).

The Gates-MacGinitie tests measure two different aspects of reading. The first subtest, *Vocabulary*, involves simple word recognition. The last subtest, *Comprehension*, measures ability to understand written passages. Both Vocabulary and Comprehension scores tend to be lower when verbal functioning is impaired. When verbal functions remain essentially intact but higher-level conceptual and organizing activities are impaired, a marked differential favoring Vocabulary over Comprehension may appear between the scores of these two subtests. The two tests have generous time limits. They can be administered as untimed tests without much loss of information since most very slow patients fail a large number of the more difficult items they complete outside the standard time limits.

SRA Reading Index (Science Research Associates, 1968)

This multiple-choice reading test provides brief assessments of five levels of reading skill: (1) *Picture–Word Association* (nine items) requires the subject to recognize the word that goes with a picture of a common object (*cow, car*); (2) *Word Decoding* (13 items) asks the subject to identify the one-word definition or description that completes short, incomplete sentences such as, "Apples grow on a . . . "; (3) in *Phrase Comprehension* (13 items) the subject must complete a sentence by choosing the correct phrase among similar phrases which differ in such aspects of grammar as prepositions or adverbs; (4) *Sentence Comprehension* (12 items) presents a sentence with four similar sentences, of which only one gives the target sentence's meaning correctly; (5) *Paragraph Comprehension* (13 items) consists of three sets of explanatory paragraphs (e.g., one gives the rules for a card game), each followed by a number of questions about the material it contains. This untimed test reportedly takes intact adults about 25 minutes to complete. With a vocabulary level that is quite basic, the breakdown into levels of reading skills may offer useful insights when reading impairment reflects neuropsychological dysfunction. Normative data are keyed to a variety of mostly blue-collar occupations, such as electrician or heavy equipment operator.

Reading Index-12 tests reading ability up to the 12th grade. Like the Reading Index, it is in a multiple-choice format. Its 72 items ask for comprehension of written materials ranging in length from phrases to paragraphs. Normative data are provided for workers in office/clerical and manufacturing positions.

Understanding Communication (T.G. Thurstone, 1992)

This reading comprehension test comprises 40 statements consisting of one to three sentences with the final wording incomplete. Four one-word or short phrase choices are offered to complete each statement, of which one makes good sense. As the test progresses, the statements become more difficult due to greater ideational complexity and more demanding vocabulary. Norms are provided for the 15-minute time limit, but examiners interested in how well patients slowed by brain dysfunction perform should allow them to complete as many items as they can. When performance on this test drops significantly below measured vocabulary level, the possibility of impaired reasoning and/or verbal comprehension may be considered.

National Adult Reading Test (NART) (H.E. Nelson and O'Connell, 1978); *National Adult Reading Test, 2nd ed. (NART-2)* (H.E. Nelson and Willison, 1991)

The NART list consists of 50 phonetically irregular words (see Table 13.9). Correct pronunciation of these words implies prior knowledge of them. This test is often used to estimate premorbid mental ability in adults because vocabulary correlates best with overall ability level and is relatively unaffected by most nonaphasic brain disorders (see pp. 92–94, 515). However, until recently, little direct evidence existed to support the assumption that current reading vocabulary is a good measure of prior intellectual ability. To assess whether NART scores correspond to premorbid mental ability, Crawford, Deary, and colleagues (2001) compared NART scores of a group of older adults (mean age 77 years) without dementia to their scores on an intelligence test taken at age 11 and found a high (.73) correlation. In contrast, NART scores had only a modest (.25) correlation with current MMSE scores in this group.

TABLE 13.9 The National Adult Reading Test

Ache	Subtle	Superfluous	Gouge	Beatify
Debt	Nausea	Radix	Placebo	Banal
Psalm	Equivocal	Assignate	Facade	Sidereal
Depot	Naive	Gist	Aver	Puerperal
Chord	Thyme	Hiatus	Leviathan	Topiary
Bouquet	Courteous	Simile	Chagrin	Demesne
Deny	Gaoled	Aeon	Detente	Labile
Capon	Procreate	Cellist	Gauche	Phlegm
Heir	Quadruped	Zealot	Drachm	Syncope
Aisle	Catacomb	Abstemious	Idyll	Prelate

Adapted from H.E. Nelson and O'Connell (1978)

Crawford (1992) and his colleagues conducted a series of studies in the United Kingdom on which they found that the NART IQ score correlates significantly with education ($r = .51$) and (not surprisingly) social class ($r = .36$); the $-.18$ correlation with age, while significant, accounted for practically none of the variance (Crawford, Stewart, Garthwaite, et al., 1988). There do not appear to be sex effects (Schlosser and Ivison, 1989). Scoring for errors, the Crawford group found a split-half reliability coefficient of .90 (Crawford, Stewart, Garthwaite, et al., 1988), interrater reliability coefficients between .96 and .98, and test–retest reliability coefficients of .98 (Crawford, Parker, Stewart, et al., 1989). In a factor analytic study combining the NART and the WAIS, they extracted a first factor, which they identified as "Verbal Intelligence", on which the NART error score had a high ($-.85$) loading (Crawford, Stewart, Cochrane, et al., 1989). In other studies comparing the NART and the WAIS IQ scores, they found that the NART predicted 72% of the VIQ variance but only 33% of the PIQ (Crawford, Parker, Stewart, et al., 1989). A correlation with demographic variables was .70 (Crawford, Allan, Cochrane, and Parker, 1990). These workers use the NART in conjunction with demographic variables for estimation of premorbid ability in deteriorating patients (Crawford, Cochrane, Besson, et al., 1990; Crawford, Nelson, et al., 1990; see also pp. 95–96).

When dementia patients have language disturbances, this procedure will underestimate premorbid ability (Stebbins, Gilley, et al., 1990; Stebbins, Wilson, et al., 1990). Alzheimer patients' reading problems were demonstrated by their decline in NART scores when examined annually over three years; the extent of decline was greatest for those with initially low Mini-Mental State Examination scores (Cockburn, Keene, et al., 2000). While NART scores do show a decrement with dementia severity, this decline is mild compared to measures of cognitive function showing marked declines (Maddrey et al., 1996). Although Spreen and Strauss (1998) recommend against using this kind of test with patients who are aphasic, dyslexic, or who have articulatory or visual acuity defects, Schlosser and Ivison (1989) pointed out that this test's sensitivity to the language deterioration in Alzheimer's disease may make it an effective early predictor of dementia.

NART variants. A short NART uses only the first half of the word list to avoid distressing patients with limited reading skills who can only puzzle through the more difficult half of the test (Crawford, Parker, Allan, et al., 1991). This format predicted WAIS IQ scores almost as well as the full word list (see p. 93).

North American Adult Reading Test (NAART, NART-R) (Blair and Spreen, 1989)[1]

This 61-word version of the NART has been modified for appropriateness for North American subjects, providing both U.S. and Canadian pronunciation guides as needed (see pp. 92–93). Twelve words from the NART generally unfamiliar to readers of North American English were replaced with 23 words more common to North Americans. Excellent interscorer reliability is reported and internal consistency is high. Like the NART, this instrument predicts WAIS-R VIQ well but not PIQ. In a large sample of healthy, well-educated adults ranging in age from 18 to 91 years, education was much more strongly related to performance than was age (Uttl, 2002). NAART scores increased with age up to 60 years and then leveled off. The correlation between NART scores and WAIS-R Vocabulary was .75. In this sample, 35 items were sufficient to predict WAIS-R Vocabulary reliably. This short version was recommended when time is limited.

American NART (AMNART) (Grober and Sliwinski, 1991)

A modification of the NART for American readers consists of 27 words from the British version and 23 new irregular American words of comparable frequency to the ones that were replaced. Grober and Sliwinski (1991) removed five words that had very low item-total correlations (see p. 93). Like the NART, this instrument predicts WAIS-R VIQ well but not PIQ.

Reading Subtest of the Wide Range Achievement Test–Revised (WRAT-R) (Jastak and Wilkinson, 1984), Wide Range Achievement Test 3 (WRAT3) (G.S. Wilkinson, 1993)

This test begins with letter reading and recognition at Level I (for children) and continues with a 75-word (WRAT-R) or 84-word (WRAT3) reading and pronunciation list. At Level II, Reading involves only the word list. The latest revision provides two forms (each a 42-item split-half) to facilitate retesting. The time limit for each response is 10 sec. The test is discontinued after ten failures. WRAT3 norms cover ages 5 to 75, but the highest WRAT-R age is "45 and over." For the WRAT3, normative data are available for the two split-half versions as well as the full 84-word list. African Americans matched for education with whites had scores about 5 points lower (Manly, Jacobs,

Touradji, et al., 2002). For the WRAT3 normative sample, correlations with WAIS-R Vocabulary was .62. WRAT-R Reading and NART correlations are strong (.82) (Wiens, Bryan, and Crossen, 1993). No sex effects were found for a group of healthy participants ages 15 to 70 years (Klimczak et al., 2000).

The word pronunciation format of this test is identical to that of the NART, but it was developed to evaluate educational achievement rather than to assess premorbid ability. Both this test and the NART are based on the same assumptions: that familiar words will be pronounced correctly, and familiarity reflects vocabulary. It is further assumed in the WRAT that reading vocabulary provides a valid measure of reading ability. However, word recognition is not the same as reading comprehension; thus this test gives only a rough measure of academic achievement. Spreen and Strauss (1998) caution against using it for academic evaluations. It has not been used much in neuropsychological research protocols. One study did find a moderate association between right temporal lesions and poor performance, and a little weaker but significant association between right parietal lesions and poor performance on this test (Egelko, Gordon, et al., 1988).

A multiple-choice version, the Wide Range Achievement Test-Expanded Version (Robertson, 2002), adds a reading comprehension test in a multiple-choice format designed for children and adults up to age 24. Reading passages include selections from textbook, recreational, and other sources, designed to test word meaning in context as well as literal and inferential reading skills.

Reading Subtest of the Kaufman Functional Academic Skills Test (K-FAST) (A.S. Kaufman and Kaufman, 1994a)

This brief 34-item test assesses reading as it relates to everyday activities such as reading signs, understanding labels on medicines, and following directions in a recipe. The normative sample was a group of 1,434 people ages 15 to 85+. No sex effects were found for a 15 to 70 year-old group (Klimczak et al., 2000). Scores strongly correlated (.82) with WRAT3 Reading in this healthy sample. Whites performed slightly better than African Americans (T.H. Chen et al., 1994).

Writing

Normal writing can be carried out only if a highly complex group of cortical zones remains intact. This complex comprises practically the whole brain and yet forms a highly differentiated system, each component of which performs a specific function . . . writing can

[1]The word list, pronunciation guide, and administration instructions are given in Spreen and Strauss (1998).

be disordered by circumscribed lesions of widely different areas of the cerebral cortex, but in every case the disorder in writing will show qualitative peculiarities depending on which link is destroyed and which primary defects are responsible for the disorder of the whole functional system.

Luria, 1966, pp. 72–73

Qualitative aspects of writing may distinguish the script of patients whose brain damage is lateralized (A. Brodal, 1973; Hécaen and Marcie, 1974). Patients with right hemisphere lesions tend to repeat elements of letters and words, particularly seen as extra loops on *m, n,* and *u,* and to leave a wider than normal margin on the left-hand side of the paper (A.W. Ellis, 1982; Roeltgen, 2003). Left visuospatial inattention may be elicited by copying tasks (see Fig. 10.8, p. 385). Difficulty in copying an address by patients with left visual inattention was significantly associated with right temporal lesions (Egelko, Gordon, et al., 1988). Generally, patients with left hemisphere lesions are more likely to have a wide right-sided margin, and they tend to leave separations between letters or syllables that disrupt the continuity of the writing line. Edith Kaplan has also noted that, frequently, aphasic patients will print when asked to write (personal communication, 1982 [mdl]). Different contributions of cortical regions to writing become apparent in the variety of writing disorders observed in patients with focal left hemisphere lesions (Coslett, Gonzalez, Rothi, et al., 1986; Roeltgen, 2003; Roeltgen and Heilman, 1985). Benson (1993) observed that "Almost every aphasic suffers some degree of agraphia." He therefore recommended that writing ability be examined by both writing to dictation and responsive writing (e.g., "What did you do this morning?").

Writing tests allow the examiner to evaluate other dysfunctions associated with brain damage, such as a breakdown in grammatical usage, apraxias involving hand and arm movements, and visuoperceptual and visuospatial abilities (Roeltgen, 2003). With brain disease, alterations in writing size (e.g., micrographia in Parkinson's disease) or writing output (diminished in dementia, increased in some conditions) may also occur. Figure 13.1 shows an attempt to write (*a*) "boat" and (*b*) "America" by a 72-year-old man with Alzheimer's disease of moderate severity and prominent apraxia. This difficulty in forming letters despite being able to spell the words orally is a form of apraxic agraphia.

In studying the writing disturbances of acutely confused patients, Chédru and Geschwind (1972) described a three-part writing test which shares some items with the Boston Diagnostic Aphasia Examination: (1) writing to command, in which patients were told to write a sentence about the weather and a sen-

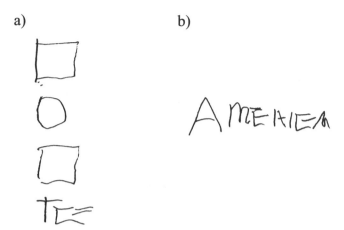

FIGURE 13.1 Alzheimer patient's attempt to write (*a*) "boat" and (*b*) "America."

tence about their jobs; (2) writing to dictation of words (business, president, finishing, experience, physician, fight) and sentences ("The boy is stealing cookies." "If he is not careful the stool will fall."); and (3) Copying a printed sentence in script writing ("The quick brown fox jumped over the lazy dog."). They found that patients' writings were characterized by dysgraphia in the form of motor impairment (e.g., scribbling), spatial disorders (e.g., of alignment, overlapping, cramping), agrammatisms, and spelling and other linguistic errors. Moreover, dysgraphia tended to be the most prominent and consistent behavioral symptom displayed by them. The authors suggested that the fragility of writing stems from its dependence on so many different components of behavior and their integration. They also noted that for most people writing, unlike speaking, is far from being an overlearned or well-practiced skill. Signatures, however, are so overpracticed that they do not provide an adequate writing sample.

When asked to write a description of "everything that is happening" in the Cookie Theft picture of the Boston Diagnostic Aphasia Examination, the responses of dementia patients were highly correlated (−.76) with ratings of dementia severity (J. Horner, Heyman, et al., 1988). Writing samples were scored according to (1) overall organization, relevance, and continuity of the writing; (2) vocabulary completeness and accuracy of word usage; (3) grammatical completeness and accuracy; (4) spelling accuracy; and (5) mechanics and legibility of writing, e.g., form, accuracy, and placement of letters and words. Evaluations were based on the sum of these scores.

Spelling

Poor spelling in adults can represent the residuals of slowed language development or childhood dyslexia, of poor schooling or lack of academic motivation, or of bad habits that were never corrected. Additionally, it may be symptomatic of adult-onset brain dysfunction. Thus, in evaluating spelling for neuropsychological purposes, the subject's background must be taken into account along with the nature of the errors. Both written and oral spelling should be examined because they can be differentially affected (McCarthy and Warrington, 1990).

Spelling Subtest of the Wide Range Achievement Test-Revised (WRAT-R) (Jastak and Wilkinson, 1984), Wide Range Achievement Test 3 (WRAT3) (Wilkinson, 1993)

This subtest calls for written responses. Young children begin with name and letter writing. The WRAT-R list consists of 46 words; the WRAT3 has 80. Normative data are available for two split-half versions of the WRAT3 containing 40 words each. The test is discontinued depending upon the subject's spelling skills. Following each word reading the examiner also reads a sentence containing the word. Fifteen seconds is allowed for each word. Ten failures is the criterion for discontinuing. No means for analyzing the nature of spelling errors is provided.

Johns Hopkins University Dysgraphia Battery (R.A. Goodman and Caramazza, 1985)

This test was developed to clarify the nature of spelling errors within the context of an information processing model (Margolin and Goodman-Schulman, 1992). It consists of three sections: I. *Primary Tasks* includes (A) Writing to dictation of material varied along such dimensions as grammatical class, word length, word frequency, and nonwords; and (B) Oral spelling. In II. *Associated Tasks,* the subject (C) writes the word depicted in a picture, (D) gives a written description of a picture, and (E, F) copies printed material either directly or as soon as it is withdrawn from sight. The subject's errors are evaluated in section III, *Error Coding,* according to one of 11 different kinds of error along with scoring categories for "Don't know" and "Miscellaneous errors." Margolin and Goodman-Schulman give examples of how these procedures can help to explicate different kinds of dysgraphic disorder.

Knowledge Acquisition and Retention

Information (Wechsler, 1955, 1981, 1997a)

Although many tests of academic achievement examine general knowledge, Information is the only one that has been incorporated into neuropsychological assessment batteries and research programs almost universally. The Information items test general knowledge normally available to persons growing up in the United States. WIS-A battery forms for other countries contain suitable substitutions for items asking for peculiarly American information. The items are arranged in order of difficulty from the four simplest, which all but severely retarded or organically impaired persons answer correctly, to the most difficult, which only few adults pass. Some Information items were dropped over the years because they became outdated. The relative difficulty of others can change with world events; e.g., the increased popular interest in Islamic culture will necessarily be reflected in a proportionately greater number of subjects in 2004 who know what the Koran is than in 1981 when this item was first used. In addition, increases in the level of education in the United States, particularly in the older age groups, probably contribute to higher mean scores on the WAIS-R version of Information and to lower mean scores on the more recently standardized WAIS-III Information (Lezak, 1988c; Quereshi and Ostrowski, 1985; see K.C.H. Parker, 1986, for a more general discussion of this phenomenon).

Administration suggestions. I [mdl] make some additions to Wechsler's instructions. I spell "Koran" after saying it since it is a word people are more likely to have read than heard, and if heard, it may have been pronounced differently. When patients who have not gone to college are given one or more of the last four items, I usually make some comment such as, "You have done so well that I have to ask you some questions that only a very few, usually college-educated, people can answer," thus protecting them as much as possible from unwarranted feelings of failure or stupidity if they are unfamiliar with the items' topics. When a patient gives more than one answer to a question and one of them is correct, the examiner must insist on the patient telling which answer is preferred, as it is not possible to score a response containing both right and wrong answers. I usually ask patients to "vote for one or another of the answers."

Although the standard instructions call for discontinuation of the test after five failures, the examiner may use discretion in following this rule, particularly with brain injured patients. On the one hand, some neurologically impaired patients with prior average or higher intellectual achievements are unable to recall once-learned information on demand and therefore fail several simple items in succession. When such patients give no indication of being able to do better on the increasingly difficult items and are also distressed by their failures, little is lost by discontinuing this task early. If there are any doubts about the patient's inability to answer the remaining questions, the next one or two questions can be given later in the session after the patient has had some success on other tests. On the other hand, bright but poorly educated subjects will often be ignorant of general knowledge but have acquired expertise in their own field, which will not become evident if the test is discontinued according to rule. Some mechanics, for example, or nursing personnel, may be ignorant about literature, geography, and religion but know the boiling point of water. When testing alert persons with specialized work experience and limited education who fail five sequential items not bearing on their personal experience, I usually give all higher-level items that might be work-related.

I have found it a waste of time to give the first few items where the usual administration begins (items 5 to 7, 8, or 9) to well-spoken, alert, and oriented persons with even as little as a tenth grade education. Thus, I begin at different difficulty levels for different subjects. Should a subject fail an item or be unable to retrieve it without the cueing that a multiple-choice format provides (see below), I drop back two items, and if one of them is failed I drop back even further; but having to drop back more than once occurs only rarely.

When giving the Information test to a patient with known or suspected brain dysfunction, it is very important to differentiate between failures due to ignorance, loss of once-stored information, and inability to retrieve old learning or say it on command. Patients who cannot answer questions at levels higher than warranted by their educational background, social and work experiences, and vocabulary and current interests have probably never known the answer. Pressing them to respond may at best waste time, at worst make them feel stupid or antagonize them. However, when patients with a high school education cannot name the capital of Italy or recognize "Hamlet," I generally ask them if they once knew the answer. Many patients who have lost information that had been in long-term storage or have lost the ability to retrieve it, usually can be fairly certain about what they once knew but have forgotten or can no longer recall readily. When this is the case, the kind of information they report having lost is usually in line with their social history. The examiner will find this useful both in evaluating the extent and nature of their impairments and in appreciating their emotional reactions to their condition.

When patients acknowledge that they could have answered the item at one time, appear to have a retrieval problem or difficulty verbalizing the answer, or have a social history that would make it likely they once knew

the answer, information storage can be tested by giving several possible answers to see whether they can recognize the correct one. I always write out the multiple-choice answers so the patient can see all of them simultaneously and need not rely on a possibly failing auditory memory. For example, when patients who have completed high school are unable to recall Hamlet's author, I write out, "Longfellow, Tennyson, Shakespeare, Wordsworth." Often patients identify Shakespeare correctly, thus providing information both about their fund of knowledge (which they have just demonstrated is bigger than the Information score will indicate) and a retrieval problem. Nonaphasic patients who can read but still cannot identify the correct answer on a multiple-choice presentation probably do not know, cannot retrieve, or have truly forgotten the answer. (The WAIS-R NI provides a prepared set of multiple-choice answers.)

The additional information that the informal multiple-choice technique may communicate about the patient's fund of knowledge raises scoring problems. Since the test norms were not standardized on this kind of administration, additional score points for correct answers to the multiple-choice presentation cannot be evaluated within the same standardization framework as scores obtained according to the standardization rules. Nevertheless, this valuable information should not be lost or misplaced. To solve this problem, I use *double scoring*; that is, I post both the age-graded standard score the patient achieves according to the standardization rules and, usually following it in parentheses, another age-graded standard score based on the "official" raw score plus raw score points for the items on which the patient demonstrated knowledge but could not give a spontaneous answer. This method allows the examiner to make an estimate of the patient's fund of background information based on a more representative sample of behavior, given the patient's impairments. The disparity between the two scores can be used in making an estimate of the amount of deficit the patient has sustained, while the lower score alone indicates the patient's present level of functioning when verbal information is retrieved without assistance.

On this and other WIS-A tests, an administration adapted to the patient's deficits with double-scoring to document performance under both standard and adapted conditions enables the examiner to discover the full extent of the neurologically impaired patient's capacity to perform the task under consideration. Effective use of this method involves both testing the limits of the patient's capacity and, of equal importance, standardized testing to ascertain a baseline against which performance under adapted conditions can be compared.

In every instance, the examiner should test the limits only after giving the test item in the standard manner with sufficient encouragement and a long enough wait to satisfy any doubts about whether the patient can perform correctly under the standard instructions.

Test characteristics.[1] Information scores hold up well with aging. When education effects are controlled (by covariance), Information scores stay steady into the 70s (A.S. Kaufman, Kaufman-Packer, et al., 1991; A.S. Kaufman, Reynolds, and McLean, 1989), and for an educationally relatively privileged group, they decline only slightly into the 90s (Ivnik, Malec, Smith, et al., 1992b). Significant sex differences of around 1 scaled score point on all forms of the WIS favor males (A.S. Kaufman, Kaufman-Packer, et al., 1991; A.S. Kaufman, McLean, and Reynolds, 1988; Snow and Weinstock, 1990). Of course, education weighs heavily in performances on this test, accounting for as much as 37 to 38% of the variance in the over-35 age ranges. After controlling for the effects of age, education, and sex, African Americans with traditional African American practices, beliefs, and experiences had significantly lower WAIS-R Information scores than African Americans who were more acculturated (Manly, Miller, et al., 1998). These authors propose that due to their educational and cultural experiences, some African Americans are not routinely exposed to item content on Information. In another study, African Americans obtained mean scores that were $1^1/_2$ to 2 scaled score points below those of whites, but education differences between these two groups were not reported (A.S. Kaufman, McLean, and Reynolds, 1988). Urban subjects over age 55 performed significantly better than their rural age peers, but this difference did not hold for younger people: "Perhaps the key variable is the impact of mass media, television . . . on the accessibility of knowledge to people who are growing up in rural areas" (A.S. Kaufman, McLean, and Reynolds, 1988, p. 238).

Test–retest reliability coefficients mostly in the .76 to .84 range have been reported, varying a little with age and neuropsychological status (Rawlings and Crewe, 1992; J.J. Ryan, Paolo, and Brungardt, 1992; Snow, Tierney, Zorzitto, et al., 1989; see also McCaffrey, Duff, and Westervelt, 2000a), with only a schizophrenic group providing an exceptional correlation coefficient of .38 (G. Goldstein and Watson, 1989). The highest reliabilities (.86–.94) are reported for samples of the normative populations (Wechsler, 1955, 1981, 1997a). Split-half reliability coefficients are high

[1]Most of the following data come from WAIS-R studies.

(.85 to .96) in clinical groups although somewhat lower (.74) in mentally retarded adults (Zhu, Tulsky, et al., 2001). TBI patients who took this test four times within a year did not gain a significantly greater number of score points than did patients who only took the first and last of the test series (Rawlings and Crewe, 1992). Older subjects retested within a half year made a significant but small gain (about 1/2 of a scaled score point) on this test (J.J. Ryan, Paolo, and Brungardt, 1992). In factor analytic studies, Information invariably loads on a Verbal Comprehension factor (see p. 650). Information's high correlations with other mental ability tests led Feingold (1982) to conclude that it can be used alone as a measure of general ability. As could be expected, correlations with measures of executive functioning are minimal (Isingrini and Vazou, 1997).

Information and Vocabulary are the best WIS-A measures of general ability, that ubiquitous test factor that appears to be the statistical counterpart of learning capacity plus mental alertness, speed, and efficiency. Information also tests verbal skills, breadth of knowledge, and—particularly in older populations—remote memory. Information tends to reflect formal education and motivation for academic achievement. It is one of the few tests in the WIS-A batteries that can give spuriously high ability estimates for overachievers or fall below the subject's general ability level because of early lack of academic opportunity or interest.

Neuropsychological findings. Glucose metabolism increases in the left temporal lobe and surrounding areas during this test, with much smaller increases also noted in the right temporal lobe (Chase et al., 1984). In brain injured populations, Information tends to appear among the least affected of the WIS-A tests (Donders, Tulsky, and Zhu, 2001; O'Brien and Lezak 1981; E.W. Russell, 1987). Although a slight depression of the Information score can be expected with brain injury of any kind, because performance on this test shows such resiliency, particularly with focal lesions or trauma, it often can serve as the best estimate of the original ability. In individual cases, a markedly low Information score suggests left hemisphere involvement, particularly if verbal tests generally tend to be relatively depressed and the patient's history provides no other kind of explanation for the low score. Thus, the Information performance can be a fairly good predictor of the hemispheric side of a suspected focal brain lesion (Hom and Reitan, 1984; A. Smith, 1966; Spreen and Benton, 1965). However, contrary to folklore that Information holds up well with dementia, it is actually one of the more sensitive of the WIS verbal tests and appears to be a good measure of dementia severity (Larrabee, Largen, and Levin, 1985; Storandt, Botwinick, and Danziger, 1986).

Information (WAIS-R NI) (E. Kaplan, Fein, et al., 1991). In the initial administration of Information, WAIS-R NI instructions recommend that all items be given unless the subject becomes too discouraged or frustrated. The multiple-choice test is given after the standardized tests. An analysis of item content (into "number facts," "directions and geography," academically related information, and responses requiring names) relates error patterns to possible interpretations of them. Using the multiple-choice technique, subjects in the 50- to 89-year age range averaged one-and-one-half raw score points more than on the standard administration (Edith Kaplan, personal communication, February, 1993 [mdl]). The WAIS-R NI benefit increased with age and was greatest (gain of 2.41 raw score points) for subjects 80–89 years old.

14 | Construction

JILL S. FISCHER AND DAVID W. LORING

Constructional activity combines perception with motor response and inevitably has a spatial component. The integral role of visuoperception in constructional activity becomes evident when persons with more than very mild perceptual deficits encounter difficulty on constructional tasks. Yet some impaired constructional performances occur without any concomitant impairment of visuoperceptual functions. Commonly used constructional tests vary considerably in their level of difficulty and in the demands that they place on other cognitive functions. Because of the complexity of functions that influence performance on a constructional test, numerical scores convey only a limited amount of information about an individual's performance. Careful observation of how patients go about doing constructional tasks and the types of errors they make is necessary to distinguish the possible contributions of perceptual deficits, spatial confusion, attentional impairments, organizational limitations, motor planning difficulties, and motivational problems: the more complex the constructional test, the less likely it is that a specific deficit can be identified.

The concept of constructional functions embraces two large classes of activities—drawing, and building or assembling. The tendency for drawing and assembling impairments to occur together—though significant—is so variable that these two types of activity need to be evaluated separately. There is ample evidence that impaired performance on constructional tests predicts limitations in important activities such as meal planning (Neistadt, 1993) and driving (Gallo et al., 1999; K. Johansson et al., 1996; Marottoli et al., 1994), yet the assessment of visuospatial abilities in clinical practice is often rather cursory. This is in no small part related to the fact that visuospatial functions—and constructional abilities in particular—lack the rich conceptual framework surrounding language abilities. Guérin, Ska, and Belleville (1999) detailed a cognitive neuropsychological model for drawing, but the applicability of this type of model to clinical practice remains to be established.

Awareness that the two cerebral hemispheres differ in their information processing capacities has brought increasing attention to the differences in how patients with unilateral lesions perform constructional tasks. A number of characteristic constructional tendencies of these patients have been described (Benton, 1967 [1985]; J.L. Mack and Levine, 1981; Walsh and Darby, 1999; McCarthy and Warrington, 1990). Patients with right hemisphere dysfunction tend to take a piecemeal, fragmented approach, losing the overall "gestalt" of the constructional task. Although some patients with right hemisphere damage produce very sparse, sketchy drawings, others create highly elaborated pictures that do not "hang together," i.e., drawings that may lack important components (e.g., the pedals on a bike), or that contain serious distortions in perspective or proportions yet simultaneously have a repetitive overdetailing that gives the drawing a not unpleasant, rhythmical quality (see Fig. 6.2, p. 141, for an example). They may even not attend to the left side of a construction or—occasionally—pile up items (e.g., lines in a drawing, blocks, or puzzle pieces) on the left.

When asked to copy a large-scale stimulus—in the shape of a letter, for example—that is made up of many smaller stimuli of a different shape (e.g., global–local stimuli such as those depicted in Fig. 3.8, p. 55), patients with right-sided lesions will typically focus on reproducing the small stimuli without appreciating the larger configuration that they form (Delis, Kiefner, and Fridlund, 1988). Patients with right hemisphere lesions often proceed from right to left on drawing or assembly tests (E. Kaplan, Fein, et al., 1991; Milberg, Hebben, and Kaplan, 1996), in contrast to the more common approach of working from left to right. This is not an infallible indicator of right hemisphere dysfunction, however, because left-handed persons and those whose language is read from right to left often draw figures from right to left as well (Vaid et al., 2002).

In contrast, patients with left-sided lesions may get the overall idea and proportions of the construction correct and their drawings may be symmetric, but they tend to omit details and generally turn out a shabby production. Unlike patients with right hemisphere dysfunction, those with lesions on the left may do better when presented with a model as opposed to drawing to command (Hécaen and Assal, 1970) and their performance will often improve with repetition (Warrington, James, and Kinsbourne, 1966). On a global–local task, these patients will tend to ignore the smaller internal stimuli and focus instead on the larger shape (Delis, Kiefner, and Fridlund, 1988). Thus the frequency of errors does not seem to differentiate patients with left and right hemisphere lesions so much as qualitative features of these errors (Gainotti and Tiacci, 1970; Hécaen and Assal, 1970; McCarthy and Warrington, 1990).

The site of the lesion along the anterior–posterior axis also affects the expression of constructional impairment (F.W. Black and Bernard, 1984; A. Smith, 1980; Walsh and Darby, 1999). While patients with right posterior lesions will, in general, be most likely to have impaired constructional functions, many fewer right hemisphere damaged patients who have anterior lesions display constructional deficits. Drawings made by patients with lateralized subcortical lesions display the same error patterns as those of cortically lesioned patients, but subcortical patients tend to have more widespread deficits (A. Kirk and Kertesz, 1993).

DRAWING

The major subdivisions within this class are copying and free drawing. The overlap between them is considerable, yet many persons whose drawing skills are impaired can copy with reasonable accuracy (Libon, Malamut, et al., 1996; Rouleau et al., 1996). Reverse instances are relatively rare (Messerli et al., 1979). This differential becomes pronounced with advancing age, as copying is relatively unaffected—particularly copying of simple or familiar material—but free drawing shows a disproportionately greater loss of details and organizational quality with aging (Ska, Desilets, and Nespoulous, 1986). Studies of children have shown that drawing ability develops in a predictable sequence—from simple closed geometric shapes, to open (three-dimensional) shapes, to segmented human figures, and finally to complete human figures (Barrett and Eames, 1996). This developmental sequence is useful to keep in mind in evaluating the drawing abilities of patients who may be able to draw simple geometric figures quite competently but then struggle to produce more complex geometric figures or common objects (Trojano and Grossi, 1998).

Drawing tasks have achieved a central position in neuropsychological testing by virtue of their sensitivity to many different kinds of deficits. This sensitivity may be the reason that the discriminating power of drawing tasks at times has assumed mythic proportions. Unfortunately, it has not been uncommon for some psychologists to think that a complete neuropsychological

examination consists of the WIS-A battery and one or two drawing tests, usually the Bender Gestalt and a human figure drawing (e.g., C. Piotrowski and Keller, 1989; C. Piotrowski and Lubin, 1990). Although they are rich sources of data, drawing tests have limits to the amount of information that they can provide. The examiner who uses them needs to remember that every kind of drawing task has been performed successfully by cognitively impaired patients, including some patients with lesions that should have kept them from drawing well. Furthermore, no matter how sensitive these tests might be to perceptual, practic, and certain types of cognitive and motor organization impairment, they still leave many cognitive functions unexamined.

In drawings, the phenomenon of spatial hemi-inattention—more common after right than after left hemisphere lesions—tends to be reflected in the omission of details on the side of the drawing opposite the lesion (see Figs. 3.13, 3.15a, 10.9, pp. 67, 69, 386; Behrmann and Plaut, 2001; Colombo et al., 1976; McCarthy and Warrington, 1990). Frederiks (1963) reported that free drawings (i.e., drawing to command) tend to elicit evidence of inattention more readily than does copying from a model. Patients with unilateral lesions tend to position their drawings on the same side of the page as their lesions, thus underutilizing the side of space that is most susceptible to inattention (Gasparrini et al., 1980; Gur et al., 1977; see Chapter 10, Fig. 10.9). This tendency was much more prominent in patients with left than with right hemisphere lesions, perhaps because those with left-sided damage were more likely to use a smaller part (typically the upper left quadrant and immediately adjacent areas) of the page, whereas patients in the right-lesioned group (whose drawings, both free and copy, tend to be larger than those of patients with left-sided lesions [Larrabee and Kane, 1983]) covered most of the page with their drawings, making the overall shift to the right of the midline less apparent.

When using drawings to test for visuospatial inattention, a complete copy in a single drawing does not rule out the possibility that the patient suffers unilateral inattention, as this phenomenon—particularly in its milder forms and with relatively simple drawings—may not show up consistently (see pp. 385–386). Examining for inattention requires a variety of tests.

When evaluating patients' drawings the integrity of primary visual and motor systems must also be assessed (Beaumont and Davidoff, 1992). The motor competence of the hand used in drawing is also relevant to the quality of the drawing. In contrast to Semenza, Denes, and their colleagues (1978) who found no differences between preferred and nonpreferred hands in the way in which normal subjects approached the task of copying a relatively simple figure, Bush (2000) noted significant differences between clock drawings done by the dominant and nondominant hands of patients on a subacute medical rehabilitation unit.

Copying

Bender-Gestalt Test (L. Bender, 1938; Hutt, 1985)

The *Bender-Gestalt* was one of the first and most widely studied tests of drawing. Conceptual approaches to the interpretation of nonobjective drawings that have evolved out of work on this test can be applied to the evaluation of drawing performances in general. This test, usually referred to as "The Bender," serves not only as a visuoconstructional task for neuropsychological assessment but also as a neuropsychological screening measure and as a projective technique for studying personality. The Bender's quick and easy administration probably contributed to its longstanding position as one of the most widely used psychological tests in the United States (C. Piotrowski and Keller, 1989; C. Piotrowski and Lubin, 1990). Recent surveys suggest that the Bender-Gestalt remains popular among clinical psychologists in independent practice, for whom it is the fifth most frequently used test, but neuropsychologists—who rank it only twenty-fifth in frequency of use—are much less likely to include it now in test batteries than previously (Camara et al., 2000; K. Sullivan and Bowden, 1997).

The Bender material is a set of nine designs originally used by Wertheimer (1923) to demonstrate the tendency of the perceptual system to organize visual stimuli into *Gestalten* (configurational wholes) (see Fig. 14.1). Lauretta Bender assembled these designs (labeled A and 1 through 8) for the study of visuoperceptual and visuomotor development in children, calling this method a "Visual Motor Gestalt Test." She standardized the test on 800 children in the 4–11 age range. Gradually, use of the test was extended from children to adolescents and then to adults.

Reliable evaluation of drawing distortions requires exact reproductions of the test stimuli. If the circles of design 2, for example, are depicted as ovals or the line quality of the model designs is uneven, then the examiner is hard put to decide whether similar distortions in a patient's copy represent distortion or finicking accuracy. Also, if the curves of design 7 do not cross in such a way that the figure can be seen as either two continuous or two overlapping sinusoidal curves, then the examiner cannot find out whether the patient would perceive the original curves in a simplified (uncrossed) or complex (crossed) manner.

Administration. Bender administration begins with the examiner laying three sharpened soft lead pencils with erasers and a small stack of unlined plain white letter-size paper so that the short side faces the patient.

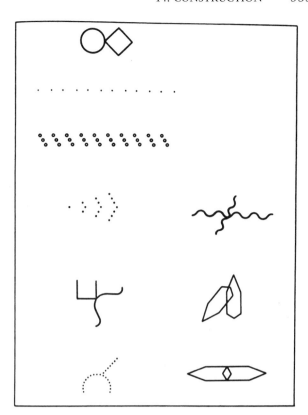

FIGURE 14.1 The Hutt adaptation of the Bender-Gestalt figures. (Hutt, 1977. Reproduced by permission)

Hard pencils tend to resist pressure so that drawing becomes more effortful and the pencil marks are less apt to reflect individual pressure differences in their shading or thickness (these materials are also appropriate for most other drawing tasks). The main purpose of putting out more than one piece of paper is to create a softer drawing surface that will increase ease of drawing and pick up pressure marks on the second sheet. Some patients set aside the top sheet of paper on completion of the first drawing or after three or four drawings. When they do, the examiner can ask them to draw all the designs on the first sheet unless no usable space remains, in which case they should complete the test on the second sheet. Forcing patients to confine their drawings to one or, at the most, two sheets provides one way to see how—or whether—they organize the designs within limited space. When not informed at the outset about placing all the designs on one page some patients will make overly large copies of the first two or three designs despite the following instructions:

I've got nine of these altogether (hold up the pack of cards with the back facing the patient). I'm going to show them to you one at a time and your job is (or "you are") to copy them as exactly as you can. The first card is then placed on the table with its length facing the patient and its edges squared with the edges of the work surface. When patients have finished the first drawing, the second card is placed on top of the first and so on to completion. When all the designs have been copied, patients can be asked to write their name and the date on the paper with no instructions about where these should be placed, and no suggestions if asked.

These instructions afford patients the barest minimum of structure and virtually no information on how to proceed. This method makes it a test of the abilities to organize activities and space as well. By letting subjects know there are nine cards, the examiner gives them the opportunity to plan ahead for their space needs. By not making reference to what is on the cards (e.g., by not calling them "designs"), subjects are less likely to demur or feel threatened because they do not consider themselves "artists." By lining the cards up with the edges of the work surface, the examiner provides an external anchoring point for the angulation of the stimulus so that, should subjects rotate their copy of the design, the examiner knows exactly how much the drawing is angled relative to the original stimulus.

Many subjects need no more instruction than this to complete the test comfortably. Others ask questions about how to draw the figures, whether they can be larger or smaller, have more or fewer dots, need to be numbered, lined up along the edge, or spread over the page, etc. To each of these questions, the answer is, "Just copy the card as exactly as you can." For subjects who continue to ask questions, the examiner should say, "I can only give you these instructions; the rest is up to you." Subjects who ask to erase are given permission without special encouragement. Those who attempt to turn either the stimulus card or the sheet of paper should be stopped before beginning to copy the card when it has been placed at an incorrect or uncommon angle, as the disorientation of the drawing might no longer be apparent when the paper is righted again. The page should not be turned more than is needed for a comfortable writing angle. Total copy usually runs from five to ten min.

In addition to variants of the standard administration, there are a number of other ways to give the test, most of which were developed for personality assessment (Hutt, 1985). Those that enable the examiner to see how well the subject can function under pressure provide interesting neuropsychological data as well. For instance, in the "stress Bender," the patient is given the whole test a second time with instructions to "copy the designs as fast as you can. You drew them in ___ seconds (any reasonable time approximation will do) the first time; I want to see how much faster you can do them this time." The examiner then begins timing ostentatiously. Some patients who can compensate well for mild constructional disabilities when under no pressure will first betray evidence of their problem as they

speed up their performance. Interestingly, many neurologically intact subjects actually improve their Bender performance under the stress condition.

Seeking to increase the sensitivity of this task, McCann and Plunkett (1984) gave three other administrations in addition to the standard one: recall following a 10 sec delay; drawing with the nonpreferred hand; and the "perfect" method, in which subjects are shown their standard administration along with the stimulus cards and asked to make a new copy, correcting any initial errors they find. All of these methods discriminated beyond chance among 30 Korsakoff patients, 30 with paranoid schizophrenia, and 30 healthy control subjects. The "perfect" method proved to be the most sensitive, correctly identifying 93% of the patient group relative to controls, but none of the methods successfully discriminated the two patient groups from each other.

Wepman (personal communication, 1974 [mdl]) incorporated two recall procedures into his three-stage standard administration of the Bender. Each card is shown for five seconds, then removed, and the subject is instructed to draw it from memory. After this, the cards are shown again, one at a time, with instructions to copy them exactly (as in the standard copy administration). In the third stage, the subject is handed another blank sheet of paper and is asked to draw as many of the figures as can be recalled. Wepman viewed difficulty with items 1, 2, 4, and 5 as particularly suggestive of a constructional disorder. He found that healthy subjects typically recall five designs or more, and he considered recall scores under five to be suggestive of brain impairment. Data from others are consistent with Wepman's observations (Lyle and Gottesman, 1977; Pirozzolo, Hansch, et al., 1982; Schraa et al., 1983). My [mdl] experience in giving a 30-min delay trial suggests that, like the delay trial for the Complex Figure, most subjects continue to retain most if not all of what they recalled immediately. Administration and scoring procedures of the many reported studies have not been standardized, leaving important questions unanswered, such as how many designs would be recalled by healthy adults after interference or a delay and how strict the scoring criteria should be.

Scoring systems. Lauretta Bender (1946) conceived of her test as a clinical exercise in which "(d)eviate behavior . . . should be observed and noted. It never represents a test failure." Consequently, she did not use a scoring system. Potential test variables are numerous and equivocal, and their dimensions are often difficult to define. The profusion of scoring possibilities has resulted in many attempts to develop a workable system to obtain scores for diagnostic purposes.

One of the earliest scoring systems for adults was devised by Pascal and Suttell (1951), who viewed deviations in the execution of Bender drawings as reflecting "disturbances in cortical function," whether on a psychiatric or neurological basis. The Pascal-Suttell system identifies 106 different scorable characteristics of the Bender drawings, from 10 to 13 for each figure (excluding A) plus seven layout variables applied to the performance as a whole. With each deviant response given a numerical value, the examiner can compute a score indicating the extent to which the drawings deviate from normal copies. An examiner who knows the Pascal-Suttell system can score most records in two to three minutes. Despite the apparent complexity of the Pascal-Suttell scoring system, a factor analysis by E.E. Wagner and Marsico (1991) found that performance on the Bender-Gestalt was reducible to a single general factor (reproductive accuracy). The highest scores tend to be obtained by patients with known brain disorders, but the considerable overlap between groups of neurologic and psychiatric patients makes differentiation between them on the basis of the Pascal-Suttell score alone very questionable.

Hutt (1985) also examined Bender performance as a whole in designing his 17-factor Psychopathology Scale. Five of Hutt's factors relate to the organization of the drawings on the page and their spatial relationships to one another, four to changes in the overall configuration ("gestalt") of a drawing (i.e., difficulties with closure, crossing, curvature, and angulation), and eight to specific distortions (e.g., fragmentation, perseveration). He identified 11 types of deviations as likely indicators of CNS pathology, particularly if four or more are present in a given patient's record: collision (overlapping) of discrete designs; marked angulation difficulty; severe perceptual rotation; simplification; severe fragmentation; moderate to severe difficulty with overlapping figures; severe perseveration; moderate to severe elaboration; redrawing of a complete figure; line incoordination; and concreteness. A careful reading of Hutt's description and interpretation of these deviant characteristics will enhance the examiner's perceptiveness in dealing with Bender data (see Hutt and Gibby, 1970, for examples). Hutt also described a number of other characteristic distortions—such as size changes and line quality—that are not included in his 17-factor scale but may be associated with neurologic conditions affecting brain function and have been included in one or more other scoring systems.

Scores on all but one of Hutt's factors range from 10 to 1, the exception being the second factor (position of the first drawing), which has only two scale values—3.25 for Abnormal and 1.0 for Normal. Scores range from 17 for a perfect performance (or at least a performance without scorable imperfections) to 163.5 for a performance in which maximum difficulty is encountered in handling each characteristic. Criteria for scoring each factor are presented in detail and are sufficiently clear to result in reliable judgments. Hutt reported interrater reliability coefficients for the 17 factors for two judges (scoring 100 schizophrenic patient records) ranging from 1.00 to .76, with five factor correlations running above .90 and nine above .80. An interrater reliability coefficient of .96 was obtained for the total scale. Lacks (1999) subsequently elaborated upon the Hutt scoring system and also collected extensive normative data on healthy adults that are representative of the age, sex, race, and educational characteristics of the U.S. population. In a comparison of scoring procedures, the Pascal-Suttell system was slightly more accurate than Lack's adaptation of Hutt's scale in classifying patients, but the latter was easier to use (Marsico and Wagner, 1990).

Although a reliable scoring system is necessary when doing research with the Bender, qualitative inspection of the patient's designs is usually sufficient for clinical purposes. Familiarity with one or more of the scoring systems will make the examiner aware of common Bender distortions and the kinds of aberrations that tend to be associated with visuospatial impairment and other symptoms of brain dysfunction. Blind reliance on Bender test scores, without adequate attention to the qualitative aspects of a patient's performance, can lead to erroneous conclusions about the absence of brain impairment, as illustrated by normal scores obtained by E.W. Russell's (1976) aphasic patient with pronounced right hemiplegia who had sustained a severe depressed skull fracture some 17 years earlier, and Bigler and Ehrfurth's (1980) three patients with CT documented brain damage who also received scores *within normal limits*.

Test characteristics. Most nine-year-olds can copy the Bender designs with a fair degree of accuracy, and by age 12, healthy youngsters can copy all of the designs well (Koppitz, 1964). Lacks and Storandt (1982) reported decrements in Bender-Gestalt performance when individuals enter their 60s to 70s. However, a review of seven smaller studies using a modification of Hutt's scoring system (Hutt-Briskin) did not find any regular age related score decrements (J.B. Murray, 2001). Bender-Gestalt performance is also influenced by cognitive ability, as evidenced by mean score differences between high school- and college-educated populations in Pascal and Suttell's (1951) sample—significant differences also observed in more recent studies (years 1985 to 1991) (J.B. Murray, 2001).

Neuropsychological findings. Like other visuographic deficits, difficulties with the Bender are more likely to appear with parietal lobe lesions (F.W. Black and Bernard, 1984; Garron and Cheifetz, 1965); lesions of the right parietal lobe are associated with the poorest performances (Diller, Ben-Yishay, et al., 1974; Hirschenfang, 1960a). A normal appearing Bender clearly does not rule out CNS pathology, but it does reduce the likelihood of parietal involvement. Patients with right hemisphere damage are more susceptible than those with left-sided lesions to errors of rotation (Billingslea, 1963) and fragmentation (Belleza et al., 1979). Diller and Weinberg (1965) asserted that omission errors would only be made by patients with right hemisphere lesions, but in my [mdl] experience, patients with either right- or left-sided lesions—and certainly those with bilateral damage—make these errors.

Bender error scores distinguished Alzheimer patients from healthy control subjects (Storandt, Botwinick, and Danziger, 1986). For elderly psychiatric patients, Bender errors were significantly related to scores on a mental status examination ($r = .60$) (Wolber, Romaniuk, et al., 1984) and to ratings of activities of daily living ($r = .62$) (Wolber and Lira, 1981). Bender error scores also predicted the level of independent living that TBI patients would achieve approximately three to four years after their accident ($r = .40, p < .001$) (M.B. Acker and Davis, 1989). The sensitivity of this test to diffuse cortical disease and to subcortical lesions (Lyle and Gottesman, 1977) suggests that copying tasks require a high level of integrative behavior that is not necessarily specific to visuographic functions but tends to break down with many kinds of cerebral damage.

Finally, scores on the Bender-Gestalt have been sensitive to changes in neuropsychological status. They faithfully reflected the deteriorating cognitive status of Alzheimer patients over time (Storandt, Botwinick, and Danziger, 1986). They also registered improved cognitive function in alcoholics who became abstinent (R.H. Farmer, 1973).

Benton Visual Retention Test (BVRT): Copy Administration (Sivan, 1992)

The three alternate forms of this test permit the use of one of them for a copy trial (see p. 462 for a description and picture of the test). The copy trial usually precedes the memory trials, thus allowing the subject to become familiarized with the test before undertaking the more difficult memory trials. Benton's original normative population of 200 adults provides the criteria for evaluating the scores (see pp. 462–464 for scoring details). Each subject's drawings are evaluated according to the estimated original level of functioning.

Persons of *average* or better mental ability are expected to make no more than two errors. Subjects making three or four errors who typically perform at *low average* to *borderline* levels on most other cognitive tasks have probably done as well as could be expected on this test; for them, the presence of a more than ordinary number of errors does not signify a visuographic disability. In contrast, the visuographic functioning of subjects whose scores on other kinds of tasks range above *average* and who make four or five errors on this task is suspect.

Neuropsychological findings. The performance of patients with frontal lobe lesions differed with the side of injury: those with bilateral damage averaged 4.6 errors; with right-sided damage, 3.5 errors; and with left-sided damage the average 1.0 error is comparable to that of the normative group (Benton, 1968). Other studies support a right–left differential in defective copying of these designs, with right hemisphere patients two or three times more likely to have difficulties (Benton, 1969a). However, in one study that included aphasic patients in the comparisons between groups with lateralized lesions, no differences were found in the frequency with which constructional impairment was present in the drawings of right and left hemisphere damaged patients (Arena and Gainotti, 1978). Error scores for Alzheimer patients virtually skyrocketed from their initial examination when their condition was diagnosed as mild ($M = 3.3 \pm 5.1$) to two-and-one-half years later ($M = 13.5 \pm 1.7$), in sharp contrast to healthy matched subjects whose first "nearly perfect" copy error scores ($M = 0.6 \pm 0.8$) did not differ significantly from the later one ($M = 0.8 \pm 1.5$) (Storandt, Botwinick, and Danziger, 1986). Although all scores other than *Perseverative errors* were associated with dementia severity in Alzheimer patients, *Omission errors* showed the greatest increase across dementia severity (Robinson-Whelen, 1992). BVRT copy is one of the predictors of cognitive decline in Alzheimer's disease, with poorer copy associated with a faster rate of dementia progression (Rasmusson, et al., 1996).

Complex Figure Test (CFT): copy administration

A "complex figure" was devised by André Rey (1941; translated by Corwin and Bylsma, 1993b) to investigate both perceptual organization and visual memory in brain impaired subjects (Fig. 14.2; see pp. 457–461 for a discussion of CFT memory testing). Osterrieth (1944; translated by Corwin and Bylsma, 1993b) standardized Rey's procedure; developed the widely used 18-item, 36-point scoring system; and obtained nor-

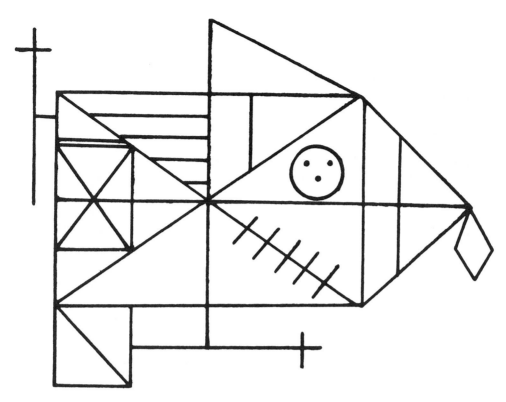

FIGURE 14.2 Rey Complex Figure (actual size). (Osterrieth, 1944)

mative data from the performances of 230 normal children ranging in age from four to 15 years and 60 adults in the 16–60-year age range. Because of Osterrieth's significant contribution, the Rey figure is also often called the Rey-Osterrieth, "Rey-O", or simply "CFT-R-O". L.B. Taylor (1979) developed an alternative complex figure for use in retesting (Fig. 14.3), which has been subsequently modified to improve its equivalence to the Rey-Osterrieth figure (Hubley and Tremblay, 2002) (Fig. 14.4).

The Medical College of Georgia (MCG) Neurology group developed four complex figures for repeated assessments (e.g., see Fig. 14.5a–d). Two of the MCG figures are rectangular in orientation—like the Rey-Osterrieth figure, and two are square—as is the Taylor figure. The MCG figures use a 36-point scoring system to facilitate comparison with the Rey-Osterrieth or Taylor figures (Loring and Meador, 2003a; Meador, Moore, Nichols, et al., 1993). A separate complex figure with a maximum score of 20 is part of the *Repeatable Brief Assessment of Neuropsychological Status (RBANS)* (C. Randolph, 1998); see pp. 696–697.

The copy task is simply that: copying the complex figure onto a sheet of paper. The figure is placed so that its length runs along the subject's horizontal plane.

The patient is not allowed to rotate either the design or the paper. Copy orientation may be less critical than originally thought, however, as one study reports no performance difference when copied at various orientations (0, 90°, 180°, or 270°) (Ferraro et al., 2002). This permits CFT use with greater confidence in less than optimal conditions such as bedside testing. Some examiners use photocopied sheets with the figure at the top portion of the page, and patients make their copies in the lower half of the paper. For persons unaccustomed to using a pencil, Dr. Harmesh Kumar recommends they be given the copy trial twice (personal communication, Feb., 2000 [mdl]).

Several methods may be used to record how the subject proceeds. Each time a portion of the drawing is completed, the examiner gives the subject a different colored pencil (or pen) while noting the order of color use. Some examiners prefer to change colors at fixed intervals (e.g., every 30 sec). Another method involves keeping a detailed record of each subject's copying sequence by copying what the subject draws and numbering each unit in the order that it is drawn, or using a "registration sheet" containing the printed Rey figure on which the examiner numbers in the order in which subjects make their copies (R.S.H. Visser, 1973;

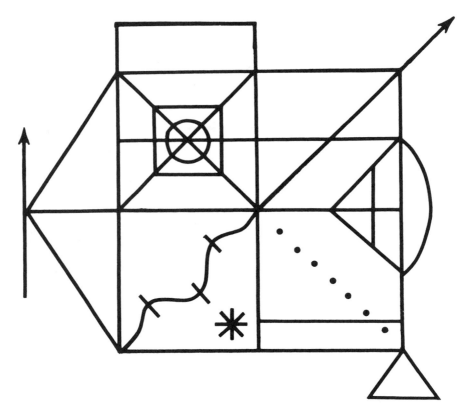

FIGURE 14.3 Taylor Complex Figure (actual size).

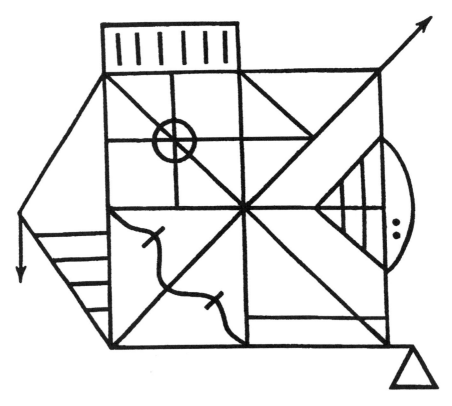

FIGURE 14.4 *Modified Taylor Figure*. (Hubley and Tremblay, 2002. © Anita Hubley. Reproduced by permission. This figure may be reproduced but may not be sold.)

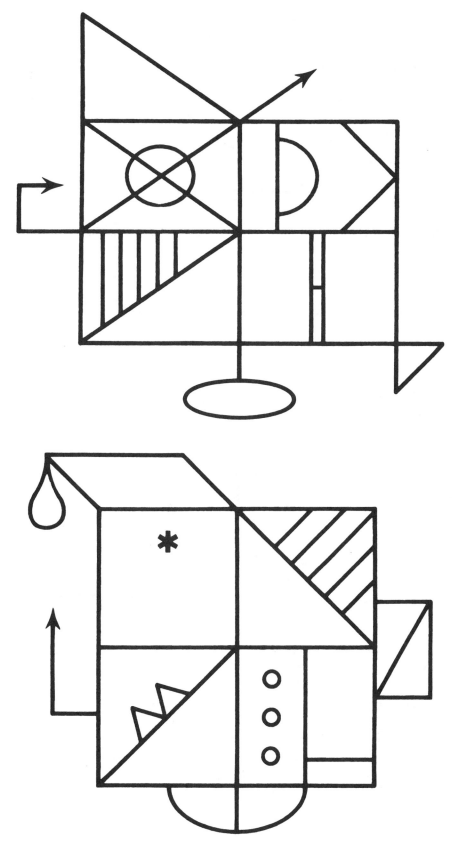

FIGURE 14.5 The four *Medical College of Georgia* (*MCG*) *Complex Figures* (actual size). (© 1988, 1989, 1990 K.J. Meador, Taylor, and Loring. Reproduced by permission.)

(continued)

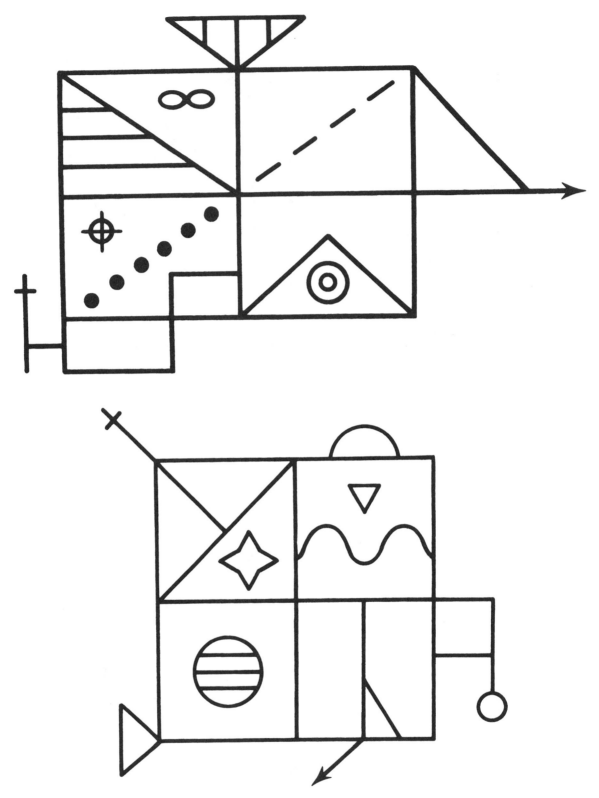

FIGURE 14.5 (Continued)

e.g., see Spreen and Strauss, 1998, pp. 342-347). For most purposes, switching colors generally affords an adequate and less cumbersome record of the subject's strategy or lack thereof. J.E. Meyers and Meyers (1995b) suggested that pen switching may be overly distracting for some patients, yet J.S. Ruffolo, Javorsky, and their colleagues (2001) found that pen switching was associated with better performance. The technique of drawing exactly what the subject draws and numbering each segment will best preserve the drawing sequence precisely (directional arrows can be useful). A registration sheet will work only for subjects whose copy is reasonably accurate; this method will not suffice for very defective copies, especially those with repeated elements or marked distortion of the basic structure (e.g., see Fig. 14.6). Some examiners also record time to completion. The copy trial is typically followed by one or more recall trials. Occasionally, subjects are dissatisfied with a poorly executed copy, others produce a copy so distorted that any examination of recall based on it would be uninterpretable, and still others begin the copy in such a manner that halfway through the task they realize they cannot make an accurate copy and ask to redo it (e.g., see Fig. 7.2, p. 240). In these cases, a second copy trial can be given if there seems to be any likelihood of improvement the second time.

Scoring systems. Although several scoring systems have been published, the most commonly used continues to be the Rey-Osterreith/Taylor/MCG unit scoring method which divides the figures into 18 scorable units (see Tables 14.1 to 14.4). These units refer to specific areas or details of the figures, with each unit numbered for scoring convenience. Since a correctly placed and proportional copy of each unit earns 2 points, the highest possible score is 36. Spreen and Strauss (1998, pp. 342–347) provide useful formats for scoring the Rey-Osterrieth, Taylor, and MCG figures using this system.

How investigators interpret and apply the scoring criteria can vary. Since subjective judgment often comes into play, whether a "strict" or "lenient" rating is used will affect the final scores. Often, a stricter scoring approach is used for the copy trial (e.g., following the

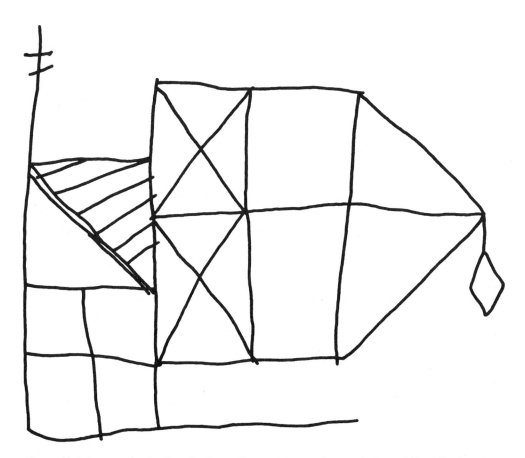

FIGURE 14.6 An example of a *Complex Figure Test Rey-Osterrieth* copy which would be difficult to document on a "registration" sheet due to fragmentation, broken configuration, and the several repetitions.

TABLE 14.1 Scoring System for the Rey Complex Figure

Units

1. Cross upper left corner, outside of rectangle
2. Large rectangle
3. Diagonal cross
4. Horizontal midline of 2
5. Vertical midline
6. Small rectangle, within 2 to the left
7. Small segment above 6
8. Four parallel lines within 2, upper left
9. Triangle above 2, upper right
10. Small vertical line within 2, below 9
11. Circle with three dots within 2
12. Five parallel lines within 2 crossing 3, lower right
13. Sides of triangle attached to 2 on right
14. Diamond attached to 13
15. Vertical line within triangle 13 parallel to right vertical of 2
16. Horizontal line within 13, continuing 4 to right
17. Cross attached to 5 below 2
18. Square attached to 2, lower left

Scoring

Consider each of the 18 units separately. Appraise accuracy of each unit and relative position within the whole of the design. For each unit count as follows:

Correct	placed properly	2 points
	placed poorly	1 point
Distorted or incomplete but recognizable	placed properly	1 point
	placed poorly	$^1/_2$ point
Absent or not recognizable		0 points
Maximum		36 points

From E.M. Taylor (1959), adapted from Osterrieth (1944)

practice at the Montreal Neurological Institute: Marilyn Jones-Gotman, personal communication, 1988 [mdl]), and a more lenient one for recall so as to not overly penalize memory performance based upon constructional accuracy alone. Bennett-Levy (1984a) offered some guidelines for "lax" scoring, and an explicit set of lenient scoring criteria was provided by Loring, Martin, and their colleagues (1990). Guyot and Rigault (1965) recommended scoring each element in terms of its relation to contiguous elements, with clearly depicted diagrams of the 18 scored Rey-Osterrieth elements and their contiguous relations. Both Loring, Martin, and colleagues, and Guyot and Rigault reminded examiners to avoid penalizing the same error twice (e.g., if the triangle above the large rectangle is misplaced, then the rectangle does not get marked down for misplacement too). Explicit scoring criteria are given by Duley and his colleagues (1993) for both the Rey-Osterrieth and Taylor figures.

TABLE 14.2 Scoring System for the Taylor Complex Figure

Units

1. Arrow at left of figure
2. Triangle to left of large square
3. Square, which is the base of figure
4. Horizontal midline of large square, which extends to 1
5. Vertical midline of large square
6. Horizontal line in top half of large square
7. Diagonals in top left quadrant of large square
8. Small square in top left quadrant
9. Circle in top left quadrant
10. Rectangle above top left quadrant
11. Arrow through and extending out of top right quadrant
12. Semicircle to right of large square
13. Triangle with enclosed line in right half of large square
14. Row of 7 dots in lower right quadrant
15. Horizontal line between 6th and 7th dots
16. Triangle at bottom right corner of lower right quadrant
17. Curved line with 3 cross-bars in lower left quadrant
18. Star in lower left quadrant

Scoring

Follow instructions given in Table 14.1 for scoring the Rey figure.

TABLE 14.3 Modified Taylor Figure

Units

1. Large square
2. Crossed diagonal lines in 1
3. Horizontal midline of 1
4. Vertical midline of 1
5. Short horizontal line in upper right quadrant
6. Short diagonal line in upper right quadrant
7. Diagonal arrow attached to corner of 1
8. Triangle in 1 on right, two vertical lines included
9. Semicircle attached to right side of 1, two dots included
10. Triangle attached to 1 by horizontal line
11. Horizontal line in lower right quadrant
12. Wavy line, includes two short lines
13. Large triangle attached to left of 1
14. Four horizontal lines within 13
15. Arrow attached to apex of 13
16. Horizontal and vertical lines in upper left quadrant
17. Circle in upper left quadrant
18. Small rectangle above 1 on left, six lines included

Modified Taylor Complex Figure (MTCF); Copyright A.M. Hubley, 1996, 1998. Reproduced by permission. This figure may be reproduced but may not be sold.

TABLE 14.4 Scoring Systems for the MCG Complex Figures

MCG COMPLEX FIGURE 1	MCG COMPLEX FIGURE 3

Units

Units

MCG COMPLEX FIGURE 1	MCG COMPLEX FIGURE 3
1. Large rectangle	1. Large rectangle
2. Vertical midline of 1	2. Vertical midline of 1
3. Horizontal midline of 1	3. Horizontal midline of 1
4. Small triangle on right hand corner of 1	4. Diagonal line in left upper quadrant of 1
5. Oval and attaching line at the bottom of 1	5. Three horizontal lines extending to 4
6. Bent arrow to the left of 1	6. Infinity sign in left upper quadrant of 1
7. Triangle above left upper quadrant of 1	7. Circle and cross in lower left quadrant of 1
8. Tilted arrow at top of 1	8. Six diagonal dots in lower left quadrant of 1
9. Diagonal in upper left quadrant of 1	9. Small rectangle in lower left quadrant of 1
10. Second diagonal in left quadrant of 1	10. Small rectangle extending from bottom of 1
11. Circle in upper left quadrant of 1	11. Cross attached to 10
12. Diagonal in lower left quadrant of 1	12. Right angle in lower right quadrant of 1
13. Five vertical lines extending above 12	13. Two concentric circles places under 12
14. Vertical lines and horizontal connection ("H") in lower right quadrant of 1	14. Four dashed lines in upper right quadrant of 1
15. Vertical line in right upper quadrant of 1	15. Triangle atop 1
16. Semicircle attached to the right of 15	16. Three vertical lines in 15
17. Diagonal line at upper right corner of 1	17. Triangle to the right of 1
18. Diagonal line extending from 17 to 3	18. Arrow attached to the right of 17

MCG COMPLEX FIGURE 2	MCG COMPLEX FIGURE 4

Units

Units

MCG COMPLEX FIGURE 2	MCG COMPLEX FIGURE 4
1. Large square	1. Large square
2. Vertical midline for 1	2. Vertical midline of 1
3. Horizontal midline for 1	3. Horizontal midline of 1
4. Asterisk in the upper left quadrant of 1	4. Rectangle to the right of 1
5. Diagonal in the lower left quadrant of 1	5. Circle with stem attached to 4
6. Two triangles attached to 5	6. Angled arrow at bottom of 1
7. Three circles in the lower right quadrant of 1	7. Small triangle outside lower left corner of 1
8. Vertical midline in the lower right quadrant of 1	8. Cross outside of upper left corner of 1
9. Horizontal line to the right of 8	9. Semicircle on top of 1
10. Diagonal line in the upper right quadrant of 1	10. Diagonal line in the upper left quadrant of 1
11. Five diagonal lines perpendicular to 10	11. Perpendicular line to 10
12. Small rectangle to the right of 1	12. Star in the upper left quadrant of 1
13. Diagonal line in 12	13. Circle in the lower left quadrant of 1
14. Semicircle at the base of 1	14. Three horizontal lines inside of 13
15. Vertical line in 14	15. Small triangle in upper right quadrant of 1
16. Angled arrow to the left of 1	16. Sine wave in upper right quadrant of 1
17. Parallelogram above 1	17. Vertical midline of the lower right quadrant
18. Teardrop attached to 17	18. Diagonal line extending to the right of 17

Medical College of Georgia Figures, © 1988–2003 K.J. Meador, D.W. Loring, & H.S. Taylor. Reproduced by permission.

Scores for copy trials of the Rey-Osterrieth, Taylor, and MCG figures tend to be comparable, although recall of the Rey-Osterrieth appears to be more difficult than that of either the Taylor or MCG figures, which tend to be roughly equivalent (see p. 458). Hamby and her colleagues (1993) note that it is easier to make a well-organized copy of the Taylor figure since its structure is simpler than that of the Rey-Osterrieth.

Fastenau, Denburg, and Hufford (1999) offer norm sets based on 211 "healthy adults" in the 30–85 age range, using the original Rey-Osterrieth scoring system (18 items, 36 points) and converted standard scores. With 43 to 102 subjects in eight overlapping age groups, these are probably the best norms currently available, at least for the U.S. Spreen and Strauss (1998) give means and standard deviations for each year from 6 to 15 and five age ranges from 16–30 to 70+.[1] The children's norms are based on hundreds of subjects, but the norms from 50–59 to 70+ must be considered only provisional because of scanty numbers. Mitrushina, Boone, and D'Elia (1999) offer a compilation of normative studies. Ingram and colleagues (1997) produced norms for older persons ages 55 to 75 for two MCG figures.

An 11-point system was developed for scoring qualitative errors most commonly made by patients with right hemisphere lesions (Loring, Lee, and Meador, 1988). Specific scoring criteria are given by Loring and his colleagues for each of 11 errors (identified by roman numerals to distinguish them from the numbered scoring elements of the Rey-Osterrieth system) (see Table 14.5). More than twice as many patients with right temporal epileptic foci made two or more of these errors than did patients whose seizure focus involved the left temporal lobe. In a cross-validation study, 66% of patients with temporal lobe epilepsy were correctly classified with respect to side of lesion on the basis of qualitative scores alone, with a sensitivity of 50% and specificity of 77% (Piguet et al., 1994). These qualitative errors, however, are also common in the recall of patients with diffuse impairment such as those with early dementia (dwl).

Denman (1987) scored the Rey figure for 24 elements, each on a 3-point scale yielding a maximum score of 72. Tombaugh, Faulkner, and Hubley (1992) produced a parallel system for scoring the Taylor figure. However, since the 18-element and the 24-element scoring systems generate virtually equivalent results (Rapport, Charter, et al., 1997; Tombaugh and Hubley, 1991), the extra time and effort required by a more complex scoring system do not appear to be justified.

Waber and Holmes (1985, 1986) used three scores to evaluate children's drawings (see p. 546 for descriptions of their *Organization* and *Style* scores). The *Objective Rating* score comprises a number of different kinds of features: Accuracy indicates the presence or absence of individual line segments belonging to one of four major structural components (base rectangle, main substructure, outer configuration, internal detail); Alignments and Intersections comprises 24 points where lines intersect or angles are formed; Continuity

TABLE 14.5 Scoring System of Qualitative Errors

I. Diamond attached by stem
II. Misplacement of the diamond
III. Rotation of horizontal lines in upper left quadrant
IV. Distortion of the overall configuration
V. Major alteration of the upper right triangle
VI. Six or more horizontal lines in upper left quadrant
VII. Parallel lines similar to those in upper left quadrant repeated elsewhere
VIII. Misplacement of either peripheral cross
IX. Major mislocation
X. Additional cross lines in either cross
XI. Incorporation of pieces into a larger element

Abbreviated from Loring, Lee, and Meador (1988)

of Lines identifies drawing style for lines that can be rendered either continuously or in separate segments; scored *Errors* are of four kinds: use of a single line to represent more than one part, rotation, perseveration, and misplacement.

Evaluating strategy. Strategy and organization when copying the complex figure are important determinants for subsequent CFT recall (L.K. Dawson and Grant, 2000; B.J. Diamond, DeLuca, and Kelley, 1997; Eslinger and Grattan, 1990; Heinrichs and Bury, 1991). Evaluation techniques use more or less complex measures of the degree to which the figure was drawn in a conceptual, fragmented, or confused manner: most of them require the examiner to record the order and direction of the drawing. Such detailed measurements are not ordinarily needed for clinical purposes if the examiner either uses the colored pencil method or keeps a record of how the subject goes about copying the figure. When quantification of strategy or organization is needed, the choice of method will probably be based on the degree of specificity required. Many of the qualitative measures in current use have been summarized and compared on such characteristics as shape of distribution, convergent and discriminant validity, and interrater reliability (Troyer and Wishart, 1997).

Osterrieth (1944; see Corwin and Bylsma, 1993a) identified seven different procedural types:

(I) Subject begins by drawing the large central rectangle and details are added in relation to it. (II) Subject begins with a detail attached to the central rectangle, or with a subsection of the central rectangle, completes the rectangle and adds remaining details in relation to the rectangle. (III) Subject begins by drawing the overall contour of the figure without explicit differentiation of the central rectangle and then adds the internal details. (IV) Subject juxtaposes details one by one without an organizing structure. (V) Subject copies discrete

---

[1]Except where noted, all studies cited here will be based on the 18-element, 36-point scoring system for each figure.

parts of the drawing without any semblance of organization. (VI) Subject substitutes the drawing of a similar object, such as a boat or house. (VII) The drawing is an unrecognizable scrawl.

In Osterrieth's sample, 83% of the adult control subjects followed procedure Types I and II, 15% used Type IV, and there was one Type III subject. Past the age of seven, no child proceeded on a Type V, VI, or VII basis, and from age 13 onward, more than half the children followed Types I and II. No one, child or adult, produced a scrawl. More than half (63%) of the TBI group also followed Type I and II procedures, although there were a few more Type III and IV subjects in this group and one of Type V. Three of four aphasic patients and one with senile dementia gave Type IV performances; one aphasic and one presenile dementia patient followed a Type V procedure.

In line with Osterrieth's observations, R.S.H. Visser (1973) noted that "brain-damaged subjects deviate from the normals mainly in the fact that the large rectangle does not exist for them . . . [Thus] since the main line clusters do not exist, [parts of] the main lines and details are drawn intermingled, working from top to bottom and from left to right" (p. 23).

Although, like all overgeneralizations, Visser's statement has exceptions, L.M. Binder (1982) showed how stroke patients tend to lose the overall configuration of the design. By analyzing how subjects draw the structural elements of the Rey-Osterrieth figure (the vertices of the pentagon drawn together, horizontal midline, vertical midline, and two diagonals) (Fig. 14.7), Binder obtained three scores: *Configural Units* is the number of these five elements that were each drawn as one unit (best score = 5). *Fragmented Units* is the number that were not drawn as a unit (this is not the inverse of the Configural score as it does not include incomplete units, i.e., those that had a part missing) (best score = 0); and *Missing Units* is the number of incomplete or omitted units (best score = 0). Fourteen patients with left hemisphere lesions tended to display more fragmentation ($M = 1.64$) than the 14 with right-sided lesions ($M = .71$), but the latter group's Missing Units score ($M = 1.71$), primarily due to left-sided inattention, far outweighed the negligible Missing Units score ($M = 0.07$) for the left CVA group. In contrast, 14 control subjects made few ($M = 0.21$) Fragmented Units and omitted none. Copying impairments were reflected in low Configural Unit scores for patients with right-sided CVAs ($M = 2.57$) and higher Configural Unit scores for those with left CVAs ($M = 3.29$); the control subjects made near-perfect scores ($M = 4.79$). An elaboration of the original system for scoring strategic sequences includes the four sides of the rectangle and takes into account whether the internal lines are drawn after the rectangle (as do most intact subjects) or before, to arrive at a 12-point sequencing score (L.M. Binder and Wonser, 1989). This score did not differentiate postacute left- and right-side damaged stroke patients, but it did document a greater tendency for fragmentation among those with damage on the left.

Using Binder's basic approach, Parkinson patients tended to copy the main structural units of the figure poorly, in contrast to healthy elderly subjects who rarely omitted main section elements (M. Grossman, Carvell, and Peltzer, 1993). Parkinson patients also tended to draw the main elements toward the end of the trial, and this in an interrupted fashion as if main elements were incidental detail rather than critical parts of the figure's structure.

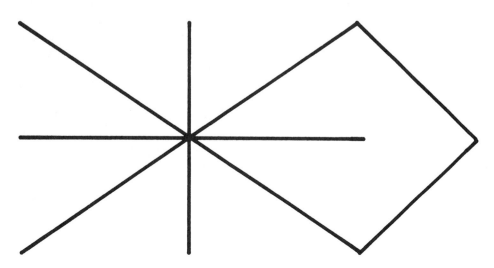

FIGURE 14.7 Structural elements of the Rey Complex Figure. (Binder, 1982)

By adding the large base rectangle to the number of main elements, Binder's method was modified slightly without compromising the attractive simplicity of a method that examines a few primary Rey-O figure features (C.R. Savage et al., 1999). Reliability coefficients are high for this modification, ranging from .69 for the vertex of the triangle to .92 for the vertical midline (Deckersbach et al., 2000). In a study of patients with obsessive-compulsive disorder (OCD), impaired complex figure recall was associated with impaired organizational strategies used during the initial copy trial (C.R. Savage et al., 1999).

Hamby and her colleagues (1993) devised a 5-point system for scoring organizational quality with criteria for both Rey and Taylor figures. They used five colors for the drawing, switching when the first element is completed, next when the subject draws a detail before the basic structure is completed or upon its completion, with the next three colors switched so that elements are divided "approximately equally" between them. Specific rules for judging *Configural mistakes, Diagonal mistakes,* and *Detail mistakes* are given. The score represents an evaluation based on the nature and number of mistakes (see Table 14.6). When Hamby and her coworkers (1993) used this score to evaluate CFT copies made by HIV positive subjects, the organization quality score of the Rey figure—but not the Taylor figure—differentiated those with AIDS related complex or AIDS from those without symptoms. This score correlated only modestly with the copy score ($r = .32$, $p < .05$).

The following three systems for evaluating strategy depend on a precise recording of the order and direction of drawing for every element.

The *perceptual cluster* score for evaluating strategy records the number of junctures (out of a possible 20) for which lines on either side are "drawn continuously or contiguously" or are fragmented into smaller parts (e.g., the two halves of the triangle on the right, the full length of each diagonal line in the left-hand box or in the major rectangle of the figure) (Shorr et al., 1992).

TABLE 14.6 Complex Figure Organizational Quality Scoring

5. No mistakes; overall organization is "excellent."
4. Detail mistakes and/or completion of upper left cross before major structures; organization is "good."
3. One configural or diagonal (e.g., lines don't cross in middle rectangle) mistake with or without detail mistakes; organization is "fair."
2. Two configural or diagonal mistakes with "poor" organization.
1. Three or more configural or diagonal mistakes; one configural or diagonal element missing, much segmentation, and "poor" organization.

Abbreviated from Hamby et al. (1993)

A *perceptual ratio* score is obtained by dividing the perceptual cluster score by the number of junctures included in the drawing. For drawings by an etiologically very mixed group of patients the perceptual ratio score's correlation with the copy score was .53, which indicates both a significant ($p < .001$) relationship with the accuracy of the copy and that the score is measuring something else besides.

Both of Waber and Holmes's (1985, 1986) two other scores reflect aspects of strategy on the drawing task. An *Organization* score is based on five closely defined levels, each with a set of sublevels (e.g., at level II, left side of base rectangle aligned; at level IV, four sides of base rectangle aligned), all of which have to be met to reach a basal level. Additional points are awarded for each higher subgoal met by the drawing. A total of 13 points can be achieved. This scale proved to be very age sensitive, as 5-year-olds had a mean organization score of $1.72 + 1.08$, while 14-year-olds' mean organization score was $9.51 + 3.93$ (1986). This score correlated quite well ($r = .60$) with one using the Rey-Osterrieth system. While these are cumbersome, labor-intensive scoring techniques, the authors found them to be useful for identifying features characteristic of stages in children's developing abilities to copy the complex figure. A third, *Style*, score is based on the relative continuity or fragmentation of the main structural elements of the figure with cut-off scores to distinguish "part" constructions from "configural" ones.

A rather complicated system proposed by Bennett-Levy (1984a) scores a maximum of 18 points for *good continuation* with a point gained wherever a line is continued—either straight or angled—at one of 18 designated juncture points. A *symmetry* score measures the number of instances (out of 18) in which the symmetry of mirrored elements is preserved, with higher scores when natural components of a symmetrical element are drawn successively. Together these scores yield a *strategy total* score which is significantly related ($p < .001$) to the copy score and a strong predictor of later recall accuracy. Statistical analyses indicated that the good continuation and symmetry scores make independent contributions to the strategy total score.

R.S.H. Visser (1973) suggested that fragmented or piecemeal copies of the complex figure that are characteristic of patients with brain disease reflect their inability to process as much information at a time as do normal subjects. Thus, brain impaired persons tend to deal with smaller visual units, building the figure by accretion. Many ultimately produce a reasonably accurate reproduction in this manner, although the piecemeal approach increases the likelihood of size and relationship errors (Messerli et al., 1979).

The *Boston Qualitative Scoring System (BQSS)* is designed to assess qualitative aspects of Rey-Osterrieth copy and memory reproduction, and also executive aspects of reproducing the complex figure (R.A. Stern, Javorsky, et al., 1999; R.A. Stern, Singer, et al., 1994). The complex figure is divided into three hierarchically arranged elements (Configural Elements, Clusters, and Details) which are scored according to specific criteria. The BQSS yields 17 qualitative scores, most of which are assessed on a 5-point scale. Visuoconstruction skills are measured by scores such as Accuracy, Placement, Rotation, and Asymmetry. Executive function scales include Planning, Fragmentation, Neatness, and Perseveration, which correlate with traditional measures of executive functioning such as the Wisconsin Card Sorting Test, Trail Making Test Part B, and WAIS-R Similarities (Somerville et al., 2000). BQSS Summary scores are generated for *Planning, Fragmentation, Neatness, Perseveration,* and *Organization*. Because scoring using the *Comprehensive Scoring Guide* may be quite time-consuming (Boone, 2000), a shorter *Quick Scoring Guide* may be used instead.

An organizational scale developed for children, the *Rey Complex Figure Organizational Strategy Score (RCF-OSS)*, appears suitable for adults as well (P. Anderson et al., 2001). It is a 7-point scale graded according to the level of organizational strategy (7 = excellent organization, 6 = conceptual organization, 5 = part-configural organization, 4 = piecemeal/fragmented organization, 3 = random organization, 2 = poor organization, 1 = unrecognizable or substitution). The focus is on how the rectangle and the vertical and horizontal midlines are rendered. In their normative sample of children ages 7 to 13, Anderson and his associates found that, surprisingly, older children used fragmented strategies more than younger ones.

Test characteristics. The mean Rey-Osterrieth copy scores for the five age groups reported by Delbecq-Dérouesné and Beauvois (1989) or by Spreen and Strauss (1998) do not differ greatly between age groups (see Table 14.7). Within an older range (from ages 65–93), copy scores do not decline significantly (see Mitrushina, Boone, and D'Elia, 1999), mostly showing about a 2-point drop from the late 60s to 80+. Fastenau, Denburg, and Hufford (1999) report that age explained 3% of the variance of their large adult sample. Ska, Dehaut, and Nespoulous (1987) compared younger (ages 40–50)

and older (ages 60–82) subjects for the quality of their Rey-Osterrieth figure copies using the Waber-Holmes scoring system and found that older and younger subjects did not differ in their organizational approach as both groups tended to build the design by accretion, but small differences favoring the younger group's accuracy and overall organization were statistically significant. Men tend to get higher scores than women (Bennett-Levy, 1984a; Rosselli and Ardila, 1991). Left-handedness of the subject or in the subject's family, plus a mathematics or science academic major, distinguished women whose copies were most accurate from women who performed less well (C.S. Weinstein et al., 1990). Education also contributes a little to success on this test (Fastenau, Denburg, and Hufford, 1999; Rosselli and Ardila, 1991). The Fastenau group found that education accounted for 2% of their sample's variance. Scores achieved by healthy Portuguese adults with less than 10 years of education were 1 to 3 points below those with 10 or more years (Bonifácio, personal communication, July, 2003 [mdl]). Moreover, illiterates' scores ran one-third (younger subjects) to two-thirds (subjects over 56 years) below persons with 10+ years of education (Ardila, Rosselli, and Rosas, 1989).

Considering that the scoring criteria are not spelled out in exacting detail, interscorer reliability for the Rey figure tends to be surprisingly high—mostly above .95 (Bennett-Levy, 1984a; Carr and Lincoln, 1988; Rapport, Charter, et al., 1997), although Frazier and his colleagues (2001) found an interrater reliability coefficient of only .80, well below that for recall which, they suggested, was due to a ceiling effect attenuating the score range. Hubley and Tombaugh (1993) report an interrater reliability coefficient of .91 for the Taylor figure. A factor analytic study of a large battery placed the copy trial among tests requiring reasoning and planning (Baser and Ruff, 1987).

Neuropsychological findings. Messerli and his colleagues (1979) looked at copies of the Rey figure drawn by 32 patients whose lesions were entirely or predominantly localized within the frontal lobes. They found that, judged overall, 75% differed significantly from the model. The most frequent error (in 75% of the defective copies) was repetition of an element that had already been copied, an error resulting from the patient's losing track of what he or she had drawn where because of a disorganized approach. In one-third of the

TABLE 14.7 High and Low Mean Rey-Osterrieth Copy Scores from Two Studies with Five Age Groups Each

Study and Age Range	High $\overline{X}$ Score: Age Group		Low $\overline{X}$ Score: Age Group	
Delbecq-Derouesné and Beauvois: 20–65+	35.26 ± 1.8	26–40	33.90 ± 2.4	65+
Spreen and Strauss: 16–70+	35.53 ± 0.8	50–59	32.90 ± 2.7	70+

defective copies, a design element was transformed into a familiar representation (e.g., the circle with three dots was rendered as a face). Perseveration occurred less often, usually showing up as additional cross-hatches (scoring unit 12) or parallel lines (scoring unit 8). Omissions were also noted.

Laterality differences in drawing strategy emerge in several ways. L.M. Binder's (1982) study showed that patients with left hemisphere damage tend to break up the design into units that are smaller than normally perceived, while right hemisphere damage makes it more likely that elements will be omitted altogether. However, on CFT recall, patients with left hemisphere damage who may have copied the figure in a piecemeal manner tended to reproduce the basic rectangular outline and the structural elements as a configural whole, suggesting that their processing of all these data is slow but, given time, they ultimately reconstitute the data as a gestalt. This reconstitution is less likely to occur with right hemisphere damaged patients who, on recall, continue to construct poorly integrated figures. Patients with right hemisphere damage produced much less accurate copies than patients with left CVAs who, although on the whole less accurate than the normal control group, still showed some overlap in accuracy scores with the control group.

Pillon (1981a) observed that the complexity of the task tends to elicit evidence of left visuospatial inattention in patients with right-sided lesions; these patients may also pile up elements on the right side of the page resulting in a jumbled drawing (see Ducarne and Pillon, 1974). However, other stroke patients showed no overall differences between laterality groups in performance accuracy, although aphasic patients were less accurate than others with left brain lesions (L.M. Binder and Wonser, 1989). These differing findings are a good reminder that severity needs to be addressed as well as age, sex, etc. when matching patient groups. Moreover, since many patients with left hemisphere lesions use their nondominant hand to draw, the issue of motor skill must be taken into account when evaluating their CFT copies or generalizing from them.

Differences between patients with parieto-occipital lesions and patients with frontal lobe impairment were demonstrated in CFT copy failures (Pillon, 1981b). Errors made by the frontal patients reflected disturbances in their ability to program the approach to copying the figure. Patients with parieto-occipital lesions, on the other hand, had difficulty with the spatial organization of the figure. When given a plan to guide their approach to the copy task, the patients with frontal damage improved markedly. The patients with posterior lesions also improved their copies when provided spatial ref-

erence points. Use of spatial reference points did not improve the copies made by the patients with frontal damage, nor did those with parieto-occipital lesions benefit from a program plan. Lesion laterality did not differentiate candidates for temporal lobe resection for epilepsy (left TLE $M = 33.31 \pm 3.20$; right TLE $M = 33.27 \pm 3.01$) (Ogden-Epker and Cullum, 2001).

The effect of TBI on the ability to copy the complex figure can vary greatly: although almost half of the 43 TBI patients in Osterrieth's (1944) sample achieved copy scores of 32 or better, one-third of this group's scores were significantly low. Interindividual variability also showed up among mildly injured patients of whom 15% performed well below the normal score range (Raskin, Mateer, and Tweeten, 1998). Another sample of mild TBI patients achieved an average score of 32.3 which was significantly below the 34.4 ± 1.2 mean control group score and their 4.0 SD was considerably larger than those documented for normal subject groups (Leininger, Grammling, et al., 1990). For skewed distributions such as generated by the Rey copy trial, this group's average score tells only part of the accuracy story: the SD indicates a wide variability among patients with many having made quite poor copies.

Of patients with progressive dementia, Alzheimer patients generally do produce very defective copies, even when many ability test scores are still within the *average* range (Brouwers et al., 1984). Huntington's disease also greatly affects ability to copy the figures but not to the same degree as Alzheimer's disease (Brouwers et al., 1984; Fedio, Cox, et al., 1979). Abnormally low scores have also been documented for "high-functioning" Parkinson patients but with wide interindividual variability ($M = 23.38 \pm 6.44$) (Ogden, Growdon, and Corkin, 1990). Many of these subjects proceeded in a piecemeal manner, with only eight of 20 patients but 13 of 14 control subjects drawing the rectangle in one step or in consecutive steps. On completion of the test some of the patients "said that they had not perceived the rectangle at all when they were copying the drawing, but when it was pointed out to them they could see it clearly" (p. 132). In a controlled prospective study examining the neuropsychological effects of carotid endarterectomy, complex figure copy differentiated patients from lumbar spine surgical controls when tested on the first post-operative day and one month later (Heyer et al., 2002).

Organizational approach is related to recall in recently detoxified alcoholic patients as assessed both by Shorr's perceptual clustering index and by measures from the Boston Qualitative Scoring System (L.K. Dawson and Grant, 2000). Not surprisingly, poor organization at baseline was related to subsequent poor recall.

Miscellaneous Copying Tasks

Since any copying task can potentially produce meaningful results, examiners should feel free to improvise tasks as they see fit. Anyone can learn to reproduce a number of useful figures—either geometric shapes or real objects—and then draw them at bedside examinations or in interviews when test stimuli not available. Strub and Black (2000) and McCarthy and Warrington (1990, p. 79) give some excellent examples of how easily drawn material for copying—such as a cube, a Greek cross, and a house—can contribute to the evaluation of visuographic disabilities (e.g., see Fig. 14.8). The Mini-Mental State Examination (M.F. Folstein et al., 1975) incorporates copying two intersecting pentagons as a standard item. The battery for the Consortium to Establish a Registry for Alzheimer's Disease (CERAD) includes four geometric figures of increasing difficulty—a circle, a diamond, intersecting rectangles, and a cube—to be copied as a measure of "constructional praxis." Normative data for white older adults (ages 50–89) who were enrolled in studies at 23 tertiary care medical centers have been published (K.A. Welsh, Butters, and Mohs, 1994), although these norms may not be applicable to African Americans or to less educated older adults seen in community practice settings (Fillenbaum, Heyman, Huber, et al., 2001).

Demographic factors such as age and education must be considered when interpreting performance on copying tasks (K.A. Welsh et al., 1994). On a copying task requiring copies of four geometric figures (circle, square, cube, and five-pointed star), the drawings of older subjects (ages 60–82) did not differ substantially from those made by two younger groups (ages 20–30 and 40–50), except that significantly fewer members of

the older group (61%) than of the younger group (76.5%) copied the most difficult figure—the star—correctly (Ska, Désilets, and Nespoulous, 1986). However, when given drawings of four objects to copy (pipe, house with fence, little man, and detailed bicycle), the oldest group scored significantly lower than the other two age groups on all four items, achieving the lowest mean score on the most complex drawing—the bicycle.[1] Older subjects appeared to have particular difficulty organizing the spatial relationships of the different parts of the figures.

Copying tasks are also sensitive to brain impairment. Bilaterally symmetrical models for copying such as the cross and the star in Figure 14.8 or the top left and bottom designs from the Stanford-Binet Scale (Terman and Merrill, 1973, see Chapter 11, Fig. 11.2), are particularly suited to the detection of unilateral inattention. Alzheimer patients perform more poorly as a group than controls on the copying tests of the CERAD battery and these tests are also sensitive to changes in the Alzheimer group over the course of one year (J.C. Morris, Heyman, et al., 1989). While difficulties with drawing are typically apparent in only a subset of patients in the early stages of Alzheimer's disease, constructional impairments often become obvious as the disease progresses such that they may be markers of disease severity (Guérin, Ska, and Belleville, 1999). Clinical lore notwithstanding, copying tasks are not effective in discriminating patients with the frontal variant of frontotemporal dementia from Alzheimer patients (Grossi et al., 2002).

Copying Drawings (Carlesimo, Fadda, and Caltagirone, 1993)

Carlesimo and his colleagues developed an array of 15 line drawings, each of which is presented individually to the patient who is asked to copy them "as exactly as possible." Seven of the drawings in this test depict flat shapes (six geometric figures and one line drawing similar to a Stanford-Binet figure (upper left, Fig. 11.2, p. 455); five are flat drawings of objects, and three are items drawn in perspective (a box, a pyramid, and a house). Each drawing is rated on a 0–4 scale. The global copying score is the mean score across all 15 drawings. These authors report high interrater reliability among three judges using this scoring system ($r > .80$). Compared with scores of 27 demographically matched non-neurologic control subjects ($M = 2.7 \pm 0.4$), 29 patients who had sustained left hemisphere or 27 with right hemisphere strokes (mostly ischemic) did signifi-

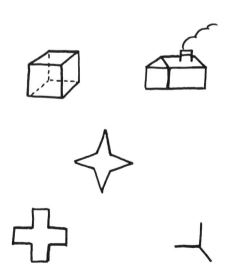

FIGURE 14.8 Sample freehand drawings for copying.

[1]Scoring systems for these eight drawings appear in an appendix to the article. Bicycle scoring follows the guidelines given below (p. 552).

cantly worse on this test, although not differently from each other ($M_L = 2.2 \pm 0.7$, $M_R = 2.2 \pm 0.5$). Using a cut-off of 2 SD below the mean for control subjects, 34.4% of the left hemisphere stroke group and 29.6% of the right hemisphere stroke group were impaired on this test. This is consistent with reports by previous investigators (e.g., Arena and Gainotti, 1978).

Different factors influenced the performance of the patient and control groups on the Copying Drawings test. For controls and patients with left hemisphere lesions who were able to copy with their right hands, constructional test performance was strongly correlated with performance on *Figure Matching* (a multiple-choice version of 10 of the items from Copying Drawings designed to assess visual perception). In contrast, motor skill (Finger Tapping speed) was the factor most strongly associated with the constructional test scores of left hemisphere lesioned patients who had to use their left hands due severe motor deficits. The drawing scores of patients with right hemisphere lesions were most strongly correlated with "manipulospatial ability" (e.g., *Visual Tracking*, drawing a line through a track composed of two parallel black lines).

Developmental Test of Visual-Motor Integration (VMI) (Beery and Buktenica, 1997)

When it is useful to evaluate test performances in terms of developmental levels, this test will provide age norms from ages 3 to 18 for accuracy in copying a set of 24 geometric figures arranged in order of developmental sequence, from less to more complex. Since development of copying accuracy levels off in the middle teen years, these norms are applicable to adults, at least into the seventh decade. The items in the fourth edition are identical to those in the third, but two supplemental standardized tests of visual perception and motor coordination, using the same stimuli, are added to the fourth edition. Some of these figures will be familiar to many examiners, such as the circle with the 45° rotated square and the overlapping hexagons of the Bender-Gestalt (Fig. 14.1, p. 533), the "tapered box" of the Stanford-Binet and Wechsler Memory Scale (Fig. 11.2, p. 455, upper right), and of course, the cube. The third and fourth editions differ in their scoring systems—especially at the older levels—and the fourth edition has expanded norms, although the absolute mean difference in scores obtained on the two editions is small (S.D. Mayes and Calhoun, 1998).

Free Drawing

The absence of a model changes the perceptual component of drawing from the immediate act of visual perception involved in copying a geometric design or object to the use of mental imagery to create a perceptual construct, a "picture in the mind," in response to an instruction to draw a particular shape or object. This difference may account for the failure of Warrington, James, and Kinsbourne (1966) to find a systematic way to sort freehand drawings on the basis of the side of the lesion, despite the many clear-cut differences between the drawings of patients with right and left hemisphere involvement. Yet some differences do persist, such as a greater likelihood of left-sided visual inattention, an increased tendency to sketch over drawings, and more details—both relevant and inconsequential—among patients with right hemisphere lesions; drawings of left hemisphere patients are more likely to have fewer details, giving the drawings an "empty" or poorly defined appearance (McFie and Zangwill, 1960). The presence of these lateralizing characteristics may enable the examiner to identify some cognitively impaired patients on the basis of their free drawings. Specific aspects of the visuographic disability may be studied by means of different drawing tasks (e.g., see also Drawing and Copying Tests for Inattention, Chapter 10, pp. 385–386). For example, the ability to draw human figures may be dissociated from other types of drawing, as in patients with Williams syndrome, whose ability to copy geometric figures (e.g., Beery and Buktenica's VMI) is deficient yet their ability to draw human figures is preserved (Dykens et al., 2001).

Human figure

Considering the number of times either the Draw-a-Person test or the House–Tree–Person test was mentioned in a recent survey on test use (Camara et al., 2000), tests involving human figure drawing come close to personality inventories in the frequency with which they are used by clinical psychologists but rank low in frequency of use by neuropsychologists. This is not surprising since human figure drawing has long been a staple in personality assessment, as well as a popular technique for evaluating children's mental ability. Among the virtues of the human figure drawing test are its simplicity of administration, requiring only pencils, paper, and the instruction to draw a person; its relative speed of administration, for few patients take more than five minutes to complete a drawing; and its applicability to all but those patients with such severe disabilities that they cannot draw.

The quality and complexity of children's drawings increase with age at a sufficiently regular pace to warrant the inclusion of drawing tests in the standard repertory of tests of cognitive development (Barrett and Eames, 1996; Fredrickson, 1985). These human figure drawing tests have been particularly prized for measuring the cognitive potential of or specific performance patterns of developmentally disabled or neurologically impaired children. Human figure drawing tests have also been used as brief cognitive screening procedures with young children.

Machover (1948) and Buck (1948) developed the best-known systems for appraising personality on the basis of human figure drawings. Both of these systems attend to dimensions and characteristics of the drawings that are, for the most part, irrelevant to neuropsychological questions. In the United States, the Goodenough "Draw a Man" test and its revision utilizing drawings of a man and a woman have provided the most popular system for estimating developmental level from human figure drawings (D.B. Harris, 1963). The subject can achieve a maximum score of 73 (man) and 71 (woman) on the Harris-Goodenough scale, which has also been modified for use with elderly subjects (Clément et al., 1996; Ericsson, Hillerås, et al., 1994).

This untimed test begins with verbal instructions to produce the desired drawing—a man or a woman, or both. The upper age norms end at 15, reflecting the normal leveling off of scores on drawing tests in the early teens. Age 15 drawing norms are applicable to adult patients. When used as a projective technique, subjects are instructed to "draw a person," leaving it up to them to determine the sex of their figure.

Test characteristics. Interscorer reliability coefficients for the Harris-Goodenough scoring system have been reported in the .80 to .96 range in children (L.H. Scott, 1981) and .89 to .96 in older adults (Clément et al., 1996; Ericsson, Hillerås, et al., 1994). Test–retest reliability is in the .61 to .91 range for children (Franzen, 1989).

The quality of human figure drawings diminishes with age, even among healthy adults (Ska, Désilets, and Nespoulous, 1986). An analysis of these drawings on the basis of the presence or absence of 26 elements (e.g., ears, clothing), and of their organization (28 items; e.g., attachment, articulation, dimensions, symmetry of limbs) suggested that organizational quality declines more rapidly than the number of elements.

Neuropsychological findings. Descriptions of human figures drawn by cognitively impaired patients with either specific visuographic disturbances or conditions of more generalized cognitive debilitation usually include such words as *childlike, simplistic, not closed, incomplete, crude,* and *unintegrated.* Several features of human figure drawings have been associated with brain impairment: lack of detail; loosely joined or noticeably shifted body parts; shortened and thin arms and legs; disproportionate size and shape of other body parts (other than the head); petal-like or scribbled fingers; and perseverative loops (Ericsson, Winblad, and Nilsson, 2001; Reznikoff and Tomblen, 1956). As on any drawing task, patients with left hemisphere lesions tend to favor the upper left portion of the page while those with right-sided lesions show a slight drift to the right side of the page (Gasparrini et al., 1980). However none of these is sufficiently pathognomonic to be diagnostic of cognitive impairment.

In evaluating human figures drawn by cognitively impaired patients, the impact of their emotional status should not be overlooked. This is particularly true for mildly impaired patients, whose sensitivity to their loss has precipitated a highly anxious or depressed mood that may lower the quality of their drawings or exaggerate the extent of their drawing impairment.

Bicycle

Most of the noncontent characteristics of the human figure drawings of cognitively impaired patients apply to other free drawings, too. Bicycle drawing can serve as a test of mechanical reasoning as well as of visuographic functioning (from Piaget, 1930, described in E.M. Taylor, 1959). The instructions are simply, "Draw a bicycle." The material consists of letter-size paper and pencils. When the drawing is completed, the examiner who is interested in ascertaining whether the patient can think through the sequential operation of a bicycle can ask, "How does it work?" This question should always be asked when the submitted drawing is incomplete. Mildly confused, distractible, and structure-dependent patients and those whose capacity for planning and organization is compromised often produce drawings lacking a necessary element—such as pedals, drive chain, or seat. They will usually note it when questioned and repair the omission. some refer to the missing component but remain satisfied with the incomplete drawing, or may overlook the missing part but add an inconsequential detail or superficial embellishments (see Figs. 3.15a,b and 6.2, pp. 69, 141). To retain the original incomplete drawing while still giving patients an opportunity to improve their performance, we [dbh, mdl] recommend handing patients a colored pen or pencil if they wish to make additions or corrections after indicating that they were done. In this way, the original omission(s) are preserved.

In order to quantify the bicycle drawing task, a 20-point scoring system was devised (Table 14.8, p. 552). Lebrun and Hoops (1974) described a 29-point scoring system devised by Van Dongen to investigate the drawing behavior of aphasic patients. This latter system

TABLE 14.8 Scoring System for Bicycle Drawings

Score 1 point for each of the following:

1. Two wheels

2. Spokes on wheels

3. Wheels approximately same size (smaller wheel must be at least three-fifths the size of the larger one)

4. Wheel size in proportion to bike

5. Front wheel shaft connected to handlebars

6. Rear wheel shaft connected to seat or seat shaft

7. Handlebars

8. Seat

9. Pedals connected to frame at rear

10. Pedals connected to frame at front

11. Seat in workable relation to pedals (not too far ahead or behind)

12. Two pedals (one-half point for one pedal)

13. Pedals properly placed relative to turning mechanism or gears

14. Gears indicated (i.e., chain wheel and sprocket; one-half point if only one present)

15. Top supporting bar properly placed

16. Drive chain

17. Drive chain properly attached

18. Two fenders (one-half point for one fender; when handlebars point down, always give credit for both fenders)

19. Lines properly connected

20. No transparencies

TABLE 14.9 Bicycle Drawing Means and Standard Deviations for 141 Blue Collar Workers in Five Age Groups

Age Group	Number	Mean	SD
20–24	21	13.95	4.03
25–34	46	13.78	3.55
35–44	37	14.22	3.63
45–54	27	12.59	3.65
55–64	10	13.90	5.51

Adapted from Nichols (1980)

includes scoring for many details (such as the tires, the taillight, or crossbars on a parcel carrier) that are infrequently drawn by normal subjects and rarely, if ever, drawn by brain damaged patients. Greenberg and colleagues (1994) recommend a 26-item scoring system organized into four categories: *Parts/Complexity* (7 items; e.g. two wheels, complete frame), *Motor Control* (5 items: e.g., pencil control, lines meet target destination), *Spatial Relationships* (9 items; e.g., placement of parts, size consistency), *Mechanical Reasoning* (five items; e.g., chain connection, steering possibility).

Test characteristics. Using the scoring system given in Table 14.8, Nichols (1980) found no pattern of age decline for five age ranges from 20–24 to 55–64 (see Table 14.9). However Ska and her colleagues (1986), using the same 20-item scoring system, did observe a decline in the quality of bicycle drawings with age, most notably between the older age groups of 40–50 and 60–82. This showed up prominently in omission of parts, although organization of the bicycle (e.g., wheel dimensions, pedals attached) showed an even steeper decline with age than loss of elements. The items most frequently left out by the older group were the front wheel shaft and the gears (each 67%), the rear wheel shaft (72%), the drive chain (78%), and the frame bars (80%). Nichols (1980) reported an interrater reliability coefficient of .97, with least agreement on items 3, 4, 6, 10, and 20 (see Table 14.8). Retesting three to five weeks after the initial examination produced a reliability coefficient of .53 with significant practice effects ($p < .003$).

Hubley and Hamilton (2002), evaluated the Greenberg scoring system on 22 men and 28 women, ages 21–80 and an education span from 10 to 21 years. They reported relatively small correlations with age (.14 to .28), with a sex difference only on Mechanical Reasoning ($p < .01$). Test–retest reliabilities for each category (.52 to .79) were satisfactory; only the Mechanical Reasoning score increased significantly on retest. Highest correlations were with Block Design (.28 to .47) and the Complex Figure (R-O, .30 to .48).

Neuropsychological findings. Comparing the accuracy of drawings of a cube, a house, and a bicycle, Messerli and his colleagues (1979) found that 56% of patients with frontal damage failed to draw an adequate bicycle, either due to a generally impoverished rendition or to poor organization, although spatial relationships overall were not likely to be distorted. Failures due to poor organization distinguished patients with frontal lesions (82% of whom demonstrated poor organization) from a group with nonfrontal lesions (25%). Frontal patients tended to draw without an apparent plan and without focusing first on the bicycle's structure before drawing details.

The bicycle drawing task may also bring out the drawing distortions characteristic of lateralized involvement. Patients with right hemisphere lesions tend to reproduce many of the component parts of the machine, sometimes with much elaboration and care, but misplace them in relation to one another, whereas left hemisphere patients are more likely to preserve the overall proportions but simplify the elements of the bicycle (Lebrun and Hoops, 1974; McFie and Zangwill,

1960). Severely impaired patients, regardless of the site of the lesion, perform this task with great difficulty, producing incomplete and simplistic drawings. In our experience, patients suffering from judgmental impairment, defective planning, difficulty with conceptual integration or accurate self-appraisal, inadequate self-monitoring, and/or impulsivity will often omit a crucial part of the bicycle's mechanism—either the drive chain or the pedals, or both.

House

This is another popular—and useful—drawing test. When giving it, the examiner asks subjects to "draw the best house you can" and specifies that it should show two sides of the house. A simple and logical scoring system is available which has demonstrated sensitivity to aging effects (Ska, Désilets, and Nespoulous, 1986, see Table 14.10). As with other items, when compared with younger subjects, older persons tend to include fewer elements and integrate them less well (Ska, Martin, and Nespoulous, 1988).

Messerli and his colleagues (1979) reported that while only 24% of patients with frontal lobe damage were unable to draw a reasonable appearing house, these failures typically represented an inability to work from structure to detail. House drawings may elicit difficulties in handling perspective that are common among cognitively deteriorated patients. An alert and otherwise bright patient who struggles with a roofline or who flattens the corner between the front and side of the house is more likely to have right hemisphere damage than left hemisphere involvement.

Clock face

Clock face drawings were originally used to expose unilateral visuospatial inattention thought to be associated with right parietal dysfunction (Battersby et al., 1956). M. Freedman, Leach, and their collaborators (1994) pointed out that clock drawing is in fact a complex task that is sensitive to a variety of focal lesions, tapping not only visuoperceptual and visuospatial abilities, but also receptive language, numerical knowledge, working memory, and executive functions (both motor and cognitive). It has come to be widely used in geriatric practice and memory disorders clinics, where it is valued for its ability to provide a quick "cognitive scan" and to demonstrate a patient's difficulties to family members.

The first systematic use of the clock test was in the *Parietal Lobe Battery,* which included both drawing a clock to command and setting clock hands (Borod, Goodglass, and Kaplan, 1980; Goodglass and Kaplan, 1983). Clock drawing to command was incorporated into the Praxis subscale of the Cambridge Cognitive Examination shortly thereafter. On *clock drawing* to command, the patient is instructed to "Draw the face of a clock showing the number and two hands, set to 10 after 11," which gives additional information about the patient's time orientation and capacity to process numbers and number–time relationships. Clock drawings are rated for accuracy of the circular shape, accuracy of numbers, and symmetry of number placement, with scores ranging from 0 to 3. For *clock setting* in the Parietal Lobe Battery, the patient is shown a sheet of paper with four blank clock faces, each of which has dashes marking the positions of the 12 numbers and is asked to draw in the two hands of the clock to make the faces read 1:00, 3:00, 9:15, and 7:30. Each clock is rated for the correct placement and relative lengths of the hands, with a total of 12 points possible.

Over a dozen administration and scoring systems have been published, a number of which are summarized in Table 14.11, p. 554. Many of these—as well as some other less commonly used systems are described in Shulman (2000). Some systems present the subject with a blank page (Goodglass and Kaplan, 1983b; see also Goodglass, Kaplan, and Barresi, 2000), whereas others present a sheet with an empty circle. The methods also differ regarding what time(s) should be set. Although "10 minutes past 11" is the most widely favored—no doubt because of its ability to elicit

TABLE 14.10 Scoring System for House Drawing

Score 1 point for each of the following:

1. One side (square or rectangular)

2. A second side

3. Perspective (each side on a different plane; the angled side must differ by more than 5° from base of the house)

4. A roof

5. Roof placed correctly on the house (with respect to the orientation of the sides)

6. Door

7. Window(s)

8. Chimney

9. Adjacent features (fence, road, steps to the door)

10. Elements connected well (no more than one excess line, no more than two lines not joined or extending beyond their connecting points)

11. Appropriate proportions (wider than tall, fence reasonably oriented)

12. No incongruities (e.g., transparencies, door "in the air," house "suspended" as if on incompletely constructed pilings

Adapted from Ska, Desilets, and Nespoulous (1986)

TABLE 14.11 Commonly Used Quantitative Scoring Systems for Clock Drawing

Method	Test Conditions	Scoring	Suggested Cut-off for Impairment	Interrater Reliability*
Shulman, Shedletsky, & Silver, 1986; Shulman, Gold et al., 1993	Predrawn circle ("Set hands to 10 past 11")	5-point global rating (5 = perfect to 0 = no resemblance to a clock)	<4	.83–.93
T. Sunderland, Hill, et al., 1989	Blank page ("Draw clock and set hands to 2:45")	10-point ordinal rating scale (1–5 cover clock face and number placement and 6–10 cover hand drawing and placement)	<6	.82–.92
Wolf-Klein et al., 1989	Predrawn circle ("Put the numbers on the clock")	10-point rating scale (comparing number placement with examples)	<7	.81–.93
Spreen & Strauss, 1991, 1998	Blank page ("Draw face of a clock with the numbers; draw hands pointing at 20 to 4")	10-point rating scale, adapted from Sunderland and Wolf-Klein scales	<7	NA
Mendez, Ala, & Underwood, 1992	Blank page ("Draw clock and set hands to 10 past 11")	20-point scale (12 for numbering, 5 for hand placement, and 3 for general impression)	<18	.92–.97
Rouleau et al., 1992	Blank page ("Draw clock and set hands to 10 after 11"); clock copy	10-point scale (2 points for clock face, 4 points each for number and hand placement); also 6-item qualitative error analysis	NA	.95–.96
Tuokko, Hadjistavropoulos, et al., 1992, 1995	Predrawn circle ("Set hands to 10 past 11"); 5 clock setting and 5 clock reading items	Presence/absence or count of 25 errors, categorized into 7 subscales; 0–3 points for each clock setting and reading	>2 errors on clock drawing	.99
Y.I. Watson et al., 1993	Predrawn circle ("Draw in the numbers")	7-point rating of number placement in each of 4 quadrants (0 = least to 7 = most impaired)	>3	.81–.98
M. Freedman, Leach, et al., 1994	Free drawing ("Draw block and set to 6:45"); also clock analysis (6:05) and 3 clock readings	15-point cumulative score on "critical items" done accurately by normal subjects; extensive normative data	NA	.98
Manos & Wu, 1994	Predrawn clock ("Set clock to 10 minutes after 11")	10-point rating, with 8 points for correct number placement and 2 for correct hand placement	<8	.94
Royall, Cordes, & Polk, 1998	Blank page ("Draw me a clock that says 1:45"); clock copy	15-point rating for each part (CLOX1, free drawing, and CLOX2, copying)	<10 (CLOX1) <12 (CLOX2)	.93–.94

*Reliability coefficients are derived from several comparative studies, including Suhr, Grace, Allen, et al. (1998), n = 71 community-based elderly and 101 stroke patients; Tuokko, Hadjistavropoulos, Rae, & O'Rourke (2000), n = 493 subjects from the Canadian Study of Health and Aging; Storey et al. (2001), n = 127 consecutive referrals to a geriatric medical outpatient clinic; and Schramm et al. (2002), n = 123 consecutive referrals to a memory disorder clinic (79 of whom were diagnosed with varied dementias).

stimulus-bound errors to the number 10—exactly what instructions are given regarding the clock hands doesn't seem to matter as all instructions elicit discriminable and neuropsychologically meaningful responses. However, including instructions to show the hands indicat-

ing a specified time can add greatly to understanding deficits—or demonstrating competencies. Edith Kaplan (1988) recommended including both drawing to command and copy trials, citing examples of failure on one form of this test and success on the other. Several investigators have heeded this suggestion and made both drawing to command and copying explicit components of their clock drawing procedures (Rouleau et al., 1992; Royall, Cordes, and Pok, 1998; Tuokko, Hadjistavropoulos, et al., 1992).

The different methods for scoring clock drawing vary substantially in their emphases and complexity. Some scoring methods rely primarily or exclusively on the accuracy of numbers and their placement, with little or no attention to the clock hands (Manos and Wu, 1994; Y.I. Watson et al., 1993; Wolf-Klein et al., 1989). Other methods provide a detailed system for analyzing errors in clock drawing (Rouleau et al., 1992; Tuokko, Hadjistavropoulos, Miller, and Beattie, 1992). Examiners interested in using the clock drawing test will want to attend to these nuances of administration and scoring to select the clock drawing method best suited to their testing situation.

Test characteristics. The psychometric properties of several of the clock drawing scoring systems have been compared in several large-scale studies (Schramm et al., 2002; Storey et al., 2001; Tuokko, Hadjistavropoulos, et al., 2000). Interrater reliability coefficients are uniformly high, irrespective of the scoring system used or the population to which it is applied (see Table 14.11, p. 554). Most scoring systems are in fact highly intercorrelated: e.g., coefficients ranging from 0.73 (Shulman's, 2000, method with Royall CLOX1) to .95 (Mendez, Ala, and Underwood's 1992 method with Royall CLOX1) in one study (Royall, Mulroy, et al., 1999). An evaluation of interscorer reliability for three systems also found high correlations, many above .91; most low interscorer agreements were on scores for "overall contour of the clock face" (South et al., 2001).

The ability to draw a clock face with reasonably good accuracy changes little over the years in cognitively intact community-dwelling elderly adults, even in those well into their 90s (M. S. Albert, Wolfe, and Lafleche, 1990; Cahn and Kaplan, 1997). This may not be the case for less educated adults, particularly those with fewer than 10 years of education, whose clock drawing ability appears to decline starting in the mid-70s (La Rue, Romero, et al., 1999; Marcopulos, McLain, and Giuliano, 1997). Education clearly has an impact on clock drawing performance and must be taken into account in interpreting results on this test (Ainslie and Murden, 1993). Clock drawing test performance is moderately correlated not only with other measures of visuoconstruction (Block Design $r = .42$) but also with several other cognitive functions, including receptive language (Token Test, $r = .54$), semantic (animal) fluency ($r = .44$), and aspects of executive function (Mattis Dementia Rating Scale, Initiation–Perseveration scale, $r = .44$). They appear to be unrelated to mem-

ory (Cahn-Weiner et al., 1999; Suhr, Grace, et al., 1998).

Neuropsychological findings. Quantitative scores from the varied clock drawing systems are often less helpful in identifying lesion location (e.g., right vs. left, anterior vs. posterior, or cortical vs. subcortical) in patients with focal lesions than are qualitative analyses of their error patterns (Suhr, Grace, et al., 1998). For example, patients with right anterior lesions often have difficulty managing the simultaneous demands of the clock drawing task (M. Freedman, Leach, et al., 1994). Patients with right posterior lesions typically show spatial inattention—leaving out numbers from the left side of the clock face, or when they do include all the numbers, spatial disorganization—bunching most of the numbers along the right margin of the clock's outline, or struggling to round out the left side of the clock (M. Freedman, Leach, et al., 1994; Suhr, Grace, et al., 1998). Patients with right parietal lesions may be more prone to distort or neglect the lower left quadrant of the clock face, whereas those whose lesions are predominantly right temporal are more likely to have difficulty with the upper left quadrant (e.g., see E. Kaplan, 1988). A few patients, all but one of whom sustained a right hemisphere stroke, have actually written numbers counterclockwise around the clock face, although this was transient (D.S. Jones, 2000; Kumral and Evayapan, 2000).

Patients with left-sided—particularly anterior—lesions may be inattentive to the right side of the clock face (Ogden, 1985a,b). They may also have difficulties with the sequencing demands of the task and are prone to perseverative errors (M.L. Albert and Sandson, 1986; M. Freedman, Leach, et al., 1994). In contrast, the errors of patients with left posterior lesions often stem from poor task comprehension and agraphia.

Patients with Alzheimer's disease consistently do much worse than healthy controls on clock drawing tests (Cahn-Weiner et al., 1999). Performance on the free drawing (CLOX1) component of Royall's clock drawing procedure can predict level of independence (independent vs. assisted living vs. skilled nursing) among residents of a comprehensive care retirement community (Royall, Chiodo, and Polk, 2000). Assumptions about the evolution of constructional impairments—namely, that clock hands and time setting are affected first, followed by number placement and shape of the clock face (T. Sunderland, Hill, et al., 1989)—have been criticized (Rouleau et al., 1992). Forstl and colleagues (1993) found that clock drawing performance was directly related to counts of large neurons in the hippocampus and in the parahippocampal gyrus but not the parietal lobe. In an MRI study, Cahn-Weiner and her colleagues (1999) reported that clock drawing performance was moderately correlated with gray matter volumes in the right anterior-superior temporal lobe but not the parietal lobe or other brain regions.

The sensitivity of clock drawing to Alzheimer's disease is sufficiently great that it is often recommended as a screening procedure, either alone or as a supplement to the Mini-Mental State Examination (Shulman, 2000). Sensitivity and specificity values will vary somewhat depending on the scoring method used and the composition of the sample. The Mendez, Shulman, and Tuokko methods appear to be the most sensitive but least specific in screening for dementia, whereas the Watson and Wolf-Klein methods are specific but relatively insensitive (Brodaty and Moore, 1997; Schramm et al., 2002; Storey et al., 2001; Tuokko, Hadjistavropoulos, et al., 2000). Interestingly the Watson and Wolf-Klein methods are the only two that do not ask examinees to place the hands on the clock. Specific error patterns on clock drawing, such as accuracy in hand drawing and placement or substitutions, may also be useful in detecting patients in the early stages of Alzheimer's disease (Cahn, Salmon, et al., 1996; Esteban-Santillan et al., 1998; O'Rourke et al., 1997) and in distinguishing early Alzheimer patients from patients who are depressed (N. Herrmann et al., 1998).

Clock drawing performance may be able to differentiate patients with Alzheimer disease from those with other forms of dementia, such as vascular dementia or frontotemporal dementia (Heinik et al., 2002; Moretti et al., 2002b). In one study vascular dementia patients were twice as likely as Alzheimer patients to adopt a segmentation strategy (i.e., using radial lines to divide the circle into segments before drawing in the numbers and the hands) (D. Meier, 1995). In another study vascular dementia patients were distinguishable from those with Alzheimer's disease because their clock drawing performance did not improve when they were allowed to copy a clock as opposed to drawing it to command (Libon, Swenson, et al., 1993; Libon, Malamut, et al., 1996). Rouleau and her colleagues (1992) made a similar observation regarding the tendency for the clock drawing performance of Alzheimer patients to improve during the copy conditions, whereas that of Huntington patients did not. Although both patient groups made visuospatial errors, graphomotor planning problems were exhibited almost exclusively by patients with Huntington's disease, whereas conceptual errors—reflecting the erosion of knowledge about the attributes, features, and meaning of a clock—were observed primarily in the drawings of patients with Alzheimer disease. Failure to draw the hands or the numbers were some of the most common conceptual errors observed. Conceptual errors were predictive of more rapid dete-

rioration over the subsequent two years (Rouleau et al., 1996).

ASSEMBLING AND BUILDING

More than any other kind of test, assembling and building tasks involve the spatial component in perception, at the conceptual level, and in motor execution. Inclusion of both assembling and drawing tests in the battery will help the examiner discriminate between the spatial and the visual aspects of a constructional disability and estimate the relative contributions of each.

With Block Design and Object Assembly, the Wechsler tests contribute two of the basic kinds of construction tasks to the neuropsychological examination, both involving two-dimensional space. Three-dimensional construction tasks call upon a somewhat different set of functions, as demonstrated by patients who can put together either the two- or the three-dimensional constructions, but not both (Benton and Fogel, 1962). Other construction tasks test the ability to execute reversals in space and to copy and reason about different kinds of visuospatial maneuvers.

Two-Dimensional Construction

Block Design (Wechsler, 1955, 1981, 1997a)

On this construction test, the subject is presented with red and white blocks: two, four, or nine, depending on the item. Each block has two white and two red sides, and two half-red half-white sides with the colors divided along the diagonal. The subject's task is to use the blocks to construct replicas of the easy block constructions made by the examiner and then designs of increasing difficulty printed in a scale smaller than the blocks (see Fig. 14.9, p. 557). The designs in the WAIS-III Block Design stimulus booklet are larger than in earlier versions, a welcome improvement for testing examinees with visual acuity problems. The WAIS-III expands the difficulty range of the Block Design test by adding five new designs to the nine WAIS-R designs: one difficult design is added at the end, and four easier designs are included at the beginning. An experienced examiner can administer the WAIS-III Block Design test in slightly over ten minutes (Axelrod, 2001). Detailed instructions are given in the test manual.

Of the 10 items above the *defective* level (< -2 SD) on WAIS-III (Designs 5–14), Designs 5 and 8 of the four-block designs and Design 10 (the first nine-block design) are relatively easier because they contain implicit grid information, as do the first four designs. When patients with visuospatial disorders, develop-

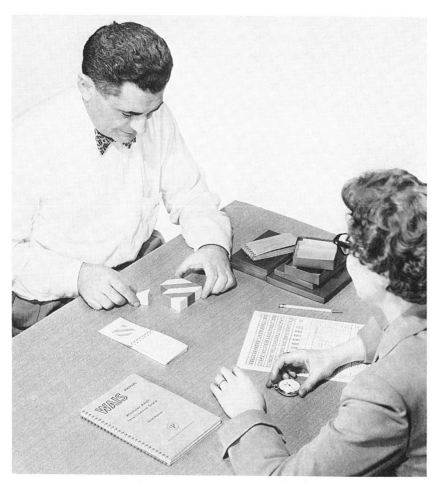

FIGURE 14.9 Block Design test. (Reproduced by permission of The Psychological Corporation)

mentally delayed individuals, or careless persons fail one of these items, it is more likely to be due to incorrect orientation of the diagonal of a red-and-white block than to errors in laying out the overall pattern. In contrast, the diagonal patterns of the other designs reach across two- and three-block spans. Concrete-minded persons and patients (particularly those with right hemisphere damage) with visuospatial deficits have particular difficulty constructing these diagonal patterns (see also Walsh and Darby, 1999).

Impaired persons sometimes do not comprehend the Block Design task when given the standard instructions alone. An accompanying verbal explanation like the following may help to clarify the demonstration:

The lower left-hand (patient's left) corner is all red, so I put an all red block here. The lower right-hand corner is also all red, so I put another all red block there. Above it in the upper right corner goes what I call a "half-and-half" block (red and white halves divided along the diagonal); the red runs along the top and inside so I'll put it above the right-hand red block this way (emphasizing the angulation of the diagonal), etc. [mdl].

Non-standard administrations of Block Design. There may be circumstances in which the examiner wishes to give the patient an opportunity to solve problems that were failed under standard conditions, or to bring out different aspects of the patient's approach to the Block Design problems. For example, following completion of the Block Design test, the examiner can return to any design that was puzzling or that elicited an atypical solution and ask subjects to try again. The examiner can then test for the nature of the difficulty by having them verbalize as they work, by breaking up the design and constructing and reconstructing it in small sections to see if simplification and practice help, or by giving a completed block design to copy instead of the smaller and unlined printed design. The examiner can test for perceptual accuracy alone by asking subjects to identify correct and incorrect block reproductions of the designs (Bortner and Birch, 1962).

The examiner who wants to know whether slow or initially confused patients can copy a design that is incomplete when the time limit is reached may choose to allow them to continue working [mdl]. When the examiner times discreetly, patients remain unaware that they have overrun the time so that if they complete the design correctly, they will have the full satisfaction of success. As on other timed tests, it is useful to obtain two scores when patients fail an item because they exceeded the time limit. Usually, permitting patients to complete the design correctly means waiting no more than an extra minute beyond the allotted time. With very slow patients, the examiner has to decide whether waiting the five or seven minutes they may take to work at a problem is time well spent in observation or providing an opportunity for success, whether the patients' struggles to do a difficult or perhaps impossible task distress them excessively, or whether they need the extra time to succeed at this kind of task at all. It is usually worthwhile to wait out very slow patients on at least one design to see them work through a difficult problem from start to finish and to gauge their persistence. However, when patients are obviously in over their depth and either do not appreciate this or refuse to admit defeat, the examiner needs to intervene tactfully before the task so upsets or fatigues them that they become reluctant to continue taking any kind of test.

The WAIS-R NI administration of Block Design called for subjects to be given 12 rather than nine blocks, making it easier for patients who did not readily conceptualize the squared 2 × 2 or 3 × 3 format to give a distorted response that demonstrates this deficiency (E. Kaplan, Fein, et al., 1991). Follow-up trials were then given for failed items, using block models drawn with a superimposed grid to see whether this level of structuring improved the patient's performance.

Qualitative aspects of Block Design performance. Block Design lends itself well to qualitative evaluation. The manner in which patients work at Block Design can reveal a great deal about their thinking processes, work habits, temperament, and attitudes toward themselves. The ease and rapidity with which patients relate the individual block sides to the design pattern give some indication of their level of visuospatial conceptualization. At the highest level is the patient who comprehends the design problem at a glance (forms a "gestalt" or unified concept) and scarcely looks at it again while putting the blocks together rapidly and correctly. Patients taking a little longer to study the design, who perhaps try out a block or two before proceeding without further hesitancy, or who refer back to the design continually as they work, function at the next lower level of conceptualization. Trial and error approaches contrast with the "gestalt" performance. In these, subjects work from block to block, trying out and comparing the positioning of each block with the design before proceeding to the next one. This kind of

performance is typical of persons in the *average* ability range. These individuals may never perceive the design as a total configuration, nor even appreciate the squared format, but by virtue of accurate perception and orderly work habits, many can solve even the most difficult of the design problems. Most people of *average* or better ability do form immediate gestalts of at least five of the easiest designs and then automatically shift to a trial and error approach at the point that the complexity of the design surpasses their conceptual level. Thus, an informal indicator of ability level on this task is the most difficult design that the subject grasps immediately.

Patients' problem-solving techniques reflect their work habits when their visuospatial abilities are not severely compromised. Orderliness and planning are among the characteristics of working behavior that the block-manipulating format makes manifest. Most examinees work systematically in the same direction—from left to right and up to down, for example—whereas others tackle whatever part of the design meets their eye and continue in helter-skelter fashion. Most examinees quickly appreciate that each block is identical, but some turn around each new block they pick up, looking for the desired side, and if it does not turn up at first they will set that block aside for another one. Some work so hastily that they misposition blocks and overlook errors through carelessness, whereas others may be slow but so methodical that they never waste a movement. Ability to perceive errors and willingness to correct them are also important aspects of work habits that can be readily seen on Block Design. Temperamental characteristics, such as cautiousness, carefulness, impulsivity, impatience, apathy, etc., appear in the manner in which patients respond to the problems. Self-deprecatory or self-congratulatory statements, requests for help, rejection of the task, and the like betray their feelings about themselves.

Examiners should record significant remarks, as well as kinds of errors (e.g., placement or position errors, rotation errors, and broken configuration) and manner of solution (e.g., location of blocks as they are placed and which blocks are correctly positioned). Most items elicit only one type of single-block error, either errors of placement or position (Joy et al., 2001). Broken configuration errors are not as rare as originally thought: slightly over one-third of the older adults in this study's sample produced one or more broken configurations on WAIS-R Block Design, mostly only one.

For quick, successful solutions, examiners usually need to note just whether the approach was conceptual or trial and error, and if trial and error, whether it was methodical or random. Time taken to solve a design will often indicate the patient's conceptual level and working efficiency since "gestalt" solutions generally take less time than those solved by methodical trial and error, which in turn are generally quicker than random trial and error solutions. It thus makes sense that high scores on this test depend to a considerable extent on speed, especially for younger subjects. Examiners can document patient difficulties such as false starts and incorrect solutions by sketching them on the blank grids in the Incorrect Designs section of the Record Form. Of particular value in understanding and describing the patient's performance, however, are sequential sketches of the evolution of a correct solution from initial errors, or of the compounding of errors and snowballing confusion of an ultimately failed design (e.g., see Fig. 3.9c–e, p. 59), which requires more space and recording flexibility than the record form allows. The number of changes made en route to a correct design is a function of both item difficulty and the introduction of new types of patterns (e.g., diagonal lines) (Joy et al., 2001).

The kinds of strategies used to solve Block Design have been the subject of a running discussion in the literature for decades (Joy et al., 2001; E. Kaplan, Fein, et al., 1991; Spelberg, 1987). There seems to be little question that most normal subjects adopt an analytic approach. Kiernan and his colleagues (1984) point out, however, that the subjects of many of these studies have been bright adults: young children, some neurologically impaired patients, and some older subjects fall back on synthetic strategies because "they have difficulty doing the mental segmenting required by designs in which some of the edge cues are not present" (Kiernan, Bower, and Schorr, 1984, p. 706).

Test characteristics. The upward drift in test scores that occurs over time (the "Flynn effect", see p. 21), appears in Block Design scores too. According to the WAIS-III manual (Wechsler, 1997a), there was a 0.7-point differential between mean WAIS-III Block Design scaled scores (10.7) and mean WAIS-R scaled scores (11.4), based on the performance of 192 subjects who took the WAIS-R and the WAIS-III in counterbalanced order.

Age has a prominent effect on Block Design performance. One need only review the normative data through the presented age ranges to appreciate how much advancing age reduces performance levels on this test (e.g., J.J. Ryan, Sattler, and Lopez, 2000; D. Wechsler, 1955, 1981, 1997a). As was observed on WAIS-R Block Design (Heaton, Grant, and Matthews, 1986; A.S. Kaufman, Reynolds, and McLean, 1989), WAIS-III Block Design performance starts to decline as early as the mid-40s and continues to worsen with each decade (J.J. Ryan, Satler, and Lopez, 2000). Much of the difference between younger and older subjects lies

in the speed with which designs are completed (Ogden, 1990; Salthouse, Fristoe, and Rhee, 1996). Among older subjects, reduced speed and accuracy are evident in the performance of the "old-old" (those over 80) when compared with the "young-old" (those in their 60s and 70s) (Howieson, Holm, et al., 1993; Joy et al., 2001). Education does not appear to contribute significantly to the decremental aging pattern (A.S. Kaufman and Lichtenberger, 1999; Salthouse, Fristoe, and Rhee, 1996). Block Design performance predicted the daily functioning of elderly (age 65–87), independently living persons as it correlated significantly with ratings on behavioral competency and several measures of the effectiveness of verbal communication (North and Ulatowska, 1981).

Men generally tend to score higher than women on Block Design, at least at younger ages (W.G. Snow and Weinstock, 1990). There is an almost one-point differential between the sexes for WAIS-R standardization population age groups within the 16– to 54 year range; from age 55 on, this difference shrinks to less than one-third of a point (A.S. Kaufman, Kaufman-Packer, et al., 1991) and is reported to be nonexistent for persons in the 65–74 and 80–100 ranges (Howieson, Holm, et al., 1993). This may in part be explained by hormonal factors. Testosterone supplementation—which also elevates estradiol levels—is associated with improved Block Design performance in older men (aged 50–80), whose baseline testosterone levels were in the low normal range for their age (Cherrier et al., 2001), but testosterone supplementation impaired performance in younger men whose baseline testosterone levels were normal (O'Connor et al., 2001). It has also been reported that younger women with higher estradiol levels do better on Block Design (Janowsky, Chavez, et al., 1998).

An approximately one-point difference in performances by whites and by African-Americans favors whites at all age levels (A.S. Kaufman, McLean, and Reynolds, 1991; Marcopulos, McLain, and Giuliano, 1997). However, deficient performances that appear at first to be attributable to race are in fact linked to disparities in education and acculturation (Ardila and Moreno, 2001; Manly, Miller, et al., 1998).

The internal consistency of the WAIS-III Block Design test is comparable to that of its WAIS-R predecessor. The manual reports split-half reliability coefficients for 13 age groups: these coefficients range from .85 to .90 in examinees under age 75, with slightly lower reliabilities (.76 to .81) observed in older examinees (Wechsler, 1997a). Slightly higher reliability coefficients (.88 to .95) were evident in most of the clinical samples, except for subjects with learning disabilities (.81) or hearing impairments (.77) (Zhu et al., 2001).

Test–retest reliabilities of the WAIS-III Block Design in 394 subjects retested over intervals of 2 to 12 weeks (with a mean of 34.6 days) ranged from .80 to .88 (corrected), depending on the age group. Similar test–retest reliability coefficients were observed in samples of adults with substance abuse disorders (J.J. Ryan, Arb, Paul, and Kreiner, 2000) and with complex partial seizures (R. Martin, Sawrie, et al., 2002).

Factor analytic studies of the WIS battery invariably demonstrate high loadings for Block Design on a Perceptual Organization factor, regardless of the number of factors derived or neuropsychological status of the subjects (J. Cohen, 1957a,b; Dickinson et al., 2002; A.S. Kaufman and Lichtenberger, 1999; J.J. Ryan and Paolo, 2001; van der Heijden and Donders, 2003; D. Wechsler, 1997c). Loading of Block Design on a Perceptual Organization factor holds across all age groups up to about age 75, at which time Block Design and other timed tests load more strongly on a Processing Speed factor. The WAIS-III manual confirms that Block Design performance correlates .48 to .52 with the predominantly verbal tests in the WAIS-III—Information, Vocabulary and Similarities.

Neuropsychological findings. Block Design is generally recognized as the best measure of visuospatial organization in the Wechsler scales. Block Design scores tend to be lower in the presence of any kind of brain impairment, suggesting that test performance is affected by multiple factors. In normal subjects, Block Design performance has been associated with increased glucose metabolism in the "posteroparietal region," particularly involving the right side (Chase et al., 1984). Studies of clinical populations corroborate the association of Block Design performance with right hemisphere, particularly parietal, function. In patients with lateralized lesions, Block Design performance is most often deficient when lesions are on the right side and involve posterior areas, particularly the parietal region (Newcombe, 1969; Warrington, James, and Maciejewski, 1986; Wilde et al., 2000), and is impaired less often when the lesion is confined to the left hemisphere—except when the left parietal lobe is involved (Benton, 1967; McFie, 1975). In Alzheimer patients, Block Design performance is strongly associated with atrophy in the right parietal region, specifically the size of the right anterior calcarine sulcus (Mega et al., 1998).

Patients with extensive right hemisphere damage that includes the parietal lobe or severe damage to prefrontal cortex and patients with considerable loss of cortical neurons as in Alzheimer's disease are all likely to perform very poorly on this test, but in different ways (e.g., Luria, 1973b). Defective Block Design performance by patients with lesions in either hemisphere

or by a "split brain" patient can use only one hemisphere, convincingly demonstrate that both hemispheres contribute to the realization of the design: "neither hemisphere alone is competent in this task" (Geschwind, 1979). The nature of the impairment tends to differ according to the side of the lesion, however (Consoli, 1979). Patients with lateralized lesions tend to make more errors on the side of the design contralateral to their lesion. Edith Kaplan has called attention to the importance of noting whether lateralized errors tend to occur more at the top or at the bottom of the constructions, as the upper visual fields have temporal lobe components while the lower fields have parietal components. Thus, a pattern of errors clustering at the top or bottom corner can also give some indication of lesion site.

Patients with left—particularly left parietal—lesions often show confusion, simplification, and concrete handling of the design. Still their approach is apt to be orderly, they typically work from left to right as do intact subjects (i.e., intact subjects whose native language is read from left to right), and their constructions usually preserve the overall configurations (square shape) of the design. When they make errors, these will involve details of the design. They may be hesitant, and their greatest difficulty may be in placing the last block (which most often will be on their right) (McFie, 1975). Time constraints contribute more to lowering scores of patients with left hemisphere involvement than of those with right-sided lesions: when allowed additional time to complete each item, many patients with left hemisphere lesions will achieve scores within or even above the *average* range (Akshoomoff et al., 1989).

In contrast, patients with right-sided lesions will often work from right to left, may have difficulty with design orientation, and may distort major elements of the design. Some patients with severe visuospatial deficits will lose sight of the overall configuration of the block pattern altogether (see Chapter 3, Fig. 3.9c–e). Left visuospatial inattention may compound these design-copying problems, resulting in two- or three-block solutions to the four-block designs, with the whole left half or one left quadrant missing. Broken configurations are a common characteristic of the constructions of patients with right-sided lesions (E. Kaplan, Fein, et al., 1991). Broken configuration errors have been observed more often in epilepsy patients whose hemisphere focus is on the right than on the left (Zipf-Williams et al., 2000), and in patients with nonpenetrating head injuries who underwent right, as opposed to left, craniotomies (Wilde et al., 2000). Patients with right hemisphere strokes typically show a small but measurable improvement in their Block Design performance during the months following their stroke, whereas patients with left hemisphere strokes may or may not improve, presumably due to differences in the reasons for their initial poor performance (T. Sunderland, Tinson, and Bradley, 1994).

Patients with severe damage to the frontal lobes may display a kind of "stickiness" (see p. 82) on this test, despite assertions that they understand the instructions. With less severe frontal involvement, patients may fail items because of impulsivity and carelessness. Unable to conduct a thorough and logical analysis of the designs, they adopt a seemingly random approach to solving the problem and fail to appreciate or correct their errors (Johanson et al., 1986). Concrete thinking often shows up on the first item, for such patients will try to make the sides as well as the top of their construction match that of the model; some will even go so far as to lift the model to make sure they have matched the underside as well. Some of these patients may be able to copy many of the designs quickly and accurately, but they tend to fail design 11 (design 7 of the WAIS-R) by laying out red and white stripes with whole blocks, rather than shifting their conceptualization of the design from the mostly squared format of the first 3×3 design to a solution based on diagonals.

Block Design performance is relatively spared in patients with mild to moderate TBI, whose processing speed deficits are much more striking (Axelrod, Fichtenberg, et al., 2001; Correll et al., 1993). Acute TBI patients with CT evidence of frontal contusions are an exception and often do poorly on this test (Wallesch, Curio, et al., 2001), as do patients with moderate to severe TBI who subsequently undergo right craniotomies (Wilde et al., 2000). There is certainly variability in the extent to which TBI patients improve over the long term, but Block Design performance often improves (Millis, Rosenthal, et al., 2001). On average, even patients with severe TBI performed Block Design similarly to controls one year after their injury (H.S. Levin, Gary, et al., 1990).

In contrast, the Block Design scores of Alzheimer patients are typically among the lowest if not the lowest in the Wechsler battery (Fuld, 1984; Larrabee, Largen, and Levin, 1985; Storandt, Botwinick, and Danziger, 1986). It has also proven to be a useful predictor of the disease as a relatively low Block Design score in the early stages, when the diagnosis is very much in question, frequently heralds the onset of the disease (Arnaiz et al., 2001; L. Berg, Danziger, et al., 1984; La Rue and Jarvik, 1987), and thus aids in the critical differential diagnosis. It is also one of the most useful neuropsychological tests for predicting which patients will deteriorate the most rapidly (B.J. Small, Viitanen, et al., 1997) and for staging dementia progression (Herlitz, Hill, et al., 1995).

Alzheimer patients will, in the very early stages of the disease, understand the task and may be able to copy several of the designs. However, with disease progression, these patients get so confused between one block and another or between their constructions and the examiner's model that they may even be unable to imitate the placement of just one or two blocks. The quality of "stickiness," often used to describe the performance of impaired patients but hard to define, here takes on concrete meaning when patients place their blocks on the design cards or adjacent to the examiner's model and appear unable to respond in any other way. Alzheimer patients and those frontal lobe patients who cannot make the blocks do what they want them to do can be properly described as having constructional apraxia. The discontinuity between intent—typically based on accurate perceptions—and action reflects the breakdown in the program of an activity that is central to the concept of apraxia.

Patients with neurodegenerative diseases that typically involve subcortical structures—such as Huntington's disease, Parkinson's disease, and multiple sclerosis—often do poorly on Block Design, although less so than patients with Alzheimer's disease (Heaton, Nelson, et al., 1985; C. Randolph, Mohr, and Chase, 1993). Processing speed deficiencies and motor problems undoubtedly contribute to the performance impairments of these patients. Chronic alcoholics also perform poorly on Block Design, even after several months of abstinence (E.V. Sullivan, Rosenbloom, and Pfefferbaum, 2000; E.V. Sullivan, Fama, et al., 2002). Unlike patients with right hemisphere damage, alcoholics benefit more from not being timed and they typically do not break the design configuration (Akshoomoff et al., 1989). Block Design is also exquisitely sensitive to the subtle neurotoxic effects of exposure to lead (A. Barth, Schaffer, Osterode, et al., 2002; Meyer-Baron and Seeber, 2000) and to other heavy metals (A. Barth, Schaffer, Konnaris, et al., 2002).

Slowness in learning new response sets may develop with a number of conditions such as aging, a dementing process, frontal lobe disease, or head injury. The Block Design format is sufficiently unfamiliar that patients capable of performing well may do poorly at first if they have this problem. Since Designs 5 to 8 are quite easy for persons with *average* or better constructional ability, they give the patient who is slow to learn a new set the opportunity to gain needed familiarity. These patients tend to display an interesting response pattern in which the first two items are failed—or at best passed only on the second trial—while the succeeding two or three or more items are passed, each more rapidly than the last. Those patients who are slow in learning a response set but whose ability to make constructions is good may succeed on most or even all the difficult items despite their early failure.

Kohs Block Design test (Kohs, 1919)

This is the original block design test, differing from the WIS Block Design in that each block has four colors—red, white, blue, and yellow—each of which appears on one face of the block, while the other two faces each have two colors, divided along the diagonal. The 17 designs are different, too, many of them being more complex than the Wechsler designs. The administration and qualitative interpretation of the test results are essentially the same as Wechsler's. The almost universal use of the Wechsler scales in North America has made the administration of the Kohs Blocks redundant in most cases, although it is still used occasionally in other parts of the world. Pontius (1997), in a fascinating series of studies, has used the Kohs Block Design Test to illustrate that certain types of constructional errors—those involving subtle intrapattern visual details—vary from culture to culture as a function of the extent to which a culture is urbanized and literate. Kohs' test has some more difficult designs than Wechsler's. It has recently been adapted for use with visually impaired individuals (Reid, 2002).

Stick construction

Stick construction is a two-dimensional task in which the examinee puts sticks together in patterns. In its usual format as a copying task, the subject is required to reproduce stick patterns arranged by the examiner (K.H. Goldstein and Scheerer, 1953). Examinees can also be asked to construct their own designs with the sticks, to copy a drawing, or to compose simple geometric figures or letters (Hécaen and Assal, 1970).

Alfano and Michel (1994) hypothesized that using a two-dimensional drawing (either realistic or schematic) as a model requires the examinee to make an extra step—first processing the drawing as an object and then processing it as a symbolic representation of the stick array. Consequently, they found that healthy young adults made more errors when working from drawings as opposed to stick models. These subjects also took more time and made more errors when the stick patterns involved diagonally placed sticks as opposed to horizontal and vertical, implicating additional processing demands for diagonally oriented stimuli.

Matute and her colleagues (2000), using a stick test consisting of four increasingly complex constructions, observed that subjects' literacy level had a significant impact on both their overall performance as well as types of errors, as illiterate subjects made more disar-

ticulation errors (inaccurately joined sticks) and reproduced fewer correct stick patterns than either literate or semiliterate subjects. Accuracy on the most complex stick pattern (an 11-stick house depicted in perspective) discriminated the performance of all three groups, with nearly all (96%) of the literates reproducing it correctly, compared with 76% of the semi-literates and only 52% of the illiterates. This study highlights the importance of considering an examinee's literacy level in interpreting performance even on ostensibly nonverbal tasks.

Twice as many right as left hemisphere impaired patients showed a severe deficit on stick construction tasks (14% vs. 7%) (Benton, 1967 [1985]). Approximately 20% of patients with lateralized lesions have some difficulty on this task regardless of the side of lesion. When attempting to construct a cube pattern with the sticks: patients with left hemisphere lesions copied stick models best, whereas right hemisphere patients copied drawings best (Hécaen and Assal, 1970).

Stick Test (Benson and Barton, 1970; N. Butters and Barton, 1970)

One version of the stick construction task includes a rotation condition as well as a standard copy condition. This ten-item test begins as a copying task. The examiner remains seated beside the patient throughout the first "match condition" part of the test. The examiner gives the patient four wooden sticks (approximately 5 inches long and 1/4-inch wide with a 1/2-inch blackened tip) and then makes a practice pattern with two other sticks, instructing the patient to copy this pattern exactly. The examiner does not proceed until convinced that the patient understands and can perform this two-stick problem. The examiner then gives the test by constructing each design in numbered order (see Fig. 14.10, p. 563), requesting the patient to make a copy directly under that of the examiner.

On completing the ten copy items, the examiner moves to the other side of the examining table to sit opposite the patient. After constructing the same two-stick practice pattern made originally, the examiner now asks the patient to "make your pattern look to you like mine looks to me." If the patient does not understand, the examiner demonstrates the right–left and up–down reversals with the practice pattern. Once again, when the examiner is confident that the patient understands what is required, the items of the test are given in the same order as the first time. Patients are encouraged to take as much time as they feel they need to be accurate. Each condition is scored for the number of failed items. On the reversal condition, the test is discontinued after five consecutive failures.

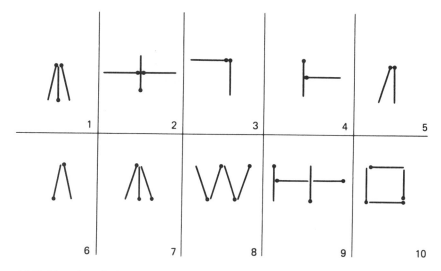

FIGURE 14.10 The 10 stick designs employed in the match and rotation conditions. (Butters and Barton, 1970. © Pergamon Press. Reprinted with permission.)

The findings on the copy task implicate postcentral lesions, particularly those localized in the right hemisphere. However, on the rotation condition, there was a significant ($p < .05$) tendency for patients with left postcentral lesions to make more errors ($M = 2.74$) than any other group. Those with right anterior lesions made the second greatest number of errors ($M = 2.13$), and the left anterior group made almost as few ($M = 1.69$) as did the 16 control subjects ($M = 1.59$) (Benson and Barton, 1970). The need for verbal mediation to handle the rotation task successfully was suggested as one possible reason for the relatively poor performance of the left posterior patients.

Object Assembly (Wechsler, 1955, 1981, 1997a)

One of the standard Performance Scale tests in previous versions of the WIS-A, Object Assembly was substantially revised and made an optional test on the WAIS-III. This test contains cut-up cardboard figures of familiar objects (see Fig. 14.11), given in order of increasing difficulty. The Mannequin (now called the Man), Profile, and Elephant have been retained from earlier versions, but the Hand item from the WAIS-R (which was similar in difficulty to the Elephant) was dropped, and two more difficult items—House and Butterfly—were added. The puzzle pieces now have numbers on the back to assist the examiner in laying them out as specified in the manual. All items are administered to every subject. Each item has a time limit (2 min for the two easiest puzzles, three min for the others), but unlike Block Design, partially complete responses receive credit too. Responses are scored for both accuracy and speed, with nearly one-third of the test's points (16 out of 52 possible points on the WAIS-III, 12 out of 41 on the WAIS-R) being awarded for speed.

Test characteristics. As in other speed-dependent tasks, performance levels on Object Assembly drop with age (Ivnik, Malec, Smith, et al., 1992b; A.S. Kaufman and Lichtenberger, 1999; J.J. Ryan, sattler, and Lopez, 2000). At ages 20–24, it takes a raw score of 34 to achieve the mean age-graded scaled score of 10, but only 26 points are needed at age 55–64 and only 18 points at age 80 and above (Wechsler, 1955, 1981, 1997). As an optional test that is no longer figures into the IQ scores and indexes, WAIS-III Object Assembly is often not administered in studies of the influence of demographic or clinical factors. WAIS-R studies of Object Assembly suggested that although there were no

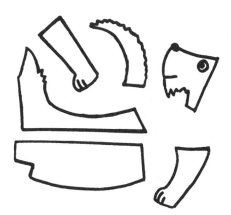

FIGURE 14.11 WIS-type Object Assembly test item.

overall sex differences, men outperformed women in some age groups and women outperformed men in others (A.S. Kaufman, Kaufman-Packer, et al., 1991; A.S. Kaufman, McLean, and Reynolds, 1988). Education accounted for no more than 10% of the variance in WAIS-R Object Assembly scores (for the 35–54 age range) and as little as 2% (for 16-19-year-olds) (A.S. Kaufman, McLean, and Reynolds, 1988). African-Americans' average scores ran about two points below those obtained by white subjects.

It is not surprising that split-half reliability coefficients for Object Assembly reported in the 1997 WAIS-III manual are the lowest among the Wechsler tests (in the .70 to .77 for subjects under age 70, and from .50 to .68 in those over 70), as items differ markedly in number of possible points that can be earned (8, 12, 11, 10, 11) and in difficulty level. Internal consistency is higher among most clinical samples, with the exception of young adults with attention deficit disorder (.58) or learning disabilities (.51) (Zhu et al., 2001). According to the manual, test–retest correlations (corrected) on Object Assembly range from .74 in 16- to 29-year-old subjects to .82 in subjects ages 55–74, with coefficients for the oldest subjects being slightly lower (.76).

Of all the WIS-A tests, Object Assembly has the lowest association with general mental ability and, in healthy individuals, performance level tends to vary relatively independently of other WIS test scores (Wechsler, 1955, 1981, 1997a). It is most strongly correlated with Block Design (.61), no doubt due to their similarity in requiring subjects to synthesize a construction from discrete parts. Object Assembly requires little abstract thinking, but subjects do need to be able to form visual concepts in order to perform adequately on this test, and they must be able to do so quickly and translate these into rapid hand responses to earn *average* or better scores. Thus, Object Assembly is as much a test of speed of visual organization and motor response as it is of the capacity for visual organization itself (Schear and Sato, 1989). Visual acuity and dexterity also make significant contributions.

Neuropsychological findings. The speed component of Object Assembly renders it relatively vulnerable to brain impairment in general. As one of the more time-consuming WIS-A tests it is typically not included in dementia batteries. However, it has proven particularly sensitive to Huntington's disease, as it is often the most difficult test in the WIS-A battery for these patients (M.E. Strauss and Brandt, 1985, 1986) and shows the steepest score declines with disease progression (Brandt, Strauss, et al., 1984).

As a test of constructional ability, Object Assembly

tends to be sensitive to posterior lesions, more so to those on the right than the left (F.W. Black and Strub, 1976). Thus, many patients, particularly those with right posterior lesions, who do poorly on Block Design are also likely to do poorly on Object Assembly. Differences in solution strategies tend to distinguish patients with left- or right-sided lesions (E. Kaplan, Fein, et al., 1991). The former are more prone to join pieces according to edge contours while ignoring internal features or relative sizes of the pieces, whereas the latter rely more on matching up surface details. To bring these differences out, Kaplan, Fein, and their colleagues developed two additional puzzles for the WAIS-R NI— a cow, which could best be solved by discriminating details, and a circle, which requires edges to be aligned for its solution. Patients with left hemisphere lesions would have more success with the circle; those with right-sided involvement would do better with the cow although, when the lesion involves the right posterior region, both puzzles would be likely to be failed.

Evaluating Block Design and Object Assembly together

The patterns of variations of Block Design and Object Assembly scores relative to one another and to other tests allow the examiner to infer the different functions that contribute to success on these tasks.

1. Impaired ability for visuospatial manipulation. The constructional rather than the perceptual component of this task is implicated when the patient performs better on such tests of visuoperceptual conceptualization and organization as the Hooper Visual Organization Test than on those requiring a constructed solution. This problem was described well by a 64-year-old logger who had had a right, predominantly temporoparietal stroke with transient mild left hemiparesis two years before taking the WAIS. When confronted with the Elephant puzzle he said, "I know what it's supposed to be but I can't do anything."

2. Impaired ability for visuospatial conceptualization. Other patients who appear unable to visualize or conceptualize what the Object Assembly constructions should be can put them together in piecemeal fashion by methodically matching lines and edges. Typically, they do not recognize what they are making until the puzzle is almost completely assembled. They are as capable of accepting grossly inaccurate constructions as correct solutions. They also tend to fail Block Design items that do not lend themselves to a verbalizable solution. Not surprisingly, these patients have difficulty with purely perceptual tasks such as the Hooper. Their ability to conceptualize what they are doing does not seem to benefit from visuomotor stimulation, although their visuomotor coordination and control may be excellent. Their damage almost invariably involves the right posterior cortex.

3. *Ability for visuospatial conceptualization dependent on visuomotor activity.* Yet another group of patients, who typically have at least some right parietal damage, perform constructional tasks such as Object Assembly and Block Design by using trial and error to manipulate their way to acceptable solutions without having to rely solely on discrete features or verbal guidance. These patients seem unable to form visuospatial concepts before seeing the actual objects, but their perceptions are sufficiently accurate and their self-correcting abilities sufficiently intact that as they manipulate the pieces they can identify correct relationships and thus use their evolving visual concepts to guide them. They too do extremely poorly on perceptual tasks such as the Hooper, on which they cannot manipulate the pieces in order to develop a visual concept.

4. *Impaired ability to appreciate details.* Patients with left hemisphere lesions who do poorly on Object Assembly usually get low scores on Block Design as well. These patients tend to rely on the overall contours of the puzzle pieces but disregard such details as internal features or the relative size of pieces.

5. *Structure dependency.* Some patients may perform satisfactorily when a framework or pattern is available—as on Block Design or Matrix Reasoning as they can follow or pick out a ready-made pattern. They tend to have much more trouble with Object Assembly, the Hooper, or drawing a bicycle since these latter tests require them to provide their own structure to conceptualize, or identify, the finished product in order to assemble it mentally or actually. These patients usually have at least some frontal lobe pathology.

6. *Concrete-mindedness.* Still other patients may perform relatively well on Object Assembly since it involves concrete, meaningful objects; they may even do all right with the first two block models on Block Design, but they have difficulty comprehending the abstract designs on the reduced-scale pictures and thus perform poorly on Block Design as a whole. Again, some frontal pathology is usually implicated in these cases.

Three-Dimensional Construction

Block construction

The simple block construction tasks described here will elicit three-dimensional visuoconstructive defects. The revision of the 1960 Stanford-Binet battery (Terman and Merrill, 1973) contains two simple block construction tasks: *Tower* at age level II is simply a four-block-high structure; *Bridge* at age level III consists of

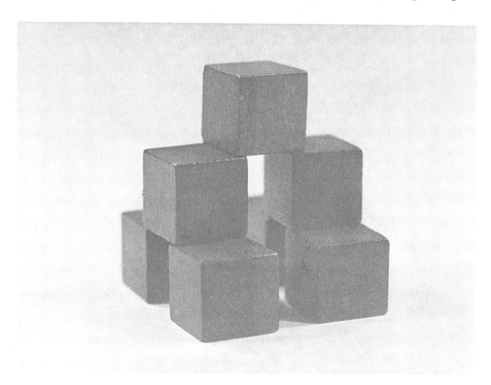

FIGURE 14.12 Block model used by Hécaen, Ajuriaguerra, and Massonnet (1951) to examine three-dimensional constructional ability.

three blocks, two forming a base with the third straddling them. The level at which age-graded tasks are failed provides a useful indicator of the severity of the impairment:

As points of reference, most three-year-olds can copy a four-block train (three blocks in a row with the fourth placed on one of the end blocks); most four-year-olds can build a six-block pyramid and a five-block gate composed of two two-block "towers," less than one inch apart, with each top block set a little back from the bottom block's edge, making room for a middle block to rest at a 45° angle. At five, most children can copy six-block steps but ten-block steps are too difficult for most six-year-olds. (E.M. Taylor, 1959)

Hécaen and his colleagues (1951) used seven blocks in their block construction task (see Fig. 14.12, p. 565). None of their six patients with severe visuoconstruc-

tive deficits associated with right parietal lesions was able to copy this construction correctly.

Test of Three-Dimensional Block Construction (Benton, Sivan, Hamsher et al., 1994)

Six block constructions are included in this test (originally called the *Test of Three-Dimensional Constructional Praxis*), three on each of two equivalent forms: a six-block pyramid, an eight-block four-level construction, and a 15-block four-level construction (see Fig. 14.13). The number of errors, namely (1) omissions, (2) additions, (3) substitutions, and (4) displacements (angular deviations greater than 45°, separations, and misplacements) that the examinee makes is subtracted from the total of 29 possible correct place-

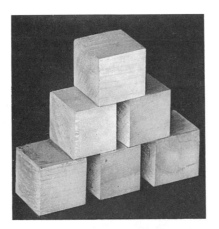
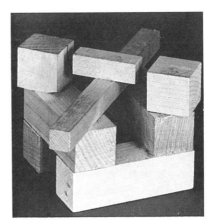
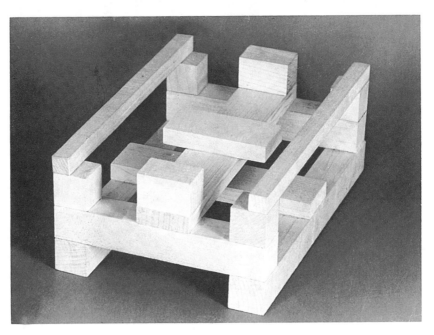

FIGURE 14.13 Test of Three-Dimensional Constructional Praxis, Form A (A.L. Benton). The three block models are presented successively to the subject.

ments. Rotations are not counted as errors, although these are noted qualitatively. The score should represent the fewest corrections needed to reproduce an accurate copy of the original construction. When the construction is so defective that it is impossible to count errors, the score is simply the number of correctly placed blocks. When the total time taken to complete all three constructions is over 380 sec, two points are subtracted from the total score. As on the Stick Test, both healthy and impaired subjects are more accurate when using a block model of the desired construction than when presented with a photograph (Benton, 1973).

Some of the construction problems exhibited by patients with impaired ability to build structures in three dimensions parallel those made on two-dimensional construction and drawing tasks. Thus, simplification (see Fig. 14.14a) and neglect of half the model are not uncommon (note also Fig. 14.14b). Failure on this task—defined as a performance level exceeded by 95% of the control group—occurred twice as frequently among patients with right hemisphere lesions (54%) as among those whose lesions were on the left (23%) (Benton, 1967 [1985]). A higher rate of defective performance on this task also distinguished right from left frontal lobe patients (Benton, 1968). Unlike other visuoconstructive tasks (e.g., block designs and stick construction), this test discriminates between groups of right and left hemisphere patients who are moderately impaired as well as between those who are severely im-

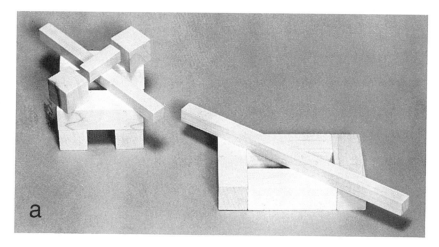

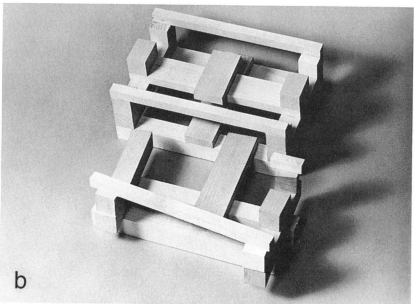

Figure 14.14 Illustrations of defective performances. (a) Simplified construction with inaccurate choice of blocks. (b) "Closing-in phenomenon" in which the patient incorporates part of the model into the construction.

paired (Benton, 1967 [1985]). One plausible interpretation of this finding is that the Test of Three-Dimensional Block Construction is more difficult and therefore better able to detect subtler visuoconstructive deficits that do not interfere with performance on less challenging tasks.

Miscellaneous three-dimensional construction tasks

In *Paper Folding: Triangle* at age level V of the revision of the 1960 Stanford-Binet (Terman and Merrill, 1973), the examinee is asked to copy a three-dimensional maneuver in which the examiner folds a square of paper along the diagonal into a triangle and folds that triangle in half. In Paper Cutting subtests at IX, XIII, and AA levels, the examiner cuts holes in folded paper so that the subject can see how the paper is cut but not how the unfolded paper looks. Subjects must then draw a picture of how they think the paper will look when unfolded. This test was included in a battery for studying the visual space perception of patients with lateralized lesions (McFie and Zangwill, 1960).

A different kind of spatial maneuver is required by Poppelreuter's test, in which the subject must cut out a four-pointed star following a demonstration by the examiner (Paterson and Zangwill, 1944). Patients with right parieto-occipital lesions were unable to perform this task. The possibility of using children's building toys (e.g., Lego type plastic blocks, erector sets, K'nex) for testing visuospatial functions should not be overlooked, even though—excepting Tinker Toys (pp. 621–626)—they have not been reported as standard assessment procedures.

15 | Concept Formation and Reasoning

If reasoning were like hauling I should agree that several reasoners would be worth more than one, just as several horses can haul more sacks of grain than one can. But reasoning is like racing and not like hauling, and a single Barbary steed can outrun a hundred dray horses.

Galileo Galilei, The Assayer, 1623 (in Sobel, 1999)

Conceptual dysfunctions and impaired reasoning tend to be affected by brain injury almost regardless of site (Luria, 1966; Mesulam, 2000b; A.C. Roberts, Robbins, and Weiskrantz, 1998, *passim*). This is not surprising since conceptual activities always involve at least (1) an intact system for organizing perceptions even though specific perceptual modalities may be impaired; (2) a well-stocked and readily accessible store of remembered learned material; (3) the integrity of the cortical and subcortical interconnections and interaction patterns that underlie "thought"; and (4) the capacity to process two or more mental events at a time. In addition, the translation of cognitive activity into overt behavior requires (5) a response modality sufficiently integrated with central cortical activity to transform conceptual experience into manifest behavior; and (6) a well-functioning response feedback system for continuous monitoring and modulation of output.

Concrete thinking is the most common sign of impaired conceptual functions. It usually appears as an inability to think in useful generalizations, at the level of ideas, or about persons, situations, events not immediately present (past, future, or out of sight). The patient may have difficulty forming concepts, using categories, generalizing from a single instance, or applying procedural rules and general principles, be they rules of grammar or conduct, mathematical operations, or good housekeeping practices. Difficulty in assuming an abstract attitude often results in a preference for obvious, superficial solutions. The patient may be unaware of subtle underlying or intrinsic aspects of a problem and thereby be unable to distinguish what is relevant from what is irrelevant, essential from unessential, and appropriate from outlandish. To the extent that the patient cannot conceptualize abstractly, each event is dealt with as if it were novel, an isolated experience with a unique set of rules.

Conceptual concreteness and mental inflexibility are sometimes treated as different aspects of the same disability. When they occur together they tend to be mutually reinforcing in their effects. However, they can be separated (Kimberg et al., 2000; Sohlberg and Mateer, 2001). Although both are associated with extensive or diffuse damage, significant conceptual inflexibility can be present without much impairment of the ability to form and apply abstract concepts, particularly when there is frontal lobe involvement (A.R. Damasio and Anderson, 2003; Stuss, Benson, Kaplan, et al., 1983). Furthermore, conceptual concreteness does not imply impairment of specific reasoning abilities. Thinking may be concrete even when the patient can perform many specific reasoning tasks well, such as solving arithmetic problems or making familiar practical judgments. On the other hand, thinking is likely to be concrete when the patient has specific reasoning disabilities.

Most tests of conceptual functions are designed to probe for concrete thinking in one form or another, usually testing concept formation by itself or in conjunction with mental flexibility. Tests of other cognitive functions, such as planning and organizing, or problem solving, and reasoning, do not treat concrete thinking as the primary examination object, but they often supply information about it. Tests that deal with mental flexibility per se are discussed in Chapter 16, pp. 627–635.

CONCEPT FORMATION

Tests of concept formation differ from most other mental tests in that they focus on the *quality* or *process* of thinking more than the content of the response. Many of these tests have no "right" or "wrong" answers. Their scores stand for qualitative judgments of the extent to which the response was abstract or concrete, complex or simple, apt or irrelevant. Tests with right and wrong answers belong in the category of tests of abstract conceptualization to the extent that they provide information about *how* the patient thinks.

Patients with moderate to severe focal or multiple lesions or with significant diffuse injury tend to do poorly on all tests of abstract thinking, regardless of their mode of presentation or channel of response (e.g., see Grafman, Jonas, and Salazar, 1990). However, patients with mild, modality specific, or subtle organic defects may not engage in concrete thinking generally, but only on those tasks that directly involve an impaired modality, are highly complex, or touch upon emotionally arousing matters. Furthermore, concrete thinking takes different forms with different patients, and varies in its effect on mental efficiency with the type of task. Examiners who are interested in finding out how their patients think will use more than one kind of concept formation test involving more than one sensory or response modality.

Concept Formation Tests in Verbal Formats

Proverbs

Tests of interpretation of proverbs are among the most widely used techniques for evaluating the quality of thinking. They require the subject to translate a concrete statement into its abstract, metaphorical meaning. The Wechsler tests, the L-M edition of the Stanford-Binet scales, and mental status examinations include proverb interpretation items (see also Luria, 1966, pp. 453–454). Their popularity rests on their usefulness as an indicator of conceptual dysfunction (W.S. Brown and Paul, 2000; Van Lancker, 1990). Moreover, most patients can offer some response without a loss of dignity.

The patient's familiarity with a proverb can be important in obscuring conceptual deficits, particularly among elderly persons. Several generations ago proverbs were common conversational coin so that many elderly patients can express suitable meanings for familiar ones while being unable to think abstractly. This pattern may be observed in patients with mild Alzheimer's disease (S.B. Chapman, 1997). On the other hand, proverbs really test abstract verbal reasoning in young people, particularly those with little interest in or exposure to the ways of older generations. Van Lancker (1990) noted that, "What makes a proverb difficult is that it is unfamiliar, not that it is more abstract."

Although it is assumed that the abstract–concrete dimension is a continuum, interpretations of proverbs are usually evaluated dichotomously, as either abstract or concrete. The commonly used 3-point scoring system preserves this dichotomy (e.g., M.S. Albert, Wolfe, and Lafleche, 1990; Strub and Black, 2000; D. Wechsler, 1955, 1981, 1997a). It is also implicit in informal evaluations of patients' responses in mental status examinations. In this system, appropriate abstract interpretations earn two points (e.g., A rolling stone gathers no moss: "You will have nothing if you keep on moving"); concrete interpretations earn one point (e.g., "Most turning objects never gather anything" or "Because of moss will fall off"), or no points if the response misses the gist of the proverb or misinterprets it (e.g., "If you

keep busy you will feel better"). Usually this scoring system creates no problems, but occasionally patients' interpretations will be borderline or difficult to classify.

Proverbs Test (Gorham, 1956a,b)

This test formalizes the task of proverb interpretation, presenting it as an important source of information about the quality of thinking in its own right rather than as part of another examination. Its standardization reduces variations in administration and scoring biases and provides norms that take into account the difficulty level of individual proverbs. The Proverbs Test has three forms, each containing 12 proverbs of equivalent difficulty. It is administered as a written test in which the subject is instructed to "tell what the proverb means rather than just tell more about it." The 3-point scoring system provides a maximum score of 36. Mean scores for each form of the test do not differ significantly, and the scoring scheme has a high test–retest reliability ($r = .96$). A multiple-choice version of the Proverbs Test (the Best Answer Form) contains 40 items, each with four choices of possible answers. Only one of the choices is appropriate and abstract; the other three are either concrete interpretations or common misinterpretations.

In addition to standard scoring procedures, M.S. Albert, Wolfe, and Lafleche (1990) used a six category system to evaluate response quality: besides *abstract* and *totally concrete* these include *partially abstract, abstract tangential, partially concrete,* and *concrete tangential.* Age differences do not appear until the 60s, but then performance averages drop substantially (M.S. Albert, Wolfe, and Lafleche, 1990). The free format elicited significantly more concrete responses from older subjects; on the multiple-choice trial both abstract and concrete tangential responses as well as totally concrete ones were given more frequently by the older groups. Bromley (1957) also documented a pronounced tendency for the relative number of concrete responses to increase with age on both kinds of test format. Proverbs Test scores vary with education level (and probably social class) (Gorham, 1956b).

Using the multiple-choice version in a study of frontal lobe functions, Benton (1968) reported very poor performance by seven patients with bilateral frontal lobe disease ($M = 11.4 \pm 6.1$), a somewhat better performance by eight patients with right frontal lobe disease ($M = 20.1 \pm 6.8$), and unexpectedly adequate scores achieved by ten patients with left frontal lobe disease ($M = 26.4 \pm 9.4$). On the multiple-choice form of the Proverbs Test, the scores of groups of schizophrenic and organic patients are significantly lower than those of normal control subjects, but they do not differ significantly among one another (Fogel, 1965). Patients with mild Alzheimer's disease perform adequately, which suggests that impairment in concept formation is not an early feature of this disease (Lafleche and Albert, 1995).

California Proverb Test (CPT) (Delis, Kramer, and Kaplan, 1988; Delis, Kaplan, and Kramer, 2001)

The 1988 version of this test takes advantage of the relatively greater sensitivity of unfamiliar than familiar proverbs by providing five of each (e.g., familiar: "Don't count your chickens before they are hatched;" unfamiliar: "The used key is always bright") (see also Delis, Kramer, Fridlund, and Kaplan, 1990). All ten proverbs are administered in both an oral, free-response trial and a printed, four-choice format in which two choices are correct but one is abstract and the other concrete, plus one incorrect phonemic response in which similar sounding words have semantically different meanings, and a completely incorrect response. Seven scoring categories were devised to classify the varieties of common errors (e.g., partial abstraction, specific instance, correct concrete, etc.). The 1988 CPT correlated well (.70 to .81) with Similarities and Vocabulary (WAIS-R). Split-half reliabilities were .88 and .77 for the free-response and multiple-choice formats, respectively.

The newer version of this multiple-choice test consists of eight proverbs of varying degrees of familiarity (e.g., "Rome was not built in a day" and "Too many cooks spoil the broth;" L.C. Henry, 1945). The four response alternatives for each item consist of two abstract interpretations—one correct and one incorrect, and two concrete interpretations—also one correct and one incorrect. Each proverb is scored 0 to 2 points for accuracy and 0 or 1 point for abstractness. Thus, a response may be scored as incorrect for abstractness yet receive 2 points for accuracy if it is a correct concrete interpretation, weighting the overall score toward accuracy rather than abstractness.

Word usage tests

Tests calling for abstract comparisons between two or more words provide a sensitive measure of concrete thinking. However, word usage is also very dependent upon both the integrity of the patient's communication system and level of verbal skills. Thus, patients who have even a mild aphasic disorder and those who have always been mentally dull or educationally underprivileged will do poorly on these tests, regardless of the extent to which their conceptual abilities have been preserved.

When the ability to form verbal concepts is evaluated, the patient's verbal skill level must always be taken into account. Easy items can be used with most adults who have completed the sixth grade. Difficult items may elicit evidence of cognitive dysfunction in bright, well-educated adults when their performance on easier words would seem to indicate that their ability to make verbal abstractions is intact.

Similarities (Wechsler, 1955, 1981, 1997a)

In this test of verbal concept formation the subject must explain what each of a pair of words has in common. The word pairs range in difficulty from the simplest ("orange-banana" in the first three editions; "fork-spoon" in the WAIS-III), which only retarded or seriously impaired adults fail, to the most difficult ("praise-punishment" on the WAIS-R; "enemy-friend" on the WAIS-III). Items are passed at the 2-point level if an abstract generalization is given and at the 1-point level if a response is a specific concrete likeness. One- or 2-point variations between scorers can occur. Deteriorated patients as well as persons whose general functioning is *borderline defective* or lower, sometimes respond with likenesses to the first few items but name a difference, which is generally easier to formulate, when the questions become difficult for them. The question can be repeated emphasizing the word "alike" the first time this happens. Sometimes this extra questioning will help the patient attend to the demand for a likeness on the next and subsequent questions. Both the erroneous and correct response will be recorded but only the latter should be scored.

The age-graded WAIS-R Similarities scaled scores are skewed in the direction of leniency for individuals 70 and older. A scaled score of 8, at the lower end of the *average* range, is relatively easy to earn at ages 70–74 since only 8 raw score points suffice (e.g., with 14 items, two to three good abstractions and two to four concrete responses) for a scaled score of 8 at ages 65 to 69. The Mayo norms for elderly people are more stringent at the lower levels; for example, awarding only 5 scaled score points—at the *borderline* level—for a raw score of 8 (Ivnik, Malec, Smith, et al., 1992b). The WAIS-III Similarities has more items, including five very easy pairs which earn only one point but are given only to persons unable to succeed on 2-point pairs. Persons in the 70–74 age group must achieve a raw score of 15 or 16 points to obtain a scaled score of 8, suggesting that this standardization is more realistic than previous ones.

Test characteristics. An age-related decline tends to show up in the 70s (Axelrod and Henry, 1992; A.S. Kaufman, Kaufman-Packer, et al., 1991) but education may account for much of it (Finlayson, Johnson, and Reitan, 1977; Heaton, Ryan, Grant, and Matthews, 1996). Education contributes to more than 25% of the variance at ages 35 and above, 24% in the 20–34 year range (A.S. Kaufman, McLean, and Reynolds, 1988). Small age and relatively large education effects continue into the 80s and 90s (Ivnik, Malec, Smith, et al., 1992b; Malec, Ivnik, Smith, et al., 1992a). Following a large group of identical twins, Jarvik (1988) found that those who gave no evidence of dementia had relatively unchanged performances until age 75 but experienced a fairly sharp drop in their Similarities scores between ages 75 and 86 (see also Whelihan and Lesher, 1985). The WAIS-III normative sample shows an age-related decline beginning with the 55 to 64 age group and proceeding slowly. At the age range 85–89, only 16 raw score points are needed for a scaled score of 10 compared to a required 23 raw score points for this scaled score level for middle-age persons.

On the WAIS-R Similarities sex effects are virtually nonexistent (A.S. Kaufman, Kaufman-Packer, et al., 1991; W.G. Snow and Weinstock, 1990). Average differences between whites and African Americans run about 2 scaled score points up through age 34 but increase to 2.5 points in the 35–54 age range (A.S. Kaufman, McLean, and Reynolds, 1988; Manly et al., 1998). When elders 65 years of age and older were matched for educational attainment, the difference between African Americans and whites was reduced to 1.2 points and was statistically significant. However, the factor structure for the two races is the same (A.S. Kaufman, McLean, and Reynolds, 1991).

Retesting subsamples from the WAIS-III standardization population after several weeks to months produced correlation coefficients from .83 to .88 for ages 30 and older (The Psychological Corporation, 1997). TBI patients who took the WAIS-R Similarities test four times in a 10-month span made a small but significant gain of almost one scaled score point compared with patients who took the test only twice with a 10-month interval (Rawlings and Crewe, 1992). Test–retest correlation coefficients for both older subjects (75+) and neurologically impaired patients were in the .70 to .80 range with intervals of one to five months (J.J. Ryan, Paolo, and Brungardt, 1992) or years (G. Goldstein and Watson, 1989), with no significant score improvement. Overall, few score gains are documented on retest (McCaffrey, Duff, and Westervelt, 2000a).

Similarities is an excellent test of general mental ability. In WIS-A batteries it reflects the verbal factor to a moderate degree (J. Cohen, 1957a,b) and often is included in short forms (e.g., J.J. Ryan and Ward, 1999). The WAIS-R verbal factor loading (3-factor solutions) runs from .63 to .70 for all ages 18 and older (K.C.H.

Parker, 1983). A higher verbal factor loading (.73) was reported for stroke patients with lateralized damage (Zillmer, Waechtler, et al., 1992), but a much lower one (.56) for a diagnostically heterogeneous group of brain impaired patients (J.J. Ryan and Schneider, 1986). The WAIS-III verbal comprehension loadings (4-factor solutions) range from .69 to .83, depending upon the age group (The Psychological Corporation, 1997).

Neuropsychological findings. Similarities was found to be sensitive to the effects of brain injury regardless of localization (Hirschenfang, 1960b). Exceptions have been reported for postacute trauma patients (Correll et al., 1993; J.T.L. Wilson, Hadley, et al., 1996) and for polysubstance abusers during detoxification (J.A. Sweeney et al., 1989) or four years after (Tapert and Brown, 1999) as the highest average score for each of these groups was on Similarities, suggesting that for some conditions this test may serve as an indicator of premorbid ability. However, these findings cannot be generalized but rather appear to characterize some subgroups within a diagnostic category but not others (e.g., Crosson, Greene, et al., 1990; G. Goldstein and Shelly, 1987).

Similarities' vulnerability to brain conditions that affect verbal functions compounds its vulnerability to impaired concept formation such that a relatively depressed Similarities score tends to be associated with left temporal and frontal involvement (McFie, 1975; Newcombe, 1969). These areas show increased glucose metabolism when normal subjects take the Similarities test (Chase et al., 1984). It is one of the best indicators of left hemisphere disease in the WIS-A battery (Warrington, James, and Maciejewski, 1986). For patients with anterior lesions on the right, Similarities scores tend to be unaffected (Bogen, DeZure, et al., 1972; McFie, 1975). Lower Similarities scores are also associated with bilateral frontal lesions (S.M. Rao, 1990; Sheer, 1956). As might be expected, Similarities is vulnerable to dementia (R.P. Hart, Kwentus, Taylor, and Hamer, 1988; Whelihan and Lesher, 1985). Some studies have found that performance decline is predictive of the development of Alzheimer's disease (D.M. Jacobs, Sano, and Dooneief, et al., 1995; Fabrigoule et al., 1998), while others have not shown any decline in the very early stage of the disease (Lafleche and Albert, 1995) or only a small scaled score point drop (Larrabee, Largen, and Levin, 1985). Relatively large losses on this test have been among the early predictors of abnormal cognitive decline in middle-aged persons (La Rue and Jarvik, 1987).

An occasional concrete-minded patient—usually one suffering from a diffuse dementing process—will do surprisingly well on this test, despite its usual independence from memory functions. Since these are almost always persons who had once enjoyed excellent verbal skills, it appears that in these cases the patient is calling upon old, well-formed verbal associations so that the test is actually eliciting old learning.

WAIS-R NI. This addition to the WIS-A examination provides a multiple-choice format offering four responses for each item. One of the four is a good (2-point) generalization; one is a concrete response (e.g., they [fruits] both have calories); and one is appropriate for only one of the two items (e.g., they both are round). Of course this version would typically be given only to subjects whose poor performance on the standard form of the test suggested that their free responses may not be indicative of their potential or to patients incapable of making a verbal response. The instructions also direct the examiner to evaluate responses for intratest scatter, although the degree of scatter on this test did not discriminate between control subjects and patients with either head injuries or focal lesions (Mittenberg, Hammeke, and Rao, 1989).

Luria's methods for examining concept formation (Luria, 1966; A.-L. Christensen, 1979; see also pp. 679–680)

Luria (1966, pp. 467–469) used a number of tasks involving words to examine conceptual thinking. In addition to questions about similarities and differences between verbal concepts, he gave subjects tasks of identifying "logical relationships." These relationships include general categories for specific ideas (e.g., "tool" for "chisel"), specific ideas for general categories (e.g., "rose" for "flower"), parts of a whole (e.g., "leg" of a "table"), and the whole from a part (e.g., "house" from "wall"). Luria also asked subjects to give opposites (e.g., "healthy—sick"), to find analogies (e.g., "table : leg :: bicycle : wheel"), and to identify "the superfluous fourth" word of a series in which three words are similar and one is different (e.g., "spade, saw, ax, log"). Luria did not give many examples of each category of concept formation problems, nor did Christensen. However, it would not be difficult for the examiner interested in using this technique to make up items for these tasks. More extensive samples of similar items are represented in the Stanford-Binet scales (see next section) where they also have the advantage of age norms.

Stanford-Binet subtests (Terman and Merrill, 1973; Thorndike et al., 1986)

The Stanford-Binet Form L-M (and earlier Forms L and M) tests verbal abstraction in a number of ways. All of the Binet items are scored on a pass–fail basis. Unlike more complex scoring systems (see pp. 570, 571), both concrete interpretations and misinterpretations of words and proverbs receive no credit.

There are three Similarities subtests: *Two Things* at age level VII contains such questions as, "In what way are wood and coal alike?" *Three Things* at age level XI is identical with the lower level similarities test except that likenesses have to be found for three words; i.e., "In what way are *book, teacher,* and *newspaper* alike?" *Essential Similarities* at the SA (*superior adult*) I level is a two-word similarities test requiring a high level of abstraction for credit.

There are also three Differences subtests in the Binet L-M. At age VI, *Differences* consists of three items asking for the differences between two words with fairly concrete referents, i.e., "What is the difference between a bird and a dog?" Differences between *Abstract Words* at the AA (*average adult*) level and *Essential Differences* at levels AA and SA II both ask for the differences between two abstract words. The only change distinguishing these two subtests, besides the content of the word pairs, is the insertion of the word "principal" in the question. "What is the (principal) difference between . . . ?" on the Essential Differences subtest.

Three *Similarities and Differences* vary in difficulty from year IV-6 to VIII. The simplest, *Pictorial Similarities and Differences I,* requires the subject to point to the one of four figures that is unlike the others (e.g., three crosses and a dash). At year V, *Pictorial Similarities and Differences II,* the subject must tell whether two figures (e.g., a circle and a square) are the same or different. The most difficult, *Similarities and Differences,* is completely verbal: the subject has to tell how two familiar objects, such as a baseball and an orange, are alike and how they differ.

In addition to the word comparison subtests, the 1973 Binet scales contain three subtests asking for definitions of *Abstract Words,* with scoring standards for years X and XII (*Abstract Words I*), XI and XIII (*Abstract Words II*), and the AA level (*Abstract Words III*). Word difficulty ranges from words of emotion, such as "pity" at the X and XII year levels to relatively abstract words, like "generosity" and "authority." The definitions, too, are scored on a 2-point pass–fail basis.

Opposite Analogies is another form of a word abstraction test. The Binet scales carry it in five versions spread over six age and ability levels from age level IV ("Brother is a boy; sister is a . . . ?") to SA III ("Ability is native; education is . . . ?").

The fourth edition of the *Stanford-Binet Intelligence Scale* (Thorndike et al., 1986) includes a series of orally presented analogy items, *Verbal Relations.* In each four-word item, the first three are similar (e.g., tools) and the fourth different. The subject's task is to tell how the first three words are similar to one another but differ from the fourth. The age-equivalent range begins at 11–9 and goes up to 17–1, making it unsuitable for discriminating examination of dull or deteriorating adults.

Concept Formation Tests in Visual Formats

Category Test (HCT) (Halstead, 1947; Reitan and Wolfson, 1993); *Booklet Category Test, 2nd ed. (BCT)* (DeFilippis and McCampbell, 1997)

This test of conceptual and spatial reasoning consists of 208 visually presented items. Six item sets, each organized on the basis of different principles, are followed by a seventh set made up mostly of previously shown items. The subject's task is to figure out the principle presented in each set and signal the answer. For example, the first set shows roman numerals from I to IV, guiding the subject to the use of a response system with four possible answers, "one" to "four". In the third set, one of the four figures of each item differs from the others (e.g., three squares and a circle) and must be identified by its position in a row. The fifth set shows geometric figures made up of solid and dotted lines for which the proportion in solid lines is the correct answer (e.g., one-fourth, two-fourths, etc.). The seventh set tests the subject's recall. The score is the number of errors.

Besides the original (and very expensive and cumbersome) mechanized screen display version in which a pleasant chime rewards correct answers and errors receive a buzz (see Fig. 15.1), both a booklet (DeFilippis and McCampbell, 1997; DeFilippis, McCampbell, and Rogers, 1979) and a new computer version (DeFilippis and PAR Staff, 2002) are available. A handy card form was developed by S.D. Kimura (1981), who distributed several hundreds of these sets, but it is no longer available. Studies of these formats indicate they are essentially interchangeable (Holtz et al., 1996). The booklet and card forms use verbal responses—"right, wrong"—to provide feedback, with no apparent effect on performances (Ivins and Cunningham, 1989; Mercer et al., 1997).

A problem that has plagued the mechanized administration is the amount of time it takes. Several brain injured groups, all with average performances within the impaired range, had mean times in the 32 to 40 minute range with 42% taking longer than 40 minutes and two patients finishing in less than 20 minutes (Finlayson, Sullivan, and Alfano, 1986). Reitan and Wolfson (1993) suggest that a set may be discontinued for subjects who seem unlikely to solve it, which is one solution to the time problem. The card format, which allows a rapid flipping through when subjects have worked out the principle to a set, rarely takes more than 15 minutes (except for patients with very slow response times) as item exposure is not tied to a preset speed. The format of the Booklet Category Test would

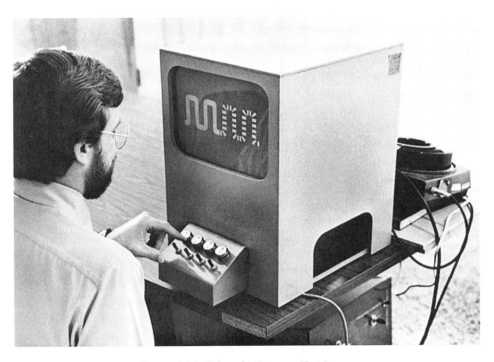

FIGURE 15.1 Halstead's Category Test in use.

also seem to lend itself to a more rapid administration. The examiner may discontinue a set when repeated failures discourage or frustrate a patient. For those subjects who demonstrate a quick and clear comprehension of the principle early in a set, a subsequent "sampling" administration of every third may be used for clinical examinations but not when research requires rigorously standardized procedures. W.G. Snow (1987b) questioned the rigor of HCT procedures, noting the variety of instructions available regarding both discontinuing a difficult set and the allowable amount of examiner cuing when subjects get stuck.

Test characteristics. In the last two decades norms have been developed by a number of workers (Heaton, Grant, and Matthews, 1991 [these data are presented in *T*-scores]; Leckliter and Matarazzo, 1989; Spreen and Strauss, 1998; see Mitrushina, Boone, and D'Elia, 1999, for 16 other norm sets). They all concur in finding age 40 to be a turning point after which error scores climb, at first slowly but rapidly after age 60, excepting subjects with less than a high school education, who show a steep increase in errors from age 40. Mitrushina, Boone, and D'Elia (1999) cite 14 studies demonstrating "a highly consistent relationship . . . between age and Category Test scores in both normal and patient samples" (p. 455). In the largest sample (*n* = 486) appropriately scaled for age, Heaton, Grant, and Matthews (1991) report an age variance of 38%. Education's contribution is smaller, with variances from 43% to 63% reported for age and education combined (see also Prigatano and Parsons, 1976). However, education effects may not show up among brain damaged persons (Corrigan, Agresti, and Hinkeldey, 1987; Finlayson, Johnson, and Reitan, 1977). Analyses of performances between sets indicate that both older healthy subjects and brain damaged patients (Bertram et al., 1990; Ernst, 1987) perform significantly worse on sets III and IV than the others. No sex differences have been reported for total error scores (Filskov and Catanese, 1986; Leckliter and Matarazzo, 1989; Yeudall, Reddon, et al., 1987). African-American and white men who were young and educationally limited did not differ in their HCT performances (means of 22.4 and 22.5, respectively), but a small group of young Hispanic men made significantly more errors (Bernard, 1989). Degree of acculturation appears to influence performance (Arnold et al., 1994).

Retest data for control subjects show lower error scores on the second testing (McCaffrey, Duff, and Westervelt, 2000b). The range of second testing scores differs from a low of 10 fewer errors to more than 30 with the exception of two small (9, 18) groups of mostly middle-aged subjects examined 5.8 and 5.6 years apart whose average error differentials were +3.9 and +0.2, respectively (Elias, Schultz, et al., 1989). In several studies cited by McCaffrey and his colleagues, mean control group scores went from near abnormal to well *within normal limits.*

Along with measuring abstract concept formation (Pendleton and Heaton, 1982) and ability to maintain attention to a lengthy task, the HCT has a visuospatial component, correlating most highly with Block Design and Picture Arrangement (P.C. Fowler, Zillmer, and Newman, 1988; Golden, Kushner, et al., 1998; B. Johnstone, Holland, and Hewett, 1997; Lansdell and Donnelly, 1977). Corrigan, Agresti, and Hinkeldey (1987) report relatively high correlations with Object Assembly as well. Leonberger and his colleagues (1991) interpreted their factor analysis data as "suggesting visual concentration and visual memory" are important components of the HCT performance. Sets III and IV rely on spatial reasoning, while sets V and VI depend on proportional reasoning (D.N. Allen et al., 1999; B. Johnstone, Holland, and Hewett, 1997). Perseverative errors occur most commonly on set IV as subjects maintain the set III pattern despite repeated failures when they have difficulty making conceptual shifts (Perrine, 1985). Boll (1981) noted that the test is also "a learning experiment" that requires learning skills for effective performance—particularly rule learning (Perrine, 1985). Yet Bertram and his colleagues (1990) consider the role of learning on this test as of only "modest importance."

Neuropsychological findings. Of the tests in Halstead's battery, HCT is generally recognized as the most sensitive to the presence of brain damage regardless of its nature or location (Cullum and Bigler, 1986; G. Goldstein and Ruthven, 1983; M.C. King and Snow, 1981). This test was originally identified as especially sensitive to frontal lobe disorders by its originator (Halstead, 1947) who reported poorer performances by patients with frontal lobe lesions (Shure and Halstead, 1958). However, a reevaluation of the 1958 data indicates that the HCT's greatest sensitivity in this study was to left frontal lesions, but "35% to 41%" of nonfrontal patients also performed abnormally (P.L. Wang, 1987). TBI patients without frontal lesions performed as poorly as those with evidence of frontal damage, supporting the interpretation that the test measures nonspecific cerebral dysfunction (C.V. Anderson, 1995). Different studies report different lateralization effects: Hom and Reitan (1984) found poorer performances by patients with right-sided tumors, but Cullum and Bigler's (1986) head trauma patients made more errors when they had greater left than right hemisphere involvement (as measured by volumetric ventricle–

brain ratios). Moreover, stroke patients showed no lateralization effects, getting high error scores regardless of the side of focal lesions or presence of diffuse damage (Hom, 1991; J.M. Taylor et al., 1984). The Category Test has enjoyed good documentation of its discriminative sensitivity to brain disorders from a variety of etiologies (Mercer et al., 1997), to schizophrenia (D.N. Allen et al., 1999), and to alcoholism (K.M. Adams and Grant, 1986; W.R. Miller and Saucedo, 1983).

Short forms of the Category Test. The practical drawbacks of the original mechanized format have enticed many workers to remedy these defects by devising paper-and-pencil substitutes and by shortening the test. Although not every HCT short form is presented here, the following review should give a general idea of their variety and usefulness.

A 128-item form using all of sets I through IV and 20 items from set V was tested on adults with diffuse brain disorders and controls (Charter et al., 1997). It produced a score that correlated highly ($r = .94$) with the long form. The authors offered a formula to convert the short form score (X) to an age- and education-corrected standardized score (Y) in which $M = 100 \pm 15$:

$$Y = \frac{-15 \ (X - .457 \ [\text{age}] + .950 \ [\text{education}] - 31.465)}{15.686 + 100}$$

Comparing the findings from this form with the original item set, Hogg and his coworkers (2001) found that while the variance overlap ($R^2 = 0.93$) was "very strong," this formula generated deviations in the error score of "nearly 10 points or more" for 25% of the 100 TBI patients in this study. In recommending against using this form with TBI patients, the Hogg group point out the risks inherent in estimated scores drawn from short forms. This study also demonstrates that statistics based on group data are not predictive for the individual case.

Dropping the last items from subtests II to V and all of subtests VI and VII resulted in a 120-item short form (Gregory et al., 1979). The authors reported a correlation between the long and short forms of .95. The short form's cutoff score of 35 errors classified three of 80 subjects differently than did the long form's cutoff score of 51 errors. However, in two of these cases the short form made the correct classification. A second study of this form found an even higher correlation with the HCT long form (.98), with 87% of cases making (converted) scores within 10% of their HCT comparison score, thus producing a relatively low standard error of estimate (± 7.5) (Sherrill, 1985).

A 108-item short form of the Category Test uses just the first four sets of the test (Calsyn et al., 1980). Correlations of error scores of the Category Test and this abbreviated version were .89 and .88, respectively, suggesting that subtests V and VI add little to the value of this test. In cross-validation studies, correlations between the score based on the first four subtests and the total HCT score ranged from .83 to .94, further supporting use of this abbreviated format (Golden, Kuperman, et al., 1981; Sherrill, 1985; J.M. Taylor et al., 1984). However, this form generates a lower prediction accuracy than the 120-item form with false negative classifications of right brain damaged patients particularly (J.M. Taylor et al., 1984). Sherrill (1985) suggests that the classification discrepancy between this and the 120-item short form may be due to omission of items from set V, thus reducing the number of principles to be inferred.

Another short form, *The Short Category Test, Booklet Format (SCT)*, is packaged in five small booklets (Wetzel and Boll, 1987). It consists of 100 items, 20 from each of five of the original subtests (I, III, IV, V, VI). Instructions are printed at the beginning of each subtest booklet so that a standardized administration can be assured throughout. Standardization is based on 120 normal volunteers whose average years of education were 15.07 ± 7.83. Almost one-third of these subjects had professional or managerial occupations. SCT scores of this relatively privileged group were compared with those made by 70 VA hospital patients with either neurologic or psychiatric diagnoses who differed significantly ($p < .001$) from the normative group in both age (older) and education (lower). These authors found that using an error score of 41 as a cutoff score for persons "aged 45 and under" and an error score of 46 for those over 45 correctly classified 83% of all subjects, both normal volunteers and patients; but they do not report the classification rates for patients and control subjects separately. An odd–even split-half reliability coefficient of .81 is reported in the manual; but only test-retest data on the full HCT format are offered. Correlations with the full test differed according to which form was given first: when HCT preceded SCT, $r = .93$; reversing administrations resulted in $r = .80$ when two outliers were excluded. A table for converting raw error scores from ≤ 4 to ≥ 63 into "Normalized" T-scores and percentile ranks is given in an appendix. In a study of 30 patients with acute TBI the cutoff scores suggested by Wetzel and Boll were less sensitive than they had reported (G.J. Horn and Kelly, 1996).

A 95-item "revision" (*RCAT*) developed by E.W. Russell and Levy (1987) halved each of the first four subtests, selectively halved V and VI, and dropped VII. The error score is multiplied by 2.2 "to retain equivalence with the full CAT." The correlation between the two total error scores was a very respectable .97. E.W. Russell and Levy continue to use the original cutting score of 50/51 errors. Their disregard for demographic variables probably accounts for a 37% false positive rate for their control subjects.

The shortest form—84 items—was proposed by G.J. Boyle (1986) who selected items to allow for two parallel forms. Sets I and II contribute four and eight items, respectively; 20 come from sets III, IV, and V + VI combined; and VII consists of 10 items chosen randomly from already included items. A cutoff score of 38 errors produced a misclassification rate of 14%. Boyle found that the error pattern paralleled that of the full HCT. However, set V/VI did not discriminate between patients with brain dysfunction and intact subjects, leading Boyle to propose that a 64-item version might suffice as he appears to use this test simply for screening.

The *Victoria Revision of the Category Test* uses sets I and II for orientation only and eliminates all items that are redundant in content and all memory items from set VII, resulting in an 81-item form (Labreche, 1983). This shortens administration time to 15 to 20 min. Cross-validations of this form on patient populations show results close to those of the full length test (Kozel and Meyers, 1998; Sherrill, 1987). Moehle and his colleagues (1988) used a similar approach, making a short form of sets III, IV, and VI, as these sets are the most discriminating. This version accounted for 77% of the variance of scores on the long form. The recommended cutoff of 26 errors had a misclassification rate of 16%. The Moehle group noted that, as the base rate for brain damage among the persons they examine in their medical center is 92%, simply diagnosing every person examined as "brain damaged" would increase the accuracy of their predictions. Rather, they argue for continued use of this test, not as a screening device, but to examine "adaptive abilities."

Brixton Spatial Anticipation Test
(Burgess and Shallice, 1996)

This test of concept formation uses 56 nearly identical visual items to test ability to recognize a rule that accounts for slight pattern variations from item to item. Each item is a card printed with ten (two rows of five each) circles, one of which is colored while the others are white. The position of each succeeding colored circle is determined by one of nine rules based on the positions of the colored circle on preceding cards. On being told that the colored circle "moves around according to various patterns that come and go without warning," the subject is asked to state the expected position of the colored circle on the next card. For the first and simplest rule the colored circle advances one position clockwise on successive cards—this is also the rule for two other test sections; a later rule has the circle alternating from place 5 to place 10. Since some rules continue for as few as three item sequences and others for as many as eight, the subject cannot anticipate rule changes. As such, the task would seem to place a heavy demand on working memory to recall the relation between previous card sequences.

An age effect has been reported: a group of 60 to 70-year-olds performed significantly poorer than a group in their 20s (Andres and Van der Linden, 2000). Patients with frontal lobe lesions made more errors than patients with posterior lesions; this latter group performed as well as control subjects (Burgess and Shallice, 1996). The frontal patients' errors tended to be random or unconstrained and even bizarre, but their perseveration error rate was as low as that of patients with posterior lesions.

"Twenty Questions" task

This familiar parlor game format has been used in several studies of conceptual problem solving. The task requires the subject to identify an object the examiner has in mind by asking questions that can only be answered by "yes" or "no." The original game begins with players being told whether the object is "animal, vegetable, or mineral," and ends when a player either guesses the answer or has not figured it out by the twentieth question. For neuropsychological assessment, the task can be scored both for the number of questions required to identify the target and for three kinds of questions: *constraint-seeking* questions refer to a class of two or more objects that help to identify the target by narrowing down alternatives (e.g., "Is it something you wear?" "Does it come in pairs?"), *pseudoconstraint* questions refer to a specific object as if it were constraint-seeking without reducing alternatives (e.g., "Does it have five fingers?"), and *hypothesis testing* questions ask about a specific object (e.g., "Is it a glove?"). This technique can bring to light the subject's ability for hypothesis generating and testing, for discriminating relevant from irrelevant information, for logical judgments, for maintaining a conceptual direction, and—for some patients—short-term memory deficits will show up when they repeat a question that has been asked or ask a question that has been answered (e.g., after being told "no" to the question, "is it bigger than a dog?" asking later if it is a cow).

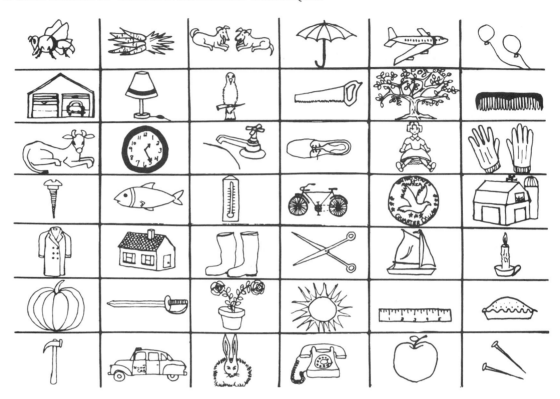

FIGURE 15.2 Identification of Common Objects stimulus card (reduced size). (Courtesy of Nelson Butters)

Identification of Common Objects
(Laine and Butters, 1982)

This test has also been called the *Object Identification Task* (Heindel, Salmon, and Butters, 1991) and is familiarly referred to as "20 Questions" although the target is usually identified long before the twentieth question is reached. The subject is shown an 8" × 10" card displaying an array of 42 drawings of objects representing such overlapping classes as animals, clothing, toys, manufactured objects, paired objects, round objects, etc. (see Fig. 15.2). First the subject is asked to name all the pictures, a procedure that both serves as a test of confrontation naming and ensures that subject and examiner apply the same name to each picture. Using each of three items in successive administrations (e.g., saw, doll, sun), the subject is then told that this is a kind of game in which, "I am thinking of one of these objects. Your task is to find it by asking questions. You can ask any kind of questions you like, but I can answer only by saying 'yes' or 'no.' The whole idea of the game is that you should find the object I am thinking of with as few questions as possible. There is no time limit so you can start whenever you are ready" (Laine and Butters, 1982, pp. 237–238). The

authors recommended that examiners should stop questioning at about 15 responses by telling their patients that a hypothesis testing question is right whether it is or not as only the subject's first five questions are scored in this system.

A 52-year-old woman in the early stage of frontotemporal dementia approached the task with familiarity. Following standard instructions in which she was told to ask only yes/no questions, she asked, "Is it animal, vegetable, or mineral?" After conforming to instructions by asking one high-level question, "Is it an animal?," she began a series of questions asking whether the designated object was a "shoe" and so forth, naming items on the page until she identified the correct one. Interestingly, she never repeated a question, which was consistent with data from other memory tests showing relatively good memory at this stage of her dementia.

Alcoholics with and without Korsakoff's syndrome ask many fewer constraint-seeking questions than control subjects (J.T. Becker et al., 1986; Laine and Butters, 1982) with Korsakoff patients' pattern of questioning being the most inefficient (Heindel, Salmon, and Butters, 1991). In a study of patients with epileptic foci in a variety of locations, those who made the most errors and had the least effective strategies were those with bifrontal lesions (Upton and Thompson, 1999). Poor strategy also was demonstrated in patients who have had severe TBI (F.C. Goldstein and Levin, 1991). However, control subjects used significantly more constraint-seeking questions than did the TBI patients. Redundant questions were rarely asked by either group.

Following the traditional oral format of the game, Klouda and Cooper (1990) used animals for their target class to compare responses of five patients with frontal lobe damage to those of matched control subjects. Only 50% of the patients' questions were constraint seeking, compared to 80% of the control subjects' questions. Moreover, many of the patients' constraint-seeking questions were relatively inefficient in eliminating alternatives (e.g., "Is it white?"). Wide variations in the number of questions to solution occurred in both groups, but only three of the five frontal patients solved both problems.

California Twenty Questions Test (Delis, Kaplan, and Kramer, 2001)

On this 30-picture version, the subject is asked to identify a different target item on each of four trials. An alternate version uses the same pictures and four different targets. The first time subjects ask a question that is not constraint-seeking (refers to only one picture), e.g., "Is it an apple?" they are reminded to ask as few questions as possible. Trials are discontinued when either subjects identify the target or have asked 20 questions. In addition to scoring the total number of questions used to identify the targets, the first three questions for each target are scored in terms of the number of objects identified by the question. If, "Is it living?" is true for 15 pictures this question receives a score of 15. The higher the score, the better the conceptual strategies. At the time of this writing, data from this test have not yet been published.

Raven's Progressive Matrices (RPM) (J. Raven, Court et al., 1995; J. Raven, Raven, and Court, 1995; J. Raven, Summers et al., 1990; J.C. Raven, 1996)

This multiple-choice paper-and-pencil test was developed in England in the 1930s and has received widespread use in the U.S. and abroad as well as in its home territory. It consists of a series of visual pattern matching and analogy problems pictured in nonrepresentational designs (see Fig. 15.3). It requires the subject to conceptualize spatial, design, and numerical relationships ranging from the very obvious and concrete to the very complex and abstract. As such it is relatively language free.

The Raven's Matrices is easy to administer. A secretary or clerk can give or demonstrate the instructions. It has no time limit; most people take from 40 minutes to an hour. The 60 items are grouped into five sets. Each item contains a pattern problem with one part removed and from six to eight pictured inserts of which one contains the correct pattern. Subjects point to the pattern piece they select as correct or write its number on an answer sheet. Norms are available for ages 6.5 to 65+ and for several national groups and ethnic populations (J. Raven, Court, et al., 1995; Spreen and Strauss, 1998). Score conversion is to percentiles. *Research Supplement 3* (J. Raven et al., 1990) provides norms for a large group of American students, as well as international norms. A somewhat more difficult version of the Standard test format is available (see Manual section 3).

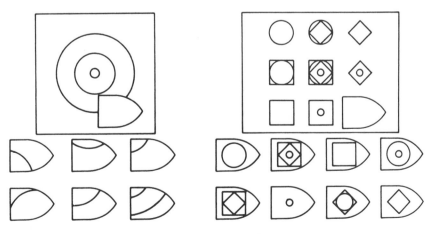

FIGURE 15.3 Examples of two levels of difficulty of Progressive Matrices type items.

Test characteristics. The age group changes that appear in normative studies (H.R. Burke, 1985; D.F. Peck, 1970) were found in other studies of the vicissitudes of conceptual thinking through the adult years (see p. 300). Performance declines begin in the 50s. Since the RPM was first published in 1938, scores have risen considerably (J.R. Flynn, 1987; see p. 21). Most studies showing score increases have examined schoolchildren, but one study of adults in the 20 to 30 age range documented an average score increase of 7.07 "IQ" points. Although this test was intended to be a "culture fair" test of general ability, and even though it requires neither language nor academic skills for success, education influences performance to a small degree (H.R. Burke, 1985; Colonna and Faglioni, 1966; P.E. Vernon, 1979). Sex differences do not appear to be significant (Llabre, 1984; Persaud, 1987).

Internal consistency coefficients tend to cluster around .90 for adults (Llabre, 1984). However, the item sequence does not provide a uniform progression in order of difficulty as there are some reversals in that order and difficulty differences between items are quite irregular even though the overall trend is from easy to hard (Franzen, 1989). Retest reliability correlations run in the range of .7 to .9 (Eichorn, 1975; Llabre, 1984), even when retesting involves three administrations six and 12 months apart (Lezak, 1982c). Score increases may average as little as 0.4 with average gains of 4.0 recorded; yet after a four year interval no improvement was found (McCaffrey, Duff, and Westervelt, 2000b). RPM validity as a measure of general ability has been consistently supported in correlational studies with other ability measures (Llabre, 1984; Spreen and Strauss, 1998).

The first (A) set of 12 items consists of incomplete figures; the missing part is depicted in one of the six response alternatives given below the figure. All of the items call for pattern matching (e.g., the left-hand item in Fig. 15.3) and test the kind of visuoperceptual skills associated with normal right hemisphere functioning (Denes et al., 1978). In the other sets, the task shifts from one of pattern completion to reasoning by analogy at levels ranging from quite simple (a few in Set B) to increasingly difficult (in the subsequent sets) and ultimately to very complex (see Llabre, 1984; J. Raven, Raven, and Court, 1995). These analogical reasoning problems appear to call upon left hemisphere functions predominantly (Denes et al., 1978). The example on the right in Figure 15.3 is similar to some of the problems in Set D. Many of the more difficult analogy problems involve mathematical concepts. Most of the analogy problems in Set B and the three more difficult sets (C–E) have nameable features so it makes sense that some factor analytic studies have demonstrated a significant verbal component in this test (Bock, 1973; H.R. Burke, 1985).

Neuropsychological findings. Given the differences in the nature of the sets, it is not surprising to find that patients with right-sided lesions perform less well than left-lesioned patients on the visuospatial problems of set A but the reverse is true for the more verbally conceptual set B (Villardita, 1985). Following "split-brain" surgery, four patients exhibited a small left hemisphere advantage overall, although analysis by sets indicated a significant right hemisphere advantage for set B (E. Zaidel, Zaidel, and Sperry, 1981). Moreover, the two commissurotomy patients achieved their best scores when exposure was not restricted to a single hemisphere. Evaluation of these findings in light of other lateralization studies and factor analytic studies led Zaidel and his colleagues to conclude that

the seeming visuospatial and nonverbal character of RPM is misleading and the test is a poor tool for discriminating right and left brain-damaged patients . . . or for assessing lateralized, e.g., visuospatial abilities . . . not because each hemisphere alone is deficient on this test but rather because each is relatively competent on it. (p. 178)

This conclusion agrees with other data showing that the standard RPM does not discriminate well between undifferentiated groups of patients with right and left hemisphere damage (Arrigoni and De Renzi, 1964; L.D. Costa and Vaughan, 1962; Sturm and Willmes, 1991). PET activation occurs in the posterior visual association areas of the inferolateral temporal cortex bilaterally during this test (Esposito, Kirkby, et al., 1999).

The effectiveness of the Progressive Matrices in identifying patients with brain disorders appears to be related to the extent of the damage (M.B. Acker and Davis, 1989). This was demonstrated nicely in D.N. Brooks and Aughton's study (1979) of traumatically injured patients whose RPM scores decreased quite regularly with increases in the duration of posttraumatic amnesia. Most of a group of 11 patients with suspected Alzheimer's disease achieved scores *within normal limits* in the early stages with almost half of them showing a decline over the first two to three years after diagnosis (Grady, Haxby, Horwitz, et al., 1988). Alcoholics, particularly long-term alcoholics, are likely to perform poorly on this test (W.R. Miller and Saucedo, 1983). However, the RPM's usefulness in screening for brain damage is limited (Heaton, Smith, et al., 1978; Newcombe, 1969). Newcombe and Artiola i Fortuny (1979) attribute some of its insensitivity to a tendency for the old (from the 1950s) norms to overestimate performance slightly, citing one case in which a socially incompetent trauma patient achieved a score above the 95th percentile.

Positional preferences in selecting a response can affect performance on this test. Bromley (1953) found that both middle-aged to elderly psychiatric patients and a group of schoolgirls tended to choose top line alternatives more than those on the bottom line and the first and last positions were also favored, but no consistent pattern of right–left preferences emerged. However, patients with lateralized lesions—particularly those who have demonstrated unilateral visuospatial inattention—show a consistent tendency to prefer alternatives on the side of the page ipsilateral to the lesion, neglecting answers on the side opposite the lesion (D.C. Campbell and Oxbury, 1976; Colombo et al., 1976; L.D. Costa, Vaughn, Horwitz, and Ritter, 1969). This phenomenon occurs with both right- and left-sided lesions, but much more so with lesions on the right, and particularly when the patient with right hemisphere damage also has a visual field defect (De Renzi and Faglioni, 1965). Thus, the presence of unilateral inattention may be elicited by this test. Other kinds of error patterns can also provide insight into the patient's mishandling of conceptual problems. Error tendencies may be determined in an item-by-item inspection of errors in which the examiner looks for such error patterns as choosing a whole for a part response (on set A), choosing a response that repeats a part of the matrix, performing a simplified abstraction (e.g., by attending to only one dimension of patterns involving both vertical and horizontal progressions), and perseverating (the direction of pattern progression, a solution mode, a position). Some patients' errors will make no sense at all. Questioning them about their choices may reveal tendencies to personalized, symbolic, or concrete thinking; incomprehension; or confusion.

Raven's Coloured Progressive Matrices (RCPM) (J.C. Raven, 1995)

The RCPM provides a simplified 36-item format with norms for children in the five to 11-year-old range, and for adults 65 years and older. It consists of sets A and B of the RPM and an intermediate set, Ab, that, like set B, contains both gestalt completion items and some simple analogies. Each item is printed with a bright background color which may make the test more appealing to children and does not seem to detract from its clarity.

Test characteristics. Adult data for the RCPM show no age effects at least to the 40th year (Yeudall, Fromm, et al., 1986). However, both age ($r = -.35$) and edu-

cation ($r = +.31$) effects were significant for older (mean ages from 51 to 55) groups of patients with lateralized brain damage (Gainotti, D'Erme, Villa, and Caltagirone, 1986). In a study of rural older adults with education ≤10 years, education accounted for 16% of the variance in the sample, while age and race (white and African-American) had no effect (Marcopulos, McLain, and Giuliano, 1997). Sex differences do not appear (Gainotti et al., 1986; Yeudall, Fromm, et al., 1986). It has satisfactory reliability (Esquivel, 1984). Education corrected norms are available for an abbreviated version using only sets A and B for ages 55 to 85 (Smits et al., 1997).

Neuropsychological findings. The RCPM has been frequently used in neuropsychological studies, probably because it is both much shorter and easier. However, it is important to be aware that *the RPM and RCPM are not interchangeable;* nor may the derived scores for the two tests mean the same thing. Patients with left hemisphere damage perform better on the colored matrices than on the standard format (Archibald, Wepman, and Jones, 1967; L.D. Costa, 1976). This finding is consistent with data from split-brain studies indicating a trend toward a right hemisphere advantage on the RCPM in contrast to a trend favoring the left hemisphere on the RPM (E. Zaidel, Zaidel, and Sperry, 1981). This is not surprising since only one-fifth of the RPM items test visuoperceptual skills almost exclusively, while more than one-third of the RCPM items are predominantly visuospatial. An analysis of poor performance by Parkinson patients suggested that the deficit was more related to the visuospatial requirements of the task than the problem solving component (Cronin-Golomb and Braun, 1997). As further evidence of its visuospatial demands, patients with dementia with Lewy bodies have more difficulty on this task than Alzheimer patients with a similar level of dementia as measured by the Mini-Mental State Examination. This finding is consistent with other evidence of a more severe visuospatial component in dementia with Lewy bodies (Shimomura et al., 1998).

A within set analysis of the patterns of performances by patients with lateralized lesions suggested a trend by right damaged patients to perform less well on the predominantly perceptual items and better on those that are more conceptual (L.D. Costa, 1976). This trend may be due, at least in part, to the significant bias toward right-sided responses shown by patients with right cortical lesions in the territory of the middle cerebral artery (Kertesz and Dobrowolski, 1981). Visual field defects exacerbate this problem (Egelko, Simon, et al., 1989).

This test is more vulnerable to posterior than anterior lesions (Berker and Smith, 1988; L.D. Costa, 1976). Patients with receptive or mixed aphasia also do poorly on it (Gainotti, D'Erme, Villa, and Caltagirone, 1986). However, severely affected aphasic patients whose comprehension is preserved may perform within one to two standard deviations below the average for control subjects and far better than those with compromised comprehension (Kertesz, 1988).

Miceli and his colleagues (1981) used a modified format in which the response choices are presented in a vertical array to minimize the effects of visuospatial inattention. A similar procedure showed that when response choices were vertically aligned patients with visuospatial inattention improved their performances significantly, but alignment made no difference to patients who did not have this problem (B. Caplan, 1988). Overall, laterality effects disappeared when response choices were vertically aligned: patients with left-sided damage but no aphasia performed much like normal subjects, while those with right-sided lesions and aphasic patients made virtually identical scores (Gainotti, D'Erme, Villa, and Caltagirone, 1986).

Advanced Progressive Matrices (J.C. Raven, 1994)

This version was developed to test adolescents and adults of *above average* intellectual ability. While the entire test takes approximately 40 minutes, Set I can be used for brief screening as it contains only 12 items which vary from easy to extremely difficult. Patients performing well on this set are likely to perform well on the Standard version.

Matrix Reasoning (Wechsler, 1997a)

This test was added to the examiner-administered WIS-A battery in the WAIS-III edition. It has the same basic features as the RPM in that it presents a series of increasingly difficult visual pattern completion and analogy problems. The subject must choose from a multiple-choice array the item that best completes the pattern. The examiner must be careful to make sure the horizontal layout of the response set does not penalize subjects with lateralized brain lesions and corresponding left or right visual inattention (see pp. 376–377 for a discussion of this problem). This test has no time limit but frequently takes 20 min or less if discontinued when an impaired or dull patient misses four out of five consecutive items. However, a slow or deliberate subject may need 40 min or more.

Age has a large effect on performance. A raw score of 11 (which includes 3 easy points for items not usually given to comprehending adults) in the *low average*

range for a young adult is *high average* for ages 85–89. *Matrix Reasoning* has a strong association with the RPM ($r = .80$) (The Psychological Corporation, 1997). A moderate association with the Halstead Category Test ($r = -.58$) due to shared reasoning requirements, and associations with verbal abstract reasoning and verbal fluency tests have been documented by Dugbartey and his colleagues (1999). These workers also report associations with verbal abstract reasoning and verbal fluency. Its utility with patient populations has yet to be established. Patients with either mild or moderate to severe TBI performed as well as control subjects (Donders, Tulsky, and Zhu, 2001).

Symbol Patterns

Deductive reasoning combines with ability for conceptual sequencing in symbol pattern tests, exemplified by the Thurstones' *Reasoning Tests* in the *Primary Mental Abilities* (*PMA*) battery (1962). These tests are composed of such number or letter patterns as 1-2-4-2-4-8-3- — or A-B-D-C-E-F-H- —. The subject must indicate, usually by selecting one of several choices, what symbol should follow in the sequence. The PMA has norms for different age and education levels. The *Numerical Reasoning* subtest of the *Employee Aptitude Survey* gives norms for different occupational groups (Ruch et al., 1963). *Number Series* in *The Stanford-Binet Intelligence Scale: Fourth Edition* contains 26 of these problems for the childhood range of age 5–11 to 17–8 (Thorndike et al., 1987). This kind of reasoning problem seems to require an appreciation of temporal or consequential relationships for success.

Abstraction Subtest, Shipley Institute of Living Scale (Shipley, 1946; Zachary, 1986)

A series of 20 such sequential completion items comprises the Abstraction subtest of the Shipley Institute of Living Scale. They include variations on word meanings and constructions, and number and letter patterns. They are paired with a vocabulary test under the assumption that since vocabulary represents the level of well-established learning and skills that are relatively resistant to brain damage and the Abstraction subtest tests concept formation which is vulnerable to many kinds of brain damage, a comparison between them will yield a ratio indicating whether mental deterioration is present (Zachary, 1986). Normative data for adults aged 20–79 are available (Harnish et al., 1994). A relatively high abstraction score may also be interpreted as representing intellectual potential. Two short forms have been developed which are equated for level of difficulty (Nixon, Parsons, et al., 1995).

A pronounced aging decrement occurs after age 45 (Zachary, 1986; Shelton, Parsons, and Leber, 1982). No sex differences have shown up (Nixon, Parsons, et al., 1995). Patients with multiple sclerosis (Beatty, Hames, and Blanco, 1995) and other diffuse brain disorders are likely to be impaired on this test as are detoxified alcoholics (Nixon, Parsons, et al., 1995). In a group of heart transplant candidates, 9% also displayed problems on the Abstraction subtest (Putzke et al., 2000). The expected relative drop in the Abstraction score appeared in a study of Huntington's disease in which the average score for patients when still unaffected by the disease was *within normal limits,* but was 25% lower at a later premorbid stage (Lyle and Gottesman, 1979).

Sorting

Sorting tests are the most common form of tests of abstraction and concept formation. The subject must sort collections of objects, blocks, tokens, or other kinds of items into subgroups following instructions such as "sort out the ones that go together" or "put together the ones that have the same thing in common." Most sorting tests assess the ability to shift concepts as well as the ability to use them. The manner in which subjects proceed will give some indication of their ability to form and handle abstract concepts. Few sorting tests produce numerical scores, for it is more patients' procedures than their solutions that are of interest. Attention is paid to whether patients sort according to a principle, whether they can formulate the principle verbally, whether it is a reasonable principle, and whether they follow it consistently.

On scored sorting tests, significant differences may not show up between the mean scores obtained by groups of brain injured patients and normal control subjects (De Renzi, Faglioni, Savoiardo, and Vignolo, 1966; McFie and Piercy, 1952; Newcombe, 1969). This does not invalidate sorting tests except for screening purposes. It does suggest, however, that deficits registered by these tests occur only mildly or infrequently in many brain injured populations. When marked impairment of performance does appear, brain dysfunction is likely.

Kasanin-Hanfmann Concept Formation Test
(Hanfmann, 1953; Hanfmann, Kasanin, Vigotsky, and Wang, no date)

This test is sometimes called the *Vigotsky* or *Vygotsky Test.* Its purpose is to "evaluate an individual's ability to solve problems by the use of abstract concepts and provide information both on the subject's level of ab-

stract thinking and on his preferred type of approach to problems" (Hanfmann, 1953). It consists of 22 different blocks varying in color, size, shape, and height. On the underside of each is printed one of four nonsense correcting clues given following each incorrect attempt, until they combine both the principles of shape and height to achieve the correct sorting solution. This may take anywhere from five min to one hour. They are words (or a number, in a variant of the test) designating the group to which the block belongs when the blocks are sorted by both shape and height (see Fig. 15.4, p. 584). Subjects continue to group and regroup the blocks, with encouragement to "think aloud" as they work, and the examiner is encouraged to keep a detailed record of both performance and verbalizations.

A modification of this test, the *Modified Vygotsky Concept Formation Test* (MVCFT) (P.L. Wang, 1984), divides it into two parts and introduces a shifting request: In the *Convergent Thinking Test* the examiner selects a target block and asks the subject to identify all other blocks that would belong with it (e.g., CEV blocks, see Fig. 15.4), telling subjects whether a choice is right or wrong. When a complete set has been identified the examiner asks subjects to explain the sorting principle and then moves on to the next set. The *Divergent Thinking Test* begins with the examiner sorting by color and asking subjects to state the principle. The test then proceeds as originally designed. Scoring methods are provided for each subtest. Patients with frontal damage made considerably more errors than those with nonfrontal damage (P.L. Wang, 1987). Although no significant lateralized differences appeared for either group, right anterior patients tended to do less well than patients with left anterior lesions. Patients with bilateral or diffuse damage made more errors than those with focal lesions. Wang interpreted these data as suggesting that "concept formation and divergent thinking, as measured by the MVCFT, are not lateralized cognitive functions" (p. 194).

Card Sorting (Caine, Ebert, and Weingartner, 1977)

This sorting task uses two sets of 32 3 × 5 cards with a word printed on each card. Four cards from each of eight categories (e.g., clothes, animals, etc.) make up one set; the second set consists of random words. The subject is simply asked to group the shuffled cards. Performance is evaluated on the basis of the number and appropriateness of the sorts.

The ability to think in categories can also be examined with sets of pictures of many different kinds of plants, animals, or other classes of entities that have hierarchically organized subclasses. For example, the

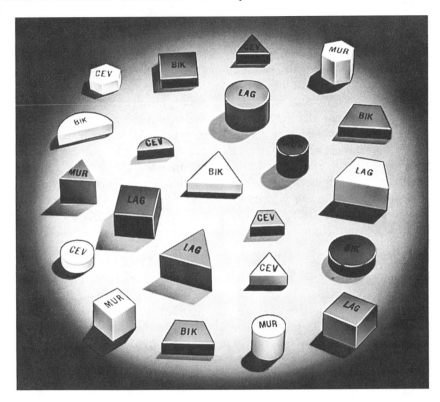

FIGURE 15.4 The Kasanin-Hanfmann Concept Formation Test. (Courtesy of The Stoelting Co.)

animal set may contain pictures of different kinds of mammals, such as felines, canines, primates, hooved animals, etc.; different kinds of birds (fowl, shorebirds, birds of prey); different kinds of dogs (St. Bernards, dachshunds), and so on. The patient's task is simply to sort the set of randomized pictures as they deem appropriate. Upon completing the task, patients should be asked for an explanation of their sorting array.

Sort and Shift

Sorting tests that include a requirement to shift concepts spread a wider screening net than simple sorting tests. Observation will clarify whether the patient's primary difficulty is in sorting or in shifting. For those sort and shift tests that produce a numerical score, the need to augment numerical data with behavioral description is obvious.

Color Form Sorting Test (K.H. Goldstein and Scheerer, 1941, 1953; Weigl, 1941)

This test has also been called *Weigl's Test* or the *Weigl-Goldstein-Scheerer Color Form Sorting Test*. It consists of 12 tokens or blocks, colored red, blue, yellow, or green on top and all white underneath, which come in

one of three shapes—square, circle, or triangle. Patients are first asked to sort the test material. On completion of the first sort, they are told to "group them again, but in a different way." On completion of each sort, the examiner asks, "Why have you grouped them this way?" or "Why do these figures go together?" When patients have difficulty in their second attempt at sorting, the examiner can give clues such as turning up the white sides for patients who spontaneously sorted by color, or showing patients who sorted by form a single grouping by color and asking if they can see why the three blocks belong together.

Neuropsychological findings. Inability to sort is rarely seen in persons whose premorbid functioning was much above *borderline defective*. Walsh and Darby (1999), for example, reported that this part of the Color Form Sorting Test task was failed by only three of 13 patients who had had orbitomedial leucotomy (psychosurgery involving the severing of thalamofrontal connections near the tip of the frontal horn of the lateral ventricle). Inability to shift from one sorting principle to another is seen more often, particularly among patients with frontal lobe damage (e.g., five of Walsh's patients needed help to make the shift). Inability to shift is evidence of impaired mental functioning in persons who were operating at a better than *dull normal* level premorbidly. Frontal lobe lesions are often implicated in failures on the Color Form Sorting Test, but aging also takes its toll (N.A. Kramer and Jarvik, 1979). More patients with left than right frontal lesions are likely to fail this test; the presence or absence of aphasia did not appear to affect the ratio of poor performances among patients with left hemisphere brain disease (Benton, 1968; McFie and Piercy, 1952). More than half of chronic alcoholics examined with this test were unable to shift after their first sort (Tamkin and Dolenz, 1990) although only five of 30 psychiatric patients (diagnosed as neurotic) failed the test (Tamkin, 1983). For patients with dementia this test has high diagnostic specificity but low sensitivity (Byrnes et al., 1989).

Object Sorting Test (K. Goldstein and Scheerer, 1941, 1953; Weigl, 1941)

This test is of historic interest but can be assembled from mostly household objects for use now. Its design to measure "abstract attitude" is based on the same principles as the block and token sorting tests and generally follows the same administration procedures, except that the materials consist of 30 familiar objects, many different but some similar in different sizes or materials (e.g, nails, forks; see Fig. 15.5). The objects can be grouped according to such principles as use, situation in which they are normally found, color, pairedness, material, etc. Variations on the basic sorting task require the patient to find objects compatible with the one preselected by the examiner, to sort objects ac-cording to a category named by the examiner, to figure out a principle underlying a set of objects grouped by the examiner, or to pick out one object of an examiner-selected set of objects that does not belong to the set. Most variations also ask for a verbal explanation. By providing a wider range of responses than most sorting tests, the Object Sorting Test allows the examiner more flexibility in the conduct of the examination and more opportunities to observe the patient's conceptual approach. The use of common objects also eliminates any need to familiarize the patient with the test material or devise names for unfamiliar objects.

Most examiners (A.-L Christensen, 1979; K. Goldstein and Scheerer, 1941, 1953; Luria, 1966) focused on the qualitative aspects of the patient's performance, but Tow (1955) emphasized the number of different solutions. Preoperatively, his frontal leucotomy patients averaged 2.5 spontaneous solutions for a total of 3.2 solutions including both spontaneous ones and those achieved with cues. Postoperatively, these same patients' average number of spontaneous solutions was 1.8, and the average number of combined solutions was 2.1. Tow concluded that frontal leucotomy interfered with concept formation.

Sorting Test (ST) (Delis, Kaplan, and Kramer, 2001)

This version of the older sort and shift formats is a component of the Delis-Kaplan Executive Function System. It was designed to provide separate measures of initiation, concept formation, problem solving, cognitive flexibility, perseverative responding, and regulation

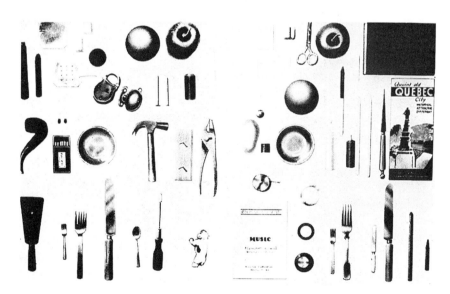

FIGURE 15.5 The Object Sorting Test. This version consists of a set of objects for men (left half) and a second set for women (on the right). (K. Goldstein and Scheerer, 1953, in A. Weidner [Ed.], *Contributions to Medical Psychology*. © Ronald Press, New York)

TABLE 15.1 Performance Components of the Sorting Test

Component of Performance
Initiation
Number of free sorts attempted
Concept formation
Number of correct free sorts
Number of correct identifications of examiner's sorts
Correct descriptions of sorts
Abstract thinking
Use of abstract sorts and descriptions
Cognitive flexibility
Number of free sorts
Number of correct identifications of examiner's sorts
Total perseveration score
Regulation of behavior
Number of unusual sorts
Number of nonmatch descriptions

of behavior (see Table 15.1). It incorporates features of other card sorting tests, particularly Weigl's Test and its modifications. Instead of tokens or blocks the subject sorts cards with a single word printed on them. With two versions, each containing two sets of cards, the examiner can avoid some of the practice effect problems that affect other sorting tests (e.g., pp. 588–589). The cards in each set can be sorted into two groups of three each based on eight different sorting rules. Within each set half of the rules involve verbal or semantic properties of the words and half involve perceptual properties (e.g., HAT-glove, HAT-APPLE). Card size, shape, and color are among the other rules governing sorting possibilities. Studies published in the 1990s used a version containing three sets of six stimulus cards, the *California Card Sorting Test* (CCST) (Delis, Squire, et al., 1992)

The *Free Sorting* condition requires the subject to sort the cards according to as many self-determined rules as possible, and to state each rule. It is scored for the total number of sorts, the number of correct sorts, the number of each of several kinds of erroneous sorts, as well as the quality of the subject's explanations (correct, overly abstract, incorrect, or perseverative). In *Structured Sorting*, the examiner sorts according to each rule and asks the subject to identify them, scoring for the same four categories as in Free Sorting. Each hypothesized behavioral *component of performance* is based on one or more scores (Table 15.1).

Test characteristics. In a group of highly educated persons, those 60 years and older made fewer free sorts than younger groups although differences in total sorts were slightly less (Beatty, 1993). In a study involving college students, women made fewer verbal sorts than

men in the Free Sorting condition (Greve et al., 1995). The data in this study correlated well with other measures of conceptual abstraction but did not discriminate between the hypothesized components, a finding the authors attribute to the cognitive competency of the student population.

Neuropsychological findings. Case study data suggest that the Sorting Test may be useful in dissociating verbal and nonverbal concept formation abilities (Crouch et al., 1996), a finding consistent with the college student study (Greve et al., 1995). Patients with Parkinson's disease perform relatively well except for perseverative tendencies (Dimitrov et al., 1999). Beatty and Monson (1996) found that multiple sclerosis patients generated and identified fewer concepts than controls. Alcoholics had measurable deficits compared to controls in both concept generation and identification on this task (Beatty, Katzung, et al., 1993).

Comparing patients with frontal lesions with nonfrontal amnesic patients, frontal damage accounted for 26% of the variance while amnesia explained nearly 10% (Delis, Squire, et al., 1992). Both patients with frontal lobe lesions and those with Korsakoff's syndrome were impaired in initiating accurate sorts and identifying sorting rules, and they made a large number of perseverative sorts, perseverative descriptions, and rule naming errors. Dimitrov and his colleagues (1999) noted that patients with frontal lesions have difficulty with many aspects of the test: strategy planning, strategy initiation, concept formation, and flexibility (i.e., evidence of perseveration).

Wisconsin Card Sorting Test (WCST)[1] (E.A. Berg, 1948; D.A. Grant and Berg, 1948)

This widely used test was devised to study "abstract behavior" and "shift of set." In its original format the subject is given a pack of 60 cards on which are printed one to four symbols—triangle, star, cross, or circle—in red, green, yellow, or blue. No two cards are identical (see Fig. 15.6). The original cards have one irrelevant stimulus dimension, placement of the symbols on the card (see p. 588). Heaton (1981) modified the cards so that the placement of the designs was the same and he numbered the cards on the back so that they could be administered in the same order to each subject.

The patient's task is to place the cards one by one under four stimulus cards—one red triangle, two green stars, three yellow crosses, and four blue circles—according to a principle that the patient must deduce

---

[1]The cards may be ordered from Wells Print and Digital Services, 3121 Watford Way, Madison, WI 53713.

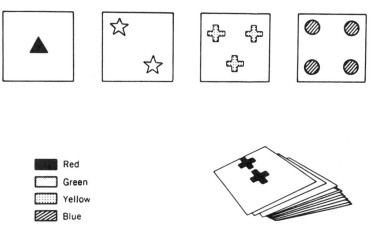

Red
Green
Yellow
Blue

FIGURE 15.6 The Wisconsin Card Sorting Test. (From Milner, 1964)

from the pattern of the examiner's responses to the patient's placement of the cards. For instance, if the principle is color, the correct placement of a red card is under *one red triangle,* regardless of the symbol or number, and the examiner will tell the subject whether the response was "right" or "wrong". The subject simply begins placing cards and the examiner states whether each placement is correct. The placement may be correct for a nontarget category as well as a target category, such as matching both color and form, so that the feedback is ambiguous without more trials. After a run of ten correct placements in a row, the examiner shifts the principle, indicating the shift only in the changed pattern of "right" and "wrong" responses. The test begins with color as the basis for sorting, shifts to form, then to number, returns again to color, and so on. The examiner continues until the subject has made six runs of ten correct placements, has placed more than 64 cards in one category, or spontaneously reports the underlying principle (e.g., "You keep changing what is correct—from the number of spots to their shape or color and back again"). If the pack is exhausted before six successful runs, the card order is rearranged and the pack is used again.

It is typically unnecessary—and perhaps unkind—to continue if 30 or 40 cards have been misplaced and the patient seems unlikely to comprehend the task. Patients who perform poorly are likely to experience frustration by the lack of rule disclosure so that it may be necessary to discontinue the test to maintain the patient's further cooperation. Also, the test can take a long time when the patient is failing. Conversely, if the patient makes four correct runs of ten consecutively (not counting the one or two trials between runs for determining the new principle), and can correctly identify the general principle, discontinuing at that point seems appropriate. B. Milner (1963) used a double pack and

discontinued after six runs or when all the cards were placed. She counted both the number of categories achieved and the number of erroneous responses for scores.

Wisconsin Card Sorting Test performances can be scored in a number of ways (e.g., see Haaland, Vranes, et al., 1987; Heaton, Chelune, Talley, et al., 1993). The most widely used scores are for *Categories Achieved, Perseverative Responses,* and *Perseverative Errors.* Following Milner's (1963) criteria, Categories Achieved refers to the number of correct runs of ten sorts, ranging from 0 for the patient who never gets the idea at all to 6, at which point the test is normally discontinued. Using a double pack of 128 cards, which allows for an optimal number of 11 runs of ten correct sorts each, most adults, including older adults under the age of 75, achieve at least four categories (Paolo, Tröster, Axelrod, and Koller, 1995). Perseverative errors occur either when the subject continues to sort according to a previously successful principle or, in the first series, when the subject persists in sorting on the basis of an initial erroneous guess. The Perseverative Error score is useful for documenting problems in forming concepts, profiting from correction, and conceptual flexibility. A correct response may be classified as a Perseverative Response if it also matches a previously correct category. Scoring perseveration takes time because the criteria change depending upon the subject's response (S. Berry, 1996). Other errors may represent guessing, losing track of the current sorting principle, or occasionally an effort to devise a complex scheme, which usually indicates that a verbally clever person has failed to keep track of the pattern of the examiner's responses or to accept the simplicity of the solution. Performances can also be scored for the number of trials required to achieve the first category, and "learning to learn" as reflected in increased rapidity in achieving subsequent

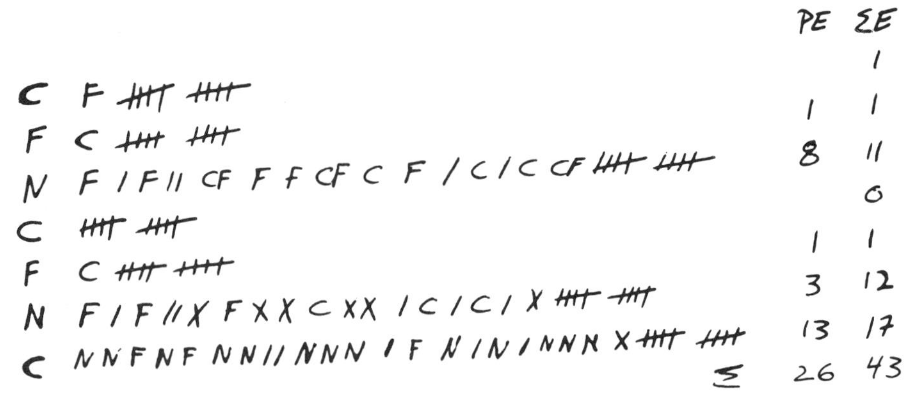

FIGURE 15.7 A simple method for recording the Wisconsin Card Sorting Test performance.

sets (see Spreen and Strauss, 1998, pp. 220–221). Variations in scoring perseverative errors—a critical category in interpreting the WCST performance—may be considerable, particularly for clinicians who do not work with this test intensively: "errors seemed to be based on idiosyncrasies and unique interpretations of the scoring rules that were easily corrected with feedback" (Greve, 1993, p. 516).

Published record forms are available but not necessary. Recording a performance, particularly if the patient works rapidly, must be efficient. Figure 15.7 shows a system that allows the examiner to keep an accurate record without undue effort, to evaluate the performance at a glance, and to make score counts as needed. This simplified system involves identifying the category to be achieved at the left of a line of note paper and marking a slash for each correct sort, the category initial of each incorrect sort (C, F, N; CF, CN, etc., when an erroneous sort satisfies two categories), and an X when none of the categories matches the sort (e.g., when three blue circles are placed under the card with two green stars). When the category has been achieved (i.e., when there are ten consecutive slash marks), the new category will begin at the left of the next line and recording will continue as before.

Test characteristics. Age effects showed up in the original study (E.A. Berg, 1948) and are documented in normative studies (Mitrushina, Boone, and D'Elia, 1999; Heaton, Grant, and Matthews, 1991; Spreen and Strauss, 1998) but generally are inconsequential before the 70s (Boone, Ghaffarian, et al., 1993; Boone, Miller, et al., 1990; Haaland, Vranes, et al., 1987). An 80+ group also achieved significantly fewer categories (1.5 ± 1.3) with a single set of cards than younger subjects (Haaland, Vranes, et al., 1987). Age-related effects on WCST performance have been attributed to poor use of feedback information, impaired working memory, and reductions in speed of processing for adults 60 to 86 years of age (Fristoe et al., 1997). Education affects performances to a small degree (Boone, Ghaffarian, et al., 1993; Heaton, Chelune, Talley, et al., 1993; Yeudall, Fromm et al., 1986). One study of adults 45 years and older found that women outperformed men on the major measures (Boone, Ghaffarian, et al., 1993).

Some scoring schemes (e.g., Heaton, Chelune, Talley, et al., 1993) derive many highly interrelated scores that appear to measure one ability in intact adults, which has been referred to as a "problem solving/ flexibility factor" (Bowden, Fowler, et al., 1998; R.S. Goldman, Axelrod, Heaton, et al., 1996). Studies using heterogeneous samples of patients with brain disorders have often reported a second factor based on a *Failure to Maintain Set* score (R.S. Goldman, Axelrod, Heaton, et al., 1996; Greve, Brooks, et al., 1997); however, the reliability of this score is low (Paolo, Axelrod, and Tröster, 1996; R.L. Tate, Perdices, and Maggiotto, 1998). Since success on this test depends upon discovery of the sort and shift principle, once this has been achieved many persons are unlikely to fail again or even use up many cards while figuring out the solution except if they have sustained brain damage between administrations or were brain impaired initially (McCaffrey, Duff, and Westervelt, 2000b). Thus the WCST is not a reliable measure of the problem-solving abilities of subjects who have solved it once and whose memory has remained reasonably intact: it is a "one-shot" test unless used perhaps as a measure of retention, or of improvement in severely damaged patients (Ferland et al., 1998). Retest scores using an alternate form for young adults and the same form for nonclinical samples and TBI patients retested more than eight months later reflect this improvement (M.R. Basso, et al., 1999; Paolo, Axelrod, and Tröster, 1996; R.L. Tate, Perdices, and Maggiotto, 1998). Moreover, using an alternate form, retest correlations were at best .63, with half of the correlations at or below .34, leading Bowden, Fowler, and their colleagues (1998) to caution that, "clinicians should not employ the Wisconsin until such times as the test is shown to be of adequate reliability" (p. 253). When given to neurologically intact Spanish subjects, findings paralleled those of the North American standardization sample (Artiola i Fortuny and Heaton, 1996).

Neuropsychological findings. The WCST appears to have first earned its reputation as a measure of frontal dysfunction in studies by B. Milner (1963, 1964) who documented defective performances by patients with frontal damage. Functional neuroimaging studies have supported the major role of the frontal lobes in performing this task (Berman et al., 1995; Esposito et al., 1999; Fallgatter and Strik, 1998; Ragland et al., 1997). There is little question that, when compared with control subjects, frontal patients make more perseverative errors (Grafman, Jonas, and Salazar, 1990; Janowsky, Shimamura, Kritchevsky, and Squire, 1989; A.L. Robinson et al., 1980). Some studies also reported that patients with frontal damage achieved the fewest categories (Drewe, 1974; Grafman, Vance, et al., 1986), but others found that frontal patients did not differ from control subjects on this measure (Janowsky, Shimamura, et al., 1989; Stuss, Benson, Kaplan, et al., 1983). In this latter study, a series of schizophrenic patients who had undergone frontal leucotomy approximately 25 years prior to examination with the WCST achieved as many categories on the first 64 cards as did normal control subjects. All subjects were then told about the three possible sorting categories. With this information, the control subjects' performances improved significantly while the patients' performances deteriorated: although they now knew the principle, they appeared unable to maintain it for more than three to five sorts.

WCST findings with respect to lesion lateralization lack consistency. One study reported that patients with temporal lobe epilepsy were impaired on the WCST but no laterality effect appeared on perseverative responses, number of categories achieved, or number of perseverative errors (M.D. Horner et al., 1996). Similar conclusions were reached in a study of patients with focal frontal lesions resulting mostly from strokes at least six months earlier (Stuss, Levine, et al., 2000). Yet an older study (L.B. Taylor, 1979) associated perseverative errors with dorsolateral lesions of the frontal lobes, but reported that more patients with left-sided lesions displayed permanent impairments on this task after lobectomy (usually for epilepsy control or excision of a tumor) than did those with right lobectomies. This finding appeared as a tendency in a series of patients with missile wounds (Grafman, Jonas, and Salazar, 1990), but in this study the most perseverative errors were made by patients whose predominantly left frontal lesions *were not confined* to that lobe, and by patients with wounds in an anterior temporal lobe (i.e., nonfrontal). A.L. Robinson and her colleagues (1980) reported just the opposite, using as supporting evidence Drewe's (1974) study, which suggested a tendency for patients with right frontal damage to make slightly more perseverative errors than those with left-sided lesions (see also Hermann, Wyler, and Ritchey, 1988, whose findings were similar).

Age of onset of the lesion may be an important determinant of lateralized dysfunction. One study found that perseverative errors are most common in patients with seizure disorders when a left hemisphere lesion exists from before one year and that these errors are also common, but less so, with right hemisphere brain injury regardless of age of onset (E. Strauss, Hunter, and Wada, 1993). The question of whether this difference arises from differences in the nature of the lesions or other patient variables needs exploration.

Perhaps most important for users of this test are findings from studies comparing test scores of patients with frontal lesions to those of patients whose lesions are nonfrontal. One report, comparing patients with focal brain lesions, identified those with frontal lesions as making more perseverative and loss-of-set errors than patients with posterior lesions (Stuss, Levine, et al., 2000). The most impaired were those with superior medial frontal lesions, the least impaired frontal patients had inferior medial lesions. However, at least some of these comparisons indicate no privileged WCST competency in differentiating anterior from posterior lesions (S.W. Anderson, Damasio, Jones, and Tranel, 1991; Axelrod, Goldman, Heaton, et al., 1996; Grafman, Jonas, and Salazar, 1990). Moreover, the test appears to be equally sensitive to diffuse damage (Axelrod, Goldman, Heaton, et al., 1996; A.L. Robinson, 1980). And at the other extreme, four patients with frontal lesions achieved significantly more categories and made significantly fewer errors of any kind than larger groups of patients with right or left temporal seizure foci (M.D. Horner, Flashman, et al., 1996; see also Heck and Bryer, 1986). In another study patients with posterior missile wounds examined by Teuber, Battersby, and Bender (1951) made considerably more errors and achieved fewer concepts than those with anterior lesions. A review of the literature led Mountain and Snow (1993) to caution against using the WCST to identify lesion sites or as "a marker of frontal dysfunction." Lombardi and her colleagues (1999) summarized the reported discrepancies by arguing for obtaining both structural and functional data regarding brain integrity when considering localization of cognitive processes. They found that patients with and without frontal structural lesions on MRI had abnormally high perseverative responses on the WCST, while PET data suggested that perseverative responding had a strong association with right dorsolateral frontal–subcortical circuit dysfunction.

Patients with many other conditions have difficulty solving the WCST. Since A.L. Robinson and her colleagues (1980) observed that patients with diffuse damage have high levels of perseveration, and the vulnerability of frontal structures to TBI is well known, it should come as no surprise to learn that perseverative errors may distinguish TBI patients from normal control subjects (Segalowitz, Unsal, and Dywan, 1992; Stuss, 1987; Stuss, Ely, et al., 1985). However, of 20 TBI patients whose anosmic condition was highly suggestive of frontal damage, only eight made more perseverative errors than a cut-off score set at the 5th percentile for normal subjects (Martzke et al., 1991), again reminding us that while sensitive to frontal damage, this test neither localizes lesions nor is it a reliable brain damage screen.

Another condition in which damage can be both relatively diffuse and particularly involve frontal lobe structures is multiple sclerosis. Patients with the relapsing–remitting form of MS, which is more common in the earlier stages of the disease, did not differ from control subjects on any of nine WCST scoring criteria; but those with chronic–progressive MS (who had had the disease longer and were more disabled physically) achieved significantly fewer categories and perseverated more than their matched control group (S.M. Rao, Hammeke, and Speech, 1987). MS patients with high frontal white matter burden achieved fewer categories and made more total errors than those with low white matter burden or patients with nonfrontal white matter lesions (Arnett, Rao, Bernardin, et al., 1994). Difficulty on this task appears to be based, at least in part, on MS patients' conceptual impairments demonstrated on a variety of tasks (Beatty, Hames, Blanco, et al., 1995). The WCST has also been useful in the analysis of executive disorders in Parkinson's disease (Bowen, 1976; Paolo, Tröster, Axelrod, and Koller, 1995; A.E. Taylor and Saint-Cyr, 1992). For some patients the problem was an abnormal number of perseveration errors (Beatty and Monson, 1990); for others it was not excessive perseveration errors (Lees and Smith, 1983), but rather showed up in nonperseverative errors and a low level of concept attainment (Bowen, 1976; A.E. Taylor, Saint-Cyr, and Lang, 1986). In two studies Parkinson patients' degree of rigidity significantly correlated with perseverative re-

sponding (Alevriadou et al., 1999; Van Spaendonck et al., 1996a).

Perseveration characterizes the performance of long-term alcoholics (Parsons, 1975; Tarter and Parsons, 1971). Their third most common error (after difficulty in forming concepts and in shifting) is difficulty in maintaining a set. (Fig. 15.7, p. 588, is an example of this phenomenon in a 55-year-old inventory control clerk who had completed 13 years of schooling and had a 20-year history of alcohol abuse. This erratic error pattern illustrates the interruptions and impersistence described by Parsons that characterize the performance of chronic alcoholics.) Schizophrenia typically produces deficits on this test (M.D. Bell et al., 1997; Gold et al., 1997). Depressed patients may make excessive perseverative errors (Channon, 1996).

Variants of the Wisconsin Card Sorting Test

The figures on the original cards are unevenly positioned relative to the cards' edges, and also to one another on cards with two or more figures. This erratic distribution lures some subjects into attempts to include positional relationships in their sorting hypotheses (these are likely to be bright subjects who distrust the obviousness of the three simple sorting solutions). In the card set developed by Heaton (1981), all cards with the same number of figures have the figures positioned in the same balanced patterns displayed by the stimulus cards (see Fig. 15.6). A manual with very explicit scoring instructions plus norms for ages 6.5 to 89 has been prepared for use with this card set (Heaton, Chelune, et al., 1993).

E.A. Berg's (1948) original card set contained 60 "response" cards plus the four "stimulus" cards; but the standard set of response cards has grown to 64, or 128 when the double pack is used. An effort to reduce the amount of time required when following Heaton's (1981) instructions to use 128 cards cut the time in half by using only 64 (Axelrod, Henry, and Woodard, 1992). These workers report that these two versions of the test give comparable results for six scoring categories. Comparisons of scores on just the first 64 responses of a standard (128-card) administration with the full performance scores found a pattern of age-related performance decrements appearing on the short form that was similar to age-related changes on the standard administration (Axelrod, Jiron, and Henry, 1993). This study includes norms for the 64-card format based on 20 well-educated subjects in each of the seven decades from the 20s to the 80s. This short version was successful in demonstrating poorer performance for most of the major variables, including number of categories and perseverative errors, in dementia patients with Alzheimer's plus Parkinson's disease compared to Parkinson patients without dementia and to control subjects (Paolo, Axelrod, and Tröster, 1996). When the WCST was used with a mixed sample of neurologically and psychiatrically impaired patients, the first 64 cards produced results similar to the full 128-card version in 86% of the patients (short version impairment was defined as at least 15 perseverative responses; long version impairment definition was a perseveration standard score of 70 or below using published norms [Heaton, Chelune, et al., 1993]) (Smith-Seemiller et al., 1997).

Classification errors with the abbreviated version tend to be in the direction of indicating that patients were impaired when they achieve normal performances in the full version. However, poor consistency across versions for individuals has led to a warning against simply extrapolating scores from the shorter version to the full one (Axelrod, Paolo, and Abraham, 1997). When short and long form comparisons were made with a mixed sample of neurologically and psychiatrically impaired patients, fewer than 60% of the cases had demographically corrected standard scores within ±5 points for the two versions. With a more liberal acceptability criterion, the two versions had standard scores within ±10 standard score points in 77% of cases for perseverative errors and 82% for perseverative responses. The authors note that the short version data most closely matched full version data when the subjects obtained at least four categories within 64 cards.

Modified Card Sorting Test (MCST)
(H.E. Nelson, 1976)

This modification of the WCST eliminates all cards from the pack that share more than one attribute with a stimulus card. For example, all red triangle cards would be removed, leaving only yellow, blue, and green triangles, and of these the two green, three yellow, and four blue triangle cards would also be removed. Only 24 of the original 64-card deck satisfy the requirement of being correct for only one attribute at a time. This method removes ambiguity in the examiner's responses, thereby simplifying the task for the patient and clarifying the nature of errors for the examiner.

Nelson uses a 48-card pack with the four stimulus cards set up as in the WCST. Whatever category the patient chooses first is designated "correct" by the examiner, who then proceeds to inform the patient whether each choice is correct or not until the patient has achieved a run of six correct responses. At this point, the patient is told that the rule has changed and is instructed to "find another rule." This procedure

continues until six categories are achieved or the pack of 48 cards is used up. Nelson noted that her pilot studies indicated that explicitly announcing each shift did not seem to affect the tendency to perseverate. However, letting the patient know that the rule had changed made it easier for patients to deal with being told their answers were wrong.

Besides a score for the number of categories obtained, Nelson derived a score for the total number of errors (TE) and scored as perseverative errors (PN) only those of the same category as the immediately preceding response. A third score ([PN/TE] × 100%) gives the percentage of errors that are perseverative. Two normative studies of intact individuals show that performance is affected by age and education (Lineweaver et al., 1999; Obonsawin et al., 1999). Nelson's data (1976) also suggested that this method is sensitive to aging effects.

Comparison of the 53 patients with unilateral lesions and 47 control subjects in the pilot study sample on number of categories achieved readily separated patients from controls. The pilot study demonstrated a tendency for patients with posterior lesions to perform better than patients whose lesions involved the frontal lobes, with considerable overlap between these two groups and no difference with respect to side of lesion. Analyses using either the number or the proportion of perseverative errors resulted in the same pattern of significance: frontal patients performing less well than those with posterior lesions, and control subjects doing best on both counts. Both the number of categories attained on the MCST and perseveration errors successfully separated normal subjects from a larger group of Alzheimer patients with mild to more severe stages of dementia, and these scores were almost equally accurate in identifying normal subjects in comparisons with mildly demented patients (Bondi, Monsch, et al., 1993).

The advantages and disadvantages of this method probably carry different weight according to population and purpose. The shorter run may not give frontal patients an adequate opportunity to develop a strong response set. In one of their original papers, D.A. Grant and Berg (1948) compared requiring 3, 4, 5, 6, 7, 8, and 10 trials correct before shifting and found that increasing the amount of reinforcement of original modes of response reduced the amount of perseveration of these responses when they suddenly became incorrect. Moreover, the advantage that a shorter run requirement has in reducing fatigue and keeping the patient attentive may be more than counterbalanced in some populations—such as chronic alcoholics—by interruptions that can come after six or more correct sorts (see Parsons, 1975). The MCST procedure has the advantage of eliminating distress that some patients experience when a category shifts with no more warning than an unexpected "wrong" called out by the examiner in the other versions. However, alerting patients to a shift in sorting principle changes the task radically as the need to appreciate the fact of change is no longer present. In one study 83% of intact individuals completed all six categories and made no more than one perseverative error, suggesting that the task is easy for well-educated adults (Obonsawin et al., 1999).

Yet the MCST may be sufficiently sensitive for clinical applications. A comparison of it with the WCST found that the two versions produced similar numbers of perseverative errors relative to total trials in two patient populations, one with dementia of the Alzheimer's type or vascular dementia, the other with HIV-1 infection (van Gorp, Kalechstein, et al., 1997). The dementia group produced a large ratio of perseverative errors to total number of responses on both tests, while the HIV group produced a small ratio on both tests.

Halstead's Category Test and Wisconsin Card Sorting Test: similarities and differences

Both of these tests require many of the same mental operations for successful completion (J.A. Bond and Buchtel, 1984; M.C. King and Snow, 1981; J.P. O'-Donnell, Macgregor, et al., 1994). Both display fairly similar levels of sensitivity to brain damage, mostly in the range of 69 to 88% accuracy in discriminating brain damaged from control groups (M.C. King and Snow, 1981; Pendleton and Heaton, 1982). Yet reported shared variances run from as little as 12% (Donders and Kirsch, 1991) to at most about one-third (Pendleton and Heaton, 1982; Perrine, 1993).

Analyses of verbalizations of normal subjects taking these tests (J.A. Bond and Buchtel, 1984) brought out similarities that had been inferred, for the most part, by experienced examiners (e.g., M.C. King and Snow, 1981). Both tests require subjects to perceive and abstract relevant attributes and ignore irrelevant ones. Subjects must recognize that two or more attributes may overlap in an item and single out the relevant one. Hypothesis generation, testing, and remembering requirements are identical. King and Snow also point out that the ability to abandon an irrelevant hypothesis or principle is also necessary. Perrine's (1985) research supported this inference in identifying failure to abandon a previously relevant principle as the source of most of the similarity between the two tests.

The obvious difference between them lies in the scoring procedures as most examiners rely on a single summary score for the HCT, but use at least three scores

to distinguish aspects of the WCST performance. Differences in the nature of these tests, following Bond and Buchtel's analyses, come from the greater complexity of the HCT due to its having more dimensions and therefore a higher level of difficulty; and from the WCST procedure of shifting principles without warning the subject. Because of the multidimensionality of the HCT, feedback has less clarity than WCST feedback which provides more precise information. Moreover, recall of previous HCT feedback is also more difficult. The chief distinguishing feature of the WCST is absence of a warning that a shift in principle has occurred thus requiring the subject to recognize a shift and, after having recognized that the principle may change, the subject must also keep in mind the need to stick with a principle for a number of trials and gauge what that number might be. A study that examined both of these tests along with tests of concept formation (attribute identification) and rule learning reported that the HCT had a significant rule learning component, while perseveration on the WCST was strongly related to attribute identification (Perrine, 1993). Perrine uses these tests to demonstrate the multifaceted nature of concept formation.

Differences have even shown up in order effects when both tests are administered as giving the WCST first may significantly increase HCT errors (Franzen, Smith, et al., 1993). The reverse order tended to decrease WCST errors but this tendency did not reach a significant level for fairly small groups (20 to 36) of psychiatric and neurological patients and healthy elderly persons. These authors suggest that because of these effects—whether likely or probable—a wise examiner will give only one of the tests.

Several considerations should help decide which test to use in the individual case. The HCT appears to be a better measure of abstraction and concept formation, while the WCST will elicit perseverative tendencies (Pendleton and Heaton, 1982) at least in a more obvious and scorable way. Most bright and relatively intact subjects breeze through the WCST, but for patients who get stuck or lose their way, it becomes even more frustrating than the HCT, particularly since a section that has become frustrating and unlikely to be achieved cannot be dropped without discontinuing the test altogether, as it can on the HCT. Moreover, because the WCST once solved becomes a measure of long-term procedural memory and little else, it is a questionable addition to a baseline battery when repeated examinations are anticipated. On the other hand, the complex scoring system of the WCST can provide insights into the nature of a thinking/problem-solving disability by distinguishing important response characteristics as elegantly illustrated in research on the nature of executive dysfunction in Parkinson's disease (e.g., A.E. Taylor and Saint-Cyr, 1992).

REASONING

Reasoning is thinking with a conscious intent to reach a conclusion. Its methods are logically justifiable (Wharton and Grafman, 1998); such as syllogistic paradigms, comprehension of relationships, and practical judgments. The WIS battery furnishes examples of different kinds of reasoning tests in Comprehension, Arithmetic, Picture Completion, and Picture Arrangement. The Stanford-Binet scales contain a varity of reasoning tests, some of which have counterparts in other tests. Many tests of problem solving and concept formation—even drawing tests such as bicycle drawing—require reasoning for success. Reasoning about content-independent situations based on formal logical operations (e.g., if A > B and B > C, then A > C) appears to be mediated by left hemisphere brain regions, while reasoning influenced by information based on previous beliefs, values, or goals is mediated by regions of the right hemisphere and the bilateral ventromedial frontal cortex (Wharton and Grafman, 1998).

Verbal Reasoning

Comprehension (Wechsler, 1955, 1981, 1997a)

This test includes two kinds of open-ended questions: common sense judgment/practical reasoning, and the meaning of proverbs. Comprehension items range in difficulty from a commonsense question passed by all nondefective adults to a proverb that is fully understood by fewer than 22% of adults (Matarazzo, 1972). It is important to recognize that Comprehension scores are not necessarily equatable across test versions. The average scaled score difference between the WAIS and WAIS-R versions may be a little more than 2 points (L.L. Thompson, Heaton, Grant, and Matthews, 1989), a finding supported by other studies. However, one small sample of neuropsychiatric outpatients with retest intervals from two to 15 years averaged less than 1 point lower on the WAIS-R, a statistically negligible difference (E.E. Wagner and Gianakos, 1985). The WAIS-III retains 12 of the 16 WAIS-R items and adds six new ones, yet scores are comparable: WAIS-III scaled scores run an average of only one-half point below WAIS-R scores, but the correlation of .76 between these two forms of Comprehension is lowest for all tests

on the "Verbal" scale (The Psychological Corporation, 1997).

Since most of the items are lengthy the examiner must make sure that patients whose immediate verbal memory span is reduced have registered all of the elements of an item. The instructions call for this test to be discontinued after four failures, but the examiner needs to use discretion in deciding whether to terminate early or continue beyond four "near misses."

Except for the easiest WAIS (first two) and WAIS-III (first three) items which are scored on a pass–fail basis, the subject can earn 1 or 2 points for each question depending on the extent to which the answer is fully relevant (for the practical reasoning questions) or abstract (for the proverbs). Scoring Comprehension can create a judgment problem for the examiner since so many answers are not clearly of 1- or 2-point quality but somewhere in between (R.E. Walker et al., 1965). There are even answers that leave the examiner in doubt as to whether to score 2 points or 0! Scores for the same set of answers by several psychologists or psychology trainees may vary from two to four points in raw score totals [mdl]. When converted to scaled scores, the difference is not often more than 1 point, which is of little consequence so long as the examiner treats individual test scores as likely representatives of a range of scores.

Test characteristics. Age alone changes virtually nothing in the Comprehension performance as, for the WAIS-R, average scores vary within a point or two across the age range from 18 to 74 (A.S. Kaufman, Reynolds, and McLean, 1989). Even from the mid-70s to late 80s and older, no changes in overall performance levels show up in intact subjects (Ivnik, Malec, and Smith, 1992b). Stability also characterized the scores of an elderly control group retested over a two-and-one-half year period (Storandt, Botwinick, and Danziger, 1986). The same stability shows up on the WAIS-III as average scores differ no more than ±1 point for all age groups from 25–29 to 75–79. Education, however, does make a significant difference in performance at every age level (Heaton, Ryan, Grant, and Matthews, 1996; A.S. Kaufman, McLean, and Reynolds, 1988). Several WAIS and WAIS-R studies reported a male superiority on this test (W.G. Snow and Weinstock, 1990). Above age 35, men's WAIS-R Comprehension score average runs a bit more than a half point higher than women's, a difference that is statistically significant though practically of little consequence (A.S. Kaufman, McLean, and Reynolds, 1988); but the pattern of factor loadings is similar for the two sexes (A.S. Kaufman, McLean, and Reynolds, 1991).

On racial comparisons a 2-point scaled score difference favoring whites appears up to age 34, after which African Americans fall behind a little more than two-and-one-half points (A.S. Kaufman, McLean, and Reynolds, 1988). The factor patterns of the two races are essentially the same (A.S. Kaufman, McLean, and Reynolds, 1991).

Practice effects were nonexistent after two to twelve weeks for subjects in the standardization groups for the WAIS-R (Matarazzo and Herman, 1984) and WAIS-III (The Psychological Corporation, 1997); nor did practice effects appear for a group of elderly subjects taking the test twice at an average interval of two months (J.J. Ryan, Paolo, and Brungardt, 1992). However, with three examinations in two-and-one-half years, a small elderly control group made a 1-point gain (Storandt, Botwinick, and Danziger, 1986). Moreover, in the first year postinjury, TBI patients who took the test four times gained significantly more than those having only the first and last administration indicating that practice effects, while small (just under 1 scaled score point), were operative (Rawlings and Crewe, 1992; see also McCaffrey, Duff, and Westervelt, 2000a). Split-half correlations for the WAIS-R are substantial, in the .78 to .87 range, and from age 35 are all .85 or higher (Wechsler, 1981). For the WAIS-III, assessing reliability by the split-half method, the average correlation was .84 with four of the 13 age groups varying from the average by 3 or more points (The Psychological Corporation, 1997). WAIS split-half reliability coefficients are at the low end of this range (.77–.79) (Wechsler, 1955). Retesting a group of healthy elderly subjects after one year produced the lowest of all the WIS-A reliability coefficients (.51) (W.G. Snow, Tierney, Zorzitto, et al., 1989).

Comprehension is only a fair test of general ability (Wechsler, 1955, 1981) but the verbal factor is influential (J. Cohen, 1957a,b; K.C.H. Parker, 1983; J.J. Ryan and Schneider, 1986). Like Information, it appears to measure remote memory in older persons. Comprehension scores also reflect the patient's social knowledgeability and judgment (Sipps et al., 1987). In evaluating Comprehension performances it is important to distinguish between the capacity to give reasonable-sounding responses to these structured questions dealing with single, delimited issues and the judgment needed to handle complex, multidimensional, real-life situations. In real life, the exercise of judgment typically involves defining, conceptualizing, structuring, and making adaptive modifications of the issue requiring judgment as well as rendering an action-oriented decision about it. Thus, it is not surprising to find that WISC-R or WAIS-R Comprehension scores

of children and young adults did not correlate with measures of social competence and social skills (J.M. Campbell and McCord, 1999). As demonstrated most vividly by many patients with right hemisphere lesions, high scores on Comprehension are no guarantee of practical common sense or reasonable behavior.

A 62-year-old retired supervisor of technical assembly work achieved a Comprehension age-graded scaled score of 15 two years after sustaining a right hemisphere CVA that paralyzed his left arm and weakened his left leg. He was repeatedly evicted for not paying his rent from the boarding homes his social worker found for him because he always spent his pension on cab fares within the first week of receiving it. On inquiry into this problem, he reported that he likes to be driven around town. During one hospitalization, when asked about future plans, he announced that upon discharge he would buy a pickup truck, drive to the beach, and go fishing.

Another 62-year-old patient obtained a Comprehension age-graded scaled score of 13 a year after having an episode of left-sided weakness that dissipated within days, leaving minimal sensory and motor residual effects and an identifiable right frontotemporal lesion on CT scan. This man with two graduate degrees had enjoyed a distinguished career in an applied science until, beginning several months after the stroke, he made over 70 decisions in blatant violation of the regulations he was responsible for carrying out. When confronted with possible criminal action against him, he defended himself quite guilelessly by explaining that he had been conducting his own independent experiments to test the appropriateness of the regulations.

Thus, high scores may not reflect social competence but low scores may predict social incompetence. Of a variety of mental ability tests, Comprehension was the best predictor of functional independence of TBI patients completing a rehabilitation program (Smith-Knapp, Corrigan, and Arnett, 1996).

Of all the WIS-A tests, Comprehension best lends itself to interpretation of content because the questions ask for the patient's judgment or opinion about a variety of socially relevant topics, such as marriage or taxes, which may have strong emotional meanings for the patient. Tendencies to impulsivity or dependency sometimes appear in responses to questions about dealing with a found letter or finding one's way out of a forest.

Because the proverbs appear to test somewhat different abilities—and experiences—than do the other items of this test, when evaluating a performance it can be useful to look at responses to the practical reasoning questions separately from responses to the proverbs. Most usually, when there is a disparity between these two different kinds of items, the quality of performance on proverbs (i.e., abstract reasoning) will be akin to that on Similarities. The WAIS-RNI (E. Kaplan, Fein, et al., 1991) provides a five-choice recognition test format for each of the two (WAIS-III) or three (WAIS-R) proverbs which, by bypassing possible verbal expression problems, is more likely to bring into clear focus the ability to comprehend abstract and metaphoric verbal material.

Occasionally a patient, usually elderly, whose reasoning ability seems quite defective for any practical purposes will give 2-point answers to many of the questions related to practical aspects of everyday living or to business issues, such as the need for taxes or the market value of property. In such instances, a little questioning typically reveals a background in business or community affairs and suggests that their good responses represent recall of previously learned information rather than on-the-spot reasoning. For those patients, Comprehension has become a test of old learning. The same holds true for good interpretation of one or more proverbs by a mentally dilapidated elderly patient.

Neuropsychological findings. When damage is diffuse, bilateral, or localized within the right hemisphere, the Comprehension score is likely to be among the best test indicators of premorbid ability, whereas its vulnerability to verbal defects makes it a useful indicator of left hemisphere involvement (Crosson, Greene, et al., 1990; P.C. Fowler, Richards, and Boll, 1980; Hom and Reitan, 1984; McFie, 1975; Zillmer, Waechtler, et al., 1992). A high loading on the verbal factor often shows up for neuropsychologically impaired patients, and these patients make lower scores on Comprehension than on Information and Similarities, a pattern that may reflect the verbally demanding explanatory responses required by many Comprehension items in contrast to most items on the other two tests which can be answered in a word or two. The left hemisphere contribution to success on Comprehension was further demonstrated by increased levels of glucose metabolism in the left hemisphere during the test, although some right-sided increase in areas homologous to left hemisphere speech and language centers was also documented (Chase et al., 1984).

This test reflects the evolution of Alzheimer's disease in mean scores that drop significantly—from 13.2 to 7.2 for 22 patients—over the first two years after diagnosis (Storandt, Botwinick, and Danziger, 1986). It also appears to be vulnerable to multiple sclerosis with lower scores accompanying disease progression (Filley, Heaton, Thompson, et al., 1990); Comprehension scores of multiple sclerosis patients were significantly associated (partial correlation of .38) with size of the corpus callosum as measured by MRI (S.M. Rao, 1990).

Stanford-Binet subtests (Terman and Merrill, 1973)

Although these reasoning tests have not had enough neuropsychological use to result in published studies, they are effective in drawing out defects in reasoning. The verbal reasoning tests of the 1973 edition of the Binet cover a sufficiently broad range of difficulty to provide suitable problems for patients at all but the highest and lowest levels of mental ability. For example, Problem Situations I and II at ages VIII and XI and Problems of Fact at age XIII involve little stories for which the patient has to supply an explanation, such as "My neighbor has been having queer visitors. First a doctor came to his house, then a lawyer, then a minister (preacher, priest, or rabbi). What do you think happened there?"

The Verbal Absurdities (VA) subtest items call for the subject to point out the logical impossibilities in several little stories. At the IX year old level, for example, one item is, "Bill Jones's feet are so big that he has to pull his trousers on over his head." There are four forms of Verbal Absurdities with scoring standards for five age levels: VIII (VA I), IX (VA II), X (VA III), XI (VA IV), and XII (VA II). Verbal Absurdities can sometimes elicit impairments in the ability to evaluate and integrate all elements of a problem that may not become evident in responses to the usual straightforward questions testing practical reasoning and common sense judgment, particularly when the mature patient with a late-onset condition has a rich background of experience to draw upon.

Three-and-a-half months after surgical removal of a left temporal hematoma incurred in a fall from a bar stool, a 48-year-old manufacturers' representative who had completed one year of college achieved age-graded scaled scores ranging from *average* to *superior* ability levels on the WAIS. However, he was unable to explain "what's funny" in a statement about an old gentleman who complained he could no longer walk around a park since he now went only halfway and back (at age level VIII). The patient's first response was, "Getting senile." (Examiner: "Can you explain . . . ") "Because he is still walking around the park; whether he is still walking around the park or not is immaterial." Another instance of impaired reasoning appeared in his explanation of "what's funny" about seeing icebergs that had been melted in the Gulf Stream (at age level IX), when he answered, "Icebergs shouldn't be in the Gulf Stream."

Codes at AA (Form M, 1937 revision) and SA II is another kind of reasoning task. Each difficulty level of Codes contains one message, "COME TO LONDON," printed alongside two coded forms of the message. The patient must find the rule for each code. This task requires the subject to deduce a verbal pattern and then translate it. Codes can be sensitive to mild verbal dysfunctions that do not appear on tests involving well-practiced verbal behavior but may show up when the task is complex and unfamiliar.

Word Finding Test (Reitan, 1972)

This test was developed to evaluate the ability of patients with cerebral damage to infer the meaning of a nonsense word through appreciation of its verbal context. The nonsense word was substituted for a meaningful word in sets of five sentences. For example, "I use my *widgit* daily at work." Patients are instructed to guess the meaning of the nonsense word based on the context in which the word was used in the sentences. Performing the task requires generating hypotheses about the meaning of the word, then refining the hypotheses to select a word that is correct for the multiple applications. Patients with a variety of cerebral disorders performed worse than matched controls in 94% of the cases (Reitan, 1972). Both patients with left hemisphere lesions (19% of whom had signs of aphasia) and those with right hemisphere lesions performed below controls on this task (Reitan, Hom, and Wolfson, 1988). Although the left hemisphere impaired group scored below the right hemisphere impaired group, another study failed to find a laterality effect (Pendleton, Heaton, Lehman, et al., 1985).

Word Context Test (Delis, Kaplan, and Kramer, 2001)

In a manner similar to the Word Finding Test, five sentences are provided as clues to the meaning of each of ten nonsense words, and the patient is asked to guess the meaning of the word after each sentence. Five scores are obtained: the first trial on which a correct meaning is given, first trial of a consistently correct response, number of times an incorrect response follows a correct response, number of "don't know" responses, and number of repetitions of an incorrect response. This is one of the tests in the Delis-Kaplan Executive Function System (see pp. 637–638).

Sentence Arrangement (E. Kaplan, Fein et al., 1991)

As a proposed verbal analogue to the Picture Arrangement test, Sentence Arrangement examines both abilities to perform sequential reasoning with verbal material and to make syntactically correct constructions. The individual words (infinitives are treated as one word) of a sentence are laid out in a scrambled order with instructions to rearrange them "to make a good

sentence." The length and complexity of the ten sentences increase from first to last. A 3-point scoring system (0 to 2) provides evaluations of correctness. Correct responses achieved after a three min time limit are noted but not included in the raw score. A sequence score can be computed for all correct sequences within the ten responses, whether or not the solutions were correct. This latter score provides credit for partial solutions thus indicating the extent to which even subjects who have failed a number of items can reason in a sequential manner. Neurologically impaired patients, most of whom had sustained a TBI an average of six years earlier, had difficulty on this task compared with controls (Mercer et al., 1998).

Verbal Reasoning (R.J. Corsini and Renck, 1992)

This set of 12 "brain teasers" presents questions of relationship between four "siblings," Anne, Bill, Carl, and Debbie, with three multiple-choice answer sets for each question. Questions are on the order of: "The siblings owed money. Anne owed ten times as much as Bill. Debbie owed half as much as Anne but twice as much as Carl. Bill had $4.00." The subject must figure out which sibling owed $40.00, which owed $20,00, and which owed $10.00. Norms are based on a 15-minute time limit. Although advertised for use in industry, this test shows promise for neuropsychological evaluations in which a patient's handling of complex conceptual relationships is of interest. For this purpose, the timed norms may not be relevant.

A 45-year-old advertising executive diagnosed with multiple sclerosis 20 years earlier and now wheelchair-bound with only clumsy use of his right hand was attempting to continue as CEO of his large business operation despite complaints about his work. His reading vocabulary and Comprehension test scores were at the *superior* level. He received a score of 1 (of 3 possible points) on an easy item such as:

"Amy is younger than Bob. Bob is younger than Curt. Curt is younger than Dot. Which sibling is: Youngest?___ Oldest?___ Second youngest?___"

He scored two points on the next item, 1 point on the following one, and handed back the test saying, "I can't track this" when confronted with the fifth item:

"Curt plays raquetball and squash. Bob plays badminton and raquetball. Amy plays ping-pong and golf. Dot plays raquetball and golf. If ping-pong is easier than golf, and golf is easier than badminton, and badminton is easier than raquetball, and raquetball is easier than squash, which sibling plays: Easiest games?___ Next most easy games?___ Most difficult games?___"

His standard score ($M = 50 \pm 10$) based on a normative population of 5,000+ "industrial employees" was 33, placing him at the 4th percentile.

Reasoning about Visually Presented Material

Picture Completion (Wechsler, 1955, 1981, 1997a)

To give this test, the examiner shows the subject incomplete pictures of human features, familiar objects, or scenes, arranged in order of difficulty with instructions to tell what important part is missing (see Fig. 15.8). While the WAIS and WAIS-R pictures are black-and-white line drawings, these pictures are in color and larger in the WAIS-III. The test difficulty ranges from items most mentally retarded persons pass and continues through the last picture (a profile lacking an eyebrow on the WAIS, snow missing from a woodpile on the WAIS-R and WAIS-III). WAIS-R average scores tend to run about six-tenths of a point below those of the WAIS (L.L. Thompson, Heaton, Grant, and Matthews, 1989; E.E. Wagner and Gianakos, 1985). WAIS-III scores run about one-half point below the WAIS-R (The Psychological Corporation, 1997). Correlation between these two versions of Picture Completion was .50, the lowest of all intertest correlations.

Twenty seconds are allowed for each response. When testing a slow responder, the examiner should note the time of completion and whether the response was correct so that both timed and untimed scores can be obtained. The patient's verbatim responses on failed items may yield useful clues to the nature of the underlying difficulty. For example, the response "somebody to row the boat" to the picture of a rowboat is a common error of persons with little initiative who respond to the obvious or who tend to think in simple, concrete terms; but the response "the house" to the drawing for a fire-place and chimney represents very concrete and uncritical thinking. Therefore a record of the patient's words is useful for documenting the seriousness of errors rather than merely noting whether or not the answer was correct. Patients who have difficulty verbalizing a response may indicate the answer by pointing (e.g., to the rim of the rowboat where an oarlock would normally be found). Verbal responses are not required if the patient can indicate a response unequivocally by pointing. Doubts about the subject's intentions in pointing can usually be clarified by multiple-choice questioning (e.g., for the missing oarlock, the examiner can ask if the subject is pointing to a missing "oar, paddle, oarlock, anchor holder").

Test characteristics. Age effects occur but quite modestly until the middle 70s (Compton et al., 2000; A.S. Kaufman, Kaufman-Packer, et al., 1991; A.S. Kaufman, Reynolds, and McLean, 1989; D. Wechsler, 1955, 1981) when the performance decline becomes relatively steep into the late 80s+ (Howieson, Holm, et al., 1993; Ivnik, Malec, Smith, et al., 1992b; The Psychological Corporation, 1997). Education, however, accounts for 14% to 17% of the variance from ages 20 to 74 (A.S. Kaufman, McLean, and Reynolds, 1988) and interacts significantly with age (A.S. Kaufman, Reynolds, and McLean, 1989). Its contribution was less for a relatively privileged older sample (Malec, Ivnik, Smith, et al., 1992a). A sex bias favoring males does not appear until age 35+ on the WAIS-R and even then accounts for less than 5% of the variance until age 74 (A.S. Kaufman, McLean, and Reynolds, 1988; see also W.G. Snow and Weinstock, 1990). A breakdown of mean scores by age and sex suggests a slightly steeper rate of declining scores for women than men (A.S. Kaufman, Kaufman-Packer, et al., 1991). Malec and colleagues (1992a) found that sex made only a 2% contribution to Picture Completion variance in a 56 to 97 age group; and no sex differences appeared in either a 65–74 year-old or an 84–100 year-old group (Howieson, Holm et al., 1993). Whites tended to outperform African Americans by about 2 points on the average throughout the WAIS-R age ranges (A.S. Kaufman, McLean, and Reynolds 1988). Only the factor pattern for African American women differs from the typical pattern (see below) in that the verbal component is even stronger than the contribution by the perceptual organization factor (A.S. Kaufman, McLean, and Reynolds, 1991). This test does not discriminate well between *superior* and *very superior* ability levels.

Split-half reliability measured on subsets of the normative population for the WAIS-R is .82 and higher for all ages 25 and older, dropping into the .70s for

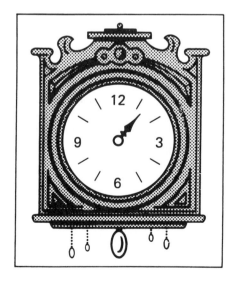

FIGURE 15.8 WIS-type Picture Completion test item.

the three younger age groups (Wechsler, 1981) and ranging from .76 to .88 for various age groups tested on the WAIS-III (The Psychological Corporation, 1997). Test–retest reliability coefficients for two other subsets of this population were .86 and .89 (Matarazzo and Herman, 1984), and .79 and .82 for the WAIS-III (The Psychological Corporation, 1997). For healthy elderly persons, retesting with an average 2-month interval produced a reliability coefficient of .76 (J.J. Ryan, Paolo, and Brungardt, 1992) and a significant gain of a little more than one-half of a scaled score point; with an interval of a year, the reliability coefficient for a similar age group was lower (.65) (W.G. Snow, Tierney, Zorzitto, et al., 1989). The average test–retest gain for the younger subjects examined by Matarazzo and Herman was 1.1 scaled score point. This was most comparable to the higher (and significant) practice effects gain (1.50) made by TBI patients in a well-controlled study (Rawlings and Crewe, 1992; see also McCaffrey, Duff, and Westervelt, 2000a). Retesting a subset of the normative sample an average of 35 days later produced a 2.4 scaled score point gain, the highest gain of any of the tests in the battery (The Psychological Corporation, 1997).

Factor analyses which extract a "general" factor found that Picture Completion (WAIS) had relatively high weightings on it, with modest weightings on both the verbal and visuospatial factors (Lansdell and Smith, 1975; A.E. Maxwell, 1960). Three-factor solutions tend to elicit moderate loadings on both Verbal Comprehension and Perceptual Organization factors with the perceptual loadings typically exceeding the verbal ones by ten to 20 points but for some age groups they are almost equal or reversed (A.S. Kaufman, McLean, and Reynolds, 1991; K.C.H. Parker, 1983). A four-factor solution of the WAIS-III showed the greatest loading on Perceptual Organization with minimum Verbal Comprehension for ages less than 75 years. For the older age groups the greatest loading was on Processing Speed (The Psychological Corporation, 1997). This latter finding suggests that examiners who want to find out about their elderly patients' perceptual organization abilities will allow these patients more than 20 secs. to figure out a solution, recording—of course—the time overtime responses take.

At its most basic level, Picture Completion tests visual recognition and thus is somewhat vulnerable to reduced visual acuity (Schear and Sato, 1989), with visual acuity accounting for 16% of the variance in elderly subjects (Howieson, Holm, et al., 1993). The kinds of visual organization and reasoning abilities needed to perform Picture Completion differ from those required by other WIS-A Performance Scale tests as the subject must supply the missing part from long-term

memory but does not have to manipulate anything. On the WAIS, Picture Completion correlates higher (.67) with the Information test than any other except Comprehension, thus reflecting the extent to which it also tests remote memory and general information. Its highest correlation on the WAIS-R, .55, is with Vocabulary, indicating the relevance of verbal functions in Picture Completion performance. This test also has reasoning components involving judgments about both practical and conceptual relevancies (Saunders, 1960b). J. Cohen (1957b) considers it to be a nonverbal analogue of Comprehension. Of the WAIS-III verbal tests, Picture Completion correlates highly (.48) with Similarities. The likeness between these tests is their susceptibility to concrete thinking such as, on the pitcher item ("hand holding the pitcher") and the leaf item ("tree"). When more than one of these occur, the possibility of abnormally concrete thinking should be further explored.

Neuropsychological findings. The verbal and visuoperceptual contributions to this test, identified by factor analysis, are faithfully reflected in the bilateral metabolic increases noted on PET scanning as right posterior hemispheric involvement is most prominent but left parietal metabolism also increases (Chase et al., 1984). Picture Completion consistently demonstrates resilience to the effects of brain damage. Lateralized lesions frequently do not have any significant differentiating effect (Boone, Miller, Lee, et al., 1999; Crosson, Greene, et al., 1990; Hom and Reitan, 1984; McFie, 1975). When brain impairment is lateralized, the Picture Completion score is usually higher than the scores on the tests most likely to be vulnerable to that kind of damage. For example, a patient with a left-sided lesion is likely to do better on this test than on the four highly verbal ones; with right-sided involvement, the Picture Completion score tends to exceed that of the other tests in the Performance Scale. Thus Picture Completion may serve as the best test indicator of previous ability, particularly when left hemisphere damage has significantly affected the ability to formulate the kinds of complex spoken responses needed for tests calling for a verbal response.

One example of the sturdiness of Picture Completion is given by the WAIS age-graded test score pattern of a 50-year-old retired mechanic. This high school graduate had a right superficial temporal and middle cerebral artery anastomosis two months after a right CVA and three years before the neuropsychological examination. A little more than one year after he had undergone the neurosurgical procedure he reported seizures involving the right arm and accompanied by headache and right-sided numbness. An EEG showed diffuse slowing, which agreed with a history that implicated bilateral brain damage. Bilateral damage was also suggested by WAIS age-graded scores of 7 on Information, Similarities, and Object Assembly, and of 5 on Block Design and Picture Arrangement. His highest score—10—was on Picture Completion.

With diffuse damage, Picture Completion also tends to be relatively unaffected although it is somewhat depressed in the acute stages of TBI, particularly for patients with moderate to severe injuries (Correll et al., 1993). In mild to moderate Alzheimer type dementia, the Picture Completion score tends to be at or near the higher end of the WIS score range, along with Information and Vocabulary (Logsdon et al., 1989). Multiple sclerosis patients showed no changes on retesting after one-and-one-half years and no significant differences between groups with different levels of disease severity (Filley, Heaton, Thompson, et al., 1990). Of the visuoperceptual tests, diffusely damaged stroke patients had their highest average score on Picture Completion (Zillmer, Waechtler, et al., 1992). However, disease in which the primary involvement is subcortical tends to be quite vulnerable on this test (Cummings and Huber, 1992; M.E. Strauss and Brandt, 1986), although newly diagnosed Huntington patients made higher scores on this test than on other visuoperceptual ones (Brandt, Strauss, Larus, et al., 1984).

Picture Arrangement (Wechsler, 1955, 1981, 1997a)

This test consists of sets of black-and-white line drawings of cartoon pictures that can be arranged into stories. Each set is presented to the subject in scrambled order with instructions to rearrange the pictures to make the most sensible story (see Fig. 15.9). Each set consists of three to six pictures. Presentation is in order of increasing difficulty or nearly so. All but seriously retarded adults can do the first set (Matarazzo, 1972). WAIS-R item 2 (FLIRT) may be disproportionately difficult and WAIS-R item 5 (ENTER) may be disproportionately easy (J.A. Heath and Leathem, 1998). WAIS-R item 5 was moved to item 3 in the WAIS-III, and it may be too difficult in this position

(J.J. Ryan and Lopez, 1999). WAIS-R and WAIS-III Picture Arrangement testing is discontinued after four consecutive failures. Time limits range from one minute on the easiest items to two minutes on the two most difficult ones. As on other timed tests, the examiner should note correct solutions completed outside the time limits. Some sets in each edition of this test provide two levels of accuracy: the most apt arrangement earns 2 points, while an alternatively correct arrangement earns only 1. Average performance levels for the WAIS and WAIS-R versions of this test are virtually identical (L.L. Thompson, Heaton, Grant, and Matthews, 1989; E.E. Wagner and Gianakos, 1985). Scaled score points, however, are approximately six-tenths of a point lower on the WAIS-III compared to the WAIS-R; a correlation between these two versions was .63 (The Psychological Corporation, 1997).

The age-graded scaled scores for Picture Arrangement, like those for Similarities, appear to be overly lenient at older age levels. From age 55 on, a person can fail all but the three easiest items on the WAIS or WAIS-R and still obtain a score within the *average* range. On the WAIS-III, for someone 85 to 89 years old, a raw score of 1 yields an age-graded scaled score of 6, raw scores of 4 or 5 (succeeding on two or three of the 11 items) fall within the *average* range! Therefore, discretion is recommended in interpreting the WIS-A Picture Arrangement age-graded scaled scores for older persons.

It is good practice to have subjects "tell the story" of their arrangement of the cartoons. This will provide a sample of the subject's ability for verbal organization of complex sequentially ordered visual data. Sometimes patients arrange the correct sequence but misinterpret the point of the story, while the reverse may also be true in which the gist of the story is reported correctly but the sequence contains an error. In order to prevent subjects from noticing an error while telling the story, the examiner can remove the cards first. Since this makes the storytelling requirement a test of immediate memory as well, stories given by those few patients whose memory defects involve confabulation are likely

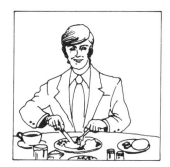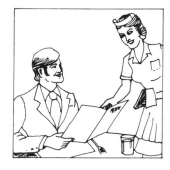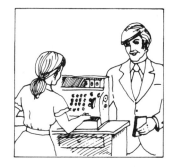

FIGURE 15.9 WIS-type Picture Arrangement test item.

to deviate from their arrangements considerably, but they are also likely to contain extraneous intrusions that, in themselves, will be of interest. Absence of the pictures does not seem to affect the stories given by most subjects. To save time, the examiner may request stories for only two or three items and, preferably, include at least one passed and one failed item. Having the patient tell the story immediately following each item does not appear to affect the score (Gaudette and Smith, 1998).

The ENTER item, whether passed or failed, is recommended for inclusion among the requests for stories because it can be misinterpreted in ways that may show patients' preoccupations, tendencies for interpreting the character's problem as under internal or external control, along with their difficulties comprehending visual information or integrating sequential material. The most common erroneous solution to this item (OPESN) was explained by a 31-year-old construction worker with a high school education who had incurred a TBI in an accident ten months earlier:

It looks like the man is trying a door. He walks up to the door and tries to open it. He just tries to open it and he walks away and another man follows just behind him and just opens the door and doesn't have any trouble opening it.

This patient's age-graded scaled score for Picture Arrangement was 12.

A 49-year-old investment counselor with graduate training in Business Administration was examined approximately one year after he had a cardiac arrest and fell to the ground, receiving a right frontal injury. He obtained a WAIS Picture Arrangement scaled score of 5. His sequencing of this item was correct, but not his explanation:

Looks like it was locked there. But there must be room for more than one. There's three darned people involved. One guy with the black hat went into wherever it was and then he came out and then the other gentleman entered.

Not surprisingly, this once highly organized patient was having a great deal of difficulty appreciating his changed situation and dealing with it reasonably. Another patient, an architectural draftsman aged 35, had sustained a severe left frontal head injury with coma and transient right-sided weakness ten years before being seen for neuropsychological assessment. He too made a correct arrangement for this item, which he interpreted as, "A guy tried to break into the house and the owner was coming home. Then he walked away."

Test characteristics. A steep age gradient appears after 65 for the normative population (Wechsler, 1955,

1981, 1997a) giving highly significant age effects (A.S. Kaufman, Kaufman-Packer, et al., 1991; A.S. Kaufman, Reynolds, and McLean, 1989). The Mayo group also reports a sharp decline beginning in the late 60s but that average raw scores for these subjects tend to run 1 point higher than the Wechsler norms (Ivnik, Malec, and Smith, 1992b). Education makes a significant contribution, amounting to an average $2^1/_2$- to 4-point score differential, depending upon the subject's age; between ages 20 and 54 it accounts for $15+\%$ of the variance, 13% for 55–74 year olds (A.S. Kaufman, McLean, and Reynolds, 1988). For subjects in a 55 to 97 year range, education effects dropped to just 6% of the variance (Malec, Ivnik, Smith, et al., 1992a). Women's scores generally run a little lower than men's (scaled score difference = .14) with no age differential (A.S. Kaufman, Kaufman-Packer, et al., 1991; A.S. Kaufman, McLean, and Reynolds, 1991). Only teenagers (A.S. Kaufman, McLean, and Reynolds, 1988) and older persons (Malec et al., 1992a) did not show this sex bias. However, women treat this test more like a verbal problem while men handle it more as a visuoperceptual test—except after age 55 when both sexes use a visuoperceptual approach (A.S. Kaufman, McLean, and Reynolds, 1991). A review of many studies found that sex biases on the WAIS tended to be very small (W.G. Snow and Weinstock, 1990). Differences between whites and African Americans favor the former with youngsters in the late teens showing only about a 1 scaled score point difference, while the difference is more on the order of 1.5 to 1.9 points in the adult years (A.S. Kaufman, McLean, and Reynolds, 1988). Factor patterns differ for the two races, and for African American men and women, as the former rely heavily on a visuoperceptual approach, while the latter use both visuoperceptual and verbal approaches to about the same degree (A.S. Kaufman, McLean, and Reynolds, 1991).

Among the tests in the battery it has the lowest reliability and stability coefficients (The Psychological Corporation, 1997). Reliability coefficients based on split-half studies range from .66 for the 16–17 year range to .82 for a 45–54 age group for the WAIS-R (Wechsler, 1981) and are similar on the WAIS-III (.66–.81) (J.J. Ryan, Arb, Paul, and Kreiner, 2000). Retesting two small subject groups after several weeks produced correlations of .69 and .76 with an average scaled score gain of 1.3 (Matarazzo and Herman, 1984). One group of elderly persons retested after approximately two months showed a low degree of stability (.49) although their retest gains—while only .41 of a scaled score point—were significant (J.J. Ryan, Paolo, and Brungardt, 1992). However, other older subjects examined after an interval of a year showed a Picture Arrangement reliability coefficient of .74, in line with most other reported studies (W.G. Snow, Tierney, Zorzitto, et al., 1989). Significant practice effects, amounting to .63 of a scaled score point, showed up when two TBI groups were compared, one having four examinations during a year and the other examined only at the first and last times (Rawlings and Crewe, 1992).

On a general ability factor, Picture Arrangement loadings are mostly in the .60s, with higher correlations on the WAIS-III with Verbal Comprehension and Perceptual Organization than with Working Memory and Processing Speed (The Psychological Corporation, 1997). For groups 75 years and older in the normative sample of the WAIS-III, the greatest factor loading was on Processing Speed (The Psychological Corporation, 1997). For all but the three oldest age groups in the WAIS-R normative population, factor loadings on the Verbal Comprehension factor exceeded those on the Perceptual Organization factor, and for three of the younger groups, the highest loadings were on the Freedom from Distractibility factor; yet no one of these factor loadings exceeded .54 (K.C.H. Parker, 1983). Picture Arrangement on the WAIS version, was shown to depend to a small degree on visual acuity (Schear and Sato, 1989). This test tends to reflect social sophistication so that, in unimpaired subjects, it serves as a nonverbal counterpart of that aspect of Comprehension (Sipps et al., 1987). Its humorous content not only enhances its sensitivity to socially appropriate thinking, but also provides an opportunity for a particular kind of social response and interplay within the test setting. Sequential thinking—including the ability to see relationships between events, establish priorities, and order activities chronologically—also plays a significant role in this test (see the procedures for measuring sequencing accuracy in the WAIS-RNI: E. Kaplan, Fein et al., 1991).

Neuropsychological findings. The absence of a distinctively verbal or visuoperceptual factor bias for normal subjects parallels a bilateral parietal pattern of increased glucose metabolism during the Picture Arrangement performance (Chase et al., 1984). Although Picture Arrangement tends to be vulnerable to brain injury in general, right hemisphere lesions have a more depressing effect on these scores than left hemisphere lesions (Boone, Miller, Lee, et al., 1999; Warrington, James, and Maciejewski, 1986; Zillmer, Waechtler, et al., 1992). A low Picture Arrangement score in itself is likely to be associated with right temporal lobe damage (Dodrill and Wilkus, 1976; Piercy, 1964).

McFie (1975) and Walsh (1987) called attention to tendencies displayed by some patients with frontal damage to shift the cards only a little if at all and to

present this response (or nonresponse) as a solution. Walsh suggested that this behavior is akin to the tendency of patients with frontal lobe lesions, described by Luria (1973a), to make hypotheses impulsively and uncritically based on first impressions or on whatever detail first catches the eye, without analyzing the entire situation.

This test is relatively sensitive to the effects of diffuse damage, whether it be due to stroke (Zillmer, Waechtler, et al., 1992), Alzheimer's disease (E.W. Sullivan, Sagar, Gabrieli, et al., 1989), or multiple sclerosis (Beatty and Monson, 1994; Filley, Heaton, Thompson, et al., 1990). Yet Logsdon and her colleagues (1989) found only a modest drop in Picture Arrangement scores (of approximately 3 scaled score points when compared with control groups) for Alzheimer patients in their 70s. Patients with vascular dementia have more difficulty on this task than Alzheimer patients (Kertesz and Clydesdale, 1994). With an approximate mean scaled score of 7.5, it was the second lowest WAIS score (next to Digit Symbol) for a group of TBI patients within the first month postinjury (Correll et al., 1993). Not surprisingly, schizophrenic patients have difficulty with Picture Arrangement, which requires interpretation of social cues (Toomey et al., 1997).

Deficits on Picture Arrangement distinguished Huntington patients from subjects at risk for the disease and control subjects (M.E. Strauss and Brandt, 1986) but the scores did not drop sharply with disease progression (Brandt, Strauss, Larus, et al., 1984). Parkinson patients perform poorly on this test, displaying a prominent gap between their normal Vocabulary scores and their Picture Arrangement scores, regardless of the presence or absence of dementia or whether or not the test was timed, thus implicating a specific sequencing deficit elicited by this test (E.V. Sullivan, Sagar, Gabrieli, et al., 1989). Poor scores differentiated Parkinson patients with preclinical dementia from those who remained dementia free (Mahieux et al., 1998). The Picture Arrangement performance of patients with Parkinson's disease may be improved by medications that reduce the disease's motor symptoms (Ogden, Growdon, and Corkin, 1990).

Picture Problems

On the Stanford-Binet Form L-M (Terman and Merrill, 1973), the visual analogue of Verbal Absurdities is *Picture Absurdities I* which consists of five picture items and II which is a one-item subtest at years VII and XIII (see Fig. 15.10, p. 602). These subtests depict a logically or practically impossible situation which the patient must identify. In studies of patients with known or suspected dementia, Picture Absurdities was shown

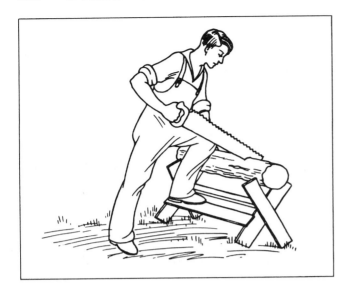

FIGURE 15.10 Picture Absurdities I, Card B. (Terman and Merrill, 1973. Courtesy of Houghton Mifflin Co.)

to correlate significantly with cerebral atrophy (−.35) and EEG slowing (−.50) (Kaszniak, Garron, Fox, et al., 1979; Bondi, Salmon, and Kaszniak, 1996). A significant correlation (.36) also occurred with age and education effects too, were significant (.33). Further analysis indicated that EEG slowing primarily, and age secondarily, made significant contributions to the Picture Absurdities performance. While Alzheimer patients differed significantly from normal control subjects on this test, depressed elderly patients did not (R.P. Hart, Kwentus, Taylor, and Hamer, 1988).

In the 1986 revision of the Stanford-Binet (Thorndike, Hagen, and Sattler), *Absurdities*, one of the 15 tests, presents 32 items of increasing difficulty, each depicting a silly or impossible situation. Items in the upper range (the ceiling age for this test is 15 years 11 months) are appropriate for adults. Visual reasoning is called for by the *Paper Folding and Cutting* test, developed for mental ability levels at ages 16 and higher. This is a multiple-choice version of the *Paper Cutting* items of earlier editions of the Stanford-Binet. Only the sample items involve actual folding and cutting of pieces of paper. In the test itself, the folds and cuts of each of the 18 items are pictured.

Focusing on functions involved in the appreciation of humor, Wapner and her colleagues (1981) reported patient responses to a three-frame funny cartoon. In contrast to control subjects and aphasic patients who "invariably" saw the humor, those whose lesions were in the right hemisphere did not even realize that a joke was intended. Their responses suggested difficulty in spontaneous integration of all the elements of the story; particular elements were taken out of context and in-

terpreted as inappropriate in some way. Howard Gardner and his associates (1975) found patients with right hemisphere disease impaired in comprehending cartoons. Captioning improved their appreciation of the humor, while captions seemed to interfere with the otherwise good understanding of patients with left-sided lesions. Even TBI patients with severe injuries could "get the joke" of captioned cartoons, but were unable to evaluate the cartoons appropriately (Braun, Lussier, et al., 1989).

MATHEMATICAL PROCEDURES

Arithmetic Reasoning Problems

Arithmetic (Wechsler, 1955, 1981, 1997a)

This test consists of arithmetic problems presented in story format arranged according to level of difficulty. Nearly all adults can answer the simplest item, which calls for block counting, and 20% of the adult population can figure out the last item (Matarazzo, 1972), which is like, "Four men can finish a job in eight hours. How many men will be needed to finish it in a half hour?" The WAIS and WAIS-R versions of this test differ by one item as a more difficult one replaced an easy one, while the WAIS-III has four new items.

When giving the WAIS-III, the four simplest Arithmetic items are not presented unless either of the first two items is missed. Subjects who cannot do the simplest addition and subtraction are asked to count blocks. For subjects who have already demonstrated generally good mental competence (they may already have performed serial subtractions and several other tests by the time this one comes up), the examiner can begin with item 5, 6, or 7, depending on an estimate of the subject's level of mental efficiency. This saves time and some boring questions which do not add much to an understanding of a bright patient's condition. Should they fail the first item (5, 6, or 7), testing can go back two items or back to the beginning if need be, but this will be unlikely with a well-educated, articulate patient. Testing is discontinued after four consecutive failures. When patients are distressed by their failures or are very unlikely to improve their performance, it may be prudent to discontinue after a second or third consecutive failure.

When recording test data using the WAIS test form, the examiner will obtain more information by noting the patient's exact responses on the Record Form. Every answer should be written in, the correct ones as well as the incorrect, so that the subject gets no hint of failure from the pace or amount of the examiner's writing. Although all Arithmetic failures receive the same zero score, some approach correctness more closely than others, and a record of the response will preserve this information. On the example above that is similar to the last item an incorrect response of "32" indicates that the patient has sorted out the elements of the problem and used the appropriate operation, but has failed to carry it through to the proper conclusion. An answer of "48" suggests that the patient performed the correct operations but miscalculated one step, whereas an answer of "$1^1/_2$" or "16" reveals ignorance or confusion. Thus, although "32," "48," "$1^1/_2$" and "16" are equally incorrect as far as scoring is concerned, only a person with a reasonably good grasp of arithmetic fundamentals and ability to reason about a complex arithmetic idea could get "32' as an answer; persons who say "48" can handle mathematical concepts well but either are careless or have forgotten their multiplication tables.

Arithmetic items have time limits ranging from 15 sec on the first items to 120 sec on the last. A subject can earn raw score bonus points for particularly rapid responses on the last four items of the WAIS-R and the last two on the WAIS-III. The total Arithmetic score of a bright intact person will usually be compounded of both number correct and time credit points. In the case of slow responders who take longer than the time limit to formulate the correct answer, the total Arithmetic score may not reflect their arithmetic ability so much as their response rate. It is important for the examiner to find out whether the subject can answer these questions correctly regardless of time limits. Two people may get the same number of responses correct—say, 11—but the intact subject could earn a raw score of 12 and a scaled score of 11, whereas a neurologically impaired patient whose arithmetic skills are comparable might receive a raw score of only 8 or 9 and a scaled score of 7 or 8, losing both time points and credit for solvable problems that were not scored because the answer came after the time limit. Thus, the examiner should obtain two Arithmetic scores: one based on the sum of correct responses given within time limits plus time bonuses, and the other on the sum of correct responses regardless of time limits. The first score can be interpreted in terms of the test norms and the second gives a better indication of the patient's ability to solve these kinds of problems. Recording and interpreting only the score dictated by the test developers does an injustice to patients whose processing may be slowed, who need to have the question repeated several times before grasping it in its entirety, or who self-correct an error only after the arbitrarily defined time limit. When testing for maximum productivity, the examiner will not interrupt patients to give another item until they have indicated that they cannot do it or they become too restless or upset to continue working on the unanswered item.

Arithmetic has one of the highest correlations with Working Memory of all the tests in the WAIS-III battery (The Psychological Corporation, 1997). Difficulties in immediate memory, concentration, or conceptual manipulation and tracking can prevent even very mathematically skilled patients from doing well on this oral test. These patients typically can answer the first several questions quickly and correctly, since they involve only one operation, few elements, and simple, familiar number relationships. When the question contains more than one operation, several elements, or less common number relationships requiring "carrying," these patients lose or confuse the elements or goal of the problems. They may succeed with repeated prompting but only after the time limit has expired, or they may be unable to do the problem "in their head" at all, regardless of how often the question is repeated. The length of WAIS-III item 19, for example, is unusually challenging and unlikely to be grasped immediately and correctly by many patients. Item 12 which calls for adding one tax to a set of purchases before concluding the solution with division is so frequently misinterpreted that failure on it is rarely due to inability to perform the required arithmetic.

A 40-year-old college graduate lay-out artist with most WAIS-III scaled scores between 11 and 13 and performances *within normal limits* on Auditory Consonant Trigrams, Sentence Repetition, Digits Span (both forward and reversed), immediate recall of stories, and first AVLT trial had difficulty grasping (only) this item. She asked, "$1.60 each or $1.60 total," commenting, "It [i.e., $1.60 for all six] doesn't come out even." A 35-year-old auto mechanic whose three high WAIS-R scaled scores were 12, 13, and 14, but who did have a pronounced auditory span deficit, mused over this problem (which was reread twice): "Six pieces of chocolate at $1.60 each" (first rereading), "That makes it more difficult . . . I have to divide by six and add sales tax into it." His final answer was $1.83.

After discovering how poorly some patients perform when they have to rely on immediate memory, the examiner can find out how well they can do these problems by giving them paper and pencil so that they can work out the problems while looking at them. It is often necessary to repeat the question so that the patient can write down the numbers in the problem. Using unlined paper has two advantages: spatial orientation problems are more apt to show up if there are no guide lines, and there is no visual interference to distract vulnerable patients. By providing only one sheet of paper, the examiner forces the patient to organize the two or three and sometimes more problems on the one page, a maneuver that may reveal defects in spatial organization, ordering, and planning. An alternate method used in the WAIS-RNI (E. Kaplan, Fein, et al., 1991) and suitable for patients who also have difficulty writing, is to give patients the problem printed out on a card which they can study as long as they wish. The WAIS-RNI also provides a worksheet printed with the numerical form of the problems for direct computation. In either case—as when dealing with responses given after the time limits—the examiner should obtain two scores: one based on the patient's performance under standard conditions will give a good measure of the extent to which memory and mental efficiency problems are interfering with the ability to handle problems mentally; the other, summing all correct answers regardless of timing or administration format, will give a better estimate of the patient's arithmetic skills per se.

Test characteristics. Until the mid 70s Arithmetic performance remains essentially the same (D.M. Compton et al., 2000; Wechsler, 1955, 1981, 1997a; A.S. Kaufman, Reynolds, and McLean, 1989) and continues to be fairly stable into the late 80s and beyond (Ivnik, Malec, Smith, et al., 1992b). Education effects, however, are prominent (Finlayson, Johnson, and Reitan, 1977) with an average gain of 4 or more scaled score points from grade school to 16+ years (A.S. Kaufman, McLean, and Reynolds, 1988). Yet education appears to contribute only a little to elderly subjects' performances (Malec, Ivnik, Smith et al., 1992a). From age 20, men outperform women to a significant degree ($p < .001$), with average scaled score differences ranging from 0.9 to 1.3 depending on the age group (A.S. Kaufman, Kaufman-Packer, et al., 1991; A.S. Kaufman, McLean, and Reynolds, 1988; see also W.G. Snow and Weinstock, 1990). As might be expected of an education-dependent test, racial differences favoring whites average 2 scaled score points for teenagers and gradually increase to 2.5 points for the 55–74 age range (A.S. Kaufman, McLean, and Reynolds, 1988).

Using the split-half technique to examine reliability, correlations of .81 to .87 were obtained for subjects 20 years and older except for a drop to .77 for the 85 to 89-year-old group (The Psychological Corporation, 1997; Wechsler, 1955, 1981). Two groups taken from the normative population who were retested within several weeks showed an average scaled score gain of up to .6 with reliability coefficients of .80 and .90 (Matarazzo and Herman, 1984; The Psychological Corporation, 1997). Retest reliability was in this general range for two groups of elderly subjects with virtually no score gain (J.J. Ryan, Paolo, and Brungardt, 1992; W.G. Snow, Tierney, Zorzitto, et al., 1989). TBI patients too showed no gain in a carefully controlled

retesting program (Rawlings and Crewe, 1992; see also McCaffrey, Duff, and Westervelt, 2000a).

Arithmetic scores are of only mediocre value as measures of general ability in the population at large, but they do reflect concentration and "ideational discipline" (Saunders, 1960a). In early adulthood, the memory component plays a relatively small role in Arithmetic, but it becomes more important with age. Arithmetic performance may suffer from poor early school attitudes or experiences.

When evaluated for the WAIS-R normative population in a three-factor solution, generally the highest factor loading is on Freedom from Distractibility (.55), with the verbal factor contributing somewhat less (.44) and Perceptual Organization still less (.33) (K.C.H. Parker, 1983; see also A.S. Kaufman, McLean, and Reynolds, 1991). Digit Span's highest correlation (.56) is with Arithmetic, pointing up the importance of the Freedom from Distractibility component of this test (The Psychological Corporation, 1997).

Under ordinary circumstances Arithmetic should not be considered a verbal test because it does not load on the Verbal Comprehension factor. The WIS-A tests that are heavily weighted with the verbal factor (Information, Comprehension, Similarities, and Vocabulary) correlate less with Arithmetic (.49 to .66) than comparable correlations with the Performance Scale test, Picture Completion (.56 to .67) (Wechsler, 1958, 1981). In WAIS-III factor analytic studies it loads mostly under Working Memory (The Psychological Corporation, 1997). However, McFie (1975) noted that subjects who have some kind of difficulty with verbal comprehension may be confused by the wording of some of the problems and fail for this reason; and the WAIS-III version does have a modest loading (.22) under Verbal Comprehension (The Psychological Corporation, 1997). McFie recommended that when the examiner suspects that impaired verbal comprehension is blocking understanding of the problem, the question should be restated. As one example, McFie reworded item 8 (7 on the WAIS-R, 9 on the WAIS-III) to say, "If you walk at three miles an hour, how long would it take you to walk 24 miles?" Also, when patients give unusual answers, it is wise to ask them to state the question. It may be that the question was misunderstood.

A lowered Arithmetic score should lead the examiner to suspect an immediate memory or concentration problem and to raise questions about verbal functions, but it does not necessarily reflect the patient's arithmetic skills, particularly if there are other indications of impairment of relevant functions. To evaluate the patient's arithmetic skills, the examiner must turn to the untimed Arithmetic score, the paper-and-pencil score, qualitative aspects of the patient's performance, and other arithmetic tests.

Neuropsychological findings. When obtained from neurologically impaired patients following standard procedure, the Arithmetic score may be more confusing than revealing. The problem lies in the oral format, which emphasizes the considerable memory and concentration components of oral arithmetic. This results in a tendency for Arithmetic scores to drop in the presence of brain damage generally (Hom and Reitan, 1984; Newcombe, 1969; Sivak et al., 1981). In addition, using the oral format, the examiner may overlook the often profound effects of the spatial type of dyscalculia that become apparent only when the patient must organize arithmetic concepts on paper (i.e., spatially). In other cases, the examiner may remain ignorant of a figure or number alexia that would show up if the patient had to look at arithmetic symbols on paper (Hécaen, 1962).

Further, a distinct verbal component emerges from the Arithmetic performances of brain impaired persons (P.C. Fowler, Richards, et al., 1987; Zillmer, Waechtler, et al., 1992) which may account for the slight but regular tendency for left hemisphere patients to do worse on this test than those whose lesions are located within the right hemisphere (Spreen and Benton, 1965; Warrington, James, and Maciejewski, 1986). McFie (1975) found that patients with left parietal lesions tended to have significantly lowered Arithmetic scores. A strong left hemisphere increase in glucose metabolism occurred when taking this test along with a small increase localized to the right frontal lobe (Chase et al., 1984). Alzheimer patients showed a significant correlation between glucose metabolism in the left hemisphere and performance (Hirono et al., 1998). Basic language measures accounted for 30% of the variance on Arithmetic in TBI patients (R.K. Lincoln et al., 1994). Some right hemisphere damaged patients also do poorly on this test, particularly relative to their scores on the verbal tests. Here the difficulty may be due to an impaired ability to organize the elements of the problems, or to memory or attention deficits. Langdon and Warrington (1997) found that patients with right as well as left unilateral lesions performed below controls on an arithmetic reasoning task similar to the number sequences in the Shipley Abstraction subtest. They speculated that the right hemisphere impaired group might have difficulty with a general appreciation of numerical magnitudes.

Arithmetic's vulnerability to so many different cognitive problems shows up in a number of diseases as more or less impaired performances. It tends to be ab-

normally low in acutely injured TBI patients (Correll et al., 1993) and tends to remain low chronically (Crosson, Greene, et al., 1990). Arithmetic scores of multiple sclerosis patients are likely to run one-half to two scaled score points lower than the predominantly verbal tests in the WIS-A (Filley, Heaton, Thompson, et al., 1990). Relatively early in the course of Alzheimer's disease the Arithmetic score is typically in the middle to lower ranges of the WIS-A test scores (Logsdon et al., 1989); its decline reflects the severity of the dementia (J.V. Bowler et al., 1997; Rosselli, Ardila, Arvizu, et al., 1998). Arithmetic scores remain more stable in patients with vascular dementia compared with Alzheimer's disease (J.V. Bowler et al., 1997). In early Huntington's disease, the average Arithmetic score dropped below all other WIS-A scores except Digit Symbol, and in later stages continued to be much below the verbal tests and even Digit Span (Brandt, Strauss, Larus, et al., 1984). Chronic alcoholics also tend to be relatively impaired on Arithmetic (W.R. Miller and Saucedo, 1983).

Arithmetic story problems

Luria (1973b, pp. 336–337) used arithmetic problems of increasing difficulty to examine reasoning abilities. These problems do not involve much mathematical skill. They implicitly require the subject to make comparisons between elements of the problem, and they contain intermediate operations that are not specified. An easy example would be, "The green basket contains three apples; the blue basket has twice as many. How many apples are there altogether?" A more difficult problem of the type suggested by Luria is "Two baskets together contain 24 apples. The blue basket has twice as many apples as the green basket. How many apples in each basket?" The most difficult problem format of this series requires the "inhibition of the impulsive direct method" for solution: "There are 12 apples in the green basket; the blue basket contains 36 apples more than the green basket. How many times more apples are in the blue than the green basket?" Luria pointed out that the tendency to set the problem up as a "direct operation" must be inhibited in favor of the more complex set of operations required for solution. Arithmetic problems were also used by Luria (1966) to examine conceptual flexibility (see also A.-L. Christensen, 1979). He set up familiar problems in unfamiliar ways—for example, placing the smaller number above rather than below the larger one in a written subtraction problem.

Seven "complex arithmetical problems" were offered by Walsh (1991) to assess various aspects of reasoning (e.g., logical, sequential) along with the abilities for sustained mental activity, to perform the mathematical operations, and to self-monitor and self-correct one's performance. These are similar to Luria's problems but some are quite difficult, calling for several operations on numbers which do not allow for obvious solutions (e.g., "If a ship can steam 16 miles an hour against a stream which runs at the rate of $2^1/_2$ miles per hour, how far could the ship steam in four hours with the stream?" p. 238).

Another set of arithmetic story problems comes in four parallel series each containing eight problems presented in order of increasing complexity (Fasotti, Bremer, and Eling, 1992). The items in each set differ from the corresponding items in the other three sets in the names of the subjects, the objects being manipulated, alternation of operations (addition–subtraction, multiplication–division), and numbers to be manipulated (from 3 to 30) (see Table 15.2). For the first set, given to assess how the patient performs this task, the patient receives each problem printed on a card with instructions to read and solve it aloud and then write

down all the required operations. The other series can be given with cueing for training purposes and then without cues to evaluate whether training was helpful. Of course, these equated series can simply be used for repeat examinations to reduce the possibility of practice effects. Successful solutions were inversely related to the complexity level of the problems. This technique discriminated between patient groups with focal lesions and also brought out deficits in cue utilization in patients with frontal lesions (see also Fasotti, 1992, for an extended treatment of arithmetic story problems in neuropsychological assessment).

Besides the usual Arithmetic story problems, the 1973 Stanford-Binet scales contain some interestingly complex reasoning problems involving arithmetic operations and concepts (Terman and Merrill 1973). These problems may expose subtle difficulties in formulating problems or in conceptual tracking that are not readily apparent in patients whose well-ingrained thinking patterns suffice for handling most test reasoning tasks. *Ingenuity I* and *II* are arithmetic "brain

TABLE 15.2 First Series of Uncued Arithmetic Word Problems

Word Problems	Number of Operations
1. Paul has been jogging for 11 miles Frank has been jogging 4 miles less than Paul How many miles have they jogged together?	2
2. Ellen has 5 apples Karen has 4 times more apples How many apples do they have together?	2
3. Company A has 20 employees Company B has 3 employees less than company A Company C has 5 employees more than company A How many employees do the 3 companies have in total?	3
4. Grandmother A has 18 grandchildren Grandmother B has 7 grandchildren less than grandmother A Grandmother C has one-third of the number of grandmother A's grandchildren How many grandchildren do the grandmothers have in total?	3
5. Peter has 10 marbles. His sister has 21 marbles more Peter's brother has 5 marbles less than Peter and his sister together How many marbles do the 3 children have together?	4
6. Peter is 12 years old His brother is 5 years younger His grandfather is 4 times older than Peter and his brother together How old are the 3 together?	4
7. Ann has $22 Maud has $17 less Sarah has $9 more than Ann and Maud together How many $ does every girl have on average?	5
8. A shopkeeper has sold 11 bottles of milk A second shopkeeper has sold 3 bottles less A third shopkeeper has sold 4 bottles more than the first and second shopkeepers together Together the 3 shopkeepers have 11 bottles of milk left How many bottles did they buy together?	5
Total score	28

Reprinted by permission from Fasotti, Bremer, and Eling, 1992.

teasers," such as "(A boy) has to bring back exactly 13 pints of water. He has a 9-pint can and a 5-pint can. Show me how he can measure out exactly 13 pints of water using nothing but these 2 cans and not guessing at the amount." This type of question, which calls for a process rather than a content answer, elicits information about how the patient reasons. The *Enclosed Box Problem* at the SA I level is also a mathematical brain teaser. It is a serial reasoning task that begins with, "Let's suppose that this box has 2 smaller boxes inside it, and each one of the smaller boxes contains a little tiny box. How many boxes are there altogether, counting the big one?" The next three items elaborate on the first, compounding the number of boxes at each step. *Induction* at year XIV involves a serial paper folding and cutting problem in which the number of holes cut increases at an algebraic ratio to the number of folds. After observing the folding and cutting procedure, subjects are asked to state the rule that will enable them to predict the number of holes from the number of folds. *Reasoning I* and *II* are brain teasers, too, requiring the patient to organize a set of numerical facts and deduce their relationship in order to solve the problem.

Block Counting

The *Block Counting* task at age level X of the Stanford-Binet (Terman and Merrill, 1973), sometimes called *Cube Analysis* (Newcombe, 1969) or *Cube Counting* (McFie and Zangwill, 1960) is another test that lends itself well to the study of reasoning processes. The material consists of two-dimensional drawings of three-dimensional block piles (see Fig. 15.11). The subject must count the total number of blocks in each pile by taking into account the ones hidden from view. Comparing right and left hemisphere patients on this task, McFie and Zangwill (1960) found more impaired performances by right hemisphere patients relative to those with left hemisphere lesions; Newcombe's (1969) right and left hemisphere patients' scores did not differ significantly, though right hemisphere patients were slower. Warrington and Rabin (1970) reported that patients in both groups may be impaired on this task: those with right-sided lesions who failed had problems with spatial analysis, while failure when lesions were

on the left was associated with aphasia (McCarthy and Warrington, 1990). Moreover, among patients with right hemisphere lesions, those who exhibited left visuospatial inattention made many more errors on a 25-item modification of the Binet drawings than patients with right-sided damage who did not display the inattention phenomenon (D.C. Campbell and Oxbury, 1976). Luria (1966, pp. 369–370) described a similar block counting task that he ascribed to Yerkes. He gives four examples of "Yerkes's test" that, in turn, are available in A.-L. Christensen's (1979) test card material. Although use of these block pictures should give some idea of whether patients can perform this kind of spatial reasoning operation and how they go about it, lack of norms and of a large enough series of graded problems limit the usefulness of this material. A set of block counting problems calling upon similar abilities to reason about spatial projections is one of the subtests of the MacQuarrie Test for Mechanical Ability (MacQuarrie, 1953). Although not presented in a graded manner, individual items are of different difficulty levels and subtest norms are provided.

Estimations

Estimations of sizes, quantities, etc., also test patients' ability to apply what they know, to compare, to make mental projections, and to evaluate conclusions. Some questions calling for estimations are in the WIS-A Information test, such as those that ask the height of the average American (or other nationality, depending upon the country in which the test is given) woman (WAIS only), the distance from New York to Paris (WAIS, WAIS-R), or the population of the United States. The examiner can make up others as appropriate, using familiar subjects such as the height of telephone poles or the number of potatoes in a ten-pound sack.

Shallice and Evans (1978) constructed a set of *Cognitive Estimation* questions for examining practical judgment. They found that patients with anterior lesions tended to give more bizarre responses than those with posterior lesions, supporting observations that patients with frontal lobe damage often use poor judgment, particularly in novel situations. Of the 15 questions, the four which elicited more bizarre responses from frontal lobe patients were, "How fast do race horses gallop?" ($p < .10$, >40 mph is scored as an error); "What is the largest object normally found in a house?" ($p < .10$, > a carpet is scored as an error); "What is the best paid occupation in Britain today?" ($p < .05$, any blue collar work is scored as an error); and "How tall is the average English woman?" ($p < .01$, $\geq 5'11"$ is scored as an error). However, on one

FIGURE 15.11 Sample items from the Block Counting task. (Terman and Merrill, 1973. Courtesy of Houghton Mifflin Co.)

of the questions, "What is the length of a pound note?" the percentage of patients with posterior lesions who gave bizarre answers exceeded that of the anterior group. Normative data for 150 healthy controls have been published. Performance was moderately related to general intellectual ability with males outperforming females (O'Carroll, Egan, and MacKenzie, 1994). These authors found poor internal reliability for this test. Among patients with a wide range of brain diseases, Korsakoff patients were particularly impaired in one study but no difference was observed between patients with frontal and nonfrontal lesions (R. Taylor and O'Carroll, 1995). An earlier study found Korsakoff patients' scores mostly within the control subjects' score range but poor performances by postencephalitic amnesia patients (Leng and Parkin, 1988).

Several American versions of *Cognitive Estimations* have been developed. Using a 10-item format, Axelrod and Millis (1994) developed deviation scores from control group responses to questions such as, "How tall is the Empire State Building?" and "How long is the average necktie?" They reported that patients with severe TBI tended to give responses that deviated significantly from those of the controls. On a 16-item test patients with both Alzheimer's disease and frontotemporal dementia were impaired relative to controls (Mendez, Doss, and Cherrier, 1998). Performance in the dementia groups correlated with their calculations and memory scores, suggesting that deficits in either or both of these areas may have contributed to their extreme estimates.

Calculations

An assessment of cognitive functions that does not include an examination of calculation skills is incomplete. An adequate review for neuropsychological purposes should give patients an opportunity to demonstrate that they recognize the basic arithmetic symbols (plus, minus, times, division, and equals) and can use them to calculate problems mentally and on paper. Story problems, like those given in the Wechsler tests, while assessing knowledge of and ability to apply arithmetic operations, do not test symbol recognition or spatial dyscalculia. Nor do the Wechsler Arithmetic problems test whether more advanced mathematical concepts (e.g., fractions, decimals, squares, algebraic formulations) that are mastered by most adults who complete high school have survived a cerebral insult (e.g., see Grafman, Kampen, et al., 1989; McCloskey et al., 1985). Converging evidence, largely from functional imaging studies, suggests that the left hemisphere is particularly involved in the knowledge of numbers and arithmetic rules, while the parietal lobes bilaterally are

implicated in appreciation of numerical magnitudes and approximations (Dehaene et al., 1999; Langdon and Warrington, 1997; Rickard et al., 2000; Stanescu-Cosson et al., 2000). The general interpretation is that arithmetic knowledge is a form of symbolic processing for which the left hemisphere specializes, plus a sense of numerical magnitudes that involves visuospatial processing.

Many examiners use the *Arithmetic* subtest of the *Wide Range Achievement Test* (*WRAT*) (see pp. 664–665) to examine arithmetic and calculation skills. A test with a larger proportion of problems at lower (grade school) difficulty levels, which makes it more suitable than the WRAT for neuropsychological evaluations, is *Calculations* of the *Woodcock-Johnson III Tests of Achievement* (*WJ-III*) (Woodcock, McGrew, and Mather, 2001b) (see pp. 666–667). Moreover, the WJ-III Calculations test also includes problems dealing with concepts and operations usually studied in advanced high school or college mathematics courses involving, for example, logarithms, exponents, and other mathematical functions. Thus, the average score for senior high school students, reported with its standard deviation, can be meaningfully applied to adults taking the test. Unfortunately, like the WRAT, the layout of the WJ-III does not allow much space for calculations, although the typeface is bigger and thus easier to read. The Calculations test also does not provide for a large enough sampling of performances on arithmetic problems involving two- and three-place numbers in the four basic operations, to meet the needs of neuropsychological assessment, particularly when spatial dyscalculia, carelessness in handling details, or impaired ability to perceive or correct errors is suspected. In the latter circumstances, the examiner may wish to make up a graded set of arithmetic problems. Most of them should require carrying, some of the multiplication and division problems should involve decimals, and at least a few of them should have zeros in the multiplier and in the dividend (e.g., see Fig. 15.12). In addition to giving the patient a sheet with the problems already laid out, the examiner can dictate some problems representing each of the four kinds of operation to see how well the patient can set them up.

Luria (1966) recounted a series of questions designed to test various aspects of arithmetic ability in an orderly manner (pp. 436–438; see also A.-L. Christensen, 1979; Grafman and Boller, 1989). The first questions involved addition and subtraction of one-digit numbers; the size and complexity of the problems gradually increased. At the simplest levels, many of the problems, such as multiplication of numbers memorized in times tables, have a virtually automatic character for most adults. Inability to respond accurately at these low

CALCULATIONS

25	172	249	750	6712	628
18	65	6418	- 419	- 456	413
+ 42	+ 33	+ 354			27
					54
					+ 248

62	713	472	928	3.56
x 5	x 4	x 16	x 53	x 2.8

54.85	72384	6.3915
x 6.25	x 503	x 48.72

24/480   16/1770   48/503890

Find the average: 35, 18, 42, 26

A newsboy collected $4.45, $3.60, $8.75, $12.30, and $5.85 from five customers,. What is the average amount he collected?

A man bought three cans of paint costing $12.65 each and a brush for $4.98. He paid for them with a fifty dollar bill. How much change did he receive?

FIGURE 15.12 Example of a page of arithmetic problems laid out to provide space for written calculations.

levels signals an impairment in symbol formulation characteristic of aphasic disturbances, or a severe breakdown in conceptual functions. More complex problems involving arithmetic operations with two- and three-place numbers test the immediate auditory memory span, attention, and mental tracking functions as well as the integrity of arithmetic skills. The examiner may be able to identify the nature of the failure on these problems by comparing solutions calculated mentally with paper-and-pencil solutions to similar kinds of problems. A similar sequence of arithmetic problems, ranging from "Verbal Rote Examples" such as 2 + 5, 4 × 4, 8 − 2, and 42 ÷ 7, to "Verbal Complex Examples," e.g., 15 + 18, 18 × 4, 52 − 27, and 126 ÷ 9, is part of the mental status examination rec-ommended by Strub and Black (2000). These authors also include two-, three-, and four-place number problems in their "Written Complex Examples." Norms for five age groups from 40–49 to 80–89 for "Verbal Rote" (eight items), "Verbal Complex" (four items) and "Written" problems (four items) vary little from decade to decade. However, for four stages of Alzheimer's disease, variations are pronounced, going from virtually identical with age norms at (an undefined) Stage 1 to 0 at Stage IV.

M. Jackson and Warrington (1986) developed an orally presented *Graded Difficulty Arithmetic test (GDA)* which contains 12 addition and 12 subtraction items presented in order of increasing difficulty from "very easy" (e.g., 16 + 12, 18 − 5) to "very difficult" (e.g., 234 + 129, 245 − 168), the latter problems involving both three places and carrying. A table provides for conversion of raw scores to standard scores. Performances by normal control subjects correlated significantly with WAIS Arithmetic (r = .76) and Digit Span (r = .65). This test proved effective in distinguishing a right from left hemisphere damaged group when WAIS Arithmetic did not, as patients with left lateralized lesions failed more items to a significant degree (Langdon and Warrington, 1997).

One great value of written calculation problems is that errors are preserved on paper. The analysis of errors rather than the score will usually provide an understanding of the patient's calculation problem. Spiers (1987) considered five calculation error types with detailed descriptions of each: *Place-holding errors* include misinterpretation of the decimal point or the size of the number, sequence reversals or partial reversals, transposition of a number. *Digit errors* involve substituting the wrong digit—which can occur as an analogue of the misspeaking often but not necessarily associated with aphasia, or as a perseveration from another part of the problem; or omission of one or more digits as frequently seen with hemi-inattention; both substitutions and omissions can come from carelessness or distractibility. *Borrow and carry errors* may be due to failure to borrow or carry, or performing these operations erroneously. *Basic fact errors* may be multiplication table slip-ups or involve confusion about use of zero or 1 in a problem. *Algorithm errors* show up in failure to carry out all the steps in a procedure, misaligning numbers, following an incorrect sequence (directional or priority) through the problem, or substituting one operation for another.

Many patients with brain dysfunction, typically associated with mild diffuse damage (e.g., TBI, multiple sclerosis), make errors due to impaired ability to self-monitor automatically (i.e., to do two things at once, in this case, to monitor the performance while working out the calculations). These errors typically show up as substitutions, misplacements (of numbers, decimals), omissions that are not always on one side or the other of the problem, multiplication table slip-ups, and not completing all steps of an operation. They are easily recognized as more problems are completed correctly than incorrectly and there is no regular error pattern. Patients with frontal damage also produce these kinds of errors in which the underlying problem is self-monitoring, but it simply does not occur to some frontal patients to monitor their performance—they are relatively unconcerned about its quality, in contrast to those who do care but do not appreciate that their once automatic self-monitoring abilities are now compromised. Alzheimer patients' problems with written calculations have been attributed to self-monitoring deficits rather than to faulty knowledge about arithmetic rules (Mantovan et al., 1999).

16 | Executive Functions and Motor Performance

THE EXECUTIVE FUNCTIONS

As the most complex of behaviors, executive functions are intrinsic to the ability to respond in an adaptive manner to novel situations and are also the basis of many cognitive, emotional, and social skills. The executive functions can be conceptualized as having four components: (1) volition; (2) planning; (3) purposive action; and (4) effective performance. Each involves a distinctive set of activity-related behaviors. All are necessary for appropriate, socially responsible, and effectively self-serving adult conduct. Moreover, it is rare to find a patient with impaired capacity for self-direction or self-regulation who has defects in just one of these aspects of executive functioning. Rather, defective executive behavior typically involves a cluster of deficiencies of which one or two may be especially prominent. Paradoxically, such profound changes in behavior are sometimes missed in a highly structured examination (Lezak, 1982a).

A medically retired financial manager whose cardiac arrest was complicated by a hard fall onto his right temple was very responsive to his own needs and energetic in attempts to carry out plans. Unfortunately, he could no longer formulate plans well because of an inability to take all aspects of a situation into account and integrate them. His lack of awareness of his mistakes further aggravated this disability. Problems arising from his emotional lability and proneness to irritability were overshadowed by crises resulting from his efforts to carry out inappropriate and sometimes financially hazardous plans.

In these cases and in much of the literature concerning the executive functions, frontal lobe damage is implicated. This is not surprising since most patients who have had significant injury or disease of the prefrontal regions, particularly when orbital or medial structures are involved, experience behavioral and personality changes stemming from defective executive functions. The classic tale of Phineas Gage is the first careful documentation of a person whose personality was strikingly altered from conforming and productive to irresponsible and unruly when a misfired tamping iron lodged in his head "passing back of the left eye, and out at the top of his head," thus running through his left frontal lobe (Macmillan, 2000).

However, the executive functions are also sensitive to damage in other parts of the brain (E. Goldberg and Bilder, 1987; E. Goldberg, Bilder, and Hughes, 1989; Lezak, 1994). Subcortical as well as cortical damage can be involved (Dujardin et al., 2000; Eslinger and Grattan, 1993; Hashimoto et al., 1995). Disturbances in executive functions may result from anoxic conditions that involve limbic structures (Januzzi and Mc-Khann, 2002) and can be among the sequelae of alcohol abuse (Munro et al., 2000) or inhalation of organic solvents (Arlien-Søborg et al., 1979; Hawkins, 1990; Tsushima and Towne, 1977). Korsakoff patients with lesions primarily in thalamic nuclei and other subcortical components of the limbic system typically exhibit profound disturbances in executive behavior. Many of them are virtually immobilized by apathy and inertia. Some Parkinson patients display diminished conceptual flexibility and impaired initiative and spontaneity. Moreover, patients with right hemisphere damage who can "talk a good game" and are neither inert nor apathetic may be ineffective because limitations in organizing conceptually all facets of an activity and integrating it with their behavior may keep them from carrying out their many intentions.

Executive functions can break down at any stage in the behavioral sequence that makes up planned or intentional activity. Systematic examination of the capacities that enter into the four aspects of executive activity will help to identify the stage or stages at which a breakdown in executive behavior takes place. Such a review of a patient's executive functions may also bring to light impairments in self-direction or self-regulation that would not become evident in the course of the usual examination or observation procedures.

A major obstacle to examining the executive functions is the paradoxical need to structure a situation in which patients can show whether and how well they can make structure for themselves. Typically, in formal examinations, the examiner determines what activity the subject is to do with what materials, when, where, and how. Most cognitive tests, for example, allow the subject little room for discretionary behavior, including many tests thought to be sensitive to executive— or frontal lobe—disorders (Frederiksen, 1986; Lezak, 1982a; Shallice and Burgess, 1991b). The problem for clinicians who want to examine the executive functions becomes how to transfer goal setting, structuring, and decision making from the clinician to the subject within the structured examination. A limited number of established examination techniques give the subject sufficient leeway to think of and choose alternatives as needed to demonstrate the main components of executive behavior.

The following review covers techniques that may be useful in exploring and elucidating this most subtle and central realm of human activity (see also Lezak, 1989; A.C. Roberts et al., 1998). Other instruments presented in this chapter test more peripheral but equally important executive capacities, such as those that enter into self-regulation and self-correction.

Volition

> The distinction between an action that is intentional and one that is not seems to have something to do with the consciousness of the goal of the action.
>
> J.W. Brown, 1989

Volition refers to the complex process of determining what one needs or wants and conceptualizing some kind of future realization of that need or want. In short, it is the capacity for intentional behavior. It requires the capacity to formulate a goal or, at a lower conceptual level, to form an intention. Motivation, including the ability to initiate activity, is one necessary precondition for volitional behavior. The other is awareness of oneself psychologically, physically, and in relation to one's surroundings. Each aspect of volition can be examined separately. Deficiencies in self-initiated behavior may occur because of disturbances in cognitive/affective processes due to damage to frontal/subcortical or frontolimbic circuitry (Stuss, Van Reekum, and Murphy, 2000), to the right hemisphere, or in diffuse conditions such as Alzheimer's disease (R.S. Marin et al., 1994).

Persons who lack volitional capacity simply do not think of anything to do. In extreme cases they may be apathetic, or unappreciative of themselves as distinctive persons (much as an infant or young child), or both. They may be unable to initiate activities except in response to internal stimuli such as bladder pressure or external stimuli, for example, an annoying mosquito. Such persons may be fully capable of performing complex activities and yet not carry them out unless instructed to do so. For instance, although able to use eating utensils properly, some will not eat what is set before them without continuing explicit instructions. Less impaired persons may eat or drink what is set before them, but will not seek nourishment spontaneously, even when hungry. Patients whose volitional capacity is only mildly impaired can do their usual chores and engage in familiar games and hobbies without prompting. However, they are typically unable to assume responsibilities requiring appreciation of long-term or abstract goals and do not enter into new activities independently. Without outside guidance, many wander aimlessly or sit in front of the television or at the same neighborhood bar or coffee shop when they have finished their routine activities.

In some cases, particularly when deficits are subtle, it becomes important to identify the presence of a volitional defect. In others, where passivity or apparent withdrawal are obvious behavioral problems, the examiner must try to distinguish the unmotivated, undirected, and disinterested anergia occurring on an organic basis from characterological (e.g., laziness, childish dependency) or psychiatric (e.g., depression, schizophrenia) disorders that superficially appear similar. However, there are no formal tests for examining volitional capacity. The examiner must rely instead on observations of these patients in the normal course of day-to-day living and reports by caregivers, family, and others who see them regularly. These reports are often the best sources of information about the patient's capacity for generating desires, formulating goals, and forming intentions. Thus the examination should include both the patient and those who know the patient best.

Examining motivational capacity

The direct examination of motivational capacity should inquire into patients' likes and dislikes, what they do for fun, and what makes them angry, as many volitionally impaired patients are apathetic with diminished or even absent capacity for emotional response. The patient's behavior in the examination can also provide valuable clues to volitional capacity. Volitionally competent persons make spontaneous—and appropriate—conversation or ask questions; or they participate actively in the examination proceedings by turning test cards or putting caps back on pens. Patients whose volitional capacity is seriously impaired typically volunteer little or nothing, even when responsive to what the examiner says or does. Some patients report what sound like normal activity programs when asked how they spend their leisure time or how they perform chores. Then the examiner needs to find out when they last dated or went on a camping trip, for example, or who plans the meals they cook. A patient may report that he likes to take his girlfriend to the movies but has not had a "girlfriend" since before his accident three years ago and has not gone to a theater since then either. Another who talks about her competence in the kitchen actually prepares the same few dishes over and over again exactly as taught since being impaired.

Excerpts from an interview with a physically competent 26-year-old woman two years after she had become fully dependent as a result of massive frontal lobe damage incurred in a car vs. train accident shows how an interview can document a severe motivational impairment.
Q: What kind of work did you do? P: In a state park.
Q: Did you like that work? P: It was OK.
Q: How come you stopped doing that work? P: I don't know.
Q: Have you thought of going back to do it? P: I really don't care. . . .
Q: What would you do if your mother got sick and had to go to the hospital? P: If it was late I would put on my pyjamas and go to bed and go to sleep.
Q: And then what would you do the next day when no one was home? P: I would have to get up and eat breakfast and then go and get dressed.
Q: And then what would you do? P: Come in and turn on the TV and sit down.
Q: And then what would you do? P: After I watched TV, I would put on my shoes and socks and go back into the bedroom and sit down because I don't know anyone else to call.

Examination techniques can require the patient to initiate activity. Heilman and Watson (1991) scatter pennies on the table in front of patients, then blindfold them and tell them to pick up as many pennies as they can. The task thus requires exploratory behavior which may be lacking in patients whose capacity to initiate responses is impaired.

Examining the capacity for self-awareness

Assessment of self-awareness and awareness of one's surroundings also depends upon observations and interviews. Like other aspects of executive functioning, defective self-awareness occurs to varying degrees. Moreover, self-awareness is multifaceted as it includes physical awareness, awareness of self and of other persons, and social awareness. Mature self-awareness requires an integrated appreciation of one's physical status and ongoing physical relationship with the immediate external environment; an appreciation of being a distinctive person in a world which mainly exists outside of one's immediate awareness and is inhabited by many other distinctive individuals; and appreciation

of oneself as an interactive part of the network of social relationships. Each of these facets of self-awareness can be disturbed by brain damage and each can be examined in its own right. Stuss and Alexander (2000) propose that the right frontal lobe with its hypothalamic limbic, posterior cortical, and cingulate connections plays an essential role in self-awareness.

Awareness of one's physical status. Inaccurate body images can occur as distortions, perceptions of more severe impairment than is the case, or as feelings of being intact when actually impaired. The most direct method for examining body image is to request a human figure drawing. Inquiry into vocational or career plans, or just plans for going home can elicit defective self-perceptions, as when a visually impaired youngster says he plans to be a pilot, or a wheelchair-bound patient assures the examiner he will be able to walk the flight of stairs to his apartment. An associated deficit can show up in impaired appreciation of one's physical strengths and limitations. Reduced or even absent appreciation of physical states and bodily functions usually involves loss of appetite or loss of satiation cues, sexual disinterest, with sleep disturbances not uncommon. Interviews with patient and family or other caregivers, and sensitive observation typically bring these problems to light.

Awareness of the environment and situational context. The extent to which patients are aware of and responsive to what goes on around them is likely to be reflected in their use of environmental cues. This can be examined with questions about the time of day, the season of the year, or other temporal events or situational circumstances (e.g., Christmas time, the dining hall, office, or waiting room, etc.) that can be easily deduced or verified by alert patients who are attentive to their surroundings.

A 58-year-old woman with mild frontotemporal dementia carried an armful of possessions to her appointment and placed them on the examination table. The examiner explained that the table must be clear for the examination and stood up to find somewhere to put the belongings. While the examiner's back was turned, the patient announced that she had found a place for her things—in the examiner's chair. Formal testing did not show many deficits, but numerous behaviors during the examination demonstrated impaired situational awareness.

Story and picture material from standard tests can also be used to examine the patient's ability to pay attention to situational cues. The Problems of Fact items of the 1973 revision of Terman and Merrill's Stanford-Binet scales require the patient to use cues to interpret a situation. The Cookie Theft picture from the Boston Diagnostic Aphasia Examination (Goodglass, Kaplan, and Barresi, 2000) or Picture Arrangement items from the WIS-A are excellent for testing the patient's ability to infer a story from a picture. The complexity and richness of responses may range from a single integrated story involving the important elements of the picture, to a bit-by-bit description of the picture that raises questions about whether the patient can integrate what is seen, to a disregard of all but one or two items because of impaired capacity to attend systematically or persevere in an activity.

Social awareness. Assessment of social awareness also depends upon observations and interviews. Lack of normal adult self-consciousness may show up in reports or observations of poor grooming and childish or crude behavior that contrast sharply with a premorbid history of social competence.

The same woman described above with frontotemporal dementia (autopsy confirmed) startled strangers in a grocery store by punching them on the shoulder and saying in a loud voice, "My daughter went to Cal Tech." Obviously proud of her daughter, the woman was unable to appreciate the inappropriateness of her behavior.

At the other extreme, excessive politeness may also expose impaired social awareness.

A very bright Vietnam veteran who had sustained a blow that crushed the anterior portion of his right frontal lobe was still able to complete a university level accounting program and qualify as a CPA. Even after working for more than ten years in his profession and in a major metropolis he continued to address women as "Ma'am," including those with whom he worked, as he had been taught to do as a child. Loneliness and feeling out of touch socially were persistent problems for him.

How patients dress and groom themselves, how they relate to the examiner or to other clinical staff, and how they interact with their family members can provide important information regarding their appreciation of social roles and accepted codes of social behavior. Interviews with the patient and family members can be invaluable in making social disturbances evident. Test responses, too, may offer insight into the patient's social understandings. For example, patients who say they would "shout fire" in a theater (WAIS and WAIS-R item) are out of touch with what is both socially acceptable and socially responsible behavior.

Planning

The identification and organization of the steps and elements (e.g., skills, material, other persons) needed to carry out an intention or achieve a goal constitute planning and involve a number of capacities. In order to plan, one must be able to conceptualize changes from present circumstances (i.e., look ahead), deal objectively with oneself in relation to the environment, and view the environment objectively (i.e., take the abstract attitude; see p. 84). The planner must also be able to conceive of alternatives, weigh and make choices, and entertain both sequential and hierarchical ideas necessary for the development of a conceptual framework or structure that will give direction to the carrying out of a plan. Good impulse control and reasonably intact memory functions are also necessary. Moreover, all of this conceptual activity requires a capacity for sustained attention. Patients who are unable to form a realistic intention also cannot plan. However, some patients who generate motives and initiate goal-directed activity spontaneously fail to achieve their goals because one or more of the abilities required for effective planning is impaired.

Use of standard examination procedures

There are few formal tests of planning ability per se. However, the patient's handling of many of the standard psychological tests will provide insight into the status of these important conceptual activities.

Responses to storytelling tasks, such as the Thematic Apperception Test, reflect the patient's handling of sequential verbal ideas. Stories told to these pictures may be complex and highly organized, have simple and straight story lines, be organized by accretion, or consist of loose or disjointed associations or descriptions (W.E. Henry, 1947). How patients address such highly structured tests as Picture Arrangement and Block Design will provide information about whether they order and plan ahead naturally and effectively, laboriously, inconsistently, or not at all. Sentence Arrangement of the WAIS-RNI affords a good opportunity to see whether patients can organize their thoughts into a sensible and linguistically acceptable construct.

The Complex Figure Test also elicits planning behavior. Osterrieth's (1944) analysis of how people go about copying the complex figure provides standards for evaluating how systematic is the patient's response to this task. A haphazard, fragmented mode of response suggests poor planning; while a systematic approach beginning with the basic structure of the figure is generally the hallmark of someone who plans well. Some examiner techniques capture the sequence of the drawing and a representation of the plan (see pp. 544–547). Several scoring systems assess the organizational approach used to copy the figure (e.g., Deckersbach et al., 2000). A time-consuming system, the Boston Qualita-

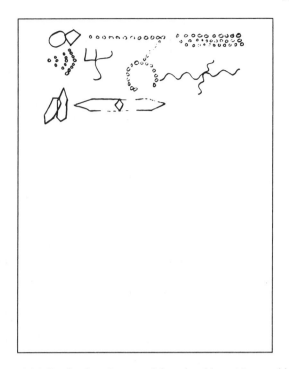

FIGURE 16.1 Bender-Gestalt copy trial rendered by a 42-year-old interior designer a year after she had sustained a mild anterior subarachnoid hemorrhage. Note that although the design configurations are essentially preserved, she used only one-third of the page, drawing several of the designs as close to each other as to elements within these designs.

but show poor judgment in unrealistic, confused, often illogical, or nonexistent plans for themselves, or lack the judgment to recognize that they need to make plans if they are to remain independent (Lezak, 1994).

Working memory tasks

Efficient planning entails decision making and developing strategies for setting priorities. Atkinson and Shiffrin (1968) described working memory as involving, among other processes, decision making. Using a similar model, Baddeley and Hitch (1974) proposed that working memory depends on an attentional controller, which they called the *central executive* and later the *supervisory attentional system* (Baddeley, 1986; Norman and Shallice, 1986). In this model, the supervisory attentional system selects and operates strategies for maintaining and switching attention as needs arise.

Executive processes include various kinds of judgments made on stimuli held in short-term memory (e.g., comparison of the relative recency of stimuli, judgments of the relative saliency or novelty of stimuli, etc.) and active (voluntary) retrieval of specific information held in long-term form. (Petrides, 1994, p. 73)

Failure of this sytem produces the *dysexecutive syndrome* (Baddeley, 1986; Baddeley and Wilson, 1988).

tive Scoring system, includes Planning as one of its main scores (Somerville et al., 2000; R.A. Stern et al., 1999).

The patient's use of space in drawings can provide a concrete demonstration of planning defects. The Bender-Gestalt designs are particularly well-suited to this purpose (see Fig. 16.1); but free drawings (e.g., human figures, house, etc.) may also elicit planning problems (see Fig. 16.2).

Questioning can bring out defective planning. How patients who are living alone or keeping house describe food purchasing and preparation may reveal how well they can organize and plan. Other issues that may bring out organizing and planning abilities concern personal care, appreciation of how disability affects the patient's activities and family, what accommodations the patient has made to disability, to altered financial and vocational status, etc. Hebb (1939) offered a pertinent question used by his colleague, Dr. W.T.B. Mitchell: "What should you do before beginning something important?" (to which a patient who had undergone a left frontal lobectomy replied, after some delay, "I can't get it into my head"). Some patients, particularly those whose lesions are in the right hemisphere, may give lucid and appropriate answers to questions involving organization and planning of impersonal situations or events

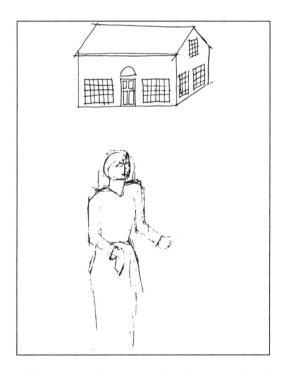

FIGURE 16.2 House and Person drawings by the interior designer whose Bender-Gestalt copy trial is given in Figure 16.1. Note absence of chimney on a highly detailed house drawing and placement and size of woman too low and too large to fit all of her on the page.

The dorsal prefrontal cortex appears critical for allocating attentional resources during working memory tasks (Koechlin, Basso, et al., 1999; Koechlin, Corrado, et al., 2000; Petrides, 1994).

Self-Ordered Pointing Test (Petrides and Milner, 1982)

Tests calling for self-ordered responses assess strategy use and self-monitoring. In the *Self-Ordered Pointing Test*, the examiner asks subjects to point to a stimulus (e.g., abstract designs, line drawings; see Spreen and Strauss, 1998, pp. 209 and 210) not seen on previous trials in an array of stimuli on each trial. The position of the stimuli shifts from trial to trial so that the subject must try to monitor previous choices from memory. Patients with frontal lesions were impaired on this task compared to those with temporal lesions; the authors attributed this relative impairment to poor organizational strategies, poor monitoring of responses, or both. Age effects have been reported for this task (Daigneault and Braun, 1993). Deficits also have been observed in patients with Huntington's disease (Rich, Blysma, and Brandt, 1996) and Parkinson's disease (Gabrieli et al., 1996; West et al., 1998). West and his colleagues observed that most errors of Parkinson patients occurred toward the end of a trial regardless of set size, which they suggested resulted from failure to monitor how far they had proceeded in the trial.

Maze tracing

The maze tracing task was designed to yield data about the highest levels of mental functioning involving planning and foresight, i.e., "the process of choosing, trying, and rejecting or adopting alternative courses of conduct or thought. At a simple level, this is similar to solving a very complex maze" (Porteus, 1959, p. 7). The ideal approach to finding the path through the maze is by making a preliminary investigation of the maze in order to envisage a path that does not go down blind alleys. Despite the sensitivity of maze tests in eliciting planning deficits, these tests are not commonly used, perhaps because the original set requires considerable time and some administration challenges.

Porteus Maze Test (Porteus, 1959, 1965)

Three sets of this test are currently in use: the Vineland Revision, which contains 12 mazes for years III through XII, year XIV, and Adult; the eight-maze Porteus Maze Extension, covering years VII through XII, year XIV, and Adult; and the Porteus Maze Supplement, which also has eight mazes for years VII through XII, XIV, and Adult (Porteus, 1965; see Fig. 16.3). The latter two series were developed to compensate for practice effects in retesting so that the maze at each year of the Porteus Maze Extension is a little more difficult than its counterpart in the Vineland Revision and each year of the Porteus Maze Supplement is more difficult than its corresponding test in the Extension series.

To achieve a successful trial, the subject must trace the maze without entering any blind alleys. The mazes range in difficulty from the simplest at year III to the most complex developed for adults. The rule for the number of failures required to discontinue the test varies with the difficulty level, with up to four trials

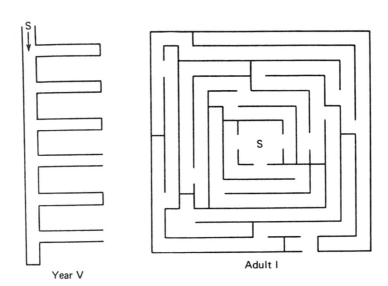

Year V   Adult I

FIGURE 16.3 Two of the Porteus mazes. (Reproduced by permission. © 1933, 1946, 1950 by S.D. Porteus, published by The Psychological Corporation. All rights reserved.)

given on the most difficult mazes. The test is not timed and may take some patients an hour or more to complete all the mazes given to them.

Scores are reported in terms of test age (TA), which is the age level of the most difficult maze the patient completes successfully minus a half-year for every failed trial. The upper score is 17 for success on the adult level maze. Porteus also used eight qualitative error scores: *First Third Errors, Last Third Errors, Wrong Direction, Cut Corner, Cross Line, Lift Pencil, Wavy Line,* and *Total Qualitative Errors.* Other kinds of score have been used. Time to completion scores of frontal leucotomy patients pre- and postoperatively showed that psychosurgery resulted in slowing, and more errors occurred postoperatively as well (Tow, 1955). Subtracting the time to trace over an already drawn path on a similar maze from the time to solution produced a time score free of the motor component of this task (H.S. Levin, Goldstein, Williams, and Eisenberg, 1991). The number of repeated entries into the same blind alley can measure perseverative tendencies (Daigneault et al., 1992).

Test characteristics. Ardila and Rosselli (1989) reported education effects but as many as one-third of their subject group had four or fewer years of school, which raises some question as to the generalizability of these findings. Age effects have shown up in 45- to 65-year-olds as these subjects made more perseverative errors than younger ones (Daigneault et al., 1992). Age effects have also appeared in the 55 to over 76 age range (Ardila and Rosselli, 1989).

Studying older persons, Daigneault and her colleagues (1992) used a battery composed of tests selected for their supposed sensitivity to frontal lobe damage and found that the Porteus Mazes loaded on a "planning" factor. In a much larger battery that included several construction tasks, the Maze test was associated with "visuospatial and visuomotor tasks" (Ardila and Rosselli, 1989). While these findings are suggestive regarding the nature of the Maze tracing task, they also illustrate how much the outcome of factor analyses depends on their input. A moderate correlation ($r = .41$) exists between performances by children and young adults on the Porteus Maze and the Tower of London, another task with a large planning component (Krikorian et al., 1994). With a young TBI group, Maze test error and time scores correlated significantly with both an untimed test contributing to Daigneault's "planning factor" (Wisconsin Card Sorting Test) and tests of visuomotor tracking (Trail Making Test A and B), implicating sensitivity to executive disorders in all three tasks (Segalowitz, Unsal, and Dywan, 1992). The Mazes error score, along with the other tests, correlated significantly ($p \leq .05$) with a physiological measure of frontal dysfunction.

Neuropsychological findings. The Porteus Maze Test can be quite sensitive to brain disorders. Perhaps the most notable research was undertaken by A. Smith (1960), who did an eight-year follow-up study of psychosurgical patients comparing younger and older groups who had undergone superior or orbital topectomy with younger and older patient controls. Following a score rise in a second preoperative testing, scores on tests taken within three months after surgery were lower than the second preoperative scores in all cases. The superior topectomy group's scores dropped still lower during the eight-year interval to a mean score significantly ($p \leq .05$) lower than the original mean. The control group mean scores climbed slightly following the first and second retest but the eight-year and the original Maze test scores were essentially the same.

Maze test scores have successfully predicted the severity of brain disease (Meier, Ettinger, and Arthur, 1982). Those patients who achieved test age (TA) scores of VIII or above during the first week after a stroke made significant spontaneous gains in lost motor functions, whereas those whose scores fell below this standard showed relatively little spontaneous improvement. In another study, a set of Maze test performances including both brain damaged and intact subjects correlated significantly ($r = .77$) with scores on actual driving tasks (Sivak et al., 1981). A small group of TBI patients with severe frontal lobe injuries solved the Porteus Mazes more slowly than either TBI patients with severe posterior damage or matched control subjects, this difference holding up even when motor speed was taken into account (H.S. Levin, Goldstein, Williams, and Eisenberg, 1991). Yet 15 of 20 anosmic TBI patients achieved scores above the failure level defined by Porteus (1965); although all of them displayed psychosocial deficits, 16 were reported to have planning problems, and only four were employed two or more years postinjury (Martzke et al., 1991; see p. 626 for a fuller description). Most patients with mild to moderate Alzheimer's disease had low Test Age scores compared to control subjects, although some overlap of scores existed between groups (Mack and Patterson, 1995). Alzheimer patients' Test Age scores correlated with ratings on activities of daily living. These patients also had higher *First Third Errors* and *Last Third Errors.*

Mazes in the Wechsler Intelligence Scales for Children (WISC-R, WISC-III) (Wechsler, 1974, 1991)

These test batteries contain a shorter maze test with time limits and an error scoring system. The most difficult item is almost as complex as the most difficult items in the Porteus series. The highest (15 years 10 months) norms allow the examiner to make a rough estimate of the adequacy of the adult patient's performance. Moreover, the format and time limits make these mazes easy to give. For most clinical purposes, they are a practical and satisfactory substitute for the lengthier Porteus test.

Tower Tests: London, Hanoi, and Toronto

These "brain teasers," familiar to puzzle lovers, get to the heart of planning disorders. To arrive at the best (most direct, fewest moves) solution of the *Tower of London* test, the subject must look ahead to determine the order of moves necessary to rearrange three colored rings or balls from their initial position on two of three upright sticks to a new set of predetermined positions on one or more of the sticks (Shallice, 1982) (see Fig. 16.4). The constraints are that only one piece may be moved at a time, each piece may be moved only from peg to peg, and only a specified number of pieces may be left on each peg at a time. The original task consists of 12 test items of graded levels of difficulty. Levels of difficulty of the test items depend on the number and complexity of subgoals required to achieve the desired arrangement. A problem is scored correct if the solution is achieved with the minimum number of moves necessary. Three trials are allowed for each problem.

Young adults (mean age 21.6 years) correctly solved 92.2% of the problems (Krikorian et al., 1994). Functional imaging has shown a major role for the prefrontal cortex during task performance (S.C. Baker et al., 1996; Lazeron, Rombouts, et al., 2000). Although this test is typically used to measure ability to plan ahead, other factors are important for successful performance such as working memory, response inhibition, and visuospatial memory (D. Carlin et al., 2000; L.H. Phillips et al., 1999; M.C. Welsh et al., 2000).

In an early study of brain injured persons in which the score was the number of correct solutions, patients with predominantly left anterior lesions performed least well while those with either left or right posterior lesions did as well as normal control subjects (Shallice,

1982; Shallice and Burgess, 1991a). Patients in the right anterior lesion group performed less well than control subjects only on the 5-move (most difficult) problems. A more recent study found that patients with frontal lobe lesions and those with frontal lobe dementia had normal planning times (D. Carlin et al., 2000). However, compared to control subjects, patients with focal lesions made more moves, used a trial and error strategy, and were slower to arrive at a solution, while patients with frontal lobe dementia made more moves, committed more rule violations, made more incorrect solutions, and were slower in executing moves. Patients with Huntington's disease also tend to be impaired on this task (L.H. Watkins et al., 2000). TBI patients with anterior lesions performed at essentially the same level as control subjects and, on the most complex item (5 moves), better than those with nonfrontal lesions (H.S. Levin, Goldstein, Williams, and Eisenberg, 1991). The relative insensitivity of this test to the cognitive impairment associated with TBI has been replicated in a sample of patients with severe TBI (Cockburn, 1995).

The *Tower of Hanoi* puzzle is more complex in that, instead of same size pieces, the objects to be rearranged are five rings of varying sizes. The goal and general procedures are the same as for the Tower of London: rings are moved from peg to peg to achieve a final goal with as few moves as possible. As with the Tower of London, only one ring may be moved at a time and any ring not being currently moved must remain on a peg. Instead of a restriction on the number of rings allowed for each peg as for the Tower of London, the restriction for the Tower of Hanoi is that a larger ring may not be placed on a smaller ring. Multiple forms of this puzzle are used and it can be computer-administered. A number of strategies work for achieving the goal; the common strategy requires establishing subgoals and a counterintuitive backward move (Goel and Grafman, 1995; a *subgoal* involves a move that is essential for the solution of the puzzle but does not place a ring into its goal position. A computerized program for this task comes from the U.S. Military Personnel Assessment Battery [Samet and Marshall-Mies, 1987]).

The Towers of London and Hanoi do not measure precisely the same skills (Goel and Grafman, 1995),

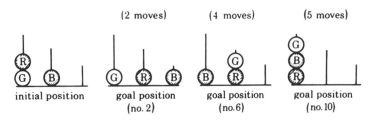

FIGURE 16.4 Tower of London examples. (From Shallice, 1982. Reproduced by permission.)

and correlation between performances on the two tasks is correspondingly low ($r = .37$) (Humes et al., 1997). Goel and Grafman (1995) propose that the Tower of Hanoi does not assess planning as much as it assesses inhibiting a prepotent response (the goal–subgoal conflict). This hypothesis was supported by structural equation modeling data from normal subjects showing that response inhibition contributes to performance (Miyake et al., 2000). Working memory contributes to solutions for medium and hard problems as more subgoal information needs to be kept in mind (Goel, Pullara, and Grafman, 2001; R.G. Morris, Miotto, et al., 1997). Information processing speed also appears to play a role in performances of normal young adults (Bestawros et al., 1999) and patients with multiple sclerosis (Arnett, Rao, Grafman et al., 1997).

At least in the 40- to 79-year age range, neither age nor education appears to affect performance on this task, whether measured by the number of moves required for solution or the number of errors (Glosser and Goodglass, 1990). Participants in their 70s and 80s were significantly impaired compared to those in their 20s and 30s (H.P. Davis and Klebe, 2001). A follow-up of 6.6 years after their first test showed a decline in Tower of Hanoi performance in the elderly group that was not seen on the Rey Auditory Verbal Learning Test. This suggested that for elderly people problem solving declines at a faster rate than some forms of memory. In this same study, patients with anterior lesions tended to do less well than those with posterior lesions. Lateralization differences have also been described. In one study patients with left frontal and right temporal lesions performed worse than control subjects and patients with right frontal and left temporal lesions on four-move problems (R.G. Morris, Miotto, et al., 1997). The left frontal group had larger lesions than the other patient groups, which may have contributed to their poor performance. When Goel and Grafman (1995) compared patients with focal frontal lobe lesions to control subjects they found no differences associated with lesion lateralization. The frontal patients made more errors and appeared to have difficulty choosing a counterintuitive backward move to reach a subgoal. On a simplified version of the Tower of London given to early- and middle-stage Alzheimer patients, along with a lower success rate than their matched control subjects, rule breaking was a prominent feature (Rainville et al., 2002).

The *Tower of Toronto* adds one more layer of complexity—a fourth ring (Saint Cyr and Taylor, 1992). Rather than using rings of different sizes, here the same-size rings have different colors: white, yellow, red, and black. The instructions require the subject to keep lighter colored rings on top of darker ones as they move the set of four blocks from the left one of three pegs to the peg on the right. Saint Cyr and Taylor used this puzzle to examine planning (the development of strategies), learning, and memory for previously developed strategies, by following the initial set of five trials with a second five-trial set $1^{1}/_{2}$ hours later. Parkinson patients tended to develop a solution plan slowly, taking and learning an inefficient path that led to a correct solution, and retained that solution on later testing. Amnesic patients performed normally on both learning and retention test trials. Some patients with early stage Huntington's disease also had consistently normal performances, others dealt with the tasks like the Parkinson patients. Late stage Huntington patients' performances were defective on both sets of trials.

Tower of London. Drexel University (TOL_{DX}) (Culbertson and Zillmer, 2001)

This formalized test version provides instructions and norms for both children and adults. It uses two boards—one on which the examiner places three colored wooden balls (red, blue, green) in the goal position, and the other containing the three colored wooden balls that the subjects rearrange from a standard "start" position to the examiner's model. Ten problems at each level—child, adult—are given in order of increasing difficulty. Two minutes are allowed for each trial. All ten problems are given. Seven different scores ("indexes") can be obtained for both number of moves and successful completions, and timing aspects. The standardization sample consisted of 264 adults (ages 20–77), of whom 192 were in the 20–29 year old group and only 21 in the 60–77 age range; many of the younger subjects were college students. Theory and interpretation are based on the extensive TOL literature. The format—copying the wooden ball set-up rather than pictures—appears practical; the difficulty levels were essentially defined in prior studies. The instructions are clear and well-detailed as are scoring sheets. Since computerized formats generate data equivalent to older picture-copying formats (Mataix-Cols and Bartres-Faz, 2002), it seems reasonable to expect that this adminstration variation will work well too.

Other tests of planning abilities

Based primarily on theory, several tests in a battery of *Cognitive Processing Tasks* were identified as involving planning (Das and Heemsbergen, 1983; Naglieri and Das, 1988). They include *Visual Search* in which the score is the time to find the target figure (located in a central circle) among many figures (objects, letters) scattered around it; *Trails,* an alternative version of the

Trail Making Test; and *Matching Numbers,* in which subjects have three minutes to find as many pairs of identical numbers as they can on a page with 20 number pairs. Indirect support for the assumption that these are tests of planning comes from factor analyses of this battery in which these three tests cluster together. Also offered as evidence of their sensitivity to planning are correlations with academic achievement tests which are at chance levels for grade 2 but gradually increase to reach the .42 to .55 range at grade 10, presumably reflecting the development of planning ability (Naglieri and Das, 1987).

A more direct approach is to give the patient a task in which planning is a necessary feature. Helm-Estabrooks and her colleagues (1985) played checkers with unilaterally brain damaged patients, recording each move onto "individual checkerboard flow sheets." None of the patients won. Of particular interest were differences between left- and right-lesioned patients as the former made fewer bad moves (losing a checker without taking the opponent's checker in return), appreciated sooner that they would lose, and kept their finger on a moved checker to evaluate the move before committing themselves to it.

Everyday tasks

The abstract nature of many standard tests is different from the planning requirements of ordinary daily activities, such as planning to meet friends, to prepare a meal, or to accomplish a set of errands. These activities present important challenges to many patients with brain disorders. Several methods have been developed to assess the everyday planning skills of patients. Channon and Crawford (1999) devised a series of brief videotapes and stories of everyday awkward situations, such as negotiating a solution with a neighbor about a problem dog. Compared to patients with posterior lesions, anterior patients were more impaired in generating a range of possible solutions to solve the problem and in the quality of the solutions. In another study, patients with focal lesions to the prefrontal cortex and control subjects were asked to plan a response for a hypothetical couple engaged in making real-world financial decisions (Goel, Grafman, Tajik, et al., 1997). The patients with frontal lesions took much longer than control subjects to identify the information that was missing from the problem scenario and less time on the problem-solving phase. They also showed poor judgment regarding the adequacy and completeness of their plans.

Goel and Grafman (2000) examined an architect with a right prefrontal lesion, giving him an architectural task that required him to develop a new design for a lab space. The authors concluded that the patient was impaired in his ability to explore possible alternatives for solutions because of the imprecise and ambiguous characteristics of the design problem. By contrast, he performed well on most standard problem-solving tests, which are more structured with definite rules.

Another patient, this one having sustained a moderate TBI, was asked to devise an emergency management plan in case of weather-related flooding for a hypothetical county (Satish et al., 1999). Using an elaborate interactive computer simulation, a variety of executive skills were assessed. Although the patient was able to plan short-term goals, her decision making and limited use of strategy impaired her overall performance. Her responses on this simulation appeared to explain her postinjury vocational failures and demonstrated specific difficulties that limited her potential.

Script generation (Grafman, Thompson, et al., 1991)

This technique was originally developed to study memory functions but a more recent application investigates the ability to plan a sequence of routine actions. It also appears to have potential value when looking for evidence of breakdown in executive functioning. Applicable "script" topics are those that involve relatively frequent activities undertaken by almost everyone, such as "going to a movie," "eating at a restaurant," or "visiting the doctor." Grafman and his colleagues instructed their probable Alzheimer patients to tell or write "all the things that you do when you get up in the morning until you leave the house or have lunch." Patients' responses were scored for the total number of events in the script, their importance (on a predetermined scale), whether this was a likely event (yes or no), and repetitions (which may or may not be true perseverations).

Dementia patients differed from both depressed elderly patients and normal control subjects in producing many fewer events ($p < .0001$), and more script items given out of order (19% compared to 5% for control subjects with no out of order items for the depressed patients). Dementia patients also made significantly more errors in the other scoring categories. Frontal patients also were impaired on this task. Compared to patients with posterior lesions and control subjects, frontal patients made errors in ordering action in the correct temporal sequence, failed to carry out the script to the stated end point and to remain within the stated boundaries, and made deviant estimates of the importance of specific actions (Sirigu et al., 1995).

More recently these investigators extended the real-world nature of the task by asking subjects to plan actions to be carried out in a "virtual" apartment presented on an interactive computer screen (Zalla et al.,

2001). Comparisons between performance on this condition and the verbal script condition found that the realistic context in the "virtual" condition improved the responses of frontal patients. However, in both conditions the frontal group made more errors than control subjects. Frontal patients persisted in carrying out habitual action sequences when inappropriate for the situation at hand and also persisted in including personally relevant but intrusive actions rather than adapting to the test environment.

Allain and his colleagues (2001) not only asked severely injured TBI patients to generate scripts (shop at a supermarket, prepare a salad) following Grafman's model, but then observed them as they engaged in these activities in real life. They found that executive functioning of these patients, all of whom had significant frontal lesions, was impaired, both in script generation and in actual behavior. However, these two aspects of what seemed to be the same task involved different subsets of the executive functions. These patients generated significantly fewer script actions than control subjects and made more script errors, especially sequencing errors. Moreover, when actually performing the tasks, sequencing errors diminished but problems in following regulations, of dependence on help from others, and of distractibility increased. The authors conclude that the cognitive and behavioral responses generated in laboratory studies differ from those elicited by real life.

Purposive Action

The translation of an intention or plan into productive, self-serving activity requires the actor to initiate, maintain, switch, and stop sequences of complex behavior in an orderly and integrated manner. Disturbances in the programming of activity can thwart the carrying out of reasonable plans regardless of motivation, knowledge, or capacity to perform the activity. However, such disturbances are less likely to impede impulsive actions which bypass the planning stages in the action sequence and thereby provide an important distinction between impulsive and consciously deliberate actions. Similarly, Shallice (1982) noted that programming functions are necessary for the successful performance of nonroutine tasks but are not needed when the action sequence is routine. Thus, overlearned, familiar, routine tasks and automatic behaviors can be expected to be much less vulnerable to impaired brain functioning than are nonroutine or novel activities, particularly when the impairment involves the frontal lobes.

Patients who have trouble programming activity may display a marked dissociation between their verbalized intentions and plans and their actions.

Hospitalized Korsakoff patients, severely impaired TBI patients who do not always know where they are, and others with profound executive disorders may still talk repeatedly about wanting to leave (to get some money, return to a wife, visit parents, etc.). When informed that they are free to go whenever they wish and even given an explanation of how they might do so, they either quickly forget what they were told, change the subject, or ignore the message. One youthful TBI victim repeatedly announced his very reasonable intention to get a much-needed haircut. Although he knew the way to the barbershop and was physically capable of going there, he never did get his hair cut on his own.

Programming difficulties may affect large-scale purposive activities or the regulation and fine-tuning of discrete intentional acts or complex movements. Patients who have trouble performing discrete actions also tend to have difficulty carrying out broader purposive activities. For example, youthful offenders who displayed an inability to switch ongoing activity by making errors on an untimed trial of the Trail Making Test Part B also tended to be those whose self-report of their criminal activities contained evidence of an inability to make appropriate shifts in the "principle of action" during the commission of the crime (Pontius and Yudowitz, 1980).

Tinkertoy Test (TTT)[1] (Lezak, 1982a)

This construction test gives patients an opportunity—within the necessarily highly structured formal examination—to demonstrate executive capacities. The Tinkertoy Test makes it possible for them to initiate, plan, and structure a potentially complex activity, and to carry it out independently. In the normal course of most neurological or neuropsychological examinations such functions are carried out by the examiner or are made unnecessary (or even unwelcome) by the structured nature of the test material and the restricted number of possible responses in most tests of cognitive functions. Thus, these functions typically remain unexamined, although they are absolutely essential to the maintenance of social independence in a complex society.

The Tinkertoy Test also gives the patient an opportunity to make a "free" construction without the constraints of a model to copy or a predetermined solution. The interplay between executive and constructional functions will more or less limit the extent to which this examination technique tests the constructional capacity of any individual patient. Its usefulness as a constructional test will vary, largely with the patient's productivity.

[1]This combination of 50 wooden pieces comes from "The Classic Tinkertoy Construction Set," Junior size (66 pieces), manufactured by Hasbro, Pautucket, RI 02862. (e-mail: www.tinkertoy.com) It is available in many toy and department stores.

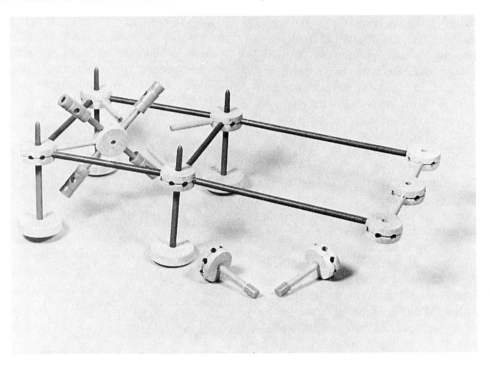

FIGURE 16.5 A 23-year-old craftsman with a high school education made this Tinkertoy "space platform" after he had first tried to construct "a design" and then "a new ride at the fair" (see text).

For example, Figure 16.5 was put together by a youthful TBI patient whose constructional abilities had remained relatively intact (WAIS scaled scores for Block Design = 10, Object Assembly = 14) but whose capacity for integrating complex stimuli was impaired (Picture Arrangement = 6). The ambitiousness, complexity, and relative symmetry of this "space platform" reflect his good constructional skills, although its instability, lack of integration (he could not figure out how to put the two little extra constructions onto the main construction), growth by accretion rather than plan, and the inappropriateness of the name given to it provide concrete evidence of defective executive functioning.

Administration of this test is simple. Fifty pieces of a Tinkertoy set (Table 16.1) are placed on a clean surface in front of the subject, who is told, "Make whatever you want with these. You will have at least five minutes and as much more time as you wish to make something." The necessity for a 5-min minimum time

limit became evident when, without such a limit, bright competitive-minded control subjects did a slapdash job thinking this was a speed test, and poorly motivated or self-deprecating patients gave up easily. Deteriorated patients may stop handling the items after two or three minutes, but should be allowed to sit for several minutes more before being asked whether they have finished with the material. Except for the 5-min minimum, the test is not timed since a pilot study involving both patients and control subjects showed that the amount of time taken may vary without regard to neuropsychological status or with the quality of the performance. Encouragement is given as needed.

Most patients find this test interesting or amusing. Of the 35 subjects with diagnosed neurological disorders who participated in the pilot study, many seemed to enjoy the constructional activity and none raised any objections. Even the one patient who made no construction played with a few pieces, fitting them together and taking them apart, before his attention drifted away. Only blind patients and those sighted patients who cannot manipulate small objects with both hands are unable to take this test.

On completion, the examiner asks what the construction represents (e.g., "What is it?"). If it does represent something (usually a named object), the construction is evaluated for its appropriateness to the indicated name (or concept). In the original scoring system, each of the following criteria earned points, as

TABLE 16.1 Items Used in the Tinkertoy Test*

Wooden Dowels	Rounds	Others
Green (4)	Knobs (10)	Connectors (4)
Orange (4)	Wheels (4)	Caps (4)
Red (4)		Points (4)
Blue (6)		
Yellow (6)		

*Since first used as a test, Tinkertoys have been through several reincarnations and manufacturers. The current sets are colored wood, like the original set. The pieces called for here are the same as those pictured but a little larger.

TABLE 16.2 Tinkertoy Test: Scoring for Complexity

Variable	Scoring Criteria	Points
1. *mc*	Any combination of pieces	1
2. *nc*	$n < 20 = 1, < 30 = 2, < 40 = 3, \leq 50 = 4$	1–4
3. *name*	Appropriate = 3; vague/inappropriate = 2; post hoc naming, description = 1; none = 0	0–3
4. *mov*	Mobility = 1, moving parts = 1	0–2
5. *3d*	3-dimensional	1
6. *stand*	Free-standing, stays standing	1
7. *error*	For each error (misfit, incomplete fit, drop and not pick up)	−1
Highest score possible		12
Lowest score possible		−1 or less

noted in Table 16.2 (Lezak, 1982a): (1) whether the patient made any construction(s) (*mc*); (2) total number of pieces used (*np*); (3) whether the construction was given a name appropriate to its appearance and when (*name*); (4a) mobility (wheels that work) and (4b) moving parts (*mov*); (5) whether it has three dimensions (*3d*); (6) whether the construction is freestanding (*stand*); and (7) whether there is a performance error such as misfit in which parts of pieces are forced together that were not made to be combined, incomplete fit in which connections are not properly made, or dropping pieces on the floor without attempting to recover them. The complexity score (*comp*) is based on all of these performance variables (see Table 16.2). A modified complexity score (*mComp*) does not include the number of pieces used. This complexity score (*comp-r*) differs slightly from the one on which the original research is based (*comp-o*). Bayless and his coworkers (1989) suggested the more sensitive 4-point scale for the name category; James L. Mack (personal communication, 1994 [mdl]) identified the poor discriminability of a symmetry score in the original protocol leading to its removal from the scoring system. Regardless of which complexity score is used, findings tend to support the complexity score's sensitivity to impaired executive functions.

An examination of the validity and reliability of the TTT compared the scores from Alzheimer patients and control subjects given by two independent raters (Koss, Patterson, Mack, et al., 1998). Interrater reliability was high. All patient scores were lower than those of control subjects except for *mc* and *error*. Scores also differentiated patients with mild and moderate dementia. They were relatively independent of one another as—for patient performances—only four of 15 possible correlations between scores were significant: *3d* with *np* ($r = .30$), *3d* with *name* ($r = .25$), *3d* with *stand* ($r = .51$), and *np* with *stand* ($r = .30$).

Neuropsychological findings. An initial evaluation of the effectiveness of the Tinkertoy Test in measuring executive capacity was made using the *np* and *comp* scores of 35 unselected patients with cerebral pathology and ten normal control subjects. On the basis of history, records, or family interviews, 18 patients who required total support and supervision were classified as Dependent (D), and 17 were classified as Not Dependent (ND) as the latter managed daily routines on their own and could drive or use public transportation, and five of them were capable of working independently. The two patient groups did not differ in age, education, or scores on Information (WAIS). The control subjects tended to be younger and better educated than the patients.

Both *np* and *comp* scores differentiated the constructions of these three groups (see Table 16.3). All

TABLE 16.3 Comparisons Between Groups on *np* and Complexity Scores

Group Measure	PATIENT		Control	F
	Dependent	Nondependent		
np				
Mean ± SD	13.5 ± 9.46	30.24 ± 11.32	42.2 ± 10.03	26.91*
Range	0–42	9–50	23–50	
Complexity				
Mean ± SD	2.22 ± 2.10	5.47 ± 1.77	7.8 ± 1.99	28.27*
Range	−1–8	2–9	5–12	

*One-way ANOVA, $p < .001$.

but one of the Dependent patients used fewer than 23 pieces; those who were Not Dependent used 23 or more. Half of the control group used all 50 pieces but none used fewer than 30. The *np* and *comp* scores of the control subjects and the 19 patients who had age-graded scaled scores of 10 or higher on WAIS Information or Block Design differed significantly. The lower Tinkertoy Test scores of the patients whose cognitive performances were relatively intact suggest that this test taps into more than cognitive abilities. As measured by correlations with the Block Design scaled scores, constructional ability contributes to the complexity of the construction ($r_{comp \times BD} = .574$, $p < .01$) but has a weaker association with the number of pieces used ($r_{np \times BD} = .379$, $p < .05$).

Other studies also looked at how TTT performances related to tests in common use. For a group of patients with TBI in the mild to moderate range, no relationship appeared between the *comp-r* score and performance on the test of Three-Dimensional Constructional Praxis (Bayless et al., 1989). Among elderly subjects ($M_{age} = 85.4$ years), of whom half were demented, the TTT performance correlated significantly ($p < .005$) with scores on the Wisconsin Card Sorting Test ($r = .54$) as well as the Trail Making Test ($r = .67$); but correlations between the TTT and tests of visuoperceptual accuracy, psychomotor speed, and vocabulary were in the .21 to .28 range (Mahurin, Flanagan, and Royall, 1993). Differences in levels of correlation between the two sets of tests were interpreted as demonstrating the

sensitivity of the TTT as a measure of executive functioning. Mahurin and his colleagues also observed that frail elderly patients whose physical and motivational limitations can preclude most formal testing may still be responsive to the TTT.

A number of executive functions appear to contribute to high scoring constructions, including the abilities to formulate a goal and to plan, initiate, and carry out a complex activity to achieve the goal. In Figure 16.6), "space vehicle," depicts the product of a distinguished neuropsychologist, well known for innovative research. She had never seen Tinkertoys before. Her construction reflects her technical competence, creativity, and well-organized and systematic thinking.

Patients who have difficulty initiating or carrying out purposive activities tend to use relatively few pieces although some make recognizable and appropriately named constructions (e.g., see Fig. 16.7, p. 625), the construction of a 60-year-old, left-handed but right-eyed medically retired plumbing contractor who had had a cerebrovascular accident involving a small area of the left parietal lobe that resulted in transient aphasic symptoms. Those who have an impaired capacity for formulating goals or planning but can initiate activity and are well motivated may use relatively more pieces, but their constructions are more likely to be unnamed or inappropriate for their names and poorly organized (e.g., Fig. 16.5, p. 622). Patients with extensive impairment involving all aspects of the executive functions may pile pieces together or sort them into

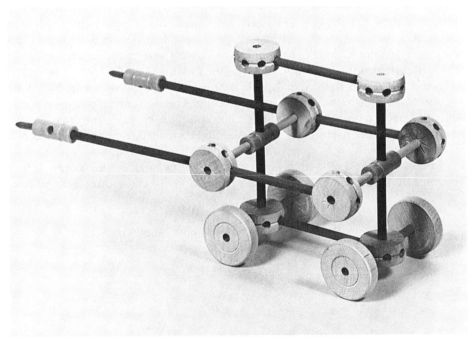

FIGURE 16.6 "Space vehicle" was constructed by a neuropsychologist unfamiliar with Tinkertoys. Although she used only 34 pieces, her complexity score is 11, well above control subjects' mean.

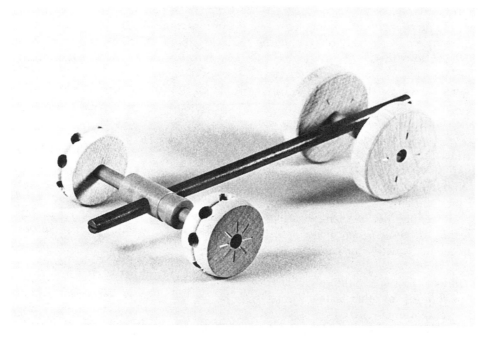

FIGURE 16.7 The creator of this "cannon" achieved WAIS age-graded scaled scores of 16 and 17 on Comprehension and Block Design, respectively (see p. 624).

groups without attempting any constructions, or they use a few pieces to make unnamed and unplanned constructions. For example, Figure 16.8 was the product of a 40-year-old appliance salesman who had suffered a bout of meningitis following a left endarterectomy and thrombectomy undertaken several days after an initial right-sided cerebrovascular accident had resulted in a mild left hemiparesis and slurred speech. Four months after the meningitis had subsided his WAIS Information, Comprehension, and Block Design scaled scores

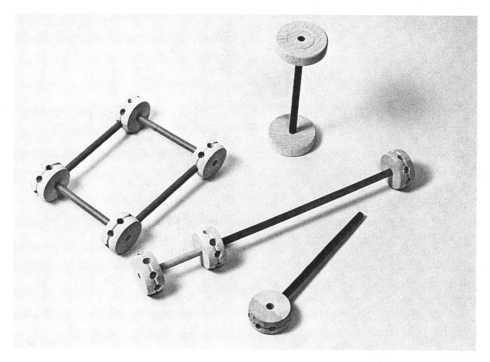

FIGURE 16.8 This patient said he was trying to make "a car" (see text p. 625). He has been totally dependent since the initial illness. Speech is dysfluent; he feeds and toilets himself and walks with a Parkinson-like gait.

were 10, 9, and 6, respectively. Pathologically inert patients, who can usually be coaxed into giving some response to standard test items, are likely to do nothing with as open-ended a task as this.

Studies using the Tinkertoy Test have found the complexity score (original or revised) to be quite sensitive to disorders of executive functions in TBI patients although, for mildly to moderately impaired patients, the score for number of pieces by itself may not be discriminating (Cicerone and DeLuca, 1990). Patients rendered anosmic by TBI typically also sustain orbitofrontal damage with consequent executive function disorders. All 20 such patients examined by Martzke and his colleagues (1991) had psychosocial deficits involving, in most instances, "poor empathy, poor judgment, absent-mindedness," with impaired initiation showing up in many ways. Twelve of them failed this test with *comp-r* scores of 6 or less, although most performed *within normal limits* on other tests purporting to be sensitive to executive functions.

The Tinkertoy Test can be a useful predictor of employability. Only 25 of 50 TBI patients with no physical disabilities were working when examined two or more years after being considered fit to return to work. All but one working patient made scores at or better than the lowest *comp-r* score (7) obtained by 25 normal control subjects; yet 13 of the 25 unemployed patients scored below the lowest control score (Bayless et al., 1989). Tinkertoy Test *comp-o* scores were significantly correlated ($r = .44$, $p < .005$) with postrehabilitation employment status in a study which found that, excepting a correlation of .45 for Trail Making Test-B, the other tests in a representative neuropsychological test battery ran correlations of .35 or less with employment status (Cicerone and DeLuca, 1990). As none of these 87 patients were working or living independently prior to rehabilitation, compared to 38% in supported employment and 40% working competitively afterwards, the Tinkertoy Test and Trail Making Test-B findings suggest that performances on these tests reflect the patients' rehabilitation potential. The Tinkertoy Test also documented improvements made by a patient receiving remediation training for a planning disorder, although scores on Maze tracing and several WAIS-R tests remained essentially unchanged (Cicerone and Wood, 1987).

Tinkertoy constructions may be useful for differentiating between dementia types as 18 patients with multi-infarct dementia achieved a lower *comp-o* score than 18 patients with probable Alzheimer's disease. On most structured tasks, both patient groups performed at the same level, much lower than that of intact elderly subjects (Mendez and Ashla-Mendez, 1991). Their performances differed qualitatively as well: the Alzheimer patients used most pieces but in separate combinations made up of a few pieces, while the multi-infarct patients' constructions were single, simple, and had the fewest pieces. This test is also sensitive to severity of dementia (Koss, Patterson, et al., 1998): mildly impaired Alzheimer patients obtained significantly higher *3d* and *comp* scores than moderately impaired ones.

Self-Regulation

Assessment of self-regulation: 1. productivity

Reduced or erratic productivity can be due to a dissociation between intention and action as well as to weak or absent development of intentions or to a planning defect. This productivity—or inactivity—problem becomes readily apparent in patients who "talk a good game," may even give the details of what needs to be done, but do not carry out what they verbally acknowledge or propose. Patients who do one thing while saying or intending another also display this kind of dissociation. The initiation of an activity may be slow or may require a series of preparatory motions before the patient can make a full response. These patients may make stuttering sounds preparatory to speaking, for example, or agitate the body part that will be undertaking the intended activity before it becomes fully activated. This too is not an intention defect but one of translation from thought to action.

Defective productivity, like many other executive disorders, can usually be observed in the course of an interview or tests of other functions. This requires the examiner to be alert to qualitative aspects of behavior, such as stuttering that heralds the onset of speech, or comments about an error without correction.

Use of standard examination procedures

Slowed responding is probably the most common cause of low productivity in people with brain disorders. It can occur on almost any kind of test, in response latencies and/or performances that are slowed generally or only when certain kinds of functions or activities are called upon. Slowing can and should be documented as it may provide cues to the nature of a disorder which are not apparent in the patient's responses in themselves.

An example of the kind of documentation that provides valuable information about slowing involves responses to a picture shown to elicit a story, the Cookie Theft Picture. Typically responses are evaluated for their linguistic attributes, but timing the rate of responding (words per minute) demonstrated significant differences between patients with multi-infarct dementia, those with probable Alzheimer's disease, and elderly controls (Mendez and Ashla-Mendez, 1991). Response sluggishness also shows up in correct but over-time responses on timed tasks (e.g., Picture Completion, Picture Arrangement, Block Design, and others of the WIS-A batteries.

Patients who are slow to develop a set but whose cognitive functions are intact may achieve quite respectable test scores. Their problem appears only in the first one or two items of a new test, after which they perform well and rapidly. It is typical of these patients when given tests from the WIS-A battery to be slow to solve the easy items of Block Design, to have long latencies on the first few items of Picture Completion or Picture Arrangement, and to give only a few words on the first trial of a word fluency task but perform other trials well. Patients slow to form a set are likely to have a relatively limited recall on the first trial of either the Auditory–Verbal Learning Test or the California Verbal Learning Test word learning tests, but to do well on the interference list since by this time they are familiar with the format.

Another pattern of slowing appears in dwindling responses. The patient begins performing tasks at a rapid enough rate but loses speed and may ultimately stop responding altogether in the course of a trial or set of trials. Tests which require many similar responses to be given rapidly for a minute or more, such as verbal fluency or symbol substitution tasks, are best suited to bring out this production defect.

Assessment of self-regulation: 2. Flexibility and the capacity to shift

The ability to regulate one's own behavior can be demonstrated on tests of flexibility that require the subject to shift a course of thought or action according to the demands of the situation. The capacity for flexibility in behavior extends through perceptual, cognitive, and response dimensions. Defects in mental flexibility show up perceptually in defective scanning and inability to change perceptual set easily. Conceptual inflexibility appears in concrete or rigid approaches to understanding and problem solving, and also as stimulus-bound behavior in which these patients cannot dissociate their responses or pull their attention away from whatever is in their perceptual field or current thoughts (e.g., see Lhermitte, 1983). It may appear as inability to shift perceptual organization, train of thought, or ongoing behavior to meet the varying needs of the moment.

Inflexibility of response results in perseverative, stereotyped, nonadaptive behavior and difficulties in regulating and modulating motor acts. Each of these problems is characterized by an inability to shift behavior readily, to conform behavior to rapidly chang-

ing demands on the person. This disturbance in the programming of behavior appears in many different contexts and forms and is typically associated with lesions in the frontal lobes (Luria, 1966; Truelle, Le Gall, et al., 1995). Its particular manifestation depends at least in part on the site of the lesion.

When evaluating performances in which the same response occurs more than once, it is important to distinguish between *perseveration* and *repetitions* due to attentional deficits. As an "involuntary continuation or recurrence of ideas, experiences, or both without the appropriate stimulation" (M.L. Albert, 1989), perseveration involves a "stickiness" in thinking or response due to a breakdown in automatic regulatory mechanisms. Perseverations result from an inability to terminate an activity or switch into another activity (E. Goldberg, 1986). Repetitions made by patients whose abilities for mental and motor flexibility are intact but who have difficulty keeping track of immediately previous or ongoing actions—as for example patients with diffusely impaired brain functioning whose ability to do or think of more than one thing at a time is limited—are not perseverations and should not be labeled as such. This kind of repetition occurs in formal testing, most commonly on word generation tasks: tests of semantic memory (word fluency) or learning ability (word list learning). These patients repeat a word when they have forgotten (lost out of short-term storage or lost to working memory) that they said it 10 or 20 sec before, or they cannot perform a mental task and keep track of what they are doing at the same time. Repetitions will typically differ qualitatively from perseverations as the latter appear in repeated repeating of one word or several, or repeated use of the same word or action with stimuli similar to those that initially elicited the word or action.

By and large, techniques that tend to bring out defects in self-regulation do not have scoring systems or even standardized formats. Neither is necessary or especially desirable. Once perseveration or inability to shift smoothly through a movement, drawing, or speaking sequence shows up, that is evidence enough that the patient is having difficulty with self-regulation. The examiner may then wish to explore the dimensions of the problem: how frequently it occurs, how long it lasts, whether the patient can self-recover (for instance, when perseverating on a word or movement, or when an alternating sequence breaks down), and what conditions are most likely to bring out the dysfunctional response (kind of task, laterality differences [e.g., design copying vs. writing], stress, fatigue, etc.). An efficient examination should be different for each patient as the examiner follows up on the unique set of dysfunctional responses displayed at each step in the course of the examination. When a subtle defect is suspected, for example, the examiner may give a series of tasks of increasing length or complexity. When a broad, very general defect is suspected, it may be unnecessary to give very long or complex tasks but, rather, for planning and rehabilitation purposes, it may be more useful to expose the patient to a wide range of tasks.

At the conceptual level, mental inflexibility can be difficult to identify, shading into personality rigidity on the one hand and stupidity on the other. Tests of abstraction that emphasize shifts in concept formation touch upon mental flexibility (see pp. 574–577, 584–592).

Uses of Objects and Alternate Uses Test (AUT)[1]

This is another kind of test that assesses inflexibility in thinking and has also served to identify creativity in bright children (Getzels and Jackson, 1962; see also Guilford et al., 1978). The printed instructions for the Uses of Objects test ask subjects to write as many uses as they can for five common objects: brick, pencil, paper clip, toothpick, sheet of paper. Two examples are given for each object, such as "Brick—build houses, doorstop," or "Pencil—write, bookmark," with space on the answer sheet for a dozen or more uses to be written in for each object. The Alternate Uses Test version of Uses of Objects provides two sets of three objects each: shoe, button, key; pencil, automobile tire, eyeglasses. One AUT format allows the subject four minutes in which to tell about as many uncommon uses for the three objects in a set as come to mind (Grattan and Eslinger, 1989). Acceptable responses must be conceivable uses that are different from each other and from the common use. Another format allows one minute for each of the six target objects and evaluates performance on the basis of the sum of acceptable responses using the Guilford group's (1978) criteria (R.W. Butler, Rorsman, et al., 1993). Following these scoring rules 17 control subjects ($M_{age} = 40 \pm 8$, $M_{educ} = 14.5 \pm 2$) gave an average of 22 ± 9.5 responses.

The tendency to give obvious, conventional responses such as for Brick "to build a wall," or "to line a garden path," reflects a search for the "right" or logical solution, which is called *convergent* thinking. In *divergent* thinking, on the other hand, the subject generates many different and often unique and daring ideas without evident concern for satisfying preconceived notions of what is correct or logical. The divergent thinker, for example, might recommend using a brick as a bedwarmer or for short people to stand on at a parade. Divergent thinking is a sign of cognitive flexibility. Age-

related decline in number of uses has been observed in a comparison of younger and older adults (mean ages 48 and 72, respectively) (Parkin and Lawrence, 1994).

Neuropsychological findings. In recommending Uses of Objects to evaluate mental inflexibility, Zangwill (1966) noted that "frontal lobe patients tend to embroider on the main or conventional use of an object, often failing to think up other, less probable uses. This is somewhat reminiscent of the inability to switch from one principle of classification to another" (p. 397).

A 28-year-old man awaiting trial on murder charges had a history of several TBIs in car accidents, untreated and occasionally out-of-control Type 1 diabetes since his teen years, and heavy alcohol and street drug use. Despite only ten years of formal education he achieved scaled scores of 9 and 10 on WAIS-III Information and Comprehension, scores of 12, 11, and 10 on Picture Completion, Picture Arrangement, and Block Design, respectively. His responses to Alternate Uses for *Shoe* were: "*play catch,* look at it, admire it, make footprints, can't think of other things;" for *Button,* responses were "throw it up and down—play catch, magic tricks to make it disappear, collect them, can't think of others." Among other *defective* performances were his bicycle drawing (no spokes, no chain), *Identification of Common Objects* (concrete and premature responses), and *Design Fluency* (seven scorable designs—he named two others "lamp").

None of the Alternate Uses scores achieved by patients with frontal lobe tumors reached the mean of control subjects, and the patients' produced only about half as many acceptable responses as the control subjects ($p < .001$) (R.W. Butler, Rorsman, et al., 1993). Yet 10 of 17 patients in this study performed *within normal limits* on a verbal fluency task (FAS) but the other seven gave far fewer responses ($p < .02$) than control subjects. In a comparison of patients with focal lesions, 89% of control subjects' responses to Uses of Objects were acceptable, patients with posterior cortical lesions gave 68% acceptable responses, and for those with basal ganglia lesions the acceptable response rate was 60% (Eslinger and Grattan, 1993). The worst performers were patients with frontal lesions who gave only 12% acceptable responses. Scores on Alternate Uses correlated significantly ($r = .61$) with a measure of empathy, which was interpreted as demonstrating a relationship between empathy and cognitive flexibility in persons with brain lesions (Grattan and Eslinger, 1989). Productivity in this kind of test tends to decrease with anxiety (Kovacs and Pléh, 1987).

Most studies have reported large standard deviations for group scores. For example, despite large mean differences on this test, between 20 Parkinson patients ($M = 2.9 \pm 9.55$) and their 20 control subjects ($M = 11.3 \pm 10.76$) (Raskin et al., 1992), the even larger

---

[1]This is one of Guilford's *Measures of Creativity,* which can be ordered from Consulting Psychologists' Press.

standard deviations appear to have obscured some real differences that nonparametric techniques might have documented.

In another set of fluency tasks, *Possible Jobs*, subjects are asked to name jobs associated with pictured objects (e.g., safety pin) or designs (e.g., setting sun) (R.W. Butler, Rorsman, et al., 1993). Another task in this set asks for descriptions of the consequences of unusual situations (e.g., if food were not needed to sustain life). Another calls for drawing elaborations, i.e., adding lines to copies of a figure to make as many different recognizable objects as possible. These tasks, which were identified as "complex" in comparison to the "simple" fluency tasks (Controlled Oral Word Association Test, Design Fluency), proved to be more sensitive to the presence of a frontal lobe tumor than the more traditional "simple" tests of fluency.

Homophone Meaning Generation Test (Warrington, 2000)

This test of flexibility of thinking asks the subject to generate different meanings for common words. Each of the eight words (*form, slip, tick, tip, bear, cent, right,* and *bored*) has at least three distinct meanings. The generation of multiple meanings of these words requires switching among dissimilar verbal concepts. For example, the word "tick" could mean a clock sound or a small insect. The score is the total number of correct meanings produced. The normative sample consisted of 170 participants ages 19 to 74 with a minimum of ten years of education. The total number of words generated ranged from 10 to 35, $M = 23.7$. The test has satisfactory reliability (Crawford and Warrington, 2002). Patients with anterior lesions performed worse than those with posterior lesions but no significant laterality effects appeared (Warrington, 2000). These data are consistent with data from fluency tests in showing that patients with frontal lesions have deficits in generation of concepts and in cognitive flexibility.

Cognitive Bias Task (CBT) (E. Goldberg, Harner, et al., 1994)

On each trial the subject must look at the top one of three vertically placed designs and then choose one of the two designs below it that "you like best." The designs differ on the basis of five binary dimensions: shape (circle/square), color (red/blue), number (one/two identical components), size (large/small), and contour (outline/filled with a homogeneous color). The two lower designs always have different degrees of similarity to the target. Low or high similarity scores indicate that subjects allowed the target to influence their choice (context dependent response), while middle range scores are less clear in revealing subjects' response patterns. There are no right or wrong answers as this procedure asks the subject to indicate a preference.

Despite subjects' freedom to choose any response criterion, a study of 15 healthy subjects found high test–retest reliability ($r = .88$) (E. Goldberg, Harner, et al., 1994). Right-handed male control subjects tended to be more "target-driven" (context dependent) than right-handed women. Response bias in nonright-handed women is comparable with that of right-handed men, i.e., context dependent. Data from small samples of male patients showed that right frontal lesions produced target-driven responses while left frontal lesions gave responses based on perceptual preferences independent of the target. Response bias in female patients was independent of lesion laterality: both right and left frontal lesioned women produced more target-driven responses than their control subjects (E. Goldberg and Podell, 2000). Target-driven behavior may represent a form of stimulus-boundedness.

Item generation

This technique is an effective means of exploring executive functioning. While productivity and the ability to vary one's responses rapidly are essential to success on these tests, other aspects of executive functioning also contribute to good performances, such as self-monitoring (to avoid repeating a response), remembering and following rules, use of strategies, and—of course—creative imagination. The major difference between the two main approaches to this kind of task lies in the degree of structure provided for the subject. See pp. 519–523 for verbal fluency tests.

Design Fluency (Jones-Gotman and Milner, 1977)

This test was developed as a nonverbal counterpart of Thurstone's Word Fluency Test. In the first—free condition—trial, the subject is asked to "invent drawings" that represent neither actual objects nor nameable abstract forms (e.g., geometric shapes) and that are not merely scribbles. After being shown examples of acceptable and unacceptable (e.g., a star is nameable, a scribble or an amoeboid shape requires no thought) drawings made by the examiner, subjects are given five minutes in which to make up as many different kinds of drawings as they can, "many" and "different" being emphasized in the instructions. The first of each type of unacceptable drawing or too similar a drawing is pointed out as is a drawing so elaborate as to decrease the quantity produced. The second, four-minute trial is the fixed (four-line) condition in which acceptable drawings are limited to four lines, straight or curved. Again the subject is shown acceptable and unacceptable examples and the instructions place emphasis on the subject's making as many different drawings as possible. The control subjects' average output on the free five-minute condition was 16.2 designs and on the fixed (four-minute) condition it was 19.7. Approximately 10% of the responses were judged perseverative. Jones-Gotman reported that the free condition is more sensitive than the fixed one (unpublished ms., no date).

Each condition is scored separately but following essentially the same rules. First, all perseverative responses are identified and subtracted from the total. These "include rotations or mirror-imaging versions of previous drawings, variations on a theme, complicated drawings that differ . . . (in) small details, and scribbles. (They) must be scored harshly" (Jones-Gotman, no date). All nameable drawings (in examiner's judgment or named by subject) and four-line condition drawings with more or fewer lines are also removed. The novel output score is then the number of remaining drawings. A perseveration score can be computed by subtracting all other erroneous responses from the total and determining the percentage of perseverative responses out of the remaining subtotal. Reported reliability correlations for interjudge scoring are in the .74 to .87 range (Jones-Gotman, 1991a). Examining the performance of college students, S.L. Carter and her colleagues (1998) reported interrater reliabilities from .66 to .99 except for lower coefficients for nameable errors and the incorrect number of lines in the fixed condition. Good to excellent interrater reliability coefficients also have been reported for a sample of older subjects (ages 51.5 to 89.6 years) (Woodard, Axelrod, and Henry, 1992). However, with some severe impairments, scoring is not only not necessary but not possible (see Fig. 16.9).

A 62-year-old man, born and raised in an Asian country but living in the West for the last 25 years, displayed a radical personality change after a heavy flower pot had fallen on his head from a display shelf. Before the accident he had been a lively, cheerful man, enjoying retirement with other elderly men from his country who frequently fished together and visited with one another. He had been interested in his family, politics, and current events. Since the accident he has been morose, withdrawn, and lacking in spontaneity and interests.

Significant in the history of this graduate engineer was two years' imprisonment after his country's government was overturned. The adjacent cell had been occupied by an army officer who was tortured so severely that he committed suicide by hanging in that cell.

When brought to a psychiatrist for treatment the patient was diagnosed as depressed and put into a six-month outpatient program (in English, in which he was not fluent!) for depressed elderly patients which proved to be ineffectual. In planning the neuropsychological assessment, frontal damage was suspected and Design Fluency included in the battery prepared for him (see Fig. 16.9). He was examined in his second language in which he was fully fluent. After producing the first design (upper left) the instructions were repeated with emphasis on drawing designs that could not be named. His next drawing was to the right of the first. When asked what it was, he said, "bombe." After the third try the test was discontinued: the patient had demonstrated an inability to make up a design due to impaired inventiveness and mental fluency and—even more important for understanding his condition and his obvious misery—loss of the ability to repress his painful, and now obsessive, memories. His personality change seemed best understood as reflecting a compromised capacity for repression plus diminished spontaneity due to a frontal lobe injury. His morbid depression was a symptom, not the cause of this change.

Test characteristics. Several studies used the free condition to examine aging effects on functions associated with the frontal lobes. For the novel output score, Daigneault and her colleagues (1992) found no age effects for subjects in the 15 to 65-year range, but the later study reported a significant tendency ($p = .038$) for perseverative responses to increase with age. With an age range extending up to 75 years, productivity of another group of healthy subjects diminished signifi-

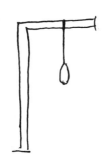
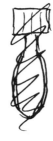
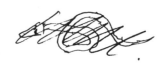

Figure 16.9 *Figural Fluency Test* responses by 62-year-old man described on p. 630.

cantly with age (Mittenberg, Seidenberg, et al., 1989), a change interpreted as reflecting a decline in prefrontal functioning.

Neuropsychological findings. TBI patients produced fewer novel designs in the free condition compared to control subjects (Varney, Roberts, et al., 1996). A small sample of TBI patients with frontal lesions made many more nonperseverative errors (rule-breaking) than nonfrontal patients and normal control subjects on the free condition and many more perseverative errors on the fixed condition (H.S. Levin, Goldstein, Williams, and Eisenberg, 1991). Frontal lobe patients tended to have reduced output on both free and fixed conditions relative to normal subjects and patients with posterior lesions. Patients with right-sided lesions generally tended to have lower productivity (except right posterior patients on the free condition), and those with right frontal lesions were least productive. Patients with frontal—particularly right frontal—and right central lesions showed the greatest tendency to perseveration relative to the control group on both free and fixed conditions (Jones-Gotman, 1991a). Studies using the fixed four-line condition found no differences in either novel output score or perseverations for patients with right or left (aphasic) hemisphere disease (M.L. Albert and Sandson, 1986) or Parkinson's disease (Sandson and Albert, 1987). Only a production lag by aphasic patients compared with normal control subjects proved significant at the 5% level.

Five-point Test (Regard, Strauss, and Knapp, 1982)

The use of a structured background for examining response fluency was introduced in the Five-point Test, which consists of a page on which are printed 40 contiguous squares in a 5×8 array, each square containing five symmetrically and identically arranged dots (see example I, Fig. 16.10). The examiner asks the subject to make "as many different figures as possible within 5 minutes by connecting [any number of] the dots with straight lines" without repeating any figure. That the figures should be *different* is emphasized in the instructions.

Age but not sex differences appeared in the 6- to 12-year age range for total production and rotated figures

(an indicator of strategy), but from age 10 production levels were in the adult score range. Self-monitoring and self-correcting first appeared among the 10- and 12-year-olds. Patients with psychiatric disorders produced more designs and made fewer perseverative errors than patients with brain disorders on a 3-minute version (G.P. Lee, Strauss, et al., 1997). The number of designs produced did not distinguish frontal from nonfrontal lesioned patients.

Ruff Figural Fluency Test (RFFT)[1] (R.W. Evans et al., 1985; Ruff, Light, and Evans, 1987)

This expanded version of Regard's Five-point Test consists of five sheets of paper, each containing 40 squares. The first is identical in appearance to the Five-point Test sheet. Of the other four, II and III retain dots in the original position but contain interference patterns; the dots on trials IV and V are asymmetrically positioned, with all squares alike on each page (see Fig. 16.10). The instructions are essentially the same as those of the Five-point Test except that the RFFT provides a three-square practice page for each trial, and the allotted time is one minute. In instructing patients, I [mdl] always ask for "patterns" rather than "designs," as used by Ruff and his colleagues, as many people think a design requires artistic talent and may feel unequal to the task. Also, my instructions include emphasizing that the subject can connect *any two or more* dots, as many persons assume that they need to connect all five dots—which precludes development of strategies and slows productivity. Patients who tend to be concrete in their thinking and/or sluggish in altering a response set may continue to connect all five dots in each frame through the first and even the second and third set, despite continuing repetition of "any two or more dots." Performances are scored for number of unique patterns and for number of repetitions of a pattern. Unlike the Five-point Test, rotations are not scored but should be noted, for a series of orderly, nonrepeating rotations is the hallmark of a strategic approach.

Test characteristics. For adults, no sex differences have appeared. However, both age and education affected productivity to a significant degree ($p < .001$) but not accuracy (Ruff, Light, and Evans, 1987). Interrater reliability correlations for unique designs and repetitions are high, .93 and .74, respectively (Berning et al., 1998). Motor skill (as measured by the Finger Tapping Test) may also contribute to a higher productivity rate on the RFFT (R.W. Evans et al., 1985).

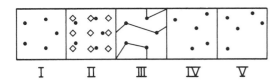

FIGURE 16.10 Ruff Figural Fluency Test (Parts I–V). (From R.W. Evans, Ruff, and Gualtieri, 1985. Reproduced by permission.)

[1]This test can be ordered from Psychological Assessment Resources.

A practice effect can be expected on repeat administrations (M.R. Basso, Bornstein, and Lang, 1999).

Neuropsychological findings. The RFFT production score discriminated mild from severe head trauma patients and both groups from normal control subjects (Ruff, Evans, and Marshall, 1986). Inspection of the data shows that the number of repeated patterns increased from control subjects (5.8 ± 7.3) to mildly injured (8.8 ± 14.9) to severely injured (10.1 ± 12.5) patients but intragroup variability was too large for these differences to reach significance using a parametric evaluation. Patients may have difficulty complying with the two key requirements at once: to be productive and to avoid repetitions (which call for continuous self-monitoring). If they are conscientious they produce either many patterns with a few repetition errors or relatively fewer but nonrepeating patterns; if they are not conscientious they go as fast as they can with frequent repetitions and occasional omissions. Generally, the greatest productivity with fewest perseverations is achieved by persons who quickly develop and then maintain a strategy so that each square no longer calls for a unique solution but rather, the pattern for a long series of squares has been predetermined by the strategy. This test also allows the examiner to see concretely the development and/or the disintegration of strategy. Both Alzheimer patients with mild to moderate dementia and Parkinson patients without dementia have reduced Figural Fluency scores (Fama, Sullivan, Shear, et al., 1998).

Design Fluency Test (Delis, Kaplan, and Kramer, 2001)

This design fluency test has three conditions, each allowing one minute for completion (see also p. 637). The first consists of squares with five asymmetrically positioned filled dots. The second condition introduces interference with five additional unfilled dots to be ignored. The third is a switch condition in which the patient is shown squares with five filled and five unfilled dots and asked to draw four straight lines alternating between filled and unfilled dots. Patients with frontal lobe lesions produced fewer designs than control subjects (Baldo et al., 2001). All participants produced fewer designs in the switch condition in which frontal patients did not show a disproportionate cost. No performance differences in side of lesion appeared for frontal patients.

Assessment of perseveration

Perseveration is one of the hallmarks of impaired capacity to shift responses easily and appropriately. Spe-

cific types of perseveration tend to appear within one response modality or kind of examination technique but may not show up in a different kind of examination or with a patient whose problems do not involve the modality in question (M.L. Albert and Sandson, 1986; E. Goldberg, 1986; E. Goldberg and Costa, 1986). For example, aphasic patients often produce word substitution errors that are perseverations of a previous response (N. Martin et al., 1998). When perseveration is suspected, or has been observed but needs concrete documentation, many tests can be useful, especially those which involve impaired response modalities.

To test for perseveration, the patient can be asked to copy and maintain alternating letters or patterns (see Fig. 16.11) or repetitive sequential patterns of hand movements with separate trials for each hand to determine whether there are laterality differences in hand control (e.g., see A.-L. Christensen, 1979; Luria, 1966, pp. 677–678). Luria (1966) gave patients a sheet of paper with several word series typed in rows such as "circle, circle, circle, cross, circle" or "square, cross, circle, cross, cross," with instructions to draw the indicated figure below each word as fast as possible (see E. Goldberg, 1986; E. Goldberg and Costa, 1986). Similar chains of verbal commands may also elicit perseverative tendencies. A variety of figures can be named in this manner, including the simple geometric forms, letters, and numbers (e.g., see Sandson and Albert's, 1987, *Stuck in Set Test*). E. Goldberg and Bilder (1987) described seven parameters of graphic figures that can enhance susceptibility to perseveration in subsequent copies of the figures: e.g., *closed/openness* refers to the

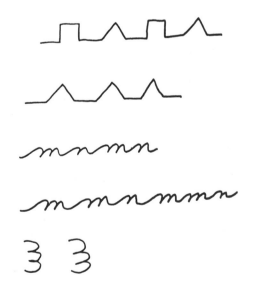

FIGURE 16.11 Repetitive patterns which subject is asked to maintain. Placing these patterns on the left side of a horizontally positioned letter-size sheet of paper allows ample space for the subject's drawings.

tendency to close an open figure (such as a cross) if drawn after a closed one (such as a circle); *straightness/curvedness,* a straight figure (a cross) drawn after a curved one (crescent moon) may be given curved features. Goldberg and Bilder also described four types of perseveration that can occur in simple drawing responses to these kinds of chained verbal commands: (1) *Hyperkinetic-like motor perseveration* refers to inability to terminate an elementary movement that continues in multiple overdrawings of single elements or continuation until stopped by the edge of the page. (2) In *perseveration of elements,* the patient can reproduce discrete elements but introduces elements of previously drawn figures into subsequent ones. (3) *Perseveration of features* involves the perpetuation of some characteristic of a previously drawn figure, such as "openness." (4) In *perseveration of activities,* different categories of stimuli, for example, words and numbers, mathematical and geometrical symbols, become confounded. These authors considered only type 1 to be a true motor perseveration.

Copying and drawing. Tasks that contain within them repeated elements tend to bring out perseverative tendencies; e.g., petals of a flower or many randomly placed lines (as in M.L. Albert's Test of Visual Neglect, p. 379; Sandson and Albert, 1984), rows of dots or circles (Bender-Gestalt Test, particularly cards 1, 2, and 6), or geometric figures (Benton Visual Retention Test). Also sensitive to perseveration are tasks involving writing to command or copying letters, numbers, or words. Perseverative patients often have difficulty in just writing the alphabet, a number series, or their address. Perseveration is least likely to show up in signatures as they are so overpracticed as to be automatic for almost all but the most impaired patients (see Fig. 16.12).

Perseveration in response set. The careful examiner will review all behavior samples, including responses to True-False and multiple-choice tests such as many personality inventories. Frankle (1996) identified a response set, "acquiescent perseveration," that characterized patients with cerebral damage as they tend to

have more runs of four or more True responses, including runs of nine or more, than do intact subjects or psychiatric patients without known brain disease. These latter groups rarely even reach, much less exceed, runs of nine.

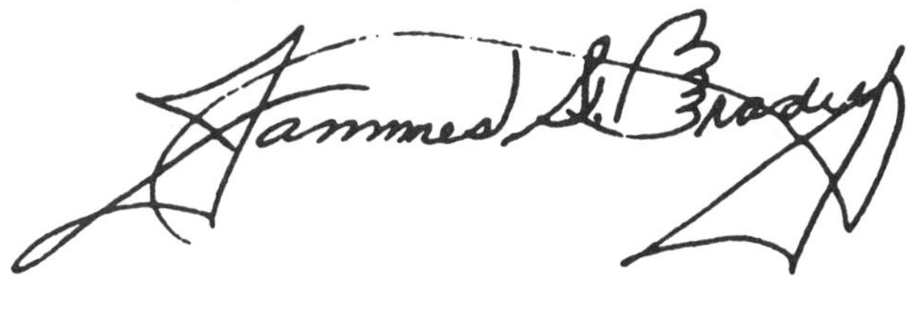

Examining motor regulation

Luria techniques. Many of the examination techniques in use today were described by Luria (1966), reported by A.-L. Christensen (1979), and incorporated into test protocols (e.g., Grigsby and Kaye, 1996 [see below]; Truelle, Le Gall, et al., 1988). When giving tasks designed to examine the capacity for motor regulation, the examiner must continue them long enough for defective responses to show up. Frequently, patients can maintain the correct response set for the first few sequences and only become confused or slip into a perseverative pattern after that. For example, Malloy, Webster, and Russell (1985) found that when giving Luria's alternating response tests, more than two-thirds of the errors occurred on the last five trials. They caution against giving few trials. If the patient's response deteriorates, the examiner should ask the patient to recall the instructions as patients with frontal lobe damage may be able to repeat the instructions accurately while continuing to respond incorrectly, thus demonstrating a dissociation between comprehension and action.

Of Luria's motor examination tasks, rapid finger sequencing (piano playing) and hand sequencing (fist–edge–palm,[1] see A.L. Christensen, 1979, p. 44) and successive oral movements (e.g., show teeth, stick out tongue, place tongue between lower teeth and lip; ibid., p. 46) were the most sensitive to frontal damage (Truelle, Le Gall, et al., 1995). Copying a series of rapidly presented, paced (by a metronome) hand movements (palm down, one finger out; palm up, all fingers out; fist with hand resting on side) was also sensitive to frontal damage and to temporal lesions (Jason, 1986). Patients with left hemisphere lesions due to stroke tended to have difficulty controlling hand postures, moving rapidly through a repetitive or mixed-movement sequence, and ordering mixed movements sequentially as they were prone to error and perseverations (Harrington and Haaland, 1991a).

Impaired regulation of motor responses can be elicited by tests in which the patient must make converse responses to the examiner's alternating signals (A.-L. Christensen, 1979; Luria, 1966; Luria and Homskaya, 1964). For example, if the examiner taps once, the patient must tap twice and vice versa; or if the ex-

FIGURE 16.12 Signature of middle-aged man who had sustained a gunshot wound to the right frontal lobe.

[1]A.S. Kaufman and Kaufman (1983) provide graded difficulty levels from age 2½ by varying position presentation and length of sequences (from 2 to 5).

aminer presses a buzzer to give a long signal, the patient must press for a short signal. Patients with self-regulation problems may irresistibly follow the examiner's response pattern.

Withholding responses (the "Go/no-go" paradigm) also examines motor regulation. In these formats the subject must respond to only one of two signals (e.g., squeeze the examiner's hand at the word "red," with instructions to not react when the examiner says "green") (A.-L. Christensen, 1979). This technique and one requiring converse responses (Competing Programs) brought to light motor regulation deficits in Parkinson patients (Raskin, Borod, and Tweedy, 1992).

Behavioral Dyscontrol Scale (BDS)[1] (Grigsby, Kaye, and Robbins, 1992; Grigsby and Kaye, 1996)

This brief bedside examination was designed to measure ability to regulate purposeful behavior, based on the work of Luria. Seven of the nine items measure motor control (including motor sequencing and a go/no-go challenge), one item consists of alphanumeric sequencing, and one rates insight. With the exception of the 4-point scale for the item rating insight, each item is scored on a 3-point scale. The manual provides detailed administration and scoring descriptions. Normative data are based on 1310 adults with a mean age of 74 years. Test–retest reliability, though high, was computed on a sample too small to carry much weight. Interrater reliabilities (obtained on several small samples) ranged from .84 to .98 for individual items, .98 for the total score. Of a large-scale sample (1,313 persons in the 60 to 99 age range), correlations for age and education were −.36 and .52, respectively (Grigsby, Kaye, Shetterly, et al., 2002).

Neuropsychological findings. Although originally designed to assess deficits that trouble many elderly persons, these brief tasks have demonstrated problems in younger patients with chronic progressive multiple sclerosis (Grigsby, Kravcisin, et al., 1993). Studies have related BDS scores to the everyday functional competence of elderly persons. BDS scores correlated significantly with poststroke patients' activities of daily living (ADLs) (e.g., −.38 Using the toilet; −.37 Bathing; −.36 Bed and chair transfers) (Grigsby, Kaye, Kowalsky, and Kramer, 2002). Similar findings (with somewhat higher correlations) are reported for elderly medical and surgical patients (Grigsby, Kaye, Eilertsen, and Kramer, 2000). The BDS also predicted functional independence

for a group of 68 mostly geriatric patients who had either orthopedic or neurological disorders three months after hospital discharge (Suchy et al., 1997).

Executive Control Battery (ECB) (E. Goldberg, Podell, Bilder, and Jaeger, 2000)

The four tests in this battery derive from the work of Luria. The *Graphical Sequences Test* involves drawing sequences of simple figures following verbal commands. The items include circle–square–triangle–cross, numerals, and other overlearned objects such as a flower, a car, or a house. Subjects might be asked to "write a number" or "write a number in words." Productions are scored for the presence of four types of perseveration: hyperkinetic motor perseveration and perseveration of elements, features, and activities. The *Manual Postures Test* assesses ability to imitate various asymmetrical hand postures. Errors are scored according to whether they are *echopraxic* (reproducing what is seen rather than making the called-for left–right switch to duplicate the examiner's posture) or visuospatial distortions. The *Motor Sequence Test* requires rapid alteration of both simple and complex unimanual and bimanual motor sequences. Performance is judged for motor perseverations, stereotypies, and other deficits of sequential motor organization. The *Competing Programs Test* examines ability to respond to commands under conflict conditions. Like other tests in the battery, responses are scored for echopraxia, behavioral sterotypies, and disinhibition.

A shortened version of the Graphical Sequences Test has been used to study perseverative behavior in patients with mild dementia from Alzheimer's disease and vascular disease (Lamar et al., 1997). While both groups produced more perseverations than control subjects, the group with vascular disease made more perseverations than the Alzheimer patients.

Frontal Assessment Battery (FAB) (Dubois, Slachevsky, et al., 2000)

This brief set of tests consists of a few items examining each of the following: conceptualization (similarities on three items: *banana–orange, table–chair, tulip–rose–daisy*), item generation (letter fluency: *S*), motor sequencing (Luria's "fist–edge–palm"), sensitivity to interference (conflict task), inhibitory control (go/no-go task), and environmental autonomy (i.e., testing for imitation or utilization behavior). Tasks are described in an appendix to the article. The estimated examination time is 10 minutes. The authors reported good interrater reliability and internal consistency. Total score differentiated patients with frontal lobe dis-

---

[1]The manual can be ordered from Jim Grigsby, Ph.D., University of Colorado Health Sciences Center, 1355 S. Colorado Blvd, #306, Denver, CO 80222. (e-mail: jim.grigsby@uchsc.edu tasks)

orders from control subjects with 89% accuracy. No comparison was made between patients with anterior and posterior lesions, so the "frontal" sensitivity of this test has not been examined.

Perseverance

Problems with perseverance may also compromise any kind of mental or motor activity. Inability to persevere can result from distractibility, or it may reflect impaired self-control usually associated with frontal lobe damage. In the former case, ongoing behavior is interrupted by some external disturbance; in the latter, dissolution of ongoing activity seems to come from within as the patient loses interest, slows down, or gives up. *Motor impersistence*, the inability to sustain discrete voluntary motor acts on command, tends to occur in those patients with right hemisphere or bilateral cortical damage who display fairly severe mental impairment, although some patients with left hemisphere lesions may also display the phenomenon (Joynt et al., 1962; Kertesz, Nicholson, et al., 1985; Pimental and Kingsbury, 1989). Motor impersistence of Alzheimer patients did not correlate with any specific cognitive domain, such as attention, memory, language, visuoperception, or visuoconstructional abilities (O.L. Lopez, Becker, and Boller, 1991).

The *Motor Impersistence* battery contains eight brief tests with origins in the neurological examination (Joynt et al., 1962; Benton, Siran, Hamsher, et al., 1994): (1) keeping eyes closed; (2) protruding tongue, blindfolded; (3) protruding tongue, eyes open; (4) fixating gaze in lateral visual fields; (5) keeping mouth open; (6) fixating on examiner's nose (during confrontation testing of visual fields); (7) sustaining "ah" sound; and (8) maintaining grip. Motor impersistence may also show up when patients are asked to hold their breath. Of course, not all impersistent patients will fail all eight tests. Only three patients of 24 left hemiplegic patients failed tongue protrusion while 20 could not maintain a fixated gaze (Ben-Yishay, Diller, Gerstman, and Haas, 1968). The proportion of patients failing these tasks increased in the same order as task difficulty, as determined by Joynt and his coworkers (1962). Such an orderly progression suggests a common underlying deficit that occurs with varying degrees of severity. The number of tests failed also reflected severity of impairment as documented by measurements of cognitive abilities, visuomotor efficiency, and functional competence (Ben-Yishay, Diller, Gerstman, and Haas, 1968). Limb impersistence, demonstrated when the patient cannot maintain arm extension for 20 secs., may be lateralized (Heilman and Watson, 1991). When impersistence is pronounced in patients with right

hemisphere dysfunction, rehabilitation prospects are poor (Joynt and Goldstein, 1975).

Effective Performance

A performance is as effective as the performer's ability to monitor, self-correct, and regulate the intensity, tempo, and other qualitative aspects of delivery. Patients with brain disorders often perform erratically and unsuccessfully since abilities for self-correction and self-monitoring are vulnerable to many different kinds of brain damage. Some patients cannot correct their mistakes because they do not perceive them. Patients with pathological inertia may perceive their errors, even identify them, and yet do nothing to correct them. Defective self-monitoring can spoil any kind of performance, showing up in such diverse ways as unmowed patches in an otherwise manicured lawn, one or two missed numbers in an account book, or shoelaces that snapped and buttons that popped from too much pressure.

Testing performance effectiveness

While few examination techniques have been developed for the express purpose of studying self-monitoring or self-correcting behavior, all test performances provide information about how the subject responds. The nature of the patient's errors, attitudes (including awareness and judgment of errors), idiosyncratic distortions, and compensatory efforts will often give more practical information about the patient than test scores that can mask either defects or compensatory strengths. In a neuropsychological examination, self-monitoring defects may appear in cramped writing that leaves little or no space between words or veers off the horizontal; in missed or slipped (e.g., answers to item 9 on line 10) responses on paper-and-pencil tests; in speech that comes in quick little bursts or a monotonic, unpunctuated delivery; and in incomplete sentences and thoughts that trail off or are disconnected or easily disrupted by internal or external distractions. Tests in which subjects can check their written responses for accuracy as they are working on them, such as arithmetic calculations, symbol substitution tests, and drawing fluency tasks, will readily expose poor self-monitoring.

Random Generation Task (Baddeley, 1966, 1986)

The subject is asked to generate a sequence of 100 letters of the alphabet in random order. Initial studies used four rates of generation: 0.5, 1.0, 2.0, and 4.0 sec. Although the task may sound easy, even normal subjects find it difficult to avoid either stereotyped sequences (e.g., X–Y–Z) or common combinations (e.g.,

F–B–I) or omitting responses. Output was measured in three ways: the frequency of each letter, which detected redundancy in the output; the frequency of letter pairs (*digrams*), again looking for redundancy; and the frequency of letter pairs in alphabetical sequence (*stereotyped digrams*). A small group of control subjects consistently increased randomness of output as generation rates slowed. As in fluency tests which forbid repetition, self-monitoring is necessary for success on this task; when self-monitoring fails, this task will be failed.

Other random generation tasks include random generation of numbers based on the work of F.J. Evans (1978). In the initial version, subjects are instructed to say numbers from 1 to 10 in random order at the same rate as a metronome's beat (1/sec). The sequence of 100 numbers is recorded. A significant practice effect has been reported (Marisi and Travlos, 1992). Since most subjects develop a strategy after a brief experience with this task, the authors recommend discarding first trial data. Another variation is the *Mental Dice Task* in which subjects are asked to "call out digits (from 1 to 6) in a sequence as random as possible" such as might appear when rolling a die repeatedly (Brugger, Monsch, et al., 1996). Even moderately demented patients were able to understand this instruction. As with letter generation, the task requires suppression of habitual and stereotyped responses plus response monitoring (Miyake et al., 2000).

Various random generation tasks have been used to examine patients with brain disorders. Clinical studies suggest that patients with frontal lobe dysfunction are impaired on these tasks as they demonstrate a strong sequential response bias (Brugger, 1997). Deficits have been observed in patients with anterior communicating artery aneurysms (Leclercq et al., 2000), Korsakoff's syndrome (Pollux et al., 1995), and degenerative diseases such as Alzheimer's (Brugger, Monsch, et al., 1996) and Parkinson's (R.G. Brown, Soliveri, and Jahanshahi, 1998). Transcranial magnetic stimulation over the left dorsolateral prefrontal cortex interfered with randomness on a letter generation task (Jahanshahi and Dirnberger, 1999).

Executive Functions: Wide Range Assessment

Some techniques for examining executive functions involve so many of them that they defy classification under any one of the subdivisions. Of course, naturalistic observation is chief among these; but since few examiners have the time and resources to spend the hours or days needed to know the status of their patients' executive behavior, these clinical methods may serve as useful substitutes for the real thing.

Behavioural Assessment of the Dysexecutive Syndrome (BADS) (B.A. Wilson, Alderman, et al., 1996)

This set of tests was developed to examine performance on a wide range of real-world tasks. All but one of the six tests are question-and-answer or paper-and-pencil tests; much of the content will be familiar to most subjects. The *Rule Shift Cards* test assesses flexibility by having subjects view playing cards and respond under two "rule" conditions: in the first condition the subject is instructed to say "yes" if a presented card is red and "no" if it is black. After a series of cards has been shown, the instructions change such that, for each card, the subject should say "yes" if it is the same color as the previous card and "no" if it is not. The *Action Program Test* instructs subjects to figure a way to get a cork out of a tube with a variety of objects at their disposal. Subjects must develop a plan and then try to get the cork out by manipulating materials such as water in a beaker and a metal hook. The *Key Search Test* asks the subject to draw a plan for finding a lost key in a square-shaped area (see also *Plan of Search* [Terman and Merrill, 1973]). The *Temporal Judgement Test* asks four questions concerning estimations on how long activities take. Planning an effective route through a zoo in order to visit certain sites is assessed with the *Zoo Map Test*. Planning and priority setting are also assessed with the *Modified Six Elements Test* in which subjects are instructed to complete as many paper-and-pencil tasks (e.g., simple calculations, naming pictures) as possible in a brief time while attempting at least something from each of the test's six parts. Performance is judged by how well subjects organize their time. The *Dysexecutive Questionnaire* (DEX) is a 20-item symptom checklist which both the patient and a collateral source complete. The manual reports very high inter-rater reliability (ranging from .88 on Temporal Judgement to 1.00 on the number of tasks passed independently). Test–retest reliability was best for the Action Program, Key Search, and Temporal Judgement tests (*r* = .64–.71), lower for the other tests.

Neuropsychological findings. Comparing means and standard deviations of a group of patients with brain disorders (primarily TBI) with a group of control subjects, all of the tests showed group differences although the Key Search difference was only marginal. Norris and Tate (2000) also compared a patient group with control subjects using nonparametric analysis because the variables were not normally distributed. Group differences appeared for Action Program, Zoo Map, Modified Six Elements, and the total profile. The remaining three tests did not show group differences. These groups differed on only two of the commonly used tests purporting to examine executive skills: the Porteus Mazes and Controlled Oral Word Association Test. They showed no differences on the Wisconsin Card Sorting Test (WCST), Trail Making Test, Complex Figure Test, and Cognitive Estimation Test. The BADS total score correctly classified 84% of control subjects and 64% of patients, which compared favorably with the commonly used tests (81% and 64%, respectively). Concurrent validity was adequate for the Rule Shift and Action Plan tests and the total profile score. Schizophrenic patients also are impaired on the BADS (Krabbendam et al., 1999; B.A. Wilson, Evans, Emslie, et al., 1998).

Delis-Kaplan Executive Function System (D-KEFS) (Delis, Kaplan, and Kramer, 2001)

The D-KEFS is a set of nine tests, each intended to stand alone. There is no composite score. The authors state that tests were selected to be sensitive to many of the types of executive impairment seen in patients with brain disorders. However, no theoretical rationale, other than inclusion of both verbal and nonverbal tests, is provided for their selection. D-KEFS's *Trail Making Test, Verbal Fluency* (letter and category), *Design Fluency, Color-Word Interference Test* (Stroop conflict task), *Sorting Test, Twenty Questions Test, Tower Test,* and *Proverb Test* are, for the most part, variations on the most commonly used tests purporting to examine executive function. The *Word Context Test* was developed by Dr. Kaplan in the 1940s to test children's understanding of words. Card-Sorting, Twenty Questions, Proverb, and Word Context tests are discussed in Chapter 15; Design Fluency is reviewed in this chapter. The authors state that one advantage of the D-KEFS tests is that they are co-normed on 1750 participants ranging in age from 8 to 89. An alternate form with normative data from a sample of 295 subjects is available for Verbal Fluency, Sorting, and Twenty Questions. Raw scores can be converted to standard scores or, in some cases, cumulative percentile ranks. Scoring software is available for $163.

Many of the standard tests have been lengthened in this version, with additional easy and difficult items to avoid ceiling and floor effects, and with subtests that break down performances into the fundamental components required for success on these complex tasks. One can compute an astounding number of scores for many of the tests. The Trail Making Test alone has 12 primary measures and 12 optional ones. The Sorting Test has five primary measures and 29 additional ones. Whether the many additional features are worth the patient's extra effort and the examiner's extra time for administration and scoring has not been established.

Whereas the principal scores generally have acceptable reliability, the additonal D-KEFS scores often have low reliability which varies across age groups. For example, the manual reports that the newly added switching condition of the Design Fluency test has test–retest reliabilities varying with age groups from .13 to .58. Scores on the second testing were higher and appear to represent a practice effect. Although scores from the more standard conditions for this test also showed a practice effect, test–retest correlations were considerably higher (ranging from .43 to .73). For some of the nine tests, standard deviations of test–retest scores were larger for the second testing, which suggests weak reliability. Internal consistency scores, calculated for some tests, varied by age group. Some examples of the median internal consistency scores for the entire normative group are: Verbal Fluency Test, Category Switching condition = .54; Sorting Test, Free Sorting Confirmed condition = .78; Twenty Questions Test, Total Weighted Achievement score = .45; Tower Test, Total Achievement score = .61; and Proverb Test, Total Achievement score, Free Inquiry condition = .78. Overall, the internal consistency reliability coefficients are lower than might be desired. Correlations between performances of a small sample on the D-KEFS tests and the Wisconson Card Sorting Test produced coefficients ranging from .30 to .60 for WCST "categories achieved" and .20 to .71 for WCST "perseverative responses." The strongest correlation was between the Proverb Test Total Achievement score and the WCST perseverative responses.

The clinical usefulness of these modifications of familiar tests is largely unknown. The manual presents data for nine Alzheimer and nine Huntington patients. In a study using the verbal and design fluency tests, participants were tested in the standard manner and for their ability to switch back and forth between different sets (e.g., alternating between naming exemplars of fruit and furniture for the verbal fluency tests) (Baldo, Shimamura, Delis, et al., 2001). Patients with focal frontal lobe lesions did not have more difficulty than control subjects with the new switching condition for either fluency test. By far the most studied of the tests is the Card Sorting Test; a similar version—the California Card Sorting Test—has been in use since 1992 (Delis, Squire, et al., 1992; see also pp. 585–586). Compared to control subjects, multiple sclerosis patients made fewer attempted sorts and fewer correct sorts (Beatty and Monson, 1996). In this study, Correct Free Sorts showed a modest correlation (.64) with categories achieved on the WCST. Perseverative responding on the two tests did not appear to be related ($r = .15$). Patients with frontal lesions produced fewer attempted sorts, correct sorts, and correct sort descriptions than control subjects, while Parkinson patients differed from control subjects only in making more perseverative sorts (Dimitrov et al., 1999).

Standard versions of the Trail Making Test, verbal fluency, twenty questions, and proverb interpretation are in the public domain.

Executive Function Route-Finding Task (EFRT) (Boyd and Sautter, 1993)

To accomplish this task subjects must find their way from a starting point to a predetermined destination within the building complex in which the examination is given (see also Sohlberg and Mateer, 2001). For a practical level of difficulty, the final destination must be a minimum of five choice points and one change in floor level away from the starting place. Ideally, there will be signs giving directions for the destination.

For example, my [mdl] patients begin on the third floor of the clinic building and have as their goal the cafeteria in University Hospital South across a street (by way of the street or an enclosed bridge) and at least five choice points away (first corridor: right, left, or straight; if right, elevator, stairs, or corridor, etc.) and, while also on a third floor, this cafeteria is seven floors below the clinic third floor (the hospital and clinics are built on a hill). The clinic building has numerous signs indicating the direction to Hospital South; Hospital South has signs for the cafeteria. Halls and elevators are full of both visitors and medical center personnel providing ample opportunities for the patient to ask directions.

While accompanying the patient the examiner records the path taken and how the patient gets there. The examiner also answers questions and gives encouragement and advice as needed, noting these too. After reaching the destination, the examiner may need to question the patient further to clarify whether moves were made by chance, what cues the patient used to find the way, etc. Performances are rated on a 4-point scale to measure the degree to which the patient was dependent on the examiner for (1) understanding the task; (2) seeking information; (3) remembering instructions; (4) detecting errors; (5) correcting errors; and (6) ability to stick with the task (on-task behavior).

Two examiners participated in the feasibility study with high ($r = .94$) interrater reliability indicating that this is a very scorable task. Scores obtained by 31 rehabilitation patients with varying degrees of TBI severity correlated well ($p < .01$) with both the Verbal Comprehension and Perceptual Organization factor scores of the WAIS-R and a shortened form of the Booklet Category Test. In general, these patients were mostly dependent on nonspecific executive cues (e.g., examiner questioning guided patients on how they might begin or what information they needed next) but they also required directed cueing.

Spikman and her colleagues (2000) used this task to study planning by patients with chronic TBI of at least moderate severity. The two scores they obtained were the number of times patients needed cues and a score combining the adequacy of information seeking, error detection, and error correction. Like the original study, they found high interrater reliability ($r > .90$). The EFRT was the only one of a number of executive tasks on which the patients performed significantly worse than control subjects. Patients with documented frontal lesions had even more difficulty than those without frontal damage. The authors attributed this test's sensitivity to its lack of structure and the need for participants to seek information and to detect and correct errors.

Behavioral Assessment for Vocational Skills (BAVS): Wheelbarrow Test (R.W. Butler, Anderson, et al., 1989)

This ingenious and quite naturalistic examination technique requires the subject to assemble the parts of a mail-order wheelbarrow within a 45 minute period. The clinicians who rate the performance also play the role of job supervisor and, although they offer as little structure as possible, they can become more directive if the subject's limitations require help to stay on task or complete it. Distractibility problems are elicited by interjecting a "brief alternate task" and then redirecting the subject's attention back to the wheelbarrow. A rater/supervisor also gives one constructive criticism in response to an error to see how the subject deals with criticism. Performances are rated on a 5-point scale for 16 vocationally relevant aspects, such as following directions, problem solving, emotional control, judgment, and dependability.

Ratings on this task did not correlate significantly with visuospatial test scores, visual tracking (Trail Making Test), or the Wisconsin Card Sorting Test. However, they did predict the levels of three categories of work performances by 20 TBI patients in volunteer trial work settings: work quantity ($r = .74$), work quality ($r = .75$), and work-related behavior ($r = .64$) (all correlations were significant at $p < .01$).

MOTOR PERFORMANCE[1]

Distinctions between disturbances of motor behavior resulting from a supramodal executive dysfunction and specific disorders of motor functions are clearer in the telling than in fact. A defective sequence of alternating

[1]We are grateful to Kathleen Y. Haaland for her helpful contributions to this section.

hand movements, for example, may occur—with a cortical lesion—as a specific disability of motor coordination or it may reflect perseveration or inability to sustain a motor pattern; or it may be a symptom of subcortical rather than cortical pathology (Heilman and Rothi, 2003). Some diagnostic discriminations can be made from observations of the defective movement, but the classification of a particular disability may also depend on whether the pattern of associated symptoms implicates a cerebellar or a frontal lesion, whether the disorder appears bilaterally or involves one side only, or whether it may reflect a sensory deficit or motor weakness rather than a disorder of movement per se. Many motor disorders that accompany cerebral brain damage cannot, by themselves, necessarily be linked with particular anatomic areas.

Examining for Apraxia

The examination for apraxia reviews a variety of learned movements of the face, the limbs, and—less often—the body (Goodglass, Kaplan, and Barresi, 2000; Heilman and Rothi, 2003; Strub and Black, 2000). The integrity of learned movements of the face and limbs, particularly the hands, is typically examined under two conditions: *imitation* of the examiner (*a*) making symbolic or communicative movements, such as familiar gestures; (*b*) using actual objects; or (*c*) pantomiming their use without objects; and *to command* for each of these three kinds of activity. A tactile modality can be introduced by blindfolding patients and handing them such familiar objects as a glass, a screwdriver, a key, or a comb, with instructions to "show me how you would use it" (De Renzi, Faglioni, and Sorgato, 1982). Table 16.4 lists activities that have been used in examinations for apraxia. The examiner may demonstrate each activity for imitation or direct its performance,

asking the subject to "do what you see me doing" or "show me how you . . . . " Some of these activities should involve the use of objects, either with the object or in pantomime . The examiner should be alert to those patients who are not apraxic but, when pantomiming to command, use their hand as if it were the tool (e.g., hammering with their fists, cutting with fingers opening and closing like scissors blades). The concreteness of their response reflects their concreteness of thought. This use of a body part as object occurs more commonly among brain damaged patients without regard to lesion laterality than in neurologically intact persons (Mozaz et al., 1993).

The difficulty in knowing just what to score and how to score it probably explains why no scoring system has achieved general acceptance. Five different systems give some idea of the range of scoring possibilities:

1. Haaland and Flaherty (1984) developed a scoring system for a 15-item battery of movements to imitation: five transitive movements (e.g., brush teeth), five intransitive movements (e.g., salute), and five meaningless movements (e.g., index finger to ear lobe). They recorded errors in hand position, arm position, and target. Patients are designated "apraxic" if they make four or more errors on this 15-item battery (i.e., 2 SD below control subjects' mean) (Haaland, Harrington, and Knight, 2000). Normative data for 75 control subjects are available.

2. A 14-category scoring system which takes into account errors of content, of timing (including sequencing), of a spatial nature (e.g., change in amplitude of movements, body-part-as-object), and of "other" error (including no response) brought out six error types occurring most typically with left cortical lesions: they involved spatial distortions—including body-part-as-object; incorrect spatial relationships between the hand and fingers; incorrect spatial relationships between the hand and the imagined object; incorrect movement with the imagined object; changes in number of movements normally called for; and correct response to the wrong target

TABLE 16.4 Activities for Examining Practic Functions

	Use of Objects	Symbolic Gestures	Other
Face (Buccofacial)	Blow out match	Stick out tongue	Whistle
	Suck on straw	Blow a kiss	Show teeth
Upper Limb	Use toothbrush	Salute	Snap fingers
	Hammer nail	Hitchhike	Touch ear with index finger
	Cut paper	"OK" sign	Hold up thumb and little finger
	Flip coin	"Stop" sign	Make a fist
Lower Limb	Kick ball		
	Put out cigarette		
Whole Body	Swing baseball bat	Bow	Stand (or sit)
	Sweep with broom	Stand like boxer	Turn around
Serial Acts (can be done in pantomine or with real objects)	Preparing a letter for mailing (fold letter, put in envelope, seal and stamp envelope)		

(e.g., combing movements for "hairbrush") (Rothi, Mack, Verfaellie, et al., 1988).

3. Poeck (1986) offered a five-part assessment scheme based on a qualitative analysis of errors for a lengthy series of movements: correct execution, augmentation phenomena, fragmentary movement, perseveration, and other types of errors. The number of perseverations is not scored as they tend to occur as intrusive motor elements of the perseverated movement rather than in the original complete form of the movement. (This observation may account for Rothi, Mack, and their colleagues' report that perseveration errors occurred too rarely for consideration, since they did not provide a scoring category for partial perseverations.)

4. Another scoring system gives 3, 2, or 1 points to a correct imitation made on a first, second, or third trial, respectively, and no points when the patient does not achieve the correct movement within three trials (De Renzi, Motti, and Nichelli, 1980). Thus, with a 24-item protocol, the maximum possible score is 72.

5. Based on good interrater agreement, and most practical for clinical work, Goodglass, Kaplan, and Baressi (2000) offer a 3-point judgment of "normal," "partially adequate," and "failed" which can be expanded to four points: "perfect," "adequate," "partially adequate," and "inadequate" (Borod, Fitzpatrick, et al., 1989).

Task characteristics. Age tends to have some effect on the quality of pantomimed movements as a substantial portion of over-60 healthy subjects may make body-part-as-object responses (L. Willis et al., 1998). The number of these and other, less frequent errors varies with the task (Ska and Nespoulos, 1987, 1988b); for example, some movements (e.g., scratching one's back) become more difficult as flexibility diminishes (Ska and Nespoulos, 1986). That R.J. Duffy and Duffy (1989) found no difference in the frequency of body-part-as-object responses between patients with right and those with left lateralized brain lesions and normal control subjects, all compared in groups in which the average age was over 60, suggests that age may be more of a determinant in the appearance of this error type than lesion presence or lateralization. The range of activities tested enables the examiner to assess the extent and severity of the disorder. Apraxia is more common for transitive movements (object use) than other movements (intransitive, meaningless), which may relate to the complexity of these movements or their dependence on object use (Haaland and Flaherty, 1984).

Neuropsychological findings. Apraxia may occur as the result of focal lesions or degenerative diseases. Among patients with unilateral lesions, most apraxias of use and gesture affect both sides of the body but typically occur with lesions in the left cerebral cortex (De Renzi, 1990; Schnider et al., 1997). Studying stroke patients with lesions in anterior or posterior regions, Haaland, Harrington, and Knight (2000) found that those

with *ideomotor limb apraxia* (inability to make correct gestures on command) "had damage lateralized to a left hemispheric network involving the middle frontal gyrus and intraparietal sulcus region." This finding supports the importance of the frontoparietal circuits in reaching and grasping movements (Heilman and Rothi, 2003). In an earlier study, Haaland and Yeo (1989) noted that patients with left parietal lesions are impaired on hand posture tasks, whether single or sequenced, but impaired performances by frontal patients were reported only in some studies.

Degenerative disorders such as Alzheimer's disease, Parkinson's disease, Huntington's disease, and corticobasal degeneration may also produce apraxia (Hamilton et al., 2003; D.H. Jacobs et al., 1999; Leiguarda et al., 1997; R.L. Schwartz, 2000; L. Willis et al., 1998).

Apraxia may occur in only one or two modalities, usually with visual (imitation) or verbal (command) presentation; rarely will apraxia be purely tactile (De Renzi, Faglioni, and Sorgato, 1982). While failure is more likely in the command than the imitation condition (Goodglass and Kaplan, 1983), the opposite can occur (Rothi, Mack, and Heilman, 1986; Rothi, Ochipa, and Heilman, 1991). Patients exhibiting apraxia on a test will also tend to have reduced recourse to gestural communication (Borod, Fitzpatrick, et al., 1989). Testing for movement imitation and oral apraxia over periods greater than two years from onset, A. Basso and her colleagues (2000) reported that all but one of 14 patients improved significantly during the first year after onset. Little further improvement occurred and six worsened after the first year.

Florida Apraxia Screening Test-Revised (FAST-R)
(Rothi, Raymer, and Heilman, 1997)

This revision of the original test consists of 30 verbal commands to demonstrate gestures. Twenty items involve object use (transitive) and ten require meaningful, tool-free gestures (intransitive) such as , "Show me how you salute." All items can be completed with one arm/hand; usually, the dominant hand is examined. A practice trial shows the patient the expected degree of precision and elaboration of movement. Productions are scored for content, temporal features, and spatial features. The score is the number of items performed correctly.

Florida Action Recall Test (FLART)
(R.L. Schwartz et al., 2000)

In some cases apraxia may represent a loss of knowledge about the action necessary to use an object. The FLART was designed to assess this type of conceptual apraxia. It consists of 45 drawings of objects placed in scenes implying an action, such as a slice of toast with a pad of just melting butter on top. Instructions include asking subjects to imagine what tool would be needed to act upon the object and to pantomime the action associated with that tool in relation to the drawing. Patients are instructed to pantomime tool use and told that using a hand to complete the action without the assistance of a tool (hand error) is unacceptable. The total score is the number of items for which the pantomime was interpretable and deemed correct. Interrater reliability was very good (*Kappa* = .97). Patients with mild to moderate Alzheimer's disease scored significantly worse than control subjects. With no time limit, the control group's time to completion was approximately 12 min; for patients with mild to moderate Alzheimer's disease, time to completion ranged from 10 to 43 min. Using 32/45 as a cut-off score, nine of the 12 Alzheimer patients were impaired while none of the 21 control subjects performed below this score. Conceptual apraxia has been found in other studies of Alzheimer patients using different tasks (Dumont et al., 2000).

Test for Apraxia (van Heugten, Dekker, Deelman, et al., 1999)

This test is based on the seminal work by De Renzi in evaluating patients with apraxia. Nine objects are used in testing the ability to pantomime their use on verbal command: first with objects absent and then with objects present, plus demonstration of the actual use of objects. Also included are six items asking for imitation of the examiner's gestures, oral (e.g., blowing out a candle) and hand (e.g., making a fist) gestures as well as closing eyes. A study of 44 stroke patients with apraxia, 35 stroke patients without apraxia, and 50 control subjects demonstrated good construct validity for this test. Its sensitivity and specificity in detecting apraxia were greater than 80%. Assessing object use was more sensitive than imitation of gestures.

Neuropsychological Assessment of Motor Functions

The motor dysfunctions within the purview of neuropsychology are those that can occur despite intact capacity for normal movement. They also have an intentional component that makes them psychological data, unlike reflex jerks, for example, or the random flailing of a delirious patient.

Motor tasks have long been used as indicators of lesion lateralization (G. Goldstein, 1974; Reitan, 1966). On speed or strength tests, it has been assumed that pronounced deviation below a 10% advantage for the dominant hand reflects lateralized brain damage on the side contralateral to the dominant hand, while a much larger dominant hand advantage may implicate a brain lesion contralateral to the nondominant hand (Jarvis and Barth, 1994; Reitan and Wolfson, 1993; see pp. 642, 645). A recommendation that lateralized brain damage is likely when either the nonpreferred hand performance exceeds that of the preferred hand or the preferred hand performance exceeds that of the nonpreferred hand by 20% (e.g., Golden, 1978a) has been seriously questioned. L.L. Thompson, Heaton, Matthews, and Grant (1987) found that this rule would misclassify as having lateralized hemisphere dysfunction up to 18% of left-handed normal subjects on the Finger Tapping Test, as many as 36% of this group on the Grooved Pegboard, and almost 50% of them on the Hand Dynamometer (Grip Strength) test. While misclassifications were greatest for left-handed subjects, around 20% of intact right-handed subjects would be labeled as having "Dominant hemisphere dysfunction" on the basis of the Hand Dynamometer and Grooved Pegboard scores, and 18% would fall into the "Nondominant hemisphere dysfunction" category (see also pp. 305–306). Moreover, mean variations for 26 normal subject groups (*n*s from 10 to 1,128) on the Hand Dynamometer have ranged from dominant > nondominant by 16.5% to nondominant > dominant by 3.3% (for five groups, mean nondominant strength exceeded dominant), leading Bohannon (2003) to conclude that, "Available information may be insufficient to justify using between-side comparisons to make judgments about grip-strength impairment" (p. 728).

Thus findings on speed and strength tests have to be interpreted with caution. Bornstein (1986b,c) found that 25% to 30% of right-handed normal subjects had intermanual discrepancies that exceeded these expectations on at least one speed or strength test; 26% of the normal males and 34% of the females showed no difference or a nondominant hand advantage, again on at least one test; but virtually none of the control subjects had significantly discrepant performances on two or three different motor tests. Right-handed patients with lateralized lesions also displayed considerable variability: those with right brain damage generally conformed to discrepancy expectations (i.e., slowed left hand) more consistently than those with left lateralized lesions, and more than half of the right-damaged patients displayed the intermanual discrepancies expected with lateralized lesions on at least two of the three tests. These findings suggest that more than one motor skill test is required for generating hypotheses about lateralization; and when left hemisphere disease is suspected, the examiner must look to "other nonmotor tasks" (Bornstein, 1986b; see also Spreen and Strauss, 1998).

Further complicating the issue is R.[F.] Lewis and Kupke's (1992) report that patients with nonlateralized lesions tend to perform relatively less well with their nondominant hand because of sluggishness of that hand to adapt to a new task. Moreover, Bornstein (1986c) found sex differences in patterns of performance variability. And on the other hand—literally—Grafman, Smutok, and their colleagues (1985) reported that left-handers who had missile wounds to the brain displayed few residual motor skill deficits long after the injury, a finding that may reflect a less stringent pattern of functional lateralization which allows for greater functional plasticity.

Manual dexterity and strength

Many neuropsychologists include tests of manipulative agility in their examination batteries. These are timed speed tests[1] that either have an apparatus with a counting device or elicit a countable performance. These tests may aid in the detection of a lateralized disability, as may strength testing.

Finger Tapping Test (FTT) (Halstead, 1947; Reitan and Wolfson, 1993; Spreen and Strauss, 1998)

Probably the most widely used test of manual dexterity, this was originally—and by some is still—called the *Finger Oscillation Test*. It is one of the tests Halstead chose for his battery, and its score contributes to the Impairment Index. It consists of a tapping key with a device for recording the number of taps. Each hand makes five 10-sec trials with brief rest periods between trials. The score for each hand is the average for each set of five trials although some examiners give fewer or more trials (Mitrushina, Boone, and D'Elia, 1999; W.G. Snow, 1987b). Reitan and Wolfson (1993) recommend the average of five consecutive trials within a five tap range which may require more than five trials and even "as many as 10 trials in cases of extreme variability" (Jarvis and Barth, 1994). With normal control subjects, Gill and his colleagues (1986) found no fatigue effects on 10-trial administrations but did observe a small but significant increment for men—but not women—retested weekly for ten weeks.

Rosenstein and Van Sickle (1991) called attention to variations in finger tapping instruments which can result in significant performance differences. For example, the manually recording instrument sold with the Halstead-Reitan Battery (HRB) differs from the elec-

tronic tapper offered by Western Psychological Services (WPS) in that both the distance the tapper moves and the force required are greater for the former than the latter so that tapping rates run higher for the electronic model (Brandon et al., 1986). Moreover, the lever on the HRB tapper is to the right of the counting box, forcing the left hand into a relatively awkward posture compared with the right hand position. As a result, a right–left hand discrepancy shows up for left-handed persons who do not display the expected left-hand advantage with the HRB instrument (see also L.L. Thompson, Heaton, Matthews, and Grant, 1987), but do show it with the electronic tapper. Like the electronic tapper, a finger tapping program for computers (Loong, 1988) generated somewhat higher tapping scores than the HRB tapper (Whitfield and Newcombe, 1992).

Test characteristics. The 28 subjects who comprised Halstead's control group (see p. 673) averaged 50 taps per 10-second period for their right hand and 45 taps for their left. They provided the cut-off score standard (impaired ranges: ≤50 for the dominant hand, ≤44 for the nondominant hand) for more than a generation of HRB examinations. Some normative studies vary widely from these scores (see Mitrushina, Boone, and D'Elia, 1999), perhaps in part because different instruments were used, but also because demographic variables influence finger tapping speed significantly. Although faster tapping with the preferred hand is expected, Bornstein (1986c) found that 30% of males and 20% of females from the general population had faster nonpreferred to preferred hand tapping.

Both age and sex exert powerful effects on tapping speed: men consistently tap faster than women (Heaton, Grant, and Matthews, 1991;[2] Heaton, Ryan, et al., 1996; Mitrushina, Boone, and D'Elia, 1999). Slowing with age becomes prominent from about the fifth decade with greatly increasing decrements through subsequent decades. (See Ruff and Parker (1993[2]) for age × sex norms for four age groups from 16–24 to 55–70.) When applied to normal populations over age 60, the traditional cutting scores correctly identified as normal only 2% to 12% of women and 8% to 10% of men among healthy subjects in the 55 to 70 age range (Bornstein, Paniak, and O'Brien, 1987[2]) and produced similar proportions of false positive classifications—increasing with age and weighing heavily against women—in another large-scale normative study (Trahan, Patterson, et al., 1987[2]). Bornstein and his colleagues (1987) recommended lowering the cut-off scores to ≤33 and ≤32 for men's dominant and non-

---

[1] I [mdl] do not give speed-dependent motor tests to motorically slowed patients as I know in advance that they will do poorly and prefer to use our time for more informative testing—and thus also avoid frustrating or embarrassing these patients unnecessarily.

[2] Data reproduced in Mitrushina, Boone, and D'Elia, 1999.

dominant hands, respectively, and to ≤20 and ≤25 for women. These cutting scores would minimize false positive classifications greatly but also increase false negative cases.

Education effects are small, with privileged groups tending to perform a little better on average than is usually reported (Fromm-Auch and Yeudall, 1983[1]), while low levels of schooling are associated with slower tapping performances (Bernard, 1989; Bornstein, 1985[1]; Bornstein and Suga, 1988[1]; Heaton, Grant, and Matthews, 1991[1]; Heaton, Ryan, et al., 1996). Bornstein's (1985) age × education norms are also reported in Spreen and Strauss (1998). Higher education was associated with faster tapping in the oldest but not the youngest group (Bornstein, 1985). Averaged WAIS scores were not related to tapping speed in a large sample of normal subjects ranging in age from 19 to 71 years (Horton, 1999).

Reliability reports vary from study to study. Test–retest study data demonstrate this variability (McCaffery, Duff, and Westervelt, 2000b). The FTT appeared to be highly reliable ($r = .94$ for men, .86 for women) for a small sample of normal subjects retested in ten weekly sessions (Gill et al., 1986). Good but less impressive reliabilities were found for more than 60 healthy adults retested after six months ($r = .71, .76$, for preferred and nonpreferred hands, respectively) (Ruff and Parker, 1993) and for 384 healthy adults retested after two to 12 months ($r = .77, -.78$) (Dikmen, Heaton, et al., 1999). Retesting clinical samples (alcohol/trauma, schizophrenia, vascular disorder) at an average of two years between tests (interval range was 4 to 469 weeks) found reliability coefficients in the .64 to .87 range, with the higher coefficients for the nondominant hand (G. Goldstein and Watson, 1989). Four retests of epilepsy patients over six to 12 month intervals found the lowest correlation between the first two tests ($r = .77$, dominant hand), with correlations between retests 2, 3, and 4 all .90 or higher, suggesting a practice effect (Dodrill and Troupin, 1975). Even with Alzheimer patients, a small (ultimately, a 12% increase) but consistently growing practice effect appeared over five assessments at weekly intervals (Teng, Wimer, et al., 1989).

Neuropsychological findings. Brain disorders often, but not necessarily, tend to have a slowing effect on finger tapping rate (Haaland, Cleeland, and Carr, 1977; Reitan and Wolfson, 1996b; Stuss, Ely, et al., 1985). Lateralized lesions usually slow the tapping rate of the contralateral hand (G.G. Brown, Spicer, Robertson, et al., 1989; Haaland and Delaney, 1981; Reitan and Wolfson, 1994). However, these effects do not appear consistently because patients with posterior lesions may not show slowing. Because of inconsistent finger tapping findings, this test cannot be used as a sole indicator of the side of lesion.

Diffuse brain injury impedes rate of tapping, even one year after injury (Haaland, Temkin, Randahl, and Dikmen, 1994). In contrast, grip strength recovered to the normal range in this group of TBI patients with varying injury severity. These findings were interpreted as indicating that slowed processing, frequently reported with TBI, underlies slow finger tapping in these patients. Some TBI patients also have difficulty inhibiting movement of other fingers while tapping, this problem increasing in frequency with severity (Prigatano and Borgaro, 2003). Epilepsy patients generally perform poorly on this test (Dodrill, 1978b), but in evaluating their performances the slowing effects of some anticonvulsive medications must be taken into account. Diseases that involve the spinal cord as well as the brain, such as multiple sclerosis, have a significant slowing effect on FTT scores (Heaton, Nelson, et al., 1985). Some alcoholics may tap more slowly than normal control subjects, but from almost half to 75% of the reported studies showed no group differences between alcoholics and normal subjects (Leckliter and Matarazzo, 1989; Parsons and Farr, 1981). In evaluating this material, one should keep in mind that the studies reviewed in these reports on alcoholics used the original cutting scores which tend to have the high false positive rates discussed above.

Purdue Pegboard Test (Purdue Research Foundation, 1948; Tiffin, 1968)

This neuropsychologically sensitive test was developed to assess manual dexterity for employment selection. It has been applied to questions of lateralization of lesions (L.D. Costa, Vaughan, et al., 1963) and motor dexterity (Diller, Ben-Yishay, Gerstman, et al., 1974) among brain-damaged patients. Following the standard instructions, the patient places the pegs first with the preferred hand, then the other hand, and then both hands simultaneously (see Fig. 16.13). A practice trial for each condition is recommended. Each condition lasts for 30 sec so that the total actual testing time is 90 sec. Although the standard instructions call for only one trial for each condition, when examining patients with known or suspected brain damage, three cycles are recommended. The score is the number of pegs placed correctly.

Average scores of normative groups, consisting of production workers and applicants for production work jobs, ranged from 15 to 19 for the right hand, from 14.5 to 18 for the left hand, from 12 to 15.5 for both hands, and from 43 to 50 for the sum of the first

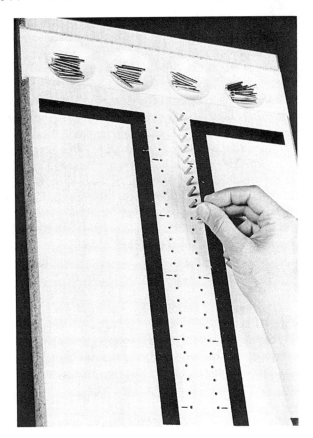

FIGURE 16.13 The Purdue Pegboard Test. (Courtesy of the Lafayette Instrument Co.)

three scores (Tiffin, 1968). As would be expected, handedness significantly affects performance. A study of 30 left-handers and 30 right-handers found that both groups placed approximately four more pegs with the preferred hand than the nonpreferred hand during three trials (Triggs et al., 2000). (For normative data, see Agnew and her coworkers, 1988; Spreen and Strauss, 1998; and Yeudall, Fromm, et al., 1986.)

Test characteristics. Averages for groups of women tend to run one-half to two or more points above the averages for men's groups (Spreen and Strauss, 1998). Scores drop with advancing age, at a slightly greater rate for men than for women (Agnew et al., 1988; Spreen and Strauss, 1998). Agnew and her colleagues also reported that the disparity between hands tends to increase with age as the nondominant hand shows greater slowing over time, a finding that appears to be supported even in the relatively small data sample presented by Spreen and Strauss. Five repeated weekly testings for right hand, left hand, and both hands trials correlated on the average in the .63 to .81 range, but correlations as low as .35 and as high as .93 were recorded (Reddon, Gill, et al., 1988). Practice effects

occurred as performances became faster from week to week, with the 12 men in the Reddon study showing a significant increase in speed for trials with each hand (but not both hands); increases in speed shown by the 14 women did not reach significance (see also McCaffery, Duff, and Westervelt, 2000b). Reliability is better for the three-trial than the one-trial administration (Buddenberg and Davis, 2000).

Neuropsychological findings. In a study of the efficiency of the Purdue Pegboard Test in making diagnostic discriminations, the accuracy of cutting scores was 70% in predicting a lateralized lesion in the validation sample, 60% in predicting lateralization in the cross-validation sample, and 89% in predicting brain damage in general for both samples (L.D. Costa, Vaughan, et al., 1963). Since the base rate of brain damaged patients in this population was 73%, the Pegboard accuracy score represented a significant ($p < .05$) prediction gain over the base rate even without taking sex into account. Two separate sets of cutting scores were developed for older and younger age groups. Further, for patients of all ages, a brain lesion is likely to be present whenever the left (or nonpreferred) hand score exceeds that of the right (preferred) hand, or the right (preferred) hand score exceeds that of the left (or nonpreferred hand) by 3 points or more. One-sided slowing suggests a lesion on the contralateral hemisphere; bilateral slowing occurs with diffuse or bilateral brain damage. However, ratio scores comparing the two hands are so unreliable that even large lateralized differences may only have diagnostic value when similar differences show up on other tests (Reddon, Gill, et al., 1988).

Grooved Pegboard[1] (Kløve, 1963)

This test adds a dimension of complex coordination to the pegboard task. It consists of a small board containing a 5×5 set of slotted holes angled in different directions. Each peg has a ridge along one side, requiring it to be rotated into position for correct insertion. It is part of the Repeatable Cognitive-Perceptual-Motor Battery (R. Lewis and Kupke, 1992) and the Wisconsin Neuropsychological Test Battery (Harley, Leuthold, et al., 1980). The score is time to completion. For most clinical purposes both hands should be tested, but one hand may suffice for studying changes in motor speed per se, as can occur with medication (e.g., R.F. Lewis and Rennick, 1979). Mitrushina, Boone, and D'Elia (1999) provide normative data from 16 studies.

[1]Lafayette Instruments offers the lowest price.

Test characteristics. Bornstein (1985[1]); Heaton, Grant, and Matthews (1991[1]); Heaton, Ryan, et al., (1996); and Ruff and Parker (1993[1]) examined demographic variables. Age effects appeared in all of these studies with slowing increasing with advancing age. Bornstein (1985) reported education differences for the dominant hand only, but the Heaton group found no education effects. Bornstein and Suga (1988[1]) attributed the discrepancy in education findings to differences in sample composition as their subjects' education levels were lower than the levels in the Heaton, Grant, and Matthews samples. Bornstein (1985) also reported small but significant sex differences for both hands with considerable overlap between groups. For a large sample ages 16 to 70 (180 of each sex), using the dominant hand, men took on the average 5 sec longer to complete the test than women, with considerable overlap (70.2 ± 13.2 sec, 65.2 ± 12.3 sec, respectively); nondominant hand mean time differences were a bit smaller with greater overlap (76.3 ± 15.3 sec, 72.0 ± 15.1 sec, respectively) (Ruff and Parker, 1993). Similar sex differences were found in a study of 102 young adults: women outperformed men in the dominant hand condition but differences between groups were not significant with the nondominant hand (S.L Schmidt et al., 2000). Substantial test–retest reliabilities have been found ($r \geq .82$) (Dikmen, Heaton, et al., 1999), although practice effects do not appear consistently when control subjects are retested (McCaffery, Duff, and Westervelt, 2000b). When each hand has three trials, performance improves significantly over trials (S.L. Schmidt et al., 2000).

Bornstein, Paniak, and O'Brien (1987) showed that previously established cutting scores misclassified 66% of dominant hand performances and 72% of nondominant ones by intact subjects, although virtually no brain damaged patients were misclassified. They recommended a new set of cutting scores ($\geq$92 dominant, $\geq$99 nondominant) which misclassified only 11% and 9%, respectively, of normal subjects but more patients (27% and 40%, respectively).

Neuropsychological findings. This test can aid in identifying lateralized impairment (Haaland, Cleeland, and Carr, 1977). Bornstein (1986b) suggested that a right/left hand score ratio greater than 1.0 suggests right hemisphere disease, and a ratio less than 1.0 may be indicative of damage involving the left hemisphere; but he cautioned that these ratios are too variable to rely on without supporting data from other tests. However, deficits on the ipsilateral hand trial after stroke or tumor to either hemisphere suggest that both hemi-

spheres are equally important for performance on this task (Haaland and Delaney, 1981). Its complexity makes this a sensitive instrument for measuring general slowing whether due to medication (R.F. Lewis and Rennick, 1979; C.G. Matthews and Harley, 1975), diffuse brain dysfunction (Nathan et al., 2001), or progression of disease processes such as parkinsonism (Matthews and Haaland, 1979) or HIV infection (E.N. Miller, Selnes, et al., 1990; Y. Stern, McDermott, Albert, et al., 2001). Slowing on this test may also appear with toxic effects of microorganism excretions (Grattan, Oldach, et al., 1998) and environmental lead (Bleecker, Lindgren, and Ford, 1997).

Hand Dynamometer or Grip Strength Test (Reitan and Wolfson, 1993; Spreen and Strauss, 1998)

This technique detects differences in hand strength under the assumption that lateralized brain damage may affect strength of the contralateral hand. The standard neuropsychological administration calls for two trials for each hand alternating between hands. The score is the force exerted in kilograms for each hand averaged for the two trials. A testing protocol for occupational therapy evaluations recommended three trials for each hand and found the average score to be more reliable than the best score (Mathiowetz et al., 1984). James L. Mack pointed out that this test requires effort and that the degree of voluntary effort a subject puts forth may vary for any number of reasons (personal communication [mdl], September 1991). He therefore recommended that the standard administration be compared with a second one in which attention is diverted from the task by performing a little sensory test, such as two-point discrimination, on the other arm. A number of workers have developed norms for this task (Mitrushina, Boone, and D'Elia, 1999). Differences between the reported mean scores are all within a one to two kilogram range.

Test characteristics. Sex differences are unequivocal (Dodrill, 1979); the sexes differ further in that men show a greater intermanual discrepancy than do women (Bornstein, 1986c[1]). Significant age effects appear (Bornstein, 1986c; Ernst et al., 1987), but men and women do not show them in the same way or in all studies. In one, men's scores held up until age 40 and then decreased (Fromm-Auch and Yeudall, 1983); however, they did not begin dropping until after age 60 in the 1986 Heaton, Grant, and Matthews[1] study. Fromm-Auch and Yeudall's data do not show a corresponding pattern of weakening with age for women, although Koffler and Zehler (1985) documented lower scores from age 40. Data on education effects are equiv-

[1]Data reproduced in Mitrushina, Boone, and D'Elia, 1999.

ocal: Bornstein (1985[1]) found that education contributed significantly to grip strength scores, but Ernst (1988) did not for an elderly sample, nor did Heaton and his colleagues. What education effects have been reported for grip strength tend to be relatively slight (Leckliter and Matarazzo, 1989) and may be more related to such other variables as healthful nutrition and/or good working conditions than to each other.

This is a highly reliable technique. With ten trials, some fatigue effects occur, but not on the first two trials (Reddon, Stefanyk, et al., 1985). Using a two-minute rest between trials, Dunwoody and coworkers (1996) found that performance actually improved over the first three trials, presumably as the subjects became more familiar with the task and, perhaps, as their muscles warmed up. Over ten weeks of weekly retesting, some increase in strength appeared, but not within the first three weeks. For both hands, the Reddon group found good average test–retest reliability for men (r = .91) and women (r = .94). R. Lewis and Kupke (1992)

---

[1]Data reproduced in Mitrushina, Boone, and D'Elia, 1999.

reported almost perfect test–retest reliability (r = .98). A comparison of women's test–retest scores on the two-trial condition showed that reliability correlations for right hand performances were somewhat lower than for the left (r = .79, r = .86, respectively) (Mathiowetz et al., 1984). (For other test–retest data, see McCaffery, Duff, and Westerveld, 2000b.)

Neuropsychological findings. As in other tests of manual abilities, strength between hands varies widely in patients with lateralized brain disorders as well as in normal control subjects (Bornstein, 1986b; Dodrill, 1978a). Using a classification criterion of −2 SD, Koffler and Zehler (1985) found 27% of normal subjects misclassified as brain damaged when dominant hand strength exceeded that of the nondominant hand by 5 kg: 21% were called "brain damaged" because the strength of the dominant hand was not greater than that of the nondominant hand. Like finger tapping, similar contralateral deficits were seen after damage in a variety of locations to the left or right hemisphere (Haaland and Delaney, 1981).

17 | Neuropsychological Assessment Batteries

Two purposes guide the development of most neuropsychological test batteries.[1] One is diagnostic accuracy, and the other is functional assessment in patients with documented neurologic diagnoses. For diagnostic accuracy, tests are chosen—or test data are handled—on the basis of their sensitivity and specificity to a particular condition or disease state. Thus, the battery not only has to have good positive predictive power (i.e., positive findings when the condition or disease is present), but also have negative predictive power (i.e., negative findings that suggest disease absence when none exists). Diagnosis was once an important assessment goal, but few neuropsychological examinations today are primarily diagnostic due to significant advances in other laboratory procedures, particularly neuroimaging. Notable exceptions are for conditions in which no other reliable diagnostic markers exist, such as mild TBI or early dementia. (See p. 5 for a discussion of how neuropsychology's role has changed over the last five decades.)

Batteries for understanding the disabilities experienced by patients with known diagnoses provide for standardized data collection that samples a broad range of behavior and assesses the major cognitive functions. Numerous test batteries, including screening batteries, elicit behaviors that are relevant to the patient's condition and needs (e.g., functional limitations, prognosis). These are reviewed in this chapter.

The strengths and limitations of set batteries for neuropsychological assessment were aptly stated by Davison (1974, p. 354):

Utilization of a standardized battery, particularly when it is administered by someone other than the neuropsychologist who will interpret it, presents great advantages for research in that the objective data can be evaluated without contaminating influences, and all subjects secure scores on the same variables. However, this method also presents great liabilities for *some* clinical diagnostic problems, among them adequate specification of an individual's characteristics for the purpose of predicting behavior in his ambient existence. For this pur-

pose the data collector must have a clear idea of the practical problem to which he is predicting and the freedom, knowledge, and ingenuity to add tests to the battery for individual cases and to *improvise* individualized assessment when necessary. . . . The clinician must recognize his responsibility not simply for addressing the referral problem, but toward the patient as a whole.

Several formalized batteries for general clinical use have been published while many others were constructed to address specific clinical or research needs. Among formalized batteries, the best known are those developed by David Wechsler (pp. 648–659). Although the Wechsler scales were originally developed as measures of "intelligence," they are widely used for neuropsychological assessment, either as an intact battery, or as a pool of reasonably well-normed tests available for judicious selection. Of those batteries designed explicitly for neuropsychological assessment, the most widely used is the Halstead-Reitan Battery (HRB) (pp. 670–676; M. Butler et al., 1991; C. Piotrowski and Lubin, 1990). Many other batteries have been constructed for specific neuropsychological purposes, such as examining for dementia and following its progression (e.g., CERAD, p. 689), examining possible effects of toxic exposure (California Neuropsychological Screening Battery, 687), or evaluating rehabilitation potential (Sohlberg and Mateer, 2001).

In these cases, tests are selected based upon the needs of a particular patient sample and the characteristics of the individual test.

The examiner's orientation to clinical assessment is often characterized as following either a "fixed battery" or "flexible" approach. Many neuropsychologists assemble their own batteries and, typically, use a flexible approach to assessment. Flexible batteries are usually based on a core set of tests that remain fairly uniform within specific diagnostic categories, with additional tests selected in response to the patient's condition or examination issues (e.g., Milberg, Hebben, and Kaplan, 1996; Tranel, 1996). This procedure is employed by approximately 70% of North American neuropsychologists (Sweet, Moberg, and Suchy, 2000). Only 15% of neuropsychologists surveyed by Sweet

---

[1]Except for updating, this section (pp. 647–648) remains essentially unchanged from the 1976 edition of this book.

and his coworkers use a fixed battery (e.g., the Halstead-Reitan or Luria-Nebraska batteries). Another 15% use a fully flexible approach in which all tests given to any one patient have been selected to be most responsive to that patient's condition and the questions raised (e.g., P. McKenna and Warrington, 1996; Stringer, 1996). Most flexible batteries contain elements from one of the Wechsler Intelligence Scales. Although "flexible" procedures contrast with rigid adherence to a fixed battery of tests given regardless of the referral question or patient characteristics, "flexible" may imply examination procedures that are idiosyncratic or experimental. Perhaps "tailored battery" better describes flexible battery procedures.

In deciding whether to use an existing battery, to develop one's own, or to modify one already in use, the clinician needs to evaluate the battery for suitability, practicality, and usefulness. A battery that is deficient in one of these areas, no matter what its other virtues, will be inadequate for general clinical purposes although it may satisfy the requirements for some individual cases or research designs.

A *suitable* battery provides an examination that is appropriate to the patient's needs, whether they call for a baseline study, differential diagnosis, rehabilitation planning, or any other type of assessment. Thus, the examination of a patient who seeks help for a memory complaint should contain tests of visual and verbal learning and of various aspects of attention plus measures of retention and retrieval. Suitability also extends to the needs of patients with limited sensory or motor function. For these patients a suitable battery allows for test variations that can provide data on the major cognitive functions by using patients' remaining sensory and response modalities.

A *practicable* battery is relatively easy to administer and, ideally, has inexpensive equipment. It can be adapted to the limitations of a wheelchair, can be moved by one person, and is transportable by car. Further, a practicable battery does not take so much time as to be prohibitive in cost, exhaust the patient, or severely limit the number of patients who can be tested by a single examiner.

A *useful* battery provides the information needed by the examiner. If the examiner relies on a single battery of tests for unselected clinical patients, then it must be multipurpose, aiding diagnosis, giving baselines, and supplying data for planning and treatment.

We know of no batteries that fully satisfy all these criteria. Such a battery is no more likely to be constructed than can physicians develop a fixed examination that includes the same clinical procedures and laboratory tests for all patients. Further, although standardized procedures are at the heart of reliable assessment, not enough is yet known to enshrine any set of tests with an unquestioned standardization. Batteries—both informal test collections and those with fully formalized evaluation procedures—have their place in neuropsychological examinations. They are, however, necessarily incomplete solutions for addressing subtle and complex problems of neuropsychological assessment (see also Bornstein, 1990; Lezak, 2002).

ABILITY AND ACHIEVEMENT

Many tests integrated into the neuropsychological assessment repertoire were originally designed to measure mental abilities in the context of school, work counseling, or placement. Increasing familiarity with these tests coupled with an evolving appreciation of what functions need to be examined have given them a valued role in neuropsychological assessment. The tests reviewed here include both those often employed in neuropsychological assessment plus some others offering less well known techniques for examining specific aspects of cognitive functioning.

Individual Administration

Wechsler Intelligence Scales for adults (WIS-A) (Wechsler, 1939, 1944, 1955, 1981, 1997a&c)

Early psychological theorists treated cognitive functioning, then called "intelligence," as a unitary phenomenon. Test makers, however, acknowledged the multidimensionality of mental ability by producing composite tests that included a variety of skills and capacities (e.g., French et al., 1963; Thurstone, 1938). In developing his set of tests, David Wechsler followed both traditions: he maintained the notion of intelligence as a global—unitary—entity (thus the IQ score) but based on an aggregate of specific abilities that are more or less complex and qualitatively distinct (Boake, 2002; Tulsky, Saklofske, and Ricker, 2003; Wechsler, 1939). Consequently, the Wechsler Intelligence Scales for adults are actually test batteries since each test within the scale assesses specific aspects of cognition and can be used independently from other tests in the battery.

The earliest Wechsler batteries were the *Wechsler-Bellevue Intelligence Scales,* Forms I and II (*WB-I, -II*) (Wechsler, 1939, 1944). Tests that had been developed for many purposes—e.g., anthropometrics, examination of children's mental abilities (Binet-Simon Scales), and tests for World War I army recruits and for immigrant screening which called for nonverbal responses—were adopted by Wechsler for his new mental ability scales (Boake, 2002). The Wechsler Adult

Intelligence Scale (*WAIS*) was first published in 1955; its revision, the *WAIS-R*, appeared in 1981. The *Wechsler Adult Intelligence Scale-Third Edition* (*WAIS-III*) was published in 1997 (The Psychological Corporation, 1997). This review is mostly limited to the WAIS-R and WAIS-III batteries; the term WIS-A refers to the Wechsler batteries generally or to more than one (see also Tulsky, Saklofske, Chelune, et al., 2003).

A significant strength of the WIS-A batteries lies in their *relatively* complete and representative standardizations. The WAIS-R included 1880 subjects ranging in age between 16 and 74 years; 2450 subjects between 16 and 89 years of age comprised the WAIS-III standardization sample. Thus, the most recent WIS-A tests appear to have better psychometric characterization of healthy, cognitively intact persons than do most other tests used in neuropsychology.

The WIS-As often contribute a substantial portion of the tests used for neuropsychological assessment of persons 16 years and older (e.g., J. Green, 2000; Milberg, Hebben, and Kaplan, 1996; Vanderploeg, 1994; Walsh, 1995). Including tests of basic communication, arithmetic, and drawing skills plus tests of attention in its various aspects, recent memory, learning, and executive functioning with tests from one of the WIS-A batteries provides an assessment of the most important aspects of cognitive functioning. Moreover, the examiner will also acquire considerable information about how the patient behaves. Such a survey of cognitive functions, in which WIS-A tests serve as the core instruments, is usually sufficient to demonstrate an absence of significant cognitive impairment or to provide clues of altered neuropsychological functions.

All WIS-A editions have the same bifurcated structure. Eleven tests made up the original scales. Wechsler classified six of them as "Verbal" tests: Information (I), Comprehension (C), Arithmetic (A), Similarities (S), Digit Span (DSp), and Vocabulary (V). The other five, called "Performance" tests, include Digit Symbol (DSy), Picture Completion (PC), Block Design (BD), Picture Arrangement (PA), and Object Assembly (OA). The WAIS-III adds three new tests: Letter-Number Sequencing (LNS), Symbol Search (SS), and Matrix Reasoning (MR). Excepting Block Design, which was adapted from the Kohs Block Design Test, the tests selected by Wechsler were derived from the Army Alpha and Army Beta batteries, with the terms "Verbal" and "Performance" already in common use (Boake, 2002; Wechsler, 1939).

Most WIS-A tests contain similar items at different levels of difficulty. This permits relatively fine gradations in item scaling and development of standardized individual test norms for comparing test performances. Each WIS-A test is individually reviewed in the chapter of the predominant function assessed by that test. Thus, *Digit Span, Digit Symbol, Symbol Search,* and *Letter–Number Sequencing* appear in Chapter 9; Orientation and Attention; *Information* and *Vocabulary* are in Chapter 13; Verbal Functions and Language Skills; *Block Design* and *Object Assembly* are in Chapter 14; Constructional Functions; and *Arithmetic, Comprehension, Picture Arrangement, Picture Completion, Matrix Reasoning,* and *Similarities* are in Chapter 15, Concept Formation and Reasoning.

Each WIS-A revision has "recentered" norms so that every test has a true mean score of 10. However, comparisons of test data from different WIS-A editions suggests an apparent decrease in difficulty levels since WIS-A scores have risen over time (e.g., the WAIS-III sample was tested in the early 1990s, while WAIS-R testing took place around 1970). This phenomenon, known as the "Flynn effect," is not limited to WIS-A but has been observed in longitudinal ability testing generally (Crawford, Allan, Besson, et al., 1990; J.R. Flynn, 1987, 1998b; Neisser et al., 1996) and is independent of genetic factors (Rushton, 2000). Many different explanations have been proposed for this performance increase, including better education, improved nutrition, and exposure to television, computers, and video games.

Differences in item content and statistical properties across test generations limit strict comparisons for the different editions, but increases from WAIS-R to WAIS-III tend to be smaller than for previous revisions; from WAIS to WAIS-R, scaled score equivalents on nine of 11 tests changed by at least one point, and four changed by 1.8 points (Wechsler, 1981). Of the 11 tests in both WAIS-R and WAIS-III batteries, only Digit Symbol changed more than one scaled score point from the previous edition.

Several other changes incorporated into the WAIS-III merit special mention because they improve the battery for neuropsychological assessment. Because of age-related slowing, the number of items with time-based bonus points was decreased. Matrix Reasoning, which is similar to the Raven Progressive Matrices, replaces Object Assembly in the computation of summary "Index" scores (see p. 650). The "floors" for each test were lowered to allow greater performance discrimination for patients with mild to moderate impairments. In addition, 1200 subjects took both WAIS-III and Wechsler Memory Scale-III (WMS-III) batteries, allowing more direct comparison of performances across tests from the two batteries since they were normed together. Thus, when using tests from either battery, the examiner should be able to assume that systematic differences in the normative sample composition are negligible. However, experience with possible WAIS-R sample distortions suggests the need for further study before relying unquestioningly on the new set of norms.[1]

WIS-A factors and Index Scores

Despite content and standardization differences, which preclude exact cross-generational comparisons between scores on the different WIS-A batteries, three functionally distinct factors have consistently emerged on all of its forms (L. Atkinson, Cyr, et al., 1989; J. Cohen, 1957a,b; A.S. Kaufman, 1990; The Psychological Corporation, 1997; Tulsky, Sakalofske, Chelune, et al., 2003). The first, a verbal factor usually called *Verbal Comprehension*, has its highest weightings on Information, Comprehension, Similarities, and Vocabulary. Block Design and Object Assembly always load on the *Perceptual Organization* factor with limited contributions from Digit Symbol; some studies have also included Picture Completion or Picture Arrangement under this factor, although these latter two tests have moderate verbal components as well as unique characteristics that distinguish them from the other tests in factorial analyses. On WAIS-III, Block Design, Matrix Reasoning, and Picture Completion make the predominant contributions to this factor. A *Freedom from Distractibility* factor weights significantly on Arithmetic, Digit Span, Letter–Number Sequencing (WAIS-III), and to some extent, Digit Symbol. Digit Symbol has never been strongly associated with any of the three factors, but the addition of Symbol Search to WAIS-III provides enough shared variance with Digit Symbol to form an independent factor, *Processing Speed*. As is true for all WIS-A factor analytic studies, the relative strength and distribution of elicited factors vary somewhat with demographic and clinical differences between the groups contributing to the analysis (e.g., Bornstein, Drake, and Pakalnis, 1988; P.C. Fowler, Zillmer, and Macciocchi, 1990), but the overall pattern remains much the same.

Scoring issues

Interpretation of WIS-A scores involves many issues such as item scaling, interexaminer reliability, and the influence of testing conditions (A.S. Kaufman and Lichtenberger, 1999). Those most important for neuropsychological assessment involve IQ and Index scores, effects of age, sex differences, and the evaluation of the significance of score discrepancies, scatter, and normative data sets that differ from those generated by the batteries' publisher.

[1]Note differences between the samples published by The Psychological Corporation and other sample sets (e.g., Heaton, Grant, and Matthews, 1991; Ivnik, Malec, Smith, et al., 1992c).

IQ scores. The WAIS-III still preserves the IQ score and the test alignment into Verbal and Performance Scales in the face of the body of literature that contradicts the assumptions underlying conglomerate scores and Wechsler's pre-1939 classification of the tests as either "Verbal" or "Performance" in nature (Boake, 2002). The Full Scale IQ score of a WIS-A battery, which is calculated from the sum of the Scaled Scores for 11 individual tests (or their prorated values if fewer than 11 tests are given), is a good predictor of academic achievement (Anastasi and Urbina, 1997; N. Brody, 1997; Suzuki and Valencia, 1997). However, neither the Full Scale IQ, nor the IQ scores calculated on the basis of the so-called Verbal or Performance tests, are useful for neuropsychological analysis (see pp. 20–22; Crawford, Johnson, et al., 1997; Lezak, 1988b). As Ward Halstead (1947, p. 108) noted, this type of approach "averages out peaks and troughs of ability and thus obscures these important details."

The individual tested makes an unspoken plea to the examiner not to summarize his or her intelligence in a single, cold number; the goal of profile interpretation should be to respond to that plea by identifying hypothesized strengths and weaknesses that extend well beyond the limited information provided by the FS-IQ, and that will conceivably lead to practical recommendations that help answer the referral questions. (A.S. Kaufman, 1990; see also A.S. Kaufman and Lichtenberger, 1999)

Much early neuropsychological research focused on comparisons between Wechsler Verbal and Performance Scale IQ scores (*VIQ, PIQ*) under the assumption that differences between these scores would reflect selective verbal or nonverbal impairment (e.g., Kløve, 1974; Warrington, James, and Maciejewski, 1986). Factor analytic studies have repeatedly shown, however, that VIQ and PIQ scores are each based on averages of quite dissimilar functions with relatively low intercorrelations and no regular neuroanatomical or neuropsychological relationship to one another (J. Cohen, 1957a; The Psychological Corporation, 1997). Moreover, functions contributing to VIQ and PIQ overlap considerably (Crawford, Jack, et al., 1990; A.S. Kaufman, 1990; Maxwell, 1960). These findings are not surprising since Wechsler assigned the individual tests to either Verbal or Performance scales in accordance with the existing Army Alpha and Beta scales rather than on an empirical basis (Boake, 2002; Wechsler, 1932; Yerkes, 1921).

Although the VIQ score tends to be reduced relative to the PIQ score following left hemisphere injury, this does not occur with sufficient regularity to permit diagnostic inferences in individual patients (Bornstein, 1983c; Hermann, Gold, et al., 1995; Larrabee, 1986).

A PIQ score relatively lower than the VIQ score is even less useful as an indicator of right hemisphere dysfunction since it contains time-dependent tests that are sensitive to any disorder that impairs mental processing efficiency. Moreover, the constructional deficits of many patients with left-sided lesions result in relatively low scores on Block Design and Object Assembly tests, lowering the PIQ (Damasio, Tranel, and Rizzo, 2000; Strub and Black, 2000). Thus, although relative lowering of PIQ is most pronounced for patients with extensive right hemisphere damage, other cerebral disorders—including left hemisphere or bilateral brain lesions, degenerative disorders, and affective disorders—can lower the PIQ score relative to the VIQ or depress both scores equally (K.B. Boone, Swerdloff, et al., 2001; Bornstein, 1983c; Chelune, Ferguson, and Moehle, 1986; Kluger and Goldberg, 1990). On reviewing VIQ-PIQ scores reported in 12 WAIS-R studies with TBI patients, Hawkins, Plehn, and Borgara (2002) advise that, "the lack of a VIQ–PIQ difference should never be used to infer that a TBI has not occurred" (p. 49).

Tests contributing to the PIQ score call upon more unfamiliar activities than do tests with high verbal weightings. The familiar/unfamiliar difference has led some authors to interpret the VIQ vs. PIQ scores as measures of crystallized and fluid intelligence, respectively (D.E. Boone, 1995; A.S. Kaufman, Kaufman-Packer, et al., 1991). This interpretation, however, has come under question (Daniel, 1997). When examining different factor weightings using the WAIS-III normative database, Caruso and Cliff (1999) found a two factor solution that corresponded more to the crystallized vs. fluid model of intelligence than do the tests organized in VIQ or PIQ scales (e.g., high crystallized [Gc component weights >.20]: Vocabulary, Information, Similarities; high fluid [Gf component weights >.20]: Digit Span [.62!], Matrix Reasoning, Arithmetic, Block Design). They conclude, "it may seem to be a radical suggestion, but the two factor scores defined in this way [crystallized vs. fluid] may well represent a more realistic, and therefore more clinically useful, bifurcation of ability" (p. 204). Moreover, tests within each scale differ in their sensitivity both to general effects of brain dysfunction—such as slowing or concrete thinking—and to specific effects associated with focal lesions in areas subserving particular verbal, mathematical, visuospatial, memory, or other functions (Hawkins, Plehn, and Borgaro, 2002). Wechsler's (1939) view of the Performance tests as reflecting "temperamental and personality factors" including "the subject's interest in doing the task set, his persistence in attacking them and his zest and desire to succeed," (p. 10) rather than strictly cognitive ability, may have contributed to his including bonus points for rapid completion.

The magnitude and direction of VIQ vs. PIQ discrepancies also vary systematically with the Full Scale IQ score (Matarazzo and Herman, 1985; The Psychological Corporation, 1997). Healthy subjects with FSIQs above 100 tend to have higher VIQ than PIQ scores, with a reverse tendency in favor of higher PIQ scores when FSIQ scores are much below 100 (A. Smith, 1966), a finding that continues to be observed (Hsu, et al., 2000; Mitrushina and Satz, 1995a). Normative data from WAIS-R and WAIS-III standardizations alone should make the clinician wary of basing judgments about a patient on this discrepancy since slightly more than 20% of both normative samples obtained VIQ–PIQ score discrepancies of 14 scaled score points or more (F.M. Grossman et al., 1985; Matarazzo and Herman, 1985; Psychological Corporation, 1997). This finding, however, may underestimate the extent of pronounced VIQ–PIQ differences in the normative sample as the test score range used to ascertain these discrepancy rates "was based unfortunately on normal scaled scores rather than age-graded scores . . . [making it] highly probable that the range necessary to be significantly abnormal will be less when age-graded scores are employed" (Crawford, 1992, p. 29).

Demographic variables are associated with VIQ–PIQ differences. Education contributes more to VIQ than PIQ (A.S. Kaufman, McLean, and Reynolds, 1988). As the percentage of men in samples of patients with lateralized brain disease increased so did the magnitude of the VIQ–PIQ discrepancy (Bornstein and Matarazzo, 1982, 1984). Lawson and Inglis (1983) suggested that this reflects a tendency for females to rely more on verbal processing of all kinds of material than males; others attribute women's smaller VIQ–PIQ differences to their relatively reduced functional asymmetry between hemispheres (McGlone, 1976; Witelson, 1991; see pp. 301–303). Cultural patterns may also contribute to wide disparities between VIQ and PIQ scores (Dershowitz and Frankel, 1975; A.S. Kaufman, 1979; Tsushima and Bratton, 1977).

When brain injury impairs performance on only one or two tests in a scale, it is not uncommon for the lower score(s) to be obscured when averaged in with the other tests measuring capacities spared by the damage (Crawford, Johnson, et al., 1997). Botez, Etheir, and their colleagues (1977) demonstrated this problem when they found a number of patients with normal pressure hydrocephalus who achieved Performance Scale IQ scores within the *average* ability range. These patients did poorest on Block Design and also on Kohs' Block Design Test, which is essentially identical to Block Design but contains many more items. In this study, impaired design copying ability was immediately obvious when communicated as a discrete score on Kohs' test, but was lost to sight in the aggregate PIQ score. Consequently, test data reported only as IQ scores are not presented in this book.

Index scores. A novel addition to WAIS-III offers *Index Scores* derived from their respective formal factor indices; these Index Scores are computed without the IQ score. Index scores are ascertained by "summing each individual's actual age-corrected scaled scores on the relevant tests" (The Psychological Corporation, 1997, p. 42), relevant defined by the tests contributing to the factor represented by an individual Index score (i.e., Information, Similarities, Vocabulary enter into the *Verbal Comprehension Index* [*VCI*]; Picture Completion, Block Design, and Matrix Reasoning comprise the *Perceptual Organization Index* [*POI*]; Arithmetic, Digit Span [including Digits Forward!] make up *Working Memory* [*WMI*]; Digit Symbol, Symbol Search constitute *Processing Speed* [*PSI*].

Some consistent performance biases may compromise the usefulness of these new Index scores. Although the WAIS-III Technical Manual includes cumulative frequency information for Index difference scores for five different ranges of FSIQ, the manual fails to distinguish the direction of the difference (The Psychological Corporation, 1997). When creating the tables, the authors treated both tails of the difference distribution as equivalent in shape. Yet, subjects with higher FSIQ scores will tend to score higher on the Verbal Comprehension Index than on the Index for Perceptual Organizational, with this pattern reversed for individuals whose FSIQ scores fall much below 100 (see above, pp. 650–651). Failure to report the direction of factor score differences raises serious questions about the clinical utility of these tables since these tables suggest that a Verbal Comprehension > Perceptual Organization difference would occur as frequently as a Perceptual Organization > Verbal Comprehension] difference for each of the five criterion ability levels. Yet a Perceptual Organization Index 20 points higher than the Verbal Comprehension Index is not equally likely at each ability level. Moreover, when presenting similar cumulative frequency differences between WAIS-III and WMS-III indices, the frequency data are based upon WAIS-III scores being higher than the memory scores. While this appears to reflect an expectation that memory scores will be more vulnerable to brain impairment than WAIS-III indices, the opposite pattern is certainly possible. For example, subjects with lower FSIQs tend to have WMS-III general memory scores that are higher than their FSIQ, and those at higher FSIQ levels tend to have lower WMS-III scores (Hawkins and Tulsky, 2001).

Age-graded scores. The WAIS-R and earlier batteries adjusted for age in the computation of the IQ scores but not in the scaled (standard) scores for each test. WAIS-R standard scores were based on a randomized sample of 500 persons from ages 20 to 34, and are therefore not appropriate for evaluating individual test performances. WAIS and WAIS-R manuals provide tables of age-adjusted "scaled score equivalents of raw scores" for the full gamut of ages 16 to 74. WAIS-R norms for the 55-and-over age groups are slightly less adequate than for younger age groups since each norm set was developed on only 160 subjects and, consequently, has the psychometric problems associated with smaller sample sizes. Older adult WAIS-R norms developed on a somewhat better educated population than the WAIS-R normative sample are available for ages 56–66 to 88+ (Ivnik, Malec, Smith, et al., 1992b). Heaton, Grant, and Matthews (1991) provide WAIS test norms, expressed in *T*-scores and stratified by age group, sex, and years of education (6–8 to 18+).

For the WAIS and the WAIS-R, when making test comparisons for subjects younger than 20 or older than 34, age-graded scaled scores are necessary. For ages outside the large, 20 to 34-year-old standardization group, it becomes difficult to interpret many of the test scores and virtually impossible to compare them or to attempt pattern analysis unless test performance has been graded according to age-appropriate norms (A.S. Kaufman, 1990). The WAIS-III reports normative data for each test for 13 age groups from 16–17 to 85–89.

WAIS-III score limitations. Despite the many welcome additions to Wechsler's tests, the WAIS-III still has several important shortcomings. Perhaps the largest deficiency is failure to include demographic corrections such as education and—when relevant—sex. Based upon WAIS-R studies, education accounts for more of the performance variance than does age (A.S. Kaufman, 1990), particularly for the more education-dependent tests such as Information and Vocabulary (A.S. Kaufman, Reynolds, and McLean, 1989). Even for Block Design, education alone accounts for approximately 24% of the variance with age accounting for an additional 7%. Similarly, education contributes to about 30% of the variance on Digit Symbol compared to an age contribution of an additional 14%. Thus, the most appropriate norms would be based upon both education and age (see M.J. Taylor and Heaton, 2001). These corrections are included in the "Scoring Assistant" computer program which can be purchased from the publisher (for $199 in 2003) but are not available to those who calculate WAIS-III scores manually.

A second problem lies in the messages implied by the factor-based index scores: that the neuropsychologist examiner need not pay much attention to the pattern of individual test performances; that variations between tests are irrelevant; and that patterns for grouped data, from which the Index scores are derived, can be assumed for the individual case, i.e., in clinical practice. In this context, the tables of discrepancy scores presented in the different appendices of the manual employ Index Scores exclusively rather than individual WAIS-III tests. The manual fails to remind WAIS-III users that these four factors are derived on the aggregated performances of hundreds of presumably cognitively intact subjects. While some neuropsychologically impaired persons' performances on these tests will follow pattern expectations raised by the four-index paradigm, for many other patients, an understanding of the cognitive strengths and weakness and the nature of their neuropsychological disorder will be only available through test by test analysis. Moreover, the use of factor scores is particularly questionable when there are large score discrepancies between the tests that comprise a particular factor (Sattler and Ryan, 1999).

For example, all WAIS-III test scores were compared for two patient groups (moderate–severe TBI, mild TBI), and healthy controls (Donders, Tulsky, and Zhu, 2001). Letter-number sequencing (LNS) scores, one of the new WAIS-III tests, varied as a function of injury severity, indicating the potential usefulness of this new WAIS-III measure. In contrast, scores on the Arithmetic and Digit Span tests, which are combined with Letter-number sequencing to form the Working Memory Index, did not relate to injury severity so that the association of LNS with severity was obscured by being combined with two less sensitive tests. Thus, relying on the Working Memory Index alone may lead the examiner to conclude erroneously that a patient had no deficits in higher order processing capability when in fact such a deficit may exist.

Clinical cases demonstrate this problem: A 40-year-old structural engineer was struck by a pipe propelled onto his forehead and between the eyes. Age-graded scaled scores were 12 for both Object Assembly and Block Design, but his Picture Completion score was 5, due to both response slowing and concrete thinking. Following the manual's prescription, the Index score would be 9.67, muting the visuospatial strengths shown in *high average* performances on construction tasks while obscuring his serious problems with concrete thinking and mental sluggishness.

Similar performance disparities were given by a 45-year-old lawyer with a metabolic disorder whose age-graded scaled scores were 12 on Information, 10 on Vocabulary, but only 7 on Similarities, giving a VCI score of 9.67, just about at the standardization mean. This Index score would indicate neither his *high average* knowledge level, nor an ability for verbal abstractions so impaired as to disable him from practising law.

Evaluating significance

The diagnostic meaningfulness of test score deviations typically depends on the extent to which they exceed expected chance variations in the subject's test performance. Consensus is lacking, however, about the appropriate standard against which deviations should be measured.

Some comparison standards that have been used for WIS-A tests include the mean scaled score, which is 10 for all tests; the patient's average test performance, which can be broken down into separate Verbal and Performance scores (A.S. Kaufman, 1990; Silverstein, 1982, 1984; Wechsler, 1958); and the average of two fairly resilient scores, Vocabulary and Picture Completion (McFie, 1975). For neuropsychological purposes, the most meaningful comparison standard is the one that gives the best estimate of the original ability level based on the patient's test scores, history, and demographic data (see Chapter 4). Which method for estimating premorbid ability will be best depends upon severity of impairment, laterality or localization of injury, and the patient's educational and occupation history. Of course, the variability across WIS-A tests reflecting the differing patterns of normal strengths and weaknesses shown by most intact subjects needs to be taken into account when estimating premorbid abilities. The WAIS-III Technical Manual notes that it is "very uncommon for a 'normal' person to function at the same level in every ability area" (The Psychological Corporation, 1997, p. 207).

With significant injury in someone who has not yet acquired distinguishing demographic markers, such as a TBI patient in his late teens or early 20s, the highest WIS-A score may give the best estimate of premorbid general ability and, even so, may underestimate premorbid function. There are two important exceptions, however, to using the highest WAIS test score as the comparison standard. First, evidence that the patient once enjoyed a level of cognitive competency higher than that indicated by the Wechsler scores, such as life history information, non-Wechsler test data, or isolated Wechsler item responses, takes precedence over Wechsler test scores in the determination of the comparison standard (Orsini, Van Gorp, and Boone, 1988).

A 52-year-old real estate developer with severe multi-infarct dementia had successfully completed two years of the Business Administration program at an outstanding private university just after World War II when this school had a highly selective admissions policy. On the verbal tests, his highest age-graded scaled score was 9, suggesting no better than an *average* original ability level. Knowledge of his previous academic experience led to an estimated premorbid ability level as having been at least in the *superior* range, at the 90th percentile or above. The WAIS test scaled score of 14 at this level became the comparison standard against which obtained test scores were measured for significance. This patient achieved an age-graded scaled score of 9 on Arithmetic by giving an erratic arithmetic performance in which he betrayed his original higher ability level by answering one difficult problem correctly while failing many easier items.

The second exception is that high scores on Digit Span, Digit Symbol, Object Assembly, or Letter Number Sequencing are less likely to reflect premorbid level than other WIS-A tests. Their lower intercorrelations with other WIS-A tests show that these tests do not predict performance on most tests of cognitive abilities or academic skills. Moreover, Object Assembly is no longer used for computation of either IQ or Index scores, a decision based in part on the test's low reliability. Knowledge of the astonishing feats of memory of patients with autistic savant syndrome—and the mild memory problems of fully competent older persons (see pp. 298–299)—should also make the examiner wary of using attention span and immediate memory scores as a basis for estimating original ability level.

A caution about using the best performance criterion concerns patients with mild injuries. On the WAIS-III, approximately 71% of the normative sample displayed discrepancies between high and low scores ≥6 scaled score points on the 11 tests used to calculate FSIQ (The Psychological Corporation, 1997). Thus, using the highest WAIS-III test performance as an estimate of premorbid functioning to evaluate a patient who had sustained minimal injury could suggest substantial decline on a number of tests when, in fact, performance differences simply reflect normal test variability and the highest scores will overestimate other aspects of premorbid ability (see also p. 99).

Wechsler originally recommended that a test score deviation measured from the subject's mean should be two scaled score units to be considered a possibly meaningful deviation and that a deviation of 3 be considered significant. For the WAIS-R, Silverstein (1987, 1988) found that age-graded scale score differences of 9 or more between WAIS-R tests appeared for fewer than 10% but more than 5% of the normative sample, a difference far greater than what Wechsler had recommended for determining statistically significant score differences. Matarazzo and Prifitera (1989) reported a much higher percentage of cases with a 9-point intertest scatter range, but they used the 20–34 year-old reference group data for determining all their test scores, thus necessarily exaggerating differences between tests which vary little with age (e.g., Vocabulary) and those most age-sensitive (e.g., Block Design, Digit Symbol) (see p. 655). For example, using the Matarazzo and Prifitera (1989) subject data from Table 3 (p. 189),

a 74-year-old who achieved a scaled score of 12 on Vocabulary and a scaled score of 5 on Digit Symbol when the scores were derived from the norms for 20-34 year olds, would score 13 on Vocabulary and 10 or 11 on Digit Symbol when compared with her own age norms so that her actual scaled score discrepancy is 2 or 3, not 7 as Matarazzo and Prifitera would have calculated.

Silverstein's (1982) statistical analyses indicated that an age-graded scaled score difference from the mean of all 11 WAIS-R tests of ±3 or more points is significant at the 5% level except for Vocabulary which requires only a ±2 point discrepancy, and Object Assembly which requires a difference from the mean of 4 age-graded scaled score points. Silverstein's data for the WAIS differed somewhat from the WAIS-R significances although the general pattern was similar.

The WAIS-III revision includes two tables for evaluating test score deviations. Derived from the normative sample, the first table compares differences between individual test scores and the average score of either six Verbal tests, five Performance tests, 11 tests making up the IQ score, or 11 tests contributing to the Index scores. Differences are reported at the .15 and .05 levels of statistical probability; test score differences are presented with a cumulative percentage table. The inclusion of cumulative percentage information is a significant improvement over previous WIS-A editions because it provides base rate information, although as discussed below, this information has limitations.

Application of the second set of tables becomes questionable. The Psychological Corporation authors list the size differences between individual tests that are significant at the .15 and .05 levels of statistical probability. However, here too the direction of the discrepancy was not accounted for, implying that a given size difference between scores on any two tests can occur with the same frequency regardless of which score is higher. Thus, an assumption inherent in these tables is that a difference between a score on a test relatively impervious to the effect of brain injury (i.e., a "hold" test) and the score on a test vulnerable to brain dysfunction (i.e., a "don't hold" test) will occur as frequently as a "don't hold" minus "hold" difference (e.g., that Vocabulary performance will be compromised by a brain disorder as often as Block Design or Digit Symbol—an assumption that has been consistently disproven; see pp. 655–656).

As examiner sophistication grows and funding for assessments shrinks, it is becoming less common for all WIS-A tests to be given. In these cases—as in all cases—no one score can be evaluated on its own. Diagnostic conclusions cannot be based on a single outlying score, no matter how deviant, because with all possible score combinations, chance alone may yield at least one large discrepancy between score pairs (L. Atkinson, 1991). What becomes exceptionally low will depend to some extent on the number of discrepant scores as increases in their number reduce the magnitude of difference required to infer a nonchance deviation. McFie's (1975) suggestion that *patterns* [italics added] of discrepancies should be considered by the clinician even when the score differences are not large enough to reach the 5% level reflects a not uncommon practice among experienced clinicians.

Test interpretation

Indices, ratios, and quotients. Most early neuropsychological studies of WIS-A sensitivity included mixed neuropsychiatric populations, with little or no attention paid to etiology, location, or extent of a brain lesion. Of course, prior to neuroimaging availability, the site and extent of many structural lesions could not be identified. A consistent pattern emerged in these early studies, however, in which tests requiring immediate memory, concentration, response speed, and abstract concept formation were more likely to show the effects of brain injury. Performance on tests of previously learned information and verbal skills tended to be less affected. While recognizing the inconstancy of relationships between WIS-A test patterns and various brain lesions, Wechsler and others also noted similarities in test sensitivity to neurologic injury and to age-related changes. Efforts to apply this apparent patterning to differential diagnosis resulted in a number of ratio formulas for cutting scores.

Wechsler (1958) devised a *deterioration quotient* (*DQ*) to compare scores on those tests that are relatively insensitive to aging ("hold" tests) with those that are more likely to decrease over the years ("don't hold" tests).[1] He assumed that deterioration exceeding *normal limits* indicated "senility" (now called dementia), an abnormal brain process, or both. For the WAIS, the Deterioration Quotient uses age-graded scores to compare "hold" tests (Vocabulary, Information, Object Assembly, and Picture Completion) with "don't hold" tests (Digit Span, Similarities, Digit Symbol, and Block Design) in the formula: (*hold − don't hold*)/*Hold*. Unfortunately, neither an earlier mental deterioration ratio calculated on Wechsler-Bellevue test scores (Wechsler, 1939) nor the WAIS DQ have proven effective in identifying neurologically impaired patients. Other formulas for detecting neurologic deterioration involved rather slight variations on Wechsler's basic theme (Gonen, 1970; Norman, 1966).

Recognizing the heterogeneity of clinical samples, Hewson (1949) developed a set of ratios in hopes of using WAIS test scores to identify neurologic patients. This method shuffled test scores into seven different formulas, each of which discriminated with more or less accuracy between normal control subjects, "neurotic", and postconcussion patients. A. Smith (1962) claimed relatively good success in identifying brain tumor patients by means of Hewson's ratios, classifying 81% of 128 subjects correctly. Compared to other WIS-A-based indices and ratios, Hewson's screened for brain impairment relatively well, but they misclassified too many cases for clinical application. Today, of course, the MRI with its high degree of sensitivity and specificity, has essentially replaced neuropsychological assessment as a means for identifying many kinds of structural brain changes.

In a variation of Wechsler's "Hold vs. Don't Hold" hypothesis, Fuld (1984) proposed a WIS-A-based formula for a test profile to identify Alzheimer's disease in patients for whom a differential diagnosis was unclear (Table 17.1). This formula was sensitive to drug-induced cholinergic depletion in 10 of 19 healthy subjects, and to presumed cholinergic deficiency in one-third to more than one-half of several groups of Alzheimer patients, but occurred in fewer than 15% of patients with nonAlzheimer dementias (Fuld, 1984). On finding Fuld's test profile in 13 of 26 Alzheimer patients but only two of 39 patients with multi-infarct dementia, Brinkman and Braun (1984) concluded that it is "somewhat specific to Alzheimer's disease."

This profile does not always show up, however, calling into question its usefulness (R.S. Goldman, Axelrod, Giordani, et al., 1992; Massman and Bigler, 1993; Randolph, Mohr, and Chase, 1993). Although it was not sensitive to two other patient groups (positive Fuld profiles: TBI-14%; Parkinson's disease-24%), Nolan and Burton (1998) suggest that "it may serve as an indicator of cholinergic deficiency." Given the Fuld profile loading on verbal tests, it is not surprising to find pronounced education effects (J.J. Ryan, Paolo,

[1]It should be noted that Wechsler's older age samples were not as well screened for neurologic or other health conditions as the current samples offering a more benign view of aging.

TABLE 17.1 WAIS and WAIS-R Formula for the Cholinergic Dysfunction Profile Based on Age-Graded Scores

A > B > C < D

Where

A = [Information + Vocabulary] ÷ 2,

B = [Similarities + Digit Span] ÷ 2,

C = [Digit Symbol + Block Design] ÷ 2,

D = Object Assembly

Adapted from Fuld (1984)

Oehlert, and Coker, 1991; Satz, Hynd, D'Elia, et al., 1990).

On observing that Vocabulary was the only test in the WAIS battery that did not discriminate between a diagnostically mixed group of dementia patients and patients suffering depression, while Block Design scores distinguished the two groups best, Coolidge and his colleagues (1985) recommended comparing just these two test scores. If the Vocabulary score is equal to or greater than twice the Block Design score, then the patient is more likely to have dementia. For 148 patients with questionable diagnoses a one-year follow-up evaluation found that this formula had a 74% accuracy rate for predicting both dementia and depression.

Pattern analysis. From its first applications in neuropsychology, Wechsler and others have looked to the pattern of WIS-A test score deviations for clues to the presence and type of brain injury (Donders, Tulsky, and Zhu, 2001; D.C. Fisher et al., 2000; C.G. Matthews, Guertin, and Reitan, 1962; McFie, 1975). A pattern of clear-cut differences between tests involving primarily verbal functions and those involving primarily visuospatial functions may suggest lateralized brain injury. However, even with lateralized damage, one or more tests in the "vulnerable" group may not necessarily be depressed, pointing up the necessity of integrating all of the examination data to understand the nature of the brain dysfunction and the patient's experience of it.

Other WIS-A test patterns are more likely to appear when focal or lateralized impairment is minimal or absent. Immediate memory, attention, and concentration problems show up in poor performances on Digit Span, Arithmetic, and Letter-Number Sequencing, whereas problems involving attention and response speed primarily affect Digit Symbol and Symbol Search scores. Not only are these tests sensitive to brain impairment due to a variety of etiologies, but patients with psychomotor slowing due to depression or taking antiepileptic medications may score lower on them (Aldenkamp, Baker, Mulder, et al., 2000; R. Martin, Meador, et al., 2001; Pagliaro and Pagliaro, 1999). The widespread tissue swelling that often accompanies an acute TBI or rapidly expanding tumor results in confusion, general dulling, and significant impairment of memory and concentration which lower scores on almost all tests, except perhaps time-independent verbal tests of old, well-established speech and thought patterns (S.W. Anderson, Damasio, and Tranel, 1990; Hom and Reitan, 1984).

An additional feature associated with many types of brain dysfunction is concrete thinking. Concrete thinking—or absence of the abstract attitude—may be reflected in lowered scores on Similarities and Picture Completion, and in failures or one-point answers on proverb items of Comprehension when responses to the other Comprehension items are of good quality. Concrete behavior can show up on Block Design, too, as inability to conceptualize the squared format or to appreciate the size relationships of the blocks relative to the pictured designs. Concrete thinking alone does not suggest brain damage in patients of low intellectual endowment or in long-term chronic psychiatric patients.

Patients with lesions primarily involving prefrontal structures may be quite impaired in their capacity to handle abstractions or to take the abstract attitude and yet do not show pronounced deficits on the close-ended, well-structured Wechsler test questions (Shallice and Burgess, 1991b). However, brain injured persons whose approach to problem solving tends to be concrete usually show some specific cognitive deficits.

A 26-year-old who had sustained a right anterior communicating artery aneurysm rupture shortly after graduating with honors from medical school was examined because he was unable to carry out to completion even basic medical duties and his wife complained of significant personality change. On the WAIS-R he achieved scaled scores of 14 and 15 on Information, Digit Span (8 forward, 6 reversed), Arithmetic, Picture Arrangement, and Block Design. His two lowest scores (10) were Similarities (five 1-point responses) and Picture Completion (woodpile: "fence should continue") suggestive of concrete thinking, but still of *average* calibre. However, recall on non-Wechsler tests—word lists, stories, designs—was *defective*.

Other than a few fairly distinctive but not mutually exclusive patterns of lateralized and diffuse damage, the WIS-A-based inquiry into the presence of brain injury depends on whether the test score pattern makes neuropsychological sense within the context of the patient's complaints, demography, and history. Of course, interpreting findings based on whether they make neuropsychological sense is the hallmark of neuropsychological evaluations in general since, with a large battery of tests, one always runs the risk of having a few performances in the *impaired* range that reflect nothing more than chance fluctuation (Type I errors) or normal variability. WIS-A pattern analysis applies best to patients with recent or ongoing brain changes and is probably least effective in identifying neurologic impairments in patients with psychiatric conditions, particularly those whose mental disorders have been longstanding.

Administering the WIS-A battery

All WIS-A manuals provide standard administration instructions for each test in excellent detail (Wechsler, 1955, 1981, 1997a).[1] Although the manuals present

---

[1]Many of the tests present special administration or scoring problems. These are noted in the discussion of each test.

the tests in a specified order, the actual order of administration need not follow the suggested sequence. Rather, the examiner may wish to vary the order and interweave other tests to meet the patient's needs and limitations. Patients who fatigue easily can be given more taxing tests, such as Arithmetic or Block Design, early in the session. Anxious patients can be given tests on which they are most likely to succeed before confronted with more difficult material. When all WIS-A tests are given, testing time can run from one and one-quarter to two hours or more.

Examiners must guard against their own very natural memory lapses. In the interest of maintaining a standardized administration, the examiner should not attempt to memorize the questions but rather should read from the manual. When questions have been memorized, the examiner is liable to insert a word here or change one there from time to time without being aware of these little changes. Ultimately they add up so that the examiner may be asking questions that differ not only in a word or two but in their meaning as well.

A verbatim record of patients' answers and comments provides permanent documentation of such important dimensions of examination behavior as qualitative aspects of speech (e.g., stuttering? grammatical errors? verbosity?), nature of failure on Arithmetic items (cannot recall all elements of problem? misheard what was said?), dependence on verbal analysis to solve visuospatial problems (e.g., "the white block goes to the right of the red one"), and others.

WAIS-R and WAIS-III alternate tests that call for verbal responses with vision-dependent tests on which verbal responses are not needed so that patients who may have function-specific deficits are not faced with a series of failures but rather can enjoy some successes throughout the examination. Alternating between the school-like question-and-answer items of the verbal tests and the visually presented puzzle-and-games items also affords a change in pace that helps maintain the interest of patients whose insight, motivation, or capacity to cooperate is deficient.

It is not necessary to complete all WIS-A tests in one sitting. To enable patients to perform at their best, the examination can be completed later when patients become restless or fatigued. In most instances, the examiner calls the recess after completing a test. Occasionally, a patient's energy or interest gives out in the middle of a test. For most tests, this creates no problem; the test can be resumed where it had been stopped. However, the easy items on Similarities, Block Design, Picture Arrangement, and Matrix Reasoning provide some people the practice they need to succeed on more difficult items. If the examination must be stopped in the middle of any of these four tests, the first few items should be repeated at the next session so that the pa-

tient can reestablish the cognitive set necessary for the harder items.

People over the age of 70 tended to be uncomfortably sensitive to failures (Savage et al., 1973). These authors found that negative reactions tended to show up when the examiner followed the requirement that tests be continued for a given number of failures. Since many older people enjoy doing "puzzles," they tolerated failure better on visually presented than on verbal tests. Thus, when faced with the choice of giving the required number of items or discontinuing early to reduce an elderly patient's discomfort, the examiner may choose to discontinue. In most cases, even if the patient could succeed on one or two of the more difficult items, continuation would not make a significant difference in the score. When patients appear capable of performing at a higher level than they seem willing to attempt, it is important to document this information so that the omitted items can be given at a later time, after they have had some obvious successes or when they seem more relaxed.

Many examiners routinely administer nine to ten or fewer tests. Substituted tests may be more quickly administered or scored (e.g., for Vocabulary, see pp. 514–515), or will provide more information (e.g., for Digit Symbol, see p. 371). The number of WIS-A tests given should depend upon the examination questions, the needs of the patient, and the circumstances of the examination rather than on the a priori, convention-based, and psychometric decisions of the test developers (Lezak, 2002).

Neuropsychologically important information can be gained by incorporating the face sheet identification and personal information questions into the examination proper. These questions allow the examiner to evaluate the patient's orientation in a naturalistic—and thus inoffensive—manner and ensure that important employment and education data have been obtained. Only the examiner who routinely asks patients about the date, their age and date of birth, and similar kinds of information usually taken for granted, can appreciate how often neurologically impaired patients fail to answer these question reliably and how important it is to know when patients cannot report this basic information about themselves.

WIS-A short forms

Under time pressure, the examiner may use only three, four, or five WIS-A tests selected to give the most relevant estimates of a patient's functioning. Short forms were originally developed to produce a quick estimate of FSIQ (e.g., see R.G. Hoffman and Nelson, 1988; Randolph, Mohr, and Chase, 1993; Silverstein, 1985). Since estimation of an aggregate IQ score is not the goal of neuropsychological examinations, selection of tests for brief neuropsychological screening should suit the patient's needs and abilities and the requirements of the examination.

The Satz-Mogel format. *Split-half* administrations, in which only every other test item is given, also save time but at the expense of accuracy and reliability. Satz and Mogel (1962) devised an abbreviated set of scales that includes all the original WIS-A scales and takes half the time of the full battery (R.L. Adams, Smigielski, and Jenkins, 1984). It uses mostly odd items ("split-half" format) except for Information, Vocabulary, and Picture Completion, in which every third item is given. Digit Span and Digit Symbol administrations are unchanged. These authors reported that only Information ($r = .89$), Comprehension ($r = .85$), Block Design ($r = .84$), and Object Assembly ($r = .79$) correlate below .90 with the complete test. G.G. Marsh (1973) obtained fairly comparable correlations in a cross-validation study of the Satz-Mogel format and concluded that it "is an adequate substitute for the long-form WAIS when it is used as a test of general intelligence with neurology or psychiatry patients." Since a significant number of both psychiatric (18%–30%) and neurologic (15%–20%) patients had Satz-Mogel scores that deviated at least three scaled scores from their whole test performances, Marsh cautioned against using this format for pattern analysis.

When evaluated for psychiatric inpatients with a variety of diagnoses, individual test score means obtained by this method differed from the whole test score mean by 1.1 scaled score point at most (Picture Arrangement), while six of the nine abbreviated tests differed by .4 or less (Dinning and Kraft, 1983). With TBI patients one mean scaled score difference as large as 1.7 (Picture Arrangement—again) showed up between Satz-Mogel and whole test scores on the WAIS-R, but average scaled scores for four tests differed no more than .14 of a scaled score point from the whole test (Robiner et al., 1988). However, five correlations between test forms fell below .90, and the amount of scatter led these workers to recommend that when patterns of interest or intratest scatter appear unusual, complete tests should be given.

Stability coefficients for an elderly sample of normal subjects retaking the Satz-Mogel short form of the WAIS-R after an average two-month delay were in the acceptable range for Verbal Scale tests (.66 to .83) but unacceptably low for Picture Arrangement (.28), Block Design (.38), and Object Assembly (.48). Thus, it is generally preferable to select and administer in their entirety tests that are the best measures of the constructs of interest and relevant to the referral question than to give more but abbreviated tests with questionable psychometric properties.

Other abbreviating techniques. Several other procedures to shorten test administration have been formalized (e.g., see individual test sections; Cargnello and Gurekas, 1987; Vincent, 1979). One version ("WAIS-M") is used with subjects who answer the first 10 items of Information correctly, in which case the examiner begins Comprehension at item 6, Arithmetic at 10, Vocabulary at 13, Block Design at 4, and Picture Arrangement at 2. Full credit is given for all earlier items when the first tested item is passed. If failed, the examiner goes back succeeding items one by one until an item is passed, scores any earlier items not given, and follows standard procedure from the new "first" item. Applying this technique to a male geriatric group, Cargnello and Gurekas (1987) found that the mean individual test scores and summary scores all differed significantly from standard administration scores, but all test score differences were within the .10 to .39 standard score range and thus of little practical consequence. The lowest correlation between the abbreviated and standard administrations was .973 (Comprehension). Cargnello and Gurekas (1988) later added Similarities (beginning at item 7) and Picture Completion (beginning at item 6) to the set of abbreviated tests (now called "WAIS-SAM"), with recommendations to begin Comprehension at 7, Arithmetic at 9, and Picture Completion at 3, leaving the "first" items for Vocabulary and Block Design as they were. These "first" items are applicable only when Information is ≥ 7; lower Information scores require lower starting points. Cella and colleagues' (1985) "first" item for the WAIS-R differs a little but his findings for the "WAIS-RM" are similar.

In a record review, the WAIS-SAM produced slightly larger discrepancies between whole and abbreviated tests (.14 to .53) than did the WIS-M; the lowest correlation was .958. Comparing this method with the Satz-Mogel technique found that WAIS-RM generated significantly smaller mean differences from the full test scores (Cella et al., 1985). However, an entry criterion based on the verbally loaded Information score limits its applicability to patients with significant left hemisphere damage (B. Caplan, 1983). For examiners who abbreviate the WIS-A tests on an ad hoc basis, these findings support the clinical impression that not administering but crediting items that are highly likely to be passed does not invalidate the examination.

Combining WAIS-III and WMS-III data

The overlapping standardization of these batteries permits data integration for the ever ongoing search to identify brain impairment reliably. M.J. Taylor and Heaton (2001) combined the four factor-based index scores from the WAIS-III with the Auditory and Visual Memory indices from the WMS-III to examine sensitivity of all measures to the six clinical samples presented in the WAIS-III/WMS-III Technical Manual, after adjusting the index scores for age, education, sex, and ethnicity. Visual Memory and Processing Speed followed by Auditory Memory were the factors most affected by the clinical conditions studied. Using a criterion of −1 SD on at least one of these three factors resulted in a diagnostic specificity of 73% and sensitivity of 90%. Although such an approach may be sufficient for identifying the presence of an abnormal condition, such a three-factor approach will not prove satisfactory for describing the range of functional capabilities and limitations required by most assessments.

WAIS-R as a Neuropsychological Instrument (WAIS-RNI) (E. Kaplan, Fein, et al., 1991)

This is a collection of adjunctive techniques designed to elicit, demonstrate, or clarify the neuropsychological and other contributions to failures on the WAIS-R specifically. The insights and recommendations for the WAIS-R examination are also applicable to the other WIS-A batteries, and several of the modifications have been adapted for the WAIS-III.

In addition to providing interpretative suggestions regarding neuropsychologically relevant aspects of performance on each of the 11 WIS-A tests, multiple-choice items are offered for the four predominantly verbal tests (Information, Vocabulary, Comprehension proverb items, Similarities); this format is thought to provide a more valid measure of premorbid attainment since it is less vulnerable to the effects of brain injury (Joy et al., 1999). Tests in the complementary modality have been developed for Digit Span (Spatial Span) and Picture Arrangement (Sentence Arrangement), three items have been added to Object Assembly, and a technique for assessing time to copy the Digit Symbol figures is also included. Poor performance on Sentence Arrangement has been correlated with other measures of frontal lobe dysfunction (Gard et al., 1999). Three rows of Digit Symbol are completed so that incidental memory for both the digit–symbol pairs and the symbols themselves can be tested. The standard discontinue rules have been extended so that a larger sample of performance is obtained. Both timed and untimed scores are obtained for Picture Completion, Picture Arrangement, Arithmetic, and Object Assembly.

Tables for evaluating the significance of intratest scatter are given for all tests but Digit Span, Digit Symbol, and Object Assembly, along with tables of Digit Span frequencies and frequency of the range of differences between the forward and reversed span; the data in these tables come from the standardization sample and are presented in the nine standardized age groups. Techniques for formalizing error analysis are also included. Using them can give invaluable learning experience as these techniques require the user to observe, distinguish, and try to make sense out of seemingly anomalous responses and abnormal behavior in a systematic manner.

Wechsler Abbreviated Scale of Intelligence (WASI) (The Psychological Corporation, 1999)

This WIS-A-based brief battery fills an important niche. It is designed to be a short form with parallel tests that yields Full Scale, Verbal, and Performance IQ scores. The four tests in the battery are Vocabulary, Similarities, Block Design, and Matrix Reasoning. Because it is a valid measure of the constructs that it purports to assess, it frees the clinician up from having to administer an entire WAIS-III battery and, thus, provides more time for tests specifically designed to examine brain–behavior relationships. Although WIS-A Vocabulary is often omitted from neuropsychological assessments, the test developers may have included it here because of its high correlations with the VIQ and FSIQ scores rather than its ability to measure any discrete neuropsychological functions.

Each of these tests is similar in form and content to its WAIS-III counterpart but contains different stimuli. The difference in item content allows them to be administered to patients who have previously been given the WAIS-III. The absolute practice effect due simply to test exposure (i.e., learning how to learn), however, is not known. Although the WAIS-III and WASI were administered in a counterbalanced order during the battery development, the possibility of order effects is not addressed in the WASI manual. Test performances are reported as T-scores rather than the familiar scaled scores of the WIS-As to facilitate the computation of IQ summary scores. Although the scaled scores can be obtained by a simple transformation, this does require an extra step.

The time to administer the four WASI tests is longer than for their WAIS-III counterparts since each WASI test contains more items. For adults who begin at the recommended normal difficulty level, the WASI item increases are four for Vocabulary, one for Block Design, and six each for Similarities and Matrix Reasoning.

In describing the potential applications of the WASI, the manual states that it should not be used for legal, judicial, or quasi-legal purposes. Of course, this leaves one to wonder if evaluations that are not intended for legal, judicial, or quasi-legal in nature are somehow less important or less significant than their forensic counterparts.

Kaufman Batteries

A.S. Kaufman and his associates have made a number of testing contributions that have potential applications in neuropsychological assessment. With the exception of the Kaufman Functional Academic Skills Test, which measures academic achievement in reading and arithmetic, the various batteries are reviewed together, in part because they share the same normative samples (11 to 85 years), but also because there has been little independent neuropsychological research on the tests in these batteries.

The Kaufman Brief Intelligence Test (K-BIT) (A.S. Kaufman and Kaufman, 1990) consists of only three tests—*Expressive Vocabulary* and *Definitions* (which are combined into a Vocabulary Standard Score), and *Matrices* (for which a Standard Score is computed). Expressive Vocabulary is essentially a confrontation naming task which, for most adult assessments, contains 15 items; Definitions requires the subject to think up a name that best fits two cues—a partial spelling of the word (e.g., B R _ W _) and a description of the word (e.g., a dark color). For most adults, 32 items are administered. Matrices contains visual analogies, 2 × 2 or 3 × 3 matrices that rely on pattern completion; 39 items are typically administered. The test has norms for ages 4–90.

Both split-half and test–retest reliabilities are high for subjects at least 20 years of age, ranging from .86 to .97. Donders (1995) failed to observe any correlation between K-BIT indexes and coma duration in a sample of children with TBI although there was a relationship with several Wechsler indexes which suggests that K-BIT may not be particularly sensitive to TBI effects. Nevertheless, K-BIT has been used by neuropsychologists to measure overall intellectual function (Bier et al., 1997; Suchy and Chelune, 2001). Not surprisingly, subjects who are poor readers tend to prefer K-BIT to the verbally based Shipley Institute of Living Scale (T.L. Bowers and Pantle, 1998).

The Kaufman Adolescent and Adult Intelligence Test (KAIT) (A.S. Kaufman and Kaufman, 1993) combines several theoretical influences: Horn and Cattell's (1966) model of fluid and crystallized intelligence, Luria's conceptualization of planning, and Piaget's (1967) stage of formal operations. It contains six subtests making up a core battery with four supplemental tests. The battery is organized into *Crystallized* and *Fluid Scales*.

In the core battery, the three Crystallized Scale tests

include *Definitions* using the same format as the K-BIT. *Auditory Comprehension* involves hearing a news story from a tape recorder followed by questions testing both literal and inferential content. *Double Meanings* items present two sets of word clues leading to the same to-be-discovered word.

The three Fluid Scale tests in the core battery are *Rebus Learning,* testing the ability to learn a word or concept associated with a particular rebus (drawing) and then apply these associations to "read" rebus phrases and sentences. In *Logical Steps* logical premises are presented both visually and aurally followed by questions based upon a given premise. *Mystery Codes* requires the subject to identify codes associated with a set of pictorial stimuli and then figure out the code for a novel pictorial stimulus.

The supplemental tests all have a memory component. *Famous Faces* requires the subject to name individuals of historical or current fame; it is also considered a test of crystallized intelligence. *Memory for Block Designs* examines the ability to construct a two-dimensional design after a brief exposure to a picture of that design. Both Auditory Comprehension and Rebus Learning are reexamined after approximately 45 minutes in *Auditory Recall* and *Rebus Recall*.

The Kaufman Short Neuropsychological Assessment Procedure (K-SNAP) (A.S. Kaufman and Kaufman, 1994) screening battery purportedly follows Luria's conceptualization of brain function as comprising three different functional units, although the individual tests are characterized by level of complexity rather than specific Lurian constructs. The tests and their various combinations generate three summary scores for the two medium- and one high-complexity tests, several composite measures, and an 8-point Impairment Index defined as a screening score to identify patients who should receive a more comprehensive evaluation.

The "low complexity" part of the battery is a mental status examination which, in addition to the usual mental status items, also assesses basic number skills such as counting, subtraction, and telling time. Basic reading skills are also tested. As with most mental status examinations, all but a few healthy patients perform at near perfect levels, giving the distribution a pronounced negative skew.

Two "medium complexity" tasks are *Gestalt Closure* and *Number Recall*. Gestalt Closure is akin to the Gestalt Completion tests developed by Street (1931), which test the ability to perceive objects or a scene from a partially completed silhouette; it is supposed to measure simultaneous processing. *Number Recall*, i.e., forward digit span, is considered a measure of successive processing. Four-Letter Words, designed to examine higher level planning, is the "high complexity" test and the only one that is timed. The subject is asked to develop strategies to figure out secret letters or secret words by generating and evaluating hypotheses.

In a study of patients with either left or right hemisphere CVAs, the K-SNAP Impairment Index discriminated left CVA patients from controls, but did not effectively identify those with right-sided lesions (Donders, 1998). Not surprisingly, patients with right cerebral lesions did significantly better than patients with left hemisphere involvement on K-SNAP Number Recall. Thus K-SNAP is a poor screening device for patients with focal right hemisphere vascular lesions. Its sensitivity in other populations remains to be established.

Peabody Individual Achievement Test–Revised (PIAT-R) (Markwardt, 1989); PIAT-R-Normative Update (PIAT-R/NU) (Markwardt, 1998)

This test battery measures academic achievement for school grades K to 12. Its wide coverage of achievement levels makes it a valuable instrument for measuring the residual cognitive competency of brain injured adults. The PIAT primarily tests verbal conceptual functions and thus handicaps patients with left hemisphere damage (Heaton, Schmitz, et al., 1987). However, the stimulus material is mostly visual—both verbal and pictorial in content—so that a variety of visuoperceptual functions enter into the PIAT performance (Fig. 17.1). No complex motor responses are required of the subject, making this available for physically handicapped patients. It was standardized on a carefully randomized national population. The PIAT is an untimed test designed to take about an hour to administer. Adult norms into the 70s are given by Heaton, Grant, and Matthews (1991). The 1998 norms show changes from earlier norms that vary on tests and at different grade levels. A computerized scoring system (ASSIST) can be purchased which can also provide a "personalized narrative report."

The six tests in the battery can each be used separately. *Mathematics* is a multiple-choice test on which patients with impaired speech need only point to an answer. It begins with simple number and symbol recognition and ends with algebra and geometry problems. On *Reading Recognition*, the subject answers the

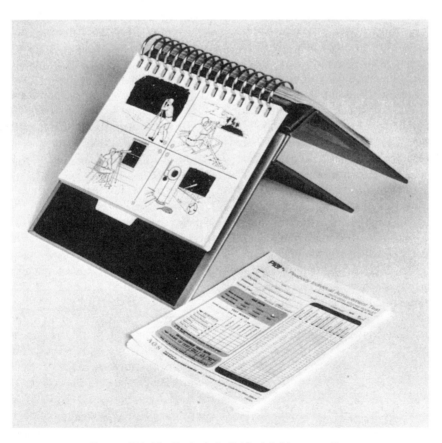

FIGURE 17.1 *The Peabody Individual Achievement Test.*

first nine items by pointing, but the remaining items require a verbal response. Items 10 to 17 present single letters, and the remaining items call for correct pronunciation of increasingly difficult words. Word difficulty ranges from "run," to "apophthegm." *Reading Comprehension* requires the subject to select which of four line drawings is described in a printed sentence. Items range in difficulty from a simple, straightforward sentence containing six one-syllable words to a complex sentence with several modifying clauses and 31 words of which 12 are at high school and college reading levels. *Spelling* is also multiple-choice and covers the full range of difficulty levels. The first 14 items test letter and word recognition; the remainder present the correct spelling and three incorrect alternatives for words in a sentence read aloud by the examiner. *General Information* is a question-and-answer test of common information. *Written Expression* requires subjects from the second grade on to write a story in response to a picture stimulus.

Each test has 100 items except Reading Comprehension, which has 82. Each test has its own norms for converting raw scores into grade and age equivalents, as well as percentile ranks for each grade level, K to 12, and percentile ranks for each age level "5-3 to 5-5" to "18-0 to 18-3." The PIAT's variety of norms facilitates comparisons of PIAT performance with that of almost any other test. Reliability and validity studies have not been done on adult populations (see Franzen, 1989).

In a group of normal older adults, a significant but virtually irrelevant age effect ($r = .17$) showed up on Reading Recognition. Education effects accounted for 20% to 46% of the variance on the reading and spelling tests for all subjects (Heaton, Schmitz, et al., 1987). Regardless of the side on which damage was lateralized, stroke patients performed below normal control subjects on Reading Comprehension and Spelling, although the scores of those with right-sided damage were not significantly lower than those of control subjects. For patients with left-sided strokes, reading and spelling scores dropped significantly as extent of damage increased. This set of tests distinguished the contributions of left hemisphere lobes as temporal and occipital damage affected reading and spelling more than damage to the other lobes. No such interlobe differences were found for the right hemisphere stroke patients.

Snijders-Oomen Nonverbal Intelligence Test–Revised 5½-17 (SON-R 5½-17) (P.J. Tellegen, M. Winkel, B.J. Wijnberg-Williams, et al., 1998)

This "intelligence test" requires neither verbal comprehension nor spoken responses although it can be given verbally. Originally developed for examining deaf children, it is not only well-suited for any communication problem but contains tests that can be used in exploring a number of neuropsychological deficits. As detailed age norms are available for each test, they can be used independently. Norms for 17-year-olds are appropriate for adults, probably well into the sixth decade, and older subjects find the tests to be user-friendly (Gerritsen et al., 2001). Norms are given as standard scores with a mean of 100 ± 15. Performances can be reported in terms of the age range at which the obtained scores are at the mean for that age. Thus, since a raw score of 13 on the Categories test converts to a standard score mean of 101 at age range 9-9 to 9-11 or 99 at age range 10-0 to 10-3, one can conclude that a person achieving this score is functioning at about the level of a 10-year-old. Standardization and normalization of the score distributions for tests by age permit comparability of intratest items and comparability across tests. An "IQ" score can be derived from a summation score. The SON-R 5½-17 is distinct from most other tests because feedback is provided to the subject and because test items are presented using an adaptive procedure.

Tests were designed to examine four areas of cognitive functioning: abstract reasoning, concrete reasoning, spatial abilities, and visuoperception. Abstract reasoning is measured by two tests: *Categories* requires the subject to recognize a class of objects (e.g., dogs) and select the two of five pictured objects that are in that category. *Analogies* requires analogic reasoning by presenting a pair of geometric figures in which the second differs from the first in some respect; another figure is depicted along with a set of four, of which the one to be identified has been altered in the same manner as the second of the model pair.

Concrete (practical and social) reasoning includes two tests: *Situations* consists of drawings of situations such as a man holding something on a leash—that something obscured by an empty square; below the picture, four or more squares contain drawings that could fit into the square from which the subject must choose the sensible fill-in picture(s). As the items get more difficult, two, three, and four responses are required for an item such that the subject must relate each possible choice to the others and the depicted situation, many of which deal with social relationships. *Stories* is a 20-item form of Picture Arrangement. Psychologists will be amused at the keys to the correct sequences as they form such famous names as WUNDT, FISHER, MASLOW, and that of the Dutch philosopher SPINOZA.

There are also two spatial tests: *Mosaics* is a flattened version of Kohs blocks (Block Design), which consists of plastic squares with six different surface patterns (all red, all white, red and white halved into triangles, red and white halved into rectangles, white with a red quarter corner, and red with a white quarter corner). These can be combined into 2 × 2 or 3 × 3 square designs. *Patterns* is a drawing test requiring the subject to continue a horizontally presented printed line and angle pattern on graphed paper. The single perceptual test, *Hidden Pictures,* consists of four items in which a target figure (e.g., a kite) must be found in the objects drawn in an accompanying picture (e.g., in a bird's beak, a man's vest, a boat's sail, etc.). All tests are introduced with examples. Norms for Hidden Pictures, Mosaics, Patterns, and Stories are based on time-restricted administrations.

Stanford-Binet Intelligence Scale (Thorndike et al., 1986)

This edition of the Stanford-Binet differs radically from its predecessors. Gone are the relatively brief items that made testing young and hyperactive children more of an athletic contest than a standardized procedure; but with them went many of the neuropsychologically valuable techniques described in this book that can enrich the neuropsychological examination. In their stead are 15 tests, some of which will be applicable to adult assessment, but few provide test formats that are both distinctive and appropriate for adult use. Among those deserving exploration for adult neuropsychological assessment purposes are *Paper Folding and Cutting, Number Series* (requiring the subject to complete a number sequence), *Equation Building* (requiring mathematical ingenuity as well as reasoning), *Verbal Relations* (identifying which of four items differs from the others), and *Memory for Objects* (in which the target figures must be identified and recalled in their proper sequence). *Absurdities* and *Bead Memory,* although limited in difficulty level, could also be of neuropsychological interest. The other tests have counterparts in tests and batteries with adult norms that are already well-integrated into neuropsychological assessment repertoires: *Vocabulary, Quantitative* (items 13–40 are arithmetic story problems), *Pattern Analysis* (at upper levels is similar to Block Design), *Comprehension, Copying* (simple geometric shapes with a limited difficulty level), *Matrices* (resemblance to Raven's Matrices), *Memory for Digits* (forward and reversed), and *Memory for Sentences.*

The tests in this battery were designed to measure abilities in four areas: Verbal Reasoning, Abstract/Visual Reasoning, Quantitative Reasoning, and Short-Term Memory. Factor analysis of the standardization data essentially supported these dimensions and the assignment of tests to them (G.J. Boyle, 1989). A Profile Analysis sheet provides for a test profile organized by these four areas; an Inferred Abilities and Influences Chart, also arranged by tests within these four areas, allows for analysis of the test performance into areas of Strengths ("S") or Weaknesses ("W"). The summary sheet provides for score conversions into age-graded standard scores for each test (called Standard Age Scores, or SAS), a Composite Score (which is another name for an IQ score with a mean of 100 ± 16), and area scores. Norms go up to age 23, although no test has an age-equivalent over 17 years 8 months. Although the Stanford-Binet continues to be used primarily with children (J.R. Smith et al., 2001; Sulzbacher et al., 1999), its sensitivity at the lower end of the age distribution makes it also appropriate for cognitively impaired adults (Dacey et al., 1999; W.S. Matthews et al., 1999; W.M. Nelson and Dacey, 1999). Reliability and validity studies relevant to adult neuropsychology are not presently available.

Stanford-Binet Intelligence Scales, 5th ed. (SB5) (G.H. Roid, 2003)

This newest mental ability battery retains some of the valuable test formats of the first three editions while adding many new ones. One striking similarity with the first three editions is the rotating assessment of different kinds of abilities through difficulty levels. The overall format and examination plan differ from any of its predecessors as the battery is organized into five factor-related "Domains": *Fluid Reasoning, Knowledge, Quantitative Reasoning, Visual–Spatial Processing,* and *Working Memory.* These Domains and the test material itself show a greater influence of neuropsychological experience and cognitive theory in the development of this battery than in previous editions. Each domain is examined by a verbal and a nonverbal subtest. These subtests are divided into difficulty—or maturity—levels: six nonverbal, five verbal (since there are no verbal tests at the lowest level, age 2). Examination at each level is conducted by a brief "testlet" for each of the five domains. The examination begins with two "Routing Subtests," *Vocabulary* and *Matrices.* Performances on these direct the examiner to proceed with the examination at the appropriate verbal and nonverbal levels. Testing continues through each level until the subject scores fewer than three points (always out of a possible six) on a testlet in each domain. It is possible to examine only one or two domains or only the verbal or nonverbal divisions.

This system permits continued testing in areas of strength after the subject has failed lower level items in other domains. Raw scores are converted into "Scaled Score Equivalents" for each domain for 70 different age ranges (1-month intervals to age 5, 3-month intervals to age 17, then two 2-year, then 5-year intervals to age 89+). Scaled Score Equivalents, in turn, are converted into "Standard Score Equivalents of Sums of Scaled Scores." Although Roid manages to pull "IQ scores" out of this essentially factor-based examination schedule, he does suggest that should the "Nonverbal IQ (NVIQ)" differ considerably from the "Verbal IQ (VIQ)", the examiner "should be cautious about evaluating FSIQ as a summary of an individual's general ability level," although he gives no such caution regarding possible large differences between domains when computing the NVIQ and VIQ. He does acknowledge that the terms "nonverbal" and "verbal" are "relative, comparative terms" in that the nonverbal tests "have lower language demands." Five factor Indexes are also computed and should be entered into test interpretation.

The SB5 normative population consisted of 4,800 persons in the 2 to 85+ age range and demographically matched to percentages defined by the U.S. Census Bureau (2001). A review of the different reliability and stability tables show ranges mostly in the .80s and .90s. Validity correlations with other editions of the Stanford-Binet, with Wechsler child and adult tests, and with the Woodcock-Johnson III Achievement battery are respectable.

Psychological examiners today are used to the single-test format of the Wechsler batteries and many other batteries in common use, including the SB5's immediate predecessor, and may find it difficult to shift gears to a shifting test pattern. However, the serial variations in tasks may well help to maintain interest and attention, especially of younger subjects. While the domains are well-substantiated statistically, since the testlets vary somewhat (e.g., Level 3 Working Memory is Memory for Sentences; but Level 4 Working Memory is a short-term word memory test), the Domain scores will be less useful for neuropsychological interpretations than would one longer assessment of the same task (e.g., Sentence Repetition, p. 358). Thus this battery does not appear to be suitable for in-depth study of specific cognitive functions although it will give an overall perspective on a subject's mental ability levels in general. Both the administration and technical manuals are clearly written, but each lacks an index.

Wide Range Achievement Test–Revised, 3rd ed.
(WRAT-R, WRAT-3) (G.S. Wilkinson, 1993)

This battery format instrument earns its "wide range" title by its applicability from early childhood to the later adult years. It tests three academic skills—spelling, single word reading, and arithmetic—and parallel forms for the WRAT-3 are available to facilitate repeated assessment. The WRAT is standardized with a full set of norms for each test, plus each parallel form has its own set of norms. Raw scores are converted to standard scores or percentiles and, if necessary, grade equivalents although they tend to be least useful. The two versions of the WRAT-3 can be administered to ages 5 to 64, but with different starting levels according to item difficulty. One or more of the tests in this battery is often included in a comprehensive neuropsychological assessment.

Alternative form correlations range from .82 to .99, with coefficients for Reading and Spelling slightly higher than for Arithmetic. The manual provides data for the different age ranges. This is a significant improvement over its predecessor which did not give a breakdown for age groups. Like previous versions of the test, however, validity information is generally lacking (Franzen, 1989; Spreen and Strauss, 1998).

This is a popular battery, in part because it is easy to administer and interpret, and it has the increasingly rare virtue of being relatively inexpensive. However, cautions against relying on its use for much more than crude screening have been raised on the basis both of the narrowness of its content—particularly on the Reading test (Spreen and Strauss, 1998)—and of the lack of satisfactory reliability and validity studies (Franzen, 1989).

With the increased interest in measures of premorbid ability, the Reading subtest has found a specialized application in neuropsychology. All measures of premorbid function are simply estimates, although this one relies on the principle that unless there is profound cognitive deterioration or focal left perisylvian lesions, single word reading should be relatively unaffected. Thus, if a patient can properly pronounce a phonetically irregular word such as "paradigm," then it is reasonable to infer that the patient has had previous experience with that word. Use of the WRAT-R Reading for premorbid prediction compares favorably to regression-based procedures (Kareken et al., 1995).

In comparison to the National Adult Reading Test–Revised (NART-R), the WRAT-R Reading score gave a more accurate premorbid estimate of *average* and lower WAIS-R scores, although both the WRAT-R Reading and NART-R underestimated WAIS-R IQ scores at the higher end of the distribution (Wiens, Bryan, and Crossen, 1993), a pattern that was confirmed in a subsequent study using the WRAT-R Reading test and the North American Adult Reading Test (NAART) (B. Johnstone, Callahan, et al., 1996). WRAT Reading has been effective in estimating premorbid abilities for patients with TBI (B. Johnstone, Hexum, et al., 1995), drug abuse (Ollo, Lindquist, et al., 1995), and schizophrenia (Weickert et al., 2000).

Woodcock-Johnson III (WJ III) (Woodcock, McGrew, and Mather, 2001a)

This is the recently developed and enlarged edition of a set of tests, originally designed for evaluation of cognitive ability and academic achievement, which continues to assess both. WJ III is actually two distinct test sets: tests in *WJ III COG* measure relatively discrete aspects of cognitive functioning (Mather and Woodcock, 2001; Woodcock, McGrew, and Mather, 2001c); *WJ III ACH* contains academic achievement measures (Woodcock, McGrew, and Mather, 2001b).

WJ III COG. This test set is of most interest to neuropsychologists. Its predecessor, *WJ-R Tests of Cognitive Ability*, was theoretically grounded in cognitive psychology theory of crystallized (*Gc*) and fluid (*Gf*) mental abilities (McArdle et al., 2002; Woodcock, 1990). This revision represents a conceptual reorganization integrating two different ways of analyzing cognition by means of factor analysis (McGrew and Woodcock, 2001). Tests are grouped into three overarching cognitive categories defined by factor analysis: *Verbal Ability, Thinking Ability,* and *Cognitive Efficiency.* Analysis along the crystallized/fluid dimension (referred to as CHC factors for the psychologists R.B. Cattell, J.L. Horn, and J.B. Carroll who developed this conceptual formulation) generated seven different factors which are considered to be "broad abilities:" *Comprehension-Knowledge* (*Gc*), *Long-Term Retrieval* (*Glr*), *Visual-Spatial Thinking* (*Gv*), *Auditory Processing* (*Ga*), *Fluid Reasoning* (*Gf*), *Processing Speed* (*Gs*), and *Short-Term Memory* (*Gsm*). Within each cognitive category are two to four tests measuring a narrow aspect of a broad ability, thus each loads on a different CHC factor (e.g., 6. *Visual Matching* and 7. *Numbers Reversed* are both in the Cognitive Efficiency category, the former also loads on Fluid Reasoning, the latter on Short-Term Memory). Additional analysis identified seven *Clinical Clusters: Phonemic Awareness, Working Memory, Broad Attention, Cognitive Fluency, Executive Processes, Delayed Recall,* and *Knowledge.*

WJ III COG tests and scoring. The COG battery contains two sets of ten tests, the *Standard Battery* and the *Extended Battery,* each set including at least one test in each of the three Cognitive Categories. Six tests in the Standard Battery and seven in the Extended Battery plus two WJ III ACH tests contribute to the Clinical Clusters, each of which is based on two to four tests. A table, identifying the Cognitive Category, CHC factor, and Clinical Cluster(s) for each test, enables the examiner to select the tests appropriate for each examination.

Age and education equivalents are provided in the Test Record booklet for all but *10. Visual-Auditory Learning-Delayed,* which assesses speed of relearning previously learned symbol–word associations (in *2. Visual-Auditory Learning*); its scoring requires the computerized "*Compuscore and Profiles Program*". Age and education ranges vary from test to test. Most age ranges for most tests begin at 2 or within age 2, with few exceptions (e.g., age 5 for Numbers Reversed). Ceilings, however, vary from 12-1 (*20. Pair Cancellation,* testing visuoperceptual speed and accuracy) to 40 (*11. General Information,* which asks "Where" named items can be found, and "What" one does with other named items). The education range for all but two tests is K.0 to 18.0, the exceptions being Pair Cancellation and *18. Rapid Picture Naming* with ceilings of 8.5 and 7.3, respectively. The authors take care to point out that these score equivalents are only estimates. The computerized scoring program provides more exact score equivalents, taking the age range up to 90. Many different scores are generated by the computer program including percentile ranks, CHC factor scores, and cluster scores (see Wendling and Mather, 2001, *Examiner Training Workbook*). Of course, when using these tests selectively, scores requiring combinations and comparisons of discrete test scores cannot be obtained. For most purposes, experienced neuropsychologists should be able to rely on the age and education equivalents.

Administration. Most of the stimulus material is contained in two Test Books which are easy to handle. Test instructions accompany the stimulus material in the Test Books. Although the authors recommend following the published test sequence, they explicitly state that, except for the immediate and delayed Visual-Auditory Learning tests, the examiner can decide the presentation order. The complete battery package for the WJ III COG comes with a record booklet for *Tests of Cognitive Abilities: BIA* (i.e., Brief Intellectual Ability). Included are one test from each of the three Cognitive Categories: Verbal Comprehension (Verbal Ability), Concept Formation (Thinking Ability), and Visual Matching (Cognitive Efficiency), presumably to provide a quick across-the-board sampling of cognitive performance.

Many of the tests are presented visually, in pictures, symbols, or words or phrases (e.g., *1. Verbal Comprehension* which has three parts together yielding one score: *Picture Vocabulary,* picturing the response to a question such as, "On what does an apple grow?", and *Synonyms* and *Antonyms,* in each of which the response is given to a word displayed in print). The administration of six tests is on tape (e.g., *4. Sound Blending*, in which words are presented as discrete syllables or phonemes to be repeated fluently as a word; yet even on this test, "in rare cases" the first 16 items can be spoken by the examiner). Other taped tests, such as Numbers Reversed, *9. Auditory Working Memory* (in which strings of mixed digits and words must be sorted out and repeated in the order in which they were heard), and *17. Memory for Words* (a straightforward word repetition test in which the longest string is seven) have counterparts elsewhere (e.g., WIS-A Digit Span, Letter-Number Sequencing), lending themselves to direct administration by an experienced examiner accustomed to maintaining appropriately paced speech. Five tests have time limits (e.g., Visual Matching has two parts: #1- for preschoolers shows 26 sets of three to five common geometric symbols with two symbols the same to be pointed out within two minutes; #2 presents a page with two printed columns of 30 rows of five nonconsecutive numbers, the subject must circle with a pencil as many row pairs of identical numbers as possible within three minutes). Acknowledging that not all examiners use stop watches, the test record booklet provides a place to record starting and stopping times for these tests.

Of tests similar to those developed elsewhere some differ a little; for example, *18. Rapid Picture Naming*, which tests confrontation naming to pictures, timing (2 min.) is for the whole test and—unfortunately, unlike the Boston Naming Test, cueing is not an option for determining whether the unspoken word is unknown or simply difficult to retrieve. Yet *12. Retrieval Fluency* tests semantic verbal fluency in three common categories: "things to eat or drink, first names of people, and animals," maintaining its similarity to most verbal fluency tests in the one min time limit per trial.

Several tests are unique to this battery and deserve special mention, especially since all but the two learning tests can be given independently of any other. *3. Spatial Relations* reversed the Minnesota Paper Form Board format by requiring the subject to identify which two or three of six pictured part pieces together form a pictured geometric figure. In *5. Concept Formation*, the subject must identify the characteristic(s) (size, shape, number, color) distinguishing one set of simple geometric shapes from another set. *15. Analysis-Synthesis* asks the subject to generalize from given color–pattern relationships to incomplete patterns in a series of increasingly complex relationship patterns. *16. Decision Speed* is a variant of timed picture or symbol matching tasks differing in that the objects to be matched are not identical but come from the same category (e.g., cat–dog, moon–sun), thus requiring not just

rapid scanning and response but a conceptual search. The authors call *19. Planning*, "a test of executive functioning" in that subjects must plan as they trace a series of increasingly complex designs without repeating a line.

Neuropsychological applications. Like its predecessor—the *Woodcock Johnson Tests of Cognitive Ability–Revised (WJ-R COG)* (Woodcock and Johnson, 1989), this set of tests was developed with neuropsychological assessment in mind. Its cognitive foundations certainly appear to fit in with a neuropsychological perspective in analyzing and interpreting test data. The free-standing but statistically equatable nature of the tests also encourages exploration of cognitive functioning on a very individualized basis. Whether these tests test what they purport to test remains to be seen. If, as they appear and as they are described, each test measures effectively the abilities associated with it, then this battery will be a valued addition to neuropsychological assessment practice (see also, Binks and Gold, 1998).

Batería Woodcock-Muñoz: Pruebas de habilidad cognitiva-Revisada (BAT-R COG) (Woodcock, 1998; Woodcock and Muñoz-Sandoval, 1996b; Woodcock and Muñoz-Sandoval, 2001). This Spanish language battery consists of tests parallel to the WJ-R COG set (Pontón and Léon Carrión, 2001). Its norms are derived from the original English-speaking normative population. "Calibration-equating data for each test" used test performances of almost 4,000 mostly monolingual native Spanish speakers tested in Latin America, the United States, and Spain. Subjects took one or more of the battery tests. Rescaling was done to equate the "empirical difficulty" of each Spanish test to its English counterpart. While acknowledging that this battery does not provide a fully comprehensive neuropsychological examination, Pontón and Léon Carrión consider this the most comprehensive Spanish language set of tests available and provide several case examples to demonstrate the battery's neuropsychological applicability.

Woodcock-Johnson III Tests of Achievement (WJ III ACH)

These tests were developed for "all age levels from preschool through geriatric." They are organized into two batteries, a *Standard Battery* containing 12 tests, and a ten test *Extended Battery;* each test has two equivalent forms, A and B. The tests cover four specific academic areas: *Reading* (three tests), *Oral Language* (four tests), *Mathematics* (three tests), and *Written Language* (three tests)—plus six supplemental topics (e.g., Academic Knowledge, Phoneme/Grapheme Knowledge). Like the WJ III COG, tests should be selected for use as needed. Although each test in an academic area examines a discrete aspect of performance in that area, the authors recommend that interpretation rest on clustered data for that area. Tables are provided indicating the kinds of discrepancies that can arise within academic areas and between academic performance (i.e., WJ III ACH scores) and ability (i.e., WJ III COG scores). Crystallized/fluid abilities theory also informs interpretation recommendations. The WJ III Compuscore and Profiles Program provides computerized scoring. When academic performance questions arise in neuropsychological assessment, tests in this battery may be particularly useful since WJ III ACH data can be related directly to WJ III COG performance levels.

Batería Woodcock-Muñoz: Pruebas de aprovechamienta–Revisada (BAT-R APR) (Woodcock, 1998; Woodcock and Muñoz-Sandoval, 1996a). This is the Spanish language battery that parallels the *WJ-R Tests of Achievement–Revised* (Woodcock and Johnson, 1989). Its development also paralleled that of the BAT-R COG, making possible comparisons between tests in the two Spanish language batteries (Woodcock, 1998; Pontón and Leon-Carrión, 2001).

Paper-and-Pencil Administration

MacQuarrie Test for Mechanical Ability (MacQuarrie, 1925, 1953)

This little set of tests was developed to aid in employee selection and job placement. Although it is a paper-and-pencil test designed for group administration, it examines a variety of functions of neuropsychological interest, such as simple visuomotor speed and accuracy, visuospatial estimation, and visual tracking. Moreover, standardized test norms enable the examiner to make informative intertest comparisons.

This test set differs from most paper-and-pencil formats in that six of the seven tests require visuomotor responses. Each test is preceded by a practice trial which enables the subject to establish a set and the examiner to make sure the subject understands the task.

The first three tests measure manual speed and more or less fine motor control. *Tracing* allows 50 sec. during which the subject must draw a continuous line through irregularly placed tiny gaps in small vertical lines is a speed test in which accuracy is equally important. The next two tests last 30 sec. *Tapping* requires the subject to make three pencil dots in each of a series of small circles and disregards accuracy. In contrast, accuracy is primary in *Dotting* as the subject must place one dot in each of a series of very small circles placed irregularly along a zig-zagging pathway.

The next three tests involve visuospatial functions. *Copying* presents 20 figures to copy onto a grid of dots with a $2^1/_2$ min. time limit (see Fig. 17.2). *Location* consists of a large square containing a 6×6 array of letters arranged so that no two of the 12 duplicated letters are in the same quadrant. Along its sides are eight smaller squares, each containing five dots scattered in the same relative positions as five corresponding letters in the large square. The subject is given two min to write in the letter corresponding to each dot. *Blocks* is a block-counting test consisting of line representations of six three-dimensional constructions made up of one size of block (e.g., see Fig. 15.11, p. 607, for a similar but easier test item). The task is to figure out the number of blocks touched by the five designated blocks in each construction within the allotted $2^1/_2$ mins. The last test, *Pursuit*, measures speed and accuracy of visual tracking by presenting a line-tracing format that requires the subject to follow lines visually through a tangle of other lines with a $2^1/_2$ min time limit. The entire test takes about 30 min. Subtests can be given or omitted as appropriate for the examination.

The test manual provides separate percentile norms for each test for men and women "aged sixteen up," based on test performances of 1000 adults of each sex. It also gives some data showing how well these tests correlated with performance on a variety of industrial jobs.

Hubley and Jassal (unpublished manuscript) examined this set of tests with 51 normal adults (ages 20 to 82, $M = 50 \pm 18$; education 9–21 years, $M = 14.7 \pm 2.6$).

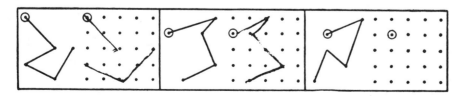

FIGURE 17.2 Practice items of the *MacQuarrie* Copying subtest. The subject who made the responses shown here performed poorly on the test items as well (see text).

TABLE 17.2 Mean Performances on the *MacQuarrie Tests of Mechanical Ability* by Age Group (Preliminary [4-4-03] Version, Small Groups)

Subtest	Maximum Score Possible	20–39 years (n = 18)	40–59 years (n = 18)	60+ years (n = 17)
Tracing	80	44.0 ± 10.8*	34.1 ± 11.4	30.1 ± 6.4
Tapping	70	41.5 ± 7.0	40.3 ± 8.5	31.6 ± 6.0
Dotting	33	21.5 ± 3.7	19.1 ± 3.5	15.8 ± 3.7
Copying	80	46.2 ± 15.4	35.7 ± 11.7	28.9 ± 18.2
Location	40	28.6 ± 10.2	25.6 ± 9.2	18.2 ± 5.8
Blocks	30	17.8 ± 5.9	11.7 ± 5.6	6.8 ± 4.4
Pursuit	40	26.7 ± 6.3	20.6 ± 6.9	13.3 ± 4.9

*S.D. rounded to one place.
Reproduced courtesy of Anita M. Hubley.

Scores decreased as age advanced but correlations with education were small and not significant (see Table 17.2). One week test–retest correlations ranged from .69 (Tracing) to .91 (Blocks). A few subtests showed insignificant retest gains. Intercorrelations between subtests were all significant at the $p < .01$ level (ranging from .45 to .73). This range was similar to subtests' correlations with WAIS-III Block Design (range .30 [Tapping] to .64 [Location]), although correlations with Vocabulary were all insignificant (range −.16 to .02). Hubley notes, "the least surprising result is that all subtests are significantly correlated with Trails A ($r = .46$ to .56) and Trails B ($r = .45$ to .63)" (personal communication, April 2003 [mdl]).

Patterns of differences in test performance levels can be clinically relevant. Patients whose visuospatial abilities are intact but who have poor regulation or coordination of fine motor activity will perform less well on the first three tests than on Tracing or Location. When visuospatial functions are impaired but motor activity remains intact and under good control, large differences in performance levels will appear in low Copying and Location scores and high scores on the motor speed and accuracy tasks. The sample Copying task items, for example (see Fig. 17.2), show the failed responses of a 30-year-old surveyor two years after he fell eight feet onto the side of his head sustaining right temporoparietal injuries. He performed in the first to fifth percentiles on this test and on Location, but Tracing, Tapping, and Dotting were all above the 90th percentile.

Multidimensional Aptitude Battery (MAB)
(D.N. Jackson, 1986)

This paper-and-pencil battery parallels the Wechsler scales but in a multiple-choice format. It is being used in a variety of research studies such as genetic contri-

butions to cognition (Luciano et al., 2001) and for measures of "practical intelligence" (Taub et al., 2001). It is divided into two scales, "Verbal" and "Performance" (although no more "performance" is required than moving a pencil). The five tests in each of these scales have such familiar-sounding names as *Information, Comprehension, Digit Symbol, Picture Arrangement,* etc. Only *Spatial* differs in name and content from the WAIS: it requires the subject to identify which of five inverted or rotated figures is identical to a target figure. Each test has a 7 min time limit which penalizes slow responders, but this restriction allows for group testing.

Performances on all ten tests can be converted into individual scaled scores (actually, T-scores with a mean of 50 ± 10), summarized into "Verbal," "Performance," and "Full Scale" scores in which the mean is 500 ± 100. The test was designed for ages 16 to 74. Sample sizes at most but not all age levels are adequate. Individual test reliability and stability coefficients range from satisfactory to excellent but may be spuriously high because of the time limitation (P.A. Vernon, 1985). Much of its validation comes from correlational studies with the WAIS-R: not surprisingly, the Spatial test correlates least well with its Wechsler mate, Block Design (.44) while Arithmetic and Vocabulary correlate best, at .89 each with their WAIS-R counterparts. Moreover, the MAB factor pattern appears similar to that of the WIS-A tests, although the individual tests should not be treated as equivalent to their Wechsler counterparts (Carless, 2000).

This set of tests may provide supplemental or comparison information to the WIS-A tests, and the spatial test appears to be interesting in its own right. Unfortunately, the timing requirement may limit the MAB's usefulness as a neuropsychological test adjunct as with it, slow subjects will not be satisfactorily examined; without timing, the examiner faces the question of applicability of the norms. So long as the tests need to be timed, they cannot be a real time saver—someone has to watch the clock. However, for examiners who are interested in how well a patient can perform without regard to speed, and who can use judgment in applying the norms, tests in this battery may be useful for some patients with motor or speech impairments. The MAB appears to have been adopted into the assessment of Air Force pilots and Space Shuttle astronaut candidates (Bishop et al., 1996; Carretta et al., 1998; R.E. King and Flynn, 1995).

Shipley Institute of Living Scale (SILS) (Shipley, 1940; Shipley and Burlingame, 1941), Revised Manual (Zachary, 1986)

This easily administered paper-and-pencil test is included here because, like the K-BIT or the Wechsler Individual Achievement Test (WIAT) Screener (see below), it has been used to screen for brain dysfunction. It was originally developed to identify mentally deteriorated psychiatric patients but was soon applied to other patient groups. It consists of two subtests that are fully reproduced with the original scoring key and normative tables in Pollack (1942). Based on the assumption that, with mental deterioration, the ability to form abstract concepts will erode sooner than vocabulary, this instrument compares scores on a 40-item multiple-choice vocabulary subtest and a 20-item subtest requiring concept formation and solution-finding on abstract verbal and arithmetic problems.

Using a normative group of 1,046 students from fourth grade through college, Shipley (1940) devised age-equivalent (and IQ score equivalent) tables for each subtest's scores. The ratio of these age equivalent scores (the vocabulary age-equivalent score is the denominator) is the *Conceptual Quotient* (*CQ*), the "index of impairment." Shipley (1940) warned that "quotients obtained from vocabulary scores below 23 are of doubtful validity." Yet in one sample of 38 relatively young male psychiatric outpatients, eight (21%) received scores below 23. That so many of these clinic patients did not achieve vocabulary scores within the acceptable range is not surprising. Many of the words (e.g., 26-rue, 32-lissom, 40-pristine) rarely appear in print and are heard even less frequently. Moreover, the "correct" responses to several items (inexorable, abet, pristine) do not appear in either Webster's 1989 *Encyclopedic Unabridged Dictionary* or Roget's *Thesaurus,* which can create a problem for persons who really know what these words mean as there is no good definition for any of these three words among the four choices.

Other workers have devised norms and scores to correct for the original failure to take account of adult ages or education (none of the norms is stratified for sex) (see Zachary, 1986). This correction is presumably accomplished by means of a regression equation based on the Vocabulary score, education, and age from which is derived a *predicted* Abstraction score which, in turn, is subtracted from the *obtained* Abstraction score; the difference is converted into a standard score called the *Abstraction Quotient* (*AQ*). The AQ is interpreted like a CQ. This formula was developed in 1964 on 198 persons associated with a Veterans Administration hospital; subjects who scored below 23 on Vocabulary were excluded from the study. The Abstraction Quotient is reported to account for 38% of the variance in Abstraction scores.

Despite its long history, the use of the CQ as an index of cognitive impairment has not received consistent experimental support.

> Most of the available research does not support use of the CQ as a screening measure to assess intellectual impairment or deterioration. Although the concept of a discrepancy index based on a ratio of "no hold" to "hold" tasks has a strong theoretical basis and persists in clinical practice, the efforts to quantify this approach have not been met with much success. (Zachary, 1986, p. 62)

The revised manual also offers age-corrected *T*-score conversion tables for the three raw scores, presumably to help examiners make a more appropriate evaluation of older (up to age 64) subjects' performances. However the "revised normative sample" is a "mixed (undefined) sample of 290 psychiatric patients" with sex evenly divided, used in a study reported in 1970. Only the mean age (34.9) is mentioned leaving unreported how many subjects contributed to each of the 11 age groups or how many age by score cells generated the smoothed-out age-corrected *T*-score tables. Obviously, not only are norms developed on psychiatric patients not applicable for many persons receiving a screening examination for neuropsychological disorders; but the diagnostic techniques and criteria and the psychiatric treatments used in 1970 make a 1970 psychiatric population an unknown quantity. It is hardly suited for the development of neuropsychological screening criteria.

Additionally, the revised manual provides for prediction of WAIS or WAIS-R IQ scores from Shipley *Total* scores. Although the Shipley is a highly verbal test, formulas are given for estimating Wechsler Full Scale IQ scores; but the examiner can look up approximated IQ score estimates in tables stratified by age. Like the original manual, the revised manual also reports *mental age equivalents* (from 8.4 to 20.8—these derived from the original set of student subjects) for the three raw scores.

In using the Shipley to obtain an estimated WAIS-R IQ score, one study found a .79 correlation between the Shipley estimate and the actual WAIS-R Full Scale IQ score for patients with a sixth grade or better reading ability (Frisch and Jessop, 1989). Another study reported correlations of .30 to .45 with the FSIQ (Fowles and Tunick, 1986); the conversion formula overestimated IQ scores for this sample, more for lower level than for higher scoring subjects. Zachary (1986) reported that the Shipley underestimates IQ scores that are either under 85 or over 120.

Both the mean Vocabulary Age and Abstractions Age of a group of alcoholics were significantly lower than those of a middle-aged control group (M.D. Shelton et al., 1984). These authors warned that Shipley scores may lead to the erroneous conclusion that patients with low scores on both subtests have generalized decrements when their losses may be quite specific. Older research studies reported that the Shipley failed to discriminate between neurologic patients and normal control subjects as well as between different categories of neuropsychiatric patients (Aita, Armitage, et al., 1947; Savage, 1970). Another study did identify patients with cognitive impairment and suggested that this test may be useful for coarse screening of thought disorders without distinguishing between neurologic and functional problems (Prado and Taub, 1966). Most of the recent studies employing the Shipley for neuropsychological evaluations, however, tend to use the Vocabulary and Abstraction scores independently (Beatty, Tivis, et al., 2000; Leckey, 2002; Putzke et al., 2000).

Wechsler Individual Achievement Test (WIAT) (The Psychological Corporation, 1992)

This set of eight tests, if given in its entirety, yields 13 scores (*Basic Reading, Reading Comprehension, Total Reading, Mathematics Reasoning, Numerical Operations, Total Mathematics, Listening Comprehension, Oral Expression, Total Language, Spelling, Written Expression, Total Writing,* and *Total Composite*). Thus, outside of academic applications, the entire battery is unlikely to be used with many adult neuropsychological assessments. A *WIAT Screener,* similar to the Wide Range Achievement Tests (WRAT) and consisting of *Basic Reading, Mathematics Reasoning,* and *Spelling,* is also available. Among these three, the test that differs most from the WRAT is Mathematics Reasoning, which contains word problems related to money, time, numerical order, and graphs. For both the complete and screening applications, the test developers include a summary scale that collapses performance across all measures into a single score, which will provide no clarification of any deficit under investigation;

nor tell any parent or teacher in what subjects a child excels or needs remedial assistance. As normative data are available through 19 years, the oldest age norms can probably be used when evaluating young adults. The advantage of this battery is its direct link to the *Wechsler Intelligence Scale for Children, Third Edition* (*WISC-III,* Wechsler, 1991), WISC-IV (Wechsler, 2003), and WAIS-R, allowing the examiner to compare test scores directly from one battery to another. In addition, the Mathematics Reasoning test likely assesses more applied mathematics than simple computational ability and, hence, may ultimately be a more ecologically valid method for assessing mathematical skills than WRAT-3 Arithmetic.

BATTERIES DEVELOPED FOR NEUROPSYCHOLOGICAL ASSESSMENT

Batteries for General Use

Halstead-Reitan Battery (HRB) (Halstead, 1947; Reitan, 1955c; Reitan and Wolfson, 1993)

Ward Halstead (1947) developed the core tests of the HRB in the 1940s as part of a larger series of tests sensitive to "brain damage;" these were subsequently combined into a fixed battery by Ralph Reitan (undated; Reitan and Wolfson, 1993). Since its inception, the set of tests that comprise the Halstead-Reitan battery has grown by accretion and revision.

The HRB core battery includes: (1) *Category Test* (CT); (2) *Tactual Performance Test* (TPT); (3) *Seashore Rhythm Test* (SRT); (4) *Speech Sounds Perception Test* (SSPT); and (5) *Finger Tapping Test* (FTT) (or *Finger Oscillation*). These five tests yield seven scores, three of which come from the Tactual Performance Test (*Total Time, Memory, Location*), which are used to calculate the Impairment Index. Additional tests in the HRB include the *Aphasia Screening Test, Grip Strength, Sensory-Perceptual Examination, Tactile Form Recognition,* and *Trail Making Test.* A WAIS and Minnesota Multiphasic Personality Inventory (MMPI) are also typically administered (Reitan and Wolfson, 1993).

Halstead's contribution. Some tests in this battery were developed by Halstead himself (e.g., Category Test; Halstead and Settlage, 1943), others were adopted without significant change from their use as ability measures, (e.g., Speech Sounds Perception—no citation other than "supplied to writer by Professor Louis D. Goodfellow"), while others were modified substantially from existing procedures (e.g., Seguin-Goddard formboard used for the Tactual Performance Test). It was typical for psychologists at that time to modify and incorporate existing tests into a battery, as was also done by David Wechsler when he developed the Wechsler-Bellevue battery (Boake, 2002).

Halstead's (1947) initial battery contained 27 neuropsychological measures and averaged 15 hours to administer and score. From this battery, Halstead selected seven tests yielding 10 scores for an *Impairment Index* based upon the tests' ability to discriminate nine patients with "a definite history of acute head injury with an interval of unconsciousness" from six subjects "without a definite history of head injury." Halstead subsequently cross-validated the Impairment Index on a sample of 25 mixed neuropsychiatric patients whose symptoms were "more marked" than the initial group and 25 control subjects. The Impairment Index ranges from 0.0 when no performance is impaired, to 1.0, indicating that all 10 scores are in the impaired range. Unlike a summary IQ measure, which is based upon test scores that are normally distributed, tests contributing to the Impairment Index have skewed distributions requiring nonparametric data handling. In this way Halstead's tests are similar to neurological examination techniques in which various reflexes or signs are often characterized as "normal" or "abnormal"— or "present" or "absent"—or rated on a 4- or 5-point scale on which most ratings are in the normal or near-normal part of the range. Halstead considered the Impairment Index to reflect the "empirical odds out of ten chances that a given individual has an impairment of cortical brain functions" (p. 110).

Halstead was aware that factors other than brain injury could contribute to Impairment Index elevations, and considered performances on other tests to be relevant. "Normal performance on [non-Impairment Index measures] supplies control information concerning such variables as co-operation, attention, malingering, and level of effort" (p. 108). Three of Halstead's 14 healthy control subjects had elevations that Halstead attributed to either "the presence of mild clinical depression" or "acute 'test' anxiety."

Unfortunately, Halstead's methods have led to confusion regarding certain "fixed battery" aspects of the Impairment Index and raise questions about the validity of his norms and recommended cutting scores. As told by Reitan (1996) "with respect to [Halstead's] data collection . . . the tests were not necessarily given in the same way to all subjects and all subjects didn't necessarily get the same tests." According to Table 16 of Halstead's 1947 book, only 14 of 50 neurosurgical patients received the Speech Sounds Perception test, and only 18 took the Category Test. Halstead's norms and cutting scores, however, continue to be used for group classification by many examiners (e.g., Dodrill, 1999; Jarvis and Barth, 1994; Reitan and Wolfson, 1996c).

Reitan's contributions. Reitan (1955c) published the first independent validity study of Halstead's seven tests (10 scores), which is the landmark paper that laid the foundation for the battery's clinical use. Based on this study, Reitan discarded two of Halstead's tests because of their poor sensitivity to brain injury (*Critical Flicker Fusion Test* and *Time Sense Test*). Without these tests, which had contributed three scores, the Impairment Index became the proportion of the remaining seven scores that fell into the impaired range (Reitan, 1955c, no date). Halstead had established an Impairment Index cutting score to infer brain impairment at 0.5, with scores of 0.4 and lower interpreted as normal; Reitan applied this same cutting score to the remaining seven of Halstead's scores.

Reitan (1955c) apparently modified two of the tests entering into the Impairment Index for his validation study. Halstead's (1947) Category Test had consisted of nine different subtests containing 360 trials. Halstead also administered the entire *Seashore Measures of Musical Talent* testing pitch, loudness, time, timbre, rhythm, and tonal memory. Although Reitan did not report raw scores, he presented data from this study in several subsequent HRB manuals (Reitan, 1979). The 1955 battery included the shortened 208-item Category Test and retained only the Rhythm subtest of the Seashore battery.

Reitan also added several tests to the remaining battery. "One of the principal aims . . . has been to effect a meaningful subdivision of the concept of 'brain damage' as such subdivisions relate differentially to psychological measurements" (Reitan, 1966, p. 159). To achieve this goal, Reitan included the Wechsler-Bellevue Scale, the Trail Making Test, a modification of Wepman's Aphasia Screening Test, a "Sensory-Perceptual" examination using neurological techniques, a measure of Grip Strength using a hand dynamometer, and the MMPI. The Impairment Index, however, remained unchanged as it did not incorporate performance on the newer measures but continued to be based solely on the five tests from Halstead's original battery. Administration time for the complete HRB, including Reitan's additional tests, runs from six to eight hours. "Our initial decision was to press for a battery that could be administered to the most impaired patient in two days. We find that the battery can be completed in one day for most patients" (Reitan, 1966, p. 161).

The original goal of the HRB protocol was to collect research data, not to provide clinical information. Studies were "not principally oriented toward determining the ability of Halstead's battery to effect binary diagnostic classifications of subjects into groups with and without cerebral damage . . . but rather to determine whether the battery was adequate to do justice to the complex range of disturbances resulting from cerebral lesions" (Reitan, 1966, p. 171).

Because of research considerations, HRB data came to be interpreted blindly without knowledge of patient history or neurological findings, and apparently, feedback was not given to the referral source much less the patient. "This procedure . . . assures a complete absence of cross reference or contamination between the psychological and neurological results." The same tests were administered to all patients, greatly increasing sample sizes. This practice differed from the "more conventional procedure of performing one problem-oriented study after another . . . . As a result, we have not been able to modify or manipulate the test battery in order to learn experimentally what the tests measure or the particular requirements of the tests which might be more sensitive to cerebral dysfunction" (Reitan, 1966, p. 163). Thus, one of the advantages of the HRB approach, which provides information from the same battery of tests for all patients regardless of diagnosis or referral question, is also one of its greatest liabilities.

A problem for early HRB research—or any other neuropsychological studies performed at that time— was the "primitive" state of neurologic diagnostic tools. Reitan (1966) was keenly aware of the limited sensitivity of these diagnostic procedures when he commented on the high false positive and false negative rates associated with EEG data. To ensure that patients with genuine brain impairment were studied, he included only those cases with clear and unambiguous evidence of brain injury. He chose neurosurgical patients as his primary patient pool since "neurological surgeons and neuropathologists represent the two professional disciplines from which the most accurate information can be obtained regarding the characteristics of brain lesions in human beings" (Reitan, 1966, p. 154). Patients with less clear and less consistent evidence of brain impairment, i.e., those with milder brain impairment whose neurological status could not be confirmed by the then current diagnostic procedures, were excluded; yet many of them would likely have had brain abnormalities identifiable by current imaging techniques. Further, it must be noted, on the Wechsler-Bellevue Intelligence Scale the brain damaged group that Reitan used to validate Halstead's tests averaged 18 FSIQ points lower than the control group (Reitan, 1959). All of these issues raise serious question about Reitan's original cutting score recommendations.

Other HRB summary scores. Because only seven scores contribute to the Halstead Impairment Index, other summary scales have been introduced that incorporate

performances on a larger number of HRB tests. For example, E.W. Russell, Neuringer, and Goldstein (1970) modified the HRB following the late Philip M. Rennick's HRB adaptation. Their *Average Impairment Index (AIR)* is based on 12 scores each rated on a 6-point scale (0 to 5): the seven scores comprising the Impairment Index, Trail Making Part B, Digit Symbol from the original WAIS, Wepman's Aphasia Screening Test with scoring differences for language and spatial errors, and the number of Perceptual Errors on the Sensory-Perceptual Examination. Rating performances on a 6-point scale contrasts with Halstead's system of scores, dichotomized as "normal" or "impaired" for the calculation of the Impairment Index. Rather than include dominant hand Finger Tapping speed in the AIR calculation, as does the Halstead Impairment Index, Russell and his colleagues chose speed of the most impaired hand. They made this change because right-handed patients with focal right hemisphere lesions, for example, can often obtain normal tapping rates in their unaffected dominant right hand. The 0-5 point ratings are not norms in a strict sense since they were developed from scores of "a group of patients tested in Reitan's laboratory," rules of thumb, and numerical weightings for the Aphasia Screening Test based upon clinical experience. E.W. Russell and his associates also rescaled the Trail Making Test norms "since the available norms tended to overestimate the severity of deficit relative to other tests in the battery" (p. 36). AIR scores of 1.55 or greater presumably identify "brain damage."

The *Alternative Impairment Index* and *Alternative Impairment Index–Revised* are shorter alternatives to the Halstead Impairment Index (A.M. Horton, Jr., 1995). They are based on scores from the Category Test, Seashore Rhythm Test, Speech Sounds Perception Test, bilateral Finger Tapping, and Trail Making A and B. Normal range is 0.0 to 0.2; the impaired range runs from mild—0.3–0.4 to severe—0.8–1.0. Little formal research on these scores has been conducted. Significant limitations include the criteria of normal, mild, moderate, and severe impairment being "based on published guidelines and clinical experience" (A.M. Horton, Jr., 1995, p. 337) rather than empirically derived. Further, this index was originally developed using Reitan and Wolfson's (1993) teaching cases, many of which date from the 1950s; a subsequent reevaluation used another collection of teaching cases (Golden, Osmon, et al., 1981). Since teaching cases may not be representative of the patient population at large, caution in using this index should be exercised.

The *General Neuropsychological Deficit Score (GNDS)* (Reitan and Wolfson, 1993) summarizes 42 HRB measures divided into four areas: (1) *Level of Performance* (19 variables), (2) *Pathognomonic Signs* (12 variables), (3) *Patterns and Relationships Among Test Results* (two variables), and (4) *Right-Left Differences* (nine variables). Excepting pathognomonic signs, test performances are rated on a 4-point scale (0–3), but the scoring criteria were not empirically derived. Scores of 0 and 1 represent normal performance, and scores of 2 and 3 refer to impaired and more impaired performances, respectively. The 4-point range for each item contributing to the GNDS presumably affords much more sensitivity to the HRB than does Halstead's dichotomously determined Impairment Index. The GNDS score ranges are 0–25 = normal, 26–40 = mild impairment, 41–67 = moderate impairment, and >68 = severe impairment. The maximum possible score is 168.

A GNDS user will find that some variables are overrepresented and thus may bias the evaluation. For example, the Impairment Index, which is the average of seven other HRB variables is itself a variable (#4) to be scored and counted. A dyscalculia (variable 25) that is real and not simply diagnosed because of difficulty with mental arithmetic (see Aphasia Screening Test, p. 507) will both receive a score of 2 on this variable (no gradations for "pathognomonic signs") and lower the Verbal IQ score (variable 1). Other potential biases include the extent of right–left discrepancies on tests using both hands and involving a number of variables.

HRB standardization issues. Despite its research origins, the HRB is used in many clinical neuropsychological assessment practices. However, the battery was never standardized on a representative, stratified sample of healthy subjects. As with other procedures lacking appropriate standardization and a set of widely accepted norms, there is much variability both in how HRB data are obtained as well as in their interpretation. With so many available norms, it is possible to choose ones based on desired outcomes (Marcopulos, 1999; see Mitrushina, Boone, and D'Elia, 1999, for many different norm sets for seven of the HRB tests, including the five in Halstead's Impairment Index).

The HRB does not meet the basic requirements of test standardization.

Although [Halstead] sat down and wrote a set of instructions, they were really very inadequate. He was experimenting with the development of the tests and he did not accumulate an extensive body of systematic data on brain-damaged patients. (Reitan, 1996, p. 12)

Reitan first published a manual for administering and scoring the HRB in 1979, yet many variations of HRB tests are in use. Neuropsychologists have typically learned about the administration and interpretation of the HRB either through courses offered by Reitan or his students, or in laboratories and training sites that employ some or all of the HRB tests. Without a single set of formalized instructions, differences in test materials and their administration have developed. In addition to Halstead's (1947) sample, other major sources of norms and test administration include E.W. Russell, Neuringer, and Goldstein (1970), Heaton, Grant, and Matthews (1991), and Reitan and Wolfson (1993). Although not intended to be a comprehensive norm book for the HRB, Mitrushina, Boone, and D'Elia (1999) lists 37 sets of possible norms for the Finger Tapping test alone!

W.G. Snow (1987b) observed that two versions of the Category Test (booklet or machine); four versions of the finger tapping apparatus; and two versions each of the Speech Sounds Perception Test, Seashore Rhythm Test, and Aphasia Screening Test, together give 64 possible different combinations of stimulus materials from which to choose. In the 21st century, the number is even higher since now several computerized Category Tests and a second Booklet Category Test are available. This estimate does not consider the test instruction differences, and the variety of administration and discontinuation rules. Thus, although the HRB is often touted as a "fixed battery" with known sensitivity and specificity given its supposedly standardized administration and scoring procedures, this claim cannot be substantiated. Moreover, while it was developed to be a single integrated set of tests, many neuropsychologists today choose not to use the complete battery but incorporate HRB tests selectively into their assessments.

Normative data. Halstead (1947) developed the original cutting scores on a group of "normals" consisting of 28 subjects (eight women) who yielded 30 scores! Ten of these subjects were servicemen who were under care for "minor" psychiatric disturbances, some of whom had had military combat experience. One subject was a military prisoner "who was facing imminent sentence, either life-imprisonment or execution" (p. 37). Three other "control" subjects were awaiting lobotomies because of behavioral problems (two had homicidal impulses, one had suicidal impulses and strong homosexual [!] trends). Two of these subjects each contributed two sets of scores, before and after their lobotomies.

Another significant limitation of Halstead's normative group is its relative youth as it ranged from 14 to 50 years of age ($M = 28.3$). Yet, performance on most HRB tests declines with advancing age (Cullum, Thompson, and Heaton, 1989; Heaton, Ryan, et al., 1996; Prigatano and Parsons, 1976). Reitan (1955b) reported that after age 45, normal subjects often score in the impaired range. Thus, "average" performance by an elderly subject may be interpreted as abnormal, with an incorrect suggestion of impairment in roughly 25% of Reitan's (1955b) series. In another example, "alarmingly high percentages" of healthy volunteers ages 55 to 67 were classified as brain impaired using the original cutting scores—0.5 on the Impairment Index misclassified 53% and 1.55 on the Average Impairment Index misclassified 38% (Elias, Podraza, et al., 1990).

In addition to HRB theory and test description, Reitan and Wolfson (1993) provide case examples on 29 patients. Reitan (1959) had previously reported 14 of these cases when they were given the Wechsler-Bellevue Scale, not the WAIS. Comparing the clinical vignettes from 1959 and 1993 for the same patients nicely illustrates the difference between retrospective and prospective interpretation. For example, one patient (WM, #6) was described in 1993 as having "a neoplastic, relatively posterior lesion [that] would account for all of the findings." Blind analysis of this patient in 1959 concluded that "the best inference . . . is probably that the lesion represents some type of vascular difficulty" p. 126.

Reitan's (1955c) sample, of which the average scores appeared in several subsequent publications, included 50 control subjects who averaged 32 years of age and just under 12 years of education. These same control subjects have appeared in multiple research reports examining different aspects of the same data set (e.g., Reitan, 1959; Reitan and Wolfson, 1988b; 1992). When deciding what norms to apply to the Halstead tests, it is important to note that the 1955 "brain damaged" group used to validate Halstead's tests had a Wechsler-Bellevue Intelligence Scale FSIQ 18 points lower than their "no brain damage" control counterparts (Reitan, 1959). Also significantly lower for the "brain damage" group were 10 of the 11 individual Wechsler-Bellevue test scores. It would appear that the significant cognitive differences between the two groups Reitan used to validate Halstead's tests were sufficient to have discriminated these groups regardless of what tests were used (HRB or other). Thus, when interpreting HRB data, it is prudent to heed Reitan's warning that a "finding should not be generalized indiscriminately to groups different from those on which they were obtained" (Reitan, 1959, p. 285).

Age- and education-graded norms broken down by sex are available in the manual of Comprehensive Norms for an Expanded Halstead-Reitan Battery (Heaton, Grant, and Matthews, 1991). These authors pooled data from healthy subjects who had participated as research controls in different studies over the years. This novel approach may partially compensate for the absence of formal HRB standardization. For the core HRB tests and the original WAIS, 378 subjects were used to develop the normative tables and the values

were subsequently validated on another 108 subjects. The entire group averaged 13.6 ± 3.5 years of education; 65.5% of the sample was male. Normative values are expressed as T-scores in separate tables for men and women. The relatively few subjects with low education and at higher age levels, make these norms questionable for persons in these categories. Only a little more than 100 women filled the 60 age × education categories. Since the women comprising the normative sample were, on average, relatively well-educated, the "norms" for women at lower education levels become even more questionable than for men. To generate their normative tables, the authors used regression-based norms to statistically correct for potential demographic mismatches and small cell sizes, a debatable procedure (Fastenau, 1998; Heaton, Avitable, et al., 1999).

The GNDS norms provided by Reitan and Wolfson (1993) come from 41 control subjects in an earlier study (Reitan, 1985). This group had an average age of 30 with an education average of 12 years. It included 12 subjects with spinal injuries, 16 patients hospitalized for psychiatric reasons, eight patients hospitalized for various other medical conditions such as rheumatoid arthritis or cancer, and five patients "with no significant medical or psychiatric condition." These same 41 control subjects also appeared in Reitan and Wolfson's (2000) report examining the effects of TBI severity. Failure to include separate, independent control groups with each new report introduces the possibility that cohort effects from using the same group biasing the findings. Since many HRB studies—Reitan's and others'—are retrospective with subjects pulled from a larger database, it is not clear how many subjects may have appeared in multiple reports, decreasing the robustness of reported findings.

Reitan and Wolfson (1996a, 1997c) have asserted that age and education corrections are generally unnecessary because the more sensitive a measure is to brain damage, the less it is affected by age and education. Although it may be necessary to adjust scores in a healthy population, Reitan and Wolfson argue that it is unnecessary to make such adjustments for brain impaired persons as the GNDS did not correlate significantly with age or education in their sample (Reitan and Wolfson, 1995b). However, other studies have shown correlations between age, education, and performance in clinical samples (e.g., between age, education, and HRB summary scores: GNDS, Halstead's Impairment Index, or AIR) (Vanderploeg, Axelrod, et al., 1997; see also Prigatano and Parsons, 1976; Shuttleworth-Jordan, 1997). (It is interesting to note that a correlation between age and the Impairment Index using Halstead's 1947 neurosurgical patient data (his Table 16) is statistically significant ($rho = .44$, $p =$

.002). Moreover, the assertion that age and education corrections are unnecessary in a brain damaged population does not take into account the phenomenon of brain reserve capacity formulated by Satz (1993).

Neuropsychological findings. Tests of HRB effectiveness in identifying lesion laterality have produced equivocal results. Early reports suggest differential performance patterns associated with left and right hemisphere lesions (Kløve and Matthews, 1974; Reitan, 1955a). However, without the sensory examination developed by Kløve, which is based on standard neurologic examination practices, HRB test scores alone do not identify lateralized lesion differences with sufficient consistency to warrant clinical decisions regarding lesion localization (e.g., G. Goldstein, 1974; Schreiber et al., 1976). Hom and Reitan (1990) studied patients with cerebrovascular lesions and reported no difference between the left and right focal lesion groups on any HRB measure with the exception of finger tapping. When including both the sensory and motor examinations, lesion localization may be relatively successful (K.M. Adams, Rennick, and Rosenbaum, 1975).

Several studies have reported that the WIS-A battery and the HRB have equivalent diagnostic sensitivity for detecting "brain damage" (Kane, Parsons, and Goldstein, 1985; Sherer, Scott, et al., 1994). This diagnostic equivalence comes from the nearly complete factor identity and overlap between the two batteries (Larrabee, 2000).

Most evaluations of the HRB that have focused on its effectiveness in correctly distinguishing neurologic patients from intact control subjects have reported good rates of correct classification (Reitan, 1955c; G. Goldstein and Shelly, 1984; Kane, Parsons, and Goldstein, 1985), although one study found many of the HRB tests to be relatively weak discriminators in themselves (Klesges et al., 1984). As with all other psychological tests, however, prediction rates are significantly lower when the discrimination is between neurology and psychiatry patients (G. Goldstein and Shelly, 1987; Heaton, Baade, and Johnson, 1978; Sherer and Adams, 1993). The Halstead Impairment Index did not differentiate between patients with temporal lobe epilepsy (II = .59 ± .06) from patients with affective disorders (II = .59 ± .05) (Donnelly et al., 1972). In another study, the Halstead Impairment Index classified 61% of patients with nonepileptic pseudoseizures, diagnosed by EEG/video monitoring, as having neurologic impairment (Kalogjera-Sackellares and Sackellares, 1999). Moreover, the WAIS alone discriminated between neurologic and psychiatric patients as well as or better than the HRB (DeWolfe et al., 1971; Kane, Parsons, and Goldstein, 1985). Barnes and Lucas (1974) stated that

"one intriguing conclusion could then be that age, IQ, TPT Time, and Aphasic Symptoms were the only variables of importance in differentiating the organic and psychogenic groups" in their study. Lenzer (1980) reviewed the HRB literature on the battery's efficacy in discriminating neurological patients from severely impaired psychiatric patients, examining this question in both methodological and theoretical detail. She recommended that HRB validation studies should be "of construct validation type and not of the criterion-oriented type" (p. 611).

Findings of studies examining the reliability of the Halstead Impairment Index have been mixed. One group reported high test–retest reliability coefficients (.82, .83) for a small group of CVA patients (Matarazzo, Wiens, et al., 1974) and schizophrenia patients, respectively (J.D. Matarazzo, Matarazzo, et al., 1976), but the earlier study found no test–retest correlation ($r = .08$) for 29 healthy young men—probably because score differences between the subjects were so slight that small variations greatly altered the order of scores from test to retest. After a two-year interval, retest correlations for the measure of overall impairment used by G. Goldstein and Watson (1989) varied from a low of .48 for schizophrenics to a high of .84 for patients with cerebrovascular disorders. Dodrill and Troupin (1975) observed a gradual drop in the Impairment Index, however, from .60 ± .24 to .45 ± .28 when four examinations were given at 6- to 12-month intervals to epilepsy patients, apparently reflecting practice effects. Practice effects probably account for the lowered average Impairment Index for the normal young men examined by Matarazzo, Wiens, and their coworkers—from .10 to .05 after a 20-week interval. A recent reliability study of the HRB, which included "384 normal or neurologically stable [post TBI] adults," found significant ($p < .001$) ten-month test–retest correlations of .81 for the Halstead II, .92 for the AIR (Dikmen, Heaton, et al., 1999). Small but statistically significant (<.02) improvements appeared on all but the Seashore Rhythm Test.

Although Bornstein (1990) concluded, after reviewing a number of HRB studies, that "the available data [mostly for individual tests] indicate adequate reliability," he also noted that "It is a telling commentary that . . . the 500-page text-manual [Reitan and Wolfson, 1985] contains no information whatsoever on the psychometric properties of the tests" (p. 295). This criticism is also applicable to the second edition published in 1993. See this book (passim) and McCaffrey, Duff, and Westervelt (2000b) for reliability studies for each of the HRB tests.

HRB summary. The HRB affords a reasonably reliable psychometric means of distinguishing patients with brain injury from healthy subjects. However, its greatest contribution may not be to diagnostic efficiency but rather to the practice of neuropsychological assessment. Reitan has been singularly instrumental in making psychologists aware of the need to test many different kinds of behavior when addressing neuropsychological questions. This procedure stands in stark contrast to the early practice of making inferences of "organic brain damage" based upon a single test (Bigler and Ehrfurth, 1981).

Yet the HRB has practical limitations in that it is unwieldy, takes a relatively long time to administer, and is not suitable for thorough examination of patients with sensory or motor handicaps. It contains no formal memory test, and its language assessment consists only of a very rudimentary and ineffective language screening that was rejected by its author. Its standard cutting scores misclassify older subjects as impaired at a high rate. Even with the Heaton, Grant, and Matthews' (1991) older age norms, some neuropsychologists consider it inappropriate for elderly persons because of its length and difficulty level (Holden, 1988b; Kaszniak, 1989).

Of course, none of the summary scores can be used to identify areas of strength and weakness. Yet, for some examiners they are the only numbers addressed. This is not a criticism of the battery, but rather a criticism of some test users. Any technique that reduces the complexities and nuances of brain functioning to a single score or even several summation scores, without incorporating a detailed analysis of the patient's performance on specific assessment areas, does disservice to both the patient and to the practice of neuropsychology. Unfortunately, the Halstead Impairment Index and the other summary scores, like the Wechsler FSIQ, appear so deceptively scientific that some neuropsychologically naïve clinicians believe that they may rely on them alone when offering diagnostic conclusions and recommendations for patient disposition.

Halstead-Reitan Battery modifications

Modifications of this battery tend to reflect the interests of their creators. The *Wisconsin Neuropsychological Test Battery* (Harley, Leuthold, et al., 1980) has been used in studies of parkinsonism (C.G. Matthews and Haaland, 1979) and to help elucidate motor disturbances associated with other brain disorders (e.g., Haaland, Cleeland, and Carr, 1977; C.G. Matthews and Harley, 1975). In addition to the HRB tests, the Wisconsin battery includes the *Wisconsin Motor Battery,* which contains five measures of motor proficiency besides Finger Tapping. Dodrill (1978b, 1988) developed a *Neuropsychological Battery for Epilepsy,* which

includes tests of memory, motor control, concentration, and mental ability. These additions provide greater sensitivity to the test performances of epilepsy patients than do most of the tests in the basic HRB.

Repeatable Cognitive-Perceptual-Motor Battery (RCPMB) (R.F. Lewis and Rennick, 1979)[1]

This battery (originally called the *Lafayette Clinic Repeatable Neuropsychological Test Battery*) includes a number of the tests from the HRB (Trail Making Test, Finger Tapping, Grip Strength, and the Digit Symbol and Digit Span tests of the WAIS), the Critical Flicker Fusion test from the original Halstead Battery, and a variety of other, all time-dependent, tests measuring such neuropsychologically relevant behavior as verbal fluency, visual scanning, and fine hand coordination. Because those of its tests that are susceptible to practice effects come in different versions, it is well suited to studies using repeated measurements (Carey and Maisto, 1987; Kelland and Lewis, 1994; Townes et al., 1986) as well as clinical patient evaluation (I. Grant, Prigatano, et al., 1987; Kupke and Lewis, 1989; Tracy, Oesterling, and Josiassen, 1995). In fact, the battery was initially developed to examine differential cognitive effects of antiepileptic drugs (R.F. Lewis, Rennick, Clifford, et al., 1976, cited in Kelland and Lewis, 1994).

In a sample of 40 healthy control subjects, test–retest reliability coefficients for RCPMB tests ranged from a low of .04 for Finger Tapping to the .90s for Digit Symbol and Grip Strength and the .80s for Digit Vigilance, Color Naming, and Grooved Pegboard (Kelland and Lewis, 1994). Two factors have been identified: a *Motor* factor, on which Finger Tapping, Grooved Pegboard, and Grip Strength load; and a *Cognitive-Perceptual* factor which has a large attentional component and involves the six other tests (R. [F.] Lewis, Kelland, and Kupke, 1990). Age and education correlated significantly with both groups of tests. The reduced alertness effects of diazepam were documented in lowered RCPMB scores. It has been used with a modified HRB (K.M. Adams, Rennick, et al., 1975), but offered as a complete battery in itself.

Halstead Russell Neuropsychological Evaluation System (HRNES) (E.W. Russell and R.I. Starkey, 1993)

This is an expanded system relying solely on actuarial evaluations. This battery consists of the usual HRB, a WAIS battery (this system will accept either the WAIS or the WAIS-R—excepting Comprehension—without regard to differences between these batteries in raw

---

[1]To order this battery or any components, contact Ronald F. Lewis, Ph.D., 2209 Rhine Rd., West Bloomfield, MI 48323. (e-mail: tblew@aol.com)

score values), and one of the versions of the Wechsler Memory Scale. In addition it includes a selective reminding word-learning test, the Corsi blocks, written verbal fluency, a verbal analogies test, the Peabody Picture Vocabulary Test, Boston Naming Test, Gestalt Identification Test, a variation of the Design Fluency Test, and the Reading test of the Wide Range Achievement Test. The time required to complete the whole battery for a bright healthy young adult is about ten hours—most patients will take longer.

E.W. Russell and Starkey indicate that this system was developed to facilitate examination flexibility by providing "coordinated norming" among the tests, with all derived scores based on the same reference scale so that individual test scores can be readily compared. The different numbers of subjects contributing to the norms of different tests, however, raises questions about how "coordinated" and comparable scores can be across tests. Subjects contributing to this study were patients in the Veterans Administration system, a few from Cincinnati (examined in 1968 to 1971), the rest from the Miami area (examined since 1971). Thus most are male, most had been referred for neuropsychological assessment (the manual alludes to some patients who had not been referred but were sought out for the "comparison" group). The referred "comparison" patients were presumed to have no brain injury on the basis of a neurological examination given because brain dysfunction had been suspected. The brain injured patients carry a variety of diagnoses; all were classified as having either left-sided, right-sided, or diffuse damage. Only those most recently examined could have had their lateralization classification checked by MRI but the manual does not indicate that this was done.

Test scores are corrected for age and the Wechsler IQ score, and then converted into HRNES Scale Scores with a mean of 100 + 10. A *Lateralization Index* can be computed. The user is presumably aided in the diagnostic enterprise by diagrams of each half of the brain with labels spotted here and there carrying the name of the putatively sensitive test for that discrete area—something like the old phrenology maps, only instead of seeing "Honesty" or "Miserliness" gracing a convolution, one finds "Grooved Pegboard (R)," "Category Test," or "Design Fluency;" the anterior portion of the frontal lobes is relatively bare and nothing is attributed to the underpinnings of the cortex.

No reliability studies have been conducted with these data; the authors refer the clinician to reliability studies performed by other researchers on other groups with other variations of the HRB. Validity is based on hit rates resulting from the cutting scores used to determine impairment. The level of cognitive functioning of the population contributing to these scores is reflected

in a Category Test cutting score that is 10 points higher than the one developed on Halstead's normative group.

Test-wise examiners who understand test development will be hesitant to use the scoring system or its derivatives. Experienced clinicians who understand the nature of brain–behavior variability will not be interested in what appears to be a rather naively programmed set of interpretations. Practical examiners will not want to spend their time on a very lengthy set of tests normed on a population sufficiently unique that generalizations to most other patient groups is not possible and for which little foundation is provided for interpreting the scores that the system generates.

Kaplan-Baycrest Neurocognitive Assessment (KBNA) (Leach, Kaplan, Rewilak, Richards, and Proulx, 2000)

This battery, called the "Kaplan-Baycrest Neuropsychological Assessment" in the text of the manual, was developed by Edith Kaplan in conjunction with the staff at the Baycrest Centre for Geriatric Care in Toronto. The authors combine the methods of behavioral neurology and psychometric testing to assess major cognitive domains in two hours or less. Behavioral neurology characterizes performance with respect to traditional brain–behavior nosology, while the psychometric methodology identifies levels of impairment as well as providing measurements of test reliability and validity.

As many of the tests that comprise the KBNA were adapted from current tests and assessment techniques, the battery will have a familiar feel to clinicians from a variety of backgrounds. The battery contains behavioral neurology staples such as Clock Drawing and Praxis tests, for example, while many neuropsychological batteries include a Complex Figure and verbal fluency. According to the authors, this battery assesses six primary cognitive domains: *Attention/Concentration, Declarative Memory, Visuoconstruction/Visuoperception, Praxis, Language,* and *Reasoning/Problem Solving.* An additional noncognitive test examines the *Expression of Emotion.*

Seven formal index scores can be obtained in addition to the *Total Index,* although these only loosely correspond to the cognitive domains listed above. The summary scores were developed for *Attention/Concentration, Immediate Memory-Recall, Delayed Memory-Recall, Delayed Memory-Recognition, Spatial Processing, Verbal Fluency,* and *Reasoning/Conceptual Shifting.* A welcome feature of the KBNA is that all test scores are not forced into different composite summary measures—many tests and their subcomponents are interpreted individually. Evaluation of test performance at the test level rather than as part of summary scores decreases the likelihood of automatic cookbook score interpretation of a few summary indexes and increases the likelihood that subtle or focal deficits will be noticed. Examiners must consider individual test performances when formulating their clinical opinions. The evaluation can also utilize *Process scores* developed for each test which, for various psychometric reasons, are scored as either *average, equivocal,* or *below average.*

A major strength of this battery is its relatively comprehensive coverage of language, an area that is surprisingly underrepresented in many neuropsychological test batteries. In fact, the language tests alone offer a comprehensive *Aphasia Screening Test* that would probably be superior to most neuropsychological language assessments.

The KBNA manual encourages the examiner to accept slang and regional variations and responses. For example, in a digit span test, although the examiner is told to pronounce 0 as "zero," a patient's response of "0" is accepted as a correct response. However, "coke" is not an acceptable verbal fluency response because it is a "proper name," although in southern US, any carbonated beverage may be referred to as "coke." Similarly, on word lists, "pop" cannot be substituted for "soda" and "lemon juice" is an incorrect recall of "lemonade." These minor concerns, however, are not likely to alter scores significantly, and do not detract from what appears to be a well-developed battery of tests for neuropsychological assessment.

Battery characteristics. The normative database covers ages from 20 to 89 years, with 100 subjects in each of seven age groups. Each test yields a scaled score with a mean of 10 and SD of 3. Index Scores are expressed as *T*-scores (mean = 50, SD = 10), which is a potential source of confusion for the very many clinicians accustomed to standard scores based on a mean of 100 and a SD of 15. Although lacking a rationale for reporting the Indexes in these *T*-scores, this does follow a trend seen in other recent tests from the same publisher (e.g., California Verbal Learning Test; Wechsler Abbreviated Scale of Intelligence). The norms appear adequate, although the screening process for potential subjects relied on self-report of their neurologic or psychiatric histories.

Attention/Concentration Tests. Orientation and *Sequences* are similar to the Orientation and Mental Control tests of the Wechsler Memory Scale. Two items from other mental status examinations appear in *Sequences,* one of which requires the subject to state which letters of the alphabet rhyme with "key" (e.g., "D") and another in which letters that have curved elements when forming capital letters are identified (e.g.,

"B" or "S"). *Numbers,* a type of forward digit span, will be less threatening to some patients since it asks for telephone numbers to be repeated on both oral and written trials for each number sequence. In *Auditory Signal Detection* the patient listens to 194 tape-recorded randomly ordered sequences of alphabet letters with instructions to tap the table each time the letter "A" is heard. Accuracy on the first and second halves of the test can be compared for performance decrement. *Symbol Cancellation* consists of many little symbols scattered over a page with instructions to draw a line through all of a specified kind. The scoring breaks the stimulus array into left- and right-side components to facilitate identification of hemispatial differences.

Visuoconstruction/Visuoperception. Several commonly used techniques assess these functions. *Clocks* is a structured variant of the bedside clock drawing task (M. Freedman, Leach, et al., 1994). Not only does it require a free drawing of a clock, including placement of the numbers and hands, but the patient is also asked to indicate given times on predrawn circles, and to copy a clock face with hands indicating a time. The ability to tell time is measured with printed clock faces showing numbers as well as clock faces with only hands and no numbers. A new *Complex Figure* is offered. It is like the original Complex Figure (p. 537) in that it is used to assess both constructional ability and memory, and several of its elements are highly verbalizable (e.g., a roman numeral ten [X], a spiked circle like a sun with rays, a reverse "S"). *Spatial Location* examines spatial memory/attention by briefly exposing a series of grids with black dots printed in specific locations. The patient must reproduce the dots' locations with small disks.

Praxis. Several tests can come under this heading. Formal tests of *Praxis* contain both transitive and intransitive commands plus tests of buccofacial movements such as blowing out a candle. Although not necessarily a measure of "praxis" narrowly defined, *Motor Programming* tests the ability to alternate hands by opening and closing them simultaneously and rapidly.

Language. The language tests may seem like a short version of the Boston Diagnostic Aphasia Examination, which should not be surprising given Edith Kaplan's involvement in the development of both tests. *Picture Naming* is a 20-item analogue of the *Boston Naming Test* (pp. 511–513) that employs semantic and phonemic cueing in addition to spontaneous naming. A *Sentence Reading-Arithmetic* task presents arithmetic problems in printed sentences. Subjects read some but not all of them aloud and then, for all of them, use paper and pencil to calculate the answers. In *Reading Single Words* the subject must read real and pseudowords aloud. *Verbal Fluency* tests the ability to generate words that begin with the letter "C" (for phonemic fluency), as well as animals and first names (for semantic fluency). One minute trials are obtained for each. Both phonemic and semantic fluency scores contribute to the *Verbal Fluency* summary index. *Picture Description* of "Joe's Grocery" is an analogue of the "Cookie Theft" picture in the Boston Diagnostic Aphasia Examination. Oral responses are scored for content, phrase length, melodic range, and grammatical form. *Auditory Comprehension* tests the ability to comprehend simple yes/no questions such as "If the lion was killed by the hunter, is the hunter dead?"

Declarative Memory. Memory tests include word list learning, picture recognition, and memory for the Complex Figure. *Word Lists*, a 12-word serial word learning task, contains semantically related items (e.g., four vegetables), making it similar to the California Verbal Learning Test. The primary measure is the sum of words recalled in all four learning trials. A variety of qualitative response characteristics can also be evaluated, such as type of intrusion, repetitions, and serial position effects. After a delay, free recall, cued recall, and yes/no recognition are tested. Unlike many list learning tests, there is no interference list nor a short-term delayed recall. *Picture Recognition* assesses recognition of the 20 items seen earlier in Picture Naming, again using a yes/no format with 40 pictures. As with the original Complex Figure Test, no forewarning is given about immediate and delayed recall trials. A delayed recognition format tests recall of both specific figure elements and their location in the figure.

Reasoning/Problem Solving. *Practical Problem Solving* asks the subject to respond to possible real-world problems that might be reasonably encountered (e.g., "What would you do if you forgot where you parked your car after a shopping trip?"). A *Conceptual Shifting* task is similar to classic card sorting tests. It consists of four line drawings that can be grouped according to two physical attributes, with three of the drawings having at least three attributes in common.

Expression of Emotion. To test for deficits in affective expression, the examiner requests the subject to make facial expressions for anger, happiness, surprise, and sadness. If unable to do so, the patient is asked to imitate the examiner's expression of these emotions.

Neuropsychological considerations. This is a new test battery as yet lacking independent clinical evalua-

tions. Little helpful information for clinical interpretations can be found in the manual in which "clinically mixed" patient samples are reported without diagnoses or performance levels on the different tasks. Further, sample sizes for the nine correlational "comparison studies" with other tests (e.g., the Dementia Rating Scale, California Verbal Learning Test) range between nine and 15 subjects, which is woefully inadequate for the calculation of correlation coefficients or any determination of shared variances. Thus, although a large number of correlation coefficients fill two separate tables in the manual, these are better left ignored.

Luria's Neuropsychological Investigation (A.-L. Christensen, 1979, 1989)

Luria's neuropsychological examination techniques were brought together in a single set of materials comprising a text, manual of instructions, and test cards. Included are the testing instructions and test material for examining the full range of functions—both neurosensory and cognitive—that Luria studied. The techniques and test materials in this battery are identical with techniques and materials that Luria describes in his work (e.g., *Higher Cortical Functions in Man*, 1966; *The Working Brain*, 1973b). Christensen made this material readily accessible to those who wish to use the methods that were so fruitful in Luria's hands. She did this in two ways: by replicating Luria's techniques in card form, using his detailed directions for administration; and, perhaps more importantly, by presenting the items in a *framework* that follows Luria's conceptualization of the roles and relationships of the brain's cortical functions and guides the course of the examination.

This collection of Luria's material is organized into ten sections according to specific functions (*motor functions, acoustico-motor organization, higher cutaneous and kinesthetic functions, higher visual functions, impressive [receptive] speech, expressive speech, writing and reading, arithmetical skill, mnestic processes,* and *investigation of intellectual processes;* see Luria, 1966). The examination techniques and test fragments making up this battery reflect the range of methods Luria incorporated into his neuropsychological investigations. For example, he used familiar psychological tests such as Kohs Blocks, Raven's Matrices, and Gottschaldt's Hidden Figures. A few items from each of these tests are included. In addition, many of Luria's tasks have the same format as items in popular tests of mental abilities or speech disorders (e.g., building a sentence using three given words, following instructions that involve prepositional relationships such as "Draw a cross beneath a circle," or arranging a set of pictures to make a story). A number of items in this battery come from the mental status examination (e.g., recitation of months forward and backward, serial sevens, telling how two verbal concepts such as boat and train are similar or different, retention of three or four words following an interference activity). Some tasks are procedures usually undertaken in neurological examinations (e.g., rapid alternating hand movements, discrimination of sharp or dull pressure on the skin, testing limb position sense). This assessment battery contains most of the techniques needed for examining most aphasic patients (A.L. Christensen, Jensen, and Risberg, 1989).

Some of the most interesting items or item sequences are those developed by Luria. These include a series of tasks involving "speech regulation of the motor act:" "conflict" commands to which the patient makes a hand response that is the alternate of the examiner's movement (e.g., "Tap once when the examiner taps twice and vice versa," "Show a fist when the examiner points a finger and vice versa"); "go/no-go" instructions which test the patient's capacity to respond to one cue and withhold response to another (e.g., squeeze the examiner's hand at the word "red"; do nothing at the word "green"); alternating commands, which examines the patient's ability to establish a stereotyped motor pattern (e.g., "Raise the right hand in response to one signal, the left to two signals") or to break out of it (e.g., continue the alternating pattern of cue presentation until the stereotyped response pattern is established, and then change the pattern, repeating one or the other signal at random). These techniques are particularly sensitive to frontal lobe damage (Truelle, Le Gall, Joseph, et al., 1995). Another interesting set of items tests arithmetic skills by systematically varying the task in terms of stimulus (written, oral), response (written in Roman or Arabic numbers, oral), operation (addition, subtraction, etc.), difficulty level (one-, two-place numbers), and complexity (serial sequences using different operations). Many of the unique features of this battery may be found in Luria's variations on conventional examination practices, such as testing short-term retention of rhythmic taps or hand position, writing (in addition to repeating) dictated phonemes, indicating differences between phoneme pairs by gesture, and solving arithmetic story problems that require several steps.

In keeping with the spirit of what Luria referred to as an "experimental" approach to the clinical examination, Christensen pointed out the value of adapting the many brief examination procedures that comprise this battery to each patient's capacity. While acknowledging the benefits that standardized procedures afford, she also stressed the need for the examiner to modify these procedures in whatever manner will most likely challenge patients without defeating them. In this respect she faithfully retained the qualitative aspects of Luria's examination procedures.

The battery's strengths and limitations. Among the advantages of this battery are its measurement of actual patient behavior rather than inferred cognitive processes and test items that are based upon Luria's theoretical principles of brain–behavior relationships. Not least of its virtues is that it is relatively inexpensive, flexible, and brief to administer.

This battery cannot satisfy all neuropsychological examination requirements. For one thing, it was not intended to be comprehensive. Among its more obvious omissions are tests of attention, concentration, and mental tracking. Few techniques are offered for assessing nonverbal memory or nonverbal concept formation nor is fund of information assessed. Another problem is that many of the subtests examine functions such as speech or simple finger and hand coordination that all intact adults can perform. Deficits elicited by these subtests may reflect either very circumscribed or relatively severe conditions. However, these same techniques are often not useful in detecting most mild or diffuse impairments, such as the residuals of a mild concussion or stroke or changes associated with early dementia. The verbal memory and learning tests are not of sufficient difficulty to pick up subtle learning deficits, particularly in bright persons. Moreover, absence of normative data makes performance on the learning tests and a number of other items in this battery difficult to evaluate.

Examiners often use subtests in this battery selectively. Many of the routines for investigating motor functions have found their way into neuropsychological assessments since they test aspects of the integration and effectiveness of motor performance and motor control that are not otherwise addressed in most neurological or neuropsychological examination procedures. Because of its incompleteness, when this battery comprises the core of the neuropsychological examination, supplemental testing is needed for most patients. Christensen typically includes a (Danish version) WAIS and uses standardized memory tests in her clinical examinations (personal communication, 1982 [mdl]).

Luria's structured format and scoring system. For an outline of Luria's neuropsychological assessment procedures, the interested reader is directed to his assessment outline (Luria, 1999), translated from one of his teaching pamphlets which, according to Tupper (1999), was also used for many years in Luria's Moscow clinics. A 6-point scoring system that attempts to capture some of the qualitative features of patient performance is also available (Glozman, 1999).

Examining special populations. Holden (1988b) considered these tests to be especially appropriate for elderly patients as they lend themselves to a flexible and highly personalized examination that can protect elderly persons from becoming frustrated, distressed, or resistive to testing. Using Lurian techniques, Äystö (1988) was able to identify elderly patients at risk for dementia with greater success than with a traditional test battery (five WAIS tests, the Wechsler Memory Scale, Benton's Visual Retention and Face Recognition Tests, and a Scandinavian memory test).

When this battery has been adapted for non-Western cultures, it has brought out ways that persons in these cultures tend to think and problem-solve that differ from Western expectations. Even for tasks that seem simple or matter-of-fact, cultural differences need to be taken into account. Although Christensen's material and manual could be translated quite accurately into Zulu, Tollman and Msengana (1990) found that tasks involving "the higher mental processes," i.e., speech, reading and writing, memory, and mathematical and grammatical rules, gave Zulu subjects the greatest difficulty, along with abstract visual problems. "The most problematic task seemed to be . . . [copying] a circle somewhere in a parallelogram. Patients were observed plotting these circles haphazardly" (p. 21), this despite a rich design tradition.

Lurian neuropsychology has become influential in the Spanish-speaking world in part, according to Ardila (1999b), because most of Luria's books were translated into Spanish in the 1970s and 1980s; but North American and Western European authors have not yet been translated. Using the Spanish adaptation of the Luria/Christensen battery, Ostrosky, Canseco, and their colleagues (1985) examined more than 100 Mexican subjects. In addition to finding a sex difference favoring males for subjects of low socioeconomic status (SES), this set of tests elicited problems for the lower SES subjects in particular in dealing with language structure and verbal concepts, and in the organization of motor sequences and motor programming generally—a somewhat different pattern of functional strengths and weaknesses than presented by the Zulu subjects. Yet despite—or perhaps because of—this battery's sensitivity to cultural differences in the development of mental processes, it may be the most appropriate means available for the neuropsychological examination of non-Western patients—so long as the examiner appreciates cultural differences (see Nell, 1999).

Concerning Luria's work. Discussion of Luria's work often cites its theoretical foundations, either explicitly or implicitly maintaining that because it is theory-based, Luria's examination practices and interpreta-

tions have a higher order of validity than purely empirical assessment approaches. A. Smith (1983) questioned validation by theory, noting that Teuber (quoted in Smith's chapter) considered Luria's theories to be "bold generalizations," while Smith refers to them as "extravagant overinterpretations and speculations" (p. 467). Absence of modern imaging techniques makes his hypothesized relationships between damage sites and specific behavioral impairments more speculative than one would wish, and perhaps accounts for some reports of irreproducibility of his findings (A.R. Damasio and Anderson, 2003; see also Bornstein, 1990).

Luria-Nebraska Neuropsychological Battery (LNNB) (Golden, Purisch, and Hammeke, 1985, 1991)

The title of this battery is somewhat of a misnomer. To the extent that the examination techniques used by A.R. Luria, as collected and organized by A.-L. Christensen (see above), have been converted into test items in this battery, it traces its lineage to that preeminent Russian neuropsychologist. However, as Spiers (1981) so aptly stated:

> It is not these items, per se, but the manner in which Luria made use of them as a means of testing hypotheses concerning various abilities, deficits or functions which is his method and his unique contribution to neuropsychological assessment. Consequently, the incorporation of items drawn from Luria's work into a standardized test should not be interpreted to mean that the test is an operationalization or standardization of Luria's method. (p. 339)

Golden and his colleagues selected items from Christensen's manual on the basis of whether they discriminated between normal subjects and an unspecified group of neurologically impaired patients. Items were assigned to 11 clinical scales according to their placement among the test procedures presented by Christensen, differing from Christensen's categorization only in that "Reading" and "Writing" are separate scales in Golden's battery. Form II, "largely a parallel form," contains a twelfth scale, Intermediate Memory, which assesses delayed recall of some of the previously administered short-term memory items. For the 70% of items on which the two forms differ, instructions for Form II are provided alongside those for Form I. Performance on each item is evaluated on a 3-point scale, from 0 for no impairment to 2 for severely impaired. Score values were also determined on the basis of how well scores separated control and neurologically impaired groups and do not necessarily bear significant relationships to any neurological disorders or patterns of neuropsychological dysfunction. The summed scores for each of these scales produce 11 (or 12 for Form II) scoring indices. Although early versions of the LNNB named each scale (e.g., *Motor Functions, Rhythm*, etc.), like the MMPI, subsequent editions refer to each scale by number, probably because all of the scales are multiply determined so that function or specialization names are meaningless. Hence, the LNNB clinical scales are now C1–C12. Two optional scales for *Spelling* and *Motor Writing*, are numbered 01 and 02.

Five *summary* scales, now referred to by a number–letter code, are made up of items from the clinical scales: *Pathognomonic, Right Hemisphere, Left Hemisphere, Profile Elevation*, and *Impairment*. The Pathognomonic scale consists of items that best discriminated patients with brain impairment from healthy controls; it may also be sensitive to acuteness of an injury. The lateralized Right and Left hemisphere scales are composed of all the tactile and motor function items. The authors suggested that the Profile Elevation and Impairment scales together register level of present functioning ("degree of behavioral compensation") and degree of overall impairment. "General validation in terms of external criteria is still left to be done" (Golden, Purisch, and Hammeke, 1985, p. 146).

Other scales have proliferated since the battery was first published. They include eight *localization* scales, four for each side of the brain, organized into Frontal, Sensorimotor, Parietal–Occipital, and Temporal scales; and 28 separate *factor* scales (e.g., four for reading which together derive from 22 separate scores). As with the basic clinical scales, letter–number labels are also used for both the Summary (S) and Localization (L) scales, a particularly welcome change that will discourage the inference of focal brain impairment (e.g., "temporal lobe dysfunction") based upon poor performance on a single scale.

Regarding the 28 scales developed from factor analytic studies, "although the reliabilities of these scales have been questioned because of the small number of items for some of the factors, their replication across different patient samples supports their utility" (Franzen, 1999, p. 5). The battery's authors caution that "considerable care must be used in their interpretation" (Golden, Purisch, and Hammeke, 1991, p. 1), but also observe that this is less of a problem if "the factor scale profile is used to *supplement* the finding of the more stable patterns" (p. 162), the process appropriate for all clinical assessments.

Another important addition is the 66-item list of qualitative aspects (*categories*) of test performance to aid the examiner in evaluating the nature of failure and not merely its fact. Knippa and his colleagues (1984) stressed the importance of the qualitative evaluation. These are organized into ten groups: *Motor, Sustained Performance, Self-Monitoring, Self-Cueing, Visual-Spatial, Peripheral Impairment, Expressive Language, Dysarthria, Receptive Language*, and *Speed*. A sum-

mary table is provided in which the examiner can indicate the number of abnormal performances and compare this with cutting scores based on normal control performances.

Although scores for the various scales can be worked out by hand, the large number of operations required would make the computerized scoring service offered by the battery's publisher an attractive alternative. In addition, hand scoring cannot be performed for Form II; computer scoring is the only available option.[1] These give score profiles for all of the scales which are reportedly "corrected" for age and education (see *Battery characteristics below*) with abnormal levels clearly identified, charted "relative strengths and weaknesses" for all of the scales, plus an estimate for the three WAIS summary IQ scores derived from performance on this battery.

Battery characteristics. The norms for Form I were provided by 50 subjects (26 women and 24 men) hospitalized for "a variety of medical problems, including back injuries, infectious diseases, and chronic pain" (p. 264), and Form II was standardized on 51 normal individuals (Golden, Purisch, and Hammeke, 1991). The average age of the Form I sample was 42 ± 14.8; their education level was 12.2 ± 2.9. The *critical level*, which gives the cutting score value for the clinical scales plus Writing/Arithmetic and the Pathognomonic scale, is found by multiplying the subject's age by .214 for every year between 25 and 70. Thus the age correction assumes a simple linear increase in number of errors in every examined function or skill, an assumption that runs contrary to every responsible study made on cognitive changes with aging. For example, Vannieuwkirk and Galbraith (1985) found no age effects for Rhythm, Receptive Speech, and Writing; and yet these scales would be subject to the same age "correction" as those that are age sensitive. Education too is treated in a similarly simplistic manner such that the number of years of education (from 0 to 20) is multiplied by 1.47 and this number is subtracted from the critical level. Again, no accommodation is made for the very considerable differential effects that education may have on different functions, nor is there even a hint that education effects may be nonlinear, affecting different scales differently. Sex is not dealt with in the scoring or interpretive system although Vannieuwkirk and Galbraith (1985) found that males outperformed females on both the Motor and Visual scales.

The manual reports a range of split-half reliabilities from .89 to .95. However, it seems logically improbable to perform split-half reliability studies on a test in which each item differs from its neighbor—some dif-

---

[1]Scoring disks, "good for 25 uses" cost $280 or $260 for more than one.

fering considerably in content and functions involved (e.g., Item 164 scores for the *number of seconds* taken by the subject to begin telling a story in response to a picture, Item 165 scores for the *number of words* spoken within the first five sec of that response; or Item 111 asks the subject to point to named body parts, Item 112 asks the subject to define some common words). Item intercorrelations determined the allocation of items to a scale (i.e., scales are collections of those items that correlated most highly with one another), although many items also had significant correlations with items on other scales. Internal consistency coefficients from .40 to .94 have been reported, with most in the .80s. On retesting, Golden, Purisch, and Hammeke (1985) reported that scores on the clinical scales tend to drop a very little and correlations are mostly in the .80s and low .90s. McCaffrey, Dunn, and Westervelt (2000b) list only two test–retest studies, both conducted by Golden and his group in 1982, one on psychiatric inpatients ($n = 30$, 8 month interval), the other on patients with diffuse brain disorders ($n = 27$, 14 month interval). Eyeballing the data suggests relatively inconsequential test–retest differences.

Validation has rested primarily on distinguishing groups of brain injured patients from other groups. As with most tests of complex functions, the LNNB will separate brain injured from normal control subjects with a relatively high level of accuracy (Golden, Purisch, and Hammeke, 1985, 1991; Kane, Parsons, and Goldstein, 1985; Sears et al., 1984). A number of studies also reported good discrimination between chronic psychotic patients and patients with neurologic disease. For example, Moses, Cardellino, and Thompson (1983) had "hit rates" of 73% to 74% with a base rate of 50%. The neurologic diagnoses were all of serious conditions that would have profound cognitive effects on many of these subjects such that one may suspect that their condition would probably be documented as well with a good mental status examination. The real test of differentiation is not whether these groups can be identified by examining a variety of neuropsychological functions, but whether subjects with subtle damage can be identified. Of the 50 subjects in the Moses study, only four had TBI, one sufficiently severe to interfere with normal motor function. Yet it is the mild TBI case or mild multiple sclerosis patient that can present diagnostic questions, and probably not the postencephalitic (herpes) or (already diagnosed) Alzheimer patients, or the patient with "alcoholic amnestic disorder" who were part of the "brain-damaged" group.

Moreover, the LNNB does not identify lesion laterality to any satisfactory degree (Sears et al., 1984). G. Goldstein, Shelly, McCue, and Kane (1987) used cluster analyses to explore LNNB diagnostic efficiency and found that the patient clusters generated by this technique bore little relationship to diagnoses generally, nor specifically to lesion lateralization, nor to discriminating laterally lesioned patients from those with diffuse damage. Many patients with right hemisphere disease produced normal records while patients with left-sided lesions tended to have LNNB profiles like those of diffusely damaged patients.

Factor analyses of the Intellectual Processes, Motor, and Memory scales with the WAIS-R and other memory and motor skill tests found a considerable overlap between the three LNNB scales and the WAIS-R: "Each set of procedures is assessing much the same aspects of general (crystallized) intelligence" (P.C. Fowler, Macciocchi, and Ranseen, 1986, p. 633). This same group examined similar data for a different set of patients by means of trait analysis and found that each of these three LNNB scales fits into its appropriate factor slot, with Intellectual Processes showing the strongest relationship (to an "Intelligence" factor), which they interpreted as support for the constructs for these three scales. They also note that "performance on the LNNB's *Memory* and *Motor Function Scales* depends heavily on general cognitive ability" (Macciocchi, Fowler, and Ranseen, 1992; see also Chelune, 1983).

The Memory scale deserves mention because of its potential for misleading users of the LNNB. A factor analytic study of just the Memory scale with several memory tests and five WAIS tests showed that this short-term memory scale has a major attentional component (Larrabee, Kane, Schuck, and Francis, 1985). These authors note that because of the heterogeneity of tasks (verbal, visual, visuospatial, verbal-visual, auditory) and the absence of any clear assessment of attentional functions in other parts of the battery, not only is clinical interpretation virtually impossible, but many kinds of memory disorders may not become apparent (see also Spiers, 1981). This problem of scale heterogeneity shows up elsewhere, confounding the data entering into a scale's score and rendering the scores confusing if not meaningless for purposes of clinical interpretation.

Neuropsychological findings. In the 1985 LNNB manual, Golden, Purisch, and Hammeke reported discriminable diagnostic characteristics generated by this battery for more than ten diagnostic categories (including "Aging"). However, in some instances, replications have not had the same success. Although R.A. Berg and Golden (1981) reported significant differences for epilepsy patients on nine of the 11 clinical scales in the first LNNB version, with an overall 82.5% hit rate in separating seizure patients from "nonneurological patients," Hermann and Melyn (1985) found that only

41% of their epilepsy patients had scores that warranted an LNNB classification of cerebral dysfunction. They suggested that "the primary reason for the different hit rates was that Berg and Golden unwittingly obtained a sample that would maximize the possibility of obtaining a high hit rate, not just for the LNNB, but for any neuropsychological measure that might have been used" (p. 309).

A similar problem occurred with an attempt to replicate findings by Golden (1979) that multiple sclerosis patients performed "worse" on some LNNB items and "better" on others than other brain injured subjects, and that the LNNB discriminated MS patients from psychiatric patients and normal subjects. Golden reported a "100%" success rate in making this discrimination. However, when patients with definitely diagnosed multiple sclerosis were compared with a matched group of normal control subjects and a demographically similar sample of brain impaired patients, Stanley and Howe (1983) found that not only did Golden's predictions regarding "worse" and "better" performances not hold up but the MS patients performed as well as the normal subjects on Golden's "worse" items; and in the right direction but not significantly differentiable from the brain impaired group on the "better" items.

The LNNB's most consistent source of classification problems comes from patients with language deficits generally, aphasia most specifically. The considerable verbal demands made by many of the items—regardless of their scale location—biases this test against persons whose language skills are deficient for whatever reason (Franzen, 1989; G. Goldstein, 1986b), although bright but brain damaged persons whose language skills have remained essentially intact may appear "normal" on these scales (F.R.J. Fields, 1987; G. Goldstein, Shelly, McCue, and Kane, 1987). With respect to aphasia—despite the nice graphic depiction of discrete functional areas in the left hemisphere (p. 159 of the LNNB manual), and some descriptions of speech and language dysfunctions related to these areas—when given to aphasic patients the LNNB localization scales not only fail to discriminate between patients with different types of aphasia (J.J. Ryan, Farage, et al., 1988), but in one study every patient with aphasia due to temporal lobe damage was misclassified as having a frontal lesion (Mittenberg, Kasprisin, and Farage, 1985). Crosson and Warren (1982) had predicted these problems in their review of the items and construction of the battery.

Critical considerations. Because it was taken directly from A.-L. Christensen's work, this battery has the same content limitations. It has also acquired a serious one of its own. By limiting scorable response times to no more than ten sec for the questions in 54 items (of 269) and to longer times (15 to 120 sec) on 41 other items, with 24 items scoring just reaction times, this test penalizes slow responders without providing the means for evaluating the quality of their performance or distinguishing between failures due to generalized slowing or to impairment of specific functions associated with an item. The timing issue is actually greater than suggested by the numbers here since many of the items for which response times are limited to ten or 15 seconds are made up of three or four subitems. For example, scores for a story recall task are given in items 166 and 167 (on the Receptive Speech scale), which grossly measure response time and number of correct words repeated by the patient. With a slowed response counted in the same category as verbal memory impairment, a 6-second delay receives the same score (2) as inability to recite even one word correctly, regardless of how accurately or completely the slow responder recalls the story. This verbal recall item, which requires a spoken response and yet is scored on the "Receptive Speech" scale, is an excellent example of the confounded items, items that overlap scales, and misplaced items that create insoluble psychometric and interpretation problems.

A considerable gap separates the evaluations of this battery by Golden and his colleagues from many of those by neuropsychologists not affiliated with them. Golden and his coworkers, without exception, offer data supporting their claims that this battery is a diagnostically efficient instrument (Golden, 1981, 1984; Golden, Purisch, and Hammeke, 1991, passim; and see also G.L. Hutchinson, 1984). Moses, Cardellino, and Thompson (1983) reported that the Pathognomonic scale alone separated psychotic patients from a neurologically impaired group at a better than chance rate. The Memory scale (C10) may be useful for "gross screening" for memory dysfunction (Larrabee, Kane, Schuck, and Francis, 1985), with which Mayes and Warburg (1992) concur but add the caveat that "the norms provided in the manual and the construction of the test are not sufficient for confident interpretation of the significance of failures" (pp. 85–86). Other neuropsychologists have concluded that this battery is diagnostically unreliable (e.g., K.M. Adams, 1980a,b, 1984; Bornstein, 1990; Crosson and Warren, 1982; Delis and Kaplan, 1982, 1983; Spiers, 1984; Stambrook, 1983).

Clinical evaluations by other neuropsychologists have focused on the battery's diagnostic accuracy in the individual case. K.M. Adams and Brown (1980) examined scores from this battery obtained by six patients with cerebral vascular disease. They found that these "tests either overestimate the degree of pathology in certain areas, or fail to detect critical focal deficit." Moreover, they noted that the Intellectual Processes scale (which Golden [1980] says "represents an evaluation of a subject's intellectual level") is "highly unstable" and produces ability estimates that are widely at variance with WAIS scores. Crosson and Warren (1982) reported that this battery misidentified the side of lesion of an aphasic patient with a posterior lesion while another patient with two right-sided CVAs had significant scale elevations indicating left hemisphere damage as well as right. They identified several items that are sensitive to left visuospatial inattention, but none is on the Visual scale. Failure due to left visuospatial inattention will show up on other scales (e.g., Receptive Speech, Memory) so that "a relatively low [i.e., nonpathological] score on the Visual scale does not guarantee that visual problems do not exist." Crosson and Warren also pointed out that many items that are purportedly nonverbal involve verbal skills.

Of course, this battery discriminates between brain damaged patients and normal control subjects at a better than chance rate. Any collection of tests of sensory, motor, and assorted cognitive functions would do the same. Moreover, when given with the HRB, each of these batteries identifies some subjects with neurologic impairment who were not accurately diagnosed by the other, although both batteries made the same discriminations most of the time (Kane, Sweet, et al., 1981). Still, given its many psychometric defects, the examiner must be extremely cautious about drawing conclusions based on the scores and indices of this battery as presently constituted.

Golden, Ariel, and their colleagues (1982) also advise against indiscriminate use of this battery, noting that simplistic interpretations of this or "any test . . . are limited, at best." They cite the importance of behavioral observations in interpreting scores obtained on this battery, of testing hypotheses by looking for internal consistency in the response pattern, and of making evaluations within the context of the patient's background and history. In pointing out that the effectiveness of this battery depends on knowledge about neuropsychology and neurology as well as an understanding of Luria's theory, they remind potential users that this instrument is not suitable for use by any examiner who does not have a good grounding in neuropsychology and its related disciplines.

An LNNB short form. McCue and colleagues (1985, 1989), proposed a short form of the LNNB for elderly patients. This form retains the complete Memory and Intellectual Processes scales and all items contributing to the Pathognomonic scale, drops the Rhythm scale altogether, and trims all other scales, resulting in a 141 item total. When given to a large sample of elderly, mostly male, patients, the greatest differences in average scale scores between the standard and the short forms were in Expressive Speech with lower (better) short-form scores, and Reading, with higher (worse) ones. The short form identified a little more than 75% of all Alzheimer patients and more than 90% of depressed elderly subjects correctly when the LNNB age and education corrections were entered into scale calculations.

Neuropsychological Assessment Battery (NAB) (R.A. Stern and T. White, 2003)

This is a broad-ranging battery. Its 36 different tests come in two equivalent forms and examine five areas (called "modules") of cognitive functioning: Attention, Language, Memory, Spatial, and Executive. Norms are provided for ages 18 to 97. A sixth—Screening—module is composed of two or more of the same or abbreviated tests in the other five modules so chosen as to test both high and low ability levels. All 1,400 of the standardization subjects participated in all of the tests allowing for reliable test comparability. The battery was developed for flexible use: each module, including the screening module, can stand alone; and norms are given for individual tests as well. Data are provided on studies of patients with dementia, TBI, aphasia, multiple sclerosis, ADHD, HIV/AIDS among others. The authors note that the easily transported test material is well organized in that each module's tests are contained in its own Stimulus Book. A computerized scoring program comes with each NAB set. Although the draft announcement of this battery (5-19-03) does not include a price, the authors estimate that its cost per administration should be "only $22.40."

Giving the complete battery should take less than four hours. When, as recommended, testing begins with the Screening Module, exceptionally good performances on one or more cognitive functions may allow the examiner to forgo further testing in that (those) area(s). Exceptionally poor performances on the Screening Module should alert the examiner to particular problem areas. Many of the tests are identical or similar to tests in general use: e.g., visual confrontation naming, list learning (12 semantically related words in three trials), copying two-dimensional designs with plastic pieces, seven mazes of increasing difficulty. Others are unique and look interesting; e.g., *Driving Scenes* shows scenes such as might be seen from the driver's seat, each followed by a similar scene with questions regarding what is "new, different, or missing"; *Bill Payment* displays a bill statement, check ledger, check, and envelope with a series of instructions involving reading, writing, calculations, and spoken responses.

It will take a number of years before studies show whether this battery lives up to its promise of "excellent psychometric properties . . . provid[ing] clinical information that satisfies a broad range of modern referral sources and questions." On the face of it, the chances appear good that it will meet its goals and enter into the standard neuropsychological assessment repertory.

Batteries Composed of Preexisting Tests

Many batteries contain tests brought together to meet their creators' (or compilers') criteria for an effective neuropsychological examination. They typically consist of both published tests that can be purchased and some developed for the batteries. Unlike the big commercially available batteries, no large-scale standardization studies have been undertaken; rather, examiners can use the standardization and normative data developed for the individual tests. The following battery illustrates this common procedure.

University of South Dakota (USD) Battery
(Volbrecht et al., 2000)

In response to E.W. Russell's (1998) criticism that the only "validated" batteries were the HRB and LNNB, Volbrecht and her colleagues examined the sensitivity of a battery of tests to TBI severity. Russell asserted that if a "battery has not been validated as a unit then its known validity is only equivalent to the validity of the most accurate single test that is utilized in the battery" (p. 370). In addition, the USD battery examined patients with other diagnoses and healthy control subjects.

This battery includes the WIS-A (Rev. or III), Trail Making A and B, Judgment of Line Orientation (JLO), Finger Tapping, Finger Localization, Token Test, Sentence Repetition, Controlled Oral Word Association Test (COWAT), Animal Naming, Auditory–Verbal Learning Test (AVLT), Complex Figure Test-RO (CFT), and Booklet Category Test. Since part of this study's goal was to evaluate the battery as a whole rather than simply to look at individual tests, the authors performed multivariate and discriminant function analyses. Patients with loss of consciousness ≤24 hours differed from those with longer LOC durations: the discriminant function accounted for 47.7% of the variance and correctly classified 61.5% of the sample. The most discriminating individual tests were the AVLT recall and total words; WIS-A variables; CFT immediate and delayed recall, and recognition; Judgment of Line

Orientation; nondominant finger tapping; Trails A and B; and the Category Test. In the mixed patient groups, these same tests still correctly classified 71.6% of the sample, although the group with longer LOC was relatively difficult to differentiate from the stroke group, and patients with various psychiatric diagnoses were most often misclassified as TBI with a short LOC.

BATTERIES FOR ASSESSING SPECIFIC CONDITIONS

HIV+

NIMH Core Neuropsychological Battery
(N. Butters, Grant, et al., 1990)

Faced with the problem of identifying early evidence of cognitive deterioration in HIV+ patients, a number of clinical neuroscientists together developed recommendations for a standardized set of tests that would be clinically useful and applicable to research. They included both tests of relatively sturdy functions, such as vocabulary, that tend to withstand at least the early depredations of the AIDS virus; and tests of vulnerable functions, such as tests involving response speed and attentional capacity. To assess ten defined domains (*Premorbid Intelligence, Attention, Speed of Processing, Memory, Abstraction, Language, Visuospatial, Construction Abilities, Motor Abilities, Psychiatric*), this battery includes tests from the WAIS-R and WMS-R, and about 15 other tests familiar to most neuropsychologists plus several computerized techniques for assessing speed of processing and working memory, plus the Mini-Mental State Examination and three measures of psychiatric and emotional status. The entire battery takes from seven to nine hours.

An abbreviated battery that requires only one to two hours is composed of Vocabulary, Visual Span (WMS-R), Paced Auditory Serial Addition Test, California Verbal Learning Test, Visual Search, the Hamilton Depression Scale, and the State-Trait Anxiety Inventory (STAI). The authors note the importance of using this battery to assess individuals and to treat the data individually to provide reliable reporting on the epidemiological aspects of this disease. They acknowledge that group means are necessary for reliability and validity studies, but also state that "on any particular test the 'normal' performances of the unaffected individuals may tend to mask the impaired scores of the affected individuals" when test data across individuals are combined. K.M. Adams and Heaton (1990) also point out the need for cross-study comparisons and demographically based norms for HIV+ patients. With repeated administrations (at least five assessments over a two-year interval) practice effects appeared on the

CVLT, PASAT, and STAI State Scale with no significant changes on five other measures (McCaffrey, Westervelt, and Haase, 2001).

Multicenter AIDS Cohort Study Battery (MACS) (Selnes, Jacobson, et al., 1991)

This battery consists of seven familiar tests: Digit Span Forward and Reversed, Auditory Verbal Learning Test, Symbol Digit Modalities Test, Verbal Fluency, Grooved Pegboard, and the Trail Making Test. Like the other battery for presymptomatic AIDS, it concentrates on attention, memory, and speed tasks. It was standardized on 969 homosexual and bisexual men tested to be free of the HIV virus, with scores reported for three age groups: 25–34, 35–44, and 45–54. Both age and education affected performances significantly, and both age and education norms are provided but not integrated. Age × education correlations for each measure are given.

Neurotoxicity

No other area of neuropsychological interest, perhaps excepting dementia, has seen a greater proliferation of test batteries than that involving the assessment of persons exposed to neurotoxins. Concerns about occupational exposure to toxins originally prompted the development of these batteries, but the use and development of batteries sensitive to neurotoxicity have been extended to toxic environmental exposure as well.

These batteries all have similar conceptual schemas of what functional areas should be included in the neurotoxicity examination (Anger, 1990; Cone et al., 1990; Schaumburg, 2000b; R.F. White and Proctor, 1992). Thus, they all include one or more tests of general mental ability (usually these are tests of verbal skills or knowledge that tend to be fairly resilient to toxicity effects), and most of them contain one or more tests of memory, attention, motor speed and coordination, visuospatial abilities, and abstract reasoning. Like the informal batteries discussed above, these are primarily compilations of other tests; most of them rely on standardization data for those tests. Lists of the contents of several other batteries that have been used in or recommended for toxicological studies can be found in Anger (1990) and Cone and his colleagues (1990).

Agency for Toxic Substances and Disease Registry (ATSDR) Battery (L.J. Hutchinson et al., 1992)

This is a core neuropsychological battery that can be used in the field as well as clinically and is considered to be appropriate for evaluating neuropsychological effects of exposure to many different kinds of airborne toxic substances. This battery, also called the *Adult Environmental Neurobehavioral Test Battery (AENTB)*, is divided into four domains, each examined by a subset of tests: *Cognitive* is examined by the Auditory Verbal Learning Test, Simple Reaction Time, Raven's Progressive Matrices, plus computerized versions of the Serial Digit Learning format, the Symbol-Digit Modalities Test, and Vocabulary; *Motor* domain tests include the Hand Dynamometer, a test of fine motor skills or the Grooved Pegboard, and a computerized test of tapping speed; for the *Sensory* domain, tests of visual acuity, contrast sensitivity, and the Lanthony desaturated 15 Hue test examine visual functions, and the vibrotactile threshold is also measured; the status of *Affect* is examined by a computerized Mood Scale. Total testing time averages approximately an hour but varies with age (Amler et al., 1994).

California Neuropsychological Screening Battery-Revised (CNS-R) (Bowler, Thaler, Law, and Becker, 1990)

Nineteen tests of cognitive functions taking about $1^1/_2$ hours to complete comprise the CNS-R. Rather than developing normative data for the battery, evaluations of toxic effects have been based on comparisons with matched control groups using published test norms. The authors suggest that the CNS-R is an appropriate screening instrument for both individual evaluation and clinical studies. It is pertinent to note that with new test versions plus augmented knowledge about tests used in neuropsychology, the 1991 revision has again been updated (Bowler, Lezak, et al., 2001). The latest revision consists of most of the tests used in 1991 but in updated versions (e.g., WAIS-III, WMS-III), a few tests have been added (e.g., Boston Naming Test; Symbol Search; tests of visual competency) or substituted (e.g., Grooved Pegboard instead of Purdue Pegboard). Also included are six questionnaires covering aspects of emotional distress and symptoms frequently reported by toxin-exposed persons.

Pittsburgh Occupation Exposures Test (POET) (C.M. Ryan, Morrow, Parkinson, and Bromet, 1987)

This battery contains 16 cognitive tests, of which several were developed by this group for automated administrations. It may be given with the MMPI (Morrow, Ryan, Hodgson, and Robin, 1991) or not (Morrow, Steinhauer, Condray, and Hodgson, 1997). Administration time is reported as typically less than 90 minutes, not including the MMPI. Age-stratified normative data for blue collar workers were published in 1987. A more recent version, using 14 of the original tests (mostly from WAIS-R and WMS-R) plus six new tests is given with a structured interview based on the *Diagnostic and Statistical Manual-IV* criteria (Morrow, Stein, et al., 2001).

Tests in this recent POET revision are organized into five categories: Learning and Memory, Spatial, Attention, Motor Speed, and General Intelligence. An interesting—and apparently useful—addition is incidental recall of the symbols in the WAIS-R Digit Symbol test as recall discriminated solvent exposed from control subjects at a significant level ($p = <.01$).

Two European batteries

These test sets have influenced battery development in neuropsychotoxicology. The nine-test *TUFF-Battery* was developed in Sweden from both American tests (e.g., Block Design, Benton Visual Retention Test) and examination techniques used in Swedish neuropsychology (Ekberg and Hane, 1984). The *London School of Hygiene* test battery consists of seven tests, most coming from the west side of the Atlantic (e.g., Trail Making Test, an early form of the selective reminding technique), simple reaction time, a speeded two-handed coordination test, and the National Adult Reading Test (Cherry, Venables, and Waldron, 1984a,b).

World Health Organization-Neurobehavioral Core Test Battery (WHO-NCTB) (B.L. Johnson et al., 1987)

The NCTB consists of seven neurobehavioral tests including Digit Symbol, Digit Span, Benton Visual Retention Test (recognition form), Santa Ana Dexterity Test, Simple Reaction time, Pursuit Aiming II, and Profile of Mood States. Tests were selected that previously has been reported to be sensitive to neuropsychological deficits from chemical exposure in workplace research. Other criteria for test selection were that they had to be administered by technicians with minimal training, the materials had to be inexpensive, and they could be given in remote settings. Total testing time averages approximately one hour but varies with age (Amler et al., 1994).

As would be expected from a WHO-supported battery, this set of tests has been used throughout the world to assess cognitive impairment associated with a variety of neurotoxic agents and exposures (e.g., Escalona et al., 1995; Guo et al., 1998; Kang, 2000; J.E. Myers, 1999; B.S. Schwartz et al., 2001). This battery is sensitive to education effects and is not recommended for subjects with less than 12 years of education (Anger,

Liang, et al., 2000; Kang, 2000). Pursuit Aiming II reportedly is difficult to score reliably (Anger, Liang, et al., 2000).

Dementia: Batteries Incorporating Preexisting Tests

Among the many dementia examination formats, the line between mental status and examinations can get very blurry if not disappear altogether. Thus, while some of the test sets discussed in this section are clearly batteries consisting of several or more distinct tests, others may seem to be more like complex or expanded mental status examinations. A similar indistinctiveness characterizes some of the mental status examinations reviewed in the next chapter. The decision as to where to place a few of these tests at least bordered on arbitrariness. We hope our decisions will not lead to either misuse or disuse of these examination formats.

Addenbrooke's Cognitive Examination (ACE) (Mathuranath, Nestor, and Berrios, 2000)

This screening instrument, named after the hospital where it was developed, is a prime example of an assessment instrument that may be considered a battery as it consists of six different sections which, theoretically, could generate scores for evaluating of each section separately and thus provide a profile of cognitive functioning. Yet it can be seen essentially as a mental status examination producing a single score. Although reviewed here as a screening instrument for dementia evaluation (see pp. 700–701), its division into six cognitive components can also be viewed (and dealt with, clinically and statistically) as subtests.

Arizona Battery for Communication Disorders of Dementia (ABCD) (Bayles and Tomoeda, 1990)

This 14-test battery mostly examines speech and language skills and verbal memory but includes a drawing and a copying task as well. Although described as a battery for examining the linguistic communication deficits of Alzheimer's disease, its breadth (mental status, story recall, word learning, description and naming tests, verbal comprehension, along with drawing and copying) make it generally appropriate for dementia evaluations, and particularly so when communication deficits are a concern. Summary scores are computed for five domains: *Mental Status, Episodic Memory, Linguistic Expression, Linguistic Comprehension,* and *Visuospatial Construction.* A reliability study showed that the evaluated subtests discriminated

Alzheimer patients from both normal subjects and aphasic stroke patients effectively, and also separated out early from middle-stage Alzheimer patients (Bayles, Boone, Tomoeda, et al., 1989). When administered to Alzheimer patients and control subjects in the United Kingdom, cultural differences in pictures and vocabulary produced no notable effects on test performance (Armstrong et al., 1996). For MS patients, poorer performance was seen on five of the 14 subtests (Wallace and Holmes, 1993).

CERAD Battery (J.C. Morris, Heyman, et al., 1989)

Probably the best known of the dementia batteries is that developed by the *Consortium to Establish a Registry for Alzheimer's Disease* (CERAD). The core battery consists of seven tests—most in general use and reviewed in this book: *Verbal Fluency–Animals* is the easiest of the fluency formats; 15 of the *Boston Naming Test* items are presented with five words each of low, medium, and high frequency of occurrence; the *Mini-Mental State;* three learning trials of a ten-word list constitute the *Word List Memory* test; *Constructional Praxis* asks for drawn copies of four geometric figures; *Word List Recall* is the delayed recall trial for Word List Memory; and *Word List Recognition* gives the target ten word list words plus ten distractors to test simple retention. Most Alzheimer centers now give this core battery.

The battery is sufficiently brief that other tests can be added without fear of taxing the strength or patience of most elderly subjects. Standardization procedures were rigorous. Clinically the CERAD is used both as a diagnostic aid and to follow patients' course, but it is also well-suited for research protocols. In general, performance on this battery is affected by age and education, and to a lesser degree, sex (Berres et al., 2000; Fillenbaum et al., 2001). Evidence about the effects of ethnicity is conflicting (Fillenbaum et al., 2001; Unverzagt, Morgan, et al., 1999; K.A. Welsh, Fillenbaum, et al., 1995).

Delayed recall when adjusted for initial recall appears to be a good predictor of Alzheimer's disease (K.A. Welsh, Butters, Mohs, et al., 1994). This battery identifies Alzheimer subtypes including one with prominent naming difficulty but relatively intact figure copying, one with relatively intact naming but poor copying ability, and one with both naming and copying impairments (N.J. Fisher et al., 1999). The wide appeal of the CERAD is reflected in part by its translation into Chinese (Liu et al., 1998), French (Demers et al., 1994), German (Berres et al., 2000), Hindi (Ganguli, Chandra, et al., 1996), Korean (J.H. Lee et al., 2002), Span-

ish (Velasquez et al., 2000), and Yoruba (Guruje et al., 1995).

Cognitive Scales for Dementia (K.J. Christensen, 1989; K.J. Christensen, Multhaup, Nordstrom, and Voss, 1990, 1991a,b)

In response to the need to distinguish levels and patterns of dysfunction in Alzheimer patients as well as to make diagnostic discriminations, the range of this set of six scales goes from normal elderly persons to mild and moderate levels of deterioration. Each scale was developed according to classical test construction theory, beginning with a pool of items and selecting and ordering them on the basis of difficulty. The completed scales each contain from 48 to 122 items. *Vocabulary, Verbal Reasoning, Visual-Spatial Reasoning, Verbal Memory,* and *Object Memory* items are all in a four-choice format; items presumably measuring executive functions consist of a series of Mazes (see K.J. Christensen, 1989). For each scale, the examiner judges which of several starting points are appropriate, and discontinues testing with that scale when six of eight consecutive items are failed. Testing may take as long as two hours. By lowering the floor generally, this test allows for gradations in Alzheimer patient performances that standard tests cannot provide. The low range dips deepest on the Verbal Memory scale.

Dementia Assessment Battery (Teng, Wimer, et al., 1989)

Most of the ten tests in this battery are in general use but have been modified for dementia patients and to provide for four repeatable versions of the battery (Teng, Chui, Saperia, 1990; Teng, Wimer, et al., 1989). Thus, *Finger Tapping* involves four 15 sec trials; *Forward Digit Span* begins with two-digit sets; four 15-item sets from the 60 Boston Naming Test items were developed for *Naming; Visual Memory* has four three-item sets of geometric designs similar to those of the Benton Visual Retention Test; *Verbal Memory* consists of four nine-item grocery lists to be repeated three times with repeated recall trials and a final recognition trial; four simplified versions of the *Token Test* came from the Multilingual Aphasia Examination Battery as did the four sets of *Word Fluency;* a five-symbol form of Digit Symbol became the *Symbol–Digit Substitution Test; Copying Designs* uses Benton Visual Retention Test figures for models; and a *Number Cancellation* task appears to have been developed for this battery. The parallel forms produce reasonably comparable data; the greatest practice effects appear on the memory tests. Each form takes about 45 minutes to administer.

Fuld Object-Memory Evaluation (FOME)
(Fuld, 1980, 1981)

This set of procedures was designed to assess several aspects of learning and retrieval in elderly persons and also provides information about tactile recognition, right–left discrimination, and verbal fluency. The test material consists of a bag containing ten small common objects that can be identified by touch (ball, bottle, button, card, cup, key, matches, nail, ring, and scissors). The procedures must be given in the prescribed order.

In the first task the patient is asked to name or describe each of the ten objects while feeling it in the bag (*tactile naming*), using the right and left hands alternately. After each response, the object is shown and the patient is asked its name if tactile naming was failed. Item naming maximizes stimulus processing by the patient.

The next task is a verbal fluency test (called *rapid semantic retrieval*), which serves as a distractor and requires patients to say as many given names (same sex as the patient) as they can think of in one min (see Table 17.3). This is followed by recall of the bag items and then by four learning and recall trials of these items using the selective reminding method introduced by Buschke (1973). The examiner reminds the patient of omitted items at the slow rate of one item every five sec. A 30-sec "rapid semantic retrieval" trial comes after each learning trial as a distractor for the next recall trial. The categories for these distractor trials are, respectively, foods, "things that make people happy," vegetables, and "things that make people sad." A recall trial follows this series of learning, recall, and distractor trials, and a delayed recall trial comes 15 min later. If the patient names all ten items after this delay, the test is terminated. If not, recognition of each item not named is tested in a three-choice recognition format: e.g., "In the bag is there a stone, a block, or a *ball*?"

Several shortened versions of the test have been developed. In a shortened version (Fuld, Masur, et al.,

TABLE 17.3 *Rapid Semantic Retrieval* Mean Scores for 1-min Trial

	Foods + Vegetables	Names
Men	15.6 ± 6.1	13.2 ± 6.1
Women	21.9 ± 4.2	16.4 ± 3.0

Data from Fuld (1980)

1990), only two learning trials are administered with a 10 min delayed recall. Other shortened versions include three trials, and different delay times have been used (e.g., Marcopulos, Gripshover, et al., 1999). The FOME has also been reduced to a single learning trial, a distractor fluency task, and a 20 min. delayed recall and recognition (La Rue, Romero, et al., 1999). Thus, much like the Selective Reminding Procedure upon which the FOME was based, the many procedural alterations may result in noncomparable data.

In the longer versions of the battery, several memory scores can be derived: *Total Recall* is the sum of items correctly named in all five trials. *Storage* refers to the total number of items (of ten) that have been recalled at least once during the first five recall trials. *Repeated Retrieval* is the sum of items named without reminding and is offered as a measure of retrieval efficiency. *Ineffective Reminders*, the sum of instances in which reminding was not followed by recall on the next trial, measures the extent to which the patient does not use feedback and is dependent, in part, on the amount of reminding required.

Test characteristics. A distinct advantage of the FOME is that the main memory components are relatively immune to the potentially confounding effects of education or cultural influences. In repeated studies from varied populations, few significant educational, cultural, or SES effects have been reported (Loewenstein, Duara, et al., 1995; Marcopulos, McLain, and Giuliano, 1997; Mast et al., 2001; Ortiz et al., 1997); and when reported, they have not been considered clinically significant (e.g., Fuld, Muramato et al., 1988). There is, however, a relationship between semantic fluency performance and education (e.g., Marcopulos, Gripshover, et al., 1999) and, not surprisingly, with cultural background (e.g., Fuld, Muramato et al., 1988). Fuld (1980) reported that of 15 persons residing in the community who were in their eighth decade, 14 recalled seven of the ten words on the delay trial and that 13 of 15 in their ninth decade recalled six. When used to compare moderately impaired with unimpaired elderly nursing home residents, these procedures elicited higher storage and recall scores for the latter group. Intact residents also tended to improve recall scores on each trial while impaired subjects' span of recall leveled off at the second trial. Normative data for the affectively neutral "rapid semantic retrieval" categories were developed on 32 unimpaired community residents in the 70 to 93 age range. The women performed significantly better than did the men.

The FOME is intended for patients who are at least

70 years of age; consequently ten items are likely to have ceiling effects for middle-aged patients. A modified and more difficult version was developed for younger subjects (Davenport et al., 1988). Difficulty level was raised by increasing the number of items to 15.

Neuropsychological findings. The verbal fluency tests in this set of procedures may aid in discriminating "pseudodementia" from a genuine dementia process, particularly when the patient is depressed since a significant reduction in verbal productivity is more likely in Alzheimer's disease than in depression. Moreover, the "happy" and "sad" categories may identify severely depressed patients, as Fuld (1980) observed that unlike most people, depressed patients tend to make more sad than happy associations. Dementia patients performed significantly poorer than depressed ones on all measures of this test, this differential holding for both young-old (60–79) and old-old (80–90) patients in each group (La Rue, 1989). However, the overlap in scores made by elderly depressed patients and those with other neurologic disorders (e.g., multi-infarct dementia) was considerable, particularly in the oldest group. In contrast, comparisons of three groups of ten elderly persons found depressed patients' scores were closer to those of normal control subjects on the FOME measures (particularly Storage and Ineffective Reminders) than to dementia patients' scores (La Rue, D'Elia, Clark, et al., 1986).

Fuld, Masur, and their colleagues (1990) used a two-trial version of the test to examine its effectiveness for predicting subsequent dementia development in healthy persons. Although three different FOME measures were examined, the best predictor of subsequent dementia development was six or fewer items on Trial 1 recall, which had a sensitivity of .57 and a specificity of .84%. This finding suggests that La Rue, Romero, and their colleagues' (1999) use of a single learning trial may provide clinically sufficient discrimination, at least when comparing one- and two-trial versions although a single trial may be less sensitive than longer forms (Loewenstein, Duara, et al., 1995). Using the original length FOME in conjunction with the Selective Reminding Test, semantic fluency, and WAIS Digit Symbol tests, 80% of healthy subjects could be identified as having an 85% probability of developing dementia after 4 years or as having a 95% probability of remaining seizure free (Masur, Sliwinski, et al., 1994). Interestingly, the FOME was among the most sensitive measures to nimodipine treatment in patients with subcortical vascular disease (Pantoni et al., 2000) or mixed cerebrovascular disease (Sze et al., 1998).

Iowa Screening Battery for Mental Decline (Eslinger, Damasio, and Benton, 1984; Eslinger, Damasio, Benton, and Van Allen, 1985)

This battery is the shortest for dementia, consisting of just the three tests—*Temporal Orientation, Benton Visual Retention Test (BVRT),* and *Controlled Oral Word Association Test (COWAT)*—that best discriminated patients with dementia due to a variety of etiologies (degenerative, vascular, degenerative and vascular mixed, and other etiologies and etiologic combinations) from normal elderly subjects. Either a discriminant function formula for the BVRT and COWAT scores or an abnormally low Temporal Orientation score provide the classification criteria. The authors use this strictly as a screening test on which to base decisions concerning further evaluation of elderly patients presenting with possible dementia symptoms. This battery's effectiveness was comparable to that of the Mini-Mental State Exam in a study of genetic and education contributions to cognitive performance in elderly persons (Carmelli et al., 1995).

Neuropsychological Screening Battery (Filley, Davis et al., 1989)

With 18 tests, most taken from the general neuropsychology test repertoire and either used in their original or an abbreviated form, this battery covers the major areas of cognitive functioning "in 30 to 45 minutes." Cutting scores for each test were developed for a middle-aged sample and used with multiple sclerosis patients (G.M. Franklin, Heaton, Nelson, et al., 1988). In applying this battery to Alzheimer patients, evaluation of impairment was made by both comparing the patients to a group of normal elderly control subjects and by the already developed cut-off scores: both techniques discriminated these groups effectively. This battery has been useful in the rapid assessment of substance abuse patients (Fals-Stewart, 1996, 1997).

Protocol d'Evaluation Neuropsychologique Optimal (PENO, Protocol for the Optimal Neuropsychological Evaluation) (Joanette, Ska, Poissant, et al., 1995a)

The diversity of cognitive profiles that appear in the early stages of Alzheimer's disease led to the development of a 20-task battery, which covers five functional areas: *Memory, Language, Visual and visuospatial perception, Praxis* (including design copy), and *Executive functions* (Joanette, Ska, Poissant, et al., 1995a). Five principles for construction of such a set of subtests guided this project: (1) The notion of a general intellectual function ("fonctionnement intellectuel général") is meaningless in cognitive neuropsychology. (2) The battery must examine all the essential components and subcomponents of cognitive functioning that may be involved in dementia. (3) The battery must be relatively brief—this one takes about three hours. (4) The battery must be generally applicable both with respect to demographic differences, and in eliciting cognitive aberrations regardless of the area of malfunction: no specific behavioral disorder(s) will be considered pathognomonic of dementia; (5) The battery must be sensitive to the earliest cognitive deficits heralding the onset of dementia. These authors demonstrate that for early identification of as many Alzheimer patients as possible, each of these areas must be examined (Joanette, Ska, Poissant et al., 1995b).

Severe Impairment Battery (SIB) (Saxton, McGonigle-Gibson, et al., 1990; Saxton and Swihart, 1989)

The SIB was developed to identify areas of relatively greater impairment when disease progression is not uniform as well as to provide documentation of residual cognitive functions at the lowest levels. It consists of a series of one-step questions and commands accompanied, as needed, by gestural cues. It takes at most 20 minutes to administer. Where possible, item formats take advantage of residual automatic responses that may be elicited only in familiar, well-structured contexts. Adequate near vision and binaural hearing are required for some items.

The test has nine subscales which each receive a subscale score total: *Social interaction* (e.g., shake hands); *Orientation* (for time, place, and person); *Visuospatial ability* (e.g., matching colors, shapes); *Constructional ability* (e.g., drawing, copying); *Language* (e.g., simple reading, writing, naming); *Memory* (e.g., examiner's name, object, sentence recall); *Attention* (e.g., digit span, counting taps); *Orienting to name*; and *Praxis* (use of cup and spoon). An elaborate scoring system provides partial credits for partial responses.

The preliminary standardization population consisted of dementia patients who met accepted criteria for probable Alzheimer's disease, had Mini-Mental State scores of 13 or less, and whose average disease duration was 5.7 years. Interrater reliability coefficients for the subscales were in the .87 to 1.00 range with no total score discrepancy greater than 6 points (out of a possible 152). With an average two-week interval, the test–retest correlation overall was .85 but the range of correlations for subscales was from .22 (Construction) to .87 (Praxis). The SIB total score correlated significantly with the MMSE ($r = .71$). The only SIB item failed by all of these very deteriorated patients was the date.

The SIB appears sensitive to disease progression over a one year period in patients with moderate to severe dementia, and has been suggested as a possible outcome measure in clinical drug trials (Schmitt, Ashford, et al., 1997). For example, the SIB demonstrated that the anticholinesterase inhibitor donepezil benefited patients with severe dementia (H. Feldman et al., 2001), although these patients had been excluded from earlier studies due to disease severity. Using the SIB to assess patients with more severe dementia showed that their rate of cognitive decline is similar to that of less severely impaired patients at initial evaluation (Wild and Kaye, 1998).

Traumatic Brain Injury

Assessment of Individuals with Cognitive Impairment (Sohlberg and Mateer, 2001)

This is a focused battery that utilizes mostly published tests, but some of the instruments were developed especially for evaluating rehabilitation candidates and their progress. It covers four major domains relevant for TBI patients with significant deficits requiring rehabilitation: *Attention; Memory/new learning; Executive functions;* and *Behavior, adjustment, and outcome measures.* Tests are allocated to components within each domain (e.g., Memory/new learning contains within it: General memory scales, Verbal learning measures, Nonverbal memory measures, Recognition memory, and Additional memory measures). The authors are aware that the multifaceted nature of many components is such that allocation of a test to a specific component may be somewhat arbitrary. Tests were selected that had proven sensitivity to *acquired brain injury (ABD)*.

San Diego Neuropsychological Test Battery (Baser and Ruff, 1987)

This battery covers a broad range of functions, appropriate for documenting both residual competencies and problem areas among the many different kinds of deficit patterns commonly exhibited by head trauma patients. It is an elaboration of the core battery developed for the multicenter National Traumatic Coma Data Bank program. It consists of some 21 procedures (counting all scorable trials of a test as one procedure) which together yield 38 scores. Most of these are well-standardized tests in general use (e.g., four WAIS-R tests, four tests from the expanded HRB); several have been developed by Ruff and his colleagues (e.g., 2 and 7 Test, Ruff Figural Fluency Test). Factor analysis produced five factors: *Complex Intelligence, Mnestic,*

Planning-Flexibility, Arousal, and *Planning Organization.* It is interesting to note that two of the five factors involved aspects of executive functioning. Baser and Ruff interpret this analysis within a Lurian framework, seeing the factors as providing "sound evidence for the construct validity of Luria's three *primary* [sic] functional units (arousal, analyzing and coding, and planning)." They report good diagnostic discrimination (80% accuracy) between normal subjects, head-injured patients, and schizophrenic patients.

Right Hemisphere Disease

Although hemi-inattention can occur with left hemisphere lesions, it is sufficiently rare with left-sided disease that the *Behavioral Inattention Test* may be rightfully considered a test for patients with right hemisphere disease. As all the items involve visuoperception, it is described in some detail in Chapter 10, p. 386.

Mini Inventory of Right Brain Injury, 2nd ed. (MIRBI-2) (Pimental and Knight, 2000)

This set of tasks and behavior criteria provides a review of those areas of functioning that are most likely to be affected by right brain impairment. Four subsections each contain a number of subtests or tasks: *Visuoperceptual/Visuospatial and Attentional Processing* includes Visual Scanning; Integrity of Gnosis (e.g., finger naming, tactile recognition); Integrity of Body Image (evidence of inattention to left-side body parts or stimuli). *Lexical Knowledge and Processing* contains tests/tasks for Visuoverbal Processing (reading, writing); Visuosymbolic Processing (four serial sevens subtractions); Integrity of Visuomotor Praxis (clock drawing). *Affective Processing* asks patients to repeat a simple sentence in a happy and then a sad voice. *Lexical Knowledge Processing* involves Higher-Level Language Skills (e.g., identifying humor in puns, identifying verbal incongruities, explaining proverbs, and similarities, plus an examiner evaluation of "general expressive language ability"). Examiner observations are reported under *Affective Processing* for presence of flat affect and under *General Behavior Processing* for evidence of impulsivity, distractibility, and poor eye contact.

The authors estimate typical testing time to take from 15 to 30 minutes. Scoring criteria are provided. Scores for each subsection are converted into percent correct scores and also contribute to a test profile. A total score can be evaluated on a 7-point severity scale ranging from Profound to Normal. A Right–Left Differentiation Subscale Score can also be computed; low scores are associated with right brain damage. The manual gives some standardization data in stanine scores. Un-

fortunately, the left and right hemisphere groups contributing to these data differed in disease chronicity as mean testing time for the right hemisphere patients took place approximately 5 months postinjury but the mean time post onset for left hemisphere group testing was almost two years. These same groups provided the normative data for the first edition of this test (Pimental and Kingsbury, 1989). Validity was supported by CT-scan evidence and agreement with MIRBI-2 test performance. Correlation studies—most showing significant relationships—between a number of scores from commonly used tests (e.g., WAIS-R, WMS-R, Halstead's Impairment Index) and MIRBI-2 Total Score were based on 14 patients with right brain injuries and six with injuries on the left.

Little in this battery appears to have changed since the first edition, except the names and numbering of test and task items. This battery's greatest value may be for training clinicians in that it directs the examiner to review a variety of potential problem areas associated with right hemisphere dysfunctions. Since each task not only is quite simple but consists of at most two items (e.g., two proverbs, one easy similarity, two lines of letters for visual scanning, one trial for astereognosis), this collection of tasks and observations is best suited for identifying deficits in more severely affected patients, although many of these deficits will be obvious. The MIRBI-2 appears likely to miss the milder, subtler deficits that are more common and frequently create serious problems for patient and family because, while not obvious, they have practical importance.

SCREENING BATTERIES FOR GENERAL USE

Relatively rapid patient screening is often needed, whether for planning and disposition or to determine whether/what further assessments or treatments must be considered. Many examiners rely on one or more of the many mental status types of examinations for this purpose (see Chapter 18), or add some brief neuropsychological tests to a favorite screener. The tests discussed here were developed specifically as brief screening instruments. Being brief, they are more like truncated batteries or test samplers than full-fledged batteries. The instruments reviewed here are all portable and can be administered at bedside.

BNI Screen for Higher Cerebral Functions (BNIS) (Prigatano, 1991a; Prigatano, Amin, and Rosenstein, 1991)

This test responds to four assessment needs not addressed by most screening instruments: (1) to determine when a patient is capable of taking neuropsychological tests; (2) to provide qualitative information about mental functioning; (3) to screen the range of higher cerebral functions; (4) to examine patients' self-awareness. To accomplish these goals the BNIS contains 38 scorable items examining 16 areas of neuropsychological interest that contribute variously to seven subscales: A. *Speech and Language Functions*; B. *Orientation*; C. *Attention/Concentration*; D. *Visuospatial and Visual Problem Solving*; E. *Memory*; F. *Affect*; and G. *Awareness*. A perfect performance receives 50 points.

The test material consists of 19 cards that contain instructions for evaluating aspects of the patient's responses and behavior for which there are no tests, such as conversational fluency, hypoarousal, and cooperativeness; stimuli for specific tasks such as object naming and sentence repetition; and administration directions along with test contents such as numbers dictated for calculations and verbal memory word sets. For example, one stimulus card of particular interest is used for examining both visual scanning and visual sequencing. It contains five lines of nine numbers each, of which two lines have the same numbers although placed in different sequences. To find these two lines requires both visual search and perseverance. The scanning task asks the subject to count the number of 2s in these lines thus examining both the capacity to maintain attention and visuospatial aspects of attention. The examination was designed to take no more than 30 min and most patients are reported to require only 10 to 15 min to complete it. A total score and a percent correct score can be computed. Examiners may drop items they deem unnecessary and evaluate items or subscales in themselves.

Test–retest reliability of the BNIS was investigated with 32—mostly TBI—patients, but other cerebral disorders were also represented. Retesting after an average of three days produced a reliability coefficient of .94, but reliability was higher (.97) for a subgroup examined by the same person each time. Test–retest coefficients for the seven subscales ranged from .31 (Awareness) to .93 (Speech and Language). An interrater reliability coefficient of .998 was found for a group of ten patients. Validation studies found an average difference of 10 points between patients and control subjects ($p < .001$) (Prigatano, Amin, and Rosenstein, 1993). A correlation of .81 with the MMSE was reported.

While sensitivity to brain dysfunction was good (92%), specificity was undesirably low when a cutting score of 47 was used (Prigatano, Amin, and Rosenstein, 1993; Rosenstein, Prigatano, and Nayak, 1997). Patients with right-sided lesions received significantly lower scores on the Visuospatial and Affect subscales ($p < .02$, $< .001$, respectively) while those with left-sided lesions performed markedly poorer on the Speech and Language subscale ($p < .001$). For a group of rehabilitation patients, performance on the BNIS—especially on the visual-spatial subtest—was related to ability to achieve specific goals (Prigatano and Wong, 1999).

Cognistat: The Neurobehavioral Cognitive Status Examination (Kiernan, Mueller, and Langston, 1995)

Now called "Cognistat," this battery was originally published under the name of *Neurobehavioral Cognitive Status Examination*. A guiding principle in the development of this screening battery has been "the importance of assessing independent areas of cognitive functioning" (Schwamm et al., 1987). Thus, rather than providing the single summation score which is the end product of most mental status screening examinations, Cognistat findings are summarized in a profile of scores for each of the domains it assesses (see Fig. 17.3).

A "screen and metric" approach is used in which an initial item at a near-normal level of difficulty is tested first; patients who fail this general screening item are given easier tasks within that domain in an effort to establish a floor level and to identify gradations of impairment. For example, Digit Repetition, one of two tasks for assessing attention, gives a 6-digit sequence for the general screen. Patients who cannot repeat six digits on the initial try are given 3- to 6-digit sequences with two opportunities to pass at each level. As in most digit recall formats, the task is discontinued with two failures at any level. Possible points that can be earned differ for each domain as domains differ in the number of items that contribute to the graded score. Thus, the different levels of competence—*average, mild impairment, moderate impairment, severe impairment*—are defined by different score levels for each of the different domains (see Fig. 17.3).

Comparisons between two age groups of normal subjects (20–39, 40–66) found no significant score differences on any scale, thus permitting the same score interpretation for persons within either age group (Kiernan, Mueller, et al., 1987). A geriatric group (ages 77–92) did perform significantly lower on Construction, Memory, and Similarities, making it necessary to broaden *average* range values for older persons. Another group of healthy persons ages 60 to 96 ($M = 79.3 \pm 11.6$) also received scores below the *average* range on the same three subtests plus Attention and Calculations (Drane and Osato, 1997). Some evidence suggests caution should be exercised when employing this battery with patients with low educational levels (Ruchinskas et al., 2001).

Validity was examined on 30 neurosurgical patients who had confirmed lesions (Schwamm et al., 1987).

COGNITIVE STATUS PROFILE

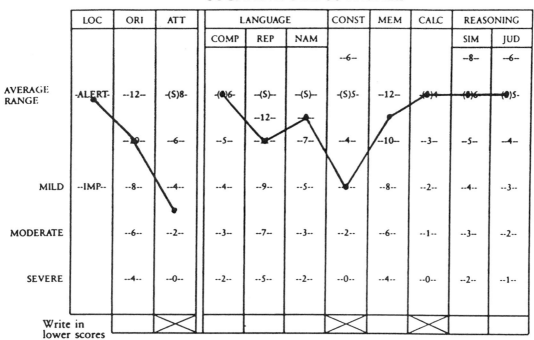

FIGURE 17.3 The *Neurobehavioral Cognitive Status Examination* (*Cognistat*) record form showing the performance profile of a 42-year-old male chronic alcoholic who had mild deficits on the Attention and Construction sections of the test. LOC = Level of Consciousness; ORI = Orientation; ATT = Attention; COMP = Comprehension; REP = Repetition; NAM = Naming; CONST = Construction; MEM = Memory; CALC = Calculations; SIM = Similarities; JUD = judgment. Screening items are identified with an *S*. IMP (in the LOC column) = Impaired. (Reprinted from the test booklet by permission. © 1988, The Northern California Neurobehavioral Group, Inc.)

Cognistat identified impairments in 28 of them, thus performing better than two mental status examination instruments that each generate only a single score and missed 12 and 15 patients identified as abnormal by the Cognistat. Moreover, when compared with a geriatric sample, the neurosurgery patients scored significantly lower in all areas except Judgment (which did not differ much between any of the study groups) (Kiernan, Mueller, et al., 1987). In a TBI sample, correlations were observed between Cognistat Memory and the California Verbal Learning Test and Logical Memory, Cognistat Construction with Block Design, and Cognistat Attention with Trail Making Part A (Nabors et al., 1997).

Because it tests a variety of functions and scores them discretely, the Cognistat profile is well suited to documenting the specific cognitive changes—and constancies—that can occur with treatment (Cammermeyer and Evans, 1988) or disease progression (Margolin, 1992c). Dementing elderly patients differed from their healthy counterparts in lower scores on Orientation, Comprehension, Repetition, Memory, and Calculations (Drane and Osato, 1997). Cognistat was reportedly superior to other tests, including the MMSE, in

identifying brain disease in patients being evaluated for late-onset psychiatric disorders (Fladby et al., 1999). But perhaps it identified it too well in 866 sequentially admitted adult psychiatric patients (ages 15–92) who scored well below the *average* range on all subtests, with very low scores on so many subtests that the Cognistat was judged to have "minimal utility as screens for this particular sample" (Logue, Tupler, et al., 1993). These authors suggested many items were vulnerable to attentional disorders and thus were not adequately assessed. However, in using this test with a series of patients with mild to moderate TBI, our [mdl] mild TBI clinic group found that Attention, and Speech and Language tasks in particular had to be supplemented with a few more difficult items in order to record the relatively subtle but troublesome problems that can occur in these areas.

Neuropsychological Screening Battery for Hispanics (NeSBHIS) (Pontón, Satz, Herrera, et al., 1996)

Responding to the problem of providing adequate assessment tools for the many persons of Hispanic background in the United States whose first—and in some cases, only—language is Spanish, Pontón and his coworkers (1996) identified a set of tests of neuropsychological functions in common use. These workers developed norms for these tests stratified by sex, age, and education. The norms are based on a sample of 300 Spanish speaking persons in the Los Angeles area (and therefore mostly of Mexican background).

This brief battery consists of 11 tests classified in six functional areas: *Memory*—Auditory Verbal Learning Test (Spanish version) plus the Rey-O Complex Figure Test; *Psychomotor*—Pin Test (measure of fine dexterity; Satz and D'Elia, 1989); *Language*—Boston Naming Test (Spanish version) plus the FAS verbal fluency form; *Mental Control*—Digit Span and Digit Symbol from a 1968 Spanish WAIS [EIWA]) plus Color Trails 1 & 2; *Visuospatial*—Block Design (EIWA) and Rey-O CFT Copy; and *Reasoning*—Raven's Progressive Matrices. These tests displayed the expected correlations for age and education, warranting the stratified norms. Sources for these tests are listed in Pontón (2001, p. 51).

Repeatable Battery for the Assessment of Neuropsychological Status (RBANS) (Randolph, 1998)

Although this brief battery was designed to screen elderly patients with possible dementia, it also serves as a general use screening battery. RBANS consists of two equivalent forms for repeated assessments. It contains ten subtests that contribute to five index scores (*Immediate Memory, Visuospatial/Constructional, Language, Attention,* and *Delayed Memory*) and a summary measure. Each index is reported as standard score with a mean of 100 ± 15. Normative data are available for patient ages 20–89. The battery can usually be administered within a half hour.

This battery contains a variety of tests likely to be familiar to most neuropsychologists. Recent memory and learning (immediate and delayed recall) are tested with word list and prose passage recall. Language assessment includes both confrontation naming and semantic fluency (fruits and vegetables) tasks. Visuospatial processing is examined with the Complex Figure—which also provides a measure of visual memory—and a modification of the Benton Judgment of Line Orientation. Forward digit span and a coding task similar to the Wechsler version measure attention. It is rare that additional memory testing is needed for elderly persons. In contrast to test sets such as the WMS-III, the difficulty level for the memory tests was targeted for the elderly population. As the WMS-III was designed to avoid ceiling effect in younger subjects, it does not leave much range for performances on the lower end of the distribution.

One of the limitations of the published version of the RBANS is that normative information for individual tests was not included, in part, because the psychometric stability of the composite indices is greater. Although forward digit span and coding, which make up the Attention Index, tend to covary with neurologic disease, these independent tests would be expected to have differential sensitivity to more subtle effects such as those associated with medications. Fortunately, the author has provided this information to individuals upon request, and these data are presented in Table 17.4.

Since the tests contain stimuli that are familiar, skilled clinicians may be able to make clinical judgments based upon their experience with similar tests. The tests are

TABLE 17.4 Repeatable Battery for the Assessment of Neuropsychological Status Test Means ± Standard Deviation by Age Groups

	AGE GROUP (YEARS)					
Test	*20–39*	*40–49*	*50–59*	*60–69*	*70–79*	*80–89*
List Learning	30.7 ± 4.3	27.6 ± 4.4	27.5 ± 4.7	28.0 ± 4.5	26.5 ± 5.0	23.2 ± 4.5
Story Memory	19.1 ± 3.3	16.9 ± 3.2	17.5 ± 3.7	18.4 ± 3.5	17.4 ± 3.6	15.3 ± 3.9
Figure Copy	19.1 ± 1.3	18.3 ± 1.4	18.2 ± 1.4	18.1 ± 1.7	17.8 ± 1.8	17.3 ± 2.0
Line Orientation	16.8 ± 3.0	15.4 ± 3.0	16.4 ± 2.9	16.6 ± 2.9	16.4 ± 2.8	15.7 ± 2.6
Picture Naming	9.6 ± 0.7	9.4 ± 1.1	9.4 ± 0.9	9.7 ± 0.5	9.6 ± 0.7	9.1 ± 1.0
Semantic Fluency	21.6 ± 3.7	20.8 ± 5.0	21.0 ± 5.0	21.0 ± 4.6	19.8 ± 5.2	17.4 ± 3.7
Digit Span	11.7 ± 2.5	10.6 ± 2.2	10.5 ± 2.4	10.2 ± 2.1	10.4 ± 2.5	9.2 ± 2.2
Coding	56.5 ± 8.8	49.8 ± 8.1	46.3 ± 8.9	46.1 ± 7.9	41.3 ± 9.0	34.0 ± 6.8
List Recall	7.5 ± 1.8	6.3 ± 1.9	6.0 ± 2.1	6.0 ± 2.2	4.9 ± 2.5	3.9 ± 2.3
List Recognition	19.8 ± 0.7	19.7 ± 0.6	19.5 ± 1.0	19.4 ± 1.2	19.2 ± 1.2	18.8 ± 1.4
Story Recall	10.1 ± 2.1	8.9 ± 1.8	9.1 ± 2.2	9.3 ± 2.1	9.0 ± 2.2	7.4 ± 2.8
Figure Recall	16.1 ± 2.9	13.5 ± 3.3	13.5 ± 3.3	13.6 ± 4.0	12.5 ± 4.2	11.4 ± 4.1

Data courtesy of C.M. Randolph.

grouped to yield summary measures for common neuropsychological constructs which can delineate distinctive performance patterns. For example, Randolph and his colleagues (1998) distinguished patients with early probable Alzheimer's disease from Huntington patients—Alzheimer patients performed poorly on Language and Delayed Memory whereas Huntington patients performed poorly on Attention and the Visuospatial-Constructional index—lending support for the use of these indexes for profile-type analyses.

This battery appears to be more appropriate for the assessment of mild dementia than the Dementia Rating Scale or the MMSE. Patients who scored in the "unimpaired" range on these two instruments nevertheless performed at lower levels than healthy controls on the RBANS (J.M. Gold, Queern, et al., 1999). Unlike other screening procedures, the RBANS addresses very few "crystallized" skills, which may contribute to its overall sensitivity to dementia or schizophrenia.

It would have been preferable to label the first memory recall factor as something other than "Immediate Memory" to avoid confusion with digit span, which is called "immediate memory" by many cognitive psychologists. Neuropsychologists may choose to add several additional tests when giving the RBANS to provide a more comprehensive assessment without unduly lengthening the process since there are several areas that are not covered by the battery (Hobart et al., 1999). What may be most important among missing areas are executive functions, category fluency, and motor responses. Additionally, more difficult levels of confrontation naming and mental tracking would increase this battery's sensitivity to milder forms of dementia and brain dysfunction. However, the RBANS provides a welcome addition to assessment resources. It is particularly useful for inpatient evaluations when comprehensive testing is not practical.

18 | Observational Methods, Rating Scales, and Inventories

JILL S. FISCHER, H. JULIA HANNAY, DAVID W. LORING, AND MURIEL D. LEZAK

The techniques presented in this chapter tend to be relatively brief. Most are based on observations. Many are not rigorously standardized. Among them are formalized mental status examinations (MSE), elaborations of components of the MSE for identified patient groups or specific diagnostic or treatment questions, screening tests, and schedules for directing and organizing behavioral observations and diagnostic interviews. Some have evolved out of clinical experience, and others were developed for specific assessment purposes. They all provide behavioral descriptions that can amplify or humanize test data and may be useful in following a patient's course or forming gross diagnostic impressions.

THE MENTAL STATUS EXAMINATION

The MSE, a semistructured interview, usually takes place during the examiner's initial session with the patient. It is the only formal procedure for assessing cognitive functions in psychiatric or neurologic examinations. Psychologists often dispense with it since most of the data obtained in the mental status examination are acquired in the course of a thorough neuropsychological evaluation. However, by beginning the examination with the brief review of cognitive and social behavior afforded by the mental status examination, the psychologist may be alerted to problem areas that will need much more detailed study. The MSE will usually indicate whether the patient's general level of functioning is too low for standard adult assessment techniques. It is also likely to draw out personal idiosyncrasies or emotional problems that may interfere with the examination or require special attention or procedural changes. The MSE, whether given as a semistructured interview or as a structured examination using one of the many standardized MSE formats, may be the chief source of data on which determination of a patient's competency for self-care or of legal issues is made (M.P. Alexander, 1988; M. Freedman, Stuss, and Gordon, 1991; S.Y. Kim et al., 2002). However, formalized methods are rapidly evolving to evaluate patients' competency for self-care, management of personal finances (H.R. Griffith et al., 2003; Marson, Sawrie, et al., 2000), or decision making regarding medical treatment (Dymek et al., 2001; Karlawish et al., 2002; Saks et al., 2002).

Mental status information comes from both direct questioning and careful observation of the patient during the course of the interview. Almost every clinical textbook or manual in psychiatry and neurology contains a model mental status examination. Examples of a variety of questions that touch upon many different areas of cognitive and social/emotional functioning and guidelines for reviewing the areas covered by the mental status examination are given in Cummings and Mega (2003), Ovsiew (2002), and Strub and Black (2002, 2003). Different authors organize the components of the mental status examination in different ways and different examiners ask some of the questions differently, but the examination always covers the following aspects of the patient's behavior.

1. *Appearance.* The examiner notes the patient's dress, grooming, carriage, facial expressions and eye contact, mannerisms, and any unusual movements.

2. *Orientation.* This concerns patients' appreciation of time, place, person, and their present situation. Some examiners also inquire about patients' awareness of the examiner's role.

3. *Speech.* Observations are made of both delivery and content of speech. The examiner looks for deviations from normal rate, tone quality, articulation, phrasing, and smoothness and ease of delivery as well as for misuse or confusion of words, grammatical and syntactical errors, perseverations, dysnomia, and other defects in word production and organization.

4. *Thought process.* In patients with aphasic disorders or verbal dyspraxias, and in some with severe func-

tional disturbances such as profound depression with motor slowing, it can be difficult to distinguish speech and thought disorders. In most patients, speech can be evaluated separately from such characteristics of thinking as mental confusion, quality and appropriateness of associations, logic, clarity, coherence, rate of thought production, and such specific thinking problems as blocking, confabulation, circumstantiality, or rationalization.

5. *Attention, concentration, and memory.* In this review of attention span, and of immediate, recent, and remote memory, the examiner inquires about the patient's early and recent history, asking for names, dates, places, and events. Digits forward and reversed, serial subtraction, recall of three or four words immediately and again after an intervening task or five more minutes of interview are typically included in the examination of concentration and memory. Visual memory can be examined by hiding objects or with brief drawing tests (e.g., see Petersen, 1991).

6. *Cognitive functioning.* Estimation of the level of general mental ability is based on quality of vocabulary, reasoning, judgment, and organization of thought as well as answers to questions about topics of general information, fairly simple arithmetic problems, and abstract reasoning tasks. Usually the patient is asked to explain one or two proverbs and to give "similarities" and "differences." When examining patients with known or suspected neurological impairment, the examiner should include simple drawing and copying tasks (e.g., draw a clock and a house, copy a cube or geometric design drawn by the examiner) and a brief assessment of reading and writing.

7. *Emotional state.* Mood (the patient's prevailing emotional tone) and *affect* (the range and appropriateness of the patient's emotional response) need to be distinguished and reported. Mood constitutes the "ground," affect the "figure" of emotional behavior.

8. *Special preoccupations and experiences.* The examiner looks for reports or expressions of bodily concerns, distortions of self-concept, obsessional tendencies, phobias, paranoidal ideation, remorse or suicidal thoughts, delusions, hallucinations, and strange experiences such as dissociation, fugue states, and feelings of impersonalization or unreality.

9. *Insight and judgment.* Questions concerning patients' self-understanding, appreciation of their condition, and their expectations of themselves and for their future elicit information regarding insight. Judgment requires realistic insight. Beyond that, practical judgment can be examined with questions about patients' plans, finances, health needs, and pertinent legal issues (e.g., see Feher, Doody, et al., 1989).

The mental status examination of a reasonably cooperative, verbally intact patient takes 20 to 30 minutes. The examiner's experience and training provide the standards for evaluating much of the patient's responses and behavior, for outside of questions drawn from standardized tests there are no quantitative norms. Thus, the data obtained in the MSE are impressionistic and tend to be coarse-grained, compared with the fine scaling of psychometric tests. It does not substitute for formal testing; rather, it adds another dimension. For many seriously impaired patients, particularly those who are bedridden, who have significant sensory or motor deficits, or whose level of consciousness is depressed or fluctuating, the mental status examination may be not only the examination of choice but also the only examination that can be made of their neuropsychological condition. For example, for severely injured head trauma victims, the mental status examination is often the best tool for following the course during the first six to eight weeks after return of consciousness.

Many of the mental status items can be integrated into an introductory interview covering the patient's history, present situation, and future plans. For example, patients' knowledge about their present income—where it comes from, how much they get from what sources, and their most recent living arrangements—reflects the integrity of recent memory. Patients must make calculations and thus demonstrate how well they can concentrate and perform mental tracking operations if asked to tell the amount of their total income when it comes from several sources, their annual rent or house payments based on the monthly cost, or the amount of monthly income left after housing is paid. Some patients who are concerned about being "crazy" or "dumb" are very touchy about responding to the formal arithmetic questions or memory tests of the MSE. These same patients often remain cooperative if they do not perceive the questions as challenging their mental competence.

RATING SCALES AND INVENTORIES

The content of most scales, inventories, and other patient rating schemes falls into one of three categories: (1) more or less complete mental status examinations that have been given scoring systems; (2) observations by a trained person of some specified class of behavior (e.g., activities, psychiatric symptoms); and (3) observations or reactions of nonprofessional persons familiar with the patient, usually family members. Most of these instruments have been devised with a particular population or diagnostic question in mind and therefore have become associated with that population or question. Moreover, the problems that some of these scales measure are unique to the population for which they were developed. Therefore, scales and inventories are grouped for review here according to the purpose for which they were originally dedicated.

Rating scales and inventories—particularly ones that were developed early on—typically include scoring schemes that, as likely as not, were devised without benefit of psychometric scaling techniques or substantial reliability or cross-validational studies. Most of the behavioral characteristics that are scored in these instruments tend to separate members of the target population from the population at large at sufficiently respectable rates to warrant their use for gross clinical screening or documentation in research. For clinical purposes, the value of a scale or inventory is more likely to be in the framework it gives to the conduct and evaluation of a brief examination than in its scores.

DEMENTIA EVALUATION

The often very difficult problem of differentiating elderly patients with cognitive or behavioral disturbances due to a progressive dementing disease from those with other neurologic conditions or a psychiatric disorder has inspired many clinicians to systematize the observational schemes that seem to work for them. Most of these instruments were developed to aid in making these difficult discriminations. Thus some contain questions that are best suited for middle-aged and older people or include simplified forms of tasks used in examinations for the general population. Most of them have general applicability including competency evaluations.

Without exception, scales and inventories designed to screen for dementia contain orientation items as these test functions that are sensitive to the most common dementing processes, such as both recent and remote memory, mental clarity, and some aspects of attention. Other areas of common interest are fund of knowledge and language skills. Only the longest scales examine most of the relevant functions; none examines them all. Diagnostic accuracy may be enhanced by combining data from several of these instruments (Eisdorfer and Cohen, 1980; Whelihan, Lesher, et al., 1984).

Thirteen scales for the evaluation of "organic mental status" were briefly described by Kochansky in 1979. Since then, many more have been described in the literature (see Lorentz et al. [2002] and Ruchinskas and Curyto [2003] for reviews). A number of these cognitive screening instruments consist solely of mental status type questions asked of the patient; a few combine such questions with observational ratings. Other scales depend solely upon examiner observations or observer reports. Some scales have had such limited

use that they are not in the general assessment repertoire. Only scales in relatively common use are reviewed here. Our focus is on instruments that primarily assess cognitive function, although a few noteworthy measures that assess either the impact of cognitive deficits on daily functioning, or affective and behavioral disturbances associated with common neurologic disorders, will also be featured. For a review of measures—some discussed here—used in Alzheimer's disease drug trials, see Demers et al. (2000a,b). Readers can find rating scales of neurologic function per se in Herndon (1997).

Mental Status Scales for Dementia Screening and Rating

Addenbrooke's Cognitive Examination (ACE)
(Mathuranath, Nestor, and Berrios, 2000)

This screening examination is essentially an elaboration of the Mini-Mental Status Examination (MMSE) that was designed to be more sensitive to amnestic syndromes and to isolated frontal or linguistic deficits than most mental status examinations, yet not as complex to administer as the Mattis Dementia Rating Scale or the cognitive section (CAMCOG) of the Cambridge Examination for Mental Disorders of the Elderly. In fact, the ACE bears many similarities to the *Quantitative Mental Status Examination* described by Mahler, Davis, and Benson (1989), which was never widely disseminated.

The ACE consists of six sections—*orientation* (10 items from the MMSE); *attention/mental tracking* (8 points: repetition of three words—*lemon, key,* and *ball*—and five serial seven subtractions); *episodic and semantic memory* (35 points: recall of three words after distraction, learning of a seven-element name and address over three trials, recall of the name and address after a 5-minute delay, and giving the names of four government figures); *verbal fluency* (up to 7 points each for phonemic ["P" words] and semantic ["animals"] fluency); *language* (28 points: naming items depicted in 12 line drawings; comprehension of three simple commands [two spoken and one written], two complex commands, and a three-step command; repeating three words and two phrases; reading two five-item lists composed of either regular and irregular words [each scored all or none]; and writing a sentence); and *visuospatial ability* (5 points: copying intersecting pentagons, copying a cube, and drawing a clock face with numbers and hands set to ten past five). Some of the recent and remote memory items would be more familiar to British citizens than to others, but this instrument could easily be adapted for use elsewhere. The authors estimate that the ACE takes about 15 to 20 minutes to administer. Scores range from 0 to 100, and an MMSE score can also be calculated.

Test characteristics. The psychometric properties of the ACE were evaluated in a sample of 139 memory clinic attenders (69 with Alzheimer's dementia, 29 with frontotemporal dementia, 14 with vascular dementia, and 27 with other degenerative neurologic disorders) and 127 age- and education-matched patients with non-neurologic illnesses or patient family members (Mathuranath et al., 2000). The ACE had very good internal consistency reliability in this sample (Cronbach's *alpha* = .78). Patients with various forms of dementia earned a mean ACE composite score of 64.8 ± 18.9; the control group's mean score was 93.8 ± 3.5.

Neuropsychological findings. Two ACE cut-off scores were derived. The first (88) was selected because it is two standard deviations below the control group mean. With excellent sensitivity (93%) but only modest specificity (71%), it might be used most appropriately in clinical settings when one wants to avoid overlooking potential dementia cases. Applying this criterion, the ACE identified an impressive 98% of patients with very mild dementia (Clinical Dementia Ratings [CDRs] = 1.0) and 100% of those with moderate to severe dementia. The second cut-off (83) was determined by estimating the probability of diagnosing dementia in the 139 clinic patients; it optimizes sensitivity (82%) and specificity (96%) across a range of dementia prevalence rates and therefore might be useful in identifying subjects for research studies.

Not only was the ACE sensitive to very mild dementia, but it also proved useful in differentiating patients with Alzheimer's dementia from those with frontotemporal dementia based on their patterns of performance on ACE subtests. Mathuranath and colleagues (2000) suggest that calculation of a VL/OM ratio, consisting of the sum of points on the verbal fluency plus language subtests to the sum of points earned on the orientation plus memory tests. Based on the mix of cases in their sample, a VL/OM of >3.2 best differentiated Alzheimer patients from those with other dementias, and a VL/OM of <2.2 as more likely to identify frontotemporal as opposed to other forms of dementia.

Cognitive Capacity Screening Examination (CCSE) (J.W. Jacobs et al., 1977)

This 30-item scale was devised to identify medical patients with brain disorders. In contrast to other brief mental status examinations, items involving attention, mental tracking, and working memory play a prominent role in the CCSE. Consequently, although much less widely used than the Mini-Mental State Examination, this scale is less prone to ceiling effects in higher functioning patients (Hershey et al., 1987). Five CCSE items cover orientation questions (four pertaining to time); 11 involve simple attention (two items) and mental tracking (digits and days of the week reversed and serial subtractions of 7 from 100); three are easy arithmetic problems (e.g., "9 + 3 is ___"); six are memory items (two of very short-term recall following a Peterson-Brown type of distraction—scored all or none—and four requiring recall of words after five intervening test items—each word scored individually); these intervening items are five very easy differences (e.g., "The opposite of **up** is ___") or similarities (e.g., "**Red** and **blue** are both ___").

Test characteristics. A study of a large heterogeneous sample of male veterans referred for psychological consultation or substance abuse treatment found 11 factors for the CCSE, of which three—digit span with interference, complex mental arithmetic, and verbal memory—accounted for the lion's share of the variance in total test scores (D.A. Anderson et al., 2001). The test–retest reproducibility of the CCSE is ±2 points in healthy subjects (J.S. Meyer, Li, and Thornby, 2001).

Based on the scores obtained by samples of medical patients referred for psychiatric consultation, psychiatric inpatients, a consecutive series of medical patients, and 25 hospital staff members, the authors defined a cut-off score of 20, interpreting scores of 19 or lower as indicating cognitive dysfunction. Using this cut-off, from 16% of a psychiatric sample (Beresford et al., 1985) to 53% of neurosurgery patients (Schwamm et al., 1987) had scores in the impaired range, with neurological patients (Hershey et al., 1987; D.M. Kaufman et al., 1979) falling in between.

False positive findings tend to be relatively infrequent and are most likely to occur in patients with hearing or language comprehension deficits associated with focal lesions, relatively mild or circumscribed cognitive deficits, developmental disabilities, or limited education. By raising the cut-off score to 25 and 27 for subjects age ≥50 and <50, respectively, Heaton, Thompson, Nelson, and their coworkers (1990) obtained a false positive rate of 15% in samples of multiple sclerosis patients and normal control subjects. The mean scores for these two groups differed by just 1 point (27.1–28.1), yet this difference was significant (*p* < .02). False negative results are more common and more likely to occur in patients who have focal lesions or relatively mild or circumscribed cognitive deficits.

Neuropsychological findings. In a sample of patients with migraine or cluster headaches (about two-thirds of whom were less than 50 years old), J.S. Meyer and colleagues set the CCSE cut-off at 27 and obtained 83% sensitivity in detecting cognitive decline (defined as a sustained decrease of >3 points) during headache intervals and 92% specificity for cognitively normal headache-free periods—much greater than the MMSE, with a sensitivity of 49%. Moreover, data from a longitudinal study of patients with memory complaints and a family history of stroke or dementia suggest that a cut-off of 26 works reasonably well in identifying patients who develop dementia in any form over a 3-year period (88% sensitivity and 83.5% specificity)—again considerably better than the MMSE, which has a sensitivity of only 57.1% in identifying these patients.

Cambridge Cognitive Examination (CAMCOG)[1]
(Huppert, Brayne, et al., 1995)

This mental status examination is the objective test portion of an instrument developed for the early diagnosis and monitoring of dementia in the elderly, the *Cambridge Mental Disorders of the Elderly Examination-Revised (CAMDEX)* (M. Roth, Tym, et al., 1999; M. Roth, Huppert, et al., 1999). The other two portions of the CAMDEX comprise structured interviews with the patient and—separately—with an informant regarding the patient's current psychiatric status, medical history, and family history. Although used primarily in England and Europe, an early study demonstrated that the CAMDEX can be used as effectively in the U.S. (Hendrie et al., 1988). It has been translated into other languages such as Hebrew (Heinik, Werner, et al., 1999).

The CAMCOG's 67 items are grouped into eight subscales: *Orientation* (ten items dealing with time and place); *Language* (seven comprehension items, six naming items, category fluency ["animals"], and four word definitions); *Memory* (recall and recognition of six pictured objects, name and address recall, and ten WIS-A Information type items [e.g., "When did World War I start?"]); *Attention* (counting from 20 to 1 and serial sevens [five subtractions]); *Praxis* (copying geometric figures and following commands); *Calculation; Abstract thinking* (similarities between pairs of items); and *Perception* (e.g., recognition of objects depicted from unusual angles and stereognosis). Eight items do not contribute to the total score but are included to permit calculation of an MMSE total score (five items) or to acquire additional qualitative information (three items).

[1]CAMCOG and CAMDEX are sold by Cambridge Cognition, Tunbridge Ct., Tunbridge Lane, Bottisham, Cambridge CB5 9DU, UK. (e-mail: info@camcog.com)

The CAMCOG also incorporates Hodkinson's (1972) modification of the Blessed Dementia Rating Scale. The full CAMCOG takes about 25 minutes and yields a maximum score of 107.

Test characteristics. Unfortunately, no age- and education-stratified norms are currently available. Some investigators have recommended using regression-based formulas to predict CAMCOG scores—with age, social class, marital status, education (or estimated premorbid intellectual level), and "general knowledge" (i.e., performance on 10 WIS Information-type items from the CAMCOG) as predictors—and defining impairment as a predetermined degree of discrepancy between actual and predicted CAMCOG scores (e.g., K. Andersen et al., 1999). Like many other mental status examinations, the CAMCOG is influenced by age and education and, to a lesser extent, sex (Huppert, Brayne, et al., 1995). Of these, age exerts the broadest effects, influencing the total score and all subscale scores—excepting Attention—whereas education principally affects performance on Language and Abstract Thinking. Thus classification errors are inevitable if a single cut-point is used without regard for a patient's age and education (Huppert et al., 1995; Lindeboom et al., 1993).

The CAMCOG correlates strongly with the MMSE—.87 in one study (Blessed, Black, et al., 1991)—as expected, given that all of the MMSE items are embedded in the CAMCOG. Unlike the MMSE though, CAMCOG total scores distribute across a wide range for patients with dementia (Huppert, Brayne, et al., 1995), Parkinson's disease (Hobson and Meara, 1999), and stroke (de Koning, van Kooten, et al., 1998). Interrater reliability on the CAMCOG is high, with an intraclass correlation coefficient of .87 for 10 examiners in one large-scale Danish study (K. Andersen et al., 1999). Test–retest reliability of the CAMCOG is also high—.97 in a sample composed of 53 Alzheimer patients and healthy elderly controls (Lindeboom et al., 1993).

Neuropsychological findings. A cut-off score of 80 was originally recommended when screening for dementia; this cut-off yielded a sensitivity of .92 and a specificity of .96 in a heterogeneous sample of inpatients and outpatients in a geriatric medicine and psychogeriatrics department (M. Roth, Tym, et al., 1986). This cut-off also did quite well in identifying Parkinson patients with dementia, with a sensitivity of .95 and a specificity of .94 in a sample in which close to half of the subjects met the *Diagnostic and Statistical Manual-IV* (DSM-IV) criteria for dementia (Hobson and Meara, 1999). Defining impairment as a total score at least 1.25 standard errors below the predicted score or a CAMCOG below 74, since none of the nondemented individuals in their pilot study of community-dwelling elderly had scored lower than this, yielded optimal sensitivity (.89) and specificity (.88) (K. Andersen et al., 1999).

Four CAMCOG composite variables—category fluency, memory, general knowledge, and attention—combined with age predicted which subjects were likely to meet criteria for dementia two years later (Nielsen, Lolk, Andersen, et al., 1999). Similarly, other investigators have found that relatively poorer performance on CAMCOG memory items than on nonmemory items predicts who would become demented over the subsequent three years (Schmand, Walstra, Lindeboom, et al., 2000). Among stroke patients, three variables heightened the risk of meeting criteria for dementia three months after a stroke: poorer CAMCOG scores, a right hemisphere stroke, and a hemorrhagic stroke (de Koning et al., 1998).

Other CAMCOG formats. A revised version (CAMCOG-R) adds ideational fluency items ("How many different uses can you think of for a bottle?") and a matrix reasoning test similar to Raven's Progressive Matrices or the WAIS-III Matrices (M. Roth, Huppert, et al., 1999). These can be summed to give an Executive Function score, with a maximum of 28. However, at least in a stroke population, these tests were strongly correlated with the tests of executive function included in the original CAMCOG (category fluency and abstract reasoning), raising questions about the necessity of including them in a screening examination (Leeds et al., 2001). Also included in the revised version are remote memory alternative questions from the 1950s and 1960s to assess more recently born cohorts.

De Koning, Dippel, and their colleagues (2000) developed a 25-item short form to use in screening for poststroke dementia by removing items subject to floor and ceiling effects, removing subscales that did not improve diagnostic accuracy, and eliminating items that diminished subscale homogeneity. With subscales for orientation, memory, perception, and abstraction, this version performs with comparable diagnostic accuracy but takes only about 10 minutes to administer. However promising this shortened instrument might be, it still must be cross-validated in other samples of stroke patients and—if it is to be used in other populations—these patients as well.

Dementia Rating Scale (DRS) (Mattis, 1976, 1988)

This widely used dementia screening scale is also known by the author's name: *Mattis Dementia Rating Scale (MDRS).* The MDRS examines five areas that are particularly sensitive to the behavioral changes that characterize senile dementia of the Alzheimer type. Five areas are covered: (I) *Attention* (37 possible points): digits forward and backward up to four; follow two successive commands (e.g., "Open your mouth and close your eyes"); (II) *Initiation and Perseveration* (37 points): name items in a supermarket; repeat series of one-syllable rhymes; imitate double alternating hand movements; copy a row of alternating O's and X's; (III) *Construction* (6 points): copy a diamond in a square; copy a set of parallel lines; write name; (IV) *Conceptual:* four WIS-A type Similarities items; identify which of three items is different; sentence generation; and (V) *Memory:* delayed recall of a five-word sentence; personal orientation; word recognition memory; design recall. A scoring system permits test–retest comparisons of both individual subscales and a total score.

An interesting feature of this scale is that, instead of giving items in the usual ascending order of difficulty, the most difficult item is given first (digit span items excepted). Since the most difficult items on the Dementia Rating Scale are within the capacity of most intact older persons, this feature can be a time-saver. An intact subject would only have to give three abstract answers on the first subtest (Similarities) of the Conceptualization section, for example; the other 26 items in this section would be skipped. Administration with an intact subject can take as little as 20 minutes, whereas with demented patients it is likely to require 30–45 minutes. Comparability between subscales is limited by their differences in the number of items and potential score points.

Test characteristics. Like scores on other mental status instruments, MDRS scores are negatively correlated with age and positively correlated with education (A.L. Bank et al., 2000; Lucas, Ivnik, Smith, et al., 1998b; G. Smith, Ivnik, Malec, and Kokmen, 1994; Vangel and Lichtenberg, 1995). Age effects are most striking in patients with moderately severe dementia (Vitaliano, Breen, Russo, et al., 1984). Appropriate interpretation of individual patients' test scores has been greatly facilitated by the publication of age- and education-stratified normative databases for well-educated healthy older Caucasian adults (Lucas et al., 1998b; Monsch, Bondi, Salmon, et al., 1995), community dwelling older adults with a range of educational backgrounds (R. Schmidt, Freidl, et al., 1994), rural community dwelling older adults with limited education (Marcopulos, McLain, and Giuliano, 1997), and less educated urban medical patients (A.L. Bank et al., 2000; see also Spreen and Strauss, 1998).

Sex (A.L. Bank et al., 2000; Vangel and Lichtenberg, 1995) and race (Woodard, Auchus, et al., 1998) affect

MDRS performance to a much lesser extent than age and education. However, interesting cultural differences have emerged in studies using translated versions of the MDRS. For example, Hispanic Alzheimer patients performed significantly worse than their nonHispanic counterparts on the total MDRS and especially the Conceptualization and Memory subscales (Hohl et al., 1999). As a group, elderly adults from Hong Kong did better than age- and education-matched persons in San Diego on the Construction subscale, whereas those in San Diego had more success on the Initiation-Perseveration and Memory subscales (Chan, Choi, et al., 2001). It is prudent for the examiner to be sensitive to cultural factors that may affect MDRS performance.

For normal older adults, MDRS scores remain reasonably stable over one to two years, although any given individual's scores may fluctuate as much as one standard deviation during this period (G. Smith, Ivnik, Malec, and Kokmen, 1994). Smith and colleagues suggest that MDRS total score declines of more than 10 points are rare, occurring in fewer than 5% of healthy older adults, and should be suspect.

The reliability of the MDRS has been extensively investigated. Test–retest reliability is excellent (.97 for the total score) (Mattis, 1988). Early studies with small patient samples reported a split-half reliability of .90 (R. Gardner et al., 1981) and coefficient *alphas* for individual subscales ranging from .95 (Attention and Conceptualization) to .75 (Memory) (Vitaliano, Breen, Russo, et al., 1984). When a larger, more heterogeneous patient sample (i.e., Alzheimer's disease, vascular dementia, or mild cognitive impairment) was examined, the internal consistency of the MDRS was somewhat lower: coefficient *alpha* for the MDRS total score was .82, while those for most subscales fell into the .75 to .84 range (G. Smith, Ivnik, Malec, and Kokmen, 1994). Initiation-Perseveration was considerably less cohesive (coefficient *alpha* = .44), which should not be surprising given the varied items on this subscale, but raises questions about its interpretability as an individual subscale.

The construct validity of the Attention, Conceptualization, and Memory subscales has been supported in studies of their correlations with Wechsler scale indices (G. Smith, Ivnik, Malec, and Kokmen, 1994) and other tests of similar cognitive functions (Marson, Dymek, et al, 1997). Interpretation of the Construction subscale becomes questionable, however, given that it correlates more strongly with attentional tests than it does with other visuoconstructional measures (Marson, Dymek, et al., 1997; G. Smith et al., 1994). Some authors have pointed out that the MDRS is limited in its assessment of visual construction and suggest that it be supplemented with additional visuoconstructional items when assessing patients who commonly have deficits in this domain, such as Parkinson patients (G.G. Brown, Rahill, et al., 1999).

Factor analyses of the MDRS have yielded varied results. For example, H.R. Kessler, Roth, and their colleagues (1994) found that a two-factor solution gave the best fit for a heterogeneous patient sample with varied neurological and psychiatric diagnoses. Studying Alzheimer patients, Colantonio and colleagues (1993) had derived three factors: memory, construction and conceptualization. Woodard, Salthouse and colleagues (1996) reported that after collapsing Attention with Initiation-Perseveration into a single factor, a modified four-factor version of Mattis' rationally derived subscales provided the best description. And yet a rather different set of five factors has been reported (Hofer et al., 1996). However, this sample was small and included more healthy subjects than dementia patients—which raises questions about factor stability. G. Smith and his colleagues (1994) advised caution in interpreting subscales other than Memory and Conceptualization which, in light of the findings reported here, appears to be wise. A recently revised MDRS manual provides additional reliability and validity data and guidelines for clinical interpretation (Jurica et al., 2002).

Neuropsychological findings. Unlike some other brief mental status examinations, the MDRS total score does well in identifying Alzheimer patients, separating mildly impaired Alzheimer patients from control subjects with perfect accuracy in one study (Prinz, Vitaliano, et al., 1982). Originally, a cut-off score of 137 (out of 144) was proposed as a "red flag" for suspected impairment, but this was based on a small sample consisting of 11 healthy adults and 20 patients with heterogeneous neurological conditions affecting brain function. This cut-off was later revised downward to 123, a score two standard deviations below the mean score of Montgomery and Costa's sample of 85 healthy older adults (cited in Mattis, 1988). This revised cut-off performed reasonably well (83% sensitivity; 100% specificity) in a sample of 41 patients with Alzheimer-type or vascular dementia and 22 healthy controls (van Gorp, Marcotte, et al. 1999).

The danger of using cut-off scores derived from demographically dissimilar samples was amply illustrated in a study which found that close to half of a sample of older rural community-dwelling adults were misclassified as impaired when the conventional cut-off of 123 was used (Marcopulos, McLain, and Giuliano, 1997). Vangel and Lichtenberg (1995) reported that a cut-off score of 125 produced acceptable sensitivity (.85) and specificity (.90) in a sample of urban elderly medical patients, but higher cut-off scores may be appropriate when well-educated patients are evaluated. For example applying a cut-off score of 129 to a sample with a 2:1 ratio of Alzheimer patients to healthy controls yielded optimal sensitivity (.98) and specificity (.97) in a highly educated, predominantly Caucasian sample (Monsch, Bondi, Salmon, et al., 1995). This cut-off score also performed well when cross-validated in a separate community-dwelling sample of older adults, about 15% of whom had Alzheimer's disease (91% of patients and 93% of healthy controls correctly classified). An even higher cut-off (133) was necessary to achieve optimal sensitivity (.96) and specificity (.92) in separating another highly educated sample of mildly impaired Alzheimer patients (those with "intact" MMSEs of 24 or higher) from matched healthy persons (Salmon, Thomas, et al., 2002).

MDRS total scores have been used to stage dementia patients in terms of level of impairment (Salmon, Thal, et al., 1990; Shay et al., 1991). Different patterns of subscale performance may help distinguish control subjects from mildly impaired Alzheimer patients (Hochberg et al., 1989; Vitaliano, Breen, Russo, et al., 1984) and mildly impaired patients from moderately impaired patients (Hochberg et al., 1989). In one study, three MDRS subscales (Initiation-Perseveration, Construction, and Memory) discriminated significantly between control subjects and mildly impaired patients and between mildly and moderately impaired patients, whereas Attention and Conceptualization discriminated only between mildly and moderately impaired patients (Vitaliano, Breen, Russo, et al., 1984). Hochberg and her colleagues (1989) found that the high degree of sensitivity of the Initiation-Perseveration subscale to Alzheimer's disease severity depended mostly on verbal fluency (articles of clothing), accounting for 78% of the variance in predicting patients' self-care behavior; adding verbal imitation raised the amount of variance accounted for to 92%.

The pattern of MDRS subscale performance may also help differentiate patients with differing neuropathological conditions. In fact, neuroimaging studies have demonstrated differential correlations between specific MDRS subscales (e.g., Memory) and brain regions known to be associated with these functions (e.g., hippocampal volumes) (Fama, Sullivan, Shear, et al., 1997). In an early study, patients with frontal involvement were impaired only on the Initiation-Perseveration subscale, whereas Korsakoff patients did most poorly on the Memory subscale (Janowsky, Shimamura, Kritchevsky, and Squire, 1989). As a group, Alzheimer patients are almost always more impaired on the MDRS Memory subscale than patients with any other dementia etiology. Autopsy studies have shown that Alzheimer patients without evidence of Lewy bodies performed significantly worse in life on the MDRS Memory subscale than did either Alzheimer patients with Lewy body pathology (D.J. Connor et al., 1998) or frontotemporal dementia patients (Rascovsky et al., 2002). In contrast, Alzheimer patients with Lewy body pathology did worse on the Initiation-Perseveration subscale (D.J. Connor et al., 1998).

Alzheimer patients also do worse on the MDRS Memory subscale than patients with so-called subcortical pathologies, such as those with Parkinson's disease (Cahn-Weiner, Grace, et al., 2002; Paolo et al., 1995) or vascular dementia, who typically perform poorly on Construction (Lukatela et al., 2000), or patients with progressive supranuclear palsy (Rosser and Hodges, 1994) or Huntington's disease (Paulsen, Butters, et al., 1995; Rosser and Hodges, 1994; Salmon, Kwo-on-Yuen, et al., 1989) who do worst on the Initiation-Perseveration subscale. These observations fit nicely with a neuroimaging study demonstrating that MDRS Memory performance was most strongly related to whole brain volume, whereas Construction and Initiation-Perseveration subscale performances were more closely linked with subcortical hyperintensities (Paul, Cohen, et al., 2001).

Both total scores and subscale scores on the MDRS were positively related to the ability to perform basic and instrumental activities of daily living—although not behavior problems—in Alzheimer patients (Teri, Borson, et al., 1989; Vitaliano, Breen, Russo, et al., 1984). The MDRS has also been shown to predict rehabilitation outcome (e.g., return to prior living situation) (MacNeill and Lichtenberg, 1997). Total MDRS scores have been used to predict length of survival in Alzheimer patients (G. Smith, Ivnik, Malek, and Kokmen, 1994) and medically ill patients (Arfken et al., 1999).

The Extended Scale for Dementia (ESD). This revision of the DRS divides up the orientation item so that time, place, and age are scored separately and it adds several items: "Information" (e.g., "How many weeks [months] are there in a year?"); "Count Backwards" and "Count by 3's"; "Simple Arithmetic"; a "simple" paired-association learning test; a "simple version" of Block Design taken from the Wechsler Intelligence Scale for Children; and the two graphomotor items of the original test combined, making a total of 23 items (Hersch, 1979). After six weeks, test–retest correlations were .94 for 24 dementia patients.

However, the ESD's sensitivity of .93 in distinguishing dementia patients from normal control subjects in the 65 and older age range dropped to .75 for persons under age 65 (Lau et al., 1988). Age-dependent cut-off scores were applied to maintain the specificity rate at

.96 for both age groups. Over six months, both Alzheimer and vascular dementia patient groups had significant score declines even though the groups were small. Another small study suggested that dementia patients deteriorated at similar rates, regardless of the underlying pathology (Alzheimer's disease, dementia with Lewy bodies, and a combination of the two) (Helmes, Bowler, et al., 2003).

Based on a factor analysis of the responses of 219 outpatients with Alzheimer's disease that yielded three factors (conceptualization, construction, and memory), Colantonio and colleagues (1993) devised an abbreviated 86-item test with a reorganized scoring system. The full scale remains much more widely used however. The MDRS has also been adapted for use with diverse populations, including Spanish-speaking and Chinese adults.

Mini-Mental State (MMS) or Mini-Mental Status Examination (MMSE) (M.F. Folstein, Folstein, and McHugh, 1975)

This formalized mental status examination is probably the most widely used brief screening instrument for dementia whether used either alone or as a component of such examination protocols as the CERAD battery (J.C. Morris, Heyman, et al., 1989). Originally devised to facilitate differential diagnosis of hospitalized psychiatric patients, it is routinely used to assess cognitive abilities in epidemiological studies—both cross-sectional and longitudinal (Crum et al., 1993; Kase, Wolf, et al., 1998). It is also routinely used to select patients for dementia treatment trials (M.J. Knapp et al., 1994; Raskind et al., 2000; S.L. Rogers, Farlow, et al., 1998). The MMSE assesses a restricted set of cognitive functions simply and quickly (see Fig. 18.1). The standardized administration and scoring procedures are easily learned, with administration by a seasoned examiner taking about five to ten minutes. A total of 30 points are possible.

Early factor analyses of the MMSE together with other tests identified three factors, labeled differently but essentially consisting of verbal functions, memory abilities, and construction (Giordani et al., 1990; J.C. Morris, Heyman, et al., 1989). When MMSE item responses of a large sample of older adults were analyzed independently, five distinct though related domains emerged: concentration or working memory (serial 7s and spelling 'world' backwards); language and praxis (naming, following commands, and construction); orientation; memory (delayed recall of three items); and attention span (immediate recall of three items) (R.N. Jones and Gallo, 2000). Very similar factors were derived in an analysis of the MMSE item responses of

psychiatric inpatients (Banos and Franklin, 2002), providing empirical support for Folstein's rational groupings of MMSE items (M.F. Folstein, Folstein, and McHugh, 1975).

Test characteristics. MMSE scores are strongly influenced by both age and education, decreasing with age and increasing with education (J.C. Anthony et al., 1982; Tombaugh and McIntyre, 1992). Individuals with less education tend to make errors on the first serial subtraction, spelling "world" backwards, repeating phrases, writing, naming the season, and copying (R.N. Jones and Gallo, 2002). Clinically useful age- and education-stratified norms have been published for the MMSE (Bravo and Hebert, 1997; Crum et al., 1993; Tombaugh, McDowell, et al., 1996). Sex has a negligible impact on overall MMSE scores (Tombaugh and McIntyre, 1992), although differences are evident on a few individual MMSE items (e.g., women are more likely to err on serial 7s, whereas men are more prone to errors on spelling "world" backwards and other language items) (R.N. Jones and Gallo, 2002).

Ethnicity also affects MMSE performance. For example, African Americans and Hispanics are more likely than European Americans to be erroneously identified as demented (J.C. Anthony et al., 1982; Auerbach and Faibish, 1989; Espino et al., 2001; Mulgrew et al., 1999). Ethnic differences—at least in Mexican Americans—appear to be largely a function of acculturation: barrio-residing Mexican Americans score lower than their counterparts who live in transitional or suburban neighborhoods (Espino et al., 2001).

Test–retest reliability over a 24-hour period in the original standardization sample of nondemented psychiatric inpatients was high, whether the examiner was the same both times ($r = .89$) or different ($r = .83$) (M.F. Folstein, Folstein, and McHugh, 1975). Test–retest reliability over a 4-week period was nearly perfect for the dementia patients in Folstein's sample ($r = .99$). (For more test–retest reliability data, see McCaffrey, Duff, and Westervelt, 2000b.)

Neuropsychological findings. By and large, the effectiveness of the MMSE in identifying cognitively compromised patients depends upon the composition of the groups under study (Tombaugh and McIntyre, 1992). In the original MMSE validation study, none of the 63 normal elderly patients scored below 24, which subsequently became the de facto criterion for identifying cognitive impairment. The MMSE is most effective in distinguishing patients with moderate or severe deficits from control subjects (Filley, Davis, et al., 1989; M.F. Folstein, Folstein, and McHugh, 1975). It is less effective in separating mildly demented patients from nor-

Patient _____

Examiner _____

Date _____

<u>MINI MENTAL STATE</u>

<u>Score</u>   <u>Orientation</u>

( )   What is the (year) (season) (month) (date) (day)? (5 points)

( )   Where are we? (state) (county) (town) (hospital) (floor)
           (5 points)

           <u>Registration</u>

( )   Name 3 objects: 1 second to say each. Then ask the patient
                            to repeat all three after you have said
                            them. 1 point for each correct. Then re-
                            peat them until he learns them. Count
                            trials and record _____.
                            (3 points)

           <u>Attention and Calculation</u>

( )   Serial 7's. 1 point for each correct. Stop at 5 answers.
           <u>Or</u> spell "world" backwards. (Number correct equals letters
           before first mistake - i.e., d l o r w = 2 correct).
           (5 points)

           <u>Recall</u>

( )   Ask for the objects above. 1 point for each correct. (3 points)

_____

           <u>Language Tests</u>

( )   name - pencil, watch (2 points)

( )   repeat - no ifs, ands or buts (1 point)

( )   follow a 3 stage command: "Take the paper in your right hand,
                                      fold it in half, and put it on the
                                      floor." (3 points)

FIGURE 18.1 Mini-Mental State. (From Folstein et al., 1975)

(continued)

mal subjects (Galasko et al., 1990; R.G. Knight, 1992), identifying cognitively impaired medical inpatients (J.C. Anthony et al., 1982; Auerbach and Faibish, 1989), or identifying patients with focal or lateralized lesions (Dick et al., 1984; Naugle and Kawczak, 1989; Schwamm et al., 1987).

Applying a cut-off score of 24 without regard for the examinee's age or educational background, or to pa-tients with subtle or focal cognitive deficits, is bound to lead to classfication errors. When the conventional cut-off of 24 was applied to samples of patients referred for dementia evaluations, the MMSE had good speci-ficity but limited sensitivity: .90 and .69 in one study (Feher and Martin, 1992) and .96 and .63 in another (Kukull et al., 1994), respectively. The ideal *screening* test should emphasize sensitivity even if this comes at

```
Mini Mental State
Page 2


Score

                Read and obey the following:
(   )           CLOSE YOUR EYES.  (1 point)

(   )           Write a sentence spontaneously below.  (1 point)


(   )           Copy design below.  (1 point)
```

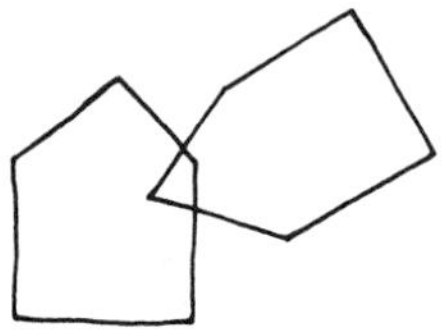

```
(   )           TOTAL 30 POINTS



_____

The above test does not include abstraction.  You may want to test this
for your own information:

                Proverbs
                Similarities
```

FIGURE 18.1 Mini-Mental State (continued).

the expense of specificity, in contrast to *diagnostic* tests which should favor specificity over sensitivity. Toward this end, Kukull and colleagues recommended raising the MMSE cut-off to 26 or 27 to increase the MMSE's sensitivity in symptomatic populations.

The MMSE is sensitive to dementia severity (J.C. Morris, Heyman, et al., 1989; Teng, Chui, Schneider, and Metzger, 1987), although individual MMSE items perform differently at earlier and later stages of the illness (Fillenbaum, Wilkinson, et al., 1994). For example, performance on the three-word delayed recall item of the MMSE predicted which community-dwelling older adults would develop Alzheimer's disease in one study (Small et al., 2000) and was the most sensitive item for distinguishing mild to moderate dementia (Galasko et al., 1990; Teng, Chui, Schneider, and Metzger, 1987). Language items—excepting the 3-stage command, which also has mental tracking and sequencing components—had the least sensitivity in the early stages of dementia (Feher, Mahurin, and Doody, 1992). These findings suggest that, in some contexts, a very brief two-item screen—using three-word recall and either orientation to time (the second most sensitive

item in the Galasko and Fillenbaum studies) or copying (the second most sensitive item in the Teng study)—might perform as well as the full MMSE. Similarly, another study identified six MMSE items that did nearly as well as the entire scale in identifying patients with dementia (Callahan et al., 2002).

The MMSE performance of healthy older adults is reasonably stable over time, following a slight improvement between the first and second testings as a result of experience with the test (Jacqmin-Gadda et al., 1997). In contrast, the MMSE performance of patients with Alzheimer's disease deteriorates over time—at an average rate of 3.26 points per year (95% confidence interval: 3.06 to 3.46) in one study (R.S. Wilson, Gilley, et al., 2000b). MMSE change is not linear across the range of test scores as it is subject to both ceiling and floor effects (Mungas and Reed, 2000). Moreover, MMSE change is not consistent from one Alzheimer patient to the next (Doody et al., 2001; Mendiondo et al., 2000) though the rate of decline for a specific patient at a given stage of dementia is reasonably predictable (Doody et al., 2001).

MMSE total scores do not differentiate patients with

Alzheimer's disease from patients with other dementias, but some investigators suggest that patterns of performance on individual MMSE items may help distinguish patients with different dementia etiologies. Thus patients with pathologically confirmed dementia with Lewy bodies performed poorly relative to patients with pathologically confirmed Alzheimer's disease on the attention and construction items of the MMSE and did relatively better on the MMSE memory items (Ala et al., 2001). Parkinson patients struggled the most with construction (both mechanics of writing a sentence and copying), while patients with ischemic vascular disease had difficulty with both attention and construction, and Alzheimer patients did worst on temporal orientation and delayed recall (Jefferson et al., 2002). Orientation to date and three-word delayed recall also distinguished Alzheimer patients from Huntington patients with early disease who had relatively greater difficulty with serial sevens (Brandt, Folstein, and Folstein, 1988). However Huntington patients with advanced disease did worse than Alzheimer patients on registration (immediate recall) of three words and writing.

MMSE performance predicts important functional outcomes such as medication adherence (Salas et al., 2001), length of hospital and rehabilitation stay, rehabilitation course and outcome, and risk of death (see reviews by Ruchinskas and Curyto, 2003 and Tombaugh and McIntyre, 1992). MMSE scores have also been used to model the costs of care in Alzheimer's disease, estimated to be approximately $2000 (in 1995 dollars) for each 1-point decrement in MMSE scores in one study (L. Jonsson et al., 1999).

Variants of the Mini-Mental State Examination. Numerous modifications of the MMSE have been proposed, some minor and others more extensive. For example, the Galasko group (1990) and others have observed that spelling "world" backwards and performing serial 7s are not interchangeable tasks, so they suggested replacing both with the "months backward task." Leopold and Borson (1997) proposed retaining the "world" item and having higher functioning individuals not only spell it backwards, but also put its letters in alphabetical order. On finding that the addition of cumulative recall over two delayed recall trials at five minute intervals improved the detection of patients with mild cognitive impairment substantially (sensitivity of 96.2% with a specificity of 90.4%) Loewenstein, Barker, and their colleagues (2000) suggested adding delayed recall trials to the MMSE.

The *Modified Mini-Mental State (3MS)* is the most widely used revision of the MMSE (Teng and Chui, 1987). These authors added four new items (listing four-legged animals and identifying similarities be-

tween three pairs of items), modified the administration order and content of other items (e.g., adding cued recall and recognition items to the memory assessment), and developed a more detailed scoring system (e.g., copying pentagons is allotted up to 10 points rather than a simple "pass/fail"). These additions extend the score range to 0–100. The 3MS is slightly more sensitive than the MMSE to cognitive impairment in stroke patients, though not appreciably better in terms of overall classification accuracy when conventional cut-offs are used (i.e., below 79 on the 3MS and below 24 on the MMSE) (Grace et al., 1995). Age and education adjusted norms for the 3MS have been developed (Bravo and Hebert, 1997; Tombaugh, McDowell, et al., 1996). The 3MS itself has been revised (*3MS-R*) with publication of normative data on the 3MS-R for 2913 healthy individuals spanning a broad age range that includes subjects more than 100 years old.

The *Cognitive Abilities Screening Instrument (CASI)* was developed for use in cross-national studies of community-dwelling older adults (Teng, Hasegawa, et al., 1994). Its 25 items come from the MMSE, the 3MS, and the Hasegawa Dementia Rating Scale. The CASI can be administered in 15–20 minutes. It has been translated into Japanese, Chinese, Vietnamese, and Spanish and has been used in a number of international studies. Nine domain subscale scores can be calculated, although the authors caution about the limited range and potential unreliability of most subscale scores. Total scores range from 0 to 100, and an MMSE score can be derived as well. A CASI cut-off score of <86 has both high sensitivity (96.5%) and specificity (92%); a slightly lower cut-off score (<81) optimizes specificity (98.9%) while still maintaining an acceptable sensitivity (82.5%) (Graves, Teng, et al., 1992). Age-stratified norms are available.

The *Severe Mini-Mental State Examination (SMMSE)* was designed to facilitate the testing of more severely impaired patients (Harrell et al., 2000). This 30-point instrument can be used until patients become mute or have no functional language. It consists of personal information (giving one's first name, last name, and complete birth date); three-word repetition; two single-step commands; three naming items; two construction items (drawing a circle to command, copying a square); writing one's name; category fluency ("animals"); and spelling "cat". Interrater reliability was exceptionally high (.99). Test–retest reliability over a 5-month period was quite good (.80), considering the long interval with deteriorating patients. The SMMSE appears to be particularly useful in assessing patients whose MMSE scores are below 10 or who are considered to have at least "moderately severe" dementia (Global Deterioration Scale of 5 or higher, or Clinical

Dementia Rating of 4 or higher). It tests a restricted set of cognitive functions simply and quickly.

The 7-Minute Screen (7MS) (P.R. Solomon, Hirschoff, et al., 1998)

The 7MS was designed as a rapid screening procedure for identifying those in the early stages of Alzheimer's disease. Rather than taking an existing mental status examination as its starting point, the 7MS combines four tests: a 16-item enhanced cued recall procedure initially described in longer form by Grober and Buschke (1987); a semantic fluency task (animal naming); the Benton Temporal Orientation Test (Benton, Sivan, Hamsher, et al., 1994); and clock drawing (setting the hands to "twenty to four"), with a simplified 7-point version of the Freedman scoring procedure (M. Freedman, Leach, et al., 1994).

Age, education, and sex had no appreciable effects on test scores. A complex algorithm was developed for combining scores from the four tests into a single score that can be interpreted as the odds of having Alzheimer's dementia. Both interrater reliability for the overall score and test-retest reliability over a one to two month interval were high in 25 randomly selected Alzheimer patients and 25 control subjects (.92 and .91, respectively). Sensitivities and specificities for detecting dementia were also impressive in the larger sample of 60 patients with Alzheimer's disease and 30 healthy control subjects (>.90), even for patients with less severe Alzheimer's disease. The major limitations of the 7MS appear to be the small, homogeneous sample on which it was validated and the complex scoring algorithm required to obtain the total score.

Short Portable Mental Status Questionnaire (SPMSQ) (Pfeiffer, 1975)

This brief screening measure was published the same year as the MMSE but it was developed specifically for use with geriatric patients. The SPMSQ has played a key role in large-scale epidemiological studies designed to identify risk factors for cognitive and functional impairment, such as the National Institute of Aging's program, Established Populations for Epidemiological Studies of the Elderly (EPESE) (Chodosh, Reuben, et al., 2002; Fillenbaum, Landerman, Blazer, et al., 2001). The SPMSQ is a ten-question, ten-point test that is even more heavily weighted toward orientation than the MMSE: seven of its items involve orientation (e.g., date, place, mother's maiden name), two tap memory for current and previous presidents, and the last assesses concentration and mental tracking with serial threes.

Test–retest reliability was .82 and .83 for two small groups of elderly control subjects (Pfeiffer, 1975) and .85 for nursing home patients (Lesher and Whelihan, 1986). A telephone version of the SPMSQ has been developed (Roccaforte et al., 1994). (The SPMSQ is not to be confused with the similarly structured and titled "Mental Status Questionnaire" [R.L. Kahn and Miller, 1978], also a ten item brief screening measure composed of orientation and general information items, but one that has been used much less in recent years.)

Test characteristics. Age affects SPMSQ performance, as it does performance on most brief screening instruments. Between ages 65–69 and 85–89, the average number correct for community-dwelling subjects dropped from 7.8 to 6.05 (Scherr et al., 1988); others have also shown that age has a pronounced effect on SPMSQ scores in these later years (Fillenbaum, Landerman, and Simonsick, 1998). Criteria for discriminating between intact subjects and three levels of impairment severity were based on a sample of almost 1,000 community-dwelling elderly Caucasian and African-American persons from the southern U.S, taking both education and race into account.

The specificity of the SPMSQ is very high (e.g., 96% in a clinical sample of 133 elderly patients, 40% of whom carried a diagnosis of dementia) (Pfeiffer data cited in Lorentz et al., 2002). However, like most screening instruments, its sensitivity is limited—peaking at 67% when the 10th percentile cut-off was applied to the clinical sample but dropping to 26% in an institutionalized sample. In a regression analysis, 47% of the variance in the SPMSQ was explained by only three items (date of birth, naming the previous president, and naming the day of the week), leading to the conclusion that these three items might well do the job of all ten (Fillenbaum, 1980).

Neuropsychological findings. Given its almost exclusive focus on orientation, the SPMSQ does not identify mildly impaired or early dementia patients to any reliable degree (G. Berg, Edwards, et al., 1987; Fillenbaum, 1980; Pfeiffer, 1975). One large epidemiological study demonstrated that community-dwelling elderly individuals who scored <7 on the SPMSQ were 2.60 (women) to 2.72 (men) times as likely to develop limitations in their ability to perform basic activities of daily living over the subsequent three years as those with higher scores (Moritz et al., 1995). In a study of over 2,500 hospitalized patients, those whose SPMSQ performance was mildly impaired were 2.8 times as likely as unimpaired individuals to have a first time admission to a nursing home within three months of discharge, while those whose SPMSQ performance was moderately to severely impaired were 6.7 times as likely to be admitted to a nursing home (Sands et al., 2003). These findings suggest that the SPMSQ may be better suited to population-based screening to identify individuals at risk for functional impairment, who can then be closely monitored, than it is to the clinical assessment of individual patients.

Telephone Interview for Cognitive Status (TICS) (Brandt, Spencer, and Folstein, 1988)

This test was the first of several telephone instruments developed to provide follow-up documentation on patients who had been seen in clinic or for research but who had not returned for later examinations. Other telephone screening instruments for dementia such as the *Minnesota Cognitive Acuity Screen* (*MCAS*) (Knopman, Knudson et al., 2000) and the *TELE* (Gatz, Reynolds, et al., 2002; Jarvenpaa et al., 2002), have been published but have not yet seen widespread use. The TICS has been incorporated into several large epidemiological studies, including the National Academy of Sciences Registry of Aging Twin Veterans (Brandt, Welsh, et al., 1993; Gallo and Breitner, 1995) and the Nurses' Health Study beginning in 1995 (Grodstein, Chen, Pollen, et al., 2000; Grodstein, Chen, Wilson, et al., 2001). It has also been used to screen patients for a recent clinical trial of rofecoxib for amnestic mild cognitive impairment (Lines et al., 2003).

The TICS covers domains similar to the MMSE but affords a more sensitive assessment of memory. In its original form the TICS had 11 items and included an assessment of immediate—but not delayed—recall as none of the Alzheimer's dementia patients in the pilot study could recall any items after a delay. A subsequent modification of the instrument (TICS-m) incorporated delayed recall to increase its sensitivity in early dementia (K.A. Welsh, Breitner, and Magruder-Habib, 1993). Several items on the TICS-m test for orientation and general fund of knowledge (name, date, telephone number, President, and Vice President, for a total of 14 points); three items involve language (following a command to tap the phone five times, repetition, responsive naming, for a total of 8 points); two are mental tracking tasks (counting backwards and subtraction, for a total of 7 points); one requires the subject to generate word opposites (of "west" and of "generous", for 2 points); and one involves immediate and delayed recall of a 10-word list (20 points total). The maximum score is 51. A computer-assisted telephone interview version of the TICS-m has recently been developed (Buckwalter et al., 2002).

Test characteristics. TICS scores were modestly correlated with education for patients but not for control subjects, whose range of scores was more restricted. Test–retest reliability of the TICS after one to six weeks was .96 for 34 Alzheimer patients (Brandt, Spencer, and Folstein, 1988) and was comparably high in stroke patients over a one month retest interval (D.W. Desmond et al., 1994). A factor analysis of TICS-m responses in 4000 twin pairs identified four factors: memory (20 points); language/attention (17 points); personal orientation (10 points); and general information (4 points) (Brandt, Welsh, et al., 1993). A subsequent factor analysis of the TICS-m responses of over 6000 subjects responding to an advertisement for those with memory complaints yielded similar findings, excepting that the personal orientation and general information factors combined into a single factor (Lines et al., 2003).

In the original validation study, the TICS was given to both normal subjects and previously diagnosed Alzheimer patients who had scored at least 20 points on the Mini-Mental State. Not surprisingly, TICS scores were strongly correlated with MMSE scores ($r = .94$) (Brandt, Spencer, and Folstein, 1988), a finding that was later replicated in an Italian sample (Ferrucci et al., 1998). In the Brandt group's study, patient scores ranged from 0 to 31, those for control subjects were in the 31 to 39 range: applying a cutting score of 30, only one patient was misclassified, for a sensitivity of 94% and a specificity of 100%. Subsequent studies confirmed the ability of the TICS to detect Alzheimer patients with excellent accuracy (>99% sensitivity and 86% specificity when a cut-off of <28 was used), even in population studies with low base rates of Alzheimer's disease (Gallo and Breitner, 1995). With the data evaluated both cross-sectionally and longitudinally, the TICS differentiated healthy controls from those with mild or ambiguous cognitive impairment and from patients with dementia (Plassman, Newman, et al., 1994). The validity of the TICS-m was further substantiated in a recent study of patients three months after they had sustained subarachnoid hemorrhages (Mayer et al., 2002). Patients who scored <30 on the TICS-m were rated as significantly more handicapped overall and less independent in performing daily activities. They also reported greater anxiety, more depression, and poorer overall quality of life.

Briefer screening instruments

The introduction of medications for dementia in the mid-1990s heightened interest in very brief screening instruments, ones that could be administered in less than five minutes and might be suitable for primary care and general neurology practices. The briefest of these—taking under two min—include three word recall, clock drawing tests (pp. 553–556), the Time and Change Test, which consists of clock reading and making change for a dollar (Froehlich et al., 1998), and the WORLD Test (Leopold and Borson, 1997), which asks subjects to spell "world" forward and backward and then arrange its letters in alphabetical order (Cullum, Thompson, and Smernoff, 1993). Unfortunately, none of these very brief tests has acceptable psychometric properties as a stand-alone screen for dementia (Lorentz et al., 2002).

The following two slightly longer screens are more promising.

Memory Impairment Screen (MIS). This is a four-item delayed free and cued recall procedure that incorporates category cues to facilitate acquisition and recall (Buschke, Kuslansky, et al., 1999). Subjects are shown a standard sheet of $8^1/_2 \times 11$" paper on which four words appear in large (24-point) uppercase letters, with each word derived from a different category. The subject is asked to read the items aloud and, when the examiner gives a category cue, to point to and read the item belonging to that category. After a two or three minute distraction period during which the subject counts from 1 to 20 forward and backward, the subject is asked to recall the four words in any order. Category cues are given for any items that are not spontaneously recalled. The total MIS score is twice the number of items retrieved on free recall (because it is assumed that these items would be retrieved on cued recall as well), plus the number of items retrieved on cued recall, for a total of 8 possible points. Two reasonably comparable ($r = .69$) alternate forms are available.

In a validation study with 483 community-dwelling elderly individuals, of whom 50 (10.4%) had dementia (Alzheimer's disease diagnosed in 39), the MIS proved surprisingly accurate in identifying patients with any form of dementia (sensitivity = .80 and specificity = .96 using a cut-off score of 4) or with Alzheimer's dementia (sensitivity = .87 and specificity = .96, also with a cut-off score of 4). Age, education, and gender did not significantly affect performance. In contrast, a standard three-word recall test had considerably poorer sensitivity (.65) and specificity (.85) as a screen for Alzheimer's dementia (Kuslansky et al., 2002). Buschke and his coworkers (1999) provide detailed tables on the performance of different cut-off scores as well as the probability of accurately identifying patients with dementia given differing base rates in the population. This enables clinicians and researchers to select the cut-off score that best meets their needs for optimizing sensitivity or specificity in a given population.

The Mini-Cog. This test combines uncued recall of three unrelated words (using words from the Cognitive Abilities Screening Instrument) with a clock drawing test (Borson, Scanlon, et al., 2000). The clock drawing test serves as the distractor between subjects' initial registration of the words (scored 0–3) and their subsequent recall of these words (also scored 0–3). Clock drawing is scored using the CERAD templates, yielding scores ranging from 0 (*normal*) to 3 (*severely impaired*) (Borson, Brush, et al., 1999). Scanlan and Borson (2001) found that inexperienced raters did nearly as well as experienced raters in scoring clock drawing. They suggested that any differences could be minimized with training in identifying clocks meeting criteria for mild impairment. Unlike the MMSE and the CASI, performance on the Mini-Cog was not influenced by education.

A classification algorithm for the Mini-Cog assigns subjects who recall none of the words to the "demented" group, those who recall all three words to the "nondemented" group, and those who recall one or two words as either "nondemented" if they perform normally (i.e., score 0) on the clock drawing test or "demented" if they exhibit any impairment (i.e., score 1–3) on clock drawing (Borson, Scanlon, et al., 2000). The Mini-Cog was initially validated in a heterogeneous sample of 249 community-dwelling older adults, about half of whom spoke—and were tested in—languages other than English and about half of whom met standard criteria for dementia (71% probable Alzheimer's dementia). Using this algorithm, the Mini-Cog demonstrated excellent sensitivity (99%) and specificity (93%), outperforming either test on its own. The sensitivity and specificity of the Mini-Cog were less impressive (approximately .75 and close to .90, respectively) in an epidemiological sample of over 1000 older adults in which the dementia prevalence was much lower (6.3%), but it performed as well as either the MMSE or a standard neuropsychological battery, identifying many subjects whose impairments were not recognized by their physicians (data reported in Lorentz et al., 2002).

Mental Status and Observer Rating Scale Combinations

Some assessment instruments include both a mental examination and a standardized observer- or informant-based rating format. In some instruments these two kinds of examination approaches are offered in separate sections. Structured patient interviews, however, may provide examiners the opportunity of rating their observations while assessing specific cognitive functions.

Alzheimer Disease Assessment Scale (ADAS)
(W.G. Rosen, Mohs, and Davis, 1984, 1986)

The *ADAS-Cognitive* subscale (*ADAS-Cog*) was the primary cognitive outcome measure in clinical trials that led to U.S. Food and Drug Administration approval of tacrine, the first medication approved for treatment of Alzheimer's disease (K.L. Davis et al., 1992). It soon replaced other clinical trial outcome measures that were either psychometrically deficient (e.g., Sandoz Clinical Assessment Geriatric [SCA-G] scale: Shader et al., 1974) or restricted in scope (e.g., the Selective Reminding Test), and has been used in all the major dementia treatment trials. In fact, the ADAS-Cog is one of two primary outcome measures required for clinical trials of new medications for Alzheimer's disease in the United States, the other being a clinician rating of global function. (The entire ADAS is usually administered in clinical trials, but the *ADAS-Noncognitive* subscale is considered a secondary outcome measure.) Numerous translations are available. For an overview of issues in selecting clinical outcome measures for dementia clinical trials, see Demers et al. (2000a,b) and Winblad et al. (2001).

ADAS-Cognitive subscale. W.G. Rosen and her colleagues (1984) selected items for the ADAS-Cog based on what they perceived to be the principal features of cognitive dysfunction in Alzheimer patients. Items cover *language ability* (25 possible points for naming objects and fingers and observer-rated comprehension of spoken language, expressive language, and word finding); *memory* (27 points for recall of instructions, word list recall and recognition); *praxis* (10 points), consisting of "constructional praxis" (copying geometric figures) and "ideational praxis" (preparing envelope to send to oneself); and *orientation* (8 points). Factor analyses of large data sets have essentially confirmed the conceptual framework underlying the ADAS-Cog, identifying three reproducible factors: memory, language, and praxis (Y.S. Kim et al., 1994; Talwalker et al., 1996).

The ADAS-Cog takes about 30–35 minutes to administer. Individual item scores are based on errors and generally range from 1 to 5, although some items have smaller or larger score ranges. The total ADAS-Cog score ranges from 0 to 70, with higher scores indicating greater impairment. The addition of a digit cancellation task, word learning with delayed recall, and a maze task has been recommended to improve sensitiv-

ity of the ADAS-Cog in assessing patients with mild Alzheimer's disease or those with mild cognitive impairment considered at risk of developing Alzheimer's disease (Mohs et al., 1997).

ADAS-Noncognitive subscale. The noncognitive portion of the ADAS consists of 10 items covering concentration, motor disturbances (tremors, pacing, and motor restlessness), appetite change, mood disturbance (tearfulness and depressed mood), behavioral disturbance ("uncooperativeness"), and psychotic symptoms (delusions and hallucinations). Some investigators have suggested dropping three of these items: concentration (beause of its high correlation [.78] with the ADAS-Cog), appetite disturbance (because it is not one of the cardinal behavioral disturbances in Alzheimer's disease), and tremor (because it is not characteristic of Alzheimer's disease). This would create a seven-item ADAS-Noncog that more purely reflects behavioral disturbances typical of Alzheimer's disease (D.B. Marin et al., 1997).

Ratings on the ADAS-Noncognitive are based on a clinician's observations, interview with the patient, and interview with a caregiver or other knowledgeable informant. Scores on individual items are rated from 0 (no impairment) to 5 (greatest impairment) for the week preceding the assessment; behavioral descriptors anchor the scale. With a maximum summation score of 50 on the full ADAS-Noncog, higher scores reflect more aberrant behavior. The ADAS-Noncognitive takes about four to six minutes to complete.

Test characteristics. Age and education had statistically significant effects on ADAS-Cog performance (Doraiswamy et al., 1995, 1997b). Scores declined with increasing age most noticeably in less educated subjects.

Interrater reliability coefficients for individual ADAS items ranged from .65 to .99 in Rosen's original sample (W.G. Rosen, Mohs, and Davis, 1986). The interrater reliability of the total ADAS was .82 to .83 in a subsequent study, with the ADAS-Cog subscale being considerably more reliable (.82–.90) than the ADAS-Noncognitive subscale (.42–.45) (Standish et al., 1996). Standardization of test administration and scoring, along with rigorous examiner training, substantially improved the interrater reliability of the ADAS-Noncognitive subscale (.85–.89). Over a one-month interval, test–retest item reliability coefficients for Alzheimer patients were in the .51 to 1.0 range in the Rosen group's original sample, with the ADAS-Noncognitive subscale producing the lower coefficients. In a separate study, test–retest reliability for the ADAS-Cog subscale alone was excellent (.91 over a 6-week period) (Talwalker et al., 1996). As expected, the

ADAS-Cog total score correlated strongly (−.76) with the MMSE; moreover, it did a better job than the MMSE in separating patients with different levels of cognitive impairment.

Neuropsychological findings. The ADAS in general—and the ADAS-Cog in particular—easily differentiated 15 Alzheimer patients from 15 elderly controls (W.G. Rosen, Mohs, and Davis, 1984). In fact, each individual ADAS-Cog item on its own successfully differentiated these groups. Group differences on the ADAS-Noncognitive were smaller in magnitude and statistically significant on only three items. The ability of the ADAS-Cog to differentiate patients with Alzheimer's disease from elderly controls was subsequently replicated by Zec, Landreth, and colleagues (1992) in a larger sample. The ADAS-Cog subscale can also successfully distinguish patients who differ in their dementia severity: for example, it discriminated patients with moderate dementia (GDS = 4) from those with moderately severe dementia (GDS = 5), with the orientation item being the best discriminator at these levels of dementia severity.

Alzheimer patients obtained consistently higher (i.e., worse) scores on both ADAS subscales at 12- and 18-month retests, while normal elderly patients' scores remained essentially unchanged (W.G. Rosen, Mohs, and Davis, 1986). The rate of deterioration is more pronounced on the ADAS-Cog as opposed to the ADAS-Noncognitive subscale and is greatest among patients with moderate to severe—as opposed to mild or very severe—impairment at baseline.

Blessed Dementia Scale (BDS) (Blessed, Tomlinson, and Roth, 1968)

This two-part scale was originally called simply the "Dementia Scale," but many users added the senior author's name to avoid confusion with other similarly named instruments. It was originally designed to evaluate the relationship between mental deterioration in the elderly and pathological changes in brain tissue observed on autopsy. The first part, the *Blessed Rating Scale* (BRS), registers changes in behavior and daily functioning reported by informants. The second part, the *Blessed Information-Memory-Concentration Test* (BIMC), consists of many of the most commonly used mental status questions examining the areas announced in the test's title (see below). A six-item mental status test taken from this portion of the BDS—(the *Orientation-Memory-Concentration Test*—also usually carries Blessed's name (see p. 715). All three instruments have had wide application, but only occasionally are the rating scale and one of the two mental status tests

used together. In recent years, Mungas and Reed (2000) used sophisticated psychometric methods to produce a 25-item cognitive screening instrument composed of 10 items from the Blessed Rating Scale, 12 from the Blessed Information-Memory-Concentration Test, and three from the MMSE. This new instrument is not only brief and easy to administer but also statistically reliable. Unfortunately, it has not been widely adopted despite its obvious psychometric appeal.

Blessed Rating Scale (BRS). This scale has been variously referred to in the literature as the "Dementia Score" (Hachinski, Iliff, et al., 1975; see Table 18.1), the "Dementia Rating Scale (DRS)" (Eastwood et al., 1983), "Part I of the Blessed Dementia Rating Scale (BDRS)" (Y. Stern, Mayeux, Sano, et al., 1987), and the "Blessed Dementia Scale (BDS)" (J.C. Morris, Heyman, et al., 1989). Here it is called the *Blessed Rating Scale* (BRS) as the most descriptive and least confusing title.

TABLE 18.1 Dementia Score

Feature	Score
CHANGES IN PERFORMANCE OF EVERDAY ACTIVITIES	
1. Inability to perform household tasks	1
2. Inability to cope with small sums of money	1
3. Inability to remember short list of items, e.g., in shopping	1
4. Inability to find way about indoors	
5. Inability to find way about familiar streets	1
6. Inability to interpret surroundings	1
7. Inability to recall recent events	1
8. Tendency to dwell in the past	1
CHANGES IN HABITS	
9. Eating	
Messily with spoon only	1
Simple solids, e.g., biscuits	2
Has to be fed	3
10. Dressing	
Occasionally misplaced buttons, etc.	1
Wrong sequence, commonly forgetting items	2
Unable to dress	3
11. Sphincter control	
Occasional wet beds	1
Frequent wet beds	2
Doubly incontinent	3
12. Increased rigidity	1
13. Increased egocentricity	1
14. Impairment of regard for feelings of others	1
15. Coarsening of affect	1
16. Impairment of emotional control	1
17. Hilarity in inappropriate situations	1
18. Diminished emotional responsiveness	1
19. Sexual misdemeanor (appearing de novo in old age)	1
20. Hobbies relinquished	1
21. Diminished initiative or growing apathy	1
22. Purposeless hyperactivity	1

From Hachinski et al. (1975) *Archives of Neurology 32*, p. 633. © 1975, American Medical Association.

The BRS measures how well patients have functioned in their usual environment during the preceding six months. Information typically comes from family informants or caregivers, but medical records can be used as well. Summing the 22 items together yields scores ranging from 0 to 28, with higher scores indicating greater incapacity. As a rule of thumb, persons receiving scores less than 4 are considered to be unimpaired, scores of 4 to 9 indicate mild impairment, and scores of 10 and higher are in the moderate to severe impairment range (Eastwood et al., 1983). Based on clinical experience, a slightly higher threshold (15) for moderate impairment has been suggested (Y. Stern, Mayeux, Sano, et al., 1987).

Test characteristics. The test–retest stability of the BRS over 4 weeks in a sample of 68 nondemented elderly subjects was estimated to be .79 (Erkinjuntti et al., 1988). The first 11 items alone show a satisfactory test–retest reliability over 4 weeks ($r = .68$). These items can be used alone to distinguish those with dementia of varying severities. This version of the BRS was adopted for CERAD (*BDRS-CERAD version:* J.C. Morris, Heyman, et al., 1989), with each item phrased positively instead of negatively (e.g., "1. *ability* to perform household tasks," as opposed to "*inability* to perform household tasks") for a total possible score of 17.

Neuropsychological findings. In the original study of 60 elderly persons who had come to autopsy, some had functional psychiatric diagnoses, some were delirious, some were demented, and a small number of physically ill patients served as control subjects (Blessed, Tomlinson, and Roth, 1968). Patients diagnosed with senile dementia were more impaired on the BRS than those in the other groups, with the correlation between the BRS total score and the mean senile plaque count reaching .77.

When repeated over time, the BRS can be used to monitor dementia progression (J.C. Morris, Heyman, et al., 1989; Y. Stern, Mayeux, Sano, et al., 1987) by documenting the behavioral alterations that accompany cognitive deterioration (Van Gorp and Cummings, 1989). A longitudinal study using the BRS documented the variability that is often observed clinically in the timing and magnitude of change across different aspects of behavior (Y. Stern, Hesdorffer, Sano, and Mayeux, 1990). Examining changes on four BRS factor scores derived from a principal components analysis of patients' individual item scores (i.e., Cognitive, Personality Change, Apathy/Withdrawal, and Basic self-care), the Stern group noted that cognitive deficiencies affecting instrumental ADLs were evident early and worsened throughout the disease course, whereas changes in Basic self-care did not occur until four to five years into the illness. Increases in Personality Changes and in Apathy/Withdrawal became more common as the disease progressed but these behavioral changes tended to fluctuate more than the cognitive symptoms.

Information-Memory-Concentration Test (BIMC). This part of the Blessed scale contains three sections. The "Information Test" (15 points) inquires into the patient's personal orientation. "Memory" (16 points) asks for recall of remote memories—both "personal" (e.g., school attended) and "non-personal" (e.g., date of World War II)—and includes a name and address to be learned for recall five minutes later. "Concentration" consists of three items, months backwards, and counting from 1 to 20 and 20 to 1, with each scored 0–2 for a total of 6 possible points. A perfect performance earns a score of 37.

When given to nursing home patients, both two to four week test–retest and split-half reliability coefficients were very satisfactory (.88 and .89, respectively). Blessed and his colleagues (1968) reported that the BIMC score had a correlation of $-.59$ with senile plaque count in their population of elderly patients. This finding was replicated exactly in a study that also included mentally intact subjects along with Alzheimer patients and other demented patients (Katzman, Brown, Fuld, et al., 1983). Among Alzheimer patients, an average annual decline in the BIMC score of 4.4 was found, independent of age, except for the most intact whose initial rate of decline was less (Katzman, Brown, Thal, et al., 1988). For individual patients, however, the rate at which scores declined was quite variable.

Orientation-Memory-Concentration Test (OMC). Upon observing that six items from the BIMC and the Mental Status Questionnaire (MSQ) correlated more highly with the total BIMC than the total MSQ score, Katzman, Brown, Fuld, and their colleagues (1983) selected them for a brief mental status screening test. They include orientation for time (month, year, and time of day), counting from 20 to 1, months backward, and repeating a brief phrase. Points are given for failures—with individual items differentially weighted—for a total possible score of 24. Calling this test the *Short Orientation-Memory-Concentration Test (SOMCT),* Lesher and Whelihan (1986) reported limited internal consistency (split-half correlation of .37, not surprising for such a brief and heterogeneous set of items) but good test–retest reliability ($r = .80$). The Katzman group found that over 90% of intact elderly subjects earned weighted error scores of 6 or less; error scores greater than 10 are strong indicators of dementia.

Brief Cognitive Rating Scale (BCRS) (Reisberg, Schneck, Ferris, et al., 1983)

This two-part scale rates both responses to mental status questions and qualitative characteristics observed in a semistructured assessment interview. Whenever possible, the interview is conducted with a spouse or caregiver present to provide realistic information when the patient's self-reports are inaccurate. The first part consists of five "Axes": I. Concentration and calculating ability; II. Recent memory; III. Remote memory; IV. Orientation; V. Functioning and self-care. Each axis has a 7-point rating scale with descriptors ranging from "No objective or subjective evidence of deficit . . . " to descriptions of severe impairment in that domain. Scores of 1 and 2 are considered to be within the range of intact functioning, while scores of 4 or greater indicate moderate to severe dementia. Scores for the five axes in the first part of the BCRS can be averaged and interpreted on a 7-point *Global Deterioration Scale (GDS)* for which each score level indicates the same degree of severity as the axis score level (Reisberg and Ferris, 1982; Reisberg, Ferris, de Leon, and Crook, 1982). Intercorrelations among the first five axes ranged from .83 to .97, indicating considerable overlap in ratings of these functions (Reisberg, Ferris, Borenstein, et al., 1986). On the basis of assessments of 50 subjects (a relatively intact sample heavily skewed toward lower GDS scores), correlations of Axes I through V with neuropsychological tests and test items in common use were all positive and significant ($p < .001$).

The second part of the BCRS—"Language, Motoric, and Mood Concomitants"—is named for each of its three "axes" which also have 7-point rating scales ranging from highest, "No subjective or objective [problems in that area]," to lowest, "Inability to perform the functions under consideration." (W.G. Rosen and her coworkers [1986] cautioned that the language scale does not adequately cover speech and language, noting that speech comprehension is not included among the descriptors, for example.) The three axes comprising the second part of the BCRS are separated from the first five because the authors did not consider them to be as closely or regularly associated with disease progression in Alzheimer patients as the first five axes. Individual correlations of Axes VI, VII, and VIII with the summed score for Axes I through V (GDS) were in the .71–.88 range.

The principal application of the BCRS has been the use of its first five axes to derive the Global Deterioration Scale. The assumption underlying the development of the GDS and other global rating scales is that all of the functions covered in Part I of the BCRS will deteriorate at a similar rate in Alzheimer's disease, an assumption that does not hold in many individual cases. Nonetheless, the GDS and other global rating scales are widely used in clinical dementia research and clinical trials of antidementia medications to provide an index of overall level of functioning, or stage of dementia, and change over time. (For an astute review of the psychometric properties of the GDS and two other commonly used global rating scales for dementia, the Clinical Global Impression (CGI) scales and Clinical Dementia Rating (CDR), see Oremus et al., 2000.)

Scales for Rating Observations

These scales can focus on many different aspects of mood, behavior, and functional abilities. Behavioral and mood problems in Alzheimer's disease are common and have a profound effect on the level of care that a patient must have and caregiver burden, not to mention the cost of such care. Assessment of mood, behavior, and functional abilities in Alzheimer patients is complicated by the fact that the patient may not be able to provide reliable responses, particularly in the later stages of the disease. Consequently, the clinician must base ratings on direct observation of the patient's behavior (as on the ADAS-Noncognitive subscale or the Blessed Rating Scale described earlier), or on information derived from an interview with a relative or other knowledgeable informant. A review of measures of functional abilities is beyond the scope of this book. For interested readers, two frequently used instruments are the *Barthel Index* (Mahoney and Barthel, 1965) with its recent modification (Novak et al., 1996) and the *Functional Independence Measure + the Functional Assessment Measure (FIM/FAM)* (Uniform Data Systems, 1987, 1993).

Behavioral Pathology in Alzheimer Disease Rating Scale (BEHAVE-AD) (Reisberg, Borenstein, Franssen, et al., 1987)

Potentially remediable behavioral disturbances common in Alzheimer's disease are the subject of this rating scale which reviews seven categories of behavior symptoms: Paranoid and Delusional Ideation: Hallucinations; Activity Disturbances (e.g., wandering); Aggressivity; Diurnal Rhythm Disturbances; Affective Disturbances; Anxieties and Phobias. The symptoms in these categories often create problems for caregivers but may be ameliorated pharmacologically. Each of the 25 symptoms is rated on a 4-point scale (from 0 = Not present, to 3 = Present—at a level intolerable to caregiver). The rating form also provides space for elaborating details of some of these problems. Information for ratings comes from patients' spouses and caregivers, and from clinical observations. Unlike many scales, the BEHAVE-AD rates the impact of behavior on caregivers. Five factors accounting for 40% of the variance were identified: agitation/anxiety, psychosis, aggression/fear of being left alone, depression, and activity disturbance/delusion that one's house is not one's home (Harwood, Ownby, et al. 1998). A version is available with a symptom frequency-weighted score, the *BEHAVE-AD-FW*, which measures both the magnitude and prevalence of behavioral symptoms (Monteiro et al., 2001).

Ratings of a group of 120 Alzheimer patients at different stages of the disease, from mild to dilapidated, brought out the typical course of development and eventual disappearance of these symptoms, with most having their peak occurrence in the late middle stages of the disease (Reisberg, Franssen, et al., 1989). A longitudinal study using the BEHAVE-AD showed that activity disturbance was a common and relatively persistent symptom in the mild stages of Alzheimer's disease (Eustace et al., 2002). Anxiety, paranoid ideation, and aggression were moderately persistent; but depressive symptoms usually lasted less than one year. Patients with frontotemporal dementia had significantly worse global BEHAVE-AD scores with more verbal outbursts and inappropriate activity compared to Alzheimer patients (Mendez, Perryman, Miller, and Cummings, 1998). The BEHAVE-AD often is used as an outcome measure in dementia treatment trials (Brodaty et al., 2003).

Geriatric Evaluation by Relative's Rating Instrument (GERRI) (G.E. Schwartz, 1983)

This scale was conceived to assess behavioral functioning in elderly persons showing signs of mental decline. The 49 items cover a broad spectrum of behaviors observable in the home. Persons in close contact with the patient (usually a relative or caregiver) rate the patient on each item by means of a 5-point scale ranging from "Almost All the Time" to "Almost Never" with a "Does Not Apply" option. Correlational analyses identified three item clusters: Cognitive Functioning (21 items), Social Functioning (18 items), and Mood (10 items). Using two sets of informants for 45 dementia patients at different severity levels, the total score interrater reliability was .94; for the three clusters, it was .96, .92, and .66, respectively. GERRI scores varied significantly with severity rating scores (Global Deterioration Score), the Cognitive and Social clusters discriminating significantly between three levels of dementia severity ($p < .0001$). In a large sample of dementia patients, GERRI scores correlated significantly

($r = .40$) with ADAS-Cog scores (Doraiswamy, Bieber, et al., 1997b).

The GERRI has been used as an outcome measure in treatment trials with geriatric and dementia patients (Le Bars et al., 2002). R.S. McDonald (1986) cautioned that untrained and emotionally close observers such as relatives may be biased in their observations, but acknowledged the advantages of an observer reporting on patient behavior—and behavioral changes—in the natural setting of the home.

The Neuropsychiatric Inventory (NPI) (Cummings, Mega, Gray, et al., 1994)

Developed to assess a wide range of behaviors common in dementia patients, ten behavior domains are evaluated: delusions, hallucinations, dysphoria, anxiety, euphoria, agitation/aggression, apathy, irritability/lability, disinhibition, and aberrant motor behavior. An informant, preferably the daily caregiver, is asked scripted questions about the patient's behavior during the previous month. Each section has screening questions and if the behavior has occurred, more detailed questioning probes the *frequency* on a 4-point scale and *severity* on a 3-point scale. Two additional scales were later added to assess sleep and appetite/eating disorders (Cummings, 1997). Also, added to each domain is a 6-point caregiver distress scale which ranges from 0 (no distress) to 5 (very severe distress). It was suggested for the original scale that the interview can be brief (7–10 min), but some caregivers elaborate their answers and require considerably more time.

Test characteristics. Interrater reliability and internal consistency of the scale were high (Cummings, Mega, Gray, et al., 1994). Test–retest reliability by a second interviewer within 3 weeks generally was adequate, with the lowest correlations (.53 for frequency, .51 for severity) for Irritability/lability. The NPI's correlation with the BEHAVE-AD was .66 for the total score. Most subscales correlated well with the corresponding BEHAVE-AD subscale except NPI dysphoria which had a .33 correlation with BEHAVE-AD Affective Disturbances. The authors state that the Dysphoria scale items were selected to represent core psychological and behavioral manifestations of depression and to exclude dementia symptoms. Three factors characterized the behavior symptoms of a large group of dementia patients: mood/apathy, psychosis, and hyperactivity (Aalten et al., 2003).

Neuropsychological findings. All behavior problems assessed by the NPI were greater in Alzheimer patients compared to age-matched control subjects (Mega,

Cummings, et al., 1996). The most common was apathy, which was exhibited by 72% of patients, followed by agitation, which was displayed by 60%. The NPI differentiated the behavioral symptoms of Alzheimer's and Parkinson's diseases (Aarsland et al., 2001) as Alzheimer patients had more aberrant motor behavior, agitation, disinhibition, irritability, euphoria, and apathy, while more hallucinations were reported for the Parkinson patients. The NPI has also been used to assess psychiatric symptoms in patients with multiple sclerosis (Diaz-Olavarrieta et al., 1999). Symptoms were present in 95% of patients, the most common being depression (79%) and agitation (40%). Although euphoria was once described as a common characteristic of patients with multiple sclerosis, only 13% showed this symptom. Euphoria was more common in patients with moderately severe frontotemporal MRI abnormalities. The NPI has also been used to assess psychiatric symptoms in other, mostly subcortical, neurodegenerative disorders (Litvan, Cummings, and Mega, 1998).

A self-administered NPI. A paper-and-pencil caregiver questionnaire, the *NPI-Q,* has been developed (Kaufer, Cummings, et al., 2000). The questionnaire format saves time for the examiner as, the authors say, most caregivers can complete the form in five minutes or less. Adequate convergent valdity and test–retest reliability were obtained. Correlations between the NPI and the NPI-Q were high (.90). More symptoms were reported on the NPI-Q than the NPI.

TRAUMATIC BRAIN INJURY

Although behavioral rating scales and inventories in general use can be adapted for traumatically brain injured patients, many of their particular issues have led to the development of specialized assessment instruments. Perhaps the most important of these issues is predicting outcome, since most TBI victims have their future before them. Many aspects of outcome are closely associated with the severity of damage such that particular attention has been given to assessing initial severity on the basis of clinical observations. Some measures can be used both to define severity of injury and to establish improvement and/or deterioration over time (e.g., Glasgow Coma Scale). A second issue has been the assessment of a condition in which rapid change is the rule, as is the case particularly in the first few months after return to consciousness. Not infrequently an examiner will have begun an examination of such a patient on a Thursday or Friday and had to discontinue a test before completing it only to find, on the following Monday or Tuesday, that the patient's

new performance level has rendered the original data obsolete. Moreover, in the early stages, the rate of change becomes an important feature in itself. Still another issue concerns the enormous intraindividual variability in performance levels that characterizes so many head injury patients. A thorough neuropsychological examination of some patients may require use of many different measures ranging in complexity and sophistication from infant scales to college aptitude tests, depending on severity and time since injury. Social adjustment is another issue that must be dealt with in assessments as some TBI patients, especially those who survived a severe injury, regain most of their premorbid physical competencies and many of their original cognitive abilities while judgment, self-control, and social skills and sensitivity remain impaired. The disparities between what these patients are capable of doing and what they are competent to do result in patterns of social maladaptation peculiar to them which the usual inventories of behavioral or social problems do not handle well.

Recent changes in the World Health Organization (WHO) system for evaluation of diseases and disorders are likely to affect our choice of outcome measures for TBI. The *International Classification of Impairments, Disabilities, and Handicaps* (ICIDH; World Health Organization, 1980) resulted from the need to assess the effectiveness of health care. Gray and Hendershot (2000) note that such evaluation was relatively uncomplicated when the health care system was dealing with acute disease or when the patient was cured or died. Now many patients live with chronic diseases and disorders, and the consequences need evaluation. "Impairments, disabilities, and handicaps" were thus included in the medical model. This classification has met with criticism for a variety of reasons, including overlap and ambiguity in the relationships between impairment, disability, and handicap, and not enough consideration of environmental and other factors (Gray and Hendershot, 2000; Pfeiffer, 1998; Fougeyrollas, 1995; Whiteneck, Fougeyrolloas, and Gerhart, 1997). Also the model emphasized the negative aspects of disease and disorders, not the competencies of individuals.

The current model, the *International Classification of Functioning, Disability, and Health* (ICFDH) (World Health Organization, 2001) emphasizes health and health-relevant components of well-being. It has two parts: Part 1. *Functioning and disability* incorporates the components "body functions and structures" and "activities and participation". Part 2. *Contextual factors* include the components "environmental factors" and "personal factors". Domains, constructs, positive aspects, and negative aspects are described for each of these four components with qualifiers for some components. The component "body functions and structures" is associated with changes in body functions and body structures: the positive aspect is functional and structural *integrity,* the negative aspect is *impairments. Localization* is a qualifier. The component "activities and participation" is associated with life tasks and actions; *capacity* (executing tasks in a standard environment) and *performance* (executing tasks in the current environment). The positive aspects are activities and participation; the negative aspects are activity limitation and participation restriction. *Assistance* is a qualifier. The component "environmental factors" involves external influences in functioning and disability; specifically, the facilitating or hindering impact of features of the physical, social, and attitudinal world: the positive aspect is *facilitators* and the negative aspect is *barriers/hindrances.* A qualifier is *extent* or *magnitude* and a second qualifier is *subjective satisfaction.* The first three components are quantified on the same scale from 0 (no problem) to 4 (complete problem). Finally, the component "personal factors" is associated with internal influences on functioning and disability respectively, that is, the impact of attributes of the person. However, positive and negative aspects of personal factors are termed "nonapplicable." It is puzzling that personal factors are defined as ". . . the particular background of an individual's life and living, and comprise features of the individual that are not part of a health condition or health states;" yet these features include age, sex, race, even coping style, overall behavior pattern, psychological assets, and other variables that are clearly related to health condition and health states, similar to environmental factors. No classification of personal factors is attempted, just as positive and negative aspects and qualifiers are not given. Assessing personal factors and integrating them into this evaluation are to be done by the clinician. Much work still needs to be done on the ICF but the emphasis on environmental factors is one of many improvements (Gray and Hendershot, 2000) and the discussion of personal factors is a beginning. Response to the ICF has been generally positive, although problems are being noted in its application (Chopra et al., 2002; Dahl, 2002; Willems and de Kleijn-de Vrankrijker, 2002). New measures are likely to be developed (Steiner et al., 2002) and changes will be made to current outcome measures in order for them to be consistent with this classification (Stineman et al., 2003).

Evaluating Severity

Glasgow Coma Scale (Teasdale and Jennett, 1974)

Although it has "coma" in its title, this brief assessment technique can be used to describe all posttraumatic states of altered consciousness from the mildest

TABLE 18.2 Glasgow Coma Scale

The Glasgow Coma Scale Response Chart (GCS)		
Examiner's Test	*Patient's Response*	*Score*
Eye opening		
Spontaneous	Opens eyes normally	4
Speech	Opens eyes when asked in loud voice	3
Pain	Opens eyes to pain (e.g., pinch)	2
Pain	Does not open eyes	1
Verbal		
Speech	Carries on a conversation correctly and demonstrates intact orientation	5
Speech	Speaks, seems confused and disoriented	4
Speech	Talks to examiner but speech makes no sense	3
Speech	Makes unintelligible sounds	2
Speech	Makes no noise	1
Best motor response		
Commands	Follows simple commands	6
Pain	Pulls examiner's hand away on painful stimuli (localizes pain source)	5
Pain	Pulls a part of body away on painful stimuli (withdraws)	4
Pain	Flexes body inappropriately to pain (abnormal flexion)	3
Pain	Decerebrate posturing (abnormal extension)	2
Pain	No motor response to pain	1
		Range 3–15

confusional state to deep coma (see Table 18.2). A coma score, the sum of the highest score in each dimension, can be calculated. In evaluating injury severity, a GCS range of 3 to 8 is considered severe, 9 to 12 is moderate, and 13 to 15 is mild (Rimel, Giordani, et al., 1982; see Table 18.3). Coma has been defined as occurring when the GCS is ≤8 in a patient without spontaneous eye opening, ability to obey commands, or comprehensible speech (H.S. Levin, Williams, et al., 1988). The simplicity of the GCS allows it to be used reliably by emergency medical technicians in the field as well as by nursing personnel and doctors (Menegazzi et al., 1993). The inclusion of three response dimensions makes it possible to evaluate level of conscious-

TABLE 18.3 Severity Classification Criteria for the Glasgow Coma Scale (GCS)

Classification	*GCS*		*Coma Duration*
Mild	≥13	or	≤20 minutes
Moderate	9–12	or	No longer than within 6 hours of admission
Severe	≤8*	or	>6 hours after admission

*Patients with GCS ≤8 are considered to be in coma (M.R. Bond, 1986).

TABLE 18.4 Frequency of "Bad" and "Good" Outcomes Associated with the Glasgow Coma Scale (24-Hour Best Response)

Coma Response Sum	n	Dead/ Vegetative (%)	Moderate Disability/Good Recovery (%)
≥11	57	7	87
8–10	190	27	68
5–7	525	53	34
3, 4	176	87	7

Adapted from Jennett (1979)

ness when vision or speech, for example, is compromised by factors other than impaired consciousness. Moreover, it can be used repeatedly to provide longitudinal data on the course of improvement during the earliest posttrauma period. Its greatest virtue is that it has proven to be a good predictor of outcome (e.g., Jennett, Teasdale, and Knill-Jones, 1975; H.S. Levin, Grossman, Rose, and Teasdale, 1979; see Table 18.4), albeit not always a strong predictor (Zafonte, Hammond, et al., 1996). It is also useful in predicting outcome from other medical conditions (Bhagwanjee et al., 2000; Gotoh et al., 1996; Mullie et al., 1988; Plum and Carona, 1975).

The Glasgow Coma Scale has been just about universally accepted as the standard measure for determining severity of injury in patients whose consciousness is compromised. The mortality rates for patients (seen at medical centers) with a GCS score ≤8 for more than four hours run in the 50 to 88% range (Eisenberg, 1985; Teasdale and Mendelow, 1984). Older age at injury is highly related to mortality and morbidity among those having a GCS of 3–8 (Kilaru et al., 1996; Quigley et al., 1997). GCS scores are significantly related to depth of lesions. Lesions in deep central gray matter or the brain stem tend to be associated with a lower GCS than cortical or subcortical white matter lesions (H.S. Levin, Williams, et al., 1988). In children and adolescents with moderate to severe TBI, depth of lesion was most predictive of the Disabilty Rating Scale (DRS) score at time of discharge from rehabilitation, while GCS better predicted the one year DRS score (Grados et al., 2001). At one month postinjury, of patients given a neuropsychological test battery, those with moderately severe injuries (GCS = 8–10) performed, on the average, less well than those with milder injuries (GCS ≥ 11) who, in turn, performed below levels obtained by matched control subjects; most coma survivors were still untestable at one month (Dikmen, McLean, Temkin, and Wyler, 1986). However, after three months, the GCS did not distinguish between

mildly and moderately injured patients with respect to rates of return to employment (Rimel, Giordani, et al., 1982). Community integration and vocational outcome (J. Fleming et al., 1999) as well as patient and family reports of quality of life and social adjustment (P.S. Klonoff, Costa, and Snow, 1986) relate directly to initial GCS measures.

Despite its demonstrated usefulness, questions arise as to which GCS measurement indicates severity of injury: the emergency medical service GCS (taken at the scene or in the ambulance), the initial Emergency Room GCS (frequently called the postresuscitation GCS), the Best Day-1 GCS, the Worst Day-1 GCS, the Best Day-1 motor score, or GCS 6 hours post injury? All of these have been used in studies. Often rehabilitation researchers use the GCS on admission to their facility to indicate severity of injury but this GCS may or may not represent the initial severity of injury. Each of these measures provides a "snapshot" of what may happen during the critical first 48 to 72 hours postinjury, especially with the more serious injuries. J.M. Williams (1992) noted that differences in scale range for the three tested response modalities can bias the evaluation, depending on which modalities are operative. It would be fair to say that clinicians such as intensivists and neurosurgeons treating these patients do not rely on one GCS but often on hourly GCS scores, continuous clinical monitoring data, and serial CT scans to determine the status of the patient and necessary treatment on an ongoing basis during this period.

The GCS also has some inherent problems. Some trauma patients are lucid initially at the scene of the accident but have to be sedated for agitation or anesthetized and intubated for medical emergencies. These circumstances artificially lower their GCS on admission to the ER. Others deteriorate on transport to the hospital or in the ER or in neurosurgery intensive care, and earlier scores may not be representative of the eventual severity of injury. If a patient goes to surgery and is anesthetized, the GCS drops to 3 for several hours. A patient with a relatively mild head injury that would not produce a low GCS score may have a period of time on the record when the GCS score is low, suggesting to the naive reader that there was some neurological deterioration. Moreover, intoxicated patients may produce unreliable GCS scores with impaired consciousness attributed inappropriately to head trauma severity in some cases, to alcoholic stupor in others. Alcohol reduces admission GCS (M.P. Kelly, Johnson, et al., 1997; Sloan et al., 1989). The effects of alcohol are likely to be seen in the first six hours after injury. Our [hjh] experience with drugs given to patients while they are in intensive care suggests that some drugs do not affect the GCS (e.g., mannitol), some have large effects (e.g., entomidate), and some have additive effects (e.g., hydrocodeine). Drug use by patients and metabolic alterations due to injuries not directly involving the brain can also affect level of consciousness resulting in a misleading GCS score (Stambrook, Moore, Lubrusko, et al., 1993). All of these effects need to be taken into account in trying to understand variations in the GCS of a patient over time.

Eisenberg (1985) noted two other important problems with the GCS: Some examination modalities may not be measurable during the first few days when patients who are intubated or have a tracheotomy cannot talk, eyes swollen from facial injuries (*ecchymosis*) will not open, and paralysis or immobilization for treatment purposes precludes limb movement. Of real concern is the way in which components of the GCS are scored under such circumstances in various medical centers. A national telephone survey of Level I trauma centers (Buechler et al., 1998) found that 26% of centers gave intubated patients 1 point for the verbal component added to the eye and motor scores, 23% scored a total GCS of 3, 16% estimated GCS with "T" given for the verbal component (16%), 10% gave "unknown" as the score, another 10% gave a score of 15, and for 15% the method of scoring was unknown. Such wide GCS scoring variations even among Level I trauma centers raises questions about institutional, state, and national databases; epidemiological and outcome research could be adversely affected by such scoring variations. The second problem noted by Eisenberg concerns the sacrifice of a richer data base for higher interexaminer and intersite reliability; but loss of information about when and how the GCS was scored will lower predictive accuracy. While it is a generally useful guideline to injury severity, the times that the GCS was measured and the circumstances surrounding the first few hours and days after injury must be taken into account in determining how much weight to give it as a predictor in the individual case.

Rancho Los Amigos Scale: Levels of Cognitive Functioning (Hagen, 1984; Hagen, Malkmus, et al., 1979)

This scale, typically referred to as the "Rancho scale," has been used to track improvement (Kay and Lezak, 1990), for evaluating potential (Story, 1991), for planning and placement purposes (Mysiw et al., 1989), and to measure outcome and treatment effects (Lal et al., 1988; Razack et al., 1997). Its main focus is on cognitive functioning in the broadest behavioral sense. It differentiates eight levels of functioning covering much of the observable range of psychosocially relevant behaviors following TBI (see Table 18.5). An often implicit

TABLE 18.5 The Eight Levels of Cognitive Functioning of the "Rancho Scale"

1. *No Response:* The patient is in deep coma and completely unresponsive.

2. *Generalized Response:* The patient reacts inconsistently and nonpurposefully to stimuli in a nonspecific manner.

3. *Localized Response:* The patient reacts specifically but inconsistently to stimuli, orienting, withdrawing, or even following simple commands.

4. *Confused-Agitated:* The patient is in a heightened state of activity with severely decreased ability to process information.

5. *Confused, Inappropriate, Non-agitated:* The patient appears alert and is able to respond to simple commands fairly consistently; however, with increased complexity of commands or lack of any external structure, responses are nonpurposeful, random, or at best fragmented toward any desired goal.

6. *Confused-Appropriate:* The patient shows goal-directed behavior but is dependent on external input for direction.

7. *Automatic-Appropriate:* The patient appears appropriate and oriented within hospital and home settings, goes through daily routine automatically, but frequently robot-like, with minimal to absent confusion, and has shallow recall of what he/she has been doing.

8. *Purposeful and Appropriate:* The patient is alert and oriented, is able to recall and integrate past and recent events, and is aware of and responsive to his environment.

Reprinted from Kay and Lezak (1990)

assumption that clinicians make about this scale is that the course of improvement following head trauma will follow the levels outlined therein. It was developed for use by clinical and rehabilitation staff.

The three highest levels of the Rancho scale tend to reflect cognitive improvement as measured by language skills (Wiig et al., 1988). Thus, patients at level VI were less able to understand metaphoric expressions or to compose sentences from sets of words than those at level VII, but these language tests did not differentiate level VII from level VIII patients. Low Rancho scale levels on admission to rehabilitation hospitals indicate patients at risk for abnormal swallowing, aspiration, delay in initiation of oral feeding, and delay in total oral feeding (L.E. MacKay et al., 1999a,b). The Rancho scale can discriminate between patients returning to competitive employment and those requiring vocational training or supported work but is not sensitive to differences in lower levels of vocational potential (Mysiw et al., 1989). Sohlberg and Mateer (1989) observed that while useful in giving a general indication of a patient's cognitive and behavioral status, the actual details of the patient's functioning cannot be deduced from the patient's level. They further note that this scale implies similar rates of improvement on different kinds of functions, when this is more often not the case.

Name _____   Date of Test |__|__|__|
                                                        mo day yr
Age _____ Sex   M   F   Day of the week s m t w th f s
Date of Birth |__|__|__| Time   AM   PM
              mo day yr
Diagnosis _____   Date of injury |__|__|__|
                                                        mo day yr

GALVESTON ORIENTATION & AMNESIA TEST (GOAT)   Error Points

1. What is your name? (2) _____   When were you born? (4) _____ |__|__|

    Where do you live? (4) _____

2. Where are you now? (5) city_____   (5) hospital _____ |__|__|
    (unnecessary to state name of hospital)

3. On what date were you admitted to this hospital? (5) _____ |__|__|

    How did you get here? (5) _____

4. What is the first event you can remember after the injury? (5)_____ |__|__|

    Can you describe in detail (e.g., date, time, companions) the first event you can recall after injury? (5) _____

    _____

5. Can you describe the last event you recall before the accident? (5) _____ |__|__|

    _____ Can you describe in detail (e.g., date, time, companions)

    the first event you can recall before the injury? (5) _____

6. What time is it now? _____ (−1 for each ½ hour removed from correct time to maximum of −5) |__|__|

7. What day of the week is it?_____(−1 for each day removed from correct one) |__|__|

8. What day of the month is it?_____(−1 for each day removed from correct date to maximum of −5) |__|__|

9. What is the month?_____(−5 for each month removed from correct one to maximum of −15) |__|__|

10. What is the year? _____(−10 for each year removed from correct one to maximum of −30) |__|__|

                                        Total Error Points |__|__|

                            Total Goat Score (100-total error points) |__|__|

                        76-100 = NORMAL
                        66-75 = BORDERLINE
                        ≤65 = IMPAIRED

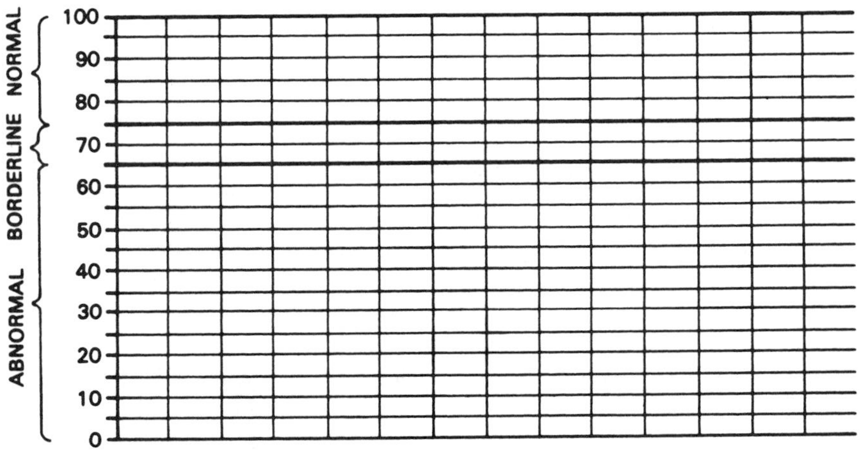

FIGURE 18.2 Galveston Orientation and Amnesia Test (GOAT) record form.

Galveston Orientation and Amnesia Test (GOAT)
(H.S. Levin, O'Donnell, and Grossman, 1979)

The GOAT is a short mental status examination devised to assess the extent and duration of confusion and amnesia following TBI (see Fig. 18.2). Like the GCS, it was designed for repeated measurements and can be used many times a day and repeated over days or weeks as necessary. Eight of the ten questions involve orien-

tation for time, place, and person. The two questions asking for the first event the patient can remember "after injury" and the last event "before the accident" relate specifically to anterograde and retrograde amnesia, respectively. The error scoring system has a score range from −8 to 100. This test can serve two purposes. In light of the relationship between early return of orientation and good outcome—and its converse—it can serve as an outcome predictor. It also provides a fairly sensitive indicator of level of responsivity in recently brain injured patients.

H.S. Levin and colleagues (1979) recommend that formal mental ability testing begin only after the patient achieves a GOAT score of 75 or better (within the "normal" range), i.e., when orientation is relatively intact. However, Hannay and Sherer (1996) found that most of their severely injured patients (at least 70%) could complete relatively simple tests (sentence comprehension; auditory and visual attention tasks; digit span) once their GOAT reached 40 but completion rates were lower for tests such as Trail Making A (50%) and B (29%). When these patients reach a GOAT of 40 (on the average at one month postinjury), a high percentage of them have recovered remote memory for personal information (name, date of birth, street address, and city) and the year, but not knowledge for events surrounding the injury or other items of temporal orientation (Hannay and Sherer, 1996). Levin and his coworkers noted that problems with amnesia are apt to persist after orientation has returned to normal. They suggested showing a calendar to aphasic and intubated patients when asking about temporal orientation. A preliminary study of the use of a multiple-choice GOAT with aphasic patients suggests that this response format results in a noticeably easier task for nonaphasic TBI patients and additionally, that the GOAT can underestimate the level of orientation and memory of aphasic TBI patients (Jain et al., 2000).

The cut-off score actually represents a level of orientation exceeded by 92% of a standardization sample of patients aged 16–50 with mild TBI (H.S. Levin, O'Donnell, and Grossman, 1979). This sample was chosen because it would control for demographic and personal characteristics that predispose one to closed head injury. Neurological examination was normal but 32% had a linear skull fracture and 24% had surgery for a depressed skull fracture. Interrater reliability in the original study was reported as .99, but it takes some training for examiners to be consistent in obtaining the information for and then scoring the amnesia items correctly.

GOAT measurements of posttraumatic amnesia (PTA) show strong associations with the severity of injury (GCS), and with a measure of long-term outcome (Glasgow Outcome Scale, GOS) (H.S. Levin, O'Donnell, and Grossman, 1979; Ellenberg et al., 1996), and the Disability Rating Scale and Functional Independence Measure (Zafonte, Mann, et al., 1997). This instrument's usefulness was supported by a study that found that only 52 of 102 head injury patients could estimate the duration of their PTA; and of these, only 30 of the 50 with mild injuries made this estimation (C.A. Bailey et al., 1984). However, those who made these estimations tended to be reasonably accurate as

the correlation between GOAT data and patients' estimations was .85. The most typical sequence of reorientation is for person, place, and time, in that order (High et al., 1990). Eighty-eight percent of acutely hospitalized head injury patients showed a "backward displacement of the date," believing it was earlier than it actually was.

Oxford Test (Artiola i Fortuny, Briggs, Newcombe, et al., 1980); Westmead PTA Scale (Shores, Marosszeky, Sandaman, and Batchelor, 1986)

The Oxford Test for measuring the duration of PTA was probably the first quantitative test that involved formal testing of memory as well as a questionnaire about personal demographics (e.g., age, marital status, number of children, occupation), orientation in time and space, and last memories before the accident and first memories after the accident. Each day the patient is shown a different set of three colored pictures and asked to recall them or recognize them among a set containing five distractor items. The patient is also tested each day for recall and, if necessary, recognition of the examiner's first name and face ("Have you seen me before?"), using a photograph of the previous day's examiner when there is a change. Recognition of the examiner's name involves three names, two phonologically similar or with the same number of syllables as that of the examiner. A perfect score for three consecutive days signals the end of PTA on the first of the three days. The authors noted that this daily examination technique also identified mental status changes indicating deterioration in the patient's condition.

Success on the formal memory testing was as effective in determining the status of PTA as were the usual questions about personal history, orientation, and events surrounding the accident, in this case by neurosurgeons (Artiola i Fortuny et al., 1980). However, formal testing is less open to misinterpretation than questions such as the first event remembered after the injury. This procedure is recommended for research, especially multicenter trials in which the examiners at different centers have slightly different training and criteria for judging the correctness of the response to such questions.

The *Westmead Scale* (Shores et al., 1986) was based on the Oxford Test and provided a standardized set of procedures and a scoring form that tracked daily performance. The scale first asks seven questions about age, date of birth, month, time of day, day of week, year, and name of place, giving 1 point for each correct answer. A point is given for correct recall or recognition of the examiner's face and name and for each of the three pictures of objects, producing a total possible score of 12. As with the examiner's name, recognition of the face involves pictures of the original examiner and two other faces. Recognition of objects involves six distractors, rather than the five of the Oxford Test. The same three object pictures are used every day until a perfect score of 12 is achieved. Thereafter, the object pictures are changed daily until the patient's recall is perfect for three consecutive days. This procedure was designed to ensure that new learning is taking place. PTA is judged to have ended on the first of three consecutive days for which the patient scores 12.

Patients who were in PTA on the Westmead, out of PTA, and orthopedic control subjects were given the Selective Reminding Test to assess learning and memory as part of the initial validation study (Shores et al., 1986). Patients still in PTA showed essentially no learning of the word list over trials while patients out of PTA learned but were still somewhat amnesic and exhibited poorer learning over trials than the orthopedic controls. The duration of PTA as measured by the Westmead was a significant predictor of severe TBI outcome in terms of verbal learning ($r = .44$) and nonverbal problem solving ($r = .37$), slightly better than the GCS on admission, and markedly better than duration of coma, which did not predict cognitive outcome (Shores, 1989). In another study, PTA duration predicted learning and memory on the Rey Auditory–Verbal Learning Test ($r = .34$), especially using a square root transformation of PTA duration ($r = .44$), and information processing speed measured by the Paced Auditory Serial Addition Test and Symbol Digit Modalities Test ($r = .29$), prediction again being better with a square root transformation ($r = .35$) (Haslam et al., 1994). With the exception of the GCS on admission and subarachnoid hemorrhage, no injury variables, including the nature of the trauma, hemorrhages, hematomas, or coma duration, were related to verbal learning or to information processing speed. Also, the duration of PTA minus coma duration (*postcoma disturbance* [PCD]) proved to be a good a predictor. A study with hospitalized children indicated that relatively few normal 6 to 7 year-olds (15%) met the Westmead's PTA criteria in four days of testing whereas over 90% of children in age groups from 8 to 15 did, suggesting that the adult Westmead procedure can be used with children over 7 years old (Marosszeky et al., 1993). Indices for consistency of "recovery" and duration to "recovery" have been developed for charting improvement of different components of orientation and memory (K. McFarland et al., 2001).

Choosing Outcome Measures

All health care professionals understandably would prefer to have brief measures of outcome that they can administer at bedside, in the office, or over the telephone.

However, the focus of outcome evaluation of the TBI patient changes over time, especially for the severely injured patient who may start in a coma and must be evaluated by relatively simple measures that involve basic visual, verbal, and motor responses, such as the Glasgow Coma Scale (Teasdale and Jennett, 1974); and who later resumes a relatively normal life but continues to have some difficulties. Long-term follow-up measures for assessing the patient some time after return to the community will differ in their format and content from measures used when the patient leaves the acute care or rehabilitation hospital. Not only does the content change, but items included in tests used earlier can have ceiling effects. K.M. Hall, Bushnik, and their coworkers (2001) determined which of 10 outcome measures were useful for long-term follow-up (an average of five years postinjury), i.e., do not have marked ceiling effects. They found that the Functional Independence Measure memory item and the Functional Assessment Measure employment item (Uniform Data Systems, 1987, 1993; see also K.M. Hall, Hamilton, Gordon, et al., 1993), the Disability Rating Scale level of functioning and employability items (Rappaport, Hall, et al., 1982), all of the Neurobehavioral Functioning Inventory scales (depression, somatic difficulties, memory/attention, communication, aggression, motor) (Kreutzer, Marwitz, et al., 1996), the Patient Rating Competency Scale (Prigatano and Altman, 1990; Fordyce and Rouche, 1986), all Community Integration Questionnaire scales (home integration, social integration, productivity) (Willer, Rosenthal, and Kreutzer, 1993), and the Craig Handicap and Reporting Technique (Whiteneck, Charlifue, Gerhart, et al., 1992) cognition and occupation scales provided a useful range of scores across patients (defined as <25% of the data at any one score). Scores from the Glasgow Outcome Scale (Jennett and Bond, 1975), the Supervision Rating Scale (Boake, 1996b), and the Level of Cognitive Functioning Scale (Hagen, Malkmus, et al., 1979) did not have enough variability to be useful for the variety of outcomes that occur. Ideal measures will have good reliability and predictive validity and document motor, cognitive, psychosocial, and behavioral changes; strengths and weaknesses; ability to carry out activities in various environments; integration and participation in society; the environmental and personal factors that act as facilitators and hindrances; and quality of life (well-being and life satisfaction) at different times after injury. For these reasons, evaluation of TBI and other patients is likely to include some of the instruments discussed below at different times in the patient's course. Measures of severity and global measures are appropriate for assessing level of functioning when a TBI patient is in the acute and postacute stages, and later on to measure changes (progress or deterioration). Measures of reintegration and participation in society, psychosocial adaptations, and quality of life are introduced later on. Representative measures from these somewhat different domains have been included here.

Outcome Evaluation

Global measures

The choice of a global measure of outcome for following the progress of a TBI patient as well as determining the effectiveness of treatments in randomized controlled trials and clinical research in general continues to be controversial. Much of the discussion focuses on the relative merits of the Glasgow Outcome Scale and the Disability Rating Scale (S.C. Choi et al., 1998; Contant et al., no date; Narayan, et al., 2002; Teasdale, Pettigrew, et al., 1998). Neither measure is particularly good at characterizing individual outcomes with less serious TBI or residual subtle impairments and disabilities.

Glasgow Outcome Scale (GOS) (Jennett and Bond, 1975; M.R. Bond, 1990)

This scale complements the Glasgow Coma Scale by providing criteria for evaluating the "goodness" of outcome. It has five levels: (1) *Death* (due to brain damage. This typically occurs within the first 48 hours after injury. It is rare that death after 48 hours, of persons who improved to an outcome level of 4 or 5, will be attributable to primary brain damage); (2) *Persistent vegetative state* (PVS) (absence of cortical function); (3) *Severe disability* (conscious but disabled; these patients are "dependent for daily support."); (4) *Moderate disability* (disabled but independent); (5) *Good recovery* (resumption of "normal life" is the criterion rather than return to work which, the authors noted, can be misleading when economic factors prevent an able person from finding employment or particularly favorable circumstances allow a relatively disabled person to earn money). Sometimes 1 is assigned to death and 5 to good outcome and sometimes the numbers have been assigned in the reverse direction. The clinician and researcher must be careful to find out which way the numbers are assigned to categories before interpreting a score of 2 as PVS or as moderate disability, a problem that has contributed to some misunderstandings in the literature (Contant et al., in press).

Although the GOS is attractive in its simplicity, this same quality makes it difficult to categorize many patients who are semidependent or independent. Inter-rater reliability is obviously not a problem for the Death and PVS categories. Valid ratings may not be obtained for the other categories if examiners do not ask appropriate questions of the patient, caretakers, or family [hjh]. Disagreements between raters are most likely to occur for the "moderate disability" rating (D.N. Brooks, Hosie, et al., 1986), which has been considered too inclusive (H.S. Levin, Benton, and Grossman, 1982) and too coarse-grained (Walsh, 1991) to provide more than suggestive categorization. Even with an expanded format (to eight categories, by adding an extra level each to the categories Severe, Moderate, and Good [Jennett, Snoek et al., 1981]), the *extended GOS* (*GOSE*) is insufficiently refined to accommodate the varieties and complexities of posttraumatic outcomes (*Lancet* Editors, 1986; B. [A.] Wilson, 1988). Moreover, an examination of interrater reliability indicated that agreement between experienced patient observers was considerably higher for the original five category scale (*Kappa* GOS = .77, *Kappa* GOSE = .48) (Maas et al., 1983). Intraobserver reliability was also better for the five category scale, but these higher *Kappa* values varied from .89 to .40 while those for the eight category scale were in the .82 to .22 range.

Structured interviews are now available for both the GOS and GOSE (J.T.L. Wilson, Pettigrew and Teasdale, 2000) with explicit criteria for categorizing individuals. The inclusion of a series of specific information-gathering questions and criteria for classifying patients should improve the agreement between ratings made by the different clinicians seeing these patients as well as the validity of the ratings. For example, data on agreement in the ratings made by a nurse and a psychologist produced a weighted *Kappa* of .89 for the GOS and .85 for the GOSE. J.T. Wilson, Edwards, et al. (2002) reported rating reliabilities a *Kappa* of .82 and .94 for the GOS, *Kappa* and repeated rating reliabilities of .89 for the GOS and .98 for the GOSE with a two week interval. They also compared the ratings obtained from a structured interview of patients conducted on the telephone by an experienced nurse and a postal version filled out by the patients about one week later with much lower agreement for the GOS than the GOSE. This is perhaps not surprising since TBI patients may be unaware of the severity of their difficulties or even that they have those difficulties.

Jennett and Bond (1975) advised that, "aspects of social outcome should be included . . . such as leisure activity and family relationships" in making outcome determinations. However, they did not offer a solution to the complex classification problem presented by so many patients whose level of social or emotional functioning is very different from the level of their cognitive skills, sensory-motor competence, or daily activities. Neither the GOS nor the GOSE has the gradation of scores necessary to provide information about the changes that take place within the severe, moderate, and good outcome categories. Especially, these scales cannot register the subtle deficits and changes that are experienced by less severely injured patients and that continue to interfere to some degree with many aspects of their lives, even though they appear to be doing well on the surface, having returned to work or school and looking after themselves independently.

Disability Rating Scale (DRS) (Rappaport, Hall, Hopkins, et al., 1982)

The DRS was designed to assess disability in severe TBI patients as they progress from coma back to the community (Rappaport, Hall, et al., 1982). It is not very sensitive to preinjury demographic variables (Hedrick

et al., 1995). The total score ranges from 30 (death) to 0 (no disability) and represents the sum of scores for eight items (Table 18.6). The first three items are almost identical to the GCS and thus allow for the assessment of an individual with compromised consciousness. There are some important differences, however. While the best response for an item on the GCS is given the highest number, the same response on the DRS is given the lowest number. Also, the motor response item of the GCS ranges from 6 (obeying commands to 1 (none) while the same response on the DRS ranges from 0 (obeying commands) to 5 (none). Since the GCS is ordinarily determined just before the DRS by clinicians in the acute or subacute situation, it is important that they be careful in translating scores from the GCS to scores on similar items on the DRS. Furthermore, the verbal response is evaluated in a slightly different way on the DRS. An intubated patient or one

TABLE 18.6 Disability Rating Scale

Arousability, Awareness, and Responsibity		
Eye Opening	Communication Ability (Verbal, Written, Letterboard or Sign)	Best Motor Response
0 Spontaneous	0 Oriented	0 Obeying
1 To speech	1 Confused	1 Localizing
2 To pain	2 Inappropriate	2 Withdrawing
3 None	3 Incomprehensible	3 Flexing
	4 None	4 Extending
		5 None

Cognitive Ability for Self-Care Activities (Does patient know how and when? Ignore motor disability?)		
Feeding	Toileting	Grooming
0 Complete	0 Complete	0 Complete
1 Partial	1 Partial	1 Partial
2 Minimal	2 Minimal	2 Minimal
3 None	3 None	3 None

Level of Functioning (Consider Both Physical and Cognitive Disability)	"Employability" (As a Full-time Worker, Homeworker, or Student)
0 Completely independent	0 Not restricted
1 Independent in special environment	1 Selected job, competitive
1 Mildly dependent	2 Sheltered workshop, noncompetitive
2 Moderately dependent	3 Not employable
3 Markedly dependent	
4 Totally dependent	

Categorizations of Outcome Scores (Limitations, Severity)		
0 None	4–6 Moderate	17–21 Extremely severe
1 Mild	7–11 Moderately severe	22–24 Vegetative state
2–3 Partial	12–16 Severe	25–29 Extreme vegetative state
		30 Dead

From Rappaport, Hall, Hopkins, et al. (1982)

with a tracheotomy is given a score of 1 on the verbal response of the GCS but could earn any possible score for the analogous communication ability item of the DRS since a written, letter board, or sign response is credited. As the patient comes out of coma and begins to be able to complete basic activities of daily living, items evaluate the level of these abilities, ignoring motor disabilities but taking into account demonstrated knowledge of how and when. Dependence is assessed with the level of functioning item which considers both physical and cognitive ability to be independent. Finally, the employability item refers to functioning as a full-time worker, homemaker, or student depending on which is most appropriate to rate. More detailed information is provided for each of these items than was originally provided in the description of each GOS category. However, a list of appropriate questions to ask the patient, caretakers, and family members in order to obtain valid information would be helpful as well and would likely increase interrater reliability.

Test characteristics: comparing DRS and GOS. The DRS has some advantages over the GOS, in part because it has a range of scores for seven of the ten suggested levels of disability, with only death, mild, and none each represented by a single score. The range is particularly wide in the severe disability category. In contrast, the GOS has a single score for each category. The measure that has a finer gradation of scores is likely to provide better prediction (Contant et al., in press). The DRS has shown better predictive success than the GOS in a number of studies: predictions from acute care variables to outcome at three and six months postinjury (Struchen et al., 2001); prediction from outcome at discharge from acute care one, three, and six months postinjury to psychosocial outcome at six months (McCauley, Hannay and Swank, 2001); and change during rehabilitation (K. Hall, Cope, and Rappaport, 1985; Rappaport, Hall, et al., 1982). Neither measure is particularly good at depicting outcome in individuals with less serious TBI or residual subtle deficits (Pender and Fleminger, 1999).

Neuropsychological findings. DRS scores are correlated with auditory, visual, and somatosensory evoked potentials (Rappaport, Hemmerle and Rappaport, 1990, 1991; Rappaport, Herrero-Backe, et al., 1989). The DRS admission score in rehabilitation (Ponsford, Olver, et al., 1995; Cifu, et al., 1997; Gollaher et al., 1998) and the DRS discharge score (Cifu et al., 1997; Gollaher et al., 1998) are predictive of later employment. Interrater reliabilities of .97–.98 (Gouvier, Blanton, et al., 1987; Rappaport et al., 1982) and a test–retest reliability of .95 (Gouvier et al., 1987) have

been reported. Predictive validity (Eliason and Topp, 1984; Gouvier et al., 1987) and concurrent validity (Gouvier et al., 1987; K. Hall, Cope, and Rappaport, 1985; K.M. Hall, Hamilton, et al., 1993) with other functional measures are high. DRS scores at six months after rehabilitation are strongly related to executive functioning and memory (Hanks, Rapport, et al., 1999). Anosmia occurs with longer coma, more neuropsychological deficits, and greater functional problems on the DRS (Callahan and Hinkebein, 1999).

Evaluation of the Psychosocial Consequences of Head Injury

An appreciation of the effects of TBI on personal and social adjustment and of their impact on family, friends, and the community has led a number of workers to develop schedules and scales for standardizing the examination and documentation of these problems. Some were designed as questionnaires for relatives, some as clinical rating scales, and for some the information is obtained from all possible sources. Although most of these scales were developed for research purposes but may be useful in the individual case for tracking the evolution of problems or their solutions, the Mayo-Portland Adaptability Inventory (see pp. 729–731) in particular was also developed for the individual case, to bring to light psychosocial issues that may be overlooked without the guidelines it provides [mdl]. Lacking comparative studies, no "best" scale or rating method has been identified, leaving examiners to decide which one(s) seems to suit their needs. The inventories reviewed here are among those most used with TBI and represent the variety of approaches to documenting these problems.

Katz Adjustment Scale: Relative's Form (KAS-R) (M.M. Katz and Lyerly, 1963)

The original purpose of this scale was the assessment of the personal, interpersonal, and social adjustment of psychiatric patients in the community, but much of it is appropriate for neuropsychologically impaired patients as well (e.g., Hanks, Rapport, et al., 1999; McSweeny et al., 1985). The issues this scale deals with are particularly relevant to TBI survivors living with their families or in noninstitutionalized settings. The authors' rationale for assessing the patient's adjustment from a relative's perspective is that "the patient's overall functioning is . . . intimately linked with the working out of mutually satisfactory relationships within the family." Additionally, the informant can provide an intimate view of the patient's day-to-day activities. Moreover, as is the case with psychiatric patients, some brain impaired patients cannot respond reliably to a self-rating inventory or may be unable to cooperate with this kind of assessment at all. Thus the only way to get dependable information about them is through an informant. The questionable objectivity of a close relative led to the development of items concerning specific behaviors.

The scale consists of five inventories, or subscales, each designed to assess a different aspect of the patient's life or the relatives' perception of it. Form R1 asks for "Relatives Ratings of Patient Symptoms and Social Behavior." It includes 127 questions about such indicators of patient adjustment as sleep, fears, quality of speech, and preoccupations, for rating on a scale ranging from "1–almost never" to "4–almost always." Forms R2 and R3, "Level of Performance of Socially-expected Activities" and "Level of Expectations for Performance of Social Activities," use the same 16 items dealing with such ordinary activities as helping with household chores, going to parties, and working. Form R2 requires the informant to indicate the patient's level of activity for each item on a 3-point scale on which a rating of 1 is given for "not doing," 2 for "doing some," and 3 for "doing regularly." A 3-point scale is used for Form R3 too, but the rating criteria are reworded to include the informant's expectations of the patient, i.e., 1–"did not expect him [sic] to be doing," etc. The 22 items of Forms R4 and R5 have to do with how patients spend their free time. Like Forms R2 and R3, these two inventories share the same items which list specific leisure activities such as watching television, shopping, or playing cards, plus a 23rd item asking for activities to be listed that were not included in the previous items. These too are on 3-point scales. Form R4 asks for the frequency of activity (1–"frequently" to 3–"practically never"). R5 inquires about the relative's level of satisfaction with the patient's activities (1–"satisfied with what he does here" to 3–"would like to see him do less"). McSweeny and his colleagues added a "does not apply" response alternative to each scale except R1.

Test characteristics. Three major factors yielding 12 factor scales have been extracted from Form 1 (M.M. Katz and Lyerly, 1963; see Table 18.7). For both relatives and patients (using an appropriately reworded version of Form R1), with an eight week interval, test–retest correlations were significant (.65–.88) on three global factors (I. Social Obstreperousness, II. Acute Psychoticism, II. Withdrawn Depression), with the lowest correlations occurring on Factors II and III, which contain only 14 and 10 items, respectively (Ruff and Niemann, 1990).

TABLE 18.7 Item Clusters and Factors from Part 1 of the Katz Adjustment Scale

Item Clusters	Factors
Belligerence (BEL)	
Verbal expansiveness (EXP)	I. Social Obstreperousness
Negativism (NEG)	
General psychopathology (PSY)	
Anxiety (ANX)	
Bizarreness (BIZ)	II. Acute Psychoticism
Hyperactivity (HYP)	
Withdrawal (WDL)	III. Withdrawn Depression
Helplessness (HEL)	
Suspiciousness (SUS)	
Nervousness (NER)	
Confusion (CON)	
Stability (STA)	

Reprinted from Grant and Alves (1987)

Neuropsychological findings. The KAS-R can provide discriminating information about TBI patients, although not always on the same factor scales or to the same degree. Eight factor scales differentiated severely head-injured patients from patients without TBI, identifying 75% and 96% of these patients, respectively (W.A. Goodman et al., 1988). TBI patients had higher average scores on those factor scales that did not discriminate statistically between the two groups: Belligerence, Negativism, Bizarreness, and Hyperactivity (Fordyce et al., 1983). A group of TBI patients whose average injury duration was 25 months had significantly higher scores than recently injured patients (≤ 6 months) on the Belligerence score, along with higher scores on the Withdrawal and Retardation and the General Psychopathology scales. Hinkeldey and Corrigan (1990) found a similar pattern of abnormal ratings for patients one to five years postinjury. Looking at patients two to four years postinjury, P.S. Klonoff, Snow, and Costa (1986) also found Belligerence—and Negativism—among others, to be significant problem areas as reported by relatives of TBI patients. Klonoff and her colleagues calculated a dissatisfaction index (R3 − R2) which characterized these patients' relatives' responses although responses on KAS-R forms R2 to R5 did not, in themselves, differ significantly from age-graded norms. The form R1 scales that correlated significantly with employment status were Belligerence (−.22), Verbal expansiveness (0.29), Helplessness (−.21), and Confusion (−.19) (Stambrook, Moore, et al., 1990). Of these, Belligerence contributed significantly to a step-wise equation for predicting vocational status. Form R2, in which social performance is reported, had the highest correlation (.30) with ratios of employment status. Hanks, Temkin, et al. (1999) obtained data on the KAS for 157 TBI (78% mild) and 125 general trauma controls. At one year postinjury, the TBI group reported many adjustment problems, typical of TBI, compared to the normative sample (M.M. Katz and Lyerly, 1963), but they did not differ from the trauma control group. Moderate TBI patients had more problems than those with mild or severe TBI. Within the TBI group, cognitive clarity, dysphoric mood, and emotional stability improved while anger management, antisocial behaviors, and self-monitoring worsened. Pender and Fleminger (1999) consider the KAS-R gives more information on post TBI personality change than on outcome.

Revisions of the KAS-R. H.F. Jackson and his coworkers (1992) modified the KAS-R so that two ratings were made for each item: how the injured persons were before the injury and how they are now (*KAS-R1*). An analysis of change scores generated 30 first order and seven second order factors. Classification of TBI patients with varying degrees of severity of injury and of spinal cord patients proved to be more accurate with their factors (60.9%) than with those of the authors (47.2%). Goran and Fabiano (1993) removed redundant items from the KAS-R1 and those not contributing to the stability of previously established psychological factors. The remaining 79 items had internal consistency *alpha* values of .75 to .93 for the component groups. With the exception of the components—Belligerence, Verbal Expansiveness, and Emotional Sensitivity—internal consistency was the same or better for relatives of TBI patients. More research is needed to establish the usefulness of this revision (see also Pender and Fleminger, 1999).

The Mayo-Portland Adaptability Inventory (MPAI) (Lezak and Malec, 2003)[1]

The MPAI is a revision and elaboration of the *Portland Adaptability Inventory (PAI)* (Lezak, 1987b; Lezak and O'Brien, 1988, 1990), developed to increase the sensitivity of its parent inventory. This set of three subscales was constructed to provide a systematic record of the personal and social maladaptations that tend to prevent many patients with *acquired brain injuries (ABI)* from resuming normal family relationships and social activities. While the MPAI retains the three-subscale format of the PAI, subscale names and contents differ somewhat from the original inventory but include the 24 PAI items. The original items were reworded as necessary to ensure that all ratings were made on the basis of current functioning. Now the 29 items (of which one, #28, comes in two parts) make up the three subscales (*Ability, Adjustment,* and *Participation;* see Table 18.8). Six additonal items which ask about "Preexisting and associated conditions" (e.g., drug and alcohol use) do not enter into the scoring or statistical evaluations of the MPAI. The *Manual for the Mayo-Portland Adaptability Inventory* (Malec and Lezak, 2003) provides detailed scoring criteria for each item.

Items are rated on a 5-point scale, from 0 (e.g., Item 16, **Pain and headache:** "0—No significant pain reported" to "4—Pain complaints are totally or almost totally disabling"). Wording of the scale varies according to the issue under consideration, but most ratings follow the same pattern in which 1 indicates a mild

[1]Copies of the MPAI may be obtained from the web site for the Center for Outcome Measures in Brain Injury (www.tbims.org/combi/mpai) or from James F. Malec, Ph.D., PM&R-1D-St. Mary's, Mayo Clinic Rochester, MN 55905. The MPAI is in the public domain and may be copied freely.

TABLE 18.8 Mayo-Portland Adaptability Inventory (MPAI) Items by Subscales

Ability Index	Adjustment Index	Participation Index
Mobility	Anxiety	Initiation
Use of Hands	Depression	Social Contact
Vision	Irritability/Anger	Leisure/Recreational
Motor Speech	Pain and Headache	Self Care
Communication	Fatigue	Residence
Attention/Concentration	Sensitivity to Mild Symptoms	Transportation
Memory	Inappropriate Social Interaction	Work/School
Fund of Information	Impaired self-awareness	Money Management
Novel Problem-Solving	Family/Significant relationships	
Visuospatial Abilities		
Dizziness		

From Malec and Lezak (2003)

problem or condition that "does *not* interfere" with functioning; 2 indicates a mild problem that interferes "5% to 24% of the time;" and 3 is given for a "moderate" problem or condition that interferes "25% to 75% of the time." For some items, the 5-point scale is worded to be parallel to the "% of time" scaling (e.g., Item 28a, **Paid employment**: 0-Full time [>30 hrs/wk], 1-Part-time [3–30 hrs/wk] without support; 2-Full-time or part-time with support; 3-Sheltered work; 4-Unemployed; employed < 3 hrs/wk).

When the MPAI is given to patients or personal associates (significant others [SO])—usually a spouse, partner, parent, or adult child—a clinical staff person should review the guidelines with the rater and be availale for questions. Patients with severe cognitive deficits should give MPAI ratings only with a staff person writing in the responses. Clinical staff ratings can provide information on patient progress. Ratings by patients and their families can alert clinicians to specific problems and achievements. As an outcome measure, the MPAI covers the full range of issues relevant to patient functioning after rehabilitation and in the community.

Test characteristics. The MPAI has undergone multiple revisions, based on analyses of responses from several large samples. Two data sets formed the bases for evaluating MPAI (MPAI-4th revision). One was a national sample of 386 patients with acquired brain injuries (ABI) (M_{age} = 38 ± 12.4, 73% male, 88% ABI, 23% < 12 years education, 80% white, with a severity range of mild [5%], moderate [29%], severe [44%], and unknown [15%]). A Mayo sample consisted of 134 ABI patients (M_{age} = 39 ± 13.5, 61% male, 65% TBI, 18% <12 years' education, 92% white, with a severity range of mild [29%], moderate [12%], severe [44%], and unknown [15%]). Total raw scores can be converted to *T*-scores (*M* = 50, *SD* =10) by using tables for staff ratings from either of these samples. Subscale tables based on Mayo staff ratings are included in the manual as are *T*-score tables for both Total and subscale raw scores made by both the brain-injured patients and their significant other derived from the Mayo samples.

Subscale items were identified following Rasch analysis of previous (and very similar) versions of the MPAI (Malec, Moessner, et al., 2000), selected on a "rational" basis; i.e., items that corresponded to clinical experience (Malec and Lezak, 2003; see Table 18.8). Item reliability for a three-rater composite (patient, SO, staff) was .99 for a sample of 134 Mayo clinic ABI outpatients. For each subscale, item reliabilities derived from the National sample were .99 for Total, Ability, and Adjustment subscales, .98 for Participation. For each subscale index for the Mayo Sample of 134 ABI outpatients, the three-rater composite was .99 for To-

tal, Ability, and Participation, .97 for Adjustment. On the Mayo sample, for the first 29 items, item agreement (±1 point) between all rating group pairs was ≥66% on all but one item (impaired self-awareness) and ≥70% on 20 items. Concurrent validity of staff responses to the MPAI was demonstrated in moderately high correlations with the Disability Rating Scale and the Rancho Scale (Malec and Thompson, 1994). Factor analysis demonstrated "an underlying unitary dimension representing outcome after TBI that includes indicators of ability, activity, and participation" (Malec, Kragness, et al., 2003). Principal components identified by factor analysis (Bohac et al., 1997) may be informative in interpreting the multifactorial structure of ABI outcome (see Malec and Lezak, 2003). However, for practical purposes, the strong internal consistency of the rational subscales (R_{xx} [*Alpha*] = .80 for Ability, .76 for Adjustment, .83 for Participation) recommends that subscale integrity be maintained. The considerable interdependence between capacity and function was reflected in some items correlating highly with two subscale indices (e.g., Self-care correlation with Participation was .61, with Ability it was .57).

Other MPAI versions. Rasch analysis of the MPAI refined prediction of outcome by removing items that did not contribute to the total score (Malec, Moessner, et al., 2000). This resulted in a *22-item MPAI* that had similar predictive validity to the 30-item MPAI. The MPAI-22 has since been shown to be sensitive to change in rehabilitation and prediction from preadmission score to level of initial vocational placement and vocational status one year later (Malec, 2001; Malec, Buffington, Moessner, et al., 2000).

The *M2PI* is just the eight-item Participation subscale (Malec and Lezak, 2003). A series of correlations (mostly above .70) with different group evaluators (patients, SOs, and staff) and with the full-scale 3-Rater Composite Index suggest that it can be used as an outcome measure. Its brevity requires minimal personal or telephone contact thus lending itself to treatment follow-up or research programs.

A French version, *Inventaire d'Adaptabilité Sociale de Mayo-Portland,* is being developed in collaboration with Drs. Pierre North and Jean-Michel Mazaux. In a preliminary study involving 15 young (ages 21–36) rehabilitation patients with severe TBI, MPAI scores identified as significant problems with fatigue, dizziness, attention and concentration, recall of old information, problem solving, anxiety and irritability, return to work or school, social contact, and participation in leisure activities (Selmaoui, 2002). A comparison with the Neurobehavioral Rating Scale-R (French version) showed that these two instruments appear to be "complementary, the NRS-R looking mostly at impairments . . . the MPAI looks mostly at cognitive and behavioral disability and handicaps" (J.-M. Mazaux, personal communication, June, 2003). Specific differences between these scales were in "fatigue" which in the MPAI referred to physical fatigue, in the NRS-R to "mental fatigability;" planning capacity was not examined in this French version; variables concerning work, social contact, and leisure were not examined in the NRS-R. The author concludes that the clinical utility of the MPAI resides in its "global evaluation of the diversity of problems—physical, cognitive, emotional, behavior, and social of TBI patients" (trans., mdl).

Neurobehavioral Rating Scale (NRS)
(H.S. Levin, High, Goethe, et al., 1987; see also I. Grant and Alves, 1987)

This 27-item modification of the *Brief Psychiatric Rating Scale* (BPRS) (Overall and Gorham, 1962) was developed specifically for TBI patients. Its use requires a trained examiner to follow detailed guidelines (given in H. S. Levin, Overall, et al., 1984). BPRS items more appropriate for a psychiatric population were dropped (e.g., mannerisms and posturing, grandiosity), and others particularly relevant to head injury were added (e.g., Inaccurate Insight, Poor Planning, Decreased Initiation/motivation). Like its parent instrument, ratings are made on a 7-point scale from "not present" to "extremely severe." The format allows for profiles to be drawn for each patient, for groups or group comparisons, or for a single patient over time. Unfortunately, the items are listed in what appears to be a random order (e.g., 16. Suspiciousness; 17. Fatigability; 18. Hallucinating Behavior; 19. Motor Retardation, etc.) so that commonalities between these characteristics and symptoms cannot be grasped at a glance. Some of the items are based on a short interview while the rest are derived from patient observation during the interview and formal examination. It would be best to complete this scale after the examination. The NRS has proved to be useful in studies of Alzheimer's disease (Sultzer et al., 2003; B.G. Pollock et al., 2002; Harwood, Sultzer, and Wheatley, 2000). Dombovy and Olek (1996) included items of the NRS in a telephone follow-up procedure involving an interview with the caregiver, a cost-effective way of determining the status of many TBI survivors.

Interrater reliability examined with two pairs of observers rating either 43 or 34 patients proved to be high in an initial study ($r = .90$, $.88$, respectively) (H.S. Levin, High, Goethe, et al., 1987). A replication of this study involving 44 TBI patients produced an interrater reliability coefficient of .78; a repeated evaluation of 37 of these patients one week later found a similar level of interrater reliability ($r = .76$) (Corrigan, Dickerson, et al., 1990). Four factors emerged on analysis of a group of patients examined at different times postinjury and with different severity levels: I. Cognition/Energy, II. Metacognition, III. Somatic/Anxiety, IV. Language. Five items either loaded on more than one factor (Inattention/Reduced Alertness and Decreased Initiative) or did not load on any (Guilt, Hallucinations, Lability of Mood) (H.S. Levin, High, Goethe, et al., 1987). The item cluster of Factors II and IV differentiated the mildly injured groups from patients with moderate and severe injuries but not the latter two groups. Factor I items differentiated only mildly from severely impaired patients. The Cognitive/Energy item was a predictor of social outcome in Vilkki, Ahola, et al. (1994). Pender and Fleminger (1999) recommend the NRS as "probably the standard" measure against which all newcomers to behavior change scale development should be compared.

The *Neurobehavioral Rating Scale–Revised* (NRS-R) (H.S. Levin, Mazaux, et al., 1990) was developed to increase reliability and content validity. Several changes were made (H.S. Levin et al., 1990; McCauley, Levin, et al., 2001). Items on difficulty with mental flexibility and irritability were added; tension and anxiety were merged into one item; and inattention became reduced alertness and attention. The Likert rating scale was reduced to four categories (absent, mild, moderate, and severe). Answers to a structured interview of 15–20 min provide rating for about two-thirds of the items; one-third are based on examiner observations, unlike the GOS and DRS which use all available information.

Interrater reliability by item on data from 70 patients ranged from a *Kappa* of .22 for difficulty in planning to .77 for memory difficulties (median *Kappa* = .40). Factorial validity of NRS-R data on 286 TBI patients assessed at least one month (mild) or three months (moderate and severe) postinjury produced five factors: Intentional Behavior, Emotional State, Survival-Oriented Behavior/Emotional State, Arousal State, and Language (Vanier, Mazaux, et al., 2000). Interrater reliability for the factor scores was reasonable (.56 to .81). Associations of factor scores with GCS and coma duration, while significant in many cases, were fairly low (.12–.33). An exploratory factor analysis (McCauley, Levin, et al., 2001) of data from 210 moderate or severe TBI patients six months postinjury identified five factors: Executive/Organization, Positive Symptoms, Negative Symptoms, Mood/Affect, and Oral/Motor. These factors had good internal consistency (.62–.88) and modest but significant correlations with GCS scores (.17–.24) once again. Correlations of the Executive/Organization and Oral/Motor factors and to some degree Mood/Affect and Negative Symptoms with several domains of neuropsychological functioning (verbal and visual memory, speed dependent visuomotor tracking, manual dexterity, and speeded language production were significant (.24–.70). The NRS-R total score correlated at .72 with the GOS and at .74 with the DRS at 6 months postinjury. A principal components analysis (Rapoport, McCauley, et al., 2002) of three month follow-up data from 115 mild/moderate patients from Toronto and the 392 patients from the McCauley, Levin, et al. (2001) study produced three factors: Cognitive, Emotional, and Hyperarousal. Severity of injury was significantly related to NRS-R total score as was the three month GOS score. Postresuscitation GCS scores were significantly related to the cognitive factor (.47) and weakly to the hyperarousal factor (.27).

Community participation

Craig Handicap Assessment and Reporting Technique (CHART) (Whiteneck, Charlifue, Gerhart, et al., 1992)

The CHART was designed to quantify the extent of handicap (community participation). It assesses the six dimensions of handicap, now referred to as "participation" (World Health Organization, 1980, 2001): (1) Physical independence—ability to sustain a customarily effective independent existence; (2) Mobility—ability to move about effectively in surroundings; (3) Occupation—ability to occupy time in the manner customary to that person's age, gender, and culture; (4) Social integration—ability to participate in and maintain customary social relationships; (5) Economic self-sufficiency—ability to sustain customary socioeconomic activity and independence. The original CHART consisted of 27 items but the addition of dimension (6) "Cognitive independence" brought it to 32 items (Mellick et al., 1999). This dimension, involving ability to orient in relation to surroundings, was not included in the original version because it was considered difficult to quantify.

The CHART assesses each dimension based on reports of how the individual functions from day to day. While the GOS estimates the capacity to work, for instance, the CHART directly asks how many hours a week the individual works. Each dimension is scored from 0–100, with 100 representing no handicap compared to a sample of able-bodied individuals. Ponsford, Olver, Nelms, and their colleagues (1999) find the CHART useful with TBI patients but have dropped the "Economic self-sufficiency" items because some patients find them intrusive, and further because this scale is not informative when patients receive substantial benefits (as in Australia). The CHART was designed as an interview that can be done in person or by telephone and takes about 15 min to give. The CHART was developed for use with spinal cord–injured (SCI) individuals but has been applied to TBI survivors. It is used when the individual is in the community, not in a hospital, since it is a measure of participation in the community.

The CHART was originally normed on 88 able-bodied individuals and 100 spinal cord injured (SCI) persons (Whiteneck, Charlifue, et al., 1992). For 135 SCI patients, one week test–retest reliability was .93 overall with the coefficients ranging from .80 for economic self-sufficiency to .95 for mobility. Patient–SO agreement ranged from .84 for mobility to .28 for social integration (total score agreement of .84). The latter coefficient rose to .57 when only patients with spouses were considered, presumably because the spouse was more knowledgeable of this aspect. (Patient–proxy agreement for the CHART total score was .70 in Cusick et al., 2001.) CHART scores for subgroups rated as having low or high handicap by rehabilitation professionals differed significantly, providing an indication of its validity. Rausch analysis of CHART items produced 11 handicap strata with a .99 item separation reliability. Corrigan, Smith-Knapp, and Granger (1998) found that inpatient rehabilitation discharge scores on the CHART were moderately predictive of CHART scores (.45) over a 5-year period as opposed to the Uniform Data Systems' (1987) Functional Independence Measure motor (.77) and cognitive (.69) scores (which were less likely to change over time as might be expected since they mainly refer to physical status).

With TBI patients, Boake and High (1996) compared the association of CHART scales and DRS and GOS scores to four outcome indicators (self-care independence, travel, employment, and friendship). CHART physical independence and DRS and GOS scores were strongly related to self-care. CHART scales have a strong association only to the related outcome indicator, although it was less for mobility and travel (.22) than for physical independence and self-care (.43), occupation and employment (.33), and social integration and friendship (.32). DRS and GOS scores had strong associations only with self-care and travel. O'Neill, Hibbard, Brown, et al. (1998) found that TBI patients' levels of employment, education, marital status, and sex were related to social integration scores on the CHART one year postinjury. C.A. Curran and colleagues (2000) found orthopedic and TBI patients with serious injuries to be similar in physical independence, mobility, occupation, and social integration but the TBI patients had significantly lower cognition scores. These groups also had similar depression, state, and trait anxiety scores. In general, higher depression and trait anxiety were associated with lower mobility and cognition scores and, to a lesser degree, with lower occupation and social integration scores.

Community Integration Questionnaire (CIQ) (Willer, Rosenthal, Kreutzer, et al., 1993)

The CIQ was specifically designed as a telephone interview to evaluate community integration in TBI survivors. The CIQ consists of 15 questions that assess Home integration (H), Social integration (S), and Productive activities (P). Six questions have a 3-point scale, ranging from "doing the activity yourself alone" to "yourself and someone else" to "someone else." Six questions have a 3-point scale for times per month from "5 or more," "1–4 times" or "never." The remaining three items have individualized ratings. The total score range is 0 to 29 for maximum integration. The patient can also give written responses to the CIQ, although help may be needed; a significant other can complete it if necessary. Normative data for various demographic groups are needed. A revised CIQ-2 is in development.

Test characteristics. The authors' initial small study ($n = 16$) with a 10-day interval produced a test–retest reliability of .91 for patients and .97 for SO assessment of the patient. The same study measured concurrent validity with the CHART and CIQ. CHART Occupation was significantly related to CIQ Productive activities (for the patient, $r = .66$; for the SO, $r = .75$), as might be expected since they involve the same domains. The Social integration scale was not significantly related, perhaps because of the CHART's low ceiling in this area. Patient–SO agreement was evaluated by Sander, Seel, et al. (1997), who reported *Kappa* coefficients of .42 (shopping) to .94 (school) on the 15 items for 122 patients with a range of injury severity. The Home integration scale produced differences that were attributable to two items, "meal preparation" and "housekeeping," the patients rating themselves higher than did SOs. Agreement was lower for an earlier study of 148 TBI patients and SOs using the intraclass coefficient (Tepper et al., 1996). Acceptable internal consistency has been reported (Corrigan and Deming, 1995; Willer, Ottenbacher, and Coad, 1994). Factor analysis on data from 312 patients with primarily severe TBI found the same three factors (H, S, P) but two items were moved: "financial management" from Social integration to Home integration and "travel" from Productive activities to Social integration (Sander, Fuchs, et al., 1999). This study also established concurrent validity as CIQ total score and scale scores had significant correlations with DRS level of functioning (.25–.47) and employability (.37–.58), Uniform Data Systems' (1987) Functional Assessment Mea-

sure Community access (.27–.47) and Employability (.41–.60) scales, and Functional Independence Measure Social interaction (.24–.34) scale. Questions about the distribution of CIQ scores have arisen (Corrigan and Deming, 1995) and not resolved satisfactorily (Willer, Ottenbacher, and Coad, 1994).

Neuropsychological findings. Patients with more severe injuries have lower CIQ scores (Colantonio, Dawson, and McLellan, 1998). CIQ scores are related to premorbid factors, severity of injury, disability level, and cognition (J. Fleming et al., 1999; C.P. Kaplan, 2001; Novack et al., 2001; Rosenthal, Dijkers, et al., 1996) as well as measures of executive functioning and verbal memory (Hanks, Rapport, et al., 1999) and depression (H.S. Levin, Brown, et al., 2001). The Trail Making Test and Rey's Auditory–Verbal Learning Test predicted outcome on the CIQ (S.R. Ross, Millis, and Rosenthal, 1997). TBI patients' communication problems appear in the CIQ's numerous aspects of discourse related to social integration (Galski, Tompkins, and Johnston, 1998). The CIQ is sensitive to time of initiation for treatment (Seale et al., 2002). Some change over time in CIQ scores has been noted by K.M. Hall, Mann, et al. (1996) and Corrigan, Smith-Knapp, and Granger (1998).

Environmental factors

Craig Hospital Inventory of Environmental Factors (CHIEF), CHIEF Manual (Craig Hospital Research Department, 2001)

The CHIEF was developed to assess the frequency and magnitude of perceived *barriers/hindrances* that interfere with the lives of disabled individuals. The 25 questions cover five domains: Physical and structural (e.g., design and layout of buildings, temperature, terrain, noise), Work and school (e.g., availability of education and training, format of material, special adapted devices), Attitudes and support (e.g., community attitudes towards disabled persons, encouragement or support at school or work), Services and assistance (e.g., programs and services in the community), and Policies (in government, education, and employment). Frequency of a problem is rated on a 5-point scale from "never" to "daily;" magnitude is rated as "little" or "big problem." Only the patient is supposed to respond to the CHIEF, not a significant other. It takes about ten minutes, can be self-administered or done as an interview in person or by telephone.

A sample of 409 disabled individuals (124 patients with SCI, 120 with TBI, 165 with other disabilities) was recruited for a validation study of the psychometric characteristics of the test. A two-week test–retest reliability study with a subset of 103 participants found an internal consistency correlation of .93 for the TBI group ($n = 44$). Family members or friends of 125 individuals not included in the test–retest reliability study completed the CHIEF in order to determine patient–SO agreement. The TBI sample's internal consistency correlation was .59 for barrier frequency and .72 for magnitude for 54 subject pairs. Factor analysis generated the five factors given above. Differences in frequency and magnitude of environmental barriers between groups with various impairments and activity limitations are reported in the manual as well as norms for disabled, non-disabled, SCI, TBI, and other diagnoses. A CHIEF short form of 12 items has been created with norms also in the manual. It remains to be seen how useful this measure of environmental barriers will be. The study of how the environment can affect outcome is a newly developing area which should see increasing development in the future.

EPILEPSY PATIENT EVALUATIONS

Scales and inventories for documenting the behavior of epilepsy patients have been used for two quite different purposes. One has been to document the behavioral and psychosocial consequences of epilepsy surgery. The other is for behavioral description, often in evaluating outcomes of clinical drug trials (Kline Leidy et al., 1998). Although some studies have used instruments from the general psychometric repertoire (e.g., R. Martin, Meador, et al., 2001), specialized questionnaires and scales have been developed specifically for this population. A brief survey of different representative instruments is presented below.

A-B Neuropsychological Assessment Schedule (ABNAS) (Aldenkamp, Baker, Pieters, et al., 1995)

This self-administered measure, previously called the Neurotoxicity Scale (Aldenkamp, Baker, Pieters, et al., 1995), enables patients to report on the adverse effects of antiepileptic drugs on cognition. The 24 questions are rated from 0 (no problem) to 3 (a serious problem). The inventory was originally validated on healthy control subjects taking a benzodiazepine and endorsing items relating to "fatigue and slowing" (Aldenkamp et al., 1995). "Fatigue and slowing" was also the dominant area endorsed by patients with poorly controlled epilepsy but this finding was unrelated to seizure frequency, drug dosing (high vs. low), or monotherapy vs. polytherapy (Aldenkamp and Baker, 1997). In general, the global ABNAS score is considered to be the primary

variable reflecting perceived cognitive effects, with excellent reliability (Cronbach's *alpha* = .96) (J. Brooks et al., 2001).

Epilepsy Foundation of America (EFA) Concerns Index (Gilliam, Kuzniecky, Faught, et al., 1997)

This scale was developed by asking patients with chronic epilepsy to list in order of importance their concerns about living with recurrent seizures. Twenty questions assess different domains including driving, autonomy, work, education, family, seizure effects, medication effects, mood and anxiety, and social activities. Ratings are made on a 5-point scale, then summed to yield an overall *Concerns Index* which ranges from 20 to 100. Cronbach's *alpha* was .94, indicating a highly reliable instrument.

For patients who had previously undergone surgery for poorly controlled epilepsy, reponses regarding mood, employment, driving, and antiepileptic drug cessation were related to quality of life perception (Gilliam, Kuzniecky, Meador, et al., 1999). In contrast to studies using the Quality of Life in Epilepsy questionnaire, seizure freedom was not a predictor of postoperative quality of life. The EFA Concerns Index provides disease-specific quality of life information that is complementary to that obtained using more generic health related quality of life scales (Viikinsalo et al., 1997).

Liverpool Assessment Battery (G.A. Baker, Smith, et al., 1993)

This battery of measures assesses health related quality of life in epilepsy using eight different instruments of which four predate this battery and have been used elsewhere with different kinds of groups. The four developed by the test authors are the *Seizure Severity–PERCEPT* and *Seizure Severity–ICTAL* scales which ask for the patient's perception of the physical characteristics of seizure severity (G.A. Baker, Smith, et al., 1991); an *Adverse Events Profile* enquiring about medication side effects; and *The Impact of Epilepsy* scales concerning the social aspects of epilepsy and treatment on everyday functioning (Jacoby et al., 1993). Mood and other psychological factors are examined with the *Affect Balance Scale* (Bradburn, 1969) and the *Hospital Anxiety and Depression Scale* (Zigmond and Snaith, 1983), both of which are independently established tests. Coping ability is tested with the *Rosenberg Self-Esteem Scale* (SES) (M. Rosenberg, 1965) and the *Mastery Scale* (Pearlin and Schooler, 1978), which is designed to measure the degree to which patients feel in control of their own life as opposed to being fatalistically determined. The *Impact of Epilepsy* scales emphasize the social aspects of epilepsy and treatment on everyday functioning (Jacoby et al., 1993). Portions of this battery have been reported in different combinations in the literature, both in clinical drug trials (G.A. Baker, Smith, et al., 1993) and patient studies (Jacoby et al., 1993; Kellett et al., 1997).

Quality of Life in Epilepsy (QOLIE)
(Devinsky et al., 1995)

This questionnaire was developed using the Epilepsy Surgery Inventory as its base (Vickrey et al., 1992), which itself includes the Rand Study 36-item Healthy Survey (Ware and Sherbourne, 1992), with additional specific epilepsy related questions. Thus, it follows the current practice for quality of life measures to use a generic instrument with disease-specific additions (G.A. Baker, 2001). In addition to assessing general quality of life, the QOLIE includes epilepsy specific domains: attention, concentration, memory, seizure worry, medication effects, and work and driving limitations.

The three versions of the QOLIE differ in length: The 89-item version containing 17 scales is intended primarily for research; the 31-item test is applicable to either research or clinical evaluations; the ten-item scale is intended for clinical practice. Although copyrighted, all versions of the test are available without charge. For the 89-item version, reliability coefficients using Cronbach's *alpha* for the 17 scales ranged from .78 to .92, with test–retest reliabilities from .58 to .86. The only scales below $r = .70$ were the two involving role limitation: pain and medication effects. Intraclass correlations ranged from .58 to .85.

To determine the magnitude of change needed to infer improved quality of life, QOLIE scores were compared to patient ratings; a 10.1 point change was required for the QOLIE-89 and an 11.8 point change for the QOLIE-31 (Wiebe, Matijevic, et al., 2002). Moreover, both measures discriminated medium from large changes in quality of life. In a surgical population, patients who became seizure free reported higher QOLIE scores (31 and 89 forms) than those who did not (Birbeck et al., 2002; Markand et al., 2000). The QOLIE-89 can be reliably administered by telephone (Leidy et al., 1999).

Side Effect and Life Satisfaction (SEALS)
(Gillham, Baker, et al., 1996)

The SEALS inventory is a 38-item, questionnaire for patients designed to measure satisfaction with medications for seizure control. Questions ask for responses based upon feelings and behavior experienced during the previous week. Answers are placed on a 4-point Likert scale ranging from 0 (never) to 3 (many times). The questionnaire yields five summary measures—worry, temper, cognition, dysphoria, and tiredness—in addition to an overall SEALS score. The SEALS appears sensitive to differential cognitive side effects of drugs; e.g., patients taking carbamazepine had more side effects than those taking lamotrigine, which led to greater patient dropout on the former medication (Gillham, Kane, et al., 2000). In a validation study comparing responses of 307 patients with poorly controlled seizures on SEALS and on two scales measuring emotional status and one for cognitive functioning, significant correlations ranging from .51 to .84 were present for all SEALS scores with the other questionnaires. The authors concluded that this is a valid test for both clinical investigations of antiepileptic drugs and long-term epilepsy management (Gillham, Bryant-Comstock, and Kane, 2000).

Washington Psychosocial Seizure Inventory (WPSI)
(Dodrill, 1986; Dodrill, Batzel, et al., 1980)

This 132-item True–False patient questionnaire was developed to document social maladaptations that tend to be associated with chronic epilepsy. The seven psychosocial scales relate closely to important aspects of the patient's life: Family Background (primarily pertaining to family and predisposing influences), Emotional Adjustment; Interpersonal Adjustment; Vocational Adjustment; Financial Status; Adjustment to Seizures; and Medicine and Medical Management. Using responses by 100 adult seizure patients, these scales were based upon item relationships with professional ratings (Dodrill, Batzel, et al., 1980). Higher scores indicate more problems.

Reliability coefficients were calculated for each scale and for an "Overall Psychosocial Functioning" scale, which includes some of the items contributing to other scales (Dodrill, Batzel et al., 1980). On 30-day follow-up, test–retest reliability coefficients were in the .66 to .87 range, split-half reliabilities ranged from .68 to .95; "Medicine and Medical Management" had the lowest correlations. Responses were evaluated by comparing them with ratings made by significant others and by professional examiners. The highest correlations between ratings and scale scores appeared for the Vocational scale ($r = .69$ with significant others' ratings, $r = .74$ with professional examiners' ratings); the lowest (.11, .33, for significant others and professional examiners, respectively) were on the "Adjustment to Seizures" scale.

Higher WPSI scores were associated with poorer neuropsychological test performance (Dodrill, 1986).

Seizure patients had significantly higher scores on the Emotional Adjustment scale than control subjects and also reported a great deal of difficulty adjusting to their illness (Tan, 1986). Invalid profiles were produced by approximately one-third of the epilepsy patients (24/68) and one-sixth of the control subjects (7/42), raising questions about the appropriateness of the validity measures. Moreover, of the normal control subjects whose inventory profiles were valid, 46% met the criterion for problems in "Emotional Adjustment," suggesting that this scale may not meet generally accepted standards for emotional disorders.

Using this scale, Trostle and colleagues (1989) found that community-dwelling people who were not seeking professional assistance for epilepsy-related problems obtained significantly lower scores on the WPSI than seizure patients seen in the clinic. The degree of psychosocial difficulty documented by the WPSI depends not only on patients' seizure frequency but also on the culture of their community (Swinkels et al., 2000). In patients undergoing surgery for poorly controlled seizures, better psychosocial functioning predicts better postoperative seizure control (Wheelock et al., 1998). Depression following anterior temporal lobectomy can be predicted, in part, by baseline WPSI emotional adjustment scores (Derry and Wiebe, 2000).

QUALITY OF LIFE

Satisfaction With Life Scale (SWLS)
(Diener, Emmons, Larsen, et al., 1985)

Subjective well-being seems to have two components: an affective component (pleasant and unpleasant affect) and a cognitive component (life satisfaction) (Andrews and Withey, 1976; Corrigan, Bogner, et al., 2001; Pavot and Diener, 1993). The SWLS is designed to measure life satisfaction which has been defined as "a global assessment of a person's quality of life according to his chosen criteria" (Shin and Johnson, 1978, p. 478). Diener et al. (1985) suggested that life satisfaction derives from the individual's judgment of what is important, not what the examiner considers important. Even if two individuals value the same aspects of life (e.g., health, energy, finances), they may differ in their emphasis on them. On this basis, the authors developed a simple five-item scale that uses a Likert rating going from 1 (strongly disagree) to 7 (strongly agree) and results in a score from 5 (low satisfaction) to 35 (high satisfaction) (Table 18.9).

Normative data are available in many studies and include samples of American, French-Canadian, Russian, Chinese, and Korean groups; disabled college students;

TABLE 18.9 Satisfaction With Life Scale (SWLS)

1. In most ways my life is close to my ideal
2. The conditions of my life are excellent
3. I am satisfied with my life
4. So far I have gotten the important things I want in life
5. If I could live my life over, I would change almost nothing

From Diener et al. (1985)

nurses and health workers; older Americans and French-Canadians; religious women (nuns); printing trade workers; military wives and nurses; VA inpatients; Dutch medical outpatients; abused women; clinical clients seeing psychologists (inpatients and outpatients); and elderly caregivers (Pavot and Diener, 1993). Concerns have been raised that self-report measures of well-being can be influenced by transient factors such as momentary mood, physical surroundings, and even the item that precedes a single-item measure of well-being and life satisfaction; but such effects have not been found for multi-item measures (Pavot, Diener, et al., 1991).

In an initial study of 176 undergraduates the mean score was 23.5 ± 6.43 (Diener et al., 1985). The two-month test–retest reliability for 76 students was .82, similar to the correlations of .89 reported for a two-week retest (Alfonso and Allison, 1996). Criterion validity was moderately strong as measured by correlations between SWLS and other measures of well-being and life satisfaction for samples of 176 and 163 undergraduates. Ratings of life satisfaction by 53 elderly individuals based on interview produced strong inter-rater reliability (.73). Internal consistency (item-total correlations) for the five items in the scale was also good (.61–.81). Others have reported substantial item-factor loadings (Arrindell et al., 1999). Factor analyses of the SWLS consistently produce a single factor accounting for over 60% of the variance (cf. Pavot and Diener, 1993; Arrindell et al., 1999).

Many different variables relate to SWLS scores (e.g., sex, marital status, health, and such personality variables as self-esteem, euphoria, dysphoria, and neuroticism) (Arrindell et al., 1999). Higher life satisfaction at one and two years postinjury has been associated with not having a preinjury history of substance abuse, having gainful employment, and a higher GCS score in 218 TBI patients (Corrigan, Bogner, et al., 2001). At one year it was associated with trauma admission GCS score and at two years, with depressed mood and social integration. Life satisfaction was relatively stable for two years, only changing significantly with marital status and depressed mood over time. Mean scores of 20.3 and 20.8 for the first and second years, respectively, represent a neutral rating in the scale. Bogner and coworkers (2001) reported similar effects of substance abuse with telephone interviews of 168 TBI patients one year after injury. Much lower mean life satisfaction scores have been found for TBI patients with PTSD (12.88) than those without it (19.07) (Bryant, Marosszeky, et al., 2001). Lowered life satisfaction in spinal cord patients two years after injury was associated with being male, unemployed, having poor perceived health, decreased mobility, and decreased social integration (Putzke, Richards, et al., 2002).

PSYCHIATRIC SYMPTOMS

Brief Psychiatric Rating Scale (BPRS) (Overall and Gorham, 1962)

This 18-item instrument has enjoyed wide use with psychiatric disorders (e.g., Belanoff et al., 2002; Umbricht et al., 2002). Although the BPRS had been used with TBI patients (e.g., H.S. Levin and Grossman, 1978), the Neurobehavioral Rating Scale modification is usually preferred for these patients (see pp. 731–732). Each item of the BPRS represents a "relatively discrete symptom area"; most of the items were derived from psychiatric rating data. Ratings are made on a 7-point scale from "Not Present" to "Extremely Severe." The scale is intended for use by psychiatrists and psychologists. Although many of the items are more appropriate for a psychiatric population than for brain impaired patients (e.g., Guilt feelings, Grandiosity), there are also items involving symptoms that are prominent features of some neurological conditions (e.g., Motor retardation, Conceptual disorganization, Blunted affect). Others, although usually considered psychiatric symptoms, also appear in many patients with organic brain damage (e.g., Uncooperativeness, Depressive mood, Suspiciousness).

Interrater reliabilities have ranged from .67 to .75 (Hafkenscheid, 2000). Five factors were reported on ratings of a large number of schizophrenic patients: Anxiety–Depression, Anergia, Thought Disturbance, Activation, and Hostile–Suspiciousness (R.S. McDonald, 1986). A four factor model was reported for a group of recent-onset schizophrenics (Van der Does et al., 1993): Positive Symptoms, Negative Symptoms, Disorganization, and Depression described a group of recent-onset schizophrenics. A similar model identified factors derived from a sample of more chronic patients as Thought Disturbance, Anergia, Disorganization, and Affect (Mueser et al., 1997). A factor analysis for geropsychiatric inpatients came up with a somewhat different factor pattern: Withdrawn Depression, Agitation, Cognitive Dysfunction, Hostile-Suspiciousness, and Psychotic Distortion. This pattern was attributed to the prominence of "conceptual disorganization and disorientation" among these patients (McDonald, 1986). Conceptual Disorganization, Disorientation, and Motor Retardation were the most frequently scored items for severely and moderately TBI patients, while mildly injured patients received ratings within the normal range on these items (H.S. Levin, 1985). These scores differentiated each severity group from the others to a significant degree.

19 | Tests of Personal Adjustment and Emotional Functioning

The assessment of personality, personal adjustment, and emotional functioning contributes to the neuropsychological examination in several important ways. To evaluate a patient's cognitive performance, the examiner often needs a basis for estimating the extent to which emotional state and characterological predisposition may affect the patient's efficiency. In some cases, emotional and social behavior patterns that are symptomatic of particular brain disorders may play a role in the formulation of a diagnosis. Furthermore, subtle aspects of cognitive dysfunction sometimes show up in the patient's responses to relatively unstructured tests of personal adjustment when they are masked by the more familiar and well-structured formats of the cognitive tests.

Assessing mood and personality variables is an important part of the neuropsychological assessment. It can be particularly challenging when interpreting self-report measures, since many patients with many different kinds of brain disorders may lack adequate awareness of themselves or their situation. In addition, self-report measures are susceptible to symptom exaggeration (see pp. 780–783).

This chapter follows the conventional classification of personality measures and tests of affect/emotion into "objective" or "projective." *Projective tests* contain relatively less structured stimulus material and provide for open-ended responses. Questionnaire-type tests that restrict the range of response are called *objective tests* without regard to the extent to which the test responses may also register projection (Anastasi and Urbina, 1997; Cronbach, 1984).

PROJECTIVE PERSONALITY TESTS

Projective tests are based on the assumption that when confronted with an ambiguous or unstructured stimulus situation, people tend to *project* onto it their own needs, experiences, and idiosyncratic ways of interacting with the world. In other words, people perceive external stimuli through a reflection of their attitudes, understandings, and perceptual and response tendencies,

and interpret the compounded percept as external reality (S.J. Beck, 1981). Projective testing uses this principle to elicit the patient's characteristic response tendencies.

Projective responses tend to differ among persons, diagnostic groups, age groups, the sexes, and cultures. These differences show up in both the *content* of the responses and the *formal*—structural and organizational—qualities of the content: in the *how* as much as in the *what* of a response. Analysis of these complementary aspects of projective productions may give the examiner a look at the inner workings of the subject's mind that would be difficult to obtain as quickly or as distinctively by any other method.

The effects of brain injury can influence patients' perceptions of the world by compromising the ease and flexibility with which they sort, select, organize, or critically evaluate their own mental contents. Close and extensive observation of patients as they go about their daily affairs is the best method of finding out when and how mental impairments affect their behavior. Short of such exacting procedures, projective testing may be the most effective means of answering many of these questions, a conclusion apparently held by practising neuropsychologists surveyed in 1989 who used the Rorschach (38%) or the Thematic Apperception Test (33%) (M. Butler et al., 1991).

Much of the research looking into how well projective test scores and score patterns identify specific diagnostic categories, personality traits, or emotional disorders has been inconclusive (Anastasi and Urbina, 1997). This may well be, in part, because projective test data tell only part of the story. Projective techniques can be compared to the EEG or any other diagnostic technique that may contribute to the evaluation of a highly complex system in which multiple variables are interacting. No single instrument can provide definitive answers to all questions about such a system. By themselves, positive EEG findings are of only limited usefulness, but in the context of a complete neurological study, they can be invaluable. Moreover, the high rate of negative EEG findings in brain disorders does not invalidate the technique. The same holds true for the

738

data of a projective study. When taken out of context of interviews, history, and medical findings, projective test data become insubstantial and unreliable. When used appropriately, projective material complements other kinds of examination data. Also, like the EEG, a normal-appearing record can be given by brain impaired or psychiatrically disturbed patients.

A number of projective response tendencies characterize the behavior of brain-injured persons. Regardless of the technique employed, these response tendencies show up in the *protocols* (the record of test responses) of some brain injured patients and occur much less frequently in the responses of neurologically intact subjects:

1. *Constriction.* Responses become reduced in size and in quantity. If they are verbal, the patient employs few words, a limited vocabulary, and a decreased range of content. If the responses are graphic, drawings are small, unelaborated, and important details may be left out. There will be little if any evidence of creativity, spontaneity, or playfulness.

2. *Stimulus-boundedness.* Responses tend to stick closely to the bare facts of the stimulus (i.e., to a storytelling task with a picture stimulus, "This is a man, this is a woman and a young woman, and there is a horse. It's a farm," or to an inkblot, "This is an ink splotch; that's all I see. Just an ink splotch"). There may be a "sticky" quality to patients' handling of the test material in that once they attend to one part of the stimulus or give one association, they seem helpless to do much more than reiterate or elaborate on the initial response.

3. *Structure-seeking.* These patients have difficulty in spontaneously making order or sense out of their experiences. They search for guidance anywhere they can and depend on it uncritically. Structure-seeking is reflected in tendencies to adhere to the edge of the page or to previously drawn figures when drawing, or to seek an inordinate amount of help from the examiner.

4. *Response rigidity.* Difficulty in shifting, in being flexible, and in adapting to changing instructions, stimuli, and situations shows up in projective tests as response perseverations (e.g., mostly "bat" or "butterfly" responses to the inkblot cards). Response rigidity may also show up in failure to produce any response at all in a changing situation, or in poorer quality of response under changing conditions than when repetitively dealing with a similar kind of task or working in the same setting.

5. *Fragmentation.* Fragmented responses are related to tendencies to concreteness and poor organization. Many brain injured patients are unable to take in the whole of a complex situation and to make unified sense out of it, and therefore can respond only in a piece-meal, pedantically matter-of-fact manner. This can be seen in responses that comprehend only part of a total stimulus situation normally grasped as one whole percept (i.e., human figure drawing constructed by accretion of the parts; an inkblot response, "leg," to what is commonly perceived, not as an isolated leg, but as the leg of a whole person).

6. *Simplification.* Simplified responses are poorly differentiated or detailed whole percepts and responses (such as "bat" without details, or "leaf" or "tree stump" to inkblot stimuli; or crudely outlined human figure drawings with minimal elaborations; or six- or eight-word descriptions instead of a creative response on a storytelling task).

7. *Conceptual confusion* and *spatial disorientation.* Both neurological and psychiatric patients may give responses reflecting logical or spatial confusion. Differential diagnosis depends on such other response characteristics as symbolic content, expansiveness, variability of quality, and emotional tone.

8. *Confabulated responses.*[1] Illogical or inappropriate compounding of otherwise discrete percepts or ideas is a response characteristic common to both neurologic and psychiatric populations. Brain impaired patients are most likely to produce confabulated responses in which naturally unrelated percepts or ideas become irrationally linked because of spatial or temporal contiguity, giving them a stimulus-bound or "sticky" quality. Confabulations in which the linkage is based on a conceptual association are more typical of functionally disordered thinking.

9. *Hesitancy and doubt (perplexity).* Regardless of performance quality or the amount and appropriateness of reassurance, many brain injured patients exhibit continuing uncertainty and dissatisfaction about their perceptions and productions (Lezak, 1978b).

It is uncommon for cognitively intact and emotionally stable adults to make any of these kinds of responses. It is rare to find the protocol of a brain-injured patient in which all of these characteristics occur. However, many brain injured persons display at least a few of them.

---

[1]"Confabulated" responses to projective test stimuli needs to be distinguished from the term "confabulation" as it applies to the often quite elaborated fabrications that some patients with memory disorders offer as responses to questions or in statements, particularly in reference to personal facts to which they no longer have reliable access (R.J. Campbell, 1981). S.J. Beck and his coworkers (1961) defined *confabulated responses* as those in which the subject "seldom engages in any directed organizing activity. The details happen to be seen in relation and eventually all are included. The [response] is accidental, not intellectual work" (p. 22). For example, card III consists of two black side patches frequently seen as profiles of "bowing waiters" and a big central red splotch that can easily be interpreted as a "bow tie:" a typical confabulated response would be, "waiters with bow ties."

Rorschach Technique (S.J. Beck et al., 1961; Exner, 1993)[1]

The Rorschach test is probably the best known of the projective techniques. Hermann Rorschach, a Swiss psychiatrist who was interested in how his patients' mental disorders affected their perceptual efficiency, developed it in the early 1920s. The subject is shown the inkblots one at a time and invited to "Tell what the blot looks like, reminds you of, what it might be; tell about everything you see in the blot."

Scoring systems in general use are all variants of Rorschach's original system and all effective in the hands of a skilled examiner (S.J. Beck et al., 1961; Exner, 1993; B. Klopfer and Davidson, 1962). The scoring systems permit categorization and quantification of the responses in terms of mode of approach and subject matter.

The scoring pattern and the verbatim content of the responses are then interpreted in terms of actuarial frequencies and the overall configuration of category scores and content. A number of rules of thumb and statistical expectancies have evolved over the years that suggest relationships between category scores or score proportions and behavioral or emotional characteristics. These rules and expectancies are only suggestive. No single Rorschach response or set of responses, taken alone, has any more or less meaning or diagnostic value than any other single statement or gesture taken by itself.

Variables that contribute to the *formal* aspect of the Rorschach performance include the number and appropriateness (form quality) of the responses; use of shape, color, shading, and movement (the *determinants*) in the formulation of a response; and the location, relative size, and frequency of use of identifiable parts of the blots (see Table 19.1). In analyzing the *content* of the responses, the examiner notes their appropriateness and usualness as well as any repetition or variation of topics, the presence and nature of elaborations on a response, emotional tone, and evidence of thought disorder or special preoccupations. Gratuitous (i.e., unnecessary for clear communication) or extraneous elaborations of a percept may reflect the patient's special preoccupations and concerns. Unusual or idiosyncratic elaborations, particularly of the most common and easily formed percepts (i.e., the whole blot animal—bat or crab—of card I, the "dancing" figures of card III, the "flying" creature of card V, the pink animals at the sides of card VIII, and the tentacled blue creatures of card X) sometimes convey the patient's self-image. Thus, it is not uncommon for a brain in-

jured patient to perceive the "bat" or "butterfly" of card V or the blue "crab" of card X as dead or injured, or to volunteer descriptions of these creatures as "crazy" or "dumb," e.g., a "crazy bat," a "dumb bunny."

Rorschach response characteristics given more often by brain impaired than intact subjects were offered as impairment "signs" by Z. Piotrowski (1937) who found that they tended to appear with relative frequency (five or more) in protocols of brain impaired patients (see Table 19.2). Although others have devised sign sets, this set appears to have been relatively successful in separating brain impaired from intact subjects (e.g., C. Meyers et al., 1982).

Test characteristics. Large-scale normative studies are lacking. Spreen and Strauss (1998) note that what normative data are available "are of limited value for the interpretation of individual cases because of the

TABLE 19.1 Major Response Variables Appearing in Every Rorschach Scoring System

1. Number of responses
2. Portion of the inkblot involved in a response: whole, obvious part, or obscure part
3. Color and shading (including texture)
4. Movement (e.g., "*dancing*" bears," "*bowing* waiters"
5. Percentage of percents that are "good," i.e., commonly perceived
6. Figure–ground reversals
7. Content, such as human, animal, anatomy, or landscape
8. Very great popularity or rarity of the response

TABLE 19.2 Z. Piotrowski's Signs for Identifying Brain Impairment

1. *R.* Less than 15 responses in all.
2. *T.* Average *time* per response is greater than 1 min.
3. *M.* There is but one *movement* response if any.
4. *Cn.* The subject *names colors* (e.g., "a pinkish splotch") instead of forming an assocation (e.g., "pinkish clouds").
5. *F%.* Percentage of *good form* responses is below 70.
6. *P%.* Percentage of *popular* responses is below 25.
7. *Rpt. Repetition* refers to perseveration of an idea in responses to several inkblots.
8. *Imp. Impotence* is scored when the patient recognizes his response is unsatisfactory but neither withdraws nor improves it.
9. *PLx. Perplexity* refers to the hesitancy and doubt displayed by many organic [*sic*] patients about their perceptions.
10. *AP.* The examiner must determine when a pet expression is repeated so often and indiscriminately as to qualify as an *automatic phrase.*

From Z. Piotrowski (1937)

---

[1]Several test publishers sell the Rorschach plates. In the U.S., Psychological Assessment Resources charges the least (2003 catalogue).

large variability of Rorschach responses" (p. 650). Poitrenaud and Moreaux (1975) found no sex differences in their older subjects' responses. Brighter persons tend to give more creative, richer responses (Ames et al., 1973; Hayslip and Lowman, 1986).

Relatively few Rorschach studies have been conducted with normal elderly persons, and of those few, most involved small groups or provided data on too wide an age range to be useful in any individual case (Hayslip and Lowman, 1986; Lezak, 1987a). One study comparing independently living persons in three age groups from 50–61 to 71–80 indicated that responses become somewhat simplified and unimaginative with advancing age (Prados and Fried, 1947). In a sample of elderly patients followed over 10 years, responses within two years of death contained less animal movement, with higher form quality and human content compared to surviving patients (Shimonaka and Nakazato, 1991). Yet studies with adequate age gradations and range indicate few age changes if any (Poitrenaud and Moreaux, 1975; Reichlin, 1984). Hassinger and her colleagues (1989) pointed out that the visual problems suffered by many elderly persons could alter their responses to this test.

Stringent reliability studies are difficult because of the variety of scoring systems and the somewhat subjective character in which some scores are determined. Interscorer reliability may be reasonably high (93% in one study) when judges have had practice using the same system (Kleinmuntz, 1982). Test–retest reliability, too, presents special problems because most protocols will contain only one or two responses in many of the scoring categories so that a little change on retesting makes a big statistical difference. Moreover, normal day-to-day shifts in subjects' moods, interest in the task, energy level, etc., will also be reflected in small differences (usually), which again have large statistical repercussions. Despite these frailties, many scoring categories show acceptable reliability coefficients (Exner, 1986).

Validity studies too present problems that personality questionnaires and inventories with limited response options do not have. Not least of these is the lack of one fully standardized scoring system (Kleinmuntz, 1982). A second problem lies in the nature of the behavior under investigation, as it is difficult to develop external criteria for such important Rorschach constructs as "apperceptive bias," "richness of emotional responsivity," or level of "mental energy." These problems have not kept investigators away from the validity issue, but they have had mixed results. Validation studies that have attempted to relate one or a cluster of scores to clinically defined groups or to predict behavior have produced inconsistent findings (Anastasi

and Urbina, 1997; Kleinmuntz, 1982). Consequently, the Rorschach continues to be a somewhat controversial assessment technique. Several research strategies have been described to provide a more scientific foundation for its use (Bornstein, 2001; Weiner, 2000).

Neuropsychological findings. M.M. Hall and G.C. Hall (1968) evaluated the Rorschach response characteristics of right and left hemisphere damaged patients using such response variables as perplexity, *fabulizing* (making story elaboration), the total number of responses, and the sum of movement responses. Patients with right hemisphere lesions tended to be uncritically free in the use of determinants and overexpansive; they created imaginative responses by opportunistically combining parts into wholes, thus generating many bizarre or preposterous responses. In contrast, patients with left-sided lesions expressed a great deal of perplexity, frequently rejected cards, and tended to give "correct" and unelaborated form-dependent responses.

Rorschach protocols of TBI patients show some consistent response characteristics. Prominent among these are a reduction in number of responses, a relatively greater number of idiosyncratic and poor form responses, loose associations, stereotypy (repetition, perseveration), and concreteness (D.W. Ellis and Zahn, 1985; Klebanoff et al., 1954; Vigouroux et al., 1971). Exner, Colligan, and their colleagues (1996) observed five distinct patterns in TBI patients: impoverished responses relative to available cognitive resources, a more simplistic approach when attending to details of the world, inconsistent coping and decision-making strategies, poor capacity or ability to deal directly and effectively with feelings and emotional situations, and finally poor social skills for promoting and maintaining meaningful interpersonal relations. The Vigouroux group also noted that, "Twelve to 18 months after the injury . . . the profound disturbances of personality which appeared in the first months remained with little change." De Mol (1975/1976) found that these characteristics increased with severity of damage.

Elderly patients with suspected dementia gave significantly fewer human movement responses, and those they gave involved much less energy (e.g., "sitting," "kneeling") than the movement responses given by normal elderly persons (e.g., "dancing," "fighting") (Insua and Loza, 1986). Patients with probable Alzheimer's disease tend to make more linguistic and perseverative errors in their responses compared to healthy controls (W. Perry et al., 1996).

It is difficult to cast much of the data on which clinical inferences are based, or the inferences themselves, into a form suitable for statistical analysis. For clinical purposes, however, the integration of inferences drawn from both the sign and clinical interpretation is apt to yield the most information, with each kind of interpretation serving as a check on the appropriateness of conclusions drawn from the other. By this means, symptomatic cognitive and behavioral aberrations can be viewed in interaction with personality predispositions so that the broader social and personal implications of the patient's brain injury may be illuminated.

Storytelling Techniques

Storytelling is a particularly rich test medium since it elicits the flow of verbal behavior, brings out the quality of the patient's abilities to organize and maintain ideas, and may reveal characteristic attitudes and behavioral propensities. Of the several storytelling projective tests for adults, the *Thematic Apperception Test (TAT)* (Murray, 1938) has been the most widely used (C. Piotrowski and Keller, 1989). Although the familiar test pictures of the TAT have the advantage of known expectations for the kinds and characteristics of stories each elicits, the examiner without TAT or other story test material can easily improvise with illustrations from magazine stories or with photographs. Asking for stories can be a relatively nonthreatening examination method that is particularly suited for elderly patients (Hassinger et al., 1989). As noted by Spreen and Strauss (1998), "the TAT is not a diagnostic instrument, but a projective technique suitable for the exploration of specific problems, conflicts, fears, and needs of the individual at the conscious and at a more subliminal level" (p. 655).

Substantial TAT normative data for any age group simply do not exist for the same reasons as for the Rorschach: there is no common scoring system and clinical judgment enters into what score determinations can be made—to an even greater extent than Rorschach scoring. In addition, the systems (including concept names) used to classify responses differ more among themselves than do Rorschach systems. Further complicating the normative situation are clinicians' preferences for different combinations of the 31 cards so that it would be rare to find two clinicians using the same set of cards in the same order for all their patients. (I [mdl] was taught to select cards according to patient characteristics and assessment issues.) Reliability studies, of course, suffer from all of these problems, although some workers suggest that training scorers in the use of specific scoring criteria can result in satisfactory interrater reliability findings (Hayslip and Lowman, 1986). These authors observed that, "External and cross-validation are badly needed" (p. 73).

Stories composed by brain injured patients possess the same response qualities that characterize Rorschach protocols. Thus, brain impaired patients are likely to use fewer words and ideas in telling stories (R).[1] Response times are apt to be longer with many punctuating pauses (T). Brain injured patients are more likely to describe the picture than make up a story; or if they make up a story, its content is apt to be trite with few characters and little action (M). These patients may be satisfied with simple descriptions of discrete elements of the picture and unable to go beyond this level of response when encouraged to do so (Cn). A more than ordinary number of misinterpretations of either elements of the picture or the theme may occur due to tendencies toward confusion, simplification, or vagueness $(F\%)$. The patient may give relatively few of the most common themes $(P\%)$. Perseveration of theme (Rpt) and automatic repetition of certain phrases or words (AP) rarely appear in stories of subjects without brain injury. Inability to change an unsatisfactory response (Imp) and expressions of self-doubt (Plx) may be present. Inflexibility, concrete responses, catastrophic reactions, and difficulties in dealing with the picture as a whole are often associated with a neurologic etiology (Fogel, 1967).

A tendency for responses with less emotional expression and reflecting increasing social isolation and passivity has been reported to occur with aging (Hayslip and Lowman, 1986; Kahana, 1978), and is most prominent among the institutionalized elderly. Kahana reported that the TAT productivity of elderly persons also tends to be relatively lowered and may be limited to descriptions. As pointed out by Spreen and Strauss (1998) when describing its use in neuropsychological assessment, the "TAT may reflect the personal reaction to injury or deficit, 'catastrophic reactions,' indications of a posttraumatic stress disorder, feelings of failure, as well as insights into premorbid or postmorbid reactive mechanisms, and it may guide the examiner into current problem content" (pp. 655–656).

Drawing Tasks

Although popular as projective techniques (C. Piotrowski and Keller, 1989), it is much more difficult to interpret drawings of brain impaired patients than their verbal products. When perceptual, motor, or constructional defects interfere with the ability to execute a drawing, the resultant distortions make doubtful any interpretations based on the projective hypothesis. Even when distortions are slight, the examiner cannot tell whether paucity of details, for instance, reflects a barren inner life or is due to low energy or feelings of uncertainty and self-consciousness or whether reduced

---

[1]The symbols in parentheses refer to the corresponding Piotrowski "organic sign" for Rorschach responses (see p. 740).

drawing size is a product of lifelong habits of constriction or of efforts to compensate for tendencies to spatial disorientation or motor unsteadiness or some interaction between them. Thus, the use of drawings as personality tests for brain injured persons is too precarious an enterprise for most cases.

OBJECTIVE TESTS OF PERSONALITY AND EMOTIONAL STATUS

Objective tests are self-report instruments: patients (or their surrogates) describe symptoms and feelings by checking those items they believe (or claim) to be true. On these tests, the effects of impairment may be manifested directly through responses to items concerning cognitive disabilities or personality and mood changes related to the impairment; indirectly, for example, in absence of complaints or indications of distress which give an inappropriately benign self-report when the patient is significantly impaired; or in conflicting responses or a wildly aberrant response pattern which suggests confusion or impaired understanding of the task. The applicability of self-report scales and inventories to brain injured patients may be limited by the patients' often restricted capacity to take paper-and-pencil tests when the level of cognitive impairment is severe or they have sensory or motor disabilities. For example, many stroke patients are unable to respond to paper-and-pencil tests appropriately because of either visuospatial inattention and visual tracking problems or compromised reading and/or writing due to aphasia (W.A. Gordon et al., 1991).

Depression Scales and Inventories

Beck Depression Inventory (BDI/BDI-II) (A.T. Beck, 1987; A.T. Beck, Steer, and Brown, 1996)

The BDI is an easily administered and scored 21-item scale that, although originally developed for research, enjoys widespread clinical use (C. Piotrowski and Lubin, 1990). Kivela (1992) reported that it has been translated into at least ten other languages. According to Richter and his colleagues (1998), it has been used in over 2000 empirical studies. The BDI was revised in 1996 (BDI-II) to bring the items more into compliance with the *Diagnostic and Statistical Manual of Mental Disorders (DSM)-IV* criteria (American Psychiatric Association, 2000) while still retaining its 21-question format. The BDI-II was designed to be applicable to subjects up to age 80.

Each item deals with a particular aspect of the experience and symptoms of depression (e.g., Mood,

Sense of Failure, Indecisiveness, Work Inhibition, and Appetite). Agitation was assessed in the original scale; sleep and eating disorders were only partially addressed. Items that dealt with symptoms of weight loss, body image changes, and somatic preoccupation were replaced on the revised scale. "Work difficulty" was changed to "loss of energy," and new items measuring agitation, worthlessness, and concentration difficulty were included. The BDI-II rates sleep and appetite disturbances for either behavioral increases or decreases, and the time that is covered was increased from one week to two weeks to bring the scale in line with DSM-IV criteria.

Each BDI/BDI-II item contains four statements of graded severity expressing how a person might feel or think about the aspect of depression under consideration. The statements carry scores ranging from 3 for most severe to 0 for absence of problem in that area. For example, the range of statements under Self-Hate is "3–I hate myself," "2–I am disgusted with myself," "1–I am disappointed in myself," "0–I don't feel disappointed in myself." This simple format may not elicit valid responses from patients unwilling to acknowledge their distress or from those who may be prone to exaggeration. When the order of benign and distressed statements within items was randomized, for example, scores were higher on the randomized format than on the standard format (Dahlstrom, Brooks, and Peterson, 1990).

The score is the sum of all the selected statements unless more than one statement from a single group is chosen, in which case the higher statement is scored. Few patients select items scoring higher than 2, however, even in psychiatric populations (Richter et al., 1998). The higher the overall score, the more depressed is the patient likely to be. Classification of depression severity by original BDI scores has been variously defined. Formal cutting scores are included in the BDI-II manual (minimal ≤13, mild = 14–19, moderate = 20–28, severe ≥29); but even here the authors indicate that different cutting scores may be needed "based on the unique characteristics of the sample and the purpose for using the BDI-II" (A.T. Beck, Steer, and Brown, 1996). This amount of variation in classification criteria indicates that these criteria are only guidelines: clinical judgment must be exercised in the individual case.

Test characteristics. Two potential problems inherent in the original BDI are especially applicable to many older subjects. Kaszniak and Allender (1985) pointed out that seven of the 21 items refer to somatic symptoms (e.g., weight loss, fatigability) making misinterpretations possible when the patient has a physical ailment. A factorial analysis of responses given by Parkinson patients to the original BDI, however, indicated that the somatic items were associated with depression rather than parkinsonian symptoms (B.E. Levin, Llabre, and Weiner, 1988). Elderly but otherwise healthy depressed patients' scores are comparable to those of younger depressed patients (Steer et al., 2000). BDI scores of medical patients were unrelated to cognitive competency as measured by the Mini-Mental State Examination, although a nonsignificant trend showed up for patients over age 65 (Cavanaugh and Wettstein, 1983). These over-65 patients also showed a trend ($p <$ .06) for BDI scores to increase with age. Neither sex nor ethnicity appeared to affect BDI response patterns when given to elderly white and Mexican-American volunteers (Gatewood-Colwell et al., 1989), although Kivela (1992) cited research indicating that ethnic styles may influence responses.

Test–retest reliabilities reported for a variety of subject groups range from .74 to .93 (Kaszniak and Allender, 1985). W.A. Gordon and his coworkers (1991) noted, however, that the somatic items correlated less well with the total scale than did all other items, leading them to suggest that stroke patients' reports of somatic problems should be somewhat discounted in making a diagnosis of depression. A number of concurrent validity studies have been reported (e.g., see Kivela, 1992; Spreen and Strauss, 1998). When correlated with other self-report measures, coefficients ranged from .81 for psychiatric patients (the Zung Self-Rating Depression Scale) to .57 for patients on a chemical dependency ward (the Depression scale of the Minnesota Multiphasic Personality Inventory) (Schaefer et al., 1985). When compared with clinical ratings, validity coefficients were in the .66 range. For elderly patients, the BDI's correlation with the Geriatric Depression Scale (Yesavage, 1986) was .79 (Gatewood-Colwell et al., 1989). However, much lower validity coefficients have also been reported (Spreen and Strauss, 1998). The correlation between the BDI and BDI-II is reportedly high (.93), although the average BDI-II score is approximately 3 points higher (A.T. Beck et al., 1996).

Neuropsychological findings. BDI scores did not discriminate between patients with right- or left-sided strokes (W.A. Gordon et al., 1991). The presence and intensity of depression reported on the BDI were unrelated to Parkinson's disease severity (A.E. Taylor, Saint-Cyr, Lang, and Kenny, 1986). In a sample of TBI outpatients administered the BDI-II, 59% scored in the depressed range (14 or greater), 34% of which were at moderate or severe levels (M.B. Glenn, O'Neil-Pirozzi,

et al., 2001). For elderly patients asking for psychological help, a BDI cutting score of 11 misclassified only 17%: patients with minor depressive disorders had the greatest number (22.2%) of misclassifications; severely depressed patients, the least (8.8%) (Gallagher et al., 1983).

Geriatric Depression Scale (GDS) (Brink, Yesavage, Lum, et al., 1982; Yesavage, Brink, Rose, et al., 1982)[1]

This 30-item self-administered test was constructed for brief (taking no more than ten min) screening of depression in elderly persons. Its "yes/no" statements may be easier for some elderly patients to answer than other test formats which call for ratings along a continuum of increasing severity (Brink et al., 1982; V.K. Dunn and Sacco, 1989). The questions can be read to patients who cannot respond independently. A 15-item short form is also available (Sheikh and Yesavage, 1986). As the GDS was developed for geriatric use, it does not include items concerning guilt, sexuality, or suicide.

Test characteristics. The number of endorsed critical items is summed; higher scores are associated with depression. The direction of positive response varies, with 20 "yes" items and 10 "no" items contributing to the summation score. Consequently, there is some tendency for "yea-saying" patients to obtain higher scores. As with other rating scales, suggested cutting scores are just that—suggested—since they may need to be adjusted as subject samples or patient needs differ. In general, however, scores ≤ 10 are considered normal while higher scores suggest possible depression.

Internal consistency and split-half reliability coefficients have both been reported to be .92 (Brink et al., 1982). In addition, the GDS correlates highly with well-studied measures such as the Beck Depression inventory (.73) (Hyer and Blount, 1984), Zung Depression Inventory (.84), and Hamilton Rating Scale for Depression (.83) (Yesavage et al., 1982).

Neuropsychological findings. With significant dementia, patients' rsponses become questionable, although the GDS appears to be a valid measure of depression in patients whose dementia is not severe (W.J. Burke et al., 1992; McGivney et al., 1994). However, the 15-item short form of the GDS may be more greatly affected than the full 30-item version by the presence of cognitive difficulty (W.J. Burke, Roccaforte, and Wengel, 1991).

---

[1]The GDS is in the public domain due to partial U.S. Government support for its development.

Zung Self-rating Depression Scale (SDS)
(Zung, 1965, 1967)

This 20-item scale, commonly referred to simply as "the Zung," uses a 4-point grading system on a scale ranging from "None OR a Little of the Time" to "Most OR All of the Time." Since half of the items are worded in the negative, severity is represented by "None OR a Little" in one-half of the cases and by "Most OR All" in the other half. For example, the severity scoring for item 1 ("I feel downhearted, blue and sad") runs counter to the severity scoring for item 18 ("My life is pretty full"). Like the BDI-II, the graded responses can be confusing to some elderly patients (Brink et al., 1982), and assistance in completing the test is sometimes needed.

Besides items obviously relating to depression, a number of items concerning physiological and psychological disturbances are not so obvious. Scores can be evaluated in terms of symptom groups (affect—two items; physiological disturbances, eight items; psychomotor disturbance—two items; and psychological disturbances—eight items) or in an overall "SDS Index." This index is obtained by converting scores from the raw score scale of 20 to 80 to a 25 to 100 SDS scale on which 100 represents maximum severity.

Test characteristics. Although the Zung was developed to identify depression in the general adult population, it has been frequently used with older patients. Fabry (1980) noted that this scale is best used with persons between the ages of 19 and 65 since older and younger subjects tend to get excessively elevated scores. Thus interpretation of the score, which is based on 20- to 64-year-old subjects, presents potential problems when applied to older persons (Kaszniak and Allender, 1985; Van Gorp and Cummings, 1989).

Among patients in a mental health clinic, mostly younger than 69, a reliability coefficient of .89 was obtained for ratings between patients and accompanying family members; internal reliability coefficients (*alpha*) ran from .88 to .93 (Gabrys and Peters, 1985). An internal consistency coefficient for "young-old" groups was reasonably close to these coefficients, but for older groups internal consistency became "unacceptably low" (Kaszniak and Allender, 1985). Kivela (1992) reported that reliability data for "young-old" persons are satisfactory across cultures and, in contrast to older elderly groups in the U.S., Finnish "old-old" subjects show as good internal consistency as younger ones (Kivela, 1992). The significant drop in internal consistency coefficients that appears in U.S. studies of normal elderly persons reflects the increased acknowl-

edgment of somatic problems compared to items concerning mood and attitude (Hassinger et al., 1989). Validity ratings of this instrument also differ according to subjects' ages. With psychiatric and mental health patients, mostly under age 69 years, validity criteria are generally satisfied (Gabrys and Peters, 1985; Kivela, 1992; Schaefer et al., 1985); but the Zung tends to misclassify as depressed a large number of normal persons over age 70. Yesavage (1985) reported 44% false positives for normal elderly—particularly those in the "old-old" ranges (Van Gorp and Cummings, 1989).

Three factors have been identified: Well-being/Optimism, Somatic symptoms, and Depression/anxiety; additionally, several vegetative symptom items generally associated with depression do not load on any of the factors (McGarvey et al., 1982; Steuer et al., 1980). Steuer and her colleagues observed that older and younger depressed patients responded similarly to the items associated with the Somatic symptoms and Depression/anxiety factors, but the elderly patients acknowledge many more problems on items associated with the Well-being/optimism factor.

Neuropsychological findings. The Zung has been used to explore relationships between depression and cognitive complaints and disorders in elderly persons. For example, for older normal persons (age range 60 to 90) the Zung scores did not show a positive relationship to verbal memory measures but rather to measures of attention and concentration (Digit Span, Digit Symbol) (Larrabee and Levin, 1986). In another study, Zung scores for elderly patients in the early stages of Alzheimer's disease did not differ from scores of intact control subjects either when the diagnosis was first made or a year later (Knesevich et al., 1983). Depression assessed by the Zung was more related to quality of life in patients with Parkinson's disease than other factors such as age, disease onset, or disease duration (Kuopio et al., 2000). Interestingly, Zung scores are associated with the likelihood of ischemic stroke occurring over a 10-year period (Ohira et al., 2001).

Inventories and Scales Developed for Psychiatric Conditions

Millon Clinical Multiaxial Inventory (MCMI, MCMI-II, MCMI-III) (Millon, 1977, 1987, 1994)

The Millon Clinical Multiaxial Inventory, now in its second revision (MCMI-III), is an MMPI type personality questionnaire consisting of 175 items. What distinguishes the MCMI from other objective personality measures is its focus on long-standing personality disorders, which are classified as Axis II Disorders by the DSM-IV schedule of the American Psychiatric Association (2000), a feature that contributes to its popularity. Thus, the MCMI purports not only to reflect clinical symptoms (i.e., state), but also to document enduring personality characteristics (i.e., trait).

Twenty-eight different scales are generated from the inventory, consisting of four *Modifying Indices*, 11 *Clinical Personality Patterns*, three *Severe Personality Pathology* scales, seven *Clinical Syndromes*, and three *Severe Syndromes*. The scales are designed to be consistent with DSM-IV diagnostic criteria.

Test characteristics. Although there have been slight content changes in the different MCMI versions, the general format with 175 statements remains the same. Neither items nor scales of the MCMI are independent as there are some overlapping items. This lack of scale independence reflects the overlapping characteristics of many of the conditions being assessed by the inventory.

Items are written at the eighth grade reading level. The inventory can usually be completed within a half-hour. The scales are plotted using Base Rate (BR) scores, which are adjusted to reflect the percentage of the population with that particular characteristic, a procedure that reportedly improves diagnostic accuracy compared to traditional *T*-scores. Millon set BR scores of 85 as indicating that the characteristic assessed by the scale was definitely present; a score of 75 indicates that some of the features being assessed by the scale are present. The median BR values for psychiatric and nonpsychiatric samples are 60 and 35, respectively.

According to Millon (1994), the internal consistency coefficients exceed .8 for 20 of the 26 scales, with the highest coefficient (.90) for Depression on the MCMI-III. Test–retest reliabilities range from .96 for Somatoform to .82 for Debasement. One of the questions raised by frequent revisions, however, concerns the degree to which validity studies of one version can be generalized to other forms. Some scales predict diagnoses no better than chance For example, in one study, the Disclosure scale (*X*) was insensitive to purely random responses (Charter and Lopez, 2002).

Neuropsychological findings. Although many neuropsychologists informally report that they may use the MCMI in their neuropsychological evaluations, formal research studies of its application in neuropsychology are limited. For TBI patients, scores above an adjusted base rate value of 75 were present on *Anxiety, Dysthymia, Somatoform, Narcissistic, Antisocial–Aggressive,* and *Passive–Aggressive*) (Tuokko, Vernon-Wilkinson, and Robinson, 1991). No relationship was seen between TBI severity or the amount of time postinjury and number of elevated MCMI scales.

Minnesota Multiphasic Personality Inventory (MMPI/MMPI-2) (Butcher, Dahlstrom, et al., 1989; Colligan et al., 1989; J.R. Graham, 1987, 1990; Hathaway and McKinley, 1951)

This most widely used of all paper-and-pencil "personality" tests (C. Piotrowski and Keller, 1989; C. Piotrowski and Lubin, 1990) was developed in the late 1930s in a medical setting to aid in psychiatric diagnosis; its revision was published in 1989. Cripe (2002) correctly notes the misnomer in the MMPI title as it is an inventory of many psychological and psychiatric symptoms and some psychophysiological symptoms with little that would qualify it as a personality test. When using this inventory the examiner should keep in mind that it is merely a record of the emotional, psychiatric, and medical problems (within the limited scope of the items' content) that the subject chooses to acknowledge.

Because of the relative simplicity of administration; the subsequent elaborations in the form of dozens of scales and subscales for almost every variety of emotional complaint or psychiatric symptom; books and articles on how to interpret MMPI-2 items, scores, and profiles; and the development of computerized interpretation systems which save clinicians the bother of analyzing their patients' response patterns themselves, the MMPI-2 has become a most attractive instrument for clinicians wanting information quickly and effortlessly about their patients' psychopathologic tendencies. Since this test was developed for differential diagnosis, it was soon put to the knottiest diagnostic task of all (before brain imaging was available): that of differentiating functionally psychotic patients from brain impaired patients with psychiatric presentations. By the 1960s, the use of the MMPI—for both diagnostic impressions and descriptions of emotional status—with persons known or suspected of being brain-injured became a generally accepted enterprise, which has continued despite equivocal research findings (Cripe, 1996b, 1997; Reitan and Wolfson, 1997b; Senior and Douglas, 2001).

In 1999, publication of the original MMPI and its forms was discontinued, according to distributors of the test (National Computer Systems), to be "consonant with the standards of the test publishing industry and the American Psychological Association."[1] The original MMPI was considered out of date; and, per-

---

[1]http://www.upress.umn.edu/tests/Phase_Out_of_MMPI.html

haps, having both forms of the inventory available could become confusing. To our knowledge, however, this has not been the practice with other tests (e.g., Wechsler batteries). Moreover, some neuropsychologists prefer using testing materials with which they are familiar, that have withstood the test of time, and that have acquired a large and well-studied data base.

Because the original MMPI is no longer available for clinical or research use, only some of the many, heretofore relevant, studies employing the original scale will be presented here. This is due, in part, to failure to demonstrate complete equivalence of the MMPI-2 with the original MMPI (Ben-Porath and Butcher, 1989; Colligan et al., 1989). As observed by Caldwell (1997), this violated Paul Meehl's basic actuarial prediction concepts (Dawes et al., 1989; Meehl, 1954, reprinted 1996). The reader interested in the use of the original MMPI in neuropsychology should refer to previous editions of this book for references and discussion.

Recognizing the normative weaknesses of the original MMPI, large-scale ($n = 2,600$) renorming of the MMPI was undertaken with a predominantly white sample from seven geographically scattered states; 19% of the subjects came from other racial groups (Butcher, Dahlstrom, et al., 1989; J.R. Graham, 1990). As in the original version, these norms do not take age into account. This is a serious problem because critical items are endorsed less frequently in older age groups, with an increase in the levels of L and K, which are supposed to help determine the validity of the test. Moreover, with higher levels of response to physical health items (e.g., relating to vision, hearing, etc.), older patients tend to minimize long-standing behavioral quirks. It has been suggested that critical item endorsements may have increased clinical significance for older subjects (Aaronson et al., 1996).

The average level of education for the MMPI-2 samples is 13 years. Colligan and his colleagues (1989) suggested that although 13 years is a little high for the U.S. population as a whole, it probably approximates the average education of persons taking this test. Since the MMPI-2 is also dependent on socioeconomic status, however, there have been concerns voiced about the standardization sample. According to R.L. Greene (1991):

The interpretation of the K scale changes dramatically depending on the socioeconomic class and education level of the client and the setting in which the MMPI-2 is administered (e.g., personnel selection, state hospital, university). The potential impact of these factors on the K scale becomes even more noteworthy on the MMPI-2 because of the relatively high socioeconomic class and years of education that characterized the MMPI-2 normative group. (p. 57)

As testimony to its popularity, the MMPI-2 has been translated into other languages, tape-recorded forms have been devised for the semiliterate or visually handicapped, and there is a form for patients who cannot write but may have enough motor coordination to sort item cards. It is an untimed test, suitable for older adolescents and adults. An MMPI-A is available for adolescent patients 14–18 years of age (Butcher, Williams, et al., 1992). Verbal comprehension must be *low average* or better with a minimum reading ability at the sixth grade level. Very impaired patients who have difficulty following or remembering instructions, who cannot make response shifts readily, or whose verbal comprehension is seriously compromised cannot take this test.

The original MMPI was constructed on principles of actuarial prediction, and this continues to be a major virtue of the MMPI-2. In the original scale, rigorous statistical discrimination techniques were used to select the items and construct the scales. The criterion for item selection and scale construction was the efficiency with which items discriminated between normal control subjects and persons with diagnosed psychiatric disorders. For the MMPI-2, a Restandardization Committee was formed to oversee the process (Butcher, Dahlstrom, et al., 1989). Many of the original MMPI statements were simply reworded because they were considered outdated, sexist, or difficult to understand. Repeated statements were deleted, as were items considered outmoded or psychometrically unsound. Additional items were added in the areas of family functioning, eating disorders, substance abuse, readiness for treatment, and work interference; these items were tested in an intermediate version of the test (Form AX). The inclusion/exclusion rationale resulting in the set of 567 MMPI-2 items was not made explicit in the MMPI-2 manual (R.L. Greene, 1991).

The MMPI-2 form provides for scoring of ten clinical scales and four validity scales. These latter scales give information about subjects' competence to take the test, the likelihood that they are malingering or denying real problems, and such test-taking attitudes as defensiveness or help-seeking. For the ten clinical scales, the subject's response pattern is compared with those of normal control subjects and the different diagnostic groups of psychiatric patients. Although each of the scales originally was given a name intended to reflect its content, it is now more common to refer to the scale number rather than the name to prevent misattribution of psychological characteristics based solely upon a scale's name when the name corresponds poorly with its content. MMPI/MMPI-2 interpretation is based on the overall scale *patterns*, not on any one response or the score for any one scale. It is inappropriate to interpret individual responses in isolation. For MMPI-2 a scale's *T*-score must be at least 65 to be considered elevated (i.e., of possible clinical significance); the original MMPI set a *T*-score of 70 as the critical level.

Spurred by the discriminating power of actuarial predictions (Meehl, 1996; Sines, 1966), numerous investigators have developed and refined "cookbook" programs for computerized scoring and interpretation of the MMPI and MMPI-2. The predictive prowess of these programs when applied to large samples has been demonstrated repeatedly. Their application to the individual case, however, is questionable since the programs in general use interpret the patient's highest but not lowest scores and not all of them account for age or physical condition (J.R. Graham, 1990). The difference between automated and actuarial interpretations has been stressed by J.R. Graham (1990) who notes that automated reports are based on "published research, clinical hypotheses, and clinical experience . . . a clinician generates interpretative states (which) . . . are stored in the computer and called upon as needed. . . . The validity of existing interpretative programs has not been adequately established" (p. 239). He further states that "the accuracy for even the highest ranked [computer service] was only modest" (p. 247). While modesty is appropriate for some situations, tools used to make important decisions about individuals must have better than "modest accuracy" [mdl]. With respect to "cookbook" interpretations in neuropsychological assessment, Cripe (1997) points out that, "Because so many items are potentially endorsed by neurologic patients for reasons other than personality or psychiatric dysfunction . . . the use of traditional cookbook clinical interpretations with neurologic patients is inappropriate."

Test characteristics. The most glaring oversight in the original standardization procedures was the omission of age norms (Kaszniak and Allender, 1985; Lezak, 1987a), and this is also true for the MMPI-2. A significant obstacle to collecting appropriate age norms for elderly subjects is their reluctance or inability of many to take a very lengthy test requiring fine visual discriminations, adequate reading ability, and the wherewithal to answer all 567 items. A 1961 study by Swenson reported that only 95 of 210 subjects age 60 and older (*M* = 71.4) produced completed protocols with valid profiles (70 refused, 39 began it but did not complete it, six had 110 or more "cannot say" responses).

Education effects have not often been addressed in MMPI studies concerning brain injury. In TBI patients, years of education correlated significantly with the *F*

(uncommon responses) and *K* (defensiveness) validity scales and scales 4 (*Pd*), 7 (*Pt*), 8 (*Sc*), and 9 (*Ma*), with a greater number of psychiatric symptoms associated with lower educational levels (J.M. Burke, Imhoff, and Kerrigan, 1990). Gass and Lawhorn (1991) found that for older, predominantly male stroke patients, education and scale 5 (*Mf*) correlated significantly (*r* = .43, *p* < .05).

MMPI-2 reliability and validity have been examined extensively for psychiatric or psychologically disturbed groups (Butcher, Dahlstrom, et al., 1989; J.R. Graham, 1987, 1990; Spreen and Strauss, 1998). However, these studies do not necessarily apply to neurologically impaired patients, particularly since brain injury frequently compromises patients' capacity for accurate self-appraisal and thus the validity of their responses to a self-report inventory (Cripe, 1999; Prigatano, 1987). Cripe (1988) suggested that, "Patients with better insights into their symptoms will endorse more items . . . [which will] lead to higher elevations on the scales affected by those items." For example, self-aware patients experiencing mental confusion tend to endorse a number of items on Scale 8 (*Sc*), which, if naively misinterpreted, can earn these acutely realistic patients a psychiatric diagnosis. Thus, clinical interpretation of the scales did not discriminate between patients with neurological, psychiatric, or pain disorders (Cripe, Maxwell, and Hill, 1995).

A problem that directly influences reliability is the greater likelihood that brain injured patients will respond inconsistently (J.M. Burke, Smith, and Imhoff, 1989; Krug, 1967). Not surprisingly, response inconsistency increases with the degree to which patients are confused or disoriented (Priddy et al., 1988), but only six of 21 validity scale profiles for nonoriented TBI patients met the usual MMPI criteria for invalidity in this study. Franzen (1989) noted specifically that "reliability data are lacking for neuropsychologically impaired subjects." Senior and Douglas (2001) stated more emphatically that, for forensic assessments,

MMPI-2 interpretative cookbooks, computer report-writers, adherence to the intent of the test-developers, and appeals to authority are inadequate substitutes for empirical accuracy [which is lacking], and an active hypothesis-testing interpretative approach, based upon setting-specific base-rate data, is recommended. (p. 203)

Neuropsychological findings. The question of MMPI sensitivity to the psychological ramifications of brain injury has been addressed by a variety of studies. Some early claims that MMPI response patterns differ according to the side of the lesion or its placement along the anterior/posterior dimension have not been consistently supported. Similarly, lateralization findings have been equivocal.

Elevated scores on scale 4 (*Pd*) did identify those head injured adults who had not returned to any work or school situation after going through a rehabilitation program (D.E. Walker et al., 1987). An examination of the validity of scale 2 (*D*) found significant correlations with clinical evaluations of depressed patients (.62), and with the Beck and Zung depression measures (.59 and .73, respectively) (Schaefer et al., 1985), but the MMPI scale identified depression least well of these three instruments.

Nevertheless, some very general *pattern* tendencies characterize the responses of many patients with neurological disorders. To some extent, the pattern of MMPI profiles of brain injured patients is an artifact of the test items and scale composition. Among the 51 items of the 357 scored items on a short form of the MMPI (omitting scale 0 [*Si*] and all items normally not scored) referable to symptoms of physical disease, 26 relate to central nervous system diseases and eight describe problems associated with being ill (Lezak and Glaudin, 1969). Most of the "neurological symptom" items appear on scale 8 (*Sc*), and many have double and triple scale loadings, particularly on scales 1 (*Hs*), 2 (*D*), and 3 (*Hy*). As a result, nonpsychiatric patients with central nervous system disease tend to have an elevated "neurotic triad" (1-2-3) and higher than average 8 (*Sc*) scores (see Fig. 19.1; see also, Mack, 1979).

Since so many MMPI items describe symptoms common to a variety of neurological disorders, self-aware and honest patients with these symptoms may produce MMPI profiles that could be misinterpreted as evidence of psychiatric disturbance, even when they do not have a psychiatric or behavioral disorder. This problem has been particularly recognized in protocols of multiple sclerosis patients who, almost universally, give responses that elevate the "neurotic triad" (G.G. Marsh, Hirsch, and Leung, 1982; Meyerink et al., 1988). After removing items describing multiple sclerosis symptoms (mostly from scales 1 [*Hs*], 2 [*D*], 3 [*Hy*], and 8 [*Sc*] but also a few from other scales), the profiles obtained were mainly well *within normal limits* and considered to provide a more accurate description of these patients than the psychiatrically biased profiles (S.R. Mueller and Girace, 1988). Gass (1992, 1996; Gass and Lawhorn, 1991) developed a similar MMPI-2 correction technique for use with stroke patients whose neurological problems also tend to elevate the same scales and another set of items to be removed from MMPI-2 scores of TBI patients for whom neurological symptom items showed up on these scales and on scale 7 (*Pt*) (Gass, 1991).

In TBI, scale 1 (*Hy*) shows up less frequently as one of the high scores than the two other "neurotic triad" scales and scale 8 (*Sc*), while scale 4 (*Pd*) is often one of the top three scoring scales (J.M. Burke, Imhoff, and Kerrigan, 1990; R. Diamond, Barth, and Zillmer, 1988; Leininger, Kreutzer, and Hill, 1991). The relatively higher proportion of young men among TBI victims accounts for the greater incidence of elevated scale 4 (*Pd*) scores for these patients than for persons suffering other brain disorders; women with TBI typically do not have scale 4 as one of their high scales (Alfano, Neilson, et al., 1992). However, enough variability in high points remains between reported studies (which differ in the proportion of women contributing to the average scores, in severity of injury, in time since injury—both between studies and within studies—and in patients' exposure to rehabilitation) that any two or dozen TBI patients are likely to have quite different MMPI profiles.

Moreover, although more severely injured and financially compensated patients among a large (*n* = 124) sample of TBI patients tended to register fewer somatic complaints (i.e., lower scales 1 [*Hs*] and 3 [*Hy*]) than patients who had relatively brief periods of coma or amnesia, by and large no regular relationships were found between severity of injury and personality as interpreted from MMPI profiles (Bornstein, Miller, and van Schoor, 1988). On the MMPI, these patients did not describe themselves as any more emotionally disturbed than any comparable group of noncompensated TBI patients. Cripe (1997) pointed out that patients who lack awareness of their symptoms—among TBI patients, these are usually the most severely injured—may give "flat profiles which falsely give the illusion that they are problem free and well adjusted" (p. 301).

Elevations on scales 1 (*Hs*), 2 (*D*), 3 (*Hy*), and 8 (*Sc*)

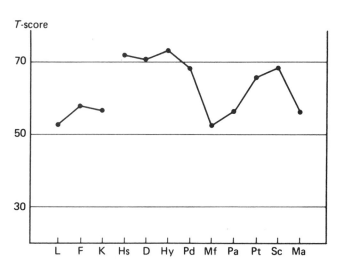

FIGURE 19.1 Mean MMPI profile for patients with diagnosed brain disease. (Lezak and Glaudin, 1969)

have also been reported for workers exposed to neurotoxic substances. This profile, which was found to characterize most of the workers coming to an occupational health clinic with complaints of cognitive dysfunction, was interpreted as indicating the "presence of somatic concerns, depression, poor concentration, and disturbances in thinking" (Morrow, Ryan, Hodgson, and Robin, 1990). More than 70% of these workers had *T*-scores >70 on at least three of these elevated scales; more than 90% of male workers had such abnormally high *T*-scores on at least two scales (Morrow, Ryan, Goldstein, and Hodgson, 1989). R.M. Bowler, Rauch, and their colleagues (1989) found the same high scores among a group of mostly women (50 of 60) workers exposed to a variety of neurotoxic substances. They identified three patterns: one they called "somatoform" (1-2-8, in order of degree of elevation), a "depression" profile (2-3-1), and a profile implicating "anxiety/phobia" (1-2-3), with specific symptom clusters associated with each profile. Among women workers exposed to organic solvents, a predominant profile emerged with *T*-scores for scales 1-2-3-8-7 (from the average highest to lowest) all above 70 (i.e., within the clinically significant range for the MMPI) (R.M. Bowler, Mergler, Rauch, et al., 1991). Here too Bowler and her coworkers found that specific elevated patterns among these high scales were associated with specific symptoms and complaints. These investigators did not attempt to separate out items concerning distinctive physical or cognitive problems from the overall scores.

In general, elevated MMPI profiles tend to be common among brain injured samples. The necessity for individualized interpretation, if the MMPI is to contribute meaningfully to an understanding of the patient, is brought out in an examination of how MMPI scores related to subjects' complaints about their mental functioning and perceptual competency (Chelune, Heaton, and Lehman, 1986). Of a large sample of control subjects and of patients referred from different sources for neuropsychological assessment, those who reported many problems or severe problems on the Patient Assessment of Own Functioning Inventory (PAF) (see Chelune, 1986) also tended to be those with the highest MMPI profile elevations; impaired performances on cognitive tests were also associated with MMPI elevations, but to a significantly lesser degree. It is thus the interpreter's responsibility to judge what and how much may be due to the patients' accurate reporting of symptoms that would indicate emotional or behavioral disturbances if they were neurologically intact, how much represents premorbid problems, how much was left unsaid because of impaired self-awareness, and just what all those numbers tell about these patients' current emotional status. When the "interpreter" is an automated scoring system, it becomes the practitioner's responsibility to determine the extent to which neurologically impaired patients' disorders might have contributed to the profile and scale patterns processed by a computer program and to assess the validity of the computer print-out for each patient.

These scales have all been evaluated for their effectiveness in discriminating between various brain injured and psychiatric patient groups. None reached a level of accuracy that would permit clinical judgments. With the increasingly common use of imaging combined with appropriate neuropsychological evaluations, neurodiagnostic applications of the MMPI have become irrelevant.

MMPI short forms. Responding to 567 items is tedious for intact adults and becomes an arduous, if not impossible, task for older persons and patients with visuomotor or visual acuity problems, or patients who can easily become fatigued or confused, or who have difficulty maintaining concentration—or the necessary posture for reading and writing—for very long. Efforts to facilitate the use of MMPI with older or brain injured subjects by reducing the number of items have produced some "short forms" with varying degrees of success when applied to groups, but they are inappropriate for clinical decisions about individuals (Butcher and Tellegen, 1978; Streiner and Miller, 1986).

In attempting to make MMPI-2 interpretations on the basis of a reduced item pool, an examiner "runs the risk of losing information or using an unreliable and unvalidated measure" (Butcher and Hostetler, 1990). These authors demonstrated this point in a review of the short form literature, summarizing the findings from 45 published studies for the three most popular short forms: The 71-item *Mini-Mult* (Kincannon, 1968), the 166-item *FAM* (*Faschingbauer Abbreviated MMPI*) (Faschingbauer, 1974), and the *MMPI-168* (Overall and Gomez-Mont, 1974). Correlations between the Mini-Mult and the MMPI ranged from .03 to .93; and although many correlations were in the .60 to .90 range, agreement on profile types exceeded 50% in only half of the studies. The FAM's record was somewhat better: short with long form correlations ran from .50 to .93, with 12 studies showing 60% or more agreement in profile types, eight agreeing in 50 to 59% of cases, and six with agreement rates of less than 50%. The MMPI-168's range of correlations with the MMPI was .33 to .98, with 10 of 18 studies producing agreement rates of 60% or more for profile types.

With just TBI subjects, congruence between the MMPI and its short form is no better. Alfano and Finlayson (1987) reported that the Mini-Mult produced the same two high points as the MMPI for 11% of their 125 head injured patients, the FAM's 2-point agreement rate was 31%, and that of the MMPI-168 was 32%. Of six short forms, these latter two instruments had the highest agreement levels (43% to 67%) with the MMPI for high point scale. When the OBD-168, a rewritten form of the MMPI-168 developed for oral presentation (Sbordone and Caldwell, 1979), was given to postacute TBI patients, a "distress syndrome" profile frequently showed up although almost all the patients denied emotional problems. Streiner and Miller's (1986) question, "Is the short form really a new test?" has especial applicability to the OBD-168 as transformations in both length and wording may well have made the OBD-168 quite different from the parent MMPI-168 and the grandparent MMPI. Like other short forms, one may suspect that the rules and traditions for MMPI interpretation have only partial applicability to the OBD-168; and, unfortunately, one can never know which are the protocols to which MMPI interpretation does not apply.

Personality Assessment Inventory (PAI) (Morey, 1991)

This instrument is similar in format to the MMPI, but with 344 items it takes on average between 45 to 50 minutes to complete. For a variety of reasons such as ease of administration and a fourth-grade reading level, the PAI is an increasingly popular method among psychologists for personality testing (C. Piotrowski, 2000).

The inventory yields four validity scales, 11 clinical scales, five treatment consideration scales, and two interpersonal scales. In contrast to other tests, such as the MMPI, the scales do not overlap. Thus, scale elevations are not due to overlapping item content. The test can be scored by hand or computer.

Test characteristics. The PAI can be used for patients who are at least 18 years old. Although stratified, the normative sample combined those 65 to 89 years old into one age range. Separate norms for age (or for sex or race) are not available as, Morey suggests, this would alter the reported prevalence rates for clinical entities and thus generate data that "would not be consistent with available epidemiologic data" (p. 50). Thus, as with the MMPI, there is the potential for scales with items concerning physical dysfunction to be disproportionately elevated, although this has not yet been formally studied.

There are four validity scales: *Inconsistency* and *Infrequency* are designed to reflect deviations from conscientious responding. *Negative Impression* and *Positive Impression* assess response bias. Negative Impression is a measure of "faking bad" by including items that are infrequently endorsed while Positive Impression elicits tendencies to deny minor flaws.

As the PAI can usually be completed within an hour this may obviate the need for a short form. However, persons who complete at least 160 items but may have discontinued taking the test due to fatigue or other factors can still be evaluated: content for all of the scales is sampled in the first 160 items, and statements with higher scale correlations are presented before items with lower scale correlations. Internal consistency *alpha*s and test–retest reliabilities across samples are in the .80s. One advantage of the PAI relative to the MMPI-2 is that it appears less likely to "overpathologize," at least for epilepsy patients (Brewer et al., 2002).

Profile of Mood States (POMS) (McNair et al., 1981)

This test consists of a list of 65 adjectives (e.g., *happy, helpless*, etc.) that subjects can use to describe how they have felt "during the past week including today." Responses are rated on a 5-point scale (0 = "not at all," 4 = "extremely"). Other time periods can be used as specified by the examiner. Ratings are scored for six mood states: *Tension-anxiety, Depression-dejection, Anger-hostility, Vigor-activity, Fatigue-inertia*, and *Confusion-bewilderment*. Raw scores are converted into *T*-scores with norms for male and female psychiatric outpatients and for a healthy college sample.

Test characteristics. This test enjoys wide use for the assessment of depression (C. Piotrowski and Lubin, 1990) and mood changes associated with drug effects (e.g., Meador, Loring, Allen, et al., 1991). It is part of the World Health Organization (WHO) Neurobehavioral Core Test Battery for neurotoxicology research (Anger, 1992), and has found a niche in sports psychology (e.g., P. Terry, 1995). POMS validity and reliability have satisfactory research support with adequate consistency in its factor loadings and reasonably good test–retest correlations, given the often fluid state of emotions—particularly in people under stress or otherwise disturbed (R.A. Peterson and Headen, 1984). Its obviously good face validity may also account for its popularity. Test–retest correlation after 12 to 16 weeks for 72 healthy adults (age *Mdn* = 35) was .39 (Salinsky et al., 2001). The norms are very limited, with no data on healthy adults at different educational levels nor norms for the elderly. The manual does not provide interpretation guidelines, leaving this sensitive matter up to clinicians. This may actually be an advantage since guidelines could hardly be developed for all factor patterns that would be applicable to all population groups (e.g., see Peterson and Headen, 1984).

Neuropsychological findings. The POMS has had its most extensive neuropsychological use with persons at risk for disorders due to toxic exposure since its incorporation into the WHO core and full batteries, as well as other batteries developed specifically for examining the effects of environmental and industrial toxins (Anger, 1990, 1992; R.F. White and Proctor, 1992). Workers with histories of exposure to industrial toxins had significantly higher scores on the *Tension, Vigor, Confusion,* and *Fatigue* scales than a demographically matched group of working people (Morrow, Kamis, and Hodgson, 1993).

Other neuropsychological applications have also demonstrated its sensitivity. *Tension, Confusion,* and *Depression* all correlated at low levels (.18, .24, .20, respectively) but significantly with employment status for a large number of TBI patents (Stambrook, Moore, Peters, et al., 1990). Mood responses to medication effects showed up in a large-scale study of epileptics given this test before being placed on antiepileptic drugs and one month later (D.B. Smith et al., 1986). On medication, these patients' *Tension* scores dropped but they scored higher on *Anger* and *Fatigue.* However, when given to AIDS patients and patients with AIDS-related diseases undergoing medication trials (zidovudine: [AZT]), unlike the Symptom Check List-90-R (see below), no differences in mood were registered although patients receiving the drug showed some cognitive improvements (F.A. Schmitt, Bigley et al., 1988).

Sickness Impact Profile (SIP) (Bergner et al., 1981; Department of Health Services, University of Washington, 1977, 1978)

The original purpose of this inventory was to examine the perception of patients' health in a manner sufficiently sensitive that changes "over time or between groups" would be registered (Bergner et al., 1981). Because it includes composite *Psychosocial* and *Independent* scales as well as a *Physical* scale, it has been widely used to measure quality of life as perceived by patients (P.S. Klonoff, Snow, and Costa, 1986; McSweeny et al., 1985) or their spouses or relatives (Stambrook, Moore, Peters, et al., 1990). In its final revision, the SIP contains 136 items, each associated with one of 12 categories contributing to the composite scales (see Table 19.3). Weighted scores, given to items answered "yes," are summed for each subscale; and these sums are converted to percentiles, which can be graphed as a profile (e.g., see I. Grant and Alves, 1987). An "overall" score, sometimes called a "Total" score, also cast as a percentile, can be used as an index of quality of life (e.g., see P.S. Klonoff, Snow, and Costa, 1986). The average score for normal healthy persons is about 4 (Bergner, personal communication, cited in Stampp et al., 1985) and about 11 for older adults (65 to 96 years) living in the community (Andresen et al., 1998).

TABLE 19.3 Sickness Impact Profile (SIP) Categories and Composite Scales

Categories	Composite	
Ambulation		
Mobility	Physical	
Body care and movement		
Social interaction		
Alertness	Psychosocial	SIP
Emotional behavior		TOTAL
Communication		
Sleep and rest		
Eating		
Work	Independent	
Home management		
Recreation and pastimes		

From I. Grant and W. Alves (1987). Psychiatric and psychosocial disturbances in head injury. In H.S. Levin, J. Grafman, and H.M. Elsenberg (Eds.), *Neurobehavorial Recovery from Head Injury.* New York: Oxford University Press. Reprinted with permission.

Test characteristics. The SIP can be administered as a paper-and-pencil test or in a structured interview. When self-administered (with or without an examiner present to instruct the subject and respond to questions), patients reported a higher level of dysfunction that also appeared to be more accurate than the structured interview administration (Bergner, 1981). Moreover, administration with an examiner present also produced the highest correlations with other measures, leading Bergner to recommend that if the SIP must be taken without an examiner present (e.g., mail-delivered), "careful follow-up and monitoring is necessary to assure and assess reliability and validity" (p. 794). Yet the test–retest reliability coefficient was highest (.97) when the SIP was given as a structured interview although the test–retest coefficient for self-administration (with an examiner present) was acceptably high (.87) (Bergner et al., 1981). Internal consistency correlations were identical (.94) for both administration procedures. In its most recent format, correlations with clinician assessments of sickness and dysfunction for medical patients with a variety of conditions that differed in severity were .40 and .50, respectively.

Factor analysis failed to support the 12 categories defined by the authors (de Bruin et al., 1994). Rather, a two-dimensional structure was produced consisting of a Physical dimension (sleep/rest, body care and movement, household management, mobility, ambulation, eating) and a Psychosocial dimension (emotional behavior, social interaction, alertness and intelligence, communication). Recreation and pastimes loaded significantly on both factors.

A shortened version emerged from an analysis of responses of a large number of respondents in Dutch studies (de Bruin et al., 1994). Eliminating skewed items and retaining items that performed well in a factor analysis resulted in a reduction to 68 items loaded on six factors: *Somatic Autonomy, Mobility Control, Psychic Autonomy and Communication, Social Behavior, Emotional Stability,* and *Mobility Range.* The total score correlated highly (.97) with the full SIP score.

Neuropsychological findings. For patients whose pulmonary disease had neuropsychological consequences (see p. 282), the SIP Total score and *Physical* scale had the highest correlations with a large set of cognitive test scores (Multiple $R = .53$ and .59, respectively) (McSweeny, Grant, et al., 1985). The SIP Total score for patients with mild cerebrovascular disease also correlated significantly (.35) with a summary neuropsychological test score (Baird et al., 1988).

The SIP has been used to measure quality of life at different levels of TBI severity and at different postinjury time intervals (Mellick et al., 2003). At one month, patients who had been in coma for a week or more had an average Total score of 30, with highest scores on the *Home Management* (75), *Pastimes and Recreation* (53), *Mobility* (51), and *Work* (70) subscales (McLean, Dikmen, et al., 1984). In contrast, patients whose consciousness was impaired for less than an hour had a Total score of 12, while those with periods of impaired consciousness longer than an hour but less than a week had Total score averages in between these two extremes. When relatives of TBI patients compared them six months after injury with their premorbid status, the SIP showed the greatest discrepancy for the *Ambulation* subscale with the *Body Care and Movement* score being the second most discrepant (I. Grant and Alves, 1987). For two large groups of TBI patients with varying degrees of severity examined two to four years after injury, scores on the *Psychosocial* scale and the *Recreation and Pastimes* subscale were higher than *Physical* scale scores which, by then, were mostly near normal (P.S. Klonoff, Snow, and Costa, 1986). SIP scores were also related to performance on the *Revised Strategy Application Test,* a test designed to assess problem-solving efficiency (B. Levine, Dawson, et al., 2000). Thus, the SIP can elicit a general picture of the evolution of patients' functioning after TBI.

TBI patients with moderate to severe injury tested three to four years postinjury had SIP total scores that significantly correlated ($-.40$) with performance in a test of planning and strategy (B. Levine, Dawson, et al., 2000). The relationship was stronger for the SIP *Physical* composite score ($-.50$) than the *Psychosocial* composite score ($-.34$), which was likely due to the finding that all but one of the patients with numerous physical complaints had very severe TBI. No significant correlation was found between the cognitive measure and the SIP for the mild TBI patients. Patients with and without mild TBI were examined with the SIP 6–9

months following motor vehicle accidents (J.F. Friedland and Dawson, 2001). Total SIP scores did not differ between the groups, but the TBI group had a higher *Psychosocial* composite score. Patients with PTSD from both groups had significantly higher SIP scores than patients who did not have stress symptoms at follow-up.

The SIP has also been used to study changes in quality of life of Parkinson patients treated with deep brain stimulation (Vingerhoets, Lannoo, van der Linden, et al., 1999). Before surgery, patients reported a 36% reduction in overall quality of life, with slightly more reduction in *Psychosocial* items (38%) than *Physical* items (33%). After surgery these scores improved in several categories, most dramatically on communication. No other *Psychosocial* measure changed significantly although all were lower following surgery. Of the *Physical* categories, body care and movement showed the greatest improvement. The SIP has also been used to measure treatment effects in patients with amyotrophic lateral sclerosis (Damiano et al., 1999). At least half of the patients reported one or more dysfunctions in sleep and rest, body care and movement, home management, social interaction, ambulation, alertness behavior, communication, and recreation and pastimes. Patients with slow to moderate progression of the disease reported significantly less increase in SIP scores than patients with rapid progression, except for ambulation, work, and recreation and pastimes.

Symptom Check List-90-R (SCL-90-R) (Derogatis, 1994)

The 90 items in this list of symptoms and complaints common to medical and psychiatric patients contribute to the score on one of nine "primary symptom dimensions": *Somatization (SOM), Obsessive-Compulsive (O-C), Interpersonal Sensitivity (INT or IS), Depression (DEP), Anxiety (ANX), Hostility (HOS), Phobic Anxiety (PHOB), Paranoid Ideation (PAR),* and *Psychoticism (PSY),* or to a set of "additional items," which include statements regarding problems that can arise in many psychiatric disorders or medical conditions (e.g., sleep and eating disturbances, concerns with death or guilt). Three other "global index" scores can be computed: the *Global Severity Index (GSI)* represents the overall level or intensity of distress; the *Positive Symptom Distress Index (PSDI)* is the average distress level across items; the *Positive Symptom Total (PST)* is the sum of the number of symptoms for which any level of distress is reported. Subjects rate on a 5-point scale (0—"Not at all" to 4—"Extremely") how much they were "distressed by" each of these symptoms during the past week "INCLUDING TODAY." Of course, the examiner can specify other time periods. It is advisable to stay with patients prone to confusion or who appear to need encouragement while they write their responses. For others, explanations are given as requested and the examiner shows how to fill out the first item before giving subjects the test sheet to answer on their own. When necessary, the examiner can read the items in which case the test becomes a kind of structured interview. The SCL-90 has been translated into at least 20 other languages.

Test characteristics. Separate norms are provided for male and female "nonpatients," psychiatric inpatients and outpatients, and adolescents. Internal consistency was examined with "symptomatic volunteers," but the manual does not indicate what conditions were associated with these symptoms. Test–retest reliability coefficients are based on responses by "heterogeneous psychiatric outpatients." For the nine clinical scales, coefficients range for these two reliability measures range from .77 to .90. A distinctive factor was extracted for each of the scales with males and females showing high levels of agreement on all but the PAR (Paranoid Ideation) scale. Validation studies conducted on both psychiatric and medical groups as well as on groups under abnormally stressful conditions have demonstrated sensitivity to the emotional and adjustment problems of these subject groups.

Neuropsychological findings. The SCL-90-R has been used with many different neuropsychological disorders: exposure to neurotoxins (Morrow, Kamis, and Hodgson, 1993; Uzzell, 1988), stroke (Magni and Schifano, 1984); TBI (B. Caplan and Woessner, 1992; Lezak, 1991), multiple sclerosis (Lezak, Whitham, and Bourdette, 1990), and AIDS (Schmitt, Bigley, et al., 1988). We [mdl, dbl] give this test to all patients who can take it, using the nonpatient norms. It has proven particularly useful in identifying patients with attentional and memory disorders who tend to have score elevations on the O-C (Obsessive-Compulsive) scale, as they check items having to do with mental inefficiency (problems in concentrating, drawing a mental blank), poor memory, and techniques to compensate for these problems, such as working slowly to guard against errors or double-checking their work. Of all the SCL-90-R scores, O-C was the only one that varied directly with the number of tests of attention and memory on which mild to moderate TBI or multiple sclerosis patients performed in the impaired range (Lezak, 1991; Lezak, Whitham, and Bourdette, 1990, respectively), thus providing a good measure of the extent to which attention and memory problems are distressful to these patients (see Slaughter et al., 1999, and comments under *Brief Symptom Inventory,* below). Pronounced elevations on the O-C and the Somatization (SOM) scales characterized the SCL-90-R profiles of TBI patients with dizziness complaints (Grimm et al., 1989). Other research with TBI patients also found high levels of O-C and SOM along with elevated Psychoticism (PSY) (a scale with few items, of which two involve fears that one's body or mind is impaired) (B. Caplan and Woessner, 1992). Stroke patients' most typical elevations were on the O-C and Depression (DEP) scales (Magni and Schifano, 1984).

These findings point up the importance of avoiding psychiatric interpretations of these scales when examining neuropsychologically impaired patients who have not had a history of emotional or behavioral problems prior to the onset of their neurological disorder. Rather, an item-by-item evaluation of their responses will often show that patients' responses reflect the kinds of neuropsychological or medical problems they are experiencing and can be used as a guide for counseling and remediation.

A study using only the three summary scores purported to show that scores on a measure of emotional distress that does not have built-in scales or items to detect faking or invalid response patterns can readily be distorted (Lees-Haley, 1989). Research with neurologically impaired patients has demonstrated that, at least in conditions in which attention or memory is affected, specific scale elevations are likely to occur. As summary scores obscure the pattern of responses to individual scales, they do not constitute data on which the reasonableness of a response pattern should be judged. Needless to say, however, when almost all scales are abnormally elevated, the subject's intentions become suspect.

Brief Symptom Inventory (BSI) (Derogatis, 1982)

This 53-item short form of the SCL-90-R is administered in the same manner as its parent measure and generates the same symptom dimensions and global ratings (Derogatis and Lazarus, 1994). For psychiatric outpatients, correlations between this measure and the SCL-90-R for the symptom dimensions ranged from .92 to .99. When used with severely head-injured patients, again the O-C scale was abnormally high, along with Anxiety (ANX), Phobic Anxiety (PHOB), Paranoid Ideation (PAR), and Psychoticism (PSY) (Hinkeldey and Corrigan, 1990).

One of the advantages of the BSI is that with fewer items it can be completed quickly, thereby enhancing its use for repeated assessments (e.g., Burg et al., 2000). It is very appropriate for neuropsychological assessment in that some of the item descriptions in the Obsessive-Compulsive scale reflect TBI-related cognitive impairment more than obsessive-compulsive traits (Slaughter et al., 1999). However, the lack of appropriate comparison groups limits its application to neurologic patients.

20 | Testing for Response Bias and Incomplete Effort

The study of malingering has, we fear, been somewhat neglected by the scientific Physician, who, more bent on establishing the features of true disease, has instinctively recoiled from the study of feigned disorders.

A.B. Jones and Llewellyn, 1918, p. v

Wittingly or unwittingly, persons undergoing a neuropsychological assessment may give distorted or erroneous responses not in keeping with their actual neuropsychological abilities. The direct financial benefits of illnesses and injuries related to job, military service, or accident and the indirect emotional and social rewards of invalidism can make malingering and psychogenic disabilities an attractive solution to all kinds of social, economic, and personal problems for some people. Moreover, emotional reactions to new limitations occasioned by injury or disease, or due to the primary effects of a neurologic condition itself, can bring about additional symptoms or exacerbate existing ones. Of course, neurogenic impairment may be superimposed on preexisting emotional disorders: psychiatric disturbances are not protective against brain injuries.

Identifying nonneurologic contributions to neuropsychological performance is important when providing patient care because a psychological overlay can increase the severity of the functional impairment and interfere with treatment or rehabilitation of the underlying neurologic problem. The challenge of determining whether and to what extent psychological factors contribute to the symptom picture is further complicated in that early or mild neurological disease may not be identified in the neurological examination or by laboratory studies, and many psychological disorders can be indistinguishable from neurologic disease since they may include relatively common neurological symptoms and complaints such as headaches, blackouts, and memory, concentration, or sensory problems. Moreover, neuropsychological performance levels can be lowered either deliberately or by nonconscious psychological factors, blurring the distinction between un-

conscious contributions and the conscious decision to exaggerate or feign illness for personal gain. Therefore, this chapter deals primarily with methods to determine whether aspects of the neuropsychological performance may have been distorted.

Millis and Putnam (1996) describe three factors that may limit the detection of malingering by clinical judgment alone. These include the difficulty of identifying malingering or response distortion when neuropsychological data alone are examined (e.g., Faust, Hart, and Guilmette, 1988 [this study included very few neuropsychology diplomates, see p. 138]), confirmatory bias and attribution error resulting in either under- or overdiagnosis of malingering, and the tendency of examiners to overestimate their capacity to identify malingerers when they feel they have established rapport with the patient.

Determination of whether the neuropsychological findings are valid usually rests on (1) evidence of consistency in the history or examination; (2) the likelihood that the set of symptoms and neuropsychological test profile—including validity measures—makes medical sense, i.e., fits a known disease pattern; (3) an understanding of the patient's present situation, personal/social history, and emotional predispositions; and (4) emotional reactions to these symptoms and complaints, such as patients who smile while relating their medical history. In a large-scale meta-analysis of neuropsychologists' judgment, Garb and Schramke (1996) concluded that their judgment is "reliable and moderately valid," and that inclusion of historical data enhances the validity of judgments regarding malingering.

In clinical practice, it is not infrequent to observe certain patients (particularly those involved in litigation or those who have a history of psychiatric disturbance) perform poorly on a variety of neuropsychological tests. In such cases, a patient's medical history many not correlate with his or her very poor test scores. An unsophisticated examiner might simply interpret such a performance as suggesting brain dysfunction. A sophisticated examiner, however, typically recognizes that the level and nature of neuropsychological test scores are not easily explainable based on other known facts. A great deal of confusion therefore is caused, not only in clinical practice but also in medical/legal matters, because of insufficient training in the interpretation of neuropsychological test performance. (Prigatano and Redner, 1993, p. 223)

Psychologists have assumed that the general public is unsophisticated regarding the effects of brain injury on behavior (e.g., Gouvier, Uddo-Crane, and Brown 1988; Wiggins and Brandt, 1988; Willer, Johnson, et al., 1993) as some malingerers reveal themselves by their ignorance of the clinical syndromes that they are trying to imitate. It is also true, however, that with increasing knowledge more people may be able to generate credible neuropsychological deficits (e.g., R.C. Martin, Bolter, et al., 1993).

Some examinees seen for forensic purposes appear to be quite knowledgeable about neuropsychological assessment. Attorneys dealing with claims of neuropsychological deficits will typically try to learn about neuropsychology (e.g., L. Miller, 1990). J.S. Taylor and his colleagues (1991, 1992) introduced the terms *neurolaw* and *neurolawyer* when referring to their practice specialty. Some psychologists have been concerned about the potential for attorneys to influence their clients' test performances (Lees-Haley, 1997; K.S. Pope et al., 1993, 2000; Youngjohn, 1995). Attorneys who brief clients about the tests they will be taking or—worse—tell their clients what answers to give can effectively invalidate the findings on many measures, including those used to detect response bias (e.g., Coleman et al., 1998; Rapport, Farchione, et al., 1998; Rose et al., 1998). Such coaching creates a special dilemma for the scientific community (Ben-Porath, 1994; D.T.R. Berry, Lamb et al., 1994), which relies on the free exchange of specific research methods. Fearing their data will be misused, some neuropsychologists have withheld specific details of their research from formal publications. Withholding from publication test details or cutting scores does not solve the coaching problem, however. Simply informing university students told to simulate malingering that measures of response distortion were included in the assessment produced more sophisticated "malingering" (Suhr and Gunstad, 2000; Youngjohn, Lees-Haley, and Binder 1999). Moreover, almost half of the attorneys in one survey believed that patients referred for testing should be informed that validity scales may be included in the assessment (Wetter and Corrigan, 1995).

Moreover, when addressing questions of poor cooperation or response exaggeration, it is important to realize that patients with genuine impairment often try to minimize or ignore their neuropsychological deficits as they want to appear psychologically normal (Pankratz, 1988). In our experience [mdl, dwl], this generally has been as true of most compensation claimants with independently confirmed evidence of brain injury (e.g., coma, neuroradiological abnormalities) as with other patients—most patients with brain injuries fight the loss of dignity (as wage earner, as fully independent, as physically competent and attractive) that they feel when their premorbid activities and ambitions are curtailed. These patients/claimants may seem to have less incentive to perform at suboptimum levels since the presence of brain injury is generally not in dispute (Slick, Iverson, and Green, 2000). However, many of these claims deal with the compensable extent of deficit so one could suspect that tendencies for symptom exaggeration would occur in some of these cases too. Yet the desire to maintain one's dignity and appear competent can override monetary or other considerations. This drive to appear competent in a psychological or neuropsychological examination is most often true of persons charged with crimes, even when the stakes may include the death sentence (mdl; for an example, see p. 628).

Patients/claimants without independent evidence of brain injury, in contrast, require greater scrutiny for response distortion since neuropsychological findings may be the only evidence of a genuine brain injury. "Those disorders which are largely *subjective in character* [sic] have the preference, as being the most easily feigned, the least easily detected" (A.B. Jones and Llewellyn, 1918). Such caution may be called for not only when patients request financial compensation for a claimed disability (e.g., workers' compensation, personal injury, or disability evaluations) but also when their personal situation suggests that they may be seeking to legitimize secondary psychological gains. Motivation to perform poorly may simply be due to the desire to receive attention as a patient or to play the sick role (e.g., factitious disorder) (Pankratz, 1999; Lazareth and Priollet, 1997; van Gorp and McMullen, 1997). Issues other than finances, therefore, may alert the clinician to possible response distortion. Slick, Sherman, and Iverson (1999) proposed criteria for suspecting malingering (see Table 20.1, p. 757). These authors suggest that malingering should be conceptualized as volitional and rational and that there should be no other plausible explanations of the behavior (e.g., factitious disorder or somatoform disorder, criterion D).

Paralleling the increasing use of neuropsychological data in forensic applications is the growth and refinement of methods to detect invalid test performance. Clinical neuropsychologists do not agree, however, regarding the need for routine specialized assessment of validity for all neuropsychological evaluations regard-

TABLE 20.1 Malingering Criteria Checklist

A. Presence of a substantial external incentive

B. Evidence from neuropsychological testing

   1. Definite negative response bias (below chance on a forced-choice measure of cognitive function)

   2. Probable response bias on a validity test

   3. Discrepancies between test data and known patterns of brain functioning

   4. Discrepancy between test data and observed behavior

   5. Discrepancy between test data and reliable collateral reports

   6. Discrepancy between test data and documented background history

C. Evidence from self-report

   1. Self-reported history discrepancy with documented history

   2. Self-reported symptom discrepancy with known patterns of brain functioning

   3. Self-reported symptom discrepancy with behavioral observations

   4. Self-reported symptom discrepancy with reports from close informants

   5. Evidence of exaggerated or fabricated psychological dysfunction

D. Behaviors meeting criteria from groups B or C not fully accounted for by psychiatric, neurologic, or developmental factors

From Slick, Sherman, and Iverson (1999)

less of the referral source or patient diagnosis (e.g., Van Gorp and McMullen, 1997). Some have argued that only patients with financial motivation to perform poorly on neuropsychological testing should be administered formal tests of response bias, whereas others prefer to include these tests in most, if not all, comprehensive assessments. In the interest of time and practicality, however, it is more common for specialized tests of response validity to be selectively administered based upon the referral source, the neuropsychologist's clinical judgment, and clinical referral patterns.

For example, validity testing is rarely relevant when there are no obvious secondary gains, and especially not relevant when a poor performance may actually compromise future opportunities. This is the case for some persons referred by employers because their medical history or deteriorating job performance has raised concerns about their employability. This would also appear to be the situation for athletes: a record of poor performance following a concussion will keep them out of play in the immediate future, and could affect their value when competing for places on a team. Although, as always, there will be exceptions, by and large it is unnecessary to spend much time evaluating the performance validity of persons being assessed under these circumstances.

As with other aspects of test interpretation, *findings on measures designed to assess performance validity and response bias should not be interpreted outside the context of clinical history and other measures of cognitive function.* Failure to take into account the contribution of demographic variables such as low education or advanced age to test performance, for example, might erroneously lead to the conclusion that performance is so severely impaired as to not be credible (e.g., R. Baker et al., 2000). Nonneurologic contributions to test performance are complex such that, with the exception of extreme cases, any permutation of cutting scores alone will usually be insufficient to conclude reliably that a person's performance is invalid. Thus, to reduce the likelihood of prediction error, the best use of single tests will be in combination with other validity measures and always within the context of the patient's history and clinical presentation which together reduce the likelihood of prediction error (McKinzey and Russell, 1997a). Social and medical history, always important, become critical in the evaluation of patients with mild injuries and symptoms. The following illustrates the risk created by slavish adherence to a single test cutting score without regard to other relevant considerations.

A prisoner convicted of murder was evaluated to determine if he was competent to be executed because state law prevented execution of retarded individuals. The prisoner was evaluated with a fairly representative battery of tests, including tests of response bias and response distortion. He was found to have an invalid response style on one forced-choice test of digit recognition, scoring significantly below chance levels. Some time after the assessment, but only days before the scheduled execution, another man confessed to the murders for which the condemned prisoner had been wrongly convicted. Although malingering by some definitions, this mentally retarded patient was demonstrating what for him was adaptive behavior (personal communication: the neuropsychologist involved in this case wishes to remain anonymous [mdl]).

Regardless of the referral source, a patient's report of an injury's severity should generally be verified independently through review of medical records. The examiner should no more accept a self-report of poor memory following a mild TBI than uncritically accept a patient's self-report of normal memory functioning during a dementia evaluation. When obtaining a history from a patient who reports an acute change of memory function, it should be remembered that a long-standing and well-documented literature demonstrates that memory is reconstructed and modified through recall (e.g., Bahrick, 1984; Barclay, 1988; Hilsabeck et al., 1998; Loftus, 1982). Memory is not simply retrieved in the same way that files are retrieved from a computer disk. Consequently, memory of an event may be modified through frequent retelling, even when there is no deliberate effort to deceive, and some inconsistencies may appear.

Some procedures discussed in this chapter are affected by significant memory, attention, or other neuropsychological impairment (e.g., Pachana, Boone, and Gazell, 1998). This does not mean, however, that these procedures should never be employed. Rather, they can be either used selectively or interpreted with appropriate caution. "The presence and degree of documented neurologic disease [should be considered] before interpreting the meaning of poor [malingering] scores" (Greiffenstein, Baker, and Gola, 1996a, p. 290). As with other aspects of neuropsychological test selection, one cannot adopt a "one size fits all" approach to assess validity and response bias; different procedures should be considered for different target populations or specific patients.

Moreover, it is important for the examining neuropsychologist to appreciate that "brain injury vs. malingering" is not a mutually exclusive dichotomy since some patients with neurologically based deficits may intentionally perform poorly on neuropsychological testing to exaggerate their impairments, thus trying to make sure the examiner recognizes a problem (Prigatano and Amin, 1993). Lipman (1962) described four malingering types: *Invention* is the complete generation of symptoms when none is present. *Perseveration* refers to symptoms that were initially present but no longer exist. *Exaggeration* is magnification of genuine symptoms. *Transference* involves genuine symptoms but they are not due to the particular injury in question. Thus, response bias may occur to various degrees and from different sources of response bias in a neuropsychological examination. For the examiner to be able always to distinguish among them is not realistic.

The use of neuropsychological findings as one basis for determining financial compensation following brain injury has encouraged the development of tests and techniques for the explicit purpose of identifying patients who would hope to profit from spurious or exaggerated claims of cognitive impairment. To apply these tests and techniques, however, the examiner must appreciate both their limitations as litmus tests for truth and their applications to patients who unwittingly distort their performances on a psychological basis. The practical and ethical issues surrounding the introduction of these techniques into clinical examinations undertaken for forensic purposes raise questions and concerns that go beyond the scope of this text. The interested reader can pursue this topic in books and reviews dealing explicitly with response distortion and forensic neuropsychology (e.g., H.V. Hall and Pritchard, 1996; McCaffrey, Williams, et al., 1997; Pankratz, 1998; R. Rogers, 1997; Sweet, 1999a,b).

Because cognitive and psychiatric functions reflect different neurobehavioral domains, measures sensitive to response exaggeration of cognitive impairment are not necessarily sensitive to exaggeration of psychiatric symptoms and vice versa (Greiffenstein, Gola, and Baker, 1995). Neuropsychologists doing forensic examinations will want to be acquainted with techniques sensitive to response exaggeration in both areas.

SPECIAL FORENSIC RESEARCH CONCERNS

Tests designed to detect malingering rely on statistical predictions, deviations from expected performance patterns, or response inconsistency. The validity of some of these tests has been evaluated in efforts to evade the ever present conundrum inherent in validating the validation procedures.

It is unrealistic to expect malingering patients to offer up a basis for systematic research by admitting that they had deliberately faked their responses; or that patients who lack awareness that they are underperforming or otherwise distorting their responses can give a valid report on their motivation. Even if they did, their claims cannot be independently verified (R. Rogers, Harrell, and Liff, 1993). Consequently, the study of malingering and response distortion has relied on two main procedures: healthy subjects instructed to feign neuropsychological impairment (*simulators*), and patients who are at increased risk of exaggerating deficits or who fit certain criteria of noncredible or inconsistent deficits.

These studies present an amusing paradox in that simulators are asked to comply with instructions to fake in order to study individuals who fake when asked to comply (R. Rogers and Cavanaugh, 1983). An important advantage of simulation studies, however, is that group assignment can be randomized, allowing for a true experimental design rather than relying on subject variables, which are not under direct experimental control. Simulation studies, however, have important limitations. Simulators are typically college students who may not possess the knowledge or experience to respond like patients trying to distort their test performances. The malingering tests given to simulators are often administered in isolation while, in clinical practice, these tests are embedded within a larger, comprehensive battery as part of formal neuropsychological assessment. Perhaps most importantly, simulators cannot have the same incentives to avoid detection as do genuine malingerers. Even when financial incentives are given to the simulators, these sums cannot begin to approximate the advantages a successful malingerer might obtain in litigation. Thus, for a variety of reasons, simulation designs tend to overestimate a test's sensitivity when used in clinical practice (Vickery, Berry, et al., 2001).

The other main procedure compares the test scores obtained by patients whose performance motivation has come under question with test scores of other—similar—patients who do not have the same motivation to distort their performance. Patients considered to be at risk are either identified individually from atypical performance patterns or are members of a group with an increased suspicion of response exaggeration because of financial interest (e.g., compensation claimants). With varying degrees of confidence, probable malingerers may be suspected on the basis of a pattern of improbable assessment findings (Greiffenstein, Baker, and Gola, 1994; Van Gorp, Humphrey, Kalechstein, et al., 1999) or on below chance performance on forced-choice symptom validity testing (Trueblood, 1994). The disadvantage of this approach, however, is that it is based on patients with extreme performance patterns and symptoms, and therefore may not necessarily be sensitive to more subtle response distortions.

When a subject with a mild injury performs at a more impaired level than patients with clearly documented significant brain damage, an invalid performance may be suspected. Patients with mild TBI who obtain poorer neuropsychological tests scores than groups of patients with more serious and independently established brain injury (Suhr, Tranel et al., 1997; van Gorp, Humphrey, et al. 1999), or perform at lower levels on tests of effort and response bias (e.g., P. Green, Iverson, and Allen, 1999) may be identified by the *floor effect* strategy (R. Rogers, Harrell, and Liff, 1993). The poorest performance of patients with known impairment establishes the floor—scores lower than the floor suggest invalid responses. Given the limitations inherent in each procedure for validating tests purporting to be sensitive to response distortion, those tests that have been studied with *both* simulation designs *and* application to known groups present the strongest validation evidence (R. Rogers, 1997). *When evaluating studies reporting group classification, it is important to remember that classification rates will vary according to the characteristics of the samples included.*[1]

A final point to keep in mind when using tests and cutting scores to evaluate response validity in a forensic examination is that many studies of test validity have not been replicated. Of course, scientific inquiry requires that relationships be first discovered, with sub-

sequent replication using independent samples and, ideally, by different researchers. The use of test data that have not been replicated to determine response validity has the potential of bringing inaccurate information to bear on individual cases. Since repeated research findings not infrequently fail to confirm previously reported relationships (e.g., Donders, 1999; A. Miller et al., 2000; this chapter, *passim*), many of the research findings reported here should not be considered definitive except as confirmed by other repeated studies.

Examining Response Validity with Established Tests

Distortions of test performances generally show up as inconsistencies, bizarre or unusual responses or "signs," and in performance levels *below* the usual range for persons who have the reported symptoms on a known neurologic basis. Rules of thumb, however, have not always withstood formal scrutiny. For example, Trueblood and Schmidt (1993) found that near misses or atypical performance on the easy and hard Associate Learning pairs of the original Wechsler Memory Scale were not related to suboptimal effort. Moreover, infrequent signs, although they may be specific markers of performance distortion, do not lend themselves readily to statistical analysis due to their low rate of occurrence.

The litigation process itself may also affect neuropsychological performance. Fox (1994), examining WMS-R Logical Memory performances, observed that many neuropsychologically normal workers' compensation claimants (i.e., emotional or orthopedic injury that did not involve potential neuropsychological sequelae) performed in the impaired range by normative standards. Possible explanations for these findings included both motivational and emotional factors. The contributions of pain to diminished performance levels should also not be overlooked.

A number of well-known tests used for ability and skill assessments have been examined for their sensitivity to simulated or exaggerated response errors. Many single tests can provide helpful information on whether patients' errors are reasonably typical for their complaints and in light of their medical and social histories. Some of these tests provide guidelines for the examiner assessing the validity of a performance. Examiners using these techniques need to be aware that they are like thermometers: Positive findings suggest that a problem is present but negative findings do not rule out a problem. Data from tests given in a neuropsychological examination may be less sensitive and specific to symptom exaggeration than specialized tests of response bias (Van Gorp, Humphrey, et al., 1999; Greiffenstein, Baker, and Gola, 1994).

---

[1]In personal injury law practices, whether for the plaintiff or defense, TBI claimants who are referred for neuropsychological study typically do not come with solid documentation of injury (e.g., rehabilitation data, MRI findings) and thus are not representative of all—even mild—TBI claimants.

The examiner needs to know the characteristics of the samples on which performance guidelines were developed to understand the appropriateness of measures derived to infer validity. For example, Trueblood and Schmidt (1993) found that the General Neuropsychological Deficit Scale (GNDS) of the Halstead-Reitan Battery separated mild TBI patients thought to be exaggerating from TBI patients without evidence of response exaggeration: the suspected exaggerating patients obtained higher (i.e., more impaired) GNDS scores. Thus, a high GNDS score in the context of mild TBI may raise a suspicion of response invalidity. This expectation underscores the risks of interpreting scores outside the clinical context or using techniques derived from studies with patient characteristics that differ significantly from the individual patient being evaluated. Since many scores, such as the GNDS, can be affected by motivation, ability, and demographic variables, an extra measure of interpretive caution is required.

Multiple Assessments

Neuropsychological evaluations are often repeated. It is not uncommon for a patient to be tested on two or more occasions, often within a short period of time. Practice effects from repeated testing—whether on cognitive, motor/sensory, or personality measures—may make interpretation of test results more difficult (see pp. 116–117). When evaluating a patient who has previously had a neuropsychological examination, the neuropsychologist wishing to lessen practice effects may consider administering an alternative but similar test to assess like constructs (e.g., the Rey Auditory–Verbal Learning Test rather than the California Verbal Learning Test). However, repeated performances on the same tests may have different response patterns that can shed light on response validity. With two assessments using the same tests, an inappropriately poor test-taking effort may show up as an absence of practice effects for subjects who have demonstrated some learning ability, if only inadvertently, such as knowledge of how to find the examiner's office; or as unaccountable ups and downs of scores; or as much different item responses; or as wide variations in intratest response patterns. Two assessments can give valuable information about test-taking effort since most patients will be unable to recall the specifics of their responses between the two evaluations (Hutt, 1985).

For example, when college student simulators were examined with repeated tests over a three-week period, performance on verbal tests (total CVLT recall, short and long delay memory from the CVLT, and Controlled Oral Word Association) tended to be at comparable levels across assessments but, unlike the control subjects, the experimental "malingerers" did

not display any practice effects (Demakis, 1999). Both groups, however, showed improvement on nonverbal measures (Rey Complex Figure recall, Ruff Figural Fluency). These findings support the interpretation of absent expected practice effects as possible evidence of incomplete effort.

Data are available to help determine expected practice and test–retest effects for many measures (McCaffrey, Duff, and Westervelt, 2000a,b). Cullum, Heaton, and Grant (1991) stated that, "examination of performance reliability across testings may be a powerful means by which the neuropsychologist can detect patients who are not consistently putting forth adequate effort on the examination" (p. 168). This principle formed the basis for the Retest Consistency Index (RCI) developed by Reitan and Wolfson (1997a), using tests from the Halstead-Reitan Battery. Similarly, the Victoria Symptom Validity Test utilized test–retest differences to separate college student "malingerers" from control subjects at a 95% probability level (E. Strauss, Hultsch, et al., 1999). Performance consistency has also been incorporated into some specialized validity measures used during a single assessment (e.g., P. Green, Allen, and Astner, 1996).

TEST BATTERIES AND OTHER MULTIPLE TEST SETS

Validity measures developed for traditional neuropsychological tests have the advantage of being available without the need for special testing dedicated solely to determine response bias. These measures can also be computed directly from scored protocols when reviewing the test data from a previous examination. The greatest limitation of this approach is that, since these tests were designed to assess complex aspects of cognitive functioning, they may be affected by ability more than many specialized tests examining narrowly defined abilities that all but the most severely impaired patients possess (e.g., shape recognition, repeating five or six digits). Thus, validity inferences drawn from these tests are based, in part, on the neuropsychologist's clinical skill in integrating the patient's responses with the clinical history.

Wechsler Scales

Wechsler Intelligence Scales for Adults (WIS-A)

Digit span. Because WIS-A batteries include tests that are used in many neuropsychological examinations, validity procedures derived from the Wechsler scales are of great interest. In the Wechsler batteries, Digit Span—both forward and reversed—is consistently performed less well by simulators than by neurologic patients (Bernard, 1990; Heaton, Smith,

Lehman, and Vogt, 1978; Öberg, Udesen, Thomsen, et al., 1985; Rawling and Brooks, 1990). Mild TBI patients suspected of response exaggeration also may perform more poorly on Digit Span (L.M. Binder and Willis, 1991; Suhr, Tranel, et al., 1997; Trueblood and Schmidt, 1993). Simply using an age-adjusted WAIS-R Digit Span scaled score of <7 correctly classified 82% of a sample of probable malingerers and control subjects (Trueblood, 1994). Of course, this technique would not be appropriate in populations with diminished attentional abilities (e.g., moderate to severe dementia patients).

Reliable Digit Span (RDS). Greiffenstein, Baker, and Gola (1994) developed a measure which is the sum of the longest string of digits recalled on both trials of each digit length for both forward and backward conditions. A score of 7 or less to classify probable malingerers yielded a hit rate of 18% over chance for that patient sample. In a cross-validation study comparing litigating and nonlitigating patients, only 4% of nonlitigants made scores ≤7 but 49% of litigants' scores were this low (J.E. Meyers and Volbrecht, 1998). In a simulation design, RDS correctly classified all of 21 control subjects and 14 of 20 experimental college student "malingerers" (E. Strauss, Hultsch, et al., 1999).

Vocabulary – Digit Span (VDS). A Vocabulary age-graded score considerably higher than the Digit Span age-graded score appears to suggest response distortion, as does a positive score obtained by a discriminant function formula (DFS) (Mittenberg, Theroux-Fichera, et al., 1995). This Vocabulary-Digit Span difference score correctly classified 90% of patients with moderate to severe TBI and 79% of mild TBI patients who were identified as giving incomplete effort based upon chance performance on at least one subtest of the Warrington Recognition Memory Test (Millis, Ross, and Ricker, 1998). However, the DFS may predict malingering better than the VDS; combining the two scores does not improve prediction (Greve, Bianchini, et al., 2003). This method was not as helpful as other techniques in identifying college student simulators (E. Strauss, Hultsch, et al., 1999).

Other WIS-A tests. Other WIS-A tests have produced less encouraging discriminations. Block Design scores of neurologically intact persons complaining of "serious cognitive impairment" were much better than those of severely impaired patients although not as good as those with mild dementia (Öberg, 1985). Rawling and Brooks (1990) observed that mild TBI patients seeking compensation performed almost 2 points lower on Arithmetic, about 1 point lower on Comprehension,

Picture Arrangement, and Block Design, and almost 1 point better on Picture Completion and Object Assembly compared to more severely impaired TBI patients. Trueblood and Schmidt (1993), however, found a slightly different pattern of test sensitivity to probable response distortion. In addition to Digit Span, these authors reported that the WIS-A tests sensitive to deliberate item failures or response slowing were Vocabulary, Picture Completion, and Digit Symbol.

A Simulation Index. In a more elaborate search for error types associated with exaggeration on the WAIS-R and the original Wechsler Memory Scale, Rawling and Brooks (1990) observed that their Simulation Index (SI), which is based upon errors seen only in their simulation patients and errors present only in their TBI patients, achieved a high classification rate. This high rate did not hold up in cross-validation, however (Milanovich et al., 1996). In this latter study, the most common simulation signs were distortions on Visual Reproduction, transposition errors on Verbal Paired Associates (Wechsler Memory Scale; see below), and dubious sequences on Picture Arrangement. TBI patients typically made plausible sequences on Picture Arrangement. Thus, without additional cross-validation studies, it is premature to make inferences based upon WIS-A data reports that do not include Digit Span.

Wechsler Memory Scales (WMS, WMS-R, WMS-III)

Paired Associate Learning (PAL). Prior to the publication of WMS-III, this test format included both easy and hard word associations (see pp. 440–441). Since people generally—especially patients with memory impairment—tend to learn the easy pairs more readily, Gronwall (1991) suggested that any deviation from this expected pattern is suspect. Although little difference in easy vs. hard performance level was not related to suboptimum effort in one patient series (Trueblood and Schmidt, 1993), this may simply reflect a low rate of occurrence. When present, however, it can be a fairly specific marker for an invalid performance.

Other WMS tests. All WMS-R tests except Mental Control have been manipulated in college student studies of simulation of post-TBI memory deficits (Bernard, 1990). Interestingly, Visual Memory Span discriminated groups even more effectively than did Digit Span.

General Memory vs. Attention/Concentration. Mittenberg, Arzin, and their coworkers (1993) developed an index based upon the discrepancy between the WMS-R General Memory and Attention/Concentration Index scores. The rationale these authors give for this difference score is their impression that poor attention rarely occurs without being accompanied by memory impairment, but memory impairment is often seen with reasonably intact attention. Normal volunteer "malingerers" performed better on General Memory than on Attention/Concentration, while TBI patients displayed the opposite pattern (General Memory < Attention/Concentration). The authors also generated a table, ranging from a probability of .99 that a subject is malingering (with Attention/Concentration score 35 scaled score points lower than the General Memory Index) to a 50:50 probability associated with only a 2-point difference. In a simulation study, college students instructed to fake deficits produced an average 11-point discrepancy, 13 points after being warned about techniques to uncover deception (J.L. Johnson and Lesniak-Karpiak, 1997). In a sample of substance abuse patients, the Attention/Concentration Index was lower than the General Memory Index by at least 25 points in only 5% of the sample (Iverson, Slick, and Franzen, 2000), and only 6% of TBI patients with injuries from mild to severe showed this same, or a greater, magnitude of discrepancy (Iverson and Slick, 2003). Thus, discrepancy of this magnitude is not a frequent occurrence in clinical populations with no external incentive to malinger. (In using this formula, it is important to realize that many patients with mild, diffuse cerebral lesions—e.g., mild TBI, multiple sclerosis—whose memory is relatively intact but whose span of immediate acquisition is constricted may get better scores on the tests of memory. The relative insensitivity of WMS tests of attention and their administration and scoring procedures may have contributed to the impression that many of these patients suffer memory disorders: the General Memory Index is based on tests with complex stimuli that are read or shown only once, so that patients with attentional disorders—especially a reduced attention span—will perform less well than on memory tests with repeated stimuli and/or recognition trials).

Logical Memory. Forced choice recognition trials for Logical Memory have correctly classified 85% of college student simulators without misclassifying any control or memory impaired subjects (Iverson and Franzen, 1996). Denney (1999) reported that a similar forced-choice recognition test for Logical Memory was successful when applied on an individual patient basis. R.C. Martin, Franzen, and Orey (1998) administered recognition tests designed for WMS-R Logical Memory and Visual Reproduction and found that both college student simulators and suspected malingerers were more likely to choose foils with a low probability of selection (i.e., grossly incorrect items).

On the WMS-III, Killgore and DellaPietra (2000a,b)

TABLE 20.2 Wechsler Memory Scale-III *Rarely Missed Index (RMI)* for Logical Memory Recognition

Item Number	RMI Point Value
12	−22
16	55
18	84
22	67
24	13
29	7

A cutting score of 136 or below has been used to suggest possible deliberate failure.
From Killgore and DellaPietra (2000a,b)

found six items from the delayed yes/no Logical Memory recognition trial for which most people (70%–80%) can make correct guesses without hearing the stories based upon question phrasing or conventional cues (see Table 20.2). These items were weighted to form the *Rarely Missed Index (RMI)*, which effectively discriminated neurological patients from college student simulators with greater than 98% accuracy (see Table 20.2). Simple supplemental testing such as this provides a method for testing response validity that is piggybacked on an existing neuropsychological test.

BATTERIES AND TEST SETS DEVELOPED FOR NEUROPSYCHOLOGICAL ASSESSMENT

Halstead-Reitan Battery (HRB)

Concerns about identifying response distortions in a neuropsychological examination were first raised in an HRB study, "Prospects for faking believable deficits on neuropsychological testing" (Heaton, Smith, et al., 1978). Discriminant function analysis obtained better rates of classification than did "blind" interpretations (i.e., viewing only test scores) by neuropsychologists, which ranged from chance to only 20% better than chance. Prior to this report experienced neuropsychologists tended to believe that they could generally identify patients who were not putting forth their best effort on testing. This paper was followed by a similar one showing the difficulty in classifying college student "malingerers" by HRB scores alone (Goebel, 1983). The two groups of simulators from the above studies differed on some tests—not always in the same direction—on the degree of performance impairment displayed. Subject differences may have accounted for the discrepancies between these two studies.

In both studies, the simulators underestimated impairment on the Category Test and all measures of the Tactile Performance Test. The simulators in Goebel's group performed significantly better than the patients on Part B of the Trail Making Test; the simulators in Heaton's study also completed this part of the test much faster than the patients and had significantly fewer errors. Both groups in this latter study had very large standard deviations on Part B, which accounts for the statistical nonsignificance despite there being a more than 30 sec difference between groups. Goebel's patients were significantly slower than the simulators on Part A of this test as well; he suggested that the ratio of Part B to Part A might be smaller in patients who were exaggerating their deficits. In fact, a separate report found that patients thought to be malingering on the basis of other tests had A/B ratios that were nearly one-half the size of those for patients with mild and moderate/severe TBI (Ruffolo, Guilmette, and Willis, 2000). These authors caution that although the Trail Making Test may provide useful information when malingering is suspected, no definitive cutting scores have been established and therefore classification decisions should not be based on this technique alone.

In both of these early studies, simulators overestimated the Speech Sounds Perception impairment. The simulators studied by Heaton and his group made many more inattention ("suppression") and finger recognition errors than did the trauma patients, were significantly slower than the patients on the Finger Tapping Test, and also feigned hand grip weakness relative to the patient group's much higher hand strength scores. Goebel found that simulators made significantly more errors on the Seashore Rhythm Test, a finding that has been independently observed (Gfeller and Cradock, 1998). Further, Gfeller and Cradock found that a cutting score of ≥9 errors on the Seashore Rhythm Test gave a 48% true positive and 98% true negative classification rate for TBI patients who were not in litigation compared with a sample of student simulators.

Bolter, Picano, and Zych (1985) identified 18 Category Test items that were infrequently missed by patients. These items discriminated simulators from TBI patients and healthy controls at a satisfactory level since simulators tended to underestimate how poorly patients would perform. Tenhula and Sweet (1996) added five more Category Test items to Bolter's 18 which together produced high rates of correct malingering and TBI classification. DiCarlo, Gfeller, and Oliveri (2000) have also replicated this finding with student simulators.

Several measures of response exaggeration and malingering using the entire Halstead-Reitan battery have been proposed. A discriminant function formula based upon performances by healthy control simulators and TBI patients was subsequently validated on a separate series of subjects (Mittenberg, Rotholc, et al., 1996). These authors then applied the formula to previously published HRB data sets reporting malingering and

were successful in correctly identifying 88% of their samples; but McKinzey and Russell (1997b), using this formula with other clinical samples including 120 TBI patients plus normal subjects, did not get quite as good results: their overall false positive rate was 27%; the TBI patients alone had a 22.5% false positive rate. This research group appropriately caution that a positive HRB index of malingering should not be the only score upon which that judgment is based. They also make an important point that is generalizable to most severely impaired performances on tests of neuropsychological functioning: Patients "with a highly elevated HRB [or other neuropsychological] profile ought to have corresponding etiology, course, symptoms, and neurological findings" (McKinzey and Russell, 1997b, p. 588).

Reitan and Wolfson (1997a) examined 40 TBI patients, half involved in litigation and half not, who were given the HRB on two occasions approximately one year apart. Finding that as a group the patients involved in litigation scored lower on the second test and those who were not litigants scored higher, Reitan and Wolfson concluded that "excess intersession variability"— such as lower scores on the second testing on each test—is a marker for nonreliable data. After comparing the groups statistically on each score, a conversion score for six test–retest differences was constructed by dividing the performance differences roughly into five equal levels and awarding scores of 1 to 5 for each test–retest difference (1 reflects considerable improvement, 5 indicates much poorer retest performance). Using a cutting score of 16 and below to separate groups, 90% of the litigants and 95% of the nonlitigants were correctly classified.

In order to develop guidelines for determining invalid responses on the HRB, Trueblood and Schmidt (1993)—using samples of eight probable malingerers and eight TBI patients and their matched controls—identified five HRB and two non-HRB tests which differentiated the groups statistically. Suspected malingerers gave lower performances. Trueblood and Schmidt then defined a cutting score (≥3 extreme scores) to infer probable malingering (see Table 20.3, p. 764). This criterion identified seven of the malingerers and six patients with questionable validity without misclassifying any control subjects. When reapplying these criteria to a larger sample, a 14% false positive rate was observed. A cross-validation study using only the five HRB measures from Trueblood and Schmidt misclassified 32% of a mixed patient group as probable malingerers, and the same error rate was present when limiting the sample to TBI patients (McKinzey and Russell, 1997a). A significant correlation between the severity of neuropsychological impairment as measured by the Average Impairment Rating and misclassification reflected a greater tendency toward misclassi-

TABLE 20.3 Halstead-Reitan Battery, Digit Span, and California Verbal Learning Test (CVLT) Scores Suggesting Response Invalidity

General Neuropsychological Deficit Scale	>44
Finger Agnosia	>3*
Finger Tip Number Writing	>5*
Seashore Rhythm Test	>8*
Speech Sounds Perception Test	>17*
WAIS-R Digit Span Scaled Score	<7
CVLT Recognition Score	<13

*Number of errors
From Trueblood and Schmidt (1993)

fication of patients with more serious brain impairment (McKinzey and Russell, 1997a). It should be noted that McKinzey and Russell's 1997a sample of patients was used to cross-validate the Mittenberg HRB malingering formula (McKinzey and Russell, 1997b, p. 487).

In addition to formal attempts to develop measures sensitive to response exaggeration, responses on several HRB measures can be compared to chance responding; as is the case with forced-choice symptom validity testing, a score lower than chance suggests intentional response distortion (Charter, 1994; see Table 20.4).

Luria-Nebraska Neuropsychological Battery (LNNB)

Simulated malingering on the LNNB was first investigated by Mensch and Woods (1986), who instructed healthy subjects to appear "brain damaged" and offered a small financial incentive for successful faking. Under the "malingering" condition, subjects performed more poorly on sensorimotor tasks and, in particular, were slow to complete motor tasks and to draw simple geometric designs, but their responses were generally accurate.

McKinzey, Podd, and their colleagues (1997) gathered data on college student "malingerers" from several studies, including those of Mensch and Woods (1986), and compared these responses to responses from a mixed group of neurological patients. They then identified and weighted items selectively associated with either the "malingering" or a patient group. The items were either simple tasks (e.g., simple motor and tactile skills, defining simple words, and phoneme writing) or more complex tasks (e.g., rearranging words to form a sentence, speed of picture arrangement type tasks, filling in the missing words in a sentence, rapid paragraph reading, performing serial 7s subtraction, understanding complex grammatical construction, and list learning). The sum of the simple tasks was compared to that of the more complex ones for group assignment: the "malingerers" did relatively poorly on the motor/simple tasks enabling the authors to correctly classify 30 of 34 college student "malingerers" and all 34 patients; cross-validation with similar samples had a comparable level of success.

Golden and Grier (1998) claim that poor motivation and malingering can be identified on the LNNB using specific scores and formulae, analysis of the 55 forced-choice items, internal consistency of the scores, and test–retest comparisons for both scales and items. As is true for all techniques to detect malingering, they also emphasize the need to put LNNB scores in the context of neurological and historical information.

Other test combinations

Investigations of other combinations of existing tests have searched for more reliable ways to assess performance validity. J.E. Meyers, Galinsky, and Volbrecht (1999) examined four tests that they use routinely in clinical examinations (Judgment of Line Orientation, Token Test, Dichotic Listening, and a 20-item forced-choice memory test). They drew their subject samples from patient files (moderate/severe TBI, TBI in litigation, mild TBI not in litigation) and also included healthy volunteers and simulators ("normally functioning individuals"). They obtained their classification criterion by subtracting 1 point from the lowest performance of the moderate/severe injury group. Thus, the cutting score was lower than the poorest score made by their most severely impaired patients. A criterion of at least one of four test scores below the "lower than

TABLE 20.4 Confidence Intervals (CIs) for Random Responses for Several Halstead-Reitan Battery Tests

	90% CI	95% CI	99% CI
Category Test	146–167	145–169	141–173
Subtests II, VII	13–19	12–19	12–21
Subtests III, VI	26–35	26–36	24–38
Speech Sounds Perception Test	40–51	39–52	38–55
Seashore Rhythm Test	11–19	10–20	8–22

From Charter (1994)

low criterion" misclassified none of the nonlitigating sample (healthy controls, mild TBI patients who were not claimants). In contrast, 24% of the litigating patients "failed" at least one of the four tests, yielding a 100% specificity and 95% sensitivity in their sample of litigants, nonlitigants, and simulators. An extension of this procedure involves nine tests—adding Finger Tapping, Rey Complex Figure, "Reliable Digit Span" (longest span forward plus longest span reversed), Sentence Repetition, Auditory Verbal Learning Test (J.E. Meyers and Volbrecht, 2003). Two or more performances below cut-off scores placed at levels well in the *defective* range was predictive of patients suspected of malingering and graduate students instructed to "fake" a brain injury. It is interesting to note that none of the 32 normal control subjects provided a false positive record.

Suhr, Tranel, and their colleagues (1997) used cut-off scores derived from Digit Span, the Benton Visual Retention test, and two Auditory-Verbal Learning Test measures (recognition score, atypical recognition failures). The cut-off score for each test was selected so that nonlitigating patients with mild or moderate TBI would not be misclassified as malingerers. When two or more cut-off scores were exceeded, the classification rate for probable malingering was only 25%, insufficient for clinical use.

Basing a discriminant analysis on Digit Span, the Knox Cube Test, and Warrington's Recognition Memory Test, Iverson and Franzen (1994) reported very high rates of correct classification (98%!) of TBI patients, college students simulating malingering, and healthy controls. These authors note, however, that they made no attempt to discourage the simulators from producing unbelievable memory deficits, which likely inflated the correct classification rates.

E. Strauss, Hultsch, and their colleagues (1999) studying the Reliable Digit Span (see p. 761), Victoria Symptom Validity Test (see pp. 775–776), and Vocabulary − Digit Span difference in college student "malingerers" and controls found good classification rates for the "malingering" (80%) and control (100%) groups. However, only accuracy on the Victoria "hard" items made a unique contribution to group prediction.

Memory Tests

Auditory-Verbal Learning Test (AVLT)

Many verbal memory tests, when used to identify poorly motivated or malingering subjects, rely on the well-documented advantage of recognition over recall in memory testing. For the AVLT, recognition of as few

or fewer words than recalled immediately following the distraction trial (trial VI) or after the delayed recall trial (VII) should raise the examiner's suspicions regarding the patient's effort (Bernard, 1990; Bernard, Houston, and Natoli, 1993; Chouinard and Rouleau, 1997). Most healthy subjects recalling 12 or fewer words will recognize three or four more than they pulled up in free recall (M. Schmidt, 1996). With significant brain injury, moreover, normal expectations no longer hold, leaving open the possibility that the patient's performance could be misjudged with painful consequences for the patient if the scores are interpreted outside the context of the entire patient history and presentation.

L.M. Binder, Villaneuva, and their coworkers (1993) observed that mild TBI patients who performed poorly on the Portland Digit Recognition Test (PDRT, see pp. 772–773) made lower scores on the 50-word recognition format (see pp. 425–426) than did mild TBI patients in whom motivation was not suspect. Similarly, Suhr, Tranel, and their colleagues (1997) found mild TBI compensation-seeking patients (those whose records indicated contradictory or excessive symptoms or who had ≥25% failures on Hiscock and Hiscock's [1989] Symptom Validity Technique, suggesting that they were probably malingering) performed worse than other head injury (including compensation seekers with injury-consistent records) and psychiatric groups. In addition, suspected malingers were less likely to recognize words after demonstrating some free recall (recalled on at least three learning trials) for those words. In a separate study, simulators (age range 18 to 59) performed poorly on the AVLT recognition trial (K.A. Flowers, Sheridan, and Shadbolt, 1996). Yet college students offered a monetary incentive to "malinger" successfully recognized more items than they recalled, about as many as control subjects, suggesting that this may not be a universally sure technique for identifying malingerers (K. Sullivan, Deffenti, and Keane, 2002).

Analysis of the serial position of words in the list recalled may be a potentially useful technique for evaluating the validity of list-learning tasks (see p. 422). Brandt (1988) demonstrated that amnesic patients recalled virtually none of the first words on the list but 40% of those most recently given. Although simulators gave fewer responses overall, both controls and simulators showed the expected primacy and recency effects. Brandt's observations have been replicated (K.A. Flowers, Sheridan, and Shadbolt, 1996; K. Sullivan, Deffenti, and Keane, 2002), but others have either not seen this effect (Bernard, Houston, and Natoli, 1993; Suhr, Tranel, et al., 1997) or have observed an opposite pattern (Bernard, 1991). Thus, this promising technique is not as yet reliably validated.

In a college student simulation study examining the

effects of warning the subject about validity testing, Suhr and Gunstad (2000) found that a combination of multiple AVLT measures was less sensitive to the warning than the Portland Digit Recognition Test (see p. 773). The pattern analysis measures included Learning vs. Recognition, Recognition vs. Recall, Learning Span, and Delayed Recall (within 30 to 60 mins). A score on even one of these four measures that was below threshold (i.e., just under the lowest score obtained by a group of mild TBI patients) correctly classified as "malingerers" 74% of simulators not warned and 85% of warned simulators.

California Verbal Learning Test (CVLT)

This popular test generates more opportunities for detecting suspect performances than the AVLT since so many different scores are available. As with the AVLT, recognition testing by itself can be quite informative. In one report, CVLT recognition testing was lower in patients who displayed below chance performance on a modified form of the Hiscock and Hiscock Symptom Validity Technique (Trueblood and Schmidt, 1993); and in fact, recognition memory testing for the CVLT produced hit rates that were as good as derived malingering measures (Trueblood, 1994). On replication, however, this method misidentified as malingering 32% of a mixed clinical sample with no financial incentive to perform poorly (McKinzey and Russell, 1997a).

Another study examined multiple CVLT measures made by a sample of litigating mild TBI patients (no loss of consciousness [LOC] or LOC <5 mins) and compared their performances with those of TBI patients who had sustained significant injuries (Millis, Putnam, et al., 1995). Identification of mild TBI patients thought to be underresponding was based on chance or below chance performance on at least one of Warrington's two recognition memory tests (see pp. 495–497) on which no severely injured TBI patients had performed at or below chance. Mild TBI patients with suspected incomplete effort gave poorer performances than more severely injured patients on CVLT score categories for Total Trials 1–5, Recognition Discriminability, Recognition Hits, and Long-Delay Cued Recall. These scores separated the groups but Recognition Hits differentiated groups better than any other, again demonstrating the value of recognition testing for assessing the validity of memory performances. These findings have been cross-validated in independent samples with acceptable sensitivity and specificity levels (R. Baker et al., 2000; Coleman et al., 1998; Sweet, Wolfe et al., 2000). Coaching subjects how to perform did negate the tendency of college student simulators to overesti-

mate the memory impairment associated with mild TBI on the CVLT (Coleman, et al., 1998). Coaching was less effective, however, on derived CVLT scores such as Recognition Discriminability.

The CVLT revision contains a two-item forced-choice recognition trial for the 16 words in the primary list (Delis, Kramer, Kaplan, and Ober, 2000). Scores of 4/16 or fewer correct are significantly lower than would be expected if a person were responding randomly ($p <$ .05). However, future studies may demonstrate a range of scores that, although not statistically different from chance responding (e.g., 5/16), suggest incomplete effort.

Benton Visual Retention Test (BVRT)

Benton and Spreen (1961) investigated the effects of deliberate faking on the 10-sec recall administration (A) of this test by comparing the performances of brain injured patients with those of college student simulators. The simulators made more distortion errors than did the patients but fewer omission errors; this finding has been replicated (Suhr, Tranel, et al., 1997). Patients were more likely to forget the small peripheral figures and to perseverate than were the simulators. In a similar study, the overall error profile of students faking "feeble-mindedness" was like that of mentally retarded patients (Spreen and Benton, 1963), with simulators making more errors and giving fewer correct responses than patients (see Sivan, 1992). More recently, probable malingerers again gave fewer correct responses and made significantly more errors that did nonmalingering patients with diagnoses of mild/moderate or severe TBI, or of Somatization Disorder or Depression (Suhr, Tranel, et al., 1997).

Complex Figure Test (CFT)

Bernard (1990), studying only college student simulators, found that they obtained scores 4 points lower than students not told to simulate on copy and 6 to 8 points lower on recall (30 min delay) trials of the Rey-Osterrieth CFT (RCFT). A simulating group with a $50 incentive to simulate effectively and one without such an incentive performed similarly. Slightly greater differences showed up in a subsequent study of college student simulators (6 points for RCFT copy, 10 points for RCFT recall) (Bernard, Houston, and Natoli, 1993). In contrast, no relationship was found between the CFT recall trials of TBI patients and their classification (by AVLT recognition) as probable malingerers in a study including TBI patients of varying severity and patients with either depression or somatization disorders (Suhr, Tranel, et al., 1997).

Specific patterns suggestive of poor performance emerged when comparing immediate and delayed CFT recall trials with recognition (J.E. Meyers and Volbrecht, 1999). For litigating and nonlitigating patients with mild TBI, those seeking compensation produced more attention and storage error patterns, a pattern that is more consistent with significant TBI than typical mild injury. The litigating patients also performed less well on standard CFT memory measures, including immediate and delayed recall, as well as delayed recognition. Of course, some patients were litigating because their injuries had been more severe and disabling. CFT recall scores were lower for college student simulators, yet they showed a normal practice effect over a three-week period (Demakis, 1999).

Recognition Memory Test (RMT)

Warrington's RMT lends itself to symptom validity testing since it is based on a 50-item forced two-choice recognition format for both words and faces. As with all tests in which probability levels for chance responding can be established, scores significantly below chance provide strong evidence that correct responses are actively being avoided (see Symptom Validity Testing, pp. 770–772). As with other forced-choice formats, low performance levels on the RMT that do not meet the "significantly below chance" criterion raise suspicions of suboptimal performance.

Millis (1992) reported that ten litigating patients with mild TBI obtained lower scores than patients with severe TBI, but their scores were not statistically below chance. Using Warrington's norms, 50% of the moderate/severe TBI patients' performances fell below the fifth percentile on both the Words and Faces tests; 90% of the claimants scored at this level on Words, and 78% were below the fifth percentile on Faces. In contrast, 25% of the moderately/severely injured group performed above the 50th percentile on Words and 10% on Faces, although none of the claimant group achieved scores that high. Millis and Putnam (1994) cross-validated this study and again achieved good group separation between the poorer performing mild TBI claimants and severe trauma patients. A discriminant function analysis yielded an overall correct classification rate of 83% (85% mild TBI in litigation, 82% moderate/severe TBI). Iverson and Franzen (1994) reported good classification rates with this procedure.

Since the RMT is a memory test, it is possible that patients with severe memory deficits may perform at chance levels. Fortunately, few in an independent sample of moderate/severe TBI patients scored 25 or lower on either the Words or Faces subtest, suggesting that chance performance on this test occurs infrequently when due to neurological impairment alone (Millis and Putnam, 1996).

Memory Assessment Scales (MAS)

Beetar and Williams (1995) assigned college students to either a malingering or control condition and administered computerized versions of the MAS, Dot Counting, Rey 15-item Memory Test, and a forced-choice symptom validity test. Overall, college student "malingerers" performed below students not told to simulate, in the *low average* range on MAS tests. Interestingly, they did best on free recall measures (e.g., List Acquisition and Visual Recall) but worse on recognition tests and delayed measures. The forced-choice test developed by these authors also included a free recall component, and a similar pattern was observed— no difference between groups on recall but a statistically significant difference on recognition trials. Unfortunately, this study did not include patients with neurologic injuries.

Single Tests

Bender-Gestalt

Hutt (1985) recommended that the copy administration of the Bender be readministered if malingering or poor motivation is suspected and, if possible, given after a delay of several days. The longer the delay between the initial testing and the retest, the more likely it will be that subjects who have deliberately altered their reproductions will have forgotten what changes they had made, resulting in inconsistent errors. If a question remains about the patient's willingness to perform well after a delayed retest, Hutt suggests that the cards be readministered for copying in the inverse position as few persons would be able to maintain the same deliberate distortions with the changed gestalt.

Four general criteria identified college students attempting to produce "organic" Bender responses (A.R. Bruhn and Reed, 1975): (1) Patients with genuine impairments tend to simplify, not complicate, their drawings. (2) When a patient markedly distorts an element in one design, similar elements in other designs will show the same kind of distortion. (3) Patients are unlikely to make both good and poor copies of designs at the same difficulty level. (4) Some kinds of distortion are made only by brain injured patients, such as rotations and difficulty with the intersection of card 6.

Loretta Bender (1938) alluded to distinct response patterns associated with malingering when describing the performance of six patients who were asked to feign "mental impairment." These patterns occurred more frequently in drawings by patients feigning schizophrenia than in schizophrenia patients or nonpsychotic inpatients.

A somewhat different and more closely elaborated set of Bender faking criteria was used by Schretlen, Wilkins, and their colleagues (1992): (a) inhibited figure size (the entire figure is no larger than 3.2 cm^2); (b) changed position (figures rotated more than 45°); (c) distorted relationship (figure in which the relationship between correctly copied parts has been altered); (d) complex additions (figures given additional complex or bizarre details); (e) gross simplification (figures drawn at a developmental level of six years or less [see Bender, 1938]); and (f) inconsistent form quality (within a complete set of drawings, figures drawn both at developmental levels of six years or less and nine years or more). The score is 1 point for each figure meeting the criteria a to e plus 1 point if f is satisfied. With these criteria, prison inmates instructed to fake insanity obtained significantly higher scores (8.8 ± 5.2 in one study, 10.8 ± 2.8 in another) than a group of mixed, mostly psychotic, psychiatric patients (3.9 ± 2.8) and one of mostly schizophrenic patients (3.2 ± 2.0). Scores on changed position, distorted relationship, and gross simplification best discriminated faking subjects from the psychiatric group. The optimal discriminant function identified only 50% of the simulators although almost all nonfakers were correctly classified. How well these criteria identify patients exaggerating cognitive rather than psychiatric impairment remains to be established.

Paced Auditory Serial Addition Test (PASAT)

Gronwall (1977) described two PASAT response patterns that suggest possible incomplete effort or response bias. Concussion patients and healthy subjects are more efficient—fewer errors and omissions—on the first third of each trial. In addition, the number of correct responses decreases as the rate at which numbers are given increases. It is therefore unlikely for response accuracy to remain at its initial level throughout a trial, particularly throughout all trials given in a session. It is perhaps even more unlikely for the score not to drop noticeably as administration speed increases. Gronwall also indicated that it would be unusual for time-per-response to remain the same at all levels of test difficulty.

As is the case with many cognitive ability tests, the level of performance may raise suspicion of performance invalidity. In a simulation study, college student "malingerers" achieved lower scores on the PASAT than patients with mild to moderate TBI (E. Strauss, Spel-

lacy, et al., 1994). Simple reaction time, however, provided better group differentiation than did the PASAT.

Wisconsin Card Sorting Test (WCST)

Reasoning that the number of obtainable WCST categories would be readily apparent to potential malingerers, less obvious measures—such as response perseveration—appeared more likely to discriminate TBI patients from college students instructed to simulate such injuries (Bernard, McGrath, and Houston, 1996). As predicted, simulators achieved significantly fewer categories than TBI patients who were mildly to moderately impaired based upon the HRB Average Impairment Rating or had documented cerebral disorders. Further, comparing these simulators' scores to just the scores of the TBI group showed that the latter group made more perseveration errors, as anticipated. Random error responses did not distinguish groups. Discriminant function analysis using Categories and Perseverative Errors correctly classified 98% of the validation sample of TBI patients and college student simulators and 91% of a cross-validation sample. Similar analyses comparing college student simulators to a mixed-etiology sample of neurology patients yielded similar classification accuracy rates for both the initial and cross-validation samples.

Suhr and Boyer (1999) also found that the number of WCST categories was reduced, both in patients thought to be malingering and in college student simulators. Rather than Perseverative Errors, however, "failing to maintain set" was the critical variable that distinguished brain injured subjects from the others with an 82% sensitivity and 93% specificity. The student malingerers obtained half as many categories as controls and failed to maintain set twice as often. Failure to maintain set occurs infrequently in patients with neurologic impairment, including those with frontal lobe involvement. One cross-validation study found that Bernard, McGrath, and Houston's (1996) malingering formula, based on the discriminant function analysis, misclassified only 5% of a well-screened sample of TBI patients to exclude those with external incentives to perform poorly as malingering (Donders, 1999). However, neither the procedures of Bernard and his colleagues nor those of Suhr and Boyer proved sensitive to response exaggeration defined by poor performance on forced-choice symptom validity testing (see pp. 770–772) (A. Miller et al., 2000).

Raven's Progressive Matrices (RPM)

Because this test's difficulty increases across the five problem sets, accuracy tends to decrease across the sets.

By comparing the first two sets (A, B) to the last two sets (D, E) for three groups—nursing student and military volunteers instructed to perform normally and again to "fake substantially and convincingly," a second group of military volunteers tested only once under normal instructions, and patients with neurological impairments—Gudjonsson and Shackleton (1986) developed a formula to indicate suboptimal effort: $(2A + B) - (D + 2E)$. They observed that faking subjects had a flatter rate of decay across the sets resulting from missing too many items in the easier series. Different cutting scores were derived as a function of total correct scores across all five test sets from the non-faking sample and from Table 1 in Raven's 1960 manual. These cutting scores identified 83% of the simulators and 95% of the patient and healthy volunteer groups. Applying this formula to 381 subjects from the RPM 1998 standardization sample and 46 patients classified as malingerers, McKinzey, Podd, and their colleagues (1999) identified 74% of the malingering group with only a 5% false positive rate. This formula will have poorer sensitivity for patients with very low overall scores whose false positive rate will be greater. Moreover, the technique for identifying "malingerers" was not reported and the standardization group clearly took the test in a different setting and under different circumstances than the "malingering" group. Other studies using college student simulators have produced less impressive results (Wogar et al., 1998).

Knox Cube Test (KCT)

The usefulness of this test for identifying response bias was examined by Iverson and Franzen (1994). Both the total number of reproduced sequences and the longest series of taps correctly reproduced were sensitive to the effects of simulated malingering by college students and penitentiary inmates. Compared to patients with mild or moderate TBI, the "malingering" subjects had significantly reduced scores for both total raw score and memory span. The cutting scores which best identified subjects in the "malingering" sample were *total correct* <3 (72% correctly identified) and *span length* <4 (42% correctly identified).

Tests with a Significant Motor Component

Motor performance is an area in which deliberate failures tend to be obvious. In extreme cases, patients may obtain scores close to zero when their grip strength is tested with a dynamometer. Heaton, Smith, and their colleagues (1978) found that the simulating group gave distinctly inferior responses on tests of motor functioning and of sensory and perceptual awareness, a finding that has been replicated (L.M. Binder and Willis, 1991).

Grip strength, finger tapping, and Grooved Pegboard Test scores for moderate to severe TBI patients were compared to scores of probable malingerers who had performed poorly on at least one motor test (Greiffenstein, Baker, and Gola, 1996b). The brain injured patients displayed the expected physiological complexity gradient across tasks proposed by Haaland and Yeo (1989): grip strength > finger tapping > Grooved Pegboard. Suspected malingerers produced the opposite pattern, with poorest scores on grip strength—the test requiring the simplest kind of response—and the best scores on Grooved Pegboard. This pattern was interpreted as a nonneurologic contribution to the probable malingering group performance. These findings were not observed in a simulation design using college students whose performances displayed a normal gradient according to task complexity (Rapport, Farchione, et al., 1998).

Reaction Time (RT)

Several authors have commented on the potential utility of speed of response for identifying exaggerated disability (Goebel, 1983; Resnick, 1984). Brandt (1988) noted the potential of reaction time in that efforts to respond incorrectly would require slower reaction times. Thus, unusually long reaction times may reflect deliberately reduced performances. In some cases, response times may exceed the norm by several hundred percent (E. Strauss, Spellacy, et al., 1994).

Reaction time offers the potential for sophisticated assessment of the validity of the performance since it typically involves several conditions of differing complexity for comparisons and requires a response that is difficult to manipulate consistently. For example, it is unlikely that a patient attempting to perform poorly could unfailingly add 300–500 msec to each response—or even to know how much delay is realistic.

Wogar and her colleagues (1998) used this technique in a matching-to-sample reaction time task with eight levels of graded complexity. Reaction time generally increases linearly, with brain impaired patients showing a greater proportional increase in latency as stimulus complexity increases. As predicted, TBI patients with a PTA of at least 12 hours had increasingly slower reaction times than control subjects as the task's information content and stimulus complexity increased. Healthy volunteers instructed to simulate cognitive impairment did not respond with a similarly sharp and steady increase in response time; while their responses were slower, their score profile was essentially parallel to that of a nonsimulating group of healthy volunteers from the community. The proportionate latency discrepancies identified 14/20 simulators while misclassifying 2/20 nonsimulators and 2/25 patients. A similar "performance curve" technique for group classification using scores for each of the increasingly difficult five sets of Raven's Matrices correctly classified only six of these simulators.

Reaction time scores can be obtained with many of the computer-based symptom validity digit recognition tests (see pp. 776–777), but few studies have formally investigated these reaction time data to identify insufficient test-taking motivation. Although reaction time by itself did not effectively discriminate between groups, detection of coached college student "malingerers" increased from 47% to 70% by including a reaction time measure with a computerized version of the Portland Digit Recognition Test (Rose et al., 1995). In this study, coached and uncoached student simulators did not differ in their reaction times; both groups had longer and more variable reaction times compared to student control subjects, but patients in the moderate to severe TBI group showed considerable overlap with the "malingering" groups.

As part of the Victoria Symptom Validity Test, which is a forced-choice digit recognition task, separate reaction time measures are obtained for the easy items—in which the target number is readily identified since it differs from its foil on all five digits—and the hard items—in which the target and foil differ only by the interposition of two different digits in the string of five (see pp. 772–773). Control subjects performed faster than "malingerers"—all college students—on both the easy and hard digit sequences, but the magnitude of the difference was greater for the hard digit series (E. Strauss, Hultsch, et al., 1999). Beetar and Williams (1995) recorded response times from a number of different computerized neuropsychological tests and observed that college student "malingerers" performed more slowly than their control counterparts. These authors caution, however, that patients' increased response times may simply reflect neurologic impairment or factors such as test-related anxiety or depression. Fortunately, for tests with different levels of difficulty or complexity, the interaction between response speed and difficulty level will aid in interpreting the findings.

SPECIAL TECHNIQUES TO ASSESS RESPONSE VALIDITY

Symptom Validity Testing (SVT)

Not infrequently questions arise concerning the extent to which patients' symptoms or complaints accurately reflect a disability, especially when compensation claims are involved. Thus it is not surprising that a number of techniques for assessing response bias have been developed. Pankrantz (1979), who introduced the term "Symptom Validity Testing" (SVT), used this technique for basing validity judgments on statistical probability, always testing the symptoms of which the patient complained. Many examiners now reserve the term *SVT* to describe tests that employ forced-choice responding without regard for the nature of the patient's complaints.

Although this technique is most often used to examine complaints of impaired memory, it can readily be adapted to sensory and perceptual complaints as well, such as, "blindness, color blindness, tunnel vision, blurry vision, deafness, paresthesias" (Pankratz, 1988; see also L.M. Binder, 1992). In applying this technique to questions of malingering or psychogenic complaints, it is important to focus on the problems presented by the patients themselves: to use the same technique regardless of patients' complaints may be inappropriate. *"Test exactly what the patient says that he can't do. You devise a test for each person—an individual strategy for each patient. In this way you motivate the patient to demonstrate the deficiency in what he says or believes he can't do"* (Pankratz, personal communication [mdl], July 1993).

This technique requires patients to make a series of forced-choice decisions about a simple, two-alternative problem involving their symptoms or complaints (Pankratz, 1979, 1998; Pankratz, Fausti, and Peed, 1975). By chance alone, approximately 50% of the choices will be correct. This is the expected result when patients' complaints are valid, e.g., when they are deaf, have a severe memory impairment, or have lost position sense in their toes. Since many trials are conducted, even quite small deviations from the expected value become statistically significant. For example, the occurrence of a number correct of 41 or fewer in 100 trials is worse than chance at the $P < .05$ level, allowing the examiner to infer that correct answers may have been actively avoided. If doubt remains, a second set of 100 trials will clarify the question since the likelihood of occurrence of two independent trials each having a probability below the .05 level is $P = .0025$ $(.05 \times .05)$.

The adaptability of this approach to perceptual and memory complaints is limited only by the examiner's imagination. The task is presented as a straightforward test of the claimed disability. Loss of feeling on the hand, for example, can be tested by having patients tell whether they were touched on the palm or the back, or on the thumb or middle finger. A patient with a visual complaint, such as eyesight too blurry for reading, can be shown two cards, each containing a different simple word or phrase. For testing "blurred" vision, the examiner can make up cards printed in small type with the statements "This card is number one" and "Number two is this card." The examiner asks the patient to identify the card shown as "one" or "two."

SVT confronts exaggerating patients quite directly since it is difficult to maintain a properly randomized response pattern over many trials that will result in a chance performance. When the examiner provides item feedback, patients may get the impression that they are doing better than they thought they could as they often hear that they are correct. The impression of doing well can have an unsettling effect on subjects exaggerating their deficits. Patients who attempt to avoid the confrontation by giving most or all of one kind of answer are obviously uncooperative. Those who naively give a wrong answer more often than chance betray their ability to identify correct answers. To avoid the dilemma presented by this technique, patients may attempt to subvert the procedure by circumventing it or withdrawing altogether. Pankratz (1979) recommended providing the patient with a "neurological" rationale for regaining the function in question by means of this technique. For example, in treating patients with numb and paralyzed limbs, he explains the procedure is an attempt to determine whether any "nerve pathways" are "still available."

The statistical probabilities underlying SVT interpretations are based on the assumption that the patient is unbiased and responding randomly. Consequently, the probabilities alone lead to a conservative inference. Patients with genuine cognitive or somatosensory deficits, unless very severely impaired, typically do not display a random response pattern and therefore perform at better than chance levels. Nor do most patients who exaggerate their complaints perform worse than chance. These findings have led to procedures for making comparisons to specific reference groups, such as patients with well-documented brain disorders (e.g., see R.C. Martin, Bolter, and their colleagues, 1993). When patients with mild TBI, for example, perform less well on a procedure examining memory complaints than do patients with severe TBI, insufficient effort can be suspected. Excepting the more complex and cognitively demanding Portland Digit Recognition Test, all two-choice SVTs involving simple number recognition show a remarkable performance consistency, with a "90% correct" rule often being effective in discriminating subjects who are not performing appropriately from those with genuine brain injuries (Sweet, 1999b).

Since SVT techniques—especially those purportedly examining "memory"—for evaluating response validity have their origins in many traditional neuropsychological tests, these techniques risk confounding cognitive ability with validity assessment. Due to this limitation, van Gorp, Humphrey, Kalechstein, and their coworkers (1999) have argued that independent measures of "validity test" validity must be obtained.

In comparisons of several procedures to assess response distortion, forced-choice recognition tests were superior to others (Vickery et al., 2001). L.M. Etcoff and Kampfer (1996) evaluated studies of 23 validity indicator scores for use in forensic TBI cases, including measures of memory and five HRB tests (SVTs with forced-choice visual stimuli were not considered). Each measure was rated for "level of certainty." Those receiving a rating of "definite" were the 72-item and 36-item versions of the Hiscocks' test, the Portland Digit Recognition Test (72- and 54-item versions), MMPI *F/F-K*, WAIS-R Digit Span <4, and Speech Sounds Perception errors ≥24. Given the additional information provided by more recent studies—and especially studies including visual SVTs and clinical reports—Etcoff and Kampfer's conclusions should be considered useful but only advisory.

Many patients with known or suspected brain dysfunction have memory impairments, and lay persons frequently interpret the mental inefficiency associated with attention disorders as "memory problems." Thus poor memory is among the most common complaints of persons seeking or referred for neuropsychological assessment (B. Gordon, 1995). For this reason, many symptom validity techniques developed for general use preserve face validity as "memory" tests. Some memory-based techniques for assessing response validity are too easy for most patients to fail. Sophisticated persons who appreciate how simple these tests are will perform at acceptable levels. Guilmette, Whelihan, and their coworkers (1996) studied whether the timing of validity testing of memory would affect patients' performances. Disability claimants made higher scores on validity tests when they were given last. The Guilmette group hypothesized that this order effect resulted from previous exposure to the clinical memory tests, which served to highlight the difference in difficulty levels between them and the easier SVT memory procedures.

For some examinees a systematic evaluation of performance validity is necessary. Including SVT assessment benefits most patients who do not exaggerate or fabricate their neuropsychological symptoms. The formal assessment of performance validity allows the neuropsychologist to make inferences about cognitive or emotional impairment that can best withstand questioning by others, as can occur in litigation or compensation claim evaluations.

To use these techniques responsibly, the examiner must appreciate that patients whose scores fall into suspected ranges may not be intentionally malingering.

Cripe (2002) documents the conditions and attitudes that may

> . . . result in a person shutting down and not performing at maximum effort. These include: illness, pain, fatigue, avoidance of concentrating, frustration with the doctor–patient relationship, psychological defenses, unhappiness with the evaluation situation, depression, or brain dysfunction itself. To conclude that poor performance on a task of effort excludes the presence of a genuine medical condition and is solid evidence of malingering is a biased leap of faith not supported by either the facts or common sense. (p. 104)

Cripe also demonstrates the fallacy in assuming that responses above the chance level necessarily rule out malingering: he had 12 persons each respond randomly to 36 Portland Digit Recognition Test cards; of the 12, only three scored at or below chance level. He points out that, especially with this low a number of trials, a randomly responding subject could perform as well above chance as below.

Forced-Choice Tests

Forced-Choice Test (Hiscock and Hiscock, 1989)[1]

This is the first widely adopted digit recognition test procedure for examining the validity of memory complaints. The Forced-Choice Test requires subjects to identify which of two five-digit numbers shown on a card was the same as a number seen prior to a brief delay. Each of eight target numbers differs by two or more digits from its foil, including either the first or the last digit. Three sets of 24 trials have delays of 5, 10, and 15 sec, for a total of 72 trials. Before beginning the second and third trial sets with the longer delays, the examiner tells patients that because they have done so well the test will be made more difficult. Since there is no evidence that the longer delays increase the likelihood of failure, Prigatano and Amin (1993) recommend that, rather than suggesting that the task becomes more difficult, the examiner should explain before giving the second and third trial sets that the delays will be longer "to see if you are still able to remember the numbers after longer periods of time" (p. 545).

Both postconcussional patients and patients suffering from other brain disorders averaged over 99% correct responses, in contrast to a group of suspected malingerers whose correct responses averaged only 74% (Prigatano and Amin, 1993). Administering this technique to groups of brain injured patients in acute rehabilitation, psychiatric inpatients, nonpatients under standard conditions, and nonpatients asked to simulate memory impairment, Guilmette, Hart, and Giuliano (1993) found that both patient groups made almost perfect scores, nonpatients made no errors, while college student simulators made an average of 44 ± 15 correct responses with 34% of their scores falling below chance. These authors concluded that even a few errors should raise the suspicion of poor motivation on a test this easy. In a separate study, Prigatano, Smason, and their colleagues (1997) suggested that, in the absence of a frank dementia, scores below 95% should be considered suggestive of incomplete effort. Patients with aphasia, frontal lobe injury, temporal lobe dysfunction, and TBI consistently displayed accuracy levels of at least 95%, but patients with probable Alzheimer's disease performed at levels comparable to suspected malingerers.

With a 36-item version of this test, Guilmette, Hart, Giuliano, and Leininger (1994) reported that a criterion of 90% correctly classified all 20 patients with brain injury, 19/20 psychiatric patients, and 17/20 student simulators. A comparison of these findings with the same groups' performances on Warrington's Recognition Memory Test found that this version of the Forced-Choice Test was more effective in classifying these patients and simulators correctly. D'Arcy and McGlone (2000) observed that all 14 patients with profound amnesia who were tested with the 36-item version obtained perfect scores. In this same sample, two patients performed below the cutting score on the Rey 15-Item Memory Test.

Portland Digit Recognition Test (PDRT)[1]

To increase the sensitivity of the Forced-Choice Test, L.M. Binder (1993b; with Willis, 1991) developed a technique incorporating a series of distraction procedures. The PDRT also consists of 72 trials in each of which a five-digit number is spoken at a one-per-second rate followed—at different time intervals—by a card on which is printed both the target number and a different five-digit number. The numbers are printed one above the other on a card with the target position varied randomly. This administration differs from the Hiscock and Hiscock procedures not only in its auditory presentation but also because the time intervals are longer—5 and 15 sec for the first two blocks of 18 trials each (the Easy set), 30 sec for the last two 18-trial blocks (the Hard set)—and because the subject counts backwards from 20 when the delay is 5 sec, from 50 when it is 15 sec, and from 100 for the 30 sec intervals.

---

[1]For instructions on making up this test material, write to Merrill C. Hiscock, Ph.D., Dept. of Psychology, Heyne Bldg., #126, University of Houston, Houston, TX 77204-5022.

[1]PDRT materials can be purchased from Laurence M. Binder, Ph.D., 4900 SW Griffith Dr., #244, Beaverton, OR 97005-2913.

The interposed distraction task incorporates a working memory component into the procedure, increasing the likelihood that performance may be affected by patients with frontal lobe injuries and/or pronounced attentional deficits (Stuss, Ely, et al., 1985; Stuss, Stetham, Hugenholtz, and Richard, 1989). Amnesic patients also performed poorly when a distraction activity (e.g., counting backwards from a three-digit number for 20 sec) was interposed between exposure to the stimuli and recall, although they performed as well as control subjects when not distracted during the 20 sec delay period (G.A. Baker et al., 1993). As noted by L.M. Binder and Willis (1991), "the PDRT may measure, in addition to motivation, divided attention and recent memory, particularly on the hard items" (p. 179). This confounding effect of the PDRT showed up in 13 patients—mostly TBI, but several with toxic exposures and one with history of an anoxic episode—as 11 of these patients performed the same on both the PDRT and Consonant Trigrams (five *within normal limits*, six in the *impaired* range). Of the two who performed differently on these tests, one did well on the PDRT and poorly on Consonant Trigrams, the other showed the opposite success/failure pattern. These proportions are at a .05 probability level (tested by a 2×2 Contingency Table: Finney et al., 1963). These findings suggest that the interference format may make this technique as much a measure of working memory as anything else (mdl: sample from private practice).

Cut-off scores (19 correct for the Easy set, 18 correct for the Hard set, 39 correct for the test as a whole) were derived from the lowest scores of a group of brain injured patients in the Veteran's Affairs system who may or may not have had memory or attentional complaints (these data were not published) and who were not seeking financial compensation (some already had it) (L.M. Binder and Willis, 1991). L.M. Binder (1993b) reported that 33% of a select group of mild head trauma patients with compensation claims—mostly screened and referred by defense lawyers—made PDRT scores that fell below cut-off scores, but that only 17% performed below chance levels, a finding that has been observed elsewhere (e.g., Wiggins and Brandt, 1988). In patients with more significant TBI, 18% performed below the cut-off score and 3% performed below chance levels.

PDRT administration is very time consuming, taking the better part of an hour which, as Larrabee (1990) notes, provides no information about the patient's neuropsychological status. Moreover, patients who have performed at their best on all other tests have reported becoming sufficiently annoyed—either because it is a protractedly boring test to take or because they feel that it insults their intelligence—that after a while they give answers without attending to the task. These problems may be alleviated by using a shortened procedure when compensation claimants' responses to the 36 easy items give no reason for the examiner to suspect their motivation (Binder, 1993a). In these cases, Binder advises that the test can be discontinued for patients who get 7 of 7 or 7 of 8 of the first nine items correct on the 30-sec delay trial. Coached and uncoached "malingerers" differed in their overall scores on the PDRT, with better scores associated with coaching (Rose et al., 1995), a finding that has been replicated (Suhr and Gunstad, 2000).

Other Forced-Choice Tests

Amsterdam Short-Term Memory Test (Schagen et al., 1997)

This forced-choice task does not use the typical two-choice recognition format. The subject sees a card containing five words from the same semantic category (e.g., *pants, skirt, shirt, sweater, coat*) with instructions to read them aloud and to remember them. The patient next sees a second—distractor—card with a simple addition or subtraction problem to solve. A third card is then displayed which contains five words from the semantic category of the first card, three of which are repeated and two are new (e.g., *cape, pants, skirt, knickers, sweater*). The subject's task is to indicate which three words appeared on the first card. Since three of the five words are target stimuli, the patient must choose at least one target on each recognition trial. Thirty word series are presented, yielding a maximum score of 90.

This test may be too difficult for patients with early dementia or Korsakoff's syndrome. Using a cutting score of either "<85 or <86 points" [*sic*] (out of 90), 20 severe TBI patients, 10 patient relatives, and 10 simulators—also patient relatives—were all correctly classified. The authors anecdotally observed that two of the subjects in the simulation group were familiar with tests and memory impairment (remedial teacher, experimental psychologist) and they too performed in the malingering range. Using these same criteria for whiplash patients, 61% of patients referred as litigants obtained invalid performance levels, whereas only 29% of the sample referred through medical channels were classified as invalid (Schmand, Lindeboom, et al., 1998). However, 60 out of the 72 patients included in the medical referral group were also engaged in some damage or compensation claim.

This measure has several distinct advantages. The first is that having to select only three of the five target words on each trial minimizes the obvious 50–50 chance component and thus improves face validity. The second is that the use of high frequency words for targets and low frequency words for foils increases the likelihood of correct selections for patients giving good effort. Finally, the task has appeal since it is a forced-choice test that does not employ a computer and will blend in with other measures in the test battery.

Coin-in-the-Hand Test (Kapur, 1994)

This simple procedure was developed as a bedside screen for exaggerated memory complaints. It is based upon the same principles as two-item forced-choice testing but simply involves showing the patient a coin in the extended palm of the hand for several seconds. Patients then close their eyes and count backward from 10 to 1. Upon opening their eyes, they indicate in which of the examiner's two clenched hands the coin is held. Ten trials are given, five for each hand randomly alternated.

Kapur (1994) observed that two suspected malingerers scored at the chance level, although five patients with dense amnesia due to herpes encephalitis obtained perfect scores. In a simulation study, Cochrane and her colleagues (1998) reported that the Coin-in-the-Hand Test, in conjunction with Wiggins and Brandt's (1988) Autobiographical Interview, correctly classified 19/20 community volunteers instructed to simulate memory impairment without misclassifying any subjects in either the control or memory impairment groups.

48-Pictures Test (Signoret, 1979)

This two-choice task shows the subject 48 line drawings of recognizable items, half of which are tested for immediate recognition and the others are tested following a 15-minute delay using a paired forced-choice format in which each recognition item contains a target and a foil. Despite the delay, memory impaired patients typically perform well on this test, in part because the stimuli can be encoded both verbally and visually. The delayed recognition component increases the face validity of this test since retention over time is assessed. When comparing suspected malingerers and simulators to clinical samples, 90% of the patients in the clinical group scored above 77% correct whereas 74% of the simulating groups scored below this level (Chouinard and Rouleau, 1997).

Hopkins Recall/Recognition Test

Brandt, Rubinsky, and Lassen (1985) compared free recall of 20 words to two-item forced-choice recognition in attempts to isolate performance discrepancies when malingering was suspected. Patients with TBI or Huntington's disease simulating amnesia routinely underestimated the amnesics' problems with recall but overestimated the difficulty of recognition for such patients. Patients with genuine memory deficits improved most on the recognition procedure whereas simulators improved least. Even patients with seriously compromised memory functions (in this study, Huntington patients) can recognize words from a list they have just heard at chance and better levels. When normal control subjects and TBI patients also took this test, six of ten college students simulating memory impairment and a man claiming amnesia for the murder of his wife were the only ones who scored below chance levels. In applying this principle to amnesic patients and assumed malingerers, Brandt (1988) found that two-choice recognition of 20 words was at least 9 points higher than free recall by the amnesic patients but none of the four suspected malingerers made gains this great.

Test of Memory Malingering (TOMM) (Tombaugh, 1996; see also Spreen and Strauss, 1998)

This validity test is really a recognition memory test, so it ranks very high on face validity. The TOMM contains two learning trials, each followed by recognition memory testing, and an optional delayed retention trial. Each learning trial contains the same 50 line drawings of common objects shown for three sec each; forced-choice recognition testing presents 50 paired pictures of which each has one target item plus a new line-drawn object. Subjects are told whether their answers are correct. An optional retention trial is given after 15 minutes and contains another 50 forced-choice pairs, each containing one target item. The stimuli are similar to those of the Boston Naming Test, and Tombaugh consequently recommends that the TOMM be given prior to the Boston Naming Test if both instruments are administered to avoid contamination of the TOMM memory items by prior exposure to similar stimuli.

The TOMM is relatively unaffected by age, education, or moderate cognitive impairment. A criterion of 90% (45/50) on the second recognition trial is suggested to identify patients with suboptimal effort. This cutting score yielded both a sensitivity and specificity of 100% in an initial validation study with student simulators and controls (Tombaugh, 1997). It is noteworthy that this student sample, also tested with an abbreviated version of the Hiscocks' test, thought that the Hiscock procedure was too easy to be a genuine memory test but considered the TOMM to be a valid one.

Applying the 45/50 criterion on the second recognition trial to litigating and nonlitigating patients also produced impressive results (L.M. Rees, Tombaugh,

Gansler, and Moczynski, 1998). Of 13 nonlitigating TBI patients ranging the gamut of injury severity, none scored below 47. Of 13 litigating TBI patients, also ranging from mild to severe, 11 scored below 47, and ten scored below 45. A sample of 26 patients hospitalized for depression obtained average scores of 49.9 (of 50) on both the second and delayed recognition trials (L.M. Rees, Tombaugh, and Boulay, 2001). The recommended cutting score of 45 generated no false positive classifications in this sample, even for the 12 patients with severe depression as indicated by their Beck Depression Inventory scores.

One minor personal dissatisfaction with this test is its name. I [dwl] have encountered one patient who spontaneously remarked "Oh, the TOMM" as I began administering the test. Since he was referred for a second neuropsychological opinion by a plaintiff's attorney and had not taken the TOMM as part of his first neuropsychological evaluation, I became concerned about coaching regarding the types of test that the patient might encounter. I have taken advantage of laser printing technology and have renamed this procedure on the test booklet.

The 21 Item Test (Iverson, Franzen, and McCracken, 1991)

Although free recall is obtained, this procedure relies on forced-choice word recognition for a list of 21 nouns read to the patient (Iverson, Franzen, and McCracken, 1991). A forced-choice recognition trial with each target word paired with an unrelated foil follows an initial free recall of the list. An advantage of this procedure, like the Rey Memory Test, is that it takes less than 5 minutes to complete. Although both the free recall and forced-choice trials appear sensitive to poor effort, forced-choice proved to be superior (Iverson, Franzen, and McCracken, 1994). Using simulation designs, a cutting score of <12 resulted in a 2.5% false positive rate in memory impaired patients with a 70% sensitivity to simulators recruited from the community (Iverson, Franzen, and McCracken, 1994); a cutting score of <13 resulted in a 5% false positive rate in memory impaired subjects with an 80% sensitivity (Iverson and Franzen, 1996). While the more conservative criterion of <9 produced no false positives, sensitivity to experimental malingerers decreased significantly (22.5 to 38%).

Validity Indicator Profile (VIP) (Frederick, 1997)

This technique applies a two-alternative forced-choice method to a set of nonmemory tests to assess response validity. The tests contain 100 nonverbal abstraction items and 78 word definition problems, both of which are in a two-choice recognition format. The nonverbal stimuli consist of an incomplete design matrix similar to those in Matrix Reasoning or Raven's Matrices. These nonverbal items were modified from the *Test of Nonverbal Intelligence (TONI)* (L. Brown et al., 1982).

Although the items are not ordered from easy to hard, they vary in difficulty, creating the impression that this is an ability test. A comparison of performances across difficulty levels is the primary means of group classification, a strategy first advocated by André Rey (1941). Performance levels that do not drop or even improve as items become more difficult represents malingering.

Test response patterns are classified into four groups reflecting the interaction of effort (high vs. low) and motivation (to excel vs. to fail). Valid performance results from high effort to excel and is termed "compliant", whereas "malingering" reflects high effort to perform badly. Two other invalid categories are termed "careless" due to poor effort to respond correctly, and "irrelevant" indicating effort to respond incorrectly.

Since the verbal and nonverbal tests are independent measures, using both raises the possibility of a valid response on one and an invalid response on the other. Of course, this is also the case if more than one SVTs are administered: the examiner is left with the potentially difficult decision of determining what relationship, if any, should be inferred (i.e., is this a pattern of domain-specific exaggeration or one of differences in test sensitivity?). S.R. Ross and Adams (1999) note that the classification accuracy of the VIP reported in the manual is based on 50 computer generated random response protocols in addition to "honest" control subjects and brain injured patients, coached control subjects, suspected malingerers, and a group with diagnosed mental retardation. Exclusion of the computer generated protocols resulted in 51% sensitivity for the verbal subtest and 60% for the nonverbal one.

Because of scoring complexities, the author recommends a scoring service for which the cost may range from $13 to $16, depending on quantity scored. This high cost will decrease the routine use of the VIP for most clinicians and thereby reduce the number and quality of clinical research studies on this instrument.

The Victoria Symptom Validity Test (VSVT) (Slick, Hopp, Strauss, and Spellacy, 1996; Slick, Hopp, Strauss, and Thompson, 1997; see also Spreen and Strauss, 1998)

Although published reports of this test deal with the computerized version, it also lends itself to individual administration using printed index cards. The VSVT adds an additional component to the digit recognition procedure since item difficulty—either easy or hard—is obvious. The easy condition contains foils with completely different numbers; the hard condition foils are very similar to the target, as just the second and third or third and fourth numbers are different. In reality, the hard condition still remains a fairly simple task, although the procedure appears to be more difficult. Given that one of the criticisms of other symptom validity tests using digits is that many patients become insulted or bored because the procedure appears too easy and a waste of time, the two difficulty levels tend to decrease patient annoyance with the test and thus reduce the likelihood of a negative attitude affecting the performance or spilling over into other areas of assessment.

In one clinical sample, compensation claimants—most mildly injured—performed significantly less well on hard VSVT items than did patients with well-documented neurological impairment (Doss et al., 1999). Patients obtaining either Questionable or Invalid VSVT scores for the hard items were over seven times more likely to be seeking compensation than not. In another study of experimental malingering, the hard VSVT items correctly predicted group membership in 88% of the control group and 89% of the malingering sample (E. Strauss, Hultsch, et al., 1999). Grote and his colleagues (2000) reported similar findings, with all patients undergoing evaluation for epilepsy surgery obtaining VSVT hard item scores in the valid range (i.e., at least 16/24), while only 59% of the compensation seeking patients—referred from both plaintiff and defense attorneys—obtained valid scores. In fact, since all of the intractable epilepsy patients obtained scores of at least 18/24 correct on the hard series, these authors suggest that scores in the 16–20 range should probably not be considered valid.

The usefulness of these technique is illustrated in a case from clinical files involving a middle-aged electrician who had passed out at work due to a heat stroke. He was evaluated to determine if the residual memory difficulty was sufficiently severe to preclude his return to work. Across all three delay sets for the easy items of the Victoria Symptom Validity Test this man had 24/24 recognition. In contrast, he gave only three correct responses on the 24 "hard" items. Because 24/24 easy items were correct but only 3/24 hard items were correct, this did not suggest a random response pattern. Normal, above chance performance on the easy items demonstrated the patient's understanding of the instruction and that he was not confused about how to respond. The below chance performances for the three hard conditions have corresponding statistical probabilities of .14, .004, and .004. Thus, when treated as independent samples, the probability of occurrence is .0000022 (.14 × .004 × .004). This success/failure pattern cannot be explained away as due to confusion or misunderstood instructions.

Word Memory Test (WMT) (P. Green, Allen, and Astner, 1996)

This test assesses response bias in the context of memory assessment. A list of 20 word pairs with strong semantic associations (e.g., *dog–cat*) is presented twice. Forced-choice recognition testing is obtained for each of the 40 words comprising the 20 word pairs. On the recognition trial, each target word is paired with a word with much lower association (e.g., *dog, rat*) and subjects are not told whether their responses are correct. A second recognition trial, in which targets are paired with new foils, follows a 30-min delay, to examine response consistency. After the delayed two-choice recognition, a multiple-choice trial presents the target words in a list of eight words. Paired associate recall is tested next in which the examiner says the first word (e.g., *dog*) for the subject to recall its pair (i.e., *cat*). This is followed by a test of free recall and, after an additional 20 minutes, a second free recall test.

One advantage of the WMT is that it was developed for administration either individually or by computer. When given in its entirety, the WMT contains separate validity and ability measures. It has a gradient of difficulty across measures: thus, the performance decrement across tasks provides an additional way to examine performance validity.

In one study, patients with clearly documented brain injuries performed better than patients with less severe injuries who were engaged in litigation (P. Green, Iverson, and Allen, 1999). Significantly higher scores on the three primary measures of effort (immediate recognition, delayed recognition, and test–retest consistency) obtained by patients with well-documented TBI indicate the relative insensitivity of these measures to injury severity. When applied to simulators (mostly psychologists) who were instructed to simulate memory impairment, 14 of the 15 subjects obtained scores on delayed recognition suggesting response distortion (P. Green, Allen, and Astner, 1996).

Computerized two-choice tests for validity of memory complaints

The forced-choice digit recognition procedure has been adapted for the computer, which lends itself to the task because it streamlines the administration procedure significantly. The examiner no longer presents cards every few seconds while scoring the patient response, and the computer allows precise timing of stimulus delay intervals. Three representative computerized versions of digit recognition tests are the *Multi-digit Memory Test* (Niccolls and Bolter, 1991), the *Computerized Assessment of Response Bias* (L.M. Allen et al., 1997; Condor et al., 1992) and the *Victoria Symptom Validity Test* (Slick, Hopp, Strauss, and Thompson, 1997) including one version containing both digits and letters (Beetar and Williams, 1995). The interested reader should consult these references as the details of these computerized tests are beyond the scope of this book.

Other Special Examination Techniques

Priming tests

Using the phenomenon of memory priming (see pp. 29–30), Wiggins and Brandt (1988) hoped to demonstrate that malingering simulators would fail to demonstrate any beneficial priming effect. They reasoned that since implicit memory performance is typically preserved in patients with amnesia, failure to demonstrate a priming effect may suggest intentional response distortion. Contrary to expectations, simulators showed priming effects too.

Despite Wiggins and Brandt's (1988) failure, several other reports have suggested that this technique has potential clinical utility for identifying malingerers. K.D. Horton and his colleagues (1992) observed that completion rates in student simulators for word and fragment completion tasks were well below those of controls. Similar results have been reported in other simulator studies using either student simulators (H.P. Davis et al., 1997) or nonneurologic patients simulating amnesia (B.E. McGuire and Shores, 1998).

Dot Counting (A. Rey, 1941)

Dot counting measures poor motivation for task performance by examining whether time to completion is associated with increasing task difficulty. Although Rey originally presented the Ungrouped and Grouped dots as two separate tasks to detect poor responding, both tests are typically employed in tandem as a two-tiered assessment of response motivation.

The first portion of the test consists of six serially numbered 3 × 5 inch cards on which are printed (1) 7, (2) 11, (3) 15, (4) 19, (5) 23, and (6) 27 randomly arranged dots, respectively. The cards are shown to the patient one at a time, in the following order: 2, 4, 3, 5, 6, 1. The patient is told to count and tell the number of the dots as quickly as possible. The cooperative patient's time will increase gradually with the increased number of dots (see Table 20.5). More than one pronounced deviation from this pattern raises the likelihood that the patient is not acting in good faith. The second portion of the test adds six more numbered cards to the Dot Counting task. These cards contain (1) 8, (2) 12, (3) 16, (4) 20, (5) 24, and (6) 28 dots

TABLE 20.5 Percentile Norms for Time (in Seconds) Taken to Count Ungrouped Dots

Card	Dots	PERCENTILE				
		100	*75*	*50*	*25*	*0*
1	7	1	2	4	5	11
2	11	2	3	4	5	17
3	15	3	4	6	7	17
4	19	4	6	7	9	19
5	23	5	8	10	12	30
6	27	6	9	11	16	30

Adapted from Rey (1941)

arranged as follows: (1) two four-dot squares; (2) two five-dot squares and two separate dots; (3) four four-dot diamonds: (4) four five-dot squares; (5) four six-dot rectangles; and (6) four five-dot squares and two four-dot squares. Again, the cards are presented in the order 2, 4, 3, 5, 6, 1. For this set of cards, however, since the dots are arranged geometrically and can be counted as groups, the time taken to count the dots is much less than for the ungrouped dots which need to be counted more or less individually (see Table 20.6). Performance is evaluated in terms of the difference between the total time for the two performances. When there is little difference or the time taken to count the grouped dots exceeds that for the ungrouped dots, the subject's cooperation becomes suspect.

Paul and his colleagues (1992) evaluated the reliability of both the ungrouped and grouped dot techniques using three subject groups: community-residing volunteers without a history of head injury (retest at two weeks), psychiatric inpatients, and patients with diagnosed brain disorders. Both "best" performances and performances under simulation instructions were obtained from the control and psychiatric groups. Test–retest reliability coefficients for response times were high (.75 to .96) but lower for accuracy (.51 to .70). This technique was validated in several ways: Under "best performance" conditions the two patient

TABLE 20.6 Percentile Norms for Time (in Seconds) Taken to Count Grouped Dots

Card	Dots	PERCENTILE				
		100	*75*	*50*	*25*	*0*
1	8	0.5	1	1	2	3
2	12	1	2	2	2	3
3	16	1	2	2	4	5
4	20	1	1	2	4	5
5	24	2	2	2	5	6
6	28	2	2	3	5	7

Adapted from Rey (1941)

groups were similar in response times but significantly slower than community volunteers on both grouped and ungrouped dots, and significantly more error-prone as well. Simulators made significantly more errors than neurology patients on both grouped and ungrouped dots. The differences between expected and actual response time patterns were not great although they separated simulators and nonsimulators at a better than chance rate. A "simultaneous" application of cutoff scores for all measured dimensions yielded only 8% false positives but 40% false negatives.

Research findings on this technique are mixed. Binks, Gouvier, and Waters (1997) report that the number of cards with incorrect counts differentiated simulating and nonsimulating subjects best but the time difference between grouped and ungrouped dots also differed for subject groups. However, college student simulators who were told how to avoid detection and naive simulators did not differ from each other. Similar results were observed by Beetar and Williams (1994) using a computerized version of this test. Yet Greiffenstein, Baker, and Gola (1994), examining several tests purporting to assess malingering, noted that not only did Dot Counting fail to discriminate probable malingerers from TBI patients but no discrepancy showed up between the nongrouped and grouped performances. Similarly, of the seven measures investigated by Hiscock, Branham, and Hiscock (1994), only dot counting failed to discriminate simulators from controls.

The overall evidence suggests that Dot Counting alone is not a particularly sensitive measure of response validity. In a meta-analytic review of multiple validity testing techniques, Dot Counting, along with the Rey Memory Test for 15 items, had poorer sensitivity to questionable effort than tests using forced-choice recognition (Vickery et al., 2001). However, genuine memory impairment does not appear to affect Dot Counting (Arnett and Franzen, 1997) so that positive findings imply response distortion. In this respect, positive findings significantly strengthen the confidence with which the examiner can conclude that a patient's effort or motivation may be invalidating test performance.

A ready-made version. A 12-card preprinted format—*The Dot Counting Test*—offers a standardized version of this technique (K.B. Boone, Lu, and Herzberg, 2002). From seven to 28 dots are the stimuli; dots on the first seven cards are randomly scattered, on the last five they are neatly ordered. Subjects are instructed to count the dots quickly. Both time and errors are scored. The principles underlying interpretation of this test are the same as Rey's for the original version of the test. Cut-off scores are provided for various clinical and nonclinical groups based on sensitivity/specificity statistics. It will be interesting to find out whether this format has greater sensitivity than the original.

Rey 15-Item Memory Test (A. Rey, 1964)

This technique for evaluating patients' cooperation has been called variously "Rey's Memory Test" (RMT) (Bernard, 1990; Bernard and Fowler, 1990), "Rey's 3 × 5 Test" (G.P. Lee, Loring, and Martin, 1992), or "Rey 15-Item Memory Test" (Schretlen, Brandt, et al., 1991). A 16-item version has been developed (four lines of four characters each; see 3 × 5 model below) (Paul et al., 1992), as well as a modification slightly altering the original stimuli (Rey II) (G.A. Griffin et al., 1997).

The task is typically presented as a test requiring the memorization of 15 *different* items. In the instructions, the number "15" and "different" are stressed to make the test appear to be difficult. In reality, patients need remember only three or four ideas to recall most of the items. The examiner marks on a piece of paper the following, in five rows of three characters to a line:

$$
\begin{array}{ccc}
A & B & C \\
1 & 2 & 3 \\
a & b & c \\
\bigcirc & \square & \triangle \\
| & \| & \||
\end{array}
$$

Patients see this display for 10 sec whereupon the examiner withdraws it and asks them to copy what they remember. A 10- or 15-sec quiet delay period can be interpolated. Anyone who is not significantly deteriorated can recall at least three of the five character sets. Paul and his colleagues (1992) designed the 16-item set to be even easier since with four rows of four items each—A-B-C-D, 1-2-3-4, a-b-c-d, I-II-III-IIII—fewer concepts need be retained, although "16" items may sound more difficult than "15"). Besides the number of items or correct rows recalled, this test has been scored for omission or addition errors (Paul et al., 1992) as well as perseverations, substitutions, and reversals (J.O. Goldberg and Miller, 1986).

With the 16-item format and three comparison groups—community volunteers, psychiatric inpatients, and patients with diagnosed neurological conditions—on two-week retesting with standard instructions, community dwellers achieved a reliability coefficient of .48, which rose to .88 under simulation instructions (Paul et al., 1992). (The relatively low correlation under standard conditions reflects the tendency for most healthy subjects to get perfect scores so that the statistical effect of slight changes between the two trials is exaggerated.) A comparison of the average number correct for the community dwellers (15.73 ± 1.85) with the psychiatric inpatients (12.87 ± 3.69) and the neurologically impaired patients (10.80 ± 5.20) differentiated the community dwellers from the two patient groups which, due to intragroup variability, did not differ from one another. When asked to simulate brain injury, the community subjects' average number correct dropped to 6.27 ± 4.7 and the psychiatric inpatients scored an average of 7.70 ± 5.6; however, only the community subjects' score was significantly lower than that achieved by the neurologically impaired patients under standard conditions because of the wide range of variation in patient scores. On the 16-item version, a cutting score of ≤7 correct regardless of placement identified only 22.5% of college student "malingerers," a much lower percentage than distinguished by several forced-choice recognition tests, Digit Span, or the WMS-R Personal History and Orientation criteria (Iverson and Franzen, 1996).

A modification of Rey's original stimuli produced the Rey-II. Although this new version retains 15 individual stimuli, it eliminates the row of geometric shapes, changes the row orders, and adds two new 1-2-3 progressions, with the stimuli contained in either squares or circles. The new stimuli were judged to be more difficult by college students than the original stimuli. A number of interesting qualitative scoring errors were also measured, categorized as either Embellishment Errors, which included Elaboration, Wrong Item Errors, and Gestalt Errors, or Ordering Errors, which included Within Row, Between Row, and Incomplete Row Errors. The Rey II was superior to the original 15-item test in classifying student simulators or clinical patient simulators using standard quantitative scoring; two or more qualitative errors provided the best group separation.

A number of studies have evaluated either the 15- or 16-item version of this technique. Most patients, including those with memory disorders, recall nine items or more (Bernard and Fowler, 1990; G.P. Lee, Loring, and Martin, 1992; Millis and Kler, 1995; Paul et al., 1992). Howver, mental ability is related to success on this technique (Schretlen, Brandt, et al., 1991), with persons in the retarded range frequently recalling fewer than seven items (J.O. Goldberg and Miller, 1986; J.R. Hays et al., 1993). In two studies, psychiatric disorders did not seem to compromise ability to perform this test (J.O. Goldberg and Miller, 1986; J.R. Hays et al., 1993). However, Schretlen, Brandt, and their colleagues (1991) found that patients with severe psychiatric disorders were prone to poor performance, as were more severely impaired brain injury patients (Guilmette, Hart, Giuliano, and Leininger, 1994).

Several recommendations on use of this technique

came out of these studies. J.O. Goldberg and Miller (1986) suggest that malingerers are more likely to deny recall and thus make omission errors. This guideline was strongly supported by the greatly increased number of omissions made by both community volunteers and psychiatric patients when asked to simulate brain injury (Paul et al., 1992). Bernard and Fowler (1990) suggest that, given their data on brain injured patients, a cutting score of 8 may be more reasonable than the frequently used cut-off of 9. A scoring technique based on the number of correct rows in correct sequence on which more brain impaired patients than college student simulators recalled was less likely to misclassify patients with verified neurologic impairment than a simple cutting score of 9 (Arnett, Hammeke, and Schwartz, 1995). Schretlen, Brandt, and their colleagues (1991) recommend that this technique not be used with mentally dull patients or those with demonstrable neurologic disease: they believe that the most likely candidates will be patients with known or reported mild brain injury who have *borderline* or better mental ability. In their study, patients suspected of malingering amnesia performed poorly on this test but so did patients with genuine amnesia. These authors caution against an uncritical application of this procedure, although it may be helpful in some cases.

Greiffenstein, Baker, and Gola (1996a) modified the scoring to see if they could improve sensitivity. The score was the number of correct items recalled without respect to position or order. An adjusted score corrected for intrusion errors (responses that differed from the stimuli, again independent of position or order; total correct − total incorrect). A spatial accuracy score was the number of stimuli recalled in the correct placement within a row and then adjusted by subtracting spatial intrusions. Their sample consisted of TBI patients and a litigating minor head injury group claiming permanent serve disability (i.e., convergent improbable outcome selection). With dense amnesia patients excluded, spatial scoring—with or without correction—provided better discrimination than traditional scoring. A cutoff score ≤8 for the spatial score, or ≤7 for the adjusted spatial score, provided test sensitivity of 69% and a specificity of 82% for both measures. Both of these produced an incremental hit rate of 12% over a 62% base rate for this sample.

In summary, the RMTM is a popular measure, in part due to its easy and brief administration and scoring. It appears to serve best, however, for screening since it is somewhat insensitive to suspected malingerers and to simulators and likely to misclassify persons with moderate to severe cognitive impairment. In a meta-analytic review of many techniques for validity testing, Rey's 15-item format (along with Dot Counting) was less sensitive to questionable effort than tests using forced-choice recognition (Vickery et al., 2001).

The b Test (K.B. Boone, Lu, et al., 2000)

This measure is based on the authors' observation that many patients whose injuries appear questionable complain of an "acquired dyslexia" in which they report seeing letters "upside down and backwards." This test assesses letter discrimination (i.e., *b*) by giving subjects pages on which are printed rows of letters randomly distributed with instructions to "circle the *b*'s" on each page. The distractor stimuli on some pages are *d, p,* and *q;* but some other distractors are these letters with diagonal stems or double stems. In addition, the letters and distractors become smaller over the trials.

Boone and her colleagues found that, among their commission errors, likely malingerers most often circled the letter *d* (47%), followed by letters with extra stems (23%), diagonal stems (13%), *p* (11%), and *q* (5%). Using the presence of more than one letter *d* commission error to identify suspected malingerers, these authors reported a 74% sensitivity for 34 patients suspected of malingering, with none of 20 TBI patients misclassified. For patients with learning disabilities, three of 38 were misclassified. Although none of ten left CVA patients were misclassified, two of ten right CVA patients failed at this error rate due to the visuospatial impairments associated with their disease. A cutoff score of three or more commission errors of any kind correctly classified 76.5% of probable malingers, with no TBI patient misclassified. Performance was not related to education or sex.

Autobiographical Memory Interview (Wiggins and Brandt, 1988)

Because autobiographical memory tends to be preserved in amnesia, Wiggins and Brandt (1988) developed this questionnaire to explore how simulators would respond to basic autobiographical questions such as remembering one's birth date or parents' names (see Table 20.7). Comparing rewarded simulators (course credit for university students, $15 for community volunteers), control subjects, and four amnesic patients, Wiggins and Brandt found that all of the control subjects and amnesic patients answered almost all of the autobiographical questions correctly but the simulators gave from 12 to 48% erroneous responses to these questions. Moreover, student simulators had a higher rate of "memory failure" than four neurologic patients with amnesia on all questions excepting for re-

TABLE 20.7 Autobiographical Memory Interview

| What is your name? |
| What is your age? |
| What is your birth date? |
| What is your telephone number? |
| What is your mother's first name? |
| What is your mother's maiden name? |
| What is your father's first name? |
| What is your brother's/sister's name? |
| What did you have for breakfast this morning? |
| What did you have for dinner last night? |
| Tested on second day |
| What is the examiner's name (free recall)? |
| What is the examiner's name (4-choice recognition)? |

From Wiggins and Brandt (1988)

calling the experimenter's name after a day's interval. In subsequent studies, assessing the ability to recall the experimenter's name was not included in the inventory.

In another study, the Coin-in-the-Hand Test (p. 774) along with Wiggins and Brandt's Autobiographical Memory Interview correctly classified 19/20 simulators without misclassifying any control or memory impaired subjects (Cochrane et al., 1998). Using a slight modification of this method, Iverson and Franzen (1996) observed significantly poorer performance in a group of college student "malingerers," correctly classifying 78% of the "malingering" subjects while misclassifying none of the controls.

SELF-REPORT INVENTORIES AND QUESTIONNAIRES

Some examiners use patients' self-reports of symptoms on inventories and rating scales to help them judge the validity of cognitive deficits demonstrated in the examination. Self-reported symptom complaints that are consistent with the claimed pathological condition may serve as validity indicators, under the assumption that most patients are relatively unsophisticated about the psychological symptom patterns associated with the condition in question. Of course, with increasing use of neuropsychology in forensic applications and greater ease of obtaining information about all clinical syndromes via the Internet, the assumption that patients are medically naïve becomes questionable. Responses to inventories developed to identify (mostly) noncognitive symptoms of psychological disorders can also be used to judge the consistency of complaints of these noncognitive symptoms and associated behavioral disturbances.

Many symptoms associated with cerebral disorders also appear with a relatively high frequency in the normal population. College students did not differ from patients with moderate head injuries on self-reported memory problems, general interest, loss of temper, irritability, fatigue, or impatience (Gouvier, Uddo-Crane, and Brown, 1988). In a study of patients in health maintenance organizations, postconcussive symptoms were neither unique nor clustered among the different groups examined, which included patients knocked unconscious, neurology and psychiatry patients, and patients seen in family practice or internal medicine (D.D. Fox et al., 1995). Rating scales, therefore, must be interpreted with the same caution as a patient's self-report. They serve best when used to identifying patterns of symptom endorsement rather than used for diagnostic purposes.

Another difficulty when relying on self report is that a variety of situational factors can affect recall, as can the process of recall itself (Freud, 1938; Gruneberg, Morris, and Sykes, 1988, *passim;* Lezak, 1973; Schacter, 1999b). For example, several groups of patients who were not in litigation were asked to rate their premorbid and present status (Hilsabeck, Gouvier, and Bolter, 1998). TBI patients overestimated the actual degree of change they attributed to their injury by recalling fewer preinjury symptoms than control subjects. As these patients were not pressing a claim for compensation, it appears that this tendency is a normal part of memory modification associated with the injury and does not necessarily reflect an attempt at purposeful distortion in the pursuit of financial gain. Patients in litigation describing their preinjury abilities may also tend to overestimate premorbid status (Lees-Haley, Williams, and English, 1996).

Patient ratings by others do not appear to be any more discriminating. Although relatives of patients with head injuries gave lower ratings of patient memory than relatives' ratings of college students memory (Gouvier, Uddo-Crane, and Brown, 1988), no difference in many postconcussive symptoms were reported including loss of temper, visual problems, irritability, restlessness, fatigue, and impatience. Further, several "post-concussive symptoms" were rated with a higher frequency in the relatives' ratings of college students than the head injured relative ratings (often impatient: 49% vs. 35%; often irritable: 43% vs. 31%).

In general, the hallmark of functional and simulated disorders on these paper-and-pencil scales and inventories is abnormally exaggerated complaints—whether in their variety, severity, or both. Typical is the pattern of response by naïve patients to symptom inventories when, seeking recognition of complaints which may have little or no relationship to their actual physical and mental status, they report problems in most if not all areas of mental, emotional, or physical functioning (see, for example, pp. 333–334).

Questionnaires provide one way of systematically documenting claims of exaggerated memory difficulty but by themselves may not provide sufficient grounds on which to base inferences about response exaggeration. The *Memory Complaints Inventory* (P. Green and Allen, 2000) contains items describing many different types of memory impairments including some that are not typically associated with an acquired cerebral lesion (e.g. "I cannot remember whether I played any sport as a child"). It includes claims of remote memory impairment, amnesia for complex behavior, and impaired memory for antisocial behavior. Patients who perform poorly on formal symptom validity testing tend to endorse implausible memory complaints. However, some patients who appear motivated to perform well on formal measures of effort nevertheless endorse implausible memory impairments. Inventory and rating scale self-reports are less likely to make response bias evident but more likely to provide information regarding both the internal consistency of complaints and the consistency of complaints with cognitive test performance and the patient's neurological and medical status.

Personality and Emotional Status Inventories

Many neuropsychological evaluations include measures to examine how patients' personality and emotional status contribute to their cognitive performance. For example, numerous studies investigating response exaggeration and malingering have used the MMPI/MMPI-2, relying upon their built-in validity scores. Before going any further into applications of personality and related tests, however, one must appreciate that efforts to appear cognitively impaired may be independent from feigning an emotional disorder (Greiffenstein, Gola, and Baker, 1995). Consequently, one should not expect tests sensitive to cognitive malingering to be generalizable to patients exaggerating emotional disorders and, conversely, tests sensitive to emotional exaggeration should not necessarily be sensitive to the embellishment of cognitive deficits.

Minnesota Multiphasic Personality Inventory (MMPI)

Two procedures have been used to evaluate the validity of MMPI (or MMPI-2) protocols. One involves an overall review of the standard profile (three validity, ten clinical scales); the other relies on validity scales or indices. Since many of the studies examining the MMPI/MMPI-2 have been conducted on patients simulating psychiatric rather than cognitive impairment, the generalizability of MMPI findings to cognitive exaggeration must be made cautiously.

Profile analysis. In two studies concerned with the validity of MMPI responses given by TBI patients in litigation, the different subject groups produced different findings based on discriminant equations. Heaton, Smith, and their colleagues (1978) examined differences in MMPI performances between TBI patients and college student simulators. The college students produced much more disturbed-appearing profiles, exceeding the head injured patients on scales *F, 1, 3, 6, 7, 8,* and *10.* The TBI patients had *T*-scores above 70 on scales *2* and *8.* The college students, in their effort to appear impaired, achieved *T*-scores above 70 on *F, 1, 2, 3, 6, 7, 8* (93.9 ± 21.2!), and *10.* However, two other groups of TBI patients seeking compensation and differing only on whether they had appeared to give good effort or not on a neuropsychological examination were indistinguishable by their MMPI scores (Cullum, Heaton, and Grant, 1991). Clinical experience with this test has made us skeptical of any protocol in which *F* is well above 70 and three or more of the clinical scales reached 90 or higher—a profile called "Sawtooth Mountains" (Gough, 1947), especially when the elevations are on scales *2, 4, 6,* and *8.* J.R. Graham (1987) observed that this elevation pattern occurs only rarely in valid clinical profiles. Cripe (2002) cautions against interpreting the "Psychosomatic V" pattern (somewhat high scale *2* with scales *1* and *3* considerably higher) as evidence of symptom exaggeration as this is not unusual among patients with neurological disorders (see p. 749).

Validity scales and index analysis. Since malingering—or inappropriate responding—on the MMPI can occur either as exaggerated or false reporting of problems or in random responses, the MMPI-2 provides several new scales developed to be sensitive to one or the other kind of invalid response pattern (D.T.R. Berry, Wetter, et al., 1991; Wetter et al., 1992). For example, the original MMPI also contained 16 items that are repeated verbatim and may be used informally as a Test–Retest consistency measure. In preparing the MMPI-2, 67 repeated statement pairs were altered to be semantically inconsistent (e.g., responding false to both "I do not tire quickly" and "I feel tired a good deal of the time" represents response inconsistency). This set of item pairs became an additional validity indicator, the *Variable Response Inconsistency* scale

(*VRIN*) (Butcher, Dahlstrom et al., 1989; J.R. Graham, 1990).

In addition to the standard validity scales included in the MMPI/MMPI-2, other workers have developed validity scales to detect response bias and intentional symptom distortion (see D.T.R. Berry, Baer, and Harris, 1991; Franzen, Iverson, and McCracken, 1990; J.E. Meyers, Millis, and Volkert, 2002). Almost all studies using simulators asked them to "fake bad" or feign mental illness; studies of patients suspected of exaggerating their problems typically used either patients in psychiatric institutions or prisoners seeking an amelioration of their situation (e.g., pleading "not guilty" by reason of insanity). Moreover, these different studies used a wide range of cut-off scores making comparisons difficult and their findings questionable for examining test-taking validity when neuropsychological deficits are claimed.

The difference between *F* (positively related to rarely occurring experiences and attitudes) and *K* (negatively related to help-seeking tendencies) scales (*F − K* index) is often used as a measure of "faking bad." It was developed from responses of individuals instructed to appear as though they were suffering from a psychiatric abnormality (Gough, 1947, 1950). A review of the literature using meta-analytic techniques reported that although *F − K* separated subjects known (by instruction) or presumed to be "faking bad" from normal subjects or patients presumed to have responded honestly, the *F* scale alone identified these groups even more effectively (D.T.R. Berry, Baer, and Harris, 1991). Many different cutting scores have been applied to many different study subjects, such as those simulating cognitive impairment or exaggerating emotional distress or pain (e.g., see J.E. Meyers, Millis, and Volkert, 2002). However, as noted by Larrabee (1998), the *F* scale has only a single item in common with scales *1* and *3,* the two scales most often associated with somatic complaints in a neuropsychological context. Thus *F* has only limited usefulness as a measure of exaggerated somatic symptoms.

A 43-item *Fake Bad* MMPI-2 scale (*FBS*) for use with personal injury claimants was developed by Lees-Haley, English, and Glenn (1991) on the same principles as Gough's (1954) *Dissimulation* scale. A score of 20 or more identified 96% of patients seen in these authors' practice suspected of malingering while misclassifying only two of 20 personal injury claimants with "genuine injuries". These authors also estimated the mean scores of the MMPI-2 normative sample for this scale to be 13.8 for women and 11.7 for men. On the basis of 12 patients presenting evidence of malingering, of whom 11 had high FBS scores, Larrabee (1998) suggests that somatic malingering should be considered when some MMPI-2 scale elevations exceed 80 and FBS is significantly elevated.

James N. Butcher, Arbisi, and their colleagues (2003) evaluated this scale on over 20,000 persons, mostly medical and psychiatric patients but also correctional facility inmates and 157 personal injury claimants. In most samples, this scale classified almost two times as many women as "malingering" as men. Even with the most conservative cut-off score of 26, false positive rates for women and men, respectively, were for the psychiatric sample 20.7% and 6.8%, for chronic pain patients 23.7% and 8.5%, for personal injury claimants 37.9% and 16.7%, and for men in a Veterans Administration hospital 23.9%). Using the lower cut-off score of 20, which had "identified" so many malingerers in the Lees-Haley, English, and Glenn (1991) study, for women and men, respectively, 57.2% and 29.6% of psychiatric patients, 63.6% and 47% of pain patients, 49.6% and 31.6% of general medical patients, 62.1% and 44.4% of personal injury claimants, and 46.7% of hospitalized veterans would be labeled as malingerers on the FBS. Thus, it is not surprising that the FBS does not appear to have appropriate sensitivity or specificity for patients faking severe psychiatric impairment (Iverson and Binder, 2000; R. Rogers, Sewell, and Ustad, 1995).

FBS scores were found to correlate quite modestly with the total number of correct items on the Victoria Symptom Validity Test (easy correct $= -.37$; hard correct $= -.32$) and with response latencies (easy RT $= .40$; hard RT $=.41$) in a sample of malingering simulators (Slick, Hopp, Strauss, and Spellacy, 1996). Over two years after their accidents, a sample of patients sustaining mild TBI and claiming complete disability obtained an average FBS score of 25; severe TBI litigants had a group mean score of 17 even though some scored above 20 (Greiffenstein, Baker, Donders, and Miller, 2002). These contrasting scores demonstrate the paradoxical inverse correlation between magnitude of injury and magnitude of a score based on symptoms and complaints.

On the basis of their very large-scale study, Butcher and his colleagues (2003) concluded that, "The [FBS] scale is likely to classify an unacceptably large number of individuals who are experiencing genuine psychological distress as malingerers." This study was subsequently criticized on methodological grounds because no attempt had been made to establish the litigation or compensation-seeking status of the clinical samples (Larrabee, 2003).

Other derived MMPI-2 scales will not be reviewed here since they tend to be used for detection of more

psychiatric or emotional/psychological exaggeration (e.g., insanity, PTSD). These measures include the *Infrequency-Psychopathology* scale (F[p]; Arbisi and Ben-Porath, 1995, 1997), *subtle vs. obvious content* item comparison (D.N. Wiener, 1947), Dissimulation scale (Gough, 1954), and *Ego Strength* (F. Barron, 1953). A novel evaluation of chronic pain patients employed a weighted score derived from the above measures (J.E. Meyers, Millis, and Volker, 2002). This method effectively identified malingering simulators and separated litigating from nonlitigating chronic pain patients.

Personality Assessment Inventory (PAI) (Morey, 1991, 1998)

This is an increasingly used objective personality test that, in addition to clinical, treatment, and interpersonal scales, contains four measures of response bias and validity: *Inconsistency* (ICN) measures response consistency for paired items with similar content; *Infrequency* (INF) contains neutral items with very high or very low endorsement rates in statistically unlikely response patterns, which may also expose inconsistent or random responding; *Negative Impression* (NIM) picks up response exaggeration and, thus, may suggest response bias associated with malingering; and *Positive Impression* (PIM). ICN and INF are designed to assess deviations from conscientious responding, whereas NIM and PIM are considered measures of impressions management (i.e., how subjects want the examiner to see them). Unlike the MMPI and MMPI-2, items do not overlap across the scales and each item is on a 4-point Likert scale.

Several authors have developed malingering measures for the PAI (Cashel et al., 1995; Morey and Lanier, 1998; R. Rogers, Sewell, et al., 1998). However, PAI research investigating response exaggeration in neuropsychological contexts is limited, so the reader should apply appropriate caution when generalizing the research data from somatic exaggeration to cognitive deficits.

And an old classic: Rorschach

As a psychologist in the armed forces, Benton (1945) had to make diagnostic decisions about servicemen presenting pseudoneurologic symptoms. He reported that the Rorschach was particularly useful for this problem because the unfamiliar, seemingly irrational task typically aroused the malingering patient's suspicions and defenses. Consequently, their Rorschach productions tended to be very sparse, constricted, and given with characteristically slow reaction times. When this response pattern was in marked contrast to the subject's performance on the "rational and understandable" intelligence tests, Benton considered that it strongly supported a supposition of malingering. A reduction in the number of responses is also characteristic of simulated (fake bad) protocols (G.G. Perry and Kinder, 1990).

In contrast to Benton's findings with young men seriously attempting to appear neurologically impaired, research on Rorschach simulation, in which subjects are asked to respond as if they were psychiatrically disturbed, invariably shows that with these instructions most subjects—including psychiatric patients—give exaggeratedly "bad" responses, emphasizing disgusting, frightening, or hostile ideas (Lezak, 1960; G.G. Perry and Kinder, 1990). These protocols appear even more "psychotic" than those given by psychotic patients under standard administration conditions (Franzen, Iverson, and McCracken, 1990).

APPENDIX: Test Publishers and Distributors

American Guidance Service: 4201 Woodland Rd., Circle Pines, MN 55014-1796; e-mail: agsmail@agsnet.com; www.agsnet.com

Consulting Psychologists Press: 3803 Bayshore Rd., P.O. Box 10096, Palo Alto, CA 94303

Educational and Industrial Testing Service (EDITS): P.O. Box 7234, San Diego, CA 92167; e-mail: edits@k-online.com; www.edits.net

Lafayette Instrument: 3700 Sagamore Parkway North, P.O. Box 5729, Lafayette, IN 47903; e-mail: eval@lafayetteinstrument.com; www.lafayetteinstrument.com

MHS: P.O. Box 950, North Tonawanda, NY 14120-0950; www.mhs.com

NCS Assessments; P.O. Box 1416, Minneapolis, MN 55440; http://assessments.ncspearson.com

NFER-Nelson Publishing Co., Ltd.: Darville House, 2, Oxford Road East, Windsor, Berkshire 2LA 1DF, U.K.

Pearson Reid London House: 1 North Dearborn, Chicago, IL 60602; www.Pearsonreidlondonhouse.com

Pro-Ed: 8700 Shoal Creek Blvd., Austin, TX 78757-6897; www.proedinc.com

Psychological Assessment Resources (PAR): 16204 N. Florida Ave., Lutz, FL 33549; www.parinc.com

Psychological Corporation: 19500 Bulverde Rd., San Antonio, TX 78259-3701; www.Harcourtassessment.com

Riverside Publishing: 425 Spring Lake Drive, Itasca, IL 60143-2079; www.riversidepublishing.com

Stoelting: 620 Wheat Lane, Wood Dale, IL 60191; e-mail: psychtests@stoeltingco.com; http://www.stoeltingco.com

Thames Valley Test Co.: Unit 22, The Granary, Station Hill, Thurston, Bury St. Edmunds, Suffolk 1P31 3QU; e-mail: orders@tvtc.com; www.tvtc.com

Western Psychological Services: 12031 Wilshire Blvd., Los Angeles, CA 90025-1251; e-mail: custsvc@wpspublish; www.wpspublish.com

Wide Range, Inc.: P.O. Box 3410, Wilmington, DE 19804-0250; www.widerange.com

References

Aalten, P., de Vugt, M.E., Lousberg, R., et al. (2003). Behavioral problems in dementia: A factor analysis of the neuropsychiatric inventory. *Dementia and Geriatric Cognitive Disorders, 15,* 99–105.

Aaronson, A.L., Dent, O.B., Webb, J.T., & Kline, C.D. (1996). Graying of the critical items: Effects of aging on responding to MMPI-2 critical items. *Journal of Personality Assessment, 66,* 169–176.

Aarsland, D., Cummings, J.L., & Larsen, J.P. (2001). Neuropsychiatric differences between Parkinson's disease with dementia and Alzheimer's disease. *International Journal of Geriatric Psychiatry, 16,* 184–191.

Aarsland, D., Larsen, J.P., Lim, N.G., et al. (1999). Range of neuropsychiatric disturbances in patients with Parkinson's disease. *Journal of Neurology, Neurosurgery and Psychiatry, 67,* 492–496.

Abikoff, H., Alvir, J., Hong, G., et al. (1987). Logical memory subtest of the Wechsler Memory Scale: Age and education norms and alternate-form reliability of two scoring systems. *Journal of Clinical and Experimental Psychology, 9,* 435–448.

Aboitiz, F., Scheibel, A.B., & Zaidel, E. (1992). Morphometry of the Sylvian fissure and the corpus callosum, with emphasis on sex differences. *Brain, 115,* 1521–1541.

Abraham, A. & Mathai, K.V. (1983). The effect of right temporal lobe lesions on matching of smells. *Neuropsychologia, 21,* 277–281.

Abrahams, S., Pickering, A., Polkey, C.E., & Morris, R.G. (1997). Spatial memory deficits in patients with unilateral damage to the right hippocampal formation. *Neuropsychologia, 35,* 11–24.

Abrams, G.M. & Jay, C.A. (2002). Neurological manifestations of endocrine disease. In A.K. Ashbury et al. (Eds.), *Diseases of the nervous system* (3rd ed.). Cambridge, UK: Cambridge University Press.

Abrams, R. (1988). *Electroconvulsive therapy.* New York: Oxford University Press.

Abrey, L.E., DeAngelis, L.M., & Yahalom, J. (1998). Long-term survival in primary CNS lymphoma. *Journal of Clinical Oncology, 16,* 859–863.

Abu-Zeid, H.A.H., Choi, N.W., Hsu, P.-H., & Maini, K.K. (1978). Prognostic factors in the survival of 1,484 stroke cases observed for 30 to 48 months. *Archives of Neurology, 35,* 121–125.

Acevedo, A., Loewenstein, D.A., Barker, W.W., et al. (2000). Category fluency test: Normative data for English and Spanish-speaking elderly. *Journal of the International Neuropsychological Society, 6,* 760–769.

Acheson, S.K., Stein, R.M., & Swartzwelder, H.S. (1998). Impairment in semantic and figural memory by acute ethanol: Age-dependent effects. *Alcoholism: Clinical and Experimental Research, 22,* 1437–1442.

Achiron, R., Lipitz, S., & Achiron, A. (2001). Sex-related differences in the development of the human fetal corpus-callosum: in utero ultrasonographic study. *Prenatal Diagnosis, 21,* 116–120.

Achté, K.A., Hillbom, E., & Aalberg, V. (1969). Psychoses following war brain injuries. *Acta Psychiatrica Scandinavica, 45,* 5–18.

Acker, M.B. & Davis, J.R. (1989). Psychology test scores associated with late outcome in head injury. *Neuropsychology, 3,* 1–10.

Acker, W., Ron, M.A., Lishman, W.A., & Shaw, G.K. (1984). A multivariate analysis of psychological, clinical and CT scanning measures in detoxified chronic alcoholics. *British Journal of Addictions, 79,* 293–301.

Ackerman, K.D., Martino, M., Heyman, R., et al., (1998). Stressor-induced alteration of cytokine production in multiple sclerosis patients and controls. *Psychosomatic Medicine, 60,* 484–491.

Adamovich, B.B., Henderson, J.A., & Auerbach, S. (1985). *Cognitive rehabilitation of closed head injured patients: A dynamic approach.* San Diego: College-Hill Press.

Adams, H.P., Jr., Brott, T.G., Furlan, A.J., et al. (1996). Guidelines for thrombolytic therapy for acute stroke: A supplement to the guidelines for the management of patients with acute ischemic stroke. A statement for healthcare professionals from a special writing group of the Stroke Council, American Heart Association. *Circulation, 94,* 1167–1174.

Adams, J.H., Graham, D.I., & Gennarelli, T.A. (1985). Contemporary neuropathological considerations regarding brain damage in head injury. In D.P. Becker & J.T. Povlishock (Eds.), *Central nervous system trauma. Status report–1985.* Washington, D.C.: National Institutes of Health.

Adams, K.M. (1980a). An end of innocence for behavioral neurology? Adams replies. *Journal of Consulting and Clinical Psychology, 48,* 522–524.

Adams, K.M. (1980b). In search of Luria's battery: A false start. *Journal of Consulting and Clinical Psychology, 48,* 511–516.

Adams, K.M. (1984). Luria left in the lurch: Unfulfilled promises are not valid tests. *Journal of Clinical Neuropsychology, 6,* 455–465.

Adams, K.M. & Brown, S.J. (1980). *Standardized behavioral neurology: Useful concept, mixed metaphor, or commercial enterprise?* Paper presented at the 88th annual meeting of the American Psychological Association, Montreal, Quebec, Canada.

Adams, K.M. & Grant, I. (1984). Failure of nonlinear models of drinking history variables to predict neuropsychological performance in alcoholics. *American Journal of Psychiatry, 141,* 663–667.

Adams, K.M. & Grant, I. (1986). Influence of premorbid risk factors on neuropsychological performance in alcoholics. *Journal of Clinical and Experimental Neuropsychology, 8,* 362–370.

Adams, K.M., Grant, I., & Reed, R. (1980). Neuropsychology in alcoholic men in their late thirties: One-year follow-up. *American Journal of Psychiatry, 137,* 928–931.

Adams, K.M. & Heaton, R.K. (1987). Computerized neuropsychological assessment: Issues and applications. In J.N. Butcher (Ed.), *Computerized psychological assessment. A practitioner's guide.* New York: Basic Books.

Adams, K.M. & Heaton, R. (1990). The NIMH Neuropsychological Battery. *Journal of Clinical and Experimental Neuropsychology, 12,* 960–962.

Adams, K.M., Rennick, P.M., Schoof, K.G., & Keegan, J.F. (1975). Neuropsychological measurement of drug effects: Polydrug research. *Journal of Psychedelic Drugs, 7,* 151–159.

Adams, K.M., Sawyer, J.D., & Kvale, P.A. (1980). Cerebral oxygenation and neuropsychological adaptation. *Journal of Clinical Neuropsychology, 2,* 189–208.

Adams, R.D. (1980). Altered cerebrospinal fluid dynamics in relation to dementia and aging. In L. Amaducci, A. N. Davison, & P. Antuono (Eds.), *Aging of the brain and dementia.* New York: Raven Press.

Adams, R.D., Victor, M., & Ropper, A.H. (1997). *Principles of neurology.* (6th ed.). New York: McGraw-Hill.

Adams, R.L., Boake, C., & Crain, C. (1982). Bias in a neuropsychological test classification related to education, age, and ethnicity. *Journal of Consulting and Clinical Psychology, 50,* 143–145.

Adams, R.L., Smigielski, J., & Jenkins, R.L. (1984). Development of a Satz-Mogel short form of the WAIS-R. *Journal of Consulting and Clinical Psychology, 52,* 908.

Adler, N.E., Boyce, T., Chesney, M.A., et al. (1994). Socioeconomic status and health. *American Psychologist, 49,* 15–24.

Adolphs, R. & Damasio, A.R. (2000). Neurobiology of emotions at a systems level. In J.C. Borod (Ed.), *The neuropsychology of emotion.* New York: Oxford University Press.

Adolphs, R., Tranel, D., & Damasio, A.R. (1998). The human amygdala in social judgment. *Nature, 393,* 470–474.

Afifi, A.K. & Bergman, R.A. (1998). *Functional neuroanatomy.* New York: McGraw-Hill.

Agency for Healthcare Research and Quality (2001). *Management of newly diagnosed patients with epilepsy: A systematic review of the literature.* AHRQ Publication 01-E038. Rockville, MD: U.S. Department of Health and Human Services.

Aggleton, J.P. (1993). The contribution of the amygdala to normal and abnormal emotional states. *Trends in Neurosciences, 16,* 328–333.

Agid, Y. & Blin, J. (1987). Nerve cell death in degenerative diseases of the central nervous system: clinical aspects. In *Selective neuronal death. Ciba Foundation Symposium 126.* New York: Wiley.

Agid, Y., Ruberg, M., DuBois, B., & Pillon, B. (1987). Anatomo-clinical and biochemical concepts of subcortical dementia. In S.M. Stahl, S.D. Iversen, & E.C. Goodman (Eds.), *Cognitive neurochemistry.* Oxford: Oxford University Press.

Agnew, J., Bolla-Wilson, K., Kawas, C.H., & Bleecker, M.L. (1988). Purdue Pegboard age and sex norms for people 40 years and older. *Developmental Neuropsychology, 4,* 29–36.

Aguero-Torres, H. & Winblad, B. (2000). Alzheimer's disease and vascular dementia. Some points of confluence. *Annals of the New York Academy of Sciences, 903,* 547–552.

Aguirre, G. (2003). Functional imaging of normal subjects. In T.E. Feinberg & M.J. Farah (Eds.), *Behavioral neurology and cognitive neuropsychology.* New York: McGraw-Hill.

Aguirre, M., Broughton, R., & Stuss, D. (1985). Does memory impairment exist in narcolepsy-cataplexy? *Journal of Clinical and Experimental Neuropsychology, 7,* 14–24.

Aharon-Peretz, J., Kliot, D., Amyel-Zvi, E., et al. (1997). Neurobehavioral consequences of closed head injury in the elderly. *Brain Injury, 11,* 871–875.

Ahern, G.L., Herring, A.M., Tackenberg, J.N., et al. (1994). Affective self-report during the intracarotid sodium amobarbital test. *Journal of Clinical and Experimental Neuropsychology, 16,* 372–376.

Ahles, T.A., Saykin, A.J., Furstenberg, C.T., et al. (2002). Neuropsychologic impact of standard-dose systemic chemotherapy in long-term survivors of breast cancer and lymphoma. *Journal of Clinical Oncology, 20,* 485–493.

Ahlskog, J.E. (1999). Medical treatment of later-stage motor problems of Parkinson disease. *Mayo Clinic Proceedings, 74,* 1239–1254.

Ahuja, G. K., Pauranik, A., Behari, M., & Prasad, K. (1988). Eating epilepsy. *Journal of Neurology, 235,* 444–447.

Aiken, L.R. (1980). Problems testing the elderly. *Educational Gerontology, 5,* 119–124.

Aikens, J.E., Fischer, J.S., Namey, M., & Rudick, R. A. (1997). A replicated prospective investigation of life stress, coping, and depressive symptoms in multiple sclerosis. *Journal of Behavioral Medicine, 20,* 433–445.

Ainslie, N.K. & Murden, R.A. (1993). Effect of education on the clock-drawing dementia seen in non-demented elderly persons. *Journal of the American Geriatric Society, 41,* 249–252.

Aita, J.A., Armitage, S.G., Reitan, R.M., & Rabinovitz, A. (1947). The use of certain placement tests in the evaluation of brain injury. *Journal of General Psychology, 37,* 25–44.

Aita, J. A., Reitan, R. M., & Ruth, J. M. (1947). Rorschach test as a diagnostic aid in brain injury. *American Journal of Psychiatry, 103,* 770–779.

Akechi, T., Kugaya, A., & Okamura, H. (1999). Fatigue and its associated factors in ambulatory cancer patients: A preliminary study. *Journal of Pain and Symptom Management, 17,* 42–48.

Akiyama, H., Barger, S., Barnum, S., et al. (2000). Inflammation and Alzheimer's disease. *Neurobiology of Aging, 21,* 383–421.

Aks, D. J. & Coren, S. (1990). Is susceptibility to distraction related to mental ability? *Journal of Educational Psychology, 82,* 388–390.

Akshoomoff, N., Delis, D.C., & Kiefner, M.G. (1989). Block constructions of chronic alcoholic and unilateral brain-damaged patients: A test of the right hemisphere vulnerability hypothesis of alcoholism. *Archives of Clinical Neuropsychology, 4,* 275–281.

Ala, T.A., Hughes, L.F., Kyrouac, G.A., et al. (2001). Pentagon copying is more impaired in dementia with Lewy bodies than in Alzheimer's disease. *Journal of Neurology, Neurosurgery and Psychiatry, 70,* 483–488.

Alajouanine, T. (1948). Aphasia and artistic realization. *Brain, 71,* 229–241.

Alaoui, P., Mazaux, J.M., Masson, F., et al (1998). Devenir neuropsychologique à long terme des traumatisés crâniens. Évaluation à 5 ans des troubles neuropsychologiques et comportementaux par l'échelle neurocomportementale révisée. *Annales de Réadaptation Médecine Physique, 41,* 171–181.

Albers, G.W., Dalen, J.E., Laupacis, A., et al. (2001). Antithrombotic therapy in atrial fibrillation. *Chest, 119,* 194S–206S.

Albert, M.L. (1973). A simple test of visual neglect. *Neurology, 23,* 658–664.

Albert, M.L. (1978). Subcortical dementia. In R. Katzman, R.D. Terry, & K.L. Bick (Eds.), *Alzheimer's disease: Senile dementia and related disorders.* New York: Raven Press.

Albert, M.L. (1989). The role of perseveration in language disorders. *Journal of Neurolinguistics, 4,* 471–478.

Albert, M.L., Feldman, R.G., & Willis, A.L. (1974). The "subcortical dementia" of progressive supranuclear palsy. *Journal of Neurology, Neurosurgery, and Psychiatry, 37,* 121–130.

Albert, M.L. & Sandson, J. (1986). Perseveration in aphasia. *Cortex, 22,* 103–115.

Albert, M.S. (1994). Age-related changes in cognitive function. In M.L. Albert & J.E. Knoefel (Eds.), *Clinical neurology of aging* (2nd ed.). New York: Oxford University Press.

Albert, M.S. (1998). Normal and abnormal memory: Aging and Alzheimer's disease. In E. Wang & D. S. Snyder (Eds.), *Handbook of the aging brain.* San Diego: Academic Press.

Albert, M.S., Butters, N., & Brandt, J. (1980). Memory for remote events in alcoholics. *Journal of Studies on Alcohol, 41,* 1071–1081.

Albert, M.S., Butters, N., & Brandt, J. (1981). Development of remote memory loss in patients with Huntington's disease. *Journal of Clinical Neuropsychology, 3,* 1–12.

Albert, M.S., Butters, N., & Levin, J. (1979). Temporal gradients in the retrograde amnesia of patients with alcoholic Korsakoff's disease. *Archives of Neurology, 36,* 211–216.

Albert, M.S., Duffy, F.H., & McAnulty, G.B. (1990). Electrophysiologic comparisons between two groups of patients with Alzheimer's disease. *Archives of Neurology, 47,* 857–863.

Albert, M.(S.), Duffy, F.H., & Naeser, M. (1987). Nonlinear changes in cognition with age and their neuropsychologic correlates. *Canadian Journal of Psychology, 41,* 141–157.

Albert, M.S., Heller, H.S., & Milberg, W. (1988). Changes in naming ability with age. *Psychology and Aging, 3,* 173–178.

Albert, M.S. & McKhann, G.S. (2002). The aging brain: morphology, imaging and function. In E.K. Asbury et al. (Eds.), *Diseases of the nervous system* (3rd ed.). Cambridge, UK: Cambridge University Press.

Albert, M.S., Moss, M.B., & Milberg, W. (1989). Memory testing to improve the differential diagnosis of Alzheimer's disease. In K. Igbal, H.M. Wisniewski, & B. Winblad (Eds.), *Alzheimer's disease and related disorders.* New York: Alan R. Liss.

Albert, M.S., Moss, M.B., Tanzi, R., & Jones, K. (2001). Preclinical prediction of AD using neuropsychological tests. *Journal of the International Neuropsychological Society, 7,* 631–639.

Albert, M.S., Wolfe, J., & Lafleche, G. (1990). Differences in abstraction ability with age. *Psychology and Aging, 5,* 94–100.

Aldenkamp, A.P. & Baker, G.A. (1997). The Neurotoxicity Scale-II. Results of a patient-based scale assessing neurotoxicity in patients with epilepsy. *Epilepsy Research, 27,* 165–173.

Aldenkamp, A.P., Baker, G., Mulder, O.G., et al. (2000). A multicenter, randomized clinical study to evaluate the effect on cognitive function of topiramate compared with valproate as add-on therapy to carbamazepine in patients with partial-onset seizures. *Epilepsia, 41,* 1167–1178.

Aldenkamp, A.P., Baker, G., Pieters, M.S., et al. (1995). The Neurotoxicity Scale: The validity of a patient-based scale, assessing neurotoxicity. *Epilepsy Research, 20,* 229–239.

Aldrich, E., Eisenberg, H., Saydjari, C., et al. (1992). Predictors of mortality in severely head-injured patients with civilian gunshot wounds: A report from the NIH Traumatic Coma Data Bank. *Surgical Neurology, 38,* 418–423.

Alegret, M., Vendrell, P., Junque, C., et al. (2001). Visuospatial deficits in Parkinson's disease assessed by Judgment of Line Orientation test: Error analysis and practice effects. *Journal of Clinical and Experimental Neuropsychology, 23,* 592–598.

Alevriadou, A., Katsarou, Z., Bostontjopoulou, S., et al., (1999). Wisconsin Card Sorting Test variables in relation to motor symptoms in Parkinson's disease. *Perceptual and Motor Skills, 89,* 824–830.

Alexander, D. (1976). The normal sample. In J. Money (Ed.), *A Standardized Road Map Test of Direction Sense.* San Rafael, CA: Academic Therapy Press.

Alexander, M.P. (1988). Clinical determination of mental competence: A theory and a retrospective study. *Archives of Neurology, 45,* 23–26.

Alexander, M.P. (1995). Mild traumatic brain injury: pathophysiology, natural history, and clinical management. *Neurology, 45,* 1253–1260.

Alexander, M.P. (2003). Aphasia: Clinical and anatomic aspects. In T.E. Feinberg & M.J. Farah (Eds.), *Behavioral neurology and neuropsychology* (2nd ed.). New York: McGraw-Hill.

Alexander, M.P., Benson, D.F., & Stuss, D.T. (1989). Frontal lobes and language. *Brain and Language, 37,* 656–691.

Alexander, M.P. & Freedman, M. (1984). Amnesia after anterior communicating artery aneurysm rupture. *Neurology, 34,* 752–757.

Alexander, M.P., Naeser, M.A., & Palumbo, C.L. (1987). Correlations of subcortical CT lesion sites and aphasia profiles. *Brain, 110,* 961–991.

Alexopoulos, G.S., Meyers, B.S., Young, R.C., et al. (1997). "Vascular depression" hypothesis. *Archives of General Psychiatry, 54,* 915–922.

Alexopoulos, G.S., Young, R.C., Abrams, R.C., et al. (1989). Chronicity and relapse in geriatric depression. *Biological Psychiatry, 26,* 551–564.

Alfano, D.P. & Finlayson, M.A.J. (1987). Comparison of standard and abbreviated MMPI's in patients with head injury. *Rehabilitation Psychology, 32,* 67–76.

Alfano, D.P., Neilson, P.M., Paniak, C.E., & Finlayson, M.A. (1992). The MMPI and closed head injury. *The Clinical Neuropsychologist, 6,* 134–142.

Alfano, P.L. & Michel, G.F. (1994). Effect of certain task characteristics on performance of two neuropsychological tests of spatial ability. *Perceptual and Motor Skills, 78,* 379–390.

Alfonso, V.C. & Allison, D.B. (1996). Further development of the extended Satisfaction with Life Scale. *Social Indicators Research, 38,* 275–281.

Ali, S.O., Denicoff, K.D., Altshuler, L.L., et al. (2000). A preliminary study of the relation of neuropsychological performance to neuroanatomic structures in bipolar disorder. *Neuropsychiatry, Neuropsychology, and Behavioral Neurology, 13,* 20–28.

Allain, P., Joseph, P.A., Onillon, M., & Truelle, J.L. (1995). Le retour au travail des traumatisés crâniens. Angers & Suresnes, France: Le programme européen Horizon avec la participation de l'A.G.E.F.I.P.H.

Allain, P., Jouadé, A.S., Le Roch, E., et al. (2001). Exécution, génération, et arrangement de scripts après un traumatisme crânien sévère. *Annals de Réadaptation et Médecine Physique, 44,* 1–4.

Allen, C.C. & Ruff, R.M. (1990). Self-rating versus neuropsychological performance of moderate versus severe head-injured patients. *Brain Injury, 4,* 7–18.

Allen, C.C. & Ruff, R.M. (1999). Factorial validation of the Ruff-Light Trail Learning Test (RULIT). *Assessment, 6,* 43–50.

Allen, D.N., Goldstein, G., & Mariano, E. (1999). Is the Halstead Category Test a multidimensional instrument? *Journal of Clinical and Experimental Neuropsychology, 21,* 237–244.

Allen, D.N. & Goreczny, A.J. (1995). Assessment and treatment of multiple sclerosis. In A.J. Goreczny (Ed.), *Handbook of health and rehabilitation psychology.* New York: Plenum Press.

Allen, D.N., Sprenkel, D.G., Heyman, R.A., et al. (1998). Evaluation of demyelinating and degenerative disorders. In G. Goldstein, P.D. Nussbaum, & S.R. Beers (Eds.), *Neuropsychology.* New York: Plenum Press.

Allen, J.G., Lewis, L., Blum, S., et al. (1986). Informing psychiatric patients and their families about neuropsychological assessment findings. *Bulletin of the Menninger Clinic, 50,* 64–74.

Allen, J.J. (2002). The role of psychophysiology in clinical assessment: ERPs in the evaluation of memory. *Psychophysiology, 39,* 261–280.

Allen, L.M., Conder, R.L., Green, P., & Cox, D.R. (1997). *CARB '97: Computerized Assessment of Response Bias. Manual.* Durham, NC: CogniSyst.

Allender, J. & Kaszniak, A.W. (1989). Processing of emotional cues in patients with dementia of the Alzheimer's type. *International Journal of Neuroscience, 46,* 147–155.

Almli, C.R. & Finger, S. (1988). Toward a definition of recovery of function. In S. Finger et al. (Eds.), *Brain injury and recovery. Theoretical and controversial issues.* New York: Plenum Press.

Al-Sebeih, K., Karagiozov, K., & Jafar, A. (2002). Penetrating craniofacial injury in a pediatric patient. *Journal of Craniofacial Surgery, 13,* 303–307.

Alter, I., John, E.R., & Ransohoff, J. (1990). Computer analysis of cortical evoked potentials following severe head injury. *Brain Injury, 4,* 19–26.

Altieri, M., Di Piero, V., Vicenzini, E., & Lenzi, G.L. (2001). Clinical aspects and correlates of stroke recovery. In J. Bogousslavsky & L. Caplan (Eds.), *Stroke syndromes* (2nd ed.). Cambridge, UK: Cambridge University Press.

Alvarez, P. & Squire, L.R. (1994). Memory consolidation and the medial temporal lobe: A simple network model. *Proceedings of the National Academy of Sciences USA, 91,* 7041–7045.

Alves, W. & Jane, J.A. (1985). Mild brain injury: Damage and outcome. In D.P. Beck & J.T. Povlishock (Eds.), *Central nervous system trauma status report–1985.* Washington, D.C.: National Institutes of Health.

Alves, W., Macciocchi, S., & Barth, J.T. (1993). Postconcussive symptoms after uncomplicated mild head injury. *Journal of Head Trauma Rehabilitation, 8,* 48–59.

Amante, D., VanHouten, V.S., Grieve, J.H., et al. (1977). Neuropsychological deficit, ethnicity, and socioeconomic status. *Journal of Consulting and Clinical Psychology, 45,* 524–535.

Amar, K. & Wilcock, G. (1996). Vascular dementia. *British Medical Journal, 312,* 227–231.

Amato, M.P., Ponziani, G., Siracusa, G., & Sorbi, S. (2001). Cognitive dysfunction in early-onset multiple sclerosis: A reappraisal after 10 years. *Archives of Neurology, 58,* 1602–1606.

American Academy of Clinical Neuropsychology (1999). American Academy of Clinical Neuropsychology policy on the use of non-doctoral-level personnel in conducting clinical neuropsychological evaluations. *The Clinical Neuropsychologist, 13,* 385.

American Academy of Neurology (2002). Disorders of cognitive function. *Continuum. Lifelong Learning in Neurology, 8,* No. 2.

American Congress of Rehabilitation Medicine (1993). Definition of mild traumatic brain injury. *Journal of Head Trauma Rehabilitation, 8,* 86–87.

American Congress of Rehabilitation Medicine (1995). Recommendations for use of uniform nomenclature pertinent to patients with severe alterations in consciousness. *Archives of Physical Medicine and Rehabilitation, 76,* 205–209.

American Medical Association (published annually). *Drug evaluations annual.* Chicago: American Medical Association.

American Psychiatric Association (2000). *Diagnostic and statistical manual of mental disorders. Text revision* (4th ed., *DSM-IV-TR*). Washington, D.C.: American Psychiatric Association.

American Psychological Association (1999). *Standards for educational and psychological testing.* Washington, D.C.: American Psychological Association.

American Psychological Association (2002). Ethical principles of psychologists and code of conduct. *American Psychologist, 47,* 1060–1073.

American Psychological Association (2003). Guidelines on multicultural education, training, research, practice, and organizational change for psychologists. *American Psychologist, 58,* 377–402.

Ameriso, S.F. & Sahai, S. (1997). Mechanisms of ischemia in situ vascular obstructive disease. In K.M.A. Welch, et al. (Eds.), *Primer on cerebrovascular diseases.* San Diego: Academic Press.

Ames, L.B., Metraux, R.W., Rodell, J.L., & Walker, R.N. (1973). *Rorschach responses in old age.* New York: Brunner-Mazel.

Amler, R.W., Lybarger, J.A., Anger, W.K., Phifer, B.L., et al. (1994). Adoption of an adult environmental neurobehavioral test battery. *Neurotoxicology and Teratology, 16,* 525–530.

Ammons, R.B. & Ammons, C.H. (1962). The Quick Test (QT): Provisional manual. *Psychological Reports (Monograph Suppl. I-VII),* 111–161.

Amodei, N., Williams, J.F., Seale, J.P., & Alvarado, M.L. (1996). Gender differences in medical presentation and detection of patients with a history of alcohol abuse or dependence. *Journal of Addictive Diseases, 15,* 19–31.

Anastasi, A. (1965). *Differential psychology* (3rd ed.). New York: Wiley.

Anastasi, A. (1988). *Psychological testing* (6th ed.). New York: MacMillan.

Anastasi, A. & Urbina, S. (1997). *Psychological testing* (7th ed.). Upper Saddle River, NJ: Prentice-Hall.

Andersen, K., Nielsen, H., Lolk, A., et al. (1999). Incidence of very mild to severe dementia and Alzheimer's disease in Denmark: The Odense Study. *Neurology, 52,* 85–90.

Andersen, R. (1978). Cognitive changes after amygdalectomy. *Neuropsychologia, 16,* 439–451.

Anderson, B., Southern, B.D., & Powers, R.E. (1999). Anatomic asymmetries of the posterior superior temporal lobes: A postmortem study. *Neuropsychiatry, Neuropsychology, and Behavioral Neurology, 12,* 247–254.

Anderson, C.V. & Bigler, E.D. (1995). Ventricular dilation, cortical atrophy, and neuropsychological outcome following traumatic brain injury. *Journal of Neuropsychiatry and Clinical Neurosciences, 7,* 42–48.

Anderson, C.V., Bigler, E.D., & Blatter, D.D. (1995). Frontal lobe lesions, diffuse damage, and neuropsychological functioning in traumatically brain-injured patients. *Journal of Clinical and Experimental Neuropsychology, 17,* 900–908.

Anderson, D.A., Burton, D.B., Parker, J.D., & Godding, P.R. (2001). A confirmatory factor analysis of the cognitive capacity screening examination in a clinical sample. *International Journal of Neuroscience, 111,* 221–233.

Anderson, D.W., Ellenberg, J.H., Leventhal, C.M., et al. (1992). Revised estimate of the prevalence of multiple sclerosis in the United States. *Annals of Neurology, 31,* 333–336.

Anderson, J.R. & Schooler, L.L. (2000). The adaptive nature of memory. In E. Tulving & F.I.M. Craik (Eds.), *The Oxford handbook of memory.* Oxford, UK: Oxford University Press.

Anderson, N.D. & Craik, F.I.M. (2000). Memory in the aging brain. In E. Tulving & F.I.M. Craik (Eds.), *The Oxford handbook of memory.* Oxford: Oxford University Press.

Anderson, P., Anderson, V., & Garth, J. (2001). Assessment and development of organizational ability: The Rey Complex Figure Organizational Strategy Score (RCF-OSS). *The Clinical Neuropsychologist, 15,* 81–94.

Anderson, S.W., Bechara, A., Damasio, H., et al. (1999). Impairment of social and moral behavior related to early damage in human prefrontal cortex. *Nature Neuroscience, 2,* 1032–1037.

Anderson, S.W., Damasio, H., Jones, R.D., & Tranel, D. (1991). Wisconsin Card Sorting Test performance as a measure of frontal lobe damage. *Journal of Clinical and Experimental Neuropsychology, 13,* 909–922.

Anderson, S.W., Damasio, H., & Tranel, D. (1990). Neuropsychological impairments with lesions caused by tumor or stroke. *Archives of Neurology, 47,* 397–405.

Anderson, S.W., Damasio, H., Tranel, D., & Damasio, A.R. (2000). Long-term sequelae of prefrontal cortex damage acquired in early childhood. *Developmental Neuropsychology, 18,* 281–296.

Anderson, S.W. & Tranel, D. (1989). Awareness of disease states following cerebral infarction, dementia, and head trauma: Standardized assessment. *The Clinical Neuropsychologist, 3,* 327–339.

Anderson, V., Northam, E., Hendy, J., & Wrennall, J. (2001). *Developmental neuropsychology. A clinical approach.* Hove, UK: Psychology Press.

Anderson-Hanley, C., Sherman, M.L., Riggs, R., et al. (2003). Neuropsychological effects of treatments for adults with cancer: A meta-analysis and review of the literature. *Journal of the International Neuropsychological Society, 9,* 967–982.

Andersson, S. & Bergedalen, A.M. (2002). Cognitive correlates of apathy in traumatic brain injury. *Neuropsychiatry, Neuropsychology, and Behavioral Neurology, 15,* 184–191.

Andersson, S., Krogstad, J.M., & Finset, A. (1999). Apathy and depressed mood in acquired brain damage: Relationship to lesion localization and psychophysiological reactivity. *Psychological Medicine, 29,* 447–456.

Andrade, J. (2001). An introduction to working memory. In J. Andrade (Ed.), *Working memory in perspective.* Hove, UK: Psychology Press.

Andreasen, N.C. (2001). *Brave new brain. Conquering mental illness in the era of the genome.* New York: Oxford University Press.

Andreasen, N.C., Paradiso, S., & O'Leary, D.S. (1998). "Cognitive dysmetria" as an integrative theory of schizophrenia: A dysfunction in cortical–subcortical–cerebellar circuitry? *Schizophrenia Bulletin, 24,* 203.

Andreassi, J.L. (1995). *Psychophysiology: Human behavior and physiological response* (3rd ed.). Hillsdale, NJ: Erlbaum.

Andres, P. & Van der Linden, M. (2000). Age-related differences in supervisory attentional system functions. *Journal of Gerontology: Series B: Psychological Sciences and Social Sciences, 55,* 373–380.

Andresen, E.M., Rothenberg, B.M., Panzer, R., et al. (1998). Selecting a generic measure of health-related quality of life for use among older adults: A comparison of candidate instruments. *Evaluation and the health professions, 21,* 244–264.

Andrewes, D.G., Puce, A., & Bladin, P.F. (1990). Post-ictal recognition memory predicts laterality of temporal lobe seizure focus: Comparison with post-operative data. *Neuropsychologia, 28,* 957–967.

Andrewes, D.G., Schweitzer, I., & Marshall, N. (1990). The comparative cognitive side-effects of lithium, carbamazepine and combined lithium–carbamazepine in patients treated for affective disorders. *Human Psychopharmacology, 5,* 41–45.

Andrews, B.E. (1995). Structural changes after lightning strike with special emphasis on special sense orifices as portals of entry. *Seminars in Neurology, 15,* 296–303.

Andrews, B.E. & Darveniza, M. (1989). Telephone-mediated lightning injury: An Australian survey. *The Journal of Trauma, 29,* 665–671.

Andrews, F.M. & Withey, S.B. (1976). *Social indicators of well-being: America's perception of life quality.* New York: Plenum Press.

Andrikopoulos, J. (2001). Malingering disorientation to time, personal information, and place in mild head injured litigants. *The Clinical Neuropsychologist, 15,* 393–396.

Angel, J.L. (1975). Paleoecology, paleodemography, and health. In S. Polgar (Ed.), *Population, ecology, and social evolution.* Chicago: Aldine.

Anger, W.K. (1990). Worksite behavioral research: Results, sensitive methods, test batteries and the transition from laboratory data to human health. *Neurotoxicology, 11,* 629–720.

Anger, W.K. (1992). Assessment of neurotoxicity in humans. In H. Tilson & C. Mitchell (Eds.), *Neurotoxicology.* New York: Raven Press.

Anger, W.K., Cassitto, M.G., Liang, Y.-X., et al. (1993). Comparison of performance on three continents on the WHO-recommended Neurobehavioral Core Test Battery (NCTB). *Environmental Research, 62,* 125–147.

Anger, W.K., Liang, Y.X., Nell, V., et al. (2000). Lessons learned—15 years of the WHO-NCTB. A review. *Neurotoxicology, 21,* 837–846.

Anger, W.K., Rohlman, D.S., & Storzbach, D. (1999). Neurotoxicology. Neurobehavioral testing in humans. In M. Maines, L.

Costa, I.G. Sipes, et al. (Eds.), *Current protocols in toxicology.* New York: Wiley.

Anger, W.K., Storzbach, D., Amler, R.W., & Sizemore, O.J. (1998). Human behavioral neurotoxicology: Workplace and community assessments. In W.M. Rom (Ed.), *Environmental and occupational medicine* (3rd ed.). Philadelphia: Lippincott-Raven.

Anke, A.G.W., Stanghelle, J.K., Finset, A., et al. (1997). Long-term prevalence of impairments and disabilities after multiple trauma. *Journal of Trauma, 42,* 54–61.

Annegers, J.F. (1996). The epidemiology of epilepsy. In E. Wyllie (Ed.), *The treatment of epilepsy: Principles and practice* (2nd ed.). Baltimore, MD: Williams & Wilkins.

Annegers, J.F., Hauser, W.A., Coan, S.P., & Rocca, W.A. (1998). A population-based study of seizures after traumatic brain injuries. *New England Journal of Medicine, 338,* 20–24.

Annett, M. (2002). *Handedness and brain asymmetry. The right shift theory.* New York: Taylor & Francis/Psychology Press.

Anthony, J. C., LeResche, L., Niaz, U., et al. (1982). Limits of the Mini-Mental State as a screening test for dementia and delirium among hospital patients. *Psychological Medicine, 12,* 397–408.

Antonini, A., Leenders, K.L., Spiegel, R., et al. (1996). Striatal glucose metabolism and dopamine d2 receptor binding in asymptomatic gene carriers and patients with Huntington's disease. *Brain, 119,* 2085–2095.

Anttinen, E.E. (1960). On the apoplectic conditions occurring among brain-injured veterans. *Acta Psychiatrica et Neurologica Scandinavica, 35 (Suppl.),* 143, 1–150.

Appell, J., Kertesz, A., & Fisman, M. (1982). A study of language functioning in Alzheimer patients. *Brain and Language, 17,* 73–91.

Arato, M., Frecska, E., Tekes, K., & MacCrimmon, D.J. (1991). Serotonergic interhemispheric asymmetry: Gender difference in the orbital cortex. *Acta Psychiatrica Scandinavica, 84,* 110–111.

Arbisi, P.A. & Ben-Porath, Y.S. (1995). An MMPI-2 infrequent response scale for use with psychopathological populations: The Infrequency-Psychopathology Scale, F(p). *Psychological Assessment, 7,* 424–431.

Arbisi, P.A. & Ben-Porath, Y.S. (1997). Characteristics of the MMPI-2 F(p) scale as a function of diagnosis in an inpatient sample of veterans. *Psychological Assessment, 9,* 102–105.

Arbuthnott, K. & Frank, J. (2000). Trail Making Test, part B as a measure of executive control: Validation using a set-switching paradigm. *Journal of Clinical and Experimental Neuropsychology, 22,* 518–528.

Archibald, C.J. & Fisk, J.D. (2000). Information processing efficiency in patients with multiple sclerosis. *Journal of Clinical and Experimental Neuropsychology, 22,* 686–701.

Archibald, S., Mateer, C.A., & Kerns, K.A. (2001). Utilization behavior: Clinical manifestations and neurologic mechanisms. *Neuropsychology Review, 11,* 117–130.

Archibald, Y.M., Wepman, J.M., & Jones, L.V. (1967). Performance on non-verbal cognitive tests following unilateral cortical injury to the right and left hemisphere. *Journal of Nervous and Mental Disease, 145,* 25–36.

Arciniegas, D.B. & Beresford, T.P. (2001). *Neuropsychiatry. An introductory approach.* Cambridge: Cambridge University Press.

Ardila, A. (1995). Directions of research in cross-cultural neuropsychology. *Journal of Clinical and Experimental Neuropsychology, 17,* 143–150.

Ardila, A. (1999a). A neuropsychological approach to intelligence. *Neuropsychology Review, 9,* 117–136.

Ardila, A. (1999b). Spanish applications of Luria's assessment methods. *Neuropsychology Review, 9,* 63–70.

Ardila, A. (2000a). Assessment of Spanish-speaking populations. *Applied Neuropsychology, 7,* 1–2.

Ardila, A. (Ed.) (2000b). Special Issue: Assessment of Spanish-speaking populations. *Applied Neuropsychology, 7, passim.*

Ardila, A. & Moreno, S. (2001). Neuropsychological test performance in Aruaco Indians: An exploratory study. *Journal of the International Neuropsychological Society, 7,* 510–515.

Ardila, A., Ostrosky-Solis, F., Rosselli, M., & Gómez, C. (2000). Age-related cognitive decline during normal aging: The complex effect of education. *Archives of Clinical Neuropsychology, 15,* 495–513.

Ardila, A. & Rosselli, M. (1989). Neuropsychological characteristics of normal aging. *Developmental Neuropsychology, 5,* 307–320.

Ardila, A. & Rosselli, M. (1993). Language deviations in aphasia: A frequency analysis. *Brain and Language, 44,* 165–180.

Ardila, A., Rosselli, M., Ostrosky-Solis, F., et al. (2000). Syntactic comprehension, verbal memory, and calculation abilities in Spanish–English bilinguals. *Applied Neuropsychology, 7,* 3–16.

Ardila, A., Rosselli, M., & Rosas, P. (1989). Neuropsychological assessment of illiterates: Visuospatial and memory abilities. *Brain and Cognition, 11,* 147–166.

Arena, R. & Gainotti, G. (1978). Constructional apraxia and visuopractic disabilities in relation to laterality of cerebral lesions. *Cortex, 14,* 463–473.

Arenberg, D. (1978). Differences and changes with age in the Benton Visual Retention Test. *Journal of Gerontology, 33,* 534–540.

Arenberg, D. (1982). Changes with age in problem solving. In F.I.M. Craik & S. Trehub (Eds.), *Aging and cognitive processes.* New York: Plenum Press.

Arezzo, J. C. & Schaumburg, H. H. (1989). Screening for neurotoxic disease in humans. *Journal of the American College of Toxicology, 8,* 147–155.

Arfken, C., Lichtenberg, P., & Tancer, M. (1999). Cognitive impairment and depression predict mortality in medically ill older adults. *Journal of Gerontology A: Biological Sciences and Medical Sciences, 54A,* M152–M156.

Arlien-Søborg, P., Bruhn, P., Gyldensted, C., & Melgaard, B. (1979). Chronic painters' syndrome. *Acta Neurologica Scandinavica, 60,* 149–156.

Armengol, C.G., Kaplan, E., & Moes, E.J. (2001). *The consumer-oriented neuropsychological report.* Lutz, FL: Psychological Assessment Resources.

Armitage, S.G. (1946). An analysis of certain psychological tests used for the evaluation of brain injury. *Psychology Monographs, 60,* 1–47.

Armstrong, C.L., Corn, B.W., Ruffer, J.E., et al. (2000). Radiotherapeutic effects on brain function: Double dissociation of memory systems. *Neuropsychiatry, Neuropsychology, and Behavioral Neurology, 13,* 101–111.

Armstrong, C.L., Stern, C.H., & Corn, B.W. (2001). Memory performance used to detect radiation effects on cognitive functioning. *Applied Neuropsychology, 8,* 129–139.

Armstrong, L., Borthwick, S.E., Bayles, K.A., & Tomoeda, C.K. (1996). Use of the Arizona Battery for Communication Disorders of Dementia in the UK. *European Journal of Disorders of Communication, 31,* 171–180.

Arnaiz, E.J.V., Almkvist, O., Wahlund, L.O., et al. (2001). Impaired cerebral glucose metabolism and cognitive functioning predict deterioration in mild cognitive impairment. *Neuroreport, 12,* 851–855.

Arndt, S. & Berger, D.E. (1978). Cognitive mode and asymmetry in cerebral functioning. *Cortex, 14,* 78–86.

Arnett, P.A. & Franzen, M.D. (1997). Performance of substance abusers with memory deficits on measures of malingering. *Archives of Clinical Neuropsychology, 12,* 513–518.

Arnett, P.A., Hammeke, T.A., & Schwartz, L. (1995). Quantitative and qualitative performance on Rey's 15-item test in neurological patients and dissimulators. *The Clinical Neuropsychologist, 9,* 17–26.

Arnett, P.A., Higginson, C.I., & Randolph, J.J. (2001). Depression in multiple sclerosis: Relationship to planning ability. *Journal of the International Neuropsychological Society, 7,* 665–674.

Arnett, P.A., Higginson, C.I., Voss, W.D., et al. (1999a). Depression in multiple sclerosis: Relationship to working memory capacity. *Neuropsychology, 13,* 546–556.

Arnett, P.A., Higginson, C.I., Voss, W.D., et al. (1999b). Depressed mood in multiple sclerosis: Relationship to capacity-demanding memory and attentional functioning. *Neuropsychology, 13,* 434–446.

Arnett, P.A., Rao, S.M., Bernardin, L., et al. (1994). Relationship between frontal lesions and Wisconsin Card Sorting Test performance in patients with multiple sclerosis. *Neurology, 44,* 420–425.

Arnett, P.A., Rao, S.M., Grafman, J., et al. (1997). Executive functions in multiple sclerosis: An analysis of temporal ordering, semantic encoding, and planning abilities. *Neuropsychology, 11,* 535–544.

Arnold, B., Cuellar, L., & Guzman, N. (1998). Statistical and clinical investigation of the Mattis Dementia Rating Scale-Spanish administration: An initial investigation. *Journal of Gerontology B: Psychological Sciences and Social Sciences, 53B,* 364–369.

Arnold, B.R., Montgomery, G.T., Castaneda, I., & Longoria, R. (1994). Acculturation and performance of Hispanics on selected Halstead-Reitan neuropsychological tests. *Assessment, 13,* 239–248.

Arnow, B.A., Desmond, J.E., Banner, L.L., et al. (2002). Brain activation and sexual arousal in healthy, heterosexual males. *Brain, 125,* 1014–1023.

Arrigoni, G. & De Renzi, E. (1964). Constructional apraxia and hemispheric locus of lesion. *Cortex, 1,* 170–197.

Arrindell, W.A., Heesink, J., & Feij, J.A. (1999). The Satisfaction With Life Scales (SWLS): Appraisal with 1700 healthy young adults in the Netherlands. *Personality and Individual Differences, 26,* 815–826.

Arthur, G. (1947). *A Point Scale of Performance Tests* (Rev. Form II). New York: Psychological Corporation.

Artiola i Fortuny, L., Briggs, M., Newcombe, F., et al. (1980). Measuring the duration of post traumatic amnesia. *Journal of Neurology, Neurosurgery, and Psychiatry, 43,* 377–379.

Artiola i Fortuny, L. & Heaton, R.K. (1996). Standard versus computerized administration of the Wisconsin Card Sorting Test. *The Clinical Neuropsychologist, 10,* 419–424.

Artiola i Fortuny, L., Heaton, R.K., & Hermosillo, D. (1999). Neuropsychological comparisons of Spanish-speaking participants from the U.S.–Mexico border region versus Spain. *Journal of the International Neuropsychological Society, 4,* 363–379.

Artiola i Fortuny, L. & Mullaney, H.A. (1997). Neuropsychology with Spanish speakers: Language use and proficiency issues for test development. *Journal of Clinical and Experimental Neuropsychology, 19,* 615–622.

Artiola i Fortuny, L. & Mullaney, H.A. (1998). Assessing patients whose language you do not know: Can the absurd be ethical? *The Clinical Neuropsychologist, 12,* 113–126.

Asbury, A.K., McKhann, G.M., McDonald, W.I., et al. (Eds.) (2002). *Diseases of the nervous system* (3rd ed.). Cambridge: Cambridge University Press.

Asikainen, I., Kaste, M., & Sarna, S. (1996). Patients with traumatic brain injury referred to a rehabilitation and re-employment programme: Social and professional outcome for 508 Finnish patients 5 or more years after injury. *Brain Injury, 10,* 883–899.

Askin-Edgar, White, K.E., & Cummings, J.L. (2002). Neuropsychiatric aspects of Alzheimer's disease and other dementing illnesses.

In S.C. Yudofsky & R.E. Hales (Eds.), *American Psychiatric Press textbook of neuropsychiatry* (4th ed.). Washington, D.C.: American Psychiatric Press.

Astell, A.J. & Harley, T.A. (1996). Tip-of-the-tongue states and lexical access in dementia. *Brain and Language, 54,* 196–215.

Athey, G.I., Jr. (1986). Implications of memory impairment for hospital treatment. *Bulletin of the Menninger Clinic, 50,* 99–110.

Atkinson, L. (1991). On WAIS-R difference scores in the standardization sample. *Psychological Assessment, 3,* 292–294.

Atkinson, L., Cyr, J.J., Doxey, N.C.S., & Vigna, C.M. (1989). Generalizability of WAIS-R factor structure within and between populations. *Journal of Clinical Psychology, 45,* 124–128.

Atkinson, R.C. & Shiffrin, R.M. (1968). Human memory: A proposed system and its control processes. In K.W. Spence (Ed.), *The psychology of learning and motivation: Advances in research and theory* (Vol. 2). New York: Academic Press.

Au, R., Albert, M.L., & Obler, L.K. (1988). Clinical forum. The relation of aphasia to dementia. *Aphasiology, 2,* 161–173.

Auerbach, V.S. & Faibish, G.M. (1989). Mini Mental State Examination: diagnostic limitations in a hospital setting [abstract]. *Journal of Clinical and Experimental Neuropsychology, 11,* 75.

Auriacombe, S., Grossman, M., Carvell, S., et al. (1993). Verbal fluency deficits in Parkinson's disease. *Neuropsychology, 7,* 182–192.

Austen, J. (1961). *Mansfield Park.* New York: Dell.

Awad, I.A., & Chelune, G.J. (1993). Outcome and complications. In E. Wyllie (Ed.), *The treatment of epilepsy: Principles and practices.* Philadelphia: Lea & Febiger.

Awad, I.A., Spetzler, R.F., Hodak, J.A., et al. (1987). Incidental lesions noted on magnetic resonance imaging of the brain: Prevalence and clinical significance in various age groups. *Neurosurgery, 20,* 222–227.

Axelrod, B.N. (2001). Administration duration for the Wechsler Adult Intelligence Scale-III and Wechsler Memory Scale-III. *Archives of Clinical Neuropsychology, 16,* 293–301.

Axelrod, B.N., Fichtenberg, N.L., Liethen, P.C., et al. (2001). Performance characteristics of postacute traumatic brain injury patients on the WAIS-III and WMS-III. *The Clinical Neuropsychologist, 15,* 516–520.

Axelrod, B.N. & Goldman, R.S. (1996). Use of demographic corrections in neuropsychological interpretation: How standard are standard scores? *The Clinical Neuropsychologist, 10,* 159–162.

Axelrod, B.N., Goldman, R.S., Heaton, R.K., et al. (1996). Discriminability of the Wisconsin Card Sorting Test using the standardization sample. *Journal of Clinical and Experimental Neuropsychology, 18,* 338–342.

Axelrod, B.N. & Henry R.R. (1992). Age-related performance on the Wisconsin Card Sorting, Similarities, and Controlled Oral Word Association Tests. *The Clinical Neuropsychologist, 6,* 16–26.

Axelrod, B.N., Henry, R.R., & Woodward, J.L. (1992). Analysis of an abbreviated form of the Wisconsin Card Sorting Test. *The Clinical Neuropsychologist, 6,* 27–31.

Axelrod, B.N., Jiron, C.C., & Henry, R.R. (1993). Performance of adults ages 20 to 90 on the abbreviated Wisconsin Card Sorting Test. *The Clinical Neuropsychologist, 7,* 205–209.

Axelrod, B.N. & Millis, S.R. (1994). Preliminary standardization of the Cognitive Estimation Test. *Assessment, 1,* 269–274.

Axelrod, B.N., Paolo, A.M., & Abraham, E. (1997). Do normative data from the full WCST extend to the abbreviated WCST? *Assessment, 4,* 41–46.

Axelrod, B.N., Putnam, S. H., Woodard, J.L., & Adams, K.M. (1996). Cross-validation of predicted Wechsler Memory Scale-Revised scores. *Psychological Assessment, 8,* 73–75.

Axelrod, B.N., Ricker, J.H., & Cherry, S.A. (1994). Concurrent validity of the MAE Visual Naming Test. *Archives of Clinical Neuropsychology, 9,* 317–321.

Axelrod, B.N., Vanderploeg, R.D., & Schinka, J.A. (1999). Comparing methods for estimating premorbid intellectual functioning. *Archives of Clinical Neuropsychology, 14,* 341–346.

Axelrod, B.N. & Woodard, J.L. (2000). Parsimonious prediction of Wechsler Memory Scale-III memory indices. *Psychological Assessment, 12,* 431–435.

Axelsson, A. (1995). Tinnitus epidemiology. In G.E. Reich & J.A. Vernon (Eds.), *Proceedings of the Fifth International Tinnitus Seminar 1995.* Portland, OR: American Tinnitus Association.

Aylward, E.H., Anderson, N.B., Bylsma, F.W., et al. (1998). Frontal lobe volume in patients with Huntington's disease. *Neurology, 50,* 252–258.

Aylward, E.H., Brandt, J., Codori, A.M., et al. (1994). Reduced basal ganglia volume associated with the gene for Huntington's disease in asymptomatic at-risk persons. *Neurology, 44,* 823–828.

Äystö, S. (1988). Comparison between psychometric and Lurian-type neuropsychological measures as detectors of "at risk" elders among 75–84 years old people [abstract]. *Journal of Clinical and Experimental Neuropsychology, 10,* 327.

Azuma, T., Bayles, K.A., Cruz, R.F., et al. (1997). Comparing the task difficulty of letter, semantic, and name fluency tasks for normal elderly and patients with Parkinson's disease. *Neuropsychology, 11,* 488–497.

Azuma, T., Cruz, R.F., Bayles, K.A., et al. (2000). Incidental learning and verbal memory in individuals with Parkinson disease. *Journal of Medical Speech-Language Pathology, 8,* 163–174.

Babcock, H. (1930). An experiment in the measurement of mental deterioration. *Archives of Psychology, 117,* 105.

Babcock, H. & Levy, L. (1940). *The measurement of efficiency of mental functioning (revised examination). Test and manual of directions.* Chicago: Stoelting.

Babcock, R.L. & Salthouse, T.A. (1990). Effects of increased processing demands on age differences in working memory. *Psychology and Aging, 5,* 421–428.

Babikian, V.L., Kase, C.S., & Wolf, P.A. (1994). Cerebrovascular diseae in the elderly. In M.L. Albert & J.E. Knoefel (Eds.), *Clinical neurology of aging* (2nd ed.). New York: Oxford University Press.

Bach, B., Molhave, L., & Pedersen, O.F. (1987). Humane reactions during controlled exposures to low concentrations of formaldehyde—performance tests. *Indoor Air '87. Proceedings of the 4th International Conference on Indoor Air Quality and Climate.* West Berlin, Germany.

Bachman, D.L. & Albert, M.L. (1988). Auditory comprehension in aphasia. In F. Boller & J. Grafman (Eds.), *Handbook of neuropsychology* (Vol. 1). Amsterdam: Elsevier.

Bachman, D.L., Wolf, P.A., Linn, R.T., et al. (1993). Incidence of dementia and probable Alzheimer's disease in a general population: The Framingham Study. *Neurology, 43,* 515–519.

Bachman, L., Fein, G., Davenport, L., & Price, L. (1993). The Indented Paragraph Reading Test in the assessment of left hemineglect. *Archives of Clinical Neuropsychology, 8,* 485–496.

Bäckman, L. & Nilsson, L.-G. (1996). Semantic memory functioning across the adult life span. *European Psychologist, 1,* 27–33.

Bäckman, L., Small, B.J., & Fratiglioni, L (2001). Stability of the preclinical episodic memory deficit in Alzheimer's disease. *Brain, 124,* 96–102.

Backman, M.E. (1972). Patterns of mental abilities: Ethnic, socioeconomic, and sex differences. *American Educational Research Journal, 9,* 1–12.

Baddeley, A.D. (1966). The capacity for generating information by randomization. *Quarterly Journal of Experimental Psychology, 18,* 119–129.

Baddeley, A.D. (1976). *The psychology of memory.* New York: Basic Books.

Baddeley, A.D. (1978). The trouble with levels: A reexamination of Craik and Lockhart's framework for memory research. *Psychological Review, 85,* 139–152.

Baddeley, A. (1986). *Working memory.* Oxford: Clarendon Press.

Baddeley, A. (2000). Short-term and working memory. In E. Tulving & F.I.M. Craik (Eds.), *The Oxford handbook of memory.* Oxford: Oxford University Press.

Baddeley, A. (2002). The psychology of memory. In A.D. Baddeley, M.D. Kopelman, & B.A. Wilson (Eds.), *The handbook of memory disorders.* Chichester, UK: Wiley.

Baddeley, A.D., Baddeley, H.A., Bucks, R.S., & Wilcock, G.K. (2001). Attentional control in Alzheimer's disease. *Brain, 124,* 1492–1508.

Baddeley, A.D., Della Sala, S., Papagno, C., & Spinnler, H. (1996). Dual-task performance in dysexecutive and nondysexecutive patients with a frontal lesion. *Neuropsychology, 11,* 187–194.

Baddeley, A., Emslie, H., & Nimmo-Smith, I. (1988). Estimating premorbid intelligence [abstract]. *Journal of Clinical and Experimental Neuropsychology, 10,* 326.

Baddeley, A., Emslie, H., & Nimmo-Smith, I. (1993). *The Speed and Capacity of Language Processing Tests: Manual.* Bury St. Edmunds, UK: Thames Valley Test Co.

Baddeley, A., Harris, J., Sunderland, A., et al. (1987). Closed head injury and memory. In H.S. Levin, J. Grafman, & H.M. Eisenberg (Eds.), *Neurobehavioral recovery from head injury.* New York: Oxford University Press.

Baddeley, A.D. & Hitch, G. (1974). Working memory. In G.A. Bower (Ed.), *The psychology of learning and motivation.* New York: Academic Press.

Baddeley, A., Logie, R., Nimmo-Smith, I., & Brerton, N. (1985). Components of fluent reading. *Journal of Verbal Learning and Verbal Behavior, 9,* 176–189.

Baddeley, A.D. & Warrington, E.K. (1970). Amnesia and the distinction between long- and short-term memory. *Journal of Verbal Learning and Verbal Behavior, 9,* 176–189.

Baddeley, A. & Wilson, B.A. (1988). Frontal amnesia and the dysexecutive syndrome. *Brain and Cognition, 7,* 212–230.

Badinand-Hubert, N., Bureau, M., Hirsch, E., et al. (1998). Epilepsies and video games: Results of a multicenter study. *Electroencephalography and Clinical Neurophysiology, 107,* 422–427.

Baehr, M.E. & Corsini, R.J. (1980). *The Press Test.* Rosemont, IL: London House.

Baguley, I.J., Felmingham, K.L., Lahz, S., et al. (1997). Alcohol abuse and traumatic brain injury: Effect on event-related potentials. *Archives of Physical Medicine and Rehabilitation, 78,* 1248–1253.

Baguley, I., Slewa-Younan, S., Lazarus, R., & Green, A. (2000). Long-term mortality trends in patients with traumatic brain injury. *Brain Injury, 14,* 505–512.

Bahrick, H. P. (1984). Replicative, constructive, and reconstructive aspects of memory: Implications for human and animal research. *Physiological Psychology, 12,* 53–58.

Bahrick, H.P. & Karis, D. (1982). Long-term ecological memory. *Handbook of methodology for memory and cognition.* New York: Academic Press.

Bailey, B., Forget, S., & Gaudreault, P. (2001). Prevalence of potential risk factors in victims of electrocution. *Forensic Science International, 123,* 58–62.

Bailey, C.A., McLaughlin, E.J., Levin, H.S., et al. (1984). *Post- traumatic amnesia and disorientation following closed head injury.* Paper presented at the 12th annual meeting of the International Neuropsychological Society, Houston, TX.

Baird, A.D., Ausman, J.I., Diaz, F.G., et al. (1988). Neurobehavioral and life-quality changes after cerebral revascularization. *Journal of Consulting and Clinical Psychology, 56,* 148–151.

Baird, A., Podell, K., Lovell, M., & McGinty, S.B. (2001). Complex real-world functioning and neuropsychological test performance in older adults. *The Clinical Neuropsychologist, 15,* 369–379.

Bak, J.S. & Green, R.I. (1981). A review of the performance of aged adults on various Wechsler Memory subtests. *Journal of Clinical Psychology, 37,* 186–188.

Bak, T.H., Antoun, N., Balan, K.K., & Hodges, J.R. (2001). Memory lost, memory regained: Neuropsychological findings and neuroimaging in two cases of paraneoplastic limbic encephalitis with radically different outcomes. *Journal of Neurology, Neurosurgery and Psychiatry, 71,* 40–47.

Baker, E.L., Letz, R.E., Eisen, E.A., et al. (1988). Neurobehavioral effects of solvents in construction painters. *Journal of Occupational Medicine, 30,* 116–123.

Baker, G. (1956). Diagnosis of organic brain damage in the adult. In B. Klopfer (Ed.), *Developments in the Rorschach technique.* New York: World Book.

Baker, G.A. (2001). Assessment of quality of life in people with epilepsy: Some practical implications. *Epilepsia, 42,* 66–69.

Baker, G.A., Smith, D.F., Dewey, M., et al. (1991). The development of a seizure severity scale as an outcome measure in epilepsy. *Epilepsy Research, 8,* 245–251.

Baker, G.A., Smith, D.F., Dewey, M., et al. (1993). The initial development of a health-related quality of life model as an outcome measure in epilepsy. *Epilepsy Research, 16,* 65–81.

Baker, R., Donders, J., & Thompson, E. (2000). Assessment of incomplete effort with the California Verbal Learning Test. *Applied Neuropsychology, 7,* 111–114.

Baker, S.C., Rogers, R.D., Owen, A.M., et al. (1996). Neural systems engaged by planning: a PET study of the Tower of London task. *Neuropsychologia, 34,* 515–526.

Bakshi, R., Ariyaratana, S., Benedict, R. H., & Jacobs, L. (2001). Fluid-attenuated inversion recovery magnetic resonance imaging detects cortical and juxtacortical multiple sclerosis lesions. *Archives of Neurology, 58,* 742–748.

Bakshi, R., Czarnecki, D., Shaikh, Z.A., et al. (2000). Brain MRI lesions and atrophy are related to depression in multiple sclerosis. *Neuroreport, 11,* 1153–1158.

Baldini, I.M., Vita, A., Mauri, M.C., et al. (1997). Psychopathological and cognitive features in subclinical hypothyroidism. *Progress in Neuropsychopharmacology and Biological Psychiatry, 21,* 925–935.

Baldo, J.V., Delis, D., Kramer, J., & Shimamura, A.P. (2002). Memory performance on the California Verbal Learning Test-II: Findings from patients with focal frontal lesions. *Journal of the International Neuropsychological Society, 8,* 539–546.

Baldo, J.V. & Shimamura, A.P. (1998). Letter and category fluency in patients with frontal lobe lesions. *Neuropsychology, 12,* 259–267.

Baldo, J.V., Shimamura, A.P., Delis, D.C., et al. (2001). Verbal and design fluency in patients with frontal lobe lesions. *Journal of the International Neuropsychological Society, 7,* 586–596.

Ball, M.J. (1977). Neuronal loss, neurofibrillary tangles and granulovacuolar degeneration in the hippocampus with aging and dementia. A quantitative study. *Acta Neuropathologica, 37,* 111–118.

Ball, M.J. & Murdoch, G.H. (1997). Neuropathological criteria for the diagnosis of Alzheimer's disease: are we really ready yet? *Neurobiology of Aging, 18,* S3–S12.

Ball, S.S., Marsh, J.T., Schubarth, G., et al. (1989). Longitudinal P300 latency changes in Alzheimer's disease. *Journal of Gerontology, 44,* M195–M200.

Ballard, C.G., Ayre, G., O'Brien, J., et al. (1999). Simple standardised neuropsychological assessments aid in the differential diagnosis of dementia with Lewy bodies from Alzheimer's disease and vascular dementia. *Dementia and Geriatric Cognitive Disorders*, 10, 104–108.

Ballard, J.C. (1996). Computerized assessment of sustained attention: Interactive effects of task demand, noise, and anxiety. *Journal of Clinical and Experimental Neuropsychology*, 18, 864–882.

Ballenger, J.C. & Post, R.M. (1989). Addictive behavior and kindling: Relationship to alcohol withdrawal and cocaine. In T.G. Bolwig & M.R. Trimble (Eds.), *The clinical relevance of kindling*. Chichester, UK: Wiley.

Balota, D.A., Dolan, P.O., & Duchek, J.M. (2000). Memory changes in healthy older adults. In E. Tulving & F.I.M. Craik (Eds.), *The Oxford handbook of memory*. Oxford: Oxford University Press.

Baltas, I., Gerogiannis, N., Sakellariou, P., et al. (1998). Outcome in severely head injured patients with and without multiple trauma. *Journal of Neurosurgical Science*, 42, 85–88.

Baltes, P.B. & Graf, P. (1996). Psychological aspects of ageing: Facts and frontiers. In D. Magnusson et al. (Eds.), *The lifespan development of individuals: behavioral, neurobiological, and psychological perspectives*. Cambridge, UK: Cambridge University Press.

Bamford, J. (2001). Assessment and investigation of stroke and transient ischaemic attack. *Journal of Neurology, Neurosurgery, and Psychiatry*, 70, I3–I6.

Bampoe, J. & Bernstein, M. (1999). The role of surgery in low grade gliomas. *Journal of Neurooncology*, 42, 470–476.

Bandak, F.A. (1995). On the mechanics of impact neurotrauma: A review and critical synthesis. *Journal of Neurotrauma*, 12, 635–649.

Banich, M.T. (1995). Interhemispheric interaction: Mechanisms of unified processing. In F.L. Kitterle (Ed.), *Hemispheric communication: Mechanisms and models*. Hillsdale, NJ: Erlbaum.

Banich, M.T. & Nicholas, C.D. (1998). Integration of processing between the hemispheres in word recognition. In M. Beeman and C. Chiarello (Eds.), *Right hemisphere language comprehension. Perspectives from cognitive neuroscience*. Mahwah, NJ: Erlbaum.

Bank, A.L., Yochim, B.P., MacNeill, S.E., & Lichtenberg, P.A. (2000). Expanded normative data for the Mattis Dementia Rating Scale for use with urban, elderly medical patients. *The Clinical Neuropsychologist*, 14, 149–156.

Banken, J.A. (1985). Clinical utility of considering digits forward and digits backward as separate components of the Wechsler Adult Intelligence Scale–Revised. *Journal of Clinical Psychology*, 41, 686–691.

Banning, A. & Sjøgren, P. (1990). Cerebral effects of long-term oral opiods in cancer patients measured by continuous reaction time. *Clinical Journal of Pain*, 6, 91–95.

Bannister, R. (1992). *Brain and Bannister's clinical neurology* (7th ed). Oxford: Oxford University Press.

Banos, J.H. & Franklin, L.M. (2002). Factor structure of the Mini-Mental State Examination in adult psychiatric inpatients. *Psychological Assessment*, 14, 397–400.

Barat, M., Blanchard, J.Y., Darriet, D., et al. (1989). Les troubles neuropsychologiques des anoxies cérébrales prolongées. Influence sur le devenir functionnel. *Annales de Réadaptation et de Médecine Physique*, 32, 657–668.

Barbarotto, R., Capitani, E., & Laiacona, M. (1996). Naming deficit in herpes simplex encephalitis. *Acta Neurologica Scandinavica*, 93, 272–280.

Barbee, J.G., Black, F.W., Kehoe, C.E., & Todorov, A.A. (1991). A comparison of the single-dose effects of alprazolam, buspirone, and placebo upon memory function. *Journal of Clinical Psychopharmacology*, 11, 351–356.

Barber, R., Ballard, C., McKeith, I.G., et al. (2000). MRI volumetric study of dementia with Lewy bodies: A comparison with AD and vascular dementia. *Neurology*, 54, 1304–1309.

Barber, R., Panikkar, A., & McKeith, I.G. (2001). Dementia with Lewy bodies: Diagnosis and management. *International Journal of Geriatric Psychiatry*, 16, S12–S18.

Barbieri, C. & De Renzi, E. (1989). Patterns of neglect dissociation. *Behavioral Neurology*, 2, 13–24.

Barbizet, J. (1974). Rôle de l'hémisphere droit dans les perceptions auditives. In J. Barbizet, M. Ben Hamida, & Ph. Duizabo (Eds.), *Le monde de l'hémiplegique gauche*. Paris: Masson.

Barbizet, J. & Duizabo, P. (1980). *Neuropsychologie* (2nd ed.). Paris: Masson.

Barclay, C.R. (1988). Truth and accuracy in autobiographical memory. In M.M. Gruneberg, et al. (Eds.), *Practical aspects of memory: Current research and issues. Memory in everyday life* (Vol. 1). New York: Wiley.

Barclay, L.L., Zemcov, A., Blass, J.P., et al. (1985). Survival in Alzheimer's disease and vascular dementias. *Neurology*, 35, 834–840.

Baribeau, J. & Roth, R.M. (1996). La neuropsychologie de l'émotion humaine. In M.I. Botez (Ed.), *Neuropsychologie clinique et neurologie du comportement*. Montréal: Les Presses de l'Université de Montréal/Paris: Masson.

Barker, A., Prior, J., & Jones, R. (1995). Memory complaint in attenders at a self-referral memory clinic: The role of cognitive factors, affective symptoms and personality. *International Journal of Geriatric Psychiatry*, 10, 777–781.

Barker, L.H., Bigler, E.D., Johnson, S.C., et al. (1999). Polysubstance abuse and traumatic brain injury: Quantitative magnetic resonance imaging and neuropsychological outcome in older adolescents and young adults. *Journal of the International Neuropsychological Society*, 5, 593–608.

Barkhof, F. (1999). MRI in multiple sclerosis. Correlation with Expanded Disability Status Scale (EDSS). *Multiple Sclerosis*, 5, 283–286.

Barkley, R.A. (1997). Behavioral inhibition, sustained attention, and executive functions: constructing a unifying theory of ADHD. *Psychological Bulletin*, 121, 65–94.

Barlow, J.S. (2002). *The cerebellum and adaptive control*. New York: Cambridge University Press.

Barncord, S.W. & Wanlass, R.L. (1999). Another ecological consideration in neuropsychological assessment. *Applied Neuropsychology*, 6, 121–122.

Barnes, G.W. & Lucas, G.J. (1974). Cerebral dysfunction vs. psychogenesis in Halstead-Reitan tests. *Journal of Nervous and Mental Diseases*, 158, 50–60.

Barnett, H.J., Meldrum, H.E., Eliasziw, M., & North American Symptomatic Carotid Endarterectomy Trial (2002). The appropriate use of carotid endarterectomy. *Canadian Medical Association Journal*, 166, 1169–1179.

Baron, I.S., Fennell, E.B., & Voeller, K.K.S. (1995). *Pediatric neuropsychology in the medical setting*. New York: Oxford University Press.

Baron-Cohen, S. (1995). *Mindblindness. An essay on autism and theory of mind*. Cambridge, MA: MIT Press.

Baron-Cohen, S., Ring, H.A., Bullmore, E.T., et al. (2000). The amygdala theory of autism. *Neuroscience amd Biobehavioral Reviews*, 24, 355–364.

Barona, A. & Chastain, R.L. (1986). An improved estimate of premorbid IQ for blacks and whites on the WAIS-R. *International Journal of Clinical Neuropsychology*, 8, 169–173.

Barona, A., Reynolds, C.R., & Chastain, R. (1984). A demographically based index of premorbid intelligence for the WAIS-R. *Journal of Consulting and Clinical Psychology*, 52, 885–887.

Barr, A., Benedict, R., Tune, L., & Brandt, J. (1992). Neuropsychological differentiation of AD from vascular dementia. *International Journal of Geriatric Psychiatry*, 7, 621–627.

Barr, W.B. (1997). Receiver operating characteristic curve analysis of Wechsler Memory Scale–Revised scores in epilepsy surgery candidates. *Psychological Assessment*, 9, 171–176.

Barr, W.B., Chelune, G.J., Hermann, B.P., et al. (1997). The use of figural reproduction tests as measures of nonverbal memory in epilepsy surgery candidates. *Journal of the International Neuropsychological Society, 3,* 435–443.

Barr, W.B., Goldberg, E., Wasserstein, J., & Novelly, R.A. (1990). Retrograde amnesia following unilateral temporal lobectomy. *Neuropsychologia,* 243–255.

Barr, W.B. & McCrea, M. (2001). Sensitivity and specificity of standardized neurocognitive testing immediately following sports concussion. *Journal of the International Neuropsychological Society, 7,* 693–702.

Barrash, J., Kealey, G.P., & Janus, T.J. (1996). Neurobehavioral sequelae of high voltage electrical injuries: Comparison with traumatic brain injury. *Applied Neuropsychology, 3,* 75–81.

Barrash, J., Tranel, D., & Anderson, S.W. (2000). Acquired personality disturbances associated with bilateral damage to the ventromedial prefrontal region. *Developmental Neuropsychology, 18,* 355–381.

Barrett, M. & Eames, K. (1996). Sequential developments in children's human figure drawing. *British Journal of Developmental Psychology, 14,* 219–236.

Barrett-Connor, E. & Kritz-Silverstein, D. (1999). Gender differences in cognitive function with age: The Rancho Bernardo study. *Journal of the American Geriatrics Society, 47,* 159–164.

Barron, F. (1953). An ego strength scale which predicts response to psychotherapy. *Journal of Consulting Psychology, 17,* 327–333.

Barron, J., Whiteley, S.J., Horn, A.C., et al. (1980). A new approach to the early detection of dialysis encephalopathy. *British Journal of Disorders of Communication, 15,* 75–85.

Barrows, D.M. (1995). Functional capacity evaluations of persons with chronic fatigue immune dysfunction syndrome. *American Journal of Occupational Therapy, 49,* 327–337.

Barry, J.J. & Sanborn, K. (2001). Etiology, diagnosis, and treatment of nonepileptic seizures. *Current Neurology and Neuroscience Reports, 1,* 381–389.

Barth, A., Bogousslavsky, J., & Caplan, L.R. (2001). Thalamic infarcts and hemorrhages. In J. Bogousslavsky & L.R. Caplan (Eds.), *Stroke syndromes* (2nd ed.). Cambridge, UK: Cambridge University Press.

Barth, A., Schaffer, A.W., Konnaris, C., et al. (2002). Neurobehavioral effects of vanadium. *Journal of Toxicology and Environmental Health A, 65,* 677–683.

Barth, A., Schaffer, A.W., Osterode, W., et al. (2002). Reduced cognitive abilities in lead-exposed men. *International Archives of Occupational and Environmental Health, 75,* 394–398.

Barth, J.T., Alves, W.M., Ryan, T.V., et al. (1989). Mild head injury in sports: Neuropsychological sequelae and recovery of function. In H.S. Levin, H.M. Eisenberg, & A.L. Benton (Eds.), *Mild head injury.* New York: Oxford University Press.

Barth, J.T., Pliskin, N., Axelrod, B., et al. (2003). Introduction to the NAN 2001 Definition of a Clinical Neuropsychologist. *Archives of Clinical Neuropsychology, 18,* 551–555.

Barth, J.T., Ryan, T.V., & Hawk, G.L. (1992). Forensic neuropsychology: A reply to the method skeptics. *Neuropsychology Review, 2,* 251–266.

Barth, J.T., Varney, N.R., Ruchinskas, R.A., & Francis, J.P. (1999). Mild head injury: The new frontier in sports medicine. In N.R. Varney & R.J. Roberts (Eds.), *The evaluation and treatment of mild traumatic brain injury.* Mahwah, NJ: Erlbaum.

Barton, J.J.S. & Caplan, L.R. (2001). Cerebral visual dysfunction. In J. Bogousslavsky and L.R. Caplan (Eds.). *Stroke syndromes* (2nd ed.). Cambridge, UK: Cambridge University Press.

Baser, C.A. & Ruff, R.M. (1987). Construct validity of the San Diego Neuropsychological Test Battery. *Archives of Clinical Neuropsychology, 2,* 13–32.

Basford, J.R., Chou, L.S., Kaufman, K.R., et al. (2003). An assess-ment of gait and balance deficits after traumatic brain injury. *Archives of Physical Medicine Rehabilitation, 84,* 343–349.

Basso, A. (1989). Spontaneous recovery and language rehabilitation. In X. Seron & G. Deloche (Eds.), *Cognitive approaches in neuropsychological rehabilitation.* Hillsdale, NJ: Lawrence Erlbaum.

Basso, A. (2003). *Aphasia and its therapy.* New York: Oxford University Press.

Basso, A., Burgio, F., & Caporali, A. (2000). Acalculia, aphasia and spatial disorders in left and right brain-damaged patients. *Cortex, 36,* 265–280.

Basso, A., Burgio, F., Paulin, M., & Prandoni, P. (2000). Long-term follow-up of ideomotor apraxia. *Neuropsychological Rehabilitation, 10,* 1–13.

Basso, A., Capitani, E., Laiacona, M., & Zanobio, M.E. (1985). Crossed aphasia: One or more syndromes? *Cortex, 21,* 25–45.

Basso, A., Capitani, E., & Moraschini, S. (1982). Sex differences in recovery from aphasia. *Cortex, 18,* 469–475.

Basso, A., Della Sala, S., & Farabola, M. (1987). Aphasia arising from purely deep lesions. *Cortex, 18,* 29–44.

Basso, M.R. & Bornstein, R.A. (1999). Relative memory deficits in recurrent versus first-episode major depression on a word-list learning task. *Neuropsychology, 13,* 557–563.

Basso, M.R., Bornstein, R.A., & Lang, J.M. (1999). Practice effects on commonly used measures of executive function across twelve months. *The Clinical Neuropsychologist, 13,* 283–292.

Basso, M.R., Bornstein, R.A., Roper, B.L., & McCoy, V.L. (2000). Limited accuracy of premorbid intelligence estimators: A demonstration of regression to the mean. *The Clinical Neuropsychologist, 14,* 325–340.

Basso, M.R., Harrington, K., Matson, M., & Lowery, N. (2000). Sex differences on the WMS-III: Findings concerning verbal paired associates and faces. *The Clinical Neuropsychologist, 14,* 231–235.

Batchelor, J., Harvey, A.G., & Bryant, R.A. (1995). Stroop Colour Word Test as a measure of attentional deficit following mild head injury. *The Clinical Neuropsychologist, 9,* 180–187.

Bate, A.J., Mathias, J.L., & Crawford, J.R. (2001). Performance on the Test of Everyday Attention and standard tests of attention following severe traumatic brain injury. *The Clinical Neuropsychologist, 15,* 405–422.

Battersby, W.S., Bender, M.B., Pollack, M., & Kahn, R.L. (1956). Unilateral "spatial agnosia" ("inattention") in patients with cerebral lesions. *Brain, 79,* 68–93.

Bauer, R.M. (1998). Physiologic measures of emotion. *Journal of Clinical Neurophysiology, 15,* 388–396.

Bauer, R.M. & Demery, J.A. (2003). Agnosia. In K.M. Heilman & E. Valenstein (Eds.), *Clinical neuropsychology* (4th ed.). New York: Oxford University Press.

Bauer, R.M., Grande, L., & Valenstein, E. (2003). Amnesic disorders. In K.M. Heilman & E. Valenstein (Eds.), *Clinical neuropsychology* (4th ed.). New York: Oxford University Press.

Bauer, R.M. & McDonald (2003). Auditory agnosia and amusia. In T.E. Feinberg and M.J. Farah (Eds.). *Behavioral neurology and neuropsychology.* New York: McGraw-Hill.

Bayles, K.A. (1988). Dementia: The clinical perspective. *Seminars in Speech and Language, 9,* 149–165.

Bayles, K.A., Boone, D.R., Tomoeda, C.K., et al. (1989). Differentiating Alzheimer's patients from the normal elderly and stroke patients with aphasia. *Journal of Speech and Hearing Disorders, 54,* 74–87.

Bayles, K.A., Salmon, D.P., Tomoeda, C.K., et al. (1989). Semantic and letter category naming in Alzheimer's patients: A predictable difference. *Developmental Neuropsychology, 5,* 335–347.

Bayles, K.A. & Tomoeda, C.K. (1983). Confrontation naming impairment in dementia. *Brain and Language, 19,* 98–114.

Bayles, K.A. & Tomoeda, C.K. (1990). *Arizona Battery for Communication Disorders of Dementia (ABCD)*. Tucson: Canyonlands.

Bayles, K.A., Tomoeda, C.K., & Boone, D.R. (1985). A view of age-related changes in language function. *Developmental Neuropsychology, 1,* 231–264.

Bayles, K.A., Tomoeda, C.K., Kaszniak, A.W., et al. (1985). Verbal perseveration of dementia patients. *Brain and Language, 25,* 102–116.

Bayles, K.A., Tomoeda, C.K., Wood, J.A., et al. (1996). Change in cognitive function in idiopathic Parkinson disease. *Archives of Neurology, 53,* 1140–1146.

Bayles, K.A., Trosset, M.W., Tomoeda, C.K., et al. (1993). Generative naming in Parkinson's disease patients. *Journal of Clinical and Experimental Neuropsychology, 15,* 547–562.

Bayless, J.D., Varney, N.R., & Roberts, R.J. (1989). Tinker Toy Test performance and vocational outcome in patients with closed head injuries. *Journal of Clinical and Experimental Neuropsychology, 11,* 913–917.

Bayley, P.J., Salmon, D.P., Bondi, M.W., et al. (2000). Comparison of the serial position effect in very mild Alzheimer's disease, mild Alzheimer's disease, and amnesia associated with electroconvulsive therapy. *Journal of Clinical and Experimental Neuropsychology, 6,* 290–298.

Baynes, K. & Eliassen, J.C. (1998). The visual lexicon: Its access and organization in commissurotomy patients. In M. Beeman, & C. Chiarello, (Eds.), *Right hemisphere language comprehension. Perspectives from cognitive neuroscience.* Mahwah, NJ: Erlbaum.

Baynes, K. & Gazzaniga, M.S. (2000). Consciousness, introspection, and the split brain: The two minds/one body problem. In M.S. Gazzaniga (Ed.), *The new cognitive neurosciences* (2nd ed.). Cambridge, MA: MIT Press.

Bazarian, J.J., Wong, T., Harris, M., et al. (1999). Epidemiology and predictors of post-concussive syndrome after minor head injury in an emergency population. *Brain Injury, 13,* 173–189.

Beal, M.F. (1995). Aging, energy, and oxidative stress in neurodegenerative diseases. *Annals of Neurology, 38,* 357–366.

Bear, D. (1977). Position paper on emotional and behavioral changes in Huntington's disease. *Report: Commission for the control of Huntington's disease and its consequences* (Vol. 3, Part 1). Washington, D.C.: U.S. Department of Health, Education, and Welfare.

Bear, D.M. (1983). Hemispheric specialization and the neurology of emotion. *Archives of Neurology, 40,* 195–202.

Bear, D., Schiff, D., Saver, J., et al. (1986). Quantitative analysis of cerebral asymmetries. Fronto-occipital correlation, sexual dimorphism and association with handedness. *Archives of Neurology, 43,* 598–603.

Beardsall, L. & Brayne, C. (1990). Estimation of verbal intelligence in an elderly community: A prediction analysis using a shortened NART. *British Journal of Clinical Psychology, 29,* 83–90.

Beardsall, L. & Huppert, F.A. (1991). A comparison of clinical, psychometric and behavioural memory tests: Findings from a community study of the early detection of dementia. *International Journal of Geriatric Psychiatry, 6,* 295–306.

Beaton, A.A. (1997). The relation of planum temporale asymmetry and morphology of the corpus callosum to handedness, gender, and dyslexia: A review of the evidence. *Brain and Language, 60,* 255–322.

Beatty, W.W. (1988). The Fargo Map Test: A standardized method for assessing remote memory for visuospatial information. *Journal of Clinical Psychology, 44,* 61–67.

Beatty, W.W. (1989a). Geographical knowledge throughout the lifespan. *Bulletin of the Psychonomic Society, 27,* 379–381.

Beatty, W.W. (1989b). Remote memory for visuospatial information in patients with Huntington's disease. *Psychobiology, 17,* 431–434.

Beatty, W.W. (1992). Memory disturbances in Parkinson's disease. In S.J. Huber & J.L. Cummings (Eds.), *Parkinson's disease.* New York: Oxford University Press.

Beatty, W.W. (1993). Age differences on the California Card Sorting Test: Implications for the assessment of problem solving by the elderly. *Bulletin of the Psychonomic Society, 31,* 511–514.

Beatty, W.W. & Bernstein, N. (1989). Geographical knowledge in patients with Alzheimer's disease. *Journal of Geriatric Psychiatry and Neurology, 2,* 76–82.

Beatty, W.W., Blanco, C.R., Wilbanks, S.L., et al. (1995). Demographic, clinical, and cognitive characteristics of multiple sclerosis patients who continue to work. *Journal of Neurologic Rehabilitation, 9,* 167–173.

Beatty, W.W. & Goodkin, D.E. (1990). Screening for cognitive impairment in multiple sclerosis: An evaluation of the Mini-Mental State Examination. *Archives of Neurology, 47,* 297–301.

Beatty, W.W., Goodkin, D.E., Hertsgaard, D., & Monson, N. (1990). Clinical and demographic predictors of cognitive performance in multiple sclerosis. *Archives of Neurology, 47,* 305–308.

Beatty, W.W., Goodkin, D.E., Monson, N., et al. (1988). Anterograde and retrograde amnesia in patients with chronic progressive multiple sclerosis. *Archives of Neurology, 45,* 611–619.

Beatty, W.W., Goodkin, D.E., Monson, N., & Beatty, P.A. (1989). Cognitive disturbances in patients with relapsing remitting multiple sclerosis. *Archives of Neurology, 46,* 1113–1119.

Beatty, W.W., Goodkin, D.E., Monson, N., & Beatty, P.A. (1990). Implicit learning in patients with chronic progressive multiple sclerosis. *International Journal of Clinical Neuropsychology, 12,* 166–172.

Beatty, W.W., Hames, K.A., Blanco, C.R., et al. (1995). Verbal abstraction deficit in multiple sclerosis. *Neuropsychology, 9,* 198–205.

Beatty, W.W., Katzung, V.M., Nixon, S.J., & Moreland, V.J. (1993). Problem-solving deficits in alcoholics: Evidence from the California Card Sorting Test. *Journal of Studies on Alcohol, 54,* 687–692.

Beatty, W.W., Krull, K.R., Wilbanks, S.L., et al. (1996). Further validation of constructs from the Selective Reminding Test. *Journal of Clinical and Experimental Neuropsychology, 18,* 52–55.

Beatty, W.W. & Monson, N. (1989). Geographical knowledge in patients with Parkinson's disease. *Bulletin of the Psychonomic Society, 27,* 473–475.

Beatty, W.W. & Monson, N. (1990). Problem solving in Parkinson's disease: Comparison of performance on the Wisconsin and California Card Sorting Tests. *Journal of Geriatric Psychiatry, Psychology and Neurology, 3,* 163–171.

Beatty, W.W. & Monson, N. (1991). Metamemory in multiple sclerosis. *Journal of Clinical and Experimental Neuropsychology, 13,* 309–327.

Beatty, W.W. & Monson, N. (1994). Picture and motor sequencing in multiple sclerosis. *Journal of Clinical and Experimental Neuropsychology, 16,* 165–172.

Beatty, W.W. & Monson, N. (1996). Problem solving by patients with multiple sclerosis: Comparison of performance on the Wisconsin and California Card Sorting Tests. *Journal of the International Neuropsychological Society, 2,* 134–140.

Beatty, W.W., Paul, R.H., Blanco, C.R., et al. (1995). Attention in multiple sclerosis: Correlates of impairment on the WAIS-R Digit Span Test. *Applied Neuropsychology, 2,* 139–144.

Beatty, W.W., Salmon, D.P., Butters, N., et al. (1988). Retrograde amnesia in patients with Alzheimer's disease or Huntington's disease. *Neurobiology of Aging, 9,* 181–186.

Beatty, W.W., Tivis, R., Stott, H.D., et al. (2000). Neuropsychological deficits in sober alcoholics: Influences of chronicity and recent alcohol consumption. *Alcoholism, Clinical and Experimental Research, 24,* 149–154.

Beatty, W.W. & Tröster, A.I. (1987). Gender differences in geographical knowledge. *Sex Roles, 16,* 565–590.

Beatty, W.W., Wilbanks, S.L., Blanco, C.R., et al. (1996). Memory disturbance in multiple sclerosis: Reconsideration of patterns of performance on the Selective Reminding Test. *Journal of Clinical and Experimental Neuropsychology, 18,* 56–62.

Beatty, W.W., Winn, P., Adams, R.L., et al. (1994). Preserved cognitive skills in dementia of the Alzheimer's type. *Archives of Neurology, 51,* 1040–1046.

Beauchamp, N.J. & Bryan, R.N. (1997). Neuroimaging of stroke. In K.M. Welch, L.R. Caplan, et al. (Eds.), *Primer on cerebrovascular diseases.* San Diego: Academic Press.

Beaumont, J.G. (1997). Future research directions in laterality. *Neuropsychology Review, 7,* 107–126.

Beaumont, J.G. & Davidoff, J.B. (1992). Assessment of visuo-perceptual dysfunction. In J.R. Crawford, D.M. Parker, & W.W. McKinlay (Eds.), *A handbook of neuropsychological assessment.* Hove, UK: Erlbaum.

Beaumont, J.G., Marjoribanks, J., Flury, S., & Lintern, T. (2002). *Putney Auditory Comprehension Screening Test (PACST).* Bury St. Edmunds, UK: Thames Valley Test Co.

Beauvois, M.-F. & Dérousné, C. (1981). Lexical or orthographic agraphia. *Brain, 104,* 21–49.

Beauvois, M.-F. & Saillant, B. (1985). Optic aphasia for colours and colour agnosia: A distinction between visual and visuo-verbal impairments in the processing of colours. *Cognitive Neuropsychology, 2,* 1–48.

Bechara, A., Damasio, H., & Damasio, A.R. (2000). Emotion, decision making and the orbitofrontal cortex. *Cerebral Cortex, 10,* 295–307.

Bechara, A., Damasio, A.R., Damasio, H., & Anderson, S.W. (1994). Insensitivity to future consequences following damage to human prefrontal cortex. *Cognition, 50,* 7–15.

Bechara, A., Damasio, H., Damasio, A.R., & Lee, G.P. (1999). Different contributions of the human amygdala and ventromedial prefrontal cortex to decision-making. *Journal of Neuroscience, 19,* 5473–5481.

Bechara, A., Damasio, H., Tranel, D., & Anderson, S.W. (1998). Dissociation of working memory from decision making within the human prefrontal cortex. *Journal of Neuroscience, 18,* 428–437.

Beck, A.T. (1987). *Beck Depression Inventory.* San Antonio: Psychological Coporation.

Beck, A.T., Steer, R.A., & Brown, G.K. (1996). *Beck Depression Inventory-II. Manual.* San Antonio, TX: Psychological Corporation.

Beck, S.J. (1981). Reality, Rorschach, and perceptual theory. In A.I. Rabin (Ed.), *Assessment with projective techniques: A concise introduction.* New York: Springer.

Beck, S.J., Beck, A. G., Levitt, E. E., & Molish, H. B. (1961). *Rorschach's test. I: Basic processes* (3rd ed.). New York: Grune & Stratton.

Becker, J.T. (1988). Working memory and secondary memory deficits in Alzheimer's disease. *Journal of Clinical and Experimental Neuropsychology, 10,* 739–753.

Becker, J.T., Butters, N., Hermann, A., & D'Angelo, N. (1983). Learning to associate names and faces. *Journal of Nervous and Mental Disease, 171,* 617–623.

Becker, J.T., Butters, N., Rivoira, P., & Miliotis, P. (1986). Asking the right questions: Problem solving in male alcoholics and male alcoholics with Korsakoff's syndrome. *Alcohol Clinical and Experimental Research, 10,* 641–646.

Becker, J.T., Huff, F.J., Nebes, R.D., et al. (1988). Neuropsychological function in Alzheimer's disease: Pattern of impairment and rates of progression. *Archives of Neurology, 45,* 263–268.

Becker, K.G., Simon, R.M., Bailey-Wilson, J.E., et al. (1998). Clustering of non-major histocompatibility complex susceptibility candidate loci in human autoimmune diseases. *Proceedings of the National Academy of Sciences USA, 95,* 9979–9984.

Beckwith, B.E. (2001). Thyroid disorders. In R.E. Tarter, M. Butters, & S.R. Beers (Eds.), *Medical neuropsychology* (2nd ed.). New York: Kluwer Academic/Plenum Press.

Bédard, M-A., Lévesque, M., Lemay, S., & Paquet, F. (2003). Nondopaminergic influences on cognition in Parkinson's disease. In M-A. Bédard et al. (Eds.), *Mental and behavioral dysfunction in movement disorders.* Totowa, NJ: Humana Press.

Bédard, M., Montplaisir, J., Malo, J., et al. (1993). Persistent neuropsychological deficits and vigilance impairment in sleep apnea syndrome after treatment with CPAP. *Journal of Clinical and Experimental Neuropsychology, 15,* 330–341.

Beeman, M. (1998). Coarse semantic coding and discourse comprehension. In M. Beeman, & C. Chiarello (Eds.), *Right hemisphere language comprehension. Perspectives from cognitive neuroscience.* Mahwah, NJ: Erlbaum.

Beeman, M. & Chiarello, C. (Eds.) (1998). *Right hemisphere language comprehension. Perspectives from cognitive neuroscience.* Mahwah, NJ: Erlbaum.

Beery, K.E. & Buktenica, N.A. (1997). *Developmental Test of Visual-Motor Integration.* Odessa, FL: Psychological Assessment Resources.

Beetar, J.T. & Williams, J.M. (1995). Malingering response styles on the Memory Assessment Scales and symptom validity tests. *Archives of Clinical Neuropsychology, 10,* 57–72.

Begley, C.E., Famulari, M., Annegers, J.F., et al. (2000). The cost of epilepsy in the United States: An estimate from population-based clinical and survey data. *Epilepsia, 41,* 342–351.

Behrmann, M. & Plaut, D.C. (2001). The interaction of spatial reference frames and hierarchical object representations. Evidence from figure copying in hemispatial neglect. *Cognitive, Affective, and Behavioral Neuroscience, 1,* 307–329.

Belanoff, J.K., Rothschild, A.J., Cassidy, F., et al. (2002). An open label trial of C-1073 (mifepristone) for psychotic major depression. *Biological Psychiatry, 52,* 386–392.

Belger, A., & Banich, M.T. (1998). Costs and benefits of integrating information between the cerebral hemispheres: A computational perspective. *Neuropsychology, 12,* 380–398.

Bell, B.D. & Davies, K.G. (1998). Anterior temporal lobectomy, hippocampal sclerosis, and memory: Recent neuropsychological findings. *Neuropsychology Review, 8,* 25–41.

Bell, B.D., Davies, K.G., Hermann, B.P., & Walters, G. (2000). Confrontation naming after anterior temporal lobectomy is related to age of acquisition of the object names. *Neuropsychologia, 38,* 83–92.

Bell, B.D., Primeau, M., Sweet, J.J., & Lofland, K.R. (1999). Neuropsychological functioning in migraine headache, nonheadache chronic pain, and mild traumatic brain injury patients. *Archives of Clinical Neuropsychology, 14,* 389–399.

Bell, B.D. & Roper, B.L. (1998). "Myths of Neuropsychology:" Another view. *The Clinical Neuropsychologist, 12,* 237–244.

Bell, M.D., Greig, T.C., Kaplan, E., & Bryson, G. (1997). Wisconsin Card Sorting Test dimensions in schizophrenia: Factorial, predictive, and divergent validity. *Journal of Clinical and Experimental Neuropsychology, 19,* 933–941.

Bell, N.L., Lassiter, K.S., Matthews, T.D., & Hutchinson, M.B. (2001). Comparison of the Peabody Picture Vocabulary Test-Third Edition and Wechsler Adult Intelligence Scale-Third Edition with university students. *Journal of Clinical Psychology, 57,* 417–422.

Bell, W.L. (1998). Ictal cognitive assessment of partial seizures and pseudoseizures. *Archives of Neurology, 55,* 1456–1459.

Bell-McGinty, S., Podell, K., Franzen, M., et al. (2002). Standard measures of executive function in predicting instrumental activities of daily living in older adults. *International Journal of Geriatric Psychiatry, 17,* 828–834.

Bellas, D.N., Novelly, R.A., Eskenazi, B., & Wasserstein, J. (1988). The nature of unilateral neglect in the olfactory sensory system. *Neuropsychologia, 26,* 45–52.

Belleville, S., Peretz, I., & Malenfant, D. (1996). Examination of the working memory components in normal aging and in dementia of the Alzheimer type. *Neuropsychologia, 34,* 195–207.

Belleza, T., Rappaport, M., Hopkins, H.K., & Hall, K. (1979). Visual scanning and matching dysfunction in brain-damaged patients with drawing impairment. *Cortex, 15,* 19–36.

Bellugi, U., Poizner, H., & Klima, E.S. (1983). Brain organization for language: Clues from sign aphasia. *Human Neurobiology, 2,* 155–170.

Benbadis, S.R., Agrawal, V., & Tatum, W.O.T. (2001). How many patients with psychogenic nonepileptic seizures also have epilepsy? *Neurology, 57,* 915–917.

Benbow, C.P. (1988). Neuropsychological perspectives on mathematical talent. In L.K. Obler & D. Fein (Eds.), *The exceptional brain. Neuropsychology of talent and special abilities.* New York: Guilford Press.

Benbow, C.P., Lubinski, D., Shea, D.L., & Eftekhari-Sanjani, H. (2000). Sex differences in mathematical reasoning ability at age 13: Their status 20 years later. *Psychological Science, 11,* 474–480.

Benbow, C.P. & Stanley, J.C. (1982). Consequences in high school and college of sex differences in mathematical reasoning ability. A longitudinal perspective. *American Educational Research Journal, 19,* 598–622.

Bender, L. (1938). A visual motor Gestalt test and its clinical use. *American Orthopsychiatric Association, Research Monographs 3.*

Bender, L. (1946). *Instructions for the use of the Visual Motor Gestalt Test.* New York: American Orthopsychiatric Association.

Bender, M.B. (1979). Defects in reversal of serial order of symbols. *Neuropsychologia, 17,* 125–138.

Bendixen, B.H. & Benton, A.L. (1997). Cognitive and linguistic outcome. In H.S. Levin, A.L. Benton, J.P. Muizelaar, & H.M. Eisenberg (Eds.), *Catastrophic brain injury.* New York: Oxford University Press.

Benedetti, M.D., Bower, J.H., Maraganore, D.M., et al. (2000). Smoking, alcohol, and coffee consumption preceding Parkinson's disease: A case-control study. *Neurology, 55,* 1350–1358.

Benedict, R.H.B., Fischer, J.S., Archibald, C.J., et al. (2002). Minimal neuropsychological assessment of MS patients: A consensus approach. *The Clinical Neuropsychologist, 16,* 381–397.

Benedict, R.H.B., Priore, R.L., Miller, C., et al. (2001). Personality disorder in multiple sclerosis correlates with cognitive impairment. *Journal of Neuropsychiatry and Clinical Neurosciences, 13,* 70–76.

Benedict, R.H.B., Schretlen, Groninger, L., & Brandt, J. (1998). Hopkins Verbal Learning Test-Revised: Normative data and analysis of inter-form and test–retest reliability. *The Clinical Neuropsychologist, 12,* 43–55.

Benedict, R.H.B., Shapiro, A., Priore, R., et al. (2000). Neuropsychological counseling improves social behavior in cognitively-impaired multiple sclerosis patients. *Multiple Sclerosis, 6,* 391–396.

Benedict, R.H.B. & Zgaljardic, D.J. (1998). Practice effects during repeated administrations of memory tests with and without alternate forms. *Journal of Clinical and Experimental Neuropsychology, 20,* 339–352.

Benke, T., Gasse, T., Hittmair-Delazer, M., & Schmutzhard, E. (1995). Lyme encephalopathy: Long-term neuropsychological deficits years after acute neuroborreliosis. *Acta Neurologica Scandinavica, 91,* 353–357.

Benke, T., Hohenstein, C., Poewe, W., & Butterworth, B. (2000). Repetitive speech phenomena in Parkinson's disease. *Journal of Neurology, Neurosurgery and Psychiatry, 69,* 319–325.

Benke, T., Kurzthaler, I., Schmidauer, C., et al. (2002). Mania caused by a diencephalic lesion. *Neuropsychologia, 40,* 245–252.

Bennett, T.L. (2001). Neuropsychological evaluation in rehabilitation planning and evaluation of functional skills. *Archives of Clinical Neuropsychology, 16,* 237–253.

Bennett, T.L. & Raymond, M.J. (1997a). Emotional consequences and psychotherapy for individuals with mild brain injury. *Applied Neuropsychology, 4,* 55–61.

Bennett, T.L. & Raymond, M.J. (1997b). Mild brain injury: An overview. *Applied Neuropsychology, 4,* 1–5.

Bennett, T.L. and Raymond, M.J. (Eds.) (1997c). Mild brain injury. *Applied Neuropychology, 4* (Special issue).

Bennett-Levy, J. (1984a). Determinants of performance on the Rey-Osterrieth Complex Figure Test: An analysis, and a new technique for single-case assessment. *British Journal of Clinical Psychology, 23,* 109–119.

Bennett-Levy, J. (1984b). Long-term effects of severe closed head injury on memory: Evidence from a consecutive series of young adults. *Acta Neurologica Scandinavica, 70,* 285–298.

Bennett-Levy, J., Klein-Boonschate, M.A., Batchelor, J., et al. (1994). Encounters with Anna Thompson: The consumer's experience of neuropsychological assessment. *The Clinical Neuropsychologist, 8,* 219–238.

Bennett-Levy, J., Polkey, C.E., & Powell, G.E. (1980). Self-report of memory skills after temporal lobectomy: The effect of clinical variables. *Cortex, 16,* 543–557.

Bennett-Levy, J. & Powell, G. E. (1980). The Subjective Memory Questionaire: An investigation into the self-reporting of "real-life" memory skills. *British Journal of Social and Clinical Psychology, 19,* 177–188.

Benowitz, L.I., Bear, D.M., Rosenthal, R., et al. (1983). Hemispheric specialization in nonverbal communication. *Cortex, 19,* 5–11.

Ben-Porath, Y.S. (1994). The ethical dilemma of coached malingering research. *Psychological Assessment, 6,* 14–15.

Ben-Porath, Y.S. & Butcher, J.N. (1989). The comparability of MMPI and MMPI-2 scales and profiles. *Psychological Assessment, 1,* 345–347.

Benson, D.F. (1988). Classical syndromes of aphasia. In F. Boller & J. Grafman (Eds.), *Handbook of neuropsychology* (Vol. 1). Amsterdam: Elsevier.

Benson, D.F. (1989). Disorders of visual gnosis. In J.W. Brown (Ed.), *Neuropsychology of visual perception.* New York: IRBN Press.

Benson, D.F. (1991). The Geschwind syndrome. *Advances in Neurology, 55,* 411–421.

Benson, D.F. (1993). Aphasia. In K.M. Heilman & E. Valenstein (Eds.), *Clinical neuropsychology* (3rd ed.). New York: Oxford University Press, pp. 17–36.

Benson, D.F. & Ardila, A. (1996). *Aphasia: A clinical perspective.* New York: Oxford University Press.

Benson, D.F. & Barton, M.I. (1970). Disturbances in constructional ability. *Cortex, 6,* 19–46.

Benson, D.F., Davis, R.J., & Snyder, B.D. (1988). Posterior cortical atrophy. *Archives of Neurology, 45,* 789–793.

Benson, D.F., Djenderedjian, A., Miller, B.L., et al. (1996). Neural basis of confabulation. *Neurology, 46,* 1239–1243.

Benton, A.L. (1945). Rorschach performance of suspected malingerers. *Journal of Abnormal and Social Psychology, 40,* 94–96.

Benton, A.L. (1967). Constructional apraxia and the minor hemisphere. *Confinia Neurologica (Basel)*, 29, 1–16; reprinted in L. Costa & O. Spreen (Eds.) (1985). *Studies in neuropsychology. Selected papers of Arthur Benton.* New York: Oxford University Press.

Benton, A.L. (1968). Differential behavioral effects in frontal lobe disease. *Neuropsychologia*, 6, 53–60.

Benton, A.L. (1969a). Constructional apraxia: Some unanswered questions. In A.L. Benton (Ed.), *Contributions to clinical neuropsychology.* Chicago: Aldine.

Benton, A.L. (1969b). Disorders of spatial orientation. In P.J. Vinken & G.W. Bruyn (Eds.), *Handbook of clinical neurology. Disorders of higher nervous activity* (Vol. 3). New York: Wiley.

Benton, A.L. (1972). Hemispheric cerebral dominance and somesthesis. In M. Hammer, K. Salzinger, & S. Sutton (Eds.), *Psychopathology: Essays in honor of Joseph Zubin.* New York: Wiley-Interscience; reprinted in L. Costa & O. Spreen (Eds.) (1985). *Studies in neuropsychology.* New York: Oxford University Press.

Benton, A.L. (1973). Test de praxie constructive tridimensionnelle: Forme alternative pour la clinique et la recherche. *Revue de Psychologie Appliquée*, 23, 1–5.

Benton, A.L. (1974). *Revised Visual Retention Test* (4th ed.). New York: Psychological Corporation.

Benton, A.L. (1977a). The amusias. In M. Critchley & R.A. Henson (Eds.), *Music and the brain.* London: William Heinemann.

Benton, A.L. (1977b). Reflections on the Gerstmann syndrome. *Brain and Language*, 4, 45–62; reprinted in L. Costa & O. Spreen (Eds.) (1985). *Studies in neuropsychology.* New York: Oxford University Press.

Benton, A.L. (1980). The neuropsychology of facial recognition. *American Psychologist*, 35, 176–186.

Benton, A.L. (1981). Focal brain damage and the concept of localization of function. In C. Loeb (Ed.), *Studies in cerebrovascular disease.* Milan: Masson Italia Editore; reprinted in L. Costa & O. Spreen (Eds.) (1985). *Studies in neuropsychology.* New York: Oxford University Press.

Benton, A.L. (1982). Spatial thinking in neurological patients: Historical aspects. In M. Potegal (Ed.), *Spatial abilities: Development and physiological foundations.* New York: Academic Press.

Benton, A.L. (1984). Constructional apraxia: An update. *Seminars in Neurology*, 4, 220–222.

Benton, A. (2000). *Exploring the history of neuropsychology. Selected papers.* New York: Oxford University Press.

Benton, A.L., Eslinger, P.J., & Damasio, A.R. (1981). Normative observations on neuropsychological test performance in old age. *Journal of Clinical Neuropsychology*, 3, 33–42.

Benton, A.L. & Fogel, M.L. (1962). The assumption that a common disability underlies failure in copying drawing and in copying two- and three-dimensional block patterns is not justified. *Archives of Neurology*, 7, 347.

Benton, A.L. & Hamsher, K. deS. (1989). *Multilingual Aphasia Examination.* Iowa City: AJA Associates.

Benton, A.L., Hamsher, K., & Sivan, A.B. (1994). *Multilingual Aphasia Examination* (3rd ed.). Iowa City: AJA.

Benton, A.L., Hannay, H.J., & Varney, N.R. (1975). Visual perception of line direction in patients with unilateral brain disease. *Neurology*, 25, 907–910; reprinted in L. Costa & O. Spreen (Eds.) (1985). *Studies in neuropsychology. Selected papers of Arthur Benton.* New York: Oxford University Press.

Benton, A.L. & Hécaen, H. (1970). Stereoscopic vision in patients with unilateral cerebral disease. *Neurology*, 20, 1084–1088.

Benton, A.L. & Sivan, A.B. (1984). Problems and conceptual issues in neuropsychological research in aging and dementia. *Journal of Clinical Neuropsychology*, 6, 57–64.

Benton, A.L., Sivan, A.B., Hamsher, K. deS., et al. (1994). *Contri-butions to neuropsychological assessment. A clinical manual* (2nd ed.). New York: Oxford University Press.

Benton, A.L. & Spreen, O. (1961). *Visual memory test:* The simulation of mental incompetence. *Archives of General Psychiatry*, 4, 79–83.

Benton, A.L., Van Allen, M.W., & Fogel, M.L. (1964). Temporal orientation in cerebral disease. *Journal of Nervous and Mental Disease*, 139, 110–119.

Ben-Yishay, Y. & Diller, L. (1993). Cognitive remediation in traumatic brain injury: Update and issues. *Archives of Physical Medicine and Rehabilitation*, 74, 204–213.

Ben-Yishay, Y., Diller, L., Gerstman, L., & Haas, A. (1968). The relationship between impersistence, intellectual function and outcome of rehabilitation in patients with left hemiplegia. *Neurology*, 18, 852–861.

Ben-Yishay, Y., Silver, S.M., Piasetsky, E., & Rattok, J. (1987). Relationship between employability and vocational outcome after intensive holistic cognitive rehabilitation. *Journal of Head Trauma Rehabilitation*, 2, 35–48.

Berch, D.B., Krikorian, R., & Huha, E.M. (1998). The Corsi block-tapping task: Methodological and theoretical considerations. *Brain and Cognition*, 38, 317–338.

Berenbaum, S.A., Baxter, L., Seidenberg, M., & Hermann, B. (1997). Role of the hippocampus in sex differences in verbal memory: Memory outcome following left anterior temporal lobectomy. *Neuropsychology*, 11, 585–591.

Berendse, H.W., Booij, J., Francot, C.M.J.E., et al. (2001). Subclinical dopamine dysfunction in asymptomatic Parkinson's disease patients' relatives with a decreased sense of smell. *Annals of Neurology*, 50, 34–41.

Berent, S., Giordani, B., Lehtinen, S., et al. (1988). Positron emission tomographic scan investigations of Huntington's disease. *Annals of Neurology*, 23, 541–546.

Beresford, T.P., Holt, R.E., Hall, R.C.W., & Feinsilver, D.L. (1985). Cognitive screening at the bedside: Usefulness of a structured examination. *Psychosomatics*, 26, 319–324.

Berg, A.T. & Shinnar, S. (1997). Do seizures beget seizures? An assessment of the clinical evidence in humans. *Journal of Clinical Neurophysiology*, 14, 102–110.

Berg, E.A. (1948). A simple objective treatment for measuring flexibility in thinking. *Journal of General Psychology*, 39, 15–22.

Berg, G., Edwards, D.F., Danziger, W.L., & Berg, L. (1987). Longitudinal change in three brief assessments of SDAT. *Journal of the American Geriatrics Society*, 35, 205–212.

Berg, L., Danziger, W.L., Storandt, M., et al. (1984). Predictive features in mild senile dementia of the Alzheimer type. *Neurology*, 34, 563–569.

Berg, L., McKeel, D.W., Jr., Miller, J.P., et al. (1998). Clinicopathologic studies in cognitively healthy aging and Alzheimer's disease: Relation of histologic markers to dementia severity, age, sex, and apolipoprotein E genotype. *Archives of Neurology*, 55, 326–335.

Berg, L. & Morris, J.C. (1990). Aging and dementia. In A.L. Pearlman & R.C. Collins (Eds.), *Neurobiology of disease.* New York: Oxford University Press.

Berg, R.A. & Golden, C. (1981). Identification of neuropsychological deficits in epilepsy using the Luria-Nebraska Neuropsychological Battery. *Journal of Consulting and Clinical Psychology*, 49, 745–757.

Berger, J.-M. & Perret, E. (1986). Interhemispheric integration of information in a surface estimation task. *Neuropsychologia*, 24, 743–746.

Berger, J.-M., Perrett, E., & Zimmermann, A. (1987). Interhemispheric integration of compound nouns: Effects of stimulus arrangement and mode of presentation. *Perceptual and Motor Skills, 65,* 663–671.

Berger, S. (1998). The WAIS-R factors: Usefulness and construct validity in neuropsychological assessments. *Applied Neuropsychology, 5,* 37–43.

Berglund, M., Hagstadius, S., Risberg, J., et al. (1987). Normalization of regional cerebral blood flow in alcoholics during the first seven weeks of abstinence. *Acta Psychiatrica Scandinavica, 75,* 202–208.

Bergner, M., Bobbitt, R.A., Carter, W.B., & Gilson, B.S. (1981). The Sickness Impact Profile: Development and final revision of a health status measure. *Medical Care, 19,* 787–805.

Bergner, M., Bobbit, R.A., & Pollard, W.E. (1981). The Sickness Impact Profile. Validation of a health status measure. *Medical Care, 14,* 57–67.

Berker, E.A., Berker, A.H., & Smith, A. (1986). Translation of Broca's 1965 report. Localization of speech in the third left frontal convolution. *Archives of Neurology, 43,* 1065–1072.

Berker, E. & Smith, A. (1988). Diaschisis, site, time and other factors in Raven performances of adults with focal cerebral lesions. *International Journal of Neuroscience, 38,* 267–285.

Berkovic, S.F., Howell, R.A., Hay, D.A., & Hopper, J.L. (1998). Epilepsies in twins: Genetics of the major epilepsy syndromes. *Annals of Neurology, 43,* 435–445.

Berliner, R. (2000). Cocaine. In P.S. Spencer & H.H. Schaumburg (Eds.), *Experimental and clinical neurotoxicology* (2nd ed.). New York: Oxford University Press.

Berman, K.F., Ostrem, J.L., Randolph, C., et al. (1995). Physiological activation of a cortical network during performance of the Wisconsin Card Sorting Test: A positron emission tomography study. *Neuropsychologia, 33,* 1027–1046.

Bernard, L.C. (1989). Halstead-Reitan neuropsychological test performance of black, Hispanic, and white young adult males from poor academic backgrounds. *Archives of Clinical Neuropsychology, 4,* 267–274.

Bernard, L.C. (1990). Prospects for faking believable memory deficits on neuropsychological tests and the use of incentives in simulation research. *Journal of Clinical and Experimental Neuropsychology, 12,* 715–728.

Bernard, L.C. (1991). The detection of faked deficits on the Rey Auditory Verbal Learning Test: The effect of serial position. *Archives of Clinical Neuropsychology, 6,* 81–88.

Bernard, L.C. & Fowler, W. (1990). Assessing the validity of memory complaints: Performance of brain-damaged and normal individuals on Rey's task to detect malingering. *Journal of Clinical Psychology, 46,* 432–435.

Bernard, L.C., Houston, W., & Natoli, L. (1993). Malingering on neuropsychological memory tests: Potential objective indicators. *Journal of Clinical Psychology, 49,* 45–53.

Bernard, L.C., McGrath, M.J., & Houston, W. (1996). The differential effects of simulating malingering, closed head injury, and other CNS pathology on the Wisconsin Card Sorting Test: Support for the "Pattern of Performance Hypotheses." *Archives of Clinical Neuropsychology, 11,* 231–245.

Bernardin, L., Rao, S.M., Lucchetta, T.L., et al. (1993). A prospective, long-term, longitudinal study of cognitive dysfunction in multiple sclerosis [abstract]. *Journal of Clinical and Experimental Neuropsychology, 15,* 17.

Berning, L.C., Weed, N.C., & Aloia, M.S. (1998). Interrater reliability of the Ruff Figural Fluency Test. *Assessment, 5,* 181–186.

Bernstein, T. (1994). Electrical injury: Electrical engineer's perspective and an historical review. *Annals of the New York Academy of Sciences, 720,* 1–10.

Berres, M., Monsch, A.U., Bernasconi, F., et al. (2000). Normal ranges of neuropsychological tests for the diagnosis of Alzheimer's disease. *Studies in Health Technology and Informatics, 77,* 195–199.

Berridge, C.W., España, R.A., & Stalnaker, T.A. (2003). Stress and coping: Asymmetry of dopamine efferents within the prefrontal cortex. In K. Hugdahl & R.J. Davidson (Eds.), *The asymmetrical brain.* Cambridge, MA: MIT Press.

Berrios, G.E., Wagle, A.C., Markova, I.S., et al. (2001). Psychiatric symptoms and CAG repeats in neurologically asymptomatic Huntington's disease gene carriers. *Psychiatry Research, 102,* 217–225.

Berrol, S. (1989). Moderate head injury. In P. Bach y Rita (Ed.), *Traumatic brain injury.* New York: Demos.

Berry, D.T., Allen, R.S., & Schmitt, F.A. (1991). The Rey-Osterrieth Complex Figure: Psychometric characteristics in a geriatric sample. *The Clinical Neuropsychologist, 5,* 143–153.

Berry, D.T.R., Baer, R.A., & Harris, M.J. (1991). Detection of malingering on the MMPI: A meta-analysis. *Clinical Psychology Review, 11,* 585–598.

Berry, D.T.R. & Carpenter, G.S. (1992). Effect of four different delay periods on recall of the Rey-Osterrieth Complex Figure by older persons. *The Clinical Neuropsychologist, 6,* 80–84.

Berry, D.T.R., Lamb, D.G., Wetter, M.W., et al. (1994). Ethical considerations in research on coached malingering. *Psychological Assessment, 6,* 16–17.

Berry, D.T.R., McConnell, J.W., Phillips, B.A., et al. (1989). Isocapnic hypoxemia and neuropsychological functioning. *Journal of Clinical and Experimental Neuropsychology, 11,* 241–251.

Berry, D.T.R., Webb, W.B., Block, A.J., et al. (1986). Nocturnal hypoxia and neuropsychological variables. *Journal of Clinical and Experimental Neuropsychology, 8,* 229–238.

Berry, D.T.R., Wetter, M.W., & Baer, R. A. (1991). Detection of random responding on the MMPI-2: Utility of *F*, back *F*, and VRIN scales. *Psychological Assessment, 3,* 418–423.

Berry, S. (1996). Diagrammatic procedure for scoring the Wisconsin Card Sorting Test. *The Clinical Neuropsychologist, 10,* 117–121.

Berthoz, A. (2000). *The brain's sense of movement* (trans. G. Weiss). Cambridge, MA: Harvard University Press.

Bertram, K.W., Abeles, N., & Snyder, P.J. (1990). The role of learning on Halstead's Category Test. *The Clinical Neuropsychologist, 4,* 244–252.

Besson, J.A.O., Crawford, J.R., Parker, D.M., et al. (1989). Brain imaging techniques in Alzheimer's disease (CT, NMR, SPECT and PET). In J.R. Crawford & D.M. Parker (Eds.), *Developments in clinical and experimental neuropsychology.* New York: Plenum Press.

Bestawros, A., Langevin, J.-P., LaLonde, R., & Botez-Marquard, T. (1999). Relationship between choice reaction time and the Tower of Hanoi test. *Perceptual and Motor Skills, 88,* 355–362.

Betancourt, H. & Lopez, S.R. (1993). The study of culture, ethnicity, and race in American psychology. *American Psychologist, 48,* 629–637.

Betz, A.L. (1997). Vasogenic brain edema. In K.M.A. Welch, et al. (Eds.), *Primer on cerebrovascular diseases.* San Diego: Academic Press.

Bever, T.G. & Chiarello, R.J. (1974). Cerebral dominance in musicians and nonmusicians. *Science, 185,* 537–539.

Bhagwanjee, S., Paruk, F., Moodley, J., & Muckart, D.J. (2000). Intensive care unit morbidity and mortality from eclampsia: an evaluation of the Acute Physiology and Chronic Health Evaluation II score and the Glasgow Coma Scale score. *Critical Care Medicine, 28,* 120–124.

Bhatia, K.P., & Marsden, C.D. (1994). The behavioural and motor consequences of focal lesions of the basal ganglia in man. *Brain, 117,* 859–876.

Bherer, L., Belleville, S., & Peretz, I. (2001) Education, age, and the Brown-Peterson technique. *Developmental Neuropsychology, 19,* 237–251.

Biber, C., Butters, N., Rosen, J., et al. (1981). Encoding strategies and recognition of faces by alcoholic Korsakoff and other brain-damaged patients. *Journal of Clinical Neuropsychology, 3,* 315–330.

Bieliauskas, L.A. & Glantz, R.H. (1989). Depression type in Parkinson disease. *Journal of Clinical and Experimental Neuropsychology, 11,* 597–604.

Bieliauskas, L.A. & Lamberty, G. (1995). Simple reaction time and depression in the elderly. *Aging and Cognition, 2,* 128–131.

Bier, J.A., Morales, Y., Liebling, J., et al. (1997). Medical and social factors associated with cognitive outcome in individuals with myelomeningocele. *Developmental Medicine and Child Neurology, 39,* 263–266.

Bigler, E.D. (1990a). Neuropathology of traumatic brain injury. In E.D. Bigler (Ed.), *Traumatic brain injury.* Austin, TX: Pro-Ed.

Bigler, E.D. (1990b). Neuropsychology and malingering: Comment on Faust, Hart, and Guilmette (1988). *Journal of Consulting and Clinical Psychology, 58,* 244–247.

Bigler, E.D. (1995). Brain morphology and intelligence. *Developmental Neuropsychology, 11,* 377–403.

Bigler, E.D. (Ed.) (1996). *Neuroimaging. I Basic science; II Clinical applications.* New York: Plenum Press.

Bigler, E.D. (1999). Neuroimaging in mild TBI. In N.R. Varney & R.J. Roberts (Eds.), *The evaluation and treatment of mild traumatic brain injury.* Mahwah, NJ: Erlbaum.

Bigler, E.D. (2001a). The lesion(s) in traumatic brain injury: Implications for clinical neuropsychology. *Archives of Clinical Neuropsychology, 16,* 95–131.

Bigler, E.D. (2001b). Quantitative magnetic resonance imaging in traumatic brain injury. *Journal of Head Trauma Rehabilitation, 16,* 117–134.

Bigler, E.D., Blatter, D.D., Johnson, S.C., et al. (1996). Traumatic brain injury, alcohol and quantitative neuroimaging: Preliminary findings. *Brain Injury, 10,* 197–206.

Bigler, E.D. & Ehrfurth, J.W. (1980). Critical limitations of the Bender-Gestalt test in clinical neuropsychology. *Clinical Neuropsychology, 2,* 88–90.

Bigler, E.D. & Ehrfurth, J.W. (1981). The continued inappropriate singular use of the Bender Visual Motor Gestalt test. *Professional Psychology: Research and Practice, 12,* 562–569.

Bigler, E.D., Kurth, S.M., Blatter, D., & Abildskov, T.J. (1992). Degenerative changes in traumatic brain injury: Post-injury magnetic resonance identified ventricular expansion compared to pre-injury levels. *Brain Research Bulletin, 28,* 651–653.

Bigler, E.D., Rosa, L., Schultz, F., et al. (1989). Rey-Auditory Verbal Learning and Rey-Osterrieth Complex Figure Design performance in Alzheimer's disease and closed head injury. *Journal of Clinical Psychology, 45,* 277–280.

Bigler, E.D. & Snyder, J.L. (1995). Neuropsychological outcome and quantitative neuroimaging in mild head injury. *Applied Neuropsychology, 10,* 159–174.

Bigner, S.H., Rasheed, K., Wiltshire, R.N., & McLendon, R. (1999). Morphologic and molecular genetic aspects of oligodendroglial neoplasms. *Neurooncology, 1,* 52–60.

Billingslea, F.Y. (1963). The Bender Gestalt. A review and a perspective. *Psychological Bulletin, 60,* 233–251.

Binder, J., Marshall, R., Lazar, R., et al. (1992). Distinct syndromes of hemineglect. *Archives of Neurology, 49,* 1187–1194.

Binder, J.R., Swanson, S.J., Hammeke, T.A., et al. (1996). Determination of language dominance using functional MRI: A comparison with the Wada test. *Neurology, 46,* 978–984.

Binder, L.M. (1982). Constructional strategies on Complex Figure drawings after unilateral brain damage. *Journal of Clinical Neuropsychology, 4,* 51–58.

Binder, L.M. (1986). Persisting symptoms after mild head injury: A review of the postconcussive syndrome. *Journal of Clinical and Experimental Neuropsychology, 8,* 323–346.

Binder, L.M. (1992). Malingering detected by forced choice testing of memory and tactile sensation: A case report. *Archives of Clinical Neuropsychology, 7,* 155–163.

Binder, L.M. (1993a). An abbreviated form of the Portland Digit Recognition Test. *The Clinical Neuropsychologist, 7,* 104–107.

Binder, L.M. (1993b). Assessment of malingering after mild head trauma with the Portland Digit Recognition Test. *Journal of Clinical and Experimental Neuropsychology, 15,* 170–182.

Binder, L.M. (1997). A review of mild head trauma. Part II: Clinical implications. *Journal of Clinical and Experimental Neuropsychology, 19,* 432–457.

Binder, L.M., Howieson, D., & Coull, B.M. (1987). Stroke: Causes, consequences, and treatment. In B. Caplan (Ed.), *Rehabilitation psychology desk reference.* Rockville, MD: Aspen.

Binder, L.M., Tanabe, C.T., Waller, F.T., & Wooster, N.E. (1982). Behavioral effects of superficial temporal artery to middle cerebral artery bypass surgery: Preliminary report. *Neurology, 32,* 422–424.

Binder, L.M. & Thompson, L.L. (1995). The Ethics Code and neuropsychological assessment practices. *Archives of Clinical Neuropsychology, 10,* 27–46.

Binder, L.M., Villanueva, M.R., Howieson, D., & Moore, R.T. (1993). The Rey AVLT Recognition Memory Task measures motivational impairment after mild head trauma. *Archives of Clinical Neuropsychology, 8,* 137–147.

Binder, L.M. & Willis, S.C. (1991). Assessment of motivation after financially compensable minor head trauma. *Psychological Assessment, 3,* 175–181.

Binder, L.M. & Wonser, D. (1989). Constructional strategies on Rey Complex Figure drawings of stroke patients in rehabilitation [abstract]. *Journal of Clinical and Experimental Neuropsychology, 11,* 45.

Binet, A. & Simon, Th. (1908). Le developpement de l'intelligence chez les enfants. *L'Année Psychologique, 14,* 1–94.

Binetti, G., Cappa, S.F., Magni, E., et al. (1998). Visual and spatial perception in the early phase of Alzheimer's disease. *Neuropsychology, 12,* 29–33.

Binetti, G., Magni, E., Cappa, S.F., et al. (1995). Semantic memory in Alzheimer's disease: an analysis of category fluency. *Journal of Clinical and Experimental Neuropsychology, 17,* 82–89.

Binks, P., Gouvier, W.D., & Waters, W. (1997). Malingering detection with the Dot Counting Test. *Archives of Clinical Neuropsychology, 12,* 41–46.

Binks, S.W. & Gold, J.M. (1998). Differential cognitive deficits in the neuropsychology of schizophrenia. *The Clinical Neuropsychologist, 12,* 8–20.

Birbeck, G.L., Hays, R.D., Cui, X., & Vickrey, B.G. (2002). Seizure reduction and quality of life improvements in people with epilepsy. *Epilepsia, 43,* 535–538.

Bird, T.D. (1998). Genotypes, phenotypes, and frontotemporal dementia: Take your pick. *Neurology, 50,* 1526–1527.

Birren, J.E. & Schaie, K.W. (Eds.) (1989). *Handbook of the psychology of aging* (3rd ed.). New York: Von Nostrand Reinhold.

Bishop, K.M. & Wahlsten, D. (1997). Sex differences in the human corpus callosum: Myth or reality? *Neuroscience and Biobehavioral Reviews, 21,* 581–601.

Bishop, S.L., Faulk, D., & Santy, P.A. (1996). The use of IQ assessment in astronaut screening and evaluation. *Aviation Space and Environmental Medicine, 67,* 1130–1137.

Bisiach, E. (1991). Extinction and neglect: Same or different? In

J. Paillard (Ed.), *Brain and space.* Oxford: Oxford University Press.

Bisiach, E. & Geminiani, G. (1991). Anosognosia related to hemiplegia and hemianopsia. In G.P. Prigatano & D.L. Schacter (Eds.), *Awareness of deficit after brain injury: Clinical and theoretical issues.* Oxford: Oxford University Press.

Bisiach, E. & Luzzatti, C. (1978). Unilateral neglect of representational space. *Cortex, 14,* 129–133.

Bisiach, E., Perani, D., Vallar, G., & Berti, A. (1986). Unilateral neglect: Personal and extra-personal. *Neuropsychologia, 24,* 759–767.

Bisiach, E. & Vallar, G. (1988). Hemineglect in humans. In F. Boller & J. Grafman (Eds.), *Handbook of neuropsychology* (Vol. 1). Amsterdam: Elsevier.

Bisiacchi, P.S. (1996). The neuropsychological approach in the study of prospective memory. In M. Brandimonte et al. (Eds.), *Prospective memory: Theory and applications.* Mahwah, NJ: Erlbaum.

Bissessur, S., Tissingh, G., Wolters, E.C., & Scheltens, P. (1997). rCBF SPECT in Parkinson's disease patients with mental dysfunction. *Journal of Neural Transmission. 50(Suppl.),* 25–30.

Bjorkman, I.K., Fastbom, J., Schmidt, I.K., & Bernsten, C.B. (2002). Drug–drug interactions in the elderly. *Annals of Pharmacotherapy, 36,* 1675–1681.

Black, B.W. (1982). Pathological laughter. *Journal of Nervous and Mental Disease, 170,* 67–71.

Black, F.W. (1986). Digit repetition in brain-damaged adults: Clinical and theoretical implications. *Journal of Clinical Psychology, 42,* 770–782.

Black, F.W. & Bernard, B.A. (1984). Constructional apraxia as a function of lesion locus and size in patients with focal brain damage. *Cortex, 20,* 111–120.

Black, F.W. & Strub, R.L. (1976). Constructional apraxia in patients with discrete missile wounds of the brain. *Cortex, 12,* 212–220.

Black, F.W. & Strub, R.L. (1978). Digit repetition performance in patients with focal brain damage. *Cortex, 14,* 12–21.

Black, S.E. (1996). Focal cortical atrophy syndromes. *Brain and Cognition, 31,* 188–229.

Blackford, R.C. & La Rue, A. (1989). Criteria for diagnosing age-associated memory impairment: Proposed improvements from the field. *Developmental Neuropsychology, 5,* 295–306.

Blackwood, H.D. (1996). Recommendation for test administration in litigation: Never administer the Category Test to a blindfolded subject. *Archives of Clinical Neuropsychology, 11,* 93–95.

Bladin, C.F., Alexandrov, A.V., Bellavance, A., et al. (2000). Seizures after stroke: A prospective multicenter study. *Archives of Neurology, 57,* 1617–1622.

Bladin, C.F. & Norris, J.W. (1997). Stroke and seizures/epilepsy. In K.M.A. Welch et al. (Eds.), *Primer on cerebrovascular diseases.* San Diego: Academic Press.

Blain, P.G. & Lane, R.J.M. (1991). Neurological disorders. In D.M. Davies (Ed.), *Textbook of adverse drug reactions* (4th ed.). Oxford: Oxford University Press.

Blair, J.R. & Spreen, O. (1989). Predicting premorbid IQ: A revision of the National Adult Reading Test. *The Clinical Neuropsychologist, 3,* 129–136.

Blanton, P.D. & Gouvier, W.D. (1987). Sex differences in visual information processing following right cerebrovascular accidents. *Neuropsychologia, 25,* 713–717.

Blass, J.P. & Gibson, G.E. (1977). Abnormality of a thiamine-requiring enzyme in patients with Wernicke-Korsakoff syndrome. *New England Journal of Medicine, 297,* 1367–1370.

Blazer, D. (1982). The epidemiology of late life depression. *Journal of the American Geriatrics Society, 30,* 587–592.

Blazer, D.G., Kessler, R.C., McGonagle, K.A., & Swartz, M.S. (1994). The prevalence and distribution of major depression in a national community sample: The National Comorbidity Sample. *American Journal of Psychiatry, 151,* 979–986.

Blazquez, P.M., Fujii, N., Kojima, J., & Graybiel, A.M. (2002). A network representation of response probability in the striatum. *Neuron, 33,* 973–982.

Bledsoe, G.H., Schexnayder, S.M., Carey, M.J., et al. (2002). The negative impact of the repeal of the Arkansas motorcycle helmet law. *Journal of Trauma, 53,* 1078–1087.

Bleecker, M.L., Bolla, K.I., Agnew, J., et al. (1991). Dose-related subclinical neurobehavioral effects of chronic exposure to low levels of organic solvents. *American Journal of Industrial Medicine, 19,* 715–728.

Bleecker, M.L., Bolla-Wilson, K., Agnew, J., and Meyers, D.A. (1988). Age-related sex differences in verbal memory. *Journal of Clinical Psychology, 44,* 403–411.

Bleecker, M.L., Bolla-Wilson, K., Kawas, C., & Agnew, J. (1988). Age-specific norms for the Mini-Mental State Exam. *Neurology, 38,* 1565–1568.

Bleecker, M.L., Lindgren, K.N., & Ford, D.P. (1997). Differential contribution of current and cumulative indices of lead dose to neuropsychological performance by age. *Neurology, 48,* 639–645.

Bleiberg, J., Garmoe, W.S., Halpern, E.L., et al. (1997). Consistency of within-day and across-day performance after mild brain injury. *Neuropsychiatry, Neuropsychology, and Behavioral Neurology, 10,* 247–253.

Blessed, G., Black, S.E., Butler, T., & Kay, D.W. (1991). The diagnosis of dementia in the elderly. A comparison of CAMCOG (the cognitive section of CAMDEX), the AGECAT program, DSM-III, the Mini-Mental State Examination and some short rating scales. *British Journal of Psychiatry, 159,* 193–198.

Blessed, G., Tomlinson, B.E., & Roth, M. (1968). The association between quantitative measures of dementia and of senile changes in the cerebral grey matter of elderly subjects. *British Journal of Psychiatry, 114,* 797–811.

Blin, J., Baron, J.C., Dubois, B., et al. (1990). Positron emission tomography study in progressive supranuclear palsy: Brain hypometabolic pattern and clinicometabolic correlations. *Archives of Neurology, 47,* 747–752.

Blinkenberg, M., Rune, K., Jensen, C.V., et al. (2000). Cortical cerebral metabolism correlates with MRI lesion load and cognitive dysfunction in MS. *Neurology, 54,* 558–564.

Blumer, D. (1975). Temporal lobe epilepsy and its psychiatric significance. In D.F. Benson & D. Blumer (Eds.), *Psychiatric aspects of neurologic disease.* New York: Grune & Stratton.

Blumer, D. (1999). Evidence supporting the temporal lobe epilepsy personality syndrome. *Neurology, 53,* S9–S12.

Blumer, D. & Altshuler, L. (1997). Affective disorders associated with epilepsy. In J. Engel, Jr., & T.A. Pedley (Eds.), *Epilepsy: A comprehensive textbook.* Philadelphia: Lippincott-Raven.

Blumer, D. & Benson, D.F. (1975). Personality changes in frontal and temporal lobe lesions. In D.F. Benson & D. Blumer (Eds.), *Psychiatric aspects of neurologic disease.* New York: Grune & Stratton.

Blumstein, S. (1981). Neurolinguistic disorders: Language-brain relationships. In S.B. Filskov & T.J. Boll (Eds.), *Handbook of clinical neuropsychology.* New York: Wiley-Interscience.

Blumstein, S. & Cooper, W.E. (1974). Hemispheric processing of intonation contours. *Cortex, 10,* 146–158.

Blusewicz, M.J., Dustman, R.E., Schenkenberg, T., & Beck, E.C. (1977). Neuropsychological correlates of chronic alcoholism and aging. *Journal of Nervous and Mental Disease, 165,* 348–355.

Boake, C. (1996a). Do patients with mild brain injuries have post-traumatic stress disorder, too? *Journal of Head Trauma Rehabilitation, 11,* 98–100.

Boake, C. (1996b). Supervision Rating Scale: A measure of functional outcome from brain injury. *Archives of Physical Medicine and Rehabilitation, 77,* 116–124.

Boake, C. (2000). Edouard Claparède and the Auditory Verbal Learning Test. *Journal of Clinical and Experimental Neuropsychology, 22,* 286–292.

Boake, C. (2002). From the Binet-Simon to the Wechsler-Bellevue: Tracing the history of intelligence testing. *Journal of Clinical and Experimental Neuropsychology, 24,* 383–405.

Boake, C. & High, W.M. (1996). Functional outcome from traumatic brain injury. Unidimensional or multidimensional? *American Journal of Physical Medicine and Rehabilitation, 75,* 105–113.

Boake, C., Millis, S.R., High, W.M., Jr., et al. (2001). Using early neuropsychologic testing to predict long-term productivity outcome from traumatic brain injury. *Archives of Physical Medicine and Rehabilitation, 82,* 761–768.

Bock, R.D. (1973). Word and image: Sources of the verbal and spatial factors in mental test scores. *Psychometrika, 38,* 437–457.

Bode, R.K. & Heinemann, A.W. (2002). Course of functional improvement after stroke, spinal cord injury, and traumatic brain injury. *Archives of Physical Medicine and Rehabilitation, 83,* 100–106.

Boden, B.P., Kirkendall, D.T., & Garrett, W.E., Jr. (1998). Concussion incidence in elite college soccer players. *American Journal of Sports Medicine, 26,* 238–241.

Bogen, J.E. (1969a). The other side of the brain. I: Dysgraphia and dyscopia following cerebral commissurotomy. *Bulletin of the Los Angeles Neurological Societies, 34,* 73–105.

Bogen, J.E. (1969b). The other side of the brain. II: An oppositional mind. *Bulletin of the Los Angeles Neurological Societies, 34,* 135–162.

Bogen, J.E. (1985). Split-brain syndromes. In P.J. Vinken, G.W. Bruyn, & H.L. Klawans (Eds.), *Handbook of clinical neurology.* New York: Elsevier.

Bogen, J. (1993). The callosal syndrome. In K.M. Heilman & E. Valenstein (Eds.), *Clinical neuropsychology* (3rd ed.). New York: Oxford University Press.

Bogen, J.E. (1997). Memory: A neurosurgeon's perspective. In M.L.J. Apuzzo (Ed.), *Surgery of the third ventricle* (2nd ed.). Baltimore, MD: Williams & Wilkins.

Bogen, J.E., DeZure, R., Tenhouten, W.D., & Marsh, J.F. (1972). The other side of the brain IV. The A/P ratio. *Bulletin of the Los Angeles Neurological Societies, 37,* 49–61.

Bogner, J.A., Corrigan, J.D., Mysiw, W.J., et al. (2001). A comparison of substance abuse and violence in the prediction of long-term rehabilitation outcomes after traumatic brain injury. *Archives of Physical Medicine and Rehabilitation, 82,* 571–577.

Bogousslavsky, J. & Caplan, L. (Eds.) (2001). Part II. Vascular topographic syndromes. In J. Bogousslavsky & L. Caplan (Eds.), *Stroke syndromes* (2nd ed.). Cambridge, UK: Cambridge University Press.

Bogousslavsky, J., Hommel, M., & Bassetti, C. (1998). Stroke. In M. Swash (Ed.), *Outcomes in neurological and neurosurgical disorders.* Cambridge, UK: Cambridge University Press.

Bohac, D.L., Malec, J.F., & Moessner, A.M. (1997). Factor analysis of the Mayo-Portland Adaptability Inventory: Structure and validity. *Brain Injury, 11,* 469–482.

Bohannan, R.W. (2003). Grip strength: A summary of studies comparing dominant and nondominant limb measurements. *Perceptual and Motor Skills, 96,* 728–730.

Bohnen, N., Jolles, J., & Twijnstra, A. (1992). Modification of the Stroop Color Word Test improves differentiation between patients with mild head injury and matched controls. *The Clinical Neuropsychologist, 6,* 178–184.

Bolderini, P., Basaglia, N., & Calanca, M.C. (1991). Sexual changes in hemiparetic patients. *Archives of Physical Medicine and Rehabilitation, 72,* 202–207.

Boll, T.J. (1974). Right and left cerebral hemisphere damage and tactile perception: Performance of the ipsilateral and contralateral sides of the body. *Neuropsychologia, 12,* 235–238.

Boll, T.J. (1981). The Halstead-Reitan Neuropsychology Battery. In S.B. Filskov & T.J. Boll (Eds.), *Handbook of clinical neuropsychology.* New York: Wiley-Interscience.

Boll, T.J. (1985). Developing issues in clinical neuropsychology. *Journal of Clinical and Experimental Neuropsychology, 7,* 473–485.

Boll, T.J., & Barth, J. (1983). Mild head injury. *Psychiatric Developments, 3,* 263–275.

Boll, T.J., Heaton, R., & Reitan, R.M. (1974). Neuropsychological and emotional correlates of Huntington's chorea. *Journal of Nervous and Mental Disease, 158,* 61–69.

Bolla-Wilson, K. & Bleecker, M. (1986). Influence of verbal intelligence, sex, age, and education on the Rey Auditory-Verbal Learning Test. *Developmental Neuropsychology, 2,* 203–212.

Bolla-Wilson, K., Bleecker, M.L., & Agnew, J. (1988). Lead toxicity and cognitive functions: A dose response relationship [abstract]. *Journal of Clinical and Experimental Neuropsychology, 10,* 88.

Boller, F. & Duykaerts, C. (2003). Alzheimer's disease: Clinical and anatomic issues. In T.E. Feinberg & M.J. Farah (Eds.), *Behavioral neurology and neuropsychology* (2nd ed.). New York: Mc-Graw-Hill.

Boller, F. & Frank, E. (1982). *Sexual functions in neurological disorders.* New York: Raven Press.

Boller, F., Marcie, P., Starkstein, S., & Traykov, L. (1998). Memory and depression in Parkinson's disease. *European Journal of Neurology, 5,* 291–295.

Boller, F., Mizutani, T., Roessmann, U., & Gambetti, P. (1980). Parkinson disease, dementia, and Alzheimer disease. Clinicopathological correlations. *Annals of Neurology, 7,* 329–335.

Boller, F., Passafiume, D., & Keefe, N. C. (1984). Visuospatial impairment in Parkinson's disease: Role of perceptual and motor factors. *Archives of Neurology, 41,* 485–490.

Boller, F. & Vignolo, L.A. (1966). Latent sensory aphasia in hemisphere-damaged patients: An experimental study with the Token Test. *Brain, 89,* 815–831.

Bolter, J.F., Hutcherson, W.L., & Long, C.J. (1984). Speech Sounds Perception Test: A rational response strategy can invalidate the test results. *Journal of Consulting and Clinical Psychology, 54,* 132–133.

Bolter, J.F., Picano, J.J., & Zych, K. (1985). *Item error frequencies on the Halstead Category Test: An index of performance validity.* Paper presented at the National Academy of Neuropsychology, Philadelphia, PA, October 1985.

Bombardier, C.H., Rimmele, C.T., & Zintel, H. (2002). The magnitude and correlates of alcohol and drug use before traumatic brain injury. *Archives of Physical Medicine and Rehabilitation, 83,* 1765–1773.

Bombardier, C.H., Temkin, N.R., Machamer, J., & Dikmen, S.S. (2003). The natural history of drinking and alcohol-related problems after traumatic brain injury. *Archives of Physical Medicine and Rehabilitation, 84,* 185–191.

Bond, F. & Godfrey, H.P.D. (1997). Conversation with traumatically brain-injured individuals: A controlled study of behavioural changes and their impact. *Brain Injury, 11,* 319–329.

Bond, J.A. & Buchtel, H.A. (1984). Comparison of the Wisconsin Card Sorting Test and the Halstead Category Test. *Journal of Clinical Psychology, 40,* 1251–1255.

Bond, M.R. (1984). The psychiatry of closed head injury. In N.

Brooks (Ed.), *Closed head injury*. Oxford: Oxford University Press.

Bond, M.R. (1986). Neurobehavioral sequelae of closed head injury. In I. Grant & K.M. Adams (Eds.), *Neuropsychological assessment of neuropsychiatric disorders*. New York: Oxford University Press.

Bond, M.R. (1990). Standardized methods of assessing and predicting outcome. In M. Rosenthal, M.R. Bond, E.R. Griffith, & J.D. Miller (Eds.), *Rehabilitation of the adult and child with traumatic brain injury* (2nd ed.). Philadelphia: Davis.

Bondi, M.W. & Kaszniak, A.W. (1991). Implicit and explicit memory in Alzheimer's disease and Parkinson's disease. *Journal of Clinical and Experimental Neuropsychology, 13*, 339–358.

Bondi, M.W., Kaszniak, A.W., Bayles, K.A., & Vance, K.T. (1993). Contributions of frontal system dysfunction to memory and perceptual abilities in Parkinson's disease. *Neuropsychology, 7*, 89–102.

Bondi, M.W., Monsch, A.U., Butters, N., et al. (1993). Utility of a modified version of the Wisconsin Card Sorting Test in the detection of dementia of the Alzheimer type. *The Clinical Neuropsychologist, 7*, 161–170.

Bondi, M.W., Monsch, A.U., Galasko, D., et al. (1994). Preclinical cognitive markers of dementia of the Alzheimer type. *Neuropsychology, 8*, 374–384.

Bondi, M.W., Salmon, D.P., & Kaszniak, A.W. (1996). The neuropsychology of dementia. In I. Grant & K.M. Adams (Eds.), *Neuropsychological assessment of neuropsychiatric disorders* (2nd ed.). New York: Oxford University Press.

Bondi, M.W., Serody, A.B., Chan, A.S., et al. (2002). Cognitive and neuropathologic correlates of Stroop Color-Word Test performance in Alzheimer's disease. *Neuropsychology, 16*, 335–343.

Bondy, M. & Ligon, B.L. (1996). Epidemiology and etiology of intracranial meningiomas: a review. *Journal of Neurooncology, 29*, 197–205.

Bontke, C.F. (1996). Do patients with mild brain injuries have posttraumatic stress disorder, too? Conclusion. *Journal of Head Trauma Rehabilitation, 11*, 100–102.

Bookheimer, S. (2002). Functional MRI of language: New approaches to understanding the cortical organization of semantic processing. *Annual Review of Neuroscience, 25*, 151–188.

Boon, A.J., Tans, J.T. Delwel, E.J., et al. (2000). The Dutch Normal-pressure Hydrocephalus Study. How to select patients for shunting? An analysis of four diagnostic criteria. *Surgical Neurology, 53*, 201–207.

Boone, D.E. (1995). A cross-sectional analysis of WAIS-R aging patterns with psychiatric inpatients: support for Horn's hypothesis that fluid cognitive abilities decline. *Perceptual and Motor Skills, 81*, 371–379.

Boone, K.B. (2000). The Boston Qualitative Scoring system for the Rey-Osterrieth Complex Figure. *Journal of Clinical and Experimental Neuropsychology, 22*, 430–434.

Boone, K.B., Ghaffarian, S., Lesser, I.M., et al. (1993). Wisconsin Card Sorting Test performance in healthy, older adults: Relationship to age, sex, education, and IQ. *Journal of Clinical Psychology, 49*, 54–60.

Boone, K.B., Lesser, I.M., Hill-Gutierrez, E., et al. (1993). Rey-Osterrieth Complex Figure performance in healthy, older adults: Relationship to age, education, sex, and IQ. *The Clinical Neuropsychologist, 7*, 22–28.

Boone, K.B., Lesser, I.M., Miller, B.L., et al. (1995). Cognitive functioning in older depressed outpatients: Relationship of presence and severity of depression to neuropsychological test scores. *Neuropsychology, 9*, 390–398.

Boone, K.B., Lu, P., & Herzberg, D. (2002). *The Dot Counting Test.* Los Angeles: Western Psychological Services.

Boone, K.B., Lu, P., Sherman, D., et al. (2000). Validation of a new technique to detect malingering of cognitive symptoms: The *b* test. *Archives of Clinical Neuropsychology, 15*, 227–241.

Boone, K.B., Miller, B.L., Lee, A., et al. (1999). Neuropsychological patterns in right versus left frontotemporal dementia. *Journal of the International Neuropsychological Society, 5*, 616–622.

Boone, K.B., Miller, B.L., Lesser, I.M., et al. (1990). Performance on frontal lobe tests in healthy, older individuals. *Developmental Neuropsychology, 6*, 215–224.

Boone, K.B., Miller, B.L., Lesser, I.M., et al. (1992). Neuropsychological correlates of white-matter lesions in healthy elderly subjects. A threshold effect. *Archives of Neurology, 49*, 549–554.

Boone, K.B. & Rausch, R. (1989). Seashore Rhythm Test performance in patients with unilateral temporal lobe damage. *Journal of Clinical Psychology, 45*, 614–618.

Boone, K.B., Swerdloff, R.S., Miller, B.L., et al. (2001). Neuropsychological profiles of adults with Klinefelter syndrome. *Journal of the International Neuropsychological Society, 7*, 446–456.

Boring, E.G. (1950). *A history of experimental psychology.* New York: Appleton-Century-Crofts.

Borkowski, J.G., Benton, A.L., & Spreen, O. (1967). Word fluency and brain damage. *Neuropsychologia 5*, 135–140.

Bornstein, R.A. (1982). Reliability of the Speech Sounds Perception Test. *Perceptual and Motor Skills, 55*, 203–210.

Bornstein, R.A. (1983a). Construct validity of the Knox Cube Test as a neuropsychological measure. *Journal of Clinical Neuropsychology, 5*, 105–114.

Bornstein, R.A. (1983b). Reliability and item analysis of the Seashore Rhythm Test. *Perceptual and Motor Skills, 57*, 571–574.

Bornstein, R.A. (1983c). Verbal IQ-Performance IQ discrepancies on the Wechsler Adult Intelligence Scale-Revised in patients with unilateral or bilateral cerebral dysfunction. *Journal of Consulting and Clinical Psychology, 51*, 779–780.

Bornstein, R.A. (1985). Normative data on selected neuropsychological measures from a nonclinical sample. *Journal of Clinical Psychology, 41*, 651–659.

Bornstein, R.A. (1986a). Classification rates obtained with "standard" cut-off scores on selected neuropsychological measures. *Journal of Clinical and Experimental Neuropsychology, 8*, 413–420.

Bornstein, R.A. (1986b). Consistency of intermanual discrepancies in normal and unilateral brain lesion patients. *Journal of Consulting and Clinical Psychology, 54*, 719–723.

Bornstein, R.A. (1986c). Normative data on intermanual differences on three tests of motor performance. *Journal of Clinical and Experimental Neuropsychology, 8*, 12–20.

Bornstein, R.A. (1990). Neuropsychological test batteries in neuropsychological assessment. In A.A. Boulton, G.B. Baker, & M. Hiscock (Eds.), *Neuromethods. Neuropsychology* (Vol. 17). Clifton, NJ: Humana Press.

Bornstein, R.A. (1991). Report of the Division 40 Task Force on Education, Accreditation and Credentialing: Recommendations for education and training of nondoctoral personnel in clinical neuropsychology. *The Clinical Neuropsychologist, 5*, 20–23.

Bornstein, R.A. (2001). Clinical utility of the Rorschach inkblot method: Reframing the debate. *Journal of Personality Assessment, 77*, 39–47.

Bornstein, R.A., Baker, G.B., & Douglass, A.B. (1987). Short-term retest reliability of the Halstead-Reitan Battery in a normal sample. *The Clinical Neuropsychologist, 5*, 20–23.

Bornstein, R.A. & Chelune, G.J. (1989). Factor structure of the Wechsler Memory Scale-Revised in relation to age and educational level. *Archives of Clinical Neuropsychology, 4*, 15–24.

Bornstein, R.A., Drake, M.E., Jr., & Pakalnis, A. (1988). WAIS-R factor structure in epileptic patients. *Epilepsia, 29*, 14–18.

Bornstein, R.A., & Kelly, M.P. (1991). Risk factors for stroke and neuropsychological performance. In R.A. Bornstein & G. Brown (Eds.), *Neurobehavioral aspects of cerebrovascular disease.* New York: Oxford University Press.

Bornstein, R.A. & Leason, M. (1984). Item analysis of Halstead's Speech-Sounds Perception Test: Quantitative and qualitative analysis of errors. *Journal of Clinical Neuropsychology, 6,* 205–214.

Bornstein, R.A. & Matarazzo, J.D. (1982). Wechsler VIQ versus PIQ differences in cerebral dysfunction: A literature review with emphasis on sex differences. *Journal of Clinical Neuropsychology, 4,* 319–334.

Bornstein, R.A. & Matarazzo, J.D. (1984). Relationship of sex and the effects of unilateral lesions on the Wechsler Intelligence Scales. *Journal of Nervous and Mental Disease, 172,* 707–710.

Bornstein, R.A., Miller, H.B., & van Schoor, T. (1988). Emotional adjustment in compensated head injury patients. *Neurosurgery, 23,* 622–627.

Bornstein, R.A., Paniak, C., & O'Brien, W. (1987). Preliminary data on classification of normal and brain-damaged elderly subjects. *The Clinical Neuropsychologist, 1,* 315–323.

Bornstein, R.A. & Suga, L.J. (1988). Educational level and neuropsychological performance in healthy elderly subjects. *Developmental Neuropsychology, 4,* 17–22.

Bornstein, R.A., Weizel, M., & Grant, C.D. (1984). Error pattern and item order on Halstead's Speech Sounds Perception Test. *Journal of Clinical Psychology, 40,* 266–270.

Borod, J.C. (1993). Cerebral mechanisms underlying facial, prosodic, and lexical emotional expression: A review of neuropsychological studies and methodological issues. *Neuropsychology, 7,* 445–463.

Borod, J., Bloom, R.L., Brickman, A.M., et al. (2002). Emotional processing deficits in individuals with unilateral brain damage. *Applied Neuropsychology, 9,* 23–36.

Borod, J., Bloom, R.L., & Santschi-Haywood, C. (1998). Verbal aspects of emotional communication. In M. Beeman & C. Chiarello (Eds.), *Right hemisphere language comprehension. Perspectives from cognitive neuroscience.* Mahwah, NJ: Erlbaum.

Borod, J.C., Carper, M., Goodglass, H., & Naeser, M. (1984). Aphasic performance on a battery of constructional, visuospatial, and quantitative tasks: Factorial structure and CT scan localization. *Journal of Clinical Neuropsychology, 6,* 189–204.

Borod, J.C., Carper, J.M., & Naeser, M. (1990). Long-term language recovery in left-handed aphasic patients. *Aphasiology, 4,* 561–572.

Borod, J.C., Carper, M., Naeser, M., & Goodglass, H. (1985). Left-handed and right-handed aphasics with left hemisphere lesions compared on nonverbal performance measures. *Cortex, 21,* 81–90.

Borod, J.C., Cicero, B.A., Obler, L.K., et al. (1998). Right hemisphere emotional perception: Evidence across multiple channels. *Neuropsychology, 12,* 446–458.

Borod, J.C., Fitzpatrick, P.M., Helm-Estabrooks, N., & Goodglass, H. (1989). The relationship between limb apraxia and the spontaneous use of communicative gesture in aphasia. *Brain and Cognition, 10,* 121–131.

Borod, J.C., Goodglass, H., & Kaplan, E. (1980). Normative data on the Boston Diagnostic Aphasia Examination, Parietal Lobe Battery, and the Boston Naming Test. *Journal of Clinical Neuropsycholgy, 2,* 209–216.

Borod, J.C., Haywood, C.S., & Koff, E. (1997). Neuropsychological aspects of facial asymmetry during emotional expression: A review of the normal adult literature. *Neuropsychology Review, 7,* 41–60.

Borod, J.C., Kent, J., Koff, E., et al. (1988). Facial asymmetry while posing positive and negative emotions: Support for the right hemisphere hypothesis. *Neuropsychologia, 26,* 759–764.

Borod, J.C., Koff, E., & Caron, H.S. (1984). The Target Test: A brief laterality measure of speed and accuracy. *Perceptual and Motor Skills, 58,* 743–748.

Borod, J.C., Koff, E., Lorch, M.P., and Nicholas, M. (1985). Channels of emotional expression in patients with unilateral brain damage. *Archives of Neurology, 42,* 345–348.

Borod, J.C., Rorie, K.D., Pick, L.H., et al. (2000). Verbal pragmatics following unilateral stroke: emotional content and valence. *Neuropsychology, 14,* 112–124.

Borod, J.C., St. Clair, J., Koff, E., & Alpert, M. (1990). Perceiver and poser asymmetries in processing facial emotion. *Brain and Cognition, 13,* 167–177.

Borod, J.C., Tabert, M.H., Santschi, C., & Strauss, E.H. (2000). Neuropsychological assessment of emotional processing in brain-damaged patients. In J.C. Borod (Ed.), *The neuropsychology of emotion.* New York: Oxford University Press.

Borod, J.C., Welkowitz, J., Alpert, M., et al. (1990). Parameters of emotional processing in neuropsychiatric disorders: Conceptual issues and a battery of tests. *Journal of Communication Disorders, 23,* 247–271.

Borod, J.C., Welkowitz, J., & Obler, L.K. (1992). *The New York Emotion Battery.* Unpublished materials. Dept. of Neurology, Mount Sinai Medical Center, New York.

Borson, S., Brush, M., Gil, E., et al. (1999). The clock drawing test: Utility for dementia detection in multi-ethnic elders. *Journal of Gerontology A: Biological Science and Medical Science, 54,* M534–M540.

Borson, S., Scanlan, J., Brush, M., et al. (2000). The Mini-Cog: A cognitive "vital signs" measure for dementia screening in multilingual elderly. *International Journal of Geriatric Psychiatry, 15,* 1021–1027.

Bortner, M. & Birch, H. G. (1962). Perceptual and perceptual-motor dissociation in brain-damaged patients. *Journal of Nervous and Mental Disease, 134,* 103–108.

Bosma, H., van Boxtel, M.P., Ponds, R.W., et al. (2000). Pesticide exposure and risk of mild cognitive dysfunction. *Lancet, 356,* 912–913.

Boström, K. & Helander, C.G. (1986). Aspects on pathology and neuropathology in head injury. *Acta Neurochirurgica (Suppl. 36), 51–55.*

Boswell, E.B., Anfinson, R.J., & Nemeroff, C.B. (2002). Neuropsychiatric aspects of endocrine disorders. In S.C. Yudofsky & R.E. Hales (Eds.), *Textbook of neuropsychiatry and clinical neurosciences* (4th ed.). Washington, D.C.: American Psychiatric Publishing.

Botez, M.I. & Botez, T. (1996). Les amusies. In M.I. Botez (Ed.), *Neuropsychologie clinique et neurologie du comportement* (2ème ed.). Montreal: Les Presses de l'Université de Montréal.

Botez, M.I., Botez, T., Leveille, J., et al. (1979). Neuropsychological correlates of folic acid deficiency: Facts and hypotheses. In M.I. Botez & E.H. Reynolds (Eds.), *Folic acid in neurology, psychiatry, and internal medicine.* New York: Raven Press.

Botez, M.I., Botez, T., & Maag, U. (1984). The Wechsler subtests in mild organic brain damage associated with folate deficiency. *Psychological Medicine, 14,* 431–437.

Botez, M.I., Ethier, R., Leveille, J., & Botez-Marquard, T. (1977). A syndrome of early recognition of occult hydrocephalus and cerebral atrophy. *Quarterly Journal of Medicine, New Series, 46,* 365–380.

Botez, M.I., Gravel, J., Attig, E., & Vezina, J.L. (1985). Reversible chronic cerebellar ataxia after phenytoin intoxication: Possible role of cerebellum in cognitive thought. *Neurology, 35,* 1152–1157.

Botez, M.I., Lalonde, R., & Botez-Marquard, T. (1996). Le cervelet: comportement moteur et non moteur. In M.I. Botez (Ed.), *Neuropsychologie clinique et neurologie du comportement* (2ème ed.). Montreal: Les Presses de l'Université de Montréal.

Botez-Marquard, T., Leveille, J., & Botez, M.I. (1994). Neuropsychological functioning in unilateral cerebellar damage. *Canadian Journal of Neurological Sciences, 21,* 353–357.

Bottini, G., Corcoran, R., Sterzi, R., et al. (1994). The role of the right hemisphere in the interpretation of figurative aspects of language. A positron emission tomography activation study. *Brain, 117,* 1241–1253.

Botwinick, J. & Storandt, M. (1974). *Memory related functions and age.* Springfield, IL: Thomas.

Botwinick, J., Storandt, M., Berg, L., & Boland, S. (1988). Senile dementia of the Alzheimer type: Subject attrition and testability in research. *Archives of Neurology, 45,* 493–496.

Bouma, A. (1990). *Lateral asymmetries and hemispheric specialization.* Amsterdam: Swets and Zeitlinger.

Bowden, S.C. (1988). Learning in young alcoholics. *Journal of Clinical and Experimental Neuropsychology, 10,* 157–168.

Bowden, S.C., Dodds, B., Whelan, G., et al. (1997). Confirmatory factor analysis of the Wechsler Memory Scale-Revised in a sample of clients with alcohol dependency. *Journal of Clinical and Experimental Neuropsychology, 19,* 755–762.

Bowden, S.C., Fowler, K.S., Bell, R.C., et al. (1998). The reliability and internal validity of the Wisconsin Card Sorting Test. *Neuropsychological Rehabilitation, 8,* 243–254.

Bowen, A., McKenna, K., & Tallis, R.C. (1999). Reasons for variability in the reported rate of occurrence of unilateral spatial neglect after stroke. *Stroke, 30,* 1196–1202.

Bowen, F.P. (1976). Behavioral alterations in patients with basal ganglia lesions. In M.D. Yahr (Ed.), *The basal ganglia.* New York: Raven Press.

Bower, G.H. (2000). A brief history of memory research. In E. Tulving & F.I.M. Craik (Eds.), *The Oxford handbook of memory.* Oxford: Oxford University Press.

Bower, J.H., Maraganore, D.M., McDonnell, S.K., & Rocca, W.A. (1997). Incidence of progressive supranuclear palsy and multiple system atrophy in Olmsted County, Minnesota, 1976 to 1990. *Neurology, 49,* 1284–1288.

Bowers, D., Bauer, R.M., & Heilman, K. (1993). The nonverbal affect lexicon: Theoretical perspectives from neuropsychological studies of affect perception. *Neuropsychology, 71,* 433–444.

Bowers, T.L. & Pantle, M.L. (1998). Shipley Institute for Living Scale and the Kaufman Brief Intelligence Test as screening instruments for intelligence. *Assessment, 5,* 187–195.

Bowler, J.V. (2000). Criteria for vascular dementia: Replacing dogma with data. *Archives of Neurology, 57,* 170–171.

Bowler, J.V., Eliasziw, M., Steenhuis, R., et al. (1997). Comparative evolution of Alzheimer disease, vascular dementia, and mixed dementia. *Archives of Neurology, 54,* 697–703.

Bowler, J.V. & Hachinski, V. (2003). Vascular dementia. In T.E. Feinberg & M.J. Farah (Eds.), *Behavioral neurology and neuropsychology* (2nd ed.). New York: McGraw-Hill.

Bowler, R.M. & Cone, J.E. (1999). *Occupational medicine secrets.* Philadelphia: Hanley & Belfus.

Bowler, R.M., Lezak, M.D., Booty, A., et al. (2001). Neuropsychological dysfunction, mood disturbance, and emotional status of munitions workers. *Appplied Neuropsychology, 8,* 74–90.

Bowler, R.M., Mergler, D., Huel, G., et al. (1991). Neuropsychological impairment among former microelectronics workers. *NeuroToxicology, 12,* 87–104.

Bowler, R.M., Mergler, D., Rauch, S.S., et al. (1991). Affective and personality disturbances among female former microelectronics workers. *Journal of Clinical Psychology, 47,* 41–52.

Bowler, R.M., Mergler, D., Rauch, S.S., & Bowler, R.P. (1992). Stability of psychological impairment: Two year follow-up of former microelectronics workers' affective and personality disturbance. *Women and Health, 18,* 27–48.

Bowler, R.M., Rauch, S.S., Becker, C.H., et al. (1989). Three patterns of MMPI profiles following neurotoxin exposure. *American Journal of Forensic Psychology, 7,* 15–31.

Bowler, R.M., Sudia, S., Mergler, D., et al. (1992). Comparison of Digit Symbol and Symbol Digit Modalities tests for assessing neurotoxic exposure. *The Clinical Neuropsychologist, 6,* 103–104.

Bowler, R.M., Thaler, C.D., Law, D., & Becker, C.E. (1990). Comparison of the NES and CNSB neuropsychological screening batteries. *NeuroToxicology, 11,* 451–464.

Bowles, N.L., Obler, L.K., & Albert, M.L. (1987). Naming errors in healthy aging and dementia of the Alzheimer type. *Cortex, 23,* 519–524.

Bowman, M. (1997). *Individual differences in posttraumatic response. Problems with the Adversity–Distress Connection.* Mahwah, NJ: Erlbaum.

Bowman, M.L. (1996). Ecological validity of neuropsychological and other predictors following head injury. *The Clinical Neuropsychologist, 10,* 382–396.

Boyd, J.L. (1981). A validity study of the Hooper Visual Organization Test. *Journal of Consulting and Clinical Psychology, 49,* 15–19.

Boyd, T.M. & Sautter, S.W. (1993). Route-Finding: A measure of everyday executive functioning in the head-injured adult. *Applied Cognitive Psychology, 7,* 171–181.

Boyle, G.J. (1986). Clinical neuropsychological assessment: Abbreviating the Halstead Category Test of brain dysfunction. *Journal of Clinical Psychology, 42,* 615–625.

Boyle, G.J. (1989). Confirmation of the structural dimensionality of the Stanford-Binet Intelligence Scale (4th edition). *Personality and Individual Differences, 10,* 709–715.

Boysen, G. & Christensen, H. (2001). Early stroke: A dynamic process. *Stroke, 32,* 2423–2425.

Bozeat, S., Gregory, C.A., Ralph, M.A.L., & Hodges, J.R. (2000). Which neuropsychiatric and behavioural features distinguish frontal and temporal dementia from Alzheimer's disease? *Journal of Neurology, Neurosurgery, and Psychiatry, 69,* 178–186.

Bozoki, A., Giordani, B., Heidebrink, J.L., et al. (2001). Mild cognitive impairments predict dementia in nondemented elderly patients with memory loss. *Archives of Neurology, 58,* 411–416.

Bózzola, F.G., Gorelick, P.B., Freels, S. (1992). Personality changes in Alzheimer's disease. *Archives of Neurology, 49,* 297–300.

Braak, H., Del Tredici, K., Schultz, C., & Braak, E. (2000). Vulnerability of select neuronal types to Alzheimer's disease. *Annals of the New York Academy of Sciences, 924,* 53–61.

Bracco, L., Gallato, R., Grigoletto, F., et al. (1994). Factors affecting course and survival in Alzheimer's disease. A 9-year longitudinal study. *Archives of Neurology, 51,* 1213–1219.

Bracken, B. & McCallum, S. (1998). *University Nonverbal Intelligence Test (UNIT).* Itasca, IL: Riverside.

Bradburn, N. (1969). *The structure of psychological well-being.* Chicago: Aldine.

Bradley, W.G., Jr. (2001). Diagnostic tools in hydrocephalus. *Neurosurgical Clinics of North America, 12,* 661–684.

Bradshaw, J.L. (1989). *Hemispheric specialization and psychological function.* Chichester, UK: Wiley.

Bradshaw, J.L., Nettleton, N.C., Nathan, G., & Wilson, L. (1985). Bisecting rods and lines: Effects of horizontal and vertical posture on left-side underestimation by normal subjects. *Neuropsychologia, 23,* 421–425.

Bradshaw, J.L., Phillips, J.G., Dennis, C., et al. (1992). Initiation and execution of movement sequences in those suffering from and at-risk of developing Huntington's disease. *Journal of Clinical and Experimental Neuropsychology, 14,* 179–192.

Braff, D.L., Silverton, L., Saccuzzo, D.P., & Janowsky, D.S. (1981). Impaired speed of visual information processing in marijuana intoxication. *American Journal of Psychiatry, 138,* 613–617.

Brain, W.R. (1969). Disorders of memory. In W.R. Brain & M. Wilkinson (Eds.), *Recent advances in neurology and neuropsychiatry*. Boston: Little, Brown.

Branas, C.C. & Knudson, M.M. (2001). State helmet laws and motorcycle rider death rates. *LDI (Leonard Davis Institute) Issue Brief, 7,* 1–4.

Branch, C., Milner, B., & Rasmussen, T. (1964). Intracarotid sodium amytal for the lateralization of cerebral speech dominance: Observations in 123 patients. *Journal of Neurosurgery, 21,* 399–405.

Brand, N. & Jolles, J. (1987). Information processing in depression and anxiety. *Psychological Medicine, 17,* 145–153.

Brandimonte, M., Einstein, G.O., & McDaniel, M.A. (1996). *Prospective memory: Theory and applications*. Mahwah, NJ: Erlbaum.

Brandon, A.D. & Bennett, T.L. (1986). *Digital Finger Tapping Test*. Los Angeles: Western Psychological Services.

Brandon, A., Chavez, E., & Bennett, T. (1986). A comparative evaluation of two neurological finger tapping instruments: Halstead-Reitan and Western Psychological Services. *International Journal of Clinical Neuropsychology, 8,* 64–65.

Brandt, J. (1985). Access to knowledge in the dementia of Huntington's disease. *Developmental Neuropsychology, 1,* 335–348.

Brandt, J. (1988). Malingered amnesia. In R. Rogers (Ed.), *Clinical assessment of malingering and deception*. New York: Guilford Press.

Brandt, J. (1991). The Hopkins Verbal Learning Test: Development of a new verbal memory test with six equivalent forms. *The Clinical Neuropsychologist, 5,* 125–142.

Brandt, J. & Butters, N. (1996). Neuropsychological characteristics of Huntington's disease. In I. Grant & K.M. Adams (Eds.), *Neuropsychological assessment of neuropsychiatric disorders* (2nd ed.). New York: Oxford University Press.

Brandt, J., Butters, N., Ryan, C., & Bayog, R. (1983). Cognitive loss and recovery in long-term alcohol abusers. *Archives of General Psychiatry, 40,* 435–442.

Brandt, J., Bylsma, F.W., Aylward, E.H., et al. (1995). Impaired source memory in Huntington's disease and its relation to basal ganglia atrophy. *Journal of Clinical and Experimental Neuropsychology, 17,* 868–877.

Brandt, J., Bylsma, F.W., Gross, R., et al. (1996). Trinucleotide repeat length and clinical progression in Huntington's disease. *Neurology, 46,* 527–531.

Brandt, J., Corwin, J., & Krafft, L. (1992). Is verbal recognition memory really different in Huntington's and Alzherimer's disease? *Journal of Clinical and Experimental Neuropsychology, 14,* 773–784.

Brandt, J., Folstein, S.E., & Folstein, M.F. (1988). Differential cognitive impairment in Alzheimer's disease and Huntington's disease. *Annals of Neurology, 23,* 555–561.

Brandt, J., Folstein, S.E., Wong, D.F., et al. (1990). D₂ receptors in Huntington's disease: Positron emission tomography findings and clinical correlates. *Journal of Neuropsychiatry and Clinical Neurosciences, 2,* 20–27.

Brandt, J., Mellits, D., Rovner, B., et al. (1989). Relation of age at onset and duration of illness to cognitive functioning in Alzheimer's disease. *Neuropsychiatry, Neuropsychology, and Behavioral Neurology, 2,* 93–101.

Brandt, J. & Rich, J.B. (2001). Memory disorders in the dementias. In A.D. Baddeley, B.A. Wilson, & M.D. Kopelman (Eds.), *Handbook of memory disorders* (2nd ed.). Chichester, UK: Wiley.

Brandt, J., Rubinsky, E., & Lassen, G. (1985). Uncovering malingered amnesia. *Annals of the New York Academy of Sciences, 44,* 502–503.

Brandt, J., Spencer, M., & Folstein, M. (1988). The telephone interview for cognitive status. *Neuropsychiatry, Neuropsychology, and Behavioral Neurology, 1,* 111–117.

Brandt, J., Spencer, M., McSorley, P., & Folstein, M.F. (1988). Semantic activation and implicit memory in Alzheimer disease. *Alzheimer Disease and Associated Disorders, 2,* 112–119.

Brandt, J., Strauss, M.E., Larus, J., et al. (1984). Clinical correlates of dementia and disability in Huntington's disease. *Journal of Clinical Neuropsychology, 6,* 401–412.

Brandt, J., Welsh, K.A., Breitner, J.C., et al. (1993). Hereditary influences on cognitive functioning in older men. A study of 4000 twin pairs. *Archives of Neurology, 50,* 599–603.

Brandt, M.M., McReynolds, M.C., Ahrns, K.S., & Wahl, W.S. (2002). Burn centers should be involved in prevention of occupational electrical injuries. *Journal of Burn Care and Rehabilitation, 23,* 132–134.

Brannen, J.H., Badie, B., Moritz, C.H., et al. (2001). Reliability of functional MR imaging with word-generation tasks for mapping Broca's area. *American Journal of Neuroradiology, 22,* 1711–1718.

Braun, C.M.J. & Daigneault, S. (1991). Sparing of cognitive executive functions and impairment of motor functions after industrial exposure to lead: A field study with a control group. *Neuropsychology, 5,* 179–193.

Braun, C.M.J., Lussier, F., Baribeau, J.M.C., & Ethier, M. (1989). Does severe traumatic closed head injury impair sense of humour? *Brain Injury, 3,* 345–354.

Braver, T.S., Cohen, J.D., Nystrom, L.E., et al. (1997). A parametric study of prefrontal cortex involvement in human working memory. *Neuroimage, 5,* 49–62.

Bravin, J.H., Kinsella, G.J., Ong, B., & Vowels, L. (2000). A study of performance of delayed intentions in multiple sclerosis. *Journal of Clinical and Experimental Neuropsychology, 22,* 418–429.

Bravo, G. & Hebert, R. (1997). Age- and education-specific reference values for the Mini-Mental and modified Mini-Mental State Examinations derived from a non-demented elderly population. *International Journal of Geriatric Psychiatry, 12,* 1008–1018.

Bray, G.P., DeFrank, R.S., & Wolfe, T.L. (1981). Sexual functioning in stroke survivors. *Archives of Physical Medicine and Rehabilitation, 62,* 286–288.

Brazzelli, M., Colombo, N., Della Sala, S., & Spinnler, H. (1994). Spared and impaired cognitive abilities after bilateral frontal damage. *Cortex, 30,* 27–51.

Brebion, G., Smith, M.J., & Ehrlich, M.-F. (1997). Working memory and aging: Deficit or strategy differences. *Aging, Neuropsychology, and Cognition, 4,* 58–73.

Breier, J.I., Plenger, P.M., Castillo, R., et al. (1996). Effects of temporal lobe epilepsy on spatial and figural aspects of memory for a complex geometric figure. *Journal of the International Neuropsychological Society, 2,* 535–540.

Breier, J.I., Simos, P.G., Zouridakis, G., et al. (1999). Language dominance determined by magnetic source imaging: A comparison with the Wada procedure. *Neurology, 53,* 938–945.

Breitling, D., Guenther, W., & Rondot, P. (1987). Auditory perception of music measured by brain electrical activity mapping. *Neuropsychologia, 25,* 765–774.

Breitner, J.C., Welsh, K.A., Gau, B.A., et al. (1995). Alzheimer's disease in the National Academy of Sciences-National Research Council Registry of Aging Twin Veterans. III. Detection of cases, longitudinal results, and observations on twin concordance. *Archives of Neurology, 52,* 763–771.

Brennan, M., Welsh, M.C., & Fisher, C.B. (1997). Aging and executive function skills: An examination of a community-dwelling older adult population. *Perceptual and Motor Skills, 84,* 1187–1197.

Brenner, R.P. & Snyder, R.D. (1980). Late EEG findings and clinical status after organic mercury poisoning. *Archives of Neurology, 37,* 282–284.

Breslau, N., Merikangas, K., & Bowden, C.L. (1994). Comorbidity of migraine disorders and major affective disorders. *Neurology, 44(Suppl 7),* S17–S22.

Brewer, C. & Perrett, L. (1971). Brain damage due to alcohol consumption. *British Journal of Addictions, 66,* 170–182.

Brewer, C., Westerveld, M., Loring, D.W., et al. (2002). Assessing psychological function in patients with epilepsy: A comparison of the MMPI-2 and PAI. *Archives of Clinical Neuropsychology, 17,* 73.

Brex, P.A., Ciccarelli, O., O'Riordan, J.I., et al. (2002). A longitudinal study of abnormalities on MRI and disability from multiple sclerosis. *New England Journal of Medicine, 346,* 158–164.

Brick, J. (Ed.) (2004). *Handbook of the medical consequences of alcohol and drug abuse.* New York: Haworth Press.

Briel, R.C., McKeith, I.G., Barker, W.A., et al. (1999). EEG findings in dementia with Lewy bodies and Alzheimer's disease. *Journal of Neurology, Neurosurgery and Psychiatry, 66,* 401–403.

Briellmann, R.S., Berkovic, S.F., Syngeniotis, A., et al. (2002). Seizure-associated hippocampal volume loss: A longitudinal study of temporal lobe epilepsy. *Annals of Neurology, 51,* 641–644.

Briggs, G.G. & Nebes, R.D. (1975). Patterns of hand preference in a student population. *Cortex, 11,* 230–238.

Bright, P., Jaldow, E., & Kopelman, M.D. (2002). The National Adult Reading Test as a measure of premorbid intelligence: A comparison with estimates derived from demographic variables. *Journal of the International Neuropsychological Society, 8,* 847–854.

Brink, T.L., Yesavage, J.A., Lum, O., et al. (1982). Screening tests for geriatric depression. *Clinical Gerontologist,* 37–44.

Brinkman, S.D. & Braun, P. (1984). Classification of dementia patients by a WAIS profile related to central cholinergic deficiencies. *Journal of Clinical Neuropsychology, 6,* 393–400.

Brinkman, S.D., Largen, J.W., Jr., Cushman, L., & Sarwar, M. (1986). Clinical validators: Alzheimer's disease and multi-infarct dementia. In L.W. Poon (Ed.), *Handbook for clinical memory assessment of older adults.* Washington, D.C.: American Psychological Association.

Brinkman, S.D., Largen, J.W., Jr., Gerganoff, S., & Pomara, N. (1983). Russell's Revised Wechsler Memory Scale in the evaluation of dementia. *Journal of Clinical Psychology, 39,* 989–993.

Brinton, R.D. (2001). Cellular and molecular mechanisms of estrogen regulation of memory function and neuroprotection against Alzheimer's disease: Recent insights and remaining challenges. *Learning and Memory, 8,* 121–133.

Brittain, J.L., La Marche, J.A., Reeder, K.P., et al. (1991). The effects of age and IQ on Paced Auditory Serial Addition Task (PASAT) performance. *The Clinical Neuropsychologist, 5,* 163–175.

Britton, J.W., Uitti, R.J., Ahlskog, J.E., et al. (1995). Hereditary late-onset chorea without significant dementia: Genetic evidence for substantial phenotypic variation in Huntington's disease. *Neurology, 45,* 443–447.

Britz, G.W. & Mayberg, M.R. (1997). Pathology of cerebral aneurysms and subarachnoid hemorrhage. In K.M.A. Welch et al. (Eds.), *Primer on cerebrovascular diseases.* San Diego: Academic Press.

Broadley, S.A., Deans, J., Sawcer, S.J., et al. (2000). Autoimmune disease in first-degree relatives of patients with multiple sclerosis. A UK survey. *Brain, 123,* 1102–1111.

Brodal, A. (1973). Self-observations and neuro-anatomical considerations after a stroke. *Brain, 96,* 675–694.

Brodal, A. (1981). *Neurological anatomy* (3rd ed.) New York: Oxford University Press.

Brodal, P. (1992). *The central nervous system. Structure and function.* New York: Oxford University Press.

Brodaty, H., Ames, D., Snowdon, J., et al. (2003). A randomized placebo-controlled trial of risperidone for the treatment of aggression, agitation, and psychosis of dementia. *Journal of Clinical Psychiatry, 64,* 134–143.

Brodaty, H. & Moore, C.M. (1997). The Clock Drawing Test for dementia of the Alzheimer's type: A comparison of three scoring methods in a memory disorders clinic. *International Journal of Geriatric Psychiatry, 12,* 619–627.

Broderick, J.P. (1997). Stroke and migraine. In K.M.A. Welch et al. (Eds.), *Primer on cerebrovascular diseases* (4th ed.). San Diego: Academic Press.

Broderick, J., Brott, T., Kothari, R., et al. (1998). The Greater Cincinnati/Northern Kentucky Stroke Study: Preliminary first-ever and total incidence rates of stroke among blacks. *Stroke, 29,* 415–421.

Brody, N. (1997). Intelligence, schooling, and society. *American Psychologist, 52,* 1046–1050.

Broman, S.H. & Fletcher, J.M. (Eds.) (1999). *The changing nervous system. Neurobehavioral consequences of early brain disorders.* New York: Oxford University Press.

Bromley, D.B. (1953). Primitive forms of response to the Matrices Test. *Journal of Mental Science, 99,* 374–393.

Bromley, D.B. (1957). Some effects of age on the quality of intellectual output. *Journal of Gerontology, 12,* 318–323.

Brooke, M.M., Questad, K.A., Patterson, D.R., & Bashak, K.J. (1992). Agitation and restlessness after closed head injury: A prospective study of 100 consecutive admissions. *Archives of Physical Medicine and Rehabilitation, 73,* 320–323.

Brooker, A.E. (1997). Performance on the Wechsler Memory Scale-Revised for patients with mild traumatic brain injury and mild dementia. *Journal of Clinical and Experimental Neuropsychology, 84,* 131–138.

Brookmeyer, R., Gray, S., & Kawas, C. (1998). Projections of Alzheimer's disease in the United States and the public health impact of delaying disease onset. *American Journal of Public Health, 88,* 1337–1342.

Brooks, D.J. (2001). Functional imaging studies on dopamine and motor control. *Journal of Neural Transmission–General Section, 108,* 1283–1298.

Brooks, D.N. (1972). Memory and head injury. *Journal of Nervous and Mental Disease, 155,* 350–355.

Brooks, D.N. (1974). Recognition memory and head injury. *Journal of Neurology, Neurosurgery and Psychiatry, 37,* 794–801.

Brooks, D.N. (1987). Measuring neuropsychological and functional recovery. In H.S. Levin et al. (Eds.), *Neurobehavioral recovery from head injury.* New York: Oxford University Press.

Brooks, D.N. (1991). The head-injured family. *Journal of Clinical and Experimental Neuropsychology, 13,* 155–188.

Brooks, D.N. & Aughton, M.E. (1979). Psychological consequences of blunt head injury. *International Rehabilitation Medicine, 1,* 160–165.

Brooks, D.N., Aughton, M.E., Bond, M.R., et al. (1980). Cognitive sequelae in relationship to early indices of severity of brain damage after severe blunt head injury. *Journal of Neurology, Neurosurgery, and Psychiatry, 43,* 529–534.

Brooks, D.N., Hosie, J., & Bond, M.R. (1986). Cognitive sequelae of severe head injury in relation to Glasgow Outcome Scale. *Journal of Neurology, Neurosurgery and Psychiatry, 49,* 549–553.

Brooks, J., Baker, G.A., & Aldenkamp, A.P. (2001). The A–B Neuropsychological Assessment Schedule (ABNAS): The further refinement of a patient-based scale of patient-perceived cognitive functioning. *Epilepsy Research, 43,* 227–237.

Brooks, N. (1988). Personality change after severe head injury. *Acta Neurochirurgica (Suppl. 44),* 59–64.

Brooks, N. (1989). Closed head trauma: Assessing the common cognitive problems. In M.D. Lezak (Ed.), *Assessment of the behavioral consequences of head trauma. Frontiers of clinical neuroscience* (Vol. 7). New York: Alan R. Liss.

Brooks, N., Campsie, L., Symington, C., et al. (1986). The five year outcome of severe blunt head injury—a relative's view. *Journal of Neurology, Neurosurgery and Psychiatry, 49*, 764–770.

Brooks, N., Kupshik, G., Wilson, L., et al. (1987). A neuropsychological study of active amateur boxers. *Journal of Neurology, Neurosurgery and Psychiatry, 50*, 997–1000.

Brooks, N., McKinlay, A., Symington, C., et al. (1987). Return to work within the first seven years of severe head injury. *Brain Injury, 1*, 5–19.

Brooks, N., Symington, C., Beattie, A., & Campsie, L. (1989). Alcohol and other predictors of cognitive recovery after severe head injury. *Brain Injury, 3*, 235–246.

Brooks, N., Truelle, J.-L., et al. (1994). *Document Européen d'évaluation des traumatisés crâniens.* Bruxelles: Éditions EBIS.

Brookshire, R.H. (1978). *An introduction to aphasia* (2nd ed.). Minneapolis: BRK.

Broshek, D.K. & Barth, J.T. (2000). The Halstead-Reitan Neuropsychological Test Battery. In G. Groth-Marnat (Ed.), *Neuropsychological assessment in clinical practice.* New York: Wiley.

Brott, T., Tomsick, T., Feinberg, W., et al. (1994). Baseline silent cerebral infarction in the asymptomatic carotid atherosclerosis study. *Stroke, 25*, 1122–1129.

Brouwer, W.H., Ponds, R.W.H.M., van Wolffelaar, P.C., & van Zomeren, A.H. (1989). Divided attention 5 to 10 years after severe closed head injury. *Cortex, 25*, 219–230.

Brouwer, W.H., van Zomeren, A.H., & van Wolffelaar, P.C. (1990). Traffic behavior after severe traumatic brain injury. In B.G. Deelman et al. (Eds.), *Traumatic brain injury: Clinical, social, and rehabilitational aspects.* Amsterdam: Swets and Zeitlinger.

Brouwer, W.H. & Withaar, F.K. (1997). Fitness to drive after traumatic brain injury. *Neuropsychological Rehabilitation, 7*, 177–193.

Brouwer, W.H., Withaar, F.K., Tant, M.L.M., & van Zomeren, A.H. (2002). Attention and driving in traumatic brain injury: A question of coping with time-pressure. *Journal of Head Trauma Rehabilitation, 17*, 1–15.

Brouwers, P., Cox, C., Martin, A., Chase, T., et al. (1984). Differential perceptual–spatial impairment in Huntington's and Alzheimer's dementias. *Archives of Neurology, 41*, 1073–1076.

Brown, E.L. & Deffenbacher, K. (1979). *Perception and the senses.* New York: Oxford University Press.

Brown, G.G., Baird, A.D., & Shatz, M.W. (1996). The effects of cerebral vascular disease and its treatment on higher cortical functioning. In I. Grant & K.M. Adams (Eds.), *Neuropsychological assessment of cerebrovascular disorders.* New York: Oxford University Press.

Brown, G.G., Baird, A.D., Shatz, M.W., & Bornstein, R.A. (1996). The effects of cerebral vascular disease on neuropsychological functioning. In I. Grant & K.M. Adams (Eds.), *Neuropsychological assessment of cerebrovascular disorders* (2nd ed.). New York: Oxford University Press.

Brown, G.G. & Kinderman, S.S. (1997). Neuropsychological aspects of stroke. In K.M.A. Welch et al. (Eds.), *Primer on cerebrovascular diseases.* San Diego: Academic Press.

Brown, G.G., Rahill, A.A., Gorell, J.M., et al. (1999). Validity of the Dementia Rating Scale in assessing cognitive function in Parkinson's disease. *Journal of Geriatric Psychiatry and Neurology, 12*, 180–188.

Brown, G.G., Spicer, K.B., Robertson, W.M., et al. (1989). Neuropsychological signs of lateralized arteriovenous malformations: Comparisons with ischemic stroke. *The Clinical Neuropsychologist, 3*, 340–352.

Brown, J.W. (1974). Language, cognition, and the thalamus. *Confinia Neurologica, 36*, 33–60.

Brown, J.W. (1975). On the neural organization of language: Thalamic and cortical relationships. *Brain and Language, 2*, 18–30.

Brown, J.W. (1987). The microstructure of action. In E. Perecman (Ed.), *The frontal lobes revisited.* New York: IRBN.

Brown, J.W. (1989). The nature of voluntary action. *Brain and Cognition, 10*, 105–120.

Brown, J.W. (1990). Psychology of time awareness. *Brain and Cognition, 14*, 144–164.

Brown, L., Sherbenou, R.J., & Johnsen, S.K. (1982). *Test of Nonverbal Intelligence.* Austin, TX: Pro-Ed.

Brown, R.G. (2003). Disorders of intention in Parkinsonian syndromes. In M-A. Bédard et al. (Eds.), *Mental and behavioral dysfunction in movement disorders.* Totowa, NJ: Humana Press.

Brown, R.G., MacCarthy, B., Jahanshahi, M., & Marsden, C.D. (1989). Accuracy of self-reported disability in patients with Parkinsonism. *Archives of Neurology, 46*, 955–959.

Brown, R.G. & Marsden, C.D. (1986). Visuospatial function in Parkinson's disease. *Brain, 109*, 987–1002.

Brown, R.G. & Marsden, C.D. (1988). "Subcortical dementia:" The neuropsychological evidence. *Neuroscience, 25*, 363–387.

Brown, R.G., Marsden, C.D., Quinn, N., & Wyke, M.A. (1984). Alterations in cognitive performance and affect-arousal state during fluctuations in motor function in Parkinson's disease. *Journal of Neurology, Neurosurgery and Psychiatry, 47*, 454–465.

Brown, R.G., Soliveri, P., & Jahanshahi, M. (1998). Executive processes in Parkinson's disease—random number generation and response suppression. *Neuropsychologia, 36*, 1355–1362.

Brown, S.C. & Craik, F.I.M. (2000). Encoding and retrieval of information. In E. Tulving & F.I.M. Craik (Eds.), *The Oxford handbook of memory.* New York: Oxford University Press.

Brown, W.S. & Paul, L.K. (2000). Cognitive and psychosocial deficits in agenesis of the corpus callosum with normal intelligence. *Cognitive Neuropsychiatry, 5*, 135–137.

Brownell, H. & Martino, G. (1998). Deficits in inference and social cognition. In M. Beeman & C. Chiarello (Eds.), *Right hemisphere language. Perspectives from cognitive neuroscience.* Mahwah, NJ: Erlbaum.

Brozgold, A.Z., Borod, J.C., Martin, C.C., et al. (1998). Social functioning and emotional expression in neurological and psychiatric disorders. *Applied Neuropsychology, 5*, 15–23.

Brugger, P. (1997). Variables that influence the generation of random sequences: An update. *Perceptual and Motor Skills, 84*, 627–661.

Brugger, P., Monsch, A.U., Salmon, D.P., & Butters, N. (1996). Random number generation in dementia of the Alzheimer type: a test of frontal executive functions. *Neuropsychologia, 34*, 97–103.

Bruhn, A.R. & Reed, M.R. (1975). Simulation of brain damage on the Bender-Gestalt test by college subjects. *Journal of Personality Assessment, 39*, 244–255.

Bruhn, P., Arlien-Søborg, P., Gyldensted, C., & Christensen, E.L. (1981). Prognosis in chronic toxic encephalopathy: A two-year follow-up study in 26 house painters with occupational encephalopathy. *Acta Neurologica Scandinavica, 64*, 259–272.

Bruhn, P. & Maage, N. (1975). Intellectual and neuropsychological functions in young men with heavy and long-term patterns of drug abuse. *American Journal of Psychiatry, 132*, 397–401.

Brun, A. & Andersson, J. (2001). Frontal dysfunction and frontal cortical synapse loss in alcoholism—the main cause of alcohol dementia? *Dementia and Geriatric Cognitive Disorders, 12*, 289–294.

Brun, A., Gustafson, L., Risberg, J., et al. (1990). Clinicopathological correlates in dementia: A neuropathological, neuropsychiatric, neurophysiological, and psychometric study. In M. Bergener & S.K. Finkel (Eds.), *Clinical and scientific psychogeriatrics. The interface of psychiatry and neurology* (Vol. 2). New York: Springer.

Brunia, C.H.M. & Van Boxtel, G.J.M. (2000). Motor preparation. In J.T. Cacioppo, L.G. Tassinary, & G.G. Berntson (Eds.), *Handbook of psychophysiology* (2nd ed.). Cambridge, UK: Cambridge University Press.

Bruno, R.L., Galski, T., & DeLuca, J. (1993). The neuropsychology of post-polio fatigue. *Archives of Physical Medicine and Rehabilitation, 74,* 1061–1065.

Brust, J.C.M. (1993). *Neurological aspects of substance abuse.* Boston: Butterworth-Heinemann.

Brust, J.C.M. (2000a). Cannabis. In P.S. Spencer & H.H. Schaumberg (Eds.), *Experimental and clinical neurotoxicology* (2nd ed.). New York: Oxford University Press.

Brust, J.C.M. (2000b). Ethanol. In P.S. Spencer & H.H. Schaumberg (Eds.), *Experimental and clinical neurotoxicology* (2nd ed.). New York: Oxford University Press.

Brust, J.C.M. (2000c). Morphine and related opiates. In P.S. Spencer & H.H. Schaumberg (Eds.), *Experimental and clinical neurotoxicology* (2nd ed.). New York: Oxford University Press.

Brust, J.C.M. (2000d). Nicotine. In P.S. Spencer & H.H. Schaumberg (Eds.), *Experimental and clinical neurotoxicology* (2nd ed.). New York: Oxford University Press.

Bruyn, G.W. (1968). Huntington's chorea. In P.J. Vinken & G.W. Bruyn (Eds.), *Handbook of clinical neurology: Disorders of the basal ganglia* (Vol. 6). Amsterdam: Elsevier, pp. 289–378.

Bryan, J. & Luszcz, M.A. (1996). Speed of information processing as a mediator between age and free-recall performance. *Psychology and Aging, 11,* 3–9.

Bryan, J. & Luszcz, M.A. (2000). Measures of fluency as predictors of incidental memory among older adults. *Psychology of Aging, 15,* 483–489.

Bryan, K.L. & Hale, J.B. (2001). Differential effects of left and right cerebral vascular accidents on language competency. *Journal of the International Neuropsychological Society, 7* 655–664.

Bryant, R.A. & Harvey, A.G. (1995). Acute stress response: a comparison of head injured and non-head injured patients. *Psychological Medicine, 25,* 869–873.

Bryant, R.A. & Harvey, A.G. (1999a). The influence of traumatic brain injury on acute stress disorder and post-traumatic stress disorder following motor vehicle accidents. *Brain Injury, 13,* 15–22.

Bryant, R.A. & Harvey, A.G. (1999b). Postconcussive symptoms and posttraumatic stress disorder after mild traumatic brain injury. *Journal of Nervous and Mental Disease, 187,* 302–305.

Bryant, R.A., Marosszeky, J.E., Crooks, J., et al. (2001). Posttraumatic stress disorder and psychosocial functioning after severe traumatic brain injury. *Journal of Nervous and Mental Disease, 189,* 109–113.

Bryden, M.P. (1978). Strategy effects in the assessment of hemispheric asymmetry. In G. Underwood (Ed.), *Strategies of information processing.* New York: Academic Press.

Bryden, M.P. (1988). Cerebral specialization: Clinical and experimental assessment. In F. Boller & J. Grafman (Eds.), *Handbook of neuropsychology* (Vol. 1). Amsterdam: Elsevier.

Bryden, M.P., Hécaen, H., & DeAgostini, M. (1983). Patterns of cerebral organization. *Brain and Language, 20,* 249–262.

Bryer, J.B., Heck, E.T., & Reams, S.H. (1988). Neuropsychological sequelae of carbon monoxide toxicity at eleven-year follow-up. *The Clinical Neuropsychologist, 2,* 221–227.

Bschor, T., Kuhl, K.P., & Reischies, F.M. (2001). Spontaneous speech of patients with dementia of the Alzheimer type and mild cognitive impairment. *International Psychogeriatrics, 13,* 289–298.

Bub, D. & Chertkow, H. (1988). Agraphia. In F. Boller & J. Graf-

man (Eds.), *Handbook of neuropsychology* (Vol. 1). Amsterdam: Elsevier.

Bublak, P., Schubert, T., Matthes-von Cramon, G., & von Cramon, D.Y. (2000). Differential demands on working memory for guiding a simple action sequence: Evidence from closed-head-injured subjects. *Journal of Clinical and Experimental Neuropsychology, 22,* 176–189.

Buck, J.N. (1948). The H-T-P Test. *Journal of Clinical Psychology, 4,* 151–159.

Buckelew, S.P. & Hannay, H.J. (1986). Relationships among anxiety, defensiveness, sex, task difficulty, and performance on various neuropsychological tasks. *Perceptual and Motor Skills, 63,* 711–718.

Buckner, R.L. (2000). Neuroimaging of memory. In M.S. Gazzaniga (ed.), *The new cognitive neuroscience* (2nd ed.). Cambridge, MA: MIT Press.

Buckner, R.L., Koutstaal, W., Schacter, D.L., et al. (1998). Functional–anatomic study of episodic retrieval. II. Selective averaging of event-related fMRI trials to test the retrieval success hypothesis. *Neuroimage, 7,* 163–175.

Buckner, R.L. & Tulving, E. (1995). Neuroimaging studies of memory: theory and recent PET results. In F. Boller & J. Grafman (Eds.), *Handbook of neuropsychology* (Vol. 10). Amsterdam: Elsevier.

Buckwalter, J.G., Crooks, V.C., & Petitti, D.B. (2002). A preliminary psychometric analysis of a computer-assested administration of the telephone interview of Cognitive Status-Modified. *Journal of Clinical and Experimental Neuropsychology, 24,* 168–175.

Buddenberg, L.A. & Davis, C. (2000). Test–retest reliability of the Purdue Pegboard Test. *American Journal of Occupational Therapy, 54,* 555–558.

Buechler, C.M., Blostein, P.A., Koestner, A., et al. (1998). Variation among trauma centers' calculation of Glasgow Coma Scale score: Results of a national survey. *Journal of Trauma, 54,* 429–432.

Burg, J.S., Williams, R., Burright, R.G., & Donovick, P.J. (2000). Psychiatric treatment outcome following traumatic brain injury. *Brain Injury, 14,* 513–533.

Burgess, C. & Lund, K. (1998). Modeling cerebral asymmetries in high-dimensional space. In M. Beeman & C. Chiarello (Eds.), *Right hemisphere language. Perspectives from cognitive neuroscience.* Mahwah, NJ: Erlbaum.

Burgess, P.W., Alderman, N., Evans, J., et al. (1998). The ecological validity of tests of executive functions. *Journal of the International Neuropsychological Society, 4,* 547–558.

Burgess, P.W. & Shallice, T. (1994). Fractionnement du syndrome frontale. *Revue de Neuropsychologie, 4,* 345–370.

Burgess, P.W. & Shallice, T. (1996). Bizarre responses, rule detection and frontal lobe lesions. *Cortex, 32,* 241–259.

Burgess, P.W., Veitch, E., de Lacy Costello, A., & Shallice, T. (2000). The cognitive and neuroanatomical correlates of multitasking. *Neuropsychologia, 38,* 848–863.

Burgess, P.W. & Wood, R.L. (1990). Neuropsychology of behavioral disorders following brain injury. In R.L. Wood (Ed.), *Neurobehavioral sequelae of traumatic brain injury.* Bristol, PA: Taylor & Francis.

Buring, J.E., Hebert, P.H., Romero, J., et al. (1995). Migraine and subsequent risk of stroke in the Physicians' Health Study. *Archives of Neurology, 52,* 129–134.

Burkart, M. & Heun, R. (2000). Psychometric analysis of the selective reminding procedure in a sample from the general elderly population. *Dementia and Geriatric Cognitive Disorders, 11,* 74–80.

Burke, H.L. & Yeo, R.A. (1994). Systematic variations in callosal morphology: The effects of age, gender, hand preference, and anatomic asymmetry. *Neuropsychology, 8,* 563–571.

Burke, H.R. (1985). Raven's Progressive Matrices: Validity, reliability, and norms. *Journal of Clinical Psychology, 41,* 231–235.

Burke, J.M., Imhoff, C.L., & Kerrigan, J.M. (1990). MMPI correlates among post-acute TBI patients. *Brain Injury, 4,* 223–232.

Burke, J.M., Smith, S.A., & Imhoff, C.L. (1989). The response styles of post-acute brain-injured patients on MMPI. *Brain Injury, 3,* 35–40.

Burke, W.J., Nitcher, R.L., Roccaforte, W.H., & Wengel, S.P. (1992). A prospective evaluation of the Geriatric Depression Scale in an outpatient geriatric assessment center. *Journal of the American Geriatrics Society, 40,* 1227–1230.

Burke, W.J., Roccaforte, W.H., & Wengel, S.P. (1991). The short form of the Geriatric Depression Scale: A comparison with the 30–item form. *Journal of Geriatric Psychiatry and Neurology, 4,* 173–178.

Burker, E., Hannay, H.J., & Halsey, J.H. (1989). Neuropsychological functioning and personality characteristics of migrainous and nonmigrainous female college students. *Neuropsychology, 3,* 61–73.

Burn, D.J., Sawle, G.V., & Brooks, D.J. (1994). Differential diagnosis of Parkinson's disease, multiple system atrophy, and Steele-Richardson-Olszewski syndrome: Discriminant analysis of striatal 18f-dopa pet data. *Journal of Neurology, Neurosurgery and Psychiatry, 57,* 278–284.

Burstein, B., Bank, L., & Jarvik, L.F. (1980). Sex differences in cognitive functioning: Evidence, determinants, implications. *Human Development, 23,* 289–313.

Burt, D.B., Zembar, M.J., & Niederehe, G. (1995). Depression and memory impairment: a meta-analysis of the association, its pattern, and specificity. *Psychological Bulletin, 117,* 285–305.

Burt, T., Lisanby, S.H., & Sackeim, H.A. (2002). Neuropsychiatric applications of transcranial magnetic stimulation: a meta analysis. *International Journal of Neuropsychopharmacology, 5,* 73–103.

Burton, D.B., Mittenberg, W., & Burton, C.A. (1993). Confirmatory factor analysis of the Wechsler Memory Scale-Revised Standardized Sample. *Archives of Clinical Neuropsychology, 8,* 467–475.

Busch, C.R. & Alpern, H.P. (1998). Depression after mild traumatic brain injury: A review of current research. *Neuropsychology Review, 8,* 95–108.

Buschke, H. (1973). Selective reminding for analysis of memory and learning. *Journal of Verbal Learning and Verbal Behavior, 12,* 543–550.

Buschke, H. (1984). Cued recall in amnesia. *Journal of Clinical Neuropsychology, 6,* 433–440.

Buschke, H. & Fuld, P.A. (1974). Evaluation of storage, retention, and retrieval in disordered memory and learning. *Neurology, 11,* 1019–1025.

Buschke, H., Kuslansky, G., Katz, M., et al. (1999). Screening for dementia with the Memory Impairment Screen. *Neurology, 52,* 231–238.

Buschke, H., Sliwinski, M., Kuslansky, G., & Lipton, R.B. (1995). Aging, encoding specificity, and memory change in the Double Memory Test. *Journal of the International Neuropsychological Society, 1,* 483–493.

Buschke, H., Sliwinski, M., Kuslansky, G., & Lipton, R.B. (1997). Diagnosis of early dementia by the Double Memory Test: Encoding specificity improves diagnostic sensitivity and specificity. *Neurology, 48,* 989–997.

Bush, S. (2000). Intermanual visuoconstructional differences in rehabilitation patients. *Journal of Cognitive Rehabilitation, 18,* 10–12.

Bush, S.S. & Drexler, M.L. (Eds.) (2002). *Ethical issues in clinical neuropsychology.* Lisse, The Netherlands: Swets and Zeitlinger.

Butcher, J.N., Arbisi, P.A., Atlis, M.M., & McNulty, J.L. (2003). The construct validity of the Lees-Haley Fake Bad Scale. Does this scale measure somatic malingering and feigned emotional distress? *Archives of Clinical Neuropsychology, 18,* 473–485.

Butcher, J.N., Dahlstrom, W.G., Graham, J.R., et al. (1989). *Manual for the restandardized Minnesota Multiphasic Personality Inventory: MMPI-2.* Minneapolis: University of Minnesota Press.

Butcher, J.N. & Hostetler, K. (1990). Abbreviating MMPI item administration: What can be learned from the MMPI for the MMPI-2? *Psychological Assessment, 2,* 12–21.

Butcher, J.N. & Tellegen, A. (1978). Common methodological problems in MMPI research. *Journal of Consulting and Clinical Psychology, 46,* 620–628.

Butcher, J.N., Williams, C.L., Graham, J.R., et al. (1992). *MMPI-A (Minnesota Multiphasic Personality Inventory-Adolescent).* Minneapolis: University of Minnesota Press.

Butler, J.M., Rice, L.N., & Wagstaff, A.K. (1963). *Quantitative naturalistic research.* Englewood Cliffs, NJ: Prentice-Hall.

Butler, M., Retzlaff, P., & Vanderploeg, R.D. (1991). Neuropsychological test usage. *Professional Psychology: Research and Practice, 22,* 510–512.

Butler, R.W., Anderson, L., Furst, C.J., & Namerow, N.S. (1989). Behavioral assessment in neuropsychological rehabilitation: A method for measuring vocational-related skills. *The Clinical Neuropsychologist, 3,* 235–243.

Butler, R.W. & Copeland, D.R. (2002). Attentional processes and their remediation in children treated for cancer: A literature review and the development of a therapeutic approach. *Journal of the International Neuropsychological Society, 8,* 115–124.

Butler, R.W., Rorsman, I., Hill, J.M., & Tuma, R. (1993). The effects of frontal brain impairment on fluency: Simple and complex paradigms. *Neuropsychology, 7,* 519–529.

Butler, S.M., Ashford, J.W., & Snowdon, D.A. (1996). Age, education, and changes in the Mini-Mental State Exam scores of older women: Findings from the nun study. *Journal of the American Geriatrics Society, 44,* 675–681.

Butter, C.M. (1987). Varieties of attention and disturbances of attention: A neuropsychological analysis. In M. Jeannerod (Ed.), *Neurophysiological and neuropsychological aspects of spatial neglect.* Amsterdam: Elsevier/North-Holland.

Butter, C.M., Mark, V.W., & Heilman, K.M. (1988). An experimental analysis of factors underlying neglect in line bisection. *Journal of Neurology, Neurosurgery and Psychiatry, 51,* 1581–1583.

Butters, M.A., Goldstein, G., Allen, D.N., & Shemansky, W.J. (1998). Neuropsychological similarities and differences among Huntington's disease, multiple sclerosis, and cortical dementia. *Archives of Clinical Neuropsychology, 13,* 721–735.

Butters, M.A., Kasniak, A.W., Glisky, E.L., et al. (1994). Recency discrimination deficits in frontal lobe patients. *Neuropsychology, 8,* 343–354.

Butters, N. (1984a). Alcoholic Korsakoff's syndrome: An update. *Seminars in Neurology, 4,* 226–244.

Butters, N. (1984b). The clinical aspects of memory disorders: Contributions from the experimental studies in amnesia and dementia. *Journal of Clinical Neuropsychology, 6,* 17–36.

Butters, N. (1985). Alcoholic Korsakoff's syndrome: Some unresolved issues concerning etiology, neuropathology, and cognitive deficits. *Journal of Clinical and Experimental Neuropsychology, 7,* 181–210.

Butters, N. & Albert, M.S. (1982). Processes underlying failures to recall remote events. In B.S. Cermak (Ed.), *Human memory and amnesia.* Hillsdale, NJ: Erlbaum.

Butters, N., Albert, M.S., Sax, D.S., et al. (1983). The effect of verbal mediators on the pictorial memory of brain-damaged patients. *Neuropsychologia, 21,* 307–323.

Butters, N. & Barton, M. (1970). Effect of parietal lobe damage on the performance of reversible operations in space. *Neuropsychologia, 8,* 205–214.

Butters, N. & Brandt, J. (1985). The continuity hypothesis. The relationship of long-term alcoholism to the Wernicke-Korsakoff syndrome. In M. Galanter (Ed.), *Recent developments in alcoholism* (Vol. 3). New York: Plenum Press.

Butters, N. & Cermak, L.S. (1976). Neuropsychological studies of alcoholic Korsakoff patients. In G. Goldstein & C. Neuringer (Eds.), *Empirical studies of alcoholism.* Cambridge, MA: Ballinger.

Butters, N. & Cermak, L.S. (1980). *Alcoholic Korsakoff's syndrome.* New York: Academic Press.

Butters, N. & Cermak, L.S. (1986). A case study of forgetting of autobiographical knowledge: Implications for the study of retrograde amnesia. In D. Rubin (ed.), *Autobiographical memory.* New York: Cambridge University Press.

Butters, N., Cermak, L.S., Jones, B., & Glosser, G. (1975). Some analyses of the information processing and sensory capacities of alcoholic Korsakoff patients. *Advances in Experimental Medical Biology, 59,* 595–604.

Butters, N. & Grady, M. (1977). Effect of predistractor delays on the short-term memory performance of patients with Korsakoff's and Huntington's disease. *Neuropsychologia, 15,* 701–706.

Butters, N., Granholm, E., Salmon, D.P., et al. (1987). Episodic and semantic memory: A comparison of amnesic and demented patients. *Journal of Clinical and Experimental Neuropsychology, 9,* 479–497.

Butters, N., Grant, I., Haxby, J., et al. (1990). Assessment of AIDS-related cognitive changes: Recommendations of the NIMH Workgroup on neuropsychological assessment approaches. *Journal of Clinical and Experimental Neuropsychology, 12,* 963–978.

Butters, N., Salmon, D.P., Cullum, C.M., et al. (1988). Differentiation of amnesic and demented patients with the Wechsler Memory Scale–Revised. *The Clinical Neuropsychologist, 2,* 133–148.

Butters, N., Salmon, D.P., Granholm, E., et al. (1987). Differentiation of amnesic and dementing states. In S.M. Stahl et al. (Eds.), *Cognitive neurochemistry.* Oxford: Oxford University Press.

Butters, N., Salmon, D.P., Heindel, W., & Granholm, E. (1988). Episodic, semantic, and procedural memory: Some comparisons of Alzheimer and Huntington disease patients. In R.D. Terry (Ed.), *Aging and the brain.* New York: Raven Press.

Butters, N., Samuels, I., Goodglass, H., & Brody, B. (1970). Short-term visual and auditory memory disorders after parietal and frontal lobe damage. *Cortex, 6,* 440–459.

Butters, N., Sax, D., Montgomery, K., & Tarlow, S. (1978). Comparison of the neuropsychological deficits associated with early and advanced Huntington's disease. *Archives of Neurology, 35,* 585–589.

Butters, N., Soeldner, C., & Fedio, P. (1972). Comparison of parietal and frontal lobe spatial deficits in man: Extrapersonal vs. personal (egocentric) space. *Perceptual and Motor Skills, 34,* 27–34.

Butters, N. & Stuss, D.T. (1989). Diencephalic amnesia. In F. Boller & J. Grafman (Eds.), *Handbook of neuropsychology* (Vol. 3). Amsterdam: Elsevier.

Butters, N., Wolfe, J., Granholm, E., & Martone, M. (1986). An assessment of verbal recall, recognition and fluency abilities in patients with Huntington's disease. *Cortex, 22,* 11–32.

Butters, N., Wolfe, J., Martone, M., et al. (1985). Memory disorders associated with Huntington's disease: Verbal recognition and procedural memory. *Neuropsychologia, 23,* 729–743.

Butterworth, B., Shallice, T., & Watson, F.L. (1990). Short-term retention without short-term memory. In G. Vallar & T. Shallice (Eds.), *Neuropsychological impairments of short-term memory.* Cambridge: Cambridge University Press.

Bylsma, F.W., Brandt, J., & Strauss, M.E. (1990). Aspects of procedural memory are differentially impaired in Huntington's disease. *Archives of Clinical Neuropsychology, 5,* 287–297.

Bylsma, F.W., Moberg, P.J., Doty, R.L., & Brandt, J. (1997). Odor identification in Huntington's disease patients and asymptomatic gene carriers. *Journal of Neuropsychiatry and Clinical Neurosciences, 9,* 598–600.

Byrne, L.M., Bucks, R.S., & Cuerden, J.M. (1998). Validation of a new scoring system for the Weigl Color Form Sorting Test in a memory disorders clinic sample. *Journal of Clinical and Experimental Neuropsychology, 20,* 286–292.

Cabeza, R. & Nyberg, L. (2000). Imaging cognition: II. An empirical review of 275 PET and fMRI studies. *Journal of Cognitive Neuroscience, 12,* 1–47.

Cacabelos, R., Rodriguez, B., Carrera, C., et al. (1996). APOE-related frequency of cognitive and noncognitive symptoms in dementia. *Methods and Findings in Experimental and Clinical Pharmacology, 18,* 693–706.

Cacioppo, J.T., Berntson, G.G., Adolphs, R., et al. (Eds.) (2002). *Foundations in social neuroscience.* Cambridge, MA: MIT Press.

Cacioppo, J.T., Tassinary, L.G., & Berntson, G.G. (Eds.) (2000). *Handbook of psychophysiology* (2nd ed.). Cambridge, UK: Cambridge University Press.

Cahill, C. & Frith, C. (1995). Memory following electroconvulsive therapy. In A.D. Baddeley, B.A. Wilson, & F.N. Watts (Eds.), *Handbook of memory disorders.* Chichester, UK: Wiley.

Cahill, L. & McGaugh, J.L. (1998). Mechanisms of emotional arousal and lasting declarative memory. *Trends in Neurosciences, 21,* 294–299.

Cahn, D.A. & Kaplan, E. (1997). Clock drawing in the oldest old. *The Clinical Neuropsychologist, 11,* 96–100.

Cahn, D.A., Salmon, D.P., Bondi, M.W., et al. (1997). A population-based analysis of qualitative features of the neuropsychological test performance of individuals with dementia of the Alzheimer type: Implications for individuals with questionable dementia. *Journal of the International Neuropsychological Society, 3,* 387–393.

Cahn, D.A., Salmon, D.P., Butters, N., et al. (1995). Detection of dementia of the Alzheimer type in a population-based sample: Neuropsychological test performance. *Journal of the International Neuropsychological Society, 1,* 252–260.

Cahn, D.A., Salmon, D.P., Monsch, A.U., et al. (1996). Screening for dementia of the Alzheimer type in the community: The utility of the clock drawing test. *Archives of Clinical Neuropsychology, 11,* 529–539.

Cahn, D.A., Sullivan, E.V., Shear, P.K., et al. (1998). Differential contributions of cognitive and motor component processes to physical and instrumental activities of daily living in Parkinson's disease. *Archives of Clinical Neuropsychology, 13,* 575–583.

Cahn-Weiner, D.A., Boyle, P.A., & Malloy, P.F. (2002). Tests of executive function predict instrumental activities of daily living in community-dwelling older individuals. *Applied Neuropsychology, 9,* 187–191.

Cahn-Weiner, D.A., Grace, J., Ott, B.R., et al. (2002). Cognitive and behavioral features discriminate between Alzheimer's and Parkinson's disease. *Neuropsychiatry, Neuropsychology, and Behavioral Neurology, 15,* 79–87.

Cahn-Weiner, D.A., Sullivan, E.V., Shear, P.K., et al. (1999). Brain structural and cognitive correlates of clock drawing performance in Alzheimer's disease. *Journal of the International Neuropsychological Society, 5,* 502–509.

Caine, D. & Watson, J.D. (2000). Neuropsychological and neuropathological sequelae of cerebral anoxia: A critical review. *Journal of the International Neuropsychological Society, 6,* 86–99.

Caine, E.D., Bamford, K.A., Schiffer, R.B., et al. (1984). A controlled neuropsychological comparison of Huntington's disease and multiple sclerosis. *Archives of Neurology, 43,* 249–254.

Caine, E.D., Ebert, M.H., & Weingartner, H. (1977). An outline for the analysis of dementia. *Neurology, 23,* 1097–1092.

Caine, E.D., Hunt, R.D., Weingartner, H., & Ebert, M.H. (1978). Huntington's dementia. *Archives of General Psychiatry, 35,* 377–384.

Caine, E.D. & Shoulson, I. (1983). Psychiatric syndromes in Huntington's disease. *American Journal of Psychiatry, 140,* 728–733.

Caldwell, A.B. (1997). Whither goest our redoubtable mentor, the MMPI/MMPI-2? *Journal of Personality Assessment, 68,* 47–68.

Calev, A., Pass, H.L., Shapira, B., et al. (1993). ECT and memory. In C.E. Coffey (Ed.), *The clinical science of electroconvulsive therapy.* Washington, D.C.: American Psychiatric Press.

Callahan, C.D. & Hinkebein, J. (1999). Neuropsychological significance of anosmia following traumatic brain injury. *Journal of Head Trauma Rehabilitation, 14,* 581–587.

Callahan, C.D. & Hinkebein, J.H. (2002). Assessment of anosmia after traumatic brain injury: Performance characteristics of the University of Pennsylvania Smell Identification Test. *Journal of Head Trauma Rehabilitation, 17,* 251–256.

Callahan, C.M., Unverzagt, F.W., & Hui, S.L. (2002). Six-item screener to identify cognitive impairment among potential subjects for clinical research. *Medical Care, 40,* 771–781.

Calne, D.B., Eisen, A., McGeer, E., & Spencer, P. (1986). Alzheimer's disease, Parkinson's disease, and motoneurone disease: abiotrophic interaction between ageing and environment? *Lancet, ii,* 1067–1070.

Calne, D.B. & Koller, W. (1998). Degenerative diseases in the CNS. In M. Swash (Eds.), *Outcomes in neurological and neurosurgical disorders.* Cambridge, UK: Cambridge University Press.

Calsyn, D.A., O'Leary, M.R., & Chaney, E.F. (1980). Shortening the Category Test. *Journal of Consulting and Clinical Psychology, 48,* 788–789.

Camara, W.J., Nathan, J.S., & Puente, A.E. (2000). Psychological test usage: Implications in professional psychology. *Professional Psychology: Research and Practice, 31,* 141–154.

Camicioli, R., Grossmann, S.J., Spencer, P.S., et al. (2001). Discriminating mild parkinsonism: Methods for epidemiological research. *Movement Disorders, 16,* 33–40.

Camicioli, R., Howieson, D., Lehman, S., & Kaye, J. (1997). Talking while walking: The effect of a dual task in aging and Alzheimer's disease. *Neurology, 48,* 955–958.

Camicioli, R., Willert, P., Lear, J., et al. (2000). Dementia in rural primary care practices in Lake County, Oregon. *Journal of Geriatric Psychiatry and Neurology, 13,* 87–92.

Cammermeyer, M. & Evans, J.E. (1988). A brief neurobehavioral exam useful for early detection of postoperative complication in neurosurgical patients. *Journal of Neuroscience Nursing, 20,* 314–323.

Camp, C.J., Foss, J.W., Stevens, A.B., & O'Hanlon, A.M. (1996). Improving prospective memory task performance in persons with Alzheimer's disease. In M. Brandimonte, G.O Einstein, & M.A. McDaniel (Eds.), *Prospective memory. Theory and applications.* Mahwah, NJ: Erlbaum.

Camp, S.J., Stevenson, V.L., Thompson, A.J., et al. (1999). Cognitive function in primary progressive and transitional progressive multiple sclerosis: A controlled study with MRI correlates. *Brain, 122,* 1341–1348.

Campbell, A.L., Jr., Bogen, J.E., & Smith, A. (1981). Disorganization and reorganization of cognitive and sensorimotor functions in cerebral commissurotomy: Compensatory roles of the forebrain commissures and cerebral hemispheres in man. *Brain, 104,* 493–511.

Campbell, A., Brown, A.P., Schildroth, C., et al. (1991). The rela-

tionship between neuropsychological measures and self-care skills in patients with cerebrovascular lesions. *Journal of the National Medical Association, 83,* 321–324.

Campbell, J.K. (1990). Manifestations of migraine. *Neurologic Clinics, 8,* 841–855.

Campbell, J.M. & McCord, D.M. (1999). Measuring social competence with the Wechsler Picture Arrangement and Comprehension subtests. *Assessment, 6,* 215–223.

Campbell, R.J. (1981). *Psychiatric dictionary* (5th ed.). New York: Oxford University Press.

Camplair, P.S., Butler, R.W., & Lezak, M.D. (2003). Providing psychological services to families of brain-injured adults and children in the present health-care environment. In G.P. Prigatano & N.H. Pliskin (Eds.), *Clinical neuropsychology and cost outcome research.* New York: Psychology Press.

Camplair, P.S., Kreutzer, J.S., & Doherty, K.R. (1990). Family outcome following adult traumatic brain injury. In J.S. Kreutzer & P. Wehman (Eds.), *Community integration following traumatic brain injury.* Baltimore: Paul H. Brookes.

Campo, P., Morales, M., & Juan-Malpartida, M. (2000). Development of two Spanish versions of the verbal selective reminding test. *Journal of Clinical and Experimental Neuropsychology, 22,* 279–285.

Campodonico, J.R., Aylward, E., Codori, A.-M., et al. (1998). When does Huntington's disease begin? *Journal of the International Neuropsychological Society, 4,* 467–473.

Canavan, A.G.M., Passingham, R.E., Marsden, C.D., et al. (1989). Sequencing ability in Parkinsonians, patients with frontal lobe lesions and patients who have undergone unilateral temporal lobectomies. *Neuropsychologia, 27,* 787–798.

Canellopoulou, M. & Richardson, J.T.E. (1998). The role of executive function in imagery mnemonics: Evidence from multiple sclerosis. *Neuropsychologia, 36,* 1181–1188.

Cannon, B.J. (1999). Relative interference on Logical Memory I story A versus story B of the Wechsler Memory Scale-Revised in a clinical sample. *Applied Neuropsychology, 6,* 178–180.

Capitani, E. (1997). Normative data and neuropsychological assessment. Common problems in clinical practice and research. *Neuropsychological Rehabilitation, 7,* 295–309.

Capitani, E., Barbarotto, R., & Laiacona, M. (1996). Does education influence the age-related cognitive decline? A further inquiry. *Developmental Neuropsychology, 12,* 231–240.

Capitani, E., Laiacona, M., & Barbarotto, R. (1999). Gender affects word retrieval of certain categories in semantic fluency tasks. *Cortex, 35,* 273–278.

Capitani, E., Scotti, G., & Spinnler, H. (1978). Colour imperception in patients with focal excisions of the cerebral hemispheres. *Neuropsychologia, 16,* 491–496.

Caplan, B. (1983). Abbreviated WAIS forms for a stroke patient. *Journal of Clinical Neuropsychology, 5,* 239–246.

Caplan, B. (1985). Stimulus effects in unilateral neglect? *Cortex, 21,* 69–80.

Caplan, B. (1987). Assessment of unilateral neglect: A new reading test. *Journal of Clinical and Experimental Neuropsychology, 9,* 359–364.

Caplan, B. (1988). Nonstandard neuropsychological assessment: An illustration. *Neuropsychology, 2,* 13–17.

Caplan, B. & Caffrey, D. (1992). Fractionating block design: Development of a test of visuospatial analysis. *Neuropsychology, 6,* 385–394.

Caplan, B. & Caffrey, D. (1996). Visual Form Discrimination as a multiple-choice visual memory test: Illustrative data. *The Clinical Neuropsychologist, 10,* 152–158.

Caplan, B., Reidy, K., Cushman, L., et al. (1990). Assessing long-term memory with the Wechsler Memory Scale-Revised: Addition of 24-hour recall [abstract]. *Journal of Clinical and Experimental Neuropsychology, 12,* 59.

Caplan, B. and Shechter, J. (1995). The role of nonstandard neuropsychological assessment in rehabilitation: History, rationale, and examples. In L. Cushman & M. Scherer (Eds.), *Psychological assessment in medical rehabilitation.* Washington, D.C.: American Psychological Association.

Caplan, B. & Woessner, R. (1992). Psychopathology following head trauma? Interpretive hazards of the Symptom Checklist-90-Revised (SCL-90-R) [abstract]. *Journal of Clinical and Experimental Neuropsychology, 14,* 78.

Caplan, D. (1987). *Neurolinguistics and linguistic aphasiology.* Cambridge: Cambridge University Press.

Caplan, D. (2003). Aphasic syndromes. In K.M. Heilman and E. Valenstein (Eds.), *Clinical neuropsychology.* New York: Oxford University Press.

Caplan, L.R. (1980). "Top of the basilar" syndrome. *Neurology, 30,* 72–79.

Caplan, L.R. (2001). Syndromes related to large artery thromboembolism within the vertebrobasilar system. In J. Bogousslavsky and L.R. Caplan (Eds.), *Stroke syndromes* (2nd ed.). Cambridge, UK: Cambridge University Press.

Caplan, L.R., Schmahmann, J.D., Kase, C.S., et al. (1990). Caudate infarcts. *Archives of Neurology, 47,* 133–143.

Caplan, P.J., MacPherson, G.M., & Tobin, P. (1985). Do sex-related differences in spatial abilities exist? A multilevel critique with new data. *American Psychologist, 40,* 786–799.

Cappa, S.F., Guariglia, C., Messa, C., et al. (1991). Computed tomography correlates of chronic unilateral neglect. *Neuropsychology, 5,* 195–204.

Capuron, L., Ravaud, A., & Dantzer, R. (2001). Timing and specificity of the cognitive changes induced by interleukin-2 and interferon-alpha treatments in cancer patients. *Psychosomatic Medicine, 63,* 376–386.

Caraceni, A., Gangeri, L., Martini, et al. (1998). Neurotoxicity of interferon-alpha in melanoma therapy: results from a randomized controlled trial. *Cancer, 83,* 482–489.

Caramata, P.J., Heros, R.C., & Latchaw, R.E. (1994). "Brain attack:" The rationale for treating stroke as a medical emergency. *Neurosurgery, 34,* 144–157.

Caramazza, A. (1984). The logic of neuropsychological research and the problem of patient classification in aphasia. *Brain and Language, 21,* 9–21.

Carey, K.B. & Maisto, S.A. (1987). Effect of a change in drinking pattern on the cognitive function of female social drinkers. *Journal of Studies on Alcohol, 48,* 236–242.

Cargnello, J.C. & Gurekas, R. (1987). The clinical use of a modified WAIS procedure in a geriatric population. *Journal of Clinical Psychology, 43,* 286–290.

Cargnello, J.C. & Gurekas, R. (1988). The WAIS-SAM: A comprehensive administrative model of modified WAIS procedures. *Journal of Psychology, 44,* 266–270.

Carhuapoma, J.R. & Hanley, D.F. (2002). Intracerebral hemorrhage. In A.K. Asbury et al. (Eds.), *Diseases of the nervous system* (2nd ed.). Cambridge: Cambridge University Press.

Carlen, P.L., Penn, R.D., Fornazzari, L., et al. (1986). Computerized tomographic scan assessment of alcoholic brain damage and its potential reversibility. *Alcoholism, Clinical and Experimental Research, 10,* 226–232.

Carlen, P.L., Wilkinson, D.A., Wortzman, G., et al. (1981). Cerebral atrophy and functional deficits in alcoholics without clinically apparent liver disease. *Neurology, 31,* 377–385.

Carlesimo, G.A. & Caltagirone, C. (1995). Components in the visual processing of known and unknown faces. *Journal of Clinical and Experimental Neuropsychology, 17,* 691–705.

Carlesimo, G.A., Fadda, L., & Caltagirone, C. (1993). Basic mechanisms of constructional apraxia in unilateral brain-damaged patients: Role of visuo-perceptual and executive disorders. *Journal of Clinical and Experimental Neuropsychology, 15,* 342–358.

Carlesimo, G.A., Mauri, M., Graceffa, A.M., et al. (1998). Memory performances in young, elderly, and very old healthy individuals versus patients with Alzheimer's disease: evidence for discontinuity between normal and pathological aging. *Journal of Clinical and Experimental Neuropsychology, 20,* 14–29.

Carlesimo, G.A., Sabbadini, M., Bombardi, P., et al. (1998). Retrograde memory deficits in severe closed-head injury patients. *Cortex, 34,* 1–23.

Carlesimo, G.A., Sabbadini, M., Fadda, L., & Caltagirone, C. (1997). Word-list forgetting in young and elderly subjects: evidence for age-related decline in transferring information from transitory to permanent memory condition. *Cortex, 33,* 155–166.

Carless, S.A. (2000). The validity of scores on the Multidimensional Aptitude Battery. *Educational and Psychological Measurement, 60,* 592–603.

Carlin, A.S. & O'Malley (1996). Neuropsychological consequences of drug abuse. In I. Grant & K.M. Adams (Eds.), *Neuropsychological assessment of neuropsychiatric disorders.* New York: Oxford University Press.

Carlin, D., Bonerba, J., Phipps, M., et al. (2000). Planning impairments in frontal lobe dementia and frontal lobe lesion patients. *Neuropsychologia, 38,* 655–665.

Carmelli, D., Swan, G.E., & Cardon, L.R. (1995). Genetic mediation in the relationship of education to cognitive function in older people. *Psychology and Aging, 10,* 48–53.

Carmichael, J.A. & MacDonald, J.W. (1984). Developmental norms for the Sentence Repetition Test. *Journal of Consulting and Clinical Psychology, 52,* 476–477.

Carmon, A. (1978). Spatial and temporal factors in visual perception of patients with unilateral cerebral lesions. In M. Kinsbourne (Ed.), *Asymmetrical function of the brain.* Cambridge, UK: Cambridge University Press.

Carmon, A. & Nachshon, I. (1971). Effect of unilateral brain damage on perception of temporal order. *Cortex, 7,* 410–418.

Carpenter, A.F., Georgopoulos, A.P., & Pellizzer, G. (1999). Motor cortical encoding of serial order in a context-recall task. *Science, 283,* 1752–1757.

Carpenter, K., Berti, A., Oxbury, S., et al. (1995). Awareness of and memory for arm weakness during intracarotid sodium amytal testing. *Brain, 118,* 243–251.

Carr, E.K. & Lincoln, N.B. (1988). Interrater reliability of the Rey figure copying test. *British Journal of Clinical Psychology, 27,* 267–268.

Carrasco, M.C., Guillem, M.J., & Redolat, R. (2000). Estimation of short temporal intervals in Alzheimer's disease. *Experimental Aging Research, 26,* 139–151.

Carretta, T.R., Retzlaff, P.D., Callister, J.D., & King, R.E. (1998). A comparison of two U.S. Air Force pilot aptitude tests. *Aviation Space and Environmental Medicine, 69,* 931–935.

Carroll, J.B. (1993). *Human cognitive abilities: A survey of factor-analytic studies.* New York: Cambridge University Press.

Carroll, J.B., Davies, P., & Richman, B. (1971). *The American Heritage Word Frequency Book.* Boston: Houghton-Mifflin.

Carson, A.J., MacHale, S., Allen, K., et al. (2000). Depression after stroke and lesion location: a systematic review. *Lancet, 356,* 122–126.

Carter, C.S., Perlstein, W., Ganguli, R., et al. (1998). Functional hypofrontality and working memory dysfunction in schizophrenia. *American Journal of Psychiatry, 155,* 1285–1287.

Carter, J.H., Nutt, J.G., Woodward, W.R., et al. (1989). Amount and distribution of dietary protein affects clinical response to levodopa in Parkinson's disease. *Neurology, 39,* 552–556.

Carter, R. (2002). *Exploring consciousness.* Berkeley: University of California Press.

Carter, S.L., Shore, D., Harnadek, M.C.S., & Kubu, C.S. (1998). Normative data and interrater reliability of the Design Fluency Test. *The Clinical Neuropsychologist, 12,* 531–534.

Carter-Saltzman, L. (1979). Patterns of cognitive functioning in relation to handedness and sex-related differences. In M.A. Wittig & A.C. Petersen (Eds.), *Sex-related differences in cognitive functioning.* New York: Academic Press.

Caruso, J.C. & Cliff, N. (1999). The properties of equally and differentially weighted WAIS-III factor scores. *Psychological Assessment, 11,* 198–206.

Cascino, G.D. (2002). Electroencephalographic recordings for epilepsy surgery. In J.R. Daube (Ed.), *Clinical neurophysiology* (2nd ed.). New York: Oxford University Press.

Caselli, R.J. (1991). Rediscovering tactile agnosia. *Mayo Clinic Proceedings, 66,* 129–142.

Caselli, R.J. & Yanagihara, T. (1991). Memory disorders in degenerative neurological diseases. In T. Yanagihara & R.C. Petersen (Eds.), *Memory disorders: Research and clinical practice.* New York: Marcel Dekker.

Casey, M.B., Winner, E., Hurwitz, I., & DaSilva, D. (1991). Does processing style affect recall of the Rey-Osterrieth or Taylor Complex Figures? *Journal of Clinical and Experimental Neuropsychology, 13,* 600–606.

Cashel, M.L., Rogers, R., Sewell, K.W., & Martin-Cannici, C. (1995). The Personality Assessment Inventory (PAI) and the detection of defensiveness. *Assessment, 2,* 333–342.

Cassel, R.H. (1962). The order of the tests in the battery. *Journal of Clinical Psychology, 18,* 464–465.

Casson, I.R., Sham, R., Campbell, E.A., et al. (1982). Neurological and CT evaluation of knocked-out boxers. *Journal of Neurology, Neurosurgery and Psychiatry, 45,* 170–174.

Casson, I.R., Siegel, O., Sham, R., et al. (1984). Brain damage in modern boxers. *Journal of the American Medical Association, 251,* 2663–2667.

Castillo, V. & Bogousslavsky, J. (1997). Brain embolism. In K.M.A. Welch et al. (Eds.), *Primer on cerebrovascular diseases.* San Diego: Academic Press.

Castro-Caldas, A., Confraria, A., Paiva, T., & Trindade, A. (1986). Contrecoup injury in the misdiagnosis of crossed aphasia. *Journal of Clinical and Experimental Neuropsychology, 8,* 697–701.

Castro-Caldas, A. & Grafman, J. (2000). Those were the (phrenological) days. *The Neuroscientist, 6,* 297–302.

Castro-Caldas, A., Petersson, K.M., Reis, A., et al. (1998). The illiterate brain. Learning to read and write during childhood influences the functional organization of the adult brain. *Brain, 121,* 1053–1063.

Cate, Y. & Richards, L. (2000). Relationship between performance on tests of basic visual functions and visual-perceptual processing in persons after brain injury. *American Journal of Occupational Therapy, 54,* 326–334.

Cattelani, R., Tanzi, F., Lombardi, F., & Mazzucchi, A. (2002). Competitive re-employment after severe traumatic brain injury: Clinical, cognitive and behavioural predictive variables. *Brain Injury, 16,* 51–64.

Cavanaugh, S. von A. & Wettstein, R.M. (1983). The relationship between severity of depression, cognitive dysfunction, and age in medical inpatients. *American Journal of Psychiatry, 140,* 495–496.

Cazalis, F., Azouvi, P., Sirigu, A., et al. (2001). Script knowledge after severe traumatic brain injury. *Journal of the International Neuropsychological Society, 7,* 795–804.

Celesia, C.G., Bushnell, D., Cone Toleikis, S., & Brigell, M.G. (1991).

Cortical blindness and residual vision: Is the "second" visual system in humans capable of more than rudimentary visual perception? *Neurology, 41,* 862–869.

Cella, D.F., Jacobsen, P.B., & Hymowitz, P. (1985). A comparison of the interest accuracy of two short forms of the WAIS-R. *Journal of Clinical Psychology, 41,* 544–546.

Centers for Disease Control and Prevention (1997). *Living well with epilepsy: Report of the 1997 national conference on public health and epilepsy.* Atlanta: Centers for Disease Control and Prevention.

Centers for Disease Control and Prevention (1997). Traumatic brain injury: Colorado, Missouri, Oklahoma, and Utah, 1990–1993. *Morbidity and Mortality Weekly Report, 46,* 8–11.

Ceranic, B. & Luxon, L.M. (2002). Disorders of the auditory system. In A.K. Asbury et al. (Eds.), *Diseases of the nervous system* (3rd ed.). Cambridge, UK: Cambridge University Press.

Cerone, L.J. & McKeever, W.F. (1999). Failure to support the right-shift theory's hypothesis of a "heterozygote advantage" for cognitive abilities. *British Journal of Psychology, 90,* 109–123.

Chafetz, M.D. (1990). *Nutrition and Neurotransmitters.* Englewood Cliffs, NJ: Prentice-Hall.

Chambers, B.R., Norris, J.W., Shurvell, B.L., & Hachinski, V.C. (1987). Prognosis of acute stroke. *Neurology, 37,* 221–225.

Chan, A.S., Choi, A., Chiu, H., & Lam, L. (2003). Clinical validity of the Chinese version of Mattis Dementia Rating Scale in differentiating dementia of Alzheimer's type in Hong Kong. *Journal of the International Neuropsychological Society, 9,* 45–55.

Chan, A.S., Choi, M.K., & Salmon, D.P. (2001). The effects of age, education and gender on the Mattis Dementia Rating Scale performance of elderly Chinese and American individuals. *Journal of Gerontology. Series B, Psychological Sciences and Social Sciences, 56,* P356–P363.

Chan, A.S. & Poon, M.W. (1999). Performance of 7- to 95-year-old individuals in a Chinese version of the Category Fluency Test. *Journal of the International Neuropsychological Society, 5,* 525–533.

Chan, R.C.K., (2001). Attentional deficits in patients with post-concussion symptoms: a componential perspective. *Brain Injury, 15,* 71–94.

Channon, S. (1996). Executive dysfunction in depression: The Wisconsin Card Sorting Test. *Journal of Affective Disorders, 39,* 107–114.

Channon, S. & Crawford, S. (1999). Problem-solving in real-life-type situations: the effects of anterior and posterior lesions on performance. *Neuropsychologia, 37,* 757–770.

Chapman, J., Vinokurov S., Achiron, A., et al. (2001). APOE genotype is a major predictor of long-term progression of disability in MS. *Neurology, 56,* 312–316.

Chapman, J.P., Chapman, L.J., & Allen, J.J. (1987). The measurement of foot preference. *Neuropsychologia, 25,* 579–584.

Chapman, L.F. & Wolff, H.G. (1959). The cerebral hemispheres and the highest integrative functions of man. *AMA Archives of Neurology, 1,* 357–424.

Chapman, S.B., Ulatowska, H.K., Franklin, L.R., et al. (1997). Proverb interpretation in fluent aphasia and Alzheimer's disease: Implications beyond abstract thinking. *Aphasiology, 11,* 337–350.

Chapman, S.B., Ulatowska, H.K., King, K., et al. (1995). Discourse in early Alzheimer's disease versus normal advanced aging. *American Journal of Speech-Language Pathology, 4,* 125–129.

Charter, R.A. (1994). Determining random responding for the Category, Speech-Sounds Perception, and Seashore Rhythm Tests. *Journal of Clinical and Experimental Neuropsychology, 16,* 744–748.

Charter, R.A. (2000). An alternate short form of the Speech-Sounds Perception Test. *Perceptual and Motor Skills, 90,* 1184–1186.

Charter, R.A. (2002). Reliability of the WMS-III discrepancy comparisons. *Perceptual and Motor Skills*, *94*, 387–390.

Charter, R.A. & Dobbs, S.M. (1998). Long and short forms of the Speech Sounds Perception Test: Item analysis and age and education corrections. *The Clinical Neuropsychologist*, *12*, 213–216.

Charter, R.A. & Dutra, R.L. (2000). Tactual Performance Test: Internal consistency reliability of the memory and location scores. *Perceptual and Motor Skills*, *91*, 143–146.

Charter, R.A. & Dutra, R.L. (2001). Tactual Performance Test: Item analysis of the memory and location scores. *Perceptual and Motor Skills*, *92*, 899–902.

Charter, R.A., Dutra, R.L., & Lopez, M.N. (1997). Speech Sounds Perception Test: Analysis of error types in normal and diffusely brain-damaged patients. *Perceptual and Motor Skills*, *84*, 1507–1510.

Charter, R.A. & Lopez, M.N. (2002). Millon Clinical Multiaxial Inventory (MCMI-III): The inability of the validity conditions to detect random responders. *Journal of Clinical Psychology*, *58*, 1615–1617.

Charter, R.A., Swift, K.M., & Bluzewicz, M.J. (1997). Age- and education-corrected standardized short form of the Category Test. *The Clinical Neuropsychologist*, *11*, 142–145.

Charter, R.A., Walden, D.K., & Padilla, S.P. (2000). Too many simple clerical scoring errors: The Rey Figure as an example. *Journal of Clinical Psychology*, *56*, 571–574.

Charter, R.A. & Webster, J.S. (1997). Psychometric structure of the Seashore Rhythm Test. *The Clinical Neuropsychologist*, *11*, 167–173.

Chase, T.N., Fedio, P., Foster, N.L., et al. (1984). Wechsler Adult Intelligence Scale performance. Cortical localization by fluorodeoxyglucose F18-positron emission tomography. *Archives of Neurology*, *41*, 1244–1247.

Chatterjee, A. (2002). Neglect: A disorder of spatial attention. In M. D'Esposito (Ed.), *Neurological foundations of cognitive neuroscience*. Cambridge, MA: MIT Press.

Chatterjee, A. & Farah, M.J. (2001). Face module, face network. The cognitive architecture of the brain revealed through studies of face processing. *Neurology*, *57*, 1151–1152.

Chaves, C.J. & Caplan, L.R. (2001). Posterior cerebral artery. In J. Bogousslavsky & L.R. Caplan (Eds.). *Stroke syndromes*. Cambridge, UK: Cambridge University Press.

Checkoway, H., Franklin, G.M., Costa-Mallen, P., et al. (1998). A genetic polymorphism of MAO-B modifies the association of cigarette smoking and Parkinson's disease. *Neurology*, *50*, 1458–1461.

Chédru, F. & Geschwind, N. (1972). Writing disturbances in acute confusional states. *Neuropsychologia*, *10*, 343–353.

Chelazzi, L. & Corbetta, M. (2000). Cortical mechanisms of visuospatial attention in the primate brain. In M.S. Gazzaniga (Ed.), *The new cognitive neurosciences* (2nd ed.). Cambridge, MA: MIT Press.

Chelune, G.J. (1983). Effects of partialing out postmorbid WAIS scores in a heterogenous sample: comment on Golden et al. *Journal of Consulting and Clinical Psychology*, *51*, 932–933.

Chelune, G.J. (1995). Hippocampal adequacy versus functional reserve: Predicting memory functions following temporal lobectomy. *Archives of Clinical Neuropsychology*, *10*, 413–432.

Chelune, G.J. & Bornstein, R.A. (1988). WMS-R patterns among patients with unilateral brain lesions. *The Clinical Neuropsychologist*, *2*, 121–132.

Chelune, G.J., Bornstein, R.A., & Prifitera, A. (1990). The Wechsler Memory Scale-Revised: Current status and applications. In J. Rosen, P. McReynolds, & G.J. Chelune (Eds.), *Advances in psychological assessment*. New York: Plenum Press.

Chelune, G.J., Ferguson, W., & Moehle, K. (1986). The role of standard cognitive and personality tests in neuropsychological assessment. In T. Incagnoli, G. Goldstein, & C.J. Golden (Eds.), *Clinical application of neuropsychological test batteries*. New York: Plenum Press.

Chelune, G.J., Heaton, R.K., & Lehman, R.A.W. (1986). Neuropsychological and personality correlates of patients' complaints of disability. In G. Goldstein & R.E. Tartar (Eds.), *Advances in clinical neuropsychology*. New York: Plenum Press.

Chelune, G.J., Naugle, R.I., Lüders, H., & Awad, I.A. (1991). Prediction of cognitive change as a function of preoperative ability status among temporal lobectomy patients seen at six-month follow-up. *Neurology*, *41*, 399–404.

Chelune, G.J., Naugle, R.I., Lüders, H., et al. (1993). Individual change after epilepsy surgery: Practice effects and base-rate information. *Neuropsychology*, *7*, 41–52.

Chen, P., Ratcliff, G., Belle, S.H., et al. (2001). Patterns of cognitive decline in presymptomatic Alzheimer disease: A prospective community study. *Archives of General Psychiatry*, *58*, 853–858.

Chen, T.H., Kaufman, A.S., & Kaufman, J.C. (1994). Examining the interaction of age × race pertaining to black–white differences at ages 15 to 93 on six Horn abilities assessed by K-FAST, K-SNAP, and KAIT subtests. *Perceptual and Motor Skills*, *79*, 1683–1690.

Cherington, M. (1995). Central nervous system complications of lightning and electrical injuries. *Seminars in Neurology*, *15*, 233–240.

Cherington, M. (2001). Lightning injuries in sports. *Sports Medicine*, *31*, 301–308.

Cherington, M., Krider, E.P., Yarnell, P.R., & Breed, D.W. (1997). A bolt from the blue: Lightning strike to the head. *Neurology*, *48*, 683–686.

Cherington, M., Kurtzman, R., Krider, E.P., & Yarnell, P.R. (2001). Mountain medical mystery: Unwitnessed death of a healthy young man, caused by lightning. *American Journal of Forensic Medical Pathology*, *22*, 296–298.

Cherington, M., Yarnell, P., & Hallmark, D. (1993). MRI in lightning encephalopathy. *Neurology*, *43*, 1437–1438.

Cherington, M., Yarnell, P.R., & London, S.F. (1995). Neurologic complications of lightning injuries. *Western Journal of Medicine*, *162*, 413–417.

Cherrier, M.M., Asthana, S., Plymate, S., et al. (2001). Testosterone supplementation improves spatial and verbal memory in healthy older men. *Neurology*, *57*, 80–88.

Cherry, K.E., & LeCompte, D.C. (1999). Age and individual differences influence prospective memory. *Psychology and Aging*, *14*, 60–76.

Cherry, N., Venables, H., & Waldron, H.A. (1984a). British studies on the neuropsychological effects of solvent exposure. *Scandinavian Journal of Work, Environment and Health*, *10*, 10–12.

Cherry, N., Venables, H., & Waldron, H.A. (1984b). Description of the tests in the London School of Hygiene test battery. *Scandinavian Journal of Work, Environment and Health*, *10*, 18–19.

Cheung, M., Chan, A.S., Law, S.C., et al. (2000). Cognitive function of patients with nasopharyngeal carcinoma with and without temporal lobe radionecrosis. *Archives of Neurology*, *57*, 1347–1352.

Chiarello, C. (1988). Lateralization of lexical processes in the normal brain: A review of visual half-field research. In H.A. Whitaker (Ed.), *Contemporary reviews in neuropsychology*. New York: Springer-Verlag.

Chipchase, S.Y. & Lincoln, N.B. (2001). Factors associated with carer strain in carers of people with multiple sclerosis. *Disability and Rehabilitation*, *23*, 768–776.

Chipman, K. & Kimura, D. (1998). An investigation of sex differences on incidental memory for verbal and pictorial material. *Learning and Individual Differences*, *10*, 259–272.

Chobor, K.L. & Brown, J.W. (1990). Semantic deterioration in Alzheimer's disease: The patterns to expect. *Geriatrics*, *45*, 68–75.

Choca, J.P., Laatsch, L., Wetzel, L., & Agresti, A. (1997). The Halstead Category Test: A fifty year perspective. *Neuropsychology Review, 7,* 61–65.

Chodosh, E.H., Foulkes, M.A., Kase, C.S., et al. (1988). Silent stroke in the NINCDS Stroke Data Bank. *Neurology, 38,* 1674–1679.

Chodosh, J., Reuben, D.B., Albert, M.S., & Seeman, T.E. (2002). Predicting cognitive impairment in high-functioning community-dwelling older persons: MacArthur Studies of Successful Aging. *Journal of the American Geriatric Society, 50,* 1051–1060.

Choi, I.S. (1983). Delayed neurologic sequelae in carbon monoxide intoxication. *Archives of Neurology, 40,* 433–435.

Choi, S.C., Marmarou, A., Bullock, R., et al. (1998). Primary end points in phase III clinical trials of severe head trauma: DRS versus GOS. The American Brain Injury Consortium Study Group. *Journal of Neurotrauma, 15,* 771–776.

Chopra, P., Couper, J., & Herrman, H. (2002). The assessment of disability in patients with psychotic disorders: An application of the ICIDH-2. *Australian and New Zealand Journal of Psychiatry, 36,* 127–132.

Chosak Reiter, J. (2000). Measuring cognitive processes underlying picture naming in Alzheimer's and cerebrovascular dementia: A general processing tree approach. *Journal of Clinical and Experimental Neuropsychology, 22,* 351–369.

Choueiri, R.N., Fayad, M.N., Farah, A., & Mikati, M.A. (2001). Classification of epilepsy syndromes and role of genetic factors. *Pediatric Neurology, 24,* 37–43.

Chouinard, M.J. & Rouleau, I. (1997). The 48-Pictures Test: A two-alternative forced-choice recognition test for the detection of malingering. *Journal of the International Neuropsychological Society, 3,* 545–552.

Christensen, A.-L. (1979). *Luria's neuropsychological investigation* (2nd ed.). Copenhagen: Munksgaard.

Christensen, A.-L. (1989). The neuropsychological investigation as a therapeutic and rehabilitative technique. In D.W. Ellis & A.-L. Christensen (Eds.), *Neuropsychological treatment after brain damage.* Norwell, MA: Kluwer.

Christensen, A.-L. & Caetano, C. (1996). Alexandr Romanovich Luria (1902–1977): Contributions to neuropsychological rehabilitation. *Neuropsychological Rehabilitation, 6,* 279–303.

Christensen, A-L., Jensen, L.R., & Risberg, J. (1989). Luria's neuropsychological and neurolinguistic testing. *Journal of Neurolinguistics, 4,* 137–154.

Christensen, A.-L. & Uzzell, B.P. (Eds.) (2000). *International handbook of neuropsychological rehabilitation.* New York: Kluwer Academic/Plenum Press.

Christensen, H., Griffiths, K., Mackinnon, A., & Jacomb, P. (1997). A quantitative review of cognitive deficits in depression and Alzheimer-type dementia. *Journal of the International Neuropsychological Society, 3,* 631–651.

Christensen, K.J. (1989). A new approach to the measurement of cognitive deficits in dementia. F.J. Pirozzola (Ed.) *Clinics in Geriatric Medicine* (Vol. 5, No. 3). Philadelphia: Saunders.

Christensen, K.J., Multhaup, K.S., Nordstrom, S., & Voss, K. (1990). Cognitive test profile analysis for the identification of dementia of the Alzheimer type. *Alzheimer Disease and Associated Disorders, 4,* 96–109.

Christensen, K.J., Multhaup, K.S., Nordstrom, S., & Voss, K. (1991a). A cognitive battery for dementia: development and measurement characteristics. *Psychological Assessment, 3,* 168–174.

Christensen, K.J., Multhaup, K.S., Nordstrom, S.K., & Voss, K.A. (1991b). A new cognitive battery for dementia: Relative severity of deficits in Alzheimer's disease. *Developmental Neuropsychology, 7,* 435–449.

Chu, N.-S., Huang, C.-C., & Calne, D.G. (2000). Manganese. In P.S. Spencer & H.H. Schaumburg (Eds.), *Experimental and clinical neurotoxicity* (2nd ed.). New York: Oxford University Press.

Chu, W.J., Mason, G.F., Pan, J.W., et al. (2002). Regional cerebral blood flow and magnetic resonance spectroscopic imaging findings in diaschisis from stroke. *Stroke, 33,* 1243–1248.

Chui, H.C. (1989). Dementia: A review emphasizing clinicopathologic correlation and brain–behavior relationships. *Archives of Neurology, 46,* 806–814.

Chui, H.C., Mack, W., Jackson, J.E., et al. (2000). Clinical criteria for the diagnosis of vascular dementia: A multicenter study of comparability and interrater reliability. *Archives of Neurology, 57,* 191–196.

Chui, H.C. & Perlmutter, L.S. (1992). Pathological correlates of dementia in Parkinson's disease. In S.J. Huber & J.L. Cummings (Eds.), *Parkinson's disease: Neurobehavioral aspects.* New York: Oxford University Press.

Chui, H.C., Victoroff, J.I., Margolin, D., et al. (1992). Criteria for the diagnosis of ischemic vascular dementia proposed by the State of California Alzheimer's Disease Diagnostic and Treatment Centers. *Neurology, 42,* 473–480.

Chukwudelunzu, F.E., Meschia, J.F., Graff-Radford, N.R., & Lucas, J.A. (2001). Extensive metabolic and neuropsychological abnormalities associated with discrete infarction of the genu of the internal capsule. *Journal of Neurology, Neurosurgery, and Psychiatry, 71,* 658–662.

Chung, C.-S. & Caplan, L.R. (2001). Pontine infarcts and hemorrhages. In J. Bogousslavsky and L.R. Caplan (Eds.), *Stroke syndromes* (2nd ed.). Cambridge, UK: Cambridge University Press.

Chung, M.K. & Bartfield, J.M. (2002). Knowledge of prescription medications among elderly emergency department patients. *Annals of Emergency Medicine, 39,* 605–608.

Chung, W.C.J., De Vries, G.J., & Swaab, D.F. (2002). Sexual differentiation of the red nucleus of the stria terminalis in humans may extend into adulthood. *Journal of Neuroscience, 22,* 1027–1033.

Cicchetti, D.V. (1994). Guidelines, criteria, and rules of thumb for evaluating normed and standardized assessment instruments in psychology. *Psychological Assessment, 6,* 284–290.

Cicchetti, D.V. (1997). Do recognition-free recall discrepancies detect retrieval deficits in closed-head injury? Demonstrating the inaccuracies of a reviewer's critique [see comments]. *Journal of Clinical and Experimental Neuropsychology, 19,* 144–148.

Cicerone, K.D. (1997). Clinical sensitivity of four measures of attention to mild traumatic brain injury. *The Clinical Neuropsychologist, 11* 266–272.

Cicerone, K.D. & DeLuca, J. (1990). Neuropsychological predictors of head injury rehabilitation outcome [abstract]. *Journal of Clinical and Experimental Neuropsychology, 12,* 92.

Cicerone, K.D. & Fraser, R.T. (1999). Counseling interactions for clients with traumatic brain injury. In R.T. Fraser & D.C. Clemmons (Eds.), *Traumatic brain injury rehabilitation,* Boca Raton, FL: CRC Press.

Cicerone, K.D. & Wood, J.C. (1987). Planning disorder after closed head injury: A case study. *Archives of Physical Medicine and Rehabilitation, 68,* 111–115.

Cicone, M., Wapner, W., & Gardner, H. (1980). Sensitivity to emotional expressions and situations in organic patients. *Cortex, 16,* 145–158.

Cifu, D.X., Keyser-Marcus, L., Lopez, E., et al. (1997). Acute predictors of successful return to work 1 year after traumatic brain injury: A multicenter analysis. *Archives of Physical Medicine and Rehabilitation, 78,* 125–131.

Cifu, D.X., Kreutzer, J.S., Marwitz, J.H., et al. (1996). Functional outcomes of older adults with traumatic brain injury: a prospective, multicenter analysis. *Archives of Physical Medicine and Rehabilitation, 77,* 883–888.

Cimino, C.R. (1994). Principles of neuropsychological interpretation. In R.D. Vanderploeg (Ed.), *Clinician's guide to neuropsychological assessment.* Hillsdale, NJ: Erlbaum.

Clark, C. & Klonoff, H. (1988). Reliability and construct validity of the Six Block Tactual Performance Test in an adult sample. *Journal of Clinical and Experimental Neuropsychology, 10,* 175–184.

Clark, C.M., Ewbank, D., Lerner, A., et al. (1997). The relationship between extrapyramidal signs and cognitive performance in patients with Alzheimer's disease enrolled in the CERAD Study. Consortium to Establish a Registry for Alzheimer's Disease. *Neurology, 49,* 70–75.

Clark, C.R., Egan, G.F., McFarlane, A.C., et al. (2000). Updating working memory for words: A PET activation study. *Human Brain Mapping, 9,* 42–54.

Clarke, J.M., McCann, C.M., & Zaidel, E. (1998). The corpus callosum and language: Anatomical–behavioral relationships. In M. Beeman & C. Chiarello (Eds.), *Right hemisphere language comprehension. Perspectives from cognitive neuroscience.* Mahwah, NJ: Erlbaum.

Clarke, S. (2001). Right hemisphere syndromes. In J. Bogousslavsky and L.R. Caplan (Eds.), *Stroke syndromes* (2nd ed.). Cambridge: Cambridge University Press.

Cleare, A.J., Miell, J., Heap, E., Sookdeo, S., et al. (2001). Hypothalamo–pituitary–adrenal axis dysfunction in chronic fatigue syndrome, and the effects of low-dose hydrocortisone therapy. *Journal of Clinical Endocrinology and Metabolism, 86,* 3545–3554.

Clément, J.P., Marchan, F., Boyon, D., et al. (1996). Utilization of the Draw a Person Test in the elderly. *International Psychogeriatrics, 8,* 349–364.

Clemons, M., Regnard, C., & Appleton, T. (1996). Alertness, cognition and morphine in patients with advanced cancer. *Cancer Treatment Reviews, 22,* 451–468.

Clifford, D.B. (1990). The somatosensory system and pain. In A.L. Pearlman & R.C. Collins (Eds.), *Neurobiology of disease.* New York: Oxford University Press.

Clifford, D.B. (2002). AIDS dementia. *Medical Clinics of North America, 86,* 537–550.

Clifton, G.L. & Hayes, R.L. (1996). Hypothermia for the treatment of head injury. In R.K. Narayan et al. (Eds.). *Neurotrauma.* New York: McGraw-Hill.

Coburn, K.L., Parks, R.W., & Pritchard, W.S. (1993). Electrophysiological indexes of cortical deterioration and cognitive impairment in dementia. In R.W. Parks, R.F. Zec, & R.S. Wilson (Eds.), *Neuropsychology of Alzheimer's disease and other dementias.* New York: Oxford University Press.

Cochrane, H.J., Baker, G.A., & Meudell, P.R. (1998). Simulating a memory impairment: Can amnesics implicitly outperform simulators? *British Journal of Clinical Psychology, 37,* 31–48.

Cockburn, J. (1995). Performance on the Tower of London test after severe head injury. *Journal of the International Neuropsychological Society, 1,* 537–744.

Cockburn, J. (1996a). Assessment and treatment of prospective memory deficits. In M. Brandimonte, G.O. Einstein, & M.A. McDaniel (Eds.), *Prospective memory. Theory and applications.* Mahwah, NJ: Erlbaum.

Cockburn, J. (1996b). Failure of prospective memory after acquired brain damage: Preliminary investigation and suggestions for future directions. *Journal of Clinical and Experimental Neuropsychology, 18,* 304–309.

Cockburn, J., Keene, J., Hope, T., & Smith, P. (2000). Progressive decline in NART score with increasing dementia severity. *Journal of the International Neuropsychological Society, 22,* 508–517.

Cockburn, J. & Smith, P.T. (1989). *Rivermead Behavioural Memory Test. Elderly people.* (Suppl. 3). Titchfield, Hants, UK: Thames Valley Test.

Cockburn, J., Wilson, B.A., Baddeley, A., & Hiorns, R. (1990a). Assessing everyday memory in patients with dysphasia. *British Journal of Clinical Psychology, 29,* 353–360.

Cockburn, J., Wilson, B.A., Baddeley, A., & Hiorns, R. (1990b). Assessing everyday memory in patients with perceptual deficits. *Clinical Rehabilitation, 4,* 129–135.

Coffey, C.E., Lucke, J.F., Saxton, J.A., et al. (1998). Sex differences in brain aging: a quantitative magnetic resonance imaging study. *Archives of Neurology, 55,* 169–179.

Coffey, C.E., Saxton, J.A., Ratcliff, G., et al. (1999). Relation of education to brain size in normal aging: implications for the reserve hypothesis. *Neurology, 53,* 189–196.

Cogan, D.G. (1985). Visual disturbances with focal progressive dementing disease. *American Journal of Ophthalmology, 100,* 68–72.

Cohadon, F., Castel, J.-P., Richer, H., et al. (2002). *Les traumatisés crâniens de l'accident à la réinsertion* (2nd ed.). Reueil-Malmaison, France: Arnette.

Cohen, G., Johnston, F.A., & Plunkett, K. (Eds.) (2000). *Exploring cognition: Damaged brains and neural networks.* Hove, UK: Psychology Press.

Cohen, H. & Levy, J. (1986). Cerebral and sex differences in the categorization of haptic information. *Cortex, 22,* 253–259.

Cohen, J. (1957a). Factor analytically based rationale for Wechsler Adult Intelligence Scale. *Journal of Consulting Psychology, 21,* 451–457.

Cohen, J. (1957b). The factorial structure of the WAIS between early adulthood and old age. *Journal of Consulting Psychology, 21,* 283–290.

Cohen, J.A. (1995). Autonomic nervous system disorders and reflex sympathetic dystrophy in lightning and electrical injuries. *Seminars in Neurology, 15,* 387–390.

Cohen, J.A., Cutter, G.R., Fischer, J.S., et al. (2002). Benefit of interferon b-1a on MSFC progression and quality of life in secondary progressive MS. *Neurology, 59,* 679–687.

Cohen, J.D., Botvinick, M., & Carter, C.S. (2000). Anterior cingulate and prefrontal cortex: Who's in control? *Nature Neuroscience, 3,* 421–423.

Cohen, M., Groswasser, Z., Barchadski, R., & Appel, A. (1989). Convergence insufficiency in brain-injured patients. *Brain Injury, 3,* 187–192.

Cohen, M.J. & Stanczak, D.E. (2000). On the reliability, validity, and cognitive structure of the Thurstone Word Fluency Test. *Archives of Clinical Neuropsychology, 15,* 267–279.

Cohen, R., Gutbrod, K., Meier, E., & Romer, P. (1987). Visual search processes in the Token Test performance of aphasics. *Neuropsychologia, 25,* 983–987.

Cohen, R.A. & Fisher, M. (1989). Amantadine treatment of fatigue associated with multiple sclerosis. *Archives of Neurology, 46,* 676–680.

Cohen, R.A., Kaplan, R.F., Moser, D.J., et al. (1999). Impairments of attention after cingulotomy. *Neurology, 53,* 819–824.

Cohen, R.F. & Mapou, R.L. (1988). Neuropsychological assessment for treatment planning: A hypothesis-testing approach. *Journal of Head Trauma Rehabilitation, 3,* 12–23.

Cohen, T.I. & Gudeman, S.K. (1996). Delayed traumatic intracranial hematoma. In R.K. Narayan et al. (Eds.). *Neurotrauma.* New York: McGraw-Hill.

Cohn, N.B., Dustman, R. E., & Bradford, D. C. (1984). Age-related decrements in Stroop Color Test performance. *Journal of Clinical Psychology, 40,* 1244–1250.

Colantonio, A., Becker, J.T., & Huff, F.J. (1993). Factor structure of the Mattis Dementia Rating Scale among patients with probable Alzheimer's disease. *The Clinical Neuropsychologist, 7,* 313–318.

Colantonio, A., Dawson, D.R., & McLellan, B.A. (1998). Head injury in young adults: Long-term outcome. *Archives of Physical Medicine and Rehabilitation, 79,* 550–558.

Colbach, E.M. & Crowe, R.R. (1970). Marijuana associated psychosis in Vietnam. *Military Medicine, 135,* 571–573.

Cole, A.J. (2000). Is epilepsy a progressive disease? The neurobiological consequences of epilepsy. *Epilepsia, 41,* S13–S22.

Cole, K.D. & Zarit, S.H. (1984). Psychological deficits in depressed medical patients. *Journal of Nervous and Mental Disease, 172,* 150–155.

Coleman, R.D., Rapport, L.J., Millis, S.R., et al. (1998). Effects of coaching on detection of malingering on the California Verbal Learning Test. *Journal of Clinical and Experimental Neuropsychology, 20,* 201–210.

Coles, R.R.A. (1995). Compensable tinnitus from causes other than noise. In G.E. Reich & J.A. Vernon (Eds.), *Proceedings of the Fifth International Tinnitus Seminar.* Portland, OR: American Tinnitus Association.

Collaer, M.L. & Nelson, J.D. (2002). Large visuospatial sex differences in line judgment: Possible role of attentional factors. *Brain and Cognition, 49,* 1–12.

Collier, A.C., Gayle, T.C., & Bahls, F.H. (1987). Clinical manifestations and approach to management of HIV infection and AIDS. *AIDS: A Guide for the Primary Physician, 13,* 27–33.

Colligan, R.C., Osborne, D., Swenson, W.M., & Offord, K.P. (1989). *The MMPI: A contemporary normative study of adults.* Odessa, FL: Psychological Assessment Resources.

Collins, J.G. (1990). Types of injuries by selected characteristics: United States, 1985–1987. *Vital Health Statistics, 175,* 1–68.

Collins, R.C. (1990). Cerebral cortex. In A.L. Pearlman & R.C. Collins (Eds.), *Neurobiology of disease.* New York: Oxford University Press.

Colombo, A., DeRenzi, E., & Faglioni, P. (1976). The occurrence of visual neglect in patients with unilateral cerebral disease. *Cortex, 12,* 221–231.

Colonna, A. & Faglioni, P. (1966). The performance of hemisphere-damaged patients on spatial intelligence tests. *Cortex, 2,* 293–307.

Coltheart, M. (1987). *The cognitive neuropsychology of language.* London: Erlbaum.

Coltheart, M., Hull, E., & Slater, D. (1975). Sex differences in imagery and reading. *Science, 253,* 438–440.

Coman, E., Moses, J.A., Jr., Kraemer, H.C., et al. (1999). Geriatric performance on the Benton Visual Retention Test: Demographic and diagnostic considerations. *The Clinical Neuropsychologist, 13,* 66–77.

Comi, G., Filippi, M., & Wolinsky, J. S. (2001). European/Canadian multicenter, double-blind, randomized, placebo-controlled study of the effects of glatiramer acetate on magnetic resonance imaging-measured disease activity and burden in patients with relapsing multiple sclerosis. European/Canadian Glatiramer Acetate Study Group. *Annals of Neurology, 49,* 290–297.

Comi, G., Leocani, L., Rossi, P., & Colombo, B. (2001). Physiopathology and treatment of fatigue in multiple sclerosis. *Journal of Neurology, 248,* 174–179. *Compendium of drug therapy* (published annually). New York: Biomedical Information.

Comijs, H., Deeg, D., Dik, M., et al. (2002). Memory complaints; the association with psycho-affective and health problems and the role of personality characteristics. A 6-year follow-up study. *Journal of Affective Disorders, 72,* 157.

Comijs, H.C., Jonker, C., Beekman, A.T., & Deeg, D.J. (2001). The association between depressive symptoms and cognitive decline in community-dwelling elderly persons. *International Journal of Geriatric Psychiatry, 16,* 361–367.

Compston, A. & Coles, A. (2002). Multiple sclerosis. *Lancet, 359,* 1221–1231.

Compton, D.M., Bachman, L.D., Brand, D., & Avet, T. L. (2000). Age-associated changes in cognitive function in highly educated adults: Emerging myths and realities. *International Journal of Geriatric Psychiatry, 15,* 75–85.

Compton, D.M., Bachman, L.D., & Logan, J.A. (1997). Aging and intellectual ability in young, middle-aged, and older educated adults: preliminary results from a sample of college faculty. *Psychological Reports 81,* 79–90.

Conant, L.L., Fastenau, P.S., Giordani, B.J., et al. (1999). Modality specificity of memory span tasks among Zairian children: A developmental perspective. *Journal of Clinical and Experimental Neuropsychology, 21,* 375–384.

Conboy, T.J., Barth, J., & Boll, T.J. (1986). Treatment and rehabilitation of mild and moderate head trauma. *Rehabilitation Psychology, 31,* 203–215.

Condon, B., Montadi, D., Wilson, J.T. L., & Hadley, D. (1997). The relation between MRI neuroactivation changes and responses rate on a word-fluency task. *Applied Neuropsychology, 4,* 201–207.

Condor, R., Allen, L., & Cox, D. (1992). *Computerized assessment of response bias test manual.* Durham, NC: CogniSyst.

Cone, J.E., Bowler, R., & So, Y. (1990). Medical surveillance for neurologic endpoints. *Occupational Medicine: State of the Art Reviews, 5,* 547–562.

Coney, J. (2002). Lateral asymmetry in phonological processing: relating behavioral measures to neuroimaged structures. *Brain and Language, 80,* 355–365.

Confavreux, C., Hutchinson, M., Hours, M.M., et al. (1998). Rate of pregnancy-related relapse in multiple sclerosis. Pregnancy in Multiple Sclerosis Group. *New England Journal of Medicine, 339,* 285–291.

Conklin, H.M., Calkins, M.E., Anderson, C.W., et al. (2002). Recognition memory for faces in schizophrenia patients and their first-degree relatives. *Neuropsychologia, 40,* 2314–2324.

Conn, D.K. (1989). Neuropsychiatric syndromes in the elderly: An overview. In D.K. Conn, A. Grek, & J. Sadavoy (Eds.), *Psychiatric consequences of brain disease in the elderly: A focus on management.* New York: Plenum Press.

Conners, C.K. (1992). *Conners' Continous Performance Test.* Toronto: Multi-Health Systems.

Conners, C.K. (2000). *Continuous Performance Test II.* Toronto: Multi-Health Systems.

Connor, A., Franzen, M., & Sharp, B. (1988). Effects of practice and differential instructions on Stroop performance. *International Journal of Clinical Neuropsychology, 10,* 1–4.

Connor, D.J., Salmon, D.P., Sandy, T.S., et al. (1998). Cognitive profiles of autopsy-confirmed Lewy body variant vs pure Alzheimer disease. *Archives of Neurology, 55,* 994–100.

Consensus Workshop on Formaldehyde (1984). Report on the Consensus Workshop on Formaldehyde. *Environmental Health Perspectives, 58,* 323–381.

Consoli, S. (1979). Étude des strategies constructives secondaires aux lésions hémispheriques. *Neuropsychologia, 17,* 303–313.

Contant, C.F., Hannay, H.J., & Pluth, S. (no date). *Analyses of the Disability Rating Scale following head injury. Journal of the International Neuropsychological Society.*

Cook, S.D. (2001). Evidence for a viral etiology of multiple sclerosis. In S.D. Cook (Ed.), *Handbook of multiple sclerosis.* (3rd ed.). New York: Marcel Dekker.

Coolidge, F.L., Middleton, P.A., & Griego, J.A. (1996). The effects of interference on verbal learning in multiple sclerosis. *Archives of Clinical Neuropsychology, 11,* 605–611.

Coolidge, F.L., Mull, C.E., Becker, L.A., et al. (1998). Hyperawareness of neuropsychological deficits in patients with mild closed head injuries: A preliminary investigation. *International Journal of Rehabilitation, 4,* 193–198.

Coolidge, F.L., Peters, B.M., Brown, R.E., & Harsch, T.L. (1985). Validation of a WAIS algorithm for the early onset of dementia. *Psychological Reports, 57,* 1299–1302.

Coonley-Hoganson, R., Sachs, N., Desai, B.T., & Whitman, S. (1984). Sequelae associated with head injuries in patients who were not hospitalized: A follow-up survey. *Neurosurgery, 14,* 315–317.

Cooper, D.B., Epker, M., Lacritz, L., et al. (2001). Effects of practice on category fluency in Alzheimer's disease. *The Clinical Neuropsychologist, 15,* 125–128.

Cooper, J.A., Sagar, H.J., Jordan, N., et al. (1991). Cognitive impairment in early, untreated Parkinson's disease and its relationship to motor disability. *Brain, 114,* 2095–2122.

Cooper, J.A. & Sagar, H.J. (1993). Incidental and intentional recall in Parkinson's disease: An account based on diminished attentional resources. *Journal of Clinical and Experimental Neuropsychology, 15,* 713–731.

Cooper, M.A. (1980). Lightning injuries: Prognostic signs for death. *Annals of Emergency Medicine, 9,* 134–138.

Cooper, M.A. (1983). Lightning injuries. *Emergency Medicine Clinics of North America, 1,* 639–641.

Cooper, M.A. (1984). Electrical and lightning injuries. *Emergency Medicine Clinics of North America, 2,* 489–501.

Cooper, M.A. (1995). Emergent care of lightning and electrical injuries. *Seminars in Neurology, 15,* 268–278.

Cooper, M.A. (2002). A fifth mechanism of lightning injury. *Academic Emergency Medicine, 9,* 172–174.

Cooper, M.A., Andrews, C.J., Holle, R.L., & Lopez, R.E. (2001). Lightning injuries. In P.S. Auerbach (Ed.), *Wilderness medicine.* St. Louis: Mosby.

Cooper, S. (1982). The post-Wechsler memory scale. *Journal of Clinical Psychology, 38,* 380–387.

Cope, D.N. (1988). Neuropharmacology and brain damage. In A.-L. Christensen & B. Uzzell (Eds.), *Neuropsychological rehabilitation.* Boston: Kluwer.

Corballis, M.C. (1991). *The lopsided ape: Evolution of the generative mind.* New York: Oxford University Press.

Corder, E.H., Saunders, A.M., Strittmatter, W.J., et al. (1993). Gene dose of apolipoprotein E type 4 allele and the risk of Alzheimer's disease in late onset families. *Science, 261,* 921–923.

Coren, S. & Porac, C. (1977). Fifty centuries of right-handedness: The historical record. *Science, 198,* 631–632.

Coren, S., Porac, C., & Duncan, P. (1979). A behaviorally validated self-report inventory to assess four types of lateral preference. *Journal of Clinical Neuropsychology, 1,* 55–64.

Coren, S. & Searleman, A. (1990). Birth stress and left-handedness: The rare trait marker model. In S. Coren (Ed.), *Left-handedness: Behavioral implication and anomalies.* Amsterdam: Elsevier/North-Holland.

Corey-Bloom, J., Wiederholt, W.C., Edelstein, S., et al. (1996). Cognitive and functional status of the oldest old. *Journal of the American Geriatric Society, 44,* 671–674.

Corkin, S. (1968). Acquisition of motor skill after bilateral medial T-lobe excision. *Neuropsychologia, 6,* 255–266.

Corkin, S. (1979). Hidden-Figures-Test performance: Lasting effects of unilateral penetrating head injury and transient effects of bilateral cingulotomy. *Neuropsychologia, 17,* 585–605.

Corkin, S. (1982). Some relationships between global amnesias and the memory impairment in Alzheimer's disease. In S. Corkin et al. (Eds.), *Alzheimer's disease: A report of progress. Aging* (Vol. 19). New York: Raven Press.

Corkin, S., Amaral, D.G., Gonzalez, R. G., et al. (1997) H.M.'s temporal lobe lesion: Findings from magnetic resonance imaging. *Journal of Neuroscience, 17,* 2964–3979.

Corkin, S., Growdon, J.H., Desclos, G., & Rosen, T.J. (1989). Parkinson's disease and Alzheimer's disease: Differences revealed by neuropsychologic testing. In T.L. Munsat (Ed.), *Quantification of neurologic deficit.* Stoneham, MA: Butterworth.

Corkin, S.H., Hurt, R.W., & Twitchell, E.T. (1987). Consequences of nonpenetrating and penetrating head injury: Retrograde amnesia, posttraumatic amnesia, and lasting effects on cognition. In H.S. Levin et al. (Eds.), *Neurobehavioral recovery from head injury.* New York: Oxford University Press.

Corkin, S., Sullivan, E.V., & Carr, A. (1984). Prognostic factors for life expectancy after penetrating head injury. *Archives of Neurology, 41,* 975–977.

Corn, B.W., Yousem, D.M., Scott, C.B., et al. (1994). White matter changes are correlated significantly with radiation dose: observations from a randomized dose-escalation trial for malignant glioma (Radiation Therapy Oncology Group 83-02). *Cancer, 74,* 2828–2835.

Cornell, D.G., Suarez, R., & Berent, S. (1984). Psychomotor retardation in melancholic and nonmelancholic depression: Cognitive and motor components. *Journal of Abnormal Psychology, 93,* 150–157.

Correia, S., Faust, D., & Doty, R.L. (2001). A re-examination of the rate of vocational dysfunction among patients with anosmia and mild to moderate closed head injury. *Archives of Clinical Neuropsychology, 16,* 477–488.

Correll, R.E., Brodginski, S.E., & Rokosz, S.F. (1993). WAIS performance during the acute recovery stage following closed-head injury. *Perceptual and Motor Skills, 76,* 99–109.

Corrigan, J.D., Agresti, A.A., & Hinkeldey, N.S. (1987). Psychometric characteristics of the Category Test: Replication and extension. *Journal of Clinical Psychology, 43,* 368–376.

Corrigan, J.D., Bogner, J.A., Mysiw, W.J., et al. (2001). Life satisfaction following traumatic brain injury. *Journal of Head Trauma Rehabilitation, 16,* 543–555.

Corrigan, J.D. & Deming, R. (1995). Psychometric characteristics of the Community Integration Questionnaire: Replication and extension. *Journal of Head Trauma Rehabilitation, 10,* 41–53.

Corrigan, J.D., Dickerson, J., Fisher, E., & Meyer, P. (1990). The Neurobehavioural Rating Scale: Replication in an acute, inpatient rehabilitation setting. *Brain Injury, 4,* 215–222.

Corrigan, J.D. & Hinkeldey, N. S. (1987). Relationships between Parts A and B of the Trail Making Test. *Journal of Clinical Psychology, 43,* 402–408.

Corrigan, J.D., Smith-Knapp, K., & Granger, C.V. (1998). Outcomes in the first 5 years after traumatic brain injury. *Archives of Physical Medicine and Rehabilitation, 79,* 298–305.

Corsini, R.J. & Renck, R. (1992). *Verbal Reasoning.* Chicago, IL: NCS London House Pearson Reid.

Corwin, J. & Bylsma, F.W. (1993a). Commentary (on Rey & Osterrieth). *The Clinical Neuropsychologist, 7,* 15–21.

Corwin, J. & Bylsma, F.W. (1993b). Translations of excerpts from André Rey's *Psychological examination of traumatic encephalopathy* and P.A. Osterrieth's *The Complex Figure Copy Test. The Clinical Neuropsychologist, 7,* 3–15.

Cory-Schlecta, D.A. & Schaumburg, H.H. (2000). Lead, inorganic. In P.S. Spencer & H.H. Schaumburg (Eds.), *Experimental and clinical neurotoxicology* (2nd ed.). New York: Oxford University Press.

Coslett, H.B. (2003). Acquired dyslexia. In K.M. Heilman & E. Valenstein (Eds.), *Clinical neuropsychology* (4th ed.). New York: Oxford University Press.

Coslett, H.B., Brashear, H.R., & Heilman, K.M. (1984). Pure word deafness after bilateral primary auditory cortex infarcts. *Neurology, 34,* 347–352.

Coslett, H.B., Gonzalez Rothi, L.J., Valenstein, E., & Heilman, K.M. (1986). Dissocations of writing and praxis: Two cases in point. *Brain and Language, 28,* 357–369.

Coslett, H.B. & Saffran, E.M. (1992). Disorders of higher visual processing: Theoretical and clinical perspectives. In D.I. Margolin (Ed.), *Cognitive neuropsychology in clinical practice*. New York: Oxford University Press.

Coslett, H.B. & Saffran, E.M. (1998). Reading and the right hemisphere: Evidence from acquired dyslexia. In M. Beeman & C. Chiarello (Eds.), *Right hemisphere language comprehension. Perspectives from cognitive neuroscience*. Mahwah, NJ: Erlbaum.

Cosmides, L. & Tooby, J. (2000). The cognitive neuroscience of social reasoning. In M.S. Gazzaniga (Ed.), *The new cognitive neurosciences* (2nd ed.). Cambridge, MA: MIT Press.

Costa, L. (1988). Clinical neuropsychology: Prospects and problems. *The Clinical Neuropsychologist, 2*, 3–11.

Costa, L.D. (1976). Interset variability on the Raven Coloured Progressive Matrices as an indicator of specific ability deficit in brain-lesioned patients. *Cortex, 12*, 31–40.

Costa, L.D., & Vaughan, H.G., Jr. (1962). Performance of patients with lateralized cerebral lesions. *Journal of Nervous and Mental Disease, 134*, 162–168.

Costa, L.D., Vaughan, H.G., Jr., Horwitz, M., & Ritter, W. (1969). Patterns of behavioral deficit associated with visual spatial neglect. *Cortex, 5*, 242–263.

Costa, L.D., Vaughan, H.G., Levita, E., & Farber, N. (1963). Purdue Pegboard as a predictor of the presence and laterality of cerebral lesions. *Journal of Consulting Psychology, 27*, 133–137.

Costa, P.T., Jr. & Shock, N.W. (1980). New longitudinal data on the question of whether hypertension influences intellectual performance. In M.F. Elias & D.H.P. Streeten (Eds.), *Hypertension and cognitive processes*. Mt. Desert, ME: Beech Hill.

Costanzo, R.M. & Zasler, N.D. (1992). Epidemiology and pathophysiology of olfactory and gustatory dysfunction in head trauma. *Journal of Head Trauma Rehabilitation, 7*, 15–24.

Cotman, C.S. & Anderson, A.J. (1995). Retention of function in the aged brain: The pivotal role of β-amyloid. In J.L. McGaugh, N.M. Weinberger, & G. Lynch (Eds.), *Brain and memory. Modulation and mediation of neuroplasticity*. New York: Oxford University Press.

Coupar, A. M. (1976). Detection of mild aphasia: A study using the Token Test. *British Journal of Medical Psychology, 49*, 141–144.

Court, J., Martin-Ruiz, C., Piggott, M., et al. (2001). Nicotinic receptor abnormalities in Alzheimer's disease. *Biological Psychiatry, 49*, 175–184.

Courville, C.B. (1942). Coup–contrecoup mechanism of cranio-cerebral injuries. *Archives of Surgery, 45*, 19–43.

Couturier, E.G., Hering, R., & Steiner, T.J. (1992). Weekend attacks in migraine patients caused by caffeine withdrawal? *Cephalalgia, 12*, 99–100.

Couturier, E.G., Laman, D.M., van Duijn, M.A., & van Duijn, H. (1997). Influence of caffeine and caffeine withdrawal on headache and cerebral blood flow velocities. *Cephalalgia, 17*, 188–190.

Covassin, T., Swanik, C.B., & Sachs, M.L. (2003). Epidemiological considerations of concussions among intercollegiate athletes. *Applied Neuropsychology, 10*, 12–22.

Cowell, P.E., Kertesz, A., & Denenberg, V.H. (1993). Multiple dimensions of handedness and the human corpus callosum. *Neurology, 43*, 2353–2357.

Cowey, C.M. & Green, S. (1996). The hippocampus: A "working memory" structure? The effect of hippocampal sclerosis on working memory. *Memory, 4*, 19–30.

Cox, D.J., Quillian, W.C., Thorndike, F.P., et al. (1998). Evaluating driving performance of outpatients with Alzheimer disease. *Journal of the American Board of Family Practice, 11*, 264–271.

Craft, S. & Newcomer, J. (2001). Cognitive neuroendocrinology. In R.E. Tarter, M. Butters, & S.R. Beers (Eds.), *Medical neuropsychology* (2nd ed.). New York: Kluwer Academic/Plenum Press.

Craft, S., Teri, L., Edland, S.D., et al. (1998). Accelerated decline in apolipoprotein E-epsilon4 homozygotes with Alzheimer's disease. *Neurology, 51*, 149–153.

Craig, S.R. (1986). When lightning strikes: Pathophysiology and treatment of lightning injuries. *Postgraduate Medicine, 79*, 109–124.

Craig Hospital Research Department (2001). *Craig Hospital Inventory of Environmental Factors (CHIEF) manual*. Englewood, CO: Craig Hospital Research Department.

Craik, F.I.M. (1977). Similarities between the effects of aging and alcoholic intoxication on memory performance, construed within a "levels of processing" framework. In I.M. Birnbaum & E.S. Parker (Eds.), *Alcohol and human memory*. Hillsdale, NJ: Erlbaum.

Craik, F.I.M. (1979). Human memory. *Annual Review of Psychology, 30*, 63–102.

Craik, F.I.M. (1990). Changes in memory with normal aging: A functional view. In R.J. Wurtman et al. (Eds.), *Advances in neurology. Alzheimer's disease* (Vol. 51). New York: Raven Press.

Craik, F.I.M. (1991). Memory functions in normal aging. In T. Yanagihara & R.C. Petersen (Eds.), *Memory disorders: Research and clinical practice*. New York: Marcel Dekker.

Craik, F.I.M. & Lockhart, R.S. (1972). Levels of processing: A framework for memory research. *Journal of Verbal Learning and Verbal Behavior, 11*, 671–684.

Craik, F.I.M., Morris, R.G., & Gick, M.L. (1990). Adult age differences in working memory. In G. Vallar & T. Shallice (Eds.), *Neuropsychological impairments of short-term memory*. Cambridge: Cambridge University Press.

Cramer, S.C., Finklestein, S.P., Schaechter, J.D., et al. (1999). Activation of distinct motor cortex regions during ipsilateral and contralateral finger movements. *Journal of Neurophysiology, 81*, 383–387.

Crawford, J.R. (1992). Current and premorbid intelligence measures in neuropsychological assessment. In J.R. Crawford, D.M. Parker, & W. W. McKinlay (Eds.), *A handbook of neuropsychological assessment*. Hove, UK: Erlbaum.

Crawford, J.R. & Allan, K.M. (1997). Estimating premorbid WAIS-R IQ with demographic variables: Regression equations derived from a UK sample. *The Clinical Neuropsychologist, 11*, 192–198.

Crawford, J.R., Allan, K.M., Besson, J.A.O., et al. (1990.) A comparison of the WAIS and WAIS-R in matched UK samples. *British Journal of Clinical Psychology, 29*, 105–109.

Crawford, J.R., Allan, K.M., Cochrane, R.H.B., & Parker, D.M. (1990). Assessing the validity of NART-estimated premorbid IQ's in the individual case. *British Journal of Clinical Psychology, 29*, 435–436.

Crawford, J.R., Allan, K.M., Jack, A.M., et al. (1991). The short NART: Cross-validation, relationship to IQ and some practical considerations. *British Journal of Clinical Psychology, 30*, 223–229.

Crawford, J.R., Cochrane, R.H.B., Besson, J.A.O., et al. (1990). Premorbid IQ estimates obtained by combining the NART and demographic variables: Construct validity. *Personality and Individual Differences, 11*, 209–210.

Crawford, J.R., Deary, I.J., Starr, J., & Whalley, L.J. (2001). The NART as an index of prior intellectual functioning: a retrospective validity study covering a 66-year interval. *Psychological Medicine, 31*, 451–458.

Crawford, J.R., Jack, A.M., Morrison, R.M., et al. (1990). The U.K. factor structure of the WAIS-R is robust and highly congruent with the U.S.A. standardization sample. *Personality and Individual Differences, 11*, 643–644.

Crawford, J.R., Johnson, D.A., Mychalkiw, B., & Moore, J.W. (1997). WAIS-R performance following closed-head injury: A comparison of the clinical utility of summary IQs, factor scores, and subtest scatter indices. *The Clinical Neuropsychologist, 11,* 345–355.

Crawford, J.R., Millar, J., & Milne, A.B. (2001). Estimating premorbid IQ from demographic variables: A comparison of a regression equation vs. clinical judgement. *British Journal of Clinical Psychology, 40,* 97–105.

Crawford, J.R., Moore, J.W., & Cameron, I.M. (1992). Verbal fluency: A NART-based equation for the estimation of premorbid performance. *British Journal of Clinical Psychology, 31,* 327–329.

Crawford, J.R., Nelson, H.E., Blackmore, L., et al. (1990). Estimating premorbid intelligence by combining the NART and demographic variables: An examination of the NART standardisation sample and supplementary equations. *Personality and Individual Differences, 11,* 1153–1157.

Crawford, J.R. , Parker, D.M., Allan, K.M., et al. (1991). The short NART: Cross-validation, relationship to IQ, and some practical considerations. *British Journal of Clinical Psychology, 30,* 1–7.

Crawford, J.R., Parker, D.M., & Besson, J.A.O. (1988). Estimation of premorbid intelligence in organic conditions. *British Journal of Psychiatry, 153,* 178–181.

Crawford, J.R., Parker, D.M., Stewart, L.E., et al. (1989). Prediction of WAIS IQ with the National Adult Reading Test: Cross-validation and extension. *British Journal of Clinical Psychology, 28,* 267–273.

Crawford, J.R., Sommerville, J., & Robertson, I.H. (1997). Assessing the reliability and abnormality of subtest differences on the Test of Everyday Attention. *British Journal of Clinical Psychology, 36,* 609–617.

Crawford, J.R., Stewart, L.E., Cochrane, R.H.B., et al. (1989). Estimating premorbid IQ from demographic variables: Regression equations derived from a UK sample. *British Journal of Clinical Psychology, 28,* 275–278.

Crawford, J.R., Stewart, L.E., Garthwaite, P.H., et al. (1988). The relationship between demographic variables and NART performance in normal subjects. *British Journal of Clinical Psychology, 27,* 181–182.

Crawford, J.R., Stewart, L.E., & Moore, J.W. (1989). Demonstration of savings on the AVLT and development of a parallel form. *Journal of Clinical and Experimental Neuropsychology, 11,* 975–981.

Crawford, J.R., Stewart, L.E., Parker, D.M., et al. (1989). Estimation of premorbid intelligence: Combining psychometric and demographic approaches improves predictive accuracy. *Personality and Individual Differences, 10,* 793–796.

Crawford, J.R. & Warrington, E.K. (2002). The Homophone Meaning Generation Test: Psychometric properties and a method for estimating premorbid intelligence. *Journal of the International Neuropsychological Society, 8,* 547–554.

Crépeau, F. & Scherzer, P. (1993). Predictors and indicators of work status after traumatic brain injury: A meta-analysis. *Neuropsychological Rehabilitation, 3,* 5–35.

Crews, W.D., Barth, J.T., Brelsford, T.N., et al. (1997). Neuropsychological dysfunction in severe accidental electrical shock: Two case reports. *Applied Neuropsychology, 4,* 208–219.

Crews, W.D., Jr., Harrison, D.W., & Rhondes, R.D. (1999). Neuropsychological test performances of young depressed outpatient women: An examination of executive functions. *Archives of Clinical Neuropsychology, 14,* 517–529.

Crick, F. & Koch, C. (1998). Consciousness and neuroscience. *Cerebral Cortex, 8,* 97–107.

Cripe, L.I. (1988). *The clinical use of the MMPI with neurologic patients. A new perspective.* Paper presented at the Army Medical Department Psychology Conference, Seattle, WA.

Cripe, L.I. (1996a). The ecological validity of executive function testing. In R.J. Sbordone & C.J. Long (Eds.), *Ecological validity of neuropsychological assessment.* Delray Beach, FL: GR Press & St. Lucie Press.

Cripe, L.I. (1996b). The MMPI in neuropsychological assessment: a murky measure. *Applied Neuropsychology, 3/4,* 97–103.

Cripe, L.I. (1997). Personality assessment of brain-impaired patients. In M.E. Maruish & J.A. Moses, Jr. (Eds.), *Clinical neuropsychology. Theoretical foundations for practitioners.* Mahwah, NJ: Erlbaum.

Cripe, L.I. (1999). Use of the MMPI with mild closed head injury. In N.R. Varney & R.J. Roberts (Eds.), *The evaluation and treatment of mild traumatic brain injury.* Mahwah, NJ: Erlbaum.

Cripe, L.I. (2002). Malady versus malingering: A tricky endeavor. In N.D. Zasler & M.F. Martelli (Eds.), *Functional disorders. Physical Medicine & Rehabilitation: State of the Art Reviews* (Vol. 16). Philadelphia: Hanley and Belfus.

Cripe, L.I. & Dodrill, C.B. (1988). Neuropsychological test performances with chronic low-level formaldehyde exposure. *The Clinical Neuropsychologist, 2,* 41–48.

Cripe, L.I., Maxwell, J.K., & Hill, E. (1995). Multivariate discriminant function analysis of neurologic, pain, and psychiatric patients with the MMPI. *Journal of Clinical Psychology, 51,* 258–268.

Criqu, M.H. & Ringel, B.L. (1994). Does diet or alcohol explain the French paradox? *Lancet, 344,* 1719–1723.

Critchley, E.M.R. (1987). *Language and speech disorders. A neurophysiological approach.* London: Clinical Neuroscience Publishers.

Critchley, M. (1934). Neurological effects of lightning and of electricity. *Lancet, 1,* 68–72.

Critchley, M. (1984). And all the daughters of musick shall be brought low. Language function in the elderly. *Archives of Neurology, 41,* 1135–1139.

Critchley, H.D. (2002). Electrodermal responses: What happens in the brain. *Neuroscientist, 8,* 132–142.

Critchley, M. & Critchley, E.A. (1998). *John Hughlings Jackson. Father of English neurology.* New York: Oxford University Press.

Crockett, D., Clark, C., Labreche, T., et al. (1982). Shortening the Speech Sounds Perception Test. *Journal of Clinical Neuropsychology, 4,* 167–172.

Crockett, D., Tallman, K., Hurwitz, T., & Kozak, J. (1988). Neuropsychological performance in psychiatric patients with or without documented brain dysfunction. *International Journal of Neuroscience, 41,* 71–79.

Croisile, B., Brabant, M.J., Carmoi, T., et al. (1996). Comparison between oral and written spelling in Alzheimer's disease. *Brain and Language, 54,* 361–387.

Croisile, B., Ska, B., Brabant, M.J., et al. (1996). Comparative study of oral and written picture description in patients with Alzheimer's disease. *Brain and Language, 53,* 1–19.

Cronbach, L.J. (1984). *Essentials of psychological testing* (4th ed). New York: Harper & Row.

Cronin-Golomb, A. (1986). Subcortical transfer of cognitive information in subjects with complete forebrain commissurotomy. *Cortex, 22,* 499–519.

Cronin-Golomb, A. (1990). Abstract thought in aging and age-related neurological disease. In F. Boller & J. Grafman (Eds.), *Handbook of Neuropsychology* (Vol. 4). Amsterdam: Elsevier.

Cronin-Golomb, A. & Braun, A.E. (1997). Visuospatial dysfunction and problems solving in Parkinson's disease. *Neuropsychology, 11,* 44–52.

Cronin-Golomb, A., Rho, W.A., Corkin, S., & Growdon, J.H. (1987). Abstract reasoning in age-related neurological disease. *Journal of Neural Transmission 24(Suppl.),* 79–83.

Croog, S.H., Levine, S., Testa, M.A., et al. (1986). The effects of antihypertensive therapy on the quality of life. *New England Journal of Medicine, 314,* 1657–1664.

Crook, T., Bartus, R.T., Ferris, S.H., et al. (1986). Age-associated memory impairment: Proposed diagnostic criteria and measures of clinical change—Report of a National Institute of Mental Health Work Group. *Developmental Neuropsychology, 2,* 261–276.

Crook, T., Ferris, S., McCarthy, M., & Rae, D. (1980). Utility of digit recall tasks for assessing memory in the aged. *Journal of Consulting and Clinical Psychology, 48,* 228–233.

Crook, T.H. & Larrabee, G.J. (1990). A self-rating scale for evaluating memory in everyday life. *Psychology and Aging, 5,* 48–57.

Crook, T.H. & Larrabee, G.J. (1992). Normative data on a self-rating scale for evaluating memory in everyday life. *Archives of Clinical Neuropsychology, 7,* 41–51.

Croot, K., Hodges, J.R., & Patterson, K. (1999). Evidence for impaired sentence comprehension in early Alzheimer's disease. *Journal of the International Neuropsychological Society, 5,* 393–404.

Crossen, J.R., Garwood, D., & Glatstein, E. (1994). Neurobehavioral sequelae of cranial irradiation in adults: a review of radiation-induced encephalopathy. *Journal of Clinical Oncology, 12,* 627–642.

Crossen, J.R. & Wiens, A.N. (1988). Residual neuropsychological deficits following head-injury on the Wechsler Memory Scale-Revised. *The Clinical Neuropsychologist, 2,* 393–399.

Crossen, J.R. & Wiens, A.N. (1994). Comparison of the Auditory-Verbal Learning Test (AVLT) and California Verbal Learning Test (CVLT) in a sample of normal subjects. *Journal of Clinical and Experimental Neuropsychology, 16,* 190–194.

Crosson, B. (1985). Subcortical functions in language: A working model. *Brain and Language, 25,* 257–292.

Crosson, B.A. (1992). *Subcortical functions in language and memory.* New York: Guilford Press.

Crosson, B. (1999). Subcortical mechanisms in language: Lexical–semantic mechanisms and the thalamus. *Brain and Cognition, 40,* 414–438.

Crosson, B., Barco, P., Velozo, C.A., et al. (1989). Awareness and compensation in post-acute head-injury rehabilitation. *Journal of Head Trauma Rehabilitation, 4,* 46–54.

Crosson, B., Greene, R.L., Roth, D.L., et al. (1990). WAIS-R pattern clusters after blunt head injury. *The Clinical Neuropsychologist, 4,* 253–262.

Crosson, B., Hughes, C.W., Roth, D.L., & Monkowski, P.G. (1984). Review of Russell's (1975) norms for the Logical Memory and Visual Reproduction subtests of the Wechsler Memory Scale. *Journal of Consulting and Clinical Psychology, 52,* 635–641.

Crosson, B., Moore, A.B., & Wierenga, C.E. (2003). Syndromes due to acquired basal ganglia damage. In T.E. Feinberg & M.J. Farah (Eds.), *Behavioral neurology and neuropsychology* (2nd ed.). New York: McGraw-Hill.

Crosson, B., Novack, T.A., Trenerry, M.R., & Craig, P.L. (1989). Differentiation of verbal memory deficits in blunt head injury using the recognition trial of the California Verbal Learning Tests: An exploratory study. *The Clinical Neuropsychologist, 3,* 29–44.

Crosson, B., Sartor, K.J., Jenny, A.B., III, et al. (1993). Increased intrusions during verbal recall in traumatic and nontraumatic lesions of the temporal lobe. *Neuropsychology, 7,* 193–208.

Crosson, B. & Warren, R.L. (1982). Use of the Luria-Nebraska Neuropsychological battery in aphasia: A conceptual critique. *Journal of Consulting and Clinical Psychology, 50,* 22–31.

Crouch, J.A., Greve, K.W., & Brooks, J. (1996). The California Card Sorting Test may dissociate verbal and non-verbal concept formation abilities. *British Journal of Clinical Psychology, 35,* 431–434.

Crovitz, H.F. & Schiffman, H. (1974). Frequency of episodic memories as a function of their age. *Bulletin of the Psychonomic Society, 4,* 517–518.

Crowe, S. (2000). Does the letter number sequence task measure anything more than digit span. *Assessment, 7,* 113–117.

Crowe, S.F., Hale, M., Dean, S., et al. (2001). The effect of heightened levels of physiological arousal on neuropsychological measures of attention in a nonclinical sample. *Australian Psychologist, 36,* 239–243.

Crowe, S.F. & Ponsford, J. (1999). The role of imagery in sexual arousal disturbances in the male traumatically brain injured individual. *Brain Injury, 13,* 347–354.

Crum, R.M., Anthony, J.C., Bassett, S.S., & Folstein, M.F. (1993). Population-based norms for the Mini-Mental State Examination by age and educational level. *Journal of the American Medical Association, 269,* 2386–2391.

Crystal, H., Dickson, D., Fuld, P., et al. (1988). Clinico-pathologic studies in dementia: Nondemented subjects with pathologically confirmed Alzheimer's disease. *Neurology, 38,* 1682–1687.

Crystal, H.A., Dickson, D.W., Sliwinski, M.J., et al. (1993). Pathological markers associated with normal aging and dementia in the elderly. *Annals of Neurology, 34,* 566–573.

Crystal, H.A. & Ginsberg, M.D. (2000). Carbon monoxide. In P.S. Spencer & H.H. Schaumberg (Eds.), *Experimental and clinical neurotoxicology* (2nd ed.). New York: Oxford University Press.

Csernansky, J.G., Leiderman, D.B., Mandabach, M., & Moses, J.A. (1990). Psychopathology and limbic epilepsy: Relationship to seizure variables and neuropsychological function. *Epilepsia, 31,* 275–280.

Culbertson, W.C. & Zillmer, E.A. (2001). *Tower of London: Drexel University (TOL$_{DX}$).* North Tonawanda, NY: Multi-Health Systems.

Cull, A., Hay, C., Love, S.B., et al. (1996). What do cancer patients mean when they complain of concentration and memory problems? *British Journal of Cancer, 74,* 1674–1679.

Cullum, C.M. & Bigler, E.D. (1986). Ventricle size, cortical atrophy and the relationship with neuropsychological status in closed head injury: A quantitative analysis. *Journal of Clinical and Experimental Neuropsychology, 8,* 437–452.

Cullum, C.M. & Bigler, E.D. (1991). Short- and long-term psychological status following stroke: Short form MMPI results. *Journal of Nervous and Mental Disease, 179,* 274–278.

Cullum, C.M., Butters, N., Troster, A.I., & Salmon, D.P. (1990). Normal aging and forgetting rates on the Wechsler Memory Scale-Revised. *Archives of Clinical Neuropsychology, 5,* 23–30.

Cullum, C.M., Heaton, R.K., & Grant, I. (1991). Psychogenic factors influencing neuropsychological performance: Somatoform disorders, factitious disorders, and malingering. In H.O. Doerr & A.S. Carlin (Eds.), *Forensic neuropsychology: Legal and scientific bases.* New York: Guilford Press.

Cullum, C.M. & Thompson, L.L. (1997). Neuropsychological diagnosis and outcome in mild traumatic brain injury. *Applied Neuropsychology, 8,* 6–15.

Cullum, C.M., Thompson, L.L., & Heaton, R.K. (1989). The use of the Halstead-Reitan Test Battery with older adults. In F.J. Pirozzola (Ed.), *Clinics in Geriatric Medicine* (Vol. 5, No. 3). Philadelphia: Saunders.

Cullum, C.M., Thompson, L.L., & Smernoff, E.N. (1993). Three-word recall as a measure of memory. *Journal of Clinical and Experimental Neuropsychology, 15,* 321–329.

Culver, C.M. & King, F.W. (1974). Neuropsychological assessment of undergraduate marihuana and LSD users. *Archives of General Psychiatry, 31,* 707–711.

Cummings, J.L. (1986). Subcortical dementia: Neuropsychology, neuropsychiatry, and pathophysiology. *British Journal of Psychiatry, 149,* 682–697.

Cummings, J.L. (1990). Introduction. In J.L. Cummings (Ed.), *Subcortical dementia*. New York: Oxford University Press.

Cummings, J. L. (1992). Depression and Parkinson's disease: A review. *American Journal of Psychiatry, 149,* 443–454.

Cummings, J.L. (1997). The Neuropsychiatric Inventory: assessing psychopathology in dementia patients. *Neurology, 48,* S10–S16.

Cummings, J.L. & Benson, D.F. (1989). Speech and language alterations in dementia syndromes. In A. Ardila & F. Ostrosky-Solis (Eds.), *Brain organization of language and cognitive processes*. New York: Plenum Press.

Cummings, J.L. & Benson, D.F. (1990). Subcortical mechanisms and human thought. In J.L. Cummings (Ed.), *Subcortical dementia*. New York: Oxford University Press.

Cummings, J.L. & Huber, S.J. (1992). Visuospatial abnormalities in Parkinson's disease. In S.J. Huber & J.L. Cummings (Eds.), *Parkinson's disease: Neurobehavioral aspects*. New York: Oxford University Press.

Cummings, J.L. & Mahler, M.E. (1991). Cerebrovascular disease. In R.A. Bornstein (Ed.), *Neurobehavioral aspects of cerebrovascular disease*. New York: Oxford University Press.

Cummings, J.L. & Mega, M.S. (2003). *Neuropsychiatry and behavioral neuroscience*. New York: Oxford University Press.

Cummings, J.L., Mega, M., Gray, K., et al. (1994). The Neuropsychiatric Inventory: comprehensive assessment of psychopathology in dementia. *Neurology, 44,* 2308–2314.

Cummings, J.L., Miller, B., Hill, M.A., & Neshkes, R. (1987). Neuropsychiatric aspects of multi-infarct dementia and dementia of the Alzheimer type. *Archives of Neurology, 44,* 389–393.

Cummings, J.L., Tomiyasu, U., Read, S., & Benson, D.F. (1984). Amnesia with hippocampal lesions after cardiopulmonary arrest. *Neurology, 34,* 679–681.

Cummings, J.L., Vinters, H.V., Cole, G.M., & Khachaturian, Z.S. (1998). Alzheimer's disease: Etiologies, pathophysiology, cognitive reserve, and treatment opportunities. *Neurology, 51,* S2–S17.

Cunningham, R.M., Maio, R.F., Hill, E.M., & Zink, B.J. (2002). The effects of alcohol on head injury in the motor vehicle crash victim. *Alcohol and Alcoholism, 37,* 236–240.

Cunningham, W.R. (1986). Psychometric perspectives: Validity and reliability. In L.W. Poon (Ed.), *Handbook for clinical memory assessment of older adults*. Washington, D.C.: American Psychological Association.

Curatolo, P.W. & Robertson, D. (1983). The health consequences of caffeine. *Annals of Internal Medicine, 98,* 641–653.

Curran, C.A., Ponsford, J.L., & Crowe, S. (2000). Coping strategies and emotional outcome following traumatic brain injury: A comparison with orthopedic patients. *Journal of Head Trauma Rehabilitation, 15,* 1256–1274.

Cushman, L.A., Como, P.G., Booth, H., & Caine, E.D. (1988). Cued recall and release from proactive interference in Alzheimer's disease. *Journal of Clinical and Experimental Neuropsychology, 10,* 685–692.

Cusick, C.P., Brooks, C.A., & Whiteneck, G.G. (2001). The use of proxies in community integration research. *Archives of Physical Medicine and Rehabilitation, 82,* 1018–1024.

Cutajar, R., Ferine, E., Candelabra, C., et al. (2000). Cognitive function and quality of life in multiple sclerosis patients. *Journal of Neurovirology, 6,* S186–S190.

Cutler, N.R., Sramek, J.J., & Gauthier, S. (2001). Review of the next generation of Alzheimer's disease therapeutics: Challenges for drug development. *Progress in Neuro-Psychopharmacology and Biological Psychiatry, 25,* 27–57.

Cutting, J. (1990). *The right cerebral hemisphere and psychiatric disorders*. Oxford: Oxford University Press.

Cwinn, A.A. & Cantrill, S.V. (1985). Lightning injuries. *Journal of Emergency Medicine, 2,* 379–388.

Dacey, C.M., Nelson, W.M., III, & Stoeckel, J. (1999). Reliability, criterion-related validity and qualitative comments of the fourth edition of the Stanford-Binet Intelligence Scale with a young adult population with intellectual disability. *Journal of Intellectual Disability Research, 43,* 179–184.

Dackis, C.A. & O'Brien, C.P. (2002). The neurobiology of drug addiction. In A.K. Asbury et al. (Eds.), *Diseases of the nervous system* (3rd ed.). Cambridge, UK: Cambridge University Press.

Daffner, K.R., Mesulam, M.M., Scinto, L.F., et al. (2000). The central role of the prefrontal cortex in directing attention to novel events. *Brain, 123,* 927–939.

Daghighian, I. (1973). Le vieillissement des anciens traumatisés du crâne. *Archives Suisses de Neurologie, Neurochururgie et de Psychiatrie, 112,* 399–447.

Dahl, T.H. (2002). International Classification of Functioning, Disability and Health: An introduction and discussion of its potential impact on rehabilitation services and research. *Journal of Rehabilitation Medicine, 34,* 201–204.

Dahlstrom, W.G., Brooks, J.D., & Peterson, C.D. (1990). The Beck Depression Inventory: Item order and the impact of response sets. *Journal of Personality Assessment, 55,* 224–233.

Daigneault, S. & Braun, C.M. (1993). Working memory and the Self-Ordered Pointing Task: Further evidence of early prefrontal decline in normal aging. *Journal of Clinical and Experimental Neuropsychology, 15,* 881–895.

Daigneault, S., Braun, C.M.J., & Whitaker, H.A. (1992). Early effects of normal aging in perseverative and non-perseverative prefrontal measures. *Developmental Neuropsychology, 8,* 99–114.

D'Alessandro, R., Ferrara, R., Benassi, G., et al. (1988). Computed tomographic scans in posttraumatic epilepsy. *Archives of Neurology, 45,* 42–43.

Dal Forno, G., Rasmusson, D.X., Brandt, J., et al. (1996). Apolipoprotein E genotype and rate of decline in probable Alzheimer's disease. *Archives of Neurology, 53,* 345–350.

Dalos, N.P., Rabins, P.V., Brooks, B.R., & O'Donnell, P. (1983). Disease activity and emotional state in multiple sclerosis. *Annals of Neurology, 13,* 573–577.

Dalton, C.M., Brex, P.A., Miszkiel, K.A., et al. (2002). Application of the new McDonald criteria to patients with clinically isolated syndromes suggestive of multiple sclerosis. *Annals of Neurology, 52,* 47–53.

Damasio, A.R. (1985). Prosopagnosia. *Trends in Neurosciences, 8,* 132–135.

Damasio, A.R. (1988). Regional diagnosis of cerebral disorders. In J.B. Wyngaarden & L.H. Smith, Jr. (Eds.), *Textbook of medicine* (18th ed.). Philadelphia: Saunders.

Damasio, A.R. (1990). Category-related recognition defects as a clue to the neural substrates of knowledge. *Trends in Neurosciences, 13,* 95–98.

Damasio, A.R. (1994). *Descartes' error. Emotion, reason, and the human brain*. New York: Avon Books.

Damasio, A.R. (2001). Neurobiological foundations of human memory. In A.D. Baddeley et al. (Eds.), *Handbook of memory disorders* (2nd ed.). Chichester, UK: Wiley.

Damasio, A.R. & Anderson, S.W. (2003). The frontal lobes. In K.M. Heilman & E. Valenstein (Eds.), *Clinical Neuropsychology* (4th ed.). New York: Oxford University Press.

Damasio, A.R. & Damasio, H. (1983). The anatomic basis of pure alexia. *Neurology, 33,* 1573–1583.

Damasio, A.R. & Damasio, H. (2000). Aphasia and the neural basis of language. In M.-M. Mesulam (Ed.), *Principles of behavioral and cognitive neurology* (2nd ed.). New York: Oxford University Press.

Damasio, A.R., Damasio, H., Rizzo, M., et al. (1982). Aphasia with nonhemorrhagic lesions in the basal ganglia and internal capsule. *Archives of Neurology, 39,* 15–20.

Damasio, A.R., Damasio, H., & Tranel, D. (1990). Impairments of visual recognition as clues to the processes of memory. In G.M. Edelman et al. (Eds.), *Signal and sense: Local and global order in perceptual maps.* New York: Wiley.

Damasio, A.R. & Geschwind, N. (1984). The neural basis of language. *Annual Review of Neuroscience, 7,* 127–147.

Damasio, A.R., Graff-Radford, N.R., Eslinger, P.J., et al. (1985). Amnesia following basal forebrain lesions. *Archives of Neurology, 42,* 263–271.

Damasio, A.R., McKee, J., & Damasio, H. (1979). Determinants of performance in color anomia. *Brain and Language, 7,* 74–85.

Damasio, A.R. & Tranel, D. (1991). Disorders of higher brain function. In R.N. Rosenberg (Ed.), *Comprehensive neurology.* New York: Raven Press.

Damasio, A.R., Tranel, D., & Damasio, H. (1989). Disorders of visual recognition. In F. Boller & J. Grafman (Eds.), *Handbook of Neuropsychology* (Vol. 2). Amsterdam: Elsevier.

Damasio, A.R., Tranel, D., & Rizzo, M. (2000). Disorders of complex visual processing. In M.-M. Mesulam (Ed.), *Principles of behavioral and cognitive neurology* (2nd ed.). New York: Oxford University Press.

Damasio, A.R. & Van Hoesen, G.W. (1983). Emotional disturbances associated with focal lesions of the limbic frontal lobe. In K. Heilman & P. Satz (Eds.), *Neuropsychology of human emotion.* New York: Guilford Press.

Damasio, A.R. & Van Hoesen, G.W. (1985). The limbic system and the localisation of herpes simplex encephalitis. *Journal of Neurology, Neurosurgery and Psychiatry, 48,* 297–301.

Damasio, A.R., Van Hoesen, G.W., & Hyman, B.T. (1990). Reflections on the selectivity of neuropathological changes in Alzheimer's disease. In M.F. Schwartz (Ed.), *Modular deficits in Alzheimer-type dementia.* Cambridge, MA: MIT Press.

Damasio, H.C. (1991). Neuroanatomy of frontal lobe in vivo: A comment on methodology. In H.S. Levin et al. (Eds.), *Frontal lobe function and dysfunction.* New York: Oxford University Press.

Damasio, H. & Damasio, A.R. (1989). *Lesion analysis in neuropsychology.* New York: Oxford University Press.

Damasio, H., Tranel, D., Spradling, J., & Alliger, R. (1989). Aphasia in men and women. In A.M. Galaburda (Ed.), *From reading to neurons.* Cambridge, MA: MIT Press.

Damiano, A.M., Patrick, D.L., Guzman, G.I., et al. (1999). Measurement of health-related quality of life in patients with amyotrophic lateral sclerosis in clinical trials of new therapies. *Medical Care, 37,* 15–26.

Danckert, J., Maruff, P., Ymer, C., et al. (2000). Goal-directed selective attention and response competition monitoring: Evidence from unilateral parietal and anterior cingulate lesions. *Neuropsychology, 14,* 16–28.

Daniel, M.H. (1997). Intelligence testing. Status and trends. *American Psychologist, 52,* 1038–1045.

Daniel, M., Haban, G.F., Hutcherson, W.L., et al. (1984). Neuropsychological and emotional consequences of accidental, high-voltage electrical shock. *International Journal of Clinical Neuropsychology, 7,* 102–106.

Dannenbaum, S.E., Parkinson, S.R., & Inman, V.W. (1988). Short-term forgetting: Comparisons between patients with dementia of the Alzheimer type, depressed, and normal elderly. *Cognitive Neuropsychology, 5,* 213–234.

D'Arcy, R.C.N. & McGlone, J. (2000). Profound amnesia does not impair performance on 36-item Digit Memory Test: A test of malingered memory. *Brain and Cognition, 44,* 54–58.

Dark, F.L., McGrath, J.J., & Ron, M.A. (1996). Pathological laughing and crying. *Australian and New Zealand Journal of Psychiatry, 30,* 472–479.

Darley, C.F., Tinklenberg, J.R., Roth, W.T., et al. (1973). Influence of marijuana on storage and retrieval processes in memory. *Memory and Cognition, 1,* 196–200.

Darley, F.L. (1967). *Apraxia of speech: 107 years of terminological confusion.* Paper presented at the annual convention of the American Speech and Hearing Society, Chicago, IL.

Dartigues, J.F., Commenges, D., Letenneur, D., et al. (1997). Cognitive predictors of dementia in elderly community residents. *Neuroepidemiology, 16,* 29–39.

Das, J.P. (1989). A system of cognitive assessment and its advantage over I.Q. In D. Vickers & P.L. Smith (Eds.), *Human information processing: Measures, mechanisms, and models.* Amsterdam: Elsevier.

Das, J.P. & Heemsbergen, D.B. (1983). Planning as a factor in the assessment of cognitive processes. *Journal of Psychoeducational Assessment, 1,* 1–15.

Daube, J.R. (Ed.) (2002). *Clinical neurophysiology* (2nd ed.). New York: Oxford University Press.

Daubert v. Merrell Dow Pharmaceuticals, 509 US 579 (1993).

Daum, I. & Quinn, N. (1991). Reaction times and visuospatial processing in Parkinson's disease. *Journal of Clinical and Experimental Neuropsychology, 13,* 972–982.

Davatzikos, C. & Resnick, S.M. (1998). Sex differences in anatomic measures of interhemispheric connectivity: Correlations with cognition in women but not men. *Cerebral Cortex, 8,* 635–640.

Davenport, L., Brown, L., Fiona, F., et al. (1988). A fifteen-item modification of the Fuld Object-Memory Evaluation: Preliminary data from healthy middle-aged adults. *Archives of Clinical Neuropsychology, 3,* 345–349.

Davidoff, D.A., Butters, N., Gestman, L.J., et al. (1984). Affective/motivational factors in the recall of prose passages by alcoholic Korsakoff patients. *Alcohol, 1,* 63–69.

Davidoff, G., Morris, J., Roth, E., & Bleiberg, J. (1985). Cognitive dysfunction and mild closed head injury in traumatic spinal cord injury. *Archives of Physical and Medical Rehabilitation, 66,* 489–491.

Davidoff, J. & Warrington, E.K. (1999). Apperceptive agnosia: A deficit of perceptual categorisation of objects. In G.W. Humphreys (Ed.), *Case studies in the neuropsychology of vision.* East Sussex, UK: Psychology Press.

Davidson, G.S. & Deck, J.H. (1988). Delayed myelopathy following lightning strike: A demyelinating process. *Acta Neuropathologica, 77,* 104–108.

Davidson, R.J. & Henriques, J. (2000). Regional brain function in sadness and depression. In J. Borod, *The neuropsychology of emotion.* New York: Oxford University Press.

Davidson, R.J. & Irwin, W. (2002). The functional neuroanatomy of emotion and affective style. In J.T. Cacioppo et al. (eds.), *Foundations in social neuroscience.* Cambridge, MA: MIT Press.

Davies, B., Andrewes, D., Stargatt, R., & Ames, D. (1990). Tetrahydroaminoacridine in Alzheimer's disease. *International Journal of Geriatric Psychiatry, 5,* 317–321.

Davies, K.G., Bell, B.D., Bush, A.J., et al. (1998a). Naming decline after left anterior temporal lobectomy correlates with pathological status of resected hippocampus. *Epilepsia, 39,* 407–419.

Davies, K.G., Bell, B.D., Bush, A.J., & Wyler, A.R. (1998b). Prediction of verbal memory loss in individuals after anterior temporal lobectomy. *Epilepsia, 39,* 820–828.

Davis, A.G. (1993). *A survey of adult aphasia* (2nd ed.). Englewood Cliffs, NJ: Prentice-Hall.

Davis, H.P., King, J.H., Klebe, K.J., et al. (1997). The detection of simulated malingering using a computerized priming test. *Archives of Clinical Neuropsychology, 12,* 145–153.

Davis, H.P. & Klebe, K.J. (2001). A longitudinal study of the performance of the elderly and young on the Tower of Hanoi puzzle and Rey recall. *Brain and Cognition, 46,* 95–99.

Davis, K.L., Thal, L.J., Gamzu, E.R., et al. (1992). A double-blind multi-center study of tacrine for Alzheimer's disease. *New England Journal of Medicine, 327,* 1253–1259.

Davis, L.E. & Johnson, R.T. (1979). An explanation for the localization of herpes simplex encephalitis? *Annals of Neurology, 5,* 2–5.

Davison, A.M., Walker, G.S., Oli, H., & Lewins, A.M. (1982). Water supply aluminum concentration, dialysis dementia, and effect of reverse-osmosis water treatment. *Lancet, i,* 785–792.

Davison, K. & Hassanyck, F. (1991). Psychiatric disorders. In *Textbook of adverse drug reactions* (4th ed.). Oxford: Oxford University Press.

Davison, L.A. (1974). Current status of clinical neuropsychology. In R.M. Reitan & L.A. Davison (Eds.), *Clinical neuropsychology: Current status and applications.* New York: Wiley.

Dawes, R.M., Faust, D., & Meehl, P.E. (1989). Clinical versus actuarial judgment. *Science, 243,* 1668–1674.

Dawson, D. & Reid, K. (1997). Fatigue, alcohol, and performance impairment. *Nature, 388,* 235.

Dawson, L.K. & Grant, I. (2000). Alcoholics' initial organizational and problem-solving skills predict learning and memory performance on the Rey-Osterrieth Complex Figure. *Journal of the International Neuropsychological Society, 6,* 12–19.

DeAngelis, L.M. (2001). Brain tumors. *New England Journal of Medicine, 344,* 114–123.

DeArmond, S.J., Fusco, M.M., & Dewey, M.M. (1976). *Structure of the human brain* (2nd ed.). New York: Oxford University Press.

Debanne, S.M., Rowland, D.Y., Riedel, T.M., & Cleves, M.A. (2000). Association of Alzheimer's disease and smoking: The case for sibling controls. *Journal of the American Geriatrics Society, 48,* 800–806.

deBenedittis, G., Lorenzetti, A., Sina, C., & Bernasconi, V. (1995). Magnetic resonance imaging in migraine and tension type headache. *Headache, 35,* 264–268.

DeBettignies, B.H., Mahurin, R.K., & Pirozzolo, F.J. (1990). Insight for impairment in independent living skills in Alzheimer's disease and multi-infarct dementia. *Journal of Clinical and Experimental Neuropsychology, 12,* 355–363.

De Bleser, R. (1988). Localisation of aphasia: Science or fiction. In G. Denes et al. (Eds.), *Perspectives on cognitive neuropsychology.* Hove, UK: Erlbaum.

de Boo, G.M., Tibben, A., Lanser, J.B., et al. (1997). Early cognitive and motor symptoms in identified carriers of the gene for Huntington disease. *Archives of Neurology, 54,* 1353–1357.

de Bruin, A.F., Buys, M., de Witte, L.P., & Diederiks, J.F. (1994). The Sickness Impact Profile: SIP68, a short generic version. First evaluation of the reliability and reproducibility. *Journal of Clinical Epidemiology, 47,* 863–871.

de Bruin, A.F., Diederiks, J.P., de Witte, L.P., et al. (1994). The development of a short generic version of the Sickness Impact Profile. Journal of Clinical Epidemiology, 47, 407–418.

Deckersbach, T., Savage, C.R., Henin, A., et al. (2000). Reliability and validity of a scoring system for measuring organizational approach in the Complex Figure Test. *Journal of Clinical and Experimental Neuropsychology, 22,* 640–648.

Dee, H.L., Benton, A.L., & Van Allen, M.W. (1970). Apraxia in relation to hemisphere locus of lesion and aphasia. *Transactions of the American Neurological Association, 95,* 147–148.

Dee, H.L. & Fontenot, D.J. (1973). Cerebral dominance and lateral differences in perception and memory. *Neuropsychologia, 11,* 167–173.

Deelman, B. & Berg, I. (2002). Evaluation of neuropsychological rehabilitation. In W. Brouwer et al. (Eds.), *Cognitive rehabilitation. A clinical neuropsychological approach.* Amsterdam: Boom.

De Filippis, N.A. & McCampbell, E. (1997). *Booklet Category Test (BCT)* (2nd ed.). Odessa, FL: Psycholgical Assessment Resources.

De Filippis, N.A., McCampbell, E., & Rogers, P. (1979). Development of a booklet form of the Category Test: Normative and validity data. *Journal of Clinical Neuropsychology, 1,* 339–342.

De Filippis, N.A. & PAR Staff (1993). *Category Test: Computer Version, Research Edition.* Odessa, FL: Psychological Assessment Resources.

De Haan, E.H.F. (2001). Face perception and recognition. In B. Rapp (Ed.), *The handbook of cognitive neuropsychology.* Philadelphia: Psychology Press.

Dehaene, S. (2000). Cerebral bases of number processing and calculation. In M.S. Gazzaniga (Ed.), *The new cognitive neurosciences* (2nd ed.). Cambridge, MA: MIT Press.

Dehaene, S. (2002). *The cognitive neuroscience of consciousness.* Cambridge, MA: MIT Press/Elsevier.

Dehaene, S., Spelke, E., Pinel, P., et al. (1999). Sources of mathematical thinking: Behavioral and brain-imaging evidence. *Science, 284,* 970–974.

Dekaban, A.S. & Sadowsky, D. (1978). Changes in brain weight during the span of the human life: Relation of brain weights to body heights and body weights. *Annals of Neurology, 4,* 345–356.

de Koning, I., Dippel, D.W., van Kooten, F., & Koudstaal, P.J. (2000). A short screening instrument for poststroke dementia : The R-CAMCOG. *Stroke, 31,* 1502–1508.

de Koning, I., van Kooten, F., & Dippel, D.W. (1998). The CAMCOG: A useful screening instrument for dementia in stroke patients. *Stroke, 29,* 2080–2086.

DeKosky, S.T. & Orgogozo, J.-M. (2001). Alzheimer's disease: Diagnosis, costs, and dimensions of treatment. *Alzheimer Disease and Associated Disorders, 15(Suppl. 1),* S3–S7.

de Kruijk, J.R., Leffers, P., Menheere, P.P., et al. (2001). S-100B and neuron-specific enolase in serum of mild traumatic brain injury patients. A comparison with health controls. *Acta Neurologica Scandinavica, 103,* 175–179.

de Lacoste, M.C., Horvath, D.S., & Woodward, D.J. (1991). Possible sex differences in the developing human fetal brain. *Journal of Clinical and Experimental Neuropsychology, 13,* 831–846.

Delacourte, A., David, J.P., Sergeant, N., et al. (1999). The biochemical pathway of neurofibrillary degeneration in aging and Alzheimer's disease. *Neurology, 52,* 1158–1165.

de la Monte, S.M. (1988). Disproportionate atrophy of cerebral white matter in chronic alcoholics. *Archives of Neurology, 45,* 990–992.

Delaney, J.S., Lacroix, V.J., Gagne, C., & Antoniou, J. (2001). Concussions among university football and soccer players: A pilot study. *Clinical Journal of Sports Medicine, 11,* 234–240.

Delaney, R.C., Prevey, M.L., Cramer, J., et al. (1992). Test-retest comparability and control subject data for the Rey Auditory Verbal Learning Test and Rey-Osterreith/Taylor complex figures. *Archives of Clinical Neuropsychology, 7,* 523–528.

Delaney, R.C., Prevey, M.L., & Mattson, R.H. (1982). Short-term retention with lateralized temporal lobe epilepsy. *Cortex, 22,* 591–600.

Delaney, R.C., Rosen, A.J., Mattson, R.H., & Novelly, R.A. (1980). Memory function in focal epilepsy: A comparison of nonsurgical, unilateral temporal lobe and frontal lobe samples. *Cortex, 16,* 103–117.

Delaney, R.C., Wallace, J.D., & Egelko, S. (1980). Transient cerebral ischemic attacks and neuropsychological deficit. *Journal of Clinical Neuropsychology, 2,* 107–114.

Delazer, M. & Bartha, L. (2001). Transcoding and calculation in aphasia. *Aphasiology, 15,* 649–679.

Delbecq-Dérouesné, J. & Beauvois, M.-F. (1989). Memory processes and aging: A defect of automatic rather than controlled processes? *Archives of Gerontology and Geriatrics (Suppl. 1),* 121–150.

Delis, D.C. (1989). Neuropsychological assessment of learning and memory. In F. Boller & J. Grafman (Eds.), *Handbook of neuropsychology* (Vol. 3). Amsterdam: Elsevier.

Delis, D.C., Freeland, J., Kramer, J. H., & Kaplan, E. (1988). Integrating clinical assessment with cognitive neuroscience: Construct validation of the California Verbal Learning Test. *Journal of Consulting and Clinical Psychology, 56,* 123–130.

Delis, D.C. & Kaplan, E.F. (1982). The assessment of aphasia with the Luria-Nebraska Neuropsychological Battery: A case critique. *Journal of Consulting and Clinical Psychology, 50,* 107–114.

Delis, D.C. & Kaplan, E. (1983). Hazards of a standardized neuropsychological test with low content validity: Comment on the Luria-Nebraska Neuropsychological Battery. *Journal of Consulting and Clinical Psychology, 51,* 396–398.

Delis, D., Kaplan, E., & Kramer, J. (2001). *Delis-Kaplan Executive Function Scale.* San Antonio: Psychological Corporation.

Delis, D.C., Kaplan, E., Kramer, J.H., & Ober, B.A. (2000). *California Verbal Learning Test–Second Edition (CVLT-II) Manual.* San Antonio: Psychological Corporation.

Delis, D.C., Kiefner, M.G., & Fridlund, A.J. (1988). Visuospatial dysfunction following unilateral brain damage: Dissociations in hierarchical and hemispatial analysis. *Journal of Clinical Neuropsychology, 10,* 421–431.

Delis, D.C., Kramer, J.H., Fridlund, A.J., & Kaplan, E. (1990). A cognitive science approach to neuropsychological assessment. In P. McReynolds et al. (Eds.), *Advances in psychological assessment* (Vol. 7). New York: Plenum Press.

Delis, D.C., Kramer, J., & Kaplan, E. (1988). *California Proverb Test.* Lexington, MA: Boston Neuropsychological Foundation.

Delis, D.C., Kramer, J.H., Kaplan, E., & Ober, B.A. (1983, 1987). *California Verbal Learning Test (CVLT). Adult Version (Research ed.).* San Antonio, TX: Psychological Corporation.

Delis, D.C., Kramer, J.H., Kaplan, E., & Ober, B.A. (2000). *California Verbal Learning Test–Second Edition (CVLT-II).* San Antonio, TX: Psychological Corporation.

Delis, D.C., Massman, P.J., Butters, N., et al. (1991). Profiles of demented and amnesic patients on the California Verbal Learning Test: Implications for the assessment of memory disorders. *Psychological Assessment, 3,* 19–26.

Delis, D.C., Massman, P.J., Butters, N., et al. (1992). Spatial cognition in Alzheimer's disease: Subtypes of global-local impairment. *Journal of Clinical and Experimental Neuropsychology, 14,* 463–477.

Delis, D.C., McKee, R., Massman, P.J., et al. (1991). Alternate form of the California Verbal Learning Test: Development and reliability. *The Clinical Neuropsychologist, 5,* 154–162.

Delis, D.C., Robertson, L.C., & Efron, R. (1986). Hemispheric specialization of memory for visual hierarchical stimuli. *Neuropsychologia, 30,* 683–697.

Delis, D.C., Squire, L.R., Bihrle, A., & Massman, P. (1992). Componential analysis of problem-solving ability: Performance of patients with frontal lobe damage and amnesic patients on a new sorting test. *Neuropsychologia, 30,* 683–697.

Delis, D.C., Wapner, W., Gardner, H., & Moses, J.A., Jr. (1983). The contribution of the right hemisphere to the organization of paragraphs. *Cortex, 19,* 43–50.

Della Malva, C.L., Stuss, D.T., D'Alton, J., & Willmer, J. (1993). Capture errors and sequencing after frontal brain lesions. *Neuropsychologia, 31,* 362–372.

Della Sala, S., Kinnear, P., Spinnler, H., & Stangalino, C. (2000). Color-to-figure matching in Alzheimer's disease. *Archives of Clinical Neuropsychology, 15,* 571–585.

Della Sala, S. & Mazzini, L. (1990). Post-traumatic extrapyramidal syndrome: Case report. *Italian Journal of Neurological Sciences, 11,* 65–69.

Deloche, G., Dellatolas, G., Vendrell, J., & Bergogo, C. (1996). Cal-

culation and number processing: Neuropsychological assessment and daily life difficulties. *Journal of the International Neuropsychological Society, 2,* 177–180.

Deloche, G., Hannequin, D., Carlomagno, S., et al. (1995). Calculation and number processing in mild Alzheimer's disease. *Journal of the International Neuropsychological Society, 17,* 634–639.

DeLuca, J.W. (1989). Neuropsychology technicians in clinical practice: Precedents, rationale and current deployment. *The Clinical Neuropsychologist, 3,* 3–21.

DeLuca, J., Barbieri-Berger, S., & Johnson, S K. (1994). The nature of memory impairment in multiple sclerosis: Acquisition versus retrieval. *Journal of Clinical and Experimental Neuropsychology, 16,* 183–189.

DeLuca, J., Gaudino, E.A., Diamond, B., et al. (1998). Acquisition and storage deficits in multiple sclerosis. *Journal of Clinical and Experimental Neuropsychology, 20,* 376–390.

DeLuca, J., Johnson, S.K., Ellis, S.P., & Natelson, B.H. (1997). Cognitive functioning is impaired in patients with chronic fatigue syndrome devoid of psychiatric disease. *Journal of Neurology, Neurosurgery and Psychiatry, 62,* 151–155.

DeLuca, J., Johnson, S.K., & Natelson, B.H. (1993). Information processing efficiency in chronic fatigue syndrome and multiple sclerosis. *Archives of Neurology, 50,* 301–304.

Demakis, G.J. (1999). Serial malingering on verbal and nonverbal fluency and memory measures: An analog investigation. *Archives of Clinical Neuropsychology, 14,* 401–410.

Demaree, H.A., DeLuca, J., Gaudino, E.A., & Diamond, B. J. (1999). Speed of information processing as a key deficit in multiple sclerosis: Implications for rehabilitation. *Journal of Neurology, Neurosurgery and Psychiatry, 67,* 661–663.

Demers, L., Oremus, M., Perrault, A., et al. (2000a). Review of outcome measurement instruments in Alzheimer's disease drug trials: Psychometric properties of functional and quality of life scales. *Journal of Geriatric Psychiatry and Neurology, 13,* 170–180.

Demers, L., Oremus, M., Perrault, A., & Wolfson, C. (2000b). Review of outcome measurement instruments in Alzheimer's disease drug trials: Introduction. *Journal of Geriatric Psychiatry and Neurology, 13,* 161–169.

Demers, P., Robillard, A., & Lafleche, G. (1994). Translation of clinical and neuropsychological instruments into French: The CERAD experience. *Age and Ageing, 23,* 449–451.

Demitrack, M.A., Szostak, C., & Weingartner, H. (1992). Cognitive dysfunction in eating disorders: A clinical psychobiological perspective. In D.I. Margolin (Ed.), *Cognitive neuropsychology in clinical practice.* New York: Oxford University Press.

De Mol, J. (1975/1976). Le test de Rorschach chez les traumatisés crâniens. *Bulletin de Psychologie, 29,* 747–757.

Démonet, J.-F. (1995). Studies of language processes using positron emission tomography. In F. Boller & J. Grafman (Eds.), *Handbook of neuropsychology* (Vol. 10). Amsterdam: Elsevier.

Denburg, N.L. & Tranel, D. (2003). Acalculia and disturbances of body schema. In K.M. Heilman & E. Valenstein (Eds.), *Clinical Neuropsychology* (4th ed.). New York: Oxford University Press.

Denes, F., Semenza, C., & Stoppa, E. (1978). Selective improvement by unilateral brain-damaged patients on Raven Coloured Progressive Matrices. *Neuropsychologia, 16,* 749–752.

Denes, G., Semenza, C., Stoppa, E., & Lis, A. (1982). Unilateral spatial neglect and recovery from hemiplegia: A follow-up study. *Brain, 105,* 543–552.

Denicoff, K.D., Ali, S.O., Mirsky, A.F., et al. (1999). Relationship between prior course of illness and neuropsychological functioning in patients with bipolar disorder. *Journal of Affective Disorders, 56,* 67–73.

Denman, S.B. (1984). *Denman Neuropsychology Memory Scale.* Charleston, SC: Sidney B. Denman.

Denman, S.B. (1987). *Denman Neuropsychology Memory Scale: Norms.* Charleston, SC: Sidney B. Denman.

Dennett, D.C. (1991). *Consciousness explained.* Boston: Little, Brown.

Denney, R.L. (1999). A brief symptom validity testing procedure for Logical Memory of the Wechsler Memory Scale-Revised which can demonstrate verbal memory in the face of claimed disability. *Journal of Forensic Neuropsychology, 1,* 5–24.

Denny-Brown, D. (1962). Clinical symptomatology in right and left hemisphere lesions. Discussion. In V.B. Mountcastle (Ed.), *Interhemispheric relations and cerebral dominance.* Baltimore: Johns Hopkins Press.

Derdeyn, C.P. & Powers, W.J. (1997). Metabolic studies using PET in stroke investigation. In K.M.A. Welch et al. (Eds.), *Primer on cerebrovascular diseases.* San Diego: Academic Press.

De Renzi, E. (1968). Nonverbal memory and hemispheric side of lesion. *Neuropsychologia, 6,* 181–189.

De Renzi, E. (Ed.) (1990). Apraxia. In F. Boller & J. Grafman (Eds.), *Handbook of neuropsychology* (Vol. 2). New York: Elsevier.

De Renzi, E. (1997a). Prosopagnosia. In T.E. Feinberg & M.J. Farah (Eds.), *Behavioral neurology and neuropsychology.* New York: McGraw-Hill.

De Renzi, E. (1997b). Visuospatial and constructional disorders. In T.E. Feinberg & M.J. Farah (Eds.), *Behavioral neurology and neuropsychology.* New York: McGraw-Hill.

De Renzi, E. (2000). Disorders of visual recognition. *Seminars in Neurology, 20,* 479–485.

De Renzi, E. (2001). The amnesic syndrome. In G.E. Berrios & J.R. Hodges (Eds.), *Memory disorders in psychiatric practice.* Cambridge, UK: Cambridge University Press.

De Renzi, E. & Faglioni, P. (1965). The comparative efficiency of intelligence and vigilance tests in detecting hemispheric cerebral damage. *Cortex, 1,* 410–433.

De Renzi, E. & Faglioni, P. (1967). The relationship between visuospatial impairment and constructional apraxia. *Cortex, 3,* 327–342.

De Renzi, E. & Faglioni, P. (1978). Normative data and screening power of a shortened version of the Token Test. *Cortex, 14,* 41–49.

De Renzi, E., Faglioni, P., Nichelli, P., & Pignattari, L. (1984). Intellectual and memory impairment in moderate and heavy drinkers. *Cortex, 20,* 525–533.

De Renzi, E., Faglioni, P., & Previdi, P. (1977). Spatial memory and hemispheric locus of lesion. *Cortex, 13,* 424–433.

De Renzi, E., Faglioni, P., Savoiardo, M., & Vignolo, L.A. (1966). The influence of aphasia and of the hemisphere side of the cerebral lesion on abstract thinking. *Cortex, 2,* 399–420.

De Renzi, E., Faglioni, P., & Sorgato, P. (1982). Modality-specific and supramodal mechanisms of apraxia. *Brain, 105,* 301–312.

De Renzi, E. & Ferrari, C. (1978). The Reporter's Test: A sensitive test to detect expressive disturbances in aphasia. *Cortex, 14,* 279–293.

De Renzi, E., Lucchelli, F., Muggia, S., & Spinnler, H. (1995). Persistent retrograde, amnesia following a minor trauma. *Cortex, 31,* 531–542.

De Renzi, E., Motti, F., & Nichelli, P. (1980). Imitating gestures. *Archives of Neurology, 37,* 6–10.

De Renzi, E., Perani, D., Carlesimo, G.A., et al. (1994). Prosopagnosia can be associated with damage confined to the right hemisphere—an MRI and PET study and a review of the literature. *Neuropsychologia, 32,* 893–902.

De Renzi, E. & Spinnler, H. (1966). Visual recognition in patients with unilateral cerebral disease. *Journal of Nervous and Mental Disease, 142,* 515–525.

De Renzi, E. & Spinnler, H. (1967). Impaired performance on color tasks in patients with hemispheric damage. *Cortex, 3,* 194–217.

De Renzi, E. & Vignolo, L.A. (1962). The Token Test: A sensitive test to detect disturbances in aphasics. *Brain, 85,* 665–678.

Derix, M.M.A. (1994). *Neuropsychological differentiation of dementing syndromes.* Lisse, The Netherlands: Swets and Zeitlinger.

Derman, H.S. (1994). Headaches: Diagnosis and treatment. In S.H. Appel (Ed.), *Current neurology* (Vol. 14). St. Louis: Mosby.

Derogatis, L.R. (1975). *BSI (Brief Symptom Inventory).* Minneapolis: National Computer Systems.

Derogatis, L.R. (1994). *SCL-R: Symptom Checklist-90-R: Administration, scoring, and procedures manual* (3rd ed.). Minneapolis: National Computer Systems.

Derogatis, L.R. & Lazarus, L. (1994). SCL-90-R, Brief Symptom Inventory, and matching clinical rating scales. In M.E. Maruish (Ed.), *The use of psychological testing for treatment planning and outcome assessment* . Hillsdale, NJ: Erlbaum.

Dérouesné, C., Lagha-Pierucci, S., Thibault, S., et al. (2000). Apraxic disturbances in patients with mild to moderate Alzheimer's disease. *Neuropsychologia, 38,* 1760–1769.

Derrer, D.S., Howieson, D.B., Mueller, E.A., et al. (2001). Memory testing in dementia: How much is enough? *Journal of Geriatric Psychiatry and Neurology, 13,* 1–6.

Derry, P.A. & Wiebe, S. (2000). Psychological adjustment to success and to failure following epilepsy surgery. *Canadian Journal of Neurological Sciences, 27,* S116–S120.

Dershowitz, A. & Frankel, Y. (1975). Jewish culture and the WISC and WAIS test patterns. *Journal of Consulting and Clinical Psychology, 43,* 126–134.

Desgranges, B., Baron, J.C., de la Sayette, V., et al. (1998). The neural substrates of memory systems impairment in Alzheimer's disease. A PET study of resting brain glucose utilization. *Brain, 121,* 611–631.

Deshpande, S.A., Millis, S.R., Reeder, K.P., et al. (1996). Verbal learning subtypes in traumatic brain injury: a replication. *Journal of Clinical and Experimental Neuropsychology, 18,* 836–842.

Desmond, D.W., Remien, R.H., Moroney, J.T., et al. (2003). Ischemic stroke and depression. *Journal of the International Neuropsychological Society, 9,* 429–439.

Desmond, D.W., Tatemichi, T.K., & Hanzawa, L. (1994). The Telephone Interview for Cognitive Status (TICS): Reliability and validity in a stroke sample. *International Journal of Geriatric Psychiatry, 9,* 803–807.

Desmond, J.E., Sum, J.M., Wagner, A.D., et al. (1995). Functional MRI measurement of language lateralization in Wada-tested patients. *Brain, 118,* 1411–1419.

Desmond, J.E., Gabrieli, J.D.E., Wagner, A.D., et al. (1997). Lobular patterns of cerebellar activation of verbal working-memory and finger-tapping tasks as revealed by functional MRI. *Journal of Neuroscience, 17,* 9675–9685.

de Sousa, R.M., Regis, F.C., & Koizumi, M.S. (1999). Traumatic brain injury: Differences among pedestrians and motor vehicle occupants. *Revista de Saude Publica, 33,* 85–94.

D'Esposito, M. (2000). Functional neuroimaging of cognition. *Seminars in Neurology, 20,* 487–498.

D'Esposito, M., Detre, J.A., Alsop, D.C., et al. (1995). The neural basis of the central executive system of working memory. *Nature, 378,* 279–281.

D'Esposito, M., Ballard, D., Aguirre, G.K., & Zarahn, E. (1998). Human prefrontal cortex is not specific for working memory: a functional MRI study. *Neuroimage, 8,* 274–282.

D'Esposito, M., Onishi, K., Thompson, H., et al. (1996). Working memory impairments in multiple sclerosis: Evidence from a dual task paradigm. *Neuropsychology, 10,* 51–56.

D'Esposito, M. & Postle, B.R. (2002). The neural basis of working memory storage, rehearsal, and control processes. Evidence from patient and functional magnetic resonance imaging studies. In L.R. Squire & D.L Schachter (Eds.), *Neuropsychology of memory* (3rd ed.). New York: Guilford Press.

desRosiers, G., Hodges, J.R., & Berrios, G. (1995). The neuropsychological differentiation of patients with very mild Alzheimer's disease and/or major depression. *Journal of the American Geriatric Society, 43*, 1256–1263.

desRosiers, G. & Ivison, D. (1986). Paired associate learning: Normative data for differences between high and low associate word pairs. *Journal of Clinical and Experimental Neuropsychology, 8*, 637–642.

DeStefano, N., Narayanan, S., Francis, S.J., et al. (2002). Diffuse axonal and tissue injury in patients with multiple sclerosis with low cerebral lesion load and no disability. *Archives of Neurology, 59*, 1565–1571.

Detre, J.A., Maccotta, L., King, D., et al. (1998). Functional MRI lateralization of memory in temporal lobe epilepsy. *Neurology, 50*, 926–932.

Deutsch, G., Bourbon, W.T., Papanicolaou, A.C., & Eisenberg, H.M. (1988). Visuospatial tasks compared via activation of regional cerebral blood flow. *Neuropsychologia, 26*, 445–452.

Deutsch, G. & Mountz, J.M. (2001). Neuroimaging evidence of diaschisis and reorganization in stroke recovery. In A.-L. Christensen & B.P. Uzzell (Eds.), *International handbook of neuropsychological rehabilitation*. New York: Kluwer Academic/Plenum Press.

Deutsch, G. & Tweedy, J.R. (1987). Cerebral blood flow in severity-matched Alzheimer and multi-infarct patients. *Neurology, 37*, 431–438.

Devanand, D.P., Folz, M., Gorlyn, M., et al. (1997). Questionable dementia: Clinical course and predictors of outcome. *Journal of the American Geriatric Society, 45*, 321–328.

Devanand, D.P., Jacobs, D.M., Tang, M.X., et al. (1997). The course of psychopathologic features in mild to moderate Alzheimer disease at follow-up. *American Journal of Psychiatry, 157*, 1399–1405.

Devanand, D.P., Michaels-Marston, K.S., Liu, X., et al. (2000). Olfactory deficits in patients with mild cognitive impairment predict Alzheimer's disease at follow-up. *American Journal of Psychiatry, 157*, 1399–1405.

Devanand, D.P., Sano, M., Tang, M.X., et al. (1996). Depressed mood and the incidence of Alzheimer's disease in the elderly living in the community. *Archives of General Psychiatry, 53*, 175–182.

Devinsky, O., Morrell, M.J., & Vogt, B.A. (1995). Contributions of anterior cingulate cortex to behaviour. *Brain, 118*, 279–306.

Devinsky, O. & Najjar, S. (1999). Evidence against the existence of a temporal lobe epilepsy personality syndrome. *Neurology, 53*, S13–S25.

Devinsky, O., Vickrey, B. G., Cramer, J., Perrine, K., et al. (1995). Development of the Quality of Life in Epilepsy Inventory. *Epilepsia, 36*, 1089–1104.

Devlin, J.T., Gonnerman, L.M., Andersen, E.S., & Seidenberg, M.S. (1998). Category-specific semantic deficits in focal and widespread brain damage: A computational account. *Journal of Cognitive Neuroscience, 10*, 77–94.

DeVolder, A.G., Goffinet, A.M., Bol, A., et al. (1990). Brain glucose metabolism in postanoxic syndrome: Positron emission tomographic study. *Archives of Neurology, 47*, 197–204.

Deweer, B., Pillon, B., Michon, A., & Dubois, B. (1993). Mirror reading in Alzheimer's disease. Normal skill learning and acquisition of item-specific information. *Journal of Clinical and Experimental Neuropsychology, 15*, 789–804.

Dewhurst, K., Oliver, J.E., & McKnight, A.L. (1970). Socio-psychiatric consequences of Huntington's disease. *British Journal of Psychiatry, 116*, 255–258.

DeWolfe, A.S., Barrell, R.P., Becker, B.C., & Spaner, F.E. (1971). Intellectual deficit in chronic schizophrenia and brain damage. *Journal of Consulting and Clinical Psychology, 36*, 197–204.

Diamond, B.J., DeLuca, J., Johnson, S.K., & Kelley, S.M. (1997). Verbal learning in amnesic anterior communicating artery aneurysm patients and in patients with multiple sclerosis. *Applied Neuropsychology, 4*, 89–98.

Diamond, B.J., DeLuca, J., & Kelley, S.M. (1997). Memory and executive functions in amnesic and non-amnesic patients with aneurysms of the anterior communicating artery. *Brain, 120*, 1015–1025.

Diamond, B.J., DeLuca, J., Kim, H., & Kelley, S.M. (1997). The question of disproportionate impairments in visual and auditory information processing in multiple sclerosis. *Journal of Clinical and Experimental Neuropsychology, 19*, 34–42.

Diamond, B.J., DeLuca, J., Rosenthal, D., et al. (2000). Information processing in older versus younger adults: Accuracy versus speed. *International Journal of Rehabilitation and Health, 5*, 55–64.

Diamond, R., Barth, J.T., & Zillmer, E.A. (1988). Emotional correlates of mild closed head trauma: The role of the MMPI. *International Journal of Clinical Neuropsychology, 10*, 35–41.

Diamond, R., White, R.F., Myers, R.H., et al. (1992). Evidence of presymptomatic cognitive decline in Huntington's disease. *Journal of Clinical and Experimental Neuropsychology, 14*, 961–975.

Diamond, S.G., Markham, C.H., Hoehn, M.M., et al. (1990). An examination of male–female differences in progression and mortality of Parkinson's disease. *Neurology, 40*, 763–766.

Diaz-Marchan, P.J., Hayman, L.A., Carrier, D.A., & Feldman, D.J. (1996). Computed tomography of closed head injury. In R.K. Narayan et al. (Eds.). *Neurotrauma*. New York: McGraw-Hill.

Diaz-Olavarrieta, C., Cummings, J.L., Velazquez, J., & Cadena, C.G. (1999). Neuropsychiatric manifestations of multiple sclerosis. *Journal of Neuropsychiatry and Clinical Neurosciences, 11*, 51–57.

DiCarlo, M.A., Gfeller, J.D., and Oliveri, M.V. (2000). Effects of coaching on detecting feigned cognitive impairment with the Category Test. *Archives of Clinical Neuropsychology, 15*, 399–413.

Dick, J.P.R., Guiloff, R.J., Stewart, A., et al. (1984). Mini-Mental State examination in neurological patients. *Journal of Neurology, Neurosurgery and Psychiatry, 47*, 496–499.

Dick, M.B., Nielson, K.A., Beth, R.E., et al. (1995). Acquisition and long-term retention of a fine motor skill in Alzheimer's disease. *Brain and Cognition, 29*, 294–306.

Dickinson, D., Iannone, V.N., & Gold, J.M. (2002). Factor structure of the Wechsler Adult Intelligence Scale-III in schizophrenia. *Assessment, 9*, 171–180.

Diener, E., Emmons, R.A., Larsen, R.J., & Griffin, S. (1985). The Satisfaction with Life Scales. *Journal of Personality Assessment, 49*, 71–75.

Diesfeldt, H.F.A. (1990). Recognition memory for words and faces in primary degenerative dementia of the Alzheimer type and normal old age. *Journal of Clinical and Experimental Neuropsychology, 12*, 931–945.

Diesfeldt, H. & Vink, M. (1989). Recognition memory for words and faces in the very old. *British Journal of Clinical Psychology, 28*, 247–253.

Diesing, T.S., Swindells, S., Gelbard, H., & Gendelman, H.E. (2002). HIV-1-associated dementia: A basic science and clinical perspective. *AIDS Reader, 12*, 358–368.

Dikmen, S.S., Donovan, D.M., Løberg, T., et al. (1993). Alcohol use and its effects on neuropsychological outcome in head injury. *Neuropsychology, 7*, 296–305.

Dikmen, S.S., Heaton, R.K., Grant, I., & Temkin, N.R. (1999). Test-retest reliability and practice effects of the expanded Halstead-

Reitan Neuropsychological Test Battery. *Journal of the International Neuropsychological Society, 5,* 346–356.

Dikmen, S., Machamer, J., Temkin, N., & McLean, A. (1990). Neuropsychological recovery in patients with moderate to severe head injury: Two-year follow-up. *Journal of Clinical and Experimental Neuropsychology, 12,* 507–519.

Dikmen, S.S., Machamer, J.E., Winn, H.R., & Temkin, N.R. (1995). Neuropsychological outcome at 1-year post head injury. *Neuropsychology, 9,* 80–90.

Dikmen, S., McLean, A., & Temkin, N. (1986). Neuropsychological and psychosocial consequences of minor head injury. *Journal of Neurology, Neurosurgery and Psychiatry, 49,* 1227–1232.

Dikmen, S.S., McLean, A., Temkin, N.R., & Wyler, A.R. (1986). Neuropsychologic outcome at one month postinjury. *Archives of Physical Medicine and Rehabilitation, 67,* 507–513.

Dikmen, S. & Reitan, R.M. (1974). MMPI correlates of localized cerebral lesions. *Perceptual and Motor Skills, 39,* 831–840.

Dikmen, S.S., Temkin, N.R., Machamer, J.E., et al. (1994). Employment following traumatic head injuries. *Archives of Neurology, 51,* 177–186.

Diller, L. (2000). Poststroke rehabilitation practice guidelines. In A.-L. Christensen & B.P. Uzzell (Eds.). *International handbook of neuropsychological rehabilitation.* New York: Kluwer Academic/Plenum Press.

Diller, L., Ben-Yishay, Y., Gerstman, L.J., et al. (1974). *Studies in cognition and rehabilitation in hemiplegia.* (Rehabilitation Monograph 50). New York: New York University Medical Center Institute of Rehabilitation Medicine.

Diller, L. & Weinberg, J. (1965). Bender Gestalt Test distortions in hemiplegia. *Perceptual and Motor Skills, 20,* 1313–1323.

Diller, L. & Weinberg, J. (1970). Evidence for accident-prone behavior in hemiplegic patients. *Archives of Physical Medicine and Rehabilitation, 51,* 358–363.

Dimitrov, M., Grafman, J., & Hollnagel, C. (1996). The effects of frontal lobe damage on everyday problem solving. *Cortex, 32,* 357–366.

Dimitrov, M., Grafman, J., Soares, A.H., & Clark, K. (1999). Concept formation and concept shifting in frontal lesion and Parkinson's disease patients assessed with the California Card Sorting Test. *Neuropsychology, 13,* 135–143.

Di Monte, D.A. & Langston, J.W. (2000). MPTP and analogs. In P.S. Spencer & H.H. Schaumburg (Eds.), *Experimental and clinical neurotoxicology* (2nd ed.). New York: Oxford University Press.

Dimopoulou, I., Korfias, S., Dafni, U., et al. (2003). Protein S-100b serum levels in trauma-induced brain death. *Neurology, 60,* 947–951.

Dinges, D.F., Pack, F., Williams, K., et al. (1997). Cumulative sleepiness, mood disturbance, and psychomotor vigilance performance decrements during a week of sleep restricted to 4–5 hours per night. *Sleep, 20,* 267–277.

Dinning, W.D. & Kraft, W.A. (1983). Validation of the Satz-Mogel Short Form for the WAIS-R with psychiatric inpatients. *Journal of Consulting and Clinical Psychology, 51,* 781–782.

Dinsdale, H.B. (1986). Hypertensive encephalopathy. In H.J.M. Bennett et al. (Eds.), *Stroke: Pathophysiology, diagnosis, and management.* New York: Churchill Livingstone.

DiPino, R.K., Kabat, M.H., & Kane, R.L. (2000). An exploration of the construct validity of the Heaton Memory Tests. *Archives of Clinical Neuropsychology, 15,* 95–103.

Direnfeld, L.K., Albert, M.L., Volicer, L., et al. (1984). Parkinson's disease: The possible relationship of laterality to dementia and neurochemical findings. *Archives of Neurology, 41,* 935–941.

Di Sclafani, V., Clark, H.W., Tolou-Shams, M., et al. (1998). Premorbid brain size is a determinant of functional reserve in absti-nent crack-cocaine and crack-cocaine–alcohol dependent adults. *Journal of the International Neuropsychological Society, 4,* 559–565.

Di Stefano, G. & Radanov, B.P. (1996). Quantitative and qualitative aspects of learning and memory in common whiplash patients: A 6-month follow-up study. *Archives of Clinical Neuropsychology, 11,* 661–676.

Divac, I. (1977). Does the neostriatum operate as a functional entity? In A.R. Cools et al. (Eds.), *Psychobiology of the striatum.* Amsterdam: Elsevier/North-Holland.

Division 40 Task Force on Education, Accreditation, and Credentialing (1989). Guidelines regarding the use of nondoctoral personnel in clinical neuropsychological assessment. *The Clinical Neuropsychologist, 3,* 23–24.

Dobbs, A.R. & Rule, B.G. (1989). Adult age differences in working memory. *Psychology and Aging, 4,* 500–503.

Dobkin, B. (1995). The economic impact of stroke. *Neurology, 45,* 56–59.

Dodrill, C.B. (1978a). The hand dynamometer as a neuropsychological measure. *Journal of Consulting and Clinical Psychology, 46,* 1432–1435.

Dodrill, C.B. (1978b). A neuropsychological battery for epilepsy. *Epilepsia, 19,* 611–623

Dodrill, C.B. (1979). Sex differences on the Halstead-Reitan Neuropsychological Battery and on other neuropsychological measures. *Journal of Clinical Psychology, 35,* 236–241.

Dodrill, C.B. (1986). Psychosocial consequences of epilepsy. In S.B. Filskov & T.J. Boll (Eds.), *Handbook of clinical neuropsychology* (Vol. 2). New York: Wiley.

Dodrill, C.B. (1988). Neuropsychology. In J. Laidlaw et al. (Eds.), *A textbook of epilepsy.* London: Churchill Livingstone.

Dodrill, C.B. (1992). Neuropsychological aspects of epilepsy. *Psychiatric Clinics of North America, 15,* 383–394.

Dodrill, C.B. (1997). Myths of neuropsychology. *The Clinical Neuropsychologist, 11,* 1–17.

Dodrill, C.B. (1999). Myths of neuropsychology: Further considerations. *The Clinical Neuropsychologist, 13,* 562–572.

Dodrill, C.B., Arnett, J.L., Shu, V., et al. (1998). Effects of tiagabine monotherapy on abilities, adjustment, and mood. *Epilepsia, 39,* 33–42.

Dodrill, C.B., Batzel, L.W., Queisser, H.R., & Temk, N.R. (1980). An objective method for the assessment of psychological and social problems among epileptics. *Epilepsia, 21,* 123–135.

Dodrill, C.B. & Temkin, N.R. (1989). Motor speed is a contaminating factor in evaluating the "cognitive" effects of phenytoin. *Epilepsia, 30,* 453–457.

Dodrill, C.B. & Thoreson, N.S. (1993). Reliability of the Lateral Dominance Examination. *Journal of Clinical and Experimental Neuropsychology, 15,* 183–190.

Dodrill, C.B., & Troupin, A.S. (1975). Effects of repeated administrations of a comprehensive neuropsychological battery among chronic epileptics. *Journal of Nervous and Mental Disease, 161,* 185–190.

Dodrill, C.B. & Troupin, A.S. (1991). Neuropsychological effects of carbamazepine and phenytoin: A reanalysis. *Neurology, 41,* 141–143.

Dodrill, C.B. & Wilkus, R.J. (1976). Relationships between intelligence and electroencephalographic epileptiform activity in adult epileptics. *Neurology, 26,* 525–531.

Dogulu, C., Kansu, T., & Karabudak, R. (1996). Alexia without agraphia in multiple sclerosis. *Journal of Neurology, Neurosurgery and Psychiatry, 61,* 528.

Dolan, R.J., Paulesu, E., & Fletcher, P. (1997). Human memory systems. In R.S.J. Frackowiak et al. (Eds.), *Human brain function.* San Diego: Academic Press.

Dollinger, S.M.C. (1995). Mental rotation performance: Age, sex, and visual field differences. *Developmental Neuropsychology, 11,* 215–222.

Dombovy, M.L. & Olek, A.C. (1996). Recovery and rehabilitation following traumatic brain injury. *Brain Injury, 11,* 305–318.

Donaghy, C.L., Chang, C.L., & Poulter, N. (2002). Duration, frequency, recency, and type of migraine and the risk of ischemic stroke in women of childbearing age. *Journal of Neurology, Neurosurgery and Psychiatry, 73,* 747–750.

Donaghy, M. (2002). *Brain's diseases of the nervous system* (12th ed.). New York: Oxford University Press.

Donaghy, S. & Williams, W. (1998). A new protocol for training severely impaired patients in the usage of memory journals. *Brain Injury, 12,* 1061–1076.

Donders, J. (1995). Validity of the Kaufman Brief Intelligence Test (K-BIT) in children with traumatic brain injury. *Assessment, 2,* 219–224.

Donders, J. (1998). Validity of the Kaufman Short Neuropsychological Assessment Procedure (KSNAP). *International Journal of Neuroscience, 94,* 275–286.

Donders, J. (1999). Specificity of a malingering formula for the Wisconsin Card Sorting Test. *Journal of Forensic Neuropsychology, 1,* 35–42.

Donders, J. & Kirsch, N. (1991). Nature and implications of selective impairment on the Booklet Category Test and Wisconsin Card Sorting Test. *The Clinical Neuropsychologist, 5,* 78–82.

Donders, J., Tulsky, D.S., & Zhu, J. (2001). Criterion validity of new WAIS-III subtest scores after traumatic brain injury. *Journal of the International Neuropsychological Society, 7,* 892–898.

Donnelly, E.F., Dent, J.K., Murphy, D.L., & Mignone, R.J. (1972). Comparison of temporal lobe epileptics and affective disorders on the Halstead-Reitan test battery. *Journal of Clinical Psychology, 28,* 61–62.

Doody, R.S., Massman, P., & Dunn, J.K. (2001). A method for estimating progression rates in Alzheimer disease. *Archives of Neurology, 58,* 449–454.

Dopson, W.G., Beckwith, B.E., Tucker, D.M., & Bullard-Bates, P.C. (1984). Asymmetry of facial expression in spontaneous emotion. *Cortex, 20,* 243–251.

Doraiswamy, P.M., Bieber, F., Kaiser, L., et al. (1997a). Memory, language, and praxis in Alzheimer's disease: Norms for outpatient clinical trial populations. *Psychopharmacology Bulletin, 33,* 123–128.

Doraiswamy, P.M., Bieber, F., Kaiser, L., et al. (1997b). The Alzheimer's Disease Assessment Scale: Patterns and predictors of baseline cognitive performance in multicenter Alzheimer's disease trials. *Neurology, 48,* 1511–1517.

Doraiswamy, P.M., Kaiser, L., Bieber, F., & Garman, R.L. (2001). The Alzheimer's Disease Assessment Scale: Evaluation of psychometric properties and patterns of cognitive decline in multicenter clinical trials of mild to moderate Alzheimer's disease. *Alzheimer Disease and Associated Disorders, 15,* 174–183.

Doraiswamy, P.M., Krishen, A., Stallone, F., et al. (1995). Cognitive performance on the Alzheimer's Disease Assessment Scale: Effect of education. *Neurology, 45,* 1980–1984.

Dörken, H., Jr. & Kral, V. A. (1952). The psychological differentiation of organic brain lesions and their localization by means of the Rorschach test. *American Journal of Psychiatry, 108,* 764–770.

Dornbush, R.L. & Kokkevi, A. (1976). Acute effects of cannabis on cognitive, perceptual, and motor performance in chronic hashish users. *Annals of the New York Academy of Sciences, 282,* 313–322.

Doss, R.C., Chelune, G.J., & Naugle, R.I. (1999). Victoria Symptom Validity Test: Compensation-seeking vs. non-compensation-seeking patients in a general clinical setting. *Journal of Forensic Neuropsychology, 1,* 5–20.

Doty, R.L. (1992). Diagnostic tests and assessment. *Journal of Head Trauma Rehabilitation, 7,* 47–65.

Doty, R.L. (2001). Olfaction. *Annual Review of Psychology, 52,* 423–452.

Doty, R.L., Applebaum, S., Zushos, H., & Settle, R.G. (1985). Sex differences in odor identification ability: A cross-cultural analysis. *Neuropsychologia, 23,* 667–672.

Doty, R.L. & Bromley, S.M. (2002). Smell. In A.K. Asbury et al. (Eds.), *Diseases of the nervous system* (3rd ed.). Cambridge: Cambridge University Press.

Doty, R.L., Li, C., Mannon, L.J., & Yousem, D. M. (1999). Olfactory dysfunction in multiple sclerosis: Relation to longitudinal changes in plaque numbers in central olfactory structures. *Neurology, 53,* 880–882.

Doty, R.L., Reyes, P.F., & Gregor, T. (1987). Presence of both odor identification and detection deficits in Alzheimer's disease. *Brain Research Bulletin, 18,* 597–600.

Doty, R.W. (1979). Neurons and memory: Some clues. In M.A.B. Brazier (Ed.), *Brain mechanisms in memory and learning: From the single neuron to man.* New York: Raven Press.

Doty, R.W. (1989). Some anatomical substrates of emotion, and their bihemispheric coordination. In G. Gainotti & C. Caltagirone (Eds.), *Emotions and the dual brain.* Heidelberg: Springer-Verlag.

Doty, R.W. (1990). Time and memory. In J.L. McGaugh et al. (Eds.), *Brain organization and memory: Cells, systems, and circuits.* New York: Oxford University Press.

Dow, R.S. (1988). Contribution of electrophysiological studies to cerebellar physiology. *Journal of Clinical Neurophysiology, 5,* 307–323.

Drachman, D.A. (1997). Aging and the brain: A new frontier. *Annals of Neurology, 42,* 8199–828.

Draelos, M.T., Jacobson, A.M., Weinger, K., et al. (1995). Cognitive function in patients with insulin-dependent diabetes mellitus during hyperglycemia and hypoglycemia. *American Journal of Medicine, 98,* 135–144.

Drake, A.I. & Hannay, H.J. (1992). Continuous recognition memory tests: Are the assumptions of the theory of signal detection met? *Journal of Clinical and Experimental Neuropsychology, 14,* 539–544.

Drane, D.L., Loring, D.W., Lee, G.P., & Meador, K.J. (1998). Trial-length sensitivity of the Verbal Selective Reminding Test to lateralized temporal lobe impairment. *The Clinical Neuropsychologist, 12,* 68–73.

Drane, D.L. & Osato, S.S. (1997). Using the Neurobehavioral Cognitive Status Examination as a screening measure for older adults. *Archives of Clinical Neuropsychology, 12,* 139–143.

Draper, B., MacCuspie-Moore, C., & Brodaty, H. (1998). Suicidal ideation and the "wish to die" in dementia patients: The role of depression. *Age and Ageing, 27,* 503–507.

Dresser, A.C., Meirowsky, A.M., Weiss, G.H., et al. (1973). Gainful employment following head injury. *Archives of Neurology, 29,* 111–116.

Dressler, W.U., Wodak, R., & Pleh, C. (1990). Gender-specific discourse differences in aphasia. In Y. Joanette & H.H. Brownell (Eds.), *Discourse ability and brain damage. Theoretical and empirical perspectives.* New York: Springer-Verlag.

Drew, R.H. & Templer, D.I. (1992). Contact sports. In D.I. Templer et al. (Eds.), *Preventable brain damage: brain vulnerability and brain health.* New York: Springer.

Drew, R.H., Templer, D.I., Schuyler, B.A., et al. (1986). Neuropsychological deficits in active licensed professional boxers. *Journal of Clinical Psychology, 42,* 520–525.

Drewe, E.A. (1974). The effect of type and area of brain lesions on Wisconsin Card Sorting Test performance. *Cortex, 10,* 159–170.

Dronkers, N.F., Redfern, B.B., & Knight, R.T. (2000). The neural architecture of language disorders. In M.S. Gazzaniga (Ed.), *The new cognitive neurosciences* (2nd ed.). Cambridge, MA: The MIT Press.

Dropcho, E.J. (2002). Remote neurologic manifestations of cancer. *Neurologic Clinics, 20,* 85–122.

Druks, J. & Masterson, J. (1999). *An Object and Action Naming Battery.* Levittown, PA: Psychology Press.

Drummond, A.E.R. (1988). Stroke: The impact on the family. *British Journal of Occupational Therapy, 51,* 193–194.

Dubas, F., Gray, F., & Escourolle, R. (1983). [Steele-Richardson-Olszewski disease without ophthalmoplegia. 6 clinico-anatomic cases]. *Revue Neurologique, 139,* 407–416.

Dubois, B., Boller, F., Pillon, B., & Agid, Y. (1991). Cognitive deficits in Parkinson's disease. In F. Boller & J. Grafman (Eds.), *Handbook of neuropsychology* (Vol. 5). Amsterdam: Elsevier.

Dubois, B., Levy, R., Verin, M., et al. (1995). Experimental approach to prefrontal functions in humans. *Annals of the New York Academy of Sciences, 769,* 41–60.

Dubois, B. & Pillon, B. (1992). Biochemical correlates of cognitive changes and dementia in Parkinson's disease. In S.J. Huber & J.L. Cummings (Eds.), *Parkinson's disease: Neurobehavioral aspects.* New York: Oxford University Press.

Dubois, B., Pillon, B., Legault, F., et al. (1988). Slowing of cognitive processing in progressive supranuclear palsy. *Archives of Neurology, 45,* 1194–1199.

Dubois, B., Pillon, B., & Sirigu, A. (1994). Fonctions intégratrices et cortex préfrontal chez l'homme. In X. Seron & M. Jeannerod (Eds.), *Neuropsychologie humaine.* Liège, Belgium: Pierre Mardaga.

Dubois, B., Pillon, B., Sternic, N., et al. (1990). Age-induced cognitive deficit in Parkinson's disease. *Neurology, 40,* 38–41.

Dubois, B., Slachevsky, A., Litvan, I., & Pillon, B. (2000). The FAB: A Frontal Assessment Battery at bedside. *Neurology, 55,* 1621–1626.

Ducarne, B. & Pillon, B. (1974). La copie de la figure complexe de Rey dans les troubles visuo-constructifs. *Journal de Psychologie, 4,* 449–470.

Duclos, P.J. & Sanderson, L.M. (1990). An epidemiological description of lightning-related deaths in the United States. *International Journal of Epidemiology, 19,* 673–679.

Dudai, Y. (1989). *The neurobiology of memory. Concepts, findings, trends.* New York: Oxford University Press.

Duff, K. & McCaffery, R.J. (2001). Electrical injury and lightning injury: A review of their mechanisms and neuropsychological, psychiatric, and neurological sequelae. *Neuropsychology Review, 11,* 101–116.

Duffy, F.H., Albert, M.S., McAnulty, G., & Garvey, A.J. (1984). Age-related differences in brain electrical activity of healthy subjects. *Annals of Neurology, 16,* 430–438.

Duffy, F.H., Iyer, V.G., & Surwillo, W.W. (1989). *Clinical electroencephalography and topographic brain mapping.* New York: Springer-Verlag.

Duffy, R.J. & Duffy, J.R. (1989). An investigation of body part as object (BPO) responses in normal and brain-damaged adults. *Brain and Cognition, 10,* 220–236.

Dugbartey, A.T., Sanchez, P.N., Rosenbaum, J.K., et al. (1999). WAIS-III Matrix Reasoning Test performance in a mixed clinical sample. *The Clinical Neuropsychologist, 13,* 396–404.

Dujardin, K., Krystkowiak, P., Defebvre, L., et al. (2000). A case of severe dysexecutive syndrome consecutive to chronic bilateral pallidal stimulation. *Neuropsychologia, 38,* 1305–1315.

Duke, L.M. & Kaszniak, A.W. (2000). Executive control functions in degenerative dementias: A comparative review. *Neuropsychology Review, 10,* 75–99.

Duley, J.F., Wilkins, J.W., Hamby, S.L., et al. (1993). Explicit scoring criteria for the Rey-Osterreith and Taylor Complex Figures. *The Clinical Neuropsychologist, 7,* 29–38.

Dumont, C., Ska, B., & Joanette, Y. (2000). Conceptual apraxia and semantic memory deficit in Alzheimer's disease: Two sides of the same coin? *Journal of the International Neuropsychological Society, 6,* 693–703.

Duncan, D. & Snow, W.G. (1987). Base rates in neuropsychology. *Professional Psychology, 18,* 368–170.

Duncan, J., Seitz, R.J., Kolodny, J., et al. (2000). A neural basis for general intelligence. *Science, 289,* 457–460.

Dunham, M.D. & Johnstone, B. (1999). Variability of neuropsychological deficits associated with carbon monoxide poisoning: four case reports. *Brain Injury, 13,* 917–925.

Dunn, L.M. & Dunn, E.S. (1981). *Peabody Picture Vocabulary Test–Revised. Technical Supplement.* Circle Pines, MN: American Guidance Service.

Dunn, L.M. & Dunn, L.M. (1997). *Peabody Picture Vocabulary Test-III.* Circle Pines, MN: American Guidance Service.

Dunn, V.K. & Sacco, W.P. (1989). Psychometric evaluation of the Geriatric Depression Scale and the Zung Self-rating Depression Scale using an elderly community sample. *Psychology and Aging, 4,* 125–126.

Dunwoody, L., Tittmar, H.G., & McClean, W.S. (1996). Grip strength and intertrial rest. *Perceptual and Motor Skills, 83,* 275–278.

Durston, S., Thomas, K.M., Worden, M.S., et al., (2002). The effect of preceding context on inhibition: An event-related fMRI study. *Neuroimage, 16,* 449–453.

Dustman, R.E., Emmerson, R.Y., Ruhling, R.O., et al. (1990). Age and fitness effects on EEG, ERP's, visual sensitivity, and cognition. *Neurobiology of Aging, 11,* 193–200.

Dustman, R.E., Emmerson, R.Y., & Shearer, D.E. (1990). Electrophysiology and aging: Slowing, inhibition, and aerobic fitness. In M.L. Howe, M.J. Stones, & C.J. Brainerd (Eds.), *Cognitive and behavioral performance factors in atypical aging.* New York: Springer-Verlag.

Dustman, R.E., Emmerson, R.Y., Steinhaus, L.A., et al. (1992). The effects of videogame playing on neuropsychological performance of elderly individuals. *Journal of Gerontology, 47,* 168–171.

Dustman, R.E., Ruhling, R.O., Russell, E.M., et al. (1984). Aerobic exercise training and improved neuropsychological function of older individuals. *Neurobiology of Aging, 5,* 35–42.

Duvoisin, R.C. (1992). Clinical diagnosis. In I. Litvan, & Y. Agid (Eds.), *Progressive supranuclear palsy: Clinical and research approaches.* New York: Oxford University Press.

Duvoisin, R.C., Eldridge, R., Williams, A., et al. (1981). Twin study of Parkinson disease. *Neurology, 31,* 77–80.

Duyao, M., Ambrose, C., Myers, R., et al. (1993). Trinucleotide repeat length instability and age of onset in Huntington's disease. *Nature Genetics, 4,* 387–392.

Dvorine, I. (1953). *Dvorine Pseudo-Isochromatic Plates* (2nd ed.). Baltimore: Waverly Press.

Dyer, F.N. (1973). The Stroop phenomenon and its use in the study of perceptual, cognitive, and response processes. *Memory and Cognition, 1,* 106–120.

Dykens, E.M., Rosner, B.A., & Ly, T.M. (2001). Drawings by individuals with Williams syndrome: Are people different than shapes? *American Journal on Mental Retardation, 106,* 94–107.

Dymek, M.P., Atchison, P., Harrell, L., & Marson, D.C. (2001). Competency to consent to medical treatment in cognitively impaired patients with Parkinson's disease. *Neurology, 56,* 17–24.

Dywan, J., Segalowitz, S.J., & Unsal, A. (1992). Speed of information processing, health, and cognitive performance in older adults. *Developmental Neuropsychology, 8,* 473–490.

Eadie, K. & Shum, D. (1995). Assessment of visual memory: A comparison of Chinese characters and geometric figures as stimulus materials. *Journal of Clinical and Experimental Neuropsychology, 17,* 731–739.

Eames, P. Haffey, W.J., & Cope, D.N. (1990). Treatment of behavioral disorders. In M. Rosenthal et al. (Eds.), *Rehabilitation of the adult and child with traumatic brain injury* (2nd ed.). Philadelphia: Davis.

Earnst, K.S., Wadley, V.G., Aldridge, T.M., et al. (2001). Loss of financial capacity in Alzheimer's disease: The role of working memory. *Aging, Neuropsychology and Cognition, 8,* 109–119.

Eastwood, M.R., Lautenschlaeger, E., & Corbin, S. (1983). A comparison of clinical methods for assessing dementia. *Journal of the American Geriatrics Society, 31,* 342–347.

Ebers, G. & Sadovnick, A.D. (1998). Epidemiology. In D.W. Paty & G. Ebers (Eds.), *Multiple sclerosis.* Philadelphia: Davis.

Echemendia, R.J. & Cantu, R.C. (2003). Return to play following sports-related mild traumatic brain injury: The role for neuropsychology. *Applied Neuropsychology, 10,* 48–55.

Echemendia, R.J. & Julian, L.J. (2001). Mild traumatic brain injury in sports: Neuropsychology's contribution to a developing field. *Neuropsychology Review, 11,* 69–88.

Echemendia, R.J., Lovell, M., & Barth, J. (2003). Neuropsychological assessment of sport-related mild traumatic brain injury. In G.P. Prigatano & N.H. Pliskin (Eds.), *Clinical neuropsychology and cost outcome research: A beginning.* New York: Psychology Press.

Eckert, G.P., Cairns, N.J., Maras, A., et al. (2000). Cholesterol modulates the membrane-disordering effects of beta-amyloid peptides in the hippocampus: Specific changes in Alzheimer's disease. *Dementia and Geriatric Cognitive Disorders, 11,* 181–186.

Edelman, G.M. (1989). *The remembered present: A biological theory of consciousness.* New York: Basic Books.

Edgeworth, J., Robertson, I., & McMillan, T. (1998). *The Balloons Test.* Bury St. Edmunds, UK: Thames Valley Test.

Edmans, J.A. & Lincoln, N.B. (1989). The frequency of perceptual deficits after stroke. *British Journal of Occupational Therapy, 52,* 266–270.

Edmans, J.A., Towle, D., & Lincoln, N.B. (1991). The recovery of perceptual problems after stroke and the impact on daily life. *Clinical Rehabilitation, 5,* 301–309.

Edwards-Lee, T., Miller, B.L., Benson, D.F., et al. (1997). The temporal variant of frontotemporal dementia. *Brain, 120,* 1027–1040.

Efron, R. & Crandall, P.H. (1983). Central auditory processing. II. Effects of anterior temporal lobectomy. *Brain and Language, 19,* 237–253.

Efron, R., Crandall, P.H., Koss, B., et al. (1983). Central auditory processing. III. The "cocktail party" effect and anterior temporal lobectomy. *Brain and Language, 19,* 254–263.

Egelko, S., Gordon, W.A., Hibbard, M.R., et al. (1988). Relationship among CT scans, neurological exam, and neuropsychological test performance in right brain-damaged stroke patient. *Journal of Clinical and Experimental Neuropsychology, 10,* 539–564.

Egelko, S., Simon, D., Riley, E., et al. (1989). First year after stroke: Tracking cognitive and affective deficits. *Archives of Physical Medical Rehabilitation, 70,* 297–302.

Ehrenreich, J.H. (1995). Normative data for adults on a short form of the Selective Reminding Test. *Psychological Reports, 76,* 387–390.

Eichenbaum, H. & Cohen, N.J. (2001). *From conditioning to conscious recollection. Memory systems of the brain.* New York: Oxford University Press.

Eichorn, D.H. (1975). The Raven Progressive Matrices (review). In W.K. Frankenburg & B.W. Camp (Eds.), *Pediatric screening tests.* Springfield, IL: Thomas.

Einstein, G.O. & McDaniel, M.A. (1990). Normal aging and prospective memory. *Journal of Experimental Psychology: Learning, Memory, and Cognition, 16,* 717–726.

Einstein, G.O., McDaniel, M.A., Richardson, S.L., et al. (1995). Aging and prospective memory: Examining the influences of self-initiated retrieval processes. *Journal of Experimental Psychology: Learning, Memory, and Cognition, 21,* 996–1007.

Einstein, G.O., Smith, R.E., McDaniel, M.A., & Shaw, P. (1997). Aging and prospective memory: The influence of increased task demands at encoding and retrieval. *Psychology and Aging, 12,* 479–488.

Eisdorfer, C. (1977). Stress, disease and cognitive change in the aged. In C. Eisdorfer & R.O. Friedel (Eds.), *Cognitive and emotional disturbance in the elderly.* Chicago: Year Book.

Eisdorfer, C. & Cohen, D. (1980). Diagnostic criteria for primary neuronal degeneration of the Alzheimer's type. *Journal of Family Practice, 11,* 553–557.

Eisenberg, H.M. (1985). Outcome after head injury. Part I: General considerations. In D.P. Becker & J.T. Povlishock (Eds.), *Central nervous system trauma. Status report.* Washington, D.C.: National Institutes of Health.

Ekberg, K. & Hane, M. (1984). Test battery for investigating functional disorders—the TUFF battery. *Scandinavian Journal of Work, Environment and Health, 10,* 14–17.

Ekman, P. & Friesen, W.V. (1975). *Pictures of facial affect.* Palo Alto, CA: Consulting Psychologists Press.

Ekstrom, R. B., French, J. W., Harman, H. H., & Dermen, D. (1976). *Manual for Kit of Factor–referenced cognitive tests.* Princeton, NJ: Educational Testing Service.

El-Awar, M., Becker, J.T., Hammond, K.M., et al. (1987). Learning deficit in Parkinson's disease. *Archives of Neurology, 44,* 180–184.

Eldad, A., Neuman, A., Weinberg, A., et al. (1992). Late onset of extensive brain damage and hypertension in a patient with high-voltage electrical burns. *Journal of Burn Care Rehabilitation, 13,* 214–217.

Elfgren, C., Passant, U., & Risberg, J. (1993). Neuropsychological findings in frontal lobe dementia. *Dementia, 4,* 214–219.

Elgerot, A. (1976). Note on selective effects of short-term tobacco abstinence on complex versus simple mental tasks. *Perceptual and Motor Skills, 42,* 413–414.

Elias, M.F., Elias, P.K., D'Agostino, R.B., et al. (1997). Role of age education, and gender on cognitive performance in the Framingham Heart Study: community-based norms. *Experimental Aging Research, 23,* 201–235.

Elias, M.F., Podraza, A.M., Pierce, T.W., & Robbins, M.A. (1990). Determining neuropsychological cut scores for older, healthy adults. *Experimental Aging Research, 16,* 209–220.

Elias, M.F., Schultz, N.R., Jr., Robbins, M.A., & Elias, P.K. (1989). A longitudinal study of neuropsychological performance by hypertensives and normotensives: A third measurement point. *Journal of Gerontology: Psychological Sciences, 44,* P25–P28.

Elias, P.K., Elias, M.F., D'Agostino, R.B., et al. (1997). NIDDM and blood pressure as risk factors for poor cognitive performance. The Framingham Study. *Diabetes Care, 20,* 1388–1395.

Eliason, M.R. & Topp, B.W. (1984). Predictive validity of Rappaport's Disability Rating Scale in subjects with acute brain dysfunction. *Physical Therapy, 64,* 1357–1360.

Ellenberg, J.H., Levin, H.S., & Saydjari, C. (1996). Posttraumatic amnesia as a predictor of outcome after severe closed head injury. *Archives of Neurology, 53,* 782–791.

Elliott, M.L. & Biever, L.S. (1996). Head injury and sexual dysfunction. *Brain Injury, 10,* 703–717.

Ellis, A.W. (1982). Spelling and writing. In A.W. Ellis (Ed.), *Normality and pathology in cognitive functions.* London: Academic Press.

Ellis, A. W., Kay, J., & Franklin, S. (1992). Anomia: Differentiating between semantic and phonological deficits. In D.I. Margolin (Ed.), *Cognitive neuropsychology in clinical practice*. New York: Oxford University Press.

Ellis, D.W. & Zahn, B.S. (1985). Psychological functioning after severe closed head injury. *Journal of Personality Assessment, 49*, 125–128.

Ellis, H.D. (1992). Assessment of deficits in facial processing. In J. Crawford et al. (Eds.), *A handbook of neuropsychological assessment*. Hove, UK: Erlbaum.

Ellis, S.J., Ellis, P.J., & Marshall, E. (1988). Hand preference in a normal population. *Cortex, 24*, 157–163.

Elwood, R. W. (1991). Factor structure of the Wechsler Memory Scale Revised (WMS-R) in a clinical sample: A methodological reappraisal. *The Clinical Neuropsychologist, 5*, 329–337.

Elwood, R.W. (1995). The California Verbal Learning Test: Psychometric characteristics and clinical application. *Neuropsychology Review, 5*, 173–201.

Elwood, R.W. (1997). Episodic and semantic memory components of verbal paired-associate learning. *Assessment, 4*, 73–77.

Emery, O.B. (2000). Language impairment in dementia of the Alzheimer type: A hierarchical decline? *International Journal of Psychiatry in Medicine, 30*, 145–164.

Emery, O.B. & Breslau, L.D. (1989). Language deficits in depression: Comparisons with SDAT and normal aging. *Journal of Gerontology, 44*, M85–M92.

Engberg, A.W. & Teasdale, T.W. (2001). Traumatic brain injury in Denmark 1979–1996. A national study of incidence and mortality. *European Journal of Epidemiology, 17*, 437–442.

Engelborghs, S. & De Deyn, P.P. (1997). The neurochemistry of Alzheimer's disease. *Acta Neurologica Belgica, 97*, 67–84.

Engert, F. & Bonhoeffer, T. (1999). Dendritic spine changes associated with hippocampal long-term synaptic plasticity. *Nature, 399*, 66–70.

Enoch, M.A., White, K.V., Harris, C.R., et al. (2001). Alcohol use disorders and anxiety disorders: Relation to the p300 event-related potential. *Alcoholism: Clinical and Experimental Research, 25*, 1293–1300.

Epstein, C.M., Meador, K.J., Loring, D.W., et al. (1999). Localization and characterization of speech arrest during transcranial magnetic stimulation. *Clinical Neurophysiology, 110*, 1073–1079.

Epstein, J.N., Johnson, D.E., Varia, I.M., & Conners, C.K. (2001). Neuropsychological assessment of response inhibition in adults with ADHD. *Journal of Clinical and Experimental Neuropsychology, 23*, 362–371.

Erber, J. T., Botwinick, J., & Storandt, M. (1981). The impact of memory on age differences in Digit Symbol performance. *Journal of Gerontology, 36*, 586–590.

Ericsson, K., Hillerås, P., Holmèn, K., et al. (1994). The short human figure drawing scale for the evaluation of suspect cognitive dysfunction in old age. *Archives of Gerontology and Geriatrics, 19*, 243–251.

Ericsson, K., Winblad, B., & Nilsson, L.-G. (2001). Human-figure drawing and memory functioning across the adult life span. *Archives of Gerontology and Geriatrics, 32*, 151–166.

Erickson, R.C. & Howieson, D. (1986). The clinician's perspective: Measuring change and treatment effectiveness. In L.W. Poon (Ed.), *Handbook for clinical memory assessment of older adults*. Washington, D.C.: American Psychological Association.

Erickson, R.C. & Scott, M.L. (1977). Clinical memory testing: A review. *Psychological Bulletin, 84*, 1130–1149.

Eriksson, P.S., Perfilieva, E., Bjork-Eriksson, T., et al. (1998). Neurogenesis in the adult human hippocampus. *Nature Medicine, 4*, 1313–1317.

Erkinjuntti, T., Hokkanen, L., Sulkava, R., & Palo, J. (1988). The Blessed Dementia Scale as a screening test for dementia. *International Journal of Geriatric Psychiatry, 3*, 267–273.

Erlanger, D.M., Kutner, K.C., Barth, J.T., & Barnes, R. (1999). Neuropsychology of sports-related head injury: Dementia pugilistica to post concussion syndrome. *The Clinical Neuropsychologist, 13*, 193–209.

Erngrund, K., Mantyla, T., & Nilsson, L.G. (1996). Adult age differences in source recall: A population-based study. *Journals of Gerontology. Series B, Psychological Sciences and Social Sciences, 51*, 335–345.

Ernst, J. (1987). Neuropsychological problem-solving skills in the elderly. *Psychology and Aging, 2*, 363–365.

Ernst, J. (1988). Language, grip strength, sensory-perceptual, and receptive skills in a normal elderly sample. *The Clinical Neuropsychologist, 2*, 30–40.

Ernst, J., Warner, M.H., Townes, B.D., et al. (1987). Age group differences on neuropsychological battery performance in a neuropsychiatric population. *Archives of Clinical Neuropsychology, 2*, 1–12.

Errebo-Knudsen, E.O. & Olsen, F. (1986). Organic solvents and presenile dementia (the painters' syndrome): A critical review of the Danish literature. *Science of the Total Environment, 48*, 45–67.

Errico, A.L., Nixon, S.J., Parsons, O.A., & Tassey, J. (1990). Screening for neuropsychological impairment in alcoholics. *Psychological Assessment, 2*, 45–50.

Escalona, E., Yanes, L., Feo, O., & Maizlish, N. (1995). Neurobehavioral evaluation of Venezuelan workers exposed to organic solvent mixtures. *American Journal of Industrial Medicine, 27*, 15–27.

Esiri, M.M. & Wilcock, G.K. (1984). The olfactory bulbs in Alzheimer's disease. *Journal of Neurology, Neurosurgery and Psychiatry, 47*, 56–60.

Eskandar, E.N., Cosgrove, G.R., & Shinobu, L.A. (2001). Surgical treatment of Parkinson disease. *Journal of the American Medical Association, 286*, 3056–3059.

Eskelinen, L., Luisto, M., Tenkanen, L., & Mattei, O. (1986). Neuropsychological methods in the differentiation of organic solvent intoxication from certain neurological conditions. *Journal of Clinical and Experimental Neuropsychology, 8*, 239–256.

Eskenazi, B., Cain, W.S., Novelly, R.A., & Mattson, R. (1986). Odor perception in temporal lobe epilepsy patients with and without temporal lobectomy. *Neuropsychologia, 24, 553–562*.

Eskenazi, B. & Maizlish, W.A. (1988). Effects of occupational exposure to chemicals in neurobehavioral functioning. In R.E. Tarter, D.H. Van Thiel, & K.L. Edwards (Eds.), *Medical neuropsychology*. New York: Plenum Press.

Eslinger, P.J. (1998a). Autobiographical memory after temporal lobe lesions. *Neurocase, 4*, 481–495.

Eslinger, P.J. (1998b). Neurological and neuropsychological bases of empathy. *European Neurology, 39*, 193–199.

Eslinger, P.J. (1999a). Orbital frontal cortex: Behavioral and physiological significance. *Neurocase, 5*, 299–300.

Eslinger, P.J. (1999b). Orbital frontal cortex: Historical and contemporary views about its behavioral and physiological significance. *Neurocase, 5*, 225–229.

Eslinger, P.J. & Benton, A.L. (1983). Visuoperceptual performances in aging and dementia: Clinical and theoretical implications. *Journal of Clinical Neuropsychology, 5*, 213–220.

Eslinger, P.J. & Damasio, A.R. (1981). Age and type of aphasia in patients with stroke. *Journal of Neurology and Psychiatry, 44*, 377–381.

Eslinger, P.J. & Damasio, A.R. (1986). Preserved motor learning in Alzheimer's disease: Implications for anatomy and behavior. *Journal of Neuroscience, 6*, 3006–3009.

Eslinger, P.J., Damasio, A.R., & Benton, A.L. (1984). *The Iowa screening battery for mental decline.* Iowa City: University of Iowa.

Eslinger, P.J., Damasio, A.R., Benton, A.L., & Van Allen, M. (1985). Neuropsychologic detection of abnormal mental decline in older persons. *Journal of the American Medical Association, 253,* 670–674.

Eslinger, P.J., Damasio, A.R. & Van Hoesen, G.W. (1982). Olfactory dysfunction in man: Anatomical and behavioral aspects. *Brain and Cognition, 1,* 259–285.

Eslinger, P.J. & Geddes, L. (2001). Behavioral and emotional changes after focal frontal lobe damage. In J. Bogousslavsky and J.L. Cummings (Eds.), *Disorders of behavior and mood in focal brain lesions.* New York: Cambridge University Press.

Eslinger, P.J. & Grattan, L.M. (1990). Influence of organizational strategy on neuropsychological performance in frontal lobe patients [abstract]. *Journal of Clinical and Experimental Neuropsychology, 12,* 54.

Eslinger, P.J. & Grattan, L.M. (1993). Frontal lobe and frontal-striatal substrates for different forms of human cognitive flexibility. *Neuropsychologia, 31,* 17–28.

Eslinger, P.J., Grattan, L.M., & Geder, L. (1995). Impact of frontal lobe lesions on rehabilitation and recovery from acute brain injury. *Neurorehabilitation, 5,* 161–182.

Eslinger, P.J., Parkinson, K., & Shamay, S.G. (2002). Empathy and social-emotional factors in recovery from stroke. *Current Opinion in Neurology, 15,* 91–97.

Eslinger, P.J., Pepin, L., & Benton, A.L. (1988). Different patterns of visual memory errors occur with aging and dementia [abstract]. *Journal of Clinical and Experimental Neuropsychology, 10,* 60–61.

Eslinger, P.J. & Reichwein, R.K. (2001). Frontal lobe stroke syndromes. In J. Bogousslavsky & L.R. Caplan (Eds.), *Stroke syndromes* (2nd ed.). Cambridge, UK: Cambridge University Press.

Eson, M.E., Yen, J.K., & Bourke, R.S. (1978). Assessment of recovery from serious head injury. *Journal of Neurology, Neurosurgery, and Psychiatry, 41,* 1036–1042.

Espino, D.V., Lichtenstein, M.J., Palmer, R.F., & Hazuda, H.P. (2001). Ethnic differences in Mini-Mental State Examination (MMSE) scores: Where you live makes a difference. *Journal of the American Geriatric Society, 49,* 538–548.

Espinosa-Fernandez, L., Miro, E., Cano, M., & Buela-Casal, G. (2003). Age-related changes and gender differences in time estimation. *Acta Psychologica, 112,* 221–232.

Esposito, G., Kirkby, B.S., Van Horn, J.D., et al. (1999). Context-dependent, neural system-specific neurophysiological concomitants of ageing: Mapping PET correlates during cognitive activation. *Brain, 122,* 963–979.

Esposito, G., Van Horn, J.D., Weinberger, D.R., & Berman, K.F. (1996). Gender differences in cerebral blood flow as a function of cognitive state with PET. *Journal of Nuclear Medicine, 37,* 559–564.

Esquivel, G.B. (1984). Coloured Progressive Matrices. In D.J. Keyser & R.C. Sweetland (Eds.), *Test critiques* (Vol. I). Kansas City, MO: Test Corporation of America.

Essman, W.B. (1987). Perspectives for nutrients and brain functions. In W.B. Essman (Ed.), *Nutrients and brain function.* Basel: Karger.

Esteban-Santillan, C., Praditsuwan, R., Ueda, H., & Geldmacher, D.S. (1998). Clock drawing in very mild Alzheimer's disease. *Journal of the American Geriatric Society, 46,* 1266–1269.

Estes, W. K. (1974). Learning theory and intelligence. *American Psychologist, 29,* 740–749.

Estol, C.J. (2001). Headache: Stroke symptoms and signs. In J. Bogousslavsky & L.R. Caplan (Eds.), *Stroke syndromes* (2nd ed.). Cambridge, UK: Cambridge University Press.

Etcoff, L.M. & Kampfer, K.M. (1996). Practical guidelines in the use of symptom validity and other psychological tests to measure malingering and symptom exaggeration in traumatic brain injury cases. *Neuropsychology Review, 6,* 171–201.

Etcoff, N.L. (1986). The neuropsychology of emotional expression. In G. Goldstein & R.E. Tarter (Eds.), *Advances in clinical neuropsychology* (Vol. 3). New York: Plenum Press.

Ettlin, T.M., Staehelin, H.B., Kischka, U., et al. (1989). Computed tomography, electroencephalography, and clinical features in the differential diagnosis of senile dementia. *Archives of Neurology, 46,* 1217–1220.

Eubanks, J. (1997). Clinical neuropsychology summary information prepared by Division 40, Clinical Neuropsychology, American Psychological Association. *The Clinical Neuropsychologist, 11,* 77–80.

Eustace, A., Coen, R., Walsh, C., et al. (2002). A longitudinal evaluation of behavioural and psychological symptoms of probable Alzheimer's disease. *International Journal of Geriatric Psychiatry, 17,* 968–973.

Eustache, F., Desgranges, B., Giffard, B., et al. (2001). Entorhinal cortex disruption causes memory deficit in early Alzheimer's disease as shown by PET. *Neuroreport, 12,* 683–685.

Eustache, F., Rioux, P., Desgranges, B., et al. (1995). Healthy aging, memory subsystems and regional cerebral oxygen consumption. *Neuropsychologia, 33,* 867–887.

Evans, D.A., Beckett, L.A., Albert, M.S., et al. (1993). Level of education and change in cognitive function in a community population of older persons. *Annals of Epidemiology, 3,* 71–77.

Evans, D.A., Funkenstein, H.H., Albert, M.S., et al. (1989). Prevalence of Alzheimer's disease in a community population of older persons. *Journal of the American Medical Association, 262,* 2551–2556.

Evans, F.J. (1978). Monitoring attention deployment by random number generation: An index to measure subject randomness. *Bulletin of the Psychonomic Society, 12,* 35–38.

Evans, J.J., Breen, E.K., Antoun, N., & Hodges, J.R. (1996). Focal retrograde amnesia for autobiographical events following cerebral vasculitis: A connectionist account. *Neurocase, 2,* 1–11.

Evans, J.J., Emslie, H., & Wilson, B.A. (1998). External cueing systems in the rehabilitation of executive impairments of action. *Journal of the International Neuropsychological Society, 4,* 399–408.

Evans, R.W. (1992). Some observations on whiplash inquiries. *Neurologic Clinics, 10,* 975–997.

Evans, R.W. (1996a). Diagnostic testing for the evaluation of headaches. *Neurologic Clinics, 14,* 1–26.

Evans, R.W. (1996b). Postconcussion syndrome and whiplash injuries. In R.K. Narayan et al. (Eds.), *Neurotrauma.* New York: McGraw-Hill.

Evans, R.W., Ruff, R.M., & Gualtieri, C.T. (1985). Verbal fluency and figural fluency in bright children. *Perceptual and Motor Skills, 61,* 699–709.

Evans, W.J. & Starr, A. (1994). Electroencephalography and evoked potentials in the elderly. In M.L. Albert & J.E. Knoefel (Eds.), *Clinical neurology of aging* (2nd ed.). New York: Oxford University Press.

Evatt, M.L., DeLong, M.R., & Vitek, J.L. (2002). Parkinson's disease. In A.K. Asbury et al. (Eds.), *Diseases of the nervous system* (3rd ed.). Cambridge, UK: Cambridge University Press.

Eviatar, Z., Hellige, J.B., & Zaidel, E. (1997). Individual differences in lateralization: Effects of gender and handedness. *Neuropsychology, 11,* 562–576.

Ewert, J., Levin, H.S., Watson, M.G., & Kalisky, Z. (1989). Procedural memory during posttraumatic amnesia in survivors of severe closed head injury. *Archives of Neurology, 46,* 911–916.

Ewing, R., McCarthy, D., Gronwall, D., & Wrightson, P. (1980). Persisting effects of minor head injury observable during hypoxic stress. *Journal of Clinical Neuropsychology, 2,* 147–155.

Exner, J.E., Jr. (1993). *The Rorschach: A comprehensive system. Basic foundations* (Vol. 1, 3rd ed.). New York: Wiley.

Exner, J.E., Jr., Colligan, S.C., Boll, T.J., et al. (1996). Rorschach findings concerning closed head injury patients. *Assessment,* 317–326.

Eysenck, M.W. (1991). Anxiety and cognitive functioning: A multifaceted approach. In R.G. Lister & H.J. Weingartner (Eds.), *Perspectives of cognitive neuroscience.* New York: Oxford University Press.

Ezrachi, O., Ben-Yishay, Y., Kay, T., et al. (1991). Predicting employment in traumatic brain injury following neuropsychological rehabilitation. *Journal of Head Trauma Rehabilitation, 6,* 71–84.

Fabbro, F. (1999). *The neurolinguistics of bilingualism.* Hove, UK: Psychology Press.

Faber-Langendoen, K., Morris, J.C., Knesevich, J.W., et al. (1988). Aphasia in senile dementia of the Alzheimer type. *Annals of Neurology, 23,* 365–370.

Fabian, M.S., Jenkins, R.L., & Parsons, O.A. (1981). Gender, alcoholism, and neuropsychological functioning. *Journal of Consulting and Clinical Psychology, 49,* 138–140.

Fabiani, M. & Friedman, D. (1997). Dissociations between memory for temporal order and recognition memory in aging. *Neuropsychologia, 35,* 129–141.

Fabrigoule, C., Rouch, I., Taberly, A., et al. (1998). Cognitive process in preclinical phase of dementia. *Brain, 121,* 135–141.

Fabry, J.J. (1980). Depression. In R.H. Woody (Ed.), *Encyclopedia of Clinical Assessment* (Vol. 2). San Francisco: Jossey-Bass.

Faglioni, P., Bertolani, L., Botti, C., & Merelli, E. (2000). Verbal learning strategies in patients with multiple sclerosis. *Cortex, 36,* 243–263.

Fahn, S., Elton, R.I., et al. (1987). Unified Parkinson's disease rating scale. In S. Fahn et al. (Eds.), *Recent developments in Parkinson's disease.* Florham Park, NJ: Macmillan Health Care Information.

Falicki, Z. & Sep-Kowalik, B. (1969). Psychic disturbances as a result of cardiac arrest. *Polish Medical Journal, 8,* 200–206.

Fallgatter, A.J. & Strik, W.K. (1998). Frontal brain activation during the Wisconsin Card Sorting Test assessed with two-channel near-infrared spectroscopy. *European Archives of Psychiatry and Clinical Neuroscience, 248,* 245–249.

Fallon, B.A., Das, S., Plutchok, J.J., et al. (1997). Functional brain imaging and neuropsychological testing in Lyme disease. *Clinical Infectious Diseases, 25,* S57–S63.

Fallon, B.A., Nields, J.A., Burrascano, J.J., et al. (1992). The neuropsychiatric manifestations of Lyme borreliosis. *Psychiatric Quarterly, 63,* 95–117.

Fals-Stewart, W. (1996). Intermediate length neuropsychological screening of impairment among psychoactive substance-abusing patients: A comparison of two batteries. *Journal of Substance Abuse, 8,* 1–17.

Fals-Stewart, W. (1997). Detection of neuropsychological impairment among substance-abusing patients: Accuracy of the Neurobehavioral Cognitive Status Examination. *Experimental and Clinical Psychopharmacology, 5,* 269–276.

Fama, R., Shear, P.K., Marsh, L., et al. (2001). Remote memory for public figures in Alzheimer's disease: Relationships to regional cortical and limbic brain volumes. *Journal of the International Neuropsychological Society, 7,* 384–390.

Fama, R., Sullivan, E.V., Shear, P.K., et al., (1997). Selective cortical and hippocampal volume correlates of Mattis Dementia Rating Scale in Alzheimer disease. *Archives of Neurology, 54,* 719–728.

Fama, R., Sullivan, E.V., Shear, P.K., et al. (1998). Fluency performance patterns in Alzheimer's disease and Parkinson's disease. *The Clinical Neuropsychologist, 12,* 487–499.

Fama, R., Sullivan, E.V., Shear, P.K., et al. (2000a). Structural brain correlates of verbal and nonverbal fluency measures in Alzheimer's disease. *Neuropsychology, 14,* 29–40.

Fama, R., Sullivan, E.V., Shear, P.K., et al. (2000b). Extent, pattern, and correlates of remote memory impairment in Alzheimer's disease and Parkinson's disease. *Neuropsychology, 4,* 265–276.

Fant, R.V., Pickworth, W.B., & Henningfield, J.E. (1999). Health effects of tobacco. In R.T. Ammerman et al. (Eds.), *Prevention and societal impact of drug and alcohol abuse.* Mahwah, NJ: Erlbaum.

Fantie, B.D. & Kolb, B. (1991). The problems of prognosis. In J. Dywan et al. (Eds.), *Neuropsychology and the law.* New York: Springer-Verlag.

Farace, E. & Alves, W.M. (2000). Do women fare worse: A meta-analysis of gender differences in traumatic brain injury outcome. *Journal of Neurosurgery, 93,* 539–545.

Farah, M.J. (1999). Relations among the agnosias. In G.W. Humphreys (Ed.), *Case studies in the neuropsychology of vision.* East Sussex, UK: Psychology Press.

Farah, M.J. (2000). The neural bases of mental imagery. In M.F. Gazzaniga (Ed.), *The new cognitive neurosciences* (2nd ed.). Cambridge, MA: MIT Press.

Farah, M.J. (2001). Consciousness. In B. Rapp (Ed.), *The handbook of cognitive neuropsychology.* Philadelphia: Psychology Press.

Farah, M.J. (2003). Disorders of visual–spatial perception and cognition. In K.M. Heilman & E. Valenstein (Eds.), *Clinical neuropsychology* (4th ed.). New York: Oxford University Press.

Farah, M.J. & Feinberg, T.E. (2000). *Patient-based approaches to cognitive neuroscience.* Cambridge, MA: MIT Press.

Farah, M.J. & Feinberg, T. E. (2003a). Perception and awareness. In T.E. Feinberg & M.J. Farah (Eds.), *Behavioral neurology and neuropsychology* (2nd ed.). New York: McGraw-Hill.

Farah, M.J. & Feinberg, T.E. (2003b). Visual object agnosia. In T.E. Feinberg & M.J. Farah (Eds.), *Behavioral neurology and neuropsychology* (2nd ed.). New York: McGraw-Hill.

Farah, M.J., Hammond, K.M., Mehta, Z., & Ratcliff, G. (1989). Category-specificity and modality-specificity in semantic memory. *Neuropsychologia, 27,* 193–200.

Farah, M.J., O'Reilly, R.C., & Vecera, S.P. (1993). Disssociated overt and covert recognition as an emergent property of a lesioned neural network. *Psychological Review, 100,* 571–588.

Farah, M.J., Wong, A.B., Monheit, M.A., & Morrow, L.A. (1989). Parietal lobe mechanisms of spatial attention: Modality-specific or supramodal? *Neuropsychologia, 27,* 461–470.

Farina, E., Fioravanti, R., Chiavari, L., et al. (2002). Comparing two programs of cognitive training in Alzheimer's disease: A pilot study. *Acta Neurologica Scandinavica, 105,* 365–371.

Farmer, J.E. & Stucky-Ropp, R. (1996). Family transactions and traumatic brain injury. In B.P. Uzzell & H.H. Stonnington (Eds.), *Recovery after traumatic brain injury.* Mahwah, NJ: Erlbaum.

Farmer, M.E., Kittner, S.J., Abbott, R.D., et al. (1990). Longitudinally measured blood pressure, antihypertensive medication use, and cognitive performance: The Framingham Study. *Journal of Clinical Epidemiology, 43,* 475–480.

Farmer, M.E., White, L.R., Abbott, R.D., et al. (1987). Blood pressure and cognitive performance. The Framingham Study. *American Journal of Epidemiology, 126,* 1103–1114.

Farmer, R.H. (1973). Functional changes during early weeks of abstinence, measured by the Bender-Gestalt. *Quarterly Journal of Studies on Alcohol, 34,* 786–796.

Farrell, D.F. & Starr, A. (1968). Delayed neurological sequelae of electrical injuries. *Neurology, 18,* 601–606.

Farrer, L.A. (1986). Suicide and attempted suicide in Huntington disease: Implications for preclinical testing of persons at risk. *American Journal of Medical Genetics, 24*, 305–311.

Faschingbauer, T.R. (1974). A 166-item short-form of the group MMPI: The FAM. *Journal of Consulting and Clinical Psychology, 42*, 645–655.

Fasotti, L. (1992). *Arithmetical word problem solving after frontal lobe damage: A cognitive neuropsychological approach.* Amsterdam: Swets and Zeitlinger.

Fasotti, L., Bremer, J.J.C.B., & Eling, P.A.T.M. (1992). Influence of improved text encoding on arithmetical word problem-solving after frontal lobe damage. *Neuropsychological Rehabilitation, 2*, 3–20.

Fassbender, K., Masters, C., & Beyreuther, K. (2000). Alzheimer's disease: An inflammatory disease? *Neurobiology of Aging, 21*, 433–436.

Fassbender, K., Schmidt, R., Moessner, R., et al. (1998). Mood disorders and dysfunction of the hypothalamic–pituitary–adrenal axis in multiple sclerosis: Association with cerebral inflammation. *Archives of Neurology, 55*, 66–72.

Fastenau, P.S. (1996a). Development and preliminary standardization of the "Extended Complex Figure Test" (ECFT). *Journal of Clinical and Experimental Neuropsychology, 18*, 63–76.

Fastenau, P.S. (1996b). An elaborated administration of the Wechsler Memory Scale-Revised. *The Clinical Neuropsychologist, 10*, 425–434.

Fastenau, P.S. (1998). Validity of regression-based norms: An empirical test of the comprehensive norms with older adults. *Journal of Clinical and Experimental Neuropsychology, 20*, 906–916.

Fastenau, P.S. (2003). *Extended Complex Figure Test (ECFT).* Los Angeles: Western Psychological Services.

Fastenau, P.S., Conant, L.L., & Lauer, R.E. (1998). Working memory in young children: Evidence for modality-specificity and implications for cerebral reorganization in early childhood. *Neuropsychologia, 36*, 643–652.

Fastenau, P.S., Denburg, N.L., & Abeles, N. (1996). Age differences in retrieval: Further support for the resource-reduction hypothesis. *Psychology and Aging, 11*, 140–146.

Fastenau, P.S., Denburg, N.L., & Hufford, B.J. (1999). Adult norms for the Rey-Osterrieth Complex Figure Test and for supplemental recognition and matching trials from the extended Complex Figure Test. *The Clinical Neuropsychologist, 13*, 30–47.

Fastenau, P.S., Denburg, N.L., & Mauer, B.A. (1998). Parallel short forms for the Boston Naming Test: Psychometric properties and norms for older adults. *Journal of Clinical and Experimental Neuropsychology, 20*, 828–834.

Faulstich, M.E. (1987). Psychiatric aspects of AIDS. *American Journal of Psychiatry, 144*, 551–556.

Faulstich, M.E., McAnulty, D.A., Carey, M.P., & Gresham, F.M. (1987). Topography of human intelligence across race: Factorial comparison of black–white WAIS-R profiles for criminal offenders. *International Journal of Neuroscience, 35*, 181–187.

Faust, D., Hart, K., & Guilmette, T.J. (1988). Pediatric malingering: The capacity of children to fake believable deficits on neuropsychological testing. *Journal of Consulting and Clinical Psychology, 56*, 578–582.

Faust, D., Hart, K., Guilmette, T.J., & Arkes, H.R. (1988). Neuropsychologists' capacity to detect adolescent malingerers. *Professional Psychology: Research and Practice, 19*, 508–515.

Fazekas, F., Barkhof, F., Filippi, M., et al. (1999). The contribution of magnetic resonance imaging to the diagnosis of multiple sclerosis. *Neurology, 53*, 448–456.

Fazekas, F., Koch, M., Schmidt, R., et al. (1992). The prevalence of cerebral damage varies with migraine type: A MRI study. *Headache, 32*, 287–291.

Fazekas, F., Strasser-Fuchs, S., Kollegger, H., et al. (2001). Apolipoprotein E epsilon 4 is associated with rapid progression of multiple sclerosis. *Neurology, 57*, 853–857.

Federal Interagency Forum on Aging-Related Statistics (2000). *Older Americans 2000: Key indicators of well-being.* Washington, D.C.: U.S. Government Printing Office.

Fedio, P., Cox, C.S., Neophytides, A., et al. (1979). Neuropsychological profile of Huntington's disease: Patients and those at risk. In T.N. Chase et al. (Eds.), *Advances in Neurology* (Vol. 23). New York: Raven Press.

Fedio, P., Martin, A., & Brouwers, P. (1984). The effects of focal cortical lesions on cognitive functions. In R.J. Porter et al. (Eds.), *Advances in epileptology: XVth Epilepsy International Symposium.* New York: Raven Press.

Fedio, P. & Van Buren, J.M. (1974). Memory deficits during electrical stimulation of the speech cortex in conscious man. *Brain and Language, 1*, 29–42.

Fedio, P. & Van Buren, J.M. (1975). Memory and perceptual deficits during electrical stimulation in the left and right thalamus and parietal subcortex. *Brain and Language, 2*, 78–100.

Feher, E.P., Doody, R., Pirozzolo, F.J., & Appel, S.H. (1989). Mental status assessment of insight and judgment. In F.J. Pirozzolo (Ed.), *Clinics in geriatric medicine* (Vol. 5, No. 3). Philadelphia: Saunders.

Feher, E.P., Larrabee, G.J., Sudilovsky, A., & Crook, T.H., 3rd (1994). Memory self-report in Alzheimer's disease and in age-associated memory impairment. *Journal of Geriatric Psychiatry and Neurology, 7*, 58–65.

Feher, E.P., Mahurin, R.K., Doody, R.S., et al. (1992). Establishing the limits of the Mini-Mental State: Examination of subtests. *Archives of Neurology, 49*, 87–92.

Feher, E.P., Mahurin, R.K., Inbody, S.B., et al. (1991). Anosognosia in Alzheimer's patients. *Neuropsychiatry, Neuropsychology, and Behavioral Neurology, 4*, 136–146.

Feher, E.P. & Martin, R.C. (1992). Cognitive assessment of long-term memory disorders. In D.I. Margolin (Ed.), *Cognitive neuropsychology in clinical practice.* New York: Oxford University Press.

Feinberg, T.E. (2003). Anosognosia and confabulation. In T.E. Feinberg & M.J. Farah (Eds.), *Behavioral neurology and neuropsychology* (2nd ed.). New York: McGraw-Hill.

Feinberg, T.E. & Farah, M.J. (2003a). *Behavioral neurology and neuropsychology* (2nd ed.). New York: McGraw-Hill.

Feinberg, T.E. & Farah, M.J. (2003b). Part 2. Aphasia and other dominant hemisphere syndromes. In *Behavioral neurology and neuropsychology* (2nd ed.). New York: McGraw-Hill.

Feinberg, T.E. & Farah, M.J. (2003c). Part 3. Disorders of perception, attention, and awareness. In *Behavioral neurology and neuropsychology* (2nd ed.). New York: McGraw-Hill.

Feinberg, T.E., Mazlin, S.E., & Waldman, G.E. (1989) Recovery from brain damage: Neurological considerations. In E. Perecman (Ed.), *Integrating theory and practice in clinical neuropsychology.* Hillsdale, NJ: Erlbaum.

Feingold, A. (1982). The validity of the Information and Vocabulary subtests of the WAIS. *Journal of Clinical Psychology, 38*, 169–174.

Feingold, A. (1988). Cognitive gender differences are disappearing. *American Psychologist, 43*, 95–103.

Feinstein, A. (1999). *The clinical neuropsychiatry of multiple sclerosis.* Cambridge: Cambridge University Press.

Feinstein, A. (2002). An examination of suicidal intent in patients with multiple sclerosis. *Neurology, 59*, 674–678.

Feinstein, A., Brown, R., & Ron, M. (1994). Effects of practice of serial tests of attention in healthy subjects. *Journal of Clinical and Experimental Neuropsychology, 16*, 436–447.

Feinstein, A. & Feinstein, K. (2001). Depression associated with multiple sclerosis. Looking beyond diagnosis to symptom expression. *Journal of Affective Disorders, 66,* 193–198.

Feinstein, A., Feinstein, K., Gray, T., & O'Connor, P. (1997). Prevalence and neurobehavioral correlates of pathological laughing and crying in multiple sclerosis. *Archives of Neurology, 54,* 1116–1121.

Feinstein, A., Hershkop, S., Ouchterlony, D., et al. (2002). Post-traumatic amnesia and recall of a traumatic event following traumatic brain injury. *Journal of Neuropsychiatry and Clinical Neurosciences, 14,* 25–30.

Feinstein, A., O'Connor, P., & Feinstein, K. (1999). Pathological laughing and crying in multiple sclerosis: A preliminary report suggesting a role for prefrontal cortex. *Multiple Sclerosis, 5,* 69–73.

Feinstein, A., O'Connor, P., Gray, T., & Feinstein, K. (1999). The effects of anxiety on psychiatric morbidity in patients with multiple sclerosis. *Multiple Sclerosis, 5,* 323–326.

Feinstein, A., Ouchterlony, D., Somerville, J., & Jardine, A. (2001). The effects of litigation on symptom expression: A prospective study following mild traumatic brain injury. *Medicine, Science and the Law, 41,* 116–121.

Feinstein, A., Ron, M., & Thompson, A. (1993). A serial study of psychometric and magnetic resonance imaging changes in multiple sclerosis. *Brain, 116,* 569–602.

Feldman, H., Gauthier, S., Hecker, J., et al. (2001). A 24-week, randomized, double-blind study of donepezil in moderate to severe Alzheimer's disease. *Neurology, 57,* 613–620.

Feldman, R.G. (1982). Neurological manifestations of mercury intoxication. *Acta Neurologica Scandinavica, 66(Suppl. 92),* 201–209.

Feldman, R.G. & White, R.F. (1992). Lead neurotoxicity and disorders of learning. *Journal of Child Neurology, 7,* 354–359.

Fel'dman, Y.G. & Bonashevskaya, T.I. (1971). On the effects of low concentrations of formaldehyde. *Hygiene and Sanitation, 36,* 174–180.

Feldstein, S.N., Keller, F.R., Portman, R.E., et al. (1999). A comparison of computerized and standard versions of the Wisconsin Card Sorting Test. *The Clinical Neuropsychologist, 13,* 303–313.

Fennell, E.B. (1986). Handedness in neuropsychological research. In H.J. Hannay (Ed.), *Experimental techniques in human neuropsychology.* New York: Oxford University Press.

Fennell, E.B. & Smith, M.C. (1990). Neuropsychological assessment. In S.M. Rao (Ed.), *Neurobehavioral aspects of multiple sclerosis.* New York: Oxford University Press.

Fenwick, P. (1989). The nature and management of aggression in epilepsy. *Journal of Neuropsychiatry and Clinical Neurosciences, 1,* 418–425.

Fenwick, P.B. & Brown, S.W. (1989). Evoked and psychogenic epileptic seizures. I. Precipitation. *Acta Neurologica Scandinavica, 80,* 535–540.

Ferber, S. & Karnath, H.-O. (2001). How to assess spatial neglect—line bisection of cancellation tasks? *Journal of Clinical and Experimental Neuropsychology, 23,* 599–607.

Ferguson, K.S. & Robinson, S.S. (1982). Life-threatening migraine. *Archives of Neurology, 39,* 374–376.

Ferguson, S.C., Blane, A., Perros, P., et al. (2003). Cognitive ability and brain structure in type 1 diabetes: Relation to microangiopathy and preceding severe hypoglycemia. *Diabetes, 52,* 149–156.

Ferland, M.B., Ramsay, J., Engeland, C., & O'Hara, P. (1998). Comparison of the performance of normal individuals and survivors of traumatic brain injury on repeat administrations of the Wisconsin Card Sorting Test. *Journal of Clinical and Experimental Neuropsychology, 20,* 473–482.

Fernaeus, S.E. & Almkvist, O. (1998). Word production: Dissociation of two retrieval modes of semantic memory across time. *Journal of Clinical and Experimental Neuropsychology, 20,* 137–143.

Fernandez, F., Ringholz, G.M., & Levy, J.K. (2002). Neuropsychiatric aspects of human immunodeficiency virus infection of the central nervous system. In S.C. Yudofsky & R.E. Hales (Eds.), *Textbook of neuropsychiatry and clinical neurosciences* (4th ed.). Washington, D.C.: American Psychiatric Publishing.

Fernandez, G., Weis, S., Stoffel-Wagner, B., et al. (2003). Menstrual cycle-dependent neural plasticity in the adult human brain is hormone, task, and region specific. *Journal of Neuroscience, 23,* 3790–3795.

Fernandez, V., Erli, H.J., Kugler, J., & Paar, O. (2001). Cognitive deficits after polytrauma. Studies of quality of life. *Unfallchirurg, 104,* 938–947.

Ferrari, M.D. & Haan, J. (2002). Migraine. In A.K. Asbury et al. (Eds.), *Diseases of the nervous system* (3rd ed.). Cambridge: Cambridge University Press.

Ferrari, R. (2001). Comment on "Nonimpact brain injury: Neuropsychological and behavioral correlates with consideration of physiological findings." *Applied Neuropsychology, 8,* 120–121.

Ferraro, F.R., Grossman, J., Bren, A., & Hoverson, A. (2002). Effects of orientation on Rey Complex Figure performance. *Brain and Cognition, 50,* 139–144.

Ferris, S., Crook, T., Sathananthan, G., & Gershon, S. (1976). Reaction time as a diagnostic measure in senility. *Journal of the American Geriatrics Society, 24,* 529–533.

Ferro, J.M. (2001). Neurobehavioural aspects of deep hemisphere stroke. In J. Bogousslavsky & L. Caplan (Eds.), *Stroke syndromes* (2nd ed.). Cambridge: Cambridge University Press.

Ferro, J.M., Kertesz, A., & Black, S.E. (1987). Subcortical neglect: Quantitation, anatomy, and recovery, *Neurology, 37,* 1487–1492.

Ferro, J.M., Santos, M.E., Caldas, A.C., & Mariano, G. (1980) Gesture recognition in aphasia. *Journal of Clinical Neuropsychology, 2,* 277–292.

Ferrucci, L., Del Lungo, I., Guralnik, J.M., et al. (1998). Is the Telephone Interview for Cognitive Status a valid alternative in persons who cannot be evaluated by the Mini Mental State Examination? *Aging, 10,* 332–338.

Fery, Y.A. & Ferry, A. (1997). Effect of physical exhaustion on cognitive functioning. *Perceptual and Motor Skills, 84,* 291–298.

Feyereisen, P., Verbeke-Dewitte, C., & Seron, X. (1986). On fluency measures in aphasic speech. *Journal of Clinical and Experimental Neuropsychology, 8,* 393–404.

Fields, F.R.J. (1987). Brain dysfunction: Relative discrimination accuracy of Halstead-Reitan and Luria-Nebraska neuropsychological test batteries. *Neuropsychology, 1,* 9–12.

Fields, S. & Fullerton, J. (1975). Influence of heroin addiction on neuropsychological functioning. *Journal of Consulting and Clinical Psychology, 43,* 114.

Filippi, M. & Grossman, R.I. (2002). MRI techniques to monitor MS evolution: The present and the future. *Neurology, 58,* 1147–1153.

Fillenbaum, G.G. (1980). Comparison of two brief tests of organic brain impairment, the MSQ and the Short Portable MSQ. *Journal of the American Geriatrics Society, 28,* 381–384.

Fillenbaum, G.G., Heyman, A., Huber, M.S., et al. (1998). The prevalence and 3-year incidence of dementia in older black and white community residents. *Journal of Clinical Epidemiology, 51,* 587–595.

Fillenbaum, G.G., Heyman, A., Huber, M.S., et al. (2001). Performance of elderly African American and white community residents on the CERAD neuropsychological battery. *Journal of the International Neuropsychological Society, 7,* 502–509.

Fillenbaum, G.G., Landerman, L.R., Blazer, D.G., et al. (2001). The relationship of APOE genotype to cognitive functioning in older

African-American and Caucasian community residents. *Journal of the American Geriatric Society, 49,* 1148–1155.

Fillenbaum, G.G., Landerman, L.R., & Simonsick, E.M. (1998). Equivalence of two screens of cognitive functioning: The Short Portable Mental Status Questionnaire and the Orientation-Memory-Concentration Test. *Journal of the American Geriatric Society, 46,* 1512–1518.

Fillenbaum, G.G., Peterson, B., Welsh-Bohmer, K.A., et al. (1998). Progression of Alzheimer's disease in black and white patients: The CERAD experience, part XVI. Consortium to Establish a Registry for Alzheimer's Disease. *Neurology, 51,* 154–158.

Fillenbaum, G.G., Wilkinson, W.E., Welsh, K.A., & Mohs, R.C. (1994). Discrimination between stages of Alzheimer's disease with subsets of Mini-Mental State Examination items. An analysis of Consortium to Establish a Registry for Alzheimer's Disease data. *Archives of Neurology, 51,* 916–921.

Filley, C.M. (1995). *Neurobehavioral anatomy.* Niwot, CO: University Press of Colorado.

Filley, C.M. (2001). *Behaviorial neurology of white matter.* New York: Oxford University Press.

Filley, C.M. & Cullum, C.M. (1993). Early detection of fronto-temporal degeneration by clinical evaluation. *Archives of Clinical Neuropsychology, 8,* 359–367.

Filley, C.M. & Cullum, C.M. (1994). Attention and vigilance functions in normal aging. *Applied Neuropsychology, 1,* 29–32.

Filley, C.M., Davis, K.A., Schmitz, S.P., et al. (1989). Neuropsychological performance and magnetic resonance imaging in Alzheimer's disease and normal aging. *Neuropsychiatry, Neuropsychology, and Behavioral Neurology, 2,* 81–91.

Filley, C.M., Heaton, R.K., Thompson, L.L., et al. (1990). Effects of disease course on neuropsychological functioning. In S.M. Rao (Ed.), *Neurobehavioral aspects of multiple sclerosis.* New York: Oxford University Press.

Filley, C.M. & Kleinschmidt-DeMasters, B.K. (2001). Toxic leukoencephalopathy. *New England Journal of Medicine, 345,* 425–432.

Filoteo, J.V., Rilling, L.M., Cole, B., et al. (1997). Variable memory profiles in Parkinson's disease. *Journal of Clinical and Experimental Neuropsychology, 19,* 878–888.

Filskov, S.B. & Catanese, R.A. (1986). Effects of sex and handedness on neuropsychological testing. In S.B. Filskov & T.J. Boll (Eds.), *Handbook of clinical neuropsychology* (Vol. 2). New York: Wiley.

Finger, S. (1994). *Origins of neuroscience. A history of explorations into brain function.* New York: Oxford University Press.

Finger, S. (1998). A happy state of mind: A history of mild elation, denial of disability, optimism, and laughing in multiple sclerosis. *Archives of Neurology, 55,* 241–250.

Finger, S. (2000). *Minds behind the brain. A history of the pioneers and their discoveries.* New York: Oxford University Press.

Finger, S., LeVere, T.E., Almli, C.R., & Stein, D.G. (1988) Recovery of function: Sources of controversy. In S. Finger et al. (Eds.), *Brain injury and recovery: Theoretical and controversial issues.* New York: Plenum Press.

Fink, G.R., Markowitsch, H.J., Reinkemeier, M., et al. (1996). Cerebral representation of one's own past: Neural networks involved in autobiographical memory. *Journal of Neuroscience, 16,* 4275–4282.

Fink, M., Green, M., & Bender, M. B. (1952). The Face–Hand Test as a diagnostic sign of organic mental syndrome. *Neurology, 2,* 46–58.

Finlayson, M.A.J., Johnson, K.A., & Reitan, R.M. (1977). Relationship of level of education to neuropsychological measure in brain-damaged and non-brain-damaged adults. *Journal of Consulting and Clinical Psychology, 45,* 536–542.

Finlayson, M.A.J., Sullivan, J.F., & Alfano, D.P. (1986). Halstead's Category Test: withstanding the test of time. *Journal of Clinical and Experimental Neuropsychology, 8,* 706–709.

Finney, D.J., et al. (1963). *Tables for testing significance in a 2 × 2 contingency table.* Cambridge: Cambridge University Press.

Finset, A. & Andersson, S. (2000). Coping strategies in patients with acquired brain injury: relationships between coping, apathy, depression and lesion location. *Brain Injury, 14,* 887–905.

Finset, A., Anke, A.W., Hofft, E., et al. (1999). Cognitive performance in multiple trauma patients 3 years after injury. *Psychosomatic Medicine, 61,* 576–583.

Finton, M.J., Lucas, J.A., Graff-Radford, N.R., & Uitti, R.J. (1998). Analysis of visuospatial errors in patients with Alzheimer's disease or Parkinson's disease. *Journal of Clinical and Experimental Neuropsychology, 20,* 186–193.

Fioravanti, M., Thorel, M., Ramelli, L., & Napoleoni, A. (1985). Reliability between the five forms of the Randt Memory Test and their equivalence. *Archives of Gerontology and Geriatrics, 4,* 357–364.

Fiore, S.M. & Schooler, J.W. (1998). Right hemisphere contributions to creative problem solving: Converging evidence for divergent thinking. In M. Beeman & C. Chiarello (Eds.), *Right hemisphere language comprehension. Perspectives from cognitive neuroscience.* Mahwah, NJ: Erlbaum.

Firsching, R., Woischneck, D., Klein, S., et al. (2001). Classification of severe head injury based on magnetic resonance imaging. *Acta Neurochirurgica, 143,* 263–271.

Fischer, J.S. (1988). Using the Wechsler Memory Scale-Revised to detect and characterize memory deficits in multiple sclerosis. *The Clinical Neuropsychologist, 2,* 149–172.

Fischer, J.S. (1989). Objective memory testing in multiple sclerosis. In K. Jensen, L. Knudsen, E. Stenager, & I. Grant (Eds.), *Current problems in neurology. Mental disorders, cognitive deficits, and their treatment in multiple sclerosis* (Vol. 10). London: Libbey.

Fischer, J.S. (1999). Assessment of neuropsychological function. In R.A. Rudick & J.A. Cohen (Eds.), *Multiple sclerosis therapeutics.* London: Martin Dunitz.

Fischer, J.S. (2003). Measure of neuropsychological functions. In R.A. Rudick & D.E. Goodkin (Eds.), *Multiple sclerosis: Experimental and applied therapeutics.* London: Martin Dunitz, in press.

Fischer, J.S. (2001). Cognitive impairment in multiple sclerosis. In S.D. Cook (Ed.), *Handbook of multiple sclerosis.* New York: Marcel Dekker.

Fischer, J.S. (2002). Assessment of neuropsychological function. In R.A. Rudick & J.A. Cohen (Eds.), *Multiple sclerosis therapeutics.* London: Martin Dunitz.

Fischer, J.S., Jacobs, L.D., Cookfair, D.L., et al. (1998). Heterogeneity of cognitive dysfunction in multiple sclerosis [abstract]. *The Clinical Neuropsychologist, 12,* 286.

Fischer, J.S., Priore, R.L., Jacobs, L., et al. (2000). Neuropsychological effects of interferon b-1a in relapsing multiple sclerosis. *Annals of Neurology, 48,* 885–892.

Fischer, J.S., Rudick, R.A., Cutter, G.R., et al. (1999). The Multiple Sclerosis Functional Composite measure (MSFC): An integrated approach to MS clinical outcome assessment. *Multiple Sclerosis, 5,* 244–250.

Fisher, C.M. (1988). Neurologic fragments. I. Clinical observations in demented patients. *Neurology, 38,* 1868–1873.

Fisher, D.C., Ledbetter, M.F., Cohen, N.J., et al. (2000). WAIS-III and WMS-III profiles of mildly to severely brain-injured patients. *Applied Neuropsychology, 7,* 126–132.

Fisher, L.M., Freed, D.M., & Corkin, S. (1990). Stroop Color-Word Test performance in patients with Alzheimer's disease. *Journal of Clinical and Experimental Neuropsychology, 12,* 745–758.

Fisher, N.J., Rourke, B.P., & Bieliauskas, L.A. (1999). Neuropsychological subgroups of patients with Alzheimer's disease: An examination of the first 10 years of CERAD data. *Journal of Clinical and Experimental Neuropsychology, 21,* 488–518.

Fisher, N.J., Tierney, M.C., Snow, W.G., & Szalai, J.P. (1999). Odd/even short forms of the Boston Naming Test: Preliminary geriatric norms. *The Clinical Neuropsychologist, 13*, 359–364.

Fisk, J.D. & Archibald, C.J. (2001). Limitations of the Paced Auditory Serial Addition Test as a measure of working memory in patients with multiple sclerosis. *Journal of the International Neuropsychological Society, 7*, 363–372.

Fisk, J.D., Pontefract, A., Ritvo, P.G., et al. (1994). The impact of fatigue on patients with multiple sclerosis. *Canadian Journal of Neurologic Sciences, 21*, 9–14.

Fisk, J.E. & Warr, P. (1996). Age and working memory: the role of perceptual speed, the central executive, and the phonological loop. *Psychology and Aging, 11*, 316–323.

Fladby, T., Schuster, M., Gronli, O., et al. (1999). Organic brain disease in psychogeriatric patients: impact of symptoms and screening methods on the diagnostic process. *Journal of Geriatric Psychiatry and Neurology, 12*, 16–20.

Fleck, D.E., Shear, P.K., & Strakowski, S. (2002). A reevaluation of sustained attention performance in temporal lobe epilepsy. *Archives of Clinical Neuropsychology, 17*, 399–405.

Fleet, W.S. & Heilman, K.M. (1986). The fatigue effect in hemispatial neglect [abstract]. *Neurology, 36*, 258.

Fleischman, D.A., Gabrieli, J.D., Reminger, S.L., et al. (1998). Object decision priming in Alzheimer's disease. *Journal of the International Neuropsychological Society, 4*, 435–446.

Fleming, J., Tooth, L., Hassell, M., & Chan, W. (1999). Prediction of community integration and vocational outcome 2–5 years after traumatic brain injury rehabilitation in Australia. *Brain Injury, 13*, 417–431.

Fleming, K., Goldberg, T.E., Gold, J.M., & Weinberger, D.R. (1995). Verbal working memory dysfunction in schizophrenia: use of a Brown-Peterson paradigm. *Psychiatry Research, 56*, 155–161.

Fletcher, C., Lovatt, C., & Baldry, C. (1998). A study of state, trait, and test anxiety, and their relationship to assessment center performance. *Journal of Social Behavior and Personality, 12*, 205–214.

Fletcher, P.C., Shallice, T., & Dolan, R.J. (1998). The functional roles of prefrontal cortex in episodic memory. I. Encoding. *Brain, 121*, episodic memory. I. Encoding. *Brain, 121*, 1239–1248.

Fletcher, P.C., Shallice, T., Frith, C.D., et al. (1998). The functional roles of prefrontal cortex in episodic memory. II. Retrieval. *Brain, 121*, 1249–1256.

Flicker, C., Ferris, S.H., Crook, T., et al. (1988). Equivalent spatial-rotation deficits in normal aging and Alzheimer's disease. *Journal of Clinical and Experimental Neuropsychology, 10*, 387–389.

Flicker, C., Ferris, S.H., & Reisberg, B. (1991). Mild cognitive impairment in the elderly: Predictors of dementia. *Neurology, 41*, 1006–1009.

Flodin, U., Edling, C., & Axelson, O. (1984). Clinical studies of psychoorganic syndromes among workers with exposure to solvents. *American Journal of Industrial Medicine, 5*, 287–295.

Flor-Henry, P. (1986). Observations, reflections and speculations on the cerebral determinants of mood and on the bilaterally asymmetrical distributions of the major neurotransmitter systems. *Acta Neurologica Scandinavica, 74(Suppl. 109)*, 75–89.

Flor-Henry, P., Koles, Z.J., & Reddon, J.R. (1987). Age and sex related EEG configurations in normal subjects. In A. Glass (Ed.), *Individual differences in hemispheric specialization*. New York: Plenum Press.

Flowers, K.A., Pearce, I., & Pearce, J.M.S. (1984). Recognition memory in Parkinson's disease. *Journal of Neurology, Neurosurgery and Psychiatry, 47*, 1174–1181.

Flowers, K.A. & Robertson, C. (1985). The effect of Parkinson's disease on the ability to maintain a mental set. *Journal of Neurology, Neurosurgery and Psychiatry, 48*, 517–529.

Flowers, K.A., Sheridan, M.R., & Shadbolt, H. (1996). Simulation of amnesia by normals on Rey's Auditory Verbal Learning Test. *Journal of Neurolinguistics, 9*, 147–156.

Flynn, F.G., Cummings, J.L., & Tomiyasu, U. (1988). Altered behavior associated with damage to the ventromedial hypothalamus: A distinctive syndrome. *Behavioral Neurology, 1*, 49–58.

Flynn, J.R. (1987). Massive IQ gains in 14 nations: What IQ tests really measure. *Psychological Bulletin, 101*, 171–191.

Flynn, J.R. (1998a). Israeli military IQ tests: gender differences small; IQ gains large. *Journal of Biosocial Science, 30*, 541–553.

Flynn, J.R. (1998b). WAIS-III and WISC-III IQ gains in the United States from 1972 to 1995: How to compensate for obsolete norms. *Perceptual and Motor Skills, 86*, 1231–1239.

Flynn, J.R. (1999). Searching for justice. The discovery of IQ gains over time. *American Psychologist, 54*, 5–20.

Fogel, B.S., Schiffer, R.B., & Rao, S.M. (Eds.) (1996). *Neuropsychiatry*. Baltimore: Williams & Wilkins.

Fogel, M.L. (1965). The Proverbs Test in the appraisal of cerebral disease. *Journal of General Psychology, 72*, 269–275.

Fogel, M.L. (1967). Picture description and interpretation in brain damaged patients. *Cortex, 3*, 433–448.

Foley, F.W. & Sanders, A. (1997a). Sexuality, multiple sclerosis, and men. *MS Management, 4, 1*, 7–15.

Foley, F.W. & Sanders, A. (1997b). Sexuality, multiple sclerosis, and women. *MS Management, 4, 1*, 3–10.

Foley, F.W., Traugott, U., LaRocca, N.G., et al. (1992). A prospective study of depression and immune dysregulation in multiple sclerosis. *Archives of Neurology, 49*, 238-244.

Folstein, M.F., Folstein, S.E., & McHugh, P.R. (1975). Mini-mental state. *Journal of Psychiatric Research, 12*, 189–198.

Folstein, S.E. (1989). *Huntington's disease*. Baltimore, MD: Johns Hopkins University Press.

Folstein, S.E., Abbott, M.H., Chase, G.A., et al. (1983). The association of affective disorder with Huntington's disease in a case series and in families. *Psychological Medicine, 13*, 537–542.

Folstein, S.E., Brandt, J., & Folstein, M.F. (1990). Huntington's disease. In J.L. Cummings (Ed.), *Subcortical dementia*. New York: Oxford University Press.

Folstein, S.E., Franz, M.L., Jensen, B.A., et al. (1983). Conduct disorder and affective disorder among the offspring of patients with Huntington's disease. *Psychological Medicine, 13*, 45–52.

Fontanarosa, P.B. (1993). Electrical shock and lightning strike. *Annals of Emergency Medicine, 22(Part 2)*, 378–387.

Foong, J., Rozewicz, L., Chong, W.K., et al. (2000). A comparison of neuropsychological deficits in primary and secondary progressive multiple sclerosis. *Journal of Neurology, 247*, 97–101.

Foong, J., Rozewicz, L., Quaghebeur, G., et al. (1997). Executive function in multiple sclerosis: The role of frontal pathology. *Brain, 120*, 15–26.

Foong, J., Rozewicz, L., Quaghebeur, G., et al. (1998). Neuropsychological deficits in multiple sclerosis after acute relapse. *Journal of Neurology, Neurosurgery and Psychiatry, 64*, 529–532.

Ford, H., Trigwell, P., & Johnson, M. (1998). The nature of fatigue in multiple sclerosis. *Journal of Psychosomatic Research, 45*, 33–38.

Forde, E.M.E. & Humphreys, G.W. (1999). Category-specific recognition impairments: A review of important case studies and influential theories. *Aphasiology, 13*, 169–193.

Fordyce, D.J. & Roueche, J.R. (1986). Changes in perspectives of disability among patients, staff, and relatives during rehabilitation of brain injury. *Rehabilitation Psychology, 31*, 217–229.

Fordyce, D.J., Roueche, J.R., & Prigatano, G.P. (1983). Enhanced emotional reactions in chronic head trauma patients. *Journal of Neurology, Neurosurgery and Psychiatry, 46*, 620–624.

Forette, F., Seux, M.L., Staessen, J.A., et al. (1998). Prevention of dementia in randomised double-blind placebo-controlled systolic hypertension in Europe (Syst-Eur) trial. *Lancet, 352,* 1347–1351.

Forstl, H., Burns, A., Levy, R., & Cairns, N. (1993). Neuropathological basis for drawing disability (constructional apraxia) in Alzheimer's disease. *Psychological Medicine, 23,* 623–629.

Fortin, D., Cairncross, J.G., & Hammond, R.R. (1999). Oligodendroglioma: An appraisal of recent data pertaining to diagnosis and treatment. *Neurosurgery, 45,* 1279–1291.

Fossum, B., Holmberg, H., & Reinvang, I. (1992). Spatial and symbolic factors in performance on the Trail Making Test. *Neuropsychology, 6,* 71–75.

Foster, J.K., Behrmann, M., & Stuss, D.T. (1999). Visual attention deficits in Alzheimer's disease: simple versus conjoined feature search. *Neuropsychology, 13,* 223–245.

Foster, N.L., Gilman, S., Berent, S., et al. (1992). Progressive subcortical gliosis and progressive supranuclear palsy can have similar clinical and PET abnormalities. *Journal of Neurology, Neurosurgery and Psychiatry, 55,* 707–713.

Fougeyrollas, P. (1995). Documenting environmental factors for preventing the handicap creation process: Quebec contributions relating to ICIDH and social participation of people with functional differences. *Disability and Rehabilitation, 17,* 145–153.

Fowler, P.C., Macciocchi, S.N., & Ranseen, J. (1986). WAIS-R factors and performance on the Luria-Nebraska's Intelligence, Memory and Motor scales: A canonical model of relationships. *Journal of Clinical Psychology, 42,* 626–635.

Fowler, P.C., Richards, H.C., & Boll, T.J. (1980). WAIS factor patterns of epileptic and normal adults. *Journal of Clinical Neuropsychology, 2,* 115–123.

Fowler, P.C., Richards, H.C., Boll, T.J., & Berent, S. (1987). A factor model of an extended Halstead Battery and its relationship to an EEG lateralization index for epileptic adults. *Archives of Clinical Neuropsychology, 2,* 81–92.

Fowler, P.C., Zillmer, E., & Macciocchi, S.N. (1990). Confirmatory factor analytic models of the WAIS-R for neuropsychiatric patients. *Journal of Clinical Psychology, 46,* 324–333.

Fowler, P.C., Zillmer, E., & Newman, A.C. (1988). A multifactor model of the Halstead-Reitan Neuropsychological Test Battery and its relationship to cognitive status and psychiatric diagnosis. *Journal of Clinical Psychology, 44,* 898–906.

Fowler, R.S. & Fordyce, W.E. (1974). *Stroke: Why do they behave that way?* Seattle: Washington State Heart Association.

Fowles, G.P. & Tunick, R.H. (1986). WAIS-R and Shipley estimated IQ correlations. *Journal of Clinical Psychology, 42,* 647–649.

Fox, D.D. (1994). Normative problems for Wechsler Memory Scale-Revised Logical Memory Test when used in litigation. *Archives of Clinical Neuropsychology, 9,* 211–214.

Fox, D.D., Lees-Haley, P.R., Earnest, K., & Dolezal-Wood, S. (1995). Base rates of postconcussion symptoms in health maintenance organization patients. *Neuropsychology, 9,* 606–611.

Fox, G.K., Bowden, S.C., Bashford, G.M., & Smith, D.S. (1997). Alzheimer's disease and driving: prediction and assessment of driving performance. *Journal of the American Geriatric Society, 45,* 949–953.

Fox, N.C., Warrington, E.K., Freeborough, P.A., et al. (1996). Presymptomatic hippocampal atrophy in Alzheimer's disease. A longitudinal MRI study. *Brain, 119,* 2001–2007.

Fozard, J.L. (1990). Vision and hearing in aging. In J.E. Birren & K.W. Schaie (Eds.), *Handbook of the psychology of aging* (3rd ed.). New York: Academic Press.

Frackowiak, R.S.J. (1997). The cerebral basis of functional recovery. In R.S.J. Frackowiak, K.J. Friston, C.D. Frith, et al. (Eds.), *Human brain function.* San Diego: Academic Press.

Frackowiak, R.S.J., Friston, K.J., Frith, C.D., et al. (1997). *Human brain function.* San Diego: Academic Press.

Francel, P.C. & Jane, J.A. (1996). Age and outcome from head injury. In R.K. Narayan et al. (Eds.), *Neurotrauma.* New York: McGraw-Hill.

Franceschi, M., Alberoni, M., Bressi, S., et al. (1995). Correlations between cognitive impairment, middle cerebral artery flow velocity and cortical glucose metabolism in the early phase of Alzheimer's disease. *Dementia, 6,* 32–38.

Francis, P.M., Harrington, T.R., Sorini, P.M., & Urbina, C.M. (1991). Helmet use and mortality and morbidity in motorcycle accidents. *BNI Quarterly, 7,* 24–27.

Frank, A.A., Blythe, L.L., & Spencer, P.S. (2000). Aspects of veterinary neurotoxicology. In P.S. Spencer & H.H. Schaumburg (Eds.), *Experimental and clinical neurotoxicology* (2nd ed.). New York: Oxford University Press.

Frank, R., Wiederholt, W.C., Kritz-Silverstein, D.K., et al. (1996). Effects of sequential neuropsychological testing of an elderly community-based sample. *Neuroepidemiology, 15,* 257–268.

Frank, R.M. & Bryne, G.J. (2000). The clinical utility of the Hopkins Verbal Learning Test as a screening test for mild dementia. *International Journal of Geriatric Psychiatry, 15,* 317–324.

Franklin, G.M., Heaton, R.K., Nelson, L.M., et al. (1988). Correlation of neuropsychological and MRI findings in chronic/progressive multiple sclerosis. *Neurology, 38,* 1826–1829.

Franklin, G.M., Nelson, L.M., Heaton, R.K., et al. (1988). Stress and its relationship to acute exacerbations in multiple sclerosis. *Journal of Neurologic Rehabilitation, 2,* 7–11.

Franssen, E.H. & Risberg, B. (1997). Neurologic markers of the progression of Alzheimer's disease. *International Psychogeriatrics, 9,* 297–306.

Franzen, M.D. (1989). *Reliability and validity in neuropsychological assessment.* New York: Plenum Press.

Franzen, M.D. (1999). Clinical interpretation of the LNNB. In C.J. Golden et al. (Eds.), *LNNB handbook: A guide to clinical interpretation and use in special settings.* Los Angeles: Western Psychological Service.

Franzen, M.D., Iverson, G.L., & McCracken, L.M. (1990). The detection of malingering in neuropsychological assessment. *Neuropsychological Review, 1,* 247–279.

Franzen, M.D., Smith, S.S., Paul, D.S. & MacInnes, W.D. (1993). Order effects in the administration of the Booklet Category Test and Wisconsin Card Sorting Test. *Archives of Clinical Neuropsychology, 8,* 105–110.

Franzen, M.D., Tishelman, A.C., Sharp, B.H., & Friedman, A.G. (1987). An investigation of the test–retest reliability of the Stroop Color-Word Test across two intervals. *Archives of Clinical Neuropsychology, 2,* 265–272.

Franzen, M.D., Tishelman, A., Smith, S., et al. (1989). Preliminary data concerning the test–retest and parallel-forms reliability of the Randt Memory Test. *The Clinical Neuropsychologist, 3,* 25–28.

Fraser, S. (Ed.). (1995). *The bell curve wars.* New York: Basic Books.

Fratiglioni, L. & Wang, H.-X. (2000). Smoking and Parkinson's and Alzheimer's disease: Review of the epidemiological studies. *Behavioral Brain Research, 113,* 117–120.

Frazier, T.W., Adams, N.L., Strauss, M.E., & Redline, S. (2001). Comparability of the Rey and Mack forms of the Complex Figure Test. *The Clinical Neuropsychologist, 15,* 337–344.

Frederick, R.I. (1997). *VIP: Validity indicator profile. Manual.* Minneapolis: National Computer Systems.

Frederiks, J.A.M. (1963). Constructional apraxia and cerebral dominance. *Psychiatria, Neurologia, Neurochirurgia, 66,* 522–530.

Frederiks, J.A.M. (1985a). Disorders of the body schema. In J.A.M. Frederiks (Ed.), *Handbook of clinical neurology. Clinical neuropsychology* (Vol. 1). Amsterdam: Elsevier.

Frederiks, J.A.M. (1985b). The neurology of aging and dementia. In J.A.M. Frederiks (Ed.), *Handbook of clinical neurology. Neurobehavioral disorders* (Vol. 2). Amsterdam: Elsevier.

Frederiksen, N. (1986). Toward a broader conception of human intelligence. *American Psychologist, 41,* 445–452.

Fredrickson, L.C. (1985). Goodenough-Harris drawing test. In D.J. Keyser & R.C. Sweetland (Eds.), *Test critiques* (Vol. II). Kansas City, MO: Test Corporation of America.

Freed, D.M., Corkin, S., Growdon, J.H., & Nissen, M.J. (1989). Selective attention in Alzheimer's disease: Characterizing cognitive subgroups of patients. *Neuropsychologia, 27,* 325–339.

Freed, D.M. & Kandel, E. (1988). Long-term occupational exposure and the diagnosis of dementia. *Neurotoxicology, 9,* 391–400.

Freedman, L. & Dexter, L.E. (1991). Visuospatial ability in cortical dementia. *Journal of Clinical and Experimental Neuropsychology, 13,* 677–690.

Freedman, M. (1990). Parkinson's disease. In J.L. Cummings (Ed.), *Subcortical dementia.* New York: Oxford University Press.

Freedman, M., Blumhardt, L.D., Brochet, B., et al. (2002). International consensus statement on the use of disease-modifying agents in multiple sclerosis. *Multiple Sclerosis, 8,* 19–23.

Freedman, M., Leach, L., Kaplan, E., et al. (1994). *Clock drawing. A neuropsychological analysis.* New York: Oxford University Press.

Freedman, M., Stuss, D.T., & Gordon, M. (1991). Assessment of competency: The role of neurobehavioral deficits. *Annals of Internal Medicine, 115,* 203–208.

Freides, D. (1978). On determining footedness. *Cortex, 14,* 134–135.

Freides, D. (1985). Desirable features in neuropsychological tests. *Journal of Psychopathology and Behavioral Assessment, 7,* 351–364.

Freides, D. (1993). Proposed standard of professional practice: Neuropsychological reports display all quantitative data. *The Clinical Neuropsychologist, 7,* 234–235.

Freides, D. (1995). Interpretations are more benign than data? *The Clinical Neuropsychologist, 9,* 248.

Freides, D. & Avery, M.E. (1991). Narrative and visual spatial recall: Assessment incorporating learning and delayed retention. *The Clinical Neuropsychologist, 5,* 338–344.

Freides, D., Engen, L., Miller, D., and Londa, J.B. (1996). Narrative and visual–spatial recall: Alternate forms, learning trial effects, and geriatric performance. *The Clinical Neuropsychologist, 10,* 407–418.

French, J.W., Ekstrom, R.B., & Price, L.A. (1963). *Kit of reference tests for cognitive factors.* Princeton, NJ: Educational Testing Service.

Freud, S. (1938). Psychopathology of everyday life. In A.A. Brill (Trans., Ed.), *The basic writings of Sigmund Freud.* New York: Modern Library.

Freund, G. (1982). The interaction of chronic alcohol consumption and aging on brain structure and function. *Alcoholism, Clinical and Experimental Research, 6,* 13–21.

Fried, I., Mateer, C., Ojemann, G., et al. (1982). Organization of visuospatial functions in human cortex. *Brain, 105,* 349–371.

Friedland, J.F. & Dawson, D.R. (2001). Function after motor vehicle accidents: A prospective study of mild head injury and post-traumatic stress. *Journal of Nervous and Mental Disease, 189,* 426–434.

Friedland, R.P. (2000). Brain imaging and cerebral metabolism. In F. Boller & J. Grafman (Eds.), *Handbook of neuropsychology* (Vol. 4). Amsterdam: Elsevier.

Friedland, R.P., Budinger, T.F., Koss, E., & Ober, B.A. (1985). Alzheimer's disease: Anterior–posterior and lateral hemispheric alterations in cortical glucose utilization. *Neuroscience Letters, 53,* 235–240.

Friedland, R.P. & Luxenberg, J. (1988). Neuroimaging and dementia. In W.H. Theodore (Ed.), *Clinical neuroimaging. Frontiers of Clinical Neuroscience* (Vol. 4). New York: Alan R. Liss.

Friedman, G., Froom, P., Sazbon, L., et al. (1999). Apolipoprotein E-4 genotype predicts a poor outcome in survivors of traumatic brain injury. *Neurology, 52,* 244–248.

Friedman, R.B., Ween, J.E., & Albert, M.L. (1993). Alexia. In K.M. Heilman & E. Valenstein (Eds.), *Clinical neuropsychology* (3rd ed.). New York: Oxford University Press.

Friend, K.B., Rabin, B.M., Groninger, L., et al. (1999). Language functions in patients with multiple sclerosis. *The Clinical Neuropsychologist, 13,* 78–94.

Friend, S.H. & Stoughton, R.B. (2002). The magic of microarrays. *Scientific American, 286,* 44–49.

Frisch, M.B. & Jessop, N.S. (1989). Improving WAIS-R estimates with the Shipley-Hartford and Wonderlic Personnel tests: need to control for reading ability. *Psychological Reports, 65,* 923–928.

Frisk, V. & Milner, B. (1990). The relationship of working memory to the immediate recall of stories following unilateral temporal or frontal lobectomy. *Neuropsychologia, 28,* 121–135.

Fristoe, N.M., Salthouse, T.A., & Woodard, J.L. (1997). Examination of age-related deficits on the Wisconsin Card Sorting Test. *Neuropsychology, 11,* 428–436.

Frith, C.D. (1998). The role of the prefrontal cortex in self-consciousness: The case of auditory hallucinations. In A.C. Roberts et al. (Eds.), *The prefrontal cortex.* Oxford: Oxford University Press.

Frith, C.D. & Dolan, R.J. (1997). Higher cognitive processes. In R.S.J. Frackowiak et al. (Eds.), *Human brain function.* San Diego: Academic Press.

Frith, C.D. & Friston, K.J. (1997). Studying brain function with neuro-imaging. In M.D. Rugg (Ed.), *Cognitive neuroscience.* Cambridge, MA: Cambridge University Press, pp. 169–195.

Fritsch, G. & Hitzig, E. (1969). On the electrical excitability of the cerebrum. In K.H. Pribam (Ed.), *Brain and behavior 2. Perception and action.* Baltimore, MD: Penguin.

Froehlich, T.E., Robison, J.T., & Inouye, S.K. (1998). Screening for dementia in the outpatient setting: The time and change test. *Journal of the American Geriatric Society, 46,* 1506–1511.

Froman, C. (1996). Whiplash. *Continuing Medical Education (South Africa), 14,* 1481–1487.

Fromm-Auch, D. & Yeudall, L.T. (1983). Normative data for the Halstead-Reitan neuropsychological tests. *Journal of Clinical Neuropsychology, 5,* 221–238.

Frost, J.A., Binder, J.R., Springer, J.A., et al. (1999). Language processing is strongly left lateralized in both sexes: Evidence from functional MRI. *Brain, 122,* 199–208.

Fuchs, K.L., Hannay, H.J., Huckeba, W.M., & Espy, K.A. (1999). Construct validity of the Continuous Recognition Memory Test. *The Clinical Neuropsychologist, 13,* 54–65.

Fugate, L.P., Spacek, L.A., Kresty, L.A., et al. (1997). Definition of agitation following traumatic brain injury: I. A survey of the brain injury special interest group of the American Academy of Physical Medicine and Rehabilitation. *Archives of Physical Medicine and Rehabilitation, 78,* 917–923.

Fujii, D.E., Lloyd, H.A., & Miyamoto, K. (2000). The salience of visuospatial and organizational skills in reproducing the Rey-Osterrieth Complex Figure in subjects with high and low IQs. *The Clinical Neuropsychologist, 14,* 551–554.

Fujimori, M., Imamura, T., Hirono, N., et al. (2000). Disturbances of spatial vision and object vision correlate differently with regional cerebral glucose metabolism in Alzheimer's disease. *Neuropsychologia, 38,* 1356–1361.

Fukuda, K., Straus, S.E., Hickie, I., et al. (1994). The chronic fatigue syndrome: A comprehensive approach to its definition and study. International Chronic Fatigue Syndrome Study Group. *Annals of Internal Medicine, 121,* 953–959.

Fuld, P.A. (1981). *Fuld Object-Memory Evaluation.* Wood Dale, IL: Stoelting.

Fuld, P.A. (1980). Guaranteed stimulus-processing in the evaluation of memory and learning. *Cortex, 16,* 255–272.

Fuld, P.A. (1983). Word intrusion as a diagnostic sign in Alzheimer's disease. *Geriatric Medicine Today, 2,* 33–41.

Fuld, P.A. (1984). Test profile of cholinergic dysfunction and of Alzheimer-type dementia. *Journal of Clinical Neuropsychology, 6,* 380–392.

Fuld, P.A., Katzman, R., Davies, P., & Terry, R.D. (1982). Intrusions as a sign of Alzheimer dementia: Chemical and pathological verification. *Annals of Neurology, 11,* 155–159.

Fuld, P.A., Masur, D.M., Blau, A.D., et al. (1990). Object-Memory Evaluation for prospective detection of dementia in normal functioning elderly: Predictive and normative data. *Journal of Clinical and Experimental Neuropsychology, 12,* 520–528.

Fuld, P.A., Muramato, O., Blau, A., et al. (1988). Cross-cultural and multi-ethnic dementia evaluation by mental status and memory testing. *Cortex, 24,* 511–519.

Fuller, K.H., Gouvier, W.D., & Savage, R.M. (1997). Comparison of list B and list C of the Rey Auditory Verbal Learning Test. *The Clinical Neuropsychologist, 11,* 201–204.

Furey-Kurkjian, M.L., Pietrini, P., Graff-Radford, N.R., et al. (1996). Visual variant of Alzheimer disease: Distinctive neuropsychological features. *Neuropsychology, 10,* 294–300.

Furman, J.M. & Cass, S.P. (2003). *Vestibular disorders. A case-study approach* (2nd ed.). New York: Oxford University Press.

Furst, H., Hartl, W.H., Haberl, R., et al. (2001). Silent cerebral infarction: Risk factor for stroke complicating carotid endarterectomy. *World Journal of Surgery, 25,* 969–974.

Furtado, S., Suchowersky, O., Rewcastle, B., et al. (1996). Relationship between trinucleotide repeats and neuropathological changes in Huntington's disease. *Annals of Neurology, 39,* 132–136.

Fuster, J.M. (1980). *The prefrontal cortex.* New York: Raven Press.

Fuster, J.M. (1985). The prefrontal cortex, mediator of cross-temporal contingencies. *Human Neurobiology, 4,* 169–179.

Fuster, J.M. (1994). La physiologie frontale et le cycle perception–action. *Revue de Neuropsychologie, 4,* 289–304.

Fuster, J.M. (1995). *Memory in the cerebral cortex: An empirical approach to neural networks in the human and nonhuman primate.* Cambridge, MA: MIT Press.

Fuster, J.M. (1999). Cognitive functions of the frontal lobes. In B.L. Miller & J.L. Cummings (Eds.), *The human frontal lobes: Functions and disorders.* New York: Guilford Press.

Fuster, J.M. (2003). *Cortex and mind. Unifying cognition.* New York: Oxford University Press.

Gabella, B., Hoffman, R.E., Marine, W.W., & Stallones, L. (1997). Urban and rural traumatic brain injuries in Colorado. *Annals of Epidemiology, 7,* 207–212.

Gabrieli, J.D.E. (1998). Cognitive neuroscience of human memory. *Annual Review of Psychology, 49,* 87–115.

Gabrieli, J.D.E., Singh, J., Stebbins, G.T., & Goetz, C.G. (1996). Reduced working memory span in Parkinson's disease: Evidence for the role of a frontostriatal system in working memory and strategic memory. *Neuropsychology, 10,* 322–332.

Gabrieli, J.D., Vaidya, C.J., Stone, M., et al. (1999). Convergent behavioral and neuropsychological evidence for a distinction between identification and production forms of repetition priming. *Journal of Experimental Psychology: General, 128,* 479–498.

Gabriels, P. (1995). Tinnitus and hyperacusis. In *Proceedings of the Fifth International Tinnitus Seminar.* Portland, OR: American Tinnitus Association.

Gabrys, J.B. & Peters, K. (1985). Reliability, discriminant and predictive validity of the Zung Self-rating Depression Scale. *Psychological Reports, 57,* 1091–1096.

Gaede, S.E., Parsons, O.A., & Berters, J.H. (1978). Hemispheric differences in music perception: Aptitude vs. experience. *Neuropsychologia, 16,* 369–373.

Gaillard, F. (1990). Synergie neuro-cognitive: Avantage dans les apprentissages en lecture et calcul. *Approche Neuropsychologique des Apprentissages chez l'Enfant, 2,* 4–9.

Gaillard, F. & Converso, G. (1988). Lecture et lateralisation: Le retour de L'homme calleux. *Bulletin d'Audiophonologie. Annales Scientifique de l'Université de Franche-Comté, 4,* 497–508.

Gaillard, F., Converso, G., & Amar, S.B. (1987). Latéralisation cérébrale et implication hémisphérique dans la réalisation de certaines tâches mathématiques. I: Revue de la littérature. *Revue Suisse de Psychologie, 46,* 173–181.

Gaillard, W.D., Balsamo, L., Xu, B., et al. (2002). Language dominance in partial epilepsy patients identified with an fMRI reading task. *Neurology, 59,* 256–265.

Gaillard, W.D., Bookheimer, S.Y., & Cohen, M. (2000). The use of fMRI in neocortical epilepsy. *Advances in Neurology, 84,* 391–404.

Gainotti, G. (1972). Emotional behavior and hemispheric side of one lesion. *Cortex, 8,* 41–55.

Gainotti, G. (1984). Some methodological problems in the study of the relationships between emotions and cerebral dominance. *Journal of Clinical Neuropsychology, 6,* 111–121.

Gainotti, G. (1993). Emotional and psychosocial problems after brain injury. *Neuropsychological Rehabilitation, 3,* 259–277.

Gainotti, G. (2000). Neuropsychological theories of emotion. In J.C. Borod (Ed.), *The neuropsychology of emotion.* New York: Oxford University Press.

Gainotti, G. (2003). Emotional disorders in relation to unilateral brain disorders. In T.E. Feinberg & M.J. Farah (Eds.), *Behavioral neurology and neuropsychology.* New York: McGraw-Hill.

Gainotti, G., Caltagirone, C., & Zoccolotti, P. (1993). Left/right and cortical/subcortical dichotomies in the neuropsychological study of human emotions. *Cognition and Emotion, 7,* 71–93.

Gainotti, G., Daniele, A., Nocentini, U., & Silveri, M.C. (1989). The nature of lexical-semantic impairment in Alzheimer's disease. *Journal of Neurolinguistics, 4,* 449–460.

Gainotti, G., D'Erme, P., & De Bonis, C. (1989). Components of visual attention disrupted in unilateral neglect. In J.W. Brown (Ed.), *Neuropsychology of visual perception.* New York: IRBN Press.

Gainotti, G., D'Erme, P., Villa, G., & Caltagirone, C. (1986). Focal brain lesions and intelligence: A study with a new version of Raven's Colored Matrices. *Journal of Clinical and Experimental Neuropsychology, 1,* 37–50.

Gainotti, G. & Marra, C. (1994). Some aspects of memory disorders clearly distinguish dementia of the Alzheimer's type from depressive pseudo-dementia. *Journal of Clinical and Experimental Neuropsychology, 16,* 65–78.

Gainotti, G., Parlato, V., Monteleone, D., & Carlomagno, S. (1992). Neuropsychological markers of dementia on visual–spatial tasks: A comparison between Alzheimer's type and vascular forms of dementia. *Journal of Clinical and Experimental Neuropsychology, 14,* 239–252.

Gainotti, G. & Tiacci, C. (1970). Patterns of drawing disability in right and left hemisphere patients. *Neuropsychologia, 8,* 379–384.

Galasko, D., Klauber, M.R., Hofstetter, C.R., et al. (1990). The Mini-Mental State Examination in the early diagnosis of Alzheimer's disease. *Archives of Neurology, 47,* 49–52.

Galbraith, S. (1985). Irritability. *British Medical Journal, 291,* 1668–1669.

Gale, J.L., Dikmen, S., Wyler, A., et al. (1983). Head injury in the Pacific Northwest. *Neurosurgery, 12,* 487–491.

Gale, S.D., Hopkins, R.O., Weaver, L.K., et al. (1999). MRI, quantitative MRI, SPECT, and neuropsychological findings following carbon monoxide poisoning. *Brain Injury, 13,* 229–243.

Gale, S.D., Johnson, S.C., Bigler, E.D., & Blatter, D.D. (1995). Nonspecific white matter degeneration following traumatic brain injury. *Journal of the International Neuropsychological Society, 1,* 17–28.

Galin, D. (1974). Implications for psychiatry of left and right cerebral specialization. *Archives of General Psychiatry, 31,* 572–583.

Galin, D., Ornstein, R., Herron, J., & Johnstone, J. (1982). Sex and handedness differences in EEG measures of hemispheric specialization. *Brain and Language, 16,* 19–55.

Gallagher, A.M., De Lisi, R., Holst, P.C., et al. (2000). Gender differences in advanced mathematical problem solving. *Journal of Experimental Child Psychology, 75,* 165–190.

Gallagher, D., Breckenridge, J., Steinmetz, J., & Thompson, L. (1983). The Beck Depression Inventory and research diagnostic criteria: Congruence in an older population. *Journal of Consulting and Clinical Psychology, 51,* 945–946.

Gallo, J.J. & Breitner, J.C. (1995). Alzheimer's disease in the NAS-NRC Registry of Aging Twin Veterans. IV. Performance characteristics of a two-stage telephone screening procedure for Alzheimer's dementia. *Psychological Medicine, 25,* 1211–1219.

Gallo, J.J., Rebok, G.W., & Lesikar, S.E. (1999). The driving habits of adults aged 60 years and older. *Journal of the American Geriatric Society, 47,* 335–341.

Galski, T., Tompkins, C., & Johnston, M.V. (1998). Competence in discourse as a measure of social integration and quality of life in persons with traumatic brain injury. *Brain Injury, 12,* 769–782.

Galton, C.J., Patterson, K., Graham, K., et al. (2001). Differing patterns of temporal atrophy in Alzheimer's disease and semantic dementia. *Neurology, 57,* 216–225.

Galuske, R.A., Schlote, W., Bratzke, H., & Singer, W. (2000). Interhemispheric asymmetries of the modular structure in human temporal cortex. *Science, 289,* 1946–1949.

Gancher, S.T. (1992). Pharmacology of Parkinson's disease. In S.J. Huber & J.L. Cummings (Eds.), *Parkinson's disease. Neurobehavioral aspects.* New York: Oxford University Press.

Ganguli, M., Chandra, V., Gilby, J.E., et al. (1996). Cognitive test performance in a community-based nondemented elderly sample in rural India: The Indo–U.S. cross-national dementia epidemiology study. *International Psychogeriatrics, 8,* 507–524.

Ganguli, M., Ratcliff, G., Huff, F.J., et al. (1991). Effects of age, gender, and education on cognitive tests in a rural elderly community sample: Norms from the Monongahela Valley Independent Elders Survey. *Neuroepidemiology, 10,* 42–52.

Ganor-Stern, D., Seamon, J.G., & Carrasco, M. (1998). The role of attention and study time in explicit and implicit memory for unfamiliar visual stimuli. *Memory and Cognition, 26,* 1187–1195.

Gao, S., Hendrie, H.C., Hall, K.S., & Hui, S. (1998). The relationships between age, sex, and the incidence of dementia and Alzheimer disease: a meta-analysis. *Archives of General Psychiatry, 55,* 809–815.

Garb, H.N. (1997). Race bias, social class bias, and gender bias in clinical judgment. *Clinical Psychology: Science and Practice, 4,* 99–120.

Garb, H.N. & Schramke, C.J. (1996). Judgment research and neuropsychological assessment: A narrative review and meta-analysis. *Psychological Bulletin, 120,* 140–153.

Garcia, J. (1981). The logic and limits of mental aptitude testing. *American Psychologist, 36,* 1172–1180.

Garcia-Monco, J.C. & Benach, J.L. (1995). Lyme neuroborreliosis. *Annals of Neurology, 37,* 691–702.

Gard, D., Harrell, E.H., & Poreh, A. (1999). Cognitive deficits in schizophrenia on the WAIS-R NI Sentence Arrangement subtest. *Journal of Clinical Psychology, 55,* 1085–1094.

Gardner, H. (1994). The stories of the right hemisphere. In W. Spaulding (Ed.), *Forty-first Nebraska symposium on motivation.* Lincoln: University of Nebraska Press.

Gardner, H., Ling, P.K., Flamm, L., & Silverman, J. (1975). Comprehension and appreciation of humorous material following brain damage. *Brain, 98,* 399–412.

Gardner, R., Jr. (1981). Mattis Dementia Rating Scale: Internal reliability study using a diffusely impaired population. *Journal of Clinical Neuropsychology, 3,* 271–275.

Garraux, G., Salmon, E., Degueldre, C., et al. (1999). Comparison of impaired subcortico-frontal metabolic networks in normal aging, subcortico-frontal dementia, and cortical frontal dementia. *Neuroimage, 10,* 149–162.

Garron, D.C. & Cheifetz, D.I. (1965). Comment on "Bender Gestalt discernment of organic pathology." *Psychological Bulletin, 63,* 197–200.

Gasparrini, B., Shealy, C., & Walters, D. (1980). Differences in size and spatial placement of drawings of left versus right hemisphere brain-damaged patients. *Journal of Consulting and Clinical Psychology, 48,* 670–672.

Gasquoine, P.G. (1997a). Emotional, cognitive, and motivational deficits in compensation-seeking, suspected brain injury cases. *Applied Neuropsychology, 4,* 99–106.

Gasquoine, P.G. (1997b). Postconcussion symptoms. *Neuropsychology Review, 7,* 77–85.

Gass, C.S. (1991). MMPI-2 interpretation and closed head injury: A correction factor. *Psychological Assessment, 3,* 27–31.

Gass, C.S. (1992). MMPI-2 interpretation of patients with cerebrovascular disease: A correction factor. *Archives of Clinical Neuropsychology, 7,* 17–27.

Gass, C.S. (1995). A procedure for assessing storage and retrieval on the Wechsler Memory Scale-Revised. *Archives of Clinical Neuropsychology, 10,* 475–487.

Gass, C.S. (1996). MMPI-2 interpretation and stroke: Cross-validation of a correction factor. *Journal of Clinical Psychology, 52,* 569–572.

Gass, C.S. & Daniel, S.K. (1990). Emotional impact on Trail Making Test performance. *Psychological Reports, 67,* 435–438.

Gass, C.S. & Lawhorn, L. (1991). Psychological adjustment following stroke: An MMPI study. *Psychological Assessment, 3,* 628–633.

Gates, J.R. (2000). Epidemiology and classification of non-epileptic events. In J.R. Gates & A.J. Rowan (Eds.), *Non-epileptic seizures* (2nd ed.). Boston: Butterworth-Heinemann.

Gates, P.C., Barnett, H.J.M., & Silver, M.D. (1986). Cardiogenic stroke. In H.J.M. Barnett et al. (Eds.), *Stroke. Pathophysiology, diagnosis, and management.* New York: Churchill Livingstone.

Gatewood-Colwell, G., Kaczmarek, M., & Ames, M.H. (1989). Reliability and validity of the Beck Depression Inventory for a white and Mexican-American gerontic population. *Psychological Reports, 65,* 1163–1166.

Gatz, M., Pedersen, N.L., Berg, S., et al. (1997). Heritability for Alzheimer's disease: the study of dementia in Swedish twins. *Journals of Gerontology. Series A, Biological Sciences and Medical Sciences, 52,* M117–M125.

Gatz, M., Reynolds, C.A., John, R., et al. (2002). Telephone screening to identify potential dementia cases in a population-based sample of older adults. *International Psychogeriatrics, 14,* 273–289.

Gaudette, M.D. & Smith, J.A. (1998). Process-oriented administration of the Picture Arrangement test does not affect the quantitative outcome. *Applied Neuropsychology, 5,* 154–158.

Gaudino, E.A., Chiaravalloti, N.D., DeLuca, J., & Diamond, B.J. (2001). A comparison of memory performance in relapsing-remitting, primary progressive and secondary progressive multiple sclerosis. *Neuropsychiatry, Neuropsychology and Behavioral Neurology, 14,* 32–44.

Gaudino, E.A., Coyle, P.K., & Krupp, L.B. (1997). Post-Lyme syndrome and chronic fatigue syndrome. Neuropsychiatric similarities and differences. *Archives of Neurology, 54,* 1372–1376.

Gaudino, E.A., Geisler, M.W., & Squires, N.K. (1995). Construct validity in the Trail Making Test: what makes Part B harder? *Journal of Clinical and Experimental Neuropsychology, 17,* 529–535.

Gaultieri, T. & Cox, D.R. (1991). The delayed neurobehavioural sequelae of traumatic brain injury. *Brain Injury, 5,* 219–232.

Gauthier, L, Dehaut, F., & Joanette, Y. (1989). The Bells Test: A quantitative and qualitative test for visual neglect. *International Journal of Clinical Neuropsychology, 11,* 49–54.

Gazzaniga, M.S. (1987). Perceptual and attentional processes following callosal section in humans. *Neuropsychologia, 25,* 119–133.

Gazzaniga, M.S. (Ed.) (2000a). *The new cognitive neurosciences* (2nd ed.). Cambridge, MA: MIT Press.

Gazzaniga, M.S. (2000b). Neuroscience. Regional differences in cortical organization. *Science, 289,* 1887–1888.

Geary, D.C. (1989). A model for representing gender differences in the pattern of cognitive abilities. *American Psychologist, 44,* 1155–1156.

Geerlings, M.I., Schoevers, R.A., Beekman, A.T., et al. (2000). Depression and risk of cognitive decline and Alzheimer's disease. Results of two prospective community-based studies in The Netherlands. *British Journal of Psychiatry, 176,* 568–575.

Geffen, G.M., Encel, J.S., & Forrester, G.M. (1991). Stages of recovery during post-traumatic amnesia and subsequent everyday deficits. *Cognitive Neuroscience and Neuropsychology, 2,* 105–108.

Geffen, G., Moar, K.J., O'Hanlon, A.P., et al. (1990). The Auditory Verbal Learning Test (Rey): Performance of 16 to 86 year olds of average intelligence. *The Clinical Neuropsychologist, 4,* 45–63.

Gehring, W.J. & Knight, R.T. (2000). Prefrontal–cingulate interactions in action monitoring. *Nature Neuroscience, 3,* 516–520.

Geidd, J.N., Snell, J.W., Lange, N., et al. (1996). Quantitative magnetic resonance imaging of human brain development: Ages 4–18. *Cerebral Cortex, 6,* 551–560.

Geisler, M.W., Sliwinski, M., Coyle, P.K., et al. (1996). The effects of amantadine and pemoline on cognitive functioning in multiple sclerosis. *Archives of Neurology, 53,* 185–188.

Gelb, L.D. (1990). Infections: bacteria, fungi, and parasites. In A.L. Pearlman & R.C. Collins (Eds.), *Neurobiology of disease.* New York: Oxford University Press.

Geldmacher, D.S. & Whitehouse, P.J. (1996). Evaluation of dementia. *New England Journal of Medicine, 335,* 330–336.

Geldmacher, D.S. & Whitehouse, P.J., Jr. (1997). Differential diagnosis of Alzheimer's disease. *Neurology, 48,* S2–S9.

Geller, A.M. (2001). A table of color distance scores of quantitative scoring of the Lanthony Desaturate Color Vision test. *Neurotoxicology and Teratology, 23,* 265–267.

Genetta-Wadley, A. & Swirsky-Sacchetti, T. (1990). Sex differences and handedness in hemispheric lateralization of tactile–spatial functions. *Perceptual and Motor Skills, 70,* 579–590.

Gennarelli, T.A. (1983). Head injury in man and experimental animals: Clinical aspects. *Acta Neurochirurgica (Suppl. 32),* 1–13.

Gennarelli, T.A. (1986). Mechanisms and pathophysiology of cerebral concussion. *Journal of Head Trauma Rehabilitation, 1,* 23–29.

Gennarelli, T.A. & Meaney, D.F. (1996). Mechanisms of primary head injury. In R.H. Wilkins & S.S. Rengachary (Eds.), *Neurosurgery.* New York: McGraw-Hill.

Gennarelli, T.A., Thibault, L.E., Adams, J.H., et al. (1982). Diffuse axonal injury and traumatic coma in the primate. *Annals of Neurology, 12,* 564–574.

Gennarelli, T.A., Thibault, L.E., & Graham, D.I. (1998). Diffuse axonal injury: An important form of traumatic brain damage. *Neuroscientist, 4,* 202–215.

Gentilini, M., Nichelli, P., Schoenhuber, R., et al. (1985). Neuropsychological evaluation of mild head injury. *Journal of Neurology, Neurosurgery and Psychiatry, 48,* 137–140.

Gentilini, N., Nichelli, P., & Schoenhuber, R. (1989). Assessment of attention in mild head injury. In H.S. Levin et al. (Eds.), *Mild head injury.* New York: Oxford University Press.

Geocadin, R.G. & Williams, M.A. (2002). Disorders of intracranial pressure. In A.A. Asbury et al. (Eds.), *Diseases of the nervous system* (3rd ed.). Cambridge: Cambridge University Press.

George, A.E., Holodny, A., Golomb, J., & de Leon, M.J. (1995). The differential diagnosis of Alzheimer's disease. Cerebral atrophy versus normal pressure hydrocephalus. *Neuroimaging Clinics of North America, 5,* 19–31.

George, M.S., Ketter, T.A., Kimbrell, T.A., et al. (2000). Neuroimaging approaches to the study of emotion. In J.C. Borod (Ed.), *The neuropsychology of emotion.* New York: Oxford University Press.

Gerritsen, M., Berg, I., & Deelman, B. (2001). Snijders-Oomen Nonverbal Intelligence Test: Useful for the elderly? [in Dutch]. *Tijdschrift voor Gerontologie en Geriatrie, 32,* 24–28.

Gerstmann, J. (1940). Syndrome of finger agnosia, disorientation for right and left agraphia, acalculia. *Archives of Neurology and Psychiatry, 44,* 398–408.

Gerstmann, J. (1942). Problem of imperception of disease and of impaired body territories with organic lesions. *Archives of Neurology and Psychiatry, 48,* 890–913.

Gerstmann, J. (1957). Some notes on the Gerstmann syndrome. *Neurology, 7,* 866–869.

Geschwind, N. (1965). Disconnexion syndromes in animals and man. *Brain, 88,* 237–294.

Geschwind, N. (1970). The organization of language and the brain. *Science, 170,* 940–944.

Geschwind, N. (1972). Language and the brain. *Scientific American, 226,* 76–83.

Geschwind, N. (1974). Late changes in the nervous system: An overview. In D.G. Stein, J.J. Rosen, & N. Butters (Eds.), *Plasticity and recovery of function in the central nervous system.* New York: Academic Press.

Geschwind, N. (1975). The apraxias: Neural mechanisms of disorders of learned movement. *American Scientist, 63,* 188–195.

Geschwind, N. (1979). Specializations of the human brain. *Scientific American, 241,* 180–199.

Geschwind, N. (1985). Mechanisms of change after brain lesions. *Annals of the New York Academy of Sciences, 457,* 1–13.

Geschwind, N. & Galaburda, A.M. (1985). Cerebral lateralization: Biological mechanisms, associations, and pathology. I. A hypothesis and a program for research. *Archives of Neurology, 42,* 428–459.

Geschwind, N. & Strub, R. (1975). Gerstmann syndrome of aphasia: A reply to Poeck & Orgass. *Cortex, 11,* 296–298.

Getz, K., Hermann, B., Seidenberg, M., et al. (2002). Negative symptoms in temporal lobe epilepsy. *American Journal of Psychiatry, 159,* 644–651.

Getzels, J.W. & Jackson, P.W. (1962). *Creativity and intelligence.* New York: Wiley.

Geula, C. (1998). Abnormalities of neural circuitry in Alzheimer's disease: Hippocampus and cortical cholinergic innervation. *Neurology, 51,* S18–S29.

Gewirtz, R.J. & Steinberg, G.K. (1997). Management of cerebral edema/ICP in stroke. In K.M.A. Welch et al. (Eds.), *Primer on cerebrovascular diseases.* San Diego: Academic Press.

Gfeller, J.D. & Cradock, M.M. (1998). Detecting feigned neuropsychological impairment with the Seashore Rhythm Test. *Journal of Clinical Psychology, 54,* 431–438.

Gfeller, J.D., Meldrum, D.L., & Jacobi, K.A. (1995). The impact of constructional impairment on the WMS-R Visual Reproduction subtest. *Journal of Clinical Psychology, 51,* 58–63.

Ghebremedhin, E., Schultz, C., Thal, D.R., et al. (2001). Gender and age modify the association between *APOE* and AD-related neuropathology. *Neurology, 56,* 1696–1701.

Ghent, L. (1956). Perception of overlapping and embedded figures by children of different ages. *Journal of Psychology, 69,* 575–587.

Ghezzi, A., Deplano, V., Faroni, J., et al. (1997). Multiple sclerosis in childhood: Clinical features of 149 cases. *Multiple Sclerosis, 3,* 43–46.

Ghika-Schmid, F. & Bogousslavsky, J. (2001). Disorders of mood behavior. In J. Bogousslavsky & L. Caplan (Eds.), *Stroke syndromes* (2nd ed.). Cambridge, UK: Cambridge University Press.

Gialanella, B. & Mattioli, F. (1992). Anosognosia and extrapersonal neglect as predictors of functional recovery following right hemisphere stroke. *Neuropsychological Rehabilitation, 2,* 169–178.

Giambra, L.M., Arenberg, D., Kawas, C., et al. (1995). Adult life span changes in immediate visual memory and verbal intelligence. *Psychology and Aging, 10,* 123–139.

Gibson, G.E., Pulsinelli, W., Blass, J.P., & Duffy, T.E. (1981). Brain dysfunction in mild to moderate hypoxia. *American Journal of Medicine, 70,* 1247–1254.

Giedd, J.N., Snell, J.W., Lange, N., et al. (1996). Quantitative magnetic resonance imaging of human brain development: Ages 4–18. *Cerebral Cortex, 6,* 551–560.

Gil, M., Cohen, M., Korn, C., & Groswasser, Z. (1996). Vocational outcome of aphasic patients following severe traumatic brain injury. *Brain Injury, 10,* 39–45.

Gilbert, J.G. (1973). Thirty-five-year follow-up study of intellectual functioning. *Journal of Gerontology, 28,* 68–72.

Gilbert, J.J. & Sadler, M. (1983). Unsuspected multiple sclerosis. *Archives of Neurology, 40,* 533–536.

Gilchrist, A.C. & Creed, F.H. (1994). Depression, cognitive impairment, and social stress in multiple sclerosis. *Journal of Psychosomatic Research, 38,* 193–201.

Gilewski, M.J., Zelinski, E.M., & Schaie, K.W. (1990). The memory functioning questionnaire for assessment of memory complaints in adulthood and old age. *Psychology and Aging, 5,* 482–490.

Gill, D.M., Reddon, J.R., Stefanyk, W.O., & Hans, H.S. (1986). Finger tapping: Effects of trials and sessions. *Perceptual and Motor Skills, 62,* 675–678.

Gilley, D.W. (1993). Behavioral and affective disturbances in Alzheimer's disease. In R.W. Parks et al. (Eds.), *Neuropsychology of Alzheimer's disease and other dementias.* New York: Oxford University Press.

Gillham, R., Baker, G., Thompson, P., Birbeck, K., et al. (1996). Standardisation of a self-report questionnaire for use in evaluating cognitive, affective and behavioural side-effects of anti-epileptic drug treatments. *Epilepsy Research, 24,* 47–55.

Gillham, R., Bryant-Comstock, L., & Kane, K. (2000). Validation of the Side Effect and Life Satisfaction (SEALS) inventory. *Seizure, 9,* 458–463.

Gillham, R., Kane, K., Bryant-Comstock, L., & Brodie, M.J. (2000). A double-blind comparison of lamotrigine and carbamazepine in newly diagnosed epilepsy with health-related quality of life as an outcome measure. *Seizure, 9,* 375–379.

Gilliam, F., Kuzniecky, R., Faught, E., Black, L., et al. (1997). Patient-validated content of epilepsy-specific quality-of-Life measurement. *Epilepsia, 38,* 233–236.

Gilliam, F., Kuzniecky, R., Meador, K., Martin, R., et al. (1999). Patient-oriented outcome assessment after temporal lobectomy for refractory epilepsy. *Neurology, 53,* 687–694.

Gilmore, G.C. & Whitehouse, P.J. (1995). Contrast sensitivity in Alzheimer's disease: a 1-year longitudinal analysis. *Optometry and Vision Science, 72,* 83–91.

Ginsberg, M.D. (1985). Carbon monoxide intoxication: Clinical features, neuropathology and mechanisms of injury. *Clinical Toxicology, 23,* 281–288.

Giordani, B., Boivin, M.J., Hall, A.L., et al. (1990). The utility and generality of Mini-Mental State Examination scores in Alzheimer's disease. *Neurology, 40,* 1894–1896.

Giovagnoli, A.R. & Avanzini, G. (1996). Forgetting rate and interference effects on a verbal memory distractor task in patients with temporal lobe epilepsy. *Journal of Clinical and Experimental Neuropsychology, 18,* 259–264.

Girelli, L. & Delazer, M. (2001). Numerical abilities in dementia. *Aphasiology, 15,* 681–694.

Girotti, F., Soliveri, P., Carella, F., et al. (1988). Role of motor performance in cognitive processes of parkinsonian patients. *Neurology, 38,* 537–540.

Gitelman, D.R. (2002). Acalculia. In M. D'Esposito (Ed.), *Neurological foundations of cognitive neuroscience.* Cambridge, MA: MIT Press.

Gladsjo, J.A., Heaton, R.K., Palmer, B.W., et al. (1999). Use of oral reading to estimate premorbid intellectual and neuropsychological functioning. *Journal of the International Neuropsychological Society, 5,* 247–254.

Gladsjo, J.A., Schuman, C.C., Evans, J.D., et al. (1999). Norms for letter and category fluency: demographic corrections for age, education, and ethnicity. *Assessment, 6,* 147–178.

Gladue, B.A. & Bailey, J.M. (1995). Spatial ability, handedness, and human sexual orientation. *Psychoneuroendocrinology, 20,* 487–497.

Glass, J.N. (1998). Differential subtest scores on the Rivermead Behavioural Memory Test (RBMT) in an elderly population with diagnosis of vascular or nonvascular dementia. *Applied Neuropsychology, 5,* 57–64.

Glatt, S.L. & Koller, W.C. (1992). Effect of antiparkinsonian drugs on memory. In S.J. Huber & J.L. Cummings (Eds.), *Parkinson's disease. Neurobehavioral aspects.* New York: Oxford University Press.

Gleason, A.C. & Meyers, C.A. (2002). Relationship between cognitive impairment and tumor grade in pre-surgical patients with primary brain tumors [abstract]. *Journal of the International Neuropsychological Society, 8,* 274.

Gleissner, U., Helmstaedter, C., & Elger, C.E. (1998). Right hippocampal contribution to visual memory: A presurgical and postsurgical study in patients with temporal lobe epilepsy. *Journal of Neurology, Neurosurgery and Psychiatry, 65,* 665–669.

Gleissner, U., Helmstaedter, C., & Elger, C.E. (2002). Memory reorganization in adult brain: Observations in three patients with temporal lobe epilepsy. *Epilepsy Research, 48,* 229–234.

Glenn, M.B., O'Neil-Pirozzi, T., Goldstein, R., et al. (2001). Depression amongst outpatients with traumatic brain injury. *Brain Injury, 15,* 811–818.

Glenn, S.W. & Parsons, O.A. (1990). The role of time in neuropsychological performance: Investigation and application in an alcoholic population. *The Clinical Neuropsychologist, 4,* 344–354.

Glick, S.D., Ross, D.A., & Hough, L.B. (1982). Lateral asymmetry of neurotransmitters in human brain. *Brain Research, 234,* 53–63.

Glioma Meta-Analysis Trialists Group (2002). Chemotherapy in adult high-grade glioma: a systematic review and meta-analysis of individual patient data from 12 randomised trials. *Lancet, 359,* 1011–1018.

Glisky, E.L. (1996). Prospective memory and the frontal lobes. In M. Brandimonte et al. (Eds.), *Prospective memory. Theory and applications.* Mahwah, NJ: Erlbaum.

Glisky, E.L., Schachter, D.L., & Tulving, E. (1986). Learning and retention of computer-related vocabulary in memory-impaired patients: Method of vanishing cues. *Journal of Clinical and Experimental Neuropsychology, 8,* 292–312.

Globus, M., Mildworf, B., & Melamed, E. (1985). Cerebral blood flow and cognitive impairment in Parkinson's disease. *Neurology, 35,* 1135–1139.

Gloning, K. & Hoff, H. (1969). Cerebral localization of disorders of higher nervous activity. In P.J. Vinken & G.W. Bruyn (Eds.), *Handbook of clinical neurology. Disorders of higher nervous activity.* (Vol. 3). New York: Wiley.

Gloning, I., Gloning, K., & Hoff, H. (1968). *Neuropsychological symptoms and syndromes in lesions of the occipital lobe and adjacent areas.* Paris: Gauthier-Villars.

Gloning, K. & Quatember, R. (1966). Statistical evidence of neuropsychological syndrome in left-handed and ambidextrous patients. *Cortex, 2,* 484–488.

Gloor, R., Olivier, A., Quesney, L.F., et al. (1982). The role of the limbic system in experiential phenomena of temporal lobe epilepsy. *Annals of Neurology, 12,* 129–144.

Gloria, L., Cravo, M., Camilo, M.E., et al. (1997). Nutritional deficiencies in chronic alcoholics: Relation to dietary intake and alcohol consumption. *American Journal of Gastroenterology, 92,* 485–489.

Glosser, G., Butters, N., & Kaplan, E. (1977). Visuoperceptual processes in brain damaged patients on the Digit Symbol Substitution Test. *International Journal of Neuroscience, 7,* 59–66.

Glosser, G., Cole, L., Khatri, U., et al. (2002). Assessing nonverbal memory with the Biber Figure Learning Test-extended in temporal lobe epilepsy patients. *Archives of Clinical Neuropsychology, 17,* 25–35.

Glosser, G. & Goodglass, H. (1990). Disorders in executive control functions among aphasic and other brain-damaged patients. *Journal of Clinical and Experimental Neuropsychology, 12,* 485–501.

Glosser, G., Goodglass, H., & Biber, C. (1989). Assessing visual memory disorders. *Journal of Consulting and Clinical Psychology, 1,* 82–91.

Glozman, J.M. (1999). Quantitative and qualitative integration of Lurian procedures. *Neuropsychology Review, 9,* 23–32.

Gnanalingham, K.K., Byrne, E.J., & Thornton, A. (1996). Clockface drawing to differentiate Lewy body and Alzheimer type dementia syndromes. *Lancet, 347,* 696–697.

Gnanalingham, K.K., Byrne, E.J., Thornton, A., et al. (1997). Motor and cognitive function in Lewy body dementia: Comparison with Alzheimer's and Parkinson's diseases. *Journal of Neurology, Neurosurgery and Psychiatry, 62,* 243–252.

Goadsby, P.J. (1997). Current concepts of the pathophysiology of migraine. *Neurologic Clinics, 15,* 115–123.

Godefroy, O., Lhullier-Lamy, C., & Rousseaux, M. (2002). SRT lengthening: role of an alertness deficit in frontal damaged patients. *Neuropsychologia, 40,* 2234–2241.

Godefroy, O. & Rousseaux, M. (1997). Novel decision making in patients with prefrontal or posterior brain damage. *Neurology, 49,* 695–701.

Godfrey, H.P.D., Marsh, N.V., & Partridge, F.M. (1987). Severe traumatic head injury and social behavior: A review. *New Zealand Journal of Psychology, 16,* 49–57.

Godfrey, H.P.D., Partridge, F.M., Knight, R.G., & Bishara, S. (1993). Course of insight disorder and emotional dysfunction following closed head injury: a controlled cross-sectional follow-up study. *Journal of Clinical and Experimental Neuropsychology, 15,* 503–515.

Godwin-Austen, R. & Bendall, J. (1990). *The neurology of the elderly.* New York: Springer-Verlag.

Goebel, R.A. (1983). Detection of faking on the Halstead-Reitan neuropsychological test battery. *Journal of Clinical Psychology, 39,* 731–742.

Goebels, N. & Soyka, M. (2000). Dementia associated with vitamin

B$_{12}$ deficiency: Presentation of two cases and review of the literature. *Journal of Neuropsychiatry and Clinical Neurosciences, 12,* 389–394.

Goel, V. & Grafman, J. (1995). Are the frontal lobes implicated in "planning" functions? Interpreting data from the Tower of Hanoi. *Neuropsychologia, 33,* 623–642.

Goel, V. & Grafman, J. (2000). Role of the right prefrontal cortex in ill-structured planning. *Cognitive Neuropsychology, 17,* 415–436.

Goel, V., Grafman, J., Tajik, J., et al. (1997). A study of the performance of patients with frontal lobe lesions in a financial planning task. *Brain, 120,* 1805–1822.

Goel, V., Pullara, S.D., & Grafman, J. (2001). A computational model of frontal lobe dysfunction: working memory and the Tower of Hanoi task. *Cognitive Science, 25,* 287–313.

Goethe, K.E., Mitchell, J.E., Marshall, D.W., et al. (1989). Neuropsychological and neurological function of human immunodeficiency virus seropositive asymptomatic individuals. *Archives of Neurology, 46,* 129–133.

Goetz, C.G., Tanner, C.M., Stebbins, G.T., & Buchman, A.S. (1988). Risk factors for the progression in Parkinson's disease. *Neurology, 38,* 1841–1844.

Goggin, K.J., Zisook, S., Heaton, R.K., et al. (1997). Neuropsychological performance of HIV-1 infected men with major depression. *Journal of the International Neuropsychological Society, 3,* 457–463.

Golanov, E.G. & Reis, D.J. (1997). Oxygen and cerebral blood flow. In K.M.A. Welch et al. (Eds.), *Primer of cerebrovascular diseases.* San Diego, CA: Academic Press.

Golbe, L.I. (1991). Young-onset Parkinson's disease. A clinical review. *Neurology, 41,* 168–173.

Golbe, L.I. (1996). The epidemiology of progressive supranuclear palsy. *Advances in Neurology, 69,* 25–31.

Golbe, L.I., Davis, P.H., Schoenberg, B.S., & Duvoisin, R.C. (1988). Prevalence and natural history of progressive supranuclear palsy. *Neurology, 38,* 1031–1034.

Gold, B.T. & Kertesz, A. (2000). Right hemisphere semantic processing of visual words in an aphasic patient: An fMRI study. *Brain and Language, 73,* 456–465.

Gold, J.M., Berman, F., Randolph, C., et al. (1996). PET validation of a novel prefrontal task: Delayed response alternation. *Neuropsychology, 10,* 3–10.

Gold, J.M., Carpenter, C., Randolph, C., et al. (1997). Auditory working memory and Wisconsin Card Sorting Test performance in schizophrenia. *Archives of General Psychiatry, 54,* 159–165.

Gold, J.M., Queern, C., Iannone, V.N., & Buchanan, R.W. (1999). Repeatable Battery for the Assessment of Neuropsychological Status as a screening test in schizophrenia I: Sensitivity, reliability, and validity. *American Journal of Psychiatry, 156,* 1944–1950.

Goldberg, E. (1986). Varieties of perseveration: A comparison of two taxonomies. *Journal of Clinical and Experimental Neuropsychology, 8,* 710–726.

Goldberg, E. (1989). Gradient approach to neocortical functional organization. *Journal of Clinical and Experimental Neuropsychology, 11,* 489–517.

Goldberg, E. (1990). Higher cortical functions in humans: The gradiental approach. In E. Goldberg (Ed.), *Contemporary neuropsychology and the legacy of Luria.* Hillsdale, NJ: Erlbaum.

Goldberg, E. (1995). Rise and fall of modular orthodoxy. *Journal of Clinical and Experimental Neuropsychology, 17,* 193–208.

Goldberg, E. (2001). *The executive brain. Frontal lobes and the civilized mind.* New York: Oxford University Press.

Goldberg, E., Antin, S.P., Bilder, R.M., Jr., et al. (1981). Retrograde amnesia: Possible role of mesencephalic reticular activation in long-term memory. *Science, 213,* 1392–1394.

Goldberg, E. & Bilder, R.M. (1986). Neuropsychological perspectives: Retrograde amnesia and executive deficits. In L.W. Poon (Ed.), *Handbook for clinical memory assessment of older adults.* Washington, D.C.: American Psychological Association.

Goldberg, E. & Bilder, R.M., Jr. (1987). The frontal lobes and hierarchical organization of cognitive control. In E. Perecman (Ed.), *The frontal lobes revisited.* New York: IRBN Press.

Goldberg, E., Bilder, R.M., Hughes, J.E., et al. (1989). A reticulofrontal disconnection syndrome. *Cortex, 25,* 687–695.

Goldberg, E. & Costa, L.D. (1981). Hemisphere differences in the acquisition and use of descriptive systems. *Brain and Language, 14,* 144–173.

Goldberg, E. & Costa, L.D. (1986). Qualitative indices in neuropsychological assessment: An extension of Luria's approach to executive deficit following prefrontal lesions. In K. Adams & I. Grant (Eds.), *Neuropsychological assessment of neuropsychiatric disorders.* New York: Oxford University Press.

Goldberg, E., Harner, R., Lovell, M., et al. (1994). Cognitive bias, functional cortical geometry, and the frontal lobes: Laterality, sex, and handedness. *Journal of Cognitive Neuroscience, 6,* 276–296.

Goldberg, E. & Podell, K. (2000). Adaptive decision making, ecological validity, and the frontal lobes. *Journal of Clinical and Experimental Neuropsychology, 22,* 56–68.

Goldberg, E., Podell, K., Bilder, R., & Jaeger, J. (2000). *The Executive Control Battery.* Melbourne, Australia: Psych Press.

Goldberg, E., Podell, K., & Lovell, M. (1994). Lateralization of frontal lobe functions and cognitive novelty. *Journal of Neuropsychiatry and Clinical Neuroscience, 6,* 371–378.

Goldberg, E. & Tucker, D. (1979). Motor perseveration and long-term memory for visual forms. *Journal of Clinical Neuropsychology, 1,* 273–288.

Goldberg, J.O. & Miller, H.R. (1986). Performance of psychiatric inpatients and intellectually deficient individuals on a task assessing the validity of memory complaints. *Journal of Clinical Psychology, 42,* 792–795.

Golden, C.J. (1978a). *Diagnosis and rehabilitation in clinical neuropsychology.* Springfield, IL: Thomas.

Golden, C.J. (1978b). *Stroop Color and Word Test.* Chicago: Stoelting.

Golden, C.J. (1979). Identification of specific neurological disorders using double discrimination scales derived from the standard Luria Neuropsychological Battery. *International Journal of Neuroscience, 10,* 51–56.

Golden, C.J. (1980). In reply to Adams' "In search of Luria's battery: A false start." *Journal of Consulting and Clinical Psychology, 48,* 517–521.

Golden, C.J. (1984). Applications of the standardized Luria-Nebraska Neuropsychological Battery to rehabilitation planning. In P.E. Logue & J.M. Schear (Eds.), *Clinical neuropsychology: A multidisciplinary approach.* Springfield, IL: Thomas.

Golden, C.J., Ariel, R.N., McKay, S.E., et al. (1982). The Luria-Nebraska Neuropsychological Battery: Theoretical orientation and comment. *Journal of Consulting and Clinical Psychology, 50,* 291–300.

Golden, C.J. & Grier, C.A. (1998). Detecting malingering on the Luria-Nebraska Neuropsychological Battery. In C.R. Reynolds (Ed.), *Detection of malingering during head injury litigation.* New York: Plenum Press.

Golden, C.J., Kuperman, S.K., MacInness, W.D., & Moses, J.A. (1981). Cross-validation of an abbreviated form of the Halstead Category Test. *Journal of Consulting and Clinical Psychology, 49,* 606–607.

Golden, C.J., Kushner, T., Lee, B., & McMorrow, M.A. (1998). Searching for the meaning of the Category Test and the Wisconson Card Sort Test: A comparative analysis. *International Journal of Neuroscience, 93,* 141–150.

Golden, C.J., Osmon, D.C., Moses, J.A., Jr., & Berg, R.A. (1981). *Interpretation of the Halstead-Reitan Neuropsychological Test Battery.* New York: Grune & Stratton.

Golden, C.J., Purisch, A.D., & Hammeke, T.A. (1991). *Luria-Nebraska Neuropsychological Battery: Forms I and II.* Los Angeles: Western Psychological Services.

Golden, C.J., White, L., Combs, T., et al. (1999). WMS-R and MAS correlations in a neuropsychological population. *Archives of Clinical Neuropsychology, 14,* 265–271.

Goldenberg, G., Mullbacher, W., & Nowak, A. (1995). Imagery without perception—a case study of anosognosia for cortical blindness. *Neuropsychologia, 33,* 1373–1382.

Goldenberg, G., Podreka, I., Muller, C., & Deecke, L. (1989). The relationship between cognitive deficits and frontal lobe functions in patients with Parkinson's disease: An emission computerized tomography study. *Behavioral Neurology, 2,* 79–87.

Goldenberg, G., Schuri, U., Gromminger, O., & Arnold, U. (1999). Basal forebrain amnesia: Does the nucleus accumbens contribute to human memory? *Journal of Neurology, Neurosurgery and Psychiatry, 67,* 163–168.

Goldfried, M.R., Stricker, G., & Weiner, I.B. (1971). *Rorschach handbook of clinical and research applications.* Englewood Cliffs, NJ: Prentice-Hall.

Goldman, H., Kleinman, K.M., Snow, M.Y., et al. (1974). Correlation of diastolic blood pressure and signs of cognitive dysfunction in essential hypertension. *Diseases of the Nervous System, 35,* 571–572.

Goldman, M.S. (1982). Reversibility of psychological deficits in alcoholics: The interaction of aging with alcohol. In A. Wilkinson (Ed.), *Symposium on cerebral deficits in alcoholism.* Toronto: Addiction Research Foundation.

Goldman, M.S. (1983). Cognitive impairment in chronic alcoholics: Some cause for optimism. *American Psychologist, 38,* 1045–1054.

Goldman, R.S., Axelrod, B.N., Giordani, B.J., et al. (1992). Longitudinal sensitivity of the Fuld cholinergic profile to Alzheimer's disease. *Journal of Clinical and Experimental Neuropsychology, 14,* 566–574.

Goldman, R.S., Axelrod, B.N., Heaton, R.K., et al. (1996). Latent structure of the WCST with the standardization samples. *Assessment, 3 3,* 73–78.

Goldman, R.S., Axelrod, B.N., & Taylor, S.F. (1996). Neuropsychological aspects of schizophrenia. In I. Grant & K.M. Adams (Eds.), *Neuropsychological assessment of neuropsychiatric disorders* (2nd ed.). New York: Oxford University Press.

Goldman, W.P., Baty, J.D., Buckles, V.D., et al. (1998). Cognitive and motor functioning in Parkinson disease: Subjects with and without questionable dementia. *Archives of Neurology, 55,* 674–680.

Goldman-Rakic, P.S. (1993). Specification of higher cortical functions. *Journal of Head Trauma Rehabilitation, 8,* 13–23.

Goldman-Rakic, P.S. (1998). The prefrontal landscape: Implications of functional architecture for understanding human mentation and the central executive. In A.C. Roberts, T.W. Robbins, & L. Weiskrantz (Eds.), *The prefrontal cortex: Executive and cognitive functions.* New York: Oxford University Press

Goldsmith, W. (1966). The physical processes producing head injury. In W.F. Cavaness & A.E. Walker (Eds.), *Head Injury Conference proceedings.* Philadelphia: Lippincott.

Goldstein, D., Mercury, M., Azin, R., et al. (2000). *Cautionary note on the Boston Naming Test: cultural considerations.* Paper presented at the 28th annual meeting of the International Neuropsychological Society, Denver, CO.

Goldstein, F.C., Gary, H.E., Jr., & Levin, H.S. (1986). Assessment of the accuracy of regression equations proposed for estimating premorbid intellectual functioning on the Wechsler Adult Intelligence Scale. *Journal of Clinical and Experimental Neuropsychology, 8*, 405–412.

Goldstein, F.C. & Levin, H.S. (1991). Question-asking strategies after severe closed head injury. *Brain and Cognition, 17*, 23–30.

Goldstein, F.C., Levin, H.S., Goldman, W.P., et al. (2001). Cognitive and neurobehavioral functioning after mild *versus* moderate traumatic brain injury in older adults. *Journal of the International Neuropsychological Society, 7*, 373–383.

Goldstein, F.C., Levin, H.S., Presley, R.M., et al. (1994). Neurobehavioral consequences of closed head injury in older adults. *Journal of Neurology, Neurosurgery and Psychiatry, 57*, 961–966.

Goldstein, G. (1974). The use of clinical neuropsychological methods in the lateralisation of brain lesions. In S.J. Dimond & J.G. Beaumont (Eds.), *Hemisphere function in the human brain.* New York: Halsted Press.

Goldstein, G. (1986b). An overview of similarities and differences between the Halstead-Reitan and Luria-Nebraska Neuropsychological batteries. In T. Incagnoli et al. (Eds.), *Clinical application of neuropsychological test batteries.* New York: Plenum Press.

Goldstein, G., Allen, D.N., & Seaton, B.E. (1998). A comparison of clustering solutions for cognitive heterogeneity in schizophrenia. *Journal of the International Neuropsychological Society, 4*, 353–362.

Goldstein, G. & Halperin, K.M. (1977). Neuropsychological differences among subtypes of schizophrenia. *Journal of Abnormal Psychology, 86*, 34–40.

Goldstein, G., Materson, B.J., Cushman, W.C., et al. (1990). Treatment of hypertension in the elderly: II. Cognitive and behavioral function. *Hypertension, 15*, 361–369.

Goldstein, G. & Ruthven, L. (1983). *Rehabilitation of the brain-damaged adult.* New York: Plenum Press.

Goldstein, G. & Shelly, C.H. (1973). Univariate vs. multivariate analysis in neuropsychological test assessment of lateralized brain damage. *Cortex, 9*, 204–216.

Goldstein, G. & Shelly, C.H. (1984). Discriminative validity of various intelligence and neuropsychological tests. *Journal of Consulting and Clinical Psychology, 52*, 383–389.

Goldstein, G. & Shelly, C. (1987). The classification of neuropsychological deficit. *Journal of Psychopathological and Behavioral Assessment, 9*, 183–202.

Goldstein, G., Shelly, C., McCue, M., & Kane, R.L. (1987). Classification with the Luria-Nebraska Neuropsychological Battery: An application of cluster and ipsative profile analysis. *Archives of Clinical Neuropsychology, 2*, 215–235.

Goldstein, G. & Watson, J.R. (1989). Test–retest reliability of the Halstead-Reitan Battery and the WAIS in a neuropsychiatric population. *The Clinical Neuropsychologist, 3*, 265–272.

Goldstein, G., Welch, R. B., Rennich, P. M., & Shelly, C. H. (1973). The validity of a visual searching task as an indication of brain damage. *Journal of Consulting and Clinical Psychology, 41*, 434–437.

Goldstein, K. (1939). *The organism.* New York: American Book Co.

Goldstein, K. (1944). The mental changes due to frontal lobe damage. *Journal of Psychology, 17*, 187–208.

Goldstein, K.H. (1948). *Language and language disturbances.* New York: Grune & Stratton.

Goldstein, K. (1995). *The organism* (reprinted from 1939 ed.). Cambridge, MA: MIT Press-Zone Books.

Goldstein, K.H. & Scheerer, M. (1941). Abstract and concrete behavior: An experimental study with special tests. *Psychological Monographs, 53*, (No. 2) (Whole No. 239).

Goldstein, K.H. & Scheerer, M. (1953). Tests of abstract and concrete behavior. In A. Weidner (Ed.), *Contributions to medical psychology* (Vol. II). New York: Ronald Press.

Goldstein, L.H., Canavan, A.G.M., & Polkey, C.E. (1988). Verbal

and abstract designs paired associate learning after unilateral temporal lobectomy. *Cortex, 24*, 41–52.

Gollaher, K., High, W., Sherer, M., et al. (1998). Prediction of employment outcome one to three years following traumatic brain injury (TBI). *Brain Injury, 12*, 255–263.

Gollin, E.S. (1960). Developmental studies of visual recognition of incomplete objects. *Perceptual and Motor Skills, 11*, 289–298.

Gollin, E.S., Stahl, G., & Morgan, E. (1989). The uses of the concept of normality in developmental biology and psychology. In H.W. Reese (Ed.), *Advances in child development* (Vol. 21). New York: Academic Press.

Golomb, J., Wisoff, J., Miller, D.C., et al. (2000). Alzheimer's disease comorbidity in normal pressure hydrocephalus: prevalence and shunt response. *Journal of Neurology, Neurosurgery and Psychiatry, 68*, 778–781.

Golper, L.C. & Binder, L.M. (1981). Communicative behaviors in aging and dementia. In J. Darby (Ed.), *Speech evaluation in medicine and psychiatry* (Vol. 2). New York: Grune & Stratton.

Gomez, P.A., Lobato, R.D., Boto, G.R., et al. (2000). Age and outcome after severe head injury. *Acta Neurochirurgica, 42*, 373–380.

Gómez-Isla, T., Hollister, R., West, H., et al. (1997). Neuronal loss correlates with but exceeds neurofibrillary tangles in Alzheimer's disease. *Annals of Neurology, 41*, 17–24.

Gómez-Isla, T. & Hyman, B.T. (2003). Neuropathological changes in normal aging, mild cognitive impairment, and Alzheimer's disease. In R.C. Petersen (Ed.), *Mild cognitive impairment.* New York: Oxford University Press.

Gomez-Tortosa, E., del Barrio, A., Garcia Ruiz, P. J., et al. (1998). Severity of cognitive impairment in juvenile and late-onset Huntington disease. *Archives of Neurology, 55*, 835–843.

Gomez-Tortosa, E., Ingraham, A.O., Irizarry, M.C., & Hyman, B.T. (1998). Dementia with Lewy bodies. *Journal of the American Geriatric Society, 46*, 1449–1458.

Gonen, J.Y. (1970). The use of Wechsler's Deterioration Quotient in cases of diffuse and symmetrical cerebral atrophy. *Journal of Clinical Psychology, 26*, 174–177.

Goodale, M.A. (2000). Perception and action in the human visual system. In M.A. Gazzaniga (Ed.), *The new cognitive neurosciences* (2nd ed.). Cambridge, MA: MIT Press.

Goodglass, H. (1980). Disorders of naming following brain injury. *American Scientist, 68*, 647–655.

Goodglass, H. (1986). The assessment of language after brain damage. In S.B. Filskov & T.J. Boll, *Handbook of clinical neuropsychology* (Vol. 2). New York: Wiley.

Goodglass, H. & Kaplan, E. (1983a). *Assessment of aphasia and related disorders* (2nd ed.). Philadelphia: Lea and Febiger.

Goodglass, H. & Kaplan, E. (1983b). *Boston Diagnostic Aphasia Examination (BDAE).* Philadelphia: Lea and Febiger.

Goodglass, H. & Kaplan, E. (1986). *La evaluacion de la afasia y de transfornos relacionados* (2nd ed.). Madrid: Editorial Medica Panamericana.

Goodglass, H. & Kaplan, E. (2000). *Boston Naming Test.* Philadelphia: Lippincott Williams & Wilkins.

Goodglass, H., Kaplan, E., & Barresi, B. (2000). *The Boston Diagnostic Aphasia Examination (BDAE-3)* (3rd ed.). Philadelphia: Lippincott.

Goodin, D.S. (1992). Electrophysiological correlates of dementia in Parkinson's disease. In S.J. Huber & J.L. Cummings (Eds.), *Parkinson's disease: Neurobehavioral aspects.* New York: Oxford University Press.

Goodin, D.S. & Aminoff, M.J. (1986). Electrophysiological differences between subtypes of dementia. *Brain, 109*, 1103–1113.

Goodin, D.S., Ebers, G.C., Johnson, K.P., et al. (1999). The relationship of MS to physical trauma and psychological stress: Report of the Therapeutic and Technology Assessment Subcommittee of the American Academy of Neurology. *Neurology, 52,* 1737–1745.

Goodin, D.S., Frohman, E.M., Garmany, G.P., Jr., et al. (2002). Disease modifying therapies in multiple sclerosis. Report of the Therapeutics and Technology Assessment Subcommittee of the American Academy of Neurology and the MS Council for Clinical Practice Guidelines. *Neurology, 58,* 169–178.

Goodkin, D.E. & Fischer, J.S. (1996). Treatment of multiple sclerosis with methotrexate. In D.E. Goodkin & R.A. Rudick (Eds.), *Multiple sclerosis: Advances in clinical trial design, treatment and future perspectives.* London: Springer.

Goodman, J.C. & Simpson, R.K. (1996). Biochemical monitoring in head injury. In R.K. Narayan et al. (Eds.), *Neurotrauma.* New York: McGraw-Hill.

Goodman, R.A. & Caramazza, A. (1985). *The Johns Hopkins University Dysgraphia Battery.* Baltimore, MD: Johns Hopkins University.

Goodman, W.A., Ball, J.D., & Peck, E. (1988). Psychosocial characteristics of head-injured patients: A comparison of factor structures of the Katz Adjustment Scales [abstract]. *Journal of Clinical and Experimental Neuropsychology, 10,* 42.

Goodwin, J.M., Goodwin, J.S., & Kellner, R. (1979). Psychiatric symptoms in disliked medical patients. *Journal of the American Medical Association, 241,* 1117–1120.

Goodwin, J.S., Goodwin, J.M., & Garry, P.J. (1983). Association between nutritional status and cognitive functioning in a healthy elderly population. *Journal of the American Medical Association, 249,* 2917–2921.

Goran, D.A. & Fabiano, R.J. (1993). The scaling of the Katz Adjustment Scale in a traumatic brain injury rehabilitation sample. *Brain Injury, 7,* 219–229.

Gordon, B. (1995). *Memory. Remembering and forgetting in everyday life.* New York: Mastermedia Limited.

Gordon, D.P. (1983). The influence of sex on the development of lateralization in speech. *Neuropsychologia, 21,* 139–146.

Gordon, H.W. (1990). The neurobiological basis of hemisphericity. In C. Trevarthen (Ed.), *Brain circuits and functions of the mind: Essays in honor of Roger W. Sperry.* Cambridge, UK: Cambridge University Press.

Gordon, H.W. & Bogen, J.E. (1974). Hemispheric lateralization of singing after intracarotid sodium amylobarbitone. *Journal of Neurology, Neurosurgery and Psychiatry, 37,* 727–738.

Gordon, H.W., Corbin, E.D., & Lee, P.A. (1986). Changes in specialized cognitive function following changes in hormone levels. *Cortex, 22,* 399–415.

Gordon, H.W. & Kravetz, S. (1991). The influence of gender, handedness, and performance level on specialized cognitive functioning. *Brain and Cognition, 15,* 37–61.

Gordon, H.W. & Lee, P.A. (1993). No difference in cognitive performance between phases of the menstrual cycle. *Psychoneuroendocrinology, 18,* 521–531.

Gordon, W.A., Hibbard, M.R., Egelko, S., et al. (1991). Issues in the diagnosis of post-stroke depression. *Rehabilitation Psychology, 36,* 71–87.

Gordon, W.P. (1983). Memory disorders in aphasia—I. Auditory immediate recall. *Neuropsychologia, 21,* 325–339.

Gordon, W.P. & Illes, J. (1987). Neurolinguistic characteristics of language production in Huntington's disease: A preliminary report. *Brain and Language, 31,* 1–10.

Gorham, D.R. (1956a). *Clinical manual for the Proverbs Test.* Missoula, MT: Psychological Test Specialists.

Gorham, D.R. (1956b). A Proverbs Test for clinical and experimental use. *Psychological Reports, 2,* 1–12.

Gorman, D.G. & Cummings, J.L. (1992). Hypersexuality following septal injury. *Archives of Neurology, 49,* 308–310.

Gormley, N. & Rozwan, M.R. (1998). Prevalence and clinical correlates of psychotic symptoms in Alzheimer's disease. *International Journal of Geriatric Psychiatry, 13,* 410–414.

Gotham, A.M., Brown, R.G., & Marsden, C.D. (1988). "Frontal" cognitive function in patients with Parkinson's disease "on" and "off" levodopa. *Brain, 111,* 299–321.

Gotoh, O., Tamura, A., Yasui, N., et al. (1996). Glasgow Coma Scale in the prediction of outcome after early aneurysm surgery. *Neurosurgery, 39,* 19–24.

Gottschaldt, K. (1928). Über den Einfluss der Erfahrung auf die Wahrnehmung von Figuren. *Psychologische Forschung, 8,* 18–317.

Gough, H.G. (1947). Simulated patterns on the Minnesota Multiphasic Personality Inventory. *Journal of Abnormal and Social Psychology, 42,* 215–225.

Gough, H.G. (1950). The *F* minus *K* dissimulation index for the Minnesota Multiphasic Personality Inventory. *Journal of Consulting Psychology, 14,* 408–413.

Gough, H.G. (1954). Some common misconceptions about neuroticism. *Journal of Consulting Psychology, 18,* 287–291.

Gould, E., Reeves, A.J., Fallah, M., et al. (1999). Hippocampal neurogenesis in adult Old World primates. *Proceedings of the National Academy of Sciences USA, 96,* 5263–5267.

Gould, E., Reeves, A.J., Graziano, M.S.A., & Gross, C.G. (1999). Neurogenesis in the neocortex of adult primates. *Science, 286,* 548–552.

Gould, R., Abramson, I., Galasko, D., & Salmon, D. (2001). Rate of cognitive change in Alzheimer's disease: Methodological approaches using random effects models. *Journal of the International Neuropsychological Society, 7,* 813–824.

Gould, R., Miller, B.L., Goldberg, M.A., & Benson, D.F. (1986). The validity of hysterical signs and symptoms. *Journal of Nervous and Mental Disease, 174,* 593–597.

Gould, S.J. (1981). *The mismeasure of man.* New York: Norton.

Goulet, P., Ska, B., & Kahn, H.J. (1994). Is there a decline in picture naming with advancing age? *Journal of Speech and Hearing Research, 37,* 629–644.

Gouvier, W.D., Blanton, P.D., LaPorte, K.K., & Nepomuceno, C. (1987). Reliability and validity of the Disability Rating Scale and the levels of Cognitive Functioning Scale in monitoring recovery from severe head injury. *Archives of Physical Medicine and Rehabilitation, 68,* 94–97.

Gouvier, W.D., Prestholdt, P., & Warner, M. (1988). A survey of common misconceptions about head injury and recovery. *Archives of Clinical Neuropsychology, 3,* 331–343.

Gouvier, W.D., Uddo-Crane, M., & Brown, L.M. (1988). Base rates for post-concussional symptoms. *Archives of Clinical Neuropsychology, 3,* 273–278.

Grace, J., Nadler, J.D., White, D.A., et al. (1995). Folstein vs. Modified Mini-Mental State Examination in geriatric stroke. *Archives of Neurology, 52,* 477–484.

Grace, J.B., Walker, M.P., & McKeith, I.G. (2000). A comparison of sleep profiles in patients with dementia with Lewy bodies and Alzheimer's disease. *International Journal of Geriatric Psychiatry, 15,* 1028–1033.

Graceffa, A.M., Carlesimo, G.A., Peppe, A., & Caltagirone, C. (1999). Verbal working memory deficit in Parkinson's disease subjects. *European Neurology, 42,* 90–94.

Grados, M.A., Slomine, B.S., & Gerring, J.P. (2001). Depth of lesion model in children and adolescents with moderate to severe traumatic brain injury: Use of SPGR MRI to predict severity and outcome. *Journal of Neurology, Neurosurgery and Psychiatry, 70,* 350–358.

Grady, C.L., Haxby J.V., Horwitz, B., et al. (1988). Longitudinal study of the early neuropsychological and cerebral metabolic changes in dementia of the Alzheimer type. *Journal of Clinical and Experimental Neuropsychology, 10,* 576–596.

Grady, C.L., Haxby, J.V., Schlageter, N.L., et al. (1986). Stability of metabolic and neuropsychological asymmetries in dementia of the Alzheimer type. *Neurology, 36,* 1390–1392.

Grady, C.L., Maisog, J.M., Horwitz, B., et al. (1994). Age-related changes in cortical blood flow activation during visual processing of faces and location. *Journal of Neuroscience, 14,* 1450–1462.

Grady, M.S. & McIntosh, T.C. (2002). Head trauma. In A.K. Asbury et al. (Eds.), *Diseases of the nervous system* (3rd ed.). Cambridge: Cambridge University Press.

Graf, P., Squire, L.R., & Mandler, G. (1984). The information that amnesic patients do not forget. *Experimental Psychology: Learning, Memory, and Cognition, 10,* 164–178.

Graff-Radford, N.R. (2003). Syndromes due to acquired thalamic damage. In T.E. Feinberg & M.J. Farah (Eds.), *Behavioral neurology and neuropsychology* (2nd ed.). New York: McGraw-Hill.

Graff-Radford, N.R., Damasio, H., Yamada, T., et al. (1985). Non-haemorrhagic thalamic infarction. *Brain, 108,* 485–516.

Graff-Radford, N.R., Heaton, R.K., Earnest, M.P., & Rudikoff, J.C. (1982). Brain atrophy and neuropsychological impairment in young alcoholics. *Journal of Studies on Alcohol, 43,* 859–868.

Graff-Radford, N.R., Tranel, D., Van Hoesen, G.W., & Brandt, J.P. (1990). Diencephalic amnesia. *Brain, 113,* 1–25.

Grafman, J. (1988). Acalculia. In F. Boller & J. Grafman (Eds.), *Handbook of neuropsychology* (Vol. 1). Amsterdam: Elsevier.

Grafman, J. & Boller, F. (1989). A comment on Luria's investigation of calculation disorders. *Journal of Neurolinguistics, 4,* 123–135.

Grafman, J., Jonas, B.S., Martin, A., et al. (1988). Intellectual function following penetrating head injury in Vietnam veterans. *Brain, 111,* 169–184.

Grafman, J., Jonas, B., & Salazar, A. (1990). Wisconsin Card Sorting Test performance based on location and size of neuroanatomical lesion in Vietnam veterans with penetrating head injury. *Perceptual and Motor Skills, 71,* 1120–1122.

Grafman, J., Kampen, D., Rosenberg, J., et al. (1989). The progressive breakdown of number processing and calculation ability: a case study. *Cortex, 25,* 121–133.

Grafman, J., Lalonde, F., Litvan, I., & Fedio, P. (1989). Premorbid effects upon recovery from brain injury in humans: Cognitive and interpersonal indices. In J. Schulkin (Ed.), *Preoperative events: Their effects on behavior following brain damage.* New York: Erlbaum.

Grafman, J. & Litvan, I. (1999). Importance of deficits in executive functions. *Lancet, 354,* 1921–1923.

Grafman, J., Litvan, I., Gomez, C., & Chase, T.N. (1990). Frontal lobe function in progressive supranuclear palsy. *Archives of Neurology, 47,* 553–561.

Grafman, J., Litvan, I., & Stark, M. (1995). Neuropsychological features of progressive supranuclear palsy. *Brain and Cognition, 28,* 311–320.

Grafman, J., Passafiume, D., Faglioni, P. & Boller, F. (1982). Calculation disturbances in adults with focal hemispheric damage. *Cortex, 18,* 37–50.

Grafman, J., Rao, S., Bernardin, L., & Leo, G.J. (1991). Automatic memory processes in patients with multiple sclerosis. *Archives of Neurology, 48,* 1072–1075.

Grafman, J. & Rickard, T. (1997). Acalculia. In T.E. Feinberg & M.J. Farah (Eds.), *Behavioral neurology and neuropsychology.* New York: McGraw-Hill.

Grafman, J. & Salazar, A.M. (1987). Methodological considerations relevant to the comparison of recovery from penetrating and closed head injuries. In H.S. Levin, J. Grafman, & H.M. Eisenberg (Eds.), *Neurobehavioral recovery from head injury.* New York: Oxford University Press.

Grafman, J., Salazar, A.M., Weingartner, H., et al. (1985). Isolated impairment of memory following a penetrating lesion of the fornix cerebri. *Archives of Neurology, 42,* 1162–1168.

Grafman, J., Schwab, K., Warden, D., et al. (1996). Frontal lobe injuries, violence, and aggression: A report of the Vietnam Head Injury Study. *Neurology, 46,* 1231–1238.

Grafman, J., Sirigu, A., Spector, L., & Hendler, J. (1993). Damage to the prefrontal cortex leads to decomposition of structured event complexes. *Journal of Head Trauma Rehabilitation, 8,* 73–87.

Grafman, J., Smutok, M., Sweeney, J., et al. (1985). Effects of left-hand preference on postinjury measures of distal motor ability. *Perceptual and Motor Skills, 61,* 615–624.

Grafman, J., Thompson, K., Weingartner, H., et al. (1991). Script generation as an indicator of knowledge representation in patients with Alzheimer's disease. *Brain and Language, 40,* 344–358.

Grafman, J., Vance, S.C., Weingartner, H., et al. (1986). The effects of lateralized frontal lesions on mood regulation. *Brain, 109,* 1127–1148.

Grafman, J., Weingartner, H., Lawlor, B., et al. (1990). Automatic memory processes in patients with dementia—Alzheimer's type (DAT). *Cortex, 26,* 361–372.

Grafman, J., Weingartner, H., Newhouse, P.A., et al. (1990). Implicit learning in patients with Alzheimer's disease. *Pharmacopsychiatry, 23,* 94–101.

Grafton, S. (2003). Apraxia: A disorder of motor control. In M. D'Esposito (Ed.), *Neurological foundations of cognitive neuroscience. Issues in clinical and cognitive neuropsychology.* Cambridge, MA: MIT Press.

Graham, D.I. (1996). Neuropathology of head injury. In R.K. Narayan (Ed.), *Neurotrauma.* New York: McGraw-Hill.

Graham, D.I., Adams, J.H., & Doyle, D. (1978). Ischaemic brain damage in fatal non-missile head injuries. *Journal of the Neurological Sciences, 39,* 213–234.

Graham, J.R. (1987). *The MMPI: A practical guide* (2nd ed.). New York: Oxford University Press.

Graham, J.R. (1990). *MMPI-2: Assessing personality and psychopathology.* New York: Oxford University Press.

Graham, J.R. & Wolff, H.G. (1938). Mechanism of migraine headache and action of ergotamine tartrate. *Archives of Neurology and Psychiatry, 39,* 737–763.

Graham, K.S. & Hodges, J.R. (1997). Differentiating the roles of the hippocampal complex and the neocortex in long-term memory storage: Evidence from the study of semantic dementia and Alzheimer's disease. *Neuropsychology, 11,* 77–89.

Graham, N.L. (2000). Dysgraphia in dementia. *Neurocase, 6,* 365–376.

Grandjean, E., Münchinger, R., Turrian, V., et al. (1955). Investigations into the effects of exposure to trichlorethylone in mechanical engineering. *British Journal of Industrial Medicine, 12,* 131–142.

Granérus, A.K. (1990). Update on Parkinson's disease: Current considerations and geriatric aspects. In M. Bergener & S.I. Finkel (Eds.), *Clinical and scientific psychogeriatrics. The interface of psychiatry and neurology* (Vol. 2). New York: Springer.

Granholm, E. & Butters, N. (1988). Associative encoding and retrieval in Alzheimer's and Huntington's disease. *Brain and Cognition, 7,* 335–347.

Granholm, E., Wolfe, J., & Butters, N. (1985). Affective-arousal factors in the recall of thematic stories by amnesic and demented patients. *Developmental Neuropsychology, 1,* 317–333.

Grant, D.A. & Berg, E.A. (1948). A behavioral analysis of the degree of reinforcement and ease of shifting to new responses in a Weigl-type card sorting problem. *Journal of Experimental Psychology, 38,* 404–411.

Grant, I. (1987). Alcohol and the brain: Neuropsychological correlates. *Journal of Consulting and Clinical Psychology, 55,* 310–324.

Grant, I. & Adams, K.M. (Eds.) (1996). *Neuropsychological assessment of neuropsychiatric disorders* (2nd ed.). New York: Oxford University Press.

Grant, I., Adams, K.M., Carlin, A.S., et al. (1978a). The collaborative neuropsychological study of polydrug users. *Archives of General Psychiatry, 35,* 1063–1064.

Grant, I, Adams, K.M., Carlin, A.S., et al. (1978b). Neuropsychological effects of polydrug abuse. In D.R. Wesson et al. (Eds.), *Polydrug abuse.* New York: Academic Press.

Grant, I., Adams, K.M., & Reed, R. (1979). Normal neuropsychological abilities in late thirties alcoholics. *American Journal of Psychiatry, 136,* 1263–1269.

Grant, I., Adams, K.M., & Reed, R. (1984). Aging, abstinence, and medical risk factors in the prediction of neuropsychologic deficit among long-term alcoholics. *Archives of General Psychiatry, 41,* 710–718.

Grant, I. & Alves, W. (1987). Psychiatric and psychosocial disturbances in head injury. In H.S. Levin et al. (Eds.), *Neurobehavioral recovery from head injury.* New York: Oxford University Press.

Grant, I., Brown, G.W., Harris, T., et al. (1989). Severely threatening events and marked life difficulties preceding onset or exacerbation of multiple sclerosis. *Journal of Neurology, Neurosurgery and Psychiatry, 52,* 8–13.

Grant, I., Heaton, R.K., McSweeny, A.J., et al. (1982). Neuropsychological findings in hypoxemic chronic obstructive pulmonary disease. *Archives of Internal Medicine, 142,* 1470–1476.

Grant, I. & Martin, A. (1994). Introduction: Neurocognitive disorders associated with HIV-1 infection. In I. Grant & A. Martin (Eds.), *Neuropsychology of HIV infection.* New York: Oxford University Press.

Grant, I., McDonald, W.I., Trimble, M.R., et al. (1984). Deficient learning and memory in early and middle phases of multiple sclerosis. *Journal of Neurology and Psychiatry, 47,* 250–255.

Grant, I., Olshen, R.A., Atkinson, J.H., et al. (1993). Depressed mood does not explain neuropsychological deficits in HIV-infected persons. *Neuropsychology, 7,* 53–61.

Grant, I., Prigatano, G.P., Heaton, R.K., et al. (1987). Progressive neuropsychologic impairment and hypoxemia. *Archives of General Psychiatry, 44,* 999–1006.

Grant, I., Reed, R., Adams, K., & Carlin, A. (1979). Neuropsychological function in young alcoholics and polydrug abusers. *Journal of Clinical Neuropsychology, 1,* 39–47.

Grantham-McGregor, S. & Ani, C. (2001). A review of studies on the effect of iron deficiency on cognitive development in children. *Journal of Nutrition, 131,* 649S–666S.

Grasso, P. (1988). Neurotoxic and neurobehavioral effects of organic solvents on the nervous system. *Occupational Medicine, 3,* 525–539.

Grattan, L.M. & Eslinger, P.J. (1989). Higher cognition and social behavior: Changes in cognitive flexibility and empathy after cerebral lesions. *Neuropsychology, 3,* 175–185.

Grattan, L.M., Oldach, D., Perl, T.M., et al. (1998). Learning and memory difficulties after environmental exposure to waterways containing toxin-producing Pfiesteria or Pfiesteria-like dinoflagellates. *Lancet, 352,* 532–539.

Graves, A.B., Bowen, J.D., Rajaram, L., et al. (1999). Impaired olfaction as a marker for cognitive decline: Interaction with apolipoprotein E epsilon4 status. *Neurology, 53,* 1480–1487.

Graves, A.B., Teng, E.L., Larson, E.B., & White, L.R. (1992). Education in cross-cultural dementia screening: Applications of a new instrument. *Neuroepidemiology, 16,* 271–280.

Gray, C., Cantagallo, A., Della Sala, S., & Basaglia, N. (1998). Bradykinesia and bradyphrenia revisited: patterns of subclinical deficit in motor speed and cognitive functioning in head-injured patients with good recovery. *Brain Injury, 12,* 429–441.

Gray, D.B. & Hendershot, G.E. (2000). The ICIDH-2: Developments for a new era of outcomes research. *Archives of Physical Medicine and Rehabilitation, 81(Suppl. 2),* S10–S14.

Gray, S.L., Lai, K.V., & Larson, E.B. (1999). Drug-induced cognition disorders in the elderly: Incidence, prevention and management. *Drug Safety, 21,* 101–122.

Graybiel, A.M. & Kubota, Y. (2003). Understanding corticobasal ganglia networks as part of a habit formation system. In M.-A. Bédard et al. (Eds.), *Mental and behavior dysfunction in movement disorders.* Totowa, NJ: Humana Press.

Green, B.F. (1978). In defense of measurement. *American Psychologist, 33,* 664–670.

Green, B.F. (1981). A primer of testing. *American Psychologist, 36,* 1001–1011.

Green, J. (2000). *Neuropsychological evaluation of the older adult. A clinician's guidebook.* San Diego, CA: Academic Press.

Green, P. & Allen, L.M. (2000). Patterns of memory complaints in 577 consecutive patients passing or failing symptom validity tests. *Archives of Clinical Neuropsychology, 15,* 844–845.

Green, P., Allen, L.M., & Astner, K. (1996). *The Word Memory Test: A user's guide to the oral and computer-administered forms.* Durham, NC: CogniSyst.

Green, P., Flaro, L., & Allen, L.M. III (1999). *The Emotional Perception Test.* Durham, NC: CogniSyst.

Green, P. & Iverson, G.L. (2001). Effects of injury severity and cognitive exaggeration on olfactory deficits in head injury compensation claims. *Neurorehabilitation, 16,* 237–243.

Green, P., Iverson, G. L., & Allen, L. (1999). Detecting malingering in head injury litigation with the Word Memory Test. *Brain Injury, 13,* 813–819.

Green, P. & Kramar, E. (1983). *Auditory Comprehension Tests.* Edmonton, Canada: Auditory Comprehension Tests.

Green, P., Rohling, M.L., Iverson, G.L., & Gervais, R.O. (2003). Relationships between olfactory discrimination and head injury severity. *Brain Injury, 17,* 479–496.

Green, S. (1987). *Physiological psychology.* New York: Routledge & Kegan Paul.

Greenberg, G.D., Rodriguez, N.M., & Sesta, J.J. (1994). Revised scoring, reliability, and validity investigation of Piaget's bicycle drawing test. *Assessment, 1,* 89–101.

Greene, J.D., Baddeley, A.D., & Hodges, J.R. (1996). Analysis of the episodic memory deficit in early Alzheimer's disease: Evidence from the Doors and People Test. *Neuropsychologia, 34,* 537–551.

Greene, R.L. (1991). *The MMPI-2/MMPI: An interpretive manual.* Boston: Allyn and Bacon.

Greene, Y.M., Tariot, P.N., Wishart, H., et al. (2000). A 12-week, open trial of donepezil hydrochloride in patients with multiple sclerosis and associated cognitive impairments. *Journal of Clinical Psychopharmacology, 20,* 350–356.

Greenfield, P.M. (1997). You can't take it with you: Why ability assessments don't cross cultures. *American Psychologist, 52,* 1115–1124.

Greenlief, C.L., Margolis, R. B., & Erker, G. J. (1985). Application of the Trail Making Test in differentiating neuropsychological impairment of elderly persons. *Perceptual and Motor Skills, 61,* 1283–1289.

Greenwald, M.L. & Gonzalez Rothi, L.J. (1998). Lexical acces via letter naming in a profoundly alexic and anomic patient: A treatment study. *Journal of the International Neuropsychological Society, 4,* 595–607.

Greenwood, P. & Parasuraman, R. (1991). Effects of aging on the speed of attentional cost of cognitive operations. *Developmental Neuropsychology, 7,* 421–434.

Greenwood, P.M. & Parasuraman, R. (1994). Attentional disengagement deficit in nondemented elderly over 75 years of age. *Aging and Cognition, 1,* 188–202.

Greenwood, P.M., Parasuraman, R., & Alexander, G.E. (1997). Controlling the focus of spatial attention during visual search: effects of advanced aging and Alzheimer disease. *Neuropsychology, 11,* 3–12.

Greenwood, P.M., Parasuraman, R., & Haxby, J.V. (1993). Changes in visuospatial attention over the adult lifespan. *Neuropsychologia, 31,* 471–485.

Greenwood, R., Bhalla, A., Gordon, A., & Roberts, J. (1983). Behavior disturbances during recovery from herpes simplex encephalitis. *Journal of Neurology, Neurosurgery, and Psychiatry, 46,* 809–817.

Gregg, E. W., Yaffe, K., Cauley, J.A., et al. (2000). Is diabetes associated with cognitive impairment and cognitive decline among older women? Study of Osteoporotic Fractures Research Group. *Archives of Internal Medicine, 160,* 174–180.

Gregor, A., Cull, A., Traynor, E., et al. (1996). Neuropsychometric evaluation of long-term survivors of adult brain tumours: Relationship with tumour and treatment parameters. *Radiotherapy and Oncology, 41,* 55–59.

Gregory, C.A. & Hodges, J. (1996). Frontotemporal dementia: Use of consensus criteria and prevalence of psychiatric features. *Neuropsychiatry, Neuropsychology and Behavioral Neurology, 9,* 145–153.

Gregory, C.A., Serra-Mestres, J., & Hodges, J.R. (1999). Early diagnosis of the frontal variant of frontotemporal dementia: how sensitive are standard neuroimaging and neuropsychologic tests? *Neuropsychiatry, Neuropsychology and Behavioral Neurology, 12,* 128–135.

Gregory, R. & Paul, J. (1980). The effects of handedness and writing posture on neuropsychological test results. *Neuropsychologia, 18,* 231–235.

Gregory, R.J., Paul, J.J., & Morrison, M.W. (1979). A short form of the Category Test for adults. *Journal of Clinical Psychology, 35,* 795–798.

Greiffenstein, M.F., Baker, J.W., Donders, J., & Miller, L. (2002). The Fake Bad scale in atypical and severe closed head injury litigants. *Journal of Clinical Psychology, 58,* 1591–1600.

Greiffenstein, M.F., Baker, W.J., & Gola, T. (1994). Validation of malingered amnesia measures with a large clinical sample. *Psychological Assessment, 6,* 218–224.

Greiffenstein, M.F., Baker, W.J., & Gola, T. (1996a). Comparison of multiple scoring methods for Rey's malingered amnesia measures. *Archives of Clinical Neuropsychology, 11,* 283–293.

Greiffenstein, M.F., Baker, W.J., & Gola, T. (1996b). Motor dysfunction profiles in traumatic brain injury and postconcussion syndrome. *Journal of the International Neuropsychological Society, 2,* 477–485.

Greiffenstien, M.W., Baker, W.J., & Gola, T. (2002). Brief report: Anosmia and remote outcome in closed head injury. *Journal of Clinical and Experimental Neuropsychology, 24,* 705–709.

Greiffenstein, M.F., Baker, W.J., & Johnson-Greene, D. (2002). Actual versus self-reported scholastic achievement of litigating postconcussion and severe closed head injury claimants. *Psychological Assessment, 14,* 202–208.

Greiffenstein, M.F., Gola, T., & Baker, W.J. (1995). MMPI-2 validity scales versus domain specific measures in detection of factitious traumatic brain injury and postconcussion syndrome. *The Clinical Neuropsychologist, 9,* 230–240.

Greve, K.W. (1993). Can perseverative responses on the Wisconsin Card Sorting Test be scored accurately? *Archives of Clinical Neuropsychology, 8,* 497–509.

Greve, K.W., Bianchini, K.J., Mathias, C.W., et al. (2003). Detecting malingered performance on the Wechsler Adult Intelligence Scale. Validation of Mittenberg's approach in traumatic brain injury. *Archives of Clinical Neuropsychology, 18,* 245–260.

Greve, K.W., Brooks, J., Crouch, J.A., et al. (1997). Factorial structure of the Wisconsin Card Sorting Test. *British Journal of Clinical Psychology, 36,* 283–285.

Greve, K.W., Farrell, J.F., & Besson, P.S. (1995). A psychometric analysis of the California Card Sorting Test. *Archives of Clinical Neuropsychology, 10,* 265–278.

Greve, K.W., Ingram, F., & Bianchini, K.J. (1998). Latent structure of the Wisconsin Card Sorting Test in a clinical sample. *Archives of Clinical Neuropsychology, 13,* 597–609.

Greve, K.W., Lindberg, R.F., Bianchini, K.J., & Adams, D. (2000). Construct validity and predictive value of the Hooper Visual Organization Test in stroke rehabilitation. *Applied Neuropsychology, 7,* 215–222,

Greve, K.W., Sherwin, E., Stanford, M.S., et al. (2001). Personality and neurocognitive correlates of impulsive aggression in long-term survivors of severe traumatic brain injury. *Brain Injury, 15,* 255–262.

Griffin, G.A., Glassmire, D.M., Henderson, E.A., & McCann, C. (1997). Rey II: Redesigning the Rey screening test of malingering. *Journal of Clinical Psychology, 53,* 757–766.

Griffin, S.L., Mindt, M.R., Rankin, E.J., et al. (2002). Estimating premorbid intelligence: Comparison of traditional and contemporary methods across the intelligence continuum. *Archives of Clinical Neuropsychology, 17,* 497–507.

Griffith, E.R., Cole, S., & Cole, T.M. (1990). Sexuality and sexual dysfunction. In M. Rosenthal et al. (Eds.), *Rehabilitation of the adult and child with traumatic brain injury* (2nd ed.). Philadelphia: Davis.

Griffith, E.R. & Lemberg, S. (1993). *Sexuality and the person with traumatic brain injury: A guide for families.* Philadelphia: Davis.

Griffith, H.R., Belue, K., Sicola, A., et al. (2003). Impaired financial abilities in mild cognitive impairment: A direct assessment approach. *Neurology, 60,* 449–457.

Grigsby, J., Ayarbe, S.D., Kravcisin, N., & Busenbark, D. (1994). Working memory impairment among persons with chronic progressive multiple sclerosis. *Journal of Neurology, 241,* 125–131.

Grigsby, J. & Kaye, K. (1996). *Behavioral Dyscontrol Scale: Manual* (2nd ed.). Authors.

Grigsby, J., Kaye, K., & Busenbark, D. (1994). Alphanumeric sequencing: A report on a brief measure of information processing used among persons with multiple sclerosis. *Perceptual and Motor Skills, 78,* 883–887.

Grigsby, J., Kaye, K., Eilertsen, T.B., & Kramer, A.M. (2000). The Behavioral Dyscontrol Scale and functional status among elderly medical and surgical rehabilitation patients. *Journal of Clinical Geropsychology, 6,* 259–268.

Grigsby, J., Kaye, K., Kowalsky, J., & Kramer, A.M. (2002). Association of behavioral self-regulation with concurrent functional capacity among stroke rehabilitation patients. *Journal of Clinical Geropsychology, 8,* 25–33.

Grigsby, J., Kaye, K., & Robbins, L.J. (1992). Reliabilities, norms and factor structure of the Behavioral Dyscontrol Scale. *Perceptual and Motor Skills, 74,* 883–892.

Grigsby, J., Kaye, K., Shetterly, S.M., et al. (2002). Prevalence of disorders of executive cognitive functioning among the elderly: Findings from the San Luis Valley Health and Aging Study. *Neuroepidemiology, 21,* 213–220.

Grigsby, J., Kravcisin, N., Ayarbe, S.D., & Busenbark, D. (1993). Prediction of deficits in behavioral self-regulation among persons with multiple sclerosis. *Archives of Physical Medicine and Rehabilitation, 74,* 1350–1353.

Grigsby, J., Rosenberg, N.L., & Busenbark, D. (1995). Chronic pain is associated with deficits in information processing. *Perceptual and Motor Skills, 81,* 403–410.

Grimm, R.J., Hemenway, W.G., LeBray, P.R., & Black, F.O. (1989).

The perilymph fistula syndrome defined in mild head trauma. *Acta Oto-Laryngologiac Supplement, 464,* 5–40.

Grober, E. & Bang, S. (1995). Sentence comprehension in Alzheimer's disease. *Developmental Neuropsychology, 11,* 95–107.

Grober, E. & Buschke, H. (1987). Genuine memory deficits in dementia. *Developmental Neuropsychology, 3,* 13–36.

Grober, E., Lipton, R.B., Hall, C., & Crystal, H. (2000). Memory impairment on free and cued selective reminding predicts dementia. *Neurology, 54,* 827–832.

Grober, E., Lipton, R.B., Katz, M., & Sliwinski, M. (1998). Demographic influences on free and cued selective reminding performance in older persons. *Journal of Clinical and Experimental Neuropsychology, 20,* 221–226.

Grober, E., Merling, A., Heimlich, T., & Lipton, R.B. (1997). Free and cued selective reminding and selective reminding in the elderly. *Journal of Clinical and Experimental Neuropsychology, 19,* 643–654.

Grober, E. & Sliwinski, M. (1991). Development and validation of a model for estimating premorbid verbal intelligence in the elderly. *Journal of Clinical and Experimental Neuropsychology, 13,* 933–949.

Grodstein, F., Chen, J., Pollen, D.A., et al. (2000). Postmenopausal hormone therapy and cognitive function in healthy older women. *Journal of the American Geriatric Society, 48,* 746–752.

Grodstein, F., Chen, J., Wilson, R.S., et al. (2001). Type 2 diabetes and cognitive function in community-dwelling elderly women. *Diabetes Care, 24,* 1060–1065.

Gronwall, D.M.A. (1977). Paced Auditory Serial-Addition Task: A measure of recovery from concussion. *Perceptual and Motor Skills, 44,* 367–373.

Gronwall, D.M.A. (1987). Advances in the assessment of attention and information processing after head injury. In H.S. Levin et al. (Eds.), *Neurobehavioral recovery from head injury.* New York: Oxford University Press.

Gronwall, D. (1989). Cumulative and persisting effects of concussion on attention andcognition. In H.S. Levin et al. (Eds.), *Mild head injury.* New York: Oxford University Press.

Gronwall, D. (1991). Minor head injury. *Neuropsychology, 5,* 253–265.

Gronwall, D.M.A. & Sampson, H. (1974). *The psychological effects of concussion.* Auckland: Oxford University Press.

Gronwall, D.M.A. & Wrightson, P. (1974). Delayed recovery of intellectual function after minor head injury. *Lancet, ii,* 1452.

Gronwall, D. & Wrightson, P. (1975). Cumulative effect of concussion. *Lancet, ii,* 995–997.

Gronwall, D. & Wrightson, P. (1980). Duration of post-traumatic amnesia after mild head injury. *Journal of Clinical Neuropsychology, 2,* 51–60.

Gronwall, D. & Wrightson, P. (1981). Memory and information processing capacity after closed head injury. *Journal of Neurology, Neurosurgery and Psychiatry, 44,* 889–895.

Gronwall, D., Wrightson, P. & Waddell, P. (1990). *Head injury: The facts. A guide for families and caregivers.* Oxford: Oxford University Press.

Groopman, J.E. (1998). Fatigue in cancer and HIV/AIDS. *Oncology (Huntington), 12,* 335–344.

Groot, Y.C., Wilson, B.A., Evans, J., & Watson, P. (2002). Prospective memory functioning in people with and without brain injury. *Journal of the International Neuropsychological Society, 8,* 645–654.

Groppel, G., Kapitany, T., & Baumgartner, C. (2000). Cluster analysis of clinical seizure semiology of psychogenic nonepileptic seizures. *Epilepsia, 41,* 610–614.

Gross, C.G. (1998). *Brain, vision, memory. Tales in the history of neuroscience.* Cambridge, MA: MIT Press.

Gross, L.S. & Nagy, R.M. (1992). Neuropsychiatric aspects of poisonous and toxic disorders. In S.C. Yudofsky & R.E. Hales (Eds.), *American Psychiatric Press textbook of psychiatry* (2nd ed.). Washington, D.C.: American Psychiatric Press.

Grossi, D., Fragassi, N.A., Chiacchio, L., et al. (2002). Do visuospatial and constructed disturbances differentiate frontal variant of frontotemporal dementia and Alzheimer's disease? An experimental study of a clinical belief. *International Journal of Geriatric Psychiatry, 17,* 641–648.

Grossman, A.R., Tempereau, C.E., Brones, M.F., et al. (1993). Auditory and neuropsychiatric behavior patterns after electrical injury. *Journal of Burn Care Rehabilitation, 14,* 169–175.

Grossman, F.M., Herman, D.O., & Matarazzo, J.D. (1985). Statistically inferred vs. empirically observed VIQ-PIQ differences in the WAIS-R. *Journal of Clinical Psychology, 41,* 268–272.

Grossman, M. (2001). A multidisciplinary approach to Pick's disease and frontotemporal dementia. *Neurology, 56,* S1–S2.

Grossman, M., Armstrong, C., Onishi, K., et al. (1994). Patterns of cognitive impairment in relapsing-remitting and chronic progressive multiple sclerosis. *Neuropsychiatry, Neuropsychology, and Behavioral Neurology, 7,* 194–210.

Grossman, M., Carvell, S., Peltzer, L., et al. (1993). Visual construction impairment in Parkinson's disease. *Neuropsychology, 7,* 536–547.

Grossman, M., Galetta, S., & D'Esposito, M. (1997). Object recognition difficulty in visual apperceptive agnosia. *Brain and Cognition, 33,* 306–342.

Grossman, M., Mickanin, J., Onishi, K., & Hughes, E. (1996). Verb comprehension deficits in probable Alzheimer's disease. *Brain and Language, 53,* 369–389.

Grossman, M., Payer, F., Onishi, K., et al. (1997). Constraints on the cerebral basis for semantic processing from neuroimaging studies of Alzheimer's disease. *Journal of Neurology, Neurosurgery and Psychiatry, 63,* 152–158.

Grossman, M., Payer, F., Onishi, K., et al. (1998). Language comprehension and regional cerebral defects in frontotemporal degeneration and Alzheimer's disease. *Neurology, 50,* 157–163.

Grossman, M., Robinson, K., Onishi, K., et al. (1995). Sentence comprehension in multiple sclerosis. *Acta Neurologica Scandinavica, 92,* 324–331.

Groswasser, Z., Cohen, M., & Blankstein, E. (1990). Polytrauma associated with traumatic brain injury: Incidence, nature and impact on rehabilitation outcome. *Brain Injury, 4,* 161–166.

Groswasser, Z., Reider-Groswasser, I., Soroker, N., & Machtey, Y. (1987). Magnetic resonance imaging in head injured patients with normal computed tomographic scans. *Surgical Neurology, 27,* 331–337.

Grote, C.L., Kooker, E.K., Garron, D.C., et al. (2000). Performance of compensation seeking and non-compensation seeking samples on the Victoria Symptom Validity Test: Cross-validation and extension of a standardization study. *Journal of Clinical and Experimental Neuropsychology, 22,* 709–719.

Grubb, R.L. & Coxe, W.S. (1978). Trauma to the central nervous system. In S.G. Eliasson et al. (Eds.), *Neurological pathophysiology.* New York: Oxford University Press.

Gudjonsson, G.H. & Shackleton, H. (1986). The pattern of scores on Raven's Matrices during "faking bad" and "non-faking" performance. *British Journal of Clinical Psychology, 25,* 35–41.

Guérin, F., Belleville, S., & Ska, B. (2002). Characterization of visuoconstructional disabilities in patients with probable dementia of the Alzheimer's type: A comparative and correlation study. *International Journal of Geriatric Psychiatry, 17,* 480–485.

Guérin, F., Ska, B., & Belleville, S. (1999). Cognitive processing of drawing abilities. *Brain and Cognition, 40,* 464–478.

Guilford, J.P., Christensen, P.R., Merrifield, P.R., & Wilson, R.C.

(1978). *Alternate uses: Manual of instructions and interpretation.* Orange, CA: Sheridan Psychological Services.

Guilmette, T.J., Hart, K.J., & Giuliano, A.J. (1993). Malingering detection: The use of a forced-choice method in identifying organic versus simulated memory impairment. *The Clinical Neuropsychologist, 7,* 59–69.

Guilmette, T.J., Hart, K.J., Giuliano, A.J., & Leininger, B.E. (1994). Detecting simulated memory impairment: Comparison of the Rey Fifteen-Item Test and the Hiscock Forced-Choice Procedure. *The Clinical Neuropsychologist, 8,* 283–294.

Guilmette, T.J. & Rasile, D. (1995). Sensitivity, specificity, and diagnostic accuracy in three verbal memory measures in the assessment of mild brain injury. *Neuropsychology, 9,* 338–344.

Guilmette, T.J., Whelihan, W.M., Hart, K.J., et al. (1996). Order effects in the administration of a forced-choice procedure for detection of malingering in disability claimants' evaluations. *Perceptual and Motor Skills, 83,* 1007–1016.

Gummow, S.J., Dustman, R.E., & Keaney, R.P. (1984). Remote effects of cerebrovascular accidents: Visual evoked potentials and electrophysiological coupling. *Electroencephalography and Clinical Neurophysiology, 58,* 408–417.

Gunning-Dixon, F.M. & Raz, N. (2000). The cognitive correlates of white matter abnormalities in normal aging: A quantitative review. *Neuropsychology, 14,* 224–232.

Guo, G., Ma, H., & Wang, X. (1998). Psychological and neurobehavioral effects of aluminum on exposed workers [in Chinese]. *Chung-Hua Yu Fang i Hsueh Tsa Chih [Chinese Journal of Preventive Medicine], 32,* 292–294.

Guo, Z., Cupples, L.A., Kuraz, A., et al. (2000). Head injury and the risk of Alzheimer's disease in the MIRAGE study. *Neurology, 54,* 1316–1323.

Gur, R.E., Levy, J., & Gur, R.C. (1977). Clinical studies of brain organization and behavior. In A. Frazer & A. Winokur (Eds.), *Biological bases of psychiatric disorders.* New York: Spectrum.

Gur, R.C., Schroeder, L., Turner, T., et al. (2002). Brain activation during facial emotion processing. *Neuroimage, 16,* 651–662.

Gurd, J.M. & Ward, D.D. (1989). Retrieval from semantic and letter-initial categories in patients with Parkinson's disease. *Neuropsychologia, 27,* 743–746.

Gurdjian, E.S. (1975). Recent developments in biomechanics, management, and mitigation of head injuries. In D.B. Tower (Ed.), *Nervous System. The Clinical Neurosciences.* (Vol. 2). New York: Raven Press.

Guruje, O., Unverzargt, F.W., Osuntokun, B.O., et al. (1995). The CERAD neuropsychological test battery: Norms from a Yoruba-speaking Nigerian sample. *West African Journal of Medicine, 14,* 29–33.

Guskiewicz, K.M., Weaver, N.L., Padua, D.A., & Garrett, W.E., Jr. (2000). Epidemiology of concussion in collegiate and high school football players. *American Journal of Sports Medicine, 28,* 643–650.

Gutbrod, K., Mager, B., Meter, E., & Cohen, R. (1985). Cognitive processing of tokens and their description in aphasia. *Brain and Language, 25,* 37–51.

Guthrie, A. & Elliot, W.A. (1980). The nature and reversibility of cerebral impairment in alcoholism. *Journal of Studies on Alcohol, 41,* 147–155.

Guy, W. (1976). *ECDEU assessment manual for psychopharmacology, revised.* DHEW Publication ADM 76-338. Rockville, MD: U.S. Department of Health and Human Services.

Guyot, Y. & Rigault, G. (1965). Méthode de cotation des elements de la figure complexe de Rey-Osterrieth. *Bulletin du Centre d'Études et de Recherches Psychotechniques, 14,* 317–329.

Güzeldere, G., Flanagan, O., & Hardcastle, V.G. (2000). The nature of consciousness: Lessons from blindsight. In M.S. Gazzaniga (Ed.), *The new cognitive neurosciences* (2nd ed.). Cambridge, MA: MIT Press.

Haaland, K.Y., Cleeland, C.S., & Carr, D. (1977). Motor performance after unilateral hemisphere damage in patients with tumor. *Archives of Neurology, 34,* 556–559.

Haaland, K.Y. & Delaney, H.D. (1981). Motor deficits after left or right hemisphere damage due to stroke or tumor. *Neuropsychologia, 19,* 17–27.

Haaland, K.Y. & Flaherty, D. (1984). The different types of limb apraxia error made by patients with left vs. right hemisphere damage. *Brain and Cognition, 3,* 370–384.

Haaland, K.Y. & Harrington, D.L. (1990). Complex movement behavior: Toward understanding cortical and subcortical interactions in regulating control processes. In G.R. Hammond (Ed.), *Advances in psychology: Cerebral control of speech and limb movements.* Amsterdam: Elsevier/North-Holland.

Haaland, K.Y., Harrington, D.L., & Knight, R.T. (2000). Neural representations of skilled movement. *Brain, 123,* 2306–2313.

Haaland, K.Y., Linn, R.T., Hunt, W.C., & Goodwin, J.S. (1983). A normative study of Russell's variant of the Wechsler Memory Scale in a healthy population. *Journal of Consulting and Clinical Psychology, 51,* 878–881.

Haaland, K.Y., Price, L., & LaRue, A. (2003). What does the WMS-III tell us about memory changes with normal aging? *Journal of the International Neuropsychological Society, 9,* 89–96.

Haaland, K.Y., Temkin, N., Randahl, G., & Dikmen, S. (1994). Recovery of simple motor skills after head injury. *Journal of Clinical and Experimental Neuropsychology, 16,* 448–456.

Haaland, K.Y., Vranes, L.F., Goodwin, J.S., & Garry, P.J. (1987). Wisconsin Card Sort Test performance in a healthy elderly population. *Journal of Gerontology, 42,* 345–346.

Haaland, K.Y. & Yeo, R.A. (1989). Neuropsychological and neuroanatomic aspects of complex motor control. In E.D. Bigler et al. (Eds.), *Neuropsychological function and brain imaging.* New York: Plenum Press.

Haan, J., Terwindt, G.M., & Ferrari, M.D. (1997). Genetics of migraine. *Neurologic Clinics, 15,* 43–60.

Habib, M., Gayraud, D., Oliva, A., et al. (1991). Effects of handedness and sex on the morphology of the corpus callosum: A study with brain magnetic resonance imaging. *Brain and Cognition, 16,* 41–61.

Habib, M. & Sirigu, A. (1987). Pure topographical disorientation: Definition and anatomical basis. *Cortex, 23,* 73–85.

Hachinski, V.C. & Bowler, J.V. (1993). Vascular dementia. *Neurology, 43,* 2159–2160; discussion 2160–2161.

Hachinski, V.C., Iliff, L.D., Zilhka, E., et al. (1975). Cerebral blood flow in dementia. *Archives of Neurology, 32,* 632–637.

Hachinsky, V. & Norris, J.W. (1985). *The acute stroke.* Philadelphia: Davis.

Hafkenscheid, A. (2000). Psychometric measures of individual change: An empirical comparison with the Brief Psychiatric Rating Scale (BPRS). *Acta Psychiatrica Scandinavica, 101,* 235–242.

Hagen, C. (1984). Language disorders in head trauma. In A. Holland (Ed.), *Language disorders in adults.* San Diego, CA: College-Hill Press.

Hagen, C., Malkmus, D., Durham, P., & Bowman, K. (1979). Levels of cognitive functioning. In *Rehabilitation of the head injured adult. Comprehensive physical management.* Downey, CA: Professional Staff Association of Rancho Los Amigos Hospital.

Hagstadius, S., Ørboek, P., Risberg, J., & Lindgren, M. (1989). Regional cerebral blood flow in organic solvent induced chronic toxic encephalopathy at the time of diagnosis and following cessation of exposure. In S. Hagstadius (Ed.), *Brain function and dysfunction.* Lund: University of Lund.

Hagstadius, S. & Risberg, J. (1989). Regional blood flow characteristics and variations with age in resting normal subjects. *Brain and Cognition, 10,* 28–43.

Hahn-Barma, V., Deweer, B., Duerr, A., et al. (1998). Are cognitive changes the first symptoms of Huntington's disease? A study of gene carriers. *Journal of Neurology, Neurosurgery and Psychiatry, 64*, 172–177.

Haikonen, S., Wikman, A.-S., Kalska, H., et al. (1998). Neuropsychological correlates of duration of glances at secondary tasks while driving. *Applied Neuropsychology, 5*, 24–33.

Haley, W.E., Brown, S.L., & Levine, E.G. (1987). Family caregiver appraisals of patient behavioral disturbance in senile dementia. *International Journal of Aging and Human Development, 25*, 25–34.

Haley, W.E. & Pardo, K.M. (1989). Relationship of severity of dementia to caregiving stressors. *Psychology and Aging, 4*, 389–392.

Hall, H.V. & Pritchard, D.A. (1996). *Detecting malingering and deception. Forensic distortion analysis (FDA)*. Delray Beach, FL: St. Lucie Press.

Hall, K.M., Bushnik, T., Lakisic-Kazazik, B., et al. (2001). Assessing traumatic brain injury outcome measures for long-term follow-up of community-based individuals. *Archives of Physical Medicine and Rehabilitation, 82*, 367–374.

Hall, K., Cope, D.N., & Rappaport, M. (1985). Glasgow Outcome Scale and Disability Rating Scale: Comparative usefulness in following recovery in traumatic head injury. *Archives of Physical Medicine and Rehabilitation, 66*, 35–37.

Hall, K.M., Hamilton, B.B., Gordon, W.A., & Zasler, N.D. (1993). Characteristics and comparisons of functional assessment indices: Disability Rating Scale, Functional Independence Measure, and Functional Assessment Measure. *Journal of Head Trauma Rehabilitation, 8*, 60–74.

Hall, K.M., Mann, N., High, W.M., et al. (1996). Functional measures after traumatic brain injury: Ceiling effects of FIM FAM+FAM, DRS, and CIQ. *Journal of Head Trauma Rehabilitation, 11*, 27–39.

Hall, M.M. & Hall, G.C. (1968). Antithetical ideational modes of left versus right unilateral hemisphere lesions as demonstrated on the Rorschach. In *Proceedings of the 76th Annual Convention of the American Psychological Association*. Washington, D.C.: American Psychological Association, pp. 657–658.

Hall, S. & Bornstein, R.A. (1991). Serial-position effects in paragraph recall following mild closed-head injury. *Perceptual and Motor Skills, 72*, 1295–1298.

Hall, S., Pinkston, S. L., Szalda-Petree, A. C., & Coronis, A. R. (1996). The performance of healthy older adults on the Continuous Visual Memory Test and the Visual-Motor Integration Test: Preliminary findings. *Journal of Clinical Psychology, 52*, 449–454.

Halliday, A.L. (1999). Pathophysiology. In D.W. Marion (Ed.), *Traumatic brain injury*. New York: Thieme.

Halligan, P. W., Cockburn, J., & Wilson, B. A. (1991). The behavioural assessment of visual neglect. *Neuropsychological Rehabilitation, 1*, 5–32.

Halligan, P.W. & Marshall, J.C. (1989). Is neglect (only) lateral? A quadrant analysis of line cancellation. *Journal of Clinical and Experimental Neuropsychology, 11*, 793–798.

Halligan, P.W., Marshall, J.C., & Wade, D.T. (1989). Visuospatial neglect: Underlying factors and test sensitivity. *Lancet, ii*, 908–911.

Halperin, J.M., Sharma, V., Greenblatt, E., & Schwartz, S.T. (1991). Assessment of the Continous Performance Test: Reliability and validity in a nonreferred sample. *Psychological Assessment, 3*, 603–608.

Halpern, D.F. (1997). Sex differences in intelligence: Implications for education. *American Psychologist, 52*, 1091–1102.

Halstead, W.C. (1947). *Brain and intelligence*. Chicago: University of Chicago Press.

Halstead, W.C. & Settlage, P.H. (1943). Grouping behavior of nor-

mal persons and persons with lesions of the brain. *Archives of Neurology and Psychiatry, 49*, 489–506.

Halstead, W.C. & Wepman, J.M. (1959). The Halstead-Wepman Aphasia Screening Test. *Journal of Speech and Hearing Disorders, 14*, 9–15.

Haltiner, A.M., Temkin, N.R., Winn, H.R., & Dikmen, S. S. (1996). The impact of posttraumatic seizures on 1-year neuropsychological and psychosocial outcome of head injury. *Journal of the International Neuropsychological Society, 2*, 494–504.

Hamberger, M.J., Goodman, R.R., Perrine, K., & Tamny, T. (2001). Anatomic dissociation of auditory and visual naming in the lateral temporal cortex. *Neurology, 56*, 56–61.

Hamby, S.L., Wilkins, J.W., & Barry, N.S. (1993). Organizational quality on the Rey-Osterrieth and Taylor Complex Figure tests: A new scoring system. *Psychological Assessment, 5*, 27–33.

Hamer, H.M. & Lüders, H.O. (2001). A new approach for classification of epileptic syndromes and epileptic seizures. In H. O. Lüders (Ed.), *Epilepsy surgery* (2nd ed.). New York: Lippincott Williams & Wilkins.

Hamilton, B.B., Granger, C.V., Sherwin, F.S., et al. (1987). A uniform national data system for medical rehabilitation. In M.D. Fuhrer (Ed.), *Rehabilitation outcomes: Analysis and measurement*. Baltimore: Paul H. Brooks.

Hamilton, J.M., Haaland, K.Y., Adair, J.C., & Brandt, J. (2003). Ideomotor limb apraxia in Huntington's disease: Implications for corticostriate involvement. *Neuropsychologia, 41*, 614–621.

Hammerstad, J.P. & Carter, J.H. (1995). Movement disorders in occupational and environmental neurology. In N. Rosenberg (Ed.), *Occupational neurology*. Boston: Butterworth.

Hammill, D.D., Pearson, N.A., & Wiederholt, J.L. (). *Comprehensive Test of Nonverbal Intelligence*. Circle Pines, MN: American Guidance Service.

Hammon, W.M. (1971). Analysis of 2187 consecutive penetrating head wounds of the brain from Vietnam. *Journal of Neurosurgery, 34*, 127–131.

Hammond, G.R. (1982). Hemispheric differences in temporal resolution. *Brain and Cognition, 1*, 95–118.

Hampson, E. (1990). Variations in sex-related cognitive abilities across the menstrual cycle. *Brain and Cognition, 14*, 26–43.

Hamsher, K. de S., Halmi, K.A., & Benton, A.L. (1981). Prediction of outcome in anorexia nervosa from neuropsychological status. *Psychiatry Research, 4*, 79–88.

Hamsher, K.de S. & Roberts, R.J. (1985). Memory for recent U.S. presidents in patients with cerebral disease. *Journal of Clinical and Experimental Neuropsychology, 7*, 1–13.

Hanfmann, E. (1953). Concept Formation Test. In A. Weider (Ed.), *Contributions toward medical psychology*. New York: Ronald Press.

Hanfman, E., Kasanin, J., Vigotsky, L., & Wang, P. (). *Kasanin-Hanfman Concept Formation (Vigotsky Test)*. Wood Dale, IL: Stoelting.

Hankey, G.J. (2001). Clinical types of transient ischemic attacks. In J. Bogousslavsky & L.R. Caplan (Eds.), *Stroke syndromes* (2nd ed.). Cambridge: Cambridge University Press.

Hankins, L., Taber, K.H., Yeakley, J., & Hayman, L.A. (1996). MRI in head injury. In R.K. Narayan et al. (Eds.), *Neurotrauma*. New York: McGraw-Hill.

Hanks, R.A., Rapport, L.J., Millis, S.R., & Deshpande, S.A. (1999). Measures of executive functioning as predictors of functional ability and social integration in a rehabilitation sample. *Archives of Physical Medicine and Remediation, 80*, 1030–1037.

Hanks, R.A., Temkin, N., Machamer, J., & Dikmen, S.S. (1999). Emotional and behavioral adjustment after traumatic brain injury. *Archives of Physical Medicine and Rehabilitation, 80*, 991–999.

Hanks, R.A., Wood, D.L., Millis, S., et al. (2003). Violent traumatic brain injury: Occurrence, patient characteristics, and risk factors from the Traumatic Brain Injury Model Systems Project. *Archives of Physical Medicine and Rehabilitation, 84,* 249–254.

Hanna-Pladdy, B., Berry, Z.M., Bennet, T., et al. (2001). Stress as a diagnostic challenge for postconcussive symptoms: Sequelae of mild traumatic brain injury or physiological stress response. *The Clinical Neuropsychologist, 15,* 289–304.

Hanna-Pladdy, B. & Rothi, L.J.G. (2001). Ideational apraxia: Confusion that began with Liepmann. *Neuropsychological Rehabilitation, 11,* 539–547.

Hannay, H.J. (1976). Real or imagined incomplete lateralization of function in females? *Perception and Psychophysics, 19,* 349–352.

Hannay, H.J. (1986). Psychophysical measurement techniques and their application in neuropsychology. In H.J. Hannay (Ed.), *Experimental techniques in human neuropsychology.* New York: Oxford University Press.

Hannay, H.J. (2003a). Cerebral preservation following injury: Clinical outcomes and assessment. In: *NIH and DoD Working Group on Trauma Research.* Washington, D.C.: Walter Reed Army Medical Research Institute.

Hannay, H.J. (2003b). *Developing outcome measurements.* Invited address. The 21st annual National Neurotrauma Society Symposium, Biloxi, MS, November 7.

Hannay, H.J., Bieliauskas, L., Crosson, B., et al. (1998). Policy statement. Proceedings of the Houston Conference on Specialty Education and Training in Clinical Neuropsychology. *Archives of Clinical Neuropsychology, 13,* 160–166.

Hannay, H.J., Falgout, J.C., Leli, D.A., et al. (1987). Focal right temporo-occipital blood flow changes associated with Judgment of Line Orientation. *Neuropsychologica, 25,* 755–763.

Hannay, H.J., Leli, D.A., Falgout, J.C., et al. (1983). rCBF for middle-aged males and females during right–left discrimination. *Cortex, 19,* 465–474.

Hannay, H.J. & Levin, H.S. (unpublished). *Continuous Recognition Memory Test.* Department of Psychology, University of Houston, Houston, TX.

Hannay, H.J. & Levin, H.S. (1985). Selective Reminding Test: An examination of the equivalence of four forms. *Journal of Clinical and Experimental Neuropsychology, 7,* 251–263.

Hannay, H.J. & Levin, H.S. (1989). Visual continuous recognition memory in normal and closed head-injured adolescents. *Journal of Clinical and Experimental Neuropsychology, 11,* 444–460.

Hannay, H.J., Levin, H.S., & Grossman, R.G. (1979). Impaired recognition memory after head injury. *Cortex, 15,* 269–283.

Hannay, H.J., & Sherer, M. (1996). Assessment of outcome from head injury. In R.K. Narayan et al. (Eds.), *Neurotrauma.* New York: McGraw-Hill.

Hannay, H.J., Struchen, M.A., & Contant, C.F. (1994). *Outcome measures for traumatically brain-injured patients. Report of the Outcome Measures Subcommittee of the NIH-NINDS Head Injury Centers.* Paper presented at the NINDS Investigators Meeting, UCLA, Los Angeles, CA.

Hannerz, J. & Hindmarsh, T. (1983). Neurological and neuroradiological examination of chronic cannabis smokers. *Annals of Neurology, 13,* 207–210.

Hänninen, H. (1982). Behavioral effects of occupational exposure to mercury and lead. *Acta Neurologica Scandinavica, 66(Suppl. 92),* 167–175.

Hänninen, T. & Soininen, H. (1997). Age-associated memory impairment. Normal aging or warning of dementia? *Drugs and Aging, 11,* 480–489.

Hansch, E.C. & Pirozzolo, F.J. (1980). Task relevant effects on the assessment of cerebral specialization for facial emotion. *Brain and Language, 10,* 51–59.

Hansen, L., Salmon, D., Galasko, D., et al. (1990). The Lewy body variant of Alzheimer's disease: A clinical and pathologic entity. *Neurology, 40,* 1–8.

Harden, C.L. (1997). Pseudoseizures and dissociative disorders: A common mechanism involving traumatic experiences. *Seizure, 6,* 151–155.

Harden, C.L. (2002). The co-morbidity of depression and epilepsy: Epidemiology, etiology, and treatment. *Neurology, 59,* S48–S55.

Hardie, R.J., Lees, A.J., & Stern, G.M. (1984). On–off fluctuations in Parkinson's disease. *Brain, 107,* 487–506.

Harding, A., Halliday, G., Caine, D., & Kril, J. (2000). Degeneration of anterior thalamic nuclei differentiates alcoholics with amnesia. *Brain, 123,* 141–154.

Hardman, J.G., et al. (Eds.) (2001). *Goodman and Gilman's the pharmacological basis of therapeutics* (10th ed.). New York: McGraw-Hill.

Hardy, C.H., Rand, G., & Rittler, J.M.C. (1957). *H-R-R Pseudoisochromatic Plates.* New York: American Optics.

Härkönen, H., Lindström, K., Seppäläinen, A.M., et al. (1978). Exposure–response relationship between styrene exposure and central nervous system functions. *Scandinavian Journal of Work and Environmental Health, 4,* 53–59.

Harley, J.P. & Grafman, J. (1983). Fingertip number writing errors in hospitalized non-neurologic patients. *Perceptual and Motor Skills, 56,* 551–554.

Harley, J.P., Leuthold, C.A., Matthews, C.G., & Bergs, L.E. (1980). *Wisconsin Neuropsychological Test Battery T-score norms for older Veterans Administration Medical Center patients.* Madison: Dept. of Neurology, University of Wisconsin Medical School.

Harnish, M.J., Beatty, W.W., Nixon, S.J., & Parsons, O.A. (1994). Performance by normal subjects on the Shipley Institute of Living Scale. *Journal of Clinical Psychology, 50,* 881–883.

Harrell, L.E., Marson, D., Chatterjee, A., & Parrish, J.A. (2000). The Severe Mini-Mental State Examination: A new neuropsychologic instrument for the bedside assessment of severely impaired patients with Alzheimer disease. *Alzheimer Disease and Associated Disorders, 14,* 168–175.

Harrington, D. L. & Haaland, K.Y. (1991a). Hemispheric specialization for motor sequencing: Abnormalities in levels of programming. *Neuropsychologia, 29,* 147–163.

Harrington, D.L. & Haaland, K.Y. (1991b). Sequencing in Parkinson's disease: Abnormalities in programming and controlling movement. *Brain, 114,* 99–115.

Harrington, D.L. & Haaland, K.Y. (1992). Motor sequencing with left hemisphere damage: Are some cognitive deficits specific to limb apraxia? *Brain, 115,* 857–874.

Harrington, D.L., Haaland, K.Y., Yeo, R.A., & Marker, E. (1990). Procedural memory in Parkinson's disease: Impaired motor but not visuoperceptual learning. *Journal of Clinical and Experimental Neuropsychology, 12,* 323–339.

Harris, D.B. (1963). *Children's drawings as measures of intellectual maturity.* New York: Harcourt, Brace & World.

Harris, J.G., Cullum, C.M., & Puente, A.E. (1995). Effects of bilingualism on verbal learning and memory in Hispanic adults. *Journal of the International Neuropsychological Society, 1,* 10–16.

Harris, J.K., Godfrey, H.P.D., Partridge, F.M., & Knight, R.G. (2001). Caregiver depression following traumatic brain injury (TBI): A consequence of adverse effects on family members? *Brain Injury, 15,* 223–238.

Harris, L.J. (1978). Sex differences in spatial ability. Possible environmental, genetic, and neurological factors. In M. Kinsbourne (Ed.), *Asymmetrical function of the brain.* Cambridge, UK: Cambridge University Press.

Harris, L.J. (1995). The corpus callosum and hemispheric communication: An historical survey of theory and research. In F.L. Kitterle (Ed.), *Hemispheric communication: Mechanisms and models*. Hillsdale, NJ: Erlbaum.

Harris, M.E., Ivnik, R.J., & Smith, G.E. (2002). Mayo's Older Americans Normative Studies: Expanded AVLT Recognition Trial norms for ages 57–98. *Journal of Clinical and Experimental Neuropsychology, 24,* 214–220.

Hart, R.P. & Kwentus, J.A. (1987). Psychomotor slowing and subcortical-type dysfunction in depression. *Journal of Neurology, Neurosurgery and Psychiatry, 50,* 1263–1266.

Hart, R.P., Kwentus, J.A., Taylor, J.R., & Hamer, R.M. (1988). Productive naming and memory in depression and Alzheimer's type dementia. *Archives of Clinical Neuropsychology, 3,* 313–322.

Hart, R.P., Kwentus, J.A., Taylor, J.R., & Harkins, S.W. (1987). Rate of forgetting in dementia and depression. *Journal of Consulting and Clinical Psychology, 55,* 101–105.

Hart, R.P., Kwentus, J.A., Wade, J.B., & Hamer, R.M. (1987). Digit Symbol performance in mild dementia and depression. *Journal of Consulting and Clinical Psychology, 55,* 236–238.

Hart, R.P., Martelli, M.F., & Zasler, N.D. (2000). Chronic pain and neuropsychological functioning. *Neuropsychological Review, 10,* 131–149.

Hart, S. (1988). Language and dementia: A review. *Psychological Medicine, 18,* 99–112.

Hart, S. & Semple, J.M. (1990). *Neuropsychology and the dementias.* London: Taylor & Francis.

Hart, T., Giovannetti, T., Montgomery, M.W., & Schwartz, M.F. (1998). Awareness of errors in naturalistic action after traumatic brain injury. *Journal of Head Trauma Rehabilitaion, 13,* 16–28.

Hartlage, L., Durant-Wilson, D., & Patch, P. (2001). Persistent neurobehavioral problems following mild traumatic brain injury. *Archives of Clinical Neuropsychology, 16,* 561–570.

Hartley, A.A. (2001). Age differences in dual-task interference are localized to response-generation processes. *Psychology and Aging, 16,* 47–54.

Hartley, L.L. & Jensen, P.J. (1991). Narrative and procedural discourse after closed head injury. *Brain Injury, 5,* 267–285.

Hartley, L.L. & Jensen, P.J. (1992). Three discourse profiles of closed-head-injury speakers: theoretical and clinical implications. *Brain Injury, 6,* 271–281.

Hartman, D.E. (1995). *Neuropsychological toxicology: Identification and assessment of human neurotoxic syndromes* (2nd ed.). New York: Plenum Press.

Hartman, M., Knopman, D.S., & Nissen, M.J. (1989). Implicit learning of new verbal associations. *Journal of Experimental Psychology: Learning, Memory, and Cognition, 15,* 1070–1082.

Harvey, G.T., Hughes, J., McKeith, I.G., et al. (1999). Magnetic resonance imaging differences between dementia with Lewy bodies and Alzheimer's disease: A pilot study. *Psychological Medicine, 29,* 181–187.

Harvey, J.A. & Siegert, R. (1999). Normative data for New Zealand elders on the Controlled Oral Word Association Test, Graded Naming Test, and the Recognition Memory Test. *New Zealand Journal of Psychology, 28,* 124–132.

Harvey, M.T. & Crovitz, H.F. (1979). Television questionnaire techniques in assessing forgetting in long-term memory. *Cortex, 15,* 609–618.

Harwood, D.G., Ownby, R.L., Barker, W.W., & Duara, R. (1998). The behavioral pathology in Alzheimer's Disease Scale (BEHAVE-AD): Factor structure among community-dwelling Alzheimer's patients. *International Journal of Geriatric Psychiatry, 13,* 793–800.

Harwood, D.G., Sultzer, D.L., & Wheatley, M.V. (2000). Impaired insight in Alzheimer disease: Association with cognitive deficits, psychiatric symptoms, and behavioral disturbances. *Neuropsychiatry, Neuropsychology, and Behavioral Neurology, 13,* 83–88.

Hasher, L. & Zacks, R.T. (1979). Automatic and effortful processes in memory. *Journal of Experimental Psychology: General, 108,* 356–388.

Hasher, L. & Zacks, R.T. (1988). Working memory, comprehension, and aging: A review and a new view. *Psychology of Learning and Motivation, 22,* 122–149.

Hashimoto, R., Yoshida, M., & Tanaka, Y. (1995). Utilization behavior after right thalamic infarction. *European Neurology, 35,* 58–62.

Haslam, C., Batchelor, J., Fearnside, M.R., et al. (1994). Post-coma disturbance and post-traumatic amnesia as nonlinear predictors of cognitive outcome following severe head closed head injury: Findings from the Westmead Head Injury Project. *Brain Injury, 8,* 519–528.

Hassaballa, H., Gorelick, P.B., West, C.P., et al. (2001). Ischemic stroke outcome: Racial differences in the trial of danaparoid in acute stroke (TOAST). *Neurology, 57,* 691–697.

Hassinger, M., Smith, G., & La Rue, A. (1989). Assessing depression in older adults. In T. Hunt & C.J. Lindley (Eds.), *Testing older adults: A reference guide for geropsychological assessments.* Austin, TX: Pro-ed.

Hathaway, S.R. & McKinley, J.C. (1951). *The Minnesota Multiphasic Personality Inventory manual* (rev.). New York: The Psychological Corporation.

Hatton, J. (2001). Pharmacological treatment of brain injury: A review of agents in development. *CNS Drugs, 15,* 553–581.

Haug, H., Barmwater, U., Eggers, R., et al. (1983). Anatomical changes in aging brain: Morphometric analysis of the human prosencephalon. In J. Cervós-Navarro & H.I. Sarkander (Eds.), *Brain aging: Neuropsychology and neuropharmacology. Aging.* (Vol. 21). New York: Raven Press.

Hauser, M.D. (1999). Perseveration, inhibition and the prefrontal cortex: a new look. *Current Opinions in Neurobiology, 9,* 214–222.

Hauser, R.A., Lacey, D.M., & Knight, M.R. (1988). Hypertensive encephalopathy: Magnetic resonance imaging demonstration of reversible cortical and white matter lesions. *Archives of Neurology, 45,* 1078–1083.

Hauser, W.A. & Hesdorffer, D.C. (1990). *Epilepsy: Frequency, causes and consequences.* New York: Demos.

Haut, M.W., Leach, S., Kuwabara, H., et al. (2000). Verbal working memory and solvent exposure: A positron emission tomography study. *Neuropsychology, 14,* 551–558.

Haut, M.W. & Shutty, M.S. (1992). Patterns of verbal learning after closed-head injury. *Neuropsychology, 6,* 51–58.

Hawkes, C.H., Shephard, B.C., & Daniel, S.E. (1997). Olfactory dysfunction in Parkinson's disease. *Journal of Neurology, Neurosurgery and Psychiatriy, 62,* 436–446.

Hawkes, C.H. & Thorpe, J.W. (1992). Acute polyneuropathy due to lightning injury. *Journal of Neurology, Neurosurgery and Psychiatry, 55,* 388–390.

Hawkins, K.A. (1990). Occupational neurotoxicology: Some neuropsychological issues and challenges. *Journal of Clinical and Experimental Neuropsychology, 12,* 664–680.

Hawkins, K.A., Plehn, K., & Borgaro, S. (2002). Verbal IQ-performance IQ differentials in traumatic brain injury samples. *Archives of Clinical Neuropsychology, 17,* 49–56.

Hawkins, K.A., Sledge, W.H., Orleans, J.E., et al. (1993). Normative implications of the relationship between reading vocabulary and Boston Naming Test performance. *Archives of Clinical Neuropsychology, 8,* 525–537.

Hawkins, K.A. & Tulsky, D.S. (2001). The influence of IQ stratification on WAIS-III/WMS-III FSIQ-General Memory Index discrepancy base-rates in the standardization sample. *Journal of the International Neuropsychological Society, 7,* 875–880.

Haxby, J.V., Courtney, S.M., & Clark, V.P. (1998). Functional magnetic resonance imaging and the study of attention. In R. Parasuraman (Ed.), *The attentive brain*. Cambridge, MA: MIT Press.

Haxby, J.V., Grady, C.L., Koss, E., et al. (1988). Heterogeneous anterior–posterior metabolic patterns in dementia of the Alzheimer type. *Neurology, 38*, 1853–1863.

Haxby, J.V., Raffaele, K., Gillette, J., et al. (1992). Individual trajectories of cognitive decline in patients with dementia of the Alzheimer type. *Journal of Clinical and Experimental Neuropsychology, 14*, 575–592.

Haxby, J.V., Ungerleider, L.G., Horwitz, B., et al. (1996). Face encoding and recognition in the human brain. *Proceedings of the National Academy of Science USA, 93*, 922–927.

Hayes, J.S., Hilsabeck, R.C., & Gouvier, W.D. (1999). Malingering traumatic brain injury: Current issues and caveats in assessment and classification. In N.R. Varney & R.J. Roberts (Eds.), *The evaluation and treatment of mild traumatic brain injury*. Mahwah, NJ: Erlbaum.

Haymaker, W. & Adams, R.D. (1982). *Histology and histopathology of the nervous system*. Springfield, IL: Thomas.

Hayman, L.A., Rexer, J.L., Pavol, M.A., et al. (1998). Klüver-Bucy syndrome after bilateral selective damage of amygdala and its cortical connections. *Journal of Neuropsychiatry and Clinical Neuroscience, 10*, 354–358.

Hays, J.R., Emmons, J., & Lawson, K.A. (1993). Psychiatric norms for the Rey 15-item Visual Memory Test. *Perceptual and Motor Skills, 76*, 1331–1334.

Hays, R.D., Vickrey, B.G., & Hermann, B.P. (1995). Agreement between self reports and proxy reports of quality of life in epilepsy patients. *Quality of Life Research, 4*, 159–168.

Hayslip, B., Jr. & Lowman, R.L. (1986). The clinical use of projective techniques with the aged. In T.L. Brink and L. Terry (Eds.), *Clinical gerontology: A guide to assessment and intervention*. New York: Haworth Press.

Hayslip, B., Jr. & Sterns, H.L. (1979). Age differences in relationships between crystallized and fluid intelligence and problem solving. *Journal of Gerontology, 34*, 404–414.

Headache Classification Committee of the International Headache Society. (1988). *Classification and diagnostic criteria for headache disorders, cranial neuralgias and facial pain* (1st ed.). Oslo: Norwegian University Press.

Healey, J.M., Liederman, J., & Geschwind, N. (1986). Handedness is not a unidimensional trait. *Cortex, 22*, 33–53.

Healey, J.M., Rosen, J.J., Gerstman, L., et al. (1982). *Differential effects of familial sinistrality on the cognitive abilities of males and females*. Paper presented at the 10th annual meeting of the International Neuropsychological Society, Pittsburgh, PA.

Heath, J.A. & Leathem, J.M. (1998). Order of item difficulty on the WAIS-R Picture Arrangement subtest: Data from a traumatically brain-injured sample. *Perceptual and Motor Skills, 87*, 243–250.

Heath, R.G., Llewellyn, R.C., & Rouchell, A.M. (1980). The cerebellar pacemaker for intractable behavioral disorders and epilepsy: Follow-up reports. *Biological Psychiatry, 15*, 243–256.

Heaton, R.K. (1981). *Wisconsin Card Sorting Test (WCST)*. Odessa, FL: Psychological Assessment Resources.

Heaton, R.K., Avitable, N., Grant, I., & Matthews, C.G. (1999). Further crossvalidation of regression-based neuropsychological norms with an update for the Boston Naming Test. *Journal of Clinical and Experimental Neuropsychology, 21*, 572–582.

Heaton, R.K., Baade, L.E., & Johnson, K.L. (1978). Neuropsychological test results associated with psychiatric disorders in adults. *Psychological Bulletin, 85*, 141–162.

Heaton, R.K., Chelune, G.J., Talley, J.L., et al. (1993). *Wisconsin Card Sorting Test. Manual revised and expanded*. Odessa, FL: Psychological Assessment Resources.

Heaton, R.K., Grant, I., Anthony, W.Z., & Lehman, R.A.W. (1981).

A comparison of clinical and automated interpretation of the Halstead-Reitan Battery. *Journal of Clinical Neuropsychology, 3*, 121–141.

Heaton, R.K., Grant, I., Butters, N., et al. (1995). The HNRC 500—Neuropsychology of HIV infection at different disease stages. *Journal of the International Neuropsychological Society, 1*, 231–251.

Heaton, R.K., Grant, I., & Matthews, C.G. (1991). *Comprehensive norms for an expanded Halstead-Reitan battery: Demographic corrections, research findings, and clinical applications*. Odessa, FL: Psychological Assessment Resources.

Heaton, R.K., Grant, I., McSweeny, A.J., et al. (1983). Psychologic effects of continuous and nocturnal oxygen therapy in hypoxemic chronic obstructive pulmonary disease. *Archives of Internal Medicine, 143*, 1941–1947.

Heaton, R.K., Nelson, L.M., Thompson, D.S., et al. (1985). Neuropsychological findings in relapsing-remitting and chronic-progressive multiple sclerosis. *Journal of Consulting and Clinical Psychology, 53*, 103–110.

Heaton, R.K., Ryan, L., Grant, I., & Matthews, C.G. (1996). Demographic influences on neuropsychological test performance. In I. Grant & K.M. Adams (Eds.), *Neuropsychological assessment of neuropsychiatric disorders* (2nd ed.). New York: Oxford University Press.

Heaton, R.K., Schmitz, S.P., Avitable, N., et al. (1987). Effects of lateralized cerebral lesions on oral reading, reading comprehension, and spelling. *Journal of Clinical and Experimental Neuropsychology, 9*, 711–721.

Heaton, R.K., Smith, H.H., Jr., Lehman, R.A.W., & Vogt, A.T. (1978). Prospects for faking believable deficits on neuropsychological testing. *Journal of Consulting and Clinical Psychology, 46*, 892–900.

Heaton, R.K., Taylor, M.J., & Manly, J. (2003). Demographic effects and use of demographically corrected norms with the WAIS-III and WMS-III. In D.S. Tulsky et al. (Eds.), *Clinical interpretation of the WAIS-III and WMS-III*. San Diego, CA: Academic Press.

Heaton, R.K., Thompson, L.I., Nelson, L.M., et al. (1990). Brief and intermediate-length screening of neuropsychological impairment. In S.M. Rao (Ed.), *Neuropsychological aspects of multiple sclerosis*. New York: Oxford University Press.

Hebb, D.O. (1939). Intelligence in man after large removal of cerebral tissue: Report of four left frontal lobe cases. *Journal of General Psychology, 21*, 73–87.

Hebb, D.O. (1942). The effect of early and late brain injury upon test scores and the nature of normal adult intelligence. *Proceedings of the American Philosophical Society, 85*, 275–292.

Hebb, D.O. (1949). *The organization of behavior*. New York: Wiley.

Hebert, L.E., Wilson, R.S., Gilley, D.W., et al. (2000). Decline of language among women and men with Alzheimer's disease. *Journals of Gerontology. Series B, Psychological Sciences and Social Sciences, 55B*, 354–360.

Hécaen, H. (1962). Clinical symptomatology in right and left hemispheric lesions. In V.B. Mountcastle (Ed.), *Interhemispheric relations and cerebral dominance in man*. Baltimore, MD: Johns Hopkins University Press.

Hécaen, H. (1964). Mental symptoms associated with tumors of the frontal lobe. In J.M. Warren & K. Akert (Eds.), *The frontal granular cortex and behavior*. New York: McGraw-Hill.

Hécaen, H. (1969). Cerebral localization of mental functions and their disorders. In P.J. Vinken & G.W. Bruhn (Eds.), *Handbook of clinical neurology* (Vol. III). New York: Wiley.

Hécaen, H. & Albert, M.L. (1978). *Human neuropsychology*. New York: Wiley.

Hécaen, H., de Ajuriaguerra, J., & Massonnet, J. (1951). Les troubles visuo-constructifs par lésion parieto-occipitale droite. *Encéphale, 40,* 122–179.

Hécaen, H. & Angelergues, R. (1963). *La cécité psychique.* Paris: Masson.

Hécaen, H. & Assal, G. (1970). A comparison of constructive deficits following right and left hemispheric lesions. *Neuropsychologia, 8,* 289–303.

Hécaen, H. & Lanteri-Laura, G. (1977). *Évolution des connaissances et des doctrines sur les localisations cérébrales.* Paris: Desclée de Brouwer.

Heck, E.T. & Bryer, J.B. (1986). Superior sorting and categorizing ability in a case of bilateral frontal atrophy: An exception to the rule. *Journal of Clinical and Experimental Neuropsychology, 8,* 313–316.

Hedrick, W.P., Picklelman, H.L., & Walker, W. (1995). Analysis of demographic and functional subacute (transitional) rehabilitation data. *Brain Injury, 9,* 563–573.

Heeger, D.J. & Ress, D. (2002). What does fMRI tell us about neuronal activity? *Nature Reviews Neuroscience, 3,* 142–151.

Heeren, T.J., Lagaay, A.M., von Beek, W.C., et al. (1990). Reference values for the Mini-Mental State Examination (MMSE) in octo- and nonagenarians. *Journal of the American Geriatric Society, 38,* 1093–1096.

Heilbronner, R.L. (1994). Rehabilitation of the neuropsychological sequelae associated with electrical trauma. *Annals of the New York Academy of Sciences, 720,* 224–229.

Heilbronner, R.L. & Parsons, O.A. (1989). Clinical utility of the Tactual Performance Test: Issues of lateralization and cognitive style. *The Clinical Neuropsychologist, 3,* 250–264.

Heilbronner, R.L & Pliskin, N.H. (2003). Clinical neuropsychology in the forensic area. In G.P. Prigatano & N.H. Pliskin (Eds.), *Clinical neuropsychology and cost outcome research: A beginning.* New York: Psychology Press.

Heilman, K.M. (2002). Neglect. In A.K. Asbury et al. (Eds.), *Diseases of the nervous system* (3rd ed.). Cambridge, UK: Cambridge University Press.

Heilman, K.M., Blonder, L.X., Bowers, D., & Crucian, G.P. (2000). Neurological disorders and emotional dysfunction. In J.C. Borod (Ed.), *The neuropsychology of emotion.* New York: Oxford University Press.

Heilman, K.M., Blonder, L.X., Bowers, D., & Valenstein, E. (2003). Emotional disorders associated with neurological diseases. In K.M. Heilman & E. Valenstein (Eds.), *Clinical neuropsychology* (4th ed.). New York: Oxford University Press.

Heilman, K.M., Chatterjee, A., & Doty, L.C. (1995). Hemispheric asymmetries of near-far spatial attention. *Neuropsychology, 9,* 58–61.

Heilman, K.M., Maher, L.M., Greenwald, M.L., & Rothi, L.J. (1997). Conceptual apraxia from lateralized lesions. *Neurology, 49,* 457–464.

Heilman, K.M. & Rothi, L.J.G. (2003). Apraxia. In K.M. Heilman & E. Valenstein (Eds.), *Clinical neuropsychology* (4th ed.). New York: Oxford University Press.

Heilman, K.M., Scholes, R., & Watson, R.T. (1975). Auditory affective agnosia. *Journal of Neurology, Neurosurgery and Psychiatry, 38,* 69–72.

Heilman, K.M. & Valenstein, E. (Eds.) (2003). *Clinical neuropsychology* (4th ed.). New York: Oxford University Press.

Heilman, K.M. & Van Den Abell, T. (1980). Right hemisphere dominance for attention: The mechanism underlying hemispheric asymmetries of inattention (neglect). *Neurology, 30,* 327–330.

Heilman, K.M. & Watson, R.T. (1991). Intentional motor disorders. In H.S. Levin et al. (Eds.), *Frontal lobe function and dysfunction.* New York: Oxford University Press.

Heilman, K.M., Watson, R.T., & Valenstein, E. (2003). Neglect and

related disorders. In K.M. Heilman & E. Valenstein (Eds.), *Clinical neuropsychology* (4th ed.). New York: Oxford University Press.

Heilman, K.M., Watson, R.T., & Valenstein, E. (2000). Neglect I: Clinical and anatomic issues. In M.J. Farah & T.E. Feinberg (Eds.), *Patient-based approaches to cognitive neuroscience.* Cambridge, MA: MIT Press.

Heimburger, R.T. & Reitan, R.M. (1961). Easily administered written test for lateralizing brain lesions. *Journal of Neurosurgery, 18,* 301–312.

Heindel, W.C., Salmon, D.P., & Butters, N. (1991). Alcoholic Korsakoff's syndrome. In T. Yanagihara & R.C. Petersen (Eds.), *Memory disorders: Research and clinical practice.* New York: Marcel Dekker.

Heindel, W.C., Salmon, D.P., Shults, C.W., et al. (1989). Neuropsychological evidence for multiple implicit memory systems: A comparison of Alzheimer's, Huntington's, and Parkinson's disease patients. *Journal of Neuroscience, 9,* 582–587.

Heinik, J., Solomesh, I., Shein, V., & Becker, D. (2002). Clock drawing test in mild and moderate dementia of the Alzheimer's type: A comparative and correlation study. *International Journal of Geriatric Psychiatry, 17,* 480–485.

Heinik, J., Werner, P., Mendel, A., et al. (1999). The Cambridge Cognitive Examination (CAMCOG): Validation of the Hebrew version in elderly demented patients. *International Journal of Geriatric Psychiatry, 14,* 1006–1013.

Heinrichs, R.W. (1990). Current and emergent applications of neuropsychological assessment: Problems of validity and utility. *Professional Psychology: Research and Practice, 21,* 171–176.

Heinrichs, R.W. (1993). Schizophrenia and the brain: Conditions for a neuropsychology of madness. *American Psychologist, 48,* 221–233.

Heinrichs, R.W. & Bury, A. (1991). Copying strategies and memory on the Complex Figure Test in psychiatric patients. *Psychological Reports, 69,* 223–226.

Heishman, S.J., Arasteh, K., & Stitzer, M.L. (1997). Comparative effects of alcohol and marijuana on mood, memory, and performance. *Pharmacology, Biochemistry, and Behavior, 58,* 93–101.

Heiss, W.D. (2000). Ischemic penumbra: Evidence from functional imaging in man. *Journal of Cerebral Blood Flow and Metabolism, 20,* 1276–1293.

Heiss, W.D., Kessler, J., Thiel, A., et al. (1999). Differential capacity of left and right hemispheric areas for compensation of poststroke aphasia. *Annals of Neurology, 45,* 430–438.

Heister, G., Landis, T., Regard, M., & Schroder-Heister, P. (1989). Shift of functional cerebral asymmetry during the menstrual cycle. *Neuropsychologica, 27,* 871–880.

Helgason, C.M. (1997). Mechanisms of antiplatelet agents and the prevention of stroke. In K.M.A. Welch et al. (Eds.), *Primer on cerebrovascular diseases.* San Diego: Academic Press.

Heller, A., Won, L., & Hoffman, P.C. (2000). Amphetamines and related compounds. In P.S. Spencer & H.H. Schaumburg (Eds.), *Experimental and clinical neurotoxicology* (2nd ed.). New York: Oxford University Press.

Hellige, J.B. (1988). Hemispheric differences for processing spatial information: Categorization versus distance [abstract]. *Journal of Clinical and Experimental Neuropsychology, 10,* 330.

Hellige, J.B. (1995). Coordinating the different processing biases of the left and right cerebral hemispheres. In F.L. Kitterle (Ed.), *Hemispheric communication: Mechanisms and models.* Hillsdale, NJ: Erlbaum.

Helmes, E. (1996). Uses of the Barona method to predict premorbid intelligence in the elderly. *The Clinical Neuropsychologist, 10,* 255–261.

Helmes, E., Bowler, J.V., Merskey, H., (2003). Rates of cognitive decline in Alzheimer's disease and dementia with Lewy bodies. *Dementia and Geriatric Cognitive Disorders, 15,* 67–71.

Helm-Estabrooks, N., Emery, P., & Liebergott, J. (1985). *It's how you play the game: A comparative analysis of the checker-playing performances of right and left brain damaged patients.* Paper presented at the 13th annual meeting of the International Neuropsychological Society, San Diego, CA.

Helmstaedter, C. (2002). Effects of chronic epilepsy on declarative memory systems. *Progress in Brain Research, 135,* 439–453.

Helmstaedter, C. & Elger, C. E. (1999). The phantom of progressive dementia in epilepsy. *Lancet, 354,* 2133–2134.

Helmstaedter, C., Grunwald, T., Lehnertz, K., et al. (1997). Differential involvement of left temporolateral and temporomesial structures in verbal declarative learning and memory: Evidence from temporal lobe epilepsy. *Brain and Cognition, 35,* 110–131.

Helmstaedter, C., Hauff, M., & Elger, C.E. (1998). Ecological validity of list-learning tests and self-reported memory in healthy individuals and those with temporal lobe epilepsy. *Journal of Clinical and Experimental Neuropsychology, 20,* 365–375.

Helmstaedter, C. & Kurthen, M. (2001). Memory and epilepsy: Characteristics, course, and influence of drugs and surgery. *Current Opinion in Neurology, 14,* 211–216.

Helmstaedter, C., Kurthen, M., Linke, D.B., & Elger, C.E. (1994). Right hemisphere restitution of language and memory functions in right hemisphere language-dominant patients with left temporal lobe epilepsy. *Brain, 117,* 729–737.

Helmstaedter, C., Pohl, C., Hufnagel, A., & Elger, C. E. (1991). Visual learning deficits in nonresected patients with right temporal lobe epilepsy. *Cortex, 27,* 547–555.

Hendelman, W.J. (2000). *Functional neuroanatomy.* Boca Raton, FL: CRC Press.

Henderson, A.S., & Hasegawa, K. (1992). The epidemiology of dementia and depression in later life. In M. Bergener (Ed.), *Aging and mental disorders: International perspectives.* New York: Springer.

Henderson, V.W. (1997). The epidemiology of estrogen replacement therapy and Alzheimer's disease. *Neurology, 48,* S27–S35.

Henderson, V.W., Mack, W., & Williams, B.W. (1989). Spatial disorientation in Alzheimer's disease. *Archives of Neurology, 46,* 391–394.

Hendrie, H.C., Hall, K.S., Brittain, H.M., et al. (1988). The CAMDEX: A standardized instrument for the diagnosis of mental disorder in the elderly: A replication with a US sample. *Journal of the American Geriatric Society, 36,* 402–408.

Henley, S., Pettit, S., Todd-Pokropek, A., & Tupper, A. (1985). Who goes home? Predictive factors in stroke recovery. *Journal of Neurology, Neurosurgery and Psychiatry, 48,* 1–6.

Hennekens, C.H. (1996). Alcohol and risk of coronary events. In S. Zakhari & M. Wassef (Eds.), *Alcohol and the cardiovascular system.* NIAA Research Monograph 31, NIH Publication 96-4133. Washington, D.C.: U.S. Government Printing Office.

Hennessy, M.J. & Britton, T.C. (2000). Transient ischaemic attacks: Evaluation and management. *International Journal of Clinical Practice, 54,* 432–436.

Henry, G.K., Gross, H.S., & Furst, C.F. (2001). Nonimpact brain injury: Neuropsychological and behavioral correlates with consideration of physiological findings: Reply to Ferrari. *Applied Neuropsychology, 8,* 122–123.

Henry, G.K., Gross, H.S., Herndon, C.A., & Furst, C.J. (2000). Nonimpact brain injury: Neuropsychological and behavioral correlates with consideration of physical findings. *Applied Neuropsychology, 7,* 65–75.

Henry, L.C. (1945). *Best quotations for all occasions.* New York: Doubleday.

Henson, R. (2001). Neural working memory. In J.A. Andrade (Ed.), *Working memory in perspective.* Hove, UK: Psychology Press.

Herlitz, A., Hill, R. D., Fratiglioni, L., & Backman, L. (1995). Episodic memory and visuospatial ability in detecting and staging dementia in a community-based sample of very old adults. *Journal of Gerontology A: Biological Science and Medical Science, 50,* M107–M113.

Herlitz, A., Nilsson, L.G., & Backman, L. (1997). Gender differences in episodic memory. *Memory and Cognition, 25,* 801–811.

Herlitz, A. & Viitanen, M. (1991). Semantic organization and verbal episodic memory in patients with mild and moderate Alzheimer's disease. *Journal of Clinical and Experimental Neuropsychology, 13,* 559–574.

Hermann, B.P., Gold, J., Pusakulich, R., et al. (1995). Wechsler Adult Intelligence Scale-Revised in the evaluation of anterior temporal lobectomy candidates. *Epilepsia, 36,* 480–487.

Hermann, B.P. & Melyn, M. (1985). Identification of neuropsychological deficits in epilepsy using the Luria-Nebraska Neuropsychological Battery: a replication attempt. *Journal of Clinical and Experimental Neuropsychology, 7,* 305–313.

Hermann, B.P., Seidenberg, M., & Bell, B. (2002). The neurodevelopmental impact of childhood onset temporal lobe epilepsy on brain structure and function and the risk of progressive cognitive effects. *Progress in Brain Research, 135,* 429–438.

Hermann, B. P., Seidenberg, M., Schoenfeld, J., et al. (1996). Empirical techniques for determining the reliability, magnitude, and pattern of neuropsychological change after epilepsy surgery. *Epilepsia, 37,* 942–950.

Hermann, B.P., Seidenberg, M., Schoenfeld, J., & Davies, K. (1997). Neuropsychological characteristics of the syndrome of mesial temporal lobe epilepsy. *Archives of Neurology, 54,* 369–376.

Hermann, B.P., Seidenberg, M., Wyler, A., & Haltiner, A. (1993). Dissociation of object recognition and spatial localization abilities following temporal lobe lesions in human. *Neuropsychology, 7,* 343–350.

Hermann, B.P. & Whitman, S. (1986). Psychopathology in epilepsy: A multietiologic model. In S. Whitman & B.P. Hermann (Eds.), *Psychopathology in epilepsy.* New York: Oxford University Press.

Hermann, B.P. & Whitman, S. (1992). Psychopathology in epilepsy: The role of psychology in altering paradigms of research, treatment and prevention. *American Psychologist, 47,* 1134–1138.

Hermann, B.P. & Wyler, A.R. (1988). Effects of anterior temporal lobectomy on language function: A controlled study. *Annals of Neurology, 23,* 585–588.

Hermann, B.P., Wyler, A.R., & Richey, E.T. (1988). Wisconsin Card Sorting Test performance in patients with complex partial seizures of temporal-lobe origin. *Journal of Clinical Neuropsychology, 10,* 467–476.

Hermann, B.P., Wyler, A.R., Richey, E.T., & Rea, J.M. (1987). Memory function and verbal learning ability in patients with complex partial seizures of temporal lobe origin. *Epilepsia, 28,* 547–554.

Hermann, B.P., Wyler, A.R., & Somes, G. (1992). Preoperative psychological adjustment and surgical outcome are determinants of psychosocial status after anterior temporal lobectomy. *Journal of Neurology, Neurosurgery and Psychiatry, 55,* 491–496.

Hermann, B.P., Wyler, A.R., Somes, G., et al. (1992). Pathological status of the mesial temporal lobe predicts memory outcome from left anterior temporal lobectomy. *Neurosurgery, 31,* 652–656.

Hermann, B.P., Wyler, A.R., Somes, G., & Clement, L. (1994). Dysnomia after left anterior temporal lobectomy without functional mapping: Frequency and correlates. *Neurosurgery, 35,* 52–56.

Hermann, B.P., Wyler, A.R., Somes, G., et al. (1994). Declarative memory following anterior temporal lobectomy in humans. *Behavioral Neuroscience, 108,* 3–10.

Hernán, M.A., Olek, M.J., & Ascherio, A. (1999). Geographic variation of MS incidence in two prospective studies of US women. *Neurology, 53,* 1711–1718.

Herndon, R.M. (Ed.) (1997). *Handbook of neurologic rating scales.* New York: Demos.

Herrmann, D.J. (1982). Know thy memory: The use of questionnaires to assess and study memory. *Psychological Bulletin, 92,* 434–452.

Herrmann, D.J. & Neisser, U. (1978). An inventory of everyday memory experiences. In M. M. Gruneberg et al. (Eds.), *Practical aspects of memory.* New York: Academic Press.

Herrmann, M., Jost, S., Kutz, S., et al. (2000). Temporal profile of release of neurobiochemical markers of brain damage after traumatic brain injury is associated with intracranial pathology as demonstrated in cranial computerized tomography. *Journal of Neurotrauma, 17,* 113–122.

Herrmann, N., Kidron, D., Shulman, K.I., et al. (1998). Clock tests in depression, Alzheimer's disease, and elderly controls. *International Journal of Psychiatry in Medicine, 28,* 437–447.

Herrnstein, R.J. & Murray, C. (1994). *The bell curve: Intelligence and class structure in American life.* New York: Free Press.

Hersch, E.L. (1979). Development and application of the extended scale for dementia. *Journal of the American Geriatrics Society, 27,* 348–354.

Hersch, S., Jones, R., Koroshetz, W., & Quaid, K. (1994). The neurogenetics genie: Testing for the Huntington's disease mutation. *Neurology, 44,* 1369–1373.

Hersch, S.M. & Rosas, H.D. (2001). The most commonly asked questions about Huntington's disease. *The Neurologist, 7,* 364–368.

Hershey, L.A., Jaffe, D.F., Greenough, P.G., & Yang, S.-L. (1987). Validation of cognitive and functional assessment instruments in vascular dementia. *International Journal of Psychiatry in Medicine, 17,* 183–192.

Hertel, P.T. (2000). The cognitive-initiative account of depression-related impairments in memory. In *The Psychology of Learning and Motivation* (Vol. 39). San Diego, CA: Academic Press.

Hertzog, C. (1996). Research design in studies of aging and cognition. In J.E. Birren & W.K. Schaie (Eds.), *Handbook of the psychology of aging* (4th ed.). San Diego: Academic Press.

Hestad, K., Aukrust, P., Ellertsen, B., et al. (1993). Neuropsychological deficits in HIV-I seropositive and seronegative intravenous drug users. *Journal of Clinical and Experimental Neuropsychology, 15,* 732–742.

Heun, R., Mazanek, M., Atzor, K.-R., et al. (1997). Amygdala-hippocampal atrophy and memory performance in dementia of the Alzheimer type. *Dementia and Geriatric Cognitive Disorders, 8,* 329–336.

Hewson, L. (1949). The Wechsler-Bellevue Scale and the Substitution Test as aids in neuropsychiatric diagnosis. *Journal of Nervous and Mental Disorders, 109,* 158–183; Pt. 2, 246–266.

Heyer, E. J., Sharma, R., Rampersad, A., Winfree, C. J., et al. (2002). A controlled prospective study of neuropsychological dysfunction following carotid endarterectomy. *Archives of Neurology, 59,* 217–222.

Heyer, E.J., Sharma, R., Winfree, C.J., et al. (2000). Severe pain confounds neuropsychological test performance. *Journal of Clinical and Experimental Neuropsychology, 22,* 633–639.

Heyman, A., Fillenbaum, G.G., Gearing, M., et al. (1999). Comparison of Lewy body variant of Alzheimer's disease with pure Alzheimer's disease: Consortium to Establish a Registry for Alzheimer's Disease, Part XIX. *Neurology, 52,* 1839–1844.

Heyman, A., Wilkinson, W.E., Hurwitz, B.J., et al. (1983). Alzheimer's disease: Genetic aspects and associated clinical disorders. *Annals of Neurology, 14,* 507–515.

Hibbard, M.R., Bogdany, J., Uysal, S., et al. (2000). Axis II psychopathology in individuals with traumatic brain injury. *Brain Injury, 14,* 45–61.

Hibbard, M.R., Uysal, S., Kepler, K., et al. (1998). Axis I psychopathology in individuals with traumatic brain injury. *Journal of Head Trauma Rehabilitation, 13,* 24–39.

Hickling, E.J., Gillen, R., Blanchard, E.B., et al. (1998). Traumatic brain injury and post-traumatic stress disorder: a preliminary investigation of neuropsychological test results in PTSD secondary to motor vehicle accidents. *Brain Injury, 12,* 265–274.

Hickman, S.E., Howieson, D.B., Dame, A., et al. (2000). Longitudinal analysis of the effects of the aging process on neuropsychological test performance in the healthy young-old and oldest-old. *Developmental Neuropsychology, 17,* 323–337.

Hickox, A.& Sunderland, A. (1992). Questionnaire and checklist approaches to assessment of everyday memory problems. In J.R. Crawford et al. (Eds.), *A handbook of neuropsychological assessment.* Hove, UK: Erlbaum.

Hier, D.B., Yoon, W.B., Mohr, J.P., et al. (1994). Gender and aphasia in the Stroke Data Bank. *Brain and Language, 47,* 155–167.

Higgins, J.J. & Mendez, M.F. (2000). Roll over Pick and tell Alzheimer the news! *Neurology, 54,* 784–785.

Higginson, C.I., Arnett, P.A., & Voss, W.D. (2000). The ecological validity of clinical tests of memory and attention in multiple sclerosis. *Archives of Clinical Neuropsychology, 15,* 185–204.

High, W.M., Jr., Levin, H.S., & Gary, H.E., Jr. (1990). Recovery of orientation following closed-head injury. *Journal of Clinical and Experimental Neuropsychology, 12,* 703–714.

Hildebrandt, H., Brand, A., & Sachsenheimer, W. (1998). Profiles of patients with left prefrontal and left temporal lobe lesions after cerebrovascular infarctions on California Verbal Learning Test-like indices. *Journal of Clinical and Experimental Neuropsychology, 20,* 673–683.

Hill, M.D. & Feasby, T.E. (2002). Principles of clinical neuro-epidemiology. In A.K. Asbury et al. (Eds.), *Diseases of the nervous system* (3rd ed.). Cambridge, UK: Cambridge University Press.

Hill, S.K., Ragland, J.D., Gur, R.C., & Gur, R.E. (2001). Neuropsychological differences among empirically derived clinical subtypes of schizophrenia. *Neuropsychology, 15,* 492–501.

Hill, T.D., Reddon, J.R., & Jackson, D.N. (1985). The factor structure of the Wechsler scales: a brief review. *Clinical Psychology Review, 5,* 287–306.

Hillbom, E. (1960). After-effects of brain injuries. *Acta Psychiatrica et Neurologica Scandinavica, 35(Suppl.),* 142.

Hillert, J. & Masterman, T. (2001). The genetics of multiple sclerosis. In S.D. Cook (Ed.), *Handbook of multiple sclerosis* (3rd ed.). New York: Marcel Dekker.

Hillier, S.L., Hiller, J.E., & Metzer, J. (1997). Epidemiology of traumatic brain injury in South Australia. *Brain Injury, 11,* 649–659.

Hilsabeck, R.C., Dunn, J.T., & Lees-Haley, P.R. (1996). An empirical comparison of the Wechsler Memory Scale-Revised and the Memory Assessment Scales in measuring four memory constructs. *Assessment, 3,* 417–422.

Hilsabeck, R.C., Gouvier, W. D., & Bolter, J.F. (1998). Reconstructive memory bias in recall of neuropsychological symptomatology. *Journal of Clinical and Experimental Neuropsychology, 20,* 328–338.

Hinchliffe, F.J., Murdoch, B.E., & Chenery, H.J. (1998). Towards a conceptualization of language and cognitive impairment in closed-head injury: use of clinical measures. *Brain Injury, 12,* 109–132.

Hinkeldey, N.S. & Corrigan, J.D. (1990). The structure of head-injured patients' neurobehavioral complaints: a preliminary study. *Brain Injury, 4,* 115–134.

Hinkin, C.H., van Gorp, W.G., Satz, P., et al. (1992). Depressed mood and its relationship to neuropsychological test performance in HIV-1 seropositive individuals. *Journal of Clinical and Experimental Neuropsychology, 14,* 289–297.

Hinton-Bayre, A.D., Geffen, G., & McFarland, K. (1997). Mild head injury and speed of information processing: A prospective study of professional rugby league players. *Journal of Clinical and Experimental Neuropsychology, 19,* 275–289.

Hirono, N., Mori, E., Ishii, K., et al. (1998). Regional metabolism: Associations with dyscalculia in Alzheimer's disease. *Journal of Neurology, Neurosurgery and Psychiatry, 65,* 913–916.

Hirschenfang, S. (1960a). A comparison of Bender Gestalt reproduction of right and left hemiplegic patients. *Journal of Clinical Psychology, 16,* 439.

Hirschenfang, S. (1960b). A comparison of WAIS scores of hemiplegic patients with and without aphasia. *Journal of Clinical Psychology, 16,* 351.

Hiscock, M. (1986). On sex differences in spatial abilities. *American Psychologist, 41,* 1011–1018.

Hiscock, C.K., Branham, J.D., & Hiscock, M. (1994). Detection of feigned cognitive impairment: The two-alternative forced-choice method compared with selected conventional tests. *Journal of Psychopathology and Behavioral Assessment, 16,* 95–110.

Hiscock, M. & Hiscock, C.K. (1989). Refining the forced-choice method for the detection of malingering. *Journal of Clinical and Experimental Neuropsychology, 11,* 967–974.

Hiscock, M., Inch, R., Hawryluk, J., et al. (1999). Is there a sex difference in human laterality? III. An exhaustive survey of tactile laterality studies from six neuropsychology journals. *Journal of Clinical and Experimental Neuropsychology, 21,* 17–28.

Hiscock, M., Inch, R., Jacek, C., et al. (1994). Is there a difference in human laterality? I. An exhaustive survey of auditory laterality studies from six neuropsychology journals. *Journal of Clinical and Experimental Neuropsychology, 16,* 423–435.

Hiscock, M., Israelian, M., Inch, R., et al. (1995). Is there a sex difference in human laterality? II. An exhaustive survey of visual laterality studies from six neuropsychology journals. *Journal of Clinical and Experimental Neuropsychology, 17,* 590–610.

Ho, M.R. & Bennett, T.L. (1997). Efficacy of neuropsychological rehabilitation. *Archives of Clinical Neuropsychology, 12,* 1–11.

Hobart, M.P., Goldberg, R., Bartko, J.J., & Gold, J.M. (1999). Repeatable battery for the assessment of neuropsychological status as a screening test in schizophrenia. II: Convergent/discriminant validity and diagnostic group comparisons. *American Journal of Psychiatry, 156,* 1951–1957.

Hobson, P. & Meara, J. (1999). The detection of dementia and cognitive impairment in a community population of elderly people with Parkinson's disease by use of the CAMCOG neuropsychological test. *Age and Ageing, 28,* 39–43.

Hoch, C.C. & Reynolds, C.F. (1990). Psychiatric symptoms in dementia: Interaction of affect and cognition. In F. Boller & G. Grafman (Eds.), *Handbook of neuropsychology* (Vol. 4). Amsterdam: Elsevier.

Hochberg, M.G., Russo, J., Vitaliano, P.P., et al. (1989). Initiation and perseveration as a subscale of the Dementia Rating Scale. *Clinical Gerontologist, 8,* 27–41.

Hochswender, W.J. (June, 1988). The mechanics of a knockout punch. *Popular Mechanics,* 72–73, 77, 112–113.

Hodges, J.R. (1995). Retrograde amnesia. In A.D. Baddeley et al. (Eds.), *Handbook of memory disorders.* Chichester, UK: Wiley.

Hodges, J.R. (2000). Memory in the dementias. In E. Tulving & F.I.M. Craik (Eds.), *The Oxford handbook of memory.* New York: Oxford University Press.

Hodges, J.R. & Oxbury, S.M. (1990). Persistent memory impairment following transient global amnesia. *Journal of Clinical and Experimental Neuropsychology, 12,* 904–920.

Hodges, J.R., Patterson, K., Graham, N., & Dawson, K. (1996). Naming and knowing in dementia of Alzheimer's type. *Brain and Language, 54,* 302–325.

Hodges, J.R., Patterson, K., Oxbury, S., & Funnell, E. (1992). Se-

mantic fluent aphasia with temporal lobe atrophy. *Brain, 115,* 1783–1806.

Hodges, J.R., Salmon, D.P., & Butters, N. (1991). The nature of the naming deficit in Alzheimer's and Huntington's disease. *Brain, 114,* 1547–1558.

Hodges, J.R., Salmon, D.P., & Butters, N. (1993). Recognition and naming of famous faces in Alzheimer's disease: a cognitive analysis. *Neuropsychologia, 31,* 775–788.

Hodges, J.R. & Ward, C.D. (1989). Observations during transient global amnesia. A behavioural and neuropsychological study of five cases. *Brain, 112,* 595–620.

Hodgson, C. & Ellis, A.W. (1998). Last in, first to go: Age of acquisition and naming in the elderly. *Brain and Language, 64,* 146–163.

Hodkinson, H.M. (1972). Evaluation of a mental test score for assessment of mental impairment in the elderly. *Age and Ageing, 1,* 233–238.

Hoehn, M.M. (1992). The natural history of Parkinson's disease in the pre-levodopa and post-levodopa eras. *Neurologic Clinics, 10,* 331–339.

Hoehn, M.M. & Yahr, M.D. (1967). Parkinsonism: Onset, progression and mortality. *Neurology, 17,* 427–442.

Hof, P.R., Archin, N., Osmand, A.P., et al. (1993). Posterior cortical atrophy in Alzheimer's disease: analysis of a new case and re-evaluation of a historical report. *Acta Neuropathologica, 6,* 215–223.

Hof, P.R., Giannakopoulos, P., & Bouras, C. (1996). The neuropathological changes associated with normal brain aging. *Histology and Histopathology, 11,* 1075–1088.

Hofer, S.M., Piccinin, A.M., & Hershey, D. (1996). Analysis of the structure and discriminative power of the Mattis Dementia Rating Scale. *Journal of Clinical Psychology, 52,* 395–409.

Hoffman, K.L. & McNaughton, B.L. (2002). Coordinated reactivation of distributed memory traces in primate neocortex. *Science, 297,* 2070–2073.

Hoffman, R.G. & Nelson, K.S. (1988). Cross-validation of six short forms of the WAIS-R in a healthy geriatric sample. *Journal of Clinical Psychology, 44,* 952–956.

Hoffman, R.G., Scott, J.G., Tremont, G., et al. (1997). Cross-validation of a method for predicting Wechsler Memory Scale-Revised index scores. *The Clinical Neuropsychologist, 11,* 402–406.

Hoffman, R.G., Speelman, D.J., Hinnen, D.A., et al. (1989). Changes in cortical functioning with acute hypoglycemia and hyperglycemia in type I diabetes. *Diabetes Care, 12,* 193–197.

Hogan, D.B. & Ebly, E.M. (1995). Primitive reflexes and dementia: Results from the Canadian Study of Health and Aging. *Age and Aging, 24,* 375–381.

Hogervorst, E., Combrinck, M., Lapuerta, P., et al. (2002). The Hopkins Verbal Learning Test and screening for dementia. *Dementia and Geriatric Cognitive Disorders, 13,* 13–20.

Hogg, J.R., Johnstone, B., Weishaar, S., & Petroski, G.F. (2001). Application of a short form of the Category Test for individuals with a traumatic brain injury. *The Clinical Neuropsychologist, 15,* 129–133.

Hohl, U., Grundman, M., Salmon, D.P., et al., (1999). Mini-Mental State Examination and Mattis Dementia Rating Scale performance differs in Hispanic and non-Hispanic Alzheimer's disease patients. *Journal of the International Neuropsychological Society, 5,* 301–307.

Hohol, M.J., Guttmann, C.R., Orav, J., et al. (1997). Serial neuropsychological assessment and magnetic resonance imaging analysis in multiple sclerosis. *Archive of Neurology, 54,* 1018–1025.

Hökfelt, T., Johansson, O., & Goldstein, M. (1984). Chemical anatomy of the brain. *Science, 225,* 1326–1334.

Holden, U. (1988b). Realistic assessment. In Una Holden (Ed.),

Neuropsychology and aging. New York: New York University Press.

Holden, U. (2001). Crossing the i's and dotting the t's. *Neuropsychological Rehabilitation, 11,* 197–200.

Holdwick, D.J., Jr. & Wingenfeld, S.A. (1999). The subjective experience of PASAT testing: Does the PASAT induce negative mood? *Archives of Clinical Neuropsychology, 14,* 273–284.

Holland, A.L. (1980). *Communicative Abilities in Daily Living. A test of functional communication for aphasic adults.* Baltimore, MD: University Park Press.

Holland, A.L., Frattali, C.M., & Fromm, D. (1999). *Communicative Abilities in Daily Living (CADL-2)* (2nd ed.). Negrang East, Australia: Pro-Ed.

Holmes, C., Cairns, N., Lantos, P., & Mann, A. (1999). Validity of current clinical criteria for Alzheimer's disease, vascular dementia and dementia with Lewy bodies. *British Journal of Psychiatry, 174,* 45–50.

Holmes, C.S. (1986). Neuropsychological profiles in men with insulin-dependent diabetes. *Journal of Consulting and Clinical Psychology, 54,* 386–389.

Holmes, C.S., Koepke, K.M., Thompson, R.G., et al. (1984). Verbal fluency and naming performance in type 1 diabetes at different blood glucose concentrations. *Diabetes Care, 7,* 454–459.

Holmes, C.S., Koepke, K.M., & Thompson, R.G. (1986). Simple versus complex performance impairments at three blood glucose levels. *Psychoneuroendocrinology, 11,* 353–357.

Holmes, G.L. & Engel, J., Jr. (2001). Predicting medical intractability of epilepsy in children: how certain can we be? *Neurology, 56,* 1430–1431.

Holmes, J.M., Droste, P. J., & Beck, R.W. (1998). The natural history of acute traumatic sixth nerve palsy or pareses. *Journal of the American Association of Pediatric Ophthalmology, 2,* 265–268.

Holmes, M.D., Dodrill, C.B., Wilkus, R.J., et al., (1998). Is partial epilepsy progressive? Ten-year follow-up of EEG and neuropsychological changes in adults with partial seizures. *Epilepsia, 39,* 1189–1193.

Holmes, T.H. and Rahe, R.H. (1967). The social readjustment scale. *Journal of Psychosomatic Research, 11,* 213–218.

Holodny, A.I., Waxman, R., George, A.E., et al. (1998). MR differential diagnosis of normal-pressure hydrocephalus and Alzheimer disease: significance of perihippocampal fissures. *American Journal of Neuroradiology, 19,* 813–819.

Holroyd, S. (2000). Hallucinations and delusions in dementia. *International Psychogeriatrics, 12(Suppl. 1),* 113–117.

Holsinger, T., Steffens, D.C., Phillips, C., et al. (2002). Head injury in early adulthood and the lifetime risk of depression. *Archives of General Psychiatry, 59,* 17–22.

Holtz, J.L., Gearhart, L.P., & Watson, C.G. (1996). Comparability of scores on projector- and booklet-administered forms of the Category Test in brain-impaired veterans and controls. *Neuropsychology, 10,* 194–196.

Hom, J. (1991). Contributions of the Halstead-Reitan Battery in the neuropsychological investigation of stroke. In R.A. Bornstein & G.G. Brown (Eds.), *Neurobehavioral aspects of cerebrovascular disease.* New York: Oxford University Press.

Hom, J. & Reitan, R.M. (1982). Effect of lateralized cerebral damage upon contralateral and ipsilateral sensorimotor performances. *Journal of Clinical Neuropsychology, 4,* 249–269.

Hom, J. & Reitan, R.M. (1984). Neuropsychological correlates of rapidly vs. slowly growing intrinsic cerebral neoplasms. *Journal of Clinical and Experimental Neuropsychology, 6,* 309–324.

Hom, J. & Reitan, R. M. (1990). Generalized cognitive function after stroke. *Journal of Clinical and Experimental Neuropsychology, 12,* 644–654.

Hommel, M. (1997). Small artery occlusive disease. In K.M.A. Welch et al. (Eds.), *Primer on cerebrovascular diseases.* San Diego, CA: Academic Press.

Hommel, M. & Besson, G. (2001). Midbrain infarcts. In J. Bogousslavsky & L.R. Caplan (Eds.), *Stroke syndromes.* Cambridge, UK: Cambridge University Press.

Homsakya, E.D. (2001). *Alexander Romanovich Luria. A scientific biography* (trans. D. Krotova). New York: Kluwer Academic/Plenum Press.

Hong, Y.-y., Morris, M.W., Chiu, C.-y., & Benet-Martínez, V. (2000). Multicultural minds. A dynamic constructivist approach to culture and cognition. *American Psychologist, 55,* 709–720.

Hoofien, D., Gilboa, A., Vakil, E., & Donovick, P.J. (2001). Traumatic brain injury (TBI) 10–20 years later: a comprehensive outcome study of psychiatric symptomatology, cognitive abilities and psychosocial functioning. *Brain Injury, 15,* 189–209.

Hoofien, D., Vakil E., Cohen, G., & Sheleff, P. (1990). Empirical results of a ten-year follow-up study on the effects of a neuropsychological rehabilitation program: A reevaluation of chronicity. In E. Vakil et al. (Eds.), *Rehabilitation of the brain injured.* London: Freund.

Hoofien, D., Vakil, E., & Gilboa, A. (2000). Criterion validation of premorbid intelligence estimation in persons with traumatic brain injury: "Hold/don't hold" versus "best performance" procedures. *Journal of Clinical and Experimental Neuropsychology, 22,* 305–315.

Hooker, W.D. & Raskin, N.H. (1986). Neuropsychological alterations in classic and common migraine. *Archives of Neurology, 43,* 709–712.

Hooper, H.E. (1983). *Hooper Visual Organization Test Manual.* Los Angeles: Western Psychological Services.

Hooshmand, H., Radfar, F., & Beckner, E. (1989). The neurophysiological aspects of electrical injuries. *Clinical Electroencephalography, 20,* 111–120.

Hopewell, C.A. (1983). Serial neuropsychological assessment in a case of reversible electrocution encephalopathy. *Clinical Neuropsychology, 5,* 61–65.

Hopkins, A. (1981). *Epilepsy. The facts.* Oxford: Oxford University Press.

Hopkins, A. (1998). The measurement of outcomes of health care. In M. Swash (Ed.), *Outcomes in neurological and neurosurgical disorders.* Cambridge: Cambridge University Press.

Hopkins, R.O., Abildskov, T.J., Bigler, E.D., & Weaver, L.K. (1997). Three dimensional image reconstruction of neuroanatomical structures: Methods for isolation of the cortex, ventricular system, hippocampus, and fornix. *Neuropsychology Review, 7,* 87–104.

Hopkins, R.O. & Bigler, E.D. (2001). In R.E. Tarter et al. (Eds.), *Medical neuropsychology* (2nd ed.). New York: Kluwer Academic/Plenum Press.

Horan, M., Ashton, R., & Minto, J. (1980). Using ECT to study hemispheric specialization for sequential processes. *British Journal of Psychiatry, 137,* 119–125.

Horn, G.J. & Kelly, M.P. (1996). Strengths and limitations of the Short Category Test in neuropsychological examination following acute traumatic brain injury. *Applied Neuropsychology, 3,* 58–64.

Horn, J.L. & Cattell, R.B. (1966). Refinement and test of the theory of fluid and crystallized general intelligence. *Journal of Educational Psychology, 57,* 253–270.

Horn, J.L. & Donaldson, G. (1976). On the myth of intellectual decline in adulthood. *American Psychologist, 31,* 701–719.

Hornak, J., Rolls, E.T., & Wade, D. (1996). Face and voice expression identification in patients with emotional and behavioural changes following ventral frontal lobe damage. *Neuropsychologia, 34,* 247–261.

Hornbein, T. F., Townes, B. D., Schoene, R.B., et al. (1989). The cost to the central nervous system of climbing to extremely high altitude. *New England Journal of Medicine, 321,* 1714–1719.

Horne, D.J. (1973). Sensorimotor control in parkinsonism. *Neurology, Neurosurgery, and Psychiatry, 36,* 742–746.

Horner, J., Dawson, D.V., Heyman, A., & Fish, A.M. (1992). The usefulness of the Western Aphasia Battery for differential diagnosis of Alzheimer dementia and focal stroke syndromes: preliminary evidence. *Brain and Language, 42,* 77–88.

Horner, J., Heyman, A., Dawson, D., & Rogers, H. (1988). The relationship of agraphia to the severity of dementia in Alzheimer's disease. *Archives of Neurology, 45,* 760–763.

Horner, M.D., Flashman, L.A., Freides, D., et al. (1996). Temporal lobe epilepsy and performance on the Wisconsin Card Sorting Test. *Journal of Clinical and Experimental Neuropsychology, 18,* 310–313.

Horner, M.D. & Hamner, M.B. (2002). Neurocognitive functioning in posttraumatic stress disorder. *Neuropsychology Review, 12,* 15–30.

Horton, A.M., Jr. (1995). Alternative impairment index: A measure of neuropsychological deficit. *Perceptual and Motor Skills, 80,* 336–338.

Horton, A.M., Jr. (1999). Above-average intelligence and neuropsychological test score performance. *International Journal of Neuroscience, 99,* 221–231.

Horton, K.D., Smith, S.A., Barghout, N.K., & Connolly, D.A. (1992). The use of indirect memory tests to assess malingered amnesia: A study of metamemory. *Journal of Experimental Psychology: General, 121,* 326–351.

Houlihan, J.P., Abrahams, J.P., LaRue, A.A., & Jarvik, L.F. (1985). Qualitative differences in Vocabulary performance of Alzheimer versus depressed patients. *Developmental Neuropsychology, 1,* 139–144.

House, A., Dennis, M., Warlow, C., et al.(1990). Mood disorders after stroke and their relation to lesion location. *Brain, 113,* 1113–1129.

Houston Conference on Specialty Education and Training in Clinical Neuropsychology (1998). Policy statement. *Archives of Clinical Neuropsychology, 13,* 160–165.

Houston, J.P., Schneider, N.G., & Jarvik, M.E. (1978). Effects of smoking on free recall and organization. *American Journal of Psychiatry, 135,* 220–222.

Hovestadt, A., de Jong, G.J., & Meerwaldt, J.D. (1987). Spatial disorientation as an early symptom of Parkinson's disease. *Neurology, 37,* 485–487.

Hovey, H.B. (1964). Brain Lesions and 5 MMPI items. *Journal of Consulting Psychology, 28,* 78–79.

Hovey, H.B. & Kooi, K.A. (1955). Transient disturbance of thought processes and epilepsy. *AMA Archives of Neurology and Psychiatry, 74,* 287–291.

Hovland, D. & Raskin, S.A. (2000). Anxiety and posttraumatic stress. In S.A. Raskin & C.A. Mateer (Eds.), *Neuropsychological management of mild traumatic brain injury.* New York: Oxford University Press.

Howard, D. (1997). Language in the human brain. In M.D. Rugg (Ed.), *Cognitive neuroscience.* Cambridge, MA: MIT Press.

Howieson, D.B., Dame, A., Camicioli, R., et al. (1997). Cognitive markers preceding Alzheimer's dementia in the healthy oldest old. *Journal of the American Geriatric Society, 45,* 584–589.

Howieson, D.B., Holm, L.A., Kaye, J.A., et al. (1993). Neurologic function in the optimally healthy oldest old. Neuropsychological evaluation. *Neurology, 43,* 1882–1886.

Howieson, D.B. & Lezak, M.D. (2002a). The neuropsychological evaluation. In S.C. Yudofsky & R.E. Hales (Eds.), *American Psychiatric Press textbook of neuropsychiatry* (4th ed.). Washington, D.C.: American Psychiatric Press.

Howieson, D.B. & Lezak, M.D. (2002b). Separating memory from other cognitive problems. In A. Baddeley (Eds.), *Handbook of memory disorders* (2nd ed.). Chichester, UK: Wiley.

Hsia, Y. & Graham, C. H. (1965). Color blindness. In C. H. Graham (Ed.), *Vision and visual perception.* New York: Wiley.

Hsiang, J. & Marshall, L.F. (1998). Head injury. In M. Swash (Ed.), *Outcome in neurological and neurosurgical disorders.* Cambridge, UK: Cambridge University Press.

Hsu, L. M. (2002). Diagnostic validity statistics and the MCMI-III. *Psychological Assessment, 14,* 410–422.

Hsu, L.M., Hayman, J., Kock, J., & Mandell, D. (2000). Relation of statistically significant, abnormal, and typical WAIS-R VIQ-PIQ discrepancies to full scale IQs. *European Journal of Psychological Assessment, 16,* 107–114.

Hua, M.-S., Chang, S.-H., & Chen, S.-T. (1997). Factor structure and age effects with an aphasia test battery in normal Taiwanese adults. *Neuropsychology, 11,* 147–155.

Hua, M.S., Chen, S.T., Tang, L.M., & Leung, W.M. (1998). Neuropsychological function in patients with nasopharyngeal carcinoma after radiotherapy. *Journal of Clinical and Experimental Neuropsychology, 20,* 684–593.

Hua, M.S. & Huang, C.C. (1991). Chronic occupational exposure to manganese and neurobehavioral function. *Journal of Clinical and Experimental Neuropsychology, 13,* 495–507.

Huang, C.-C., Chu, N.-S., Lu C.-S., et al. (1989). Chronic manganese intoxication. *Archives of Neurology, 46,* 1104–1106.

Huang, Q., Liu, W., Pan, C. (1990). The neurobehavioral changes of ferromanganese smelting workers. In H. Sakurai et al. (Eds.), *Occupational epidemiology.* Amsterdam: Elsevier.

Hubel, D. & Wiesel, T. (1962). Receptive fields, binocular interaction and functional architecture in the cat's visual cortex. *Journal of Physiology, 160,* 106–154.

Hubel, D. & Wiesel, T. (1968). Receptive fields and functional architecture of monkey striate cortex. *Journal of Physiology, 195,* 215–243.

Huber, S.J., Freidenberg, D.L., Shuttleworth, E.C., et al. (1989). Neuropsychological similarities in lateralized Parkinsonism. *Cortex, 25,* 461–470.

Huber, S.J. & Paulson, G.W. (1987). Memory impairment associated with progression of Huntington's disease. *Cortex, 23,* 275–283.

Huber, S.J., Rammohan, K.W., Bornstein, R.A., & Christy, J. A. (1993). Depressive symptoms are not influenced by severity of multiple sclerosis. *Neuropsychiatry, Neuropsychology, and Behavioral Neurology, 6,* 177–180.

Huber, S.J. & Shuttleworth, E.C. (1990). Neuropsychological assessment of subcortical dementia. In J.L. Cummings (Ed.), *Subcortical dementia.* New York: Oxford University Press.

Huber, S.J., Shuttleworth, E.C., & Freidenberg, D.L. (1989). Neuropsychological differences between the dementias of Alzheimer's and Parkinson's diseases. *Archives of Neurology, 46,* 1287–1291.

Huber, S.J., Shuttleworth, E.C., Paulson, G.W., et al. (1986). Cortical vs. subcortical dementia. *Archives of Neurology, 43,* 392–394.

Hubley, A.M. & Hamilton, L. (2002). Using the bicycle drawing test with adults [abstract]. *Archives of Clinical Neuropsychology, 17,* 839–840.

Hubley, A.M. & Tombaugh, T.N. (1993). *Accuracy and inter-scorer reliability of the Taylor and Tombaught scoring systems for the Taylor Complex Figure.* Unpublished manuscript. Ottowa: Carleton University, Department of Psychology.

Hubley, A.M. & Tombaugh, T.N. (2002). *Memory Test for Older Adults (MTOA).* Toronto: Multi-Health System.

Hubley, A.M. & Tremblay, D. (2002). Comparability of total score performance on the Rey-Osterrieth Complex Figure and a modified Taylor Complex Figure. *Journal of Clinical and Experimental Neuropsychology, 24,* 370–382.

Hudetz, A.G. (1997). Cerebral microcirculation. In K.M.A. Welch et al. (Eds.), *Primer on cerebrovascular diseases*. San Diego, CA: Academic Press.

Huettner, M.I.S., Rosenthal, B.L., & Hynd, G.W. (1989). Regional cerebral blood flow (fCBF) in normal readers: Bilateral activation with narrative text. *Archives of Clinical Neuropsychology, 4*, 71–78.

Huff, F.J. (1990). Language in normal aging and age-related neurological diseases. In R.D. Nebes & S. Corkin (Eds.), *Handbook of neuropsychology*. Amsterdam: Elsevier.

Huff, F.J., Becker, J.T., Belle, S.H., et al. (1987). Cognitive deficits and clinical diagnosis of Alzheimer's disease. *Neurology, 37*, 1119–1124.

Huff, F.J., Corkin, S., & Growdon, J.H. (1986). Semantic impairment and anomia in Alzheimer's disease. *Brain and Language, 28*, 235–249.

Huff, F.J., Mack, L., Mahlmann, J., & Greenberg, S. (1988). A comparison of lexical–semantic impairments in left hemisphere stroke and Alzheimer's disease. *Brain and Language, 34*, 262–278.

Hugdahl, K., Carlsson, G., Uvebrant, P., & Lundervold, A.J. (1997). Dichotic-listening performance and intracarotid injections of amobarbital in children and adolescents. Preoperative and postoperative comparisons. *Archives of Neurology, 54*, 1494–1500.

Hugdahl, K. & Davidson, R.J. (Eds.). (2003). *The asymmetrical brain*. Cambridge, MA: MIT Press.

Hugenholtz, H., Stuss, D.T., Stethem, L.L., & Richard, M.T. (1988). How long does it take to recover from a mild concussion? *Neurosurgery, 22*, 853–858.

Hughes, A.J., Ben-Shlomo, Y., Daniel, S.E., & Lees, A.J. (1992). What features improve the accuracy of clinical diagnosis in Parkinson's disease: A clinicopathologic study. *Neurology, 42*, 1142–1146.

Hughes, D. & Bryan, J. (2002). Adult age differences in strategy use during verbal fluency performance. *Journal of Clinical and Experimental Neuropsychology, 24*, 642–654.

Huisman, T.A., Sorensen, A.G., Hergan, K., et al. (2003). Diffusion-weighted imaging for the evaluation of diffuse axonal injury in closed head injury. *Journal of Computer Assisted Tomography, 27*, 5–11.

Hulicka, I.M. (1966). Age differences in Wechsler Memory Scale scores. *Journal of Genetic Psychology, 109*, 135–145.

Hulshoff Pol, H.E., Hijman, R., Tulleken, C.A., et al. (2002). Odor discrimination in patients with frontal lobe damage and Korsakoff's syndrome. *Neuropsychologia, 40*, 888–891.

Hultsch, D.F., Hertzog, C., Small, B.J., et al. (1992). Short-term longitudinal change in cognitive performance in later life. *Psychology and Aging, 7*, 571–584.

Humes, G.E., Welsh, M.C., Retzlaff, P., & Cookson, N. (1997). Towers of Hanoi and London: Reliability of two executive function tasks. *Assessment, 4*, 249–257.

Humphreys, G.W. (1999). Integrative agnosia. In G.W. Humphreys (Ed.), *Case studies in the neuropsychology of vision*. East Sussex, UK: Psychology Press.

Hunkin, N.M., Stone, J.V., Isaac, C.L., et al. (2000). Factor analysis of three standardized tests of memory in a clinical population. *British Journal of Clinical Psychology, 39*, 169–180.

Hunt, A.L., Orrison, W.W., Yeo, R.A., et al. (1989). Clinical significance of MRI white matter lesions in the elderly. *Neurology, 39*, 1470–1471.

Hunt, L., Morris, J.C., Edwards, D., & Wilson, B.S. (1993). Driving performance in persons with mild senile dementia of the Alzheimer type. *Journal of the American Geriatric Society, 41*, 747–752.

Huntzinger, J.A., Rosse, R.B., Schwartz, B.L., et al. (1992). Clock drawing in the screening assessment of cognitive impairment in an ambulatory care setting: A preliminary report. *General Hospital Psychiatry, 14*, 142–144.

Huppert, F.A. & Beardsall, L. (1993). Prospective memory impairment as an early indicator of dementia. *Journal of Clinical and Experimental Neuropsychology, 15*, 805–821.

Huppert, F.A., Brayne, C., Gill, C., et al. (1995). CAMCOG—a concise neuropsychological test to assist dementia diagnosis: Sociodemographic determinants in an elderly population sample. *British Journal of Clinical Psychology, 34*, 529–541.

Huppert, F.A. & Kopelman, M.D. (1989). Rates of forgetting in normal aging: A comparison with dementia. *Neuropsychologia, 27*, 849–860.

Huppert, F.A. & Piercy, M. (1976). Recognition memory in amnesic patients: Effect of temporal center and familiarity of material. *Cortex, 12*, 3–20.

Hurley, R.A., Bradley, W.G., Jr., Latifi, H.T., & Taber, K.H. (1999). Normal pressure hydrocephalus: Significance of MRI in a potentially treatable dementia. *Journal of Neuropsychiatry and Clinical Neurosciences, 11*, 297–300.

Hurley, R.A., Hayman, R.C., & Taber, K.H. (2002). Clinical neuroimaging in neuropsychiatry. In S.C. Yudofsky & R.E. Hales (Eds.), *The American Psychiatric Press Textbook of Neuropsychiatry* (3rd ed.). Washington, D.C.: American Psychiatric Press.

Hutchinson, G.L. (1984). The Luria-Nebraska Neuropsychological Battery controversy: A reply to Spiers. *Journal of Consulting and Clinical Psychology, 52*, 539–545.

Hutchinson, L.J., Amler, R.W., Lybarger, J.A., & Chappell, W. (1992). *Neurobehavioral test battery for use in environmental health field studies*. Atlanta, GA: Agency for Toxic Substances and Disease Registry, Public Health Service.

Hutt, M. (1977). *The Hutt adaptation of the Bender-Gestalt test* (3rd ed.). New York: Grune & Stratton.

Hutt, M.L. (1985). *The Hutt adaptation of the Bender-Gestalt Test: Rapid screening and intensive diagnosis* (4th ed.). Orlando, FL: Grune & Stratton.

Hutt, M.L. and Gibby, R.G. (1970). *An atlas for the Hutt adaptation of the Bender-Gestalt test*. New York: Grune & Stratton.

Huttenlocher, P.R. (2002). *Neural plasticity. The effects of environment on the development of the cerebral cortex*. Cambridge, MA: Harvard University Press.

Huttenlocher, P.R. & Hapke, R.J. (1990). A follow-up study of intractable seizures in childhood. *Annals of Neurology, 28*, 699–705.

Hy, L.X. & Keller, D.M. (2000). Prevalence of AD among whites: A summary by levels of severity. *Neurology, 55*, 198–204.

Hyde, J.S., Fennema, E., & Lamon, S.J. (1990). Gender differences in mathematics performance: A meta-analysis. *Psychological Bulletin, 107*, 53–69.

Hyde, J.S. & Linn, M.C. (1988). Gender differences in verbal ability. A meta-analysis. *Psychological Bulletin, 104*, 53–69.

Hyer, L. & Blount, J. (1984). Concurrent and discriminant validities of the Geriatric Depression Scale with older psychiatric inpatients. *Psychological Reports, 54*, 611–616.

Hyman, B.T. & Gomez-Isla, T. (1998). Normal aging and Alzheimer's disease. In E. Wang & D.S. Snyder (Eds.). *Handbook of the aging brain*. San Diego: Academic Press.

Hynd, G.W. & Hynd, C.R. (1984). Dyslexia: Neuroanatomical/neurolinguistic perspectives. *Reading Research Quarterly, 19*, 482–498.

Hynd, G.W. & Willis, W.G. (1987). *Pediatric neuropsychology*. Orlando, FL: Grune & Stratton.

Ibanez, V., Pietrini, P., Alexander, G.E., et al. (1998). Regional glucose metabolic abnormalities are not the result of atrophy in Alzheimer's disease. *Neurology, 50*, 1585–1593.

Iddon, J.L., Pickard, J.D., Cross, J.J., et al. (1999). Specific patterns of cognitive impairment in patients with idiopathic normal pressure hydrocephalus and Alzheimer's disease: A pilot study. *Journal of Neurology, Neurosurgery and Psychiatry, 67,* 723–732.

Iezzi, T., Archibald, Y., Barnett, P., et al. (1999). Neurocognitive performance and emotional status in chronic pain patients. *Journal of Behavioral Medicine, 22,* 205–216.

IFNB Multiple Sclerosis Study Group (1993). Interferon beta-1b is effective in relapsing-remitting multiple sclerosis. I. Clinical results of a multicenter, randomized, double-blind, placebo-controlled trial. *Neurology, 43,* 655–661.

Igarashi, H., Sakai, F., Kan, S., et al. (1991). Magnetic resonance imaging of the brain in patients with migraine. *Cephalalgia, 11,* 69–74.

Iidaka, T., Sadato, N., Yamada, H., & Yonekura, Y. (2000). Functional asymmetry of human prefrontal cortex in verbal and nonverbal episodic memory as revealed by fMRI. *Brain Research: Cognitive Brain Research, 9,* 73–83.

Illarioshkin, S.N., Igarashi, S., Onodera, O., et al. (1994). Trinucleotide repeat length and rate of progression of Huntington's disease. *Annals of Neurology, 36,* 630–635.

Incisa della Rocchetta, A. & Milner, B. (1993). Strategic search and retrieval inhibition: The role of the frontal lobes. *Neuropsychologia, 31,* 503–524.

Indefrey, P. & Levelt, W.J.M. (2000). The neural correlates of language production. In M.S. Gazzaniga (Ed.), *The new cognitive neurosciences* (2nd ed.). Cambridge, MA: MIT Press.

Ingebrigtsen, T., Romner, B., Marup-Jensen, S., et al. (2000). The clinical value of serum S-100 protein measurements in minor head injury: a Scandinavian multicentre study. *Brain Injury, 14,* 1047–1055.

Inglis, J. (1957). An experimental study of learning and "memory function" in elderly psychiatric patients. *Journal of Mental Science, 103,* 796–803.

Inglis, J. (1959). A paired-associate learning test for use with elderly psychiatric patients. *Journal of Mental Science, 105,* 440–443.

Inglis, J., Ruckman, M., Lawson, J.S., et al. (1982). Sex differences in the cognitive effects of unilateral brain damage. *Cortex, 18,* 257–276.

Ingraham, L.J. & Aiken, C.B. (1996). An empirical approach to determining criteria for abnormality in test batteries with multiple measures. *Neuropsychology, 10,* 120–124.

Ingram, F., Soukup, V.M., & Ingram, P.T.F. (1997). The Medical College of Georgia Complex figures: Reliability and preliminary normative data using an intentional learning paradigm in older adults. *Neuropsychiatry, Neuropsychology, and Behavioral Neurology, 10,* 144–146.

Insua, A.M. & Loza, S.M. (1986). Psychometric patterns on the Rorschach of healthy elderly persons and patients with suspected dementia. *Perceptual and Motor Skills, 63,* 931–936.

International League Against Epilepsy, Commission on Classification and Terminology (1989). Proposal for the classification of epilepsy and epileptic syndromes. *Epilepsia, 30,* 389–399.

Irigaray, L. (1973). *Le langage des dements.* The Hague: Mouton.

Irving, G. (1971). Psychometric assessment in a geriatric unit. In G. Stocker et al. (Eds.), *Assessment in cerebrovascular insufficiency.* Stuttgart: George Thieme Verlag.

Isaac, C.L. & Mayes, A.R. (1999). Rate of forgetting in amnesia: I. Recall and recognition of prose. *Journal of Experimental Psychology: Learning, Memory, and Cognition, 25,* 942–962.

Ishihara, S. (1983). *Ishihara's tests for color blindness.* Tokyo: Kanehara.

Ishii, N., Nishihara, Y., & Imamura, T. (1986). Why do frontal lobe symptoms predominate in vascular dementia with lacunes? *Neurology, 36,* 340–344.

Isingrini, M. & Vazou, F. (1997). Relation between fluid intelligence and frontal lobe functioning in older adults. *International Journal of Aging and Human Development, 45,* 99–109.

Iverson, G.L. (2001). Interpreting change on the WAIS-III/WMS-III in clinical samples. *Archives of Clinical Neuropsychology, 16,* 183–191.

Iverson, G.L. & Binder, L.M. (2000). Detecting exaggeration and malingering in neuropsychological assessment. *Journal of Head Trauma Rehabilitation, 15,* 829–858.

Iverson, G.L. & Franzen, M. D. (1994). The Recognition Memory Test, Digit Span, and Knox Cube Test as markers of malingered memory impairment. *Assessment, 1,* 323–334.

Iverson, G.L. & Franzen, M.D. (1996). Using multiple objective memory procedures to detect simulated malingering. *Journal of Clinical and Experimental Neuropsychology, 18,* 38–51.

Iverson, G.L., Franzen, M.D., & McCracken, L.M. (1991). Evaluation of an objective assessment technique for the detection of malingered memory deficits. *Law and Human Behavior, 15,* 667–676.

Iverson, G.L., Franzen, M.D., & McCracken, L.M. (1994). Application of a forced-choice memory procedure designed to detect experimental malingering. *Archives of Clinical Neuropsychology, 9,* 437–450.

Iverson, G.L., Lovell, M.R., & Smith, S.S. (2000). Does brief loss of consciousness affect cognitive functioning after mild head injury? *Archives of Clinical Neuropsychology, 15,* 643–648.

Iverson, G.L. & Slick, D.J. (2001). Base rates of the WMS-R malingering index following traumatic brain injury. *American Journal of Forensic Psychology, 19,* 5–14.

Iverson, G.L., Slick, D.J., & Franzen, M.D. (2000). Evaluation of a WMS-R malingering index in a non-litigating clinical sample. *Journal of Clinical and Experimental Neuropsychology, 22* 191–197.

Ivins, R.G. & Cunningham, J.L. (1989). *Comparison of verbal and nonverbal auditory reinforcement on the Booklet Category Test.* Paper presented at the 9th annual meeting of the National Academy of Neuropsychologist, Washington, D.C.

Ivison, D.J. (1977). The Wechsler Memory Scale: Preliminary findings toward an Australian standardisation. *Australian Psychologist, 12,* 303–312.

Ivison, D. (1986). Anna Thompson and the American Liner New York: Some normative data. *Journal of Clinical and Experimental Neuropsychology, 8,* 317–320.

Ivnik, R.J. (1991). Memory testing. In T. Yanagihara & R.C. Petersen (Eds.), *Memory disorders: Research and clinical practice.* New York: Marcel Dekker.

Ivnik, R.J., Malec, J.F., Sharbrough, F.W., et al. (1993). Traditional and computerized assessment procedures applied to the evaluation of memory change after temporal lobectomy. *Archives of Clinical Neuropsychology, 8,* 69–81.

Ivnik, R.J., Malec J.F., Smith, G.E., et al. (1992a). Mayo's Older Americans Normative Studies: Updated AVLT norms for ages 56–97. *The Clinical Neuropsychologist, 6,* 83–104.

Ivnik, R.J., Malec, J.F., Smith, G.E., et al. (1992b). Mayo's Older Americans Normative Studies: WAIS-R norms for ages 56–97. *The Clinical Neuropsychologist, 6,* 1–30.

Ivnik, R.J., Malec, J.F., Smith, G.E., et al. (1992c). Mayo's Older Americans Normative Studies: WMS-R norms for ages 56–94. *The Clinical Neuropsychologist, 6,* 49–82.

Ivnik, R.J., Malec, J.F., Smith, G.E., et al. (1996). Neuropsychological tests' norms above age 55: COWAT, BNT, MAE Token, WRAT-R Reading, AMNART, STROOP, TMT, and JLO. *The Clinical Neuropsychologist, 10,* 262–278.

Ivnik, R.J., Malec, J.F., Tangalos, E.G., et al. (1990). The Auditory-Verbal Learning Test (AVLT): Norms for ages 55 years and older. *Psychological Assessment, 2,* 304–312.

Ivnik, R.J., Sharbrough, F.W., & Laws, E.R., Jr. (1988). Anterior temporal lobectomy for the control of partial complex seizures: Information for counseling patients. *Mayo Clinic Proceedings, 63,* 783–793.

Ivnik, R.J., Smith, G.E., Lucas, J.A., et al. (1997). Free and cued Selective Reminding test: MOANS norms. *Journal of Clinical and Experimental Neuropsychology, 19,* 676–91.

Ivnik, R.J., Smith, G.E., Lucas, J.A., et al. (1999). Testing normal older people three or four times at 1- to 2-year intervals: Defining normal variance. *Neuropsychology, 13,* 121–127.

Ivnik, R.J., Smith, G.E., Malec, J.F., et al. (1995). Long-term stability and intercorrelations of cognitive abilities in older persons. *Psychological Assessment, 7,* 155–161.

Ivnik, R.J., Smith, G.E., Tangalos, E.G., et al. (1991). Wechsler Memory Scale: IQ-dependent norms for persons ages 65–97 years. *Psychological Assessment, 3,* 156–161.

Ivory, S.J., Knight, R.G., Longmore, B.E., & Caradoc-Davies, T. (1999). Verbal memory in non-demented patients with idiopathic Parkinson's disease. *Neuropsychologia, 37,* 817–828.

Ivry, R.B. & Fiez, J.A. (2000). Cerebellar contributions to cognition and imagery. In M.S. Gazzaniga (Ed.), *The new cognitive neurosciences* (2nd ed.). Cambridge, MA: MIT Press.

Ivry, R.B. & Lebby, P.C. (1998). The neurology of consonant perception: Specialized module or distributed processors? In M. Beeman & C. Chiarello (Eds.), *Right hemisphere language comprehension.* Mahwah, NJ: Erlbaum.

Iwata, M. (1989). Modular organization of visual thinking. *Behavioral Neurology, 2,* 153–166.

Izard, C.E. (1971). *The face of emotion.* New York: Appleton-Century-Crofts.

Jack, C.R., Petersen, R.C., Xu, Y.C., et al. (1998). Hippocampal atrophy and apolipoprotein E genotype are independently associated with Alzheimer's disease. *Annals of Neurology, 43,* 303–310.

Jack, C.R., Jr., Petersen, R.C., Xu, Y.C., et al. (1999). Prediction of AD with MRI-based hippocampal volume in mild cognitive impairment. *Neurology, 52,* 1397–1403.

Jackson, D.L. & Menges, H. (1980). Accidental carbon monoxide poisoning. *Journal of the American Medical Association, 243,* 772–774.

Jackson, D.N. (1986). *The Multidimensional Aptitude Battery.* London, Canada: Research Psychologist Press.

Jackson, H.F., Hopewell, C.A., Glass, C.A., et al. (1992). The Katz Adjustment Scale: Modification for use with victims of traumatic brain and spinal injury. *Brain Injury, 6,* 109–127.

Jackson, J.F. (1988). Brain, cognition, and grief. *Aphasiology, 2,* 89–92.

Jackson, M. & Warrington, E.K. (1986). Arithmetic skills in patients with unilateral cerebral lesions. *Cortex, 22,* 611–620.

Jacobs, A., Put, E., Ingels, M., et al. (1996). One-year follow-up of technetium-99m-HMPAO SPECT in mild head injury. *Journal of Nuclear Medicine, 37,* 1605–1609.

Jacobs, D., Tröster, A.I., Butters, N., et al. (1990). Intrusion errors on the Visual Reproduction Test of the Wechsler Memory Scale and the Wechsler Memory Scale-Revised: An analysis of demented and amnesic patients. *The Clinical Neuropsychologist, 4,* 177–191.

Jacobs, D.H., Adair, J.C., Macauley, B., et al. (1999). Apraxia in corticobasal degeneration. *Brain and Cognition, 40,* 336–354.

Jacobs, D.M., Levy, G., & Marder, K. (2003). Dementia in Parkinson's disease, Huntington's disease, and related disorders. In T.E. Feinberg & M.J. Farah (Eds.), *Behavioral neurology and neuropsychology* (2nd ed.). New York: McGraw-Hill.

Jacobs, D.M., Marder, K., Cote, L.J., et al. (1995). Neuropsychological characteristics of preclinical dementia in Parkinson's disease. *Neurology, 45,* 1691–1696.

Jacobs, D.M., Sano, M., Albert, S., et al. (1997). Cross-cultural neuropsychological assessment: A comparison of randomly selected, demographically matched cohorts of English- and Spanish-speaking older adults. *Journal of Clinical and Experimental Neuropsychology, 19,* 331–339.

Jacobs, D.M., Sano, M., Dooneief, G., et al. (1995). Neuropsychological detection and characterization of preclinical Alzheimer's disease. *Neurology, 45,* 957–962.

Jacobs, D., Sano, M., Marder, K., et al. (1994). Age at onset of Alzheimer's disease: relation to pattern of cognitive dysfunction and rate of decline. *Neurology, 44,* 1215–1220.

Jacobs, J.W., Bernhard, M.R., Delgado, A., & Strain, J.J. (1977). Screening for organic mental syndromes in the medically ill. *Annals of Internal Medicine, 86,* 40–46.

Jacobs, L.D., Cookfair, D.L., Rudick, R.A., et al. (1996). Intramuscular interferon beta-1a for disease progression in relapsing multiple sclerosis. *Annals of Neurology, 39,* 285–294.

Jacobsen, P.B., Hann, D.M., Azzarello, L.M., et al. (1999). Fatigue in women receiving adjuvant chemotherapy for breast cancer: Characteristics course, and correlates. *Journal of Pain and Symptom Management, 18,* 233–242.

Jacobson, B.H. & Thurman-Lacey, S.R. (1992). Effect of caffeine on motor performance by caffeine-naive and -familiar subjects. *Perceptual and Motor Skills, 74,* 151–157.

Jacoby, A., Baker, G., Smith, et al. (1993). Measuring the impact of epilepsy: The development of a novel scale. *Epilepsy Research, 16,* 83–88.

Jacqmin-Gadda, H., Fabrigoule, C., Commenges, D., & Dartigues, J.F. (1997). A 5-year longitudinal study of the Mini-Mental State Examination in normal aging. *American Journal of Epidemiology, 145,* 498–506.

Jager, T.E., Weiss, H.B., Coben, J.H., & Pepe, P.E. (2000). Traumatic brain injuries evaluated in U.S. emergency departments, 1992–1994. *Academic Emergency Medicine, 7,* 134–140.

Jagger, J., Fife, D., Vernberg, K., & Jane, J.A. (1984). Effect of alcohol intoxication on the diagnosis and apparent severity of brain injury. *Neurosurgery, 15,* 303–306.

Jahanshahi, M. & Dirnberger, G. (1999). The left dorsolateral prefrontal cortex and random generation of responses: studies with transcranial magnetic stimulation. *Neuropsychologia, 37,* 181–190.

Jain, N., Layton, B.S., & Murray, P.K. (2000). Are aphasic patients who fail the GOAT in PTA? A modified Galveston Orientation and Amnesia Test for persons with aphasia. *The Clinical Neuropsychologist, 14,* 13–17.

Jain, S.S., & DeLisa, J.A. (1998). Chronic fatigue syndrome: A literature review from a physiatric perspective. *American Journal of Physical Medicine and Rehabilitation, 77,* 160–167.

Jalan, R., Gooday, R., O'Carroll, R.E., et al. (1995). A prospective evaluation of changes in neuropsychological and liver function tests following transjugular intrahepatic portosystemic stent-shunt. *Journal of Hepatology, 23,* 697–705.

James, W. (1950 [1890]) *The principles of psychology.* New York: Dover.

Janati, A. & Appel, A.R. (1984). Psychiatric aspects of progressive supranuclear palsy. *Journal of Nervous and Mental Disease, 172,* 85–89.

Janke, L. & Steinmetz, H. (2003). Anatomical brain asymmetries and their relevance for functional asymmetries. In K. Hugdahl & R.J. Davidson (Eds.), *The asymmetrical brain.* Cambridge, MA: MIT Press.

Jankovic, J., Beach, J., & Ashizawa, T. (1995). Emotional and functional impact of DNA testing on patients with symptoms of Huntington's disease. *Journal of Medical Genetics, 32,* 516–518.

Janowsky, J.S., Carper, R.A., & Kaye, J.A. (1996). Asymmetrical memory decline in normal aging and dementia. *Neuropsychologia, 34,* 527–535.

Janowsky, J.S., Chavez, B., & Orwoll, E. (2000). Sex steroids modify working memory. *Journal of Cognitive Neuroscience, 12,* 407–414.

Janowsky, J.S., Chavez, B., Zamboni, B.D., & Orwoll, E. (1998). The cognitive neuropsychology of sex hormones in men and women. *Developmental Neuropsychology, 14*, 421–440.

Janowsky, J.S., Shimamura, A.P., Kritchevsky, M., & Squire, L.R. (1989). Cognitive impairment following frontal lobe damage and its relevance to human amnesia. *Behavioral Neuroscience, 103*, 548–560.

Janowsky, J.S., Shimamura, A.P., & Squire, L.R. (1989). Source memory impairment in patients with frontal lobe lesions. *Neuropsychologia, 27*, 1043–1056.

Janowsky, J.S. & Thomas-Thrapp, L.J. (1993). Complex Figure recall in the elderly: A deficit in memory or constructional strategy? *Journal of Clinical and Experimental Neuropsychology, 15*, 159–169.

Janssen, R.S., Saykin, A.J., Cannon, L., et al. (1989). Neurological and neuropsychological manifestations of HIV-1 infection. *Annals of Neurology, 26*, 592–600.

Janus, C., Pearson, J., McLaurin, J., et al. (2000). A beta peptide immunization reduces behavioural impairment and plaques in a model of Alzheimer's disease. *Nature, 408*, 979–982.

Janus, T.J. & Barrash, J. (1996). Neurologic and neurobehavioral effects of electric and lightning injuries. *Journal of Burn Care Rehabilitation, 17*, 409–415.

Januzzi, J.L., Jr. & McKhann, G.M. (2002). The brain and the cardiovascular system. In A.K. Asbury et al. (Eds.), *Diseases of the nervous system* (3rd ed.). Cambridge, UK: Cambridge University Press.

Jarvenpaa, T., Rinne, J.O., Raiha, I., et al. (2002). Characteristics of two telephone screens for cognitive impairment. *Dementia and Geriatric Cognitive Disorders, 13*, 149–155.

Jarvik, J.G., Hesselink, J.R., Kennedy, C., et al. (1988). Acquired immunodeficiency syndrome. Magnetic resonance pattern of brain involvement with pathologic correlation. *Archives of Neurology, 45*, 731–736.

Jarvik, L.F. (1988). Aging of the brain: How can we prevent it? *The Gerontologist, 28*, 739–747.

Jarvis, P.E. & Barth, J.T. (1994). *The Halstead-Reitan Neuropsychological Battery. A guide to interpretation and clinical applications.* Odessa, FL: Psychological Assessment Resources.

Jason, G.W. (1985). Gesture fluency after focal cortical lesions. *Neuropsychologia, 23*, 463–481.

Jason, G.W. (1986). Performance of manual copying tasks after focal cortical lesions. *Neuropsychologia, 24*, 181–191.

Jason, G.W. (1987). Studies of manual learning and performance after surgical excisions for the control of epilepsy. In J. Engel, Jr. (Ed.), *Fundamental mechanisms of human brain function.* New York: Raven Press.

Jason, G.W. (1990). Disorders of motor function following cortical lesions: Review and theoretical considerations. In G.R. Hammond (Ed.), *Cerebral control of speech and limb movements.* Amsterdam: Elsevier.

Jason, G. W., Suchowersky, O., Pajurkova, E.H., et al. (1997). Cognitive manifestations of Huntington disease in relation to genetic structure and clinical onset. *Archives of Neurology, 54*, 1081–1088.

Jastak, S. & Wilkinson, G.S. (1984). *Wide Range Achievement Test-Revised.* Wilmington, DE: Jastak Assessment Systems.

Javitt, D.C. (2000). Phencyclidine. In P.S. Spencer & H.H. Schaumburg (Eds.), *Experimental and clinical neurotoxicology* (2nd ed.). New York: Oxford University Press.

Jean-Bay, E. (2000). The biobehavioral correlates of post-traumatic brain injury depression. *Journal of Neuroscience Nursing, 32*, 169–176.

Jeeves, M.A. (1990). Agenesis of the corpus callosum. In F. Boller & J. Grafman (Eds.), *Handbook of neuropsychology* (Vol. 4). Amsterdam: Elsevier.

Jeeves, M.A. (1994). Callosal agenesis—a natural split brain. Overview. In M. Lassonde & M.A. Jeeves (Eds.), *Callosal agenesis: A natural split brain?* New York: Plenum Press.

Jefferson, A.L., Cosentino, S.A., Ball, S.K., et al. (2002). Errors produced on the Mini-Mental State Examination and neuropsychological test performance in Alzheimer's disease, ischemic vascular dementia, and Parkinson's disease. *Journal of Neuropsychiatry and Clinical Neurosciences, 14*, 311–320.

Jeffery, D.R., Absher, J., Pfeiffer, F.E., & Jackson, H. (2000). Cortical deficits in multiple sclerosis on the basis of subcortical lesions. *Multiple Sclerosis, 6*, 50–55.

Jeffery, D.R. & Good, D.C. (1995). Rehabilitation of the stroke patient. *Current Opinion in Neurology, 8*, 62–68.

Jelic, V., Blomberg, M., Dierks, T., et al. (1998). EEG slowing and cerebrospinal fluid tau levels in patients with cognitive decline. *Neuroreport, 9*, 157–160.

Jelicic, M., Bonebakker, A.E., & Bonke, B. (1995). Implicit memory performance of patients with Alzheimer's disease: a brief review. *International Psychogeriatrics, 7*, 385–392.

Jelicic, M., Jonker, C., & Deeg, D.J. (2001). Effects of low levels of serum vitamin B_{12} and folic acid on cognitive performance in old age: A population based study. *Developmental Neuropsychology, 20*, 565–571.

Jellinger, K.A. & Bancher, C. (1992). Neuropathology. In I. Litvan, & Y. Agid (Eds.), *Progressive supranuclear palsy: Clinical and research approaches.* New York: Oxford University Press.

Jellinger, K.A., Paulus, W., Wrocklage, C., & Litvan, I. (2001). Traumatic brain injury as a risk factor for Alzheimer disease. Comparison of two retrospective autopsy cohorts with evaluation of ApoE genotype. *BMC Neurology, 1*, 3 (www.biomedcentral.com).

Jenike, M.A. (1994). Psychiatric disorders in the elderly. In M.L. Albert & J.E. Knoefel (Eds.), *Clinical neurology of aging* (2nd ed.). New York: Oxford University Press.

Jenkyn, L.R., Reeves, A.G., Warren, T., et al. (1985). Neurologic signs in senescence. *Archives of Neurology, 42*, 1154–1157.

Jennekens-Schinkel, A., Laboyrie, P.M., Lanser, J.B.K., & van der Velde, E.A. (1990). Cognition in patients with multiple sclerosis: After four years. *Journal of the Neurological Sciences, 99*, 229–247.

Jennett, B. (1972). Some aspects of prognosis after severe head injury. *Scandinavian Journal of Rehabilitation Medicine, 4*, 16–20.

Jennett, B. (1979). Severity of brain damage, altered consciousness and other indicators. In G.L. Odom (Ed.), *Central nervous system trauma research. Status report.* Washington, D.C.: National Institutes of Health.

Jennett, B. (1990). Post-traumatic epilepsy. In M. Rosenthal et al. (Eds.), *Rehabilitation of the adult and child with traumatic brain injury* (2nd ed.). Philadelphia: Davis.

Jennett, B. & Bond, M. (1975). Assessment of outcome after severe brain damage. A practical scale. *Lancet, i*, 480–484.

Jennett, B., Snoek, J., Bond, M.R., & Brooks, N. (1981). Disability after severe head injury: Observations on the use of the Glasgow Outcome Scale. *Journal of Neurology, Neurosurgery, and Psychiatry, 44*, 285–293.

Jennett, B., Teasdale, G., & Knill-Jones, R. (1975). Prognosis after severe head injury. In *Ciba Foundation Symposium, 34 (new series). Symposium on the outcome of severe damage to the CNS.* Amsterdam: Elsevier.

Jensen, A.R. & Rohwer, W.D. (1966). The Stroop Color-Word Test: a review. *Acta Psychologica, 25*, 36–93.

Jensen, G.B. & Pakkenberg, B. (1993). Do alcoholics drink their neurons away? *Lancet, 342*, 1201–1204.

Jensen, P., Fenger, K., Bolwig, T.G., & Sorensen, S.A. (1998). Crime in Huntington's disease: A study of registered offences among patients, relatives, and controls. *Journal of Neurology, Neurosurgery and Psychiatry, 65*, 467–471.

Jeremitsky, E., Omert, L., Dunham, C.M., et al. (2003). Harbingers of poor outcome the day after severe brain injury: Hypothermia, hypoxia, and hypoperfusion. *Journal of Trauma, 54,* 312–319.

Jernigan, T.L., Butters, N., DiTraglia, G., et al. (1991). Reduced cerebral grey matter observed in alcoholics using magnetic resonance imaging. *Alcoholism: Clinical and Experimental Research, 15,* 418–427.

Jernigan, T.L., Ostergaard, A.L., & Fennema-Notestine, C. (2001). Mesial temporal, diencephalic, and striatal contributions to deficits in single word reading, word priming, and recognition memory. *Journal of the International Neuropsychological Society, 7,* 63–78.

Jernigan, T.L., Salmon, D.P., Butters, N., & Hesselink, J.R. (1991). Cerebral structure on MRI. Part II: Specific changes in Alzheimer's and Huntington's diseases. *Biological Psychiatry, 29,* 68–81.

Jernigan, T.L., Schafer, K., Butters, N., & Cermak, L.S. (1991). Magnetic resonance imaging of alcoholic Korsakoff patients. *Neuropsychopharmacology, 4,* 175–186.

Jeste, D.V., Galasko, D., Corey-Bloom, J., et al. (1996). Neuropsychiatric aspects of the schizophrenias. In B.S. Fogel et al. (Eds.), *Neuropsychiatry.* Baltimore, MD: Williams & Wilkins.

Jetter, W., Poser, U., Freeman, R.B., Jr., & Markowitsch, H.J. (1986). A verbal long-term memory deficit in frontal lobe damaged patients. *Cortex, 22,* 229–242.

Joanette, Y., Goulet, P., & Hannequin, D. (1990). *Right hemisphere and verbal communication.* New York: Springer-Verlag.

Joanette, Y., Melançon, L., Ska, B., & Lecours, A.-R. (1993). Hétérogénéité des profils cognitifs dans les démences de type Alzheimer: aspects théoriques et conséquences cliniques. *L'Union Médicale du Canada,* Novembre, 420–426.

Joanette, Y., Ska, B., Poissant, A., & Giroux (1994). Vers une multiplicité des profils des atteintes cognitives dans la démence de type Alzheimer. In M. Poncet et al. (éds.), *Actualités sur la maladie d'Alzheimer et les syndromes apparentés.* Marseille: Solal.

Joanette, Y., Ska, B., Poissant, A., et al. (1995a). Évaluation neuropsychologique dans la démence de type Alzheimer: un compromis optimal. *L'Année Gérontologique, 2,* 69–83.

Joanette, Y., Ska, B., Poissant, A., et al. (1995b). Évaluation neuropsychologique et profils cognitifs des démences de type Alzheimer: dissociations transversales et longitudinales. In F. Eustache & A. Agniel (éds.), *Neuropsychologie clinique des démences: Évaluations et prises en charges.* Marseille: Solal.

Jobst, E.E., Melnick, M.E., Byl, N.N., et al. (1997). Sensory perception in Parkinson disease. *Archives of Neurology, 54,* 450–454.

Joffe, R.T., Lippert, G.P., Gray, T.A., et al. (1987). Mood disorder and multiple sclerosis. *Archives of Neurology, 44,* 376–378.

Jog, M.S., Kubota, Y., Connolly, C.I., et al. (1999). Building neural representatives of habits. *Science, 296,* 1745–1749.

Johannsen, L.G., Stenager, E., & Jensen, K. (1996). Clinically unexpected multiple sclerosis in patients with mental disorders. A series of 7301 psychiatric autopsies. *Acta Neurologica Belgica, 96,* 62–65.

Johanson, A.M., Gustafson, L., & Risberg, J. (1986). Behavioural observations during performance of the WAIS Block Design Test related to abnormalities of regional cerebral blood flow in organic dementia. *Journal of Clinical and Experimental Neuropsychology, 8,* 201–209.

Johansson, B., Allen-Burge, R., & Zarit, S.H. (1997). Self-reports on memory functioning in a longitudinal study of the oldest old: Relation to current, prospective, and retrospective performance. *Journals of Gerontology. Series B, Psychological Sciences and Social Sciences, 52,* 139–146.

Johansson, B. & Berg, S. (1989). The robustness of the terminal decline phenomenon: Longitudinal data from the digit-span memory test. *Journal of Gerontology, 44,* 184–186.

Johansson, B.B. (1997). Hypertension. In K.M.A. Welch et al. (Eds.), *Primer on cerebrovascular diseases.* San Diego: Academic Press.

Johansson, K., Bronge, L., Lundberg, D., et al. (1996). Can a physician recognize an older driver with increased crash risk potential? *Journal of the American Geriatric Society, 44,* 1198–1204.

Johnson, B.L., Baker, E.L., El Batawi, M., et al. (Eds.) (1987). *Prevention of neurotoxic illness in working populations.* New York: Wiley.

Johnson, B.W., McKenzie, K.J., & Hamm, J.P. (2002). Cerebral asymmetry for mental rotation: Effects of response hand, handedness and gender. *Neuroreport, 13,* 1929–1932.

Johnson, J. (1969). Organic psychosyndromes due to boxing. *British Journal of Psychiatry, 115,* 45–53.

Johnson, J.L. & Lesniak-Karpiak, K. (1997). The effect of warning on malingering on memory and motor tasks in college samples. *Archives of Clinical Neuropsychology, 12,* 231–238.

Johnson, K.A., Jones, K., Holman, B.L., et al. (1998). Preclinical prediction of Alzheimer's disease using SPECT. *Neurology, 50,* 1563–1571.

Johnson, K.P., Brooks, B.R., Cohen, J.A., et al. (1995). Copolymer 1 reduces relapse rate and improves disability in relapsing-remitting multiple sclerosis: Results of a phase III multicenter, double-blind, placebo-controlled trial. *Neurology, 45,* 1268–1276.

Johnson, M.D. & Ojemann, G.A. (2000). The role of the human thalamus in language and memory: Evidence from electrophysiological studies. *Brain and Cognition, 42,* 218–230.

Johnson, M.K. (1990). Functional forms of human memory. In J.L. McGaugh et al. (Eds.), *Brain organization and memory. Cells, systems, and circuits.* New York: Oxford University Press.

Johnson, M.K., Hashtroudi, S., & Lindsay, D.S. (1993). Source monitoring. *Psychological Bulletin, 114,* 3–28.

Johnson, M.K. & Hirst, W. (1991). Processing subsystems of memory. In R.G. Lister & H.J. Weingartner (Eds.), *Perspectives on cognitive neuroscience.* New York: Oxford University Press.

Johnson, R., Jr. (Ed.) (1995). Section 14: Event-related brain potentials and cognition. In F. Boller & J. Grafman (Eds.), *Handbook of neuropsychology* (Vol. 10). Amsterdam: Elsevier.

Johnson, R., Jr., Litvan, I., & Grafman, J. (1991). Progressive supranuclear palsy: Altered sensory processing leads to degraded cognition. *Neurology, 41,* 1257–1262.

Johnson, R.T. (1998). *Viral infections of the nervous system* (2nd ed.). Philadelphia: Lippincott-Raven.

Johnson, S.C., Farnworth, T., Pinkston, J.B., et al. (1994). Corpus callosum surface area across the human adult life span: Effect of age and gender. *Brain Research Bulletin, 35,* 373–377.

Johnson, S.C., Saykin, A.J., Flashman, L.A., et al. (2001). Brain activation on fMRI and verbal memory ability: Functional neuroanatomic correlates of CVLT performance. *Journal of the International Neuropsychological Society, 7,* 55–62.

Johnson, S.K., Lange, G., DeLuca, J., et al. (1997). The effects of fatigue on neuropsychological performance in patients with chronic fatigue syndrome, multiple sclerosis, and depression. *Applied Neuropsychology, 4,* 145–153.

Johnson-Greene, D., Hardy-Morais, C., Adams, K., et al. (1997). Informed consent and neuropsychological assessment: Ethical considerations and proposed guidelines. *The Clinical Neuropsychologist, 11,* 454–460.

Johnson-Selfridge, M.T., Zalewski, C., & Aboudarham, J.-F. (1998). The relationship between ethnicity and word fluency. *Archives of Clinical Neuropsychology, 13,* 319–325.

Johnston, D. & Amaral, D.G. (1998). Hippocampus. In G.M. Shepherd (Ed.), *The synaptic organization of the brain* (4th ed.). New York: Oxford University Press.

Johnston, M.V. & Keister, M. (1984). Early rehabilitation for stroke patients. A new look. *Archives of Physical Medicine and Rehabilitation, 65,* 437–441.

Johnstone, B., Callahan, C.D., Kapila, C.J., & Bouman, D.E. (1996). The comparability of the WRAT-R Reading Test and NAART as estimates of premorbid intelligence in neurologically impaired patients. *Archives of Clinical Neuropsychology, 11,* 513–519.

Johnstone, B., Hexum, C.L., & Ashkanazi, G. (1995). Extent of cognitive decline in traumatic brain injury based on estimates of premorbid intelligence. *Brain Injury, 9,* 377–384.

Johnstone, B., Holland, D., & Hewett, J.E. (1997). The construct validity of the Category Test: Is it a measure of reasoning or intelligence. *Psychological Assessment, 9,* 28–33.

Johnstone, B., Slaughter, J., Schopp, L., et al. (1997). Determining neuropsychological impairment using estimates of premorbid intelligence: Comparing methods based on level of education versus reading score. *The Clinical Neuropsychologist, 12,* 591–601.

Johnstone, B. & Wilhelm, K.L. (1996). The longitudinal stability of the WRAT-R reading subtest: Is it an appropriate estimate of premorbid intelligence? *Journal of the International Neuropsychological Society, 2,* 282–285.

Johnstone, E.C., Crow, T.J., & Frith, C.D. (1976). Cerebral ventricular size and cognitive impairment in chronic schizophrenics. *Lancet, ii,* 924–926.

Jokeit, H., Okujava, M., & Woermann, F. G. (2001). Memory fMRI lateralizes temporal lobe epilepsy. *Neurology, 57,* 1786–1793.

Jonas, D.L., Blumenthal, J.A., Madden, D.J., & Serra, M. (2001). Cognitive consequences of antihypertensive medications. In S.R. Waldstein & M.F. Elias (Eds.), *Neuropsychology of cardiovascular disease.* Mahwah, NJ: Erlbaum.

Jonas, S. (1987). The supplementary motor region and speech. In E. Perecman (Ed.), *The frontal lobes revisited.* New York: IRBN Press.

Jones, A.B. & Llewellyn, L.J. (1918). *Malingering, or the simulation of disease.* Philadelphia: Blakiston's.

Jones, B.M. & Jones, M.K. (1977). Alcohol and memory impairment in male and female social drinkers. In I.M. Birnbaum & E.S. Parker (Eds.), *Alcohol and human memory.* Hillsdale, NJ: Erlbaum.

Jones, B.P., Duncan, C.C., Brouwers, P., & Mirsky, A.F. (1991). Cognition in eating disorders. *Journal of Clinical and Experimental Neuropsychology, 13,* 711–728.

Jones, B.P., Moskowitz, H.R., Butters, N., & Glosser, G. (1975). Psychosocial scaling of olfactory, visual, and auditory stimuli by alcoholic Korsakoff patients. *Neuropsychologia, 13,* 387–393.

Jones, D.S. (2000). Reversed clock phenomenon: A right-hemisphere syndrome. *Neurology, 55,* 1939–1942.

Jones, R.D., Tranel, D., Benton, A., & Paulsen, J. (1992). Differentiating dementia from "pseudodementia" early in the clinical course: Utility of neuropsychological tests. *Neuropsychology, 6,* 13–21.

Jones, R.N. & Gallo, J. (2000). Dimensions of the Mini-Mental State Examination among community dwelling older adults. *Psychological Medicine, 30,* 605–618.

Jones, R.N. & Gallo, J.J. (2002). Education and sex differences in the Mini-Mental State Examination: Effects of differential item functioning. *Journal of Gerontology. Series B, Psychological Sciences and Social Sciences, 57,* P548–P558.

Jones-Gotman, M. (1986). Right hippocampal excision impairs learning and recall of a list of abstract designs. *Neuropsychologia, 24,* 659–670.

Jones-Gotman, M. (1987). Commentary: Psychological evaluation—Testing hippocampal function. In J. Engel, Jr. (Ed.), *Surgical treatment of the epilepsies.* New York: Raven Press.

Jones-Gotman, M. (1991). Localization of lesions by neuropsychological testing. *Epilepsia, 32(Suppl. 5),* S41–S52.

Jones-Gotman, M. & Milner, B. (1977). Design fluency: The invention of nonsense drawings after focal cortical lesions. *Neuropsychologia, 15,* 653–674.

Jones-Gotman, M. & Zatorre, R.J. (1988). Olfactory identification deficits in patients with focal cerebral excision. *Neuropsychologia, 26,* 387–400.

Jones-Gotman, M., Zatorre, R.J., Olivier, A., et al. (1997). Learning and retention of words and designs following excision from medial or lateral temporal-lobe structures. *Neuropsychologia, 35,* 963–973.

Jonides, J. & Smith, E.E. (1997). The architecture of working memory. In M.D. Rugg (Ed.), *Cognitive neuroscience.* Cambridge, MA: MIT Press.

Jonsdottir, M.K., Magnusson, T., & Kjartansson, O. (1998). Pure alexia and word-meaning deafness in a patient with multiple sclerosis. *Archives of Neurology, 55,* 1473–1474.

Jønsson, A., Korfitzen, E.M., Heltberg, A., et al. (1993). Effects of neuropsychological treatment in patients with multiple sclerosis. *Acta Neurologica Scandinavica, 88,* 394–400.

Jonsson, L., Lindgren, P., Wimo, A., et al. (1999). Costs of Mini Mental State Examination–related cognitive impairment. *Pharmacoeconomics, 16,* 409–416.

Jordan, B.D. (1987). Neurologic aspects of boxing. *Archives of Neurology, 44,* 453–459.

Jordan, B.D. (2000). Chronic traumatic brain injury associated with boxing. *Seminars in Neurology, 20,* 179–185.

Jordan, B.D., Relkin, N.R., Ravin, L.D., et al. (1997). Apolipoprotein E ε4 associated with chronic traumatic brain injury in boxing. *Journal of the American Medical Association, 278,* 136–140.

Jordan, B.D. & Zimmerman, R.D. (1990). Computed tomography and magnetic resonance imaging comparison in boxers. *Journal of the American Medical Association, 263,* 1670–1673.

Jorge, R.E., Leston, J.E., Arndt, S., & Robinson, R.G. (1999). Cluster headaches: Association with anxiety disorders and memory deficits. *Neurology, 53,* 543–547.

Jorge, R.E. & Robinson, R.G. (2002). Behavioural manifestations of stroke. In A.K. Asbury et al. (Eds.), *Diseases of the nervous system. Clinical neuroscience and therapeutic principles* (3rd ed.). Cambridge: Cambridge University Press.

Jorge, R.E., Robinson, R.G., Starkstein, S.E., & Arndt, S.V. (1993). Depression and anxiety following traumatic brain injury. *Journal of Neuropsychiatry, 5,* 369–374.

Jorgensen, H.S., Nakayama, H., Raaschou, H.O., & Olsen, T.S. (1999). Stroke. Neurologic and functional recovery. The Copenhagen Stroke Study. *Physical Medicine and Rehabilitation Clinics of North America, 10,* 887–906.

Jorm, A.F. & Jolley, D. (1998). The incidence of dementia: a meta-analysis. *Neurology, 51,* 728–733.

Joseph, J.E. & Gathers, A.D. (2002). Natural and manufactured objects activate the fusiform face area. *NeuroReport, 13,* 935–938.

Josiassen, R.C., Curry, L.M., & Mancall, E.L. (1983). Development of neuropsychological deficits in Huntington's disease. *Archives of Neurology, 40,* 791–796.

Josiassen, R.C., Curry, L., Roemer, R.A., et al. (1982). Patterns of intellectual deficit in Huntington's disease. *Journal of Clinical Neuropsychology, 4,* 173–183.

Joy, S., Fein, D., Kaplan, E., & Freedman, M. (1999). Information multiple choice among healthy older adults: Characteristics, correlates, and clinical implications. *Clinical Neuropsychologist, 13,* 48–53.

Joy, S., Fein, D., Kaplan, E., & Freedman, M. (2000). Speed and memory in WAIS-R NI Digit Symbol performance among healthy older adults. *Journal of the International Neuropsychological Society, 6,* 770–780.

Joy, S., Fein, D., Kaplan, E., & Freedman, M. (2001). Quantifying qualitative features of Block Design performance among healthy older adults. *Archives of Clinical Neuropsychology, 16,* 157–170.

Joyce, E.M. (1987). The neurochemistry of Korsakoff's syndrome. In S.M. Stahl et al. (Eds.), *Cognitive neurochemistry.* Oxford, UK: Oxford University Press.

Joynt, R.J., Benton, A.L., & Fogel, M.L. (1962). Behavioral and pathological correlates of motor impersistence. *Neurology, 12,* 876–881.

Joynt, R.J. & Goldstein, M.N. (1975). Minor cerebral hemisphere. In W.J. Friedlander (Ed.), *Advances in Neurology* (Vol. 7). New York: Raven Press.

Judd, L.L., Squire, L.R., Butters, N., et al. (1987). Effects of psychotropic drugs on cognition and memory in normal humans and animals. In H.Y. Meltzer (Ed.), *Psychopharmacology: The Third Generation of Progress.* New York: Raven Press.

Junqué, C., Pujol, J., Vendrell, P., et al. (1990). Leuko-araiosis on magnetic resonance imaging and speed of mental processing. *Archives of Neurology, 47,* 151–156.

Juntunen, J., Hernberg, S., Eistola, P., & Hupli, V. (1980). Exposure to industrial solvents and brain atrophy. *European Neurology, 19,* 366–375.

Juottonen, K., Laakso, M.P., Insausti, R., et al. (1998). Volumes of the entrorhinal and perirhinal cortices in Alzheimer's disease. *Neurobiology of Aging, 19,* 15–22.

Jurica, P.J., Leitten, C.L., & Mattis, S. (2002). *Dementia Rating Scale-2 (DRS-2) professional manual.* Odessa, FL: Psychological Assessment Resources.

Jury, M.A. & Flynn, M.C. (2001). Auditory and vestibular sequelae to traumatic brain injury: a pilot study. *New Zealand Medical Journal, 114,* 286–288.

Kaczmarek, B.L.J. (1984). Neurolinguistic analysis of verbal utterances in patients with focal lesions of frontal lobes. *Brain and Language, 21,* 52–58.

Kaczmarek, B.L.J. (1987). Regulatory function of the frontal lobes. In E. Perecman (Ed.), *The frontal lobes revisited.* New York: IRBN Press.

Kaczmarek, L.K. (2002). *The neuron. Cell and molecular biology.* New York: Oxford University Press.

Kaemingk, K.L. & Kaszniak, A.W. (1989). Neuropsychological aspects of human immunodeficiency virus infection. *The Clinical Neuropsychologist, 3,* 309–326.

Kahana, B. (1978). The use of projective techniques in personality assessment of the aged. In M. Storandt et al. (Eds.), *The clinical psychology of aging.* New York: Plenum Press.

Kahn, R.L., Goldfarb, A.I., Pollack, M., & Peck, A. (1960). Brief objective measures for the determination of mental status in the aged. *American Journal of Psychiatry, 117,* 326–328.

Kahn, R.L. & Miller, N.E. (1978). Assessment of altered brain function in the aged. In M. Storandt et al. (Eds.), *The clinical psychology of aging.* New York: Plenum Press.

Kail, R. (1998). Speed of information processing in patients with multiple sclerosis. *Journal of Clinical and Experimental Neuropsychology, 20,* 98–106.

Kalant, H. (1975). Direct effects of ethanol on the nervous system. *Proceedings of the American Societies for Experimental Biology, 34,* 1930–1941.

Kalashnikova, L.A., Gulevskaya, T.S., & Kashina, E.M. (1999). Disorders of higher mental function due to single infarctions in the thalamus and in the area of the thalamofrontal tracts. *Neuroscience and Behavioral Physiology, 29,* 397–403.

Kalechstein, A.D., van Gorp, W.G., & Rapport, L.J. (1998). Variability in clinical classifcation of raw test scores across normative data sets. *The Clinical Neuropsychologist, 12,* 339–347.

Kales, A., Caldwell, A.B., Cadieux, R.J., et al. (1985). Severe obstructive sleep apnea—II: Associated psychopathology and psychosocial consequences. *Chronic Disease, 38,* 427–434.

Kalogjera-Sackellares, D. & Sackellares, J.C. (1999). Intellectual and neuropsychological features of patients with psychogenic pseudoseizures. *Psychiatry Research, 86,* 73–84.

Kalska, H., Punamäki, R.-L., Mäkinen-Pelli, T., & Saarinen, M.

(1999). Memory and metamemory functioning among depressed patients. *Applied Neuropsychology, 6,* 96–107.

Kaltreider, L.B., Cicerello, A.R., Lacritz, L.H., et al. (2000). Comparison of the CERAD and CVLT list-learning tasks in Alzheimer's disease. *The Clinical Neuropsychologist, 14,* 269–274.

Kaltreider, L.B., Cullum, C.M., Lacritz, L.H., & Brewer, K. (1999). Brief recall tasks and memory assessment in Alzheimer's disease. *Applied Neuropsychology, 6,* 165–169.

Kandel, E.R., Schwartz, J.H., & Jessell, T.M. (Eds.) (2000). *Principles of neural science* (4th ed.). New York: McGraw-Hill.

Kane, R.L., Parsons, O.A., & Goldstein, G. (1985). Statistical relationships and discriminative accuracy of the Halstead-Reitan, Luria-Nebraska, and Wechsler IQ scores in the identification of brain damage. *Journal of Clinical and Experimental Neuropsychology, 7,* 211–223.

Kane, R.L., Sweet, J.J, Golden, C.J., et al. (1981). Comparative diagnostic accuracy of the Halstead-Reitan and Standardized Luria-Nebraska Neuropsychological Batteries in a mixed psychiatric and brain-damaged population. *Journal of Consulting and Clinical Psychology, 49,* 484–485.

Kaneko, S., Okada, M., Iwasa, H., et al. (2002). Genetics of epilepsy: Current status and perspectives. *Neuroscience Research, 44,* 11–30.

Kanemoto, K., Kawasaki, J., & Mori, E. (1999). Violence and epilepsy: A close relation between violence and postictal psychosis. *Epilepsia, 40,* 107–109.

Kang, S.K. (2000). The applicability of WHO-NCTB in Korea. *Neurotoxicology, 21,* 697–701.

Kant, R., Smith-Seemiller, L., Isaac, G., & Duffy, J. (1997). Tc-HM-PAO SPECT in persistent post-concussion syndrome after mild head injury. Comparison with MRI/CT. *Brain Injury, 11,* 115–124.

Kantarci, O.H. & Weinshenker, B.G. (2001). Prognostic factors in multiple sclerosis. In S.D. Cook (Ed.), *Handbook of multiple sclerosis* (3rd ed.). New York: Marcel Dekker.

Kaplan, C.P. (2001). The Community Integration Questionnaire with new scoring guidelines: concurrent validity and need for appropriate norms. *Brain Injury, 15,* 725–731.

Kaplan, E. (1988). A process approach to neuropsychological assessment. In T. Boll & B.K. Bryant (Eds.) *Clinical neuropsychology and brain function: Research, measurement, and practice.* Washington, D.C.: American Psychological Association.

Kaplan, E., Fein, D., Morris, R. & Delis, D. (1991). *WAIS-R as a neuropsychological instrument.* San Antonio, TX: The Psychological Corporation.

Kaplan, E.F., Goodglass, H., & Weintraub, S. (1983). *The Boston Naming Test* (2nd ed.). Philadelphia: Lea & Febiger.

Kaplan, E.F., Goodglass, H., & Weintraub, S. (1986). *Tests de Vocabulario de Boston.* Madrid: Panamericana.

Kaplan, J. & Waltz, J.R. (1965). *The trial of Jack Ruby.* New York: Macmillan.

Kaplan, N.M. (2001). Systemic hypertension: Therapy. In Braunwald et al. (Eds.), *Heart disease* (Vol. 1, 6th ed.). Philadelphia: Saunders.

Kaplan, R.F., Jones-Woodward, L., Workman, K., et al. (1999). Neuropsychological deficits in Lyme disease patients with and without other evidence of central nervous system pathology. *Applied Neuropsychology, 6,* 3–11.

Kaplan, S.P. (1990). Social support, emotional distress and vocational outcomes among persons with brain injuries. *Rehabilitation Counseling Bulletin, 34,* 16–23.

Kaplan, S.P. (1991). Psychosocial adjustment three years after traumatic brain injury. *The Clinical Neuropsychologist, 5,* 360–369.

Kaplan, S.P. (1993). Tracking psychosocial changes in people with severe traumatric brain injury over a five year period using the

Portland Adaptability Inventory. *Rehabilitation Counseling Bulletin, 36,* 151–159.

Kappos, L., Weinshenker, B., Pozzilli, C., et al. (2004). Interferon beta-1b in secondary progressive multiple sclerosis. *Neurology, 63,* 1779–1787.

Kapur, N. (1987). Some comments on the technical acceptability of Warrington's Recognition Memory test. *British Journal of Clinical Psychology, 26,* 144–146.

Kapur, N. (1988a). *Memory disorders in clinical practice.* London: Butterworth.

Kapur, N. (1988b). Pattern of verbal memory deficits in patients with bifrontal pathology and patients with third ventricle lesions. In M.M. Gruneberg et al. (Eds.), *Practical aspects of memory: Current research and issues* (Vol. 2). New York: Wiley.

Kapur, N. (1994). The coin-in-the-hand test: A new "bed-side" test for the detection of malingering in patients with suspected memory disorder. *Journal of Neurology, Neurosurgery and Psychiatry, 57,* 385–386.

Kapur, N. & Brooks, D.J. (1999). Temporally-specific retrograde amnesia in two cases of discrete bilateral hippocampal pathology. *Hippocampus, 9,* 247–254.

Kapur, N. & Butters, N. (1977). Visuoperceptive deficits in long-term alcoholics and alcoholics with Korsakoff's psychosis. *Journal of Studies on Alcohol, 38,* 2025–2035.

Kapur, N., Millar, J., Abbott, P., & Carter, M. (1998). Recovery of function processes in human amnesia: Evidence from transient global amnesia. *Neuropsychologia, 36,* 99–107.

Kapur, N. & Pearson, D. (1983). Memory symptoms and memory performance of neurological patients. *British Journal of Psychology, 74,* 409–415.

Kapur, N., Scholey, K., Moore, E., et al. (1996). Long-term retention deficits in two cases of disproportionate retrograde amnesia. *Journal of Cognitive Neuroscience, 8,* 416–434.

Kapur, N., Thompson, S., Cook, P., et al. (1996). Anterograde but not retrograde memory loss following combined mammillary body and medial thalamic lesions. *Neuropsychologia, 34,* 1–8.

Kapur, S., Craik, F.I., Jones, C., et al. (1995). Functional role of the prefrontal cortex in retrieval of memories: A PET study. *NeuroReport, 6,* 1880–1884.

Karakas, S., Yalin, A., Irak, M., & Erzengin, Ö.U. (2002). Digit span changes from puberty to old age under different levels of education. *Developmental Neuropsychology, 22,* 423–453.

Karbe, H., Kertesz, A., & Polk, M. (1993). Profiles of language impairment in primary progressive aphasia. *Archives of Neurology, 50,* 193–201.

Kareken, D.A. (1997). Judgment pitfalls in estimating premorbid intellectual function. *Archives of Clinical Neuropsychology, 12,* 701–709.

Kareken, D.A., Gur, R.C., & Saykin, A.J. (1995). Reading on the Wide Range Achievement Test–Revised and parental education as predictors of IQ: Comparison with the Barona formula. *Archives of Clinical Neuropsychology, 10,* 147–157.

Kareken, D.A., Moberg, P.J., & Gur, R.C. (1996). Proactive inhibition and semantic organization: Relationship with verbal memory in patients with schizophrenia. *Journal of the International Neuropsychological Society, 2,* 486–493.

Kareken, D.A., Unverzagt, F., Caldemeyer, K., et al. (1998). Functional brain imaging in apraxia. *Archives of Neurology, 55,* 107–113.

Karim, A.B.M.F., Agra, D., & Cornu, P. (2002). Randomized trial on the efficacy of radiotherapy for cerebral low-grade glioma in the adult. *International Journal of Radiation, Oncology, Biology, and Physics, 52,* 316–324.

Karim, A.B.M.F., Maat, B., Hatlevoll, R., et al. (1996). A randomized trial on dose-response radiation therapy of low-grade cerebral glioma. *International Journal of Radiation Oncology, Biology, and Physics, 36,* 549–556.

Karlawish, J.H., Casarett, D.J., & James, B.D. (2002). Alzheimer's disease patients' and caregivers' capacity, competency, and reasons to enroll in an early-phase Alzheimer's disease clinical trial. *Journal of the American Geriatric Society, 50,* 2019–2024.

Karlsen, K., Larsen, J.P., Tandberg, E., & Jorgensen, K. (1999). Fatigue in patients with Parkinson's disease. *Movement Disorders, 14,* 237–241.

Karlsson, T., Backman, L., Herlitz, A., et al. (1989). Memory improvement at different stages of Alzheimer's disease. *Neuropsychologia, 27,* 737–742.

Karnaze, D.S., Weinter, J.M., & Marshall, L.F. (1985). Auditory evoked potentials in coma after closed head injury: A clinical-neurophysiologic coma scale for predicting outcome. *Neurology, 35,* 1122–1126.

Karnovsky, A.R. (1974). Sex differences in spatial abilitiy. A developmental study. *Dissertation Abstracts International, 34,* 813.

Karol, R.L. (1989). Duration of seeking help following traumatic brain injury: The persistence of symptom complaints. *The Clinical Neuropsychologist, 3,* 244–249.

Kartsounis, L.D. & Warrington, E.K. (1989). Unilateral visual neglect overcome by cues implicit in stimulus arrays. *Journal of Neurology, Neurosurgery and Psychiatry, 52,* 1253–1259.

Karzmark, P. (2001). Impact of musical experience on the Seashore Rhythm Test. *The Clinical Neuropsychologist, 15,* 305–308.

Karzmark, P., Heaton, R.K., Grant, I., & Matthews, C.G. (1985). Use of demographic variables to predict full scale IQ: A replication and extension. *Journal of Clinical and Experimental Neuropsychology, 7,* 412–420.

Kasahara, H., Yamada, H., Tanno, M., et al. (1995). Magnetic resonance imaging study of the brain in aged volunteers: T_2 high intensity lesions and higher order cortical function. *Psychiatry and Clinical Neurosciences, 49,* 273–279.

Kasamatsu, K., Suzuki, S., Anse, M., et al. (2002). Menstrual cycle effects on performance of mental arithmetic task. *Journal of Physiological Anthropology and Applied Human Science, 21,* 285–290.

Kase, C.S., Wolf, P.A., Kelly-Hayes, M., et al. (1998). Intellectual decline after stroke: The Framingham Study. *Stroke, 29,* 805–812.

Kashner, T.M., Cullum, C.M., & Naugle, R.I. (2003). Measuring the economics of neuropsychology. In G.P. Prigatano & N.H. Pliskin (Eds.), *Clinical neuropsychology and cost outcome research.* New York: Psychology Press.

Kaskie, B. & Storandt, M. (1995). Visuospatial deficit in dementia of the Alzheimer type. *Archives of Neurology, 52,* 422–425.

Kaste, M., Kuurne, T., Vilkki, J., et al. (1982). Is chronic brain damage in boxing a hazard of the past? *Lancet, ii,* 1186–1187.

Kastrup, A., Li, T.Q., Glover, G.H., et al. (1999). Gender differences in cerebral blood flow and oxygenation response during focal physiologic neural activity. *Journal of Cerebral Blood Flow and Metabolism, 19,* 1066–1071.

Kaszniak, A.W. (1987). Neuropsychological consultation to geriatricians: Issues in the assessment of memory complaints. *The Clinical Neuropsychologist, 1,* 35–46.

Kaszniak, A.W. (1989). Psychological assessment of the aging individual. In J.E. Birren & K.W. Schaie (Eds.), *Handbook of the psychology of aging.* New York: Academic Press.

Kaszniak, A.W. (1991). Dementia and the older driver. *Human Factors, 33,* 527–537.

Kaszniak, A.W. & Allender, J. (1985). Psychological assessment of depression in older adults. In G.M. Chaisson-Stewart (Ed.), *Depression in the elderly: An interdisciplinary approach.* New York: Wiley.

Kaszniak, A.W., Fox, J., Gandell, D.L., et al. (1978). Predictors of mortality in presenile and senile dementia. *Annals of Neurology, 3,* 246–252.

Kaszniak, A.W., Garron, D.C., & Fox, J.H. (1979). Differential effects of age and cerebral atrophy upon span of immediate recall and paired-associate learning in older patients suspected of dementia. *Cortex, 15,* 285–295.

Kaszniak, A.W., Garron, D.C., Fox, J.H., et al. (1979). Cerebral atrophy, EEG slowing, age, education, and cognitive functioning in suspected dementia. *Neurology, 29,* 1273–1279.

Kaszniak, A.W., Poon, L.W., & Riege, W. (1986). Assessing memory deficits: An information-processing approach. In L.W. Poon (Ed.), *Handbook for clinical memory assessment of older adults.* Washington, D.C.: American Psychological Association.

Kaszniak, A.W., Sadeh, M., & Stern, L.Z. (1985). Differentiating depression from organic brain syndromes in older age. In G.M. Chaisson-Stewart (Ed.), *Depression in the elderly: An interdisciplinary approach.* New York: Wiley.

Kaszniak, A.W., Wilson, R.S., Fox, J.H., & Stebbins, G.T. (1986). Cognitive assessment in Alzheimer's disease: cross-sectional and longitudinal perspectives. *Canadian Journal of Neurological Sciences, 13,* 420–423.

Katz, D.I., Alexander, M.P., & Mandell, A.M. (1987). Dementia following strokes in the mesencephalon and diencephalon. *Archives of Neurology, 44,* 1127–1133.

Katz, M.M. & Lyerly, S.B. (1963). Methods for measuring adjustment and social behavior in the community: I. Rationale, description, discriminative validity and scale development. *Psychological Reports, 13,* 503–535.

Katzen, H.L., Levin, B.E., & Llabre, M. (1998). Age of disease onset influences cognition in Parkinson's disease. *Journal of the International Neuropsychological Society, 4,* 285–290.

Katzman, D.K., Christensen, B., Young, A.R., & Zipursky, R.B. (2001). Starving the brain: Structural abnormalities and cognitive impairment in adolescents with anorexia nervosa. *Seminars in Clinical Neuropsychiatry, 6,* 146–152.

Katzman, R. (1997). The aging brain. Limitations in our knowledge and future approaches. *Archive of Neurology, 54,* 1201–1205.

Katzman, R., Brown, T., Fuld, P., et al. (1983). Validation of a short orientation-memory-concentration test of cognitive impairment. *American Journal of Psychiatry, 140,* 734–739.

Katzman, R., Brown, T., Thal, L.J., et al. (1988). Comparison of rate of annual change of mental status score in four independent studies of patients with Alzheimer's disease. *Annals of Neurology, 24,* 384–389.

Katzman, R., Zhang, M.Y., Ouang-Ya-Qu, et al. (1988). A Chinese version of the Mini-Mental State Examination: Impact of illiteracy on a Shanghai dementia survey. *Journal of Clinical Epidemiology, 41,* 971–978.

Kaufer, D.I. & Cummings, J.L. (2003). Dementia and delirium: An overview. In T.E. Feinberg & M.J. Farah (Eds.), *Behavioral neurology and neuropsychology* (2nd ed.). New York: McGraw-Hill.

Kaufer, D.I., Cummings, J.L., Christine, D., et al. (1998). Assessing the impact of neuropsychiatric symptoms in Alzheimer's disease: The Neuropsychiatric Inventory Caregiver Distress Scale. *Journal of the American Geriatric Society, 46,* 210–215.

Kaufer, D.I., Cummings, J.L., Ketchel, P., et al. (2000). Validation of the NPI-Q, a brief clinical form of the Neuropsychiatric Inventory. *The Journal of Neuropsychiatry and Clinical Neurosciences, 12,* 233–239.

Kaufman, A.S. (1979). *Intelligent testing with the WISC-R.* New York: Wiley.

Kaufman, A.S. (1990). *Assessing adolescent and adult intelligence.* Boston: Allyn and Bacon.

Kaufman, A.S. & Horn, J.L. (1996). Age changes on tests of fluid and crystallized ability for women and men on the Kaufman Adolescent and Adult Intelligence Test (KAIT) at ages 17–94 years. *Archives of Clinical Neuropsychology, 11,* 97–121.

Kaufman, A.S. & Kaufman, N.L. (1983). *Kaufman Assessment Battery for Children (K-ABC).* Circle Pines, MN: American Guidance Service.

Kaufman, A.S. & Kaufman, N.L. (1990). *Kaufman Brief Intelligence Test (K-BIT).* Circle Pines, MN: American Guidance Service.

Kaufman, A.S. & Kaufman, N.L. (1993). *Kaufman Adolescent and Adult Intelligence Test (KAIT).* Circle Pines, MN: American Guidance Service.

Kaufman, A.S. & Kaufman, N.L. (1994a). *Kaufman Functional Academic Skills Test. Manual.* Circle Pines, MN: American Guidance Service.

Kaufman, A.S. & Kaufman, N.L. (1994b). *Kaufman Short Neuropsychological Assessment Procedure (K-SNAP).* Circle Pines, MN: American Guidance Service.

Kaufman, A.S., Kaufman-Packer, J.L., McLean, J.E., & Reynolds, C.R. (1991). Is the pattern of intellectual growth and decline across the adult life span different for men and women? *Journal of Clinical Psychology, 47,* 801–812.

Kaufman, A.S. & Lichtenberger, E.O. (1999). *Essentials of WAIS-III assessment.* New York: Wiley.

Kaufman, A.S., McLean, J.E., & Reynolds, C.R. (1988). Sex, race, residence, region, and education differences on the 11 WAIS-R subtests. *Journal of Clinical Psychology, 44,* 231–248.

Kaufman, A.S., McLean, J., & Reynolds, C. (1991). Analysis of WAIS-R factor patterns by sex and race. *Journal of Clinical Psychology, 47,* 548–557.

Kaufman, A.S., Reynolds, C.R., & McLean, J.E. (1989). Age and WAIS-R intelligence in a national sample of adults in the 20 to 74-year age range: A cross-sectional analysis with educational level controlled. *Intelligence, 13,* 235–253.

Kaufman, D.M., Weinberger, M., Strain, J.J., & Jacobs, J.W. (1979). Detection of cognitive deficits by a brief mental status examination. The Cognitive Capacity Screening Examination, a reappraisal and a review. *General Hospital Psychiatry, 1,* 247–255.

Kaufman, H.H., Levin, H.S., High, W.M., Jr., et al. (1985). Neurobehavioral outcome after gunshot wounds to the head in adult civilians and children. *Neurosurgery, 16,* 754–758.

Kauhanen, M., Korpelainen, J.T., Hiltunen, P., et al. (1999). Poststroke depression correlates with cognitive impairment and neurological deficits. *Stroke, 30,* 1875–1880.

Kauhanen, M.L., Korpelainen, J.T., Hiltunen, P., et al. (2000a). Aphasia, depression, and non-verbal cognitive impairment in ischaemic stroke. *Cerebrovascular Diseases, 10,* 455–461.

Kauhanen, M.L., Korpelainen, J.T., Hiltunen, P., et al. (2000b). Domains and determinants of quality of life after stroke caused by brain infarction. *Archives of Physical Medicine and Rehabilitation, 81,* 1541–1546.

Kawamura, S., Hadeishi, H., Sasaguchi, N., et al. (1997). Penetrating head injury caused by chopstick: case report. *Neurologia Medico-Chirurgica, 37,* 332–335.

Kay, G.G. & Quig, M.E. (2001). Impact of sedating antihistamines on safety and productivity. *Allergy and Asthma Proceedings, 22,* 281–283.

Kay, T. (1986). *Minor head injury: Introduction for professionals.* Framingham, MA: National Head Injury Foundation.

Kay, T., Ezrachi, O., & Cavallo, M. (1986). *Plateaus and consistency: Long-term neuropsychological changes following head trauma.* Paper presented at the 94th annual convention of the American Psychological Association, Washington, D.C.

Kay, T. & Lezak, M. (1990). The nature of head injury. In D. Corthell (Ed.), *Traumatic brain injury and vocational rehabilitation.* Menomonie, WI: University of Wisconsin, Stout Research and Training Center.

Kay, T. & Silver, S.M. (1989). Closed head trauma: Assessment for rehabilitation. In M.D. Lezak (Ed.), *Assessment of the behavioral consequences of head trauma. Frontiers of clinical neuroscience* (Vol. 7). New York: Alan R. Liss.

Kaye, J.A., DeCarli, C., Luxenberg, J.S., & Rapoport, S.I. (1992). The significance of age-related enlargement of the cerebral ventricles in healthy men and women measured by quantitative computed X-ray tomography. *Journal of the American Geriatrics Society, 40,* 225–231.

Kaye, J.A., Oken, B.S., Howieson, D.B., et al. (1994). Neurologic evaluation of the optimally healthy oldest old. *Archives of Neurology, 51,* 1205–1211.

Kaye, J.A., Swihart, T., Howieson, D., et al. (1997). Volume loss of the hippocampus and temporal lobe in healthy elderly persons destined to develop dementia. *Neurology, 48,* 1297–1304.

Kear-Colwell, J.J. (1973). The structure of the Wechsler Memory Scale and its relationship to "brain damage." *Journal of Social and Clinical Psychology, 12,* 384–392.

Keenan, P.A., Ricker, J.H., Lindamer, L.A., et al. (1996). Relationship between WAIS-R Vocabulary and performance on the California Verbal Learning Test. *The Clinical Neuropsychologist, 10,* 455–458.

Keenan, J.P., Wheeler, M.A., Gallup, G.G., Jr., & Pascual-Leone, A. (2000). Self-recognition and the right prefrontal cortex. *Trends in Cognitive Sciences, 4,* 338–344.

Keene, J., Hope, T., Fairburn, C.G., & Jacoby, R. (2001). Death and dementia. *International Journal of Geriatric Psychiatry, 16,* 969–974.

Kehrer, C.A., Sanchez, P.N., Habif, U., et al. (2000). Effects of a significant-other observer on neuropsychological test performance. *The Clinical Neuropsychologist, 14,* 67–71.

Keilp, J.G., Alexander, G.E., Stern, Y., & Prohovnik, I. (1996). Inferior parietal perfusion, lateralization, and neuropsychological dysfunction in Alzheimer's disease. *Brain and Cognition, 32,* 365–383.

Kelland, D.Z. & Lewis, R. F. (1994). Evaluation of the reliability and validity of the Repeatable Cognitive-Perceptual-Motor Battery. *The Clinical Neuropsychologist, 8,* 295–308.

Kelland, D.Z. & Lewis, R.F. (1996). The Digit Vigilance Test: Reliability, validity, and sensitivity to diazepam. *Archives of Clinical Neuropsychology, 11,* 339–344.

Kellett, M. W., Smith, D. F., Baker, G. A., & Chadwick, D. W. (1997). Quality of life after epilepsy surgery. *Journal of Neurology, Neurosurgery and Psychiatry, 63,* 52–58.

Kelley, K.M., Pliskin, N., Meyer, G., & Lee, R.C. (1994). Neuropsychiatric aspects of electrical injury. The nature of psychiatric disturbance. *Annals of the New York Academy of Sciences, 720,* 213–219.

Kelly, D.F., Doberstein, C., & Becker, D.P. (1996). General principles of head injury management. In R.K. Narayan et al. (Eds.), *Neurotrauma.* New York: McGraw-Hill.

Kelly, M.D., Grant, I., Heaton, R.K., et al. (1996). Neuropsychological findings in HIV infection and AIDS. In I. Grant & K.M. Adams (Eds.), *Neuropsychological assessment of psychiatric disorders* (2nd ed.). New York: Oxford University Press.

Kelly, M.P., Johnson, C.T., & Govern, J.M. (1996). Recognition Memory Test: Validity in diffuse traumatic brain injury. *Applied Neuropsychology, 3,* 147–154.

Kelly, M.P., Johnson, C.T., Knoller, N., et al. (1997). Substance abuse, traumatic brain injury and neuropsychological outcome. *Brain Injury, 11,* 391–402.

Kelly, M.P., Kaszniak, A.W., & Garron, D.C. (1986). Neurobehavioral impairment patterns in carotid disease and Alzheimer disease. *International Journal of Clinical Neuropsychology, 8,* 163–169.

Kemp, P.M., Houston, A.S., MacLeod, M.A., & Pethybridge, R.J. (1995). Cerebral perfusion and psychometric testing in military amateur boxers and controls. *Journal of Neurology, Neurosurgery and Psychiatry, 59,* 368–374.

Kemper, T. (1994). Neuroanatomical and neuropathological changes during normal aging and dementia. In M.L. Albert & J.E. Knoefel (Eds.), *Clinical neurology of aging* (2nd ed.). New York: Oxford University Press.

Kempler, D., Teng, E.L., Dick, M., et al. (1998). The effects of age, education, and ethnicity on verbal fluency. *Journal of the International Neuropsychological Society, 4,* 531–538.

Kenealy, P.M., Beaumont, J.G., Lintern, T.C., & Murrell, R.C. (2002). Autobiographical memory in advanced multiple sclerosis: Assessment of episodic and personal semantic memory across three time spans. *Journal of the International Neuropsychological Society, 8,* 855–860.

Kennedy, P.G. & Chaudhuri, A. (2002). Herpes simplex encephalitis. *Journal of Neurology, Neurosurgery and Psychiatry, 73,* 237–238.

Kent, T.A., Gelman, B.B., Casper, K., et al. (1994). Neuroimaging in HIV infection: Neuropsychological and pathological correlation. In I. Grant & A. Martin (Eds.), *Neuropsychology of HIV infection.* New York: Oxford University Press.

Keogh, E. & Birkby, J. (1999). The effect of anxiety sensitivity and gender on the experience of pain. *Cognition and Emotion, 13,* 813–829.

Keppel, C.C. & Crowe, S.F. (2000). Changes to body image and self-esteem following stroke in young adults. *Neuropsychological Rehabilitation. 10,* 15–31.

Keren, O., Reznik, J., & Groswasswer, Z. (2001). Combined motor disturbances following severe traumatic brain injury: an integrative long-term treatment approach. *Brain Injury, 15,* 633–638.

Kertesz, A. (1979). *Aphasia and associated disorders.* New York: Grune & Stratton.

Kertesz, A. (1982). *Western Aphasia Battery.* San Antonio, TX: Psychological Corporation.

Kertesz, A. (1988). Cognitive function in severe aphasia. In L. Weiskrantz (Ed.), *Thought Without Language.* Oxford, UK: Clarendon Press.

Kertesz, A. (1989). Assessing aphasic disorders. In E. Perecman (Ed.), *Integrating theory and practice in clinical neuropsychology.* Mahwah, NJ: Erlbaum.

Kertesz, A. (1996). Les apraxies. In M.I. Botez (Ed.), *Neuropsychologie clinique et neurologie du comportement* (2ème ed.). Montréal: Les Presses de l'Université de Montréal; Paris: Masson.

Kertesz, A. (2001). Aphasia and stroke. In J. Bogousslavsky & L.R. Caplan (Eds.), *Stroke syndromes* (2nd ed.). Cambridge, UK: Cambridge University Press.

Kertesz, A. & Clydesdale, S. (1994). Neuropsychological deficits in vascular dementia vs Alzheimer's disease. Frontal lobe deficits prominent in vascular dementia. *Archives of Neurology, 51,* 1226–1231.

Kertesz, A. & Dobrowolski, S. (1981). Right-hemisphere deficits, lesion size and location. *Journal of Clinical Neuropsychology, 3,* 283–299.

Kertesz, A., Ferro, J.M., & Shewan, C.M. (1984). Apraxia and aphasia: The functional-anatomical basis for their dissociation. *Neurology, 34,* 40–47.

Kertesz, A. & Gold, B.T. (2003). Recovery of cognition. In K.M. Heilman & E. Valenstein (Eds.), *Clinical neuropsychology* (4th ed.). New York: Oxford University Press.

Kertesz, A. & Hooper, P. (1982). Praxis and language: The extent and variety of apraxia in aphasia. *Neuropsychologia, 20,* 275–286.

Kertesz, A. & Munoz, D.G. (1997). Primary progressive aphasia. *Clinical Neuroscience, 4,* 95–102.

Kertesz, A., Nadkarni, N., Davidson, W., & Thomas, A.W. (2000). The Frontal Behavioral Inventory in the differential diagnosis of frontotemporal dementia. *Journal of the International Neuropsychological Society, 6,* 460–468.

Kertesz, A., Nicholson, I., Cancelliere, A., et al. (1985). Motor impersistence: A right-hemisphere syndrome. *Neurology, 35,* 662–666.

Kesler, S.R., Hopkins, R.O., Weaver, L.K., et al. (2001). Verbal memory deficits associated with fornix atrophy in carbon monoxide poisoning. *Journal of the International Neuropsychological Society, 7,* 640–646.

Kesselring, J. & Lassmann, H. (1997). Pathogenesis. In J. Kesselring (Ed.), *Multiple sclerosis.* Cambridge, UK: Cambridge University Press.

Kessels, R.P.C., Aleman, A., Verhagen, W.I.M., et al. (2000). Cognitive functioning after whiplash injury: A meta-analysis. *Journal of the International Neuropsychological Society, 6,* 271–278.

Kessels, R.P., de Haan, E.H., Kappelle, L.J., & Postma, A. (2001). Varieties of human spatial memory: A meta-analysis on the effects of hippocampal lesions. *Brain Research Review, 35,* 295–303.

Kessels, R.P., van Zandvoort, M.J., Postma, A., et al. (2000). The Corsi Block-Tapping Task: Standardization and normative data. *Applied Neuropsychology, 7,* 252–258.

Kessler, H.R., Roth, D.L., Kaplan, R.F., & Goode, K.T. (1994). Confirmatory factor analysis of the Mattis Dementia Rating Scale. *Clinical Neuropsychologist, 8,* 451–461.

Kessler, J., Markowitsch, H.J., & Bast-Kessler, C. (1987). Memory of alcoholic patients, including Korsakoff's, tested with a Brown-Peterson paradigm. *Archives of Psychology, 139,* 115–132.

Kewman, D.G., Vaishampayan, N., Zald, D., & Han, B. (1991). Cognitive impairment in musculoskeletal pain patients. *International Journal of Psychiatry in Medicine, 23,* 253–262.

Keys, B.A. & White, D.A. (2000). Exploring the relationship between age, executive abilities, and psychomotor speed. *Journal of the International Neuropsychological Society, 6,* 76–82.

Khachaturian, Z.S. (1985). Diagnosis of Alzheimer's disease. *Archives of Neurology, 42,* 1097–1105.

Kibby, M.Y., Schmitter-Edgecombe, M., & Long, C.J. (1998). Ecological validity of neuropsychological tests: Focus on the California Verbal Learning Test and the Wisconsin Card Sorting Test. *Archives of Clinical Neuropsychology, 13,* 523–534.

Kidd, D., Barkhof, F., McConnell, R., et al. (1999). Cortical lesions in multiple sclerosis. *Brain, 122,* 17–26.

Kiehl, K.A., Liddle, P.F., Smith, A.M., et al. (1999). Neural pathways involved in the processing of concrete and abstract words. *Human Brain Mapping, 7,* 225–233.

Kiernan, R.J., Bower, G.H., & Schorr, D. (1984). Stimulus variables in the Block Design task revisited: A reply to Royer. *Journal of Consulting and Clinical Psychology, 52,* 705–707.

Kiernan, R.J., Mueller, J., & Langston, J.W. (1995). *Cognistat (Neurobehavioral Cognitive Status Examination).* Lutz, FL: Psychological Assessment Resources.

Kiernan, R.J., Mueller, J., Langston, J.W., & VanDyke, C. (1987). The Neurobehavioral Cognitive Status Examination. *Annals of Internal Medicine, 107,* 481–485.

Kilaru, S., Garb, J, Emhoff, T., et al. (1996). Long-term functional status and mortality of elderly patients with severe closed head injuries. *Journal of Trauma, 41,* 957–963.

Kilburn, K.H., Warshaw, R., & Thornton, J.C. (1987). Formaldehyde impairs memory, equilibrium, and dexterity in histology technicians: Effects which persist for days after exposure. *Archives of Environmental Health, 42,* 117–120.

Killackey, H.P. (1990). The neocortex and memory storage. In J.L. McGaugh et al. (Eds.), *Brain organization and memory: Cells, systems, and circuits.* New York: Oxford University Press.

Killcross, S. (2000). The amygdala, emotion, and learning. *Psychologist, 13,* 502–507.

Killgore, W.D. & Adams, R.L. (1999). Prediction of Boston Naming Test performance from Vocabulary scores: Preliminary guidelines for interpretation. *Perceptual and Motor Skills, 89,* 327–337.

Killgore, W.D. & DellaPietra, L. (2000a). Item response biases on the Logical Memory delayed recognition subtest of the Wechsler Memory Scale-III. *Psychological Reports, 86,* 851–857.

Killgore, W.D. & DellaPietra, L. (2000b). Using the WMS-III to detect malingering: Empirical validation of the rarely missed index (RMI). *Journal of Clinical and Experimental Neuropsychology, 22,* 761–771.

Kilpatrick, C., Murrie, V., Cook, M., et al. (1997). Degree of left hippocampal atrophy correlates with severity of neuropsychological deficits. *Seizure, 6,* 213–218.

Kim, E. (2002). Agitation, aggression, and disinhibition syndromes after traumatic brain injury. *NeuroRehabilitation, 17,* 297–310.

Kim, H. & Na, D.L. (1999). Normative data on the Korean version of the Boston Naming Test. *Journal of Clinical and Experimental Neuropsychology, 21,* 127–133.

Kim, J.K. & Kang, Y. (1999). Normative study of the Korean-California Verbal Learning Test (K-CVLT). *The Clinical Neuropsychologist, 13,* 365–369.

Kim, J.S. (2001). Sensory abnormality. In J. Bogousslavsky & L.R. Caplan (Eds.), *Stroke syndromes* (2nd ed.). Cambridge, UK: Cambridge University Press.

Kim, J.S. & Choi-Kwon, S. (2000). Poststroke depression and emotional incontinence: Correlation with lesion location. *Neurology, 54,* 1805–1810.

Kim, J.S., Lee, J.H., & Lee, M.C. (1997). Pattern of sensory dysfunction in lateral medullary infarction: Clinical-MRI correlation. *Neurology, 49,* 1557–1563.

Kim, S.H., Manes, F., Kosier, T., et al. (1999). Irritability following traumatic brain injury. *Journal of Nervous and Mental Disease, 187,* 327–335.

Kim, S.Y., Karlawish, J.H., & Caine, E.D. (2002). Current state of research on decision-making competence of cognitively impaired elderly persons. *American Journal of Geriatric Psychiatry, 20,* 151–165.

Kim, Y., Morrow, L., Passafiume, D., & Boller, F. (1984). Visuoperceptual and visuomotor abilities and locus of lesion. *Neuropsychologia, 22,* 177–185.

Kim, Y.S., Nibbelink, D.W., & Overall, J.E. (1994). Factor structure and reliability of the Alzheimer's Disease Assessment Scale (ADAS) in a multicenter trial with linopirdine. *Journal of Geriatric Psychiatry and Neurology, 7,* 74–83.

Kimball, D.R. & Holyoak, K.J. (2000). Transfer and expertise. In E. Tulving & F.I.M. Craik (Eds.), *The Oxford handbook of memory.* Oxford: Oxford University Press.

Kimberg, D.Y., D'Esposito, M.D., & Farah, M.J. (2000). Frontal lobes II: Cognitive issues. In M.J. Farah & T.E. Feinberg (Eds.), *Patient-based approaches to cognitive neuroscience.* Cambridge, MA: MIT Press.

Kimura, D. (1963). Right temporal lobe damage. *Archives of Neurology, 8,* 264–271.

Kimura, D. (1999). *Sex and cognition.* Cambridge, MA: MIT Press.

Kimura, D. & Archibald, Y. (1974). Motor functions of the left hemisphere. *Brain, 97,* 337–350.

Kimura, D., Barnett, H.J.M., & Burkhart, G. (1981). The psychological test pattern in progressive supranuclear palsy. *Neuropsychologia, 19,* 301–306.

Kimura, D. & Vanderwolf, C.H. (1970). The relation between hand preference and the performance of individual finger movements by left and right hands. *Brain, 93,* 769–774.

Kimura, S.D. (1981). A card form of the Reitan-Modified Halstead Category Test. *Journal of Consulting and Clinical Psychology, 49,* 145–146.

Kincannon, J.C. (1968). Prediction of the standard MMPI scale scores from 71 items: the Mini-Mult. *Journal of Consulting and Clinical Psychology, 32,* 319–325.

Kindermann, S.S. & Brown, G.G. (1997). Depression and memory in the elderly: a meta-analysis. *Journal of Clinical and Experimental Neuropsychology, 19*, 625–642.

King, D.A. & Caine, E.D. (1996). Cognitive impairment and major depression: Beyond the pseudodementia syndrome. In I. Grant & K.M. Adams (Eds.), *Neuropsychological assessment of neuropsychiatric disorders* (2nd ed.). New York: Oxford University Press.

King, D.A., Caine, E.D., & Cox, C. (1993). Influence of depression and age on selected cognitive functions. *The Clinical Neuropsychologist, 7*, 443–453.

King, D.A., Cox, C., Lyness, J.M., et al. (1998). Quantitative and qualitative differences in the verbal learning performance of elderly depressives and healthy controls. *Journal of the International Neuropsychological Society, 4*, 115–126.

King, G.D., Hannay, H.J., Masek, B.J., & Burns, J.W. (1978). Effects of anxiety and sex on neuropsychological tests. *Journal of Consulting and Clinical Psychology, 46*, 375–376.

King, M.C. & Snow, W.G. (1981). Problem-solving task performance in brain-damaged subjects. *Journal of Clinical Psychology, 37*, 400–404.

King, N.S. (1997). Post-traumatic stress disorder and head injury as a dual diagnosis: "Islands" of memory as a mechanism. *Journal of Neurology, Neurosurgery and Psychiatry, 62*, 82–84.

King, N.S., Crawford, S., Wenden, F.J., et al. (1999). Early prediction of persisting post-concussion symptoms following mild and moderate head injuries. *British Journal of Clinical Psychology, 38*, 15–25.

King, R.E. & Flynn, C.F. (1995). Defining and measuring the "right stuff:" Neuropsychiatrically enhanced flight screening (N-EFS). *Aviation Space and Environmental Medicine, 66*, 951–956.

Kinsbourne, M. (1988). Integrated field theory of consciousness. In A.J. Marcel & E. Bisiach (Eds.), *Consciousness in contemporary science*. Oxford: Clarendon Press.

Kinsella, G., Murtagh, D., Landry, A., et al. (1996). Everyday memory following traumatic brain injury. *Brain Injury, 10*, 499–507.

Kinsella, G., Packer, S., Ng, K., et al. (1995). Continuing issues in the assessment of neglect. *Neuropsychological Rehabilitation, 5*, 239–258.

Kircher, T.T., Senior, C., Phillips, M.L., et al. (2001). Recognizing one's own face. *Cognition, 78*, B1–B15.

Kirk, A. & Kertesz, A. (1993). Subcortical contributions to drawing. *Brain and Cognition, 21*, 57–70.

Kirkwood, S.C., Siemers, E., Stout, J.C., et al. (1999). Longitudinal cognitive and motor changes among presymptomatic Huntington disease gene carriers. *Archives of Neurology, 56*, 563–568.

Kish, S.J., Chang, L.J., Mirchandani, L., et al. (1985). Progressive supranuclear palsy: Relationship between extrapyramidal disturbances, dementia, and brain neurotransmitter markers. *Annals of Neurology, 18*, 530–536.

Kitterle, F.L. (Ed.) (1995). *Hemispheric communication: Mechanisms and models*. Hillsdale, NJ: Erlbaum.

Kittner, S.J. & Bush, T. (1997). Pregnancy, hormonal contraception, and postmenopausal estrogen replacement therapy. In K.M.A. Welch et al. (Eds.), *Primer on cerebrovascular diseases*. San Diego: Academic Press.

Kivela, S.L. (1992). Psychological assessment and rating scales: Depression and other age-related affective disorders. In M. Bergener et al. (Eds.), *Aging and mental disorders*. New York: Springer.

Kivipelto, J., Helkala, E.-L., Laakso, M.P., et al. (2001). Midlife vascular risk factors and Alzheimer's disease in later life: Longitudinal, population based study. *British Medical Journal, 322*, 1447–1451.

Kizilbash, A.H., Vanderploeg, R.D., & Curtiss, G. (2002). The effects of depression and anxiety on memory performance. *Archives of Clinical Neuropsychology, 17*, 57–67.

Klass, D.W. & Westmoreland, B.F. (2002). Electroencephalography: General principles and adult electroencephalograms. In J.R. Daube (Ed.), *Clinical neurophysiology* (2nd ed.). New York: Oxford University Press.

Klatsky, A.L. (1994). Epidemiology of coronary heart disease. Influence of alcohol. *Alcohol Clinical and Experimental Research, 18*, 88–96.

Klatsky, A.L., Armstrong, M.A., & Friedman, G.D. (1997). Red wine, white wine, liquor, beer, and risk for coronary artery disease hospitalization. *American Journal of Cardiology, 80*, 416–520.

Klebanoff, S.G. (1945). Psychological changes in organic brain lesions and ablations. *Psychological Bulletin, 42*, 585–623.

Klebanoff, S.G., Singer, J.L., & Wilensky, H. (1954). Psychological consequences of brain lesions and ablations. *Psychological Bulletin, 51*, 1–41.

Kleihues, P. & Cavenee, W. K. (2000). *Pathology and genetics of tumours of the nervous system. World Health Organization classification of tumours*. Lyon: IARC Press.

Klein, M. (1997). Cognitive aging theories and models—an overview. In *Cognitive aging, attention, and mild traumatic brain injury*. Maastricht, Netherlands: Neuropsych.

Klein, M., Ponds, R.W.H.M., Houx, P.J., & Jolles, J. (1997). The impact of aging on sustained attention: Time-on-task effects in visual search. In *Cognitive aging, attention, and mild traumatic brain injury*. Maastricht, Netherlands: Neuropsych.

Klein, M., Taphoorn, M.J., Heimans, J.J., et al. (2001). Neurobehavioral status and health-related quality of life in newly diagnosed high-grade glioma patients. *Journal of Clinical Oncology, 19*, 4037–4047.

Kleinmuntz, B. (1982). *Personality and psychological assessment*. New York: St. Martin's Press.

Kleinschmidt, J.J., Digre, K.B., & Hanover, R. (2000). Idiopathic intracranial hypertension. Relationship to depression, anxiety, and quality of life. *Neurology, 54*, 319–324.

Klesges, R.C., Fisher, L., Pheley, A., et al. (1984). A major validational study of the Halstead-Reitan in the prediction of CAT-scan assessed brain damage in adults. *International Journal of Clinical Neuropsychology, 6*, 29–34.

Klimczak, N.C., Bradford, K.A., Burright, R.G., & Donovick, P.J. (2000). K-FAST and WRAT-3: Are they really different? *The Clinical Neuropsychologist, 14*, 135–138.

Kline Leidy, N., Rentz, A. M., & Grace, E. M. (1998). Evaluating health-related quality of life outcomes in clinical trials of antiepileptic drug therapy. *Epilepsia, 39*, 965–977.

Klingberg, T. & Roland, P.E. (1998). Right prefrontal activation during encoding, but not during retrieval, in a non-verbal paired-associates task. *Cerebral Cortex, 8*, 73–79.

Klinteberg, B.A., Levander, S.E., & Schalling, D. (1987). Cognitive sex differences: Speed and problem-solving strategies on computerized neuropsychological tasks. *Perceptual and Motor Skills, 65*, 683–697.

Klonoff, D.C., Andrews, B.T., & Obana, W.G. (1989). Stroke associated with cocaine use. *Archives of Neurology, 46*, 989–993.

Klonoff, E.A. & Landrine, H. (1997). *Preventing misdiagnosis of women. A guide to physical disorders that have psychiatric symptoms*. Thousand Oaks, CA: Sage.

Klonoff, H., Clark, C., Oger, J., et al. (1991). Neuropsychological performance in patients with mild multiple sclerosis. *Journal of Nervous and Mental Disease, 179*, 127–131.

Klonoff, P.S., Costa, L.D., & Snow, W.G. (1986). Predictors and indicators of quality of life in patients with closed-head injury. *Journal of Clinical and Experimental Neuropsychology, 8*, 469–485.

Klonoff, P.S. & Lamb, D.G. (1998). Mild head injury, significant impairment on neuropsychological test scores, and psychiatric disability. *The Clinical Neuropsychologist, 12*, 31–42.

Klonoff, P.S., Snow, W.G., & Costa, L.D. (1986). Quality of life in patients two to four years after closed head injury. *Neurosurgery, 19*, 735–743.

Klopfer, B. & Davidson, H.H. (1962). *Rorschach technique: An introductory manual.* New York: Harcourt, Brace & World.

Klouda, G.V. & Cooper, W.E. (1990). Information search following damage to the frontal lobes. *Psychological Reports, 67*, 411–416.

Kløve, H. (1963). Clinical neuropsychology. In F.M. Forster (Ed.), *The medical clinics of North America.* New York: Saunders.

Kløve, H. & Matthews, C.G. (1974). Neuropsychological studies of patients with epilepsy. In R.M. Reitan & L.A. Davison (Eds.), *Clinical neuropsychology.* Washington, D.C.: Hemisphere.

Kluger, A., Gianutsos, J.G., Golomb, J., et al. (1997). Motor/psychomotor dysfunction in normal aging, mild cognitive decline, and early Alzheimer's disease: Diagnostic and differential diagnostic features. *International Psychogeriatrics, 9(Suppl. 1),* 307–316.

Knapp, M.J., Knopman, D.S., Solomon, P.R., et al. (1994). A 30-week randomized controlled trial of high-dose tacrine in patients with Alzheimer's disease. *Journal of the American Medical Association, 271*, 985–991.

Knave, B., Olson, B.Q., Elofsson, S., et al. (1978). Long-term exposure to jet fuel. *Scandinavian Journal of Work Environment and Health, 4*, 19–45.

Knecht, S., Deppe, M., Ebner, A., et al. (1998). Noninvasive determination of language lateralization by functional transcranial Doppler sonography: A comparison with the Wada test. *Stroke, 29*, 82–86.

Knecht, S., Drager, B., Deppe, M., et al. (2000). Handedness and hemispheric language dominance in healthy humans. *Brain, 123*, 2512–2518.

Kneebone, A.C., Chelune, G.J., & Lüders, H.O. (1997). Individual patient prediction of seizure lateralization in temporal lobe epilepsy: A comparison between neuropsychological memory measures and the intracarotid amobarbital procedure. *Journal of the International Neuropsychological Society, 3*, 159–168.

Knesevich, J.W., Martin, R.L., Berg, L., & Danziger, W. (1983). Preliminary report on affective symptoms in the early stages of senile dementia of the Alzheimer's type. *American Journal of Psychiatry, 140*, 233–235.

Knight, R.G. (1992). *The neuropsychology of degenerative brain diseases.* Hillsdale, NJ: Erlbaum.

Knight, R.G., Devereux, R.C., & Godfrey, H.P.D. (1997). Psychosocial consequences of caring for a spouse with multiple sclerosis. *Journal of Clinical and Experimental Neuropsychology, 19*, 7–19.

Knight, R.G. & Longmore, B.E. (1994). *Clinical neuropsychology of alcoholism.* Hillsdale, NJ: Erlbaum.

Knight, R.T. (1984). Decreased response to novel stimuli after prefrontal lesions in man. *Electroencephalography and Clinical Neurophysiology, 59*, 9–20.

Knight, R.T. & Grabowecky, M. (2000). Prefrontal cortex, time, and consciousness. In M.S. Gazzaniga (Ed.), *The new cognitive neurosciences* (2nd ed.). Cambridge, MA: MIT Press.

Knightly, J.J. & Pulliman, M.W. (1996). Military head injury. In R.K. Narayan et al. (Eds.). *Neurotrauma.* New York: McGraw-Hill.

Knippa, J., Golden, C.J., & Franzen, M. (1984). Interpretation and use of the Luria-Nebraska Battery. *Brain and Cognition, 3*, 343–348.

Knoke, D., Taylor, A.E., & Saint-Cyr, J.A. (1998). The differential effects of cueing on recall in Parkinson's disease and normal subjects. *Brain and Cognition, 38*, 261–274.

Knopman, D., Boland, L.L., Mosley, T., et al. (2001). Atherosclerosis Risk in Communities (ARIC) study investigators. Cardiovascular risk factors and cognitive decline in middle-aged adults. *Neurology, 56*, 485–493.

Knopman, D., Knudson, D., Yoes, M.E., & Weiss, D.J. (2000). Development and standardization of a new telephonic cognitive screening test: The Minnesota Cognitive Acuity Screen (MCAS). *Neuropsychiatry, Neuropsychology, and Behavioral Neurology, 13*, 286–296.

Knopman, D.S. & Ryberg, S.A. (1989). A verbal memory test with high predictive accuracy for dementia of the Alzheimer's type. *Annals of Neurology, 46*, 141–145.

Knopman, D. and Selnes, O. (2003). Neuropsychology of dementia. In K.M. Heilman & E. Valenstein (Eds.), *Clinical neuropsychology* (4th ed.). New York: Oxford University Press.

Knopman, D.S., Selnes, O.A., Niccum, N., & Rubens, A.B. (1984). Recovery of naming in aphasia: Relationship to fluency, comprehension and CT findings. *Neurology, 34*, 1461–1470.

Knopman, D.S., Selnes, O.A., Niccum, N., et al. (1983). A longitudinal study of speech fluency in aphasia: CT correlates of recovery and persistent nonfluency. *Neurology, 33*, 1170–1178.

Knowlton, B.J., Mangels, J.A., & Squire, L.R. (1996). A neostriatal habit learning system in humans. *Science, 273*, 1399–1402.

Kobari, M., Meyer, J.S., & Ichijo, M. (1990). Leuko-araiosis, cerebral atrophy, and cerebral perfusion in normal aging. *Archives of Neurology, 47*, 161–165.

Koch, C. & Crick, F. (2000). Some thoughts on consciousness and neuroscience. In M.S. Gazzaniga (Ed.), *The new cognitive neurosciences* (2nd ed.). Cambridge, MA: MIT Press.

Koch, C. & Segev, I. (2000). The role of single neurons in information processing. *Nature Neuroscience, 3(Suppl.)*, 1171–1177.

Kochansky, G.E. (1979). Psychiatric rating scales for assessing psychopathology in the elderly: A critical review. In A. Raskin & L. Jarvik (Eds.), *Psychiatric symptoms and cognitive loss in the elderly.* Washington, D.C.: Hemisphere.

Koechlin, E., Basso, G., Pietrini, P., et al. (1999). The role of the anterior prefrontal cortex in human cognition. *Nature, 399*, 148–151.

Koechlin, E., Corrado, G., Pietrini, P., & Grafman, J. (2000). Dissociating the role of the medial and lateral anterior prefrontal cortex in human planning. *Proceedings of the National Academy of Sciences of the United States of America, 97*, 7651–7656.

Koelega, H.S. (1993). Stimulant drugs and vigilance performance: A review. *Psychopharmacology, 111*, 1–16.

Koestler, J. & Keshavarz, R. (2001). Penetrating head injury in children: A case report and review of the literature. *Journal of Emergency Medicine, 21*, 145–150.

Koffler, S.P. & Zehler, D. (1985). Normative data for the hand dynamometer. *Perceptual and Motor Skills, 61*, 589–590.

Köhler, S., Black, S.E., Sinden, M., et al. (1998). Memory impairments associated with hippocampal versus parahippocampal-gyrus atrophy: An MR volumetry study in Alzheimer's disease. *Neuropsychologia, 36*, 901–914.

Köhler, S. & Moscovitch, M. (1997). Unconscious visual processing in neuropsychological syndromes: A survey of the literature and evaluation of models of consciousness. In M.D. Rugg (Ed.), *Cognitive neuroscience.* Cambridge, MA: MIT Press.

Kohs, S.C. (1919). *Kohs Block Design Test.* Wood Dale, IL: Stoelting.

Kolakowsky-Hayner, S.A., Gourley, E.V. 3rd, Kreutzer, J.S., et al. (2002). Post-injury substance abuse among persons with brain injury and persons with spinal cord injury. *Brain Injury, 16*, 583–592.

Kolb, B. (1990). Recovery from occipital stroke: A self-report and an inquiry into visual processes. *Canadian Journal of Psychology, 44*, 130–147.

Kolb, B. & Wishaw, Q. (1996). *Fundamentals of neuropsychology* (4th ed.). New York: Freeman.

Kolers, P.A. (1976). Reading a year later. *Journal of Experimental Psychology: Human Learning and Memory, 2,* 554–565.

Koller, W.C. (1984a). Disturbance of recent memory function in parkinsonian patients on anticholinergic therapy. *Cortex, 20,* 307–311.

Koller, W.C. (1984b). Sensory symptoms in Parkinson's disease. *Neurology, 34,* 957–959.

Koller, W.C., Langston, J.W., Hubble, J.P., et al. (1991). Does a long preclinical period occur in Parkinson's disease? *Neurology, 41(Suppl. 2),* 8–13.

Koller, W.C., Wilson, R.S., Glatt, S.L., & Fox, J.H. (1984). Motor signs are infrequent in dementia of the Alzheimer type. *Annals of Neurology, 16,* 514–516.

Kompoliti, K., Goetz, C.G., Litvan, I., et al. (1998). Pharmacological therapy in progressive supranuclear palsy. *Archives of Neurology, 55,* 1099–1102.

Kopelman, M.D. (1985). Rates of forgetting in Alzheimer-type dementia and Korsakoff's syndrome. *Neuropsychologia, 23,* 623–638.

Kopelman, M.D. (1986). Recall of anomalous sentences in dementia and amnesia. *Brain and Language, 29,* 154–170.

Kopelman, M.D. (1987a). Amnesia: Organic and psychogenic. *British Journal of Psychiatry, 150,* 428–442.

Kopelman, M.D. (1987b). Crime and amnesia: A review. *Behavioral Sciences and the Law, 5,* 323–342.

Kopelman, M.D. (1987c). How far could cholinergic depletion account for the memory deficits of Alzheimer-type dementia or the alcoholic Korsakoff syndrome? In S.M. Stahl et al. (Eds.), *Cognitive neurochemistry.* Oxford, UK: Oxford University Press.

Kopelman, M.D. (1989). Remote and autobiographical memory, temporal cortex memory and frontal atrophy in Korsakoff and Alzheimer patients. *Neuropsychologia, 27,* 437–460.

Kopelman, M.D. (1994). The Autobiographical Memory Interview (AMI) in organic and psychogenic amnesia. *Memory, 2,* 211–235.

Kopelman, M.D. (2002). Retrograde amnesia. In A.D. Baddeley et al. (Eds.), *Handbook of memory disorders* (2nd ed.). Chichester, UK: Wiley.

Kopelman, M.D., Christensen, H., Puffett, A., & Stanhope, N. (1994). The great escape: A neuropsychological study of psychogenic amnesia. *Neuropsychologia, 32,* 675–691.

Kopelman, M.D. & Corn, T.H. (1988). Cholinergic "blockade" as a model for cholinergic depletion. *Brain, 111,* 1079–1110.

Kopelman, M.D. & Kapur, N. (2001). The loss of episodic memories in retrograde amnesia: Single-case and group studies. *Philosophical Transactions of the Royal Society of London Series B, Biological Sciences, 356,* 1409–1421.

Kopelman, M.D., Stanhope, N., & Kingsley, D. (1999). Retrograde amnesia in patients with diencephalic, temporal lobe or frontal lesions. *Neuropsychologia, 37,* 939–958.

Kopelman, M.D., Wilson, B.A., & Baddeley, A.D. (1989). The Autobiographical Memory Interview: A new assessment of autobiographical and personal semantic memory in amnesic patients. *Journal of Clinical and Experimental Neuropsychology, 11,* 724–744.

Kopelman, M.D., Wilson, B.A., & Baddeley, A.D. (1990). *The Autobiographical Memory Interview.* Bury St. Edmunds, UK: Thames Valley Test.

Koponen, S., Taiminen, T., Portin, R., et al. (2002). Axis I and II psychiatric disorders after traumatic brain injury: A 30-year follow-up study. *American Journal of Psychiatry, 159,* 1315–1321.

Koppitz, E.M. (1964). *The Bender Gestalt test for young children.* New York: Grune & Stratton.

Korsten, M.A. & Wilson, J.S. (1999). Health effects of alcohol. In R.T. Ammerman et al. (Eds.), *Prevention and societal impact of drug and alcohol abuse.* Mahwah, NJ: Erlbaum.

Kortte, K.B., Horner, M.D., & Windham, W.K. (2002). The Trail Making Test, part B: Cognitive flexibility or ability to maintain set? *Applied Neuropsychology, 9,* 106–109.

Koss, E., Edland, S., Fillenbaum, G., et al. (1996). Clinical and neuropsychological differences between patients with earlier and later onset of Alzheimer's disease: A CERAD analysis, Part XII. *Neurology, 46,* 136–141.

Koss, E., Haxby, J.V., DeCarli, C., et al. (1991). Patterns of performance preservation and loss in healthy elderly. *Developmental Neuropsychology, 7,* 99–113.

Koss, E., Ober, B.A., Delis, D.C., & Friedland, R.P. (1984). The Stroop Color-Word Test: Indicator of dementia severity. *International Journal of Neuroscience, 24,* 53–61.

Koss, E., Patterson, M.B., Mack, J.L., et al. (1998). Reliability and validity of the Tinkertoy Test in evaluating individuals with Alzheimer's disease. *The Clinical Neuropsychologist, 12,* 325–329.

Koss, E., Weiffenbach, J.M., Haxby, J.V., & Friedland, R.P. (1988). Olfactory detection and identification performance are dissociated in early Alzheimer's disease. *Neurology, 38,* 1228–1232.

Kostandov, E.A., Arsumanov, Y.L., Genkina, O.A., et al. (1982). The effects of alcohol on hemispheric functional asymmetry. *Journal of Studies on Alcohol, 43,* 411–426.

Kotler-Cope, S. & Camp, C.J. (1995). Anosognosia in Alzheimer disease. *Alzheimer Disease and Associated Disorders, 9,* 52–56.

Kovacs, A. & Pléh, G. (1987). The effects of anxiety, success and failure in convergent and divergent, verbal and figural tasks. In L. Kardos et al. (Eds.), *Studies in creativity.* Budapest: Akademiai Kialo.

Kovacs, M., Ryan, C., & Obrosky, D.S. (1994). Verbal intellectual and verbal memory performance of youths with childhood-onset insulin-dependent diabetes mellitus. *Journal of Pediatric Psychology, 19,* 475–483.

Kozel, J.J. & Meyers, J.E. (1998). A cross-validation of the Victoria revision of the Category Test. *Archives of Clinical Neuropsychology, 13,* 327–332.

Kozora, E. & Cullum, C.M. (1994). Qualitative features of clock drawings in normal aging and Alzheimer's disease. *Assessment, 1,* 179–188.

Kozora, E. & Cullum, C.M. (1995). Generative naming in normal aging: Total output and qualitative changes using phonemic and semantic constraints. *The Clinical Neuropsychologist, 9,* 313–320.

Kozora, E., Filley, C.M., Julian, L.J., & Cullum, C.M. (1999). Cognitive functioning in patients with chronic obstructive pulmonary disease and mild hypoxemia compared with patients with mild Alzheimer disease and normal controls. *Neuropsychiatry, Neuropsychology, and Behavioral Neurology, 12,* 178–183.

Krabbendam, L., de Vugt, M.E., Derix, M.M., & Jolles, J. (1999). The behavioural assessment of the dysexecutive syndrome as a tool to assess executive functions in schizophrenia. *The Clinical Neuropsychologist, 13,* 370–375.

Kraft, J.F., Schwab, K.A., Salazar, A.M., & Brown, H.R. (1993). Occupational and educational achievements of head injured Vietnam veterans at 15-year follow-up. *Archives of Physical Medicine and Rehabilitation, 74,* 596–601.

Kramer, A.F., Hahn, S., & Gopher, D. (1999). Task coordination and aging: Explorations of executive control processes in the task switching paradigm. *Acta Psychologica, 101,* 339–378.

Kramer, J.H., Blusewicz, M.J., & Preston, K.A. (1989). The premature aging hypothesis: Old before its time? *Journal of Consulting and Clinical Psychology, 57,* 257–262.

Kramer, J.H., Delis, D.C., Blusewicz, M.J., et al. (1988). Verbal memory errors in Alzheimer's and Huntington's dementias. *Developmental Neuropsychology, 4,* 1–15.

Kramer, J.H., Delis, D.C., & Daniel, M. (1988). Sex differences in verbal learning. *Journal of Clinical Psychology, 44*, 907–915.

Kramer, J.H., Levin, B.E., Brandt, J., & Delis, D.C. (1989). Differentiation of Alzheimer's, Huntington's, and Parkinson's disease patients on the basis of verbal learning characteristics. *Neuropsychology, 3*, 111–120.

Kramer, N.A. & Jarvik, L. (1979). Assessment of intellectual changes in the elderly. In A. Raskin & L. Jarvik (Eds.), *Psychiatric symptoms and cognitive loss in the elderly.* Washington, D.C.: Hemisphere.

Kraus, J.F., McArthur, D.L., Silverman, T.A., & Jayaraman, M. (1996). Epidemiology of brain injury. In R.K. Narayan et al. (Eds.), *Neurotrauma.* New York: McGraw-Hill.

Kraus, J.F. & Nourjah, P. (1989). The epidemiology of mild head injury. In H.S. Levin et al. (Eds.), *Mild head injury.* New York: Oxford University Press.

Kraus, J.F. & Peek, C. (1995). The impact of two related prevention strategies on head injury reduction among nonfatally injured motorcycle riders, California, 1991–1993. *Journal of Neurotrauma, 12*, 873–881.

Krauss, I.K. (1980). *Assessing cognitive skills of older workers.* Paper presented at the annual meeting of the American Psychological Association, Montreal, Canada.

Krausz, Y., Bonne, O., Gorfine, M., et al. (1998). Age-related changes in brain perfusion of normal subjects detected by 99mTc-HM-PAO SPECT. *Neuroradiology, 40*, 428–434.

Kreiner, D.S. and Ryan, J.J. (2001). Memory and motor skill components of the WAIS-III Digit Symbol-Coding subtest. *The Clinical Neuropsychologist, 15*, 109–113.

Kreiter, K.T., Copeland, D., Bernardini, G.L., et al. (2002). Predictors of cognitive dysfunction after subarachnoid hemorrhage. *Stroke, 33*, 200–208.

Kremer, H.P.H., Goldberg, Y.P., Andrew, S.E., et al. (1994). Worldwide study of the Huntington's disease mutation. *New England Journal of Medicine, 330*, 1401–1406.

Kremin, H. (1988). Naming and its disorders. In F. Boller & J. Grafman (Eds.), *Handbook of neuropsychology* (Vol. 1). Amsterdam: Elsevier.

Kreuter, M., Dahllof, A.G., Gudjonsson, G., et al. (1998). Sexual adjustment and its predictors after traumatic brain injury. *Brain Injury, 12*, 349–368.

Kreutzer, J.S., Doherty, K.R., Harris, J.A., & Zasler, N.D. (1990). Alcohol use among persons with traumatic brain injury. *Journal of Head Trauma Rehabilitation, 5*, 9–20.

Kreutzer, J.S., Marwitz, J.H., Seel, R., & Serio, C.D. (1996). Validation of a Neurobehavioral Functioning Inventory for adults with traumatic brain injury. *Archives of Physical Medicine and Rehabilitation, 77*, 116–124.

Krikorian, R., Bartok, J., & Gay, N. (1994). Tower of London procedure: A standard method and developmental data. *Journal of Clinical and Experimental Neuropsychology, 16*, 840–850.

Kristof, N.D. (2003). Is race real? *New York Times, 152*, Sect A:19.

Kroencke, D.C., Denney, D.R., & Lynch, S.G. (2001). Depression during exacerbations in multiple sclerosis: the importance of uncertainty. *Multiple Sclerosis, 7*, 237–242.

Kroll, N.E., Markowitsch, H.J., Knight, R.T., & von Cramon, D.Y. (1997). Retrieval of old memories: The temporofrontal hypothesis. *Brain, 120*, 1377–1399.

Krug, R.S. (1967). MMPI response inconsistency of brain damaged individuals. *Journal of Clinical Psychology, 23*, 366.

Krull, K.R., Scott, J.G., & Sherer, M. (1995). Estimation of premorbid intelligence from combined performance and demographic variables. *The Clinical Neuropsychologist, 9*, 83–88.

Krupp, L.B. (1997). Mechanisms, measurement, and management of fatigue in multiple sclerosis. In A.J. Thompson et al. (Eds.), *Mul-* tiple sclerosis: Clinical challenges and controversies. London: Martin Dunitz.

Krupp, L.B. & Elkins, L.E. (2000). Fatigue and declines in cognitive functioning in multiple sclerosis. *Neurology, 55*, 934–939.

Krupp, L.B., Sliwinski, M., Masur, D.M., et al. (1994). Cognitive functioning and depression in patients with chronic fatigue syndrome and multiple sclerosis. *Archives of Neurology, 51*, 705–710.

Kubu, C.S., Grace, G.M., & Parrent, A.G. (2000). Cognitive outcome following pallidotomy: The influence of side of surgery and age of patient at disease onset. *Journal of Neurosurgery, 92*, 384–389.

Kuehn, S.M. & Snow, W.G. (1992). Are the Rey and Taylor Figures equivalent? *Archives of Clinical Neuropsychology, 7*, 445–448.

Kuhl, D.E., Koeppe, R.A., Minoshima, S., et al. (1999). In vivo mapping of cerebral acetylcholinesterase activity in aging and Alzheimer's disease. *Neurology, 52*, 691–699.

Kuhl, P.K. (2000). Language, mind, and brain. Experience alters perception. In M.S. Gazzaniga (Ed.), *The new cognitive neurosciences* (2nd ed.). Cambridge, MA: MIT Press.

Kujala, P., Portin, R., Revonsuo, A., & Ruutiainen, J. (1994). Automatic and controlled information processing in multiple sclerosis. *Brain, 117*, 1115–1126.

Kujala, P., Portin, R., Revonsuo, A., & Ruutiainen, J. (1995). Attention related performance in two cognitively different subgroups of patients with multiple sclerosis. *Journal of Neurology, Neurosurgery and Psychiatry, 59*, 77–82.

Kujala, P., Portin, R., & Ruutiainen, J. (1997). The progress of cognitive decline in multiple sclerosis: A controlled 3-year follow-up. *Brain, 120*, 289–297.

Kukull, W.A. (2001). The association between smoking and Alzheimer's disease: Effects of study design and bias. *Biological Psychiatry, 49*, 194–199.

Kukull, W.A., Larson, E.B., Teri, L., et al. (1994). The Mini-Mental State Examination score and the clinical diagnosis of dementia. *Journal of Clinical Epidemiology, 47*, 1061–1067.

Kulynych, J.J., Vladar, K., Jones, D.W., & Weinberger, D.R. (1994). Gender differences in the normal lateralization of the supratemporal cortex: MRI surface-rendering morphometry of Heschl's gyrus and the planum temporale. *Cerebral Cortex, 4*, 107–118.

Kumkova, E. (1990). Memory for birds' voices: Hemispheric specialization [abstract]. *Journal of Clinical and Experimental Neuropsychology, 12*, 42.

Kumral, E. (2001). Multiple, multilevel, and bihemispheric strokes. In J. Bogousslavsky & L. Caplan (Eds.), *Stroke syndromes* (2nd ed.). Cambridge: Cambridge University Press.

Kumral, E. & Evayapan, D. (2000). Reversed clock phenomenon: A right-hemisphere syndrome. *Neurology, 55*, 151–152.

Kuopio, A.M., Marttila, R.J., Helenius, H., et al. (2000). The quality of life in Parkinson's disease. *Movement Disorders, 15*, 216–223.

Kupersmith, M.J., Shakin, E., Siegel, I.M., & Lieberman, A. (1982). Visual system abnormalities in patients with Parkinson's disease. *Archives of Neurology, 39*, 284–286.

Kupke, T. & Lewis, R. (1989). Relative influence of subject variables and neurological parameters on neuropsychological performance of adult seizure patients. *Archives of Clinical Neuropsychology, 4*, 351–363.

Kurlychek, R.T. (1987). Neuropsychological evaluation of workers exposed to industrial neurotoxins. *American Journal of Forensic Psychology, 5*, 55–66.

Kurlychek, R.T. (1989). Electroencephalography (EEG) in the differential diagnosis of dementia. *Journal of Clinical Psychology, 45*, 117–123.

Kurlychek, R.T. & Glang, A.E. (1984). The use of an information letter to increase compliance and motivation in neuropsychological evaluation of the elderly. *Clinical Gerontologist, 3,* 40–41.

Kurtzke, J.F. (1983a). Epidemiology and risk factors in thrombotic brain infarction. In M.J.G. Harrison & M.L. Dyken (Eds.), *Cerebral vascular disease.* London: Butterworth.

Kurtzke, J.F. (1983b). Rating neurologic impairment in multiple sclerosis: An expanded disability status scale (EDSS). *Neurology, 33,* 1444–1452.

Kurtzke, J.F. (1984). Neuroepidemiology. *Annals of Neurology, 16,* 265–277.

Kurtzke, J.F. (2000). Multiple sclerosis in time and space—geographic clues to cause. *Journal of Neurovirology, 6,* S134–S140.

Kurylo, D.D., Corkin, S., Rizzo, J.F. III, & Growdon, J.H. (1996). Greater relative impairment of object recognition than of visuospatial abilities in Alzheimer's disease. *Neuropsychology, 10,* 74–81.

Kuslansky, G., Buschke, H., Katz, M., et al. (2002). Screening for Alzheimer's disease: The Memory Impairment Screen versus the conventional three-word memory test. *Journal of the American Geriatric Society, 50,* 1086–1091.

Kutas, M. & Dale, A. (1997). Electrical and magnetic readings of mental functions. In M.D. Rugg (Ed.), *Cognitive neuroscience.* Cambridge, MA: MIT Press.

Kuzis, G., Sabe, L., Tiberti, C., et al. (1999). Explicit and implicit learning in patients with Alzheimer disease and Parkinson disease with dementia. *Neuropsychiatry, Neuropsychology, and Behavioral Neurology, 12,* 265–269.

Kwan, P. & Brodie, M. J. (2000). Early identification of refractory epilepsy. *New England Journal of Medicine, 342,* 314–319.

Kwan, P. & Brodie, M. J. (2002). Refractory epilepsy: A progressive, intractable but preventable condition? *Seizure, 11,* 77–84.

Kwentus, J.A., Hart, R.P., Peck, E.T., & Kornstein, S. (1985). Psychiatric complications of closed head trauma. *Psychosomatics, 26,* 8–17.

Laakso, M.P., Halikainen, M., Hanninen, T., et al. (2000). Diagnosis of Alzheimer's disease: MRI of the hippocampus vs delayed recall. *Neuropsychologia, 38,* 579–584.

Laatu, S., Hamalainen, P., Revonsuo, A., et al. (1999). Semantic memory deficit in multiple sclerosis: Impaired understanding of conceptual meanings. *Journal of the Neurological Sciences, 162,* 152–161.

LaBarge, E., Balota, D.A., Storandt, M., & Smith, D.S. (1992). An analysis of confrontation naming errors in senile dementia of the Alzheimer type. *Neuropsychology, 6,* 77–95.

LaBerge, D. (2000). Networks of attention. In M.S. Gazzaniga (Ed.), *The new cognitive neurosciences* (2nd ed.). Cambridge, MA: MIT Press.

Labreche, T.M. (1983). *The Victoria Revision of the Halstead Category Test.* Victoria, Canada: University of Victoria.

LaBuda, J. & Lichtenberg, P. (1999). The role of cognition, depression, and awareness of deficit in predicting geriatric rehabilitation patients' IADL performance. *The Clinical Neuropsychologist, 13,* 258–267.

LaCalle, J.J. (1987). Forensic psychological examinations through an interpreter: Legal and ethical issues. *American Journal of Forensic Psychology, 5,* 29–43.

Lacks, P. (1999). *Bender Gestalt screening for brain dysfunction* (2nd ed.). New York: Wiley.

Lacks, P. & Storandt, M. (1982). Bender Gestalt performance of normal older adults. *Journal of Clinical Psychology, 38,* 624–627.

Lacritz, L.H. & Cullum, C.M. (1998). The Hopkins Verbal Learning Test and the CVLT: A preliminary comparison. *Archives of Clinical Neuropsychology, 13,* 623–628.

Lacritz, L.H., Cullum, C.M., Weiner, M.F., & Rosenberg, R.N. (2001). Comparison of the Hopkins Verbal Learning Test-Revised to the California Verbal Learning Test in Alzheimer's disease. *Applied Neuropsychology, 8,* 180–184.

Ladavas, E., del Pesce, M., & Provinciali, L. (1989). Unilateral attention deficits and hemispheric asymmetries in the control of visual attention. *Neuropsychologia, 27,* 353–366.

Lafargue, G. & Sirigu, A. (2002). Sensation of effort is altered in Huntington's disease. *Neuropsychologia, 40,* 1654–1661.

Lafleche, G. & Albert, M.S. (1995). Executive function deficits in mild Alzheimer's disease. *Neuropsychology, 9,* 313–320.

Laforce, R., Jr. & MacLeod, L.M. (2001). Symptom cluster associated with mild traumatic brain injury in university students. *Perceptual and Motor Skills, 93,* 281–288.

Laine, M. (1988). Correlates of word fluency performance. In P. Koivuselka-Sallinen & L. Sarajarvi (Eds.), *Studies in languages* (Vol. 12). Joensuu, Finland: University of Joensuu.

Laine, M. & Butters, N. (1982). A preliminary study of the problem-solving strategies of detoxified long-term alcoholics. *Drug and Alcohol Dependence, 10,* 235–242.

Laine, M., Vuorinen, E., & Rinne, J.O. (1997). Picture naming deficits in vascular dementia and Alzheimer's disease. *Journal of Clinical and Experimental Neuropsychology, 19,* 126–140.

Lal, S., Merbitz, C.P., & Grip, J.C. (1988). Modification of function in head injured patients with Sinemet. *Brain Injury, 2,* 225–233.

Lamar, M., Podell, K., Carew, T.G., et al. (1997). Perseverative behavior in Alzheimer's disease and subcortical ischemic vascular dementia. *Neuropsychology, 11,* 523–534.

Lamar, M., Zonderman, A.B., & Resnick, S. (2002). Contribution of specific cognitive processes to executive functioning in an aging population. *Neuropsychology, 16,* 156–162.

Lambert, J., Eustache, F., Viader, F., et al. (1996). Agraphia in Alzheimer's disease: An independent lexical impairment. *Brain and Language, 53,* 222–233.

Lamberty, G.J. & Bieliauskas, L.A. (1993). Distinguishing between depression and dementia in the elderly: A review of neuropsychological findings. *Archives of Clinical Neuropsychology, 8,* 149–170.

Lamberty, G.J., Kennedy, C.M., & Flashman, L.A. (1995). Clinical utility of the CERAD word list memory test. *Applied Neuropsychology, 2,* 170–173.

Lambon Ralph, M.A., Graham, K.S., Ellis, A.W., & Hodges, J.R. (1998). Naming in semantic dementia—what matters? *Neuropsychologia, 36,* 775–784.

Lambon Ralph, M.A., Powell, J., Howard, D., et al. (2001). Semantic memory is impaired in both dementia with Lewy bodies and dementia of Alzheimer's type: a comparative neuropsychological study and literature review. *Journal of Neurology, Neurosurgery and Psychiatry, 70,* 149–156.

Lancet Editors (1986). Psychosocial outcome of head injury. *Lancet, i,* 1361–1362.

Landis, T., Cummings, J.L., Benson, D.F., & Palmer, D. (1986). Loss of topographical familiarity. *Archives of Neurology, 43,* 132–136.

Landis, T., Cummings, J.L., Christen, L., et al. (1986). Are unilateral right posterior cerebral lesions sufficient to cause prosopagnosia? *Cortex, 22,* 243–252.

Landis, Th. & Regard, M. (1988). The right hemisphere's access to lexical meaning: A function of its release from left-hemisphere control? In C. Chiarello (Ed.), *Right hemisphere contributions to lexical semantics.* New York: Springer-Verlag.

Landis, T., Regard, M., Graves, R., & Goodglass, H. (1983). Semantic paralexia: A release of right hemispheric function from left hemisphere control? *Neuropsychologia, 21,* 359–364.

Landrø, N.I., Sletvold, H., & Celius, E.G. (2000). Memory functioning and emotional changes in early phase multiple sclerosis. *Archives of Clinical Neuropsychology, 15,* 37–46.

Landrø, N.I., Stiles, T.C., & Sletvold, H. (2001). Neuropsychological function in nonpsychotic unipolar major depression. *Neuropsychiatry, Neuropsychology, and Behavioral Neurology, 14,* 233–240.

Langdon, D.W. & Thompson, A.J. (1999). Multiple sclerosis: A preliminary study of selected variables affecting rehabilitation outcome. *Multiple Sclerosis, 5,* 94–100.

Langdon, D.W. & Warrington, E.K. (1997). The abstraction of numerical relations: A role for the right hemisphere in arithmetic? *Journal of the International Neuropsychological Society, 3,* 260–268.

Lange, K.W., Tucha, O., Steup, A., et al. (1995). Subjective time estimation in Parkinson's disease. *Journal of Neural Transmission 46(Suppl.),* 433–438.

Langston, J.W. & Koller, W.C. (1991). The next frontier in Parkinson's disease: Presymptomatic detection. *Neurology, 41(Suppl. 2),* 5–7.

Lannoo, E., Colardyn, F., Vandekerckhove, T., et al. (1998). Subjective complaints versus neuropsychological test performance after moderate to severe head injury. *Acta Neurochirurgica, 140,* 245–253.

Lannoo, E. & Vingerhoets, G. (1997). Flemish normative data on common neuropsychological tests: Influence of age, education, and gender. *Psychologica Belgica, 37,* 141–155.

Lansdell, H. & Donnelly, E.F. (1977). Factor analysis of the Wechsler Adult Intelligence Scale subtests and the Halstead-Reitan Category and Tapping tests. *Journal of Consulting and Clinical Psychology, 45,* 412–416.

Lansdell, H. & Smith, F.J. (1975). Asymmetrical cerebral function for two WAIS factors and their recovery after brain injury. *Journal of Consulting and Clinical Psychology, 43,* 923.

Lansing, A.E., Ivnik, R.J., Cullum, C.M., & Randolph, C. (1999). An empirically derived short form of the Boston Naming Test. *Archives of Clinical Neuropsychology, 14,* 481–487.

Laperriere, N., Zuraw, L., & Cairncross, G. (2002). Radiotherapy for newly diagnosed malignant glioma in adults: a systematic review. *Radiotherapy and Oncology, 64,* 259.

Laplane, D., Baulac, M., Widlocher, D., & Dubois, B. (1984). Pure psychic akinesia with bilateral lesions of basal ganglia. *Journal of Neurology, Neurosurgery and Psychiatry, 47,* 377–385.

Larcombe, N.A. & Wilson, P.H. (1984). An evaluation of cognitive-behaviour therapy for depression in patients with multiple sclerosis. *British Journal of Psychiatry, 145,* 366–371.

Larrabee, G.J. (1986). Another look at VIQ-PIQ scores and unilateral brain damage. *International Journal of Neuroscience, 29,* 141–148.

Larrabee, G.J. (1990). Cautions in the use of neuropsychological evaluation in legal settings. *Neuropsychology, 4,* 239–247.

Larrabee, G.J. (1998). Somatic malingering on the MMPI and MMPI-2 in personal injury litigants. *The Clinical Neuropsychologist, 12,* 179–188.

Larrabee, G.J. (1999). Current controversies in mild head injury: Scientific and methodological considerations. In N.R. Varney & R.J. Roberts (Eds.), *The evaluation and treatment of mild traumatic brain injury.* Mahway, NJ: Erlbaum.

Larrabee, G.J. (2003). Exaggerated MMPI-2 symptom report in personal injury litigants with malingered neurocognitive deficit. *Archives of Clinical Neuropsychology, 18,* 673–686.

Larrabee, G.J. (2000). Association between IQ and neuropsychological test performance: Commentary on Tremont, Hoffman, Scott, and Adams (1998). *The Clinical Neuropsychologist, 14,* 139–145.

Larrabee, G.J. & Crook, T.H. III (1996). Computers and memory. In I. Grant & K.M. Adams (Eds.), *Neuropsychological assessment of neuropsychiatric disorders* (2nd ed.). New York: Oxford University Press.

Larrabee, G.J. & Curtiss, G. (1985). Factor structure and construct validity of the Denman Neuropsychology Memory Scale. *International Journal of Neuroscience, 25,* 269–276.

Larrabee, G.J. & Curtiss, G. (1995). Construct validity of various verbal and visual memory tests. *Journal of Clinical and Experimental Neuropsychology, 17,* 536–547.

Larrabee, G.J. & Kane, R.L. (1983). Differential drawing size associated with unilateral brain damage. *Neuropsychologia, 21,* 173–177.

Larrabee, G.J. & Kane, R.L. (1986). Reversed digit repetition involves visual and verbal processes. *International Journal of Neuroscience, 30,* 11–15.

Larrabee, G.J., Kane, R.L., & Schuck, J.R. (1983). Factor analysis of the WAIS and Wechsler Memory Scale: An analysis of the construct validity of the Wechsler Memory Scale. *Journal of Clinical Neuropsychology, 5,* 159–168.

Larrabee, G.J., Kane, R.L., Schuck, J.R., & Francis, D.J. (1985). Construct validity of various memory testing procedures. *Journal of Clinical and Experimental Neuropsychology, 7,* 239–250.

Larrabee, G.J., Largen, J.W., & Levin, H.S. (1985). Sensitivity of age-decline resistant ("Hold") WAIS subtests to Alzheimer's disease. *Journal of Clinical and Experimental Neuropsychology, 7,* 497–504.

Larrabee, G.J. & Levin, H.S. (1986). Memory self-ratings and objective test performance in a normal elderly sample. *Journal of Clinical and Experimental Neuropsychology, 8,* 275–284.

Larrabee, G.J., McEntee, W. J., Youngjohn, J. R., & Crook, T. H. III (1992). Age-associated memory impairment: Diagnosis, research, and treatment. In M. Bergener et al. (Eds.), *Aging and mental disorders: International perspectives.* New York: Springer.

Larrabee, G.J., Trahan, D.E., & Curtiss, G. (1992). Construct validity of the Continuous Visual Memory Test. *Archives of Clinical Neuropsychology, 7,* 395–405.

Larrabee, G.J., Trahan, D.E., Curtiss, G., & Levin, H.S. (1988). Normative data for the Verbal Selective Reminding Test. *Neuropsychology, 2,* 173–182.

Larrabee, G.J., Trahan, D.E., & Levin, H.S. (2000). Normative data for a six-trial administration of the Verbal Selective Reminding Test. *The Clinical Neuropsychologist, 14,* 110–118.

Larrabee, G.J., Youngjohn, J.R., Sudilovsky, A., & Crook, T.H. III. (1993). Accelerated forgetting in Alzheimer-type dementia. *Journal of Clinical and Experimental Neuropsychology, 14,* 701–712.

Larrain, C.M. & Cimino, C.R. (1998). Alternate forms of the Boston Naming Test in Alzheimer's disease. *The Clinical Neuropsychologist, 12,* 525–530.

Larson, E. B., Reifler, B. V., Featherstone, H. J., & English, D. R. (1984). Dementia in elderly outpatients: A prospective study. *Annals of Internal Medicine, 100,* 417–423.

La Rue, A. (1989). Patterns of performance on the Fuld Object Memory Evaluation in elderly inpatients with depression or dementia. *Journal of Clinical and Experimental Neuropsychology, 11,* 409–422.

La Rue, A., D'Elia, L.F., Clarke, E.O., et al. (1986). Clinical tests of memory in dementia, depression, and healthy aging. *Journal of Psychology and Aging, 1,* 69–77.

La Rue, A. & Jarvik, L.R. (1987). Cognitive function and prediction of dementia in old age. *International Journal of Aging and Human Development, 25,* 79–89.

La Rue, A. & Markee, T. (1995). Clinical assessment research with older adults. *Psychological Assessment, 7,* 376–386.

La Rue, A., Romero, L.J., Ortiz, I.E., et al. (1999). Neuropsychological performance of Hispanic and non-Hispanic older adults: An epidemiologic survey. *The Clinical Neuropsychologist, 13,* 474–486.

Lashley, K.S. (1929). *Brain mechanisms and intelligence: A quanti-*

tative study of injuries to the brain. Chicago: University of Chicago Press.

Lashley, K.S. (1938). Factors limiting recovery after central nervous system lesions. *Journal of Nervous and Mental Disease, 88,* 733–755.

Lasker, A.G. & Zee, D.S. (1997). Ocular motor abnormalities in Huntington's disease. *Vision Research, 37,* 3639–3645.

Lassonde, M., Sauerwein, H., Chicoine, A.-J., & Geoffroy, G. (1991). Absence of disconnexion syndrome in callosal agenesis and early callosotomy: Brain reorganization or lack of structural specificity during ontogeny? *Neuropsychologia, 29,* 481–495.

Laterra, J. & Brem, H. (2002). Primary brain tumours in adults. In A.K. Asbury et al. (Eds.), *Diseases of the nervous system* (3rd ed.). Cambridge: Cambridge University Press.

La Torre, G. (2003). Epidemiology of scooter accidents in Italy: The effectiveness of mandatory use of helmets in preventing incidence and severity of head trauma. *Recenti Progressi in Medicina, 94,* 1–4.

Lau, C., Wands, K., Merskey, H., et al. (1988). Sensitivity and specificity of the Extended Scale for Dementia. *Archives of Neurology, 45,* 839–852.

Launer, L.J., Andersen, K., Dewey, M.E., et al. (1999). Rates and risk factors for dementia and Alzheimer's disease: Results from eurodem pooled analyses. EURODEM incidence research group and work groups. European studies of dementia. *Neurology, 52,* 78–84.

Lauritzen, M. (1987). Cerebral blood flow in migraine and cortical spreading depression. *Acta Scandanavica, 76(Suppl. 113),* 1–40.

Lauritzen, M. (1994). Pathophysiology of the migraine aura: The spreading depression theory. *Brain, 117,* 199–210.

Laursen, P. (1997). The impact of aging on cognitive functions. An 11 year follow-up study of four age cohorts. *Acta Neurologica Scandinanvica Supplementum, 172,* 7–86.

Lauterbach, E.C., Cummings, J.L., Duffy, J., et al. (1998). Neuropsychiatric correlates and treatment of lenticulostriatal diseases: A review of the literature and overview of research opportunities in Huntington's, Wilson's, and Fahr's diseases. A report of the ANPA committee on research. American Neuropsychiatric Association. *Journal of Neuropsychiatry and Clinical Neurosciences, 10,* 249–266.

Lavie, N. (2001). Capacity limits in selective attention: Behavioral evidence and implications for neural activity. In J. Braun et al. (Eds.), *Visual attention and cortical circuits.* Cambridge, MA: MIT Press.

Lawrence, A.D., Sahakian, B.J., Rogers, R.D., et al. (1999). Discrimination, reversal, and shift learning in Huntington's disease: Mechanisms of impaired response selection. *Neuropsychologia, 37,* 1359–1374.

Lawson, J.S. & Inglis, J. (1983). A laterality index of cognitive impairment after hemispheric damage: A measure derived from a principal-components analysis of the Wechsler Adult Intelligence Scale. *Journal of Consulting and Clinical Psychology, 51,* 832–840.

Lawton, M.P. (1986). Contextual perspectives: Psychosocial influences. In L.W. Poon (Ed.), *Handbook for clinical memory assessment of older adults.* Washington, D.C.: American Psychological Association.

Lazareth, I. & Priollet, P. (1997). Malingering in vascular disease [in French]. *Journal des Maladies Vasculaires, 22,* 229–233.

Lazarus, L.W., Newton, N., Cohler, B., et al. (1987). Frequency and presentation of depressive symptoms in patients with primary degenerative dementia. *American Journal of Psychiatry, 144,* 41–45.

Lazeron, R.H., Langdon, D.W., Filippi, M., et al. (2000). Neuropsychological impairment in multiple sclerosis patients: The role of (juxta)cortical lesions on FLAIR. *Multiple Sclerosis, 6,* 280–285.

Lazeron, R.H., Rombouts, S.A., Machielsen, W.C., et al. (2000). Visualizing brain activation during planning: The Tower of London test adapted for functional MR imaging. *American Journal of Neuroradiology, 21,* 1407–1414.

Lazzarino, L.G., Nicolai, A., Valassi, F., & Biasizzo, E. (1991). Language disturbances from mesencephalo-thalamic infarcts. Identification of thalamic nuclei by CT-reconstructions. *Neuroradiology, 33,* 300–304.

Le, T.H., Pardo, J.V., & Hu, X. (1998). 4T-fMRI study of nonspatial shifting of selective attention: cerebellar and parietal contributions. *Journal of Neurophysiology, 79,* 1535–1548.

Leach, L., Kaplan, E., Rewilak, D., et al. (2000). *Kaplan-Baycrest Neurocognitive Assessment (manual).* San Antonio, TX: The Psychological Corporation.

Leao, A.A.P. (1944). Spreading depression of activity in cerebral cortex. *Journal of Neurophysiology, 7,* 359–390.

Leathem, J. (1999). Comment. Un-earthing the IQ: in support of limited application of cognitive assessment. *New Zealand Council for Educational Research, 3,* 22–23.

Lebert, F., Pasquier, F., Souliez, L., & Petit, H. (1998). Frontotemporal behavioral scale. *Alzheimer Disease and Associated Disorders, 12,* 335–339.

Lebrun, Y. (1987). Anosognosia in aphasics. *Cortex, 23,* 251–263.

Lebrun, Y. & Hoops, R. (1974). *Intelligence and aphasia.* Amsterdam: Swets and Zeitlinger.

Le Carret, N., Lafont, S., Letenneur, L., et al. (2003). The effect of education on cognitive performance and its implications for the constitution of the cognitive reserve. *Developmental Neuropsychology, 23,* 317–337.

Lechtenberg, R. (1999). *Epilepsy and the family.* Cambridge, MA: Harvard University Press.

Leckliter, I.N. & Matarazzo, J.D. (1989). The influence of age, education, IQ, gender, and alcohol abuse on Halstead-Reitan neuropsychological test battery performance. *Journal of Clinical Psychology, 45,* 484–512.

Leclercq, M. (2002). Theoretical aspects of the main components and functions of attention. In M. Leclercq & P. Zimmerman (Eds.), *Applied neuropsychology of attention.* New York: Psychology Press.

Leclercq, M. & Azouvi, P. (2002). Attention after traumatic brain injury. In M. Leclercq & P. Zimmerman (Eds.), *Applied neuropsychology of attention.* New York: Psychology Press.

Leclercq, M., Couillet, J., Azouvi, P., et al. (2000). Dual task performance after severe diffuse traumatic brain injury or vascular prefrontal damage. *Journal of Clinical and Experimental Neuropsychology, 22,* 339–350.

Leclercq, M., Deloche, G., & Rousseaux, M. (2002). Attentional complaints evoked by traumatic brain-injured and stroke patients: Frequency and importance. In M. Leclercq & P. Zimmerman (Eds.), *Applied neuropsychology of attention.* New York: Psychology Press.

Leclercq, M. & Sturm, W. (2002). Rehabilitation of attention disorders: A literature review. In M. Leclercq & P. Zimmerman (Eds.), *Applied neuropsychology of attention.* New York: Psychology Press.

Leclercq, P.D., McKenzie, J.E., Graham, D.I., & Gentleman, S.M. (2001). Axonal injury is accentuated in the caudal corpus callosum of head injured patients. *Journal of Neurotrauma, 18,* 1–9.

Lecours, A., Mehler, J., Parente, M.A., et al. (1987). Illiteracy and brain damage: 1. Aphasia testing in culturally contrasted populations (control subjects). *Neuropsychologia, 25,* 231–245.

Lee, A.C., Robbins, T.W., Pickard, J.D., & Owen, A.M. (2000). Asymmetric frontal activation during episodic memory: The effects of stimulus type on encoding and retrieval. *Neuropsychologia, 38,* 677–692.

Lee, G.P., Bechara, A., Adolphs, R., et al. (1998). Clinical and physiological effects of stereotaxic bilateral amygdalotomy for intractable aggression. *Journal of Neuropsychiatry and Clinical Neuroscience, 10,* 413–420.

Lee, G.P., Loring, D.W., & Martin, R.C. (1992). Rey's 15 item visual memory test for the detection of malingering: Normative observations on patients with neurological disorders. *Psychological Assessment, 4,* 43–46.

Lee, G.P., Loring, D.W., Meador, K.J., & Brooks, B.B. (1990). Hemispheric specialization for emotional expression: A reexamination of results from intracarotid administration of sodium amobarbital. *Brain and Cognition, 12,* 267–280.

Lee, G.P., Loring, D.W., & Thompson, J.L. (1989). Construct validity of material-specific memory measures following unilateral temporal lobe ablations. *Psychological Assessment, 1,* 192–197.

Lee, G.P., Meador, K.J., Smith, J.R., et al. (1988). Preserved cross-modal association following bilateral amygdalotomy in man. *International Journal of Neuroscience, 40,* 47–55.

Lee, G.P., Strauss, E., Loring, D.W., & McCloskey, L. (1997). Sensitivity of figural fluency on the Five-Point Test to focal neurological dysfunction. *The Clinical Neuropsychologist, 11,* 59–68.

Lee, J.H. (1999). Test anxiety and working memory. *Journal of Experimental Education, 67,* 218–240.

Lee, J.H., Lee, K.U., Lee, D.Y., et al. (2002). Development of the Korean version of the Consortium to Establish a Registry for Alzheimer's Disease assessment packet (CERAD-K): Clinical and neuropsychological assessment batteries. *Journals of Gerontology. Series B, Psychological Sciences and Social Sciences, 57,* 47–53.

Lee, R.C. (1997). Injury by electrical forces: Pathophysiology, manifestations, and therapy. *Current Problems in Surgery, 34,* 667–764.

Lee, R.C., Cannaday, D.J., & Hammer, S.M. (1993). Transient and stable ionic permeabilization of isolated skeletal muscle cells after electric shock. *Journal of Burn Care Rehabilitation, 14,* 528–540.

Lee, T., Yuen, K., & Chan, C. (2002). Normative data for neuropsychological measures of fluency, attention, and memory measures for Hong Kong Chinese. *Journal of Clinical and Experimental Neuropsychology, 24,* 615–632.

Lee, T.G. & Solomon, G.D. (1996). Incidence of migraine during weekends vs. weekdays [abstract]. *Headache, 36,* 269.

Lee, T.M. & Chan, C.C. (2000). Are Trail Making and Color Trails tests of equivalent constructs? *Journal of Clinical and Experimental Neuropsychology, 22,* 529–534.

Lee, T.M., Yip, J.T., & Jones-Gotman, M. (2002). Memory deficits after resection from left or right anterior temporal lobe in humans: A meta-analytic review. *Epilepsia, 43,* 283–291.

Leeds, L., Meara, R.J., Woods, R., & Hobson, J.P. (2001). A comparison of the new executive functioning domains of the CAMCOG-R with existing tests of executive function in elderly stroke survivors. *Age and Aging, 30,* 251–254.

Lees, A.J. (1990). Progressive supranuclear palsy (Steele-Richardson-Olszewski syndrome). In J.L. Cummings (Ed.), *Subcortical dementia.* New York: Oxford University Press.

Lees, A.J. & Smith, E. (1983). Cognitive deficits in the early stages of Parkinson's disease. *Brain, 106,* 257–270.

Lees-Haley, P.R. (1989). Malingering emotional distress on the SCL-90-R: Toxic exposure and cancerphobia. *Psychological Reports, 65,* 1203–1208.

Lees-Haley, P.R. (1997). Attorneys influence expert evidence in forensic psychological and neuropsychological cases. *Assessment, 4,* 321–324.

Lees-Haley, P.R., English, L.T., & Glenn, W.J. (1991). A Fake Bad Scale on the MMPI-2 for personal injury claimants. *Psychological Reports, 68,* 203–210.

Lees-Haley, P.R., Williams, C.W., & English, L.T. (1996). Response bias in self-reported history of plaintiffs compared with nonlitigating patients. *Psychological Reports, 79,* 811–888.

Le Fever, F.F. (1985). A noncoding motoric equivalent measures most of what the Digit Symbol does, including age changes. *Perceptual and Motor Skills, 61,* 371–377.

Leff, A., Crinion, J., Scott, S., et al. (2002). A physiological change in the homotopic cortex following left posterior temporal lobe infarction. *Annals of Neurology, 51,* 553–558.

Le Gall, D., Joseph, P.A., & Truelle, J.L. (1987). Le syndrome frontal post-traumatique. *Neuropsychologie, 2,* 257–265.

Lehmann, J.F., DeLatour, B.J., Fowler, R.S., Jr., et al. (1975). Stroke rehabilitation: Outcome and prediction. *Archives of Physical Medicine and Rehabilitation, 56,* 383–389.

Lehmann, U., Gobiet, W., Regel, G., et al. (1997). Functional neuropsychological and social outcome of polytrauma patients with severe craniocerebral trauma. *Unfallchirurg, 100,* 552–560.

Leibson, C.L., Rocca, N.A., Hanson, V.A., et al. (1997). Risk of dementia among persons with diabetes mellitus: A population-based cohort study. *American Journal of Epidemiology, 145,* 301–308.

Leicester, J., Sidman, M., Stoddard, L.T., & Mohr, J.P. (1969). Some determinants of visual neglect. *Journal of Neurology, Neurosurgery, and Psychiatry, 32,* 580–587.

Leidy, N.K., Elixhauser, A., Rentz, A.M., et al. (1999). Telephone validation of the Quality of Life in Epilepsy Inventory-89 (QOLIE-89). *Epilepsia, 40,* 97–106.

Leiguarda, R.C., Pramstaller, P.P., Merello, M., et al. (1997). Apraxia in Parkinson's disease, progressive supranuclear palsy, multiple system atrophy and neuroleptic-induced parkinsonism. *Brain, 120,* 75–90.

Leijdekkers, M.L.A., Passchier, J., Goudswaard, P., et al. (1990). Migraine patients cognitively impaired? *Headache, 30,* 352–358.

Leiner, H.C., Leiner, A.L., & Dow, R.S. (1987). Does the cerebellum contribute to mental skills? *Behavioral Neuroscience, 100,* 443–454.

Leiner, H.C., Leiner, A.L., & Dow, R.S. (1989). Reappraising the cerebellum: What does the hindbrain contribute to the forebrain? *Behavioral Neuroscience, 103,* 998–1008.

Leininger, B.E., Gramling, S.E., Farrell, A.D., et al. (1990). Neuropsychological deficits in symptomatic minor head injury patients after concussion and mild concussion. *Journal of Neurology, Neurosurgery and Psychiatry, 53,* 293–296.

Leininger, B.E., Kreutzer, J.S., & Hill, M.R. (1991). Comparison of minor and severe head injury emotional sequelae using the MMPI. *Brain Injury, 5,* 199–205.

Leist, M. & Nicotera, P. (1997). Cell death: Apoptosis versus necrosis. In K.M.A. Welch et al. (Eds.), *Primer on cerebrovascular diseases.* San Diego: Academic Press.

Leli, D.A. & Filskov, S.B. (1984). Clinical detection of intellectual deterioration associated with brain damage. *Journal of Clinical Psychology, 40,* 1435–1441.

Leneman, M., Buchanan, L., & Rovet, J. (2001). *Where* and *what* visuospatial processing in adolescents with congenital hypothyroidism. *Journal of the International Neuropsychological Society, 7,* 556–562.

Leng, N.R.C. & Parkin, A.J. (1988a). Amnesic patients can benefit from instructions to use imagery. Evidence against the cognitive mediation hypothesis. *Cortex, 24,* 33–39.

Leng, N.R.C. & Parkin, A.J. (1988b). Double dissociation of frontal dysfunction in organic amnesia. *British Journal of Clinical Psychology, 27,* 359–362.

Leng, N.R.C. & Parkin, A.J. (1989). Aetiological variation in the amnesic syndrome: Comparisons using the Brown-Peterson task. *Cortex, 25,* 251–259.

Leng, N.R.C. & Parkin, A.J. (1990). The assessment of memory disorders: A review of some current clinical tests. *Clinical Rehabilitation, 4,* 159–165.

Lennie, P. (2001). Color coding in the cortex. In K.R. Gegenfurtner & L.T. Sharpe (Eds.), *Color vision. From genes to perception.* New York: Cambridge University Press.

Lennox, W.G. (1942). Brain injury, drugs and environment as causes of mental decay in epilepsy. *American Journal of Psychiatry, 99,* 174–180.

Lenzer, I.I. (1980). Halstead-Reitan test battery: A problem of differential diagnosis. *Perceptual and Motor Skills, 50,* 611–630.

Lenzi, G.L. & Padovani, A. (1994). The contribution of imaging techniques to current knowledge of the frontal lobes. In F. Boller & J. Grafman (Eds.), *Handbook of neuropsychology* (Vol. 9). Amsterdam: Elsevier.

Leo, G.J. & Rao, S.M. (1988). Effects of intravenous physostigmine and lecithin on memory loss in multiple sclerosis: Report of a pilot study. *Journal of Neurologic Rehabilitation, 2,* 123–129.

Leon, J., Cheng, C.K., & Neumann, P.J. (1998). Alzheimer's disease care: Costs and potential savings. *Health Affairs (Project Hope), 17,* 206–216.

Leonard, G., Jones, L., & Milner, B. (1988). Residual impairment in handgrip strength after unilateral frontal-lobe lesions. *Neuropsychologia, 26,* 555–564.

Leonberger, F.T., Nicks, S.D., Goldfader, P.R., & Munz, D.C. (1991). Factor analysis of the Wechsler Memory Scale-Revised and the Halstead-Reitan Neuropsychological Battery. *The Clinical Neuropsychologist, 5,* 83–88.

Leopold, N.A. & Borson, A.J. (1997). An alphabetical "WORLD." A new version of an old test. *Neurology, 49,* 1521–1524.

Lerner, A.J. & Whitehouse, P.J. (2002). Neuropsychiatric aspects of dementias associated with motor dysfunction. In S.C. Yudofsky & R.E. Hales (Eds.), *Textbook of neuropsychiatry and clinical neurosciences* (4th ed.). Washington, D.C.: American Psychiatric Publishing.

Leroi, I. & Michalon, M. (1998). Treatment of the psychiatric manifestations of Huntington's disease: A review of the literature. *Canadian Journal of Psychiatry, 43,* 933–940.

Lesher, E.L. & Whelihan, W.M. (1986). Reliability of mental status instruments administered to nursing home residents. *Journal of Consulting and Clinical Psychology, 54,* 726–727.

Leskela, M., Hietanen, M., Kalska, H., et al. (1999). Executive functions and speed of mental processing in elderly patients with frontal or nonfrontal ischemic stroke. *European Journal of Neurology, 6,* 653–661.

Lesnik, P.G., Ciesielski, K.T., Hart, B.L., et al., (1998). Evidence for cerebellar-frontal subsystem changes in children treated with intrathecal chemotherapy for leukemia: Enhanced data analysis using an effect size model. *Archives of Neurology, 55,* 1561–1568.

Lesser, R. (1976). Verbal and non-verbal memory components in the Token Test. *Neuropsychologia, 14,* 79–85.

Lesser, R.P. (1996). Psychogenic seizures. *Neurology, 46,* 1499–1507.

Lesser, R.P., Lüders, H., Wyllie, E., et al. (1986). Mental deterioration in epilepsy. *Epilepsia, 27,* S105–S123.

Lester, M.L. & Fishbein, D.H. (1988). Nutrition and childhood neuropsychological disorders. In R.E. Tarter et al. (Eds.), *Medical neuropsychology: The impact of disease on behavior.* New York: Plenum Press.

Lethlean, J.B. & Murdoch, B.E. (1994). Naming errors in multiple sclerosis: Support for a combined semantic/perceptual deficit. *Journal of Neurolinguistics, 8,* 207–223.

Lethlean, J.B. & Murdoch, B.E. (1997). Performance of subjects with multiple sclerosis on tests of high-level language. *Aphasiology, 11,* 39–57.

Levav, M., Mirsky, A.F., French, L.M., et al. (1998). Multinational neuropsychological testing: Performance of children and adults. *Journal of Clinical and Experimental Neuropsychology, 20,* 658–672.

Levin, B.E. (1990). Spatial cognition in Parkinson disease. *Alzheimer Disease and Associated Disorders, 4,* 161–170.

Levin, B.E., Llabre, M.M., Reisman, S., et al. (1991). Visuospatial impairment in Parkinson's disease. *Neurology, 41,* 365–369.

Levin, B.E., Llabre, M.M., & Weiner, W.J. (1988). Parkinson's disease and depression: Psychometric properties of the Beck Depression Inventory. *Journal of Neurology, Neurosurgery and Psychiatry, 51,* 1401–1404.

Levin, B.E., Llabre, M.M., & Weiner, W.J. (1989). Cognitive impairments associated with early Parkinson's disease. *Neurology, 39,* 557–561.

Levin, B.E., Tomer, R., & Rey, G.J. (1992). Clinical correlates of cognitive impairment in Parkinson's disease. In S.J. Huber & J.L. Cummings (Eds.), *Parkinson's disease: Neurobehavioral aspects.* New York: Oxford University Press.

Levin, H.S. (1983). *The Paced Auditory Serial Additon Test-Revised.* Unpublished manuscript.

Levin, H.S. (1985). Outcome after head injury. Part II. Neurobehavioral recovery. In D.P. Becker & J.T. Povlishock (Eds.), *Central nervous system trauma. Status report–1985.* Washington, D.C.: National Institutes of Health.

Levin, H.S. (1986). Learning and memory. In H.J. Hannay (Ed.), *Experimental techniques in human neuropsychology.* New York: Oxford University Press.

Levin, H.S. (1991). Aphasia after head injury. In M.T. Sarno (Ed.), *Acquired aphasia* (2nd ed.). San Diego: Academic Press, pp. 455–498.

Levin, H.S. (1995). Neurobehavioral outcome of closed head injury: Implications for clinical trials. *Journal of Neurotrauma, 12,* 601–610.

Levin, H.S., Amparo, E., Eisenberg, H.M., et al. (1987). Magnetic resonance imaging and computerized tomography in relation to the neurobehavioral sequelae of mild and moderate head injuries. *Journal of Neurosurgery, 66,* 706–713.

Levin, H.S., Benton, A.L., & Grossman, R.G. (1982). *Neurobehavioral consequences of closed head injury.* New York: Oxford University Press.

Levin, H.S., Benton, A.L., Muizelaar, J.P., & Eisenberg, H.M. (Eds.) (1996). *Catastrophic brain injury.* New York: Oxford University Press.

Levin, H.S., Brown, S.A., Song, J.X., et al. (2001). Depression and posttraumatic stress disorder at three months after mild to moderate traumatic brain injury. *Journal of Clinical and Experimental Neuropsychology, 23,* 754–769.

Levin, H.S., Gary, H.E., Eisenberg, H.M., et al. (1990). Neurobehavioral outcome 1 year after severe head injury: Experience of the traumatic coma data bank. *Journal of Neurosurgery, 73,* 699–709.

Levin, H.S., Goldstein, F.C., High, W.M., Jr., et al. (1988). Disproportionately severe memory deficit in relation to normal intellectual functioning after closed head injury. *Journal of Neurology, Neurosurgery and Psychiatry, 51,* 1294–1301.

Levin, H.S., Goldstein, F.C., Williams, D.H., & Eisenberg, H.M. (1991). The contribution of frontal lobe lesions to the neurobehavioral outcome of closed head injury. In H.S. Levin et al. (Eds.), *Frontal lobe function and dysfunction.* New York: Oxford University Press.

Levin, H.S. & Grafman, J. (Eds.) (2000). *Cerebral reorganization after brain damage.* New York: Oxford University Press.

Levin, H.S. & Grossman, R.G. (1978). Behavioral sequelae of closed head injury. *Archives of Neurology, 35,* 720–727.

Levin, H.S., Grossman, R.G., Rose, J.E., & Teasdale, G. (1979).

Long-term neuropsychological outcome of closed head injury. *Journal of Neurosurgery, 50,* 412–422.

Levin, H.S., Hamsher, K. de S., & Benton, A.L. (1975). A short form of the Test of Facial Recognition for clinical use. *Journal of Psychology, 91,* 223–228.

Levin, H.S., High, W.M., Jr., & Eisenberg, H.M. (1988). Learning and forgetting during posttraumatic amnesia in head injured patients. *Journal of Neurology, Neurosurgury and Psychiatry, 51,* 14–20.

Levin, H.S., High, W.M., Goethe, K.E., et al. (1987). The Neurobehavioral Rating Scale Assessment of the behavioural sequelae of head injury by the clinician. *Journal of Neurology, Neurosurgery and Psychiatry, 50,* 183–193.

Levin, H.S., High, W.M., Meyers, C.A., et al. (1985). Impairment of remote memory after closed head injury. *Journal of Neurology, Neurosurgery, and Psychiatry, 48,* 556–563.

Levin, H.S., Mattis, S., Ruff, R.M., et al. (1987). Neurobehavioral outcome of minor head injury: A three center study. *Journal of Neurosurgery, 66,* 234–243.

Levin, H.S., Mazaux, J.M., Vanier, M., et al. (1990). Évaluation des troubles neuropsychologiques et comportementaux des traumatisés crâniens par le clinicien: Proposition d'une échelle neurocomportementale et premiers resultats de sa version française. *Annales de Réadaptation et de Médecine Physique, 33,* 35–40.

Levin, H.S., Meyers, C.A., Grossman, R.G., & Sarwar, M. (1981). Ventricular enlargement after closed head injury. *Archives of Neurology, 38,* 623–629.

Levin, H.S., O'Donnell, V.M., & Grossman, R.G. (1979). The Galveston Orientation and Amnesia Test. A practical scale to assess cognition after head injury. *Journal of Nervous and Mental Disease, 167,* 675–684.

Levin, H.S., Overall, J.E., Goethe, K.E., et al. (1984). *Guidelines for Using the Neurobehavioral Rating Scale.* Unpublished manuscript.

Levin, H.S., Williams, D., Crofford, M.J., et al. (1988). Relationship of depth of brain lesions to consciousness and outcome after closed head injury. *Journal of Neurosurgery, 69,* 861–866.

Levine, B., Black, S.E., Cabeza, R., et al. (1998). Episodic memory and the self in a case of isolated retrograde amnesia. *Brain, 121,* 1951–1973.

Levine, B., Black, S.E., Cabeza, R., et al. (2001). Episodic memory and the self in a case of isolated retrograde amnesia: Data sheet. *Neurocase, 7,* 279.

Levine, B., Dawson, D., Boutet, I., et al. (2000). Assessment of strategic self-regulation in traumatic brain injury: Its relationship to injury severity and psychosocial outcome. *Neuropsychology, 14,* 491–500.

Levine, B., Stuss, D.T., Milberg, W.P., et al. (1998). The effects of focal and diffuse brain damage on strategy application: Evidence from focal lesions, traumatic brain injury and normal aging. *Journal of the International Neuropsychological Society, 4,* 247–264.

Levine, D.N., Lee, J.M., & Fisher, C.M. (1993). The visual variant of Alzheimer's disease: a clinicopathologic case study. *Neurology, 43,* 305–313.

Levine, D.N., Warach, J., & Farah, M. (1985). Two visual systems in mental imagery: Dissociation of "what" and "where" in imagery disorders due to bilateral posterior cerebral lesions. *Neurology, 35,* 1010–1018.

Levine, E.S. & Black, I.B. (2000). Trophic interactions and neuronal plasticity. In M.S. Gazzaniga (Ed.), *The new cognitive neurosciences* (2nd ed.). Cambridge, MA: MIT Press.

Levine, R.A. & Häusler, R. (2001). Auditory disorders in stroke. In J. Bogousslavsky & L. Caplan (Eds.), *Stroke syndromes* (2nd ed.). Cambridge, UK: Cambridge University Press.

Levine, S.C. (1995). Individual differences in characteristic arousal asymmetry: Implications for cognitive functioning. In F.L. Kitterle (Ed.), *Hemispheric communication: Mechanisms and models.* Hillsdale, NJ: Erlbaum.

Levine, S.R., Washington, J.M., Jefferson, M.F., et al. (1987). "Crack" cocaine-associated stroke. *Neurology, 37,* 1849–1853.

Levitan, I.B. & Kaczmarek, L.K. (2002). *The neuron* (3rd ed.). New York: Oxford University Press.

Levy, D.E. (1988). How transient are transient ischemic attacks? *Neurology, 38,* 674–677.

Levy, J. (1972). Lateral specialization of the brain: Behavioral manifestations and possible evolutionary basis. In J.A. Kiger, Jr. (Ed.), *The biology of behaviors.* Corvallis, OR: Oregon State University Press.

Levy, J. (1983). Language, cognition, and the right hemisphere. A response to Gazzaniga. *American Psychologist, 38,* 538–541.

Levy, J. & Gur, R.C. (1980). Individual differences in psychoneurological organization. In J. Herron (Ed.), *Neuropsychology of left-handedness.* New York: Academic Press.

Levy, J. & Heller, W. (1992). Gender differences in human neuropsychological function. In J. Herron (Ed.), *Neuropsychology of left-handedness.* New York: Academic Press.

Levy, J. & Reid, M. (1976). Variations in writing posture and cerebral organization. *Science, 194,* 337–339.

Levy, M.L., Cummings, J.L., Fairbanks, L.A., et al. (1998). Apathy is not depression. *Journal of Neuropsychiatry, 10,* 314–319.

Levy, M.L., Miller, B.L., Cummings, J.L., et al. (1996). Alzheimer disease and frontotemporal dementias. Behavioral distinctions. *Archives of Neurology, 53,* 687–690.

Levy, R.M. & Bredesen, D.E. (1988a). Central nervous system dysfunction in acquired immunodeficiency syndrome. *Journal of Acquired Immune Deficiency, 1,* 41–64.

Levy, R.M. & Bredesen, D.E. (1988b). Central nervous system dysfunction in acquired immunodeficiency syndrome. In M.L. Rosenbaum et al. (Eds.), *AIDS and the nervous system.* New York: Raven Press.

Lewine, J.D., Orrison, W.W., Jr., Davis, J.T., et al. (1996). Neuromagnetic evaluation of brain dysfunction in postconcussive syndromes associated with mild head trauma. In B.P. Uzzell & H.H. Stonnington (Eds.), *Recovery after traumatic brain injury.* Mahwah, NJ: Erlbaum.

Lewis, P. & Kopelman, M.D. (1998). Forgetting rates in neuropsychiatric disorders. *Journal of Neurology, Neurosurgury and Psychiatry, 65,* 890–898.

Lewis, R., Kelland, D.Z., & Kupke, T. (1990). A normative study of the Repeatable Cognitive-Perceptual-Motor Battery [abstract]. *Archives of Clinical Neuropsychology, 5,* 201.

Lewis, R. & Kupke, T. (1992). Intermanual differences on skilled and unskilled motor tasks in nonlateralized brain dysfunction. *The Clinical Neuropsychologist, 6,* 374–382.

Lewis, R.F. & Rennick, P.M. (1979). *Manual for the Repeatable Cognitive-Perceptual-Motor Battery.* Clinton Township, MI: Ronald F. Lewis.

Lewis, R.S. & Harris, L.J. (1990). Handedness, sex, and spatial ability. In S. Coren (Ed.), *Left-handedness: Behavioral implications and anomalies.* Amsterdam: Elsevier/North Holland.

Ley, R.G. & Bryden, M.P. (1982). A dissociation of right and left hemispheric effects for recognizing emotional tone and verbal content. *Brain and Cognition, 1,* 3–9.

Lezak, M.D. (1960). *The conscious control of Rorschach responses.* Portland, OR: University of Portland. Dissertation.

Lezak, M.D. (1978a). Living with the characterologically altered brain injured patient. *Journal of Clinical Psychiatry, 39,* 592–598.

Lezak, M.D. (1978b). Subtle sequelae of brain damage: Perplexity, distractibility, and fatigue. *American Journal of Physical Medicine, 57,* 9–15.

Lezak, M.D. (1979). Recovery of memory and learning functions following traumatic brain injury. *Cortex, 15,* 63–70.

Lezak, M.D. (1982a). The problem of assessing executive functions. *International Journal of Psychology, 17,* 281–297.

Lezak, M.D. (1982b). Specialization and integration of the cerebral hemispheres. In *The brain: Recent research and its implications.* Eugene: University of Oregon College of Education.

Lezak, M.D. (1982c). *The test–retest stability and reliability of some tests commonly used in neuropsychological assessment.* Paper presented at the 5th European conference of the International Neuropsychological Society, Deauville, France.

Lezak, M.D. (1984a). An individualized approach to neuropsychological assessment. In P.E. Logue & J.M. Schear (Eds.), *Clinical neuropsychology: A multidisciplinary approach.* Springfield, IL: Thomas.

Lezak, M.D. (1984b). Neuropsychological assessment in behavioral toxicology—developing techniques and interpretative issues. *Scandinavian Journal of Work, Environment and Health, 10(Suppl. 1),* 25–29.

Lezak, M.D. (1986). Neuropsychological assessment. In L. Teri & P. Lewinsohn (Eds.), *Geropsychological assessment and treatment.* New York: Springer.

Lezak, M.D. (1987a). Norms for growing older. *Developmental Neuropsychology, 3,* 1–12.

Lezak, M.D. (1987b). Relationships between personality disorders, social disturbances, and physical disability following traumatic brain injury. *Journal of Head Trauma Rehabilitation, 2,* 57–69.

Lezak, M.D. (1988a). Brain damage is a family affair. *Journal of Clinical and Experimental Neuropsychology, 10,* 111–123.

Lezak, M.D. (1988b). IQ: R.I.P. *Journal of Clinical and Experimental Neuropsychology, 10,* 351–361.

Lezak, M.D. (1988c). Neuropsychological tests and assessment techniques. In F. Boller & J. Grafman (Eds.), *Handbook of neuropsychology* (Vol. 1). Amsterdam: Elsevier.

Lezak, M.D. (1988d). The walking wounded of head injury: When subtle deficits can be disabling. *Trends in Rehabilitation, 3,* 4–9.

Lezak, M.D. (1989). Assessment of psychosocial dysfunctions resulting from head trauma. In M.D. Lezak (Ed.), *Assessment of the behavioral consequences of head trauma. Frontiers of clinical neuroscience* (Vol. 7). New York: Alan R. Liss.

Lezak, M.D. (1991). Emotional impact of cognitive inefficiencies in mild head trauma [abstract]. *Journal of Clinical and Experimental Neuropsychology, 13,* 23.

Lezak, M.D. (1992). Assessment of mild, moderate, and severe head injury. In N. von Steinbuchel et al. (Eds.), *Neuropsychological rehabilitation.* Berlin: Springer-Verlag.

Lezak, M.D. (1994). Domains of behavior from a neuropsychological perspective: The whole story. In W. Spaulding (Ed.), *41st Nebraska Symposium on Motivation, 1992–1993.* Lincoln: University of Nebraska Press.

Lezak, M.D. (1996). Family perceptions and family reactions: Reconsidering "denial." In H.S. Levin et al. (Eds.), *Catastrophic brain injury.* New York: Oxford University Press.

Lezak, M.D. (2002). Responsive assessment and the freedom to think for ourselves. *Psychological Rehabilitation, 47,* 339–353 .

Lezak, M.D., Bourdette, D., Whitham, R., & Hikida, R. (1989). Differential patterns of cognitive deficit in multiple sclerosis [abstract]. *Journal of Clinical and Experimental Neuropsychology, 11,* 49.

Lezak, M.D. & Glaudin, V. (1969). Differential effects of physical illness on MMPI profiles. *Newsletter for Research in Psychology, 11,* 27–28.

Lezak, M.D. & Gray, D.K. (1984a [1991]). Sampling problems and nonparametric solutions in neuropsychological research. *Journal of Clinical Neuropsychology, 6,* 101–109; also in B.P. Rourke et al. (Eds.), *Methodological and biostatistical foundations of clinical neuropsychology.* Amsterdam: Swets & Zeitlinger.

Lezak, M.D. & Malec, J.F. (2003). *Mayo-Portland Adaptability Inventory.* Rochester, MN: Mayo Clinic (PMR-ID-SMH); www.tbims.org/combi/mpai.

Lezak, M.D. & Newman, S.P. (1979). *Verbosity and right hemisphere damage.* Paper presented at the 2nd European meeting of the International Neuropsychological Society, Noordvijkerhout, Holland.

Lezak, M.D. & O'Brien, K.P. (1988). Longitudinal study of emotional, social, and physical changes after traumatic brain injury. *Journal of Learning Disabilities, 21,* 456–463.

Lezak, M.D. & O'Brien, K.P. (1990). Chronic emotional, social, and physical changes after traumatic brain injury. In E.D. Bigler (Ed.), *Traumatic brain injury.* Austin, TX: Pro-Ed.

Lezak, M.D., Whitham, R., & Bourdette, D. (1990). Emotional impact of cognitive inefficiencies in multiple sclerosis (MS) [abstract]. *Journal of Clinical and Experimental Neuropsychology, 12,* 50.

Lhermitte, F. (1983). "Utilization behaviour" and its relation to lesions of the frontal lobes. *Brain, 106,* 237–255.

Lhermitte, F. (1986). Human autonomy and the frontal lobes. Part II: Patient behavior in complex and social situations: The "environmental dependency syndrome." *Annals of Neurology, 19,* 335–343.

Lhermitte, F., Pillon, B., & Serdaru, M. (1986). Human autonomy and the frontal lobes. Part I: Imitation and utilization behavior: A neuropsychological study of 75 patients. *Annals of Neurology, 19,* 326–334.

Lhermitte, F. & Signoret, J.-L. (1972). Analyse neuropsychologique et différenciation des syndromes amnésiques. *Revue Neurologique, 126,* 164–178.

Li, D.K. & Paty, D.W. (1999). Magnetic resonance imaging results of the PRISMS trial: A randomized, double-blind, placebo-controlled study of interferon-beta1a in relapsing-remitting multiple sclerosis. *Annals of Neurology, 46,* 197–206.

Li, Y.-S., Meyer, J.S., & Thornby, J. (2001). Depressive symptoms among cognitively normal versus cognitively impaired elderly subjects. *International Journal of Geriatric Psychiatry, 16,* 455–461.

Libon, D.J., Bogdanoff, B., Cloud, B.S., et al. (1998). Declarative and procedural learning, quantitative measures of the hippocampus, and subcortical white alterations in Alzheimer's disease and ischaemic vascular dementia. *Journal of Clinical and Experimental Neuropsychology, 20,* 30–41.

Libon, D.J., Glosser, G., Malamut, B.L., et al. (1994). Age, executive functions, and visuospatial functioning in healthy older adults. *Neuropsychology, 8,* 38–43.

Libon, D.J., Malamut, B.L., Swenson, R., et al. (1996). Further analysis of clock drawings among demented and nondemented older subjects. *Archives of Clinical Neuropsychology, 11,* 193–205.

Libon, D.J., Mattson, R.E., Glosser, G., et al. (1996). A nine-word dementia version of the California Verbal Learning Test. *The Clinical Neuropsychologist, 10,* 237–244.

Libon, D.J., Swenson, R.A., Barnoski, E.J. & Sands, L.P. (1993). Clock drawing as an assessment tool for dementia. *Archives of Clinical Neuropsychology, 8,* 405–415.

Lichtenberg, P.A. & Christensen, B. (1992). Extended normative data for the Logical Memory subtests of the Wechsler Memory Scale–Revised: responses from a sample of cognitively intact elderly medical patients. *Psychological Reports, 71,* 745–746.

Lichter, D.G. & Cummings, J.L. (Eds.) (2001). *Frontal-subcortical circuits in psychiatric and neurological disorders.* New York: Guilford Press.

Licinio, J., Kling, M.A., & Hauser, P. (1998). Cytokines and brain function: Relevance to interferon-alpha-induced mood and cognitive changes. *Seminars in Oncology, 25,* 30–38.

Lieber, C.S. (2000). Ethnic and gender differences in ethanol metabolism. *Alcoholism: Clinical and Experimental Research, 24,* 417–418.

Lieberman, A. (1995a). Other forms of movement disorders. In J.P. Mohr & J.C. Gautier (Eds.), *Guide to clinical neurology.* New York: Churchill Livingstone.

Lieberman, A. (1995b). Parkinson plus conditions. In *Guide to clinical neurology.* New York: Churchill Livingstone, pp. 871–873.

Lieberman, A. (1995c). Parkinson's disease. In J.P. Mohr & J.C. Gautier (Eds.), *Guide to clinical neurology.* New York: Churchill Livingstone, pp. 865–870.

Lieberman, A. (1998). Managing the neuropsychiatric symptoms of Parkinson's disease. *Neurology, 50(Suppl. 6),* S33–S38.

Lieberman, A. & Benson, D.F. (1977). Control of emotional expression in pseudobulbar palsy. *Archives of Neurology, 34,* 717–719.

Lieberman, A., Dziatolowski, M., Neophytides, A., et al. (1979). Dementias of Huntington's and Parkinson's disease. In T.N. Chase et al. (Eds.), *Advances in neurology. Huntington's disease* (Vol. 23). New York: Raven Press.

Lieberman, P., Protopapas, A., & Kanki, B.G. (1995). Speech production and cognitive deficits on Mt. Everest. *Aviation, Space, and Environmental Medicine, 66,* 857–864.

Liepmann, H. (1988). Apraxia. In J.W. Broun (Ed.), *Agnosia and apraxia: Selected papers of Liepmann, Lange, and Potzl* (trans. George Dean). New York: Erlbaum.

Likert, R. & Quasha, W. H. (1970). *The revised Minnesota Paper Form Board Test.* New York: The Psychological Corporation.

Lincoln, R.K., Crosson, B., Bauer, R.M., et al. (1994). Relationship between WAIS-R subtests and language measures after blunt head injury. *The Clinical Neuropsychologist, 8,* 140–152.

Lindeboom, J., Ter Horst, R., Hooyer, C., et al. (1993). Some psychometric properties of the CAMCOG. *Psychological Medicine, 23,* 213–219.

Lindenberger, U. & Baltes, P.B. (1994). Sensory functioning and intelligence in old age: a strong connection. *Psychology and Aging, 9,* 339–355.

Lindley, C.J. (1989). Who is the older person? In T. Hunt & C.J. Lindley (Eds.), *Testing older adults: A reference guide for geropsychological assessments.* Austin, TX: Pro-ed.

Lines, C.R., McCarroll, K.A., Lipton, R.B., et al. (2003). Telephone screening for amnestic mild cognitive impairment. *Neurology, 60,* 261–266.

Lineweaver, T.T., Bond, M.W., Thomas, R.G., & Salmon, D.P. (1999). A normative study of Nelson's (1976) modified version of the Wisconsin Card Sorting Test in healthy older adults. *The Clinical Neuropsychologist, 13,* 328–347.

Linge, F.R. (1980). What does it feel like to be brain damaged? *Canada's Mental Health, 28,* 4–7.

Linn, R.T., Wolf, P.A., Bachman, D.L., et al. (1995). The "preclinical phase" of probable Alzheimer's disease. A 13-year prospective study of the Framingham cohort. *Archives of Neurology, 52,* 485–490.

Linscott, R.J., Knight, R.G., & Godfrey, H.P.D. (1996). The Profile of Functional Impairment in Communication (PFIC): A measure of communication impairment for clinical use. *Brain Injury, 10,* 397–412.

Linz, D.H., deGarmo, P.L., Morton, W.E., et al. (1986). Organic solvent-induced encephalopathy in industrial patients. *Journal of Occupational Medicine, 28,* 119–125.

Lipinska, B., Backman, L., Mantyla, T., & Viitanen, M. (1994). Effectiveness of self-generated cues in early Alzheimer's disease. *Journal of Clinical and Experimental Neuropsychology, 16,* 809–819.

Lipman, F.D. (1962). Malingering in personal injury cases. *Temple Law Quarterly, 35,* 141–162.

Lippa, C.F., Smith, T.W., Saunders, A.M., et al. (1995). Apolipoprotein E genotype and Lewy body disease. *Neurology, 45,* 97–103.

Lippa, R.A. (2003). Handedness, sexual orientation, and gender-related personality traits in men and women. *Archives of Sexual Behavior, 32,* 103–114.

Lipton, R.B., Ottman, R., Ehrenberg, B.L., & Hauser, W.A. (1994). Comorbidity of migraine: The connection between migraine and epilepsy. *Neurology, 44(Suppl. 7),* S28–S32.

Lipton, R.B. & Silberstein, S.D. (1994). Why study the comorbidity of migraine? *Neurology, 44(Suppl. 7),* S4–S5.

Lipton, R.B. & Stewart, W.F. (1997). Prevalence and impact of migraine. *Neurologic Clinics, 15,* 1–13.

Lishman, W.A. (1973). The psychiatric sequelae of head injury: A review. *Psychological Medicine, 3,* 304–318.

Lishman, W.A. (1997). *Organic psychiatry* (3rd ed.). Oxford, UK: Blackwell.

Lissauer, H. (1988 [1888]). A case of visual agnosia with a contribution to theory. *Cognitive Neuropsychology, 5,* 157–192.

Little, M.M., Williams, J.M., & Long, C.J. (1986). Clinical memory tests and everyday memory. *Archives of Clinical Neuropsychology, 1,* 323–333.

Litvan, I., Agid, Y., Calne, D., et al. (1996). Clinical research criteria for the diagnosis of progressive supranuclear palsy (Steele-Richardson-Olszewski syndrome): Report of the NINDS-SPSP International Workshop. *Neurology, 47,* 1–9.

Litvan, I., Agid, Y., Jankovic, J., et al. (1996). Accuracy of clinical criteria for the diagnosis of progressive supranuclear palsy (Steele-Richardson-Olszewski syndrome). *Neurology, 46,* 922–930.

Litvan, I., Cummings, J.L., & Mega, M. (1998). Neuropsychiatric features of corticobasal degeneration. *Journal of Neurology, Neurosurgery, and Psychiatry, 65,* 717–721.

Litvan, I., Grafman, J., Gomez, C., & Chase, T.N. (1989). Memory impairment in patients with progressive supranuclear palsy. *Archives of Neurology, 46,* 765–767.

Litvan, I., Mangone, C.A., McKee, A., et al. (1996). Natural history of progressive supranuclear palsy (Steele-Richardson-Olszewski syndrome) and clinical predictors of survival: A clinicopathological study. *Journal of Neurology, Neurosurgery and Psychiatry, 60,* 615–620.

Litvan, I., Mega, M.S., Cummings, J.L., & Fairbanks, L. (1996). Neuropsychiatric aspects of progressive supranuclear palsy. *Neurology, 47,* 1184–1189.

Liu, C.K., Lai, C.L., Tai, C.T., et al. (1998). Incidence and subtypes of dementia in southern Taiwan: Impact of socio-demographic factors. *Neurology, 50,* 1572–1579.

Liu, Y.K. (1999). Biomechanics of "low-velocity impact" head injury. In N.R. Varney & R.J. Roberts (Eds.), *The evaluation and treatment of mild traumatic brain injury.* Mahwah, NJ: Erlbaum.

Livingston, M.G. & Brooks, D.N. (1988). The burden on families of the brain injured: A review. *Journal of Head Trauma Rehabilitation, 3,* 6–15.

Llabre, M.M. (1984). Standard Progressive Matrices. In D.J. Keyser & R.C. Sweetland (Eds.), *Test critiques* (Vol. I). Kansas City, MO: Test Corporation of America.

Llinás, R.R. & Walton, K.D. (1998). Cerebellum. In G.M. Shepherd (Ed.), *The synaptic organization of the brain* (4th ed.). New York: Oxford University Press.

Llorente, A.M., van Gorp, W.G., Stern, M.J., et al. (2001). Long-term effects of high-dose zidovudine treatment on neuropsychological performance in mildly symptomatic HIV-positive patients: Results of a randomized, double-blind, placebo-controlled investigation. *Journal of the International Neuropsychological Society, 7,* 27–32.

Lloyd, D. (2000). Virtual lesions and the not-so-modular brain. *Journal of the International Neuropsychological Society, 6,* 627–635.

Lobotesis, K., Fenwick, J.D., Phipps, A., et al. (2001). Occipital hypoperfusion on SPECT in dementia with Lewy bodies but not AD. *Neurology, 56,* 643–649.

Locascio, D. & Ley, R. (1972). Scaled-rated meaningfulness of 319 CVCVC words and paralogs previously assessed for associative reaction time. *Journal of Verbal Learning and Verbal Behavior, 11,* 243–250.

Locascio, J.J., Growdon, J.H., & Corkin, S. (1995). Cognitive test performance in detecting, staging, and tracking Alzheimer's disease. *Archives of Neurology, 52,* 1087–1099.

Loewenstein, D.A., Arguelles, T., Arguelles, S., & Linn-Fuentes, P. (1994). Directions of research in cross-cultural neuropsychology. *Journal of Clinical and Experimental Neuropsychology, 17,* 143–150.

Loewenstein, D.A., Barker, W.W., Harwood, D.G., et al. (2000). Utility of a modified Mini-Mental State Examination with extended delayed recall in screening for mild cognitive impairment and dementia among community dwelling elders. *International Journal of Geriatric Psychiatry, 15,* 434–440.

Loewenstein, D.A., Duara, R., Arguelles, T., & Arguelles, S. (1995). Use of the Fuld Object-Memory Evaluation in the detection of mild dementia among Spanish- and English-speaking groups. *American Journal of Geriatric Psychiatry, 3,* 300–307.

Loewenstein, D.A., Duara, R., Rubert, M.P., et al. (1995). Deterioration of functional capacities in Alzheimer's disease after a 1-year period. *International Psychogeriatrics, 7,* 495–503.

Loewenstein, D.A., Wilkie, F., Eisdorfer, C., et al. (1989). An analysis of intrusive error types in Alzheimer's disease and related disorders. *Developmental Neuropsychology, 5,* 115–126.

Loftus, E.F. (1982). Memory and its distortions. In A.G. Kraut (Ed.), *G. Stanley Hall lectures.* Washington, D.C.: American Psychological Association.

Logigian, E.L., Kaplan, R.F., & Steere, A.C. (1999). Successful treatment of Lyme encephalopathy with intravenous ceftriaxone. *Journal of Infectious Diseases, 180,* 377–383.

Logsdon, R.G., Teri, L., Williams, D.E., et al. (1989). The WAIS-R profile: A diagnostic tool for Alzheimer's disease? *Journal of Clinical and Experimental Neuropsychology, 11,* 892–898.

Logue, P., Tupler, L.A., D'Amico, C., & Schmitt, F.A. (1993). The Neurobehavioral Cognitive Status Examination: Psychometric properties in use with psychiatric inpatients. *Journal of Clinical Psychology, 49,* 80–89.

Logue, P. & Wyrick, L. (1979). Initial validation of Russell's revised Wechsler Memory Scale: A comparison of normal aging versus dementia. *Journal of Consulting and Clinical Psychology, 47,* 176–178.

Lohr, J.B. & Wisniewski, A.A. (1987). *Movement disorders.* New York: Guilford Press.

Lokken, K., Ferraro, F.R., Petros, T., et al. (1999). The effect of importance level, delay, and rate of forgetting on prose recall in multiple sclerosis. *Applied Neuropsychology, 6,* 147–153.

Lombardi, W.J., Andreason, P.J., Sirocco, K.Y., et al. (1999). Wisconsin Card Sorting Test performance following head injury: Dorsolateral fronto-striatal circuit activity predicts perseveration. *Journal of Clinical and Experimental Neuropsychology, 21,* 2–16.

London, R., Wick, B., & Kirschen, D. (2003). Post-traumatic pseudomyopia. *Optometry, 74,* 111–120.

Loo, R. & Schneider, R. (1979). An evaluation of the Briggs-Nebes modified version of Annett's handedness inventory. *Cortex, 15,* 683–686.

Loong, J. (1988). *The Finger Tapping Test (computer program).* San Luis Obispo, CA: Wang Neuropsychological Laboratory.

Loonstra, A.S., Tarlow, A.R., & Sellers, A.H. (2001). COWAT metanorms across age, education, and gender. *Applied Neuropsychology, 8,* 161–166.

Lopez, F., Martinez-Lage, J.F., Herrera, A., et al. (2000). Penetrating craniocerebral injury from an underwater fishing harpoon. *Childs Nervous System, 16,* 117–119.

Lopez, O.L., Becker, J.T., & Boller, F. (1991). Motor impersistence in Alzheimer's disease. *Cortex, 27,* 93–99.

Lopez, O.L., Becker, J.T., Brenner, R.P., et al. (1991). Alzheimer's disease with delusions and hallucinations: Neuropsychological and electroencephalographic correlates. *Neurology, 41,* 906–911.

Loranger, A.W., Goodell, H., McDowell, F.H., et al. (1972). Intellectual impairment in Parkinson's syndrome. *Brain, 95,* 405–412.

Lorentz, W.J., Scanlan, J.M., & Borson, S. (2002). Brief screening tests for dementia. *Canadian Journal of Psychiatry, 47,* 723–733.

Loring, D.W. (1989). The Wechsler Memory Scale-Revised, or the Wechsler Memory Scale-Revisited? *The Clinical Neuropsychologist, 3,* 59–69.

Loring, D.W. (Ed.) (1999). *INS dictionary of neuropsychology.* New York: Oxford University Press.

Loring, D.W., Hermann, B.P., Lee, G.P., et al. (2000). The Memory Assessment Scales and lateralized temporal lobe epilepsy. *Journal of Clinical Psychology, 56,* 563–570.

Loring, D.W., Lee, G.P., Martin, R.C., & Meador, K.J. (1988). Material-specific learning in patients with partial complex seizures of temporal lobe origin: Convergent validation of memory constructs. *Journal of Epilepsy, 1,* 53–59.

Loring, D.W., Lee, G.P., Martin, R.C., & Meador, K.J. (1989). Verbal and Visual Memory Index discrepancies from the Wechsler Memory Scale-Revised: Cautions in interpretation. *Psychological Assessment, 1,* 198–202.

Loring, D.W., Lee, G.P., & Meador, K.J. (1988). Revising the Rey-Osterrieth: Rating right hemisphere recall. *Archives of Clinical Neuropsychology, 3,* 239–247.

Loring, D.W., Lee, G.P., & Meador, K.J. (1989). Issues in memory assessment of the elderly. In F.J. Pirozzolo (Ed.), *Clinics in geriatric medicine* (Vol. 5). Philadelphia: Saunders.

Loring, D.W., Lee, G.P., Meador, K.J., et al. (1991). Hippocampal contribution to verbal recent memory following dominant-hemisphere temporal lobectomy. *Journal of Clinical and Experimental Neuropsychology, 13,* 575–586.

Loring, D.W., Martin, R.C., Meador, K.J., & Lee, G.P. (1990). Psychometric construction of the Rey-Osterrieth Complex Figure: Methodological considerations and interrater reliability. *Archives of Clinical Neuropsychology, 5,* 1–14.

Loring, D.W. & Meador, K.J. (2001). Cognitive and behavioral effects of epilepsy treatment. *Epilepsia, 42,* 24–32.

Loring, D.W. & Meador, K.J. (2003a). The Medical College of Georgia (MCG) Complex Figures: Four forms for follow-up. In J. Knight & E. Kaplan (Eds.), *Rey-Osterrieth handbook.* Odessa, FL: Psychological Assessment Resources.

Loring, D.W. & Meador, K.J. (2003b). Neuropsychological aspects of temporal lobe epilepsy surgery. In T.E. Feinberg & M.J. Farah (Eds.), *Behavioral neurology and neuropsychology* (2nd ed.). New York: McGraw-Hill.

Loring, D.W., Meador, K.J., & Lee, G.P. (1989). Differential-handed response to verbal and visual spatial stimuli: Evidence of specialized hemispheric processing following callosotomy. *Neuropsychologia, 27,* 811–827.

Loring, D.W., Meador, K.J., Lee, G.P., et al. (1990). Cerebral language lateralization: Evidence from intracarotid amobarbital testing. *Neuropsychologia, 28,* 831–838.

Loring, D.W., Meador, K.J., & Lee, G.P. (1994). Effects of temporal lobectomy on generative fluency and other language functions. *Archives of Clinical Neuropsychology, 9,* 229–238.

Loring, D.W., Meador, K.J., Lee, G.P., et al. (1995). Wada memory asymmetries predict verbal memory decline after anterior temporal lobectomy. *Neurology, 45,* 1329–1333.

Loring, D.W., Meador, K.J., Lee, G.P., & King, D.W. (1992). *Amobarbital effects and lateralized brain function: The Wada test.* New York: Springer-Verlag.

Loring, D.W. & Papanicolaou, A.W. (1987). Memory assessment in neuropsychology: Theoretical consideration and practical utility. *Journal of Clinical and Experimental Neuropsychology, 9,* 340–358.

Loring, D.W., Strauss, E., Hermann, B.P., et al. (1999). Effects of anomalous language representation on neuropsychological performance in temporal lobe epilepsy. *Neurology, 53,* 260–264.

LoSasso, G.L., Rapport, L.J., & Axelrod, B.N. (2001). Neuropsychological symptoms associated with low-level exposure to solvents and (meth)acrylates among nail technicians. *Neuropsychiatry, Neuropsychology, and Behavioral Neurology, 14,* 183–189.

Lovell, M.R., Iverson, G.L., Collins, M.W., et al. (1999). Does loss of consciousness predict neuropsychological decrements after concussion? *Clinical Journal of Sports Medicine, 9,* 193–198.

Lovett, M.M. (2003). Developmental reading disorders. In T.E. Feinberg & M.J. Farah, Eds., *Behavioral neurology and neuropsychology* (2nd ed.). New York: McGraw-Hill.

Löwel, S. & Singer, W. (2002). Experience-dependent plasticity of intracortical connections. In M. Fahle & T. Poggio (Eds.), *Perceptual learning.* Cambridge, MA: MIT Press.

Lu, L. & Bigler, E.D. (2000). Performance on original and a Chinese version of Trail Making Test Part B: A normative bilingual sample. *Applied Neuropsychology, 7,* 243–246.

Lu, L.H., Crosson, B., Nadeau, S.E., et al. (2002). Category-specific naming deficits for objects and actions: Semantic attribute and grammatical role hypotheses. *Neuropsychologia, 40,* 1608–1621.

Lublin, F.D. & Reingold, S.C., for the National Multiple Sclerosis Society Advisory Committee on Clinical Trials of New Agents in Multiple Sclerosis (1996). Defining the clinical course of multiple sclerosis: Results of an international survey. *Neurology, 46,* 907–911.

Lucas, J.A. (1998). Traumatic brain injury and postconcussive syndrome. In P.J. Snyder & P.D. Nussbaum (Eds.), *Clinical neuropsychology.* Washington, D.C.: American Psychological Association.

Lucas, J.A., Ivnik, R.J., Smith, G.E., et al. (1998a). Mayo's Older Americans Normative Studies: Category fluency norms. *Journal of Clinical and Experimental Neuropsychology, 20,* 194–200.

Lucas, J.A., Ivnik, R.J., Smith, G.E., et al., (1998b). Normative data for the Mattis Dementia Rating Scale. *Journal of Clinical and Experimental Neuropsychology, 20,* 536–547.

Lucchelli, F. & De Renzi, E. (1992). Proper name anomia. *Cortex, 28,* 221–230.

Lucchinetti, C., Bruck, W., Parisi, J., et al. (2000). Heterogeneity of multiple sclerosis lesions: Implications for the pathogenesis of demyelination. *Annals of Neurology, 47,* 707–717.

Luck, S.J. & Hillyard, S.A. (2000). The operation of selective attention at multiple stages of processing: Evidence from human and monkey electrophysiology. In M.S. Gazzaniga (Ed.), *The new cognitive neurosciences* (2nd ed.). Cambridge, MA: MIT Press.

Luh, K. (1995). Line bisection and perceptual asymmetries in normal individuals: What you see is not what you get. *Neuropsychology, 9,* 435–448.

Lukas, S.E., Mendelson, J.H., Benedikt, R.A., & Jones, B. (1986). EEG, physiologic and behavioral effects of ethanol administration. In *National Institute of Drug Abuse Research Monograph Series* (Vol. 67). Washington, D.C.: National Institute of Drug Abuse Research, pp. 209–214.

Lukas, S.E. & Renshaw, P.F. (1998). Cocaine effects on brain function. In S.T. Higgins & J.L. Katz (Eds.), *Cocaine abuse: Behavior, pharmacology, and clinical applications.* New York: Academic Press.

Lukatela, K., Cohen, R.A., Kessler, H., et al. (2000). Dementia Rating Scale performance: A comparison of vascular and Alzheimer's dementia. *Journal of Clinical and Experimental Neuropsychology, 22,* 445–454.

Lukatela, K., Malloy, P., Jenkins, M., & Cohen, R. (1998). The naming deficit in early Alzheimer's and vascular dementia. *Neuropsychology, 12,* 565–572.

Lumer, E.D. (2000). Binocular rivalry and human visual awareness. In T. Metzinger (Ed.), *Neural correlates of consciousness. Empirical and conceptual questions.* Cambridge, MA: MIT Press.

Lundqvist, A., Alinder, J., Alm, H., et al. (1997). Neuropsychological aspects of driving after brain lesion: Simulator study and on-road driving. *Applied Neuropsychology, 4,* 220–223.

Luria, A.R. (1966). *Higher cortical functions in man.* New York: Basic Books.

Luria, A.R. (1970). *Traumatic aphasia.* The Hague: Mouton.

Luria, A.R. (1973a). The frontal lobes and the regulation of behavior. In K.H. Pribram & A.R. Luria (Eds.), *Psychophysiology of the frontal lobes.* New York: Academic Press.

Luria, A.R. (1973b). *The working brain: An introduction to neuropsychology* (trans. B. Haigh). New York: Basic Books.

Luria, A.R. (1999). Outline for the neuropsychological examination of patients with local brain lesions (trans. J. M. Glozman). *Neuropsychology Review, 9,* 9–22.

Luria, A.R. & Homskaya, E.D. (1964). Disturbances in the regulative role of speech with frontal lobe lesions. In J.M. Warren & K. Akert (Eds.), *The frontal granular cortex and behavior.* New York: McGraw-Hill.

Lussier, I., Peretz, I., Belleville, S., & Fontaine, F. (1989). Contribution of indirect measures of memory to clinical neuropsychology assessment [abstract]. *Journal of Clinical and Experimental Neuropsychology, 11,* 64.

Luszcz, M.A. & Bryan, J. (1999). Toward understanding age-related memory loss in late adulthood. *Gerontology, 45,* 2–9.

Lye, T.C. & Shores, E.A. (2000). Traumatic brain injury as a risk factor for Alzheimer's disease: A review. *Neuropsychology Review, 10,* 115–129.

Lyle, O.E. & Gottesman, I.I. (1977). Premorbid psychometric indicators of the gene for Huntington's disease. *Journal of Consulting and Clinical Psychology, 45,* 1011–1022.

Lyle, O.E. & Gottesman, I.I. (1979). Psychometric indicators of the gene for Huntington's disease: Clues to "ontopathogenesis." *Clinical Psychologist, 32,* 14–15.

Lynch, G. (2000). Memory consolidation and long-term potentiation. In M.S. Gazzaniga (Ed.), *The new cognitive neurosciences* (2nd ed.). Cambridge, MA: MIT Press.

Lynn, J.G., Levine, K.N., & Hewson, L.R. (1945). Psychologic tests for the clinical evaluation of late "diffuse organic," "neurotic," and "normal" reactions after closed head injury. In *Trauma of the central nervous system. Research Publication of the Association of Nervous and Mental Disease.* Baltimore, MD: Williams & Wilkins.

Lynn, R. (1991). Race differences in intelligence: A global perspective. *Mankind Quarterly, 31,* 255–296.

Lyons, F., Hanley, J.R., & Kay, J. (2002). Anomia for common names and geographical names with preserved retrieval of names of people: A semantic memory disorder. *Cortex, 38,* 23–35.

Lyons, K., Kemper, S., LaBarge, E., et al. (1994). Oral language and Alzheimer's disease: A reduction in syntactic complexity. *Aging and Cognition, 1,* 271–281.

Lyons, K.E., Hubble, J.P., Tröster, A.I., et al. (1998). Gender differences in Parkinson's disease. *Clinical Neuropharmacology, 21,* 118–121.

Maas, A.I.R., Braakman, R., Schouten, H.J.A., et al. (1983). Agreement between physicians in assessment of outcome following severe head injury. *Journal of Neurosurgery, 58,* 321–325.

Macartney-Filgate, M.S. (1990). Neuropsychological sequelae of major physical trauma. In R.Y. McMurtry & B.A. McLellan (Eds.), *Management of blunt trauma.* Baltimore, MD: Williams & Wilkins.

Macartney-Filgate, M.S. & Vriezen, E.R. (1988). Intercorrelation of clinical tests of verbal memory. *Archives of Clinical Neuropsychology, 3,* 121–126.

Macaruso, P., Harley, W., & McCloskey, M. (1992). Assessment of acquired dyscalculia. In D.I. Margolin (Ed.), *Cognitive neuropsychology in clinical practice.* New York: Oxford University Press.

Macciocchi, S. (2000). Informed consent and neuropsychological assessment. In *Newsletter 40.* Washington, D.C.: American Psychological Association, Division 40.

Macciocchi, S., Barth, J., Alves, M., et al. (1996). Neuropsychological functioning and recovery after mild head injury in college athletes. *Neurosurgery, 39,* 510–514.

Macciocchi, S., Barth, J., Alves, M., et al. (2001). Multiple concussions and neuropsychological functioning in college football players. *Journal of Athletic Training, 36,* 303–306.

Macciocchi, S.N., Fowler, P.C. & Ranseen, J.D. (1992). Trait analyses of the Luria-Nebraska Intellectual Processess, Motor Functions and Memory Scales. *Archives of Clinical Neuropsychology, 7,* 541–551.

Mace, C.J. & Trimble, M.R. (1991). Psychogenic amnesias. In T. Yanagihara & R.C. Petersen (Eds.), *Memory disorders: Research and clinical practice.* New York: Marcel Dekker.

Mace, N. & Rabins, P. (1991). *The 36-hour day: A family guide to caring for persons with Alzheimer's disease, related dementing illnesses, and memory loss later in life.* Baltimore, MD: Johns Hopkins University Press.

MacFlynn, G., Montgomery, E.A., Fenton, G.W., & Rutherford, W. (1984). Measurement of reaction time following minor head injury. *Journal of Neurology, Neurosurgery and Psychiatry, 47,* 1326–1331.

MacGinitie, W.H., MacGinitie, R.K., Maria, K., & Dreyer, L.G. (2000). *Gates-MacGinitie Reading Tests* (4th ed.). Itasca, IL: Riverside.

MacGregor, E.A. (1997). Menstruation, sex hormones, and migraine. *Neurologic Clinics, 15,* 125–142.

MacHale, S.M., O'Rourke, S.J., Wardlaw, J.M., & Dennis, M.S. (1998). Depression and its relation to lesion location after stroke. *Journal of Neurology, Neurosurgery, and Psychiatry, 64,* 371–374.

Machamer, J., Temkin, J., & Dikmen, S. (2002). Significant other burden and factors related to it in traumatic brain injury. *Journal of Clinical and Experimental Neuropsychology, 24,* 420–433.

Machover, K. (1948). Personality projection in the drawing of the human figure. Springfield, IL: Thomas.

Machulda, M.M., Bergquist, T.F., Ito, V., & Chew, S. (1998). Relationship between stress, coping, and postconcussion symptoms in a healthy adult population. *Archives of Clinical Neuropsychology, 13,* 415–424.

Mack, J.L. (1979). The MMPI and neurological dysfunction. In C.S. Newmark (Ed.), *MMPI: Current clinical and research trends.* New York: Praeger.

Mack, J.L. & Levine, R.N. (1981). The basis of visual constructional disability in patients with unilateral cerebral lesions. *Cortex, 17,* 512–532.

Mack, J.L. & Patterson, M.B. (1995). Executive dysfunction and Alzheimer's disease: Performance on a test of planning ability, the Porteus Maze Test. *Neuropsychology, 9,* 556–564.

Mack, J.L., Patterson, M.B., Schnell, A.H., & Whitehouse, D.J. (1993). Performance of subjects with probable Alzheimer's disease and normal elderly controls on the Gollin Incomplete Pictures Test. *Perceptual and Motor Skills, 77,* 951–969.

Mack, W.J., Freed, D.M., Williams, B.W., & Henderson, V.W. (1992). Boston Naming Test: shortened versions for use in Alzheimer's disease. *Journal of Gerontology, 47,* 154–158.

Mackay, A.I., Connor, L.T., Albert, M.L., & Obler, L.K. (2002). Noun and verb retrieval in healthy aging. *Journal of the International Neuropsychological Society, 8,* 764–770.

Mackay, L.E., Morgan, A.S., & Bernstein, B.A. (1999a). Factors affecting oral feeding with severe traumatic brain injury. *Journal of Head Trauma Rehabilitation, 14,* 435–447.

Mackay, L.E., Morgan, A.S., & Bernstein, B.A. (1999b). Swallowing disorders in severe brain injury: risk factors affecting return to oral intake. *Archives of Physical Medicine and Rehabilitation, 80,* 365–371.

Mackenzie, R.S. (2000). Profound retrograde amnesia following mild head injury: Organic or functional? *Cortex, 36,* 521–537.

Mackenzie, T.B., Robiner, W.N., & Knopman, D.S. (1989). Differences between patient and family assessments of depression in Alzheimer's disease. *American Journal of Psychiatry, 146,* 1174–1178.

MacKinnon, D.F. & DePaulo, J.R. (2002). Disorders of mood. In A.K. Asbury et al. (Eds.), *Diseases of the nervous system. Clinical neuroscience and therapeutic principles* (3rd ed.). Cambridge, UK: Cambridge University Press.

Mackintosh, N.J. (1998). *I.Q. and human intelligence.* Oxford: Oxford University Press.

Maclean, L.E., Collins, C.C., & Byrne, E.J. (2001). Dementia with Lewy bodies treated with rivastigmine: Effects on cognition, neuropsychiatric symptoms, and sleep. *International Psychogeriatrics, 13,* 277–288.

MacLean, P.D. (1991). Neofrontocerebellar evolution in regard to computation and prediction: Some fractal aspects of microgenesis. In R.E. Hanlon (Ed.), *Cognitive microgenesis: A neuropsychological perspective.* New York: Springer-Verlag.

MacLeod, C.M. (1985). Learning a list for free recall: Selective reminding versus the standard procedure. *Memory and Cognition, 13,* 233–240.

Macmillan, M. (2000). *An odd kind of fame. Stories of Phineas Gage.* Cambridge, MA: MIT Press.

MacNeilage, P.F. (1987). The evolution of hemispheric specialization for manual function and language. In S.P. Wise (Ed.), *Higher brain functions.* New York: Wiley.

MacNeill, S. & Lichtenberg, P. (1997). Home alone: The role of cognition in return to independent living. *Archives of Physical Medicine and Rehabilitation, 78,* 755–758.

MacQuarrie, T.W. (1925, 1953). *MacQuarrie Test for Mechanical Ability.* Monterey, CA: CTB/McGraw-Hill.

MacVane, J., Butters, N., Montgomery, K., & Farber, J. (1982). Cognitive functioning in men social drinkers. *Journal of Studies on Alcohol, 43,* 81–95.

Madden, D.J., Turkington, T.G., Provenzale, J.M., et al. (1999). Adult age differences in the functional neuroanatomy of verbal recognition memory. *Human Brain Mapping, 7,* 115–135.

Maddrey, A.M., Cullum, C.M., Weiner, M.F., & Filley, C.M. (1996). Premorbid intelligence estimation and level of dementia in Alzheimer's disease. *Journal of the International Neuropsychological Society, 2,* 551–555.

Madigan, N.K., DeLuca, J., Diamond, B.J., et al., (2000). Speed of information processing in traumatic brain injury: Modality-specific factors. *Journal of Head Trauma and Rehabilitation, 15,* 943–956.

Madureira, S., Guerreiro, J., & Ferro, J.M. (1999). A follow-up study of cognitive impairment due to inferior capsular genu infarction. *Journal of Neurology, 246,* 764–769.

Maehara, K., Negishi, N., Tsai, A., et al. (1988). Handedness in the Japanese. *Developmental Neuropsychology, 4,* 117–127.

Maghazaji, H.I. (1974). Psychiatric aspects of methylmercury poisoning. *Journal of Neurology, Neurosurgery and Psychiatry, 37,* 954–958.

Magni, G. & Schifano, F. (1984). Psychological distress after stroke. *Journal of Neurology, Neurosurgery and Psychiatry, 47,* 567–571.

Maguire, E.A., Burke, T., Phillips, J., & Staunton, H. (1996). Topographical disorientation following unilateral temporal lobe lesions in humans. *Neuropsychologia, 34,* 993–1001.

Maguire, E.A., Frackowiak, R.S.J., & Frith, C.D. (1997). Recalling routes around London: Activation of the right hippocampus in taxi drivers. *Journal of Neuroscience, 17,* 7103–7110.

Mahalick, D.M., Ruff, R.M., and Sang, H. (1991). Neuropsychological sequelae of arteriovenous malformations. *Neurosurgery, 29,* 351–357.

Maher, B.A. (1963). Intelligence and brain damage. In N.R. Ellis (Ed.), *Handbook of mental deficiency.* New York: McGraw-Hill.

Maher, E.R., Smith, E.M., & Lees, A.J. (1985). Cognitive deficits in the Steel-Richardson-Olszewski syndrome (progressive supranuclear palsy). *Journal of Neurology, 48,* 1234–1239.

Maher, N.E., Golbe, L.I., Lazzarini, A.M., et al. (2002). Epidemiologic study of 203 sibling pairs with Parkinson's disease: The gene PD study. *Neurology, 58,* 79–84.

Mahieux, F., Fenelon, G., Flahault, A., et al. (1998). Neuropsychological prediction of dementia in Parkinson's disease. *Journal of Neurology, Neurosurgery and Psychiatry, 64,* 178–183.

Mahler, M., Davis, R.J., & Benson, D.F. (1989). Screening multiple sclerosis patients for cognitive impairment. In K. Jensen et al., (Eds.), *Current problems in neurology 10. Mental disorders and cognitive deficits in multiple sclerosis.* London: Libbey, pp. 11–14.

Mahoney, F.I. & Barthel, D.W. (1965). Functional evaluation: The Barthel Index. *Maryland State Medical Journal, 14,* 61–65.

Mahurin, R.K., Feher, E.P., Nance, M.L., et al. (1993). Cognition in Parkinson's disease and related disorders. In R.W. Parks et al. (Eds.), *Neuropsychology of Alzheimer's disease and other dementias.* New York: Oxford University Press.

Mahurin, R.K., Flanagan, A.M., & Royall, D.R. (1993). Neuropsychological measures of executive function in frail elderly patients [abstract]. *Archives of Clinical Neuropsychology, 7,* 356.

Mahurin, R.K. & Pirozzolo, F.J. (1986). Chronometric analysis: Clinical applications in aging and dementia. *Developmental Neuropsychology, 2,* 345–362.

Mahurin, R. K., & Pirozzolo, F. J. (1993). Application of Hick's law of response speed in Alzheimer and Parkinson diseases. *Perceptual and Motor Skills, 77,* 107–113.

Maillard, L., Ishii, K., Bushara, K., et al. (2000). Mapping the basal ganglia: fMRI evidence for somatotopic representation of face, hand, and foot. *Neurology, 55,* 377–383.

Maj, M., D'Elia, L., Satz, P., et al. (1993). Evaluation of two new neuropsychological tests designed to minimize cultural bias in the assessment of HIV-1 seropositive persons: A WHO study. *Archives of Clinical Neuropsychology, 8,* 123–135.

Majdan, A., Sziklas, V., & Jones-Gotman, M. (1996). Performance of healthy subjects and patients with resection from the anterior temporal lobe on matched tests of verbal and visuoperceptual learning. *Journal of Clinical and Experimental Neuropsychology, 18,* 416–430.

Majeres, R.L. (1988). Serial comparison processes and sex differences in clerical speed. *Intelligence, 12,* 149–165.

Majeres, R.L. (1990). Sex differences in comparison and decision processes when matching strings of symbols. *Intelligence, 14,* 357–370.

Maki, P.M., Rich, J.B., & Rosenbaum, R.S. (2002). Implicit memory varies across the menstrual cycle: Estrogen effects in young women. *Neuropsychologia, 40,* 518–529.

Malamud, N. (1975). Organic brain disease mistaken for psychiatric disorder: A clinicopathologic study. In D.F. Benson & D. Blumer (Eds.), *Psychiatric aspects of neurologic disease.* New York: Grune & Stratton.

Malapani, C., Deweer, B., & Gibbon, J. (2002). Separating storage from retrieval dysfunction of temporal memory in Parkinson's disease. *Journal of Cognitive Neuroscience, 14,* 311–322.

Malaspina, A., Alimonti, D., Poloni, T.E., & Ceroni, M. (2002). Disease clustering: The example of ALS, PD, dementia and hereditary ataxias in Italy. *Functional Neurology, 17,* 177–182.

Malec, J.F. (1999). Mild traumatic brain injury: Scope of the problem. In N.R. Varney & R.J. Roberts (Eds.), *The evaluation and treatment of mild traumatic brain injury.* Mahwah, NJ: Erlbaum.

Malec, J.F. (2001). Impact of comprehensive day treatment on societal participation for persons with acquired brain injury. *Archives of Physical Medicine and Rehabilitation, 82,* 885–894.

Malec, J.F., Buffington, A.L.H., Moessner, A.M., & Degiorgio, L. (2000). A medical/vocational case coordination system for persons with brain injury: An evaluation of employment outcomes. *Archives of Physical Medicine and Rehabilitation, 81,* 1005–1015.

Malec, J.F., Ivnik, R.J., & Hinkeldey, N.S. (1991). Visual Spatial Learning Test. *Psychological Assessment, 3,* 82–88.

Malec, J.F., Ivnik, R.J., Smith, G.E., et al. (1992a). Mayo's older American normative studies: Utility of corrections for age and education for the WAIS-R. *The Clinical Neuropsychologist, 6(Suppl.),* 31–47.

Malec, J.F., Ivnik, R.J., Smith, G.E., et al. (1992b). Visual Spatial Learning Test: Normative data and further validation. *Psychological Assessment, 4,* 433–441.

Malec, J.F., Kragness, M., Evans, R.W., et al. (2003). Further psychometric evaluation and revision of the Mayo-Portland Adaptability Inventory in a national sample. *Journal of Brain Trauma Rehabilitation, 18,* 479–492.

Malec, J.F. & Lezak, M.D. (2003). *Manual for the Mayo-Portland Adaptability Inventory.* Rochester, MN: Mayo Clinic and Medical School.

Malec, J.F., Machulda, M.M., & Moessner, A.M. (1997). Differing problem perceptions of staff, survivors, and significant others and brain injury. *Journal of Head Trauma Rehabilitation, 12,* 1–13.

Malec, J.F., Moessner, A.M., Kragness,, M., & Lezak, M.D. (2000). Refining a measure of brain injury sequelae to predict postacute rehabilitation outcome: Rating scale analysis of the Mayo-Portland Adaptability Inventory. *Journal of Head Trauma Rehabilitation, 15,* 670–683.

Malec, J.F. & Thompson, J.M. (1994). Relationship of the Mayo-Portland Adaptability Inventory to functional outcome and cognitive performance measures. *Journal of Head Trauma Rehabilitation, 9,* 1–15.

Malec, J., Zweber, B., & DePompolo, R. (1990). The Rivermead Behavioural Memory Test, laboratory neurocognitive measures, and everyday functioning. *Journal of Head Trauma Rehabilitation, 5,* 60–68.

Malina, A.C., Bowers, D.A., Millis, S.R., & Uekert, S. (1998). Internal consistency of the Warrington Recognition Memory Test. *Perceptual and Motor Skills, 86,* 1320–1322.

Malina, A., Regan, T., Bowers, D., & Millis, S. (2001). Psychometric analysis of the Visual Form Discrimination Test. *Perceptual and Motor Skills, 92,* 449–455.

Malloy, P.F., Bihrle, A., Duffy, J., & Cimino, C. (1993). The orbitomedial frontal syndrome. *Archives of Clinical Neuropsychology, 8,* 185–201.

Malloy, P.F., Webster, J.S., & Russell, W. (1985). Tests of Luria's frontal lobe syndrome. *International Journal of Clinical Neuropsychology, 12,* 88–95.

Malone, D.R., Morris, H.H., Kay, M.C., & Levin, H.S. (1982).

Prosopagnosia: A double dissociation between the recognition of familiar and unfamiliar faces. *Journal of Neurology, 45*, 820–822.

Mangels, J.A., Gershbergs, F.B., Knight, R.T., & Shimamura, A.P. (1996). Impaired retrieval from remote memory in patients with frontal lobe damage. *Neuropsychology, 10*, 32–41.

Mankani, M.H., Abramov, G.S., Boddie, A., & Lee, R.C. (1994). Detection of peripheral nerve injury in electrical shock patients. *Annals of the New York Academy of Sciences, 720*, 206–212.

Manly, J.J., Jacobs, D.M., Sano, M., et al. (1998). Cognitive test performance among nondemented elderly African Americans and whites. *Neurology, 50*, 1238–1245.

Manly, J.J., Jacobs, D.M., Touradji, P., et al. (2002). Reading level attenuates differences in neuropsychological test performance between African American and white elders. *Journal of the International Neuropsychological Society, 8*, 341–348.

Manly, J.J., Miller, S.W., Heaton, R.K., et al. (1998). The effect of African-American acculturation on neuropsychological test performance in normal and HIV-positive individuals. The HIV Neurobehavioral Research Center (HNRC) Group. *Journal of the International Neuropsychological Society, 4*, 291–302.

Mann, D., Yates, P., & Marcyniuk, B. (1984). A comparison of changes in the nucleus basalis and locus caeruleus in Alzheimer's disease. *Journal of Neurology, Neurosurgery and Psychiatry, 47*, 201–203.

Manning, S.K., Greenhut-Wertz, J., & Mackell, J.A. (1996). Intrusions in Alzheimer's disease in immediate and delayed memory as a function of presentation modality. *Experimental Aging Research, 22*, 343–361.

Manos, P.J. & Wu, R. (1994). The ten point clock test: A quick screen and grading method for cognitive impairment in medical and surgical patients. *International Journal of Psychology in Medicine, 24*, 229–244.

Mantovan, M.C., Delazer, M., Ermani, M., & Denes, G. (1999). The breakdown of calculation procedures in Alzheimer's disease. *Cortex, 35*, 21–38.

Mäntyla, T. & Nilsson, L.-G. (1997). Remembering to remember in adulthood: a population-based study on aging and prospective memory. *Aging, Neuropsychology, and Cognition, 4*, 81–92.

Mapou, R.L. (1988). Testing to detect brain damage: An alternative to what may no longer be useful. *Journal of Clinical and Experimental Neuropsychology, 10*, 271–278.

Mapou, R.L. (1995). A cognitive framework for neuropsychological assessment. In R.L. Mapou & J. Spector (Eds.), *Clinical neuropsychological assessment. A cognitive approach.* New York: Plenum Press.

Marcopulos, B.A. (1989). Pseudodementia, dementia, and depression: Test differentiation. In T. Hunt & C.J. Lindley (Eds.), *Testing older adults: A reference guide for geropsychological assessment.* Austin, TX: Pro-Ed.

Marcopulos, B.A. (1999). So many norms, so little time. *The Clinical Neuropsychologist, 13*, 530–536.

Marcopulos, B.A., Gripshover, D.L., Broshek, D.K., et al. (1999). Neuropsychological assessment of psychogeriatric patients with limited education. *The Clinical Neuropsychologist, 13*, 147–156.

Marcopulos, B.A., McLain, C.A., & Giuliano, A.J. (1997). Cognitive impairment or inadequate norms? A study of healthy, rural, older adults with limited education. *The Clinical Neuropsychologist, 11*, 111–131.

Marcos, L.R., Alpert, M., Urcuyo, L., & Kesselman, M. (1973). The effect of interview language on the evaluation of psychopathology in Spanish-American schizophrenic patients. *American Journal of Psychiatry, 130*, 549–553.

Margolin, D.I. (1992a). Clinical cognitive neuropsychology: An emerging speciality. In D.I. Margolin (Ed.), *Cognitive neuropsychology in clinical practice.* New York: Oxford University Press.

Margolin, D.I. (1992c). Probing the multiple facets of human intelligence: The cognitive neuropsychologist as clinician. In D.I. Margolin (Ed.), *Cognitive neuropsychology in clinical practice.* New York: Oxford University Press.

Margolin, D.I. & Goodman-Schulman, R. (1992). Oral and written spelling impairments. In D.I. Margolin (Ed.), *Cognitive neuropsychology in clinical practice.* New York: Oxford University Press.

Margolin, D.I., Pate, D.S., Friedrich, F.J., & Elia, E. (1990). Dysnomia in dementia and in stroke patients: Different underlying cognitive deficits. *Journal of Clinical and Experimental Neuropsychology, 12*, 597–612.

Margolis, R.B., Dunn, E.J., & Taylor, J.M. (1985). Parallel-form reliability of the Wechsler Memory Scle in a geriatric population with suspected dementia. *Journal of Psychology, 119*, 81–86.

Margolis, R.B. & Scialfa, C.T. (1984). Age differences in Wechsler Memory Scale performance. *Journal of Clinical Psychology, 40*, 1442–1449.

Maricle, R.A. (1993). Psychiatric disorders in Huntington's disease. In A. Stoudemire & B.S. Fogel (Eds.), *Medical-psychiatric practice* (Vol. 2). Washington, D.C.: American Psychiatric Press.

Marin, D.B., Breen, C.R., Schmeidler, J., et al. (1997). Noncognitive disturbances in Alzheimer's disease: Frequency, longitudinal course, and relationship to cognitive symptoms. *Journal of the American Geriatric Society, 45*, 1331–1338.

Marin, O.S. & Gordon, B. (1979). Neuropsychologic aspects of aphasia. In H.R. Tyler & D.M. Dawson (Eds.), *Current neurology* (Vol. 2). Boston: Houghton-Mifflin.

Marin, R.S., Firinciogullari, S., & Biedrzycki, R.C. (1994). Group differences in the relationship between apathy and depression. *Journal of Nervous and Mental Diseases, 182*, 235–239.

Marisi, D.Q. & Travlos, A.K. (1992). Reliability of the random number generation test of attentional deployment. *Perceptual and Motor Skills, 74*, 1026.

Markand, O. N., Salanova, V., Whelihan, E., & Emsley, C. L. (2000). Health-related quality of life outcome in medically refractory epilepsy treated with anterior temporal lobectomy. *Epilepsia, 41*, 749–759.

Markowitsch, H.J. (1984). Can amnesia be caused by damage of a single brain structure? *Cortex, 20*, 27–45.

Markowitsch, H.J. (1988). Long-term memory processing in the human brain: On the influence of individual variations. In J. Delacour & J.C.S. Levy (Eds.), *Systems with learning and memory abilities.* Amsterdam: Elsevier.

Markowitsch, H.J. (2000). Neuroanatomy of memory. In E. Tulving & F.I.M. Craik (Eds.), *The Oxford handbook of memory.* Oxford, UK: Oxford University Press.

Markowitsch, H.J. & Calabrese, P. (1996). Commonalities and discrepancies in the relationships between behavioural outcome and the results of neuroimaging in brain-damaged patients. *Behavioral Neurology, 9*, 45–55.

Markowitsch, H.J., Calabrese, P., Neufeld, H., et al. (1999). Retrograde amnesia for world knowledge and preserved memory for autobiographic events. A case report. *Cortex, 35*, 243–252.

Markowitsch, H.J., Calabrese, P., Wurker, M., et al. (1994). The amygdala's contribution to memory—a study on two patients with Urbach-Wiethe disease. *Neuroreport, 5*, 1349–1352.

Markwardt, F.C., Jr. (1989). *The Peabody Individual Achievement Test–Revised.* Circle Pines, MN: American Guidance Service.

Markwardt, F.C., Jr. (1998). *The Peabody Individual Achievement Test. Revised–Normative Update.* Circle Pines, MN: American Guidance Service.

Marmarou, A. (1985). Progress in the analysis of intracranial pressure dynamics and application to head injury. In D.P. Becker & J.T. Povlishock (Eds.), *Central nervous system trauma. Status report–1985.* Washington, D.C.: National Institutes of Health.

Marosszeky, N.E.V., Batchelor, J., Shores, E.A., et al. (1993). The performance of hospitalized, non head-injured children on the Westmead PTA Scale. *The Clinical Neuropsychologist, 7,* 85–95.

Marottoli, R.A., Cooney, L.M., Wagner, D.R., et al. (1994). Predictors of automobile crashes and moving violations among elderly drivers. *Annals of Internal Medicine, 121,* 842–846.

Marquardt, G., Schick, U., & Moller-Hartmann, W. (2000). Brain abscess decades after a penetrating shrapnel injury. *Journal of Neurosurgery, 14,* 246–248.

Marra, C., Silveri, M.C., & Gainotti, G. (2000). Predictors of cognitive decline in the early stage of probable Alzheimer's disease. *Dementia and Geriatric Cognitive Disorders, 11,* 212–218.

Marsh, G.G. (1973). Satz-Mogel abbreviated WAIS and CNS-damaged patients. *Journal of Clinical Psychology, 29,* 451–455.

Marsh, G.G., Hirsch, S.H., & Leung, G. (1982). Use and misuse of the MMPI in multiple sclerosis. *Psychological Reports, 51,* 1127–1134.

Marsh, N.V. & Kersel, D.A. (1993). Screening tests for visual neglect following stroke. *Neuropsychological Rehabilitation, 3,* 245–257.

Marsh, N.V., Kersel, D.A., Havill, J.H., & Sleigh, J.W. (1998). Caregiver burden at 1 year following severe traumatic brain injury. *Brain Injury, 12,* 1045–1059.

Marsh, N.V., Kersel, D.A., Havill, J.H., & Sleigh, J.W. (2002). Caregiver burden during the year following severe traumatic brain injury. *Journal of Clinical and Experimental Neuropsychology, 24,* 434–447.

Marsh, N.V. & Knight, R.G. (1991). Relationship between cognitive deficits and social skill after head injury. *Neuropsychology, 5,* 107–117.

Marsh, N.V., Knight, R.G., & Godfrey, H.P.D. (1990). Long-term psychosocial adjustment following very severe closed head injury. *Neuropsychology, 4,* 13–27.

Marshall, L.H. & Magoun, H.W. (1998). *Discoveries in the human brain. Neuroscience prehistory, brain structure, and function.* Totowa, NJ: Humana Press.

Marshall, R.C. (1989). Evaluation of communication deficits of closed head injury patients. In M.D. Lezak (Ed.), *Assessment of the behavioral consequences of head trauma. Frontiers of clinical neuroscience* (Vol. 7). New York: Alan R. Liss.

Marshall, R.C., Tompkins, C.A., & Phillips, D.S. (1982). Improvement in treated aphasia: Examination of selected prognostic factors. *Folia Phoniatrica, 34,* 305–315.

Marshall, S.W., Waller, A.E., Dick, R.W., et al. (2002). An ecologic study of protective equipment and injury in two contact sports. *International Journal of Epidemiology, 31,* 587–592.

Marsico, D.S. & Wagner, E.E. (1990). A comparison of the Lacks and Pascal-Suttell Bender-Gestalt scoring methods for diagnosing brain damage in an outpatient sample. *Journal of Clinical Psychology, 46,* 868–877.

Marson, D.C., Cody, H.A., Ingram, K.K., & Harrell, L.E. (1995). Neuropsychologic predictors of competency in Alzheimer's disease using a rational reasons legal standard. *Archives of Neurology, 52,* 955–959.

Marson, D.C., Dymek, M.P., Duke, L.W., & Harrell, L.E. (1997). Subscale validity of the Mattis Dementia Rating Scale. *Archives of Clinical Neuropsychology, 12,* 269–275.

Marson, D.C., Ingram, K.K., Cody, H.A., & Harrell, L.E. (1995). Assessing the competency of patients with Alzheimer's disease under different legal standards. A prototype instrument. *Archives of Neurology, 52,* 949–954.

Marson, D.C., Sawrie, S.M., Snyder, S., et al. (2000). Assessing financial capacity in patients with Alzheimer disease: A conceptual model and prototype instrument. *Archives of Neurology, 57,* 977–884.

Martilla, R.J. (1987). Epidemiology. In W.C. Koller (Ed.), *Handbook of Parkinson's disease.* New York: Marcel Dekker.

Martin, A. (1990). Neuropsychology of Alzheimer's disease: The case for subgroups. In M.F. Schwartz (Ed.), *Modular deficits in Alzheimer-type dementia.* Boston: MIT Press.

Martin, A. (1992). Semantic knowledge in patients with Alzheimer's disease: Evidence for degraded representations. In L. Bäckman (Ed.), *Memory functioning in dementia.* Amsterdam: Elsevier.

Martin, A., Brouwers, P., Lalonde, F., et al. (1986). Towards a behavioral typology of Alzheimer's patients. *Journal of Clinical and Experimental Neuropsychology, 8,* 594–610.

Martin, A. & Fedio, P. (1983). Word production and comprehension in Alzheimer's disease: The breakdown of semantic knowledge. *Brain and Language, 19,* 124–141.

Martin, A., Haxby, J.V., Lalonde, F.M., et al. (1995). Discrete cortical regions associated with knowledge of color and knowledge of action. *Science, 270,* 102–105.

Martin, A., Ungerleider, L.G., & Haxby, J.V. (2000). Category specificity and the brain: The sensory/motor model of semantic representations of objects. In M.S. Gazzaniga (Ed.), *The new cognitive neurosciences* (2nd ed.). Cambridge, MA: MIT Press.

Martin, A., Wiggs, C.L., Ungerleider, L.G., & Haxby, J.V. (1996). Neural correlates of category-specific knowledge. *Nature, 379,* 649–652.

Martin, A., Wiggs, C.L., & Weisberg, J. (1997). Modulation of human medial temporal lobe activity by form, meaning, and experience. *Hippocampus, 7,* 587–593.

Martin, A.D. (1977). Aphasia testing. A second look at the Porch Index of Communicative Ability. *Journal of Speech and Hearing Disorders, 42,* 547–562.

Martin, E.M., Sullivan, T.S., Reed, R.A., et al. (2001). Auditory working memory in HIV-1 infection. *Journal of the International Neuropsychological Society, 7,* 20–26.

Martin, E.M., Wilson, R.S., Penn, R.D., et al. (1987). Cortical biopsy results in Alzheimer's disease: correlation with cognitive deficits. *Neurology, 37,* 1201–1204.

Martin, J.B. (1984). Huntington's disease: new approaches to an old problem. *Neurology, 34,* 1059–1072.

Martin, M.J. (1983). A brief review of organic diseases masquerading as functional illness. *Hospital and Community Psychiatry, 34,* 328–332.

Martin, N., Roach, A., Brecker, A., & Lowery, J. (1998). Lexical retrieval mechanisms underlying whole-word perseveration errors in anomic aphasia. *Aphasiology, 12,* 319–333.

Martin, N.J. & Franzen, M.D. (1989). The effect of anxiety on neuropsychological function. *International Journal of Neuropsychology, 11,* 1–8.

Martin, P. & Albers, M. (1995). Cerebellum and schizophrenia: A selective review. *Schizophrenia Bulletin, 21,* 241–250.

Martin, P., Maestu, F., & Sola, R.G. (2002). Effects of surgical treatment on intellectual performance and memory in a Spanish sample of drug-resistant partial onset-temporal lobe epilepsy patients. *Seizure, 11,* 151–156.

Martin, R., Dowler, R., & Gilliam, F. (1999). Cognitive consequences of coexisting temporal lobe developmental malformations and hippocampal sclerosis. *Neurology, 53,* 709–715.

Martin, R., Meador, K., Turrentine, L., Faught, E., et al. (2001). Comparative cognitive effects of carbamazepine and gabapentin in healthy senior adults. *Epilepsia, 42,* 764–771.

Martin, R., Sawrie, S., Gilliam, F., et al. (2002). Determining reliable cognitive change after epilepsy surgery: Development of reliable change indices and standardized regression-based change norms for the WMS-III and WAIS-III. *Epilepsia, 43,* 1551–1558.

Martin, R.C. (1990). Neuropsychological evidence on the role of short-term memory in sentence processing. In G. Vallar & T.

Shallice (Eds.), *Neuropsychological impairments of short-term memory*. Cambridge, UK: Cambridge University Press.

Martin, R.C., Bolter, J.F., Todd, M.E., et al. (1993). Effects of sophistication and motivation on the detection of malingered memory performance using a computerized forced-choice task. *Journal of Clinical and Experimental Neuropsychology, 15,* 867–880.

Martin, R.C., Franzen, M.D., & Orey, S. (1998). Magnitude of error as a strategy to detect feigned memory impairment. *The Clinical Neuropsychologist, 12,* 84–91.

Martin, R.C., Hugg, J.W., Roth, D.L., et al. (1999). MRI extrahippocampal volumes and visual memory: Correlations independent of MRI hippocampal volumes in temporal lobe epilepsy patients. *Journal of the International Neuropsychological Society, 5,* 540–548.

Martinelli, V. (2000). Trauma, stress, and multiple sclerosis. *Journal of the Neurological Sciences, 21,* S849–S852.

Martinez, B.A., Cain, W.S., de Wijk, R.A., et al. (1993). Olfactory functioning before and after temporal lobe resection for intractable seizures. *Neuropsychology, 7,* 351–363.

Martland, H.S. (1928). Punch drunk. *Journal of the American Medical Association, 91,* 1103–1107.

Martone, M., Butters, N., Payne, M., et al. (1984). Dissociations between skill learning and verbal recognition in amnesia and dementia. *Archives of Neurology, 41,* 965–970.

Martone, M., Butters, N., & Trauner, D. (1986). Some analyses of forgetting of pictorial material in amnesic and demented patients. *Journal of Clinical and Experimental Neuropsychology, 8,* 161–178.

Martzke, J.S., Swan, C.S., & Varney, N.R. (1991). Posttraumatic anosmia and orbital frontal damage: Neuropsychological and neuropsychiatric correlates. *Neuropsychology, 5,* 213–225.

Marvin, D.B., Green, C.R., Schmeideler, J., et al. (1997). Noncognitive disturbances in Alzheimer's disease: Frequency, longitudinal course, and relationship to cognitive symptoms. *Journal of the American Geriatrics Society, 45,* 1331–1338.

Massman, P.J. & Bigler, E.D. (1993). A quantitative review of the diagnostic utility of the WAIS-R Fuld profile. *Archives of Clinical Neuropsychology, 8,* 417–428.

Massman, P.J., Delis, D.C., & Butters, N. (1993). Does impaired primacy recall equal impaired long-term storage? Serial position effects in Huntington's disease and Alzheimer's disease. *Developmental Neuropsychology, 9,* 1–15.

Massman, P.J., Delis, D.C., Butters, N., et al. (1990). Are all subcortical dementias alike? Verbal learning and memory in Parkinson's and Huntington's disease patients. *Journal of Clinical and Experimental Neuropsychology, 12,* 729–744.

Massman, P.J., Delis, D.C., Butters, N., et al. (1992). The subcortical dysfunction model of memory deficits in depression: Neuropsychological validation in a subgroup of patients. *Journal of Clinical and Experimental Neuropsychology, 14,* 687–706.

Massman, P.J., Delis, D.C., Filoteo, J.V., et al. (1993). Mechanisms of spatial impairment in Alzheimer's disease subgroups: Differential breakdown of directed attention to global–local stimuli. *Neuropsychology, 7,* 172–181.

Masson, F., Maurette, P., Salmi, L.R., et al. (1996). Prevalence of impairments 5 years after a head injury, and the relationship with disabilities and outcome. *Brain Injury, 10,* 487–497.

Masson, F., Thicoipe, M., Aye, P., et al. (2001). Epidemiology of severe brain injuries: A prospective population-based study. *Journal of Trauma, 51,* 481–489.

Mast, B.T., Fitzgerald, J., Steinberg, J., et al. (2001). Effective screening for Alzheimer's disease among older African Americans. *The Clinical Neuropsychologist, 15,* 196–202.

Masur, D.M., Fuld, P.A., Blau, A.D., et al. (1989). Distinguishing normal and demented elderly with the Selective Reminding Test.

Masur, D.M., Fuld, P.A., Blau, A.D., et al. (1990). Predicting development of dementia in the elderly with the Selective Reminding Test. *Journal of Clinical and Experimental Neuropsychology, 12,* 529–538.

Masur, D.M., Sliwinski, M., Lipton, R.B., et al. (1994). Neuropsychological prediction of dementia and the absence of dementia in healthy elderly persons. *Neurology, 44,* 1427–1432.

Masure, M.C. & Tzavaras, A. (1976). Perception de figures entrecroisées par des sujets atteints de lésions corticales unilatérales. *Neuropsychologia, 14,* 371–374.

Mata, G.V., Fernandez, R.R., Aragon, A.P., et al. (1996). Analysis of quality of life in polytraumatized patients two years after discharge from an intensive care unit. *Journal of Trauma, 41,* 326–332.

Mataix-Cols, D. & Bartres-Faz, D. (2002). Is the use of the wooden and computerized versions of the Tower of Hanoi puzzle equivalent. *Applied Neuropsychology, 9,* 117–120.

Matarazzo, J.D. (1972). *Wechsler's measurement and appraisal of adult intelligence* (5th ed.). Baltimore: Williams & Wilkins.

Matarazzo, J.D., Carmody, T.P., & Jacobs, L.D. (1980). Test–retest reliability and stability of the WAIS: A literature review with implications for clinical practice. *Journal of Clinical Neuropsychology, 2,* 89–105.

Matarazzo, J.D. & Herman, D.O. (1984). Base rate data for the WAIS-R: Test–retest stability and VIQ-PIQ differences. *Journal of Clinical Neuropsychology, 6,* 351–366.

Matarrazzo, J.D. & Herman, D.O. (1985). Clinical uses of the WAIS-R: Base rates of differences between VIQ and PIQ in the WAIS-R standardization sample. In B.B. Wolman (Ed.), *Handbook of intelligence: Theories, measurements and applications.* New York: Wiley.

Matarazzo, J.D., Matarazzo, R.G., Wiens, A.N., et al. (1976). Retest reliability of the Halstead Impairment Index in a normal, a schizophrenic, and two samples of organic patients. *Journal of Clinical Psychology, 32,* 338–349.

Matarazzo, J.D. & Prifitera, A. (1989). Subtest scatter and premorbid intelligence: Lessons from the WAIS-R standardization sample. *Psychological Assessment, 1,* 186–191.

Matarazzo, J.D., Wiens, A.N., Matarazzo, R.G., & Goldstein, S.G. (1974). Psychometric and clinical test–retest reliability of the Halstead Impairment Index in a sample of healthy, young, normal men. *Journal of Nervous and Mental Disease, 158,* 37–49.

Matarazzo, R. (1995). Psychological report standards in neuropsychology. *The Clinical Neuropsychologist, 9,* 249–250.

Mateer, C.A. (2000). Attention. In S.A. Raskin & C.A. Mateer, *Neuropsychological management of mild traumatic brain injury.* New York: Oxford University Press.

Mateer, C.A. & D'Arcy, R.C.N. (2000). Current concepts and approaches to management. In S.A. Raskin & C.A. Mateer, *Neuropsychological management of mild traumatic brain injury.* New York: Oxford University Press.

Mateer, C.A., Sohlberg, M.M., & Crinean, J. (1987). Perceptions of memory function in individuals with closed-head injury. *Journal of Head Trauma Rehabilitation, 2,* 74–84.

Mather, N. & Woodcock, R.W. (2001). *Woodcock-Johnson III Tests of Cognitive Abilities. Examiner's manual.* Itasca, IL: Riverside.

Mathew, N. (2000). Migraine. In *Handbook of headache.* Philadelphia: Lippincott Williams & Wilkins.

Mathew, R.J., Wilson, W.H., Turkinton, T.G., & Coleman, R.E. (1998). Cerebellar activity and disturbed time sense after THC. *Brain Research, 797,* 183–189.

Mathiowetz, V., Weber, K., Volland, G., & Kashman, N. (1984). Reliability and validity of grip and pinch strength evaluations. *Journal of Hand Surgery, 9A,* 222–226.

Mathuranath, P.S., Nestor, P.J., Berrios, G.E., et al. (2000). A brief cognitive test battery to differentiate Alzheimer's disease and frontotemporal dementia. *Neurology, 55*, 1613–1620.

Matjucha, I.C.A. & Katz, B. (1994). Neuro-opthalmology of aging. In M.L. Albert & J.E. Knoefel (Eds.), *Clinical neurology of aging* (2nd ed.). New York: Oxford University Press.

Matotek, K., Saling, M.M., Gates, P., & Sedal, L. (2001). Subjective complaints, verbal fluency, and working memory in mild multiple sclerosis. *Applied Neuropsychology, 8*, 204–210.

Matser, J.T., De Bijl, M.A.O., & Luijtelaar, G. (1992). Is amateur boxing dangerous? *De Psycholoog (Netherlands), 12*, 515–521.

Matser, J.T., Kessels, A.G.H., Jordan, B.D., et al. (1998). Chronic traumatic brain injury in professional soccer players. *Neurology, 51*, 791–796.

Matser, J.T., Kessels, A.G., Lezak, M.D., et al. (1999). Neuropsychological impairment in amateur soccer players. *Journal of the American Medical Association, 282*, 971–973.

Matser, J.T., Kessels, A.G.H., Lezak, M.D., et al. (2000). Acute traumatic brain injury in amateur boxing. *Physician and Sports Medicine, 28*, 87–92.

Matsumoto, J.Y. (2002). Movement-related potentials and event-related potentials. In J.R. Daube (Ed.), *Clinical neurophysiology* (2nd ed.). New York: Oxford University Press.

Matthews, C.G., Guertin, W.H., & Reitan, R.M. (1962). Wechsler-Bellevue subtest mean rank orders in diverse diagnostic groups. *Psychological Reports, 11*, 3–9.

Matthews, C.G. & Haaland, K.Y. (1979). The effect of symptom duration on cognitive and motor performance in parkinsonism. *Neurology, 29*, 951–956.

Matthews, C.G. & Harley, J.P. (1975). Cognitive and motor-sensory performances in toxic and nontoxic epileptic subjects. *Neurology, 25*, 184–188.

Matthews, P.M. & Arnold, D.L. (2001). Magnetic resonance imaging of multiple sclerosis: New insights linking pathology to clinical evolution. *Current Opinion in Neurology, 14*, 279–287.

Matthews, W.S., Solan, A., Barabas, G., & Robey, K. (1999). Cognitive functioning in Lesch-Nyhan syndrome: A 4-year follow-up study. *Developmental Medicine and Child Neurology, 41*, 260–262.

Mattis, S. (1976). Mental status examination for organic mental syndrome in the elderly patient. In L. Bellak & T.B. Karasu (Eds.), *Geriatric psychiatry*. New York: Grune & Stratton.

Mattis, S. (1988). *Dementia Rating Scale (DRS)*. Odessa, FL: Psychological Assessment Resources.

Mattson, A.J., Levin, H.S., & Grafman, J. (2000). A case of prosopagnosia following moderate closed head injury with left hemisphere focal lesion. *Cortex, 36*, 125–137.

Matute, E., Leal, F., Zarabozo, D., et al. (2000). Does literacy have an effect on stick construction tasks? *Journal of the International Neuropsychological Society, 6*, 668–672.

Max, J.E., Robertson, B.A., & Lansing, A.E. (2001). The phenomenology of personality change due to traumatic brain injury in children and adolescents. *Journal of Neuropsychiatry and Clinical Neurosciences, 13*, 161–170.

Maxwell, A.E. (1960). Obtaining factor scores on the WAIS. *Journal of Mental Science, 106*, 1060–1062.

Maxwell, J.K. & Wise, F. (1984). PPVT IQ validity in adults: A measure of vocabulary, not of intelligence. *Journal of Clinical Psychology, 40*, 1048–1053.

Mayberg, H.S. (2002). Mapping mood: An evolving emphasis on frontal–limbic interactions. In D.T. Stuss & R.T. Knight (Eds.), *Principles of frontal lobe function*. New York: Oxford University Press.

Mayberg, H.S., Keightley, M., Mahurin, R.K., & Brannon, S.K. (2002). Neuropsychiatric aspects of mood and affective disorders. In S.C. Yudofsky & R.E. Hales (Eds.), *Textbook of neuropsychiatry and clinical neurosciences*. Washington, D.C.: American Psychiatric Publishing.

Mayer, S.A., Kreiter, K.T., Copeland, D., et al. (2002). Global and domain-specific cognitive impairment and outcome after subarachnoid hemorrhage. *Neurology, 59*, 1750–1758.

Mayes, A.R. (1988). *Human organic memory disorders*. New York: Cambridge University Press.

Mayes, A.R. (2000a). The neuropsychology of memory. In G.E. Berrios & J.R. Hodges (Eds.), *Memory disorders in psychiatric practice*. Cambridge, UK: Cambridge University Press.

Mayes, A.R. (2000b). Selective memory disorders. In E.Tulving & F.I.M. Craik (Eds.), *The Oxford handbook of memory*. Oxford, UK: Oxford University Press.

Mayes, A. & Warburg, R. (1992). Memory assessment in clinical practice and research. In J.R. Crawford et al. (Eds.), *A handbook of neuropsychological assessment*. Hove, UK: Erlbaum.

Mayes, S.D. & Calhoun, S.L. (1998). Comparison of scores on two recent editions of the Developmental Test of Visual-motor Integration. *Perceptual and Motor Skills, 87*, 1324–1326.

Mayeux, R., Stern, Y., Cote, L., & Williams, J.B.W. (1984). Altered serotonin metabolism in depressed patients with Parkinson's disease. *Neurology, 34*, 642–646.

Mayeux, R., Stern, Y., Rosen, J., & Benson, D.F. (1983). Is "subcortical dementia" a recognizable clinical entity? *Annals of Neurology, 14*, 278–283.

Mayeux, R., Stern, Y., Rosen, J., & Leventhal, J. (1981). Depression, intellectual impairment, and Parkinson disease. *Neurology, 31*, 645–650.

Mayeux, R., Stern, Y., Rosenstein, R., et al. (1988). An estimate of the prevalence of dementia in idiopathic Parkinson's disease. *Archives of Neurology, 45*, 260–262.

Mayeux, R., Stern, Y., Sano, M., et al. (1987). Clinical and biochemical correlates of bradyphrenia in Parkinson's disease. *Neurology, 37*, 1130–1134.

Maylor, E.A. (1997). Proper name retrieval in old age: Converging evidence against disproportionate impairment. *Aging, Neuropsychology, and Cognition, 4*, 211–226.

Maylor, E.A. (1998). Changes in event-based prospective memory across adulthood. *Aging, Neuropsychology, and Cognition, 5*, 107–128.

Mayou, R., Bryant, B., & Duthie, R. (1993). Psychiatric consequences of road traffic accidents. *British Journal of Medicine, 307*, 647–651.

Mayrhauser, R.T. von (1992). The mental testing community and validity: A prehistory. *American Psychologist, 47*, 244–249.

Mazaux, J.-M., Boisson, D., & Daverat, P. (1989). Le bilan de l'aphasie: Problèmes méthodologiques. *Annales de Réadaptation et de Médecine Physique, 32*, 585–595.

Mazaux, J.-M., Dartigues, J.F., Letenneur, L., et al. (1995). Visuospatial attention and psychomotor performance in elderly community residents: Effects of age, gender, and education. *Journal of Clinical and Experimental Neuropsychology, 17*, 71–81.

Mazaux, J.-M., Dehail, P., Orgogozo, J.M., & Deleplanque, B. (1999). Agnosie visuelle. In *Encyclopédia Médicale Chirurgicale, Neurologie*. Paris: Elsevier, 17-021-B-10.

Mazaux, J.-M., Giroire, J.M., Vanier, M., et al. (1991). Les troubles de mémoire des traumatisés crâniens graves. In J. Pélissier et al. (Eds.), *Traumatisme crânien grave et médecine de rééducation*. Paris: Masson.

Mazaux, J.-M. & Orgogozo, J.M. (1982). Étude analytique et quantitative des troubles du langage par lésion du thalamus gauche: l'aphasie thalamique. *Cortex, 18*, 403–416.

Mazaux, J.-M. & Orgogozo, J.M. (1985). *Échelle d'Évaluation de l'Aphasie*. Issy-les-Moulineaux, France: EAP.

Mazaux, J.-M. & Richer, E. (1998). Rehabilitation after traumatic brain injury in adults. *Disability and Rehabilitation, 20,* 435–447.

Mazziota, J.C., Phelps, M.E., Carson, R.E., & Kuhl, D.E. (1982). Tomographic mapping of human cerebral metabolism: Auditory stimulation. *Neurology, 32,* 921–937.

Mazziota, J.C., Toga, A., Evans, P. et al. (1997). Brain maps: Linking the present to the future. In R.S.J. Frackowiak et al. (Eds.). *Human brain function.* San Diego: Academic Press.

Mazzucchi, A. (2000). Formes cliniques actuelles de l'aphasie: Implications pour la rééducation. In J.-M. Mazaux et al. (Eds.), *Aphasie 2000. Rééducation et réadaptation des aphasies vasculaires.* Paris: Masson.

Mazzucchi, A. & Biber, C. (1983). Is prosopagnosia more frequent in males than females? *Cortex, 19,* 509–516.

McAllister, A.K., Usrey, W.M., Kriegstein, A.R., & Rayport, S. (2002). Cellular and molecular biology of the neuron. In S.C. Yudofsky & R.E. Hales (Eds.), *Textbook of neuropsychiatry and clinical neurosciences.* Washington, D.C.: American Psychiatric Publishing.

McAllister, T.W. & Flashman, L.A. (1999). Mild brain injury and mood disorders: Causal connections, assessment, and treatment. In N.R. Varney & R.J. Roberts (Eds.), *The evaluation and treatment of mild traumatic brain injury.* Mahwah, NJ: Erlbaum.

McAllister, T.W., Saykin, A.J., Flashman, L.A., et al. (1999). Brain activation during working memory 1 month after mild traumatic brain injury: a functional MRI study. *Neurology, 53,* 1300–1308.

McArdle, J.J., Ferrer-Caja, E., Hamagami, F., & Woodcock, R.W. (2002). Comparative longitudinal structural analyses of the growth and decline of multiple intellectual abilities over the life span. *Developmental Psychology, 38,* 115–142

McCaffrey, R.J., Cousins, J.P., Westervelt, H.J., et al. (1995). Practice effects with the NIMH AIDS abbreviated neuropsychological battery. *Archives of Clinical Neuropsychology, 10,* 241–250.

McCaffrey, R.J., Duff, K., & Solomon, G.S. (2000). Olfactory dysfunction discriminates probable Alzheimer's dementia from major depression: A cross-validation and extension. *Journal of Neuropsychiatry and Clinical Neurosciences, 12,* 29–33.

McCaffrey, R.J., Duff, K., & Westervelt, H.J. (2000a). *Practitioner's guide to evaluating change with intellectual assessment instruments.* New York: Kluwer Academic/Plenum Press.

McCaffrey, R.J., Duff, K., & Westervelt, H.J. (2000b). *Practitioner's guide to evaluating change with neuropsychological assessment instruments.* New York: Kluwer Academic/Plenum Press.

McCaffrey, R.J., Fisher, J.M., Gold, B.A., & Lynch, J.K. (1996). Presence of third parties during neuropsychological evaluations: Who is evaluating whom? *The Clinical Neuropsychologist, 10,* 435–449.

McCaffrey, R.J., Krahula, M.M., & Heimberg, R.G. (1989). An analysis of the significance of performance errors on the Trail Making Test in polysubstance users. *Archives of Clinical Neuropsychology, 4,* 393–398.

McCaffrey, R.J., Krahula, M.M., Heimberg, R.G., et al. (1988). A comparison of the Trail Making Test, Symbol Digit Modalities Test, and the Hooper Visual Organization Test in an inpatient substance abuse population. *Archives of Clinical Neuropsychology, 3,* 181–187.

McCaffrey, R.J., Ortega, A., & Haase, R.F. (1993). Effects of repeated neuropsychological assessments. *Archives of Clinical Neuropsychology, 8,* 519–524.

McCaffrey, R.J., Ortega, A., Orsillo, S.M., et al. (1992). Practice effects in repeated neuropsychological assessments. *The Clinical Neuropsychologist, 6,* 32–42.

McCaffrey, R.J. & Westervelt, H.J. (1995). Issues associated with repeated neuropsychological assessments. *Neuropsychology Review, 5,* 203–221.

McCaffrey, R.J., Westervelt, H.J., & Haase, R.F. (2001). Serial neuropsychological assessment with the National Institute of Mental Health (NIMH) AIDS abbreviated neuropsychological battery. *Archives of Clinical Neuropsychology, 16,* 9–18.

McCaffrey, R.J., Williams, A.D., Fisher, J.M., & Laing, L.C. (Eds.) (1997). The practice of forensic neuropsychology. Meeting challenges in the courtroom. In A.E. Puente & C.R. Reynolds (Eds.), *Critical issues in neuropsychology.* New York: Plenum Press.

McCann, R. & Plunkett, R.P. (1984). Improving the concurrent validity of the Bender-Gestalt test. *Perceptual and Motor Skills, 58,* 947–950.

McCarthy, G. (2000). Physiological studies of face processing in humans. In M.S. Gazzaniga (Ed.), *The new cognitive neurosciences* (2nd ed.). Cambridge, MA: MIT Press.

McCarthy, R.A. & Warrington, E.K. (1990). *Cognitive neuropsychology: A clinical introduction.* San Diego: Academic Press.

McCarty, S.M., Logue, P.E., Power, D.G., et al. (1980). Alternate-form reliability and age-related scores for Russell's revised Wechsler Memory Scale. *Journal of Consulting and Clinical Psychology, 48,* 196–298.

McCarty, S.M., Siegler, I.C., & Logue, P.E. (1982). Cross-sectional and longitudinal patterns of three Wechsler Memory Scale subtests. *Journal of Gerontology, 37,* 169–175.

McCauley, S.R. & Hannay, H.J. (1999). *Growth curve analyses comparing the Disability Rating Scale and Glasgow Outcome Scale scores in outcome prediction following closed-head injury.* Poster presented at the 17th annual meeting of the Neurotrauma Society, Miami, FL, October 1999.

McCauley, S.R., Hannay, H.J., & Swank, P.R. (2001). Use of the Disability Rating Scale recovery curve as a predictor of psychosocial outcome following closed-head injury. *Journal of the International Neuropsychological Society, 7,* 457–467.

McCauley, S.R., Levin, H.S., Vanier, M., et al. (2001). The Neurobehavioral Rating Scale-revised: Sensitivity and validity in closed head injury assessment. *Journal of Neurology, Neurosurgery and Psychiatry, 71,* 643–651.

McClearn, G.E., Johansson, B., Berg, S., et al. (1997). Substantial genetic influence on cognitive abilities in twins 80 or more years old. *Science, 276,* 1560–1563.

McClelland, J.L. (1994). The organization of memory. A parallel distributed processing perspective. *Revue Neurologique, 150,* 570–579.

McClelland, J.L. (2000). Connectionist models of memory. In E. Tulving & F.I.M. Craik (Eds.), *The Oxford handbook of memory.* Oxford: Oxford University Press.

McCloskey, M., Caramazza, A., & Basili, A. (1985). Cognitive mechanisms in number processing and calculation: Evidence from dyscalculia. *Brain and Cognition, 4,* 171–196.

McCormick, C.M. & Witelson, S.F. (1991). A cognitive profile of homosexual men compared to heterosexual men and women. *Psychoneuroendocrinology, 16,* 459–473.

McCormick, D.A. (1998). Membrane properties and neurotransmitter actions. In G.M. Shepherd (Ed.), *The synaptic organization of the brain* (4th ed.). New York: Oxford University Press.

McCrory, P.R. & Berkovic, S.F. (1998). Second impact syndrome. *Neurology, 50,* 677–683.

McCrory, P.R. & Berkovic, S.F. (2000). Video analysis of acute motor and convulsive manifestations in sports-related concussion. *Neurology, 54,* 1488–1491.

McCue, M., Goldstein, G., & Shelly, C. (1989). The application of a short form of the Luria-Nebraska Neuropsychological Battery to discrimination between dementia and depression in the elderly. *International Journal of Clinical Neuropsychology, 11,* 21–29.

McCue, M., Shelly, C., & Goldstein, G. (1985). A proposed short form of the Luria-Nebraska Neuropsychological Battery oriented toward assessment of the elderly. *International Journal of Clinical Neuropsychology, 7,* 96–101.

McCurry, S.M., Edland, S.D., Teri, L., et al. (1999). The Cognitive

Abilities Screening Instrument (CASI): Data from a cohort of 2524 cognitively intact elderly. *International Journal of Geriatric Psychiatry, 14*, 882–888.

McDaniel, M.A., Glisky, E.L., Rubin, S.R., 5–30 et al. (1999). Prospective memory: A neuropsychological study. *Neuropsychology, 13*, 103–110.

McDermott, K.B., Buckner, R.L., Petersen, S.E., et al. (1999). Set- and code-specific activation in frontal cortex: An fMRI study of encoding and retrieval of faces and words. *Journal of Cognitive Neuroscience, 11*, 631–640.

McDermott, K.B., Ojemann, J.G., Petersen, S.E., et al. (1999). Direct comparison of episodic encoding and retrieval of words: An event-related fMRI study. *Memory, 7*, 661–678.

McDermott, P.A., Glutting, J.J., Jones, J.N., & Noonan, J.V. (1989). Typology and prevailing composition of core profiles in the WAIS-R standardization sample. *Psychological Assessment, 1*, 118–125.

McDonald, R.S. (1986). Assessing treatment effects: Behavior rating scales. In L.W. Poon (Ed.), *Handbook for clinical memory assessment of older adults.* Washington, D.C.: American Psychological Association.

McDonald, W.I., Compston, A., Edan, G., et al. (2001). Recommended diagnostic criteria for multiple sclerosis: Guidelines from the International Panel on the Diagnosis of Multiple Sclerosis. *Annals of Neurology, 50*, 121–127.

McDowell, F. (1997). Stroke rehabilitation. In K.M.A. Welch et al. (Eds.), *Primer on cerebrovascular diseases.* San Diego: Academic Press.

McDowell, S., Whyte, J., & D'Esposito, M. (1997). Working memory impairments in traumatic brain injury: evidence from a dual-task paradigm. *Neuropsychologia, 35*, 1341–1353.

McDuff, T. & Sumi, S.M. (1985). Subcortical degeneration in Alzheimer's disease. *Neurology, 35*, 123–125.

McEntee, W.J., Mair, R.G., & Langlais, P.J. (1984). Neurochemical pathology in Korsakoff's psychosis: Implications for other cognitive disorders. *Neurology, 34*, 648–652.

McFall, R.M. & Townsend, J.T. (1998). Foundations of psychological assessment: Implications for cognitive assessment in clinical science. *Psychological Assessment, 10*, 316–330.

McFarland, K., Jackson, L., & Geffen, G. (2001). Post-traumatic amnesia: Consistency-of-recovery and duration-to-recovery following traumatic brain impairment. *The Clinical Neuropsychologist, 15*, 59–68.

McFarlin, D.E. & McFarland, H.F. (1982). Multiple sclerosis. *New England Journal of Medicine, 307*, 1183–1188.

McFie, J. (1960). Psychological testing in clinical neurology. *Journal of Nervous and Mental Disease, 131*, 383–393.

McFie, J. (1975). *Assessment of organic intellectual impairment.* London: Academic Press.

McFie, J. & Piercy, M.F. (1952). The relation of laterality of lesion to performance on Weigl's sorting test. *Journal of Mental Science, 98*, 299–305.

McFie, J. & Zangwill, O.L. (1960). Visual construction disabilities associated with lesions of the left cerebral hemisphere. *Brain, 83*, 243–260.

McGarry, L.J., Thompson, D., Millham, F.H., et al. (2002). Outcomes and costs of acute treatment of traumatic brain injury. *Journal of Trauma, 53*, 1152–1159.

McGarvey, B., Gallagher, D., Thompson, L.W., & Zelinski, E. (1982). Reliability and factor structure of the Zung Self-Rating Depression Scale in three age groups. *Essence, 5*, 141–151.

McGaugh, J.L. (1966). Time-dependent processes in memory storage. *Science, 153*, 1351–1358.

McGaugh, J.L. (2000). Memory—a century of consolidation. *Science, 287*, 248–251.

McGaugh, J.L., Weinberger, N.M., & Lynch, G. (Eds.) (1990). *Brain organization and memory: Cells, systems, and circuits.* New York: Oxford University Press.

McGaugh, J.L., Weinberger, N.M., & Lynch, G. (Eds.) (1995). *Brain and memory. Modulation and mediation of neuroplasticity.* New York: Oxford University Press.

McGivern, R.F., Mutter, K.L., Anderson, J., et al. (1998). Gender differences in incidental learning and visual recognition memory: Support for a sex difference in unconscious environmental awareness. *Personality and Individual Differences, 25*, 223–232.

McGivney, S.A., Mulvihill, M., & Taylor, B. (1994). Validating the GDS depression screen in the nursing home. *Journal of the American Geriatrics Society, 42*, 490–492.

McGlinchey-Berroth, R., Milberg, W., Verfaellie, et al. (1993). Semantic processing in the neglected visual field: Evidence from a lexical decision task. *Cognitive Neuropsychology, 10*, 79–108.

McGlone, J. (1976). Sex differences in functional brain asymmetry. Research bulletin 378. London: University of Western Ontario.

McGlone, J. (1994). Memory complaints before and after temporal lobectomy: Do they predict memory performance or lesion laterality? *Epilepsia, 35*, 529–539.

McGlone, J., Losier, B.J., & Black, S.E. (1997). Are there sex differences in hemispatial visual neglect after unilateral stroke? *Neuropsychiatry, Neuropsychology, and Behavioral Neurology, 10*, 125–134.

McGlone, J. & Young, B. (1986). Cerebral localization. In A.B. Baker (Ed.), *Clinical neurology.* Philadelphia: Harper & Row.

McGlynn, S.M. & Kaszniak, A.W. (1991). Unawareness of deficits in dementia and schizophrenia. In G.P. Prigatano & D.L. Schacter (Eds.), *Awareness of deficit after brain injury: Clinical and theoretical issues.* New York: Oxford University Press.

McGlynn, S.M. & Schacter, D.L. (1989). Unawareness of deficits in neuropsychological syndromes. *Journal of Clinical and Experimental Neuropsychology, 11*, 143–205.

McGrath, J. (1997). Cognitive impairment associated with post-traumatic stress disorder and minor head injury. A case report. *Neuropsychological Rehabilitation, 7*, 231–239.

McGrew, K.S. & Woodcock, R.W. (2001). *Technical manual. Woodcock-Johnson III.* Itasca, IL: Riverside.

McGuire, B.E. & Shores, E.A. (1998). Malingering of memory impairment on the Colorado Priming Test. *British Journal of Clinical Psychology, 37*, 99–102.

McGuire, L.C., Morian, A., Codding, R., & Smyer, M.A. (2000). Older adults' memory for medical information: Influence of elderspeak and note taking. *International Journal of Rehabilitation and Health, 5*, 117–128.

McHugh, P.R. & Folstein, M.F. (1975). Psychiatric syndromes of Huntington's chorea. In D.F. Benson & D. Blumer (Eds.), *Psychiatric aspects of neurologic disease.* New York: Grune & Stratton.

McIntosh, T.K., Juhler, M., Raghupathi, R., et al. (1999). Secondary brain injury: Neurochemical and cellular mediators. In D.W. Marion (Ed.), *Traumatic brain injury.* New York: Thieme.

McIntosh, T.K., Saatman, K.E., Raghupathi, R., et al. (1998). The molecular and cellular sequelae of experimental traumatic brain injury: pathogenetic mechanisms. *Neuropathology and Applied Neurobiology, 24*, 251–267.

McKeever, C.K. & Schatz, P. (2003). Current issues in the identification, assessment, and management of concussions in sports-related injuries. *Applied Neuropsychology, 10*, 4–11.

McKeever, W.F. (1986). The influence of handedness, sex, familial sinistrality, and androgeny on language laterality, verbal ability, and spatial ability. *Cortex, 22*, 521–537.

McKeever, W.F. (1990). Familial sinistrality and cerebral organization. In S. Coren (Ed.), *Left-handedness. Behavioral implications and anomalies.* Amsterdam: Elsevier/North-Holland.

McKeith, I.G. (2002). Dementia with Lewy bodies. *British Journal of Psychiatry, 180*, 144–147.

McKeith, I.G. & Burn, D. (2000). Spectrum of Parkinson's disease, Parkinson's dementia, and Lewy body dementia. *Neurologic Clinics, 18,* 865–902.

McKeith, I.G., Grace, J.B., Walker, Z., et al. (2000). Rivastigmine in the treatment of dementia with Lewy bodies: Preliminary findings from an open trial. *International Journal of Geriatric Psychiatry, 15,* 387–392.

McKeith, I.G., Perry, R. H., Fairbairn, A. F., et al. (1992). Operational criteria for senile dementia of Lewy body type (SDLT). *Psychological Medicine, 22,* 911–922.

McKenna, P. (1998). *The Category Specific Names Test.* Levittown, PA: Psychology Press.

McKenna, P. & Warrington, E.K. (1980). Testing for nominal dysphasia. *Journal of Neurology, Neurosurgery and Psychiatry, 43,* 781–788.

McKenna, P. & Warrington, E.K. (1996). The analytic approach to neuropsychological assessment. In I. Grant & K.M. Adams (Eds.), *Neuropsychological assessment of neuropsychiatric disorders* (2nd ed.). New York: Oxford University Press.

McKenna, P.J., Kane, J.M., & Parrish, K. (1985). Psychotic syndromes in epilepsy. *American Journal of Psychiatry, 142,* 895–904.

McKenna, P.J., Ornstein, T., & Baddeley A.D. (2002). Schizophrenia. In A.D. Baddeley et al. (Eds.), *The handbook of memory disorders.* Chichester, U.K.: Wiley.

McKeon, J., McGuffin, P., & Robinson, P. (1984). Obsessive-compulsive neurosis following head injury. *British Journal of Psychiatry, 144,* 190–192.

McKhann, G., Drachman, D., Folstein, M., et al. (1984). Clinical diagnosis of Alzheimer's disease. Report of the NINCDS-ADRDA Work Group. *Neurology, 34,* 939–944.

McKinlay, W.W., Brooks, D.N., & Bond, M.R. (1983). Postconcussional symptoms, financial compensation and outcome of severe blunt head injury. *Journal of Neurology, Neurosurgery and Psychiatry, 46,* 1084–1091.

McKinzey, R.K., Podd, M.H., Krehbiel, M.A., et al. (1997). Detection of malingering on the Luria-Nebraska Neuropsychological Battery: An initial and cross-validation. *Archives of Clinical Neuropsychology, 12,* 505–512.

McKinzey, R.K., Podd, M.H., Krehbiel, M.A., & Raven, J. (1999). Detection of malingering on Raven's Standard Progressive Matrices: A cross-validation. *British Journal of Clinical Psychology, 38,* 435–439.

McKinzey, R.K., & Russell, E.W. (1997a). A partial cross-validation of a Halstead-Reitan Battery malingering formula. *Journal of Clinical and Experimental Neuropsychology, 19,* 484–488.

McKinzey, R.K. & Russell, E.W. (1997b). Detection of malingering on the Halstead-Reitan battery: A cross validation. *Archives of Clinical Neuropsychology, 12,* 585–589.

McLatchie, G., Brooks, N., Galbraith, S., et al. (1987). Clinical neurological examination, neuropsychology, electroencephalography and computer tomographic head scanning in active amateur boxers. *Journal of Neurology, Neurosurgery and Psychiatry, 50,* 96–99.

McLean, A., Jr., Dikmen, S., Temkin, N., et al. (1984). Psychosocial functioning at one month after head injury. *Neurosurgery, 14,* 393–399.

McLean, A., Jr., Temkin, N.R., Dikmen, S., & Wyler, A.R. (1983). The behavioral sequelae of head injury. *Journal of Clinical Neuropsychology, 5,* 361–376.

McMillan, T.M. (1984). Investigation of everyday memory in normal subjects using the Subjective Memory Questionnaire (SMQ). *Cortex, 20,* 333–347.

McMillan, T.M. (1996a). Neuropsychological assessment after extremely severe head injury in a case of life or death. *Brain Injury, 11,* 483–490.

McMillan, T.M. (1996b). Post-traumatic stress disorder following minor and severe closed head injury: 10 single cases. *Brain Injury, 10,* 749–758.

McMillan, T.M. & Herbert, C.M. (2000). Neuropsychological assessment of a potential "euthanasia" case: A 5 year follow up. *Brain Injury, 14,* 197–203.

McNair, D.M., Lorr, M., & Droppleman, L.F. (1981). *EDITS manual for the Profile of Mood States.* San Diego: Educational and Industrial Service.

McNeil, J.E. & Warrington, E.K. (1993). Propopagnosia: A face-specific disorder. *Quarterly Journal of Experimental Psychology, 40A,* 561–580.

McNeil, M.R. (1979). Porch Index of Communicative Ability (PICA). In F.L. Darley (Ed.), *Evaluation of appraisal techniques in speech and language pathology.* Reading, ME: Addison-Wesley.

McPherson, S. & Cummings, J.L. (1996). Neuropsychological aspects of Parkinson's disease and parkinsonism. In I.G. Grant & K.M. Adams (Eds.), *Neuropsychological assessment of neuropsychiatric disorders* (2nd ed.) New York: Oxford University Press.

McSweeny, A.J., Becker, B.C., Naugle, R.I., et al. (1998). Ethical issues related to the presence of third party observers in clinical neuropsychology evaluations. *The Clinical Neuropsychologist, 12,* 552–559.

McSweeny, A.J., Grant, I., Heaton, R.K., et al. (1985). Relationship of neuropsychological status to everyday functioning in healthy and chronically ill persons. *Journal of Clinical and Experimental Neuropsychology, 7,* 281–291.

McSweeny, A.J. & Naugle, R.I. (2002). Competence and appropriate use of neuropsychological assessments and interventions. In S.S. Bush & M.L. Drexler (Eds.), *Ethical issues in clinical neuropsychology.* Lisse, Netherlands: Swets and Zeitlinger.

McWalter, G.J., Montaldi, D., Bhutani, G.E., et al. (1991). Paired associate verbal learning in dementia of the Alzheimer's type. *Neuropsychology, 5,* 205–211.

Mead, G.E. & Warlow, C.P. (2002). Preventive management of stroke. In A.K. Asbury et al. (Eds.), *Diseases of the nervous system. Clinical neuroscience and therapeutic principles.* Cambridge: Cambridge University Press.

Meador, K.J. (1998a). Cognitive side effects of medications. *Neurologic Clinics, 16,* 141–155.

Meador, K.J. (1998b). Cognitive and behavioral assessments in AED trials. *Advances in Neurology, 76,* 231–238.

Meador, K.J. (2001). Cognitive effects of epilepsy and of antiepileptic medications. In E. Wyllie (Ed.), *The treatment of epilepsy* (3rd ed.) Baltimore: Williams & Wilkins.

Meador, K. J. (2002). Cognitive outcomes and predictive factors in epilepsy. *Neurology, 58,* S21–S26.

Meador, K.J., Allison, J.D., Loring, D.W., et al. (2002). Topography of somatosensory processing. Cerebral lateralization and focused attention. *Journal of the International Neuropsychological Society, 8,* 349–359.

Meador, K.J., Gilliam, F.G., Kanner, A.M., & Pellock, J.M. (2001). Cognitive and behavioral effects of antiepileptic drugs. *Epilepsy and Behavior, 2,* S1–S17.

Meador, K.J., Loring, D.W., Allen, M.E., et al. (1991). Comparative cognitive effects of carbamazepine and phenytoin in healthy adults. *Neurology, 41,* 1537–1540.

Meador, K.J., Loring, D.W., Bowers, D., & Heilman, K.M. (1987). Remote memory and neglect syndrome. *Neurology, 37,* 522–526.

Meador, K.J., Loring, D.W., Feinberg, T.E., et al. (2000). Anosognosia and asomatognosia during intracarotid amobarbital inactivation. *Neurology, 55,* 816–820.

Meador, K.J., Loring, D.W., Hulihan, J.F., et al. (2003). Differential cognitive and behavioral effects of topiramate and valproate. *Neurology, 60,* 1483–1488.

Meador, K.J., Loring, D.W., Lee, G.P., et al. (1988). Right cerebral specialization for tactile attention as evidenced by intracarotid sodium amytal. *Neurology, 38,* 1763–1766.

Meador, K.J., Loring, D.W., Lee, K., et al. (1999). Cerebral lateralization: Relationship of language and ideomotor praxis. *Neurology, 53,* 2028–2031.

Meador, K.J., Loring, D.W., Ray, P.G., et al. (1999). Differential cognitive effects of carbamazepine and gabapentin. *Epilepsia, 40,* 1279–1285.

Meador, K.J., Moore, E.E., Nichols, M.E., et al. (1993). The role of cholinergic systems in visuospatial processing and memory. *Journal of Clinical and Experimental Neuropsychology, 15,* 832–842.

Meador, K.J. & Moser, E. (2000). Negative seizures. *Journal of the International Neuropsychological Society, 6,* 731–733.

Meador, K.J., Ray, P.G., Day, L.J., & Loring, D.W. (2001). Relationship of extinction to perceptual thresholds for single stimuli. *Neurology, 56,* 1044–1047.

Meador, K.J., Ray, P.G., Echauz, J.R., et al. (2002). Gamma coherence and conscious perception. *Neurology, 59,* 847–854.

Meehl, P. E. (1954, reprinted 1996). *Clinical versus statistical prediction.* Northvale, NJ: Jason Aronson.

Meehl, P.E. & Rosen, A. (1967). Antecedent probability and the efficiency of psychometric signs, patterns, on cutting scores. In D.N. Jackson & S. Messick (Eds.), *Problems in human assessment.* New York: McGraw-Hill.

Meeker, M. & Meeker, R. (1985). *Structure of Intellect Learning Abilities Test (SOI-LA).* Los Angeles: Western Psychological Services.

Mega, M.S., Cummings, J.L., Fiorello, T., & Gornbein, J. (1996). The spectrum of behavioral changes in Alzheimer's disease. *Neurology, 46,* 130–135.

Mega, M.S., Thompson, P.M., Cummings, J.L., et al. (1998). Sulcal variability in the Alzheimer's brain: Correlations with cognition. *Neurology, 50,* 145–151.

Mehta, K.M., Ott, A., Kalmijn, S., et al. (1999). Head trauma and risk of dementia and Alzheimer's disease: The Rotterdam Study. *Neurology, 53,* 1959–1962.

Mehta, Z. & Newcombe, F. (1996). Dissociable contributions of the two cerebral hemispheres to judgments of line orientation. *Journal of the International Neuropsychological Society, 2,* 335–339.

Mehta, Z., Newcombe, F. & Ratcliff, G. (1989). Patterns of hemispheric asymmetry set against clinical evidence. In J.R. Crawford & D.M. Parker (Eds.). *Developments in clinical and experimental neuropsychology.* New York: Plenum Press.

Meier, D. (1995). The segmented clock: A typical pattern in vascular dementia. *Journal of the American Geriatric Society, 43,* 1071–1073.

Meier, M.J., Ettinger, M.G., & Arthur, L. (1982). Recovery of neuropsychological functioning after cerebrovascular infarction. In R.N. Malatesha (Ed.), *Neuropsychology and cognition.* The Hague: Martinus Nijhoff.

Meier, M.J. & Story, J.L. (1967). Selective impairment of Porteus Maze Test performance after right subthalamotomy. *Neuropsychologia, 5,* 181–189.

Meier-Ruge, W., Ulrich, J., Bruhlmann, M., & Meier, E. (1992). Age-related white matter atrophy in the human brain. *Annals of the New York Academy of Sciences, 673,* 260–269.

Meiran, N. & Jelicic, M. (1995). Implicit memory in Alzheimer's disease: A meta-analysis. *Neuropsychology, 9,* 291–303.

Meiser, B. & Dunn, S. (2000). Psychological impact of genetic testing for Huntington's disease: An update of the literature. *Journal of Neurology, Neurosurgery and Psychiatry, 69,* 574–578.

Mellen, P.F., Weedn, V.W., & Kao, G. (1992). Electrocution: A review of 155 cases with emphasis on human factors. *Journal of Forensic Sciences, 37,* 1016–1022.

Mellick, D., Gerhart, K.A., & Whiteneck, G.G. (2003). Understanding outcomes based on the post-acute hospitalization pathways followed by persons with traumatic brain injury. *Brain Injury, 17,* 55–71.

Mellick, D., Walker, N., Brooks, C.A., & Whiteneck, G.G. (1999). Incorporating the cognitive independence domain into CHART. *Journal of Rehabilitation Outcomes Measurement, 3,* 12–21.

Melvold, J.L., Au, R., Obler, L.K., & Albert, M.L. (1994). Language during aging and dementia. In M.L. Albert & J.E. Knoefel (Eds.), *Clinical neurology of aging* (2nd ed.). New York: Oxford University Press.

Mendez, M.F. (1995). The neuropsychiatric aspects of boxing. *International Journal of Psychiatry in Medicine, 25,* 249–262.

Mendez, M.F., Adams, N.L., & Lewandowski, K.S. (1989). Neurobehavioral changes associated with caudate lesions. *Neurology, 39,* 349–354.

Mendez, M.F., Ala, T., & Underwood, K.L. (1992). Development of scoring criteria for the clock drawing task in Alzheimer's disease. *Journal of the American Geriatric Society, 40,* 1095–1099.

Mendez, M.F. & Ashla-Mendez, M. (1991). Differences between multi-infarct dementia and Alzheimer's disease on unstructured neuropsychological tasks. *Journal of Clinical and Experimental Neuropsychology, 13,* 923–932.

Mendez, M.F., Cherrier, M.M., & Cymerman, J.S. (1997). Hemispatial neglect on visual search tasks in Alzheimer's disease. *Neuropsychiatry, Neuropsychology, and Behavioral Neurology, 10,* 203–208.

Mendez, M.F. & Cummings, J.L. (2002). Neuropsychiatric aspects of aphasia and related disorders. In S.C. Yudofsky & R.E. Hales (Eds.), *Textbook of neuropsychiatry and clinical neurosciences* (4th ed.). Washington, D.C.: American Psychiatric Publishing.

Mendez, M.F., Doss, R.C., & Cherrier, M.M. (1998). Use of the Cognitive Estimations Test to discriminate frontotemporal dementia from Alzheimer's disease. *Journal of Geriatric Psychiatry and Neurology, 11,* 2–6.

Mendez, M.F., Martin, R.J., Smyth, K.A., & Whitehouse, P.J. (1990). Psychiatric symptoms associated with Alzheimer's disease. *Journal of Neuropsychiatry and Clinical Neurosciences, 1,* 28–33.

Mendez, M.F., Mendez, M.A., Martin, R., et al. (1990). Complex visual disturbances in Alzheimer's disease. *Neurology, 40,* 439–443.

Mendez, M.F., Perryman, K.M., Miller, B.L., et al. (1997). Compulsive behaviors as presenting symptoms of frontotemporal dementia. *Journal of Geriatrics, Psychiatry, and Neurology, 10,* 154–157.

Mendez, M.F., Perryman, K.M., Miller, B.L., & Cummings, J.L. (1998). Behavioral differences between frontotemporal dementia and Alzheimer's disease: a comparison on the BEHAVE-AD rating scale. *International Psychogeriatrics, 10,* 155–162.

Mendez, M.F., Selwood, A., Mastri, A.R., & Frey, W.H. 2nd (1993). Pick's disease versus Alzheimer's disease: a comparison of clinical characteristics. *Neurology, 43,* 289–292.

Mendiondo, M.S., Ashford, J.W., Kryscio, R.J., & Schmitt, F.A. (2000). Modelling Mini-Mental State Examination changes in Alzheimer's disease. *Statistics in Medicine, 19,* 1607–1616.

Mendola, J.D., Cronin-Golomb, A., Corkin, S., & Growdon, J.H. (1995). Prevalence of visual deficits in Alzheimer's disease. *Optometry and Vision Science, 72,* 155–167.

Menegazzi, J.J., Davis, E.A., Sucov, A.N., & Paris, P.M. (1993). Reliability of the Glasgow Coma Scale when used by emergency physicians and paramedics. *Journal of Trauma, 34,* 46–48.

Mensch, A.J. & Woods, D.J. (1986). Patterns of feigning brain damage on the LNNB. *International Journal of Clinical Neuropsychology, 8,* 59–63.

Mercer, W.N., Harrell, E.H., Miller, D.C., et al. (1997). Performance of brain-injured versus healthy adults on three versions of the Category Test. *The Clinical Neuropsychologist, 11*, 174–179.

Mercer, W.N., Harrell, E.H., Miller, D.C., et al. (1998). Performance of healthy adults versus individuals with brain injuries on the supplemental measures of the WAIS-RNI. *Brain Injury, 12*, 753–758.

Mergler, D., Baldwin, M., Belanger, S., et al. (1999). Manganese neurotoxicity, a continuum of dysfunction: results from a community based study. *Neurotoxicology, 20*, 327–342.

Mergler, D. & Blain, L. (1987). Assessing color vision loss among solvent-exposed workers. *American Journal of Industrial Medicine, 12*, 195–203.

Mergler, D., Blain, L., Lemaire, J., & Lalande, F. (1988). Colour vision impairment and alcohol consumption. *Neurotoxicology and Teratology, 10*, 255–260.

Mergler, D., Bowler, R., & Cone, J. (1990). Colour vision loss among disabled workers with neuropsychological impairment. *Neurotoxicology and Teratology, 12*, 669–672.

Mergler, D., Frenette, B., Legault-Bélanger, S., et al. (1991). Relationship between subjective symptoms of visual dysfunction and measurements of vision in a population of former microelectronic workers. *Journal of Occupational Medicine, Singapore, 3*, 75–82.

Merikangas, K.R., Fenton, B.T., Cheng, S.H., et al. (1997). Association between migraine and stroke in a large-scale epidemiological study of the United States. *Archives of Neurology, 54*, 362–368.

Merikangas, K.R. & Stevens, D.E. (1997). Comorbidity of migraine and psychiatric disorders. *Neurologic Clinics, 15*, 115–123.

Merikle, P.M., Smilek, D., & Eastwood, J.D. (2001). Perception without awareness: Perspectives from cognitive psychology. In S. Dehaene (Ed.), *The cognitive neuroscience of consciousness.* Cambridge, MA: MIT Press/Elsevier.

Merten, T. & Beal, C. (2000). An analysis of the Hooper Visual Organization Test with neurological patients. *The Clinical Neuropsychologist, 13*, 521–529.

Mesholam, R.I., Moberg, P.J., Mahr, R.N., & Doty, R.S. (1998), Olfaction in neurodegenerative disease. A meta-analysis of olfactory functioning in Alzheimer's and Parkinson's diseases. *Archives of Neurology, 55*, 84–89.

Messerli, P., Pegna, A., & Sordet, N. (1995). Hemispheric dominance for melody recognition in musicians and non-musicians. *Neuropsychologia, 33*, 395–405.

Messerli, P., Seron, X., & Tissot, R. (1979). Quelques aspects des troubles de la programmation dans le syndrome frontal. *Archives Suisse de Neurologie, Neurochirurgie et Psychiatrie, 125*, 23–35.

Mesulam, M.-M. (1981). A cortical network for directed attention and unilateral neglect. *Annals of Neurology, 10*, 309–325.

Mesulam, M.M. (1998). From sensation to cognition. *Brain, 121*, 1013–1052.

Mesulam, M.-M. (2000a). Aging, Alzheimer's disease, and dementia. Clinical and neurobiological perspectives. In M.-M. Mesulam (Ed.), *Principles of behavioral and cognitive neurology* (2nd ed.). New York: Oxford University Press.

Mesulam, M.-M. (2000b). Behavioral neuroanatomy. In M.-M. Mesulam (Ed.), *Principles of behavioral and cognitive neurology* (2nd ed.). New York: Oxford University Press.

Mesulam, M.-M. (2000c). *Principles of behavioral and cognitive neurology* (2nd ed.). New York: Oxford University Press.

Mesulam, M.-M. (2001). Primary progressive aphasia. *Annals of Neurology, 49*, 425–432.

Metter, E. J. & Wilson, R. S. (1993). Vascular dementias. In R.W. Parks et al. (Eds.), *Neuropsychology of Alzheimer's disease and other dementias.* New York: Oxford University Press.

Metzinger, T. (Ed.) (2000). *Neural correlates of consciousness. Empirical and conceptual questions.* Cambridge, MA: MIT Press.

Metzinger, T. (Ed.) (2003). *The self-model theory of subjectivity.* Cambridge, MA: MIT Press.

Meudell, P., Butters, N., & Montgomery, K. (1978). The role of rehearsal in the short-term memory performance of patients with Korsakoff's and Huntington's disease. *Neuropsychologia, 16*, 507–510.

Meyer, G.J., Finn, S.E., Eyde, L.D., et al. (2001). Psychological testing and psychological assessment: A review of evidence and issues. *American Psychologist, 56*, 128–165.

Meyer, J.S., Kawamura, J., & Terayama, Y. (1994). Cerebral blood flow and metabolism with normal and abnormal aging. In M.L. Albert & J.E. Knoefel (Eds.), *Clinical neurology of aging* (2nd ed.). New York: Oxford University Press.

Meyer, J.S., Li, Y.-S., & Thornby, J. (2001). Validating Mini-Mental Status, Cognitive Capacity screening and Hamilton Depression scales utilizing subjects with vascular headaches. *International Journal of Geriatric Psychiatry, 16*, 430–435.

Meyer, J.S., Shirai, T., & Akiyama, H. (1997). Vascular dementia. In K.M.A. Welch et al. (Eds.), *Primer of cerebrovascular diseases.* San Diego: Academic Press.

Meyer, R.E. (2001). Finding paradigms for the future of alcoholism research: An interdisciplinary perspective. *Alcoholism: Clinical and Experimental Research, 25*, 1393–1406.

Meyer-Baron, M. & Seeber, A. (2000). A meta-analysis for neurobehavioural results due to occupational lead exposure with blood lead concentrations <70 μg/100 ml. *Archives of Toxicology, 73*, 510–518.

Meyerink, L.H., Reitan, R.M., & Selz, M. (1988). The validity of the MMPI with multiple sclerosis patients. *Journal of Clinical Psychology, 44*, 764–769.

Meyers, C., Gengler, L., & Lieffring, D. (1982). L'atrophie cérébrale, diagnostiquée par la tomodensitométrie, face au psychosyndrome organique du Rorschach, dans une population psychiatrique. *Acta Psychiatrica Belgica, 82*, 168–180.

Meyers, C.A. (1985). *The perception of time passage during posttraumatic amnesia.* Paper presented at the 13th annual meeting of the International Neuropsychological Society, San Diego, CA.

Meyers, C.A. (1999). Mood and cognitive disorders in cancer patients receiving cytokine therapy. *Advances in Experimental Medicine and Biology, 461*, 75–81.

Meyers, C.A. (2000a). Cognitive deficits. In M.L. Winningham & M. Barton-Burke (Eds.), *Fatigue in cancer.* Sudbury, MA: Jones and Bartlett.

Meyers, C.A. (2000b). Neurocognitive dysfunction in cancer patients. *Oncology, 14*, 75–78.

Meyers, C.A., Byrne, K.S., & Komaki, R. (1995). Cognitive deficits in patients with small cell lung cancer before and after chemotherapy. *Lung Cancer, 12*, 231–235.

Meyers, C.A. & Cantor, S.B. (2003). Neuropsychological assessment and treatment of patients with malignant brain tumors. In G.P. Prigatano & N.H. Pliskin (Eds.), *Clinical neuropsychology and cost outcome research. A beginning.* New York: Psychology Press.

Meyers, C.A., Geara, F., Wong, P.F., & Morrison, W.H. (2000). Neurocognitive effects of therapeutic irradiation for base of skull tumors. *International Journal of Radiation Oncology, Biology, and Physics, 46*, 51–55.

Meyers, C.A., Hess, K.R., Yung, W.K., & Levin, V.A. (2000). Cognitive function as a predictor of survival in patients with recurrent malignant glioma. *Journal of Clinical Oncology, 18*, 646–650.

Meyers, C.A. & Levin, H.S. (1992). Temporal perception following closed head injury: Relationship of orientation and attention span. *Neuropsychiatry, Neuropsychology, and Behavioral Neurology, 5*, 28–32.

Meyers, C.A., Levin, H.S., Eisenberg, H.M., & Guinto, F.C. (1983). Early versus late lateral ventricular enlargement following closed head injury. *Journal of Neurology, Neurosurgery and Psychiatry, 46*, 1092–1097.

Meyers, C.A. & Scheibel, R.S. (1990). Early detection and diagnosis of neurobehavioral disorders associated with cancer and its treatment. *Oncology, 4,* 115–130.

Meyers, C.A., Scheibel, R.S., & Forman, A.D. (1991). Persistent neurotoxicity of systemically administered interferon-alpha. *Neurology, 41,* 672–676.

Meyers, C.A., Weitzner, M.A., Valentine, A.D., & Levin, V.A. (1998). Methylphenidate therapy improves cognition, mood and function of brain tumor patients. *Journal of Clinical Oncology, 16,* 2522–2527.

Meyers, J.E. & Diep, A. (2000). Assessment of malingering in chronic pain patients using neuropsychological tests. *Applied Neuropsychology, 7,* 133–139.

Meyers, J.E., Galinsky, A.M., & Volbrecht, M. (1999). Malingering and mild brain injury: How low is too low. *Applied Neuropsychology, 6,* 208–216.

Meyers, J.E. & Lange, D. (1994). Recognition subtest for the Complex Figure. *The Clinical Neuropsychologist, 8,* 153–186.

Meyers, J.E. & Meyers, K.R. (1995a). *Rey Complex Figure Test and Recognition Trial.* Odessa, FL: Psychological Assessment Resources.

Meyers, J.E. & Meyers, K.R. (1995b). Rey Complex Figure Test under four different administration procedures. *The Clinical Neuropsychologist, 9,* 63–67.

Meyers, J.E., Millis, S.R., & Volkert, K. (2002). A validity index for the MMPI-2. *Archives of Clinical Neuropsychology, 17,* 157–169.

Meyers, J.E. & Volbrecht, M. (1998). Validation of reliable digits for detection of malingering. *Assessment, 5,* 303–307.

Meyers, J.E. & Volbrecht, M. (1999). Detection of malingerers using the Rey Complex Figure and Recognition Trial. *Applied Neuropsychology, 6,* 201–207.

Meyers, J.E. & Volbrecht, M. (2003). A validation of multiple malingering detection methods in a large clinical sample. *Archives of Clinical Neuropsychology, 18,* 261–276.

Meyers, J.E., Volbrecht, M., & Kaster-Bundgaard, J. (1999). Driving is more than pedal pushing. *Applied Neuropsychology, 6,* 154–164.

Miceli, G., Caltagirone, C., Gainotti, G., et al. (1981). Neuropsychological correlates of localized cerebral lesions in nonaphasic brain-damaged patients. *Journal of Clinical Neuropsychology, 3,* 53–63.

Michiels, V. & Cluydts, R. (2001). Neuropsychological functioning in chronic fatigue syndrome: A review. *Acta Psychiatrica Scandinavica, 103,* 84–93.

Middleton, F.A. & Strick, P.L. (2000a). Basal ganglia and cerebellar loops: Motor and cognitive circuits. *Brain Research: Brain Research Reviews, 31,* 236–250.

Middleton, F.A. & Strick, P.L. (2000b). Basal ganglia output and cognition: Evidence from anatomical, behavioral, and clinical studies. *Brain and Cognition, 42,* 183–200.

Milanovich, J.R., Axelrod, B. N., & Millis, S. R. (1996). Validation of the Simulation Index-Revised with a mixed clinical population. *Archives of Clinical Neuropsychology, 11,* 53–59.

Milberg, W. & Albert, M. (1989). Cognitive differences between patients with progressive supranuclear palsy and Alzheimer's disease. *Journal of Clinical and Experimental Neuropsychology, 11,* 605–614.

Milberg, W., Cummings, J., Goodglass, H., & Kaplan, E. (1979). Case report: A global sequential processing disorder following head injury: A possible role for the right hemisphere in serial order behavior. *Journal of Clinical Neuropsychology, 1,* 213–225.

Milberg, W.P., Hebben, N., & Kaplan, E. (1996). The Boston process approach to neuropsychological assessment. In I. Grant & K.M. Adams (Eds.), *Neuropsychological assessment of neuropsychiatric disorders* (2nd ed.). New York: Oxford University Press.

Milders, M. (1998). Learning people's names following severe closed-head injury. *Journal of Clinical and Experimental Neuropsychology, 20,* 237–244.

Milders, M., Deelman, B., & Berg, I. (1999). Retrieving familiar people's names in patients with severe closed-head injuries. *Journal of Clinical and Experimental Neuropsychology, 21,* 171–185.

Milhaud, D., Bogousslavsky, J., van Melle, G., & Liot, P. (2001). Ischemic stroke and active migraine. *Neurology, 57,* 1805–1811.

Miller, A., Donders, J., & Suhr, J. A. (2000). Evaluation of malingering with the WIsconsin Card Sorting Test: A cross-validation. *Clinical Neuropsychological Assessment, 2,* 141–149.

Miller, A.E. (2001). Clinical features. In S.D. Cook (Ed.), *Handbook of multiple sclerosis* (3rd ed.). New York: Marcel Dekker.

Miller, B.L., Ikonte, C., Ponton, M., et al. (1997). A study of the Lund-Manchester research criteria for frontotemporal dementia: Clinical and single-photon emission CT correlations. *Neurology, 48,* 937–942.

Miller, D.H., Barkhof, F., & Nauta, J.J. (1993). Gadolinium enhancement increases the sensitivity of MRI in detecting disease activity in multiple sclerosis. *Brain, 116,* 1077–1094.

Miller, D.H., Grossman, R.I., Reingold, S.C., & McFarland, H.F. (1998). The role of magnetic resonance techniques in understanding and managing multiple sclerosis. *Brain, 121,* 3–24.

Miller, E. (1972). *Clinical neuropsychology.* Harmondsworth, UK: Penguin Books.

Miller, E. (1973). Short- and long-term memory in patients with presenile dementia (Alzheimer's disease). *Psychological Medicine, 3,* 221–224.

Miller, E. (1983). A note on the interpretation of data derived from neuropsychological tests. *Cortex, 19,* 131–132.

Miller, E.N., Selnes, O.A., McArthur, J.C., et al. (1990). Neuropsychological peformance in HIV-1-infected homosexual men: The Multicenter AIDS Cohort Study (MACS). *Neurology, 40,* 197–203.

Miller, G.A. (1956). The magical number seven, plus or minus two: Some limits on our capacity for processing information. *Psychological Review, 63,* 81–97.

Miller, G.A., Galanter, E., & Pribram, K.H. (1960). *Plans and the structure of behavior.* New York: Holt.

Miller, J.D. (1991). Pathophysiology and management of head injury. *Neuropsychology, 5,* 235–261.

Miller, J.D. & Jones, P.A. (1990). Minor head injury. In M. Rosenthal et al. (Eds.), *Rehabilitation of the adult and child with traumatic brain injury* (2nd ed.). Philadelphia: Davis.

Miller, J.D., Piper, I.R., & Jones, P.A. (1996). Pathophysiology of head injury. In R.K. Narayan et al. (Eds.), *Neurotrauma.* New York: McGraw-Hill.

Miller, J.D., Piper, I.R., & Stathan, P.F.X. (1996). ICP monitoring: Indications and techniques. In R.K. Narayan et al. (Eds.), *Neurotrauma.* New York: McGraw-Hill.

Miller, J.M., Chaffin, D.B., & Smith, R.G. (1975). Subclinical psychomotor and neuromuscular changes in workers exposed to inorganic mercury. *American Industrial Hygiene Association Journal, 36,* 725–733.

Miller, L. (1990). Litigating the head trauma case: Issues and answers for attorneys and their clients. *Cognitive Rehabilitation, 8,* 8–12.

Miller, L. & Milner, B. (1985). Cognitive risk-taking after frontal or temporal lobectomy—II. *Neuropsychologia, 23,* 371–379.

Miller, L.L. (1976). Marijuana and human cognition: A review of laboratory investigations. In S. Cohen & R.C. Stillman (Eds.), *The therapeutic potential of marijuana.* New York: Plenum Press.

Miller, R.E., Shapiro, A.P., King, H.E., et al. (1984). Effect of antihypertensive treatment on the behavioral consequences of elevated blood pressure. *Hypertension, 6,* 202–208.

Miller, W.R. & Saucedo, C.F. (1983). Assessment of neuropsychological impairment and brain damage in problem drinkers. In C.J.

Golden et al. (Eds.), *Clinical neuropsychology: Interface with neurologic and psychiatric disorders*. New York: Grune & Stratton.

Millis, S.R. (1992). Recognition Memory Test in the detection of malingered and exaggerated memory deficits. *The Clinical Neuropsychologist, 6*, 406–414.

Millis, S.R. (1995). Factor structure of the California Verbal Learning Test in moderate and severe closed-head injury. *Perceptual and Motor Skills, 80*, 219–224.

Millis, S.R. & Kler, S. (1995). Limitations of the Rey Fifteen-Item test in the detection of malingering. *The Clinical Neuropsychologist, 9*, 241–244.

Millis, S.R., Malina, A.C., Bowers, D.A., & Ricker, J.H. (1999). Confirmatory factor analysis of the Wechsler Memory Scale-III. *Journal of Clinical and Experimental Neuropsychology, 21*, 87–93.

Millis, S.R. & Putnam, S.H. (1994). The Recognition Memory Test in the assessment of memory impairment after financially compensable mild head injury: A replication. *Perceptual and Motor Skills, 79*, 384–386.

Millis, S.R. & Putnam, S.H. (1996). Detection of malingering in postconcussive syndrome. In M. Rizzo & D. Tranel (Eds.), *Head injury and postconcussive syndrome*. New York: Churchill Livingstone.

Millis, S.R., Putnam, S.H., Adams, K.M., & Ricker, J.H. (1995). The California Verbal Learning Test in the detection of incomplete effort in neuropsychological evaluation. *Psychological Assessment, 7*, 463–471.

Millis, S.R., Rosenthal, M., Novack, T.A., et al. (2001). Long-term neuropsychological outcome after traumatic brain injury. *Journal of Head Trauma Rehabilitation, 16*, 343–355.

Millis, S.R., Ross, S.R., & Ricker, J.H. (1998). Detection of incomplete effort on the Wechsler Adult Intelligence Scale-Revised: A cross-validation. *Journal of Clinical and Experimental Neuropsychology, 20*, 167–173.

Millon, T. (1977). *Millon Clinical Multiaxial Inventory*. Minneapolis, MN: National Computer Systems.

Millon, T. (1987). *Manual for the MCMI-II* (2nd ed.). Minneapolis, MN: National Computer Systems.

Millon, T. (1994). *Manual for the MCMI-III*. Minneapolis, MN: National Computer Systems.

Milner, B. (1954). Intellectual function of the temporal lobes. *Psychological Bulletin, 51*, 42–62.

Milner, B. (1958). Psychological deficits in temporal lobe excision. In H.C. Solomon et al. (Eds.), *The brain and human behavior*. Baltimore: Williams & Wilkins.

Milner, B. (1962). Les troubles de le memoire accompagnant des lésions hippocampiques bilaterales. In *Physiologie de l'hippocampe*. Paris: Centre National de la Recherche Scientifique.

Milner, B. (1963). Effects of different brain lesions on card sorting. *Archives of Neurology, 9*, 90–100.

Milner, B. (1964). Some effects of frontal lobectomy in man. In J.M. Warren & K. Akert (Eds.), *The frontal granular cortex and behavior*. New York: McGraw-Hill.

Milner, B. (1965). Memory disturbance after bilateral hippocampal lesions. In P.M. Milner & S. Glickman (Eds.), *Cognitive processes and the brain*. Princeton: Van Nostrand.

Milner, B. (1968). Visual recognition and recall after right temporal-lobe excision in man. *Neuropsychologia, 6*, 191–209.

Milner, B. (1970). Memory and the medial temporal regions of the brain. In K. H. Pribram & D. E. Broadbent (Eds.), *Biology of memory*. New York: Academic Press.

Milner, B. (1971). Interhemispheric differences in the localization of psychological processes in man. *British Medical Bulletin, 27*, 272–277.

Milner, B. (1972). Disorders of learning and memory after temporal lobe lesions in man. *Clinical Neurosurgery, 19*, 421–446.

Milner, B. (1974). Hemisphere specialization: Scope and limits. In F.O. Schmitt & F.G. Worden (Eds.), *The Neuroscience Third Study Program*. Cambridge, MA: MIT Press.

Milner, B. (1975). Psychological aspects of focal epilepsy and its neurological management. In D.P. Purpura et al. (Eds.), *Advances in neurology* (Vol. 8). New York: Raven Press.

Milner, B. (1978). Clues to the cerebral organization of memory. In P.A. Buser & A. Rougeul-Buser (Eds.), *Cerebral correlates of conscious experience*. INSERM Symposium 6. Amsterdam: Elsevier/North-Holland.

Milner, B., Corsi, P., & Leonard, G. (1991). Frontal-lobe contribution to recency judgements. *Neuropsychologia, 29*, 601–618.

Milner, B. & Petrides, M. (1984). Behavioural effects of frontal lobe lesions in man. *Trends in Neuroscience, 7*, 403–407.

Milner, B. & Taylor, L. (1972). Right hemisphere superiority in tactile pattern-recognition after cerebral commissurectomy. *Neuropsychologia, 10*, 1–15.

Milton, W.J., O'Dell, R.H., & Warner, E.G. (1996). MRI of lightning injury: Early white matter changes associated with cerebral dysfunction. *Journal of Oklahoma State Medical Association, 89*, 93–94.

Mimura, M., Kato, M., Sano, Y., et al. (1998). Prospective and retrospective studies of recovery in aphasia. Changes in cerebral blood flow and language functions. *Brain, 121*, 2083–2094.

Minden, S.L., Moes, E.J., Orav, J., et al. (1990). Memory impairment in multiple sclerosis. *Journal of Clinical and Experimental Neuropsychology, 12*, 566–586.

Minden, S.L., Orav, J., & Reich, P. (1987). Depression in multiple sclerosis. *General Hospital Psychiatry, 9*, 426–434.

Minden, S.L. & Schiffer, R.B. (1990). Affective disorders in multiple sclerosis. *Archives of Neurology, 47*, 98–104.

Minnaert, A.E. (1999). Individual differences in text comprehension as a function of text anxiety and prior knowledge. *Psychological Reports, 84*, 167–177.

Miranda, J.P. & Valencia, R.R. (1997). English and Spanish versions of a memory test: Word-length effects versus spoken-duration effects. *Hispanic Journal of Behavioral Sciences, 19*, 171–181.

Mirsky, A.F. (1989). The neuropsychology of attention: Elements of a complex behavior. In E. Perecman (Ed.), *Integrating theory and practice in clinical neuropsychology*. Hillsdale, NJ: Erlbaum.

Mishkin, M. & Appenzeller, T. (1987). The anatomy of memory. *Scientific American, 256*, 80–89.

Mishkin, M. & Petri, H.L. (1984). Memories and habits: Some implications for the analysis of learning and retention. In L.R. Squire & N. Butters (Eds.), *Neuropsychology of memory*. New York: Guilford Press.

Mishkin, M., Ungerleider, L.G., & Macko, K.A. (1983). Object vision and spatial vision: Two cortical pathways. *Trends in Neurosciences, 6*, 414–417.

Mitchell, K.J. & Johnson, M.K. (2000). Source monitoring. Attributing mental experiences. In E. Tulving & F.I.M. Craik (Eds.), *The Oxford handbook of memory*. Oxford: Oxford University Press.

Mitchell, M. (1987). Scoring discrepancies on two subtests of the Wechsler Memory Scale. *Journal of Consulting and Clinical Psychology, 55*, 914–915.

Mitrushina, M.N., Boone, K.B., & D'Elia, L.F. (1999). *Handbook of normative data for neuropsychological assessment*. New York: Oxford University Press.

Mitrushina, M., Drebing, C., Uchiyama, C., et al. (1994). The pattern of deficit in different memory components in normal aging and dementia of Alzheimer's type. *Journal of Clinical Psychology, 50*, 591–596.

Mitrushina, M. & Satz, P. (1991). Effect of repeated administration of a neuropsychological battery in the elderly. *Journal of Clinical Psychology, 47*, 790–801.

Mitrushina, M. & Satz, P. (1995a). Base rates of the WAIS-R inter-subtest scatter and VIQ-PIQ discrepancy in normal elderly. *Journal of Clinical Psychology, 51,* 70–78.

Mitrushina, M. & Satz, P. (1995b). Repeated testing of normal elderly with the Boston Naming Test. *Aging (Milano), 7,* 123–127.

Mitrushina, M., Satz, P., & Van Gorp, W. (1989). Some putative cognitive precursors in subjects hypothesized to be at-risk for dementia. *Archives of Clinical Neuropsychology, 4,* 323–333.

Mitrushina, M., Uchiyama, C., & Satz, P. (1995). Heterogeneity of cognitive profiles in normal aging: Implications for early manifestations of Alzheimer's disease. *Journal of Clinical and Experimental Neuropsychology, 17,* 374–382.

Mittenberg, W., Arzin, R., Millsaps, C., & Heilbronner, R. (1993). Identification of malingered head injury on the Wechsler Memory Scale-Revised. *Psychological Assessment, 5,* 34–40.

Mittenberg, W., Hammeke, T.A., & Rao, S.M. (1989). Intrasubtest scatter on the WAIS-R as a pathognomonic sign of brain injury. *Psychological Assessment, 1,* 273–276.

Mittenberg, W., Kasprisin, A., & Farage, C. (1985). Localization and diagnosis in aphasia with the Luria-Nebraska Neuropsychological Battery. *Journal of Consulting and Clinical Psychology, 53,* 386–392.

Mittenberg, W. & Motta, S. (1993). Effects of chronic cocaine abuse on memory and learning. *Archives of Clinical Neuropsychology, 8,* 477–483.

Mittenberg, W., Rotholc, A., Russell, E., & Heilbronner, R. (1996). Identification of malingered head trauma on the Halstead-Reitan Battery. *Archives of Clinical Neuropsychology, 11,* 271–281.

Mittenberg, W., Seidenberg, M., O'Leary, D.S., & DiGiulio, D.V. (1989). Changes in cerebral functioning associated with normal aging. *Journal of Clinical and Experimental Neuropsychology, 11,* 918–932.

Mittenberg, W., Theroux-Fichera, S., Zielinski, R., and Heilbronner, R.L. (1995). Identification of malingered head injury on the Wechsler Adult Intelligence Scale-Revised. *Professional Psychology: Research and Practice, 26,* 491–498.

Mittl, R.L., Grossman, R.I., Hiehle, J.F., et al. (1994). Prevalence of MR evidence of diffuse axonal injury in patients with mild head injury and normal head CT findings. *American Journal of Neuroradiology, 15,* 1583–1589.

Miyake, A., Friedman, N.P., Emerson, M.J., et al. (2000). The unity and diversity of executive functions and their contributions to complex "frontal lobe" tasks: A latent variable analysis. *Cognitive Psychology, 41,* 49–100.

Miyamoto, O. & Auer, R.N. (2000). Hypoxia, hyperoxia, ischemia, and brain necrosis. *Neurology, 54,* 362–371.

Miyazaki, Y., Isojima, A., Takekawa, M., et al. (1995). Frontal acute extradural hematoma due to contrecoup injury: A case report. *No Shinkei Geka (Neurological Surgery), 23,* 917–920.

Moberg, P.J., Pearlson, G.D., Speedy, L.J., et al. (1987). Olfactory recognition: Differential impairments in early and late Huntington's and Alzheimer's diseases. *Journal of Clinical and Experimental Neuropsychology, 9,* 650–664.

Mody, C.K., Miller, B.L., McIntyre, H.B., et al. (1988). Neurologic complications of cocaine abuse. *Neurology, 38,* 1189–1193.

Moehle, K.A., Fitzhugh-Bell, K.B., Engleman, E., & Hennon, D. (1987). Diagnostic accuracy of the Halstead Category Test and a short form [abstract]. *Journal of Clinical and Experimental Neuropsychology, 9,* 37.

Moene, F.C., Landberg, E.H., Hoogduin, K.A., et al. (2000). Organic syndromes diagnosed as conversion disorder: Identification and frequency in a study of 85 patients. *Journal of Psychosomatic Research, 49,* 7–12.

Mohr, D.C., Boudewyn, A.C., Goodkin, D.E., et al. (2001). Comparative outcomes for individual cognitive-behavior therapy, supportive-expressive group psychotherapy, and sertraline for the treatment of depression in multiple sclerosis. *Journal of Consulting and Clinical Psychology, 69,* 942–949.

Mohr, D.C. & Goodkin, D.E. (1999). Treatment of depression in multiple sclerosis: Review and meta-analysis. *Clinical Psychology: Science and Practice, 6,* 1–9.

Mohr, D.C., Goodkin, D.E., Bacchetti, P., et al. (2000). Psychological stress and the subsequent appearance of new brain MRI lesions in MS. *Neurology, 55,* 55–61.

Mohr, D.C., Goodkin, D.E., Islar, J., et al. (2001). Treatment of depression is associated with suppression of nonspecific and antigen-specific TH1 responses in multiple sclerosis. *Archives of Neurology, 58,* 1081–1086.

Mohr, J.P., Spetzler, R.F., Kistler, J.P., et al. (1986). Intracranial aneurysms. In H.J.M. Bennett et al. (Eds.), *Stroke. Pathophysiology, diagnosis, and management.* New York: Churchill Livingstone.

Mohr, J.P., Tatemichi, T.K., Nichols, F.C., et al. (1986). Vascular malformations of the brain: Clinical considerations. In H.J.M. Bennett et al. (Eds.), *Stroke. Pathophysiology, diagnosis, and management.* New York: Churchill Livingstone.

Mohr, E., Walker, D., Randolph, C., et al. (1996). Utility of clinical trial batteries in the measurement of Alzheimer's and Huntington's dementia. *International Psychogeriatrics, 8,* 397–411.

Mohs, R.C., Knopman, D., Petersen, R.C., et al. (1997). Development of cognitive instruments for use in clinical trials of antidementia drugs: Additions to the Alzheimer's Disease Assessment Scale that broaden its scope. *Alzheimer Disease and Associated Disorders, 11(Suppl. 2),* S13–S21.

Money, J. (1976). *A Standardized Road Map Test of Direction Sense. Manual.* San Rafael, CA: Academic Therapy Publications.

Monsch, A.U., Bondi, M.W., Butters, N., et al. (1992). Comparisons of verbal fluency tasks in the detection of dementia of the Alzheimer type. *Archives of Neurology, 49,* 1253–1258.

Monsch, A.U., Bondi, M.W., & Butters, N., et al. (1994). A comparison of category and letter fluency in Alzheimer's disease. *Neuropsychology, 8,* 25–30.

Monsch, A.U., Bondi, M.W., Salmon, D.P., et al. (1995). Clinical validity of the Mattis Dementia Rating Scale in detecting dementia of the Alzheimer type. A double cross-validation and application to a community-dwelling sample. *Archives of Neurology, 52,* 899–904.

Montaldi, D. & Parkin, A.J. (1989). Retrograde amnesia in Korsakoff's syndrome: An experimental and theoretical analysis. In J. Crawford & D. Parker (Eds.), *Developments in clinical and experimental neuropsychology.* New York: Plenum Press.

Monteiro, I.M., Boksay, I., Auer, S.R., et al. (2001). Addition of a frequency-weighted score to the Behavioral Pathology in Alzheimer's Disease Rating Scale: The BEHAVE-AD-FW: methodology and reliability. *European Psychiatry, 16(Suppl. 1),* 5s–24s.

Montemurro, D.G. & Bruni, J.E. (1988). *The human brain in dissection* (2nd ed.). New York: Oxford University Press.

Montgomery, K. & Costa, L. (1983). *Neuropsychological test performance of a normal elderly sample.* Paper presented at the eleventh annual meeting of the International Neuropsychological Society, Mexico City, Mexico.

Montreys, C.R. & Borod, J.C. (1998). A preliminary evaluation of emotional experience and expression following unilateral brain damage. *International Journal of Neuroscience, 96,* 269–283.

Moore, P.M. & Baker, G.A. (1996). Validation of the Wechsler Memory Scale-Revised in a sample of people with intractable temporal lobe epilepsy. *Epilepsia, 37,* 1215–1220.

Moore, P.M. & Baker, G.A. (1997). Psychometric properties and factor structure of the Wechsler Memory Scale-Revised in a sample of persons with intractable epilepsy. *Journal of Clinical and Experimental Neuropsychology, 19,* 897–905.

Moore, R.D., Bone, L.R., Geller, G., et al. (1989). Prevalence, detection, and treatment of alcoholism in hospitalized patients. *Journal of the American Medical Association, 261,* 403–407.

Moore, W.H., Jr. (1984). The role of right hemispheric information processing strategies in language recovery in aphasia: An electroencephalographic investigation of hemispheric alpha asymmetries in normal and aphasic subjects. *Cortex, 20,* 193–205.

Moossy, J., Zubenko, G.S., Martinez, A.J., et al. (1989). Lateralization of brain morphologic and cholinergic abnormalities in Alzheimer's disease. *Archives of Neurology, 46,* 639–642.

Moreno, C.R., Borod, J.C., Welkowitz, J., & Alpert, M. (1990). Lateralization for the expression and perception of facial emotion as a function of age. *Neuropsychologia, 28,* 199–209.

Moretti, R., Torre, P., Antonello, R. M., et al. (2002). Ten-point clock test: A correlation analysis with other neuropsychological tests in dementia. *International Journal of Geriatric Psychiatry, 17,* 347–353.

Morey, L.C. (1991). *Personality Assessment Inventory: Professional manual.* Odessa, FL: Psychological Assessment Resources.

Morey, L.C. & Lanier, V.W. (1998). Operating characteristics of six reponse distortion indicators for the Personality Assessment Inventory. *Assessment, 5,* 203–214.

Morgan, D.G. & Gordon, M.N. (1996). Aging and molecular biology. In D. Magnusson (Ed.), *The lifespan development of individuals. Behavioral, neurobiological, and psychosocial perspectives.* New York: Cambridge University Press.

Morgan, J.E. & Caccappolo-van Vliet, E. (2001). Advanced years and low education: The case against the comprehensive norms. *Journal of Forensic Neuropsychology, 2,* 53–69.

Morgan, M.J. (1999). Memory deficits associated with recreational use of "ecstasy" (MDMA). *Psychopharmacology, 141,* 30–36.

Morgan, S. (1992). The relationship between performance on the Symbol Digit Modalities Test and WAIS Digit Symbol [abstract]. *Journal of Clinical and Experimental Psychology, 14,* 63.

Morgen, K., Martin, R., Stone, R.D., et al. (2001). FLAIR and magnetization transfer imaging of patients with post-treatment Lyme disease syndrome. *Neurology, 57,* 1980–1985.

Mori, E., Shimomura, T., Fujimori, M., et al. (2000). Visuoperceptual impairment in dementia with Lewy Bodies. *Archives of Neurology, 57,* 489–493.

Moriarty, D.M., Blackshaw, A.J., Talabot, P.R., et al. (1999). Memory dysfunction in multiple sclerosis corresponds to juxtacortical lesion load on fast fluid-attenuated inversion-recovery MR images. *American Journal of Neuroradiology, 20,* 1956–1962.

Morita, A., Puumala, M.R., & Meyer, F.B. (1998). Intracranial aneurysms and subarachnoid hemorrhage. In M. Swash (Ed.), *Outcomes in neurological and neurosurgical disorders.* Cambridge, UK: Cambridge University Press.

Moritz, D.J., Kasl, S.V., & Berkman, L.F. (1995). Cognitive functioning and the incidence of limitations in activities of daily living in an elderly community sample. *American Journal of Epidemiology, 141,* 41–49.

Morley, G.K., Lundgren, S., & Haxby, J. (1979). Comparison and clinical applicability of auditory comprehension scores on the Behavioral Neurology Deficit Evaluation, Boston Diagnostic Aphasia Examination, Porch Index of Communicative Ability, and Token Tests. *Journal of Clinical Neuropsychology, 1,* 249–258.

Morris, J., Kunka, J.M., & Rossini, E.D. (1997). Development of alternative paragraphs for the Logical Memory subtest of the Wechsler Memory Scale-Revised. *The Clinical Neuropsychologist, 11,* 370–374.

Morris, J.C., Cyrus, P.a., Orazem, J., et al. (1998). Metrifonate benefits cognitive, behavioral, and global function in patients with Alzheimer's disease. *Neurology, 50,* 1222–1230.

Morris, J.C., Edland, S., Clark, C., et al. (1993). The Consortium to Establish a Registry for Alzheimer's Disease (CERAD). Part IV. Rates of cognitive change in the longitudinal assessment of probable Alzheimer's disease. *Neurology, 43,* 2457–2465.

Morris, J.C., Heyman, A., Mohs, R.C., et al. (1989). The Consortium to Establish a Registry for Alzheimer's Disease (CERAD). Part I. Clinical and neuropsychological assessment of Alzheimer's disease. *Neurology, 39,* 1159–65.

Morris, J.C., McKeel, D.W., Jr., Fulling, K., et al. (1988). Validation of clinical diagnostic criteria for Alzheimer's disease. *Annals of Neurology, 24,* 17–22.

Morris, J.C., McKeel, D.W., Storandt, M., et al. (1991). Very mild Alzheimer's disease: Informant-based clinical, psychometric, and pathologic distinction from normal aging. *Neurology, 41,* 469–478.

Morris, J.C. & McManus, D.Q. (1991). The neurology of aging: normal versus pathologic change. *Geriatrics, 46,* 47–48, 51–44.

Morris, R.D. & Baddeley, A.D. (1988). Primary and working memory functioning in Alzheimer-type dementia. *Journal of Clinical and Experimental Neuropsychology, 10,* 279–296.

Morris, R.D., Hopkins, W.D., & Bolser-Gilmore, L. (1993). Assessment of hand preference in two language-trained chimpanzees (Pantroglodytes): A multimethod analysis. *Journal of Clinical and Experimental Neuropsychology, 15,* 487–502.

Morris, R.G., Abrahams, S., & Polkey, C.E. (1995). Recognition memory for words and faces following unilateral temporal lobectomy. *British Journal of Clinical Psychology, 34,* 571–576.

Morris, R.G. & Kopelman, M.D. (1986). The memory deficits in Alzheimer-type dementia: A review. *Quarterly Journal of Experimental Psychology, 38A,* 575–602.

Morris, R.G. & Kopelman, M.D. (1992). The neuropsychological assessment of dementia. In J.R. Crawford et al. (Eds.), *A handbook of neuropsychological assessment.* Hillsdale, NJ: Erlbaum.

Morris, R.G., Miotto, E.C., Feigenbaum, J.D., et al. (1997). The effect of goal-subgoal conflict on planning ability after frontal- and temporal-lobe lesions in humans. *Neuropsychologia, 35,* 1147–1157.

Morrison, R.G. (1986). Medical and public health aspects of boxing. *Journal of the American Medical Association, 255,* 2475–2480.

Morrison, R.S. and Sui, A.L. (2000). Survival in end-stage dementia following acute illness. *Journal of the American Medical Association, 284,* 47–52.

Morrow, L.A. (1998). Assessment following neurotoxic exposure. In G. Goldstein et al. (Eds.), *Neuropsychology.* New York: Plenum Press.

Morrow, L.A., Furman, J.M.R., Ryan, C.M., & Hodgson, M.J. (1988). Neuropsychological deficits associated with vestibular abnormalities in solvent exposed workers [abstract]. *The Clinical Neuropsychologist, 2,* 272–273.

Morrow, L.A., Kamis, H., & Hodgson, M.J. (1993). Psychiatric symptomatology in persons with organic solvent exposure. *Journal of Consulting and Clinical Psychology, 61,* 171–174.

Morrow, L.A., Muldoon, S.B., & Sandstrom, D.J. (2001). Neuropsychological sequelae associated with occupational and environmental exposure to chemicals. In R.E. Tarter et al. (Eds.), *Medical neuropsychology* (2nd ed.). New York: Kluwer Academic/Plenum Press.

Morrow, L.A. & Ratcliff, G. (1988). The disengagement of covert attention and the neglect syndrome. *Psychobiology, 16,* 261–269.

Morrow, L.A., Robin, N., Hodgson, M.J., & Kamis, H. (1992). Assessment of attention and memory efficiency in persons with solvent neurotoxicity. *Neuropsychologia, 30,* 911–922.

Morrow, L.A., Ryan, C.M., Goldstein, G., & Hodgson, M.J. (1989). A distinct pattern of personality disturbance following exposure to mixtures of organic solvents. *Journal of Occupational Medicine, 31,* 743–746.

Morrow, L.A., Ryan, C.M., Hodgson, M.J., & Robin, N. (1990). Alterations in cognitive and psychological functioning after organic solvent exposure. *Journal of Occupational Medicine, 32,* 444–449.

Morrow, L.A., Ryan, C.M., Hodgson, M.J., & Robin, N. (1991). Risk factors associated with persistence of neuropsychological deficits in persons with organic solvent exposure. *Journal of Nervous of Mental Disease, 179,* 540–545.

Morrow, L.A., Stein, L., Bagovich, G.R., et al. (2001). Neuropsychological assessment, depression, and past exposure to organic solvents. *Applied Neuropsychology, 8,* 65–73.

Morrow, L.A., Steinhauer, S.R., & Condray, R. (1996). Differential associations of P300 amplitude and latency with cognitive and psychiatric function in solvent-exposed adults. *Journal of Neuropsychiatry and Clinical Neuroscience, 8,* 446–449.

Morrow, L.A., Steinhauer, S.R., Condray, R., & Hodgson, M. (1997). Neuropsychological performance of journeymen painters under acute solvent exposure and exposure-free conditions. *Journal of the International Neuropsychological Society, 3,* 269–275.

Morrow, L.A., Steinhauer, S.R., & Hodgson, M.J. (1992). Delay in P300 latency in patients with organic solvent exposure. *Archives of Neurology, 49,* 315–320.

Morrow, L.A., Vrtunski, P.B., Kim, Y., & Boller, F. (1981). Arousal responses to emotional stimuli and laterality of lesion. *Neuropsychologia, 19,* 65–71.

Mortensen, E.L., Gade, A., & Reinisch, J.M. (1991). "Best Performance Method" in clinical neuropsychology. *Journal of Clinical and Experimental Neuropsychology, 13,* 361–371.

Mortimer, J.A. (1988a). The dementia of Parkinson's disease. *Clinics in Geriatric Medicine, 4,* 785–797.

Mortimer, J.A. (1988b). Do psychosocial risk factors contribute to Alzheimer's disease? In A.S. Henderson & J.H. Henderson (Eds.), *Etiology of dementia of Alzheimer's type.* Chichester, UK: Wiley.

Mortimer, J.A. (1997). Brain reserve and the clinical expression of Alzheimer's disease. *Geriatrics, 52(Suppl. 2),* S50–S53.

Mortimer, J.A., Christensen, K.J., & Webster, D.D. (1985). Parkinsonian dementia. In P.J. Vinken, G.W. Bruyn, & H.L. Klawans (Eds.), *Handbook of clinical neurology* (Vol. 2 [46]). Amsterdam: Elsevier.

Mortimer, J.A., French, L.R., Hutton, J.T., & Schuman, L.M. (1985). Head injury as a risk factor for Alzheimer's disease. *Neurology, 35,* 264–266.

Mortimer, J.A. & Pirozzolo, F.J. (1985). Remote effects of head trauma. *Developmental Neuropsychology, 1,* 215–229.

Mortimer, J.A., Pirozzolo, F.J., Hansch, E.C., & Webster, D.D. (1982). Relationship of motor symptoms to intellectual deficits in Parkinson disease. *Neurology, 32,* 133–137.

Morton, M.V. & Wehman, P. (1995). Psychosocial and emotional sequelae of individuals with traumatic brain injury: A literature review and recommendations. *Brain Injury, 9,* 81–92.

Moscovitch, M. (1979). Information processing and the cerebral hemisphere. In M.S. Gazzaniga (Ed.), *Handbook of behavioral neurobiology. II. Neuropsychology.* New York: Plenum Press.

Moscovitch, M. (2000). Theories of memory and consciousness. In E. Tulving & F.I.M. Craik (Eds.), *The Oxford handbook of memory.* Oxford, UK: Oxford University Press.

Moser, R.S. & Schatz, P. (2002). Enduring effects of concussion in young athletes. *Archives of Clinical Neuropsychology, 17,* 91–100.

Moses, H. 3rd, & Kaden, I. (1986). Neurologic consultations in a general hospital. Spectrum of iatrogenic disease. *American Journal of Medicine, 81,* 955–958.

Moses, J.A., Jr., Cardellino, J.P., & Thompson, L.L. (1983). Discrimination of brain damage from chronic psychosis by the Luria-Nebraska Neuropsychological Battery: a closer look. *Journal of Consulting and Clinical Psychology, 51,* 441–449.

Moses, J.A., Jr., Pritchard, D.A., and Adams, R.L. (1996). Modal

profiles for the Wechsler Adult Intelligence Scale-Revised. *Archives of Clinical Neuropsychology, 11,* 61–68.

Mosimann, U.P., Müri, R.M., Felblinger, J., & Radanov, B.P. (2000). Saccadic eye movement disturbances in whiplash patients with persistent complaints. *Brain, 123,* 828–835.

Moss, M.B., Albert, M.S., Butters, N., & Payne, M. (1986). Differential patterns of memory loss among patients with Alzheimer's disease, Huntington's disease, and Korsakoff's syndrome. *Archives of Neurology, 43,* 239–246.

Moss, M.B., Albert, M.S., & Kemper, T.L. (1992). Neuropsychology of frontal lobe dementia. In R. F. White (Ed.), *Clinical syndromes in adult neuropsychology: The practitioner's handbook.* Amsterdam: Elsevier.

Moss, P.S., Wan, A., & Whitlock, M.R. (2002). A changing pattern of injuries to horse riders. *Emergency Medicine Journal, 19,* 412–414.

Motohashi, O., Tominaga, T., Shimizu, H., et al. (2000). Acute epidural hematoma caused by contrecoup injury. *No To Shinkei (Brain and Nerve), 52,* 833–836.

Mottaghy, F.M., Hungs, M., Brugmann, M., et al. (1999). Facilitation of picture naming after repetitive transcranial magnetic stimulation. *Neurology, 53,* 1806–1812.

Mountain, M.A. & Snow, W.G. (1993). Wisconsin Card Sorting Test as a measure of frontal pathology: A review. *The Clinical Neuropsychologist, 7,* 108–118.

Mozaz, M.J., Pena, J., Barraquer, L.L., et al. (1993). Use of body part as object in brain-damaged subjects. *The Clinical Neuropsychologist, 7,* 39–47.

Mueller, E.A., Moore, M.M., Kerr, D.C., et al. (1998). Brain volume preserved in healthy elderly through the eleventh decade. *Neurology, 51,* 1555–1562.

Mueller, H., Hasse-Sander, I., Horn, R., et al. (1997). Rey Auditory-Verbal Learning Test: Structure of a modified German version. *Journal of Clinical Psychology, 53,* 663–671.

Mueller, J.E. (1979). Test anxiety and the encoding and retrieval of information. In I.G. Sarason (Ed.), *Test anxiety: Theory, research, and applications.* Hillsdale, NJ: Erlbaum.

Mueller, J.H. & Overcast, T.D. (1976). Free recall as a function of test anxiety, concreteness and instructions. *Bulletin of the Psychonomic Society, 8,* 194–196.

Mueller, S.R. & Girace, M. (1988). Use and misuse of the MMPI, a reconsideration. *Psychological Reports, 63,* 483–491.

Muenter, M.D., Forno, L.S., Hornykiewicz, O., et al. (1998). Hereditary form of parkinsonism—dementia. *Annals of Neurology, 43,* 768–781.

Mueser, K.T., Curran, P.J., & McHugo, G.J. (1997). Factor structure of the Brief Psychiatric Rating Scale in schizophrenia. *Psychological Assessment, 9,* 196–204.

Muizelaar, J.P. (1996). CBF and patient management. In R.K. Narayan et al., (Eds.), *Neurotrauma.* New York: McGraw-Hill.

Mukamal, K.J., Conigrave, K.M., Mittleman, M.A., et al. (2003). Roles of drinking pattern and type of alcohol consumed in coronary heart disease in men. *New England Journal of Medicine, 348,* 109–118.

Mulgrew, C.L., Morgenstern, N., Shetterly, S.M., et al. (1999). Cognitive functioning and impairment among rural elderly Hispanics and non-Hispanic whites as assessed by the Mini-Mental State Examination. *Journal of Gerontology B: Psychological Sciences and Social Sciences, 54,* P223–P230.

Mullie, A., Verstringe, P., Buylaert, W., et al. (1988). Predictive value of Glasgow Coma score for awakening after out-of hospital cardiac arrest. *Lancet, i,* 137–140.

Mungas, D. & Reed, B.R. (2000). Application of item response theory for development of a global functioning measure of dementia with linear measurement properties. *Statistics in Medicine, 19,* 1631–1644.

Mungas, D., Wallace, R., & Reed, B.R. (1998). Dimensions of cognitive ability in dementia: Differential sensitivity to degree of impairment in Alzheimer's disease. *The Clinical Neuropsychologist, 12,* 129–142.

Munoz-Garcia, D. & Ludwin, S.K. (1984). Classic and generalized variants of Pick's disease: A clinico-pathological, ultrastructural, and immunocytochemical comparative study. *Annals of Neurology, 16,* 467–480.

Munro, C.A., Saxton, J., & Butters, M.A. (2000). The neuropsychological consequences of abstinence among older alcoholics: a cross-sectional study. *Alcoholism, Clinical and Experimental Research, 24,* 1510–1516.

Munro, P.T., Smith, R.D., & Parke, T.R. (2002). Effect of patients' age on management of acute intracranial haematoma: prospective national study. *British Medical Journal, 325,* 1001–1005.

Munte, T.F., Ridao-Alonso, M.E., Preinfalk, J., et al. (1997). An electrophysiological analysis of altered cognitive functions in Huntington disease. *Archives of Neurology, 54,* 1089–1098.

Murdoch, G.E. (1990). *Acquired speech and language disorders: A neuroanatomical and functional neurological approach.* New York: Chapman and Hall.

Murji, S., Rourke, S.B., Donders, J., et al. (2003). Theoretically derived CVLT subtypes in HIV-1 infection: Internal and external validation. *Journal of the International Neuropsychological Society, 9,* 1–16.

Murphy, C., Jernigan, T.L., & Fennema-Notestine, C. (2003). Left hippocampal volume loss in Alzheimer's disease is reflected in performance on odor identification: A structural MRI study. *Journal of the International Neuropsychological Society, 9,* 459–471.

Murray, H.A. (1938). *Explorations in personality.* NY: Oxford University Press.

Murray, J.B. (2001). New studies of adults' responses to the Bender Gestalt. *Psychological Reports, 88,* 68–74.

Murrey, G.J. (2000a). Appendix A. Model outline for the assessment of mild traumatic brain injury. In G.J. Murrey (Ed.), *The forensic evaluation of traumatic brain injury.* Boca Raton, FL: CRC Press.

Murrey, G.J. (2000b). Overview of traumatic brain injury: Issues in the forensic assessment. In G.J. Murrey (Ed.), *The forensic evaluation of traumatic brain injury.* Boca Raton, FL: CRC Press.

Murros, K. & Toole, J.F. (1997). Management of asymptomatic extracranial carotid artery disease. In K.M.A. Welch et al. (Eds.), *Primer on cerebrovascular diseases.* San Diego: Academic Press.

Murtha, S., Cismaru, R., Waechter, R., & Cherikow, H. (2002). Increased variability accompanies frontal lobe damage in dementia. *Journal of the International Neuropsychological Society, 8,* 360–372.

Musch, J. & Broder, A. (1999). Test anxiety versus academic skills: a comparison of two alternative models for predicting performance on a statistics exam. *British Journal of Educational Psychology, 69,* 105–116.

Mussack, T., Biberthaler, P., Kanz, K.G., et al. (2002). Immediate S-100B and neuron-specific enolase plasma measurements for rapid evaluation of primary brain damage in alcohol-intoxicated, minor head-injured patients. *Shock, 18,* 395–400.

Mychack, P., Kramer, J.H., Boone, K.B., & Miller, B.L. (2001). The influence of right frontotemporal dysfunction on social behavior in frontotemporal dementia. *Neurology, 56(Suppl. 4),* 11–15.

Myers, D.C. (1983). The psychological and perceptual-motor aspects of Huntington's disease. *Rehabilitation Psychology, 28,* 13–34.

Myers, J.E., Nell, V., Colvin, M., et al. (1999). Neuropsychological function in solvent-exposed South African paint makers. *Journal of Occupational & Environmental Medicine, 41,* 1011–1018.

Myers, J.J. & Sperry, R.W. (1985). Interhemispheric communication after section of the forebrain commissures. *Cortex, 21,* 249–260.

Myers, R.H., Vonsattel, J.P., Stevens, T.J., et al. (1988). Clinical and neuropathologic assessment of severity in Huntington's disease. *Neurology, 38,* 341–347.

Mysiw, W.J., Corrigan, J.D., Hunt, M., et al. (1989). Vocational evaluation of traumatic brain injury using the Functional Assessment Inventory. *Brain Injury, 3,* 27–34.

Myslobodsky, M., Lalone, F.M., & Hicks, L. (2001). Are patients with Parkinson's disease suicidal? *Journal of Geriatric Psychiatry and Neurology, 14,* 120–124.

Na, D.L., Adair, J.C., Kang, Y., et al. (1999). Motor perseverative behavior on a line cancellation task. *Neurology, 52,* 1569–1576.

Nabors, N.A., Millis, S.R., & Rosenthal, M. (1997). Use of the Neurobehavioral Cognitive Status Examination (Cognistat) in traumatic brain injury. *Journal of Head Trauma Rehabilitation, 12,* 79–84.

Nadler, J.D., Grace, J., White, D.A., et al. (1996). Laterality differences in quantitative and qualitative Hooper performance. *Archives of Clinical Neuropsychology, 11,* 223–229.

Naeser, M.A. (1982). Language behavior in stroke patients. Cortical vs. subcortical lesion sites on CT scans. *Trends in Neurosciences, 5,* 53–59.

Naeser, M.A., Alexander, M.P., Helm-Estabrooks, N., et al. (1982). Aphasia with predominantly subcortical lesion sites. *Archives of Neurology, 39,* 2–14.

Naeser, M.A. & Borod, J.C. (1986). Aphasia in left-handers: Lesion site, lesion side, and hemispheric asymmetries on CT. *Neurology, 36,* 471–488.

Naeser, M.A., Helm-Estabrooks, N., Haas, G., et al. (1987). Relationship between lesion extent in "Wernicke's area" on computed tomographic scan and predicting recovery of comprehension in Wernicke's aphasia. *Archives of Neurology, 44,* 73–82.

Naeser, M.A., Palumbo, C.L., Helm-Estabrooks, N., et al. (1989). Severe non-fluency in aphasia: Role of the medial subcallosal fasciculus plus other white matter pathways in recovery of spontaneous speech. *Brain, 112,* 1–38.

Nagaratnam, N., Verma, S., Nagaratnam, K., et al. (1994). Psychiatric and behavioural manifestations of normal pressure hydrocephalus. *British Journal of Clinical Practice, 48,* 122–124.

Nagi, K.S., Joshi, R., & Thakur, R.K. (1996). Cardiac manifestations of Lyme disease: A review. *Canadian Journal of Cardiology, 12,* 503–506.

Nakagawa, A., Su, C.C., Yamashita, Y., et al. (2002). A temporal head injury involving intracranial penetration by glass. *No Shinkei Geka, 30,* 529–533.

Nakayama, Y., Tanaka, A., Arita, T., et al. (1995). Penetrating head injury caused by weed: Case report. *No To Shinkei (Brain and Nerve), 47,* 1192–1194.

Namba, H., Iyo, M., Fukushi, K., et al. (1999). Human cerebral acetylcholinesterase activity measured with positron emission tomography: Procedure, normal values and effect of age. *European Journal of Nuclear Medicine, 26,* 135–143.

NAN Policy and Planning Committee (2000a). Presence of third party observers during neuropsychological testing: Official statement of the National Academy of Neuropsychology. *Archives of Clinical Neuropsychology, 15,* 379–380.

NAN Policy and Planning Committee (2000b). The use of neuropsychology test technicians in clinical practice: Official statement of the National Academy of Neuropsychology. *Archives of Clinical Neuropsychology, 15,* 381–382.

Narayan, R.K., Michel, M.E., Ansell, B., et al. (2002). Clinical trials in head injury. *Journal of Neurotrauma, 19,* 503–557.

Narayan, R.K., Wilberger, J.E., & Povlishock, J.T. (1996). *Neurotrauma.* New York: McGraw-Hill.

Nash, S.C. (1979). Sex role as a mediator of intellectual functioning.

In M.A. Wittig & A.C. Petersen (Eds.), *Sex-related differences in cognitive functioning*. New York: Academic Press.

Nathan, H.J., Wells, G.A., Munson, J.L., & Wozny, D. (2001). Neuroprotective effect of mild hypothermia in patients undergoing coronary artery surgery with cardiopulmonary bypass: A randomized trial. *Circulation, 104,* 473–479.

National Advisory Mental Health Council (1989). *Approaching the 21st century: Opportunities for NIMH neuroscience research*. Report to Congress on the decade of the brain. Rockville, MD: National Institute of Mental Health.

National Conference on Public Health and Epilepsy (1997). *Living well with epilepsy*. Atlanta: Centers for Disease Control and Prevention.

National Head Injury Foundation (1993). *Interagency Head Injury Task Force reports*. Washington, D.C.: National Institute of Neurologic Disorders and Stroke, National Institutes of Health.

National Institute of Neurological Disorders and Stroke (2002). *White House–initiated conference on epilepsy*. Bethesda, MD: NINDS/National Institutes of Health.

Naugle, R.I. (1990). Epidemiology of traumatic brain injury in adults. In E.D. Bigler (Ed.), *Traumatic brain injury*. Austin, TX: Pro-ed.

Naugle, R., Cullum, C.M., & Bigler, E.D. (1997). *Introduction to clinical neuropsychology. A casebook*. Austin, TX: Pro-ed.

Naugle, R.I. & Kawczak, K. (1989). Limitations of the Mini-Mental State Examination. *Cleveland Clinic Journal of Medicine, 56,* 277–281.

Naugle, R.I. & McSweeny, J. (1995). On the practice of routinely appending neuropsychological data to reports. *The Clinical Neuropsychologist, 9,* 245–247.

Naugle, R.I. & McSweeny, J. (1996). More thoughts on the practice of routinely appending raw data to reports: Response to Freides and Matarazzo. *The Clinical Neuropsychologist, 10,* 313–314.

Naunheim, R.S., Standeven, J., Richter, C., & Lewis, L.M. (2000). Comparison of impact data in hockey, football, and soccer. *Journal of Trauma, 48,* 938–941.

Nauta, W.J.H. (1964). Some brain structures and functions related to memory. *Neurosciences Research Progress Bulletin, II,* 1–20.

Nauta, W.J.H. (1971). The problem of the frontal lobe. *Journal of Psychiatric Research, 8,* 167–187.

Neary, D. & Snowden, J.S. (1991). Dementia of the frontal lobe type. In H.S. Levin et al. (Eds.), *Frontal lobe function and dysfunction*. New York: Oxford University Press.

Neary, D. & Snowden, J. (1996). Fronto-temporal dementia: Nosology, neuropsychology, and neuropathology. *Brain and Cognition, 31,* 176–187.

Neary, D., Snowden, J.S., Gustafson, L., et al. (1998). Frontotemporal lobar degeneration: A consensus on clinical diagnostic criteria. *Neurology, 51,* 1546–1554.

Neary, D., Snowden, J.S., Mann, D.M.A., et al. (1990). Frontal lobe dementia and motor neuron disease. *Journal of Neurology, Neurosurgery and Psychiatry, 53,* 23–32.

Neary, D., Snowden, J.S., Northen, B., & Goulding, P. (1988). Dementia of frontal lobe type. *Journal of Neurology, Neurosurgery, and Psychiatry, 51,* 353–361.

Neau, J.-P. & Bogousslavsky, J. (2001). Superficial middle cerebral artery syndromes. In J. Bogousslavsky & L. Caplan (Eds.), *Stroke syndromes* (2nd ed.). Cambridge, UK: Cambridge University Press.

Nebes, R.D. (1978). Direct examination of cognitive function in the right and left hemispheres. In M. Kinsbourne (Ed.), *Asymmetrical function of the brain*. Cambridge, UK: Cambridge University Press.

Nebes, R.D. (1992a). Cognitive dysfunction in Alzheimer's disease. In F.I.M. Craik & T.A. Salthouse (Eds.), *The handbook of aging*. Hillsdale, NJ: Erlbaum.

Nebes, R.D. (1992b). Semantic memory dysfunction in Alzheimer's disease: Disruption of semantic knowledge or information-processing limitation? In L.R. Squire & N. Butters (Eds.), *Neuropsychology of memory* (2nd ed.). New York: Guilford Press.

Nebes, R.D. & Brady, C.B. (1989). Focused and divided attention in Alzheimer's disease. *Cortex, 25,* 305–315.

Nebes, R.D. & Brady, C.B. (1992). Generalized cognitive slowing and severity of dementia in Alzheimer's disease: Implication for the interpretation of response-time data. *Journal of Clinical and Experimental Neuropsychology, 14,* 317–326.

Nebes, R.D. & Brady, C.B. (1993). Phasic and tonic alertness in Alzheimer's disease. *Cortex, 29,* 77–90.

Nebes, R.D., Vora, I.J., Meltzer, C.C., et al. (2001). Relationship of deep white matter hyperintensities and apolipoprotein E genotype to depressive symptoms in older adults without clinical depression. *American Journal of Psychiatry, 158,* 878–884.

Nehemkis, A.M. & Lewinsohn, P.M. (1972). Effects of left and right cerebral lesions on the memory process. *Perceptual and Motor Skills, 35,* 787–798.

Neils, J., Boller, F., Gerdeman, B., & Cole, M. (1989). Descriptive writing abilities in Alzheimer's disease. *Journal of Clinical and Experimental Neuropsychology, 11,* 692–698.

Neisser, U., Boodoo, G., & Bouchard, T.J., Jr. (1996). Intelligence: Knowns and unknowns. *American Psychologist, 51,* 77–101.

Neisser, U. & Libby, L.K. (2000). Remembering life experiences. In E. Tulving & F.I.M. Craik (Eds.), *The Oxford handbook of memory*. Oxford: Oxford University Press.

Neistadt, M.E. (1993). The relationship between constructional and meal preparation skills. *Archives of Physical Medicine and Rehabilitation, 74,* 144–146.

Neitz, J., Summerfelt, P., & Neitz, M. (2001). *The Neitz Test of Color Vision*. Los Angeles: Western Psychological Services.

Neitz, M. & Neitz, J. (2001). A new mass creening test for color-vision deficiencies in children. *Color Research and Application, 26(Suppl.),* S239–S249.

Nell, V. (1999). Luria in Uzbekistan: The vicissitudes of cross-cultural neuropsychology. *Neuropsychology Review, 9,* 45–52.

Nell, V. (2000). *Cross-cultural neuropsychological assessment: Theory and practice*. Mahwah, NJ: Erlbaum.

Nell, V. & Brown, S.O.D. (1991). Epidemiology of traumatic brain injury in Johannesburg: II. Morbidity, mortality and etiology. *Social Science and Medicine, 33,* 289–296.

Nelson, C.A. (Ed.) (2000). *The effects of early adversity on neurobehavioral development. The Minnesota Symposia on Child Development* (Vol. 31). Mahwah, NJ: Erlbaum.

Nelson, D.R., Martz, K.L., Bonner, H., et al. (1992). Non-Hodgkin's lymphoma of the brain: Can high dose, large volume radiation therapy improve survival? Report on a prospective trial by the Radiation Therapy Oncology Group (RTOG): RTOG 8315. *International Journal of Radiation Oncology, Biology, and Physics, 23,* 9–17.

Nelson, H.E. (1976). A modified card sorting test sensitive to frontal lobe defects. *Cortex, 12,* 313–324.

Nelson, H.E. & O'Connell, A. (1978). Dementia: The estimation of premorbid intelligence levels using the National Adult Reading Test. *Cortex, 14,* 234–244.

Nelson, H.E. & Willison, J. (1991). *The National Adult Reading Test (NART): Test manual* (2nd ed.). Windsor, UK: NFER Nelson.

Nelson, L.D., Cicchetti, D., Satz, P., et al. (1993). Emotional sequelae of stroke. *Neuropsychology, 7,* 553–560.

Nelson, P.G. & Davenport, R. (1999). Wiring the brain: Activity-dependent and activity-independent development of synaptic circuits. In S.H. Broman & J.M. Fletcher (Eds.), *The changing nervous system*. New York: Oxford University Press.

Nelson, W.M., 3rd & Dacey, C.M. (1999). Validity of the Stanford-

Binet Intelligence Scale-IV: Its use in young adults with mental retardation. *Mental Retardation, 37,* 319–325.

Nemec, R.E. (1978). Effects of controlled background interference on test performance by right and left hemiplegics. *Journal of Consulting and Clinical Psychology, 46,* 294–297.

Nemeth, A.J. (1991). Common blind spots in the diagnosis and management of minor brain trauma. *Medical Trial Technique Quarterly, 37,* 478–487.

Nemeth, A.J. (1996). Behavior-descriptive data on cognitive, personality, and somatic residua after relatively mild brain trauma: Studying the syndrome as a whole. *Archives of Clinical Neuropsychology, 11,* 677–701.

Nemetz, P.N., Leibson, C., Naessens, J.M., et al. (1999). Traumatic brain injury and time to onset of Alzheimer's disease: A population-based study. *American Journal of Epidemiology, 149,* 32–40.

Nespoulous, J.-L. & Soum, Ch. (2000). Éléments de neuropsycholinguistique cognitive: De quelques pièges à éviter dans l'évaluation et l'interprétation des symptômes aphasiques. In J.-M. Mazaux et al. (Eds.), *Aphasie 2000.* Paris: Masson.

Nestler, E.J. & Self, D.W. (2002). Neuropsychiatric aspects of ethanol and other chemical dependencies. In S.C. Yudofsky & R.E. Hales (Eds.), *Textbook of neuropsychiatry and clinical neurosciences* (2nd ed.). Washington, D.C.: American Psychiatric Publishing.

Nestor, P.J., Graham, K.S., Bozeat, S., et al. (2002). Memory consolidation and the hippocampus: Further evidence from studies of autobiographical memory in semantic dementia and frontal variant frontotemporal dementia. *Neuropsychologia, 40,* 633–654.

Netter, F.H. (1983). *The Ciba collection of medical illustrations. Nervous system. Anatomy and physiology* (Vol. 1, Part 1). West Caldwell, NJ: Ciba-Geigy.

Neugarten, B.L. (1990). The changing meanings of age. In M. Bergener & S.K. Finkel (Eds.), *Clinical and scientific psychogeriatrics. The holistic approaches.* (Vol. I). New York: Springer.

Neuger, G.J., O'Leary, D.S., Fishburne, F., et al. (1981). Order effects on the Halstead-Reitan Neuropsychological Test Battery and allied procedures. *Journal of Consulting and Clinical Psychology, 49,* 722–730.

Newcombe, F. (1969). *Missile wounds of the brain.* London: Oxford University Press.

Newcombe, F. (1982). The psychological consequences of closed head injury: Assessment and rehabilitation. *Injury, 14,* 111–136.

Newcombe, F. (1987). Psychometric and behavioral evidence: Scope, limitations, and ecological validity. In H.S. Levin et al. (Eds.), *Neurobehavioral recovery from head injury.* New York: Oxford University Press.

Newcombe, F. & Artiola i Fortuny, L. (1979). Problems and perspectives in the evaluation of psychological deficits after cerebral lesions. *International Rehabilitation Medicine, 1,* 182–192.

Newcombe, F. & Ratcliff, G. (1989). Disorders of visuospatial analysis. In F. Boller & J. Grafman (Eds.), *Handbook of neuropsychology* (Vol. 2). Amsterdam: Elsevier.

Newcombe, F. & Russell, W.R. (1969). Dissociated visual perceptual and spatial deficits in focal lesions of the right hemisphere. *Journal of Neurology, Neurosurgery and Psychiatry, 32,* 73–81.

Newhouse, P.A., Potter, A., & Lenox, R.H. (1993). The effects of nicotinic agents on human cognition: Possible therapeutic applications in Alzheimer's and Parkinson's diseases. *Medical Chemistry Research, 2,* 628–642.

Newman, M.F., Kirchner, J.L., Phillips-Bute, B., et al. (2001). Longitudinal assessment of neurocognitive function after coronary-artery bypass surgery. *New England Journal of Medicine, 344,* 395–452.

Newman, P.D. & Krikorian, R. (2001). Encoding and complex figure recall. *Journal of the International Neuropsychological Society, 7,* 728–733.

Newman, R.P., Weingartner, H., Smallberg, S.A., & Calne, D.B. (1984). Effortful and automatic memory: Effects of dopamine. *Neurology, 34,* 805–807.

Ng, C., Schweitzer, I., Alexopoulos, P., et al. (2000). Efficacy and cognitive effects of right unilateral electroconvulsive therapy. *Journal of ECT, 16,* 370–379.

Niccolls, R. & Bolter, J.F. (1991). *Multi-digit Memory Test.* San Luis Obispo, CA: Wang Neuropsychological Laboratories.

Nichelli, P., Grafman, J., Pietrini, P., et al. (1994). Brain activity in chess playing. *Nature, 369,* 191.

Nichelli, P., Grafman, J., Pietrini, P., et al. (1995). Where the brain appreciates the moral of a story. *NeuroReport, 6,* 2309–2313.

Nichelli, P. & Menabue, R. (1988). Can association between transient global amnesia and migraine tell us something about the pathophysiology of transient global amnesia? *Italian Journal of Neurological Science (Suppl. 9),* 41–43.

Nichelli, P., Venneri, A., Molinari, M., et al. (1993). Precision and accuracy of subjective time estimation in different memory disorders. *Brain Reseach: Cognitive Brain Research, 1,* 87–93.

Nicholas, L.E., MacLennan, D.L., & Brookshire, R.H. (1986). Validity of multiple-sentence reading comprehension tests for aphasic adults. *Journal of Speech and Hearing Disorders, 51,* 82–87.

Nicholas, M., Obler, L., Albert, M., & Goodglass, H. (1985). Lexical retrieval in healthy aging. *Cortex, 21,* 595–606.

Nicholas, M., Obler, L.K., Albert, M.L., & Helm-Estabrooks, N. (1985). Empty speech in Alzheimer's disease and fluent aphasia. *Journal of Speech and Hearing Research, 28,* 405–410.

Nichols, F.T. & Mohr, J.P. (1986). Binswanger's subacute arteriosclerotic encephalopathy. In H.J.M. Barnett et al. (Eds). *Stroke: Pathophysiology, Diagnosis, and Prevention.* New York: Churchill Livingstone.

Nichols, J.M. & Martin, F. (1996). The effect of heavy social drinking on recall and event-related potentials. *Journal of Studies on Alcohol, 57,* 125–135.

Nichols, M.L. (1980). *A psychometric evaluation of the bicycle drawing test and the establishment of preliminary norms.* Portland, OR: Portland State University. Thesis.

Nicolai, A. & Lazzarino, L.G. (1991). Language disturbances from paramedian thalamic infarcts: A CT method for lesion location. *Rivista di Neurologia, 61,* 86–91.

Niederehe, G. (1986). Depression and memory impairment in the aged. In L.W. Poon (Ed.), *Handbook for clinical memory assessment of older adults.* Washington, D.C.: American Psychological Association.

Nielsen, H., Knudsen, L., & Daugbjerg, O. (1989). Normative data for eight neuropsychological tests based on a Danish sample. *Scandinavian Journal of Psychology, 30,* 37–45.

Nielsen, H., Lolk, A., Andersen, K., et al. (1999). Characteristics of elderly who develop Alzheimer's disease during the next two years—a neuropsychological study using CAMCOG. The Odense Study. *International Journal of Geriatric Psychiatry, 14,* 957–963.

Nielsen, H., Lolk, A., & Kragh-Sorensen, P. (1998). Age-associated memory impairment—pathological memory decline or normal aging? *Scandinavian Journal of Psychology, 39,* 33–37.

Niemi, M.-L., Laaksonen, R., Kotila, M., & Waltimo, O. (1988). Quality of life four years after stroke. *Stroke, 19,* 1101–1107.

Niestadt, M.E. (1993). The relationship between constructional and meal preparation skills. *Archives of Physical Medicine and Rehabilitation, 74,* 144–148.

Nii, Y., Uematsu, S., Lesser, R.P. & Gordon, B. (1996). Does the central sulcus divide motor and sensory functions? *Neurology, 46,* 360–367.

Nilson, L., Barregard, L., & Backman, L. (1999). Trail making test in chronic toxic encephalopathy: Performance and discriminative potential. *The Clinical Neuropsychologist, 13,* 314–327.

Nilsson, L.-G, Nyberg, L., Klingberg, T., et al. (2000). Activity in motor areas while remembering action events. *Neuroreport, 11,* 2199–2201.

Nilson, L.N., Sallsten, G., Hagberg, S., et al. (2002). Influence of solvent exposure and aging on cognitive functioning: An 18 year follow up of formerly exposed floor layers and their controls. *Occupational and Environmental Medicine, 59,* 49–57.

Nimura, K., Chugani, D.C., Muzik, O., & Chugani, H.T. (1999). Cerebellar reorganization following cortical injury in humans: Effects of lesion size and age. *Neurology, 52,* 792–797.

Nishimoto, T. & Murakami, S. (1998). Relation between diffuse axonal injury and internal head structures on blunt impact. *Journal of Biochemical Engineering, 120,* 140–147.

Nissen, M.J. & Bullemer, P. (1987). Attentional requirements of learning: Evidence from performance measures. *Cognitive Psychology, 19,* 1–32.

Nissen, M.J., Willingham, D., & Hartman, M. (1989). Explicit and implicit remembering: When is learning preserved in amnesia? *Neuropsychologia, 27,* 341–352.

Nixon, S.J., Kiyawski, A., Parsons, O.A., & Yohman, J.R. (1987). Semantic (verbal) and figural memroy impairment in alcoholics. *Journal of Clinical and Experimental Neuropsychology, 9,* 311–322.

Nixon, S.J., Parsons, O.A., Schaeffer, K.W., & Hale, R.L. (1995). A methodological study of the Shipley Institute of Living Scale in alcoholics and non-alcoholics: Reliability, discriminating items, and alternative forms. *Applied Neuropsychology, 2,* 155–160.

N'Kaoua, B., Lespinet, V., Barsse, A., et al. (2001). Exploration of hemispheric specialization and lexico-semantic processing in unilateral temporal lobe epilepsy with verbal fluency tasks. *Neuropsychologia, 39,* 635–642.

Nobili, F., Copello, F., Burroni, F., et al. (2001). Regional cerebral blood flow and prognostic evaluation in Alzheimer's disease. *Dementia and Geriatric Cognitive Disorders, 12,* 89–97.

Noël, M.-P. (2001). Numerical cognition. In B. Rapp (Eds.), *The handbook of cognitive neuropsychology.* Philadelphia: Psychology Press.

Nolan, K.A. & Burton, L.A. (1998). Incidence of the Fuld WAIS-R profile in traumatic brain injury and Parkinson's disease. *Archives of Clinical Neuropsychology, 13,* 425–432.

Nolte, J. (1999). *The human brain: An introduction to its functional neuroanatomy.* St Louis: Mosby.

Nopoulos, P., Flaum, M., O'Leary, D., & Andreasen, N.C. (2000). Sexual dimorphism in the human brain: Evaluation of tissue volume, tissue composition and surface anatomy using magnetic resonance imaging. *Psychiatry Research: Neuroimaging, 98,* 1–13.

Nordberg, A. (2001). Nicotinic receptor abnormalities of Alzheimer's disease: Therapeutic implications. *Biological Psychiatry, 49,* 200–210.

Nores, J.M., Biacabe, B., & Bonfils, P. (2000). Olfactory disorders in Alzheimer's disease and in Parkinson's disease. Review of the literature. *Annales de Medecine Interne (Paris), 151,* 97–106.

Norman, D.A. & Shallice, T. (1986). Attention to action: Willed and automataic control of behavior. In R.J. Davison et al. (Eds.), *Consciousness and self-regulation. Advances in research and theory.* New York: Plenum Press.

Norman, M.A., Evans, J.D., Miller, W.S., & Heaton, R.K. (2000). Demographically corrected norms for the California Verbal Learning Test. *Journal of Clinical and Experimental Neuropsychology, 22,* 80–94.

Norman, R.D. (1966). A revised deterioration formula for the Wechsler Adult Intelligence Scale. *Journal of Clinical Psychology, 22,* 287–294.

Norris, C.R., Trench, J.M., & Hook, R. (1982). Delayed carbon monoxide encephalopathy: Clinical and research implications. *Journal of Clinical Psychiatry, 43,* 294–295.

Norris, G. & Tate, R.L. (2000). The Behavioural Assessment of the Dysexecutive Syndrome (BADS): Ecological, concurrent and construct validity. *Neuropsychological Rehabilitation, 10,* 33–45.

Norris, J.W. & Hachinski, V.C. (Eds.) (2001). *Stroke prevention.* New York: Oxford University Press.

North, A.J. & Ulatowska, H.K. (1981). Competence in independently living older adults: Assessment and correlates. *Journal of Gerontology, 36,* 576–582.

North American Symptomatic Carotid Endarterectomy Trial Collaborators (1991). Beneficial effect of carotid endarterectomy in symptomatic patients with high-grade carotid stenosis. *New England Journal of Medicine, 325,* 445–453.

Norton, L.E., Bondi, M.W., Salmon, D.P., & Goodglass, H. (1997). Deterioration of generic knowledge in patients with Alzheimer's disease: Evidence from the Number Information Test. *Journal of Clinical and Experimental Neuropsychology, 19,* 857–866.

Noseworthy, J.H., Lucchinetti, C., Rodriguez, M., & Weinshenker, B.G. (2000). Multiple sclerosis. *New England Journal of Medicine, 343,* 938–952.

Noseworthy, J., Paty, D., Wonnacott, T., et al. (1983). Multiple sclerosis after age 50. *Neurology, 33,* 1537–1544.

Nottebohm, F. (1979). Origins and mechanisms in the establishment of cerebral dominance. In M.S. Gazzaniga (Ed.), *Handbook of behavioral neurobiology. Neuropsychology* (Vol. 2). New York: Plenum Press.

Novack, T.A., Bush, B.A., Meythaler, J.M., & Canupp, K. (2001). Outcome after traumatic brain injury: Pathway analysis of contributions from premorbid, injury severity, and recovery variables. *Archives of Physical Medicine and Rehabilitation, 82,* 300–305.

Novack, T.A., Dillon, M.C., & Jackson, W.T. (1996). Neurochemical mechanisms in brain injury and treatment. A review. *Journal of Clinical and Experimental Neuropsychology, 18,* 685–706.

Novack, T.A., Kofoed, B.A., & Crosson, B. (1995). Sequential performance on the California Verbal Learning Test following traumatic brain injury. *The Clinical Neuropsychologist, 9,* 38–43.

Novak, S., Johnson, J., & Greenwood, R. (1996). Barthel revisited: Making guidelines work. *Clinical Rehabilitation, 10,* 128–134.

Novelly, R.A., Augustine, E.A., Mattson, R.H., et al. (1984). Selective memory improvement and impairment in temporal lobectomy for epilepsy. *Annals of Neurology, 15,* 64–67.

Nussbaum, P.D. (Ed.) (1997). *Handbook of neuropsychology and aging.* New York: Plenum Press.

Nutt, J.G. (1989). Excitatory amino acids and Huntington's disease. *Genetics Northwest, 6,* 4–5.

Nutt, J.G., Hammerstad, J.P., & Gancher, S.T. (1992). *Parkinson's disease. 100 maxims.* St. Louis, MO: Mosby Year Book.

Nutt, J.G., Woodward, W.R., Hammerstad, J.P., et al. (1984). The "on-off" phenomenon in Parkinson's disease. Relation to levodopa absorption and transport. *New England Journal of Medicine, 310,* 483–488.

Nuwer, M.R. (1989). Uses and abuses of brain mapping. *Archives of Neurology, 46,* 1134–1135.

Nyberg, L. (1998). Mapping episodic memory. *Behavioral Brain Research, 90,* 107–114.

Nyberg, L. & Cabeza, R. (2000). Brain imaging of memory. In E. Tulving & F.I.M. Craik (Eds.), *The Oxford handbook of memory.* Oxford, UK: Oxford University Press.

Nyberg, L., Winocur, G., & Moscovitch, M. (1997). Correlation between frontal lobe functions and explicit and implicit stem completion in healthy elderly. *Neuropsychology, 11,* 70–76.

Oates, J.C. (1992 Feb 13). The cruelest sport. *New York Review of Books*, 3–6.

Ober, B.A., Koss, E., Friedland, R.P., & Delis, D.C. (1985). Processes of verbal memory failure in Alzheimer-type dementia. *Brain and Cognition, 4*, 90–103.

Öberg, R.G.E., Udesen, H., Thomsen, A.M., et al. (1985). Psychogenic behavioral impairments in patients exposed to neurotoxins. Neuropsychological assessment in differential diagnosis. In *Neurobehavioural methods in occupational and environmental health. Environmental Health Document 3*. Copenhagen: World Health Organization.

Obeso, J.A., Olanow, C.W., & Nutt, J.G. (2000). Levodopa motor complications in Parkinson's disease. *Trends in Neurosciences, 23*, S2–S7.

Obler, L.K. & Albert, M.L. (1979). *The Action Naming Test (experimental ed.)*. Boston: VA Medical Center.

Obler, L.K. & Albert, M.L. (1980). *Language and communication in the elderly*. Lexington, MA: Lexington Books.

Obler, L.K. & Albert, M.L. (1985). Language skills across adulthood. In J. Birren & K.W. Schaie (Eds.), *The psychology of aging*. New York: Van Nostrand Reinhold.

Obleser, J., Eulitz, C., Lahiri, A., & Elbert, T. (2001). Gender differences in functional hemispheric asymmetry during processing of vowels as reflected by the human brain magnetic response. *Neuroscience Letters, 314*, 131–134.

Obonsawin, M.C., Crawford, J.R., Page, J., et al. (1999). Performance on the Modified Card Sorting Test by normal, healthy individuals: Relationship to general intellectual ability and demographic variables. *British Journal of Clinical Psychology, 38*, 27–41.

O'Boyle, M.W. & Benbow, C.P. (1990). Handedness and its relationship to ability and talent. In S. Coren (Ed.), *Left-handedness: Behavioral implications and anomalies*. Amsterdam: Elsevier/North-Holland.

O'Boyle, M.W., Benbow, C.P., & Alexander, J.E. (1995). Sex differences, hemispheric laterality, and associated brain activity in the intellectually gifted. *Developmental Neuropsychology, 11*, 415–444.

O'Brien, H.L., Tetewsky, S.J., Avery, L.M., et al. (2001). Visual mechanisms of spatial disorientation in Alzheimer's disease. *Cerebral Cortex, 11*, 1083–1092.

O'Brien, K. & Lezak, M.D. (1981). *Long-term improvements in intellectual function following brain injury*. Paper presented at the European meeting of the International Neuropsychological Society, Bergen, Norway.

O'Brien, T.J., So, E.L., Meyer, F.B., et al. (1999). Progressive hippocampal atrophy in chronic intractable temporal lobe epilepsy. *Annals of Neurology, 45*, 526–529.

Obrist, W.D. & Marion, D.W. (1996). Xenon techniques for CBF measurement in clinical head injury. In R.K. Narayan (Eds.), *Neurotrauma*. New York: McGraw-Hill.

Obrzut, J., Dalby, P., Boliek, C., & Cannon, G. (1992). Factorial structure of the Waterloo Handedness Questionnaire for control and learning-disabled adults. *Journal of Clinical and Experimental Neuropsychology, 14*, 935–950.

O'Carroll, R., Egan, V., & MacKenzie, D.M. (1994). Assessing cognitive estimation. *British Journal of Clinical Psychology, 33*, 193–197.

O'Carroll, R.E., Woodrow, J., & Maroun, F. (1991). Psychosexual and psychosocial sequelae of closed head injury. *Brain Injury, 5*, 303–313.

Ochsner, K.N. & Schacter, D.L. (2000). A social cognitive neuroscience approach to emotion and memory. In J.C. Borod (Ed.), *The neuropsychology of emotion*. New York: Oxford University Press.

O'Connor, D.B., Archer, J., Hair, W.M., & Wu, F.C. (2001). Activational effects of testosterone on cognitive function in men. *Neuropsychologia, 39*, 1385–1394.

O'Connor, M. & Verfaillie, M. (2002). The amnesic syndrome: Overview and subtypes. In A.D. Baddeley et al. (2002). *The handbook of memory disorders*. Chichester, UK: Wiley.

O'Connor, M., Verfaellie, M., & Cermak, L.S. (1995). Clinical differentiation of amnesic subtypes. In A.D. Baddeley et al. (Eds.), *Handbook of memory disorders*. Chichester, UK: Wiley.

O'Connor, M.G., Sieggreen, M.A., Bachna, K., et al. (2000). Long-term retention of transient news events. *Journal of the International Neuropsychological Society, 6*, 44–51.

Oder, W., Podreka, I., Spatt, J., & Goldenberg, G. (1996). Cerebral function following catastrophic brain injury: Relevance of single photon emission computed tomography and positron emission tomography. In H.S. Levin et al. (Eds.), *Catastrophic brain injury*. New York: Oxford University Press.

O'Donnell, B.F., Drachman, D.A., Lew, R.A., & Swearer, J.M. (1988). Measuring dementia: Assessment of multiple deficit domains. *Journal of Clinical Psychology, 44*, 916–923.

O'Donnell, B.F., Friedman, S., Squires, N.K., et al. (1990). Active and passive P3 latency in dementia: Relationship to psychometric, EEG, and CT measures. *Journal of Neuropsychiatry, Neuropsychology and Behavioral Neurology, 3*, 164–179.

O'Donnell, B.F., Squires, N.K., Martz, M.J., et al. (1987). Evoked potential changes and neuropsychological performance in Parkinson's disease. *Biological Psychology, 24*, 23–37.

O'Donnell, J.P., Macgregor, L.A., Dabrowski, J.J., et al. (1994). Construct validity of neuropsychological tests of conceptual and attentional abilities. *Journal of Clinical Psychology, 50*, 596–600.

O'Donoghue, J.L. (2000). Styrene. In P.S. Spencer & H.H. Schaumburg (Eds.), *Experimental and clinical neurotoxicology* (2nd ed.). New York: Oxford University Press.

Oepen, G., Mohr, U., Willmes, K., & Thoden, U. (1985). Huntington's disease: Visuomotor disturbance in patients and offspring. *Journal of Neurology, Neurosurgery and Psychiatry, 48*, 426–433.

O'Flynn, R.R., Monkman, S.M., & Waldron, H.A. (1987). Organic solvents and presenile dementia: A case referent study using death certificates. *British Journal of Industrial Medicine, 44*, 259–262.

Ogden, J.A. (1985a). Anterior–posterior interhemispheric differences in the loci of lesions producing visual hemineglect. *Brain and Cognition, 4*, 59–75.

Ogden, J.A. (1985b). Contralesional neglect of constructed visual images in right and left brain-damaged patients. *Neuropsychologia, 23*, 273–277.

Ogden, J.A. (1986). Neuropsychological and psychological sequelae of shunt surgery in young adults with hydrocephalus. *Journal of Clinical and Experimental Neuropsychology, 8*, 657–679.

Ogden, J.A. (1990). Spatial abilities and deficits in aging and age-related disorders. In F. Boller & J. Grafman (Eds.), *Handbook of neuropsychology* (Vol. 4). Amsterdam: Elsevier.

Ogden, J.A. (1993). The psychological and neuropsychological assessment of chronic organic solvent neurotoxicity: A case series. *New Zealand Journal of Psychology, 22*, 82–93.

Ogden, J.A. (1996). *Fractured minds*. New York: Oxford University Press.

Ogden, J.A., Growdon, J.H., & Corkin, S. (1990). Deficits on visuospatial tests involving forward planning in high-functioning parkinsonians. *Neuropsychiatry, Neuropsychology, and Behavioral Neurology, 3*, 125–139.

Ogden, J.A., Mee, E.W., & Henning, M. (1993). A prospective study of impairment of cognition and memory and recovery after subarachnoid hemorrhage. *Neurosurgery, 33*, 1–15.

Ogden, J.A. & Wolfe, M. (1998). Post-concussional syndrome: A preliminary study comparing young and middle-aged adults. *Neuropsychological Rehabilitation, 8,* 413–431.

Ogden-Epker, M. & Cullum, C.M. (2001). Quantitative and qualitative interpretation of neuropsychological data in the assessment of temporal lobectomy candidates. *The Clinical Neuropsychologist, 15,* 183–195.

Ogren, F.P. & Edmunds, A.L. (1995). Neuro-otologic findings in the lightning-injured patient. *Seminars in Neurology, 15,* 256–262.

Ohira, T., Iso, H., Satoh, S., et al. (2001). Prospective study of depressive symptoms and risk of stroke among Japanese. *Stroke, 32,* 903–908.

Ohry, A., Rattok, J., & Solomon, Z. (1996). Post-traumatic stress disorder in brain injury patients. *Brain Injury, 10,* 687–695.

Ojemann, R.G. (1966). Correlations between specific human brain lesions and memory changes. *Neurosciences Research Progress Bulletin, 4(Suppl.),* 1–70.

Ojemann, G.A. (1978). Organization of short-term verbal memory in language areas of human cortex: Evidence from electrical stimulation. *Brain and Language, 5,* 331–340.

Ojemann, G.A. (1979). Individual variability in cortical localization of language. *Journal of Neurosurgery, 50,* 164–169.

Ojemann, G.A. (1980). Brain mechanisms for language: Observations during neurosurgery. In J.S. Lockard & A.A. Ward, Jr. (Eds.), *Epilepsy: A window to brain mechanisms.* New York: Raven Press.

Ojemann, G.A. (1984). Common cortical and thalamic mechanisms for language and motor functions. *American Journal of Physiology, 246,* 901–903.

Ojemann, G.A., Cawthon, D.F., & Lettich, E. (1990). Localization and physiological correlates of language and verbal memory in human lateral temporoparietal cortex. In A.B. Scheibel & A.F. Wechsler (Eds.), *Neurobiology of higher cognitive function.* New York: Guilford Press.

Ojemann, G.A., Hoyenga, K.B., & Ward, A.A. (1971). Prediction of short-term verbal memory disturbance after ventrolateral thalamotomy. *Journal of Neurosurgery, 35,* 203–210.

Oka, S., Miyamoto, O., Janjua, N.A., et al. (1999). Re-evaluation of sexual dimorphism in human corpus callosum. *Neuroreport, 10,* 937–940.

Okawa, M., Maeda, S., Nukui, H., & Kawafuchi, J. (1980). Psychiatric symptoms in ruptured anterior communicating aneurysms: Social prognosis. *Acta Psychiatrica Scandinavica, 61,* 306–312.

Okazaki, S. & Sue, S. (1995). Methodological issues in assessment research with ethnic minorities. *Psychological Assessment, 7,* 367–375.

O'Keefe, J. & Nadel, L. (1978). *The hippocampus as a cognitive map.* London: Oxford University Press.

Oken, B.S. & Chiappa, K.H. (1985). Electroencephalography and evoked potentials in head trauma. In D.B. Becker & J.T. Povlishock (Eds.), *Central nervous system trauma—status report.* Washington, D.C.: NINCDS/NIH.

Oken, B.S. & Kaye, J. A. (1992). Electrophysiologic function in the healthy, extremely old. *Neurology, 42,* 519–526.

Oken, B.S., Kishiyama, S.S., Kaye, J.A., & Howieson, D.B. (1994). Attention deficit in Alzheimer's disease is not simulated by an anticholinergic/antihistaminergic drug and is distinct from deficits in healthy aging. *Neurology, 44,* 657–662.

Oken, B.S., Kishiyama, S.S., Kaye, J.A., & Jones, D.E. (1999). Age-related differences in global–local processing: Stability of laterality differences but disproportionate impairment in global processing. *Journal of Geriatric Psychiatry and Neurology, 12,* 76–81.

Oksenberg, J.R., Baranzini, S.E., Barcellos, L.F., & Hauser, S.L. (2001). Multiple sclerosis: Genomic rewards. *Journal of Neuroimmunology, 113,* 171–184.

Oksenberg, J.R. & Hauser, S.L. (1999). Emerging concepts of pathogenesis: Relationship to multiple sclerosis therapies. In R.A. Rudick & D.E. Goodkin (Eds.), *Multiple sclerosis therapeutics.* London: Martin Dunitz.

Okuda, B., Tanaka, H., Tomino, Y., et al. (1995). The role of the left somatosensory cortex in human hand movement. *Experimental Brain Research, 106,* 493–498.

Oldfield, R.C. (1971). The assessment and analysis of handedness. The Edinburgh Inventory. *Neuropsychologia, 9,* 97–113.

Olesen, J., Friberg, L., Olsen, T.S., et al. (1990). Timing and topography of cerebral blood flow, aura, and headache during migraine attacks. *Annals of Neurology, 28,* 791–798.

Olesen, J., Friberg, L., Olsen, T.S., et al. (1993). Ischaemia-induced (symptomatic) migraine attacks may be more frequent than migraine-induced ischaemic insults. *Brain, 116,* 187–202.

Olichney, J.M., Galasko, D., Salmon, D.P., et al. (1998). Cognitive decline is faster in Lewy body variant than in Alzheimer's disease. *Neurology, 51,* 351–357.

Olin, J.J. (2001). Cognitive function after systemic therapy for breast cancer. *Oncology, 15,* 613–618.

Oliver, T.M. (1999). The effects of induced and trait social anxiety on measures of fluid and crystallized intelligence. *Dissertation Abstracts International. Section B, Sciences and Engineering, 60,* 1909.

Ollo, C., Johnson, R., Jr., & Grafman, J. (1991). Signs of cognitive change in HIV disease: An event-related brain potential study. *Neurology, 41,* 209–215.

Ollo, C., Lindquist, T., Alim, T.N., & Deutsch, S.I. (1995). Predicting premorbid functioning in crack-cocaine abusers. *Drug and Alcohol Dependence, 40,* 173–175.

Olmedo, E.L. (1981). Testing linguistic minorities. *American Psychologist, 36,* 1078–1085.

Olsen, J.H. & Dossing, M. (1982). Formaldehyde induced symptoms in day care centers. *American Industrial Hygiene Association Journal, 43,* 366–370.

Olsen, T.S. (2001). Post-stroke epilepsy. *Current Atherosclerosis Reports, 3,* 340–344.

Olson, J.D., Riedel, E., & DeAngelis, L.M. (2000). Long-term outcome of low-grade oligodendroglioma and mixed glioma. *Neurology, 54,* 1442–1448.

Olson, K.R. (1984). Carbon monoxide poisoning: Mechanisms, presentation, and controversies in management. *Journal of Emergency Medicine, 1,* 233–243.

Ommaya, A.K. & Gennarelli, T.A. (1974). Cerebral concussion and traumatic unconsciousness. *Brain, 97,* 633–654.

O'Neill, J., Hibbard, M.R., Brown, M., et al. (1998). The effect of employment on quality of life and community integration after traumatic brain injury. *Journal of Head Trauma Rehabilitation, 13,* 68–79.

Oppenheimer, D.R. (1968). Microscopic lesions in the brain following head injury. *Journal of Neurology, Neurosurgery and Psychiatry, 31,* 299–306.

Optic Neuritis Study Group (1997). The 5-year risk of MS after optic neuritis: Experience of the Optic Neuritis Treatment Trial. *Neurology, 49,* 1404–1413.

Ørbaek, P., & Lindgren, M. (1988). Prospective clinical and psychometric investigation of patients with chronic toxic encephalopathy induced by solvents. *Scandinavian Journal of Work and Environmental Health, 14,* 37–44.

Oremus, M., Perrault, A., Demers, L., & Wolfson, C. (2000). Review of outcome measurement instruments in Alzheimer's disease drug trials: Psychometric properties of global scales. *Journal of Geriatric Psychiatry and Neurology, 13,* 197–205.

Orey, S.A., Cragar, D.E., & Berry, D.T.R. (2000). The effects of two motivational manipulations on the neuropsychological performance of mildly head-injured college students. *Archives of Clinical Neuropsychology, 15,* 335–348.

Orgogozo, J.M. (1976). Le syndrome de Gerstmann. *L'Encephale, II*, 41–53.

Orgogozo, J.M., Dartigues, J.F., Lafont, S., et al. (1997). Wine consumption and dementia in the elderly : A prospective community study in the Bordeaux area. *Revue Neurologique (Paris), 153*, 185–192.

Orloski, K.A., Campbell, G.L., Genese, C.A., et al. (1998). Emergence of Lyme disease in Nunterdon County, New Jersey, 1993: A case-control study of risk factors and evaluation of reporting patterns. *American Journal of Epidemiology, 147*, 391–397.

Orloski, K.A., Hayes, E.B., Campbell, G.L., & Dennis, D.T. (2000). Surveillance for Lyme disease—United States, 1992–1998. *Morbidity and Mortality Weekly Report CDC Surveillance Summaries, 49*, 1–11.

Orme, D., Ree, M.J., & Rioux, P. (2001). Premorbid IQ estimates from a multiple aptitude test battery: Regression vs. equating. *Archives of Clinical Neuropsychology, 16*, 679–688.

Ornstein, R., Herron, J., Johnstone, J., & Swencionis, C. (1979). Differential right hemisphere involvement in two reading tasks. *Psychophysiology, 16*, 398–401.

O'Rourke, N., Tuokko, H., Hayden, S., & Beattie, B.L. (1997). Early identification of dementia: Predictive validity of the Clock Test. *Archives of Clinical Neuropsychology, 12*, 257–267.

Orsini, A., Chiacchio, L., Cinque, M., et al. (1986). Effects of age, education and sex on two tests of immediate memory: A study of normal subjects from 20–99 years of age. *Perceptual and Motor Skills, 63*, 727–732.

Orsini, A., Pasquadibisceglie, M., Picone, L., & Tortora, R. (2001). Factors which influence the difficulty of the spatial path in Corsi's block-tapping test. *Perceptual and Motor Skills, 92*, 732–738.

Orsini D.L., Satz, P., Soper, H.V., & Light, R.K. (1985). The role of familial sinistrality in cerebral organization. *Neuropsychologia, 23*, 223–232.

Orsini, D.L., Van Gorp, W.G., & Boone, K.B. (1988). *The neuropsychology casebook*. New York: Springer-Verlag.

Ortiz, I.E., LaRue, A., Romero, L.J., et al. (1997). Comparison of cultural bias in two cognitive screening instruments in elderly Hispanic patients in New Mexico. *American Journal of Geriatric Psychiatry, 5*, 333–338.

Ortiz, N., Reicherts, M., Pegna, A.J., et al. (2000). Interhemispheric transfer evaluation in multiple sclerosis. *Swiss Journal of Psychology, 59*, 150–158.

Osborne, D.P., Jr., Brown, E.R., & Randt, C.T. (1982). Qualitative changes in memory function: Aging and dementia. In S. Corkin et al. (Eds.), *Alzheimer's disease: A report of progress. Aging* (Vol. 19). New York: Raven Press.

Oscar-Berman, M. (1980). Neuropsychological consequences of long-term chronic alcoholism. *American Scientist, 68*, 410–419.

Oscar-Berman, M. (1984). Comparative neuropsychology and alcoholic Korsakoff disease. In L.R. Squire & N. Butters (Eds.), *Neuropsychology of memory*. New York: Guilford Press.

Oscar-Berman, M. (1987). Alcohol-related ERP changes in cognition. *Alcohol, 4*, 289–292.

Oscar-Berman, M. & Weinstein, A. (1985). Visual processing, memory, and lateralization in alcoholism and aging. *Developmental Neuropsychology, 1*, 99–112.

Oscarsson, B. (Director) (1980). *Solvents in the work environment*. Stockholm: Swedish Work Environment Fund (Arbetarskyddsfonden).

O'Shanick, G.J. & Zasler, N.D. (1990). Neuropsychopharmacological approaches to traumatic brain injury. In J.S. Kreutzer & P. Wehman (Eds.), *Community integration following traumatic brain injury*. Baltimore: Paul H. Brooks.

Osterrieth, P.A. (1944). Le test de copie d'une figure complexe. *Archives de Psychologie, 30*, 206–356 [trans. J. Corwin and F.W. Bylsma (1993), *The Clinical Neuropsychologist, 7*, 9–15].

Ostrosky, F., Canseco, E., Quintanar, L., et al. (1985). Sociocultural effects in neuropsychological assessment. *International Journal of Neuroscience, 26*, 14–26.

Ostrosky-Solis, F., Ardila, A., & Rosselli, M. (1999). NEUROPSI: A brief neuropsychological test battery in Spanish with norms by age and educational level. *Journal of the International Neuropsychological Society, 5*, 413–433.

Ostrosky-Solis, F., Jaime, R. M., & Ardila, A. (1998). Memory abilities during normal aging. *International Journal of Neuroscience, 93*, 151–162.

Ostrosky-Solis, F., Lopez-Arango, G., & Ardila, A. (2000). Sensitivity and specificity of the Mini-Mental State Examination in a Spanish speaking population. *Applied Neuropsychology, 7*, 25–31.

O'Sullivan, M., Jones, D.K., Summers, P.E., et al. (2001). Evidence for cortical "disconnection" as a mechanism of age-related cognitive decline. *Neurology, 57*, 632–638.

Ott, A., Slooter, A.J., Hofman, A., et al. (1998). Smoking and the risk of dementia and Alzheimer's disease in a population-based cohort study: The Rotterdam Study. *Lancet, 351*, 1840–1843.

Ott, A., Stolk, R.P., van Harskamp, F., et al. (1999). Diabetes mellitus and the risk of dementia: The Rotterdam Study. *Neurology, 53*, 1937–1942.

Ott, A., van Rossum, C.T., van Harskamp, F., et al. (1999). Education and the incidence of dementia in a large population-based study: The Rotterdam Study. *Neurology, 52*, 663–666.

Ottman, R., Lee, J.H., Hauser, W.A., & Risch, N. (1998). Are generalized and localization-related epilepsies genetically distinct? *Archives of Neurology, 55*, 339–344.

Otto, M.W., Bruder, G.E., Fava, M., et al. (1994). Norms for depressed patients for the California Verbal Learning Test: Associations with depression severity and self-report of cognitive difficulties. *Archives of Clinical Neuropsychology, 9*, 81–88.

Overall, J.E. & Gomez-Mont, F. (1974). The MMPI-168 for psychiatric screening. *Educational and Psychological Measurement, 34*, 315–319.

Overall, J.E. & Gorham, D.R. (1962). The Brief Psychiatric Rating Scale. *Psychological Reports, 10*, 799–812.

Ovsiew, F. (2002). Bedside neuropsychiatry: Eliciting the clinical phenomena of neuropsychiatric illness. In S.C.Yudofsky & R.E. Hales (Eds.), *American Psychiatric Publishing textbook of neuropsychiatry and clinical neurosciences*. Washington, D.C.: American Psychiatric Publishing.

Owen, A.M., Doyon, J., Dagher, A., et al. (1998). Abnormal basal ganglia outflow in Parkinson's disease identified with PET: Implications for higher cortical functions. *Brain, 121*, 949–965.

Owen, A.M., Milner, B., Petrides, M., & Evans, A.C. (1996). Memory for object features versus memory for object location: A positron-emission tomography study of encoding and retrieval processes. *Proceedings of the National Academy of Sciences USA, 93*, 9212–9217.

Owen, A.M., Morris, R.G., Sahakian, B.J., et al. (1996). Double dissociations of memory and executive functions in working memory tasks following frontal lobe excisions, temporal lobe excisions or amygdalo-hippocampectomy in man. *Brain, 119*, 1597–1615.

Pachana, N.A., Boone, K. B., & Ganzell, S. L. (1998). False positive errors on selected tests of malingering. *American Journal of Forensic Psychology, 16*, 17–25.

Pachana, N.A., Boone, K.B., Miller, B.L., et al. (1996). Comparison of neuropsychological functioning in Alzheimer's disease and frontotemporal dementia. *Journal of the International Neuropsychological Society, 2*, 505–510.

Pachner, A.R., Duray, P., & Steere, A.C. (1989). Central nervous system manifestations of Lyme disease. *Archives of Neurology, 46,* 790–795.

Packer, R.J. (1999). Brain tumors in children. *Archives of Neurology, 56,* 421–425.

Padula, W.V. & Argyris, S. (1996). Post trauma vision syndrome and visual midline shift syndrome. *Neurorehabilitation, 6,* 165–171.

Pagani, M., Salmaso, D., Jonsson, C., et al. (2002). Regional cerebral blood flow as assessed by principal component analysis and (99m)Tc-HMPAO SPET in healthy subjects at rest. *European Journal of Nuclear Medicine and Molecular Imaging, 29,* 67–75.

Pagliaro, L.A. & Pagliaro, A.M. (1999). *Psychologists' neuropsychotropic drug reference.* Philadephia: Brunner/Mazel.

Paivio, A., Yuille, J. C., & Madigan, S. A. (1968). Concreteness, imagery, and meaningfulness values for 925 nouns. *Journal of Experimental Psychology Monographs, 76,* 1.

Pakenham, K.I. (1999). Adjustment to multiple sclerosis: Application of a stress and coping model. *Health Psychology, 18,* 383–392.

Palella, F.J., Delaney, K.M., Moorman, A.C., et al. (1998). Declining morbidity and mortality among patients with advanced human immunodeficiency virus infection. *New England Journal of Medicine, 338,* 853–860.

Palermo, D.S. & Jenkins, J.J. (1964). *Word association norms.* Minneapolis: University of Minnesota Press.

Palmer, A.M. (1996). Neurochemical studies of Alzheimer's disease. *Neurodegeneration, 5,* 381–391.

Palmer, B.W., Boone, K.B., Lesser, I.M., et al. (1996). Neuropsychological deficits among older depressed patients with predominantly psychological or vegetative symptoms. *Journal of Affective Disorders, 41,* 17–24.

Palmer, B.W., Boone, K.B., Lesser, I.M., & Wohl, M.A. (1998). Base rates of "impaired" neuropsychological test peformance among healthy older adults. *Archives of Clinical Neuropsychology, 13,* 503–511.

Palmer, B.W., Heaton, R.K., Paulsen, J.S., et al. (1997). Is it possible to be schizophrenic yet neuropsychologically normal? *Neuropsychology, 11,* 437–446.

Pandey, S., Mohanty, S., & Mandal, M.K. (2000). Tactual recognition of cognitive stimuli: Roles of hemisphere and lobe. *International Journal of Neuroscience, 100,* 21–28.

Pandya, D.N. & Barnes, C.L. (1987). Architecture and connections of the frontal lobe. In E. Perecman (Ed.), *The frontal lobes revisited.* New York: IRBN Press.

Pandya, D.N. & Yeterian, E.H. (1990). Architecture and connections of cerebral cortex: Implications for brain evolution and function. In A.B. Scheibel & A.F. Wechsler (Eds.), *Neurobiology of higher cognitive function.* New York: Guilford Press.

Pandya, D.N. & Yeterian, E.H. (1998). Comparison of prefrontal architecture and connections. In A.C. Roberts, T.W. Robbins, & L. Weiskrantz (Eds.), *The prefrontal cortex. Executive and cognitive functions.* New York: Oxford University Press.

Pang, D. (1989). Physics and pathology of closed head injury. In M.D. Lezak (Ed.), *Assessment of the behavioral consequences of head trauma. Frontiers of clinical neuroscience* (Vol. 7). New York: Alan R. Liss.

Pang, S., Borod, J. C., Hernandez, A., et al. (1990). The auditory P300 correlates with specific cognitive deficits in Parkinson's disease. *Journal of Neural Transmission, 2,* 249–264.

Paniak, C., Reynolds, S., Phillips, K., et al. (2002). Patient complaints within 1 month of mild traumatic brain injury: A controlled study. *Archives of Clinical Neuropsychology, 17,* 319–334.

Paniak, C., Reynolds, S., Toller-Lobe, G., et al. (2002). A longitudinal study of the relationship between financial compensation and symptoms after treated mild traumatic brain injury. *Journal of Clinical and Experimental Neuropsychology, 24,* 187–193.

Paniak, C.E., Shore, D.L., & Rourke, B.P. (1989). Recovery of memory after severe closed-head injury: Dissocations in recovery of memory parameters and predictors of outcome. *Journal of Clinical and Experimental Neuropsychology, 11,* 631–644.

Pankratz, L. (1979). Symptom validity testing and symptom retraining: Procedures for the assessment and treatment of functional sensory deficits. *Journal of Consulting and Clinical Psychology, 47,* 409–410.

Pankratz, L. (1983). A new technique for the assessment and modification of feigned memory deficit. *Perceptual and Motor Skills, 57,* 367–372.

Pankratz, L. (1988). Malingering on intellectual and neuropsychological measures. In R. Rogers (Ed.), *Clinical assessment of malingering and deception.* New York: Guilford Press.

Pankratz, L. (1998). *Patients who deceive.* Springfield, IL: Thomas.

Pankratz, L. (1999). Factitious disorders and factitious disorders by proxy. In S.D. Netherton et al. (Eds.), *Child and adolescent psychological disorders: A comprehensive textbook.* New York: Oxford University Press.

Pankratz, L. & Erickson, R.D. (1990). Two views of malingering. *The Clinical Neuropsychologist, 4,* 379–389.

Pankratz, L., Fausti, S.A., & Peed, S. (1975). A forced-choice treatment to evaluated deafness in the hysterical or malingering patient. *Journal of Consulting and Clinical Psychology, 43,* 421–422.

Pankratz, L. & Glaudin, V. (1980). Psychosomatic disorders. In R.H. Woody (Ed.), *Encyclopedia of clinical assessment.* San Francisco: Jossey-Bass.

Pankratz, L. & Kofoed, L. (1988). The assessment and treatment of geezers. *Journal of the American Medical Association, 259,* 1228–1229.

Pankratz, L. & Lezak, M.D. (1987). Cerebral dysfunction in the Munchausen syndrome. *Hillside Journal of Clinical Psychiatry, 9,* 195–206.

Pankratz, L.D. & Taplin, J.D. (1982). Issues in psychological assessment. In J.R. McNamara & A.G. Barclay (Eds.), *Critical issues, developments, and trends in professional psychology.* New York: Praeger.

Panse, F. (1970). Electrical lesions of the nervous system. In P.J. Vinken & G.W. Bruyn (Eds.), *Handbook of clinical neurology. Diseases of nerves* (Vol. 7). New York: Elsevier.

Pantoni, L., Rossi, R., Inzitari, D., et al. (2000). Efficacy and safety of nimodipine in subcortical vascular dementia: A subgroup analysis of the Scandinavian Multi-Infarct Dementia Trial. *Journal of the Neurological Sciences, 175,* 124–134.

Paolo, A.M., Axelrod, B.N., & Tröster, A. (1996). Test–retest stability of the Wisconsin Card Sorting Test. *Assessment, 3,* 137–143.

Paolo, A.M., Tröster, A.I., Axelrod, B.N., & Koller, W.C. (1995). Construct validity of the WCST in normal elderly and persons with Parkinson's disease. *Archives of Clinical Neuropsychology, 10,* 463–473.

Paolo, A.M., Tröster, A.I., Glatt, S.L., et al. (1995). Differentiation of the dementias of Alzheimer's and Parkinson's diseae with the Dementia Rating Scale. *Journal of Geriatric Psychiatry and Neurology, 8,* 184–188.

Paolo, A.M., Tröster, A.I., & Ryan, J.J. (1997a). California Verbal Learning Test: Normative data for the elderly. *Journal of Clinical and Experimental Neuropsychology, 19,* 220–234.

Paolo, A.M., Tröster, A.I., & Ryan, J.J. (1997b). Test–retest stability of the California Verbal Learning Test in older persons. *Neuropsychology, 11,* 613–616.

Paolo, A.M., Tröster, A.I., & Ryan, J.J. (1998a). Continuous Visual Memory Test performance in healthy persons 60 to 94 years of age. *Archives of Clinical Neuropsychology, 13,* 333–337.

Paolo, A.M., Tröster, A.I., & Ryan, J.J. (1998b). Test-retest stability of the Continuous Visual Memory Test in elderly persons. *Archives of Clinical Neuropsychology, 13,* 617–621.

Papagno, C. (1998). Transient retrograde amnesia associated with impaired naming of living categories. *Cortex, 34,* 111–121.

Papanicoloaou, A.C. (1998). *Fundamentals of functional brain imaging.* Lisse, Netherlands: Swets and Zeitlinger.

Papanicolaou, A.C., Moore, B.D., Deutsch, G., et al. (1988). Evidence for right-hemisphere involvement in recovery from aphasia. *Archives of Neurology, 45,* 1025–1029.

Papanicolaou, A.C., Moore, B.D., Levin, H.S., & Eisenberg, H.M. (1987). Evoked potential correlates of right hemisphere involvement in language recovery following stroke. *Archives of Neurology, 44,* 521–524.

Papanicolaou, A.C., Simos, P.G., Breier, J.I., et al. (2001). Brain plasticity for sensory and linguistic functions: A functional imaging study using magnetoencephalography with children and young adults. *Journal of Child Neurology, 16,* 241–252.

Papez, J.W. (1937). A proposed mechanism of emotion. *Archives of Neurology and Psychiatry, 38,* 725–744.

Papka, M., Rubio, A., Schiffer, R.B., & Cox, C. (1998). A review of Lewy body disease, an emerging concept of cortical dementia. *Journal of Neuropsychiatry and Clinical Neurosciences, 10,* 267–279.

Paque, L. & Warrington, E. (1995). A longitudinal study of reading ability in patients suffering from dementia. *Journal of the International Neuropsychological Society, 1,* 517–524.

Paradiso, S. & Robinson, R.G. (1998). Gender differences in post-stroke depression. *Journal of Neuropsychiatry and Clinical Neuroscience, 10,* 41–47.

Parashos, I.A., Wilkinson, W.E., & Coffey, C.E. (1995). Magnetic resonance imaging of the corpus callosum: Predictors of size in normal adults. *Journal of Neuropsychiatry and Clinical Neurosciences, 7,* 35–41.

Parasuraman, R. (1998). The attentive brain: Issues and prospects. In R. Parasuraman (Ed.), *The attentive brain.* Cambridge, MA: MIT Press.

Parasuraman, R. & Greenwood, P.M. (1998). Selective attention in aging and dementia. In R. Parasuraman (Ed.), *The attentive brain.* Cambridge, MA: MIT Press.

Parasuraman, R. & Haxby, J.V. (1993). Attention and brain function in Alzheimer's disease: A review. *Neuropsychology, 7,* 242–272.

Parasuraman, R., Warm, J.S., & See, J.E. (1998). Brain systems of vigilance. In R. Parasuraman (Ed.), *The attentive brain.* Cambridge, MA: MIT Press.

Parenté, F.J. & Anderson, J.K. (1984). Use of the Wechsler Memory Scale for predicting success in cognitive rehabilitation. *Cognitive Rehabilitation, 2,* 12–15.

Parizel, P.M., Ozsarlak, O., Van Goethem, J.W., et al. (1998). Imaging findings in diffuse axonal injury after closed head trauma. *European Radiology, 8,* 960–965.

Park, D.C., Smith, A.D., Lautenschlager, G., et al. (1996). Mediators of long-term memory performance across the life span. *Psychology and Aging, 11,* 621–637.

Park, N.W., Moscovitch, M., & Robertson, I.H. (1999). Divided attention impairments after traumatic brain injury. *Neuropsychologia, 37,* 1119–1133.

Park, S.M., Gabrieli, H.D.E., Reminger, S.L., et al. (1998). Preserved priming across study-test picture transformations in patients with Alzheimer's disease. *Neuropsychology, 12,* 340–352.

Parker, E.S., Birnbaum, I.M., Weingartner, H., et al. (1980). Retrograde enhancement of human memory with alcohol. *Psychopharmacology, 69,* 219–222.

Parker, E.S., Morihisa, J.M., Wyatt, R.J., et al. (1981). The alcohol facilitation effect on memory: A dose-response study. *Psychopharmacology, 74,* 88–92.

Parker, E.S. & Noble, E.P. (1977). Alcohol consumption and cognitive functioning in social drinkers. *Journal of Studies on Alcohol, 38,* 1224–1232.

Parker, K.C.H. (1983). Factor analysis of the WAIS-R at nine age levels between 16 and 74 years. *Journal of Consulting and Clinical Psychology, 51,* 302–308.

Parker, K.C.H. (1986). Change with age, year-of-birth, cohort, age by year-of-birth cohort interaction, and standardization of the Wechsler Adult Intelligence Tests. *Human Development, 29,* 209–222.

Parker, R.S. (2001). *Concussive brain trauma. Neurobehavioral impairment and maladaptation.* Boca Raton, FL: CRC Press.

Parkin, A.J. (1982). Residual learning capability in organic amnesia. *Cortex, 18,* 417–440.

Parkin, A.J. (1984). Amnesic syndrome: A lesion-specific disorder? *Cortex, 20,* 479–508.

Parkin, A.J. (1991). The relationship between anterograde and retrograde amnesia in alcoholic Wernicke-Korsakoff syndrome. *Psychological Medicine, 21,* 11–14.

Parkin, A.J. (2001). The structure and mechanisms of memory. In B. Rapp (Ed.), *The handbook of cognitive neuropsychology.* Philadelphia: Psychology Press.

Parkin, A.J. & Java, R.I. (1999). Deterioration of frontal lobe function in normal aging: Influences of fluid intelligence versus perceptual speed. *Neuropsychology, 13,* 539–545.

Parkin, A.J. & Lawrence, A. (1994). A dissociation in the relation between memory tasks and frontal lobe tests in the normal elderly. *Neuropsychologia, 32,* 1523–1532.

Parkin, A.J., Miller, J., & Vincent, R. (1987). Multiple neuropsychological deficits due to anoxic encephalopathy: A case study. *Cortex, 23,* 655–665.

Parkin, A.J., Walter, B.M., & Hunkin, N.M. (1995). Relationships between normal aging, frontal lobe function, and memory for temporal and spatial information. *Neuropsychology, 9,* 304–312.

Parkinson, J. (1817). *Essay on the shaking palsy.* London: Whittingham and Rowland.

Parkinson, R.B., Hopkins, R.O., Cleavinger, H.B., et al. (2002). White matter hyperintensities and neuropsychological outcome following carbon monoxide poisoning. *Neurology, 58,* 1525–1532.

Parkinson, S.R. (1979). The amnesic Korsakoff syndrome: A study of selective and divided attention. *Neuropsychologia, 17,* 67–75.

Parks, R.W., Duara, R., Barker, W.W., & Kaplan, E. (1987). Boston Naming Test correlates with positron emission tomography in Alzheimer's disease and normals [abstract]. *Journal of Clinical and Experimental Neuropsychology, 9,* 75.).

Parks, R.W., Levine, D.S., & Long, D.L. (Eds.). (1998). *Fundamentals of neural network modeling.* Cambridge, MA: MIT Press.

Parks, R.W., Zec, R.F., & Wilson, R.S. (Eds.) (1993). *Neuropsychology of Alzheimer's disease and other dementias.* New York: Oxford University Press.

Parnetti, L., Ambrosoli, L., Agliati, G., et al. (1996). Posatirelin in the treatment of vascular dementia: A double-blind multicentre study vs placebo. *Acta Neurologica Scandinavica, 93,* 456–463

Parsons, O.A. (1975). Brain damage in alcoholics: Altered states of unconsciousness. In M.M. Gross (Ed.), *Alcohol intoxication and withdrawal. Experimental Studies 2.* New York: Plenum Press.

Parsons, O.A. (1977). Neuropsychological deficits in alcoholics: Facts and fancies. *Alcoholism: Clinical and Experimental Research, 1,* 51–56.

Parsons, O.A. (1986). Cognitive functioning in sober social drinkers: A review and critique. *Journal of Studies on Alcohol, 47,* 101–114.

Parsons, O.A., Butters, N., & Nathan, P.E. (Eds.) (1987). *Neuropsychology of alcoholism: Implications for diagnosis and treatment.* New York: Guilford Press.

Parsons, O.A. & Farr, S.P. (1981). The neuropsychology of alcohol and drug use. In S.B. Filskov & T.J. Boll (Eds.), *Handbook of clinical neuropsychology*. New York: Wiley-Interscience.

Parsons, O.A., Vega, A., Jr., & Burn, J. (1969). Differential psychological effects of lateralized brain damage. *Journal of Consulting and Clinical Psychology, 33*, 551–557.

Parvizi, J., Anderson, S.W., Martin, C.O., et al. (2001). Pathological laughter and crying: A link to the cerebellum. *Brain, 124*, 1708–1719.

Parvizi, J. & Damasio, A. (2001). Consciousness and the brain stem. In S. Dehaene (Ed.), *The cognitive neuroscience of consciousness*. Cambridge, MA: MIT Press/Amsterdam: Elsevier.

Pascal, G.R. & Suttell, B.J. (1951). *The Bender-Gestalt Test: Quantification and validity for adults*. New York: Grune & Stratton.

Pascual-Leone, A., Dhuma, A., Altafullah, I., & Anderson, D.C. (1990). Cocaine-induced seizures. *Neurology, 40*, 404–407.

Pashler, H.E. (1998). *The psychology of attention*. Cambridge, MA: The MIT Press.

Pasquier, F., Bergego, C., & Deloche, G. (1989). Line bisection: Length of lines and performance effects in normal subjects and hemisphere damaged patients [abstract]. *Journal of Clinical and Experimental Neuropsychology, 11*, 371.

Pasquier, F., Grymonprez, L., Lebert, F., & Van der Linden, M. (2001). Memory impairment differs in frontotemporal dementia and Alzheimer's disease. *Neurocase, 7*, 161–171.

Passingham, R.E. (1987). From where does the motor cortex get its instructions? In S.P. Wise (Ed.), *Higher brain functions*. New York: Wiley.

Passingham, R. (1997). Functional organization of the motor system. In R.S.J. Frackowiak et al. (Eds.), *Human brain function*. San Diego: Academic Press.

Passingham, R.E. (1998). Attention to action. In A.C. Roberts, T.W. Robbins, & L. Weiskrantz (Eds.), *The prefrontal cortex: Executive and cognitive functions*. New York: Oxford University Press.

Pasternak, G., Becker, C.E., Lash, A., et al. (1989). Cross-sectional neurotoxicology study of lead-exposed cohort. *Clinical Toxicology, 27*, 37–51.

Pastorek, N.J., Hannay, H.J., & Contant, C.S. (2004). Prediction of global outcome with acute neuropsychological testing following closed-head injury. *Journal of the International Neuropsychological Society, 10*, 807–817.

Patchell, R.A. (2002). Brain metastases. In A.K. Asbury et al. (Eds.), *Diseases of the nervous system* (3rd ed.). Cambridge, UK: Cambridge University Press.

Paterson, A. & Zangwill, O.L. (1944). Disorders of visual space perception associated with lesions of the right cerebral hemisphere. *Brain, 67*, 331–358.

Patrick, C.L. (1998). The relations among cognitive strategy, mental rotation performance and mathematical reasoning. *Dissertation Abstracts International. Section B, Sciences and Engineering, 58*, 9-B. (University Microfilms AAT9808841).

Patten, B.M. (1992). Lightning and electrical injuries. *Neurologic Clinics, 10*, 1047–1058.

Patten, S.B. & Metz, L.M. (1997). Depression in multiple sclerosis. *Psychotherapy and Psychosomatics, 66*, 286–292.

Patterson, J.C. II & Kotrla, K.J. (2002). Functional neuroimaging in psychiatry. In S.C. Yudofsky & R.E. Hales (Eds.), *Textbook of neuropsychiatry and clinical neurosciences*. Washington, D.C.: American Psychiatric Publishing.

Patterson, K. & Hodges, J.R. (1995). Disorders of semantic memory. In A.D. Baddeley et al. (Eds.), *Handbook of memory disorders*. Chichester, UK: Wiley.

Patterson, M.B., Mack, J.L., & Schnell, A.H. (1999). Performance of elderly and young normals on the Gollin Incomplete Pictures Test. *Perceptual and Motor Skills, 89*, 663–664.

Pau, C.W.H., Lee, T.M.C., & Chan, S.-f.F. (2002). The impact of heroin on frontal executive functions. *Archives of Clinical Neuropsychology, 17*, 663–670.

Paul, D.S., Franzen, M.D., Cohen, S.H., & Fremouw, W. (1992). An investigation into the reliability and validity of two tests used in the detection of dissimulation. *International Journal of Clinical Neuropsychology, 14*, 1–9.

Paul, R.H., Beatty, W.W., Schneider, R., et al. (1998a). Impairments of attention in individuals with multiple sclerosis. *Multiple Sclerosis, 4*, 433–439.

Paul, R.H., Beatty, W.W., Schneider, R., et al. (1998b). Cognitive and physical fatigue in multiple sclerosis: Relations between self-report and objective performance. *Applied Neuropsychology, 5*, 143–148.

Paul, R.H., Blanco, C.R., Hames, K.A., & Beatty, W.W. (1997). Autobiographical memory in multiple sclerosis. *Journal of the International Neuropsychological Society, 3*, 246–251.

Paul, R.H., Cohen, R.A., Moser, D., et al. (2001). Performance on the Mattis Dementia Rating Scale in patients with vascular dementia: Relationships to neuroimaging findings. *Journal of Geriatric Psychiatry and Neurology, 14*, 33–36.

Paulesu, E., Frackowiak, R.S.J., and Bottini, G. (1997). Maps of somatosensory systems. In R.S.J. Frackowiak et al. (Eds.), *Human brain function*. San Diego: Academic Press.

Paulsen, J.S., Butters, N., Sadek, J.R., et al. (1995). Distinct cognitive profiles of cortical and subcortical dementia in advanced illness. *Neurology, 45*, 951–956.

Paulsen, J.S., Butters, N., Salmon, D.P., et al. (1993). Prism adaptation in Alzheimer's and Huntington's disease. *Neuropsychology, 7*, 73–81.

Paulsen, J.S., Heaton, R.K., Sadek, J.R., et al. (1995). The nature of learning and memory impairments in schizophrenia. *Journal of the International Neuropsychological Society, 1*, 88–99.

Paulsen, J.S., Ready, R.E., Hamilton, J.M., et al. (2001). Neuropsychiatric aspects of Huntington's disease. *Journal of Neurology, Neurosurgery and Psychiatry, 71*, 310–314.

Paulsen, J.S., Zhao, H., Stout, J.C., et al. (2001). Clinical markers of early disease in persons near onset of Huntington's disease. *Neurology, 57*, 658–662.

Paulson, G.W. & Dadmehr, N. (1991). Is there a premorbid personality typical for Parkinson's disease? *Neurology, 41(Suppl. 2)*, 73–76.

Pavot, W. & Diener, E. (1993). Review of the Satisfaction with Life Scale. *Psychological Assessment, 5*, 164–172.

Pavot, W., Diener, E., Colvin, C.R., & Sandvik, E. (1991). Further validation of the Satisfaction with Life Scale: Evidence for the cross-method convergence of well-being measures. *Journal of Personality Assessment, 57*, 149–161.

Pearlin, L.I. & Schooler, C. (1978). The structure of coping. *Journal of Health and Social Behavior, 19*, 2–21.

Pearlman, A.L. (1990). Visual system. In A.L. Pearlman & R.C. Collins (Eds.), *Neurobiology of disease*. New York: Oxford University Press.

Pearlson, G.D., Ross, C.A., Lohr, W.D., et al. (1990). Association between family history of affective disorder and the depressive syndrome of Alzheimer's disease. *American Journal of Psychiatry, 147*, 452–456.

Peatfield, R.C. (1995). Relationships between food, wine, and beer-precipitated migrainous headaches. *Headache, 35*, 355–357.

Peck, D.F. (1970). The conversion of Progressive Matrices and Mill Hill Vocabulary raw scores into deviation IQ's. *Journal of Clinical Psychology, 26*, 67–70.

Peck, E.A. & Warren, J.B. (1989). The neuropsychological and quality-of-life sequelae to severe head injury. In D.P. Becker & S.K. Gudeman (Eds.), *Textbook of head injury*. Philadelphia: Harcourt Brace Jovanovich.

Pedersen, P.M., Jorgensen, H.S., Nakayama, H., et al. (1996). Frequency, determinants, and consequences of anosognosia in acute stroke. *Journal of Neurologic Rehabilitation, 10,* 243–250.

Peek-Asa, C., McArthur, D., Hovda, D., & Kraus, J. (2001). Early predictors of mortality in penetrating compared with closed brain injury. *Brain Injury, 15,* 801–810.

Peek-Asa, C., McArthur, D.L., & Kraus, J.F. (1999). The prevalence of non-standard helmet use and head injuries among motorcycle riders. *Accident Analysis and Prevention, 31,* 229–233.

Peeke, S.C. & Peeke, H.V.S. (1984). Attention, memory, and cigarette smoking. *Psychopharmacology, 84,* 205–216.

Peirson, A.R. & Jansen, P. (1997). Comparability of the Rey-Osterrieth and Taylor forms of the Complex Figure Test. *The Clinical Neuropsychologist, 11,* 244–248.

Peled, S., Gudbjartsson, H., Westin, C.F., et al. (1998). Magnetic resonance imaging shows orientation and asymmetry of white matter fiber tracts. *Brain Research, 780,* 27–33.

Pelletier, J., Suchet, L., Witjas, T., et al. (2001). A longitudinal study of callosal atrophy and interhemispheric dysfunction in relapsing-remitting multiple sclerosis. *Archives of Neurology, 58,* 105–111.

Pelosi, A., Geesken, J. M., Holly, M., et al. (1997). Working memory impairment in early multiple sclerosis: Evidence from an event-related potential study of patients with clinically isolated myelopathy. *Brain, 120,* 2039–2058.

Pender, N. & Fleminger, S. (1999). Outcome measures on inpatient cognitive and behavioural units: An overview. *Neuropsychological Rehabilitation, 9,* 345–361.

Pendleton, M.G. & Heaton, R.K. (1982). A comparison of the Wisconsin Card Sorting Test and the Category Test. *Journal of Clinical Psychology, 38,* 392–396.

Pendleton, M.G., Heaton, R.K., Lehman, R.A.W., & Hulihan, D. (1982). Diagnostic utility of the Thurstone Word Fluency Test in neuropsychological evaluations. *Journal of Clinical Neuropsychology, 4,* 307–318.

Pendleton, M.G., Heaton, R.K., Lehman, R.A., et al. (1985). Word Finding Test performance: Effects of localization of cerebral damage, level of neuropyschological impairment, age, and education. *Journal of Clinical Psychology, 41,* 82–85.

Penfield, W. (1958). Functional localization in temporal and deep sylvian areas. *Research Publication, Association for Nervous and Mental Disease, 36,* 210–227.

Penfield, W. (1968). Engrams in the human brain. *Proceedings of the Royal Society of Medicine, 61,* 831–840.

Penfield, W. & Rasmussen, T. (1950). *The cerebral cortex of man.* New York: MacMillan.

Pennington, B.F. (2002). *The development of psychopathology. Nature and nurture.* New York: Guilford Press.

Peran, P., Rascol, O., Demonet, J.F., et al. (2003). Deficit of verb generation in nondemented patients with Parkinson's disease. *Movement Disorders, 18,* 150–156.

Perecman, E. (1987). Consciousness and the meta-functions of the frontal lobes: Setting the stage. In E. Perecman (Ed.), *The frontal lobes revisited.* New York: IRBN Press.

Peretz, I. (2001). Music perception and recognition. In B. Rapp (Ed.), *The handbook of cognitive neuropsychology.* Philadelphia: Psychology Press.

Peretz, J.A. & Cummings, J.L. (1988). Subcortical dementia. In U. Holden (Ed.), *Neuropsychology and aging.* New York: New York University Press.

Perez, S.A., Schlottmann, R.S., Holloway, J.A., & Ozolins, M.S. (1996). Measurement of premorbid intellectual ability following brain injury. *Archives of Clinical Neuropsychology, 11,* 491–501.

Pérez-Arce, P. (1999). The influence of culture on cognition. *Archives of Clinical Neuropsychology, 14,* 581–592.

Pérez-Stable, E.J., Halliday, R., Gardiner, P.S., et al. (2000). The effects of propranolol on cognitive function and quality of life: A randomized trial among patients with diastolic hypertension. *American Journal of Medicine, 108,* 359–365.

Perfect, T.J. & Maylor, E.A. (Eds.) (2000). *Models of cognitive aging.* Oxford, UK: Oxford University Press.

Perkin, G.D. (1998). *Mosby's color atlas and text of neurology.* London: Times Mirror.

Perlick, D. & Atkins, A. (1984). Variations in the reported age of a patient: A source of bias in the diagnosis of depression and dementia. *Journal of Consulting and Clinical Psychology, 52,* 812–820.

Perlmuter, L.C., Goldfinger, S.H., Shore, A.R., & Nathan, D.M. (1990). Cognitive function in non-insulin-dependent diabetes. In C.S. Holmes (Ed.), *Neuropsychological and behavioral aspects of diabetes.* New York: Springer-Verlag.

Perlmuter, L.C., Hakami, M.K., Hodgson-Harrington, C., et al. (1984). Decreased cognitive function in aging non-insulin-dependent diabetic patients. *American Journal of Medicine, 77,* 1043–1048.

Perrault, A., Oremus, M., Demers, L., et al. (2000). Review of outcome measurement instruments in Alzheimer's disease drug trials: Psychometric properties of behavioral and mood scales. *Journal of Geriatric Psychiatry and Neurology, 13,* 181–196.

Perret, E. (1974). The left frontal lobe of man and the suppression of habitual responses in verbal categorical behaviour. *Neuropsychologia, 12,* 323–330.

Perrigot, M., Fakacs, Ch., Soler, J.M., & Pradat-Diehl, P. (1991). Troubles génito-sexuels des traumatisés crâniens. In J. Pélissier et al. (Eds.), *Traumatisme crânien grave et médecine de rééducation.* Paris: Masson.

Perrine, K.R. (1985). Concept formation in the Wisconsin Card Sorting test and Halstead Category Test [abstract]. *Journal of Clinical and Experimental Neuropsychology, 7,* 299.

Perrine, K. (1993). Differential aspects of conceptual processing in the Category Test and Wisconsin Card Sorting Test. *Journal of Clinical and Experimental Neuropsychology, 15,* 461–473.

Perrine, K., Dogali, M., Fazzini, E., et al. (1998). Cognitive functioning after pallidotomy for refractory Parkinson's disease. *Journal of Neurology, Neurosurgery and Psychiatry, 65,* 150–154.

Perrine, K., Gershengorm, J., & Brown, E. R. (1991). Interictal neuropsychological function in epilepsy. In O. Devinsky & W.H. Theodore (Eds.), *Epilepsy and behavior.* New York: Wiley-Liss.

Perry, E.K., Curtis, M., Dick, D.J., et al. (1985). Cholinergic correlates of cognitive impairment in Parkinson's disease: Comparisons with Alzheimer's disease. *Journal of Neurology, Neurosurgery, and Psychiatry, 48,* 413–421.

Perry, G.G. & Kinder, B.N. (1990). The susceptibility of the Rorschach to malingering: A critical review. *Journal of Personality Assessment, 54,* 47–57.

Perry, J.R., Louis, D.N., & Cairncross, J.G. (1999). Current treatment of oligodendrogliomas. *Archives of Neurology, 56,* 434–436.

Perry, R.J. & Hodges, J.R. (1999). Attention and executive deficits in Alzheimer's disease. A critical review. *Brain, 122,* 383–404.

Perry, R.J. & Hodges, J.R. (2000). Differentiating frontal and temporal variant frontotemporal dementia from Alzheimer's disease. *Neurology, 54,* 2277–2284.

Perry, S., Belsky-Barr, D., Barr, W.B., & Jacobsberg, L. (1989). Neuropsychological function in physically asymptomatic HIV-seropositive men. *Journal of Neuropsychiatry, 1,* 296–302.

Perry, W., Potterat, E., Auslander, L., et al. (1996). A neuropsychological approach to the Rorschach in patients with dementia of the Alzheimer type. *Assessment, 3,* 351–363.

Persaud, G. (1987). Sex and age differences on the Raven's Matrices. *Perceptual and Motor Skills, 65,* 45–46.

Pestell, S., Shanks, M.F., Warrington, J., & Venneri, A. (2000). Quality of spelling breakdown in Alzheimer's disease is independent of disease progression. *Journal of Clinical and Experimental Neuropsychology, 22,* 599–612.

Peters, H.A., Levine, R.L., Matthews, C.G., et al. (1982). Carbon disulfide–induced neuropsychiatric changes in grain storage workers. *American Journal of Industrial Medicine, 3,* 373–391.

Peters, L.C., Stambrook, M., Moore, A.D., & Esses, L. (1990). Psychosocial sequelae of closed head injury: Effects on the marital relationship. *Brain Injury, 4,* 39–48

Peters, M. (1990). Subclassification of non-pathological left-handers poses problems for theories of handedness. *Neuropsychologia, 28,* 279–289.

Peters, M. (1997). Gender differences in intercepting a moving target by using a throw or button press. *Journal of Motor Behavior, 29,* 290–296.

Peters, M. & Servos, P. (1989). Performance of subgroups of left-handers and right-handers. *Canadian Journal of Psychology, 43,* 341–358.

Petersen, R.C. (1991). Memory assessment at the bedside. In T. Yanagihara & R. C. Petersen (Eds.), *Memory disorders: Research and clinical practice.* New York: Marcel Dekker.

Petersen, R.C., Smith, G.E., Ivnik, R.J., et al. (1994). Memory function in very early Alzheimer's disease. *Neurology, 44,* 867–872.

Petersen, R.C., Smith, G., Kokmen, E., et al. (1992). Memory function in normal aging. *Neurology, 42,* 396–401.

Petersen, R.C., Smith, G.E., Waring, S.C., et al. (1999). Mild cognitive impairment: Clinical characterization and outcome. *Archives of Neurology, 56,* 303–308.

Petersen, R.C. & Weingartner, H. (1991). Memory nomenclature. In T. Yanagihara & R.C. Petersen (Eds.), *Memory disorders: Research and clinical practice.* New York: Marcel Dekker.

Peterson, K., Paleologos, N., Forsyth, P., et al. (1996). Salvage chemotherapy for oligodendroglioma. *Journal of Neurosurgery, 85,* 597–601.

Peterson, L.R. (1966). Short-term memory. *Scientific American, 215,* 90–95.

Peterson, L.R. & Peterson, M.J. (1959). Short-term retention of individual verbal items. *Journal of Experimental Psychology, 58,* 193–198.

Peterson, R.A. & Headen, S.W. (1984). Profile of Mood States. In D.J. Keyser & R.C. Sweetland (Eds.), *Test critiques* (Vol. 1). Kansas City, MO: Test Corporation of America.

Petit, H., Wiart, L., Destaillats, J.M., et al. (1994). Réinsertion professionnelle des traumatisés cranio-encéphaliques. In P. Codine et al. (Eds.), *La réinsertion socio-professionnelle des personnes handicapées.* Paris: Masson.

Petit-Taboue, M.C., Landeau, B., Desson, J.F., et al. (1998). Effects of healthy aging on the regional cerebral metabolic rate of glucose assessed with statistical parametric mapping. *Neuroimage, 7,* 176–184.

Petrides, M. (1989). Frontal lobes and memory. In F. Boller & J. Grafman (Eds.), *Handbook of neuropsychology* (Vol. 3). Amsterdam: Elsevier.

Petrides, M. (1994). Frontal lobes and working memory: Evidence from investigations of the effects of cortical excisions in nonhuman primates. In F. Boller & H. Spinnler (Eds.), *Handbook of neuropsychology* (Vol. 9). New York: Elsevier.

Petrides, M. & Milner, B. (1982). Deficits on subject-ordered tasks after frontal- and temporal-lobe lesions in man. *Neuropsychologia, 20,* 249–262.

Petry, S., Cummings, J.L., Hill, M.A., & Shapira, J. (1988). Personality alterations in dementia of the Alzheimer type. *Archives of Neurology, 45,* 1187–1190.

Petry, S., Cummings, J.L., Hill, M.A., & Shapira, J. (1989). Personality alterations in dementia of the Alzhiemer type: A three-year follow-up study. *Journal of Geriatric Psychiatry and Neurology, 2,* 203–207.

Pettinati, H.M. & Bonner, K.M. (1984). Cognitive functioning in depressed geriatric patients with a history of ECT. *American Journal of Psychiatry, 141,* 49–52.

Peyser, J.M., Rao, S. M., LaRocca, N.G., & Kaplan, E. (1990). Guidelines for neuropsychological research in multiple sclerosis. *Archives of Neurology, 47,* 94–97.

Pfeffer, R.I., Kurosaki, T.T., Harrah, C.H., Jr., et al. (1981). A survey diagnostic tool for senile dementia. *American Journal of Epidemiology, 114,* 515–527.

Pfefferbaum, A., Sullivan, E.V., Hedehus, M., et al. (2000). In vivo detection and functional correlates of white matter microstructural disruption in chronic alcoholism. *Alcoholism: Clinical and Experimental Research, 24,* 1214–1221.

Pfeiffer, D. (1998). The ICIDH and the need for its revision. *Disability and Society, 13,* 503–523.

Pfeiffer, E. (1975). *SPMSQ:* Short Portable Mental Status Questionnaire. *Journal of the American Geriatric Society, 23,* 433–441.

Phadke, J.G. & Best, P.V. (1983). Atypical and clinically silent multiple sclerosis: A report of 12 cases discovered unexpectedly at necropsy. *Journal of Neurology, Neurosurgery and Psychiatry, 46,* 414–420.

Pharr, V., Litvan, I., Brat, D.J., et al. (1999). Ideomotor apraxia in progressive supranuclear palsy: A case study. *Movement Disorders, 14,* 162–166.

Pharr, V., Uttl, B., Stark, M., et al. (2001). Comparison of apraxia in corticobasal degeneration and progressive supranuclear palsy. *Neurology, 56,* 957–963.

Phillips, C.G., Zeki, S., & Barlow, H.B. (1984). Localization of function in the cerebral cortex. *Brain, 107,* 327–361.

Phillips, L.H., Wynn, V., Gilhooly, K.J., et al. (1999). The role of memory in the Tower of London task. *Memory, 7,* 209–231.

Phinney, J.S. (1996). When we talk about American ethnic groups what do we mean? *American Psychologist, 51,* 918–927.

Physician's desk reference (PDR) (published annually). Oradell, NJ: Medical Economics.

Piaget, J. (1967). *Biologie et connaissance.* Paris: Gallimard.

Piatt, A.L., Fields, J.A., Paolo, A.M., et al. (1999). Lexical, semantic, and action verbal fluency in Parkinson's disease with and without dementia. *Journal of Clinical and Experimental Neuropsychology, 21,* 435–443.

Piazza, D.M. (1980). The influence of sex and handedness in hemispheric specialization of verbal and nonverbal tasks. *Neuropsychologia, 18,* 163–176.

Picton, T.W., Bentin, S., Berg, P., et al. (2000). Guidelines for using human event-related potentials to study cognition: Recording standards and publication criteria. *Psychophysiology, 37,* 127–152.

Pieniadz, J.M., Naeser, M.A., Koff, E., & Levine, H.L. (1983). CT scan cerebral hemispheric asymmetry measurements in stroke cases with global aphasia: Atypical asymmetries associated with improved recovery. *Cortex, 19,* 371–391.

Piercy, M. (1964). The effects of cerebral lesions on intellectual functions: A review of current research trends. *British Journal of Psychiatry, 110,* 310–352.

Pietrini, P., Guazzelli, M., Gasso, G., et al. (2000). Neural correlates of imaginal aggressive behavior assessed by positron emission tomography in healthy subjects. *American Journal of Psychiatry, 157,* 1772–1781.

Pignatti, F., van den Bent, M., Curran, D., et al. (2002). Prognostic factors for survival in adult patients with cerebral low-grade glioma. *Journal of Clinical Oncology, 20,* 2076–2084.

Piguet, O., Saling, M.M., O'Shea, M.F., et al. (1994). Rey figure distortions reflect nonverbal recall differences between right and left foci in unilateral temporal lobe epilepsy. *Archives of Clinical Neuropsychology, 9*, 451–460.

Pike, G.B., De Stefano, N., Narayanan, S., et al. (2000). Multiple sclerosis: Magnetic transfer MR imaging of white matter before lesion appearance on T_2-weighted images. *Radiology, 215*, 824–830.

Pillon, B. (1979). Activités constructives et lésions cérébrales chez l'homme. *L'Année Psychologique, 79*, 197–227.

Pillon, B. (1981a). Négligence de l'hémi-espace gauche dans des épreuves visuo-constructives. *Neuropsychologia, 19*, 317–320.

Pillon, B. (1981b). Troubles visuo-constructifs et méthodes de compensation: Résultats de 85 patients atteints de lésions cérébrales. *Neuropsychologia, 19*, 375–383.

Pillon, B., Agid, Y., & Dubois, B. (1996). *Le rôle des ganglions de la base dans l'organisation cognitive et comportementale*. In M.I. Botez (Ed.), *Neuropyschologie clinique et neurologie du comportement*. Montréal: Les Presses de l'Université de Montréal.

Pillon, B., Ardouin, C., Damier, P., et al. (2000). Neuropsychological changes between "off" and "on" STN or GPi stimulation in Parkinson's disease. *Neurology, 55*, 411–418.

Pillon, B., Bazin, B., Deweer, B., et al. (1999). Specificity of memory deficits after right or left temporal lobectomy. *Cortex, 35*, 561–571.

Pillon, B. & Dubois, B. (1992). Cognitive and behavioral impairments. In I. Litvan & Y. Agid (Eds.), *Progressive supranuclear palsy: Clinical and research approaches*. New York: Oxford University Press.

Pillon, B., Dubois, B., Bonnet, A.-M., et al. (1989). Cognitive slowing in Parkinson's disease fails to respond to levodopa treatment: The 15-objects test. *Neurology, 39*, 762–768.

Pillon, B., Dubois, B., Cusimano, G., et al. (1989). Does cognitive impairment in Parkinson's disease result from non-dopaminergic lesions? *Journal of Neurology, 52*, 201–206.

Pillon, B., Dubois, B., Lhermitte, F., & Agid, Y. (1986). Heterogeneity of cognitive impairment in progressive supranuclear palsy, Parkinson's disease, and Alzheimer's disease. *Neurology, 36*, 1179–1185.

Pillon, B., Dubois, B., Ploska, A., & Agid, Y. (1991). Severity and specificity of cognitive impairment in Alzheimer's, Huntington's, and Parkinson's diseases and progressive supranuclear palsy. *Neurology, 41*, 634–643.

Pimental, P.A. & Kingsbury, N.A. (1989). The injured right hemisphere: Classification of related disorders. In *Neuropsychological aspects of right brain injury*. Austin, TX: Pro-Ed.

Pimental, P.A. & Knight, J.A. (2000). *Mini Inventory of Right Brain Injury (MIRBI-2)* (2nd ed.). Austin, TX: Pro-Ed.

Pincus, J.H. & Tucker, G.J. (2003). *Behavioral neurology* (4th ed.). New York: Oxford University Press.

Pineda, D.A., Rosselli, M., Ardila, A., et al. (2000). The Boston Diagnostic Aphasia Examination-Spanish version: The influence of demographic variables. *Journal of the International Neuropsychological Society, 6*, 802–814.

Pinho e Melo, T. & Bogousslavsky, J. (2001). Hemiparesis and other types of motor weakness. In J. Bogousslavsky & L. Caplan (Eds.), *Stroke syndromes* (2nd ed.). Cambridge: Cambridge University Press.

Pinkston, J.B., Wu, J.C., Gouvier, W.D., & Varney, N.R. (2000). Quantitative PET scan findings in carbon monoxide poisoning: Deficits seen in a matched pair. *Archives of Clinical Neuropsychology, 15*, 545–553.

Piotrowski, C. (2000). How popular is the Personality Assessment Inventory in practice and training? *Psychological Reports, 86*, 65–66.

Piotrowski, C. & Keller, J.W. (1989). Psychological testing in outpatient mental health facilties: A national study. *Professional Psychology, 20*, 423–425.

Piotrowski, C. & Lubin, B. (1990). Assessment practices of health psychologists: Survey of APA Division 38 clinicians. *Professional Psychology: Research and Practice, 2*, 99–106.

Piotrowski, Z. (1937). The Rorschach inkblot method in organic disturbances of the central nervous system. *Journal of Nervous and Mental Disease, 86*, 525–537.

Pirozzolo, F.J., Hansch, E.C., Mortimer, J.A., et al. (1982). Dementia in Parkinson disease: A neuropsychological analysis. *Brain and Cognition, 1*, 71–83.

Pirozzolo, F.J., Inbody, S.B., Sims, P.A., et al. (1989). Neuropathological and neuropsychological changes in Alzheimer's disease. In F.J. Pirozzolo (Ed.), *Clinics in geriatric medicine*. Philadelphia: Saunders.

Pishkin, V., Lovallo, W.R., & Bourne, L.E., Jr. (1985). Chronic alcoholism in males: Cognitive deficit as a function of age of onset, age, and duration. *Alcoholism: Clinical and Experimental Research, 9*, 400–405.

Pizzagalli, D., Regard, M., & Lehmann, D. (1999). Rapid emotional face processing in the human right and left brain hemispheres: An ERP study. *Neuroreport, 10*, 2691–2698.

Pizzamiglio, L. & Mammucari, A. (1989). Disturbance of facial emotional expressions in brain-damaged subjects. In G. Gainotti & C. Caltagirone (Eds.), *Emotions and the dual brain*. Berlin: Springer-Verlag.

Pizzamiglio, L., Mammucari, A., & Razzano, C. (1985). Evidence for sex differences in brain organization in recovery in aphasia. *Brain and Language, 25*, 213–223.

Plassman, B.L., Havlik, R.J., Steffens, D.C., et al. (2000). Documented head injury in early adulthood and risk of Alzheimer's disease and other dementias. *Neurology, 55*, 1158–1166.

Plassman, B.L., Newman, T.T., Welsh, K.A., et al. (1994). Properties of the telephone interview for cognitive status: Application in epidemiological and longitudinal studies. *Neuropsychiatry, Neuropsychology, and Behavioral Neurology, 7*, 235–241.

Plassman, B.L., Welsh, K.A., Helms, M., et al. (1995). Intelligence and education as predictors of cognitive state in late life: A 50-year follow-up. *Neurology, 45*, 1446–1450.

Pliskin, N.H., Capelli-Schellpfeffer, M., Law, R.T., et al. (1998). Neuropsychological symptom presentation after electrical injury. *Journal of Trauma: Injury, Infection, and Critical Care, 44*, 709–715.

Pliskin, N.H., Fink, J., Malina, A., et al. (1999). The neuropsychological effects of electrical injury. *Annals of the New York Academy of Sciences, 888*, 140–149.

Pliskin, N.H., Hamer, D.P., Goldstein, D.S., et al. (1996). Improved delayed Visual Reproduction Test performance in multiple sclerosis patients receiving interferon beta-1b. *Neurology, 47*, 1463–1468.

Pliskin, N.H., Kiolbasa, T.A., Hart, R.P., & Umans, J.G. (2001). Neuropsychological function in renal disease and its treatment. In R.E. Tarter et al. (Eds.), *Medical neuropsychology* (2nd ed.). New York: Kluwer Academic/Plenum Press.

Pliskin, N.H. & Sworowski, L.A. (2003). Neuropsychological assessment of patients with cerebrovascular accidents. In G.P. Prigatano & N.H. Pliskin (Eds.), *Clinical neuropsychology and cost outcome research*. New York: Psychology Press.

Plohmann, A.M., Kappos, L., Ammann, W., et al. (1998). Computer assisted retraining of attentional impairments in patients with multiple sclerosis. *Journal of Neurology, Neurosurgery and Psychiatry, 64*, 455–462.

Plomin, R., Pedersen, N.L., Lichtenstein, P., & McClearn, G.E. (1994). Variability and stability in cognitive abilities are largely genetic later in life. *Behavior Genetics, 24*, 207–215.

Plourde, G., Joanette, Y., Fontaine, F.S., et al. (1993). The severity of visual hemineglect follows a bimodal frequency distribution. *Brain and Cognition, 21*, 131–139.

Plum, F. & Caronna, J.J. (1975). Can one predict outcome of medical coma? In *Outcome of severe damage to the central nervous system. Ciba Foundation Symposium 34.* Amsterdam: Elsevier.

Plum, F. & Posner, J.B. (1980). *Diagnosis of stupor and coma* (3rd ed.). Philadelphia: Davis.

Poeck, K. (1983). What do we mean by "aphasic syndromes"? *Brain and Language, 20,* 79–89.

Poeck, K. (1986). The clinical examination for motor apraxia. *Neuropsychologia, 24,* 129–134.

Poeck, K. & Pietron, H.P. (1981). The influence of stretched speech presentation on Token Test performance of aphasic and right brain damaged patients. *Neuropsychologia, 19,* 133–136.

Pohjasvaara, T., Mantyla, R., Aaronen, H.J., et al. (1999). Clinical and radiological determinants of prestroke cognitive decline in a stroke cohort. *Journal of Neurology, Neurosurgery and Psychiatry, 67,* 742–748.

Pohlmann-Eden, B., Dingethal, K., Bender, H.J., & Koelfen, W. (1997). How reliable is the predictive value of SEP (somatosensory evoked potentials) patterns in severe brain damage with special regard to the bilateral loss of cortical responses? *Intensive Care Medicine, 23,* 301–308.

Poitrenaud, J. & Moreaux, C. (1975). Responses given to the Rorschach test by a group of normal aged subjects [in French]. *Revue de Psychologie Appliquée, 25,* 267–284. [From *Psychological Abstracts* (1977), *58,* Abstract Nr. 3074.]

Poizner, H., Bellugi, U., & Klima, E.S. (1990). Biological foundations of language. Clues from sign language. *Annual Review in Neuroscience, 13,* 283–307.

Pollack, B. (1942). The validity of the Shipley-Hartford Retreat Test for "deterioration." *Psychiatric Quarterly, 16,* 119-131.

Pollock, B.G., Mulsant, B.H., Rosen, J., et al. (2002). Comparison of citalopram, perphenazine, and placebo for acute treatment of psychosis and behavioral disturbances in hospitalized, demented patients. *American Journal of Psychiatry, 159,* 460–465.

Pollux, P.M., Wester, A., & De Haan, E.H. (1995). Random generation deficit in alcoholic Korsakoff patients. *Neuropsychologia, 33,* 125–129.

Poloni, M., Capitani, E., Mazzini, L., et al. (1986). Neuropsychological measures in amyotrophic lateral sclerosis and their relationship with CT scan-assessed cerebral atrophy. *Acta Neurologica Scandinavica, 74,* 257–260.

Polster, M.R. & Rose, S.B. (1998). Disorders of auditory processing: Evidence for modularity in audition. *Cortex, 34,* 47–65.

Polubinski, J.P. & Melamed, L.E. (1986). Examination of the sex difference on a symbol digit substitution test. *Perceptual and Motor Skills, 62,* 975–982.

Polyakov, G.I. (1966). Modern data on the structural organization of the cerebral cortex. In A.P. Luria (Ed.), *Higher cortical functions in man.* New York: Basic Books.

Pondal, M., Del Ser, T., & Bermejo, F. (1996). Anticholinergic therapy and dementia in patients with Parkinson's disease. *Journal of Neurology, 243,* 543–546.

Ponsford, J. (1995). *Traumatic brain injury. Rehabilitation for everyday adaptive living.* Hove, UK: Erlbaum.

Ponsford, J. & Kinsella, G. (1992). Attentional deficits following closed head injury. *Journal of Clinical and Experimental Neuropsychology. 17,* 822–838.

Ponsford, J.L., Olver, J.H., & Curran, C. (1995). A profile of outcome: 2 years after traumatic brain injury. *Brain Injury, 9,* 1–10.

Ponsford, J.L., Olver, J.H., Curran, C., & Ng, K. (1995). Prediction of employment status 2 years after traumatic brain injury. *Brain Injury, 9,* 11–20.

Ponsford, J., Olver, J., Nelms, R., et al. (1999). Outcome measurement in an inpatient and outpatient traumatic brain injury rehabilitation programme. *Neuropsychological Rehabilitation, 9,* 517–534.

Ponsford, J., Willmott, C., Rothwell, A., et al. (2000). Factors influencing outcome following mild traumatic brain injury in adults. *Journal of the International Neuropsychological Society, 6,* 568–579.

Pontius, A.A. (1997). Spatial representation in face drawing and block design by nine groups from hunter-gatherers to literates. *Perceptual and Motor Skills, 85,* 947–959.

Pontius, A.A. & Yudowitz, B.S. (1980). Frontal lobe system dysfunction in some criminal actions as shown in the Narratives Test. *Journal of Nervous and Mental Disease, 168,* 111–117.

Pontón, M.O., Gonzalez, J.J., Hernandez, I., et al. (2000). Factor analysis of the Neuropsychological Screening Battery for Hispanics (NeSBHIS). *Applied Neuropsychology, 7,* 32–39.

Pontón, M.O. & León-Carrión, J. (Eds.) (2001).*Neuropsychology and the Hispanic patient.* Mahwah, NJ: Erlbaum.

Pontón, M.O., Satz, P., Herrera, L., et al. (1996). Normative data stratified by age and education for the Neuropsychological Screening Battery for Hispanics (NeSBHIS): Initial report. *Journal of the International Neuropsychological Society, 2,* 96–104.

Pope, K.S., Butcher, J.N., and Seelen, J. (1993). *The MMPI, MMPI-2, and MMPI-A in court.* Washington, D.C.: American Psychological Association.

Pope, K.S., Butcher, J.N., and Seelen, J. (2000). *The MMPI, MMPI-2, and MMPI-A in court* (2nd ed.). Washington, D.C.: American Psychological Association.

Pöppel, E. & von Steinbüchel, N. (1992). Neuropsychological rehabilitation from a theoretical point of view. In N. von Steinbüchel et al. (Eds.), *Neuropsychological rehabilitation.* Berlin: Springer-Verlag.

Poppelreuter, W. (1990). *Disturbances of lower and higher visual capacities caused by occipital damage.* Oxford, UK: Clarendon (trans. J. Zihl, L. Weiskranz, from *Die psychischen Schädigungeng durch Kopfschuss im Kriege 1914–1916.* Leipzig: Voss, 1917.)

Porch, B.E. (1971). Multi-dimensional scoring in aphasia tests. *Journal of Speech and Hearing Research, 14,* 776–792.

Porch, B.E. (1983). *Porch Index of Communicative Ability.* Palo Alto, CA: Consulting Psychologists Press.

Poreh, A.M. (2000). The quantified process approach: An emerging methodology in neuropsychological assessment. *The Clinical Neuropsychologist, 14,* 212–222.

Porter, S.S., Hopkins, R.A., Weaver, L.K., et al. (2002). Corpus callosum atrophy and neuropsychological outcome following carbon monoxide poisoning. *Archives of Clinical Neuropsychology, 17,* 195–204.

Porteus, S.D. (1959). *The Maze Test and clinical psychology.* Palo Alto, CA: Pacific Books.

Porteus, S.D. (1965). *Porteus Maze Test. Fifty years' application.* New York: The Psychological Corporation.

Portin, R., Raininko, R., & Rinne, U.K. (1984). Neuropsychological disturbances and cerebral atrophy determined by computerized tomography in Parkinson patients with long-term levodopa treatment. In R.G. Hassler & J.F. Christ (Eds.), *Advances in neurology.* New York: Raven Press.

Portin, R. & Rinne, U.K. (1980). Neuropsychological responses of parkinsonian patients to long-term levadopa treatment. In U.K. Rinne et al. (Eds.), *Parkinson's disease—current progress, problems and management.* Amsterdam: Elsevier/North-Holland.

Poser, C.M., Paty, D.W., Scheinberg, L., et al. (1983). New diagnostic criteria for multiple sclerosis. *Annals of Neurology, 13,* 227–231.

Poser, S., Kurtzke, J.G.F., Poser, W., & Schlaf, G. (1989). Survival in multiple sclerosis. *Journal of Clinical Epidemiology, 42,* 159–168.

Posner, M.I. (1978). *Chronometric explorations of mind.* Hillside, NJ: Erlbaum.

Posner, M.I. (1988). Structures and functions of selective attention.

In T. Boll & B.K. Bryant (Eds.), *Clinical neuropsychology and brain function: Research, measurement, and practice.* Washington, D.C.: American Psychological Association.

Posner, M.I. (1990). Hierarchical distributed networks in the neuropsychology of selective attention. In A. Caramazza (Ed.), *Cognitive neuropsychology and neurolinguistics: Advances in models of cognitive function and impairment.* Hillsdale, NJ: Erlbaum.

Posner, M.I. & Rothbart, M.K. (1998). Attention, self-regulation and consciousness. *Philosophical Transactions of the Royal Society of London Series B: Biological Sciences, 353,* 1915–1927.

Posner, M.I., Walker, J.A., Friedrich, F.J., & Rafal, R.D. (1984). Effects of parietal injury on covert orienting of attention. *Journal of Neuroscience, 4,* 1863–1874.

Post, R.M. (2000). Neural substrates of psychiatric syndromes. In M.-M. Mesulam (Ed.), *Principles of behavioral and cognitive neurology* (2nd ed.). New York: Oxford University Press.

Postma, A., Izendoorn, R., & De Haan, E.H. (1998). Sex differences in object location of memory. *Brain and Cognition, 36,* 334–345.

Postma, A., Winkel, J., Tuiten, A., & van Honk, J. (1999). Sex difference and menstrual cycle effects in human spatial memory. *Psychoneuroendocrinology, 24,* 175–192.

Postma, T.J., Klein, M., Verstappen, C.C.P., et al. (2002). Radiotherapy-induced cerebral abnormalities in patients with low-grade glioma. *Neurology, 59,* 121–123.

Pottash, A.L.C., Black, H.R., & Gold, M.S. (1981). Psychiatric complications of antihypertensive medications. *Journal of Nervous and Mental Disease, 169,* 430–438.

Powell, A.L., Cummings, J.L., Hill, M.A., & Benson, D.F. (1988). Speech and language alterations in multi-infarct dementia. *Neurology, 38,* 717–719.

Powell, J.B., Cripe, L.I., & Dodrill, C.B. (1991). Assessment of brain impairment with the Rey Auditory Verbal Learning Test: A comparison with other neuropsychological measures. *Archives of Clinical Neuropsychology, 6,* 241–249.

Powell, J.W. & Barber-Foss, K.D. (1999). Traumatic brain injury in high school athletes. *Journal of the American Medical Association, 282,* 958–963.

Powers, W.J. (1990). Stroke. In A.L. Pearlman & R.C. Collins (Eds.), *Neurobiology of disease.* New York: Oxford University Press.

Pozzilli, C., Falaschi, P., Mainero, C., et al. (1999). MRI in multiple sclerosis during the menstrual cycle: Relationship with sex hormone patterns. *Neurology, 53,* 622–624.

Pradat-Diehl, P., Masure, M.C., Lauriot-Prevost, M.C., et al. (1999). Impairment of visual recognition after traumatic brain injury. *Revue Neurologique, 155,* 375–382.

Prado, W.M. & Taub, D.V. (1966). Accurate prediction of individual intellectual functioning by the Shipley-Hartford. *Journal of Clinical Psychology, 22,* 294–296.

Prados, M. & Fried, E.G. (1947). Personality structure of the older age groups. *Journal of Clinical Psychology, 3,* 113–120.

Prather, P., Jarmulowicz, L., Brownell, H., & Gardner, H. (1992). Selective attention and the right hemisphere: A failure in integration, not detection [abstract]. *Journal of Clinical and Experimental Neuropsychology, 14,* 35.

Pribram, K.H. (1987). The subdivisions of the frontal cortex revisited. In E. Perecman (Ed.), *The frontal lobes revisited.* New York: IRBN Press.

Price, B.H. & Mesulam, M. (1985). Psychiatric manifestations of right hemisphere infarctions. *Journal of Nervous and Mental Disease, 173,* 610–614.

Price, C.J. (1997). Functional anatomy of reading. In R.S.J. Frackowiak et al. (Eds.), *Human brain function.* San Diego: Academic Press.

Price, C.J., Warburton, E.A., Moore, C.J., et al. (2001). Dynamic diaschisis: Anatomically remote and context-sensitive human brain lesions. *Journal of Cognitive Neuroscience, 13,* 419–429.

Price, T.R.P., Goetz, K.L., & Lovell, M.R. (2002). Neuropsychiatric aspects of brain tumors. In S.C. Yudofsky & R.E. Hales (Eds.), *Textbook of neuropsychiatry and clinical neurosciences* (4th ed.). Washington, D.C.: American Psychiatric Publishing.

Priddy, D.A., Mattes, D., & Lam, C.S. (1988). Reliability of self report among non-oriented head-injured adults. *Brain Injury, 2,* 249–253.

Prigatano, G.P. (1987). Personality and psychosocial consequences after brain injury. In M.J. Meier et al. (Eds.), *Neuropsychological rehabilitation.* Edinburgh: Churchill Livingstone.

Prigatano, G.P. (1991a). BNI Screen for higher cerebral functions: Rationale and initial validation. *BNI Quarterly, 7,* 2–9.

Prigatano, G.P. (1991b). Disturbances of self-awareness of deficit after traumatic brain injury. In G.P. Prigatano & D.L. Schacter (Eds.), *Awareness of deficit after brain injury: Clinical and theoretical issues.* New York: Oxford University Press.

Prigatano, G.P. (1991c). The relationship of frontal lobe damage to diminished awareness: Studies in rehabilitation. In H.S. Levin, H.M. Eisenberg, & A.L. Benton (Eds.), *Frontal lobe function and dysfunction.* New York: Oxford University Press.

Prigatano, G.P. (1992). Personality disturbances associated with traumatic brain injury. *Journal of Consulting and Clinical Psychology, 60,* 360–368.

Prigatano, G.P. (1999). *Principles of neuropsychological rehabilitation.* New York: Oxford University Press.

Prigatano, G.P. (2000). Neuropsychology, the patient's experience, and the political forces within our field. *Archives of Clinical Neuropsychology, 15,* 71–82.

Prigatano, G.P. & Altman, I.M. (1990). Impaired awareness of behavioral limitations after traumatic brain injury. *Archives of Physical Medicine and Rehabilitation, 71,* 1058–1064.

Prigatano, G.P., Altman, I.M., & O'Brien, K.P. (1990). Behavioral limitations that traumatic brain-injured patients tend to underestimate. *The Clinical Neuropsychologist, 4,* 163–176.

Prigatano, G.P. & Amin, K. (1993). Digit Memory Test: Unequivocal cerebral dysfunction and suspected malingering. *Journal of Clinical and Experimental Neuropsychology, 15,* 537–546.

Prigatano, G.P., Amin, K., & Rosenstein, L. (1991). *Manual for the BNI Screen for Higher Cerebral Functions.* Phoenix: Barrow Neurological Institute.

Prigatano, G.P., Amin, K., & Rosenstein, L.D. (1993). Validity studies on the BNI Screen for Higher Cerebral Functions. *BNI Quarterly, 9,* 2–9.

Prigatano, G.P. & Borgaro, S.R. (2003). Qualitative features of finger movement during the Halstead Finger Oscillation Test following traumatic brain injury. *Journal of the International Neuropsychological Society, 9,* 128–133.

Prigatano, G.P. & Parsons, O.A. (1976). Relationship of age and education to Halstead test performance in different patient populations. *Journal of Consulting and Clinical Psychology, 44,* 527–533.

Prigatano, G.P., Parsons, O., Wright, E., et al. (1983). Neuropsychological test performance in mildly hypoxemic COPD patients. *Journal of Consulting and Clinical Psychology, 51,* 108–116.

Prigatano, G.P. & Pliskin, N.H. (Eds.) (2003). *Clinical neuropsychology and cost outcome research.* New York: Psychology Press.

Prigatano, G.P. & Pribram, K.H. (1982). Perception and memory of facial affect following brain injury. *Journal of Perceptual and Motor Skills, 54,* 859–869.

Prigatano, G.P. & Redner, J.E. (1993). Uses and abuses of neuropsychological testing in behavioral neurology. *Neurology Clinics, 11,* 219–231.

Prigatano, G.P., Smason, I., Lamb, D.G., and Bortz, J.J. (1997). Suspected malingering and the Digit Memory Test: A replication and extension. *Archives of Clinical Neuropsychology, 12,* 609–619.

Prigatano, G.P. & Schacter, D.L. (Eds.) (1991). *Awareness of deficit after brain injury.* New York: Oxford University Press.

Prigatano, G.P. & Wong, J.L. (1999). Cognitive and affective improvement in brain dysfunctional patients who achieve inpatient rehabilitation goals. *Archives of Physical Medicine and Rehabilitation, 80,* 77–84.

Prigatano, G.P., Wright, E.C., & Levin, D. (1984). Quality of life and its predictors in patients with mild hypoxemia and chronic obstructive pulmonary disease. *Archives of Internal Medicine, 144,* 1613–1619.

Primeau, M., Engelstatter, G.H., & Bares, K.K. (1995). Behavioral consequences of lightning and electrical injury. *Seminars in Neurology, 15,* 279–285.

Prinz, P.N., Dustman, R.E., & Emmerson, R. (1990). Electrophysiology and aging. In J.E. Birren & K.W. Schaie (Eds.), *Handbook of the psychology of aging* (3rd ed.). San Diego, CA: Academic Press.

Prinz, P.N., Scanlan, J.M., Vitaliano, P.P., et al. (1999). Thyroid hormones: Positive relationships with cognition in healthy, euthyroid older men. *Journals of Gerontology. Series A, Biological Sciences and Medical Sciences, 54,* M111–M116.

Pritchard, T.C., Macaluso, D.A., & Eslinger, P.J. (1999). Taste perception in patients with insular cortex lesions. *Behavioral Neuroscience, 113,* 663–671.

Pritchard, W.S. (1991). Electroencephalographic effects of cigarette smoking. *Psychopharmacology, 104,* 485–490.

Pritchard, W.S., Robinson, J.H., & Guy, T.D. (1992). Enhancement of continuous performance task reaction time by smoking in non-deprived smokers. *Psychopharmacology, 108,* 437–442.

Privitera, M.D., Morris, G.L., & Gilliam, F. (1991). Postictal language assessment and lateralization of complex partial seizures. *Annals of Neurology, 30,* 391–396.

Prognosis in penetrating brain injury: Part 2. (2001). *Journal of Trauma, 51(Suppl. 2),* S44–S86.

Proulx, G.-B. (1999). Family education and family partnership in cognitive rehabilitation. In D.T. Stuss et al. (Eds.), *Cognitive neurorehabilitation.* Cambridge, UK: Cambridge University Press.

Pryse-Phillips, W. & Costello, F. (2001). Epidemiology of multiple sclerosis. In S.D. Cook (Ed.), *Handbook of multiple sclerosis* (3rd ed.). New York: Marcel Dekker.

Psychological Corporation (The) (1992). *Wechsler Individual Achievement Test.* San Antonio, TX: The Psychological Corporation.

Psychological Corporation (The) (1997). *WAIS-III and WMS-III technical manual.* San Antonio, TX: The Psychological Corporation.

Psychological Corporation (The) (1999). *Wechsler Abbreviated Scale of Intelligence (WASI).* San Antonio, TX: The Psychological Corporation.

Puente, A.E. & Gillespie, J.B. (1991). Workers' compensation and clinical neuropsychological assessment. In J. Dywan et al. (Eds.), *Neuropsychology and the law.* New York: Springer-Verlag.

Purdon, S.E., Klein, S., & Flor-Henry, P. (2001). Menstrual effects of asymmetrical olfactory acuity. *Journal of the International Neuropsychological Society, 7,* 703–709.

Purdue Research Foundation (1948). *Purdue Pegboard Test.* Lafayette, IN: Lafayette Instrument Co.

Putnam, S.H., Millis, S.R., & Adams, K.M. (1996). Mild traumatic brain injury: Beyond cognitive assessment. In I. Grant & K.M. Adams (Eds.), *Neuropsychological assessment of neuropsychiatric disorders.* New York: Oxford University Press.

Putzke, J.D., Richards, J.S., Hicken, B.L., & DeVivo, M.J. (2002). Predictors of life satisfaction: A spinal cord injury cohort study. *Archives of Physical Medicine and Rehabilitation, 83,* 555–561.

Putzke, J.D., Williams, M.A., Daniel, J.F., et al. (2000). Neuropsychological functioning among heart transplant candidates: A case control study. *Journal of Clinical and Experimental Neuropsychology, 22,* 95–103.

Pyke, S. & Agnew, N.M.K. (1963). Digit span performance as a function of noxious stimulation. *Journal of Consulting Psychology, 27,* 281.

Qualls, C.E., Bliwise, N.G., & Stringer, A.Y. (2000). Short forms of the Benton Judgment of Line Orientation Test: Development and psychometric properties. *Archives of Clinical Neuropsychology, 15,* 159–163.

Querishi, M.Y. & Ostrowski, M.J. (1985). The comparability of three Wechsler adult intelligence scales in a college sample. *Journal of Clinical Psychology, 41,* 397–407.

Quigley, M.R., Vidovich, D., Cantella, D., et al. (1997). Defining the limits of survivorship after very severe head injury. *Journal of Trauma, 42,* 7–10.

Quinn, N., Critchley, P., & Marsden, C.D. (1987) Young onset Parkinson's disease. *Movement Disorders, 2,* 73–91.

Quintard, B., Croze, P., Mazaux, J.M., et al. (2002). Life satisfaction and psychosocial outcome in severe traumatic brain injuries in Aquitaine. *Annales de Réadaptation et de Médecine Physique, 45,* 456–465.

Qureshi, A.I., Mohammad, Y., Suri, M.F., et al. (2001). Cocaine use and hypertension are major risk factors for intracerebral hemorrhage in young African Americans. *Ethnicity and Disease, 11,* 311–319.

Qureshi, A.I., Tuhrim, S., Broderick, J.P., et al. (2001). Spontaneous intracerebral hemorrhage. *New England Journal of Medicine, 344,* 1450–1460.

Rabbitt, P., Donlan, C., Watson, P., et al. (1995). Unique and interactive effects of depression, age, socioeconomic advantage, and gender on cognitive performance of normal healthy older people. *Psychology and Aging, 10,* 307–313.

Rabinowicz, T., Petetot, J.M.C., Gartside, P.S., et al. (2002). Structure of the cerebral cortex in men and women. *Journal of Neuropathology and Experimental Neurology, 61,* 46–57.

Rabins, P.V., Brooks, B.R., O'Donnell, P., et al. (1986). Structural brain correlates of emotional disorder in multiple sclerosis. *Brain, 109,* 585–597.

Rabins, P.V., Mace, N.L., & Lucas, M.J. (1982). The impact of dementia on the family. *Journal of the American Medical Association, 248,* 333–335.

Raczkowski, D., Kalat, J.W., & Nebes, R. (1974). Reliability and validity of some handedness questionnaire items. *Neuropsychologia, 12,* 43–47.

Radanov, B.P., Begré, S., Sturznegger, M., & Augustiny, K.F. (1996). Course of psychological variables in whiplash injury—a two year follow-up with age, gender, and education in pair-matched patients. *Pain, 64,* 429–434.

Radanov, B.P. & Dvorak, J.P. (1996). Impaired cognitive functioning after whiplash injury of the cervical spine. *Spine, 21,* 392–397.

Rademacher, J., Morosan, P., Schleicher, A., et al. (2001). Human primary auditory cortex in women and men. *Neuroreport, 12,* 1561–1565.

Rafal, R. (1992). Visually guided behavior. In I. Litvan & Y. Agid (Eds.), *Progressive supranuclear palsy: Clinical and research approaches.* New York: Oxford University Press.

Rafal, R.D. (1997a). Balint syndrome. In T.E. Feinberg & M.J. Farah (Eds.), *Behavioral neurology and neuropsychology.* New York: McGraw-Hill.

Rafal, R.D. (1997b). Hemispatial neglect: Cognitive neuropsychological aspects. In T.E. Feinberg & M.J. Farah (Eds.), *Behavioral neurology and neuropsychology.* New York: McGraw-Hill.

Rafal, R.D. (2000). Neglect II: Cognitive neuropsychological issues. In M.J. Farah & T.E. Feinberg (Eds.), *Patient-based approaches to cognitive neuroscience*. Cambridge, MA: MIT Press.

Rafal, R.D., Posner, M.I., Walker, J.A., & Friedrich, F.J. (1984). Cognition and the basal ganglia. *Brain, 107,* 1083–1094.

Raff, M. (1998). Cell suicide for beginners. *Nature, 396,* 119–122.

Raghavan, S. (1961). *A comparison of the performance of right and left hemiplegics on verbal and nonverbal body image tasks*. Northampton, MA: Smith College, Thesis.

Ragland, J.D., Coleman, A.R., Gur, R.C., et al. (2000). Sex differences in brain–behavior relationships between verbal episodic memory and resting regional cerebral blood flow. *Neuropsychologia, 38,* 451–461.

Ragland, J.D., Glahn, D.C., Gur, R.C., et al. (1997). PET regional cerebral blood flow change during working and declarative memory: Relationship with task performance. *Neuropsychology, 11,* 222–231.

Ragland, J.D., Gur, R.C., Lazarev, M.G., et al. (2000). Hemispheric activation of anterior and inferior prefrontal cortex during verbal encoding and recognition: A PET study of healthy volunteers. *Neuroimage, 11,* 624–633.

Rahmani, L., Geva, N., Rochberg, J., et al. (1990). Issues in neurocognitive assessment and training. In E. Vakil, D. Hoofien, & Z. Groswasser (Eds.), *Rehabilitation of the brain injured person: A neuropsychological perspective*. London: Freund.

Raichle, M.E. (2000). The neural correlates of consciousness: An analysis of cognitive skill learning. In M.S. Gazzaniga (Ed.), *The new cognitive neurosciences* (2nd ed.). Cambridge, MA: MIT Press.

Rains, G.D. (2002). *Principles of human neuropsychology*. New York: McGraw-Hill.

Rainville, C., Amieva, H., Lafont, S., et al. (2002). Executive function deficits in patients with dementia of the Alzheimer's type: A study with a Tower of London task. *Archives of Clinical Neuropsychology, 17,* 513–530.

Rainville, C., Marchand, N., & Passini, R. (2002). Performances of patients with a dementia of the Alzheimer type in the Standardized Road-Map Test of Direction Sense. *Neuropsychologia, 40,* 567–573.

Rajamani, K. & Fisher, M. (1997). An overview of atherosclerosis. In K.M.A. Welch et al. (Eds.), *Primer on cerebrovascular diseases*. San Diego: Academic Press.

Rajput, A. H. (1992). Frequency and cause of Parkinson's disease. *Canadian Journal of Neurological Sciences, 19, 103*–107.

Rajput, A.H., Offord, K.P., Beard, C.M., & Kurland, L.T. (1984). Epidemiology of parkinsonism: Incidence, classification, and mortality. *Annals of Neurology, 16,* 278–282.

Rakic, P. (2000). Setting the stage for cognition: Genesis of the primate cerebral cortex. In M.S. Gazzaniga (Ed.), *The new cognitive neurosciences* (2nd ed.). Cambridge, MA: MIT Press.

Ramani, V. (1991). Audiogenic epilepsy induced by a specific television performer. *New England Journal of Medicine, 325,* 134–135.

Ramier, A.-M. & Hécaen, H. (1970). Rôle respectif des atteintes frontales et de la latéralisation lésionelle dans les déficits de la "fluence verbale." *Revue Neurologique (Paris), 123,* 17–22.

Ramsay, C.G., Nicholas, M., Au, R., et al. (1999). Verb naming in normal aging. *Applied Neuropsychology, 6,* 57–67.

Rand, M.B., Trudeau, M.D., & Nelson, L.K. (1990). Reading assessment post head injury: How valid is it? *Brain Injury, 4,* 155–160.

Randall, C.M., Dickson, A.L., & Plasay, M.T. (1988). The relationship between intellectual function and adult performance on the Benton Visual Retention Test. *Cortex, 24,* 277–289.

Randolph, C. (1998). *RBANS manual: Repeatable Battery for the Assessment of Neuropsychological Status*. San Antonio, TX: The Psychological Corporation.

Randolph, C., Braun, A.R., Goldberg, T.E., & Chase, T.N. (1993). Semantic fluency in Alzheimer's, Parkinson's, and Huntington's disease: Dissociation of storage and retrieval failures. *Neuropsychology, 7,* 82–88.

Randolph, C., Lansing, A.E., Ivnik, R.J., et al. (1999). Determinants of confrontation naming performance. *Archives of Clinical Neuropsychology, 14,* 489–496.

Randolph, C., Mohr, E., & Chase, T.N. (1993). Assessment of intellectual function in dementing disorders: Validity of WAIS-R short forms for patients with Alzheimer's, Huntington's & Parkinson's disease. *Journal of Clinical and Experimental Neuropsychology, 15,* 743–753.

Randolph, C., Tierney, M. C., Mohr, E., & Chase, T.N. (1998). The Repeatable Battery for the Assessment of Neuropsychological Status (RBANS): Preliminary clinical validity. *Journal of Clinical and Experimental Neuropsychology, 20,* 310–319.

Randolph, J.J., Arnett, P.A., & Higginson, C.I. (2001). Metamemory and tested cognitive functioning in multiple sclerosis. *The Clinical Neuropsychologist, 15,* 357–368.

Randt, C.T. & Brown, E.R. (1986). *Randt Memory Test*. Bayport, NY: Life Science Associates.

Randt, C.T., Brown, E.R., & Osborne, D.J., Jr. (1980). A memory test for longitudinal measurement of mild to moderate deficits. *Clinical Neuropsychology, 2,* 184–194.

Rao, N., Rosenthal, M., Cronin-Stubbs, D., et al. (1990). Return to work after rehabilitation following traumatic brain injury. *Brain Injury, 4,* 49–56.

Rao, R. & Georgieff, M.K. (2000). Early nutrition and brain development. In C.A. Nelson (Ed.), *The effects of early adversity on neurobehavioral development. The Minnesota Symposia on Child Development* (Vol. 31). Mahwah, NJ: Erlbaum.

Rao, S.M. (1990). Neuroimaging correlates of cognitive dysfunction. In S.M. Rao (Ed.), *Neurobehavioral aspects of multiple sclerosis*. New York: Oxford University Press.

Rao, S.M., Bernardin, L., Leo, G.J., et al. (1989). Cerebral disconnection in multiple sclerosis: Relationship to atrophy of the corpus callosum. *Archives of Neurology, 46,* 918–920.

Rao, S.M., Grafman, J., DiGiulio, D., et al. (1993). Memory dysfunction in multiple sclerosis: Its relation to working memory, semantic encoding and implicit learning. *Neuropsychology, 7,* 364–374.

Rao, S.M., Hammeke, T.A., McQuillen, M.P., et al. (1984). Memory disturbance in chronic progressive multiple sclerosis. *Archives of Neurology, 41,* 625–631.

Rao, S.M., Hammeke, T.A., & Speech, T.J. (1987). Wisconsin Card Sorting Test performance in relapsing-remitting and chronic-progressive multiple sclerosis. *Journal of Consulting and Clinical Psychology, 55,* 263–265.

Rao, S.M., Huber, S.J., & Bornstein, R.A. (1992). Emotional changes with multiple sclerosis and Parkinson's disease. *Journal of Consulting and Clinical Psychology, 60,* 369–378.

Rao, S.M., Leo, G.J., Bernardin, L., & Unverzagt, F. (1991). Cognitive dysfunction in multiple sclerosis. I. Frequency, patterns, and predictions. *Neurology, 41,* 685–691.

Rao, S.M., Leo, G.J., Ellington, L., et al. (1991). Cognitive dysfunction in multiple sclerosis. II. Impact on employment and social functioning. *Neurology, 41,* 692–696.

Rao, S.M., Leo, G.J., Haughton, V.M., et al. (1989). Correlation of magnetic resonance imaging with neuropsychological testing in multiple sclerosis. *Neurology, 39,* 161–166.

Rao, S.M., Leo, G.J., & St. Aubin-Faubert, P. (1989). On the nature of memory disturbance in multiple sclerosis. *Journal of Clinical and Experimental Neuropsychology, 11,* 699–712.

Rao, S.M., Mayer, A.R., & Harrington, D.L. (2001). The evolution of brain activation during temporal processing. *Nature Neuroscience, 4,* 317–323.

Rao, S.M., Mittenberg, W., Bernardin, L., et al. (1989). Neuropsychological test findings in subjects with leukoaraiosis. *Archives of Neurology, 46,* 40–44.

Rao, S.M. & National Multiple Sclerosis Society (1990). *A manual of the Brief, Repeatable Battery of Neuropsychological Tests in multiple sclerosis.* New York: National Multiple Sclerosis Society.

Rao, S.M., St. Aubin-Faubert, P., & Leo, G.J. (1989). Information processing speed in patients with multiple sclerosis. *Journal of Clinical and Experimental Neuropsychology, 11,* 471–477.

Rapaport, D., Gill, M.M., & Schafer, R. (1968). *Diagnostic psychological testing* (rev. ed.). New York: International Universities Press.

Rapcsak, S.Z., Arthur, S.A., Bliklen, D.A., & Rubens, A.B. (1989). Lexical agraphia in Alzheimer's disease. *Archives of Neurology, 46,* 65–68.

Rapcsak, S.Z., Kaszniak, A.W., Reminger, S.L., et al. (1998). Dissociation between verbal and autonomic measures of memory following frontal lobe damage. *Neurology, 50,* 1259–1265.

Rapcsak, S.Z., Nielsen, L., Littrell, L.D., et al. (2001). Face memory impairments with frontal lobe damage. *Neurology, 57,* 1168–1175.

Rapoport, J.L., Jensvold, M., Elkins, R., et al. (1981). Behavioral and cognitive effects of caffeine in boys and adult males. *Journal of Nervous and Mental Disease, 169,* 726–732.

Rapoport, M., McCauley, S., Levin, H., Song, J., & Feinstein, A. (2002). The role of injury severity in neurobehavioral outcome 3 months after traumatic brain injury. *Neuropsychiatry, Neuropsychology, and Behavioral Neurology, 15,* 123–132.

Rapoport, M.J. & Feinstein, A. (2001). Age and functioning after mild traumatic brain injury: The acute picture. *Brain Injury, 15,* 857–864.

Rapp, B. (Ed.) (2001). *The handbook of cognitive neuropsychology. What deficits reveal about the human mind.* Philadelphia: Taylor & Francis, Psychology Press.

Rapp, B., Folk, J.R., & Tainturier, M.-J. (2001). Word reading. *The handbook of cognitive neuropsychology. What deficits reveal about the human mind.* Philadelphia: Taylor & Francis, Psychology Press.

Rappaport, M., Hall, K.M., Hopkins, K., et al. (1982). Disability Rating Scale for severe head trauma: Coma to community. *Archives of Physical Medicine and Rehabilitation, 63,* 118–123.

Rappaport, M., Hemmerle, A.V., & Rappaport, M.L. (1990). Intermediate and long latency SEPs in relation to clinical disability in traumatic brain injury patients. *Clinical Electroencephalography, 21,* 188–192.

Rappaport, M., Hemmerle, A.V., & Rappaport, M.L. (1991). Short and long latency auditory evoked potentials in traumatic brain injury patients. *Clinical Electroencephalography, 22,* 199–202.

Rappaport, M., Herrero-Backe, C., Winterfield, K.M., et al. (1989). Visual evoked potential pattern abnormalities and disability in severe traumatically brain-injured patients. *Journal of Head Trauma Rehabilitation, 4,* 45–52.

Rapport, L.J., Axelrod, B.N., Theisen, M.E., et al. (1997). Relationship of IQ to verbal learning and memory: Test and retest. *Journal of Clinical and Experimental Neuropsychology, 19,* 655–666.

Rapport, L.J., Brines, D.B., Axelrod, B.N., & Thiesen, M.E. (1997). Full scale IQ as mediator of practice effects: The rich get richer. *The Clinical Neuropsychologist, 11,* 375–380.

Rapport, L.J., Charter, R.A., Dutra, R.L., et al. (1997). Psychometric properties of the Rey-Osterrieth Complex Figure: Lezak-Osterrieth versus Denman scoring systems. *The Clinical Neuropsychologist, 11,* 46–53.

Rapport, L.J., Farchione, T.J., Coleman, R.D., & Axelrod, B.N. (1998). Effects of coaching on malingered motor function profiles. *Journal of Clinical and Experimental Neuropsychology, 20,* 89–97.

Rapport, L.J., Farchione, T.J., Dutra, R.L., et al. (1996). Measures of hemi-inattention on the Rey Figure Copy for the Lezak-Osterrieth scoring method. *The Clinical Neuropsychologist, 10,* 450–454.

Rapport, L.J., Hanks, R.A., Millis, S.R., & Deshpande, S.A. (1998). Executive functioning and predictors of falls in the rehabilitation setting. *Archives of Physical Medicine and Rehabilitation, 79,* 629–633.

Rapport, L.J., Millis, S.R., & Bonello, P.J. (1998). Validation of the Warrington theory of visual processing and the Visual Object and Space Perception Battery. *Journal of Clinical and Experimental Neuropsychology, 20,* 211–220.

Rapport, L.J., Webster, J.S., & Dutra, R.L. (1994). Digit span performance and unilateral neglect. *Neuropsychologia, 32,* 517–525.

Rascovsky, K., Salmon, D.P., Ho, G.J., et al. (2002). Cognitive profiles differ in autopsy-confirmed frontotemporal dementia and AD. *Neurology, 58,* 1801–1808.

Raskin, S.A., Borod, J.C., & Tweedy, J.R. (1992). Set-shifting and spatial orientation in patients with Parkinson's disease. *Journal of Clinical and Experimental Neuropsychology, 14* 801–821.

Raskin, S.A., Borod, J.C., Wasserstein, J., et al. (1990). Visuospatial orientation in Parkinson's disease. *International Journal of Neuroscience, 51,* 9–18.

Raskin, S.A. & Mateer, C.A. (Eds.) (2000). *Neuropsychological management of mild traumatic brain injury.* New York: Oxford University Press.

Raskin, S.A., Mateer, C.A., & Tweeten, R. (1998). Neuropsychological assessment of individuals with mild traumatic brain injury. *The Clinical Neuropsychologist, 12,* 21–30.

Raskin, S.A. & Rearick, E. (1996). Verbal fluency in individuals with mild traumatic brain injury. *Neuropsychology, 10,* 416–422.

Raskin, S.A., Sliwinski, M., & Borod, J.C. (1992). Clustering strategies on tasks of verbal fluency in Parkinson's disease. *Neuropsychologia, 30,* 95–99.

Raskin, S.A. & Stein, P.N. (2000). Depression. In S.A. Raskin & C.A. Mateer, C.A. (Eds.) *Neuropsychological management of mild traumatic brain injury.* New York: Oxford University Press.

Rasmusson, D.X., Bylsma, F.W., & Brandt, J. (1995). Stability of performance on the Hopkins Verbal Learning Test. *Archives of Clinical Neuropsychology, 10,* 21–26.

Rasmusson, D.X., Carson, K.A., Brookmeyer, R., et al. (1996). Predicting rate of cognitive decline in probable Alzheimer's disease. *Brain and Cognition, 31,* 133–147.

Ratcliff, G. (1979). Spatial thought, mental rotation, and the right cerebral hemisphere. *Neuropsychologia, 17,* 49–54.

Rattock, J. (1996). Do patients with mild brain injuries have posttraumatic stress disorder, too? *Journal of Head Trauma Rehabilitation, 11,* 95–97.

Rausch, R. & Ary, C.M. (1990). Supraspan learning in patients with unilateral anterior temporal lobe resections. *Neuropsychologia, 28,* 111–120.

Rausch, R. & Babb, T.L. (1993). Hippocampal neuron loss and memory scores before and after temporal lobe surgery for epilepsy. *Archives of Neurology, 50,* 812–817.

Rausch, R. & Risinger, M. (1990). Intracarotid sodium amobarbital procedure. In A.A. Boulton et al. (Eds.), *Neuromethods. Neuropsychology* (Vol. 17). Clifton, NJ: Humana Press.

Rauschecker, J.P. & Tian, B. (2000). Mechanisms and streams for processing of "what" and "where" in auditory cortex. *Proceedings of the National Academy of Sciences USA, 97,* 11800–11806.

Ravden, L.D., Hilton, E., Primeau, M., et al. (1996). Memory functioning in Lyme borreliosis. *Journal of Clinical Psychiatry, 57,* 282–286.

Raven, J.C. (1982). *Revised manual for Raven's Progressive Matrices and Vocabulary Scales.* Windsor, UK: NFER Nelson; San Antonio, TX: The Psychological Corporation.

Raven, J., Court, J.H., et al. (1995). Summary of normative, reliability and validity studies. In *Raven Manual Research Supplement 4.* Oxford: Oxford Psychologists Press.

Raven, J., Raven, J.C., & Court, J.H. (1995). *General overview (1995 edition).* Oxford: Oxford Psychologists Press.

Raven, J., Summers, B., Birchfield, M., et al. (1990). *Manual for Raven's Progressive Matrices and Vocabulary Scales. Research Supplement No. 3: A compendium of North American normative and validity studies.* Oxford: Oxford Psychologists Press.

Raven, J.C. (1994). *Advanced Progressive Matrices. Manual Sections 1 & 4 (Sets I, II).* Oxford: Oxford Psychologists Press.

Raven, J.C. (1995). *Coloured Progressive Matrices Sets A, Ab, B. Manual Sections 1 & 2.* Oxford: Oxford Psychologists Press.

Raven, J.C. (1996). *Raven's Progressive Matrices: A perceptual test of intelligence.* Oxford: Oxford Psychologists Press.

Rawling, P. & Brooks, N. (1990). Simulation index: a method for detecting factitious errors on the WAIS-R and WMS. *Neuropsychology, 4,* 223–238.

Rawlings, D.B. & Crewe, N.M. (1992). Test–retest practice effects and test score changes of the WAIS-R in recovering traumatically brain-injured survivors. *The Clinical Neuropsychologist, 6,* 415–430.

Raz, N., Gunning-Dixon, F.M., Head, D., et al. (1998). Neuroanatomical correlates of cognitive aging: Evidence from structural magnetic resonance imaging. *Neuropsychology, 12,* 95–114.

Razack, N., Singh, R.V.P., Petrin, D., et al. (1997). Bilateral craniotomies for blunt head trauma. *Journal of Trauma, 43,* 840–843.

Razani, J., Boone, K.B., Miller, B.L., et al. (2001). Neuropsychological performance of right- and left-frontotemporal dementia compared to Alzheimer's disease. *Journal of the International Neuropsychological Society, 7,* 468–480.

Rechlin, T., Loew, T.H., & Joraschky, P. (1997). Pseudoseizure "status." *Journal of Psychosomatic Research, 42,* 495–498.

Recht, L.D., Lew, R., & Smith, T.W. (2000). Suspected low-grade glioma: Is deferring treatment safe? *Annals of Neurology, 31,* 431–436.

Reddon, J.R., Gill, D.M., Gauk, S.E., & Maerz, M.D. (1988). Purdue Pegboard: Test–retest estimates. *Perceptual and Motor Skills, 66,* 503–506.

Reddon, J.R., Schopflocher, D., Gill, D.M., & Stefanyk, W.O. (1989). Speech Sounds Perception Test: Non-random response locations form a logical fallacy in structure. *Perceptual and Motor Skills, 69,* 235–240.

Reddon, J.R., Stefanyk, W.O., Gill, D.M., & Renney, C. (1985). Hand dynamometer: Effects of trials and sessions. *Perceptual and Motor Skills, 61,* 1195–1198.

Reddy, H., Narayanan, S., Arnoutelis, R., et al. (2000). Evidence for adaptive functional changes in the cerebral cortex with axonal injury from multiple sclerosis. *Brain, 123,* 2314–2320.

Redlich, F.C. & Dorsey, J.F. (1945). Denial of blindness by patients with cerebral disease. *Archives of Neurology and Psychiatry, 53,* 407–417.

Reed, B.R., Paller, K.A., & Mungas, D. (1998). Impaired acquisition and rapid forgetting of patterned visual stimuli in Alzheimer's disease. *Journal of Clinical and Experimental Neuropsychology, 20,* 738–749.

Reed, J.M. & Squire, L.R. (1998). Retrograde amnesia for facts and events: Findings from four new cases. *Journal of Neuroscience, 18,* 3943–3954.

Rees, L.M., Tombaugh, T.N., & Boulay, L. (2001). Depression and the Test of Memory Malingering. *Archives of Clinical Neuropsychology, 16,* 501–506.

Rees, L.M., Tombaugh, T.N., Gansler, D.A., & Moczynski, N.P. (1998). Five validation experiments of the Test of Memory Malingering (TOMM). *Psychological Assessment, 10,* 10–20.

Rees, M. (1979). Symbol Digit Modalities Test (SDMT). In F.L. Darley (Ed.), *Evaluation of appraisal techniques in speech and language pathology.* Reading, ME: Addison-Wesley.

Regard, M. & Landis, Th. (1988). Procedure vs. content learning: Effects of emotionality and repetition in a new clinical memory test [abstract]. *Journal of Clinical and Experimental Neuropsychology, 10,* 86.

Regard, M., Oelz, O., Brugger, P., et al. (1989). Persistent cognitive impairment in climbers after repeated exposure to extreme altitude. *Neurology, 39,* 210–213.

Regard, M., Strauss, E., & Knapp, P. (1982). Children's production on verbal and non-verbal fluency tasks. *Perceptual and Motor Skills, 55,* 839–844.

Reichlin, R.E. (1984). Current perspectives on Rorschach performance among older adults. *Journal of Personality Assessment, 48,* 71–81.

Reichman, W.E., Coyne, A.C., & Shah, A. (1993). Diagnosis of multi-infarct dementia: Predictive value of clinical criteria. *Perceptual and Motor Skills, 76,* 793–794.

Reid, J.M. (2002). Testing nonverbal intelligence of working-age visually impaired adults: Evaluation of the Adapted Kohs Block Design Test. *Journal of Visual Impairment and Blindness, 96,* 585–595.

Reider-Groswasser, I.I., Groswasser, Z., Ommaya, A.K., et al. (2002). Quantitative imaging in late traumatic brain injury. Part I: Late imaging parameters in closed and penetrating head injuries. *Brain Injury, 16,* 517–525.

Reidy, T.J., Bowler, R.M., Rauch, S.S., & Pedroza, G.I. (1992). Pesticide exposure and neuropsychological impairment in migrant farm workers. *Archives of Clinical Neuropsychology, 7,* 85–95.

Reifler, B.V. (1982). Arguments for abandoning the term pseudodementia. *Journal of the American Geriatric Society, 82,* 665–668.

Reifler, B.V. (1986). Mixed cognitive-affective disturbances in the elderly: A new classification. *Journal of Clinical Psychiatry, 47,* 354–356.

Reifler, B.V. (1992). Dementia versus depression in the elderly. In M. Bergener (Ed.), *Aging and mental disorders: International perspectives.* New York: Springer.

Reifler, B.V., Larson, E., & Hanley, R. (1982). Coexistence of cognitive impairment and depression in geriatric outpatients. *American Journal of Psychiatry, 139,* 623–626.

Reiman, E.M., Lane, R.D., Van Petten, C., & Bandettini, P.A. (2000). Positron emission tomography and functional magnetic resonance imaging. In J.T. Cacioppo et al. (Eds.), *Handbook of psychophysiology* (2nd ed.). Cambridge, UK: Cambridge University Press.

Reinke, L.A. & McCay, P.B. (1996). Interaction between alcohol and antioxidants. In S. Zakhari & M. Wassef (Eds.), *Alcohol and the cardiovascular system.* NIAA Research Monograph 31, NIH Publication 96-4133. Washington, D.C.: U.S. Government Printing Office.

Reis, A. & Castro-Caldas, A. (1997). Illiteracy: A cause for biased cognitive development. *Journal of the International Neuropsychological Society, 3,* 444–450.

Reis, A., Guerreiro, M., & Castro-Caldas, A. (1994). Influence of educational level of non brain-damaged subjects on visual naming. *Journal of Clinical and Experimental Neuropsychology, 16,* 939–942.

Reisberg, B., Borenstein, J., Franssen, E., et al. (1987). BEHAVE-AD: A clinical rating scale for the assessment of pharmacologically remediable behavioral symptomatology in Alzheimer's disease. In H.J. Altman (Ed.), *Alzheimer's disease*. New York: Plenum.

Reisberg, B., Borenstein, J., Salob, S.P., et al. (1987). Behavioral symptoms in Alzheimer's disease: Phenomenology and treatment. *Journal of Clinical Psychiatry, 48*, 9–15.

Reisberg, B. & Ferris, S.H. (1982). Diagnosis and assessment of the older patient. *Hospital and Community Psychiatry, 33*, 104–110.

Reisberg, B., Ferris, S.H., Borenstein, J., et al. (1986). Assessment of presenting symptoms. In L.W. Poon (Ed.), *Handbook for clinical memory assessment of older adults*. Washington, D.C.: American Psychological Association.

Reisberg, B., Ferris, S.H., Borenstein, J., et al. (1990). Some observations on the diagnosis of dementia of the Alzheimer type. In M. Bergener & S.I. Finkel (Eds.), *Clinical and scientific psychogeriatrics. The interface of psychiatry and neurology* (Vol. 2). New York: Springer.

Reisberg, B., Ferris, S.H., DeLeon, M.J., & Crook, T. (1982). The Global Deterioration Scale for assessment of primary degenerative dementia. *American Journal of Psychiatry, 139*, 1136–1139.

Reisberg, B., Franssen, E., Sclan, S.G., et al. (1989). Stage specific incidence of potentially remediable behavioral symptoms in aging and Alzheimer's disease. *Bulletin of Clinical Neurosciences, 54*, 95–112.

Reisberg, B., Schneck, M.K., Ferris, S.H., et al. (1983). The Brief Cognitive Rating Scale (BCRS). Findings in primary degenerative dementia (PDD). *Psychopharmacology Bulletin, 19*, 734–739.

Reitan, R.M. (1955a). Certain differential effects of left and right cerebral lesions in human adults. *Journal of Comparative and Physiological Psychology, 48*, 474–477.

Reitan, R.M. (1955b). The distribution according to age of a psychologic measure dependent upon organic brain functions. *Journal of Gerontology, 10*, 338–340.

Reitan, R.M. (1955c). Investigation of the validity of Halstead's measures of biological intelligence. *Archives of Neurology and Psychiatry, 73*, 28–35.

Reitan, R.M. (1958). Validity of the Trail Making Test as an indicator of organic brain damage. *Perceptual and Motor Skills, 8*, 271–276.

Reitan, R.M. (1959). The comparative effects of brain damage on the Halstead Impairment Index and the Wechsler-Bellevue Scale. *Journal of Clinical Psychology, 15*, 281–285.

Reitan, R.M. (1964). Psychological deficits resulting from cerebral lesions in man. In J.M. Warren & K. Akert (Eds.), *The frontal granular cortex and behavior*. New York: McGraw-Hill.

Reitan, R.M. (1966). A research program on the neuropsychological effects of brain lesions in human beings. In N.R. Ellis (Ed.), *International review of research on mental retardation*. New York: Academic Press.

Reitan, R.M. (1972). Verbal problem solving as related to cerebral damage. *Perceptual and Motor Skills, 34*, 515–524.

Reitan, R.M. (1976). Neurological and physiological bases of psychopathology. *Annual Review of Psychology, 27*, 189–216.

Reitan, R.M. (1979). Manual for administration of neuropsychological test batteries for adults and children. Tucson: Reitan Neuropsychological Laboratory.

Reitan, R.M. (1996). On the history of neuropsychology. In *Division 40 Newsletter*. Washington, D.C.: American Psychological Association.

Reitan, R.M. & Davison, L.A. (1974). *Clinical neuropsychology: Current status and applications*. New York: Winston/Wiley.

Reitan, R.M., Hom, J., & Wolfson, D. (1988). Verbal processing by the brain. *Journal of Clinical and Experimental Neuropsychology, 10*, 400–408.

Reitan, R.M. & Wolfson, D. (1985). *The Halstead-Reitan Neuropsychological Test Battery. Theory and Clinical Interpretation*. Tucson: Neuropsychology Press.

Reitan, R.M. & Wolfson, D. (1988). *Traumatic brain injury. Recovery and rehabilitation* (Vol. 2). Tucson, AZ: Neuropsychology Press.

Reitan, R.M. & Wolfson, D. (1989). The Seashore Rhythm Test and brain functions. *The Clinical Neuropsychologist, 3*, 70–78.

Reitan, R.M. & Wolfson, D. (1992). Conventional intelligence measurements and neuropsychological concepts of adaptive abilities. *Journal of Clinical Psychology, 48*, 521–529.

Reitan, R.M. & Wolfson, D. (1993). *The Halstead-Reitan Neuropsychological Test Battery: Theory and clinical applications* (2nd ed.). Tucson, AZ: Neuropsychology Press.

Reitan, R.M. & Wolfson, D. (1994). Dissociation of motor impairment and higher-level brain deficits in strokes and cerebral neoplasms. *The Clinical Neuropsychologist, 8*, 193–208.

Reitan, R.M. & Wolfson, D. (1995a). Category Test and Trail Making Test as measures of frontal lobe functions. *The Clinical Neuropsychologist, 9*, 50–56.

Reitan, R.M. & Wolfson, D. (1995b). Influence of age and education on neuropsychological test results. *The Clinical Neuropsychologist, 9*, 151–158.

Reitan, R.M. & Wolfson, D. (1996a). Relationships of age and education to Wechsler Adult Intelligence Scale IQ values in brain-damaged and non-brain-damaged groups. *The Clinical Neuropsychologist, 10*, 293–304.

Reitan, R.M. & Wolfson, D. (1996b). Relationships between specific and general tests of cerebral functioning. *The Clinical Neuropsychologist, 10*, 37–42.

Reitan, R.M. & Wolfson, D. (1996c). Theoretical and methodological bases of the Halstead-Reitan Neuropsychological Test Battery. In I. Grant & K.M. Adams (Eds.), *Neuropsychological assessment of neuropsychiatric disorders* (2nd ed.). New York: Oxford University Press.

Reitan, R.M. & Wolfson, D. (1997a). Consistency of neuropsychological test scores of head-injured subjects involved in litigation compared with head-injured subjects not involved in litigation: Development of the Retest Consistency Index. *The Clinical Neuropsychologist, 11*, 69–76.

Reitan, R.M. & Wolfson, D. (1997b). Emotional disturbances and their interaction with neuropsychological deficits. *Neuropsychology Review, 7*, 3–19.

Reitan, R.M. & Wolfson, D. (1997c). The influence of age and education on neuropsychological performances of persons with mild head injuries. *Applied Neuropsychology, 4*, 16–33.

Reitan, R.M. & Wolfson, D. (1999). The two faces of mild head injury. *Archives of Clinical Neuropsychology, 14*, 191–202.

Reitan, R.M. & Wolfson, D. (2000). The neuropsychological similarities of mild and more severe head injury. *Archives of Clinical Neuropsychology, 15*, 433–442.

Reitan, R.M. & Wolfson, D. (2002). Using the Tactile Form Recognition Test to differentiate persons with brain damage from control subjects. *Archives of Clinical Neuropsychology, 17*, 117–121.

Reite, M., Cullum, C.M., Stocker, J., et al. (1993). Neuropsychological test performance and MEG-based brain lateralization: Sex differences. *Brain Research Bulletin, 32*, 325–328.

Reite, M., Teale, P., & Rojas, D.C. (1999). Magnetoencephalography: Applications in psychiatry. *Biological Psychiatry, 45*, 1553–1563.

Rempel-Clower, N.L., Zola, S.M., Squire, L.R., & Amaral, D.G. (1996). Three cases of enduring memory impairment after bilateral damage limited to the hippocampal formation. *Journal of Neuroscience, 16*, 5233–5255.

Renaud, S., Criqui, M.H., Farchi, G., et al. (1993). Alcohol drinking and coronary heart disease. In P.M. Verschuren (Ed.), *Health issues related to alcohol consumption*. Washington, D.C.: ILSI Press.

Rentz, D.M. & Weintraub, S. (2000). Neuropsychological detection of early probable Alzheimer's disease. In L.F.M. Scinto & K.R. Daffner (Eds.), *Early diagnosis of Alzheimer's disease.* Totowa, NJ: Humana Press, pp. 169–189.

Reschly, D.J. (1981). Psychological testing in educational classification and placement. *American Psychologist, 36,* 1094–1102.

Rescorl, D. (1995). Environmental emergencies. *Critical Care Nursing Clinics of North America, 7,* 445–456.

Resnick, P.J. (1984). The detection of malingered mental illness. *Behavioral Sciences and the Law, 2,* 21–38.

Retzlaff, P.D. & Gibertini, M. (1994). Neuropsychometric issues and problems. In R.D. Vanderploeg (Ed.), *Clinician's guide to neuropsychological assessment.* Hillsdale, NJ: Erlbaum.

Reuler, J.B., Girard, D.E., & Cooney, T.G. (1985). Wernicke's encephalopathy. *New England Journal of Medicine, 312,* 1035–1039.

Rey, A. (1941). L'examen psychologique dans les cas d'encephalopathie traumatique. *Archives de Psychologie, 28,* 286–340 (see Corwin & Bylsma, 1993b, for translation).

Rey, A. (1959). Sollicitation de la mémoire de fixation par des mots et des objets presentés simultanément. Archives de Psychologie, *37,* 126–139.

Rey, A. (1964). *L'examen clinique en psychologie.* Paris: Presses Universitaires de France.

Rey, G.J. & Benton, A.L. (1991). *Examen de Afasia Multilingue.* Iowa City: AJA Associates.

Rey, G.J., Feldman, E., Hernandez, D., et al. (2001). Application of the Multilingual Aphasia Examination-Spanish in the evaluation of Hispanic patients post closed-head trauma. *The Clinical Neuropsychologist, 15,* 13–18.

Rey, G.J., Feldman, E., & Rivas-Vazquez, R. (1999). Neuropsychological test development and normative data on Hispanics. *Archives of Clinical Neuropsychology, 14,* 593–601.

Reyes, M., Gary, H.E., Jr., Dobbins, J.G., et al. (1997). Surveillance for chronic fatigue syndrome—four U.S. cities, September 1989 through August 1993. *Morbidity and Mortality Weekly Report CDC Surveillance Summaries, 46,* 1–13.

Reyes, R.L., Bhattacharyya, A.K., & Heller, D. (1981). Traumatic head injury: Restlessness and agitation as prognosticators of physical and psychological improvement. *Archives of Physical Medicine and Rehabilitation, 62,* 20–23.

Reynolds, C. & Fletcher-Janzen, E. (Eds.) (1997). *Handbook of clinical child neuropsychology* (2nd ed.). New York: Plenum Press.

Reynolds, C.R., Hopkins, R.O., & Bigler, E.D. (1999). Continuing decline of memory skills with significant recovery of intellectual function following severe carbon monoxide exposure: Clinical, psychometric, and neuroimaging findings. *Archives of Clinical Neuropsychology, 14,* 235–249.

Reznikoff, M. & Tomblen, D. (1956). The use of human figure drawings in the diagnosis of organic pathology. *Journal of Consulting Psychology, 20,* 467–470.

Ricci, S., Vigevano, F., Manfredi, M., & Kasteleijn-Nolst Trenite, D.G. (1998). Epilepsy provoked by television and video games: Safety of 100-hz screens. *Neurology, 50,* 790–793.

Rice, E. & Gendelman, S. (1973). Psychiatric aspects of normal pressure hydrocephalus. *Journal of the American Medical Association, 223,* 409–412.

Rich, J.B., Bylsma, F.W., & Brandt, J. (1996). Self-ordered pointing performance in Huntington's disease patients. *Neuropsychiatry, Neuropsychology, and Behavioral Neurology, 9,* 99–109.

Rich, J.B., Campodonico, J.R., Rothlind, J., et al. (1997). Perseverations during paired-associate learning in Huntington's disease. *Journal of Clinical and Experimental Neuropsychology, 19,* 191–203.

Richard, I.H., Justus, A.W., & Kurlan, R. (2001). Relationship between mood and motor fluctuations in Parkinson's disease. *Journal of Neuropsychiatry and Clinical Neurosciences, 13,* 35–41.

Richards, M., Cote, L.J., & Stern, Y. (1993). Executive function in Parkinson's disease: Set-shifting or set-maintenance? *Journal of Clinical and Experimental Neuropsychology, 15,* 266–279.

Richards, P. & Persinger, M. A. (1992). Toe graphaesthesia as a discriminator of brain impairment: The outstanding feet for neuropsychology. *Perceptual and Motor Skills, 74,* 1027–1030.

Richards, P.M. & Ruff, R.M. (1989). Motivational effects on neuropsychological functioning: Comparison of depressed versus nondepressed individuals. *Journal of Consulting and Clinical Psychology, 57,* 396–402.

Richardson, E.D. & Marottoli, R.A. (1996). Education-specific normative data on common neuropsychological indices for individuals older than 75 years. *The Clinical Neuropsychologist, 10,* 375–381.

Richardson, E.D., Nadler, J.D., & Malloy, P.F. (1995). Neuropsychological prediction of performance measures of daily living skills in geriatric patients. *Neuropsychology, 9,* 565–572.

Richardson, E.D., Varney, N.R., Roberts, R.J., et al. (1997). Long-term cognitive sequelae of cerebral malaria in Vietnam veterans. *Applied Neuropsychology, 4,* 238–243.

Richardson, J.T.E. (1994). Continuous recognition memory tests: Are the assumptions of the theory of signal detection really met? *Journal of Clinical and Experimental Neuropsychology, 16,* 482–486.

Richardson, J.T.E. (2000). *Clinical and neuropsychological aspects of closed head injury* (2nd ed.). London: Taylor & Francis.

Richardson, J.T.E., Robinson, A., & Robinson, I. (1997). Cognition and multiple sclerosis: A historical analysis of medical perceptions. *Journal of the History of the Neurosciences, 6,* 302–319.

Richardson, J.T.E. & Snape, W. (1984). The effects of closed head injury upon human memory: An experimental analysis. *Cognitive Neuropsychology, 1,* 217–231.

Richer, F. & Chouinard, S. (2003). Cognitive control in frontostriatal disorders. In M.-A. Bédard et al. (Eds.), *Mental and behavioral dysfunction in movement disorders.* Totowa, NJ: Humana Press.

Richter, P., Werner, J., Heerlein, A., et al. (1998). On the validity of the Beck Depression Inventory. A review. *Psychopathology, 31,* 160–168.

Rickard, T.C., Romero, S.G., Basso, G., et al. (2000). The calculating brain: An fMRI study. *Neuropsychologia, 38,* 325–335.

Ricker, J.H. (1998). Traumatic brain injury rehabilitation: Is it worth the cost? *Applied Neuropsychology, 5,* 184–193.

Ricker, J.H. & Axelrod, B.N. (1994). Analysis of an oral paradigm for the Trail Making Test. *Assessment, 1,* 47–52.

Ricker, J.H. & Axelrod, B.N. (1995). Hooper Visual Organization Test: Effects of object naming ability. *The Clinical Neuropsychologist, 9,* 57–62.

Ricker, J.H., Müller, R.-A., Zafonte, R.D., et al. (2001). Verbal recall and recognition following traumatic brain injury: A [0–15]-water positron emission tomography study. *Journal of Clinical and Experimental Neuropsychology, 23,* 196–206.

Ricker, J.H. & Zafonte, R.D. (2000). Functional neuroimaging and quantitative electroencephalography in adult traumatic head injury: Clinical applications and interpretive cautions. *Journal of Head Trauma Rehabilitation, 15,* 859–868.

Riddell, S.A. (1962). The performance of elderly psychiatric patients on equivalent forms of tests of memory and learning. *British Journal of Social and Clinical Psychology, 1,* 70–71.

Riddoch, M.J. & Humphreys, G.W. (2001). Object recognition. In B. Rapp (Ed.), *The handbook of cognitive neuropsychology.* Philadelphia: Psychology Press.

Riedel, W.J. & Jorissen, B.L. (1998). Nutrients, age and cognitive function. *Current Opinion in Clinical Nutrition and Metabolic Care, 1,* 579–585.

Riedel-Heller, S.G., Matschinger, H., Schork, A., & Angermeyer, M.C. (1999). Do memory complaints indicate the presence of cognitive impairment? Results of a field study. *European Archives of Psychiatry and Clinical Neuroscience, 249,* 197–204.

Riese, H., Hoedemaeker, M., Brouwer, W.H., et al. (1999). Mental fatigue after very severe closed head injury: Sustained performance, mental effort, and distress and two levels of workload in a driving simulator. *Neuropsychological Rehabilitation, 9,* 189–205.

Riklan, M., Zahn, T.P., & Diller, L. (1962). Human figure drawings before and after chemosurgery of the basal ganglia in parkinsonism. *Journal of Nervous and Mental Disease, 135,* 500–506.

Rimel, R.W., Giordani, B., Barth, J.T., et al. (1981). Disability caused by minor head injury. *Neurosurgery, 9,* 221–228.

Rimel, R.W., Giordani, B., Barth, J.T., & Jane, J.A. (1982). Moderate head injury: Completing the clinical spectrum of brain trauma. *Neurosurgery, 11,* 344–351.

Ringo, J.L., Doty, R.W., Demeter, S., & Simard, P.Y. (1994). Time is of the essence: A conjecture that hemispheric specialization arises from interhemispheric conduction delay. *Cerebral Cortex, 4,* 331–343.

Rinkel, G.J., Djibuti, M., Algra, A., & van Gijn, J. (1998). Prevalence and risk of rupture of intracranial aneurysms: A systematic review. *Stroke, 29,* 251–256.

Riordan, H.J., Flashman, L.A., Saykin, A.J., et al. (1999). Neuropsychological correlates of methylphenidate treatment in adult ADHD with and without depression. *Archives of Clinical Neuropsychology, 14,* 217–233.

Ripich, D.N., Carpenter, B., & Ziol, E. (1997). Comparison of African-American and white persons with Alzheimer's disease on language measures. *Neurology, 48,* 781–783.

Risberg, J. (1989). Regional cerebral blood flow measurements with high temporal and spatial resolution. In D. Ottoson & W. Rostene (Eds.), *Visualization of brain functions.* London: MacMillan.

Risberg, J. & Hagstadius, S. (1983). Effects on the regional cerebral blood flow of long-term exposure to organic solvents. *Acta Psychiatrica Scandinavica, 67(Suppl. 303),* 92–99.

Risch, N., Burchard, E., Ziv, E., & Tang, M.-X. (2002). Categorization of humans in biomedical research: Genes, race and disease. *Online Journal of Genome Biology, 3* (http://genomebiology.com/2002/3/7/comment/2007).

Risse, G.L., Gates, J.R., & Fangman, M.C. (1997). A reconsideration of bilateral language representation based on the intracarotid amobarbital procedure. *Brain and Cognition, 33,* 118–132.

Risse, G.L., Rubens, A.B., & Jordan, L.S. (1984). Disturbances of long-term memory in aphasic patients. *Brain, 107,* 605–617.

Rivers, D.L. & Love, R.J. (1980). Language performance on visual processing tasks in right hemisphere lesion cases. *Brain and Language, 10,* 348–366.

Rixecker, H. & Hartje, W. (1980). Kimura's Recurring-Figures-Test: A normative study. *Journal of Clinical Psychology, 36,* 465–467.

Rizzo, M. & Robin, D.A. (1990). Simultanagnosia: A defect of sustained attention yields insights on visual information processing. *Neurology, 40,* 447–455.

Rizzolatti, G. & Camarda, R. (1987). Neural circuits for spatial attention and unilateral neglect. In M. Jeannerod (Ed.), *Neurophysiological and neuropsychological aspects of spatial neglect.* Amsterdam: Elsevier/North-Holland.

Rizzolatti, G. & Gallese, V. (1988). Mechanisms and theories of spatial neglect. In F. Boller & J. Grafman (Eds.), *Handbook of neuropsychology* (Vol. 1). Amsterdam: Elsevier.

Robbins, T.W. (1998). Dissociating executive functions of the prefrontal cortex. In A.C. Roberts et al. (Eds.), *The prefrontal cortex: Executive and cognitive functions.* Oxford: Oxford University Press.

Robbins, T.W., James, M., Owen, A.M., et al. (1998). A study of the performance on tests from the CANTAB Battery sensitive to frontal lobe dysfunction in a large sample of normal volunteers: Implications for theories of executive functioning and cognitive aging. *Journal of the International Neuropsychological Society, 4,* 474–490.

Roberts, A.C., Robbins, T.W., & Weiskrantz, L. (Eds.) (1998). *The prefrontal cortex: Executive and cognitive functions.* Oxford, UK: Oxford University Press.

Roberts, A.H. (1976). Long-term prognosis of severe accidental head injury. *Proceedings of the Royal Society of Medicine, 69,* 137–140.

Roberts, R.J. (1999). Epilepsy spectrum disorder in the context of mild traumatic brain injury. In N.R. Varney & R.J. Roberts (Eds.), *The evaluation and treatment of mild traumatic brain injury.* Mahwah, NJ: Erlbaum.

Roberts, R.J. & Hamsher, K.deS. (1984). Effects of minority status on facial recognition and naming performance. *Journal of Clinical Psychology, 40,* 539–545.

Roberts, R.J., Hamsher, K. deS., Bayless, J.D., & Lee, G.P. (1990). Presidents Test performance in varieties of diffuse and unilateral cerebral disease. *Journal of Clinical and Experimental Neuropsychology, 12,* 195–208.

Roberts, R.J., Paulsen, J. S., Marchman, J. N., & Varney, N. R. (1988). MMPI profiles of patients who endorse multiple partial seizure symptoms. *Neuropsychology, 2,* 183–198.

Roberts, R.J.J. & Pennington, B.F. (1996). An interactive framework for examining prefrontal cognitive processes. *Developmental Neuropsychology, 12,* 105–126.

Robertson C. & Empson, J. (1999). Slowed cognitive processing and high workload in Parkinson's disease. *Journal of the Neurological Sciences, 162,* 27–33.

Robertson, G.J. (2002). *Wide Range Achievement Test-Expanded Edition (WRAT-Expanded).* Wilmington, DL: Wide Range.

Robertson, I.H. (1990). Digit span and visual neglect: A puzzling relationship. *Neuropsychologia, 28,* 217–222.

Robertson, I.H., Manly, T., Andrade, J., et al. (1997). "Oops!": Performance correlates of everyday attentional failures in traumatic brain injured and normal subjects. *Neuropsychologia, 35,* 747–758.

Robertson, I.H., Ward, T., Ridgeway, V., & Nimmo-Smith, I. (1994). *The Test of Everyday Attention.* Bury St. Edmunds, UK: Thames Valley Test.

Robertson, I.H., Ward, T., Ridgeway, V., & Nimmo-Smith, I. (1996). The structure of normal human attention: The Test of Everyday Attention. *Journal of the International Neuropsychological Society, 2,* 525–534.

Robertson, L.C. (1995). Hemispheric specialization and cooperation in processing complex visual patterns. In F.L. Kitterle (Ed.), *Hemispheric communication: Mechanisms and models.* Hillsdale, NJ: Erlbaum.

Robertson, L.C. & Rafal, R. (2000). Disorders of visual attention. In M.S. Gazzaniga (Ed.), *The new cognitive neurosciences* (2nd ed.). Cambridge, MA: MIT Press.

Robiner, W.N., Dossa, D., & O'Down, W.K. (1988). Abbreviated WAIS-R procedures: Use and limitations with head-injured patients. *The Clinical Neuropsychologist, 2,* 365–374.

Robinson, A.L., Heaton, R.K., Lehman, R.A.W., and Stilson, D.W. (1980). The utility of the Wisconsin Card Sorting Test in detecting and localizing frontal lobe lesions. *Journal of Consulting and Clinical Psychology, 48,* 605–614.

Robinson, R.G. (1998). *The clinical neuropsychiatry of stroke.* New York: Cambridge University Press.

Robinson, R.G., Bolduc, P. L., Kubos, K. L., et al. (1985). Social functioning assessment in stroke patients. *Archives of Physical Medicine and Rehabilitation, 66,* 496–500.

Robinson, R.G. & Manes, F. (2000). Elation, mania, and mood disorders: Evidence from neurological disease. In J.C. Borod (Ed.), *The neuropsychology of emotion.* New York: Oxford University Press.

Robinson, R.G. & Starkstein, S.E. (2002). Neuropsychiatric aspects of cerebrovascular disorders. In S.C. Yudofsky & R.E. Hales (Eds.), *Textbook of neuropsychiatry and clinical neurosciences* (2nd ed.). Washington, D.C.: American Psychiatric Press.

Robinson, R.G., Starr, L.B., Kubos, K.L., & Price, T.R. (1983). A two-year longitudinal study of post-stroke mood disorders: Findings during the initial evaluation. *Stroke, 14,* 736–741.

Robinson, R.G. & Travella, J.I. (1996). Neuropsychiatry of mood disorders. In B.S. Fogel et al. (Eds.), *Neuropsychiatry.* Baltimore: Williams & Wilkins.

Robinson-Whelen, S. (1992). Benton Visual Retention Test performance among normal and demented older adults. *Neuropsychology, 6,* 261–269.

Rocca, W.A., Amaducci, L.A., & Schoenberg, B.S. (1986). Epidemiology of clinically diagnosed Alzheimer's disease. *Annals of Neurology, 19,* 415–424.

Rocca, M.A., Falini, A., Colombo, B., et al. (2002). Adaptive functional changes in the cerebral cortex of patients with nondisabling multiple sclerosis correlate with the extent of brain structural damage. *Annals of Neurology, 51,* 330–339.

Roccaforte, W.H., Burke, W.J., Bayer, B.L., & Wengel, S.P. (1994). Reliability and validity of the Short Portable Mental Status Questionnaire administered by telephone. *Journal of Geriatric Psychiatry and Neurology, 7,* 33–38.

Rockswold, G.L. (1996). Hyperbaric oxygen therapy in head injury. In R.K. Narayan et al. (Eds.), *Neurotrauma.* New York: McGraw-Hill.

Rockwell, E., Choure, J., Galasko, D., et al. (2000). Psychopathology at initial diagnosis in dementia with Lewy bodies versus Alzheimer disease: Comparison of matched groups with autopsy-confirmed diagnoses. *International Journal of Geriatric Psychiatry, 15,* 819–823.

Rodriguez, G., Warkentin, S., Risberg, J., & Rosadini, G. (1988). Sex differences in regional cerebral blood flow. *Journal of Cerebral Blood Flow and Metabolism, 8,* 783–789.

Roeltgen, D.P. (2003). Agraphia. In K.M. Heilman & E. Valenstein (Eds.), *Clinical neuropsychology* (4th ed.). New York: Oxford University Press.

Roeltgen, D.P. & Heilman, K.M. (1985). Review of agraphia and a proposal for an anatomically-based neuropsychological model of writing. *Applied Psycholinguistics, 6,* 205–230.

Roeltgen, D.P., Sevush, S., & Heilman, K.M. (1983). Pure Gerstmann's syndrome from a focal lesion. *Archives of Neurology, 40,* 46–47.

Rogers, D. (1992). Bradyphrenia in Parkinson's disease. In S.J. Huber and J.L. Cummings (Eds.), *Parkinson's disease: Neurobehavioral aspects.* New York: Oxford University Press.

Rogers, F.B., Shackford, S.R., Hoyt, D.B., et al. (1997). Trauma deaths in a mature urban vs rural trauma system. A comparison. *Archives of Surgery, 132,* 376–381.

Rogers, J.D., Brogan, D., & Mirra, S.S. (1985). The nucleus basalis of Meynert in neurological disease: A quantitative morphological study. *Annals of Neurology, 17,* 163–170.

Rogers, R. (Ed.) (1997). *Clinical assessment of malingering and deception* (2nd ed.). New York: Guilford Press.

Rogers, R. & Cavanaugh, J.L., Jr. (1983). "Nothing but the truth . . . "A reexamination of malingering. *Journal of Law and Psychiatry, 11,* 443–460.

Rogers, R., Harrell, E.H., & Liff, C.D. (1993). Feigning neuropsychological impairment: A critical review of methodological and clinical considerations. *Clinical Psychology Review, 13,* 255–274.

Rogers, R., Sewell, K.W., Cruise, K.R., et al. (1998). The PAI and feigning: A cautionary note on its use in forensic-correctional settings. *Assessment, 5,* 399–405.

Rogers, R., Sewell, K.W., & Ustad, K.L. (1995). Feigning among chronic outpatients on the MMPI-2: A systematic examination of fake-bad results. *Assessment, 2,* 81–89.

Rogers, S.L., Doody, R.S., Mohs, R.C., & Friedhoff, L.T. (1998). Donepezil improves cognition and global function in Alzheimer disease: A 15-week double-blind, placebo-controlled study. Donepezil Study Group. *Archives of Internal Medicine, 158,* 1021–1031.

Rogers, S.L., Farlow, M.R., Doody, R.S., et al. (1998). A 24-week, double-blind, placebo-controlled trial of donepezil in patients with Alzheimer's disease. *Neurology, 50,* 136–145.

Rogler, L.H. (1999). Methodological sources of cultural insensitivity in mental health research. *American Psychologist, 54,* 424–433.

Rohling, M.R., Green, P., Allen, L.M. III, & Iverson, G.L. (2002). Depressive symptoms and neurocognitive test scores in patients passing symptom validity tests. *Archives of Clinical Neuropsychology, 17,* 205–222.

Rohner, R.P. (1984). Toward a conception of culture for cross-cultural psychology. *Journal of Cross-Cultural Psychology, 15,* 111–138.

Roid, G.H. (2003). *Stanford-Binet Intelligence Scale* (5th ed.). Itasca, IL: Riverside.

Roig, M. & Placakis, N. (1992). Hemisphericity style, sex, and performance on a mirror-tracing task. *Perceptual and Motor Skills, 74,* 1143–1148.

Rolls, E.T. (1998). The orbitofrontal cortex. In A.C. Roberts et al. (Eds.), *The prefrontal cortex: Executive and cognitive functions.* Oxford: Oxford University Press.

Rolls, E.T. (1999). *The brain and emotion.* Oxford: Oxford University Press.

Rolls, E.T., Hornak, J., Wade, D., & McGrath, J. (1994). Emotion-related learning in patients with social and emotional changes associated with frontal lobe damage. *Journal of Neurology, Neurosurgery, and Psychiatry, 57,* 1518–1524.

Rolls, E.T. & Treves, A. (1998). *Neural networks and brain function.* New York: Oxford University Press.

Roman, D.D., Edwall, G.E., Buchanan, R.J., & Patton, J.H. (1991). Extended norms for the Paced Auditory Serial Addition Task. *The Clinical Neuropsychologist, 5,* 33–40.

Ron, M.A. (1983). The alcoholic brain: CT scan and psychological findings. *Psychological Medicine (Monogr. Suppl. 3),* 1–33.

Ron, M.A. (1989). Psychiatric manifestations of frontal lobe tumours. *British Journal of Psychiatry, 155,* 735–738.

Ron, M.A. (1996). Somatization and conversion disorders. In B.S. Fogel et al. (Eds.), *Neuropsychiatry.* Baltimore: Williams & Wilkins.

Ron, M.A. & Logsdail, S.J. (1989). Psychiatric morbidity in multiple sclerosis: A clinical and MRI study [abstract]. *Psychological Medicine, 19,* 887–895.

Rorschach, H. (1942). *Psychodiagnostics: A diagnostic test based on perception (trans. P. Lemkau & B. Kronenburg).* Berne: Huber.

Rose, F.E., Hall, S., & Szalda-Petree, A.D. (1995). Computerized Portland Digit Recognition Test—the measurement of response latency improves the detection of malingering. *The Clinical Neuropsychologist, 9,* 124–134.

Rose, F.E., Hall, S., & Szalda-Petree, A.D. (1998). A comparison of four tests of malingering and the effects of coaching. *Archives of Clinical Neuropsychology, 13,* 349–363.

Rosen, J. & Schulkin, J. (1998). From normal fear to pathological anxiety. *Psychological Review, 105,* 325–350.

Rosen, W.G. (1980). Verbal fluency in aging and dementia. *Journal of Clinical Neuropsychology, 2*, 135–146.

Rosen, W.G. (1989). Assessment of cognitive disorders in the elderly. In E. Perecman (Ed.), *Integrating theory and practice in clinical neuropsychology.* Hillsdale, NJ: Erlbaum.

Rosen, W.G., Mohs, R.C., & Davis, K.L. (1984). A new rating scale for Alzheimer's disease. *American Journal of Psychiatry, 141,* 1356–1364.

Rosen, W.G., Mohs, R.C., & Davis, K.L. (1986). Longitudinal changes: Cognitive, behavioral, and effective patterns in Alzheimer's disease. In L.W. Poon (Ed.), *Handbook for clinical memory assessment of older adults.* Washington, D.C.: American Psychological Association.

Rosen, W.G., Terry, R.D., Fuld, P.A., et al. (1980). Pathological verification of ischemic score in differentiation of dementias. *Annals of Neurology, 7,* 486–488.

Rosenberg, I.H. & Miller, J.W. (1992). Nutritional factors in physical and cognitive functions of elderly people. *American Journal of Clinical Nutrition, 55,* 1237–1243.

Rosenberg, J. & Pettinati, H.M. (1984). Differential memory complaints after bilateral and unilateral ECT. *American Journal of Psychiatry, 141,* 1071–1074.

Rosenberg, M. (1965). *Society and the adolescent self-image.* Princeton: Princeton University Press.

Rosenberg, N.L., Kleinschmidt-DeMasters, B.K., Davis, K.A., et al. (1988). Toluene abuse causes diffuse central nervous system white matter changes. *Annals of Neurology, 23,* 611–614.

Rosenfeld, B., Sands, S.A., & Van Gorp, W.G. (2000). Have we forgotten the base rate problem? Methodological issues in the detection of distortion. *Archives of Clinical Neuropsychology, 15,* 349–359.

Rosenstein, L.D. (1998). Differential diagnosis of the major progressive dementias and depression in middle and late adulthood: A summary of the literature of the early 1990s. *Neuropsychology Review, 8,* 109–167.

Rosenstein, L.D., Prigatano, G.P., & Nayak, M. (1997). Differentiating patients with higher cerebral dysfunction from patients with psychiatric or acute medical illness using the BNI screen for higher cerebral functions. *Neuropsychiatry, Neuropsychology, and Behavioral Neurology, 10,* 113–119.

Rosenstein, L.D. & Van Sickle, L.F. (1991). Artificial depression of left-hand finger-tapping rates: A critical evaluation of the Halstead-Reitan neuropsychological finger tapping test instrument. *International Journal of Clinical Neuropsychology, 13,* 106–110.

Rosenthal, M., Christensen, B.K., & Ross, T.P. (1998). Depression following traumatic brain injury. *Archives of Physical Medicine and Rehabilitation, 79,* 90–103.

Rosenthal, M., Dijkers, M., Harrison-Felix, C., et al. (1996). Impact of minority status on functional outcome and community integration following traumatic brain injury. *Journal of Head Trauma Rehabilitation, 11,* 40–57.

Rosenzweig, M.R. (1999). Effects of differential experience on brain and cognition throughout the life span. In S.H. Broman & J.M. Fletcher (Eds.), *The changing nervous system. Neurobehavioral consequences of early brain disorders.* New York: Oxford University Press.

Rosenzweig, M.R. & Leiman, A.L. (1968). Brain functions. *American Review of Psychology, 19,* 55–98.

Roses, A.D. & Saunders, A.M. (1997). Apolipoprotein E genotyping as a diagnostic adjunct for Alzheimer's disease. *International Psychogeriatrics, 9,* 277–288.

Ross, E.D. (2003). The aprosodias. In T.E. Feinberg & M.J. Farah (Eds.), *Behavioral neurology and neuropsychology* (2nd ed.). New York: McGraw-Hill.

Ross, E.D. (2000). Affective prosody and the aprosodias. In M.-M.

Mesulam (Ed.), *Principles of behavioral and cognitive neurology.* New York: Oxford University Press.

Ross, E.D. & Rush, A.J. (1981). Diagnosis and neuroanatomical correlates of depression in brain-damaged patients. *Archives of General Psychiatry, 38,* 1344–1354.

Ross, J.L., Roeltgen, D., Feuillan, P., et al. (2000). Use of estrogen in young girls with Turner syndrome: Effects on memory. *Neurology, 54,* 164–170.

Ross, S.R. & Adams, K.M. (1999). One more test of malingering? *Clinical Neuropsychologist, 13,* 112–116.

Ross, S.R., Millis, S.R., & Rosenthal, M. (1997). Neuropsychological prediction of psychosocial outcome after traumatic brain injury. *Applied Neuropsychology,4,* 165–170.

Ross, T.P., Lichtenberg, P.A., & Christensen, B.K. (1995). Normative data on the Boston Naming Test for elderly adults in a demographically diverse medical sample. *The Clinical Neuropsychologist, 9,* 321–325.

Rosselli, M. & Ardila, A. (1989). Calculation deficits in patients with right and left hemisphere damage. *Neuropsychologia, 27,* 607–617.

Rosselli, M. & Ardila, A. (1991). Effects of age, education, and gender on the Rey-Osterrieth Complex Figure. *The Clinical Neuropsychologist, 5,* 370–376.

Rosselli, M., Ardila, A., Arvizu, L., et al. (1998). Arithmetical abilities in Alzheimer disease. *International Journal of Neuroscience, 96,* 141–148.

Rosselli, M., Ardila, A., Florez, A., & Castro, C. (1990). Normative data on the Boston Diagnostic Aphasia Examination in a Spanish speaking population. *Journal of Clinical and Experimental Neuropsychology, 12,* 313–322.

Rosselli, M., Ardila, A., Lubomski, M., et al. (2001). Personality profile and neuropsychological test performance in chronic cocaine abusers. *International Journal of Neuroscience, 110,* 55–72.

Rosselli, M., Ardila, A., Ostrosky-Solis, F., et al. (2000). Verbal fluency and repetition skills in healthy older Spanish–English bilinguals. *Applied Neuropsychology, 7,* 17–24.

Rosser, A.E. & Hodges, J.R. (1994). The Dementia Rating Scale in Alzheimer's disease, Huntington's disease and progressive supranuclear palsy. *Journal of Neurology, 241,* 531–536.

Rossion, B., Dricot, L., Devolder, A., et al. (2000). Hemispheric asymmetries for whole-based and part-based face processing in the human fusiform gyrus. *Journal of Cognitive Neuroscience, 12,* 793–802.

Rossor, M. (1987). The neurochemistry of cortical dementias. In S.M. Stahl et al. (Eds.), *Cognitive neurochemistry.* Oxford: Oxford University Press.

Rossor, M.N. (1993). Headache, stupor, and coma. In J. Walton (Ed.), *Brain's diseases of the nervous system.* Oxford: Oxford University Press.

Rosvold, H.E., Mirsky, A.F., Sarason, I., et al. (1956). A continuous performance test of brain damage. *Journal of Consulting Psychology, 20,* 343–350.

Roth, D.L., Conboy, T.J., Reeder, K.P., & Boll, T.J. (1990). Confirmatory factor analysis of the Wechsler Memory Scale–Revised in a sample of head-injured patients. *Journal of Clinical and Experimental Neuropsychology, 12,* 834–842.

Roth, D.L. & Crosson, B. (1985). Memory span and long-term memory deficits in brain-impaired patients. *Journal of Clinical Psychology, 41,* 521–527.

Roth, G. (2000). The evolution and ontogeny of consciousness. In T. Metzinger (Ed.), *Neural correlates of consciousness.* Cambridge, MA: MIT Press.

Roth, M., Huppert, F.A., Tym, E., & Mountjoy, C.Q. (1999). *The Cambridge Examination for Mental Disorders of the Elderly-Revised.* Cambridge: Cambridge University Press.

Roth, M., Tym, E., Mountjoy, C.Q., et al. (1986). CAMDEX. A standardised instrument for the diagnosis of mental disorder in the elderly with special reference to the early detection of dementia. *British Journal of Psychiatry, 149,* 698–709.

Rothi, L.J.G. & Horner, J. (1983). Restitution and substitution: Two theories of recovery with application to neurobehavioral treatment. *Journal of Clinical Neuropsychology, 5,* 73–82.

Rothi, L.J.G., Mack, L., & Heilman, K.M. (1986). Pantomime agnosia. *Journal of Neurology, Neurosurgery and Psychiatry, 49,* 451–454.

Rothi, L.J.G., Mack, L., Verfaellie, M., et al. (1988). Ideomotor apraxia: Error pattern analysis. *Aphasiology, 2,* 381–388.

Rothi, L.J.G., Ochipa, C., & Heilman, K.M. (1991). A cognitive neuropsychological model of limb praxis. *Cognitive Neuropsychology, 8,* 443–458.

Rothi, L.J.G., Raymer, A.M., & Heilman, K.M. (1997). Limb praxis assessment. In L.J.G. Rothi & K.M. Heilman (Eds.), *Apraxia: The Neuropsychology of Action.* Hove, UK: Psychology Press.

Rothi, L.J.G., Raymer, A.M., Maher, L., et al. (1991). Assessment of naming failures in neurological communication disorders. *Clinical Communication Disorders, 1,* 7–20.

Rothrock, J.F., Rubenstein, R., & Lyden, P.D. (1988). Ischemic stroke associated with methamphetamine inhalation. *Neurology, 38,* 589–592.

Rothweiler, B., Temkin, N.R., & Dikmen, S.S. (1998). Aging effect on psychosocial outcome in traumatic brain injury. *Archives of Physical Medicine and Rehabilitation, 79,* 881–887.

Rouleau, I., Salmon, D.P., Butters, N., et al. (1992). Quantitative and qualitative analyses of clock drawings in Alzheimer's and Huntington's disease. *Brain and Cognition, 18,* 70–87.

Rouleau, I., Salmon, D.P., & Butters, N. (1996). Longitudinal analysis of clock drawing in Alzheimer's disease patients. *Brain and Cognition, 31,* 17–34.

Rounsaville, B.J., Jones, C., Novelly, R.A., & Kleber, H. (1982). Neuropsychological functioning in opiate addicts. *Journal of Nervous and Mental Disease, 82,* 209–216.

Rounsaville, B.J., Novelly, R.A., & Kleber, H.D. (1981). Neuropsychological impairment in opiate addicts: Risk factors. *Annals of the New York Academy of Sciences, 362,* 79–90.

Rourke, B.P., Costa, L., Cicchetti, D.V., et al. (Eds.) (1991). *Methodological and biostatistical foundations of clinical neuropsychology.* Amsterdam: Swets and Zeitlinger.

Rourke, S.B. & Grant, I. (1999). The interactive effects of age and length of abstinence on the recovery of neuropsychological functioning in chronic male alcoholics: A 2-year follow-up study. *Journal of the International Neuropsychological Society, 5,* 234–246.

Rourke, S.B. & Løberg, T. (1996). Neurobehavioral correlates of alcoholism. In I. Grant & K.M. Adams (Eds.), *Neuropsychological assessment of neuropsychiatric disorders.* New York: Oxford University Press.

Rousseaux, M., Beis, J.M., Pradat-Diehl, P., et al. (2001). Présentation d'une batterie de dépistage de la négligence spatiale. Normes et effets de l'âge, du niveau d'éducation, du sexe, de la main et de la latéralité. *Revue de Neurologie (Paris), 157,* 1385–1400.

Rousseaux, M., Cabaret, M., Lesoin, F., et al. (1986). Bilan de l'amnésie des infarctus thalamiques restreints—6 cas. *Cortex, 22,* 213–228.

Rousseaux, M., Fimm, B., & Cantagallo, A. (2002). Attention disorders in cerebrovascular diseases. In M. Leclercq & P. Zimmerman (Eds.), *Applied neuropsychology of attention. Theory, diagnosis and rehabilitation.* New York: Psychology Press.

Rovaris, M., Bozzali, M., Santuccio, G., et al. (2001). In vivo assessment of the brain and cervical cord pathology of patients with primary progressive multiple sclerosis. *Brain, 124,* 2540–2549.

Rovaris, M. & Filippi, M. (2000). MRI correlates of cognitive dysfunction in multiple sclerosis patients. *Journal of Neurovirology, 6,* S172–S175.

Rovaris, M., Filippi, M., Minicucci, L., et al. (2000). Cortical/subcortical disease burden and cognitive impairment in patients with multiple sclerosis. *American Journal of Neuroradiology, 21,* 402–408.

Roy, E.A. (1982). Action and performance. In A.W. Ellis (Ed.), *Normality and pathology in cognitive functions.* New York: Academic Press.

Roy, E.A. (1983). Neuropsychological perspectives on apraxia and related action disorders. In R.A. Magill (Ed.), *Memory and control of action.* Amsterdam: North-Holland.

Roy, E.A., Reuter-Lorenz, P., Roy, L.G., et al. (1987). Unilateral attention deficits and hemispheric asymmetries in the control of attention. In M. Jeannerod (Ed.), *Neurophysiological and neuropsychological aspects of spatial neglect.* Amsterdam: Elsevier/North-Holland.

Roy, E.A. & Square, P.A. (1985). Common considerations in the study of limb, verbal and oral apraxia. In E.A. Roy (Ed.), *Advances in psychology. Neuropsychological studies of apraxia and related disorders* (Vol. 23). Amsterdam: North-Holland.

Royall, D.R., Chiodo, L.K., & Polk, M.J. (2000). Correlates of disability among elderly retirees with "subclinical" cognitive impairment. *Journals of Gerontology. Series A, Biological and Medical Sciences, 55A,* M541–M546.

Royall, D.R., Cordes, J.A., & Polk, M. (1998). CLOX: An executive clock drawing task. *Journal of Neurology, Neurosurgery and Psychiatry, 64,* 588–594.

Royall, D.R., Mulroy, A.R., Chiodo, L.K., & Polk, M.J. (1999). Clock drawing is sensitive to executive control: A comparison of six methods. *Journals of Gerontology. Series B, Psychological Sciences and Social Sciences, 54B,* P328–P333.

Royall, D.R. & Roman, G.C. (2000). Differentiation of vascular dementia from AD on neuropsychological tests. *Neurology, 55,* 604–606.

Roy-Byrne, P.P. & Upadhyaha, M. (2002). Psychopharmacologic treatments for patients with neuropsychiatric disorders. In S.C. Yudofsky & R.E. Hales (Eds.), *Textbook of neuropsychiatry and clinical neurosciences* (4th ed.). Washington, D.C.: American Psychiatric Press.

Royer, F.L. & Holland, T.R. (1975). Rotational transformation of visual figures as a clinical phenomenon. *Psychological Bulletin, 82,* 843–868.

Royet, J.P., Croisile, B., Williamson-Vasta, R., & Hilbert, O. (2001). Rating of different olfactory judgements in Alzheimer's disease. *Chemical Senses, 26,* 409–417.

Rozans, M., Dreisbach, A., Lertora, J.J., & Kahn, M.J. (2002). Palliative uses of methylphenidate in patients with cancer: A review. *Journal of Clinical Oncology, 20,* 335–339.

Rubens, A.B., Froehling, B., Slater, M.D., & Anderson, D. (1985). Left ear suppression on verbal dichotic tests in patients with multiple sclerosis. *Annals of Neurology, 18,* 459–463.

Rubens, A.B. & Garrett, M.F. (1991). Anosognosia of linguistic deficits in patients with neurological deficits. In G.P. Prigatano & D.L. Schachter (Eds.), *Awareness of deficit after brain injury: Clinical and theoretical issues.* New York: Oxford University Press.

Ruberg, M., Hirsch, E., & Javoy-Agid, F. (1992). Neurochemistry. In I. Litvan & Y. Agid (Eds.), *Progressive supranuclear palsy: Clinical and research approaches.* New York: Oxford University Press.

Rubia, K., Schuri, U., von Cramon, D.Y., & Pöppel, E. (1997). Time estimation as a neuronal network property: A lesion study. *Neuroreport, 8,* 1273–1276.

Rubin, E.H. & Kinscherf, D.A. (1989). Psychopathology of very mild dementia of the Alzheimer type. *American Journal of Psychiatry, 146,* 1017–1021.

Rubin, E.H., Morris, J.C., & Berg, L. (1987). The progression of personality changes in senile dementia of the Alzheimer's type. *Journal of the American Geriatrics Society, 35,* 721–725.

Rubin, E.H., Morris, J.C., Grant, E.A., & Vendegna, T. (1989). Very mild senile dementia of the Alzheimer type. I. Clinical assessment. *Archives of Neurology, 46,* 379–382.

Rubin, E.H., Morris, J.C., Storandt, M., & Berg, L. (1987). Behavioral changes in patients with mild senile dementia of the Alzheimer's type. *Psychiatry Research, 21,* 55–62.

Rubin, E.H., Storandt, M., Miller, J.P., et al. (1998). A prospective study of cognitive function and onset of dementia in cognitively healthy elders. *Archives of Neurology, 55,* 395–401.

Ruch, F.L., Warren, N.D., Grimsley, G., & Ford, J.S. (1963). *Employee Aptitude Survey (EAS)*. San Diego: Educational and Industrial Testing Service.

Ruchinskas, R.A. & Curyto, K.J. (2003). Cognitive screening in geriatric rehabilitation. *Rehabilitation Psychology, 48,* 14–22.

Ruchinskas, R.A., Repetz, N.K., & Singer, H.K. (2001). The use of the Neurobehavioral Cognitive Status Examination with geriatric rehabilitation patients. *Rehabilitation Psychology, 46,* 219–228.

Ruckdeschel-Hibbard, M., Gordon, W.A., & Diller, L. (1986). Affective disturbances associated with brain damage. In S.B. Filskov & T.J. Boll (Eds.), *Handbook of clinical neuropsychology* (Vol. 2). New York: Wiley.

Rudick, R.A., Fisher, E., Lee, J.-C., et al. (1999). Use of the brain parenchymal fraction to measure whole brain atrophy in relapsing-remitting MS. *Neurology, 53,* 1698–1704.

Rudick, R.A., Weinshenker, B.G., & Cutter, G. (2001). Therapeutic considerations: Rating scales. In S.D. Cook (Ed.), *Handbook of multiple sclerosis* (3rd ed.). New York: Marcel Dekker.

Ruesch, J. & Moore, B.E. (1943). The measurement of intellectual functions in the acute stage of head injury. *Archives of Neurology and Psychiatry, 50,* 165–170.

Ruff, R.M., Crouch, J.A., Tröster, A.I., et al. (1994). Selected cases of poor outcome following minor brain trauma: Comparing neuropsychological and positive emission tomography assessment. *Brain Injury, 8,* 297–308.

Ruff, R.M., Evans, R.W., & Light, R.H. (1986). Automatic detection vs controlled search: A paper and pencil approach. *Perceptual and Motor Skills, 62,* 407–416.

Ruff, R.M., Evans, R., & Marshall, L.F. (1986). Impaired verbal and figural fluency after head injury. *Archives of Clinical Neuropsychology, 1,* 87–101.

Ruff, R.M. & Grant, I. (1999). Postconcussional disorder: Background to DSM-IV and future considerations. In N.R. Varney & R.J. Roberts (Eds.), *The evaluation and treatment of mild traumatic brain injury*. Mahwah, NJ: Erlbaum.

Ruff, R.M. & Jurica, P. (1999). In search of a unified definition for mild traumatic brain injury. *Brain Injury, 13,* 943–952.

Ruff, R.M., Levin, H.S., Mattis, S., et al. (1989). Recovery of memory after mild head injury: A three-center study. In H.S. Levin et al. (Eds.), *Mild head injury*. New York: Oxford University Press.

Ruff, R.M., Light, R.H., & Evans, R.W. (1987). The Ruff Figural Fluency Test: A normative study with adults. *Developmental Neuropsychology, 3,* 37–52.

Ruff, R., Light, R., & Parker, S. (1996). Visuospatial learning: Ruff-Light Trail Learning Test. *Archives of Clinical Neuropsychology, 11,* 313–327.

Ruff, R.M., Light, R.H., Parker, S.B., & Levin, H.S. (1996). Benton Controlled Oral Word Association Test: Reliability and updated norms. *Archives of Clinical Neuropsychology, 11,* 329–338.

Ruff, R.M., Light, R.H., Parker, S.B., & Levin, H.S. (1997). The psychological construct of word fluency. *Brain and Language, 57,* 394–405.

Ruff, R.M., Light, R.H., & Quayhagen, M. (1989). Selective Reminding Test: A normative study of verbal learning in adults. *Journal of Clinical and Experimental Neuropsychology, 11,* 539–550.

Ruff, R.M. & Niemann, H. (1990). Cognitive rehabilitation versus day treatment in head-injured adults: Is there an impact on emotional and psychosocial adjustment? *Brain Injury, 4,* 339–347.

Ruff, R.M., Niemann, H., Allen, C.C., et al. (1992). The Ruff 2 and 7 Selective Attention Test: A neuropsychological application. *Perceptual and Motor Skills, 75,* 1311–1319.

Ruff, R.M. & Parker, S.B. (1993). Gender and age-specific changes in motor speed and eye-hand coordination in adults: Normative values for the Finger Tapping and Grooved Pegboard tests. *Perceptual and Motor Skills, 76,* 1219–1230.

Ruff, R.M. & Richards, P.M. (2003). Neuropsychological assessment and management of patients with persistent postconcussional disorders. In G.P. Prigatano & N.H. Pliskin (Eds.), *Clinical neuropsychology and cost outcome research: A beginning*. New York: Psychology Press.

Ruff, R.M., Wylie, T., & Tennant, W. (1993). Malingering and malingering-like aspects of mild closed head injury. *Journal of Head Trauma Rehabilitation, 8,* 60–73.

Ruffalo, C.A. (2003). Advocacy in the forensic practice of neuropsychology. In R.D. Franklin (Ed.), *Prediction in forensic and neuropsychology*. Mahwah, NJ: Erlbaum.

Ruffolo, J.S., Javorsky, D.J., Tremont, G., et al. (2001). A comparison of administration procedures for the Rey-Osterrieth Complex Figure: Flowcharts versus pen switching. *Psychological Assessment, 13,* 299–305.

Ruffolo, L.F., Guilmette, T.J., & Willis, G.W. (2000). Comparison of time and error rates on the Trail Making Test among patients with head injuries, experimental malingerers, patients with suspect effort on testing, and normal controls. *The Clinical Neuropsychologist, 14,* 223–230.

Rugg, M.D. (Ed.) (1997). *Cognitive neuroscience*. Cambridge, MA: MIT Press.

Rugg, M.D. (2002). Functional neuroimaging of memory. In A.D. Baddeley et al. (Eds.), *The handbook of memory disorders*. Chichester, UK: Wiley.

Ruitenberg, A., van Swieten, J.C., Witteman, J.C., et al. (2002). Alcohol consumption and risk of dementia: The Rotterdam Study. *Lancet, 359,* 281–286.

Rund, B.R. (1998). A review of longitudinal studies of cognitive functions in schizophrenia patients. *Schizophrenia Bulletin, 24,* 425–435.

Ruoppila, I. & Suutama, T. (1997). Cognitive functioning of 75- and 80-year-old people and changes during a 5-year follow-up. *Scandinavian Journal of Social Medicine (Suppl.), 53,* 44–65.

Rush, M.C., Panek, P.E., & Russell, J.E. (1990). Analysis of individual variability among older adults on the Stroop Color Word Interference Test. *International Journal of Aging and Human Development, 30,* 225–236.

Rushton, J.P. (2000). Flynn effects not genetic and unrelated to race differences. *American Psychologist, 55,* 542–543.

Russ, M.O. & Seger, L. (1995). The effect of task complexity on reaction times in memory scanning and visual discrimination in Parkinson's disease. *Neuropsychologia, 33,* 561–575.

Russell, E.W. (1975). A multiple scoring method for the assessment of complex memory functions. *Journal of Consulting and Clinical Psychology, 43,* 800–809.

Russell, E.W. (1976). The Bender-Gestalt and the Halstead-Reitan battery: A case study. *Journal of Clinical Psychology, 32,* 355–361.

Russell, E.W. (1981). The chronicity effect. *Journal of Clinical Psychology, 37*, 246–253.

Russell, E.W. (1984). Theory and development of pattern analysis methods related to the Halstead-Reitan Battery. In P. E. Logue & J. M. Schear (Eds.), *Clinical neuropsychology: A multidisciplinary approach*. Springfield, IL: Thomas.

Russell, E.W. (1985). Comparison of the TPT 10 and 6 Hole Form Board. *Journal of Clinical Psychology, 41*, 68–81.

Russell, E.W. (1987). Neuropsychological interpretation of the WIS. *Neuropsychology, 1*, 2–6.

Russell, E.W. (1988). Renorming Russell's version of the Wechsler Memory Scale. *Journal of Clinical and Experimental Neuropsychology, 10*, 235–249.

Russell, E.W. (1998). In defense of the Halstead-Reitan Battery: A critique of Lezak's review. *Archives of Clinical Neuropsychology, 13*, 365–381.

Russell, E.W., Hendrickson, M.E., & Van Eaton, E. (1988). Verbal and figural gestalt completion tests with lateralized occipital area brain damage. *Journal of Clinical Psychology, 44*, 217–225.

Russell, E.W. & Levy, M. (1987). Revision of the Halstead Category Test. *Journal of Consulting and Clinical Psychology, 55*, 898–901.

Russell, E.W., Neuringer, C., & Goldstein, G. (1970). *Assessment of brain damage: A neuropsychological key approach*. New York: Wiley-Interscience.

Russell, E.W. & Starkey, R.I. (1993). *Halstead Russell Neuropsychological Evaluation System (HRNES)*. Los Angeles: Western Psychological Services.

Russell, W.R. (1963). Some anatomical aspects of aphasia. *Lancet, i*, 1173–1177.

Russell, W.R. (1974). Recovery after minor head injury. *Lancet, ii*, 1314.

Russell, W.R. & Nathan, P.W. (1946). Traumatic amnesia. *Brain, 69*, 280–300.

Russo, M. & Vignolo, L. A. (1967). Visual figure–ground discrimination in patients with unilateral cerebral disease. *Cortex, 3*, 118–127.

Rusted, J.M. & Warburton, D.M. (1992). Facilitation of memory by post-trial administration of nicotine: Evidence for an attentional explanation. *Psychophamaracology, 108*, 452–455.

Rutherford, W.H. (1989). Postconcussion symptoms: Relationship to acute neurological indices, individual differences, and circumstances of injury. In H.S. Levin et al. (Eds.), *Mild head injury*. New York: Oxford University Press.

Rutherford, W.H., Merrett, J.D., & McDonald, J.R. (1979). Symptoms at one year following concussion from minor head injuries. *Injury, 10*, 225–230.

Ryan, C. & Butters, N. (1980a). Further evidence for a continuum-of-impairment encompassing alcoholic Korsakoff patients and chronic alcoholics. *Alcoholism: Clinical and Experimental Research, 4*, 190–198.

Ryan, C. & Butters, N. (1980b). Learning and memory impairments in young and old alcoholics: Evidence for the premature-aging hypothesis. *Alcoholism: Clinical and Experimental Research, 4*, 288–293.

Ryan, C., Butters, N., Montgomery, K., et al. (1980). Memory deficits in chronic alcoholics: Continuities between the "intact" alcoholic and the alcoholic Korsakoff patient. In H. Begleiter & B. Kissin (Eds.), *Biological effects of alcohol*. New York: Plenum Press.

Ryan, C. & Butters, N. (1982). Cognitive effects in alcohol abuse. In B. Kissin & H. Begleiter (Eds.), *Cognitive effects in alcohol abuse*. New York: Plenum Press.

Ryan, C. & Butters, N. (1986). Neuropsychology of alcoholism. In D. Wedding, A.M. Horton, Jr., & J.S. Webster (Eds.), *The neuropsychology handbook*. New York: Springer.

Ryan, C., DiDario, B., Butters, N., & Adinolfi, A. (1980). The relationship between abstinence and recovery of function in male alcoholics. *Journal of Clinical Neuropsychology, 2*, 125–134.

Ryan, C.M. (1997). Effects of diabetes mellitus on neuropsychological functioning: A lifespan perspective. *Seminars in Clinical Neuropsychiatry, 2*, 4–14.

Ryan, C.M. & Geckle, M. (2000a). Why is learning and memory dysfunction in Type 2 diabetes limited to older adults? *Diabetes/Metabolism Research and Reviews, 16*, 308–315.

Ryan, C.M. & Geckle, M. (2000b). Circumscribed cognitive dysfunction in middle-aged adults with Type 2 diabetes. *Diabetes Care, 23*, 1486–1493.

Ryan, C.M. & Hendrickson, R. (1998). Evaluating the effects of treatment for medical disorders: Has the value of neuropsychological assessment been fully realized? *Applied Neuropsychology, 5*, 209–219.

Ryan, C.M., Morrow, L.A., & Hodgson, M. (1988). Cacosmia and neurobehavioral dysfunction associated with occupational exposure to mixtures of organic solvents. *American Journal of Psychiatry, 145*, 1442–1445.

Ryan, C.M., Morrow, L., Parkinson, D., & Bromet, E. (1987). Low level lead exposure and neuropsychological functioning in blue collar males. *International Journal of Neuroscience, 36*, 29–39.

Ryan, C.M., Williams, T.M., Finegold, D.N., & Orchard, T.J. (1993). Cognitive dysfunction in adults with type 1 (insulin-dependent) diabetes mellitus of long duration: Effects of recurrent hypoglycemia and other chronic complications. *Diabetologia, 36*, 329–334.

Ryan, G.A., McLean, A.J., Vilenius, A.T., et al. (1994). Brain injury patterns in fatally injured pedestrians. *Journal of Trauma, 36*, 469–476.

Ryan, J.J., Arb, J.D., & Ament, P.A. (2000). Supplementary WMS-III tables for determining primary subtest strengths and weaknesses. *Psychological Assessment, 12*, 193–196.

Ryan, J.J., Arb, J.D., Paul, C.A., & Kreiner, D.S. (2000). Reliability of the WAIS-III subtests, indexes, and IQs in individuals with substance abuse disorders. *Assessment, 7*, 151–156.

Ryan, J.J., Farage, C.M., Mittenberg, W., & Kasprisin, A. (1988). Validity of the Luria-Nebraska Language Scales in aphasia. *International Journal of Neuroscience, 43*, 75–80.

Ryan, J.J., Geisser, M.E., & Dalton, J.E. (1988). Construct validity of the Denman Memory for Human Faces test. *International Journal of Neuroscience, 38*, 89–95.

Ryan, J.J., Geisser, M.E., Randall, D.M., & Georgemiller, R.J. (1986). Alternate form reliability and equivalency of the Rey Auditory Verbal Learning Test. *Journal of Clinical and Experimental Neuropsychology, 8*, 611–616.

Ryan, J.J., Georgemiller, R.J., Geisser, M.E., & Randall, D.M. (1985). Test–retest stability of the WAIS-R in a clinical sample. *Journal of Clinical Psychology, 41*, 552–556.

Ryan, J.J. & Lewis, C.V. (1988). Comparison of normal controls and recently detoxified alcoholics on the Wechsler Memory Scale-Revised. *The Clinical Neuropsychologist, 2*, 173–180.

Ryan, J.J. & Lopez, S.J. (1999). Order of item difficulty on Picture Arrangement: Extending the discussion to the WAIS-III. *Perceptual and Motor Skills, 88*, 1053–1056.

Ryan, J.J., Lopez, S.J., & Paolo, A.M. (1996). Digit span performance of persons 75–96 years of age: Base rates and associations with selected demographic variables. *Psychological Assessment, 8*, 324–327.

Ryan, J.J. & Paolo, A.M. (1992). A screening procedure for estimating premorbid intelligence in the elderly. *The Clinical Neuropsychologist, 6*, 53–62.

Ryan, J.J. & Paolo, A.M. (2001). Exploratory factor analysis of the WAIS-III in a mixed patient sample. *Archives of Clinical Neuropsychology, 16*, 151–156.

Ryan, J.J., Paolo, A.M., & Brungardt, T.M. (1992). WAIS-R test–retest stability in normal persons 75 years and older. *The Clinical Neuropsychologist, 6,* 3–8.

Ryan, J.J., Paolo, A.M., Oehlert, M.E., & Coker, M.C. (1991). Relationship of sex, race, age, education, and level of intelligence to the frequency of occurrence of a WAIS-R marker for dementia of the Alzheimer's type. *Developmental Neuropsychology, 7,* 451–458.

Ryan, J.J., Prifitera, A., & Powers, L. (1983). Scoring reliability on the WAIS-R. *Journal of Consulting and Clinical Psychology, 51,* 149–150.

Ryan, J.J., Rosenberg, S.J., & Mittenberg, W. (1984). Factor analysis of the Rey Auditory-Verbal Learning Test. *International Journal of Clinical Neuropsychology, 6,* 239–241.

Ryan, J.J., Sattler, J.M., & Lopez, S.J. (2000). Age effects on Wechsler Adult Intelligence Scale-III subtests. *Archives of Clinical Neuropsychology, 15,* 311–317.

Ryan, J.J. & Schneider, J.A. (1986). Factor analysis of the Wechsler Adult Intelligence Scale–Revised (WAIS-R) in a brain-damaged sample. *Journal of Clinical Psychology, 42,* 962–964.

Ryan, J.J. & Ward, L.C. (1999). Validity, reliability, and standard errors of measurement for two seven-subtest short forms of the Wechsler Adult Intelligence Scale-III. *Psychological Assessment, 11,* 207–211.

Ryan, L., Clark, C.M., Klonoff, H., et al. (1996). Patterns of cognitive impairment in relapsing-remitting multiple sclerosis and their relationship to neuropathology on magnetic resonance images. *Neuropsychology, 10,* 176–193.

Rybash, J.M. (1996). Implicit memory and aging: A cognitive neuropsychological perspective. *Developmental Neuropsychology, 12,* 127–180.

Rypma, B. & D'Esposito, M. (1999). The roles of prefrontal brain regions in components of working memory: Effects of memory load and individual differences. *Proceedings of the National Academy of Sciences USA, 96,* 6558–6563.

Sabatini, U., Pozzilli, C., Pantano, P., et al. (1996). Involvement of the limbic system in multiple sclerosis patients with depressive disorders. *Biological Psychiatry, 39,* 970–975.

Sabel, M., Felsbert, J., Messing-Junger, M., et al. (1999). Glioblastoma multiforme at the site of metal splinter injury: A coincidence? Case report. *Journal of Neurosurgery, 91,* 1041–1044.

Sabin, J.E. (1975). Translating despair. *American Journal of Psychiatry, 132,* 197–200.

Sacco, R.L. (2001). Newer risk factors for stroke. *Neurology, 57,* S31–S34.

Sackeim, H.A., Greenberg, M.S., Weiman, A.L., et al. (1982). Hemisphere asymmetry in the expression of positive and negative emotions. *Archives of Neurology, 39,* 210–218.

Sackeim, H.A., Gur, R.C., & Saucy, M.C. (1978). Emotions are expressed more intensely on the left side of the face. *Science, 202,* 434–436.

Sackeim, H.A., Prudic, J., Devanand, D.P., et al. (2000). A prospective, randomized, double-blind comparison of bilateral and right unilateral electroconvulsive therapy at different stimulus intensities. *Archives of General Psychiatry, 57,* 425–434.

Sackellares, J.C., Giordani, B., Berent, S., et al. (1985). Patients with pseudoseizures: Intellectual and cognitive performance. *Neurology, 35,* 116–119.

Sacks, O. (1987). *The man who mistook his wife for a hat.* New York: Harper & Row.

Sacks, T.L., Clark, C. R., Pols, R., & Geffen, L. B. (1991). Comparability and stability of performance on six alternate forms of the Dodrill-Stroop Colour-Word Test. *The Clinical Neuropsychologist, 5,* 220–225.

Sadovnik, A.D., Ebers, G.C., Wilson, R.W., & Paty, D.W. (1992). Life expectancy in patients attending multiple sclerosis clinics. *Neurology, 42,* 991–994.

Sadovnick, A.D., Remick, R.A., Allen, J., et al. (1996). Depression and multiple sclerosis. *Neurology, 46,* 628–632.

Safer, M.A. & Leventhal, H. (1977). Ear differences in evaluating emotional tones of voice and verbal content. *Journal of Experimental Psychology: Human Perception and Performance, 3,* 75–82.

Saffran, E.M. (2003). Aphasia: Cognitive neuropsychological issues. In T.E. Feinberg & M.J. Farah (Eds.), *Behavioral neurology and neuropsychology* (2nd ed.). New York: McGraw-Hill.

Saffran, E.M., Dell, G.S., & Schwartz, M.F. (2000). Computational modeling of language disorders. In M.S. Gazzaniga (Ed.), *The new cognitive neurosciences* (2nd ed.). Cambridge, MA: MIT Press.

Sagar, H.J., Cohen, N.J., Sullivan, E.V., et al. (1988). Remote memory function in Alzheimer's disease and Parkinson's disease. *Brain, 111,* 185–206.

Sagar, H.J., Gabrieli, J.D., Sullivan, E.V., & Corkin, S. (1990). Recency and frequency discrimination in the amnesic patient H.M. *Brain, 113,* 581–602.

Sailer, M., Heinze, H.-J., Schoenfeld, M. A., et al. (2000). Amantadine influences cognitive processing in patients with multiple sclerosis. *Pharmacopsychiatry, 33,* 28–37.

Saint-Cyr, J.A. & Taylor, A.E. (1992). The mobilization of procedural learning: The "key signature" of the basal ganglia. In L.R. Squire & N. Butters (Eds.), *Neuropsychology of memory* (2nd ed.). New York: Guilford Press.

Saks, E.R., Dunn, L.B., & Marshall, B.J. (2002). The California Scale of Appreciation: A new instrument to measure the appreciation component of capacity to consent to research. *American Journal of Geriatric Psychiatry, 10,* 166–174.

Salas, M., In't Veld, B.A., van der Linden, P.D., et al. (2001). Impaired cognitive function and compliance with antihypertensive drugs in elderly: The Rotterdam Study. *Clinical Pharmacology and Therapeutics, 70,* 561–566.

Salat, D.H., Kaye, J.A., & Janowsky, J.S. (1999). Prefrontal gray and white matter volumes in healthy aging and Alzheimer disease. *Archives of Neurology, 56,* 338–344.

Salat, D., Ward, A., Kaye, J.A., & Janowsky, J.S. (1997). Sex differences in the corpus callosum with aging. *Neurobiology of Aging, 18,* 191–197.

Salat, D.H., Kaye, J.A., & Janowsky, J.S. (2002). Greater orbital prefrontal volume selectively predicts worse working memory performance in older adults. *Cerebral Cortex, 12,* 494–505.

Salazar, A.M., Amin, D., Vance, S.C., et al. (1987). Epilepsy after penetrating head injury: Effects of lesion location. *Advances in Epileptology, 16,* 753–757.

Salazar, A.M., Grafman, J., Jabbari, B., et al. (1987). Epilepsy and cognitive loss after penetrating head injury. *Advances in Epileptology, 16,* 627–631.

Salazar, A.M., Grafman, J., Schlesselman, S., et al. (1986). Penetrating war injuries of the basal forebrain: Neurology and cognition. *Neurology, 36,* 459–465.

Salazar, A.M., Jabbari, B., Vance, S.C., et al. (1985). Epilepsy after penetrating head injury. I. Clinical correlates: A report of the Vietnam Head Injury Study. *Neurology, 35,* 1406–1414.

Salazar, A.M., Martin, A., & Grafman, J. (1987). Mechanisms of traumatic unconsciousness. *Progress in Clinical Neurosciences, 1,* 225–239.

Saling, M.M. Berkovic, S.F., O'Shea, M.F., et al. (1993). Lateralization of verbal memory and unilateral hippocampal sclerosis: Evidence of task-specific effects. *Journal of Clinical and Experimental Neuropsychology, 15,* 608–618.

Salinsky, M.C., Binder, L.M., Oken, B.S., et al. (2002). Effects of gabapentin and carbamazepine on the EEG and cognition in healthy volunteers. *Epilepsia, 43,* 482–490.

Salinsky, M.C., Storzbach, D., Dodrill, C.B., & Binder, L.M. (2001). Test–retest bias, reliability, and regression equations for neuropsychological measures repeated over a 12–16 week period. *Journal of the International Neuropsychological Society, 7,* 597–605.

Salmaso, D. & Longoni, A.M. (1985). Problems in the assessment of hand preference. *Cortex, 21,* 533–549.

Salmon, D.P. & Butters, N. (1987). The etiology and neuropathology of alcoholic Korsakoff's syndrome: Some evidence for the role of the basal forebrain. In M. Galanter (Ed.), *Recent developments in alcoholism* (Vol. 5). New York: Plenum Press.

Salmon, D.P., Granholm, E., McCullough, D., et al. (1989). Recognition memory span in mildly and moderately demented patients with Alzheimer's disease. *Journal of Clinical and Experimental Neuropsychology, 11,* 429–443.

Salmon, D.P., Heindel, W.C., & Lange, K.L. (1999). Differential decline in word generation from phonemic and semantic categories during the course of Alzheimer's disease: Implications for the integrity of semantic memory. *Journal of the International Neuropsychological Society, 7,* 692–703.

Salmon, D.P., Jin, H., Zhang, M., et al. (1995). Neuropsychological assessment of Chinese elderly in the Shanghai Dementia Survey. *The Clinical Neuropsychologist, 9,* 159–168.

Salmon, D.P., Kwo-on-Yuen, P.F., Heindel, W.C., et al. (1989). Differentiation of Alzheimer's disease and Huntington's disease with the Dementia Rating Scale. *Archives of Neurology, 46,* 1204–1208.

Salmon, D.P., Thal, L.J., Butters, N., & Heindel, W.C. (1990). Longitudinal evaluation of dementia of the Alzheimer type: A comparison of three standarized mental status examinations. *Neurology, 40,* 1225–1230.

Salmon, D.P., Thomas, R.G., Pay, M.M., et al. (2002). Alzheimer's disease can be accurately diagnosed in very mildly impaired individuals. *Neurology, 59,* 1022–1028.

Salmoni, A.W., Richards, P.M., & Persinger, M.A. (1996). Absence of prefrontal lobe dysfunction indicators in healthy elderly participants: Comparisons with verified prefrontal lobe damage. *Developmental Neuropsychology, 12,* 201–206.

Salthouse, T.A. (1978). The role of memory in the age decline in Digit-Symbol substitution performance. *Journal of Gerontology, 33,* 232–238.

Salthouse, T.A. (1991a). Mediation of adult age differences in cognition by reductions in working memory and speed of processing. *Psychological Science, 2,* 179–183.

Salthouse, T.A. (1991b). *Theoretical perspectives on cognitive aging.* Hillsdale, NJ: Erlbaum.

Salthouse, T.A., Fristoe, N., & Rhee, S.H. (1996). How localized are age-related effects of neuropsychological measures? *Neuropsychology, 10,* 272–285.

Salthouse, T.A., Toth, J., Daniels, K., et al. (2000). Effects of aging on efficiency of task switching in a variant of the Trail Making Test. *Neuropsychology, 14,* 102–111.

Salvioli, G. & Neri, M. (1994). L-Acetylcarnitine treatment of mental decline in the elderly. *Drugs under Experimental and Clinical Research, 20,* 169–176.

Samet, M.G. & Marshall-Mies, J.C. (1987). *Expanded Complex Cognitive Assessment Battery (CCAB): Final test administrator user guide.* Alexandria, VA: Systems Research Laboratory, U.S. Army Research Institute.

Samson, S. & Zatorre, R.J. (1988). Melodic and harmonic discrimination following unilateral cerebral excision. *Brain and Cognition, 7,* 348–360.

Samson, W.N., van Duijn, C.M., Hop, W.C., & Hofman, A. (1996). Clinical features and mortality in patients with early-onset Alzheimer's disease. *European Neurology, 36,* 103–106.

Samuel, M., Ceballos-Baumann, A.O., Boecker, H., & Brooks, D.J. (2001). Motor imagery in normal subjects and Parkinson's disease patients: An $H_2^{15}O$ PET study. *NeuroReport, 12,* 821–828.

Samuel, W., Galasko, D., & Thal, L.J. (2002). Alzheimer disease: Biochemical and pharmacologic aspects. In T.E. Feinberg & M.J. Farah (Eds.), *Behavioral neurology and neuropsychology* (2nd ed.). New York: McGraw-Hill.

Samuelsson, H., Hjelmquist, E., Jensen, C., & Blomstrand, C. (2002). Search pattern in a verbally reported visual scanning test in patients showing spatial neglect. *Journal of the International Neuropsychological Society, 8,* 382–394.

Samuelsson, H., Hjelmquist, E., Naver, H., & Blomstrand, C. (1996). Visuospatial neglect and an ipsilesional bias during the start of performance in conventional tests of neglect. *The Clinical Neuropsychologist, 10,* 15–24.

Sanchez-Craig, M. (1980). Drinking pattern as a determinant of alcoholics' performance on the Trail-making Test. *Journal of Studies on Alcohol, 41,* 1083–1089.

Sander, A.M., Caroselli, J.S., High, W.M., Jr., et al. (2002). Relationship of family functioning to progress in a post-acute rehabilitation programme following traumatic brain injury. *Brain Injury, 16,* 649–657.

Sander, A.M., Fuchs, K.L, High, W.M., et al. (1999). The Community Integration Questionnaire revisited: An assessment of factor structure and validity. *Archives of Physical Medicine and Rehabilitation, 80,* 1303–1308.

Sander, A.M., Seel, R.T., Kreutzer, J.S., et al. (1997). Agreement between persons with traumatic brain injury and their relatives regarding psychosocial outcome using the Community Integration Questionnaire. *Archives of Physical Medicine and Rehabilitation, 78,* 353–357.

Sander, A.M., Sherer, M., Malec, J.F., et al. (2003). Preinjury emotional and family functioning in caregivers of persons with traumatic brain injury. *Archives of Physical Medicine and Rehabilitation, 84,* 197–203.

Sanders, G. & Wenmoth, D. (1998). Verbal and music dichotic listening tasks reveal variations in functional cerebral asymmetry across the menstrual cycle that are phase and task dependent. *Neuropsychologia, 36,* 869–874.

Sanders, H. (1972). The problems of measuring very long-term memory. *International Journal of Mental Health, 1,* 98–102.

Sanders, V.M., Iciek, L., & Kasprowicz, D.J. (2000). Psychosocial factors and humoral immunity. In J.T. Cacioppo et al. (Eds.), *Handbook of psychophysiology* (2nd ed.). Cambridge: Cambridge University Press.

Sands, L.P., Yaffe, K., Covinsky, K., et al. (2003). Cognitive screening predicts magnitude of functional recovery from admission to 3 months after discharge in hospitalized elders. *Journal of Gerontology A: Biological Sciences and Medical Sciences, 58,* 37–45.

Sandson, J. & Albert, M.L. (1984). Varieties of perseveration. *Neuropsychologia, 22,* 715–732.

Sandson, J. & Albert, M.L. (1987). Perseveration in behavioral neurology. *Neurology, 37,* 1736–1741.

Sano, M., Marder, K., & Dooneief, G. (1996). Basal ganglia diseases. In B.S. Fogel et al. (Eds.), *Neuropsychiatry* . Baltimore: Williams & Wilkins.

Sano, M., Rosen, W., Stern, Y., et al. (1995). Simple reaction time as a measure of global attention in Alzheimer's disease. *Journal of the International Neuropsychological Society, 1,* 56–61.

Sano, M., Stern, Y., Williams, J., et al. (1989). Coexisting dementia and depression in Parkinson's disease. *Archives of Neurology, 46,* 1284–1286.

Santacruz, P., Uttl, B., Litvan, I., & Grafman, J. (1998). Progressive supranuclear palsy: A survey of the disease course. *Neurology, 50,* 1637–1647.

Santamaria, J. & Tolosa, E. (1992). Clinical subtypes of Parkinson's disease and depression. In S.J. Huber & J.L. Cummings (Eds.), *Parkinson's disease: Neurobehavioral aspects.* New York: Oxford University Press.

Santos, M.E., Castro-Caldas, A., & De Sousa, L. (1998). Spontaneous complaints of long-term traumatic brain injured subjects and their close relatives. *Brain Injury, 12,* 759–767.

Saper, C.B. (1990). Hypothalamus. In A.L. Pearlman & R.C. Collins (Eds.), *Neurobiology of disease.* New York: Oxford University Press.

Saper, J.S., Silberstein, S., & Gordon, C.D. (1993). *Handbook of headache management.* Baltimore: Williams & Wilkins.

Sapienza, C. (1990). Parental imprinting of genes. *Scientific American, 263,* 52–61.

Sarason, I.G., Sarason, B.R., Keefe, D.E., et al. (1986). Cognitive interference: Situational determinants and traitlike characteristics. *Journal of Personality and Social Psychology, 51,* 215–226.

Sarazin, M., Pillon, B., Giannakopoulos, P., et al. (1998). Clinicometabolic dissociation of cognitive functions and social behavior in frontal lobe lesions. *Neurology, 51,* 142–148.

Sarno, J.E., Sarno, M.T., & Levita, E. (1971). Evaluating language improvement after completed stroke. *Archives of Physical Medicine and Rehabilitation, 52,* 73–78.

Sarno, M.T. (1969). *The Functional Communication Profile: Manual of directions.* New York: Institute of Rehabilitation Medicine, New York University Medical Center.

Sarno, M.T. (1976). The status of research in recovery from aphasia. In Y. Lebrun & B. Hoops (Eds.), *Recovery in aphasics.* Amsterdam: Swets & Zeitlinger.

Sarno, M.T. (1980). The nature of verbal impairment after closed head injury. *Journal of Nervous and Mental Disease, 168,* 685–692.

Sarno, M.T., Buonaguro, A., & Levita, E. (1985). Gender and recovery from aphasia after stroke. *Journal of Nervous and Mental Disease, 173,* 605–609.

Sarno, M.T., Buonaguro, A., & Levita, E. (1986). Characteristics of verbal impairment in closed head injured patients. *Archives of Physical Medicine and Rehabilitation, 67,* 400–405.

Sarnquist, F.H., Schoene, R.B., Hackett, P.H., & Townes, B.D. (1986). Hemodilution of polycythemic mountaineers: Effects on exercise and mental function. *Aviation, Space, and Environmental Medicine, 57,* 313–317.

Sarter, M. & Markowitsch, H.J. (1985). Involvement of the amygdala in learning and memory: A critical review, with emphasis on anatomical relations. *Behavioral Neuroscience, 99,* 342–380.

Sass, J.B., Mergler, D., & Silbergeld, E.K. (2002). Environmental toxins and neurological disease. In A.K. Asbury et al. (Eds.), *Diseases of the nervous system* (3rd ed.). Cambridge, UK: Cambridge University Press.

Sass, K.J., Buchanan, C.P., Kraemer, S., et al. (1995). Verbal memory impairment resulting from hippocampal neuron loss among epileptic patients with structure lesions. *Neurology, 45,* 2154–2158.

Sass, K.J., Sass, A., Westerveld, M., et al. (1992). Specificity in the correlation of verbal memory and hippocampal neuron loss: Dissociation of memory, language, and verbal intellectual ability. *Journal of Clinical and Experimental Neuropsychology, 14,* 662–672.

Satish, U., Streufert, S., & Eslinger, P.J. (1999). Complex decision making after orbitofrontal damage: Neuropsychological and strategic management simulation assessment. *Neurocase: Case Studies in Neuropsychology, Neuropsychiatry, and Behavioural Neurology, 5,* 355–364.

Sato, R., Bryan, R.N., & Fried, L.P. (1999). Neuroanatomic and functional correlates of depressed mood: The Cardiovascular Health Study. *American Journal of Epidemiology, 150,* 919–929.

Sattler, J.M. (2001a). *Assessment of children. Cognitive applications* (4th ed.). La Mesa, CA: Sattler.

Sattler, J.M. (2001b). *Assessment of children. Behavioral and clinical applications* (4th ed.). La Mesa, CA: Sattler.

Sattler, J.M. & Ryan, R.M. (1999). *Assessment of children: Revised and updated third edition, WAIS-III supplement.* San Diego, CA: Sattler.

Satz, P. (1993). Brain reserve capacity on symptom onset after brain injury: A formulation and review of evidence for threshold theory. *Neuropsychology, 7,* 273–295.

Satz, P., Fennell, E., & Reilly, C. (1970). Predictive validity of six neurodiagnostic tests. *Journal of Consulting and Clinical Psychology, 34,* 375–381.

Satz, P., Fletcher, J.M., & Sutker, L.S. (1976). Neuropsychologic, intellectual, and personality correlates of chronic marijuana use in native Costa Ricans. *Annals of the New York Academy of Sciences, 282,* 266–306.

Satz, P., Hynd, G.W., D'Elia, L., et al. (1990). A WAIS-R marker for accelerated aging and dementia, Alzheimer's type? Base rates of the Fuld Formula in the WAIS-R standardization sample. *Journal of Clinical and Experimental Neuropsychology, 12,* 759–765.

Satz, P. & Mogel, S. (1962). An abbreviation of the WAIS for clinical use. *Journal of Clinical Psychology, 18,* 77–79.

Satz, P., Nelson, L., & Green, M. (1989). Ambiguous-handedness: Incidence in a non-clinical sample. *Neuropsychologia, 27,* 1309–1310.

Satz, P., Orsini, D.L., Saslow, E., & Henry, R. (1985). The pathological left-handedness syndrome. *Brain and Cognition, 4,* 27–46.

Saunders, D.R. (1960a). A factor analysis of the Information and Arithmetic items of the WAIS. *Psychological Reports, 6,* 367–383.

Saunders, D.R. (1960b). A factor analysis of the Picture Completion items of the WAIS. *Journal of Clinical Psychology, 16,* 146–149.

Savage, C.R., Baer, L., Keuthen, N.J., et al. (1999). Organizational strategies mediate nonverbal memory impairment in obsessive-compulsive disorder. *Biological Psychiatry, 45,* 905–916.

Savage, R.D. (1970). Intellectual assessment. In P. Mittler (Ed.), *The psychological assessment of mental and physical handicaps.* London: Methuen.

Savage, R.D., Britton, P.G., Bolton, N., & Hall, E.H. (1973). *Intellectual functioning in the aged.* New York: Harper & Row.

Savage, R.M. & Gouvier, W.D. (1992). Rey Auditory-Verbal Learning Test: The effects of age and gender, and norms for delayed recall and story recognition trials. *Archives of Clinical Neuropsychology, 7,* 407–414.

Savola, O. & Hillbom, M. (2003). Early predictors of post-concussion symptoms in patients with mild head injury. *European Journal of Neurology, 10,* 175–181.

Sawrie, S.M., Chelune, G.J., Naugle, R.I., & Lüders, H.O. (1996). Empirical methods for assessing meaningful neuropsychological change following epilepsy surgery. *Journal of the International Neuropsychological Society, 2,* 556–564.

Sawrie, S.M., Martin, R.C., Gilliam, F.G., et al. (2000). Visual confrontation naming and hippocampal function: A neural network study using quantitative ^{1}H magnetic resonance spectroscopy. *Brain, 123,* 770–780.

Sawrie, S.M., Martin, R.C., Gilliam, F., et al. (2001). Verbal retention lateralizes patients with unilateral temporal lobe epilepsy and bilateral hippocampal atrophy. *Epilepsia, 42,* 651–659.

Saxton, J., McGonigle-Gibson, K.L., Swihart, A.A., et al. (1990). Assessment of the severely impaired patient: Description and validation of a new neuropsychological test battery. *Psychological Assessment, 2,* 298–303.

Saxton, J. & Swihart, A.A. (1989). Neuropsychological assessment of the severely impaired elderly patients. In F.J. Pirozzolo (Ed.), *Clinics in geriatric medicine* (Vol. 5, No. 3). Philadelphia: Saunders.

Saykin, A.J., Gur, R.C., Shtasel, D.L., et al. (1995). Normative neuropsychological test performance: Effects of age, education, gender, and ethnicity. *Applied Neuropsychology, 2,* 79–88.

Saykin, A.J., Janssen, R.S., Sprehn, G.C., et al. (1988). Neuropsychological dysfunction in HIV-infection: Characterization in a lymphadenopathy cohort. *International Journal of Clinical Neuropsychology, 10,* 81–95.

Saykin, A.J., Stafiniak, P., Robinson, L.J., et al. (1995). Language before and after temporal lobectomy: Specificity of acute changes and relation to early risk factors. *Epilepsia, 36,* 1071–1077.

Sbordone, R.J. (2000). The assessment interview in clinical neuropsychology. In G. Groth-Marnat (Ed.), *Neuropsychological assessment in clinical practice.* New York: Wiley.

Sbordone, R.J. & Caldwell, A.B. (1979). The OBD-168: Assessing the emotional adjustment to cognitive impairment and organic brain damage. *Clinical Neuropsychology, 4,* 36–41.

Sbordone, R.J. & Liter, J.C. (1995). Mild traumatic brain injury does not produce post-traumatic stress disorder. *Brain Injury, 9,* 405–412.

Sbordone, R.J., Liter, J.C., & Pettler-Jennings, P. (1995). Recovery of function following severe traumatic brain injury: A retrospective 10-year follow-up. *Brain Injury, 9,* 285–299.

Sbordone, R.J. & Long, C.J. (Eds.) (1996). *Ecological validity of neuropsychological assessment.* Delray Beach, FL: G.R. Press/Lucie Press.

Scanlan, J. & Borson, S. (2001). The Mini-Cog: Receiver operation characteristics with expert and naive raters. *International Journal of Geriatric Psychiatry, 16,* 216–222.

Scarisbrick, D.J., Tweedy, J.R., & Kuslansky, G. (1987). Hand preference and performance effects on line bisection. *Neuropsychologia, 25,* 695–699.

Scelsa, S.N. (2000). Nitrous oxide. In P.S. Spencer & H.H. Schaumburg (Eds.), *Experimental and clinical neurotoxicology.* New York: Oxford University Press.

Schabet, M. (1999). Epidemiology of primary CNS lymphoma. *Journal of Neurooncology, 43,* 219–226.

Schacter, D.L. (1986a). Amnesia and crime. How much do we really know? *American Psychologist, 41,* 286–295.

Schacter, D.L. (1986b). Feeling-of-knowing ratings distinguish between genuine and simulated forgetting. *Journal of Experimental Psychology, 12,* 30–41.

Schacter, D.L. (1986c). On the relation between genuine and simulated amnesia. *Behavioral Sciences and the Law, 4,* 47–64.

Schachter, D.L. (1987). Memory, amnesia, and frontal lobe dysfunction. *Psychobiology, 15,* 21–36.

Schachter, D.L. (1990b). Toward a cognitive neuropsychology of awareness: Implicit knowledge and anosognosia. *Journal of Clinical and Experimental Neuropsychology, 12,* 155–178.

Schachter, D.L. (1991). Unawareness of deficit and unawareness of knowledge in patients with memory disorders. In G.P. Prigatano & D.L. Schachter (Eds.), *Awareness of deficit after brain injury: Clinical and theoretical issues.* New York: Oxford University Press.

Schachter, D.L., Harbluk, J.L., & McLachlan, D.R. (1984). Retrieval without recollection: An experimental analysis of source amnesia. *Journal of Verbal Learning and Verbal Behavior, 23,* 591–611.

Schachter, D.L., Kaszniak, A.W., Kihlstrom, J.F., & Valdiserri, M. (1991). The relation between source memory and aging. *Psychology and Aging, 6,* 559–568.

Schachter, D.L. & Kihlstrom, J.F. (1989). Functional amnesia. In F. Boller & J. Grafman (Eds.), *Handbook of neuropsychology* (Vol. 3). Amsterdam: Elsevier.

Schachter, D.L., McAndrews, M.P., & Moscovitch, M. (1988). Access to consciousness: Dissociations between implicit and explicit knowledge in neuropsychological syndromes. In L. Weiskrantz (Ed.), *Thought without language.* Oxford, UK: Clarendon Press.

Schachter, D.L. & Nadel, L. (1991). Varieties of spatial memory: A problem for cognitive neuroscience. In R.G. Lister & H.J. Weingartner (Eds.), *Perspectives on cognitive neuroscience.* New York: Oxford University Press.

Schacter, D.L., Norman, K.A., & Koutstaal, W. (1998). The cognitive neuroscience of constructive memory. *Annual Review of Psychology, 49,* 289–318.

Schachter, D.L., Wagner, A.D., & Buckner, R.L. (2000). Memory systems of 1999. In E. Tulving and F.I.M. Craik (Eds.), *The Oxford handbook of memory.* New York: Oxford University Press.

Schachter, S.C. & Ransil, B.J. (1996). Handedness distributions in nine professional groups. *Perceptual and Motor Skills, 82,* 51–63.

Schaefer, A., Brown, J., Watson, C.G., et al. (1985). Comparison of the validities of the Beck, Zung, and MMPI depression scales. *Journal of Consulting and Clinical Psychology, 53,* 415–418.

Schaefer, R.T. (1998). *Racial and ethnic groups.* New York: Longman.

Schaeffer, J., Andrysiak, T., & Ungerleider, J.T. (1981). Cognition and long-term use of ganja (cannabis). *Science, 213,* 465–466.

Schafer, R. (1948). *The clinical application of psychological tests.* New York: International Universities Press.

Schagen, S., Schmand, B., de Sterke, S., & Lindeboom, J. (1997). Amsterdam Short-Term Memory test: A new procedure for the detection of feigned memory deficits. *Journal of Clinical and Experimental Neuropsychology, 19,* 43–51.

Schagen, S.B., van Dam, F.S., Muller, M.J., et al. (1999). Cognitive deficits after postoperative adjuvant chemotherapy for breast carcinoma. *Cancer, 85,* 640–650.

Schaie, K.W. (1974). Translations in gerontology from lab to life: Intellectual functioning. *American Psychologist, 29,* 802–807.

Schaie, K.W. (1994). The course of adult intellectual development. *American Psychologist, 49,* 304–313.

Schaie, K.W. (1995). *Intellectual development in adulthood: The Seattle Longitudinal Study.* Cambridge, UK: Cambridge University Press.

Schaumburg, H.H. (2000a). Gasoline. In P.S. Spencer & H.H. Schaumburg (Eds.), *Experimental and clinical neurotoxicology.* New York: Oxford University Press.

Schaumburg, H.H. (2000b). Human neurotoxic disease. In P.S. Spencer & H.H. Schaumburg (Eds.), *Experimental and clinical neurotoxicology.* New York: Oxford University Press.

Schaumburg, H.H. (2000c). Toluene. In P.S. Spencer & H.H. Schaumburg (Eds.), *Experimental and clinical neurotoxicology.* New York: Oxford University Press.

Schaumburg, H.H. (2000d). Water. In P.S. Spencer & H.H. Schaumburg (Eds.), *Experimental and clinical neurotoxicology.* New York: Oxford University Press.

Schaumburg, H.H. & Spencer, P.S. (2000). Organic solvent mixtures. In P.S. Spencer & H.H. Schaumburg (Eds.), *Experimental and clinical neurotoxicology.* New York: Oxford University Press.

Schear, J.M. & Craft, R.B. (1989). A replication of the factor structure of the California Verbal Learning Test [abstract]. *Journal of Clinical and Experimental Neuropsychology, 11,* 63.

Schear, J.M. & Sato, S.D. (1989). Effects of visual acuity and visual motor speed and dexterity on cognitive test performance. *Archives of Clinical Neuropsychology, 4,* 25–32.

Schear, J.M. & Skenes, L.L. (1991). The interface between clinical neuropsychology and speech–language pathology in the assessment of the geriatric patient. In D. Ripich (Ed.), *Handbook of geriatric communication disorders.* Boston: College-Hill Press.

Schear, J.M., Skenes, L.L., & Larson, V.D. (1988). Effect of simulated hearing loss on Speech Sounds Perception. *Journal of Clinical and Experimental Neuropsychology, 10,* 597–602.

Scheibel, R.S., Meyers, C.A., & Levin, V.A. (1996). Cognitive dysfunction following surgery for intracerebral glioma: Influence of histopathology, lesion location, and treatment. *Journal of Neurooncology, 30,* 61–69.

Schenkenberg, T., Bradford, D. C., & Ajax, E. T. (1980). Line bisection and unilateral visual neglect in patients with neurologic impairment. *Neurology, 30,* 509–517.

Schenker, M.B., Weiss, S.T., & Murawski, B.J. (1982). Health effects of residence in homes with urea formaldehyde foam insulation: A pilot study. *Environment International, 8,* 359–363.

Schenkman, M., Butler, R.B., Naeser, M.A., & Kleefield, J. (1983). Cerebral hemisphere asymmetry in CT and functional recovery from hemiplegia. *Neurology, 33,* 473–477.

Scherer, I.W., Winne, J.F., & Baker, R.W. (1955). Psychological changes over a 3-year period following bilateral prefrontal lobotomy. *Journal of Consulting Psychology, 19,* 291–298.

Scherr, P.A., Albert, M.A., Funkenstein, H.H., et al. (1988). Correlates of cognitive function in an elderly community population. *American Journal of Epidemiology, 128,* 1084–1101.

Schiffer, R.B. & Babigian, H.M. (1984). Behavioral disturbance in multiple sclerosis, temporal lobe epilepsy and amyotrophic lateral sclerosis: An epidemiological study. *Archives of Neurology, 41,* 1067–1069.

Schiffer, R.B., Caine, E.D., Bamford, K.A., & Levy, S. (1983). Depressive episodes in patients with multiple sclerosis. *American Journal of Psychiatry, 140,* 1498–1500.

Schiffer, R.B., Herndon, R.M., & Rudick, R.A. (1985). Treatment of pathologic laughing and weeping with amitriptyline. *New England Journal of Medicine, 312,* 1480–1482.

Schiffer, R.B. & Wineman, N.M. (1990). Antidepressant pharmacotherapy of depression associated with multiple sclerosis. *American Journal of Psychiatry, 147,* 1493–1497.

Schinka, J.A., Vanderploeg, R.D., Rogish, M., & Ordorica, P.I. (2002a). Effects of alcohol and cigarette use on cognition in middle-aged adults. *Journal of the International Neuropsychological Society, 8,* 683–690.

Schinka, J.A., Vanderploeg, R.D., Rogish, M., et al. (2002b). Effects of the use of alcohol and cigarettes on cognition in elderly adults. *Journal of the International Neuropsychological Society, 8,* 811–818.

Schlosser, D. & Ivison, D. (1989). Assessing memory deterioration with the Wechsler Memory Scale, the National Adult Reading Test, and the Shonell Graded Word Reading Test. *Journal of Clinical and Experimental Neuropsychology, 11,* 785–792.

Schluter, N.D., Krams, M., Rushworth, M.F., & Passingham, R.E. (2001). Cerebral dominance for action in the human brain: The selection of actions. *Neuropsychologia, 39,* 105–113.

Schmahmann, J.D. (2003). The role of the cerebellum in cognition and emotion. In M.-A. Bédard et al. (Eds.), *Mental and behavioral dysfunction in movement disorders.* Totawa, NJ: Humana Press.

Schmahmann, J.D. & Sherman, J.C. (1998). The cerebellar cognitive affective syndrome. *Brain, 121,* 561–579.

Schmand, B., Lindeboom, J., Schagen, S., et al. (1998). Cognitive complaints in patients after whiplash injury: The impact of malingering. *Journal of Neurology, Neurosurgery and Psychiatry, 64,* 339–343.

Schmand, B., Smit, J.H., Geerlings, M.I., & Lindeboom, J. (1997). The effects of intelligence and education on the development of dementia. A test of the brain reserve hypothesis. *Psychological Medicine, 27,* 1337–1344.

Schmand, B., Walstra, G., Lindeboom, J., et al. (2000). Early detection of Alzheimer's disease using the Cambridge Cognitive Examination (CAMCOG). *Psychological Medicine, 30,* 619–627.

Schmidley, J.W. & Maas, E.F. (1990). Cerebrospinal fluid, blood–brain barrier, and brain edema. In A.L. Pearlman & R.C. Collins (Eds.), *Neurobiology of disease.* New York: Oxford University Press.

Schmidt, J.P., Tombaugh, T.N., & Faulkner, P. (1992). Free-recall, cued-recall and recognition procedures with three verbal memory tests: Normative data from age 20 to 79. *The Clinical Neuropsychologist, 6,* 185–200.

Schmidt, M. (1996). *Rey Auditory and Verbal Learning Test. A handbook.* Los Angeles: Western Psychological Services.

Schmidt, M.M. & Coolidge, F. L. (1999). *Interference Learning Test. Manual.* Los Angeles: Western Psychological Services.

Schmidt, R., Fazekas, F., Kapeller, P., et al. (1999). MRI white matter hyperintensities: Three-year follow-up of the Austrian Stroke Prevention Study. *Neurology, 53,* 132–139.

Schmidt, R., Fazekas, F., Offenbacher, H., et al. (1991). Magnetic resonance imaging white matter lesions and cognitive impairment in hypertensive individuals. *Archives of Neurology, 48,* 417–420.

Schmidt, R., Freidl, W., Fazeka, F., et al., (1994). The Mattis Dementia Rating Scale: Normative data from 1001 healthy volunteers. *Neurology, 44,* 964–966.

Schmidt, S.L., Oliveira, R.M., Rocha, F.R., & Abreu-Villaca, Y. (2000). Influences of handedness and gender on the Grooved Pegboard Test. *Brain and Cognition, 44,* 445–454.

Schmidtke, K. & Ehmsen, L. (1998). Transient global amnesia and migraine. *European Neurology, 40,* 9–14.

Schmitt, F.A., Ashford, W., Ernesto, C., et al. (1997). The Severe Impairment Battery: Concurrent validity and the assessment of longitudinal change in Alzheimer's disease. The Alzheimer's Disease Cooperative Study. *Alzheimer Disease and Associated Disorders, 11,* S51–S56.

Schmitt, F.A., Bigley, J.W., McKinnis, R., et al. (1988). Neuropsychological outcome of zidovudine (AZT) treatment of patients with AIDS and AIDS-related complex. *New England Journal of Medicine, 319,* 1573–1578.

Schneider, E.L. (1999). Aging in the third millennium. *Science, 283,* 796–797.

Schnider, A. (2000). Spontaneous confabulations, disorientation, and the processing of "now." *Neuropsychologia, 38,* 175–185.

Schnider, A., Hanlon, R.E., Alexander, D.N., & Benson, D.F. (1997). Ideomotor apraxia: Behavioral dimensions and neuroanatomical basis. *Brain and Language, 58,* 125–136.

Schnider, A., von Daniken, C., & Gutbrod, K. (1996). Disorientation in amnesia. A confusion of memory traces. *Brain, 119,* 1627–1632.

Schoenhuber, R. & Gentilini, M. (1989). Neurophysiological assessment of mild head injury. In H.S. Levin, H.M. Eisenberg, & A.L. Benton (Eds.), *Mild head injury.* New York: Oxford University Press.

Schofield, P.W., Tang, M., Marder, K., et al. (1997). Alzheimer's disease after remote head injury: An incidence study. *Journal of Neurology, Neurosurgery and Psychiatry, 62,* 119–124.

Schomer, D.L., O'Connor, M., Spiers, P., et al. (2000). Temporolimbic epilepsy and behavior. In M.-M. Mesulam (Eds.), *Principles of behavioral and cognitive neurology* (2nd ed.). New York: Oxford University Press.

Schomer, D.L., Pegna, A., Matton, B., et al. (1998). Ictal agraphia: A patient study. *Neurology, 50,* 542–545.

Schott, B., Mauguiere, F., Laurent, B., et al. (1980). L'amnésie thalamique. *Revue Neurologique (Paris), 136,* 117–130.

Schraa, J.C., Jones, N.F., & Dirks, J.E. (1983). Bender-Gestalt recall: A review of the normative data and related issues. In J.N. Butcher & C.D. Spielberger (Eds.), *Advances in personality assessment* (Vol. 2.). Hillsdale, NJ: Erlbaum.

Schramm, U., Berger, G., Mueller, R., et al. (2002). Psychometric properties of Clock Drawing Test and MMSE or Short Performance Test (SPT) in dementia screening in a memory clinic population. *International Journal of Geriatric Psychiatry, 17,* 254–260.

Schreiber, D.J., Goldman, H., Kleinman, K.M., et al. (1976). The relationship between independent neuropsychological and neurological detection and localization of cerebral impairment. *Journal of Nervous and Mental Disease, 162,* 360–365.

Schretlen, D., Brandt, J., Krafft, L., & Van Gorp, W. (1991). Some caveats in using the Rey 15-item Memory Test to detect malingered amnesia. *Psychological Assessment, 31,* 667–672.

Schretlen, D., Pearlson, G.D., Anthony, J.C., et al. (2000). Elucidating the contributions of processing speed, executive ability, and frontal lobe volume to normal age-related differences in fluid intelligence. *Journal of the International Neuropsychological Society, 6,* 52–61.

Schretlen, D., Wilkins, S.S., Van Gorp, W.G., & Bobholz, J.H. (1992). Cross-validation of a psychological test battery to detect faked insanity. *Psychological Assessment, 4,* 77–83.

Schroder, J., Kratz, B., Pantel, J., et al. (1998). Prevalence of mild cognitive impairment in an elderly community sample. *Journal of Neural Transmission Supplementum, 54,* 51–59.

Schultheis, M.T., Caplan, B., Ricker, J.H., & Woessner, R. (2000). Fractioning the Hooper: A multiple-choice response format. *The Clinical Neuropsychologist, 14,* 196–201.

Schultheis, M.T., Garay, E., & DeLuca, J. (2001). The influence of cognitive impairment on driving performance in multiple sclerosis. *Neurology, 56,* 1089–1094.

Schum, R.L. & Sivan, A.B. (1997). Verbal abilities in healthy elderly adults. *Applied Neuropsychology, 4,* 130–134.

Schwab, K., Grafman, J., Salazar, A.M., & Kraft, J. (1993). Residual impairments and work status 15 years after penetrating head injury: Report from the Vietnam Head Injury Study. *Neurology, 43,* 95–103.

Schwamm, L.H., VanDyke, C., Kiernan, R.J., et al. (1987). The Neurobehavioral Cognitive Status Examination. *Annals of Internal Medicine, 107,* 486–491.

Schwarcz, R. & Shoulson, I. (1987). Excitotoxins and Huntington's disease. In J.T. Coyle (Ed.), *Animal models of dementia.* New York: Alan R. Liss.

Schwartz, A.F. & McMillan, T.M. (1989). Assessment of everyday memory after severe head injury. *Cortex, 25,* 665–671.

Schwartz, A.S., Frey, J.L., & Luka, R.J. (1988). Risk factors in Alzheimer's disease: Is aluminum hazardous to your health? *BNI Quarterly, 4,* 2–8.

Schwartz, A.S., Marchok, P.L., & Flynn, R.E. (1977). A sensitive test for tactile extinction: Results in patients with parietal and frontal lobe disease. *Journal of Neurology, Neurosurgery and Psychiatry, 40,* 228–233.

Schwartz, A.S., Marchok, P., & Kreinick, C. (1988). Relationship between unilateral neglect and sensory extinction. In G.C. Galbraith et al. (Eds.), *Neurophysiology and psychophysiology: Experimental and clinical applications.* Hillsdale, NJ: Erlbaum.

Schwartz, B.S., Lee, B.K., Lee, G.S., et al. (2001). Associations of blood lead, dimercaptosuccinic acid-chelatable lead, and tibia lead with neurobehavioral test scores in South Korean lead workers. *American Journal of Epidemiology, 153,* 453–464.

Schwartz, B.S., Stewart, W.F., Bolla, K.I., et al. (2000). Past adult lead exposure is associated with longitudinal decline in cognitive function. *Neurology, 55,* 1144–1150.

Schwartz, C.E., Coulthard-Morris, L., & Zeng, Q. (1996). Psychosocial correlates of fatigue in multiple sclerosis. *Archives of Physical Medicine and Rehabilitation, 77,* 165–170.

Schwartz, C.E., Foley, F.W., Rao, S.M., et al. (1999). Stress and course of disease in multiple sclerosis. *Behavioral Medicine, 25,* 110–116.

Schwartz, G.E. (1983). Development and validation of the Geriatric Evaluation by Relative's Rating Instrument (GERRI). *Psychological Reports, 53,* 479–488.

Schwartz, J. & Tallal, P. (1980). Rate of acoustic change may underlie hemispheric specialization for speech perception. *Science, 207,* 1380–1381.

Schwartz, M.F., Mayer, N.H., FitzpatrickDeSalme, E.J., & Montgomery M.W. (1993). Cognitive theory and the study of everyday action disorders after brain damage. *Journal of Head Trauma Rehabilitation, 8,* 59–72.

Schwartz, R.L., Adair, J.C., Raymer, A.M., et al. (2000). Conceptual apraxia in probable Alzheimer's disease as demonstrated by the Florida Action Recall Test. *Journal of the International Neuropsychological Society, 6,* 265–270.

Schwartz, R.S. (2001). Racial profiling in medical research. *New England Journal of Medicine, 344,* 1392–1393.

Science Research Associates (1968). *Reading Index-12.* Chicago, IL: Pearson-Reid London House.

Scott, J.G., Krull, K.R., Williamson, D.G., et al. (1997). Oklahoma Premorbid Intelligence Estimation (OPIE): Utilization in clinical samples. *The Clinical Neuropsychologist, 11,* 146–154.

Scott, L.H. (1981). Measuring intelligence with the Goodenough-Harris Drawing Test. *Psychological Bulletin, 89,* 483–505.

Scott, P.A., Pancioli, A.M., Davis, L.A., et al. (2002). Prevalence of atrial fibrillation and antithrombotic prophylaxis in emergency department patients. *Stroke, 33,* 2664–2669.

Scott, W.K., Nance, M.A., Watts, R.L., et al. (2001). Complete genomic screen in Parkinson disease: Evidence for multiple genes. *Journal of the American Medical Association, 286,* 2239–2244.

Seale, G.S., Caroselli, J.S., High, W.M., et al. (2002). Use of the Community Integration Questionnaire (CIQ) to characterize changes in funtioning for individuals with traumatic brain injury who participated in a post-acute rehabilitation programme. *Brain Injury, 16,* 955–967.

Searleman, A. (1977). A review of right hemisphere linguistic capabilities. *Psychological Bulletin, 84,* 503–528.

Searleman, A. (1980). Subject variables and cerebral organization for language. *Cortex, 16,* 239–254.

Sears, J.D., Hirt, M.L., & Hall, R.W. (1984). A cross-validation of the Luria-Nebraska Neuropsychological Battery. *Journal of Consulting and Clinical Psychology, 52,* 309–310.

Seashore, C.E., Lewis, D., & Saetveit, D.L. (1960). *Seashore Measures of Musical Talents* (rev. ed.). New York: Psychological Corporation.

See, S.T. & Ryan, E.B. (1995). Cognitive mediation of adult age differences in language performance. *Psychology and Aging, 10,* 458–468.

Seeber, A., Meyer-Baron, M., & Schaper, M. (2002). A summary of two meta-analyses on neurobehavioural effects due to occupational lead exposure. *Archives of Toxicology, 76,* 137–145.

Seex, K., Koppel, D., Fitzpatrick, M., & Pyott, A. (1997). Trans-orbital penetrating head injury with a door key. *Journal of Craniomaxillofacial Surgery, 25,* 353–355.

Segalowitz, S.J. (1986). Validity and reliability of noninvasive lateralization measures. In J.E. Obrzut & G.W. Hynd (Eds.), *Child neuropsychology* (Vol. 1). New York: Academic Press.

Segalowitz, S.J., Unsal, A., & Dywan, J. (1992). CNV evidence for the distinctiveness of frontal and posterior neural processes in a traumatic brain-injured population. *Journal of Clinical and Experimental Neuropsychology, 14,* 545–565.

Seidenberg, M., Hermann, B.P., Schoenfeld, J., et al. (1997). Reorganization of verbal memory function in early onset left temporal lobe epilepsy. *Brain and Cognition, 35,* 132–148.

Seidenberg, M., Hermann, B., Wyler, A.R., et al. (1998). Neuropsychological outcome following anterior temporal lobectomy in patients with and without the syndrome of mesial temporal lobe epilepsy. *Neuropsychology, 12,* 303–316.

Seidenwurm, D., Bird, C.R., Enzmann, D.R., & Marshall, W.H.

(1985). Left–right temporal region asymmetry in infants and children. *AJNR American Journal of Neuroradiology, 6,* 777–779.

Seidman, L.J. (1983). Schizophrenia and brain dysfunction: An integration of recent neurodiagnostic findings. *Psychological Bulletin, 94,* 195–238.

Seitz, R.J., Azari, N.P., Knorr, U., et al. (1999). The role of diaschisis in stroke recovery. *Stroke, 30,* 1844–1850.

Sekul, E.A. & Adams, R.J. (1997). Stroke and sickle cell disease. In K.M.A. Welch et al. (Eds.), *Primer on cerebrovascular diseases.* San Diego: Academic Press.

Selhub, J., Bagley, L.C., Miller, J., & Rosenberg, I.H. (2000). B vitamins, homocysteine, and neurocognitive function in the elderly. *American Journal of Clinical Nutrition, 71,* 614S–620S.

Sellal, F., Manning, L., Seegmuller, C., et al. (2002). Pure retrograde amnesia following a mild head trauma: A neuropsychological and metabolic study. *Cortex, 38,* 499–509.

Selmaoui, M.H. (2002). *Devenir des traumatisés crâniens graves: E´valuation des troubles neuropsychologiques, comportementaux et sociaux. Proposition d'un Inventaire d'Adaptation Sociale: Premiers resultats de sa version française.* Annecy, France: Departement de Psychologie, Université de Savoie.

Selnes, O.A., Jacobson, L., Machado, A.M., et al. (1991). Normative data for a brief neuropsychological screening battery. *Perceptual and Motor Skills, 73,* 539–550.

Selnes, O.A., Miller, E., McArthur, J., et al. (1990). HIV-1 infection: No evidence of cognitive decline during the asymptomatic stages. *Neurology, 40,* 204–208.

Selwa, L.M., Geyer, J., Nikakhtar, N., et al. (2000). Nonepileptic seizure outcome varies by type of spell and duration of illness. *Epilepsia, 41,* 1330–1334.

Semenza, C., Borgo, F., Mondini, S., et al. (2000). Proper names in the early stages of Alzheimer's disease. *Brain and Cognition, 43,* 384–387.

Semenza, C., Denes, G., D'Urso, V., et al. (1978). Analytic and global strategies in copying designs by unilaterally brain-damaged patients. *Cortex, 14,* 404–410.

Semenza, C. & Goodglass, H. (1985). Localization of body parts in brain injured subjects. *Neuropsychologia, 23,* 161–175.

Semmes, J. (1968). Hemispheric specialization: A possible clue to mechanism. *Neuropsychologia, 6,* 11–26.

Semmes, J., Weinstein, S., Ghent, L., & Teuber, H.-L. (1963). Correlates of impaired orientation in personal and extra-personal space. *Brain, 86,* 747–772.

Senior, G. & Douglas, L. (2001). Misconceptions and misuse of the MMPI-2 in assessing personal injury claimants. *NeuroRehabilitation, 16,* 203–213.

Sergent, J. (1984). Inferences from unilateral brain damage about normal hemispheric functions in visual pattern recognition. *Psychological Bulletin, 96,* 99–115.

Sergent, J. (1987). A new look at the human split brain. *Brain, 110,* 1375–1392.

Sergent, J. (1988a). Face perception and the right hemisphere. In L. Weiskrantz (Ed.), *Thought without language.* Oxford: Clarendon Press.

Sergent, J. (1988b). Some theoretical and methodological issues in neuropsychological research. In F. Boller & J. Grafman (Eds.), *Handbook of neuropsychology* (Vol. 1). Amsterdam: Elsevier.

Sergent, J. (1989). Structural processing of faces. In A.W. Young & H.D. Ellis (Eds.), *Handbook of research on face processing.* Amsterdam: Elsevier.

Sergent, J. (1990). Furtive incursions into bicameral minds. *Brain, 113,* 537–568.

Sergent, J. (1991a). Judgments of relative position and distance on representations of spatial relations. *Journal of Experimental Psychology: Human Perception and Performance, 91,* 762–780.

Sergent, J. (1991b). Processing of spatial relations within and between the disconnected cerebral hemispheres. *Brain, 114,* 1025–1043.

Sergent, J., Ohta, S., & MacDonald, B. (1992). Functional neuroanatomy of face and object processing: A positron emission tomography study. *Brain, 115,* 15–36.

Seshadri, S., Drachman, D.A., & Lippa, C.F. (1995). Apolipoprotein E epsilon4 allele and the lifetime risk of Alzheimer's disease. What physicians know, and what they should know. *Archives of Neurology, 52,* 1074–1079.

Seymour, S.E., Reuter-Lorenz, P.A., & Gazzaniga, M.S. (1994). The disconnection syndrome. Basic findings reaffirmed. *Brain, 117,* 105–115.

Sgaramella, T.M., Borgo, F., Fenzo, F., et al. (2000). Memory for/and execution of future intentions: Evidence from patients with herpes simplex encephalitis. *Brain and Cognition, 43,* 388–392.

Shader, R.I., Harmatz, J.S., & Salzman, C. (1974). A new scale for clinical assessment in geriatric populations: Sandoz Clinical Assessment-Geriatric (SCAG). *Journal of the American Geriatrics Society, 22,* 107–113.

Shale, H. & Tanner, C. (1996). Pharmacological options for the management of dyskinesias. *Drugs, 52,* 849–860.

Shallice, T. (1982). Specific impairments of planning. *Philosophical Transactions of the Royal Society of London, 298,* 199–209.

Shallice, T. & Burgess, P.W. (1991a). Deficits in strategy application following frontal lobe damage in man. *Brain, 114,* 727–741.

Shallice, T. & Burgess, P. (1991b). Higher-order cognitive impairments and frontal lobe lesions in man. In H.S. Levin et al. (Eds.), *Frontal lobe function and dysfunction.* New York: Oxford University Press.

Shallice, T. & Evans, M.E. (1978). The involvement of the frontal lobes in cognitive estimation. *Cortex, 14,* 294–303.

Shallice, T., Fletcher, P., Frith, C.D., et al. (1994). Brain regions associated with acquisition and retrieval of verbal episodic memory. *Nature, 368,* 633–635.

Shammi, P. & Stuss, D.T. (1999). Humour appreciation: A role of the right frontal lobe. *Brain, 122,* 657–666.

Shankweiler, D. (1966). Effects of temporal lobe damage on perception of dichotically presented melodies. *Journal of Comprehensive Physiology and Psychology, 62,* 115.

Shanon, B. (1980). Lateralization effects in musical decision tasks. *Neuropsychologia, 18,* 21–31.

Shanon, B. (1981). Classification of musical information presented to the right and left ear. *Cortex, 17,* 583–596.

Shanon, B. (1984). Asymmetries in musical aesthetic judgments. *Cortex, 20,* 567–573.

Shapiro, A.M., Benedict, R.H., Schretlen, D., & Brandt, J. (1999). Construct and concurrent validity of the Hopkins Verbal Learning Test–Revised. *The Clinical Neuropsychologist, 13,* 348–358.

Shapiro, A.P., Miller, R.E., King, H.E., et al. (1982). Behavioral consequences of mild hypertension. *Hypertension, 4,* 355–360.

Shapiro, B.E. & Danly, M. (1985). The role of the right hemisphere in the control of speech prosody in positional and affective contents. *Brain and Language, 25,* 19–36.

Shapiro, B.E., Grossman, M., & Gardner, H. (1981). Selective musical processing deficits in brain damaged populations. *Neuropsychologia, 19,* 161–169.

Shapiro, I.M., Cornblath, D.R., Sumner, A.J., et al. (1982). Neurophysiological and neuropsychological function in mercury-exposed dentists. *Lancet, i,* 1147–1150.

Shapiro, M.B. (1951). An experimental approach to diagnostic psychological testing. *Journal of Mental Science, 97,* 748–764.

Sharief, M.K. & Swash, M. (1998). Viral infections of the nervous system. In M. Swash (Ed.), *Outcomes in neurological and neurosurgical disorders.* Cambridge: Cambridge University Press.

Sharif, S., Roberts, G., & Phillips, J. (2000). Transnasal penetrating brain injury with a ball-pen. *British Journal of Neurosurgery, 14,* 159–160.

Sharma, B.P. (1975). Cannabis and its users in Nepal. *British Journal of Psychiatry, 127,* 550–552.

Sharrack, B., Hughes, R.A.C., Soudain, S., & Dunn, G. (1999). The psychometric properties of clinical rating scales used in multiple sclerosis. *Brain, 122,* 141–159.

Shatz, M.W. (1981). WAIS practice effects in clinical neuropsychology. *Journal of Clinical Neuropsychology, 3,* 171–191.

Shavelle, R.M., Strauss, D., Whyte, J., et al. (2001). Long-term causes of death after traumatic brain injury. *American Journal of Physical Medicine and Rehabilitation, 80,* 510–516.

Shaw, G.J., Jauch, E.C., & Zemlan, F.P. (2002). Serum cleaved tau protein levels and clinical outcome in adult patients with closed head injury. *Annals of Emergency Medicine, 39,* 254–257.

Shay, K.A., Kuke, L.W., Conboy, T., et al. (1991). The clinical validity of the Mattis Dementia Rating Scale in staging Alzheimer's dementia. *Journal of Geriatric Psychiatry and Neurology, 4,* 18–25.

Shaywitz, B.A., Shaywitz, S.E., Pugh, K.R., et al. (1995). Sex differences in the functional organization of the brain for language. *Nature, 373,* 607–609.

Shear, P.K., Wells, C.T., & Brock, M.A. (2000). The effect of semantic cuing on CVLT performance in healthy participants. *Journal of Clinical and Experimental Neuropsychology, 22,* 649–655.

Sheer, D.E. (1956). Psychometric studies. In N.D.C. Lewis et al. (Eds.), *Studies in topectomy.* New York: Grune & Stratton.

Sheikh, J.I. & Yesavage, J. A. (1986). Geriatric Depression Scale (GDS): Recent evidence and development of a shorter version. In *Clinical gerontology: A guide to assessment and intervention.* New York: Haworth Press.

Shelton, J.R. & Caramazza, A. (2001). The organization of semantic memory. In B. Rapp (Eds.), *The handbook of cognitive neuropsychology. What deficits reveal about the human mind.* Philadephia: Psychology Press.

Shelton, J.R., Martin, R.C., & Yaffee, L.S. (1992). Investigating a verbal short-term memory deficit and its consequences for language processing. In D.I. Margolin (Ed.), *Cognitive neuropsychology in clinical practice.* New York: Oxford University Press.

Shelton, M.D., Parsons, O.A., & Leber, W.R. (1982). Verbal and visuospatial performance and aging: A neuropsychological approach. *Journal of Gerontology, 37,* 336–341.

Shelton, M.D., Parsons, O.A., & Leber, W.R. (1984). Verbal and visuospatial performance in male alcoholics: A test of the premature-aging hypothesis. *Journal of Consulting and Clinical Psychology, 52,* 200–206.

Shepard, I. & Leathem, J. (1999). Factors affecting performance in cross-cultural neuropsychology: From a New Zealand perspective. *Journal of the International Neuropsychological Society, 5,* 83–84.

Shepherd, G.M. (1994). *Neurobiology* (3rd ed.). New York: Oxford University Press.

Shepherd, G.M. (Ed.). (1998). *The synaptic organization of the brain* (4th ed.). New York: Oxford University Press.

Shepherd, G.M. & Greer, C.A. (1998). Olfactory bulb. In G.M. Shepherd, (Ed.), *The synaptic organization of the brain* (4th ed.). New York: Oxford University Press.

Shepherd, G.M. & Koch, C. (1998). Introduction to synaptic circuits. In G.M. Shepherd (Ed.) *The synaptic organization of the brain* (4th ed.). New York: Oxford University Press.

Sherer, M. & Adams, R. L. (1993). Cross-validation of Reitan and Wolfson's Neuropsychological Deficit Scales. *Archives of Clinical Neuropsychology, 8,* 429–435.

Sherer, M., Bergloff, P., Levin, E., et al. (1998). Impaired awareness and employment outcome after traumatic brain injury. *Journal of Head Trauma Rehabilitation, 13,* 52–61.

Sherer, M. & Novack, T.A. (2003). Neuropsychological assessment after brain injury in adults. In G.P. Prigatano & N.H. Pliskin (Eds.), *Clinical neuropsychology and cost outcome research: A beginning.* New York: Psychology Press.

Sherer, M., Scott, J.G., Parsons, O.A., & Adams, R.L. (1994). Relative sensitivity of the WAIS-R subtests and selected HRNB measures to the effects of brain damage. *Archives of Clinical Neuropsychology, 9,* 427–436.

Sherman, D.G. & Lalonde, D. (1997). Anticoagulants in stroke treatment. In K.M.A. Welch et al. (Eds.), *Primer on cerebrovascular diseases.* San Diego: Academic Press.

Sherman, E.M.S., Strauss, E., Slick, D.J., & Spellacy, F. (2000). Effect of depression on neuropsychological functioning in head injury; measureable but minimal. *Brain Injury, 14,* 621–632.

Sherman, E.M.S., Strauss, E., & Spellacy, F. (1997). Validity of the Paced Auditory Serial Addition Test (PASAT) in adults referred for neuropsychological assessment after head injury. *The Clinical Neuropsychologist, 11,* 34–45.

Sherman, S.M. & Koch, C. (1998). Thalamus. In G.M. Shepherd (Ed.), *The synaptic organization of the brain.* New York: Oxford University Press.

Sherrill, R.E., Jr. (1985). Comparison of three short forms of the Category Test. *Journal of Clinical and Experimental Neuropsychology, 7,* 231–238.

Sherrill, R.E., Jr. (1987). Options for shortening Halstead's Category Test for adults. *Archives of Clinical Neuropsychology, 2,* 343–352.

Sherrington, C. (1955). *Man on his nature* (2nd ed.). Garden City, NY: Doubleday.

Shiffrin, R.M. & Schneider, W. (1977). Controlled and automatic human information processing: II. Perceptual learning, automatic attending, and a general theory. *Psychological Review, 84,* 127–188.

Shimamura, A.P. (1989). Disorders of memory: The cognitive science perspective. In F. Boller & J. Grafman (Eds.), *Handbook of neuropsychology* (Vol. 3). Amsterdam: Elsevier.

Shimamura, A.P. (2002). Memory retrieval and executive control processes. In D.T. Stuss & R.T. Knight (Eds.), *Principles of frontal lobe function.* New York: Oxford University Press.

Shimamura, A.P., Janowsky, J.S., & Squire, L.R. (1990). Memory for the temporal order of events in patients with frontal lobe lesions and amnesic patients. *Neuropsychologia, 28,* 803–813.

Shimamura, A.P., Janowsky, J.S., & Squire, L.R. (1991). What is the role of frontal lobe damage in memory disorders? In H. S. Levin et al. (Eds.), *Frontal lobe function and dysfunction.* New York: Oxford University Press.

Shimamura, A.P. & Jurica, P.J. (1994). Memory interference effects and aging: Findings from a test of frontal lobe function. *Neuropsychology, 8,* 408–412.

Shimamura, A.P., Salmon, D.P., Squire, L.R., & Butters, N. (1987). Memory dysfunction and word priming in dementia and amnesia. *Behavioral Neuroscience, 101,* 347–351.

Shimamura, A.P. & Squire, L.R. (1987). A neuropsychological study of fact memory and source amnesia. *Journal of Experimental Psychology: Learning, Memory, and Cognition, 13,* 464–473.

Shimizu, T., Nariai, T., Maehara, T., et al. (2000). Enhanced motor cortical excitability in the unaffected hemisphere after hemispherectomy. *Neuroreport, 11,* 3077–3084.

Shimoda, K. & Robinson, R.G. (1999). The relationship between poststroke depression and lesion location in long-term follow-up. *Biological Psychiatry, 45,* 187–192.

Shimonaka, Y. & Nakazato, K. (1991). Aging and terminal changes in Rorschach responses among the Japanese elderly. *Journal of Personality Assessment, 57,* 10–18.

Shimoyama, T., Keneko, T., Nasu, D., et al. (1999). A case of an electrical burn in the oral cavity of an adult. *Journal of Oral Science, 41,* 127–128.

Shin, D.C. & Johnson, D.M. (1978). Avowed happiness as an overall assessment of the quality of life. *Social Indicators Research, 5,* 475–492.

Shinedling, M.M., Shinedling, T., & Smith, A. (1990). Performance on neuropsychological tests amenable to patient manipulation in suing and non-suing closed-head-injury patients [abstract]. *Journal of Clinical and Experimental Neuropsychology, 12,* 393.

Shinkawa, A., Ueda, K., Kiyohara, Y., et al. (1995). Silent cerebral infarction in a community-based autopsy series in Japan. The Hisayama Study. *Stroke, 26,* 380–385.

Shipley, W.C. (1940). A self-administered scale for measuring intellectual impairment and deterioration. *Journal of Psychology, 9,* 371–377.

Shipley, W.C. (1946). *Institute of Living Scale.* Los Angeles: Western Psychological Services.

Shipley, W.C. & Burlingame, C.C. (1941). A convenient self-administered scale for measuring intellectual impairment in psychotics. *American Journal of Psychiatry, 97,* 1313–1325.

Shnek, Z.M., Foley, F.W., LaRocca, N.G., et al. (1995). Psychological predictors of depression in multiple sclerosis. *Journal of Neurologic Rehabilitation, 9,* 15–23.

Shores, E.A. (1989). Comparison of Westmead PTA Scale and Glasgow Coma Scale as predictors of neuropsychological outcome following extremely severe blunt head injury. *Journal of Neurology, Neurosurgery and Psychiatry, 52,* 126–127.

Shores, E.A., Marosszeky, J.E., Sandanam, J., & Batchelor, J. (1986). Preliminary validation of a clinical scale for measuring the duration of post-traumatic amnesia. *Medical Journal of Australia, 144,* 569–572.

Shorr, J.S., Delis, D.C., & Massman, P.J. (1992). Memory for the Rey-Osterrieth Figure: Perceptual clustering, encoding, and storage. *Neuropsychology, 6,* 43–50.

Shukla, S., Cook, B.L., Mukherhee, S., et al. (1987). Mania following head trauma. *American Journal of Psychiatry, 144,* 93–96.

Shulman, K.I. (2000). Clock-drawing: Is it the ideal cognitive screening test? *International Journal of Geriatric Psychiatry, 15,* 548–561.

Shulman, K.I., Gold, D.P., Cohen, C.A., & Zucchero, C.A. (1993). Clock drawing and dementia in the community. A longitudinal study. *International Journal of Geriatric Psychiatry, 8,* 487–496.

Shulman, K.I., Sheldetsky, R., & Silver, I. (1986). The challenge of time: Clock-drawing and cognitive function in the elderly. *International Journal of Geriatric Psychiatry, 1,* 135–140.

Shum, D.H.K., Harris, D., & O'Gorman, J.G. (2000). Effects of severe traumatic brain injury on visual memory. *Journal of Clinical and Experimental Neuropsychology, 22,* 25–39.

Shum, D.H.K., McFarland, K.A., & Bain, J.D. (1990). Construct validity of eight tests of attention: Comparison of normal and closed head injured samples. *The Clinical Neuropsychologist, 4,* 151–162.

Shum, D.H., McFarland, K., & Bain, J.D. (1994). Assessment of attention: Relationship between psychological testing and information processing approaches. *Journal of Clinical and Experimental Neuropsychology, 16,* 531–538.

Shum, D.H.K., Murray, R.A., & Eadie, K. (1997). Effect of speed of presentation on administration of the Logical Memory subtest of the Wechsler Memory Scale–Revised. *The Clinical Neuropsychologist, 11,* 188–191.

Shum, D.H.K., O'Gorman, J.G., & Eadie, K. (1999). Normative data for a new memory test: The Shum Visual Learning Test. *The Clinical Neuropsychologist, 13,* 121–135.

Shure, G.H. & Halstead, W.C. (1958). Cerebral localization of intellectual processes. *Psychology Monograph, 72,* No. 12 (Whole No. 465).

Shuttleworth-Jordan, A.B. (1997). Age and education effects on brain-damaged subjects: "Negative" findings revisited. *The Clinical Neuropsychologist, 11,* 205–209.

Shuttleworth-Jordan, A.B. & Bode, S.G. (1995). Taking account of age-related differences on Digit Symbol and Incidental Recall for diagnostic purposes. *Journal of Clinical and Experimental Neuropsychology, 17,* 439–448.

Sickness Impact Profile. Manual (1977). Seattle: Department of Health Services (SC-37), University of Washington.

Sickness Impact Profile. A brief summary of its purpose, uses, and administration. (1978). Seattle: Department of Health Services (SC-37), University of Washington.

Sidtis, J.J. & Price, R.W. (1990). Early HIV-1 infection and the AIDS dementia complex. *Neurology, 40,* 323–326.

Siegel, B.V., Jr., Shihabuddin, L., Buchsbaum, M.S., et al. (1996). Gender differences in cortical glucose metabolism in Alzheimer's disease and normal aging. *Journal of Neuropsychiatry and Clinical Neurosciences, 8,* 211–214.

Siegel, S. (1956). *Nonparametric statistics for the behavioral sciences.* New York: McGraw-Hill.

Siegel-Hinson, R. (2000). Laterality of mental rotation processing and its application to standardized tests of mental rotation. *Dissertation Abstracts International. Section B, Sciences and Engineering, 61,* 6-B. (University Microfilms ATT9979240.)

Siegler, I.C., McCarty, S.M., & Logue, P.E. (1982). Wechsler Memory Scale scores, selective attrition, and distance from death. *Journal of Gerontology, 37,* 176–181.

Siesling, S. van Vugt, J. P., Zwinderman, K. A., et al. (1998). Unified Huntington's Disease Rating Scale: A follow-up. *Movement Disorders, 13,* 915–919.

Siesling, S., Zwinderman, A.H., van Vugt, J.P., et al. (1997). A shortened version of the motor section of the Unified Huntington's Disease Rating Scale. *Movement Disorders, 12,* 229–234.

Signoret, J.L. (1979). *Batterie d'Efficience Mnésique BEM 144.* Unpublished test battery. Paris: La Salpetrière.

Silberstein, S.D. (1992). The role of sex in hormones in headache. *Neurology, 42(Suppl. 2),* 37–42.

Silberstein, S.D. (2001). Shared mechanisms and co-morbidities in neurologic and psychiatric disorders. *Headache,* S11–S17.

Silberstein, S.D. & Lipton, R.B. (1994). Overview of diagnosis and treatment of migraine. *Neurology, 44(Suppl. 7),* S6–S16.

Silberstein, S.D., Lipton, R.B., & Breslau, N. (1995). Migraine: Association with personality characteristics and psychopathology. *Cephalalgia, 15,* 358–369.

Silberstein, S.D., Lipton, R.B., & Breslau, N. (2002). Neuropsychiatric aspects of primary headache disorders. In S.C. Yudofsky & R.E. Hales (Eds.), *American Psychiatric Publishing textbook of neuropsychiatry and clinical neurosciences* (4th ed.). Washington, D.C.

Silver, J.M., Hales, R.E., & Yudofsky, S.C. (2002). Neuropsychiatric aspects of traumatic brain injury. In S.C. Yudofsky & R.E. Hales (Eds.), *American Psychiatric Press textbook of neuropsychiatry and clinical neurosciences* (3rd ed.). Washington, D.C.: American Psychiatric Press.

Silver, M.H. & Perls, T.T. (2000). Is dementia the price of a long life? An optimistic report from centenarians. *Journal of Geriatric Psychiatry, 33,* 71–79.

Silverman, I.E., Restrepo, L., & Mathews, G. C. (2002). Poststroke seizures. *Archives of Neurology, 59,* 195–201.

Silverstein, A.B. (1962). Perceptual, motor, and memory functions in the Visual Retention Test. *American Journal of Mental Deficiency, 66,* 613–617.

Silverstein, A.B. (1982). Pattern analysis as simultaneous statistical inference. *Journal of Consulting and Clinical Psychology, 50,* 234–249.

Silverstein, A.B. (1984). Pattern analysis: The question of abnormality. *Journal of Consulting and Clinical Psychology, 42,* 936–939.

Silverstein, A.B. (1985). Two- and four-subtest short forms of the WAIS-R: A closer look at validity and reliability. *Journal of Clinical Psychology, 41*, 95–97.

Silverstein, A.B. (1987). Accuracy of estimates of premorbid intelligence based on demographic variables. *Journal of Clinical Psychology, 43*, 493–495.

Silverstein, A.B. (1988). Estimated vs. empirical values of scaled-score ranges on Wechsler's Intelligence Scales: A correction. *Journal of Clinical Psychology, 44*, 259–261.

Silverstein, A.B. (1991). Reliability of score differences on Wechsler's intelligence scales. *Journal of Clinical Psychology, 47*, 264–266.

Simkins-Bullock, J. (2000). Beyond speech lateralization: A review of the variability, reliability, and validity of the intracarotid amobarbital procedure and its nonlanguage uses in epilepsy surgery candidates. *Neuropsychology Review, 10*, 41–74.

Simon, R.P. (1999). Hypoxia versus ischemia. *Neurology, 52*, 7–8.

Simons, J.S., Verfaellie, M., Galton, C.J., et al. (2002). Recollection-based memory in frontotemporal dementia: Implications for theories of long-term memory. *Brain, 125*, 2523–2536.

Simos, P.G., Breier, J.I., Maggio, W.W., et al. (1999). Atypical temporal lobe language representation: Meg and intraoperative stimulation mapping correlation. *Neuroreport, 10*, 139–142.

Simos, P.G., Castillo, E.M., Fletcher, J.M., et al. (2001). Mapping of receptive language cortex in bilingual volunteers by using magnetic source imaging. *Journal of Neurosurgery, 95*, 76–81.

Simpson, G., Mohr, R., & Redman, A. (2000). Cultural variations in the understanding of traumatic brain injury and brain injury rehabilitation. *Brain Injury, 14*, 125–140.

Sines, J.O. (1966). Actuarial methods and personality assessment. In B.A. Maher (Ed.), *Progress in experimental personality research*. New York: Academic Press.

Sinforiani, E., Farina, S., Mancuso, A., et al. (1987). Analysis of higher nervous functions in migraine and cluster headaches. *Functional Neurology, 2*, 69–77.

Singer, L.T. & Zeskind, P.S. (2001). *Biobehavioral assessment of the infant*. New York: Guilford Press.

Singer, R. & Scott, N.E. (1987). Progression of neuropsychological deficits following toluene diisocyanate exposure. *Archives of Clinical Neuropsychology, 2*, 135–144.

Singh, A., Black, S.E., Herrmann, N., et al. (2000). Functional and neuroanatomic correlations in poststroke depression: The Sunnybrook Stroke Study. *Stroke, 31*, 637–644.

Sinnett, E.R. & Holen, M.C. (1999). Assessment of memory functioning among an aging sample. *Psychological Reports, 84*, 339–350.

Sipps, G.J., Berry, G.W., & Lynch, E.M. (1987). WAIS-R and social intelligence: A test of established assumptions that uses the CPI. *Journal of Clinical Psychology, 43*, 499–504.

Sirigu, A., Zalla, T., Pillon, B., et al. (1995). Selective impairments in managerial knowledge following pre-frontal cortex damage. *Cortex, 31*, 301–316.

Sittinger, H., Muller, M., Schweizer, I., & Merkelbach, S. (2002). Mild cognitive impairment after viral meningitis in adults. *Journal of Neurology, 249*, 554–560.

Sivak, M., Olson, P.L., Kewman, D.G., et al. (1981). Driving and perceptual/cognitive skills: Behavioral consequences of brain damage. *Archives of Physical and Medical Rehabilitation, 62*, 476–483.

Sivan, A.B. (1992). *Benton Visual Retention Test* (5th ed.). San Antonio, TX: The Psychological Corporation.

Sivan, A.B. & Benton, A.L. (1999). Cognitive disabilities, diagnosis. In G. Adelman & B.H. Smith (Eds.), *Encyclopedia of neuroscience* (2nd ed.) Amsterdam: Elsevier.

Sjøgren, P., Olsen, A.K., Thomsen, A.B., & Dalberg, J. (2000). Neuropsychological performance in cancer patients: The role of oral opioids, pain and performance status. *Pain, 86*, 237–245.

Sjøgren, P., Thomsen, A.B., & Olsen, A.K. (2000). Impaired neuropsychological performance in chronic nonmalignant pain patients receiving long-term oral opioid therapy. *Journal of Pain and Symptom Management, 19*, 100–108.

Sjøgren, T., Sjøgren, H., & Lindgren, A.G.H. (1952). Morbus Alzheimer and morbus Pick. *Acta Psychiatrica et Neurologica Scandinavica (Suppl. 82)*, 1–152.

Ska, B., Dehaut, F., & Nespoulous, J.-L. (1987). Dessin d'une figure complexe par des sujets agés. *Psychologica Belgica, 27*, 25–42.

Ska, B., Désilets, H., & Nespoulous, J.-L. (1986). Performances visuoconstructive et vieillissement. *Psychologica Belgica, 26*, 125–145.

Ska, B., Martin, G., & Nespoulous, J-L. (1988). Image du corps et vieillissement normal: Représentation graphique et verbale. *Canadian Journal of Behavioral Science/Revue Canadienne de la Science de Comportement, 20*, 121–132.

Ska, B., Montellier, M., & Nespoulous, J.-L. (1991). Communication et vieillissement normal. In M. Habib et al. (Eds.), *Démences et syndromes démentials. Approche neuropsychologique*. Paris: Masson.

Ska, B. & Nespoulous, J.-L. (1986). Destructuration des praxies chez le sujet age normal. *Cahiers Scientifiques, 46*, 173–199.

Ska, B. & Nespoulous, J. (1987). Pantomimes and aging. *Journal of Clinical and Experimental Neuropsychology, 9*, 754–766.

Ska, B. & Nespoulous, J.-L. (1988a). Encoding strategies and recall performance of a complex figure by normal elderly subjects. *Canadian Journal on Aging, 7*, 408–418.

Ska, B. & Nespoulous, J.-L. (1988b). Gestural praxes and normal aging [abstract]. *Journal of Clinical and Experimental Neuropsychology, 10*, 316.

Ska, B., Poissant, A., & Joanette, Y. (1990). Line orientation judgment in normal elderly and subjects with dementia of Alzheimer's type. *Journal of Clinical and Experimental Neuropsychology, 12*, 695–702.

Skegg, K. (1993). Multiple sclerosis presenting as a pure psychiatric disorder. *Psychological Medicine, 23*, 909–914.

Skelton, R.W., Bukach, C.M., Laurance, H.E., et al. (2000). Humans with traumatic brain injuries show place-learning deficits in computer-generated virtual space. *Journal of Clinical and Experimental Neuropsychology, 22*, 157–175.

Skloot, F. (2003). *In the shadow of memory*. Lincoln, NE: University of Nebraska Press.

Skoog, I. & Blennow, K. (2001). Alzheimer's disease. In A. Hofman & R. Mayeux (Eds.), *Investigating neurological disease. Epidemiology for clinical neurology*. Cambridge, UK: Cambridge University Press.

Skoog, I., Lernfelt, B., Landahl, S., et al. (1996). 15-year longitudinal study of blood pressure and dementia. *Lancet, 347*, 1141–1145.

Skoraszewski, M.J., Ball, J.D., & Mikulka, P. (1991). Neuropsychological functioning of HIV-infected males. *Journal of Clinical and Experimental Neuropsychology, 13*, 278–290.

Skuster, D.Z., Digre, K.B., & Corbett, J.J. (1992). Neurologic conditions presenting as psychiatric disorders. *Psychiatric Clinics of North America, 15*, 311–333.

Slaughter, J., Johnstone, G., Petroski, G., & Flax, J. (1999). The usefulness of the brief symptom inventory in the neuropsychological evaluation of traumatic brain injury. *Brain Injury, 13*, 125–130.

Slick, D., Hopp, G., Strauss, E., & Thompson, G.B. (1997). *Victoria Symptom Validity Test*. Odessa, FL: Psychological Assessment Resources.

Slick, D.J., Hopp, G., Strauss, E., & Spellacy, F.J. (1996). Victoria Symptom Validity Test: Efficiency for detecting feigned memory impairment and relationship to neuropsychological tests and MMPI-2 validity scales. *Journal of Clinical and Experimental Neuropsychology, 18*, 911–922.

Slick, D.J., Iverson, G.L., & Green, P. (2000). California Verbal

Learning Test indicators of suboptimal performance in a sample of head injury litigants. *Journal of Clinical and Experimental Neuropsychology, 22,* 569–579.

Slick, D.J., Sherman, E.M., & Iverson, G.L. (1999). Diagnostic criteria for malingered neurocognitive dysfunction: Proposed standards for clinical practice and research. *The Clinical Neuropsychologist, 13,* 545–561.

Sliwinski, M., Buschke, H., Stewart, W.F., et al. (1997). The effect of dementia risk factors on comparative and diagnostic Selective Reminding norms. *Journal of the International Neuropsychological Society, 3,* 317–326.

Sloan, E.P., Zalenski, R.J., Smith, R.F., et al. (1989). Toxicology screening in urban trauma patients: Drug prevalence and its relationship to trauma severity and management. *Journal of Trauma, 29,* 1647–1653.

Sloan, M.A. (1997). Toxicity/substance abuse. In K.M.A. Welch et al. (Eds.), *Primer on cerebrovascular diseases.* San Diego: Academic Press.

Sloan, S. & Ponsford, J. (1995). Assessment of cognitive difficulties following TBI. In J. Ponsford (Ed.), *Traumatic brain injury. Rehabilitation for everyday adaptive living.* Hillsdale, NJ: Erlbaum.

Small, B.J., Fratiglioni, L., & Viitanen, M. (2000). The course of cognitive impairment in preclinical Alzheimer disease: Three- and 6-year follow-up of a population-based sample. *Archives of Neurology, 57,* 839–844.

Small, B.J., Herlitz, A., Fratiglioni, L., et al. (1997). Cognitive predictors of incident Alzheimer's disease: A prospective longitudinal study. *Neuropsychology, 11,* 413–420.

Small, B.J., Viitanen, M., Winblad, B., & Backman, L. (1997). Cognitive changes in very old persons with dementia: The influence of demographic, psychometric, and biological variables. *Journal of Clinical and Experimental Neuropsychology, 19,* 245–260.

Small, G.W., La Rue, A., Komo, S., et al. (1995). Predictors of cognitive change in middle-aged and older adults with memory loss. *American Journal of Psychiatry, 152,* 1757–1764.

Small, G.W., Rabins, P.V., Barry, P.P., et al. (1997). Diagnosis and treatment of Alzheimer disease and related disorders. Consensus statement of the American Association for Geriatric Psychiatry, the Alzheimer's Association, and the American Geriatrics Society. *Journal of the American Medical Association, 278,* 1363–1371.

Small, I.F., Heimburger, R.F., Small, J.G., et al. (1977). Follow-up of stereotaxic amygdalotomy for seizure and behavior disorders. *Biological Psychiatry, 12,* 401–411.

Small, J.A., Kemper, S., & Lyons, K. (2000). Sentence repetition and processing resources in Alzheimer's disease. *Brain and Language, 75,* 232–258.

Smirni, P., Villardita, G., & Zappala, G. (1983). Influence of different paths on spatial memory performance in the Block Tapping Test. *Journal of Clinical Neuropsychology, 5,* 355–360.

Smith, A. (1960). Changes in Porteus Maze scores of brain-operated schizophrenics after an eight-year interval. *Journal of Mental Science, 106,* 967–978.

Smith, A. (1962a). Ambiguities in concepts and studies of "brain damage" and "organicity." *Journal of Nervous and Mental Disease, 135,* 311–326.

Smith, A. (1962b). Psychodiagnosis of patients with brain tumors. *Journal of Nervous and Mental Disease, 135,* 513–533.

Smith, A. (1966). Intellectual functions in patients with lateralized frontal tumors. *Journal of Neurology, Neurosurgery and Psychiatry, 29,* 52–59.

Smith, A. (1967). The Serial Sevens Subtraction Test. *Archives of Neurology, 17,* 78–80.

Smith, A. (1975). Neuropsychological testing in neurological disorders. In W.J. Friedlander (Ed.), *Advances in neurology* (Vol. 7). New York: Raven Press.

Smith, A. (1979). Practices and principles of neuropsychology. *International Journal of Neuroscience, 9,* 233–238.

Smith, A. (1980). Principles underlying human brain functions in neuropsychological sequelae of different neuropathological processes. In S.B. Filskov & T.J. Boll (Eds.), *Handbook of clinical neuropsychology.* New York: Wiley-Interscience.

Smith, A. (1982). *Symbol Digit Modalities Test (SDMT). Manual* (revised). Los Angeles: Western Psychological Services.

Smith, A. (1983). Clinical psychological practice and principles of neuropsychological assessment. In C.E. Walker (Ed.), *Handbook of clinical psychology: Theory, research and practice.* Homewood, IL: Dorsey Press.

Smith, A. (1984). Early and long-term recovery from brain damage in children and adults: Evolution of concepts of localization, plasticity, and recovery. In C.R. Almli & S. Finger (Eds.), *Early brain damage* (Vol. 1). New York: Academic Press.

Smith, A. (1993). Critical considerations in neuropsychological assessments of closed head (CHI) and traumatic brain (TBI) injury. In C.N. Simkins (Ed.), *Analysis, understanding, and presentation of cases involving traumatic brain injury.* Southborough, MA: National Head Injury Foundation.

Smith, A. (1997). Development and course of receptive and expressive vocabulary from infancy to old age: Administrations of the Peabody Picture Vocabulary Test, Third Edition, and the Expressive Vocabulary Test to the same standardization population of 2725 subjects. *International Journal of Neuroscience, 92,* 73–78.

Smith, A. & Kinder, E. (1959). Changes in psychological test performance of brain-operated schizophrenics after eight years. *Science, 129,* 149–150.

Smith, B.D., Meyers, M.B., & Kline, R. (1989). For better or for worse: Left-handedness, pathology, and talent. *Journal of Clinical and Experimental Neuropsychology, 11,* 944–958.

Smith, D. & Over, R. (1987). Correlates of fantasy-induced and film-induced male sexual arousal. *Archives of Sexual Behavior, 16,* 395–409.

Smith, D.B., Craft, B.R., Collins, J., et al. (1986). Behavioral characteristics of epilepsy patients compared with normal controls. *Epilepsia, 27,* 760–768.

Smith, G., Ivnik, R., Malec, J., & Kokmen, E. (1994). Psychometric properties of the Mattis Dementia Rating Scale. *Assessment, 1,* 123–131.

Smith, G.E., Malec, J.F., & Ivnik, R.J. (1992). Validity of the construct of nonverbal memory: A factor-analytic study in a normal elderly sample. *Journal of Clinical and Experimental Neuropsychology, 14,* 211–221.

Smith, G.E., Wong, J.S., Ivnik, R.J., & Malec, J.F. (1997). Mayo's Older American Normative Studies: Separate norms for WMS-R Logical Memory stories. *Assessment, 4,* 79–86.

Smith, J.R., Brooks-Gunn, J., Kohen, D., & McCarton, C. (2001). Transitions on and off AFDC: Implications for parenting and children's cognitive development. *Child Development, 72,* 1512–1533.

Smith, J.S., Perry, A., Borell, T.J., et al. (2000). Alterations of chromosome arms 1p and 19q as predictors of survival in oligodendrogliomas, astrocytomas, and mixed oligoastrocytomas. *Journal of Clinical Oncology, 18,* 636–645.

Smith, L.M. & Godfrey, H.P.D. (1995). *Family support programs and rehabilitation. A cognitive-behavioral approach to traumatic brain injury.* New York: Plenum Press.

Smith, M.L. (1989). Memory disorders associated with temporal-lobe lesions. In F. Boller & J. Grafman (Eds.), *Handbook of neuropsychology* (Vol. 3). Amsterdam: Elsevier.

Smith, M.L. & Milner, B. (1984). Differential effects of frontal-lobe lesions on cognitive estimation and spatial memory. *Neuropsychologia, 22,* 697–705.

Smith, M.L. & Milner, B. (1988). Estimation of frequency of occurrence of abstract designs after frontal or temporal lobectomy. *Neuropsychologia, 26,* 297–306.

Smith, M.S. & Godfrey, H.P.D. (1995). *Family support programs and rehabilitation. A cognitive-behavioral approach to traumatic brain injury.* New York: Plenum Press.

Smith, P., Langolf, G.D., & Goldberg, J. (1983). Effects of occupational exposure to elemental mercury on short-term memory. *British Journal of Industrial Medicine, 40,* 413–419.

Smith, P.F. & Darlington, C.L. (1996). *Clinical psychopharmacology. A primer.* Mahwah, NJ: Erlbaum.

Smith, R.L., Goode, K.T., LaMarche, J.A., & Boll, T.A. (1995). Selective Reminding Test short form administration: A comparison of two through twelve trials. *Psychological Assessment, 7,* 177–182.

Smith, Y.R. & Zubieta, J.K. (2001). Neuroimaging of aging and estrogen effects on central nervous system physiology. *Fertility and Sterility, 76,* 651–659.

Smith-Knapp, K., Corrigan, J.D., & Arnett, J.A. (1996). Predicting functional independence from neuropsychological tests following traumatic brain injury. *Brain Injury, 10,* 651–661.

Smith-Seemiller, L., Franzen, M.D., & Bowers, D. (1997). Use of Wisconsin Card Sorting Test short forms in clinical samples. *The Clinical Neuropsychologist, 11,* 421–427.

Smits, C.H., Smit, J.H., van den Heuvel, N., & Jonker, C. (1997). Norms for an abbreviated Raven's Coloured Progressive Matrices in an older sample. *Journal of Clinical Psychology, 53,* 687–697.

Smutok, M.A., Grafman, J., Salazar, A.M., et al. (1989). The effects of unilateral brain damage on contralateral and ipsilateral upper extremity function in hemiplegia. *Physical Therapy, 69,* 195–203.

Snitz, B.E., Roman, D.D., & Beniak, T.E. (1996). Efficacy of the Continuous Visual Memory Test in lateralizing temporal lobe dysfunction in chronic complex-partial epilepsy. *Journal of Clinical and Experimental Neuropsychology, 18,* 747–754.

Snodgrass, J.G. & Vanderwart, M. (1980). A standardized set of 260 pictures: Norms for name agreement, image agreement, familiarity, and visual complexity. *Journal of Experimental Psychology: Human Learning and Memory, 6,* 174–215.

Snoek, J.S., Minderhoud, J.M., & Wilmink, J.T. (1984). Delayed deterioration following mild head injury in children. *Brain, 107,* 15–36.

Snow, P., Douglas, J., & Ponsford, J. (1998). Conversational discourse abilities following severe traumatic brain injury: A follow-up study. *Brain Injury, 12,* 911–935.

Snow, W.G. (1985). Can you tell me where I can buy the Halstead-Reitan Test Battery? *Ontario Psychologist, 17,* 4–5.

Snow, W.G. (1987a). Aphasia Screening Test performance in patients with lateralized brain damage. *Journal of Clinical Psychology, 43,* 266–271.

Snow, W.G. (1987b). Standardization of test administration and scoring criteria: Some shortcomings of current practice with the Halstead-Reitan Test Battery. *The Clinical Neuropsychologist, 1,* 250–262.

Snow, W.G. & Sheese, S. (1985). Lateralized brain damage, intelligence, and memory: A failure to find sex differences. *Journal of Clinical and Consulting Psychology, 53,* 940–941.

Snow, W.G., Tierney, M.C., Zorzitto, M.L., et al. (1988). One-year test–retest reliability of selected neuropsychological tests in older adults [abstract]. *Journal of Clinical and Experimental Neuropsychology, 10,* 60.

Snow, W.G., Tierney, M.C., Zorzitto, M.L., et al. (1989). WAIS-R test–retest reliability in a normal elderly sample. *Journal of Clinical and Experimental Neuropsychology, 11,* 423–428.

Snow, W.G. & Weinstock, J. (1990). Sex differences among non-brain-damaged adults on the Wechsler Adult Intelligence Scales: A review of the literature. *Journal of Clinical and Experimental Neuropsychology, 12,* 873–886.

Snowden, J. (2002). Disorders of semantic memory. In A.D. Baddeley et al. (Eds.), *The handbook of memory disorders* (2nd ed.). Chichester, UK: Wiley.

Snowden, J.S., Craufurd, D., Griffiths, H.L., & Neary, D. (1998). Awareness of involuntary movements in Huntington disease. *Archives of Neurology, 55,* 801–805.

Snowden, J.S., Neary, D., Mann, D.M.A., & Benson, D.F. (1996). *Fronto-temporal lobar degeneration: Fronto-temporal dementia, progressive aphasia, and semantic dementia.* New York: Churchill Livingstone.

Snowdon, D.A. (1997). Aging and Alzheimer's disease: Lessons from the Nun Study. *Gerontologist, 37,* 150–156.

Snowdon, D.A., Kemper, S.J., Mortimer, J.A., et al. (1996). Linguistic ability in early life and cognitive function and Alzheimer's disease in late life. Findings from the Nun Study. *Journal of the American Medical Association, 275,* 528–532.

Snyder, P.J. & Cappelleri, J.C. (2001). Information processing speed deficits may be better correlated with the extent of white matter sclerotic lesions in multiple sclerosis than previously suspected. *Brain and Cognition, 46,* 279–284.

Snyder, P.J., Cappelleri, J.C., Archibald, C.J., & Fisk, J.D. (2001). Improved detection of differential information-processing speed deficits between two disease-course types of multiple sclerosis. *Neuropsychology, 15,* 617–625.

Snyder, P.J., Novelly, R.A., & Harris, L.J. (1990). Mixed speech dominance in the intracarotid sodium amytal procedure: Validity and criteria issues. *Journal of Clinical and Experimental Neuropsychology, 12,* 629–643.

Snyder, T.J. (1991). Self-rated right–left confusability and objectively measured right–left discrimination. *Developmental Neuropsychology, 7,* 219–230.

So, E.L. (2000). Integration of EEG, MRI, and SPECT in localizing the seizure focus for epilepsy surgery. *Epilepsia, 41,* S48–S54.

Sobel, D. (1999). *Galileo's daughter.* New York: Walker.

Sohlberg, M.M. & Mateer, C.A. (1989). *Introduction to cognitive remediation.* New York: Guilford Press.

Sohlberg, M.M. & Mateer, C.A. (1990). Evaluation and treatment of communicative skills. In J.S. Kreutzer & P. Wehman (Eds.), *Community integration following traumatic brain injury.* Baltimore: Brooks.

Sohlberg, M.M. & Mateer, C.A. (2001). *Cognitive rehabilitation. An integrative neuropsychological approach.* New York: Guilford Press.

Soininen, H.S., Partanen, K., Pitkänen, A., et al. (1994). Volumetric MRI analysis of the amygdala and the hippocampus in subjects with age-associated memory impairment: Correlation to visual and verbal memory. *Neurology, 44,* 1660–1668.

Sokoloff, L. (1997). Anatomy of cerebral circulation. In K.M.A. Welch et al. (Eds.), *Primer on cerebrovascular diseases.* San Diego: Academic Press.

Solfrizzi, V., Pana, F., Torres, F., et al. (1999). High monounsaturated fatty acids intake protects against age-related cognitive decline. *Neurology, 52,* 1563–1569.

Solomon, G.S., Petrie, W.M., Hart, J.R., & Brackin, H.B., Jr. (1998). Olfactory dysfunction discriminates Alzheimer's dementia from major depression. *Journal of Neuropsychiatry and Clinical Neurosciences, 10,* 64–67.

Solomon, P.R., Hirschoff, A., Kelly, B., et al. (1998). A 7 minute neurocognitive screening battery highly sensitive to Alzheimer's disease. *Archives of Neurology, 55,* 349–355.

Solomon, S. (1997). Diagnosis of primary headache disorders. Validity of the International Headache Society criteria in clinical practice. *Neurologic Clinics, 15,* 15–26.

Solomon, S., Hotchkiss, E., Saraway, S.M., et al. (1983). Impairment of memory function by antihypertensive medication. *Archives of General Psychiatry, 40,* 1109–1112.

Solowij, N. (1998). *Cannabis and cognitive functioning.* New York: Cambridge University Press.

Somerville, J., Tremont, G., & Stern, R.A. (2000). The Boston Qualitative Scoring System as a measure of executive functioning in Rey-Osterrieth Complex Figure performance. *Journal of Clinical and Experimental Neuropsychology, 22,* 613–621.

Sommerfield, A.J., Deary, I.J., McAulay, V., & Frier, B.M. (2003). Moderate hypoglycemia impairs multiple memory functions in healthy adults. *Neuropsychology, 17,* 125–132.

Soper, H.V., Cicchetti, D.V., Satz, P., et al. (1988). Null hypothesis disrespect in neuropsychology: Dangers of alpha and beta errors. *Journal of Clinical and Experimental Neuropsychology, 10,* 255–270.

Soper, H.V. & Satz, P. (1984). Pathological left-handedness and ambiguous handedness: A new explanatory model. *Neuropsychologia, 22,* 511–515.

Sorgato, P., Colombo, A., Scarpa, M., & Faglioni, P. (1990). Age, sex, and lesion site in aphasic stroke patients with single focal damage. *Neuropsychology, 4,* 165–173.

Sosin, D.M., Sniezek, J.E., & Thurman, D.J. (1996). Incidence of mild and moderate brain injury in the United States, 1991. *Brain Injury, 10,* 47–54.

Sosin, D.M., Sniezek, J.E., & Waxweiler, R.J. (1995). Trends in death associated with traumatic brain injury, 1979 through 1992. Success and failure. *Journal of the American Medical Association, 273,* 1778–1780.

Soukup, V.M., Ingram, F., Grady, J.J., & Schiess, M.C. (1998). Trail Making Test: Issues in normative data selection. *Applied Neuropsychology, 5,* 65–73.

Soukup, V.M., Ingram, F., Schiess, M.C., et al. (1997). Cognitive sequelae of unilateral posteroventral pallidotomy. *Archives of Neurology, 54,* 947–950.

Soustiel, J.F., Hafner, H., Guilburd, J.N., et al. (1993). A physiological coma scale: Grading a coma by combined use of brainstem trigeminal and auditory evoked potentials and the Glasgow Coma Scale. *Electroencephalography and Clinical Neurophysiology, 87,* 277–283.

South, M., Greve, K.W., Bianchini, K.J., & Adams, D. (2001). Interrater reliability of three clock drawing test scoring systems. *Applied Neuropsychology, 8,* 174–179.

Sox, H.C., Jr., Blatt, M.A., Higgins, M.C., & Marton, K.I. (1988). *Medical decision making.* Boston: Butterworth.

Spearman, C. (1904). "General intelligence" objectively determined and measured. *American Journal of Psychology, 15,* 201–293.

Speed, W.G., III (1989). Closed head injury sequelae: Changing concepts. *Headache, 29,* 643–647.

Speedie, L., O'Donnell, W., Rabins, P., et al. (1990). Language performance deficits in elderly depressed patients. *Aphasiology, 4,* 197–205.

Spelberg, H.C.L. (1987). Problem-solving strategies on the Block Design task. *Perceptual and Motor Skills, 65,* 99–104.

Spellacy, F.J. & Spreen, O. (1969). A short form of the Token Test. *Cortex, 5,* 390–397.

Spencer, P.S. (2000a). Aluminum. In P.S. Spencer & H.H. Schaumburg (Eds.), *Experimental and clinical neurotoxicology* (2nd ed.). New York: Oxford University Press.

Spencer, P.S. (2000b). Biological principles of chemical neurotoxicity. In P.S. Spencer & H.H. Schaumburg (Eds.), *Experimental and clinical neurotoxicology* (2nd ed.). New York: Oxford University Press.

Spencer, P.S. & Schaumburg, H.H. (Eds.) (2000). *Experimental and clinical neurotoxicology* (2nd ed.). New York: Oxford University Press.

Spennemann, D.R. (1984). Handedness data on the European neolithic. *Neuropsychologia, 22,* 613–615.

Sperling, R.A., Guttmann, C.R., Hohol, M.J., et al. (2001). Regional magnetic resonance imaging lesion burden and cognitive function in multiple sclerosis: A longitudinal study. *Archives of Neurology, 58,* 115–121.

Sperry, R.W. (1974). Lateral specialization in the surgically separated hemispheres. In F.O. Schmitt & F.G. Worden (Eds.), *The neurosciences. Third study program.* Cambridge, MA: MIT Press.

Sperry, R.W. (1976). Changing concepts of consciousness and free will. *Perspectives in Biology and Medicine, 20,* 9–19.

Sperry, R. (1982). Some effects of disconnecting the cerebral hemispheres. *Science, 217,* 1223–1226.

Sperry, R. (1984). Consciousness, personal identity and the divided brain. *Neuropsychologia, 22,* 661–673.

Sperry, R.W. (1990). Forebrain commissurotomy and conscious awareness. In C.B. Trevarthen & R.W. Sperry (Eds.), *Brain circuits and functions of the mind.* Cambridge: Cambridge University Press.

Sperry, R.W., Zaidel, E., & Zaidel, D. (1979). Self-recognition and social awareness in the deconnected minor hemisphere. *Neuropsychologia, 17,* 153–166.

Spiers, P.A. (1981). Have they come to praise Luria or to bury him? The Luria-Nebraska Battery Controversy. *Journal of Consulting and Clinical Psychology, 49,* 331–341.

Spiers, P.A. (1984). What more can I say? In reply to Hutchinson, one last comment from Spiers. *Journal of Consulting and Clinical Psychology, 52,* 546–552.

Spiers, P.A. (1987). Acalculia revisited: Current issues. In F. Deloche & X. Seron (Eds.), *Mathematical disabilities: A cognitive neuropsychological perspective.* Hillsdale, NJ: Erlbaum.

Spikman, J.M., Berg, I.J., & Deelman, B.G. (1995). Spared recognition capacity in elderly and closed-head-injury subjects with clinical memory deficits. *Journal of Clinical and Experimental Neuropsychology, 17,* 29–34.

Spikman, J.M., Deelman, B.G., & van Zomeren, A.H. (2000). Executive functioning, attention and frontal lesions in patients with chronic CHI. *Journal of Clinical and Experimental Neuropsychology, 22,* 325–338.

Spikman, J.M., Kiers, H.A.L., Deelman, B.G., & van Zomeren, A.H. (2001). Construct validity of concepts of attention in healthy controls and patients with CHI. *Brain and Cognition, 47,* 446–460.

Spikman, J.M., van Zomeren, A.H., & Deelman, B.G. (1996). Deficits of attention after closed head injury: Slowness only? *Journal of Clinical and Experimental Neuropsychology, 18,* 755–767.

Spirduso, W.W. & MacRae, P.G. (1990). Motor performance and aging. In J.E. Birren & K.W. Schaie (Eds.), *Handbook of the psychology of aging* (3rd ed.). New York: Academic Press.

Spitz, H.H. (1972). Note on immediate memory for digits: Invariance over the years. *Psychological Bulletin, 78,* 183–185.

Spreen, O. & Benton, A. L. (1963). Simulation of mental deficiency on a visual memory test. *American Journal of Mental Deficiency, 67,* 909–913.

Spreen, O. & Benton, A.L. (1965). Comparative studies of some psychological tests for cerebral damage. *Journal of Nervous and Mental Disease, 140,* 323–333.

Spreen, O. & Benton, A.L. (1977). *Neurosensory Center Comprehensive Examination for Aphasia.* Victoria, BC: University of Victoria Neuropsychology Laboratory.

Spreen O. & Risser, A. (1991). Assessment of aphasia. In M.T. Sarno (Ed.), *Acquired aphasia* (2nd ed.). San Diego: Academic Press.

Spreen, O. & Risser, A. (2003). *Assessment of aphasia.* New York: Oxford University Press.

Spreen, O. & Strauss, E. (1991). *A compendium of neuropsychological tests* New York: Oxford University Press.

Spreen, O. & Strauss, E. (1998). *A compendium of neuropsychological tests* (2nd ed.). New York: Oxford University Press.

Springer, J.A., Binder, J.R., Hammeke, T.A., et al. (1999). Language dominance in neurologically normal and epilepsy subjects: A functional MRI study. *Brain, 122,* 2033–2046.

Springer, S.P. & Deutsch, G. (1989). *Left brain, right brain* (3rd ed.). New York: Freeman.

Square-Storer, P. & Roy, E.A. (1989). The apraxias: Commonalities and distinctions. In P. Square-Storer (Ed.), *Acquired apraxia of speech in aphasic adults.* Hove, UK: Erlbaum.

Squire, L.R. (1981). Two forms of human amnesia: An analysis of forgetting. *Journal of Neuroscience, 1,* 635–640.

Squire, L.R. (1986). Mechanisms of memory. *Science, 232,* 1612–1619.

Squire, L.R. (1987). *Memory and brain.* New York: Oxford University Press.

Squire, L.R., Clark, R.E., & Knowlton, B.J. (2001). Retrograde amnesia. *Hippocampus 11,* 50–55.

Squire, L.R., Haist, F., & Shimamura, A.P. (1989). The neurology of memory: Quantitative assessment of retrograde amnesia in two groups of amnesic patients. *Journal of Neuroscience, 9,* 828–839.

Squire, L.R. & Knowlton, B.J. (2000). The medial temporal lobe, the hippocampus, and the memory systems of the brain. In M.S. Gazzaniga (Ed.), *The new cognitive neurosciences* (2nd ed.). Cambridge, MA: MIT Press.

Squire, L.R. & Shimamura, A.P. (1986). Characterizing amnesic patients for neurobehavioral study. *Behavioral Neuroscience, 100,* 866–877.

Squire, L.R., Wetzel, C.D., & Slater, P.C. (1979). Memory complaint after electroconvulsive therapy: Assessment with a new self-rating instrument. *Biological Psychiatry, 14,* 791–801.

Squire, L.R. & Zola, S.M. (1996). Structure and function of declarative and nondeclarative memory systems. *Proceedings of the National Academy of Sciences USA, 93,* 13515–13522.

Stacy, M. & Jankovic, J. (1992). Clinical and neurobiological aspects of Parkinson's disease. In S.J. Huber & J.L. Cummings (Eds.), *Parkinson's disease: Neurobehavioral aspects.* New York: Oxford University Press.

Stahl, S.M. (2002). *Essential psychopharmacology of antipsychotics and mood stabilizers.* New York: Cambridge University Press.

Stallings, G., Boake, C., & Sherer, M. (1995). Comparison of the California Verbal Learning Test and the Rey Auditory Verbal Learning Test in head-injured patients. *Journal of Clinical and Experimental Neuropsychology, 17,* 706–712.

Stambrook, M. (1983). The Luria-Nebraska Neuropsychological Battery: A promise that may be partly fulfilled. *Journal of Clinical Neuropsychology, 5,* 247–269.

Stambrook, M., Gill, D.D., Cardoso, E.R., & Moore, A.D. (1993). Communicating (normal-pressure) hydrocephalus. In R.W. Parks et al. (Eds.), *Neuropsychology of Alzheimer's disease and other dementias.* New York: Oxford University Press.

Stambrook, M., Moore, A.D., Lubrusko, A.A., et al. (1993). Alternatives to the Glasgow Coma Scale as a quality of life predictor following traumatic brain injury. *Archives of Clinical Neuropsychology, 8,* 95–103.

Stambrook, M., Moore, A.D., Peters, L.C., et al. (1990). Effects of mild, moderate and severe closed head injury on long-term vocational status. *Brain Injury, 4,* 183–190.

Stampp, M., Snow, G., McMurthy, R., & Gawel, M. (1985). Quality of life in head-injured and non-head-injured trauma patients [abstract]. *Journal of Clinical and Experimental Neuropsychology, 7,* 160.

Stanczak, E.M., Stanczak, D.E., & Templer, D.I. (2000). Subject-selection procedures in neuropsychological research: A meta-analysis and prospective study. *Archives of Clinical Neuropsychology, 15,* 587–601.

Standish, T.I., Mollowy, D.W., Bedard, M., et al. (1996). Improved reliability of the Standardized Alzheimer's Disease Assessment Scale (SADAS) compared with the Alzheimer's Disease Assessment Scale (ADAS). *Journal of the American Geriatric Society, 44,* 712–716.

Stanescu-Cosson, R., Pinel, P., van De Moortele, P.F., et al. (2000). Understanding dissociations in dyscalculia: A brain imaging study of the impact of number size on the cerebral networks for exact and approximate calculation. *Brain, 123,* 2240–2255.

Stanley, B. & Howe, J.G. (1983). Identification of multiple sclerosis using double discrimination scales derived from the Luria-Nebraska Neuropsychological Battery: An attempt at cross-validation. *Journal of Consulting and Clinical Psychology, 51,* 420–423.

Stanzione, P., Semprini, R., Pierantozzi, M., et al. (1998). Age and stage dependency of P300 latency alterations in non-demented Parkinson's disease patients without therapy. *Electroencephalography and Clinical Neurophysiology: Evoked Potentials, 108,* 80–91.

Starkstein, S.E. (1992). Cognition and hemiparkinsonism. In S.J. Huber & J.L. Cummings (Eds.), *Parkinson's disease: Neurobehavioral aspects.* New York: Oxford University Press.

Starkstein, S.E., Brandt, J., Folstein, S., et al. (1988). Neuropsychological and neuroradiological correlates in Huntington's disease. *Journal of Neurology, Neurosurgery and Psychiatry, 51,* 1259–1263.

Starkstein, S.E., Leiguarda, R., Gershanik, O., & Berthier, M. (1987). Neuropsychological disturbances in hemiparkinson's disease. *Neurology, 37,* 1762–1764.

Starkstein, S.E. & Robinson, R.G. (1997). Mechanism of disinhibition after brain lesions. *Journal of Nervous and Mental Diseases, 185,* 108–114.

Starkstein, S.E., Robinson, R.G., Berthier, M.L., et al. (1988). Differential mood changes following basal ganglia vs. thalamic lesions. *Archives of Neurology, 45,* 725–730.

Starkstein, S.E., Sabe, L., Petracca, G., et al. (1996). Neuropsychological and psychiatric differences between Alzheimer's disease and Parkinson's disease with dementia. *Journal of Neurology, Neurosurgery and Psychiatry, 61,* 381–387.

St. Clair, D., Blackburn, I., Blackwood, D., & Tyrer, G. (1988). Measuring the course of Alzheimer's disease. *British Journal of Psychiatry, 152,* 48–54.

Steadman-Pare, D., Colantonio, A., Ratcliff, G., et al. (2001). Factors associated with perceived quality of life many years after traumatic brain injury. *Journal of Head Trauma Rehabilitation, 16,* 330–342.

Stebbins, G.T., Gilley, D.W., Wilson, R.S., et al. (1990). Effects of language disturbances on premorbid estimates of IQ in mild dementia. *The Clinical Neuropsychologist, 4,* 64–68.

Stebbins, G.T., Wilson, R.S., Gilley, D.W., et al. (1990). Use of the National Adult Reading Test to estimate premorbid IQ in dementia. *The Clinical Neuropsychologist, 4,* 18–24.

Steele, J.C., Richardson, J.C., & Olszewski, J. (1964). Progressive supranuclear palsy: A heterogeneous degeneration involving the brain stem, basal ganglia and cerebellum with vertical gaze and pseudobulbar palsy, nuchal dystonia and dementia. *Archives of Neurology, 10,* 333–359.

Steenhuis, R.E. & Bryden, M.P. (1989). Different dimensions of hand preference that relate to skilled and unskilled activities. *Cortex, 25,* 289–304.

Steer, R.A., Rissmiller, D.J., & Beck, A.T. (2000). Use of the Beck

Depression Inventory-II with depressed geriatric inpatients. *Behaviour Research and Therapy, 38,* 311–318.

Stein, D.G. (2000). Brain injury and theories of recovery. In A.-L. Christensen & B.P. Uzzell (Eds.), *International handbook of neuropsychological rehabilitation.* New York: Kluwer Academic/ Plenum Press.

Stein, D.G., Brailowsky, S., & Will, B. (1995). *Brain repair.* New York: Oxford University Press.

Stein, D.J. & Hugo, F.J. (2002). Neuropsychiatric aspects of anxiety disorders. In S.C. Yudofsky & R.E. Hales (Eds.), *American Psychiatric Publishing textbook of neuropsychiatry and clinical neurosciences* (4th ed.). Washington, D.C.: American Psychiatric Publishing.

Stein, J. (Ed.) (1966). *The Random House dictionary of the English language. Unabridged edition.* New York: Random House.

Stein, J.F. (1991). Space and the parietal association areas. In J. Paillard (Ed.), *Brain and space.* Oxford: Oxford University Press.

Stein, R.A. & Strickland, T.L. (1998). A review of the neuropsychological effects of commonly used prescription medications. *Archives of Clinical Neuropsychology, 13,* 259–284.

Stein, S. & Volpe, B.T. (1983). Classical "parietal" neglect syndrome after subcortical right frontal lobe infarction. *Neurology, 33,* 797–799.

Stein, S.C. (1996). Outcome from moderate head injury. In R.K. Narayan et al. (Eds.), *Neurotrauma.* New York: McGraw-Hill.

Stein, S.C. & Ross, S.E. (1992). Moderate head injury: A guide to initial management. *Journal of Neurosurgery, 77,* 562–564.

Steiner, W.A., Ryser, L., Huber, E., et al. (2002). Use of the ICF model as a clinical problem-solving tool in physical therapy and rehabilitation medicine. *Physical Therapy, 82,* 1098–1107.

Steinmetz, H., Staiger, J.F., Schlaug, G., et al. (1995). Corpus callosum and brain volume in women and men. *Neuroreport, 6,* 1002–1004.

Steinmetz, J.E., Gluck, M.A., & Solomon, P.R. (Eds.) (2001). *Model systems and the neurobiology of associative learning.* Mahwah, NJ: Erlbaum.

Stemmer, B. & Joanette, Y. (1998). The interpretation of narrative discourse of brain-damaged individuals within the framework of a multilevel discourse model. In M. Beeman & C. Chiarello (Eds.), *Right hemisphere language comprehension. Perspectives from cognitive neuroscience.* Mahwah, NJ: Erlbaum.

Steriade, M., Jones, E.G., & Llinas, R.R. (1990). *Thalamic oscillations and signaling.* New York: Wiley.

Sterling, P. (1998). Retina. In G.M. Shepherd (Ed.), *The synaptic organization of the brain* (4th ed.). New York: Oxford University Press.

Stern, R.A., Javorksy, D.J., Singer, E.A., et al. (1999). *The Boston Qualitative Scoring System for the Rey-Osterrieth Figure.* Odessa, FL: Psychological Assessment Resources.

Stern, R.A., Singer, E.A., Duke, L.M., et al. (1994). The Boston Qualitative Scoring System for the Rey-Osterrieth Complex Figure: Description and interrater reliability. *The Clinical Neuropsychologist, 8,* 309–322.

Stern, R.A. & White, T. (2003). *Neuropsychological Assessment Battery.* Lutz, FL: Psychological Assessment Resources.

Stern, R.G., Mohs, R.C., Davidson, M., et al. (1994). A longitudinal study of Alzheimer's disease: Measurement, rate, and predictors of cognitive deterioration. *American Journal of Psychiatry, 151,* 390–396.

Stern, Y. (2002). What is cognitive reserve? Theory and research applications of the reserve concept. *Journal of the International Neuropsychological Society, 8,* 448–460.

Stern, Y., Andrews, H., Pittman, J., et al. (1992). Diagnosis of dementia in a heterogeneous population: Development of a neuropsychological paradigm-based diagnosis of dementia and quan-

tified correction for the effects of education. *Archives of Neurology, 49,* 453–460.

Stern, Y., Gurland, B., Tatemichi, T.K., et al. (1994). Influence of education and occupation on the incidence of Alzheimer's disease. *Journal of the American Medical Association, 271,* 1004–1010.

Stern, Y., Hesdorffer, D., Sano, M., & Mayeux, R. (1990). Measurement and prediction of functional capacity in Alzheimer's disease. *Neurology, 40,* 8–14.

Stern, Y., Marder, K., Bell, K., et al. (1991). Multidisciplinary baseline assessment of homosexual men with and without human immunodeficiency virus infection. *Archives of General Psychiatry, 48,* 131–138.

Stern, Y., Mayeux, R., & Rosen, J. (1984). Contribution of perceptual motor dysfunction to construction and tracing disturbances in Parkinson's disease. *Journal of Neurology, Neurosurgery and Psychiatry, 47,* 983–989.

Stern, Y., Mayeux, R., Sano, M., et al. (1987). Predictors of disease course in patients with probable Alzheimer's disease. *Neurology, 37,* 1649–1653.

Stern, Y., McDermott, M.P., Albert, S., et al. (2001). Factors associated with incident human immunodeficiency virus-dementia. *Archives of Neurology, 58,* 473–479.

Stern, Y. & Sackeim, H.A. (2002). Neuropsychiatric aspects of memory and amnesia. In S.C. Yudofsky & R.E. Hales (Eds.), *American Psychiatric Publishing textbook of neuropsychiatry and clinical neurosciences* (4th ed.). Washington, D.C.: American Psychiatric Publishing.

Stern, Y., Tetrud, J.W., Martin, W.R.W., et al. (1990). Cognitive change following MPTP exposure. *Neurology, 40,* 261–264.

Sterne, D.M. (1966). The Knox Cubes as a test of memory and intelligence with male adults. *Journal of Clinical Psychology, 22,* 191–193.

Sternick, I., Gomes, R.D., Serra, M.C., et al. (2000). "Train surfers:" Analysis of 23 cases of electrical burns caused by high tension railway overhead cables. *Burns, 26,* 470–473.

Steuer, J., Bank, L., Olsen, E.J., & Jarvik, L.F. (1980). Depression, physical health and somatic complaints in the elderly: A study of the Zung Self-Rating Depression Scale. *Journal of Gerontology, 35,* 683–688.

Stevens, A. & Kircher, T. (1998). Cognitive decline unlike normal aging is associated with alterations of EEG temporo-spatial characteristics. *European Archives of Psychiatry and Clinical Neuroscience, 248,* 259–266.

Stevens, J.R. (1991). Psychosis and the temporal lobe. In D. Smith et al. (Eds.), *Advances in neurology.* New York: Raven Press.

Stevenson, J.D., Jr. (1986). Alternate form reliability and concurrent validity of the PPVT-R for referred rehabilitation agency adults. *Journal of Clinical Psychology, 42,* 650–653.

Stewart, P.A. (1997). Glial–vascular relations. In K.M.A. Welch et al. (Eds.), *Primer on cerebrovascular diseases.* San Diego: Academic Press.

Stewart, R. & Liolitsa, D. (1999). Type 2 diabetes mellitus, cognitive impairment and dementia. *Diabetic Medicine, 16,* 93–112.

Stewart, W., Breslau, N., & Keck, P.E., Jr. (1994). Comorbidity of migraine and panic disorder. *Neurology, 44(Suppl. 7),* S23–S27.

Stewart, W.F., Lipton, R., & Liberman, J. (1996). Variation in migraine prevalence by race. *Neurology, 46,* 231–238.

Stewart, W.F., Schwartz, B.S., Simon, D., et al. (1999). Neurobehavioral function and tibial and chelatable lead levels in 543 former organolead workers. *Neurology, 52,* 1610–1617.

Stewart, W.F., Shechter, A., & Rasmussen, B.K. (1994). Migraine prevalence: A review of population-based studies. *Neurology, 44(Suppl. 4),* S17–S23.

Stineman, M.G., Ross, R.N., Fiedler, R., Granger, C.V., & Maislin,

G. (2003). Functional independence staging: Conceptual foundation, face validity, and empirical derivation. *Archives of Physical Medicine and Rehabilitation, 84,* 29–37.

Stone, B.J. (1992). Prediction of achievement by Asian-American and white children. *Journal of School Psychology, 30,* 91–99.

Stone, C.P., Girdner, J., & Albrecht, R. (1946). An alternate form of the Wechsler Memory Scale. *Journal of Psychology, 22,* 199–206.

Storandt, M. (1976). Speed and coding effects in relation to age and ability level. *Developmental Psychology, 12,* 177–178.

Storandt, M. (1977). Age, ability level, and method of administering and scoring the WAIS. *Journal of Gerontology, 32,* 175–178.

Storandt, M. (1990). Longitudinal studies of aging and age-associated dementias. In F. Boller & J. Grafman (Eds.), *Handbook of neuropsychology* (Vol. 4). Amsterdam: Elsevier.

Storandt, M., Botwinick, J., Danziger, W.L., et al. (1984). Psychometric differentiation of mild senile dementia of the Alzheimer type. *Archives of Neurology, 41,* 497–499.

Storandt, M., Botwinick, J., & Danziger, W.L. (1986). Longitudinal changes: Patients with mild SDAT and matched healthy controls. In L.W. Poon (Ed.), *Handbook for clinical memory assessment of older adults.* Washington, D.C.: American Psychological Association.

Storandt, M. & Futterman, A. (1982). Stimulus size and performance on two subtests of the Wechsler Adult Intelligence Scale by younger and older adults. *Journal of Gerontology, 37,* 602–603.

Storandt, M., Kaskie, B., & Von Dras, D.D. (1998). Temporal memory for remote events in healthy aging and dementia. *Psychology and Aging, 13,* 4–7.

Storandt, M., Morris, J.C., Rubin, E., et al. (1992). Progression of senile dementia of the Alzheimer's type on a battery of psychometric tests. In L. Baeckman (Ed.), *Memory functioning in dementia.* Amsterdam: Elsevier, pp. 207–226.

Storandt, M., Stone, K., & LaBarge, E. (1995). Deficits in reading performance in very mild dementia of the Alzheimer's type. *Neuropsychology, 9,* 174–176.

Storck, P.A. & Looft, W.R. (1973). Qualitative analysis of vocabulary responses from persons aged six to sixty-six plus. *Journal of Education Psychology, 65,* 192–197.

Storey, J.E., Rowland, J.T.J., Basic, D., & Conforti, D.A. (2001). A comparison of five clock scoring methods using ROC (receiver operating characteristics) curve analysis. *International Journal of Geriatric Psychiatry, 16,* 394–399.

Story, T.B. (1991). Cognitive rehabilitation services in home and community settings. In J.S. Kreutzer and P.H. Wehman (Eds.), *Cognitive rehabilitation for persons with traumatic brain injury.* Baltimore, MD: Paul H. Brooks.

Stout, J.C., Bondi, M.W., Jernigan, T.L., et al. (1999). Regional cerebral volume loss associated with verbal learning and memory in dementia of the Alzheimer type. *Neuropsychology, 13,* 188–197.

Stout, J.C. & Paulsen, J.S. (2003). Assessing cognition in movement disorders. In M.-A. Bédard et al. (Eds.), *Mental and behavioral dysfunction in movement disorders.* Totowa, NJ: Humana Press.

Strachan, M.W., Deary, I.J., Ewing, F.M., & Frier, B.M. (1997). Is Type II diabetes associated with an increased risk of cognitive dysfunction? A critical review of published studies. *Diabetes Care, 20,* 438–445.

Strain, E., Patterson, K., Graham, N., & Hodges, J.R. (1998). Word reading in Alzheimer's disease: Cross-sectional and longitudinal analyses of response time and accuracy data. *Neuropsychologia, 36,* 155–171.

Strange, P.G. (1992). *Brain biochemistry and brain disorders.* Oxford: Oxford University Press.

Straus, S.E., Majumdar, S.R., & McAlister, F.A. (2002). New evidence for stroke prevention: Scientific review. *Journal of the American Medical Association, 288,* 1388–1395.

Strauss, D.J., Shavelle, R.M., & Anderson, T.W. (1998). Long-term survival of children and adolescents after traumatic brain injury. *Archives of Physical Medicine and Rehabilitation, 79,* 1095–1100.

Strauss, E. & Goldsmith, S.M. (1987). Lateral preferences and performance on nonverbal laterality tests in a normal population. *Cortex, 23,* 495–503.

Strauss, E., Hultsch, D.F., Hunter, M., et al. (1999). Using intraindividual variability to detect malingering in cognitive performance. *The Clinical Neuropsychologist, 13,* 420–432.

Strauss, E., Hunter, M., & Wada, J. (1993). Wisconsin Card Sorting performance: Effects of age of onset of damage and laterality of dysfunction. *Journal of Clinical and Experimental Neuropsychology, 15,* 896–902.

Strauss, E., LaPointe, J.S., Wada, J.A., et al. (1985). Language dominance: Correlation of radiological and functional data. *Neuropsychologia, 23,* 415–420.

Strauss, E., MacDonald, S.W.S., Hunter, M., et al. (2002). Intraindividual variability in cognitive performance in three groups of older adults: Cross-domain links to physical status and self-perceived affect and beliefs. *Journal of the International Neuropsychological Society. 8,* 893–906.

Strauss, E. & Moscovitch, M. (1981). Perception of facial expression. *Brain and Language, 13,* 308–332.

Strauss, E., Satz, P., & Wada, J. (1990). An examination of the crowding hypothesis in epileptic patients who have undergone the carotid amytal test. *Neuropsychologia, 28,* 1221–1227.

Strauss, E., Semenza, C., Hunter, M., et al. (2000). Left anterior lobectomy and category-specific naming. *Brain and Cognition, 43,* 403–406.

Strauss, E., Spellacy, F., Hunter, M., & Berry T. (1994). Assessing believable deficits on measures of attention and information processing capacity. *Archives of Clinical Neuropsychology, 9,* 483–490.

Strauss, E. & Spreen, O. (1990). A comparison of the Rey and Taylor figures. *Archives of Clinical Neuropsychology, 5,* 417–420.

Strauss, E. & Wada, J. (1983). Lateral preferences and cerebral speech dominance. *Cortex, 19,* 165–177.

Strauss, E. & Wada, J. (1987). Hand preference and proficiency and cerebral speech dominance determined by the carotid amytal test. *Journal of Clinical and Experimental Neuropsychology, 9,* 169–174.

Strauss, E., Wada, J., & Kosaka, B. (1984). Writing hand posture and cerebral dominance for speech. *Cortex, 20,* 143–147.

Strauss, M.E. & Brandt, J. (1985). Is there increased WAIS pattern variability in Huntington's disease. *Journal of Clinical and Experimental Neuropsychology, 7,* 122–126.

Strauss, M.E. & Brandt, J. (1986). Attempt at preclinical identification of Huntington's disease using the WAIS. *Journal of Clinical and Experimental Neuropsychology, 8,* 210–218.

Street, R.F. (1931). *A Gestalt Completion Test. Contributions to Education 481.* New York: Teachers College, Columbia University.

Streiner, D.L. & Miller, H.R. (1986). Can a good short form of the MMPI ever be developed? *Journal of Clinical Psychology, 42,* 109–113.

Strich, S.J. (1961). Shearing of nerve fibers as a cause of brain damage due to head injury. *Lancet, ii,* 446–448.

Strickland, T., Miller, B.L., Kowell, A., & Stein, R. (1998). Neurobiology of cocaine-induced organic brain impairment: Contributions from functional imaging. *Neuropsychology Review, 8,* 1–9.

Stricks, L., Pittman, J., Jacobs, D.M., et al. (1998). Normative data for a brief neuropsychological battery administered to English-

and Spanish-speaking community dwelling elders. *Journal of the International Neuropsychological Society, 4,* 311–318.

Stringer, A.Y. (1996). *A guide to adult neuropsychological diagnosis.* Philadelphia: Davis.

Stringer, A.Y., Cooley, E.L, & Christensen, A.-L. (2002). *Pathways to prominence in neuropsychology. Reflections of twentieth century pioneers.* New York: Psychology Press.

Strite, D., Massman, P.J., Cooke, N., & Doody, R.S. (1997). Neuropsychological asymmetry in Alzheimer's disease: Verbal versus visuoconstructional deficits across stages of dementia. *Journal of the International Neuropsychological Society, 3,* 420–427.

Stroop, J.R. (1935). Studies of interference in serial verbal reactions. *Journal of Experimental Psychology, 18,* 643–662.

Strub, R.L. (1989). Frontal lobe syndrome in a patient with bilateral globus pallidus lesions. *Archives of Neurology, 46,* 1024–1027.

Strub, R.L. & Black, F.W. (1988). *Neurobehavioral disorders. A clinical approach.* Philadelphia: Davis.

Strub, R.L. & Black, F.W. (2000). *The mental status examination in neurology* (4th ed.). Philadelphia: Davis.

Strub, R.L. & Black, F.W. (2003). The mental status examination. In T.E. Feinberg & M.J. Farah (Eds.), *Behavioral neurology and neuropsychology* (2nd ed.). New York: McGraw-Hill.

Strub, R.L. & Wise, M.G. (1997). Differential diagnosis in neuropsychiatry. In S.C. Yudofsky & R.E. Hales (Eds.), *Textbook of neuropsychiatry* (3rd ed.). Washington, D.C.: American Psychiatric Publishing.

Struben, E.A.M. & Tredoux, C.G. (1989). *The estimation of premorbid intelligence: The National Adult Reading Test in South Africa.* Paper presented at the 4th national congress of the Brain and Behaviour Society, Durban, South Africa.

Struchen, M.A., Hannay, H.J., Contant, C.F., & Robertson, C.S. (2001). The relation between acute physiological variables and outcome on the Glasgow Outcome Scale and Disability Rating Scale following severe traumatic brain injury. *Journal of Neurotrauma, 18,* 115–125.

Stumpf, H. & Klieme, E. (1989). Sex-related differences in spatial ability: More evidence for convergence. *Perceptual and Motor Skills, 69,* 915–921.

Sturm, W. & Willmes, K. (1991). Efficacy of a reaction training on various attentional and cognitive functions in stroke patients. *Neuropsychological Rehabilitation, 1,* 241–280.

Stuss, D.T. (1987). Contribution of frontal lobe injury to cognitive impairment after closed head injury: Methods of assessment and recent findings. In H.S. Levin, J. Grafman, & H.M. Eisenberg (Eds.), *Neurobehavioral recovery from head injury.* New York: Oxford University Press.

Stuss, D.T. (1991a). Interference effects on memory functions in postleukotomy patients: An attentional perspective. In H.S. Levin, H.M. Eisenberg, & A.L. Benton (Eds.), *Frontal lobe function and dysfunction.* New York: Oxford University Press.

Stuss, D.T. (1991b). Self-awareness and the frontal lobes: A neuropsychological perspective. In G.R. Goethals & J. Strauss (Eds.), *The self: An interdisciplinary approach.* New York: Springer-Verlag.

Stuss, D.T. (1993). Assessment of neuropsychological dysfunction in frontal lobe degeneration. *Dementia, 4,* 220–225.

Stuss, D.T. & Alexander, M.P. (1999). Affectively burnt in: A proposed role of the right frontal lobe. In E. Tulving (Ed.), *Memory, consiousness and the brain: The Tallin Conference.* Philadelphia: Psychology Press.

Stuss, D.T. & Alexander, M.P. (2000). The anatomical basis of affective behavior, emotion and self-awareness: A specific role of the right frontal lobe. In G. Hatano, N. Okada, & H. Tanabe (Eds.), *Affective minds.* Amsterdam: Elsevier.

Stuss, D.T., Alexander, M.P., Hamer, L., et al. (1998). The effects of focal anterior and posterior brain lesions on verbal fluency. *Journal of the International Neuropsychological Society, 4,* 265–278.

Stuss, D.T., Alexander, M.P., Lieberman, A., & Levine, H. (1978). An extraordinary form of confabulation. *Neurology, 28,* 1166–1172.

Stuss, D.T. & Benson, D.F. (1984). Neuropsychological studies of the frontal lobes. *Psychological Bulletin, 95,* 3–28.

Stuss, D.T. & Benson, D.F. (1986). *The frontal lobes.* New York: Raven Press.

Stuss, D.T. & Benson, D.F. (1987). The frontal lobes and control of cognition and memory. In E. Perecman (Ed.), *The frontal lobes revisited.* New York: IRBN Press.

Stuss, D.T. & Benson, D.F. (1990). The frontal lobes and language. In E. Goldberg (Ed.), *Contemporary neuropsychology and the legacy of Luria.* Hillsdale, NJ: Erlbaum.

Stuss, D.T., Benson, D.F., Kaplan, E.F., et al. (1983). The involvement of orbitofrontal cerebrum in cognitive tasks. *Neuropsychologia, 21,* 235–248.

Stuss, D.T., Binns, M.A., Carruth, F.G., et al. (1999). The acute period of recovery from traumatic brain injury: Posttraumatic amnesia or posttraumatic confusional state? *Journal of Neurosurgery, 90,* 635–643.

Stuss, D.T., Binns, M.A., Carruth, F.G., et al. (2000). Prediction of recovery of continuous memory after traumatic brain injury. *Neurology, 54,* 1337–1344.

Stuss, D.T., Bisschop, S.M., Alexander, M.P., et al. (2001). The Trail Making Test: A study in focal lesion patients. *Psychological Assessment, 13,* 230–239.

Stuss, D.T., Craik, F.I., Sayer, L., et al. (1996). Comparison of older people and patients with frontal lesions: Evidence from word list learning. *Psychology and Aging, 11,* 387–395.

Stuss, D.T. & Cummings, J.L. (1990). Subcortical vascular dementias. In J.L. Cummings (Ed.), *Subcortical dementia.* New York: Oxford University Press.

Stuss, D.T., Ely, P., Hugenholtz, H., et al. (1985). Subtle neuropsychological deficits in patients with good recovery after closed head injury. *Neurosurgery, 17,* 41–47.

Stuss, D.T., Eskes, G.A., & Foster, J.K. (1994). Experimental neuropsychological studies of frontal lobe functions. In F. Boller & J. Grafman (Eds.), *Handbook of neuropsychology* (Vol. 9). Amsterdam: Elsevier.

Stuss, D.T., Floden, D., Alexander, M.P., et al. (2001). Stroop performance in focal lesion patients: Dissociation of processes and frontal lobe lesion location. *Neuropsychologia, 39,* 771–786.

Stuss, D.T. & Gow, C.A. (1992). "Frontal dysfunction" after traumatic brain injury. *Neuropsychiatry, Neuropsychology, and Behavioral Neurology, 5,* 272–282.

Stuss, D.T., Gow, C.A., & Hetherington, C.R. (1992). "No longer Gage:" Frontal lobe dysfunction and emotional changes. *Journal of Consulting and Clinical Psychology, 60,* 349–359.

Stuss, D.T., Guberman, A., Nelson, R., & Larochelle, S. (1988). The neuropsychology of paramedian thalamic infarction. *Brain and Cognition, 8,* 348–378.

Stuss, D.T., Kaplan, E.F., Benson, D.F., et al. (1981). Long-term effects of prefrontal leucotomy—an overview of neuropsychologic residuals. *Journal of Clinical Neuropsychology, 3,* 13–32.

Stuss, D.T. & Levine, B. (2002). Adult clinical neuropsychology: Lessons from studies of the frontal lobes. *Annual Review of Psychology, 53,* 401–433.

Stuss, D.T., Levine, B., Alexander, M.P., et al. (2000). Wisconsin Card Sorting Test performance in patients with focal frontal and posterior brain damage: Effects of lesion location and test structure on separable cognitive processes. *Neuropsychologia, 38*, 388–402.

Stuss, D.T., Peterkin, I., Guzman, D.A., et al. (1997). Chronic obstructive pulmonary disease: Effects of hypoxia on neurological and neuropsychological measures. *Journal of Clinical and Experimental Neuropsychology, 19*, 515–524.

Stuss, D.T., Pogue, J., Buckle, L., & Bondar, J. (1994). Characterization of stability of performance in patients with traumatic brain injury: Variability and consistency on reaction time tests. *Neuropsychology, 8*, 316–324.

Stuss, D.T., Stethem, L.L., Hugenholtz, H., & Richard, M.T. (1989). Traumatic brain injury. *The Clinical Neuropsychologist, 3*, 145–156.

Stuss, D.T., Stethem, L.L., Hugenholtz, H., et al. (1989). Reaction time after head injury: Fatigue, divided and focused attention, and consistency of performance. *Journal of Neurology, Neurosurgery and Psychiatry, 52*, 742–748.

Stuss, D.T., Stethem, L.L., & Pelchat, G. (1988). Three tests of attention and rapid information processing: An extension. *The Clinical Neuropsychologist, 2*, 246–250.

Stuss, D.T., Stethem, L.L., & Poirier, C.A. (1987). Comparison of three tests of attention and rapid information processing across six age groups. *The Clinical Neuropsychologist, 1*, 139–152.

Stuss, D.T., Van Reekum, R., & Murphy, K.J. (2000). Differentiation of states and causes of apathy. In J. Borod (Ed.), *The neuropsychology of emotion*. New York: Oxford University Press.

Stuss, D.T., Winocur, G., & Robertson, I.H. (1999). *Cognitive neurorehabilitation*. New York: Cambridge University Press.

Suchoff, I.B., Kapoor, N., Waxman, R., & Ference, W. (1999). The occurrence of ocular and visual dysfunctions in an acquired brain-injured patient sample. *Journal of the American Optometry Association, 70*, 301–308.

Suchy, Y., Blint, A., & Osmon, D.C. (1997). Behavioral Dyscontrol Scale: Criterion and predictive validity in an inpatient rehabilitation unit population. *The Clinical Neuropsychologist, 11*, 258–265.

Suchy, Y. & Chelune, G. (2001). Postsurgical changes in self-reported mood and composite IQ in a matched sample of patients with frontal and temporal lobe epilepsy. *Journal of Clinical and Experimental Neuropsychology, 23*, 413–423.

Sue, S. (1999). Science, ethnicity, and bias. Where have we gone wrong? *American Psychologist, 54*, 1070–1077.

Suhr, J.A. & Boyer, D. (1999). Use of the Wisconsin Card Sorting Test in the detection of malingering in student simulator and patient samples. *Journal of Clinical and Experimental Neuropsychology, 21*, 701–708.

Suhr, J., Grace, J., Allen, J., et al. (1998). Quantitative and qualitative performance of stroke versus normal elderly on six clock drawing systems. *Archives of Clinical Neuropsychology, 13*, 495–502.

Suhr, J.A. & Gunstad, J. (2000). The effects of coaching on the sensitivity and specificity of malingering measures. *Archives of Clinical Neuropsychology, 15*, 415–424.

Suhr, J.A. & Jones, R.D. (1998). Letter and semantic fluency in Alzheimer's, Huntington's, and Parkinson's dementias. *Archives of Clinical Neuropsychology, 13*, 447–454.

Suhr, J., Tranel, D., Wefel, J., & Barrash, J. (1997). Memory performance after head injury: Contributions of malingering, litigation status, psychological factors, and medication use. *Journal of Clinical and Experimental Neuropsychology, 19*, 500–514.

Sullivan, E.T., Clark, W.N., & Tiegs, E.W. (1963). *California Short-Form Test of Mental Maturity* (1963 rev.). New York: McGraw-Hill.

Sullivan, E.V., Corkin, S., & Growdon, J.H. (1986). Verbal and nonverbal short-term memory in patients with Alzheimer's disease and in healthy elderly subjects. *Developmental Neuropsychology, 2*, 387–400.

Sullivan, E.V., Fama, R., Rosenbloom, M.J., & Pfefferbaum, A. (2002). A profile of neuropsychological deficits in alcoholic women. *Neuropsychology, 16*, 74–83.

Sullivan, E.V., Lim, K.O., Mathalon, D., et al. (1998). A profile of cortical gray matter volume deficits characteristic of schizophrenia. *Cerebral Cortex, 8*, 117–124.

Sullivan, E.V., Mathalon, D.H., Ha, C.N., et al. (1992). The contribution of constructional accuracy and organizational strategy to nonverbal recall in schizophrenia and chronic alcoholism. *Biological Psychiatry, 32*, 312–333.

Sullivan, E.V., Rosenbloom, M.J., & Pfefferbaum, A. (2000). Pattern of motor and cognitive deficits in detoxified alcoholic men. *Alcoholism: Clinical and Experimental Research, 24*, 611–621.

Sullivan, E.V. & Sagar, H.J. (1988). Nonverbal short-term memory impairment in Parkinson's disease [abstract]. *Journal of Clinical and Experimental Neuropsychology, 10*, 34.

Sullivan, E.V., Sagar, H.J., Cooper, J.A., & Jordan, N. (1993). Verbal and nonverbal short-term memory impairment in untreated Parkinson's disease. *Neuropsychology, 7*, 396–405.

Sullivan, E.V., Sagar, H.J., Gabrieli, J.D.E., et al. (1989). Different cognitive profiles on standard behavioral tests in Parkinson's disease and Alzheimer's disease. *Journal of Clinical and Experimental Neuropsychology, 11*, 799–820.

Sullivan, K. (1996). Estimates of interrater reliability for the Logical Memory subtest of the Wechsler Memory Scale–Revised. *Journal of Clinical and Experimental Neuropsychology, 18*, 707–712.

Sullivan, K. & Bowden, S.C. (1997). Which tests do neuropsychologists use? *Journal of Clinical Psychology, 53*, 657–661.

Sullivan, K., Deffenti, C., & Keane, B. (2002). Malingering on the RAVLT: Part II. Detection strategies. *Archives of Clinical Neuropsychology, 17*, 223–233.

Sullivan, M.J.L., Weinshenker, B., Mikail, S., & Edgley, K. (1995). Depression before and after diagnosis of multiple sclerosis. *Multiple Sclerosis, 1*, 104–108.

Sultzer, D.L., Brown, C.V., Mandelkern, M.A., et al. (2003). Delusional thoughts and regional frontal/temporal cortex metabolism in Alzheimer's disease. *American Journal of Psychiatry, 160*, 341–349.

Sultzer, D.L. & Cummings, J.L. (1994). Secondary dementias in the elderly. In M.L. Albert & J.E. Knoefel (Eds.), *Clinical neurology of aging* (2nd ed.). New York: Oxford University Press.

Sulzbacher, S., Farwell, J.R., Temkin, N., et al. (1999). Late cognitive effects of early treatment with phenobarbital. *Clinical Pediatrics, 38*, 387–394.

Sumerall, S.W., Timmons, P.L., James, A.L., et al. (1997). Expanded norms for the Controlled Oral Word Association Test. *Journal of Clinical Psychology, 53*, 517–521.

Sun, A.Y., Simonyi, A., & Sun, G.Y. (2002). The "French Paradox" and beyond: Neuroprotective effects of polyphenols. *Free Radicals Biology and Medicine, 32*, 314–318.

Sunderland, A., Harris, J.E., & Gleave, J. (1984). Memory failures in everyday life following severe head injury. *Journal of Clinical Neuropsychology, 6*, 127–142.

Sunderland, A., Stewart, F.M., & Sluman, S.M. (1996). Adaptation to cognitive deficit? An exploration of apparent dissociations between everyday memory and test performance late after stroke. *British Journal of Clinical Psychology, 35*, 463–476.

Sunderland, A., Tinson, D., & Bradley, L. (1994). Differences in recovery from constructional apraxia after right and left hemisphere stroke? *Journal of Clinical and Experimental Neuropsychology, 16*, 916–920.

Sunderland, A., Watts, K., Baddeley, A.D., & Harris, J.E. (1986). Subjective memory assessment and test performance in elderly adults. *Journal of Gerontology, 41*, 376–384.

Sunderland, T., Hill, J.L., Mellow, A.M., et al. (1989). Clock drawing in Alzheimer's disease. *Journal of the American Geriatrics Society, 37,* 725–729.

Sundet, K., Finset, A., & Reisberg, I. (1988). Neuropsychological predictors in stroke rehabilitation. *Journal of Clinical and Experimental Neuropsychology, 10,* 363–379.

Sungaila, P. & Crockett, D.J. (1993). Dementia and the frontal lobes. In R.W. Parks, R.F. Zec, & R.S. Wilson (Eds.). *Neuropsychology of Alzheimer's disease and other dementias.* New York: Oxford University Press.

Susman, M., DiRusso, S.M., Sullivan, T., et al. (2002). Traumatic brain injury in the elderly: Increased mortality and worse functional outcome at discharge despite lower injury severity. *Journal of Trauma, 53,* 219–224.

Sutton, L.R. (1983). The effects of alcohol, marijuana and their combination on driving ability. *Journal of Studies on Alcohol, 44,* 438–445.

Sutula, T. & Pitkänen, A. (2002). *Do seizures damage the brain.* Amsterdam: Elsevier.

Suutama, T., Ruoppila, I., & Stig, B. (2002). Changes in cognitive functioning from 75 to 80 years of age: A 5-year follow-up in two Nordic localities. *Aging Clinical and Experimental Research, 14,* 29–36.

Suzuki, L.A. & Valencia, R.R. (1997). Race-ethnicity and measured intelligence: Educational implications. *American Psychologist, 52,* 1103–1114.

Svetina, C., Barr, W.B., Rastogi, R., & Hilton, E. (1999). The neuropsychological examination of naming in Lyme borreliosis. *Applied Neuropsychology, 6,* 33–38.

Swaab, D.F. & Fliers, E. (1985). A sexually dimorphic nucleus in the human brain. *Science, 228,* 1112–1115.

Swaine, B.R. & Sullivan, S.J. (1996). Longitudinal profile of early motor recovery following severe traumatic brain injury. *Brain Injury, 10,* 347–366.

Swan, G.E., Carmelli, D., & Larue, A. (1998). Systolic blood pressure tracking over 25 to 30 years and cognitive performance in older adults. *Stroke, 29,* 2334–2340.

Swan, G.E., Morrison, E., & Eslinger, P. J. (1990). Interrator agreement on the Benton Visual Retention Test. *The Clinical Neuropsychologist, 4,* 37–44.

Swan, G.E., Reed, T., Jack, L.M., et al. (1999). Differential genetic influence for components of memory in aging adult twins. *Archives of Neurology, 56,* 1127–1132.

Swanson, S.J., Rao, S.M., Grafman, J., et al. (1995). The relationship between seizure subtype and interictal personality: Results from the Vietnam Head Injury Study. *Brain, 118,* 91–103.

Swartz, B.E., Halgren, E., Fuster, J.M., et al. (1995). Cortical metabolic activation in humans during a visual memory task. *Cerebral Cortex, 5,* 205–214.

Swartz, J.D. (1985). Quick Test (review). In D.J. Keyser and R.C. Sweetland (Eds.), *Test critiques* (Vol. I). Kansas City, MO: Test Corporation of America.

Swartz, J.R., Miller, B.L., Lesser, I.M., et al. (1997). Behavioral phenomenology in Alzheimer's disease, frontotemporal dementia, and late-life depression: A retrospective analysis. *Journal of Geriatric Psychiatry and Neurology, 10,* 67–74.

Swearer, J.M., Drachman, D.A., O'Donnell, B.F., & Mitchell, A.L. (1988). Troublesome and disruptive behaviors in dementia. *Journal of the American Geriatric Society, 36,* 784–790.

Sweeney, J.A., Meisel, L., Walsh, V.L., & Castrovinci, D. (1989). Assessment of cognitive functioning in poly-substance abusers. *Journal of Clinical Psychology, 45,* 346–351.

Sweeney, J.E. (1992). Nonimpact brain injury: Grounds for clinical study of the neuropsychological effects of acceleration forces. *The Clinical Neuropsychologist, 6,* 443–457.

Sweet, J.J. (1983). Confounding effects of depression on neuropsychological testing: Five illustrative cases. *Clinical Neuropsychology, 5,* 103–109.

Sweet, J.J. (Ed.) (1999a). *Forensic neuropsychology.* Exton, PA: Swets and Zeitlinger.

Sweet, J.J. (1999b). Malingering: Differential diagnosis. In J.J. Sweet (Ed.), *Forensic neuropsychology.* Exton, PA: Swets and Zeitlinger.

Sweet, J.J., Demakis, G.J., Ricker, J.H., & Millis, S.R. (2000). Diagnostic efficiency and material specificity of the Warrington Recognition Memory Test: A collaborative multisite investigation. *Archives of Clinical Neuropsychology, 15,* 301–309.

Sweet, J.J., Moberg, P.J., & Suchy, Y. (2000). Ten-year follow-up survey of clinical neuropsychologists: Part I. Practices and beliefs. *The Clinical Neuropsychologist, 14,* 18–37.

Sweet, J.J., Moberg, P.J., & Tovian, S.M. (1990). Evaluation of Wechsler Adult Intelligence Scale–Revised premorbid IQ formulas in clinical populations. *Psychological Assessment, 2,* 41–44.

Sweet, J.J., Moberg, P.J., & Westergaard, C. (1996). Five-year follow-up survey of practices and beliefs of clinical neuropsychologists. *The Clinical Neuropsychologist, 10,* 202–221.

Sweet, J.J., Newman, P., & Bell, B. (1992). Significance of depression in clinical neuropsychological assessment. *Clinical Psychology Review, 12,* 21–45.

Sweet, J.J., Suchy, Y., Leahy, B., et al. (1999). Normative clinical relationships between orientation and memory: Age as an important moderator variable. *The Clinical Neuropsychologist, 13,* 495–508.

Sweet, J.J., Wolfe, P., Sattlberger, E., et al. (2000). Further investigation of traumatic brain injury versus insufficient effort with the California Verbal Learning Test. *Archives of Clinical Neuropsychology, 15,* 105–113.

Swenson, W.M. (1961). Structured personality testing in the aged: An MMPI study of the gerontic population. *Journal of Clinical Psychology, 17,* 302–304.

Swick, D. & Knight, R.T. (1998). Cortical lesions and attention. In R. Parasuraman (Ed.), *The attentive brain.* Cambridge, MA: MIT Press.

Swihart, A.A., Panisett, M., Becker, J.T., et al. (1989). The Token Test: Validity and diagnostic power in Alzheimer's disease. *Developmental Neuropsychology, 5,* 69–78.

Swihart, A.A. & Pirozzolo, F.J. (1988). The neuropsychology of aging and dementia: Clinical issues. In H.A. Whitaker (Ed.), *Neuropsychological studies of nonfocal brain damage.* New York: Springer-Verlag.

Swinkels, W.A., Shackleton, D.P., & Trenite, D.G. (2000). Psychosocial impact of epileptic seizures in a Dutch epilepsy population: A comparative Washington Psychosocial Seizure Inventory study. *Epilepsia, 41,* 1335–1341.

Swithenby, S.J., Bailey, A.J., Brautigam, S., et al. (1998). Neural processing of human faces: A magnetoencephalographic study. *Experimental Brain Research, 118,* 501–510.

Symonds, C.P. (1937). Mental disorder following head injury. *Proceedings of the Royal Society of Medicine, 30,* 1081–1092.

Syndulko, K., Ke, D., Ellison, G.W., et al. (1996). Comparative evaluations of neuroperformance and clinical outcome assessments in chronic progressive multiple sclerosis: 1. Reliability, validity and sensitivity to disease progression. *Multiple Sclerosis, 2,* 142–156.

Szaflarski, J.P., Binder, J.R., Possing, E.T., et al. (2002). Language lateralization in left-handed and ambidextrous people: fMRI data. *Neurology, 59,* 238–244.

Sze, K.H., Sim, T.C., Wong, E., et al. (1998). Effect of nimodipine on memory after cerebral infarction. *Acta Neurologica Scandinavica, 97,* 386–392.

Szmukler, G.I., Andrewes, D., Kingston, K., et al. (1992). Neuropsychological impairment in anorexia nervosa: Before and after refeeding. *Journal of Clinical and Experimental Neuropsychology, 14,* 347–352.

Tachibana, H., Aragane, K., Kawabata, K., & Sugita, M. (1997). P3 latency change in aging and Parkinson disease. *Archives of Neurology, 54,* 296–302.

Takaoka, M., Tabuse, H., Kumura, E., et al. (2002). Semiquantitative analysis of corpus callosum injury using magnetic resonance imaging indicates clinical severity in patients with diffuse axonal injury. *Journal of Neurology Neurosurgery and Psychiatry, 73,* 289–293.

Talland, G.A. (1965). *Deranged memory.* New York: Academic Press.

Talland, G.A. & Ekdahl, M. (1959). Psychological studies of Korsakoff's psychosis: IV. The rate and mode of forgetting narrative material. *Journal of Nervous and Mental Disease, 129,* 391–404.

Talwalker, S., Overall, J.E., Srirama, M.K., & Gracon, S.I. (1996). Cardinal features of cognitive dysfunction in Alzheimer's disease: A factor-analytic study of the Alzheimer's Disease Assessment Scale. *Journal of Geriatric Psychiatry and Neurology, 9,* 39–46.

Tamkin, A.S. (1983). Impairment of cognitive functioning in alcholics. *Military Medicine, 148,* 793–795.

Tamkin, A.S. & Dolenz, J.J. (1990). Cognitive impairment in alcoholics. *Perceptual and Motor Skills, 70,* 816–818.

Tamminga, C.A., Thaker, G.K., Buchanan, R., et al. (1992). Limbic system abnormalities identified in schizophrenia using positron emission tomography with fluorodeoxyglucose and neocortical alterations with deficit syndrome. *Archives of General Psychiatry, 49,* 522–530.

Tamminga, C.A., Thaker, G.K., & Medoff, D.R. (2002). Neuropsychiatric aspects of schizophrenia. In S.C. Yudofsky & R.E. Hales (Eds.), *American Psychiatric Publishing textbook of neuropsychiatry and clinical neurosciences.* Washington, D.C.: American Psychiatric Publishing.

Tan, S.-Y. (1986). Psychosocial functioning of adult epileptic and MS patients and adult normal controls on the WPSI. *Journal of Clinical Psychology, 42,* 528–534.

Tanaka, Y., Miyazawa, Y., Akaoka, F., & Yamada, T. (1997). Amnesia following damage to the mammillary bodies. *Neurology, 48,* 160–165.

Tang, M-X., Cross, P., Andrews, H., et al. (2001). Incidence of AD in African-Americans, Caribbean Hispanics, and Caucasians in northern Manhattan. *Neurology, 56,* 49–56.

Tang, M-X., Stern, Y., Marder, K., et al. (1998). The APOE-ε4 allele and the risk of Alzheimer's disease among African Americans, whites, and Hispanics. *Journal of the American Medical Association, 279,* 751–755.

Tanner, C.M. (1989). The role of environmental toxins in the etiology of Parkinson's disease. *Trends in Neurosciences, 12,* 49–53.

Tanner, C.M. (1992). Epidemiology of Parkinson's disease. *Neurologic Clinics, 10,* 317–329.

Tanner, C.M. & Langston, J.W. (1990). Do environmental toxins cause Parkinson's disease? A critical review. *Neurology, 40(Suppl. 3),* 17–31.

Tanner, C.M., Ottman, R., Goldman, S.M., et al. (1999). Parkinson disease in twins: An etiologic study. *Journal of the American Medical Association, 281,* 341–346.

Tanridag, O. & Kirshner, H.S. (1985). Aphasia and agraphia in lesions of the posterior internal capsule and putamen. *Neurology, 35,* 1797–1801.

Tapert, S.F. & Brown, S.A. (1999). Neuropsychological correlates of adolescent substance abuse: Four-year outcomes. *Journal of the International Neuropsychological Society, 5,* 481–493.

Tapley, S.M. & Bryden, M.P. (1985). A group test for the assessment of performance between the hands. *Neuropsychologia, 23,* 215–221.

Tarter, R.E. (1976). Neuropsychological investigations of alcoholism. In G. Goldstein & C. Neuringer (Eds.), *Empirical studies of alcoholism.* Cambridge, MA: Ballinger.

Tarter, R.E. & Alterman, A.I. (1984). Neuropsychological deficits in alcoholics: Etiological considerations. *Journal of Studies on Alcohol, 45,* 1–9.

Tarter, R.E., Butters, M., & Beers, S.R. (Eds.) (2001). *Medical neuropsychology* (2nd ed.). New York: Kluwer Academic/Plenum.

Tarter, R.E., Goldstein, G., Alterman, A., et al. (1983). Alcoholic seizures: Intellectual and neuropsychological sequelae. *Journal of Nervous and Mental Disease, 171,* 123–125.

Tarter, R.E. & Jones, B.M. (1971). Motor impairment in chronic alcoholics. *Diseases of the Nervous System, 32,* 632–636.

Tarter, R.E. & Parsons, O.A. (1971). Conceptual shifting in chronic alcoholics. *Journal of Abnormal Psychology, 77,* 71–75.

Tarter, R. E. & Van Thiel (2001). Neuropsychological dysfunction due to liver disease. In R.E. Tarter et al. (Eds.), *Medical neuropsychology* (2nd ed.). New York: Kluwer Academic/Plenum.

Tate, D.F. & Bigler, E.D. (2000). Fornix and hippocampal atrophy in traumatic brain injury. *Learning and Memory, 7,* 442–446.

Tate, P.S., Freed, D.M., Bombardier, C.H., et al. (1999). Traumatic brain injury: Influence of blood alcohol level on post-acute cognitive function. *Brain Injury, 13,* 767–784.

Tate, R.L. (1998). "It is not only the kind of injury that matters, but the kind of head:" The contribution of premorbid psychosocial factors to rehabilitation outcomes after severe traumatic brain injury. *Neuropsychological Rehabilitation, 8,* 1–18.

Tate, R.L., Fenelon, B., Manning, M.L., & Hunter, M. (1991). Patterns of neuropsychological impairment after severe blunt head injury. *Journal of Nervous and Mental Disease, 179,* 117–126.

Tate, R.L., Lulham, J.M., Broe, G.A., et al. (1989). Psychosocial outcome for the survivors of severe blunt head injury. *Journal of Neurology, Neurosurgery and Psychiatry, 52,* 1128–1134.

Tate, R.L., Perdices, M., & Maggiotto, S. (1998). Stability of the Wisconsin Card Sorting Test and the determination of reliability of change in scores. *The Clinical Neuropsychologist, 12,* 348–357.

Tatemichi, T.K., Desmond, D.W., Mayeux, R., et al. (1992). Dementia after stroke: Baseline frequency, risks, and clinical features in a hospitalized cohort. *Neurology, 42,* 1185–1193.

Tatu, L., Moulin, T., Bogousslavsky, J., & Duvernoy, H. (2001). Arterial territories of human brain. In J. Bogousslavsky & L.R. Caplan (Eds.), *Stroke syndromes* (2nd ed.). Cambridge: Cambridge University Press.

Tatu, L., Moulin, T., Bogousslavsky, J., & Duvernoy, H. (2001). Arterial territories of the human brain. In J. Bogousslavsky & L. Caplan (Eds.), *Stroke syndromes* (2nd ed.). Cambridge: Cambridge University Press.

Tauboll, E., Lundervold, A., & Gjerstad, L. (1991). Temporal distribution of seizures in epilepsy. *Epilepsy Research, 8,* 153–165.

Taussig, I.M., Mack, W.J., & Henderson, V.W. (1996). Concurrent validity of Spanish-language versions of the Mini-Mental State Examination, Mental Status Questionnaire, Information-Memory-Concentration Test, and Orientation-Memory-Concentration Test: Alzheimer's disease patients and nondemented elderly comparison subjects. *Journal of the International Neuropsychological Society, 2,* 286–298.

Taylor, A.E. & Saint-Cyr, J.A. (1992). Executive function. In S.J. Huber, & J.L. Cummings (Eds.), *Parkinson's disease: Neurobehavioral aspects.* New York: Oxford University Press.

Taylor, A.E., Saint-Cyr, J.A., & Lang, A.E. (1986). Frontal lobe dysfunction in Parkinson's disease. *Brain, 109,* 845–883.

Taylor, A.E., Saint-Cyr, J.A., Lang, A.E., & Kenny, F.T. (1986). Parkinson's disease and depression: A critical reevaluation. *Brain, 109,* 279–292.

Taylor, D.C. (1989). Affective disorders in epilepsies: A neuropsychiatric review. *Behavioural Neurology, 2,* 49–68.

Taylor, E.M. (1959). *Psychological appraisal of children with cerebral deficits.* Cambridge, MA: Harvard University Press.

Taylor, H.G. & Hansotia, P. (1983). Neuropsychological testing of Huntington's patients. *Journal of Nervous and Mental Disease, 171,* 492–496.

Taylor, J.M., Goldman, H., Leavitt, J., & Kleimann, K.M. (1984). Limitations of the brief form of the Halstead Category Test. *Journal of Clinical Neuropsychology, 6,* 341–344.

Taylor, J.R. & Combs-Orne, T. (1985). Alcohol and strokes in young adults. *American Journal of Psychiatry, 142,* 116–118.

Taylor, J.R. & Jentsch, J.D. (2001). Stimulant effects on striatal and cortical dopamine systems involved in reward-related behavior and impulsivity. In M.V. Solanto et al. (Eds.), *Stimulant drugs and ADHD. Basic and clinical neuroscience.* New York: Oxford University Press.

Taylor, J.S., Harp, J.H., & Elliot, T. (1991). Neuropsychologists and neurolawyers. *Neuropsychology, 5,* 293–305.

Taylor, J.S., Harp, J.H., & Elliot, T. (1992). Preparing the plaintiff in the mild brain injury case. *Trial Diplomacy Journal, 15,* 65–72.

Taylor, L.B. (1979). Psychological assessment of neurosurgical patients. In T. Rasmussen & R. Marino (Eds.), *Functional neurosurgery.* New York: Raven Press.

Taylor, M.A. (1999). *The fundamentals of clinical neuropsychiatry.* New York: Oxford University Press.

Taylor, M.J. & Heaton, R.K. (2001). Sensitivity and specificity of WAIS-III/WMS-III demographically corrected factor scores in neuropsychological assessment. *Journal of the International Neuropsychological Society, 7,* 867–875.

Taylor, R. (1990). Relationships between cognitive test performance and everyday cognitive difficulties in multiple sclerosis. *British Journal of Clinical Psychology, 29,* 251–252.

Taylor, R. & O'Carroll, R. (1995). Cognitive estimation in neurological disorders. *British Journal of Clinical Psychology, 34,* 223–228.

Taylor, R.L. (1990). *Mind or body: Distinguishing psychological from organic disorders.* New York: Springer.

Taylor, T.N., Davis, P.H., Torner, J.C., et al. (1996). Lifetime cost of stroke in the United States. *Stroke, 27,* 1459–1466.

Teasdale, G. & Jennett, B. (1974). Assessment of coma and impaired consciousness. *Lancet, ii,* 81–84.

Teasdale, G. & Mathew, P. (1996). Mechanism of cerebral concussion, contusion, and other effects of head injury. In J.R. Youmans (Ed.), *Neurological surgery.* Philadelphia: Saunders.

Teasdale, G. & Mendelow, D. (1984). Pathophysiology of head injuries. In N. Brooks (Ed.), *Closed head injury. Psychological, social and family consequences.* Oxford: Oxford University Press.

Teasdale, G.M., Nicoll, J.R., Murray, G., & Fiddes, M. (1997). Association of apolipoprotein E polymorphism with outcome after head injury. *Lancet, 350,* 1069–1071

Teasdale, G.M., Pettigrew, L.E.L., Wilson, J.T.L., et al. (1998). Analyzing outcome of treatment of severe head injury: A review and update on advancing the use of the Glasgow Outcome Scale. *Journal of Neurotrauma, 15,* 587–597.

Teasdale, T.W., Skovdahl Hansen, H.S., Gade, A., & Christensen, A.-L. (1997). Neuropsychological test scores before and after brain-injury rehabilitation in relation to return to employment. *Neuropsychological Rehabilitation, 7,* 23–42.

Teasell, R.W. & Shapiro, A.P. (1994). Strategic-behavioral intervention in the treatment of chronic nonorganic motor disorders. *American Journal of Physical Medicine and Rehabilitation, 73,* 44–50.

Tedeschi, E., Hasselbalch, S.G., Waldemar, G., et al. (1995). Heterogeneous cerebral glucose metabolism in normal pressure hydrocephalus. *Journal of Neurology, Neurosurgery and Psychiatry, 59,* 608–615.

Teeter, P.A. & Semrud-Clikeman, M. (1997). *Child neuropsychology: Assessment and intervention for neurodevelopmental disorders.* Needham Heights, MA: Allyn and Bacon.

Teichner, G., Horner, M.D., & Harvey, R.T. (2001). Neuropsychological predictors of the attainment of treatment objectives in substance abuse patients. *International Journal of Neuroscience, 106,* 253–263.

Tellegen, P.J., Winkel, M., Wijnberg-Williams, B.J., et al. (1998). *Snijders-Oomen Non-verbal Intelligence Tests (SON-R 5^1/$_2$–17, rev. ed.).* Bury St. Edmonds, UK: Thames Valley Test.

Tellier, A., Adams, K.M., Walker, A.E., & Rourke, B.P. (1990). Long-term effects of severe penetrating head injury on psychosocial adjustment. *Journal of Consulting and Clinical Psychology, 58,* 531–537.

Templer, D.I. & Drew, R.H. (1992). Non-contact sports. In D.I. Templer, L.C. Hartledge, & W.G. Cannon (Eds.), *Preventable brain damage: Brain vulnerability and brain health.* New York: Springer.

Teng, E.L. & Chui, H.C. (1987). The Modified Mini-Mental State (MMS) examination. *Journal of Clinical Psychiatry, 48,* 314–318.

Teng, E.L., Chui, H.C., & Saperia, D. (1990). Senile dementia: Performance on a neuropsychological test battery. *Recent Advances in Cardiovascular Disease, 11,* 27–34.

Teng, E.L., Chui, H.C., Schneider, L.S., & Metzger, L.E. (1987). Alzheimer's dementia: Performance on the Mini-Mental State Examination. *Journal of Consulting and Clinical Psychology, 55,* 96–100.

Teng, E.L., Hasegawa, K., Homma, A., et al. (1994). The Cognitive Abilities Screening Instrument (CASI): A practical test for cross-cultural epidemiological studies of dementia. *International Psychogeriatrics, 6,* 45–58.

Teng, E.L., Wimer, C., Roberts, E., et al. (1989). Alzheimer's dementia: Performance on parallel forms of the Dementia Assessment Battery. *Journal of Clinical and Experimental Neuropsychology, 11,* 899–912.

Tenhula, W.M.N. & Sweet, J.J. (1996). Double cross-validation of the Booklet Category Test in detecting malingered traumatic brain injury. *The Clinical Neuropsychologist, 10,* 104–116.

Tepper, S., Beatty, P., & DeJong, G. (1996). Outcomes in traumatic brain injury: Self-report versus report of significant others. *Brain Injury, 10,* 575–581.

Teri, L., Borson, S., Kiyak, A., & Yamagishi, M. (1989). Behavioral disturbance, cognitive dysfunction, and functional skill: Prevalence and relationship in Alzheimer's disease. *Journal of the American Geriatrics Society, 37,* 109–116.

Teri, L., Larson, E.B., & Reifler, B.V. (1988). Behavioral disturbance in dementia of the Alzheimer's type. *Journal of the American Geriatrics Society, 36,* 1–6.

Teri, L., McCurry, S.M., Edland, S.D., et al. (1995). Cognitive decline in Alzheimer's disease: A longitudinal investigation of risk factors for accelerated decline. *Journals of Gerontology. Series A, Biological Sciences and Medical Sciences, 50A,* M49–M55.

Teri, L. & Wagner, A. (1992). Alzheimer's disease and depression. *Journal of Consulting and Clinical Psychology, 60,* 379–391.

Terman, L.M. (1916). *The measurement of intelligence.* Boston: Houghton-Mifflin.

Terman, L.M. & Merrill, M.A. (1937). *Measuring intelligence. A guide to the administration of the new revised Stanford-Binet Tests of intelligence.* Boston: Houghton-Mifflin.

Terman, L.M. & Merrill, M.A. (1973). *Stanford-Binet Intelligence Scale: 1972 norms edition.* Boston: Houghton-Mifflin.

Terry, P. (1995). The efficacy of mood state profiling with elite performers: A review and synthesis. *Sport Psychologist, 9,* 309–324.

Terry, R.D., DeTeresa, R., & Hansen, L.A. (1987). Neocortical cell counts in normal human adult aging. *Annals of Neurology, 21,* 530–539.

Terry, R.D. & Katzman, R. (1983). Senile dementia of the Alzheimer type. *Annals of Neurology, 14,* 497–506.

Terry, R.D., Masliah, E., Salmon, D.P., et al. (1991). Physical basis of cognitive alterations in Alzheimer's disease: Synapse loss is the major correlate of cognitive impairment. *Annals of Neurology, 30,* 572–580.

Tetrud, J.W. (1991). Preclinical Parkinson's disease: Detection of motor and nonmotor manifestations. *Neurology, 41(Suppl. 2),* 69–71.

Teuber, H.-L. (1948). Neuropsychology. In M.R. Harrower (Ed.), *Recent advances in diagnostic psychological testing.* Springfield, IL: Thomas.

Teuber, H.-L. (1955). Physiological psychology. *Annual Review of Psychology, 6,* 267–296.

Teuber, H.-L. (1959). Some alterations in behavior after cerebral lesions in man. In A.D. Bass (Ed.), *Evolution of nervous control.* Washington, D.C.: American Association for the Advancement of Science.

Teuber, H.-L. (1962). Effects of brain wounds implicating right or left hemisphere in man. In V.B. Mountcastle (Ed.), *Interhemispheric relations and cerebral dominance.* Baltimore, MD: Johns Hopkins Press.

Teuber, H.-L. (1964). The riddle of frontal lobe function in man. In J.M. Warren & K. Akert (Eds.), *The frontal granular cortex and behavior.* New York: McGraw-Hill.

Teuber, H.-L. (1968). Alterations of perception and memory in man. In L. Weiskrantz (Ed.), *Analysis of behavioral change.* New York: Harper & Row.

Teuber, H.-L. (1969). Neglected aspects of the post-traumatic syndrome. In A. Walker et al. (Eds.), *The late effects of head injury.* Springfield, IL: Thomas.

Teuber, H.-L. (1975). Effects of focal brain injury on human behavior. In D.B. Tower (Ed.), *The nervous system. The clinical neurosciences* (Vol. 2). New York: Raven Press.

Teuber, H.-L., Battersby, W.S., & Bender, M.B. (1951). Performance on complex visual tasks after cerebral lesion. *Journal of Nervous and Mental Disease, 114,* 413–429.

Teuber, H. L., Battersby, W.S., & Bender, M.B. (1960). *Visual field defects after penetrating missile wounds of the brain.* Cambridge, MA: Harvard University Press.

Teuber, H. L. & Weinstein, S. (1954). Performance on a form board task after penetrating brain injury. *Journal of Psychology, 38,* 177–190.

Thach, W.T., Jr. & Montgomery, E.B., Jr. (1990). Motor system. In A.L. Pearlman & R.C. Collins (Eds.), *Neurobiology of disease.* New York: Oxford University Press.

Tharion, W.J., Kobrick, J.L., Lieberman, H.R., & Fine, B.J. (1993). Effects of caffeine and diphenhydramine on auditory evoked cortical potentials. *Perceptual and Motor Skills, 76,* 707–715.

Thatcher, R.W. & John, E.R. (1977). *Foundations of cognitive processes.* Hillsdale, NJ: Erlbaum.

Theisen, M.E., Rapport, L.J., Axelrod, B.N., & Brines, D.B. (1998). Effects of practice in repeated administrations of the Wechsler Memory Scale Revised in normal adults. *Assessment, 5,* 85–92.

Theodore, W.H. & Gaillard, W.D. (2002). Neuroimaging and the progression of epilepsy. *Progress in Brain Research, 135,* 305–313.

Thiagarajan, J., Taylor, P., Hogbin, E., & Ridley, S. (1994). Qual-ity of life after multiple trauma requiring intensive care. *Anaesthesia, 49,* 211–218.

Thiery, E., Dietens, E., & Vandereecken, H. (1982). La récupération spontanée: Ampleur et limites. In X. Seron & C. Latere (Eds.), *Rééduquer le cerveau.* Brussels: Pierre Mardaga.

Thomas, R., O'Connor, A.M., & Ashley, S. (1995). Speech and language disorders in patients with high grade glioma and its influence on prognosis. *Journal of Neurooncology, 23,* 265-270.

Thomas, S., Iezzi, T., Duckworth, M.P., et al. (2000). Posttraumatic stress symptoms and general activity level in the prediction of neurocognitive performance in chronic pain patients. *International Journal of Rehabilitation and Health, 5,* 31–42.

Thompson, A.J. (1998). Multiple sclerosis. In M. Swash (Ed.), *Outcomes in neurological and neurosurgical disorders.* Cambridge: Cambridge University Press.

Thompson, A.J., Montalban, X., Barkhof, F., et al. (2000). Diagnostic criteria for primary progressive multiple sclerosis: A position paper. *Annals of Neurology, 47,* 831–835.

Thompson, D.C., Rivara, F.P., & Thompson, R. (2003). Helmets for preventing head and facial injuries in bicyclists. Cochrane Review. The Cochrane Library, 2. New York: Oxford. Update software (retrieved May 5, 2003, from http://www.update-software.com/abstracts/ab001855.htm).

Thompson, I.M. (1988). Communication changes in normal and abnormal aging. In Una Holden (Ed.), *Neuropsychology and aging.* New York: New York University Press.

Thompson, L.L. & Heaton, R.K. (1991). Pattern of performance on the Tactual Performance Test. *The Clinical Neuropsychologist, 5,* 322–328.

Thompson, L.L., Heaton, R.K., Grant, I., & Matthews, C.G. (1989). Comparison of the WAIS and WAIS-R using T-Score conversions that correct for age, education, and sex. *Journal of Clinical and Experimental Neuropsychology, 11,* 478–488.

Thompson, L.L., Heaton, R.K., Matthews, C.G., & Grant, I. (1987). Comparison of preferred and nonpreferred hand performance on four neuropsychological motor tasks. *The Clinical Neuropsychologist, 1,* 324–334.

Thompson, L.L. & Parsons, O.A. (1985). Contribution of the TPT to adult neuropsychological assessment: A review. *Journal of Clinical and Experimental Neuropsychology, 7,* 430–444.

Thompson, L.W., Gong, V., Haskins, E., & Gallagher, D. (1987). Assessment of depression and dementia during the late years. In K.W. Schaie (Ed.), *Annual review of gerontology and geriatrics.* New York: Springer.

Thompson, P.J. & Trimble, M.R. (1996). Neuropsychological aspects of epilepsy. In I. Grant & K.M. Adams (Eds.), *Neuropsychological aspects of neuropsychiatric disorders* (2nd ed.). New York: Oxford University Press.

Thompson, R.F. (1976). The search for the engram. *American Psychologist, 31,* 209–227.

Thompson, R.F. (1988). Brain substrates of learning and memory. In T. Boll & B.K. Bryant (Eds.), *Clinical neuropsychology and brain function: Research, measurement, and practice.* Washington, D.C.: American Psychological Association.

Thompson, S.A., Graham, K.S., Patterson, K., et al. (2002). Is knowledge of famous people disproportionately impaired in patients with early and questionable Alzheimer's disease? *Neuropsychology, 16,* 344–358.

Thompson-Schill, S.L., Gabrieli, J.D., & Fleischman, D.A. (1999). Effects of structural similarity and name frequency on picture naming in Alzheimer's disease. *Journal of the International Neuropsychological Society, 5,* 659–667.

Thompson-Schill, S.L., Swick, D., Farah, M.J., et al. (1998). Verb generation in patients with focal frontal lesions: A neuropsychological test of neuroimaging findings. *Proceedings of the National*

Academy of Sciences of the United States of America, 95, 15855–15860.

Thomsen, I.V. (1984). Late outcome of very severe blunt head trauma: A 10–15 year second follow-up. *Journal of Neurology, Neurosurgery, and Psychiatry, 47,* 260–268.

Thomsen, I.V. (1989). Do young patients have worse outcomes after severe blunt head trauma? *Brain Injury, 3,* 157–162.

Thomsen, I.V. (1990). Recognizing the development of behaviour disorders. In R.L. Wood (Ed.), *Neurobehavioral sequelae of traumatic brain injury.* Bristol, PA: Taylor & Francis.

Thorndike, R.L., Hagen, E.P., & Sattler, J.M. (1987). *Stanford-Binet Intelligence Scale* (4th ed.). Chicago: Riverside.

Thornhill, S., Teasdale, G.M., Murray, G.D., et al. (2000). Disability in young people and adults one year after head injury: Prospective cohort study. *British Medical Journal, 320,* 1631–1635.

Thornton, A.E. & Raz, N. (1997). Memory impairment in multiple sclerosis: A quantitative review. *Neuropsychology, 11,* 357–366.

Thornton, A.E., Raz, N., & Tucker, K.A. (2002). Memory in multiple sclerosis: Contextual encoding deficits. *Journal of the International Neuropsychological Society, 8,* 395–409.

Thun, M.J., Peto, R., Lopez, A.D., et al. (1997). Alcohol consumption and mortality among middle-aged and elderly U.S. adults. *New England Journal of Medicine, 337,* 1705–1714.

Thurman, D.J., Alverson, C., Browne, D., et al. (1999). Traumatic brain injury in the United States. A report to Congress. Atlanta: Centers for Disease Control and Prevention, U.S. Department of Health and Human Services.

Thurstone, L.L. (1938). *Primary mental abilities.* Chicago: University of Chicago Press.

Thurstone, L.L. (1944). *A factorial study of perception.* Chicago: University of Chicago Press.

Thurstone, L.L. (1949). *Mechanical aptitudes III. Analysis of group tests* (Vol. 2). Psychometric Laboratory Report 55. Chicago: University of Chicago.

Thurstone, L.L. & Jeffrey, T.E. (1982). *Closure Flexibility (Concealed Figures).* Rosemont, IL: London House Pearson Reid.

Thurstone, L.L. & Jeffrey, T.E. (1983). *Closure Speed (Gestalt Completion).* Rosemont, IL: London House Pearson Reid.

Thurstone, L.L. & Jeffrey, T.E. (1984). *Space Thinking (Flags).* Chicago, IL: London House Pearson Reid.

Thurstone, L.L. & Jeffrey, T.E. (1987). *Perceptual Speed (Identical Forms).* Chicago, IL: London House Pearson Reid.

Thurstone, L.L & Thurstone, T.G. (1962). *Primary Mental Abilities* (rev.). Chicago: Science Research Associates.

Thurstone, T.G. (1992). *Understanding Communication.* Chicago, IL: London House Pearson Reid.

Tierney, M.C., Fisher, R.H., Lewis, A.J., et al. (1988). The NINCDS-ADRDA work group criteria for the clinical diagnosis of probable Alzheimer's disease. *Neurology, 38,* 359–364.

Tierney, M.C., Szalai, J.P., Snow, W.G., et al. (1996). Prediction of probable Alzheimer's disease in memory-impaired patients: A prospective longitudinal study. *Neurology, 46,* 661–665.

Tiersky, L., Johnson, S.K., Lange, G., et al. (1997). Neuropsychology of chronic fatigue syndrome: A critical review. *Journal of Clinical and Experimental Neuropsychology, 19,* 560–586.

Tietjen, G.E. (1997). Transient focal neurologic events. In K.M.A. Welch et al. (Eds.), *Primer on cerebrovascular diseases.* San Diego: Academic Press.

Tiffin, J. (1968). *Purdue Pegboard Examiner's Manual.* Rosemont, IL: London House.

Timmerman, M.E. & Brouwer, W.H. (1999). Slow information processing after very severe closed head injury: Impaired access to declarative knowledge and intact application and acquisition of procedural knowledge. *Neuropsychologia, 37,* 467–478.

Tinkcom, M., Obrzut, J.E., & Poston, C.S.L. (1983). Spatial lateralization: The relationship among sex, handedness, and familial sinistrality. *Neuropsychologia, 21,* 683–686.

Tinson, D.J. & Lincoln, N.B. (1987). Subjective memory impairment after stroke. *International Disability Studies, 9,* 6–9.

Tippin, J., Adams, H.P., & Smoker, W.R.K. (1984). Early computed tomographic abnormalities following profound cerebral hypoxia. *Archives of Neurology, 41,* 1098–1100.

Tissot, R., Lhermitte, F., & Ducarne, B. (1963). État intellectuel des aphasiques. *Encéphale, 52,* 286–320.

Tobin, A.J. (1990). Genetic disorders: Huntington's disease. In A.L. Pearlman & R.C. Collins (Eds.), *Neurobiology of disease.* New York: Oxford University Press.

Toglia, M. P. & Battig, W. F. (1978). *Handbook of semantic word norms.* Hillsdale, NJ: Erlbaum.

Tognola, G. & Vignolo, L.A. (1980). Brain lesions associated with oral apraxia in stroke patients: A clinico-neuroradiological investigation with the CT scan. *Neuropsychologia, 18,* 257–272.

Tollman, S.G. & Msengana, N.B. (1990). Neuropsychological assessment: Problems in evaluating the higher mental functioning of Zulu-speaking people using traditional Western techniques. *South African Journal of Psychology, 20,* 20–24.

Tombaugh, T.N. (1996). *Test of Memory Malingering.* Los Angeles: Western Psychological Services.

Tombaugh, T.N. (1997). The Test of Memory Malingering (TOMM): Normative data from cognitively intact and cognitively impaired individuals. *Psychological Assessment, 9,* 260–268.

Tombaugh, T.N., Faulkner, P., & Hubley, A.M. (1992). Effects of age on the Rey-Osterrieth and Taylor Complex Figures: Test–retest data using an intentional learning paradigm. *Journal of Clinical and Experimental Neuropsychology, 14,* 647–661.

Tombaugh, T.N., Grandmaison, L.J., & Schmidt, J.P. (1995). Prospective memory: Relationship to age and retrospective memory in the Learning and Memory Battery (LAMB). *The Clinical Neuropsychologist, 9,* 135–142.

Tombaugh, T.N. & Hubley, A.M. (1991). Four studies comparing the Rey-Osterrieth and Taylor Complex Figures. *Journal of Clinical and Experimental Neuropsychology, 13,* 587–599.

Tombaugh, T.N. & Hubley, A.M. (1997). The 60-item Boston Naming Test: Norms for cognitively intact adults aged 25 to 88 years. *Journal of Clinical and Experimental Neuropsychology, 14,* 167–177.

Tombaugh, T.N. & Hubley, A.M. (2001). Rates of forgetting on three measures of verbal learning using retention intervals ranging from 20 min to 62 days. *Journal of the International Neuropsychological Society, 7,* 79–91.

Tombaugh, T.N., Kozak, J., & Rees, L. (1999). Normative data stratified by age and education for two measures of verbal fluency: FAS and animal naming. *Archives of Clinical Neuropsychology, 14,* 167–177.

Tombaugh, T.N., McDowell, L., Kristjansson, B., & Hubley, A.M. (1996). Mini-Mental State Examination (MMSE) and the Modified MMSE (2MS): A psychometric comparison and normative data. *Psychological Assessment, 8,* 48–59.

Tombaugh, T.N. & McIntyre, N.J. (1992). The Mini-Mental State Examination: A comprehensive review. *Journal of the American Geriatrics Society, 40,* 922–935.

Tombaugh, T.N. & Schmidt, J.P. (1992). The Learning and Memory Battery (LAMB): Development and standardization. *Psychological Assessment, 4,* 193–206.

Toni, N., Buchs, P.A., Nikonenko, I., et al. (1999). LTP promotes formation of multiple spine synapses between a single axon terminal and a dendrite. *Nature, 402,* 421–425.

Toomey, R., Wallace, C.J., Corrigan, P.W., et al. (1997). Social processing correlates of nonverbal social perception in schizophrenia. *Psychiatry, 60,* 292–300.

Torelli, P., Cologno, D., & Manzoni, G.C. (1999). Weekend headache: A retrospective study in migraine without aura and episodic tension-type headache. *Headache, 39,* 11–20.

Tovée, M.J. (1996). *An introduction to the visual system.* Cambridge, UK: Cambridge University Press.

Tow, P.M. (1955). *Personality changes following frontal leucotomy.* London: Oxford University Press.

Towle, D. & Lincoln, N.B. (1991). Use of the indented paragraph test with right hemisphere-damaged stroke patients. *British Journal of Clinical Psychology, 30,* 37–45.

Townend, W.J., Guy, M.J., Pani, M.A., et al. (2002). Head injury outcome prediction in emergency department: A role for protein S-100B? *Journal of Neurology, Neurosurgery and Psychiatry, 73,* 542–546.

Townes, B.D., Dikmen, S.S., Bledsoe, S. W., et al. (1986). Neuropsychological changes in a young, healthy population after controlled hypotensive anesthesia. *Anesthesia and Analgesia, 65,* 955–959.

Townes, B.D., Hornbein, R.B., Schoene, F.H., et al. (1984). Human cerebral function at extreme altitude. In J.B. West & S. Lahiri (Eds.), *High altitude and man.* Bethesda, MD: American Physiological Society.

Trabert, W., Betz, T., Niewald, M., & Huber, G. (1995). Significant reversibility of alcoholic brain shrinkage within 3 weeks of abstinence. *Acta Psychiatrica Scandinavica, 92,* 87–90.

Trahan, D.E. (1985). Analysis of gender differences in verbal and visual memory [abstract]. *Journal of Clinical and Experimental Neuropsychology, 7,* 640–641.

Trahan, D.E. (1992). Analysis of learning and rate of forgetting in age-associated memory differences. *The Clinical Neuropsychologist, 6,* 241–246.

Trahan, D.E., Goethe, K.E., & Larrabee, G.J. (1989). An examination of verbal supraspan in normal adults and patients with head trauma or unilateral cerebrovascular accident. *Neuropsychology, 3,* 81–90.

Trahan, D.E. & Larrabee, G.J. (1988). *Continuous Visual Memory Test.* Odessa, FL: Psychological Assessment Resources.

Trahan, D.E., Larrabee, G.J., Fritzsche, B., & Curtiss, G. (1996). Continuous Visual Memory Test: Alternate form and generalizability estimates. *The Clinical Neuropsychologist, 10,* 73–79.

Trahan, D.E., Larrabee, G.J., & Levin, H.S. (1986). Age-related differences in recognition memory for pictures. *Experimental Aging Reserch, 12,* 147–150.

Trahan, D.E., Larrabee, G.J., & Quintana, J.W. (1990). Visual recognition memory in normal adults and patients with unilateral vascular lesions. *Journal of Clinical and Experimental Neuropsychology, 12,* 857–872.

Trahan, D.E., Patterson, J., Quintana, J., & Biron, R. (1987). The Finger Tapping Test: A reexamination of traditional hypotheses regarding normal adult performance [abstract]. *Journal of Clinical and Experimental Neuropsychology, 9,* 52.

Trahan, D.E., Quintana, J., Willingham, A.C., & Goethe, K.E. (1988). The Visual Reproduction subtest: Standardization and clinical validation of a delayed recall procedure. *Neuropsychology, 2,* 29–39.

Tran, T.A., Spencer, S.S., & Spencer, D.D. (1998). Epilepsy: Medical and surgical outcome. In M. Swash (Ed.), *Outcomes in neurological and neurosurgical disorders.* Cambridge, UK: Cambridge University Press.

Tranel, D. (1996). The Iowa-Benton school of neuropsychological assessment. In I. Grant & K.M. Adams (Eds.), *Neuropsychological assessment of neuropsychiatric disorders* (2nd ed.). New York: Oxford University Press.

Tranel, D. (2000). Non-conscious brain processing indexed by psy-

chophysiological measures. *Progress in Brain Research, 122,* 317–332.

Tranel, D. (2002). Functional neuroanatomy: Neuropsychological correlates of cortical and subcortical damage. In S.C. Yudofsky & R.E. Hales (Eds.), *The American Psychiatric Publishing textbook of neuropsychiatry and clinical neurosciences* (4th ed.). Washington, D.C.: American Psychiatric Publishing.

Tranel, D., Benton, A., & Olson, K. (1997). A 10-year longitudinal study of cognitive changes in elderly persons. *Developmental Neuropsychology, 13,* 87–96.

Tranel, D. & Damasio, A.R. (2000). Neuropsychology and behavioral neurology. In J.T. Cacioppo et al. (Eds.), *Handbook of psychophysiology* (2nd ed.). Cambridge: Cambridge University Press.

Tranel, D. & Damasio, A.R. (2002). Neurobiological foundations of human memory. In A.D. Baddeley et al. (Eds.), *The handbook of memory disorders* (2nd ed.). Chichester, UK: Wiley.

Tranel, D., Damasio, A.R., & Damasio, H. (1988). Intact recognition of facial expression, gender, and age in patients with impaired recognition of face identity. *Neurology, 38,* 690–696.

Trask, T.W. & Narayan, R.K. (1996). Civilian pentetrating head injury. In R.K. Narayan et al. (Eds.), *Neurotrauma.* New York: McGraw-Hill.

Traub, G.S. & Spruill, J. (1982). Correlations between the Quick Test and Wechsler Adult Intelligence Scale–Revised. *Psychological Reports, 51,* 309–310.

Tredget, E.E., Shankowsky, H.A., & Tilley, W.A. (1999). Electrical injuries in Canadian burn care. Identification of unsolved problems. *Annals of the New York Academy of Sciences, 888,* 75–87.

Treiman, D.M. (1986). Epilepsy and violence: Medical and legal issues. *Epilepsia, 27,* S77–S104.

Treiman, D.M. (1991). Psychobiology of ictal aggression. *Advances in Neurology, 55,* 341–356.

Tremblay, F., Mireault, A.C., Letourneau, J., et al. (2002). Tactile perception and manual dexterity in computer users. *Somatosensory and Motor Research, 19,* 101–108.

Tremont, G., Hoffman, R.G., Scott, J.G., & Adams, R.L. (1998). Effect of intellectual level on neuropsychological test performance: A response to Dodrill (1997). *The Clinical Neuropsychologist, 12,* 560–567.

Trenerry, M.R. (1996). Neuropsychologic assessment in surgical treatment of epilepsy. *Mayo Clinic Proceedings, 71,* 1196–1200.

Trenerry, M.R., Crosson, B., DeBoe, J., & Leber, W.R. (1989). *The Stroop Neuropsychological Screening Test.* Odessa, FL: Psychological Assessment Resources.

Trenerry, M.R., Crosson, B., DeBoe, J., & Leber, W.R. (1990). *Visual Search and Attention Test.* Odessa, FL: Psychological Assessment Resources.

Trenerry, M.R., Jack, C.R., Jr., Ivnik, R.J., et al. (1993). MRI hippocampal volumes and memory function before and after temporal lobectomy. *Neurology, 43,* 1800–1805.

Trenerry, M.R., Westerveld, M., & Meador, K.J. (1995). MRI hippocampal volume and neuropsychology in epilepsy surgery. *Magnetic Resonance Imaging, 13,* 1125–1132.

Trevarthen, C. (1990). Integrative functions of the cerebral commissures. In F. Boller & J. Grafman (Eds.), *Handbook of neuropsychology* (Vol. 4). Amsterdam: Elsevier.

Trexler, L.E., Eberle, R., & Zappala, G. (2000). Models and programs of the Center for Neuropsychological Rehabilitation: Fifteen years experience. In A.-L. Christensen & B. Uzzell (Eds.), *International handbook of neuropsychological rehabilitation.* New York: Kluwer Academic/Plenum Press.

Trexler, L.E. & Zappala, G. (1988). Re-examining the determinants of recovery and rehabilitation of memory defects following traumatic brain injury. *Brain Injury, 2,* 187–203.

Trick, G.L., Trick, L.R., Morris, P., & Wolf, M. (1995). Visual field loss in senile dementia of the Alzheimer's type. *Neurology, 45,* 68–74.

Triebig, G. (1989), Occupational neurotoxicology of organ solvents and solvent mixures. *Neurotoxicology and Teratology, 11,* 575–578.

Triebig, G., Claus, D., Csuzda, I., et al. (1988). Cross-sectional epidemiological study on neurotoxicity of solvents in paints and lacquers. *International Archives of Occupational and Environmental Health, 60,* 233–241.

Triggs, W.J., Calvanio, R., Levine, M., et al. (2000). Predicting hand preference with performance on motor tasks. *Cortex, 36,* 679–689.

Triggs, W.J., McCoy, K.J., Greer, R., et al. (1999). Effects of left frontal transcranial magnetic stimulation on depressed mood, cognition, and corticomotor threshold. *Biological Psychiatry, 45,* 1440–1446.

Trimble, M.R. (1983). Personality disturbances in epilepsy. *Neurology, 33,* 1332–1340.

Trimble, M.R. (1986). Pseudoseizures. *Neurology Clinics, 4,* 531–548.

Trimble, M.R. (1989). Kindling, epilepsy and behavior. In T.G. Bolwig & M.R. Trimble (Eds.), *The clinical relevance of kindling.* Chichester, UK: Wiley.

Trimble, M.R., Mendez, M.F., & Cummings, J.L. (1997). Neuropsychiatric symptoms from the temporolimbic lobes. *Journal of Neuropsychiatry and Clinical Neuroscience, 9,* 429–438.

Trimble, M.R., Ring, H.A., & Schmitz, B. (1996). Neuropsychiatric aspects of epilepsy. In B.S. Fogel et al. (Eds.), *Neuropsychiatry.* Baltimore, MD: Williams & Wilkins.

Trobe, J.D., Waller, P.F., Cook-Flannagan, C.A., et al. (1996). Crashes and violations among drivers with Alzheimer disease. *Archives of Neurology, 53,* 411–416.

Trojano, L. & Grossi, D. (1998). "Pure" constructional apraxia: A cognitive analysis of a single case. *Behavioural Neurology, 11,* 43–49.

Tromp, E. & Mulder, T. (1991). Slowness of information processing after traumatic head injury. *Journal of Clinical and Experimental Neuropsychology, 13,* 821–830.

Troost, B.T. (1992). Neuro-ophthalmological aspects. In I. Litvan & Y. Agid (Eds.), *Progressive supranuclear palsy: Clinical and research approaches.* New York: Oxford University Press.

Tross, S. & Hirsch, D.A. (1988). Psychological distress and neuropsychological complications of HIV infection and AIDS. *American Psychologist, 43,* 929–934.

Tröster, A.I., Butters, N., Salmon, D.P., et al. (1993). The diagnostic utility of savings scores: Differentiating Alzheimer's and Huntington's disease with the Logical Memory and Visual Reproduction Tests. *Journal of Clinical and Experimental Neuropsychology, 15,* 773–788.

Tröster, A.I., Fields, J.A., Testa, J.A., et al. (1998). Cortical and subcortical influences on clustering and switching in the performance of verbal fluency tasks. *Neuropsychologia, 36,* 295–304.

Tröster, A.I., Jacobs, D., Butters, N., et al. (1989). Differentiating Alzheimer's disease with the Wechsler Memory Scale–Revised. In F.J. Pirozzolo (Ed.), *Clinics in geriatric medicine* (Vol. 5, No. 3). Philadelphia: Saunders.

Trostle, J.A., Hauser, W.A., & Sharbrough, F.W. (1989). Psychological and social adjustment to epilepsy in Rochester, Minnesota. *Neurology, 39,* 633–637.

Troy, L., McFarland, K., Littman-Power, S., et al. (2000). Cisplatin-based therapy: A neurological and neuropsychological review. *Psychooncology, 9,* 29–39.

Troyer, A.K. (2000). Normative data for clustering and switching on verbal fluency tasks. *Journal of Clinical and Experimental Neuropsychology, 22,* 370–378.

Troyer, A.K., Fisk, J.D., Archibald, C.J., et al. (1996). Conceptual reasoning as a mediator of verbal recall in patients with multiple sclerosis. *Journal of Clinical and Experimental Neuropsychology, 18,* 211–219.

Troyer, A.K., Moscovitch, M., & Winocur, G. (1997). Clustering and switching as two components of verbal fluency: Evidence from younger and older healthy adults. *Neuropsychology, 11,* 138–146.

Troyer, A.K., Moscovitch, M., Winocur, G., et al. (1998a). Clustering and switching on verbal fluency: The effects of focal frontal- and temporal-lobe lesions. *Neuropsychologia, 36,* 499–504.

Troyer, A.K., Moscovitch, M., Winocur, G., et al. (1998b). Clustering and switching on verbal fluency tests in Alzheimer's and Parkinson's disease. *Journal of the International Neuropsychological Society, 4,* 137–143.

Troyer, A.K. & Wishart, H.A. (1997). A comparison of qualitative scoring systems for the Rey-Osterreith Complex Figure Test. *The Clinical Neuropsychologist, 11,* 381–390.

Trueblood, W. (1994). Qualitative and quantitative characteristics of malingered and other invalid WAIS-R and clinical memory data. *Journal of Clinical and Experimental Neuropsychology, 16,* 597–607.

Trueblood, W. & Schmidt, M. (1993). Malingering and other validity considerations in the neuropsychological evaluation of mild head injury. *Journal of Clinical and Experimental Neuropsychology, 15,* 578–590.

Truelle, J.-L. (1987). Le traumatisme crânien grave: Un handicap singular. *Réadaptation, Novembre No. 344,* 6–8.

Truelle, J.-L., Le Gall, D., Joseph, P.A., et al. (1988). L'évaluation des sequelles mentales. Difficulté de l'expertise des traumatismes crâniens graves. *Revue Française de Dommage Corporel, 14,* 153–165.

Truelle, J.-L., Le Gall, D., Joseph, P.A., et al. (1995). Movement disturbances following frontal lobe lesions. *Neuropsychiatry, Neuropsychology, and Behavioral Neurology, 8,* 14–19.

Trzepacz, P.T., Meagher, D.J., & Wise, M.G. (2002). Neuropsychiatric aspects of delirium. In S.C. Yudofsky & R.E. Hales (Eds.), *American Psychiatric Publishing textbook of neuropsychiatry and clinical neurosciences.* Washington, D.C.: American Psychiatric Publishing.

Tsai, Y.J., Wang, J.D., & Huang, W.F., (1995). Case-control study of the effectiveness of different types of helmets for the prevention of head injuries among motorcycle riders in Taipei, Taiwan. *American Journal of Epidemiology, 142,* 974–981.

Tsang, H.-L. & Lee, T.M.C. (2003). The effect of ageing on confrontational naming ability. *Archives of Clinical Neuropsychology, 18,* 81–90.

Tsushima, W.T. & Bratton, J.C. (1977). Effects of geographic region upon Wechsler Adult Intelligence Scale results: A Hawaii–mainland United States comparison. *Journal of Consulting and Clinical Psychology, 45,* 501–502.

Tsushima, W.T. & Towne, W.S. (1977). Effects of paint sniffing on neuropsychological test performance. *Journal of Abnormal Psychology, 86,* 402–407.

Tucha, O.W., Smely, C.W., & Lange, K.W. (1999). Verbal and figural fluency in patients with mass lesions of the left or right frontal lobes. *Journal of Clinical and Experimental Neuropsychology, 21,* 229–236.

Tucker, Daniel M., Watson, R.T., & Heilman, K.M. (1977). Discrimination and evocation of affectively intoned speech in patients with right parietal disease. *Neurology, 27,* 947–950.

Tucker, Don M., Derryberry, & Luu, P. (2000). Anatomy and physiology of human emotion: Vertical integration of brainstem, limbic, and cortical systems. In J.C. Borod (Ed.), *The neuropsychology of emotion*. New York: Oxford University Press.

Tucker, Don M., Roth, D.L., & Bair, T.B. (1986). Functional connections among cortical regions: Topography of EEG coherence. *Electroencephalography and Clinical Neurophysiology, 63,* 242–250.

Tucker, G.J. (2002). Neuropsychiatric aspects of seizure disorders. In S.C. Yudofsky & R.E. Hales (Eds.), *American Psychiatric Publishing textbook of neuropsychiatry and clinical neurosciences* (4th ed.). Washington, D.C.

Tulsky, D.S., Saklofske, D.H., Chelune, G.J., et al. (2003). *Clinical interpretation of the WAIS-III and WMS-III.* San Diego: Academic Press.

Tulsky, D.S., Saklofske, D.H., & Ricker, J.H. (2003). Historical overview of the Wechsler scales. In D.S. Tulsky et al. (2003). *Clinical interpretation of the WAIS-III and WMS-III.* San Diego: Academic Press.

Tulsky, D.S., Zhu, J., & Ledbetter, M.F. (1997). *WAIS-III WMS-III technical manual.* San Antonio, TX: Psychological Corporation.

Tulving, E. (1985). How many memory systems are there? *American Psychologist, 40,* 385–398.

Tulving, E. (2000). Introduction (memory). In M.S. Gazzaniga (Ed.), *The new cognitive neurosciences* (2nd ed.). Cambridge, MA: MIT Press.

Tulving, E. (2002a). Episodic memory: From mind to brain. *Annual Review of Psychology, 53,* 1–25.

Tulving, E. (2002b). *Episodic memory: Yesterday and today.* Invited lecture, International Neuropsychological Society midyear meeting, Stockholm, Sweden, July.

Tulving, E. & Craik, F.I.M. (Eds.) (2000). *The Oxford handbook of memory.* New York: Oxford University Press.

Tulving, E., Kapur, S., Craik, F.I., et al. (1994). Hemispheric encoding/retrieval asymmetry in episodic memory: Positron emission tomography findings. *Proceedings of the National Academy of Sciences USA, 91,* 2016–2020.

Tulving, E. & Markowitsch, H.J. (1998). Episodic and declarative memory: Role of the hippocampus. *Hippocampus, 8,* 198–204.

Tuokko, H. & Crockett, D. (1989). Cued recall and memory disorders in dementia. *Journal of Clinical and Experimental Neuropsychology, 11,* 278–294.

Tuokko, H., Gallie, K. A., & Crockett, D. J. (1990). Patterns of memory deterioration in normal and memory impaired elderly. *Developmental Neuropsychology, 6,* 291–300.

Tuokko, H. & Hadjistavropoulos, T. (1998). *An assessment guide to geriatric neuropsychology.* Mahwah, NJ: Erlbaum.

Tuokko, H., Hadjistavropoulos, T., Miller, J.A., & Beattie, B.L. (1992). The Clock Test: A sensitive measure to differentiate normal elderly from those with Alzheimer disease. *Journal of the American Geriatrics Society, 40,* 579–584.

Tuokko, H., Hadjistavropoulos,, T., Miller, J.A., et al. (1992). *The Clock Test. Administration and scoring manual.* Toronto: Multi-Health Systems.

Tuokko, H., Hadjistavropoulos, T., Rae, S., & O'Rourke, N. (2000). A comparison of alternative approaches to the scoring of clock drawing. *Archives of Clinical Neuropsychology, 15,* 137–148.

Tuokko, H., Vernon-Wilkinson, R., & Robinson, E. (1991). The use of the MCMI in the personality assessment of head-injured adults. *Brain Injury, 5,* 287–293.

Tupler, L.A., Welsh, K.A., Asare-Aboagye, Y., & Dawson, D.V. (1995). Reliability of the Rey-Osterrieth Complex Figure in use with memory impaired patients. *Journal of Clinical and Experimental Neuropsychology, 17,* 566–579.

Tupper, D.E. (1999). Introduction: Alexander Luria's continuing influence on worldwide neuropsychology. *Neuropsychology Review, 9,* 1–7.

Turkheimer, E., Yeo, R.A., Jones, C.L., & Bigler, E.D. (1990). Quantitative assessment of covariation between neuropsychological function and location of naturally occurring lesions in humans. *Journal of Clinical and Experimental Neuropsychology, 12,* 549–565.

Turnbull, O.H., Carey, D.P., & McCarthy, R.A. (1997). The neuropsychology of object constancy. *Journal of the International Neuropsychological Society, 3,* 288–298.

Turner, M.A., Moran, N.F., & Kopelman, M.D. (2002). Subcortical dementia. *British Journal of Psychiatry, 180,* 148–151.

Turner, S.M., DeMers, S.T., Fox, H.R., & Reed, G.M. (2001). APA's guidelines for test user qualifications: An executive summary. *American Psychologist, 56,* 1099–1113.

Tweedy, J.R., Langer, K.G., & McDowell, F.H. (1982). Effect of semantic relations on the memory deficit associated with Parkinson's disease. *Journal of Clinical Neuropsychology, 4,* 235–248.

Twum, M. & Parente, R. (1994). Role of imagery and verbal labeling in the performance of paired associates tasks by persons with closed head injury. *Journal of Clinical and Experimental Neuropsychology, 16,* 630–639.

Tzavaras, A., Hécaen, H., & Le Bras, H. (1970). Le problème de la specificité du déficit de la reconnaissance du visage humain lors des lésions hémisphèriques unilatérales. *Neuropsychologia, 8,* 403–416.

Tzourio, N., Crivello, F., Mellet, E., et al. (1998). Functional anatomy of dominance for speech comprehension in left handers vs. right handers. *Neuroimage, 8,* 1–16.

Tzourio, C., Tehindrazanarivelo, A., Iglesias, S., et al. (1995). Case-control study of migraine and risk of ischaemic stroke in young women. *British Medical Journal, 310,* 830–833.

Uchiyama, C.L., D'Elia, L.F., Dellinger, A.M., et al. (1995). Alternate forms of the Auditory-Verbal Learning Test: Issues of test comparability, longitudinal reliability, and moderating demographic variables. *Archives of Clinical Neuropsychology, 10,* 133–145.

Umbricht, D.S., Wirshing, W.C., Wirshing, D.A., et al. (2002). Clinical predictors of response to clozapine treatment in ambulatory patients with schizophrenia. *Journal of Clinical Psychiatry, 63,* 420–424.

Umile, E.M., Sandel, M.E., Alavi, A., et al. (2002). Dynamic imaging in mild traumatic brain injury: Support for the theory of medial temporal vulnerability. *Archives of Physical Medicine and Rehabilitation, 83,* 1506–1513.

Umilta, C. (1995). Domain-specific forms of neglect. *Journal of Clinical and Experimental Neuropsychology, 17,* 209–219.

Uniform Data Systems (1987). *The Functional Independence Measure.* New York: State University of Buffalo.

Uniform Data System for Medical Rehabilitation (1993). *Guide for the uniform data set for medical rehabilitation (Adult FIM), version 4.0.* Buffalo: State University of New York at Buffalo. Center for Functional Assessment Research. 232 Parker Hall, SUNY South Campus, 3435 Main St., (zip) 14214–3007.

Unkenstein, A.E. & Bowden, S.C. (1991). Predicting the course of neuropsychological status in recently abstinent alcoholics: A pilot study. *The Clinical Neuropsychologist, 5,* 24–32.

Unverzagt, F.W., Hall, K.S., Torke, A.M., et al. (1996). Effects of age, education, and gender on CERAD neuropsychological test performance in an African American sample. *The Clinical Neuropsychologist, 10,* 180–190.

Unverzagt, F.W., Morgan, O.S., Thesiger, C.H., et al. (1999). Clinical utility of CERAD neuropsychological battery in elderly Jamaicans. *Journal of the International Neuropsychological Society, 5,* 255–259.

Upton, D. & Thompson, P.J. (1999). Twenty Questions Task and frontal lobe dysfunction. *Archives of Clinical Neuropsychology, 14,* 203–216.

U'Ren, R.C., Riddle, M.C., Lezak, M.D., & Bennington-Davis, M. (1990). The mental efficiency of the elderly person with Type II diabetes mellitus. *Journal of the American Geriatrics Society, 38,* 505–510.

U.S. Congress, Office of Technology Assessment (1987). *Losing a million minds: Confronting the tragedy of Alzheimer's disease and other dementias* (OTA-BA-323). Washington, D.C.: U.S. Government Printing Office.

Uttl, B. (2002). North American Adult Reading Test: Age norms, reliability, and validity. *Journal of Clinical and Experimental Neuropsychology, 24,* 1123–1137.

Uttl, B. & Pilenton-Taylor, C. (2001). Letter cancellation performance across the adult life span. *The Clinical Neuropsychologist, 15,* 521–530.

Uzzell, B.P. (1988). Neuropsychological functioning after mercury exposure. *Neuropsychology, 2,* 19–27.

Uzzell, B.P. (1999). Mild head injury: Much ado about something. In N.R. Varney & R.J. Roberts (Eds.), *The evaluation and treatment of mild traumatic brain injury.* Mahwah, NJ: Erlbaum.

Uzzell, B.P., Dolinskas, C.A., & Langfitt, T.W. (1988). Visual field defects in relation to head injury severity. A neuropsychological study. *Archives of Neurology, 45,* 420–424.

Uzzell, B.P., Dolinskas, C.A., & Wiser, R.F. (1990). Relation between intracranial pressure, computed tomographic lesion, and neuropsychological outcome. *Advances in Neurology, 52,* 269–274.

Uzzell, B.P., Langfitt, T.W., & Dolinskas, C.A. (1987). Influence of injury severity on quality of survival after head injury. *Surgical Neurology, 27,* 419–429.

Uzzell, B.P., Obrist, W.D., Dolinskas, C.A., & Langfitt, T.W. (1986). Relationship of acute CBF and ICP findings to neuropsychological outcome in severe head injury. *Journal of Neurosurgery, 65,* 630–635.

Uzzell, B.P. & Oler, J. (1986). Chronic low-level mercury exposure and neuropsychological functioning. *Journal of Clinical and Experimental Neuropsychology, 8,* 581–593.

Vaid, J., Singh, M., Sakhuja, T., & Gupta, G.C. (2002). Stroke direction asymmetry in figure drawing: Influence of handedness and reading/ writing habits. *Brain and Cognition, 42,* 597–602.

Vakil, E. & Agmon-Ashkenazi, D. (1997). Baseline performance and learning rate of procedural and declarative memory tasks: Younger versus older adults. *Journals of Gerontology. Series B, Psychological Sciences and Social Sciences, 52,* 229–234.

Vakil, E., Arbell, N., Gozlan, M., et al. (1992). Relative importance of informational units and their role in long-term recall by closed-head-injured patients and control groups. *Journal of Consulting and Clinical Psychology, 60,* 802–803.

Vakil, E. & Blachstein, H. (1993). Rey Auditory-Verbal Learning Test: Structure analysis. *Journal of Clinical Psychology, 49,* 883–890.

Vakil, E. & Blachstein, H. (1997). Rey AVLT: Developmental norms for adults and the sensitivity of different memory measures to age. *The Clinical Neuropsychologist, 11,* 356–369.

Vakil, E., Blachstein, H., & Hoofien, D. (1991). Automatic temporal order judgment: The effect of intentionality of retrieval on closed-head-injured patients. *Journal of Clinical and Experimental Neuropsychology, 13,* 291–298.

Vakil, E., Hoofien, D., & Blachstein, H. (1992). Total amount learned versus learning rate of verbal and nonverbal information, in differentiating left- from right-brain injured patients. *Archives of Clinical Neuropsychology, 7,* 111–120.

Valencia-Flores, M., Bliwise, D.L., Guilleminault, C., et al. (1996). Cognitive function in patients with sleep apnea after acute noc-

turnal nasal continuous positive airway pressure (CPAP) treatment: Sleepiness and hypoxemia effects. *Journal of Clinical and Experimental Neuropsychology, 18,* 197–210.

Valentine, A.D. & Meyers, C.A. (2001). Cognitive and mood disturbance as causes and symptoms of fatigue in cancer patients. *Cancer, 92,* 1694–1698.

Valentine, A.D., Meyers, C.A., Kling, M. A., et al. (1998). Mood and cognitive effects of interferon-alpha therapy. *Seminars in Oncology, 25,* 39–47.

Vallar, B. (1991). Current methodological issues in human neuropsychology. In F. Boller & J. Grafman (Eds.), *Handbook of neuropsychology* (Vol. 5). Amsterdam: Elsevier.

Vallar, G. & Papagno, C. (2002). Neuropsychological impairments of short-term memory. In A.D. Baddeley et al. (Eds.), *Handbook of memory disorders* (2nd ed.). Chichester, UK: Wiley.

Vallar, G. & Perani, D. (1986). The anatomy of unilateral neglect after right-hemisphere stroke lesions. A clinical/CT-scan correlation study in man. *Neuropsychologia, 24,* 609–622.

Vallar, G. & Perani, D. (1987). The anatomy of spatial neglect in humans. In M. Jeannerod (Ed.), *Neurophysiological and neuropsychological aspects of spatial neglect.* Amsterdam: Elsevier/North-Holland.

Vallar, G., Rusconi, M.L., & Bernardini, B. (1996). Modulation of neglect hemianesthesia by transcutaneous electrical stimulation. *Journal of the International Neuropsychological Society, 2,* 452–459.

van Balen, E., Jorritsma, T., Groet, E., & Vink, M. (2002). A cognitive rehabilitation approach to long-term consequences following brain injury: Dutch practice. In W. Brouwer et al. (Eds.), *Cogntivie rehabilitation. A clinical neuropsychological approach.* Amsterdam: Boom.

van Boxtel, M.P., van Beijsterveldt, C.E., Houx, P.J., et al. (2000). Mild hearing impairment can reduce verbal memory performance in a healthy adult population. *Journal of Clinical and Experimental Neuropsychology, 22,* 147–154.

van Buchem, M.A., Grossman, M., Armstrong, C., et al. (1998). Correlation of volumetric magnetization transfer imaging with clinical data in MS. *Neurology, 50,* 1609–1617.

Van Camp, L.A., Vanderschot, P.M., Sabbe, M.B., et al. (1998). The effect of helmets on the incidence and severity of head and cervical spine injuries in motorcycle and moped accident victims: A prospective analysis based on emergency department and trauma center data. *European Journal of Emergency Medicine, 5,* 207–211.

van Dam, F.S., Schagen, S.B., Muller, M.J., et al. (1998). Impairment of cognitive function in women receiving adjuvant treatment for high-risk breast cancer: High-dose versus standard-dose chemotherapy. *Journal of the National Cancer Institute, 90,* 210–218.

van den Bent, M.J. (2001). The diagnosis and management of brain metastases. *Current Opinion in Neurology, 14,* 717–723.

van den Broek, A., Golden, C.J., Loonstra, A., et al. (1998). Short forms of the Wechsler Memory Scale-revised: Cross-validation and derivation of a two-subtest form. *Psychological Assessment, 10,* 38–40.

Van den Burg, L.H., Wokke, J.H.J., & Jennekens, F.G.I. (1998). Outcome of polyneuropathies and mononeuropathies. In M. Swash (Ed.), *Outcomes in neurological and neurosurgical disorders.* New York: Cambridge University Press.

van den Burg, W., Van Zomeren, A.H., Minderhoud, J.M., et al. (1987). Cognitive impairment in patients with multiple sclerosis and mild physical disability. *Archives of Neurology, 44,* 494–501.

Van der Does, A.J., Linszen, D.H., Dingemans, P.M., et al. (1993). A dimensional and categorical approach to the symptomatology of recent-onset schizophrenia. *Journal of Nervous and Mental Disease, 181,* 744–749.

van der Heijden, P. & Donders, J. (2003). A confirmatory factor analysis of the WAIS-III in patients with traumatic brain injury. *Journal of Clinical and Experimental Neuropsychology, 25,* 59–65.

Van der Linden, M. & Collette, F. (2002). Attention and normal ageing. In M. Leclercq & P. Zimmerman (Eds.), *Applied neuropsychology of attention. Theory, diagnosis, and rehabilitation.* New York: Psychology Press/Taylor & Francis.

van der Naalt, J., van Zomeren, A.H., Sluiter, W.J., & Minderhoud, J.M. (1999). One year outcome in mild to moderate head injury: The predictive value of acute injury characteristics related to complaints and return to work. *Journal of Neurology, Neurosurgery, and Psychiatry, 66,* 207–213.

Vanderploeg, R.D. (1994). Interview and testing: The data-collection phase of neuropsychological evaluations. In R.D. Vanderploeg (Ed.), *Clinician's guide to neuropsychological assessment.* Hillsdale, NJ: Erlbaum.

Vanderploeg, R.D. (1998). Neuropsychological outcomes research: A necessity and an opportunity. *Applied Neuropsychology, 5,* 169–171.

Vanderploeg, R.D., Axelrod, B.N., Sherer, M., et al. (1997). Importance of demographic adjustments on neuropsychological test performance: A response to Reitan and Wolfson (1995). *The Clinical Neuropsychologist, 11,* 210–217.

Vanderploeg, R.D., Crowell, T.A., & Curtiss, G. (2001). Verbal learning and memory deficits in traumatic brain injury: Encoding, consolidation, and retrieval. *Journal of Clinical and Experimental Neuropsychology, 23,* 185–195.

Vanderploeg, R.D. & Schinka, J.A. (1995). Predicting WAIS-R IQ premorbid ability: Combining subtest performance and demographic variable predictors. *Archives of Clinical Neuropsychology, 10,* 225–239.

Vanderploeg, R.D., Schinka, J.A., Jones, T., et al. (2000). Elderly norms for the Hopkins Verbal Learning Test–Revised. *The Clinical Neuropsychologist, 14,* 318–324.

Vanderploeg, R.D., Schinka, J.A., & Retzlaff, P. (1994). Relationships between measures of auditory verbal learning and executive functioning. *Journal of Clinical and Experimental Neuropsychology, 16,* 243–252.

Vanderploeg, R.D., Yuspeh, R.L., & Schinka, J.A. (2001). Differential episodic and semantic memory performance in Alzheimer's disease and vascular dementias. *Journal of the International Neuropsychological Society, 7,* 563–573.

Van der Werf, Y.D., Witter, M.P., Uylings, H.B., & Jolles, J. (2000). Neuropsychology of infarctions in the thalamus: A review. *Neuropsychologia, 38,* 613–627.

Vanderzant, C.W., Giordani, B., Berent, S., et al. (1986). Personality of patients with pseudoseizures. *Neurology, 36,* 664–667.

Van de Vijver, F. & Hambelton, R.K. (1996). Translating tests: Some practical guidelines. *European Psychologist, 1,* 89–99.

Vangel, S.J. & Lichtenberg, P.A. (1995). Mattis Dementia Rating Scale: Clinical utility and the relationship with demographic variables. *The Clinical Neuropsychologist, 9,* 209–213.

van Gijn, J. & Rinkel, G.J.E. (2001). Subarachnoid hemorrhage syndromes. In J. Bogousslavsky & L. Caplan (Eds.), *Stroke syndromes* (2nd ed.). Cambridge, UK: Cambridge University Press.

van Gorp, W.G., Baerwald, J.P., Ferrando, S.J., et al. (1999). The relationship between employment and neuropsychological impairment in HIV infection. *Journal of the International Neuropsychological Society, 5,* 534–539.

Van Gorp, W.G. & Cummings, J.L. (1989). Assessment of mood, affect, and personality. In F.J. Pirozzolo (Ed.), *Clinics in Geriatric Medicine,* (Vol. 5, No. 3).

Van Gorp, W.G., Hinkin, C., Satz, P., et al. (1993). Subtypes of HIV-related neuropsychological functioning: A cluster analysis approach. *Neuropsychology, 7,* 62–72.

van Gorp, W.G., Humphrey, L.A., Kalechstein, A.L., et al. (1999). How well do standard clinical neuropsychological tests identify malingering? A preliminary analysis. *Journal of Clinical and Experimental Neuropsychology, 21,* 245–250.

van Gorp, W.G., Kalechstein, A.D., Moore, L.H., et al. (1997). A clinical comparison of two forms of the Card Sorting Test. *The Clinical Neuropsychologist, 11,* 155–160.

van Gorp, W.G. & Mahler, M. (1990). Subcortical features of normal aging. In J. Cummings (Ed.), *Subcortical dementia.* New York: Oxford University Press.

van Gorp, W.G., Marcotte, T.D., Sultzer, D., et al. (1999). Screening for dementia: Comparison of three commonly used instruments. *Journal of Clinical and Experimental Neuropsychology, 21,* 29–38.

van Gorp, W.G. & McMullen, W. (1997). Potential sources of bias in forensic neuropsychological evaluations. *The Clinical Neuropsychologist, 11,* 180–187.

Van Gorp, W.G., Mitrushina, M., Cummings, J.L., et al. (1989). Normal aging and the subcortical encephalopathy of AIDS: A neuropsychological comparison. *Neuropsychiatry, Neuropsychology, and Behavioral Neurology, 2,* 5–20.

Van Gorp, W.G., Satz, P., Kiersch, M.E., & Henry, R. (1986). Normative data on the Boston Naming Test for a group of normal older adults. *Journal of Clinical and Experimental Neuropsychology, 8,* 702–705.

van Gorp, W.G., Satz, P., & Mitrushina, M. (1990). Neuropsychological processes associated with normal aging. *Developmental Neuropsychology, 6,* 279–290.

van Heugten, C.M., Dekker, J., Deelman, B.G., et al. (1999). A diagnostic test for apraxia with stroke patients: Internal consistency and diagnostic value. *The Clinical Neuropsychologist, 13,* 182–192.

Van Hoesen, G.W. (1990). The dissection by Alzheimer's disease of cortical and limbic neural systems relevant to memory. In J.L. McGaugh et al. (Eds.), *Brain organization and memory: Cells, systems, and circuits.* New York: Oxford University Press.

Van Hoesen, G.W. & Damasio, A.R. (1987). Neural correlates of cognitive impairment in Alzheimer's disease. In F. Plum (Ed.), *Handbook of physiology. The nervous system.* (Vol. 5). New York: Oxford University Press.

Vanier, M., Gauthier, L., Lambert, J., et al. (1990). Evaluation of left visuospatial neglect: Norms and discrimination power of two tests. *Neuropsychology, 4,* 87–96.

Vanier, M., Mazaux, J.M., Lambert, J., et al. (2000). Assessment of neuropsychologic impairments after head injury: Interrater reliability and factorial and criterion validity of the Neurobehavioral Rating Scale–Revised. *Archives of Physical Medicine and Rehabilitation, 81,* 796–806.

Van Lancker, D. (1990). The neurology of proverbs. *Behavioural Neurology, 3,* 169–187.

Van Lancker, D.R., Cummings, J.L., Kreiman, J., & Dobkin, B.H. (1988). Phonagnosia: A dissociation between familiar and unfamiliar voices. *Cortex, 24,* 195–209.

Van Lancker, D.R., Kreiman, J., & Cummings, J. (1989). Voice perception deficits: Neuroanatomical correlates of phonagnosia. *Journal of Clinical and Experimental Neuropsychology, 11,* 665–674.

Van Lancker, D. & Nicklay, C.K.H. (1992). Comprehension of personally relevant (PERL) versus novel language in two globally aphasic patients. *Aphasiology, 6,* 37–61.

Van Lancker, D. & Sidtis, J. J. (1992). The identification of affective-prosodic stimuli by left and right hemisphere damaged subjects: All errors are not created equal. *Journal of Speech and Hearing Research, 35,* 963–970.

Vannieuwkirk, R.R. & Galbraith, G.G. (1985). The relationship of age to performance on the Luria-Nebraska Neuropsychological Battery. *Journal of Clinical Psychology, 41,* 527–532.

van Ravensberg, C.D., Tyldesley, D.A., Rozendal, R.H., & Whiting, H.T.A. (1984). Visual perception in hemiplegic patients. *Archives of Physical and Medical Rehabilitation, 65,* 304–309.

Van Reekum, R., Bolago, I., Finlayson, M.A.J., et al. (1996). Psychiatric disorders after traumatic brain injury. *Brain Injury, 10,* 319–327.

van Spaendonck, K.P., Berger, H.J., Horstink, M.W., et al. (1993). Impaired cognitive shifting in parkinsonian patients on anticholinergic therapy. *Neuropsychologia, 31,* 407–411.

van Spaendonck, K.P., Berger, H.J., Horstink, M.W., et al. (1996a). Executive functions and disease characteristics in Parkinson's disease. *Neuropsychologia, 34,* 617–626.

van Spaendonck, K.P., Berger, H.J., Horstink, M.W., et al. (1996b). Memory performance under varying cueing conditions in patients with Parkinson's disease. *Neuropsychologia, 34,* 1159–1164.

van't Spijker, A. & ten Kroode, H.F.J. (1997). Psychological aspects of genetic counseling: A review of the experience with Huntington's disease. *Patient Education and Counseling, 32,* 33–40.

van Walderveen, M.A., Tas, M.W., Barkhof, F., et al. (1994). Magnetic resonance evaluation of disease activity during pregnancy in multiple sclerosis. *Neurology, 44,* 327–329.

Van Zomeren, A.H. & Brouwer, W.H. (1987). Head injury and concepts of attention. In H.S. Levin et al. (Eds.), *Neurobehavioral recovery from head injury.* New York: Oxford University Press.

Van Zomeren, A.H. & Brouwer, W.H. (1990). Attentional deficits after closed head injury. In B.G. Deelman et al. (Eds.), *Traumatic brain injury: Clinical, social and rehabilitation aspects.* Amsterdam: Swets and Zeitlinger.

Van Zomeren, A.H. & Brouwer, W.H. (1992). Assessment of attention. In J.R. Crawford et al. (Eds.), *A handbook of neuropsychological assessment.* Hove, UK: Erlbaum.

Van Zomeren, A.H. & Brouwer, W.H. (1994). *Clinical neuropsychology of attention.* New York: Oxford University Press.

Van Zomeren, A.H., Brouwer, W.H., & Deelman, B.G. (1984). Attentional deficits: The riddle of selectivity, speed, and alertness. In N. Brooks (Ed.), *Closed head injury.* Oxford: Oxford University Press.

van Zomeren, A.H., ten Duis, H.J., Minderhoud, J.M., & Sipma, M. (1998). Lightning stroke and neuropsychological impairment: cases and questions. *Journal of Neurology, Neurosurgery and Psychiatry, 64,* 763–769.

Varma, A.R., Snowden, J.S., Lloyd, J.J., et al. (1999). Evaluation of the NINCDS-ADRDA criteria in the differentiation of Alzheimer's disease and frontotemporal dementia. *Journal of Neurology, Neurosurgery and Psychiatry, 66,* 184–188.

Varney, N.R. (1982). Colour association and "colour amnesia" in aphasia. *Journal of Neurology, Neurosurgery and Psychiatry, 45,* 248–252.

Varney, N.R. (1986). Somesthesis. In H.J. Hannay (Ed.), *Experimental techniques in human neuropsychology.* New York: Oxford University Press.

Varney, N.R. (1988). Prognostic significance of anosmia in patients with closed-head trauma. *Journal of Clinical and Experimental Neuropsychology, 10,* 250–254.

Varney, N.R. & Bushnell, D. (1998). NeuroSPECT findings in patients with posttraumatic anosmia: A quantitative analysis. *Journal of Head Trauma Rehabilitation, 13,* 63–72.

Varney, N.R., Ju, D., & Shepherd, J.S. (1998). Long-term neuropsychological sequelae of severe burns. *Archives of Clinical Neuropsychology, 13,* 737–749.

Varney, N.R., Martzke, J.S., & Roberts, R.J. (1987). Major depression in patients with closed head injury. *Neuropsychology, 1,* 7–9.

Varney, N.R. & Menefee, L. (1993). Psychosocial and executive deficits following closed head injury: Implications for orbital frontal cortex. *Journal of Head Trauma Rehabilitation, 8,* 32–44.

Varney, N.R., Pinkston, J.B., & Wu, J.C. (2001). Quantitative PET findings in patients with posttraumatic anosmia. *Journal of Head Trauma Rehabilitation, 16,* 253–259.

Varney, N.R. & Risse, G.L. (1993). Locus of lesion in defective color association. *Neuropsychology, 7,* 548–552.

Varney, N.R. & Roberts, R.J. (Eds.) (1999a). *The evaluation and treatment of mild traumatic brain injury.* Mahwah, NJ: Erlbaum.

Varney, N.R. & Roberts, R.J. (1999b). Forces and accelerations in car accidents and resultant brain injuries. In N.R. Varney & R.J. Roberts (Eds.), *The evaluation and treatment of mild traumatic brain injury.* Mahwah, NJ: Erlbaum.

Varney, N.R., Roberts, R.J., Struchen, M.A., et al. (1996). Design fluency among normals and patients with closed head injury. *Archives of Clinical Neuropsychology, 11,* 345–353.

Varney, N.R. & Shepherd, J.S. (1991). Predicting short-term memory on the basis of temporal orientation. *Neuropsychology, 5,* 13–17.

Varney, N.R. & Varney, R.N. (1995). Brain injury without head injury. Some physics of automobile collisions with particular reference to brain injuries occurring without physical head trauma. *Applied Neuropsychology, 2,* 47–62.

Vasterling, J.J., Seltzer, B., & Watrous, W.E. (1997). Longitudinal assessment of deficit unawareness in Alzheimer's disease. *Neuropsychiatry, Neuropsychology, and Behavioral Neurology, 10,* 197–202.

Vecchi, T. & Girelli, L. (1998). Gender differences in visuo-spatial processing: The importance of distinguishing between passive storage and active manipulation. *Acta Psychologica, 99,* 1–16.

Veiel, H.O. (1997a). A preliminary profile of neuropsychological deficits associated with major depression. *Journal of Clinical and Experimental Neuropsychology, 19,* 587–603.

Veiel, H.O. (1997b). CVLT recognition-recall discrepancies and methodological rigor: A reply. *Journal of Clinical and Experimental Neuropsychology, 19,* 942–947.

Veiel, H.O. (1997c). CVLT recognition–recall discrepancies and retrieval deficits. A comment on Wilde et al. (1995). *Journal of Clinical and Experimental Neuropsychology, 19,* 141–143.

Velasco, F., Velasco, M., Ogarrio, C., & Olvera, A. (1986). Neglect induced by thalamotomy in humans: A quantitative appraisal of the sensory and motor deficits. *Neurosurgery, 19,* 744–751.

Velasquez, M., Arcos-Burgos, M., Toro, M.D., et al. (2000). Analisis factorial y discriminante de variables neuropsicologicas en la demencia tipo Alzheimer de inicio tardio, familiar y esporadica. *Revista de Neurologia, 31,* 501–506.

Vendrell, P., Junqué, C., Pujol, J., et al. (1995). The role of prefrontal regions in the Stroop task. *Neuropsychologia, 33,* 341–352.

Venneri, A., Nichelli, P., Modonesi, G., et al. (1997). Impairment in dating and retrieving remote events in patients with early Parkinson's disease. *Journal of Neurology, Neurosurgery and Psychiatry, 62,* 410–413.

Verduyn, W.H., Hilt, J., Roberts, M.A., & Roberts, R.J. (1992). Multiple partial seizure-like symptoms following "minor" closed head injury. *Brain Injury, 6,* 245–260.

Verfaellie, M. & Cermak, L.S. (1997). Wernicke-Korsakoff and related nutritional disorders of the nervous system. In T.E. Feinberg & M.J. Farah (Eds.), *Behavioral neurology and neuropsychology.* New York: McGraw-Hill.

Verfaellie, M. & O'Connor, M. (2000). A neuropsychological analysis of memory and amnesia. *Seminars in Neurology, 20,* 455–462.

Verger, K., Junqué, C., Levin, H.S., et al. (2001). Correlation of atrophy measures on MRI with neuropsychological sequelae in children and adolescents with traumatic brain injury. *Brain Injury, 15,* 211–221.

Verhaeghen, P. & De Meersman, L. (1998). Aging and the Stroop effect: A meta-analysis. *Psychology and Aging, 13,* 120–126.

Verity, M.A. & Sarafian, T.A. (2000). Mercury and mercury compounds. In P.S. Spencer & H.H. Schaumberg (Eds.), *Experimental and clinical neurotoxicology* (2nd ed.). New York: Oxford University Press.

Vermeer, S.E., Koudstaal, P.J., Oudkerk, M., et al. (2002). Prevalence and risk factors of silent brain infarcts in the population-based Rotterdam Scan Study. *Stroke, 33,* 21–25.

Vermeulen, J., Aldenkamp, A.P., & Alpherts, W.C. (1993). Memory complaints in epilepsy: Correlations with cognitive performance and neuroticism. *Epilepsy Research, 15,* 157–170.

Vernon, M. (1989). Assessment of older persons with hearing disabilities. In T. Hunt & C.J. Lindley (Eds.), *Testing older adults: A reference guide for geropsychological assessment.* Austin, TX: Pro-Ed.

Vernon, P.A. (1985). Multidimensional Aptitude Battery. In D.J. Keyser & R.C. Sweetland (Eds.), *Test critiques* (Vol. II). Kansas City, MO: Test Corporation of America.

Vernon, P.E. (1979). *Intelligence: Heredity and environment.* San Francisco: Freeman.

Verstichel, P. & Cambier, J. (1996). Les aphasies. In M.I. Botez (Ed.), *Neuropsychologie clinique et neurologie du comportement* (2nd ed.). Montréal: Les Presses de l'Université de Montréal.

Verstraeten, E., Cluydts, R., Verbraecken, J., & De Roeck, J. (1996). Neuropsychological functioning and determinants of morning alertness in patients with obstructive sleep apnea syndrome. *Journal of the International Neuropsychological Society, 2,* 306–314.

Vickery, C.D., Berry, D.T.R., Inman, T.H., et al. (2001). Detection of inadequate effort on neuropsychological testing: A meta-analytic review of selected procedures. *Archives of Clinical Neuropsychology, 16,* 45–73.

Vickrey, B.G., Hays, R.D., Graber, J., et al. (1992). A health-related quality of life instrument for patients evaluated for epilepsy surgery. *Medical Care, 30,* 299–319.

Victor, M., Adams, R.D., & Collins, G.H. (1971). *The Wernicke-Korsakoff syndrome.* Philadelphia: Davis.

Victor, M. & Ropper, A.H. (2001). *Adams' and Victor's Principles of neurology* (7th ed.). New York: McGraw-Hill.

Vigliani, M.C., Duyckaerts, C., Hauw, J.J., et al. (1999). Dementia following treatment of brain tumors with radiotherapy administered alone or in combination with nitrosourea-based chemotherapy: A clinical and pathological study. *Journal of Neurooncology, 41,* 137–149.

Vigliani, M.C., Sichez, N., Poisson, M., & Delattre, J.Y. (1996). A prospective study of cognitive functions following conventional radiotherapy for supratentorial gliomas in young adults: 4-year results. *International Journal of Radiation Oncology, Biology, and Physics, 35,* 527–533.

Vigouroux, R.P., Baurand, C., Naquet, R., et al. (1971). A series of patients with cranio-cerebral injuries studied neurologically, psychometrically, electroencephalographically and socially. In *International symposium on head injuries.* Edinburgh: Churchill Livingstone.

Viikinsalo, M., Gilliam, F., Faught, E., & Kuzniecky, R. (1997). Development of the EFA Concerns Index: A patient-based measure of the effects of epilepsy. *Epilepsia, 38(Suppl. 8),* S241–S242.

Vilkki, J. (1979). *Effects of thalamic lesions on cognitive functions in man. A neuropsychological study of thalamic surgery.* Helsinki: University of Helsinki. Dissertation.

Vilkki, J. (1984). Visual hemi-inattention after ventrolateral thalamotomy. *Neuropsychologia, 22,* 399–408.

Vilkki, J. (1988). Problem solving deficits after focal cerebral lesions. *Cortex, 24,* 119–127.

Vilkki, J., Ahola, K., Holst, P., et al. (1994). Prediction of psychosocial recovery after head injury with cognitive tests and neurobehavioral ratings. *Journal of Clinical and Experimental Neuropsychology, 16,* 325–338.

Vilkki, J. & Holst, P. (1989). Deficient programming in spatial learning after frontal lobe damage. *Neuropsychologia, 27,* 971–976.

Vilkki, J., Holst, P., Öhman, J., et al. (1989). Cognitive deficits related to computed tomographic findings after surgery for a ruptured intracranial aneurysm. *Neurosurgery, 25,* 166–172.

Vilkki, J., Holst, P., Öhman, J., et al. (1990). Social outcome related to cognitive performance and computed tomographic findings after surgery for a ruptured intracranial aneurysm. *Neurosurgery, 26,* 579–585.

Vilkki, J., Holst, P., Öhman, J., et al. (1992). Cognitive test performances related to early and late computed tomography findings after closed-head injury. *Journal of Clinical and Experimental Neuropsychology, 14,* 518–532.

Vilkki, J. & Laitinen, L.V. (1974). Differential effects of left and right ventrolateral thalamotomy on receptive and expressive verbal performances and face-matching. *Neuropsychologia, 12,* 11–19.

Vilkki, J. & Laitinen, L.V. (1976). Effects of pulvinotomy and ventrolateral thalamotomy on some cognitive functions. *Neuropsychologia, 14,* 67–78.

Vilkki, J., Servo, A., & Surma-aho, O. (1998). Word list learning and prediction of recall after frontal lobe lesions. *Neuropsychology, 12,* 268–277.

Villardita, C. (1985). Raven's Progressive Matrices and intellectual impairment in patients with focal brain damage. *Cortex, 21,* 627–634.

Villardita, C., Smirni, P., & Zappala, G. (1983). Visual neglect in Parkinson's disease. *Archives of Neurology, 40,* 737–739.

Vincent, K.R. (1979). The modified WAIS: An alternative to short forms. *Journal of Clinical Psychology, 35,* 624–625.

Vingerhoets, G., De Soete, G., & Jannes, C. (1995). Relationship between emotional variables and cognitive test performance before and after open-heart surgery. *The Clinical Neuropsychologist, 9,* 198–202.

Vingerhoets, G., Lannoo, E., & Bauwens, S. (1996). Analysis of the Money Road-Map Test performance in normal and brain-damaged subjects. *Archives of Clinical Neuropsychology, 11,* 1–9.

Vingerhoets, G., Lannoo, E., van der Linden, C., et al. (1999). Changes in quality of life following unilateral pallidal stimulation in Parkinson's disease. *Journal of Psychosomatic Research, 46,* 247–255.

Vingerhoets, G., Lannoo, E., & Wolters, M. (1998). Comparing the Rey-Osterrieth and Taylor Complex Figures: Empirical data and meta-analysis. *Psychologica Belgica, 38,* 109–119.

Vingerhoets, G., Van Nooten, G., & Jannes, C. (1996). Effect of asymptomatic carotid artery disease on cognitive outcome after cardiopulmonary bypass. *Journal of the International Neuropsychological Society, 2,* 236–239.

Visser, P.J., Krabbendam, L., Verhey, F.R., et al. (1999). Brain correlates of memory dysfunction in alcoholic Korsakoff's syndrome. *Journal of Neurology, Neurosurgery and Psychiatry, 67,* 774–778.

Visser, P.J., Scheltens, P., Verhey, F.R., et al. (1999). Medial temporal lobe atrophy and memory dysfunction as predictors for dementia in subjects with mild cognitive impairment. *Journal of Neurology, 246,* 477–485.

Visser, P.J., Verhey, F.R., Ponds, R.W., et al. (2000). Distinction between preclinical Alzheimer's disease and depression. *Journal of the American Geriatric Society, 48,* 479–484.

Visser, R.S.H. (1973). *Manual of the Complex Figure Test.* Amsterdam: Swets and Zeitlinger.

Vitaliano, P.P., Breen, A.R., Albert, M.S., et al. (1984). Memory, attention, and functional status in community-residing Alzheimer type dementia patients and optimally healthy aged individuals. *Journal of Gerontology, 39,* 58–64.

Vitaliano, P.P., Breen, A.R., Russo, J., et al. (1984). The clinical utility of the Dementia Rating Scale for assessing Alzheimer patients. *Journal of Chronic Disorders, 37,* 743–753.

Vleugels, L., Lafosse, C., van Nunen, A., et al. (2000). Visuoperceptual impairment in multiple sclerosis patients diagnosed with neuropsychological tasks. *Multiple Sclerosis, 6,* 241–254.

Vogenthaler, D.R., Smith, K.R., & Goldfader, P. (1989). Head injury, an empirical study: Describing long-term productivity and independent living outcome. *Brain Injury, 3,* 355–368.

Voelker, J.L. & Kaufman, H.H. (1997). Clinical aspects of intracerebral hemorrhage. In K.M.A. Welch et al. (Eds.) *Primer on cerebrovascular diseases.* San Diego: Academic Press.

Volbrecht, M.E., Meyers, J.E., & Kaster-Bundgaard, J. (2000). Neuropsychological outcome of head injury using a short battery. *Archives of Clinical Neuropsychology, 15,* 251–264.

Vollhardt, B. R., Bergener, M., & Hesse, C. (1992). Psychotropics in the elderly. In M. Bergener et al. (Eds.), *Aging and mental disorders: International perspectives.* New York: Springer.

Volpato, S., Guralnik, J.M., Fried, L.P., et al. (2002). Serum thyroxine level and cognitive decline in euthyroid older women. *Neurology, 58,* 1055–1061.

Volpe, B.T. & Hirst, W. (1983). The characterization of an amnestic syndrome following hypoxic ischemic injury. *Archives of Neurology, 40,* 436–440.

Von Dras, D. D. & Lichty, W. (1990). Correlates of depression in diabetic adults. *Behavior, Health, and Aging, 1,* 79–84.

von Cramon, D.Y., Hebel, N., & Schuri, U. (1985). A contribution to the anatomical basis of thalamic amnesia. *Brain, 108,* 993–1008.

von Monakow, C. (1969 [1914]). Diaschisis. In K.H. Pribram (Ed.), *Brain and behavior. I. Mood states and mind.* Baltimore: Penguin Books.

von Schenck, U., Bender-Gotze, C., & Koletzko, B. (1997). Persistence of neurological damage induced by dietary vitamin b-12 deficiency in infancy. *Archives of Disease in Childhood, 77,* 137–139.

von Steinbüchel, N., Wittmann, M., Strasburger, H., & Szelag, E. (1999). Auditory temporal-order judgement is impaired in patients with cortical lesions in posterior regions of the left hemisphere. *Neuroscience Letters, 264,* 168–171.

Vuilleumier, P. (2001). Agnosias, apraxias, and callosal disconnection syndromes. In J. Bogousslavsky & L.R. Caplan (Eds.), *Stroke syndromes.* Cambridge, UK: Cambridge University Press.

Vukusic, S. & Confavreux, C. (2001). Natural history of multiple sclerosis. In S.D. Cook (Ed.), *Handbook of multiple sclerosis* (3rd ed.). New York: Marcel Dekker.

Waber, D.P. & Holmes, J.M. (1985). Assessing children's copy production of the Rey-Osterrieth Complex Figure. *Journal of Clinical and Experimental Neuropsychology, 7,* 264–280.

Waber, D.P. & Holmes, J.M. (1986). Assessing children's memory productions of the Rey-Osterrieth Complex Figure. *Journal of Clinical and Experimental Neuropsychology, 8,* 563–580.

Waber, D.P., Shapiro, B.L., Carpentieri, S.C., et al. (2001). Excellent therapeutic efficacy and minimal late neurotoxicity in children treated with 18 grays of cranial radiation therapy for high-risk acute lymphoblastic leukemia: A 7-year follow-up study of the Dana-Farber Cancer Institute Consortium Protocol 87-01. *Cancer, 92,* 15–22.

Wada, J. & Rasmussen, T. (1960). Intra-carotid injection of sodium amytal for the lateralization of cerebral speech dominance. *Journal of Neurosurgery, 17,* 266–282.

Wade, D.T., Hewer, R.L., & Wood, V.A. (1984). Stroke: Influence of patient's sex and side of weakness on outcome. *Archives of Physical Medicine and Rehabilitation, 65,* 513–516.

Wade, N.J. & Brozek, J. (2001). *Purkinje's vision. The dawning of neuroscience.* Mahwah, NJ: Erlbaum.

Wagner, A.D., Poldrack, R.A., Eldridge, L.L., et al. (1998). Material-specific lateralization of prefrontal activation during episodic encoding and retrieval. *Neuroreport, 9,* 3711–3717.

Wagner, A.K., Hammond, F.M., Sasser, H.C., & Wiercisiewski, D. (2002). Return to productive activity after traumatic brain injury: Relationship with measures of disability, handicap, and community integration. *Archives of Physical Medicine and Rehabilitation, 83,* 107–114.

Wagner, E.E. & Gianakos, I. (1985). Comparison of WAIS and WAIS-R scaled scores for an outpatient clinic sample retested over extended intervals. *Perceptual and Motor Skills, 61,* 87–90.

Wagner, E.E. & Marsico, D.S. (1991). Redundancy in the Pascal-Suttell Bender-Gestalt scoring system: Discriminating organicity with only one design. *Journal of Clinical Psychology, 47,* 261–263.

Wagner, M.T., Spangenberg, K.B., Bachman, D.L., & O'Connell, P. (1997). Unawareness of cognitive deficit in Alzheimer disease and related dementias. *Alzheimer Disease and Associated Disorders, 11,* 125–131.

Wahlin, A., Nilsson, E., & Fastbom, J. (2002). Cognitive performance in very old diabetic persons: The impact of semantic structure, preclinical dementia, and impending death. *Neuropsychology, 16,* 208–216.

Wahlund, L.O., Almkvist, O., Basun, H., & Julin, P. (1996). MRI in successful aging, a 5-year follow-up study from the eighth to ninth decade of life. *Magnetic Resonance Imaging, 14,* 601–608.

Waldemar, G., Hogh, P., & Paulson, O.B. (1997). Functional brain imaging with single-photon emission computed tomography in the diagnosis of Alzheimer's disease. *International Psychogeriatrics, 9,* 223–227.

Waldstein, S.R., Jennings, J.R., Ryan, C.M., et al. (1996). Hypertension and neuropsychological performance in men: Interactive effects of age. *Health Psychology, 15,* 102–109.

Waldstein, S.R., Manuck, S.B., Ryan, C.M., & Muldoon, M.F. (1991). Neuropsychological correlates of hypertension: Review and methodologic considerations. *Psychological Bulletin, 110,* 451–468.

Waldstein, S.R., Ryan, C.M., Jennings, J.R., et al. (1997). Self-reported levels of anxiety do not predict neuropsychological performance in healthy men. *Archives of Clinical Neuropsychology, 12,* 523–530.

Walker, A.E. & Blumer, D. (1989). The fate of World War II veterans with posttraumatic seizures. *Archives of Neurology, 46,* 23–26.

Walker, A.E. & Jablon, S. (1961). *A follow-up study of head wounds in World War II.* Washington, D.C.: VA Medical Monograph.

Walker, A.J., Shores, E.A., Trollor, J.N., et al. (2000). Neuropsychological functioning of adults with attention deficit hyperactivity disorder. *Journal of Clinical and Experimental Neuropsychology, 22,* 115–124.

Walker, D.E., Blankenship, V., Ditty, J.A., & Lynch, K.P. (1987). Prediction of recovery for close-head-injured adults: An evaluation of the MMPI, the Adaptive Behavior Scale, and a "Quality of Life" Rating Scale. *Journal of Clinical Psychology, 43,* 699–707.

Walker, J.A. (2000). Use of neuropsychological testing to differentiate neurologic from non-neurologic disorders. In J.R. Gates & A.J. Rowan (Eds.), *Non-epileptic seizures* (2nd ed.). Boston: Butterworth-Heinmann.

Walker, R.E., Hunt, W.A. & Schwartz, M.L. (1965). The difficulty of WAIS Comprehension scoring. *Journal of Clinical Psychology, 21,* 427–429.

Walker, S. (1992). Assessment of language dysfunction. In J.R. Crawford et al. (Eds.), *A handbook of neuropsychological assessment.* Hove, UK: Erlbaum.

Walker, Z., Allen, R. L., Shergill, S., & Katona, C. L. (1997). Neuropsychological performance in Lewy body dementia and Alzheimer's disease. *British Journal of Psychiatry, 170,* 156–158.

Walker, Z., Costa, D.C., Ince, P., et al. (1999). In-vivo demonstration of dopaminergic degeneration in dementia with Lewy bodies. *Lancet, 354,* 646–647.

Walker, Z., Costa, D.C., Walker, R.W., et al. (2002). Differentiation of dementia with Lewy bodies from Alzheimer's disease using a dopaminergic presynaptic ligand. *Journal of Neurology, Neurosurgery and Psychiatry, 73,* 134–140.

Wallace, E., Hayes, D., & Jerger, J. (1994). Neurotology of aging: The auditory system. In M.L. Albert & J.E. Knoefel (Eds.), *Clinical neurology of aging* (2nd ed.). New York: Oxford University Press.

Wallace, G.L. & Holmes, S. (1993). Cognitive-linguistic assessment of individuals with multiple sclerosis. *Archives of Physical Medicine and Rehabilitation, 74,* 637–643.

Wallesch, C.W., Curio, N., Galazky, I., et al. (2001). The neuropsychology of blunt head injury in the early postacute stage: Effects of focal lesions and diffuse axonal injury. *Journal of Neurotrauma, 18,* 11–20.

Wallesch, C.W., Kornhuber, H.-H., Brunner, R.J., & Kunz, T. (1983). Lesions of the basal ganglia, thalamus, and deep white matter: Differential effects on language functions. *Brain and Language, 20,* 286–304.

Walsh, K.W. (1985). *Understanding brain damage.* Edinburgh: Churchill-Livingstone.

Walsh, K.W. (1991). *Understanding brain damage: A primer of neuropsychological evaluation* (2nd ed.). Edinburgh: Churchill Livingstone.

Walsh, K. W. (1992). Some gnomes worth knowing. *The Clinical Neuropsychologist, 6,* 119–133.

Walsh, K.W. (1995). A hypothesis-testing approach to assessment. In R.L. Mapou & J. Spector (Eds.), *Clinical neuropsychological assessment. A cognitive approach.* New York: Plenum Press.

Walsh, K.W. and Darby, D. (1999). *Neuropsychology. A clinical approach* (4th ed.). Edinburgh: Churchill Livingstone.

Walton, J.N. (1994). *Brain's diseases of the nervous system* (10th ed.). Oxford: Oxford University Press.

Wang, J.L., Reimer, M. A., Metz, L.M., & Patten, S.B. (2000). Major depression and quality of life in individuals with multiple sclerosis. *International Journal of Psychiatry in Medicine, 30,* 309–317.

Wang, P.L. (1977). Visual organization ability in brain-damaged adults. *Perceptual and Motor Skills, 45,* 723–728.

Wang, P.L. (1984). *Modified Vygotsky Concept Formation Test manual.* Chicago: Stoelting.

Wang, P.L. (1987). Concept formation and frontal lobe function. In E. Perecman (Ed.), *The frontal lobes revisited.* New York: IRBN Press.

Wang, P.L. & Goltz, M.D. (1991). *Hypoawareness versus hyperawareness of deficits in a head injured population.* Paper presented at the annual convention of the Canadian Psychological Association, Calgary, Canada.

Wapner, W., Hamby, S., & Gardner, H. (1981). The role of the right hemisphere in the apprehension of complex linguistic materials. *Brain and Language, 41,* 15–33.

Warburton, D.M., Rusted, J.M., & Fowler, J. (1992). A comparison of the attentional and consolidation hypotheses for the facilitation of memory by nicotine. *Psychopharmacology, 108,* 443–447.

Warburton, D.M., Rusted, J.M., & Muller, C. (1992). Patterns of facilitation of memory by nicotine. *Behavioral Pharmacology, 3,* 375–378.

Ward, C.D., Hess, W.A., & Calne, D.B. (1983). Olfactory impairment in Parkinson's disease. *Neurology, 33,* 943–946.

Ward, J., Parkin, A.J., Powell, G., et al. (1999). False recognition of unfamiliar people: "Seeing film stars everywhere." *Cognitive Neuropsychology, 16,* 293–315.

Ward, L.C., Ryan, J.J., & Axelrod, B.N. (2000). Confirmatory factor analyses of the WAIS-III standardization data. *Psychological Assessment, 12,* 341–345.

Ward, L.C., Selby, R.B., & Clark, B.L. (1987). Subtest administration times and short forms of the Wechsler Adult Intelligence Scale–Revised. *Journal of Clinical Psychology, 43,* 276–278.

Warden, D.L., Labbate, L.A., Salazar, A.M., et al. (1997). Posttraumatic stress disorder in patients with traumatic brain injury and amnesia for the event? *Journal of Neuropsychiatry and Clinical Neurosciences, 9,* 18–22.

Ware, J.E., Jr. & Sherbourne, C.D. (1992). The MOS 36-item short-form health survey (SF-36): I. Conceptual framework and item selection. *Medical Care, 20,* 437–483.

Waring, S.C., Rocca, W.A., Petersen, R.C., et al. (1999). Postmenopausal estrogen replacement therapy and risk of AD: A population-based study. *Neurology, 52,* 965–970.

Warkentin, S. & Passant, U. (1993). Functional activation of the frontal lobes. Regional cerebral blood flow findings in normals and in patients with frontal lobe dementia performing a word fluency test. *Dementia, 4,* 188–191.

Warren, S., Greenhill, S., & Warren, K.G. (1982). Emotional stress and the development of multiple sclerosis: Case-control evidence of a relationship. *Journal of Chronic Disease, 351,* 821–831.

Warren, S., Warren, K.G., & Cockerill, R. (1991). Emotional stress and coping in multiple sclerosis (MS) exacerbations. *Journal of Psychosomatic Research, 35,* 37–47.

Warrington, E.K. (1982). The fractionation of arithmetical skills: A single case study. *Quarterly Journal of Experimental Psychology, 34A,* 31–51.

Warrington, E.K. (1984). *Recognition Memory Test.* Los Angeles: Western Psychological Services.

Warrington, E.K. (1986). *The Camden Memory Tests.* Hove, UK: Psychology Press.

Warrington, E.K. (1997). The Graded Naming Test: A restandardization. *Neuropsychological Rehabilitation, 7,* 143–146.

Warrington, E.D. (2000). Homophone meaning generation: A new test of verbal switching for the detection of frontal lobe dysfunction. *Journal of the International Neuropsychological Society, 6,* 643–648.

Warrington, E.K. & James, M. (1967). An experimental investigation of facial recognition in patients with unilateral cerebral lesions. *Cortex, 3,* 317–326.

Warrington, E.K. & James, M. (1986). Visual object recognition in patients with right-hemisphere lesions: Axes or features? *Perception, 15,* 355–366.

Warrington, E.K. & James, M. (1991). *Visual Object and Space Perception Battery.* Bury St. Edmunds, UK: Thames Valley Test.

Warrington, E.K., James, M., & Kinsbourne, M. (1966). Drawing disability in relation to laterality of cerebral lesion. *Brain, 89,* 53–82.

Warrington, E.K., James, M., & Maciejewski, C. (1986). The WAIS as a lateralizing and localizing diagnostic instrument. *Neuropsychologia, 24,* 223–239.

Warrington, E.K. & McCarthy, R.A. (1987). Categories of knowledge. Further fractionations and an attempted integration. *Brain, 110,* 1273–1296.

Warrington, E.K. & McCarthy, R.A. (1988). The fractionation of retrograde amnesia. *Brain and Cognition, 7,* 184–200.

Warrington, E.K. & Rabin, P. (1970). Perceptual matching in patients with cerebral lesions. *Neuropsychologia, 8,* 475–487.

Warrington, E.K. & Shallice, T. (1984). Category specific semantic impairments. *Brain, 107,* 829–854.

Warrington, E.K. & Silberstein, M. (1970). A questionnaire technique for investigating very long term memory. *Quarterly Journal of Experimental Psychology, 22,* 508–512.

Warrington, E.K. & Taylor, A.M. (1973). The contribution of the right parietal lobe to object recognition. *Cortex, 9,* 152–164.

Warrington, E.K. & Weiskrantz, L. (1968). A study of learning and retention in amnesic patients. *Neuropsychologia, 6,* 283–292.

Warrington, E.K. & Weiskrantz, L. (1982). Amnesia: A disconnection syndrome? *Neuropsychologia, 20,* 233–248.

Wasantwisut, E. (1997). Nutrition and development: Other micronutrients' effect on growth and cognition. *Southeast Asian Journal of Tropical Medicine and Public Health, 28,* 78–82.

Washton, A.M. & Stone, N.S. (1984). The human cost of chronic cocaine use. *Medical Aspects of Human Sexuality, 18,* 36–44.

Wasserstein, J. (2002). Gestalt concept of closure: A construct without closure. *Perceptual and Motor Skills, 95,* 963–964.

Wasserstein, J., Barr, W.B., Zappulla, R., & Rock, D. (2003). Facial closure: Interrelationship with Facial Discrimination, other closure tests, and subjective contour illusions. *Neuropsychologia.*

Wasserstein, J., Zappulla, R., Rosen, J., & Gerstman, L. (1984). Evidence for differentiation of right hemisphere visual-perceptual functions. *Brain and Cognition, 3,* 51–56.

Wasserstein, J., Zappulla, R., Rosen, J., et al. (1987). In search of closure: Subjective contour illusions, gestalt completion tests, and implications. *Brain and Cognition, 6,* 1–14.

Watkins, L.H., Rogers, R.D., Lawrence, A.D., et al. (2000). Impaired planning but intact decision making in early Huntington's disease: Implications for specific fronto-striatal pathology. *Neuropsychologia, 38,* 1112–1125.

Watson, C.G. & Plemel, D. (1978). An MMPI scale to separate brain-damaged from functional psychiatric patients in neuropsychiatric settings. *Journal of Consulting and Clinical Psychology, 46,* 1127–1132.

Watson, Y.I., Arfken, C.L., & Birge, S.J. (1993). Clock completion: An objective screening test for dementia. *Journal of the American Geriatric Society, 41,* 1235–1240.

Waxman, S.G. (2000). Multiple sclerosis as a neuronal disease. *Archives of Neurology, 57,* 22–24.

Waxman, S.G. & Geschwind, N. (1975). The interictal behavior syndrome of temporal lobe epilepsy. *Archives of General Psychiatry, 32,* 1580–1586.

Webbe, F.M. & Ochs, S.R. (2003). Recency and frequency of soccer heading interact to decrease neurocognitive performance. *Applied Neuropsychology, 10,* 31–41.

Weber, A.M. & Bradshaw, J.L. (1981). Levy and Reid's neurological model in relation to writing hand/posture: An evaluation. *Psychological Bulletin, 90,* 74–88.

Weber, A.M. & Bradshaw, J.L. (1987). Handwriting posture and cerebral organization. In A. Glass (Ed.), *Individual differences in hemispheric specialization.* New York: Plenum Press.

Webster, J.S., Godlewski, M.C., Hanley, G.L., & Sowa, M.V. (1992). A scoring method for Logical Memory that is sensitive to right-hemisphere dysfunction. *Journal of Clinical and Experimental Neuropsychology, 14,* 222–238.

Wechsler, D. (1932). Analytic use of the Army Alpha examination. *Journal of Applied Psychology, 16,* 254–256.

Wechsler, D. (1939). *The measurement of adult intelligence.* Baltimore, MD: Williams & Wilkins.

Wechsler, D. (1944). *The measurement of adult intelligence* (3rd ed.). Baltimore, MD: Williams & Wilkins.

Wechsler, D. (1945). A standardized memory scale for clinical use. *Journal of Psychology, 19,* 87–95.

Wechsler, D. (1955). *WAIS manual.* New York: The Psychological Corporation.

Wechsler, D. (1958). *The measurement and appraisal of adult intelligence* (4th ed.). Baltimore, MD: Williams & Wilkins.

Wechsler, D. (1974). *WISC-R manual. Wechsler Intelligence Scale for Children–Revised.* New York: Psychological Corporation.

Wechsler, D. (1981). *WAIS-R manual.* New York: The Psychological Corporation.

Wechsler, D. (1987). *Wechsler Memory Scale–Revised manual.* San Antonio: The Psychological Corporation.

Wechsler, D. (1991). *Wechsler Intelligence Scale for Children–Third Edition (WISC-III).* San Antonio: The Psychological Corporation.

Wechsler, D. (1997a). *Wechsler Adult Intelligence Scale-III.* San Antonio: The Psychological Corporation.

Wechsler, D. (1997b). *Wechsler Memory Scale. Third edition manual.* San Antonio: The Psychological Corporation.

Wechsler, D. (1997c). *WAIS-III/WMS-III technical manual.* San Antonio: The Psychological Corporation.

Wechsler, D. (2003). *Wechsler Intelligence Scale for Children–Fourth Edition (WISC-IV).* San Antonio: The Psychological Corporation.

Wechsler, D. & Stone, C.P. (1974). *Wechsler Memory Scale manual.* New York: The Psychological Corporation.

Wecker, N.S., Kramer, J.H., Wisniewski, A., et al. (2000). Age effects on executive ability. *Neuropsychology, 14,* 409–414.

Wedding, D. & Faust, D. (1989). Clinical judgment and decision making in neuropsychology. *Archives of Clinical Neuropsychology, 4,* 233–265.

Wedekind, C., Hesselmann, V., Lippert-Gruner, M., & Ebel, M. (2002). Trauma to the pontomesencephalic brainstem—a major clue to the prognosis of severe traumatic brain injury. *British Journal of Neurosurgery, 16,* 256–260.

Weder, B., Azari, N.P., & Knorr, U. (2000). Disturbed functional brain interactions underlying deficient tactile object discrimination in Parkinson's disease. *Human Brain Mapping, 11,* 131–145.

Weeramanthri, T.S., Puddey, I.B., & Beilen, L.J. (1991). Lightning strike and autonomic failure—coincidence or causally related? *Journal of the Royal Society of Medicine, 84,* 687–688.

Weickert, T., Goldberg, T.E., Gold, J.M., et al. (2000). Cognitive impairments in patients with schizophrenia displaying preserved and compromised intellect. *Archives of General Psychiatry, 57,* 907–913.

Weigl, E. (1941). On the psychology of so-called processes of abstraction. *Journal of Normal and Social Psychology, 36,* 3–33.

Weinberg, J., Diller, L., Gerstman, L., & Schulman, P. (1972). Digit span in right and left hemiplegics. *Journal of Clinical Psychology, 28,* 361.

Weinberger, D.R. (1984). Brain disease and psychiatric illness: When should a psychiatrist order a CT scan? *American Journal of Psychiatry, 141,* 1521–1527.

Weinberger, D.R., Berman, K.F., & Daniel, D.G. (1991). Prefrontal cortex dysfunction in schizophrenia. In H.S. Levin et al. (Eds.), *Frontal lobe function and dysfunction.* New York: Oxford University Press.

Weinberger, J. (2002). Stroke and TIA. Prevention and management of cerebrovascular events in primary care. *Geriatrics, 57,* 38–44.

Weiner, I.B. (2000). Making Rorschach interpretation as good as it can be. *Journal of Personality Assessment, 74,* 164–174.

Weiner, M.F. (1999). Dementia associated with Lewy bodies: Dilemmas and directions. *Archives of Neurology, 56,* 1441–1442.

Weiner, M.F., Doody, R.S., Sairam, R., et al. (2002). Prevalence and incidence of major depressive disorder in Alzheimer's disease: Findings from two databases. *Dementia and Geriatric Cognitive Disorders, 13,* 8–12.

Weiner, M.F., Risser, R.C., Cullum, C.M., et al. (1996). Alzheimer's disease and its Lewy body variant: A clinical analysis of postmortem verified cases. *American Journal of Psychiatry, 153,* 1269–1273.

Weingartner, D.H., Faillace, L.A., & Markley, H.G. (1971). Verbal information retention in alcoholics. *Quarterly Journal of the Study of Alcoholism, 32,* 293–303.

Weingartner, H. (1986). Automatic and effort-demanding cognitive processes in depression. In L.W. Poon (Ed.), *Handbook for clinical memory assessment of older adults*. Washington, D.C.: American Psychological Association.

Weingartner, H., Adefris, W., Eich, J.E., & Murphy, D.L. (1976). Encoding-imagery specificity in alcohol state-dependent learning. *Journal of Experimental Psychology, 2*, 83–87.

Weingartner, H., Burns, S., Diebel, R., & LeWitt, P.A. (1984). Cognitive impairments in Parkinson's disease: Distinguishing between effort-demanding and automatic cognitive processes. *Psychiatry Research, 11*, 223–235.

Weingartner, H., Caine, E.D., & Ebert, M.H. (1979a). Encoding processes, learning, and recall in Huntington's disease. In T.N. Chase et al. (Eds.), *Advances in neurology* (Vol. 23). New York: Raven Press.

Weingartner, H., Caine, E.D., & Ebert, M.H. (1979b). Imagery, encoding, and retrieval of information from memory: Some specific encoding-retrieval changes in Huntington's disease. *Journal of Abnormal Psychology, 88*, 52–58.

Weingartner, H., Eckardt, M., Grafman, J., et al. (1993). The effects of repetition on memory performance in cognitively impaired patients. *Neuropsychology, 7*, 385–395.

Weinshenker, B.G., Bass, B., Rice, G.P.A., et al. (1989). The natural history of multiple sclerosis: A geographically based study. I. Clinical course and disability. *Brain, 112*, 1419–1428.

Weinstein, A., Schwid, S. R., Schiffer, R.B., et al. (1999). Neuropsychological status in multiple sclerosis after treatment with glatiramer acetate (Copaxone). *Archives of Neurology, 56*, 319–324.

Weinstein, C.S., Kaplan, E., Casey, M.B., & Hurwitz, I. (1990). Delineation of female performance on the Rey-Osterrieth Complex Figure. *Neuropsychology, 4*, 117–128.

Weinstein, S. (1964). Deficits concomitant with aphasia or lesions of either cerebral hemisphere. *Cortex, 1*, 154–169.

Weisberg, L.A. (1985). Computed tomography in benign intracranial hypertension. *Neurology, 35*, 1075–1078.

Weisberg, L. (2002). Abnormal involuntary movement disorders (dyskinesias). In L.A. Weisberg, C. Garcia, & R.L. Strub (Eds.), *Essentials of clinical neurology* (4th ed.). St. Louis: Mosby.

Weisberg, L.A., Garcia, C., & Strub, R.L. (2002). *Essentials of clinical neurology* (4th ed.). St. Louis: Mosby.

Weiskrantz, L. (1986). *Blindsight*. Oxford, UK: Clarendon Press.

Weiskrantz, L. (1991). Dissociations and associates in neuropsychology. In R.G. Lister & H.J. Weingartner (Eds.), *Perspectives on cognitive neuroscience*. New York: Oxford University Press.

Weiskrantz, L. (1996). Blindsight revisited. *Current Opinions in Neurobiology, 6*, 215–220.

Weiskrantz, L. (1997). *Consciousness lost and found. Neuropsychological exploration*. New York: Oxford University Press.

Weiss, B. (1983). Behavioral toxicology and environmental health science. *American Psychologist, 38*, 1174–1187.

Weiss, G.H., Caveness, W.F., Einsiedel-Lechtape, H., & McNeel, M.I. (1982). Life expectancy and causes of death in a group of head-injured veterans of World War I. *Archives of Neurology, 39*, 741–743.

Weiss, G.H., Salazar, A.M., Vance, S.C., et al. (1986). Predicting posttraumatic epilepsy in penetrating head injury. *Archives of Neurology, 43*, 771–773.

Weissberg, E., Lyons, S.A., & Richman, J.E. (2000). Fixation dysfunction with intermittent saccadic intrusions managed by yoked prisms: a case report. *Optometry, 71*, 183–188.

Weissman, D.H. & Banich, M.T. (2000). The cerebral hemispheres cooperate to perform complex but not simple tasks. *Neuropsychology, 14*, 41–59.

Weitzner, M.A. (1999). Psychosocial and neuropsychiatric aspects of patients with primary brain tumors. *Cancer Investigation, 17*, 285–291.

Welch, K.M.A. (1994). Relationship of stroke and migraine. *Neurology, 44(Suppl. 7)*, S33–S36.

Welch, K.M.A., Caplan, L.R., et al. (Eds.) (1997). Section II. Pathogenesis and pathology. In K.M.A. Welch et al. (Eds.), *Primer on cerebrovascular diseases*. San Diego: Academic Press.

Welch, K.M.A. & Lewis, D. (1997). Migraine and epilepsy. *Neurologic Clinics, 15*, 107–114.

Welch, L.W., Doineau, D., Johnson, S., & King, D. (1996). Educational and gender normative data for the Boston Naming Test in a group of older adults. *Brain and Language, 53*, 260–266.

Welch, L.W., Nimmerrichter, A., Gilliland, R., et al. (1997). "Wineglass" confabulations among brain-damaged alcoholics on the Wechsler Memory Scale–Revised Visual Reproduction subtest. *Cortex, 33*, 543–551.

Wells, C.E. (1977). Symptoms and behavioral manifestions. In C.E. Wells (Ed.), *Dementia* (2nd ed.). Philadelphia: Davis.

Welsh, K.A., Breitner, J.C., & Magruder-Habib, K. (1993). Detection of dementia in the elderly using telephone screening of cognitive status. *Neuropsychiatry, Neuropsychology, and Behavioral Neurology, 6*, 103–110.

Welsh, K., Butters, N., Hughes, J., et al. (1991). Detection of abnormal memory decline in mild cases of Alzheimer's disease using CERAD neuropsychological measures. *Archives of Neurology, 48*, 278–281.

Welsh, K.A., Butters, N., Hughes, J.P., et al. (1992). Detection and staging of dementia in Alzheimer's disease. Use of the neuropsychological measures developed for the Consortium to Establish a Registry for Alzheimer's Disease. *Archives of Neurology, 49*, 448–452.

Welsh, K.A., Butters, N., Mohs, R.C., et al. (1994). The Consortium to Establish a Registry for Alzheimer's Disease (CERAD). Part V. A normative study of the neuropsychological battery. *Neurology, 44*, 609–614.

Welsh, K.A., Fillenbaum, G., Wilkinson, W., et al. (1995). Neuropsychological test performance in African-American and white patients with Alzheimer's disease. *Neurology, 45*, 2207–2211.

Welsh, M.C., Revilla, V., Strongin, D., & Kepler, M. (2000). Towers of Hanoi and London: Is the nonshared variance due to differences in task administration? *Perceptual and Motor Skills, 90*, 562–572.

Welsh-Bohmer, K.A., Attix, D.K., & Mason, D.J. (2003). The clinical utility of neuropsychological evaluation of patients with known or suspected dementia. In G.P. Prigatano & N.H. Pliskin (Eds.), *Clinical neuropsychology and cost outcome research: A beginning*. New York: Psychology Press.

Welsh-Bohmer, K.A., Tschanz, J.T., Norton, M.C., et al. (2000). Normative data into the ninth and tenth decades of life for a brief neuropsychological battery used in assessing community dwelling elderly [abstract]. *Journal of the International Neuropsychological Society, 6*, 143.

Wendling, B.J. & Mather, N. (2001). *Examiner training workbook. Woodcock-Johnson-III Tests of Cognitive Abilities*. Itasca, IL: Riverside.

Wepman, J.M. (1976). Aphasia: Language without thought or thought without language? *Journal of the American Speech and Hearing Association, 18*, 131–136.

Wepman, J.M. & Jones, L.V. (1967). Aphasia: Diagnostic description and therapy. In W.S. Fields & W.A. Spencer (Eds.), *Stroke rehabilitation*. St. Louis, MO: Green.

Wepman, J.M. & Reynolds, W.M. (1987). *Wepman's Auditory Discrimination Test* (2nd ed.). Los Angeles: Western Psychological Services.

Wernicke, C. (1874). [The symptom complex of aphasia. A psychological study on an anatomical basis.] [Translated from German; G.H. Eggert, Trans.]. In *Wernicke's Works on aphasia: A sourcebook and review.* The Hague, Mouton, 1977.

Wertheim, N. & Botez, M. I. (1961). Receptive amusia: A clinical analysis. *Brain, 84,* 19–30.

Wertheimer, M. (1923). Untersuchungen zur lehre von der Gestalt. *Psychol. Forsch., 4,* 301–350.

Wertz, R.T. (1979). Review of the Token Test (TT). In F.L. Darley (Ed.), *Evaluation of appraisal techniques in speech and language pathology.* Reading, ME: Addison-Wesley.

Wessely, S. (2001). Chronic fatigue: Symptom and syndrome. *Annals of Internal Medicine, 134,* 838–843.

West, R., Winocur, G., Ergis, A.-M., & Saint-Cyr, J. (1998). The contribution of impaired working memory monitoring to performance of the Self-Ordered Pointing Task in normal aging and Parkinson's disease. *Neuropsychology, 12,* 546–554.

West, R.L. (1986). Everyday memory and aging. *Developmental Neuropsychology, 2,* 323–344.

Westbrook, B.K. & McKibben, H. (1989). Dance/movement therapy with groups of outpatients with Parkinson's disease. *American Journal of Dance Therapy, 11,* 27–38.

Westbrook, L.E., Devinsky, O., & Geocadin, R. (1998). Nonepileptic seizures after head injury. *Epilepsia, 39,* 978–982.

Westerveld, M., Sass, K.J., Sass, A., & Henry, H.G. (1994). Assessment of verbal memory in temporal lobe epilepsy using the Selective Reminding Test: Equivalence and reliability of alternate forms. *Journal of Epilepsy, 7,* 57–63.

Westerveld, M., Stoddard, K., Spencer, D.D., et al. (1999). Case report of false lateralization using fMRI: Comparison of fMRI language localization, Wada testing, and cortical stimulation. *Archives of Clinical Neuropsychology, 14,* 162–163.

Westervelt, H.J. & McCaffrey, R.J. (2002). Neuropsychological functioning in chronic Lyme disease. *Neuropsychology Review, 12,* 153–177.

Wetter, M.W., Baer, R.A., Berry, D.T.R., et al. (1992). Sensitivity of MMPI-2 validity scales to random responding and malingering. *Psychological Assessment, 4,* 369–374.

Wetter, M.W. & Corrigan, S.K. (1995). Providing information to clients about psychological tests: A survey of attorneys' and law students' attitudes. *Professional Psychology: Research and Practice, 26,* 474–477.

Wetzel, L. & Boll, T.J. (1987). *Short Category Test, Booklet Format.* Los Angeles: Western Psychological Services.

Wetzel, L. & Murphy, S.G. (1991). Validity of the use of a discontinue rule and evaluation of the Hooper Visual Organization Test. *Neuropsychology, 5,* 119–122.

Wharton, C.M. & Grafman, J. (1998). Deductive reasoning and the brain. *Trends in Cognitive Sciences, 2,* 54–59.

Wheeler, M.A. (2002). Episodic memory and autonoetic awareness. In E. Tulving & F.I.M. Craik (Eds.), *The Oxford handbook of memory.* Oxford: Oxford University Press.

Wheelock, I., Peterson, C., & Buchtel, H. A. (1998). Presurgery expectations, postsurgery satisfaction, and psychosocial adjustment after epilepsy surgery. *Epilepsia, 39,* 487–494.

Whelihan, W.M. & Lesher, E.L. (1985). Neuropsychological changes in frontal functions with aging. *Developmental Neuropsychology, 1,* 371–380.

Whelihan, W.M., Lesher, E.L., Kleban, M.H., & Granick, S. (1984). Mental status and memory assessment as predictors of dementia. *Journal of Gerontology, 39,* 572–576.

Whetten-Goldstein, K., Sloan, F.A., Goldstein, L.B., & Kulas, E.D. (1998). A comprehensive assessment of the cost of multiple sclerosis in the United States. *Multiple Sclerosis, 4,* 419–425.

Whitaker, J.N. & Benveniste, E.N. (1990). Demyelinating diseases. In A.L. Pearlman & R.C. Collins (Eds.), *Neurobiology of disease.* New York: Oxford University Press.

White, A.M., Matthews, D.B., & Best, P.J. (2000). Ethanol, memory, and hippocampal function: A review of recent findings. *Hippocampus, 10,* 88–93.

White, D.A. & Murphy, C.F. (1998). Working memory for nonverbal auditory information in dementia of the Alzheimer type. *Neuropsychology, 13,* 339–347.

White, D.A., Taylor, M.J., Butters, N., et al. (1997). Memory for verbal information in individuals with HIV-associated dementia complex. HNRC Group. *Journal of Clinical and Experimental Neuropsychology, 19,* 357–366.

White, P.D., Dash, A.R., & Thomas, J.M. (1998). Poor concentration and the ability to process information after glandular fever. *Journal of Psychosomatic Research, 44,* 269–278.

White, R.F., Diamond, R., Proctor, S., et al. (1993). Residual cognitive deficits 50 years after lead poisoning during childhood. *British Journal of Industrial Medicine, 50,* 613–622.

White, R.F., Feldman, R.G., & Proctor, S.P. (1992). Neurobehavioral effects of toxic exposures. In R.F. White (Ed.), *Clinical syndromes in adult neuropsychology: The practitioner's handbook.* New York: Elsevier.

White, R.F., Feldman, R.G., & Travers, P.H. (1990). Neurobehavioral effects of toxicity due to metals, solvents, and insecticides. *Clinical Neuropharmacology, 13,* 392–412.

White, R.F. & Proctor, S.P. (1992). Research and clinical criteria for development of neurobehavioral test batteries. *Journal of Occupational Medicine, 34,* 140–148.

Whitehouse, F.W. (1997). Management of diabetes in stroke. In K.M.A. Welch et al. (Eds.), *Primer on cerebrovascular diseases.* San Diego: Academic Press.

Whitehouse, P.J., Price, D.L., Clark, A.W., et al. (1981). Alzheimer disease: Evidence for selective loss of cholinergic neurons in the nucleus basalis. *Annals of Neurology, 10,* 122–126.

Whiteneck, G.G., Charlifue, S.W., Gerhart, K.A., et al. (1992). Quantifying handicap: A new measure of long-term rehabilitation outcomes. *Archives of Physical Medicine and Rehabilitation, 73,* 519–526.

Whiteneck, G.G., Fougeyrolloas, P., & Gerhart, K.A. (1997). Elaborating the model of disablement. In M. Fuhrer (Ed.), *Assessing medical rehabilitation practices: The promise of outcomes research.* Baltimore: Paul H. Brooks.

Whitfield, K. & Newcomb, R.A. (1992). A normative sample using the Loong Computerized Tapping Program. *Perceptual and Motor Skills, 74,* 861–862.

Whiting, W.L.T. & Smith, A.D. (1997). Differential age-related processing limitations in recall and recognition tasks. *Psychology and Aging, 12,* 216–224.

Whitman, S. & Hermann, B.P. (Eds.) (1986). *Psychopathology in epilepsy. Social dimensions.* New York: Oxford University Press.

Whyte, J., Schuster, K., Polansky, M., et al. (2000). Frequency and duration of inattentive behavior after traumatic brain injury: Effects of distraction, task, and practice. *Journal of the International Neuropsychological Society, 6,* 1–11.

Wickelgren, I. (1996). For the cortex, neuron loss may be less than thought. *Science, 273,* 48–50.

Wiebe, S., Blume, W.T., Girvin, J.P., & Eliasziw, M. (2001). A randomized, controlled trial of surgery for temporal-lobe epilepsy. *New England Journal of Medicine, 345,* 311–318.

Wiebe, S., Matijevic, S., Eliasziw, M., & Derry, P. A. (2002). Clinically important change in quality of life in epilepsy. *Journal of Neurology, Neurosurgery and Psychiatry, 73,* 116–120.

Wiegner, S. & Donders, J. (1999). Performance on the California Verbal Learning Test after traumatic brain injury. *Journal of Clinical and Experimental Neuropsychology, 21,* 159–170.

Wielgos, C.M. & Cunningham, W.R. (1999). Age-related slowing on the Digit Symbol task: Longitudinal and cross-sectional analyses. *Experimental Aging Research, 25,* 109–120.

Wiener, D.N. (1947). Subtle and obvious keys for the Minnesota Multiphasic Personality Inventory. *Journal of Consulting Psychology, 12,* 164–170.

Wiens, A.N., Bryan, J.E., & Crossen, J.R. (1993). Estimating WAIS-R FSIQ from the National Adult Reading Test–Revised in normal subjects. *The Clinical Neuropsychologist, 7,* 70–84.

Wiens, A.N., Fuller, K.H., & Crossen, J.R. (1997). Paced Auditory Serial Addition Test: Adult norms and moderator variables. *Journal of Clinical and Experimental Neuropsychology, 19,* 473–483.

Wiens, A.N., McMinn, M.R., & Crossen, J.R. (1988). Rey Auditory-Verbal Learning Test: Development of norms for healthy young adults. *The Cinical Neuropsychologist, 2,* 67–87.

Wiens, A.N., Tindall, A.G., & Crossen, J.R. (1994). California Verbal Learning Test: A normative data study. *The Clinical Neuropsychologist, 8,* 75–90.

Wieser, H.G. (1986). Psychomotor seizures of hippocampal–amygdalar origin. In T.A. Pedley & B.S. Meldrum (Eds.), *Recent advances in epilepsy* (No. 3). New York: Churchill-Livingstone.

Wiggins, E.C. & Brandt, J. (1988). The detection of simulated amnesia. *Law and Human Behavior, 12,* 57–77.

Wiig, E.H., Alexander, E.W., & Secord, W. (1988). Linguistic competence and level of cognitive functioning in adults with traumatic closed head injury. In H.A. Whitaker (Ed.), *Neuropsychological studies of nonfocal brain damage.* New York: Springer-Verlag.

Wilcox, R.E. & Gonzales, R.A. (1995). Introduction to neurotransmitters, receptors, signal transduction, and second messengers. In A.F. Schatzberg and C.B. Nemeroff (Ed.), *The American Psychiatric Press textbook of pharmacology.* Washington, D.C.: American Psychiatric Association.

Wild, K.V. & Kaye, J.A. (1998). The rate of progression of Alzheimer's disease in the later stages: Evidence from the Severe Impairment Battery. *Journal of the International Neuropsychological Society, 4,* 512–516.

Wild, K.V., Kaye, J.A., & Oken, B.S. (1994). Early non-cognitive change in Alzheimer's disease and healthy aging. *Journal of Geriatric Psychiatry and Neurology,7,* 199–205.

Wild, K.V., Lezak, M.D., Whitham, R.H., & Bourdette, D.N. (1991). Psychosocial impact of cognitive impairment in the multiple sclerosis patient [abstract]. *Journal of Clinical and Experimental Neuropsychology, 13,* 74.

Wilde, M.C., Boake, C., & Sherer, M. (1995). Do recognition-free recall discrepancies detect retrieval deficits in closed-head injury? An exploratory analysis with the California Verbal Learning Test. *Journal of Clinical and Experimental Neuropsychology, 17,* 849–855.

Wilde, M.C., Boake, C., & Sherer, M. (1997). Do recognition-free recall discrepancies detect retrieval deficits? A response to Veiel. *Journal of Clinical and Experimental Neuropsychology, 19,* 153–155.

Wilde, M.C., Boake, C., & Sherer, M. (2000). Wechsler Adult Intelligence Scale–Revised Block Design broken configuration errors in nonpenetrating traumatic brain injury. *Applied Neuropsychology, 7,* 208–214.

Wilde, N., Strauss, E., Chelune, G.J., et al. (2001). WMS-III performance in patients with temporal lobe epilepsy: Group differences and individual classification. *Journal of the International Neuropsychological Society, 7,* 881–891.

Wilhelm, K.L. & Johnstone, B. (1995). Use of the Wechsler Memory Scale–Revised in traumatic brain injury. *Applied Neuropsychology, 2,* 42–45.

Wilkie, F.L., Eisdorfer, C., & Nowlin, J.B. (1976). Memory and blood pressure in the aged. *Experimental Aging Research, 2,* 3–16.

Wilkinson, D.A. & Carlen, P.I. (1981). Chronic organic brain syndromes associated with alcoholism. Neuropsychological and other aspects. In Y. Israel et al. (Eds.), *Research advances in alcohol and drug problems* (Vol. 6). New York: Plenum Press.

Wilkinson, G.S. (1993). *WRAT-3: The Wide Range Achievement Test administration manual* (3rd ed.). Wilmington, DE: Wide Range.

Wilkinson, R.T. & Allison, S. (1989). Age and simple reaction time: Decade differences for 5,325 subjects. *Journal of Gerontology: Psychological Sciences, 44,* 29–35.

Willems, H. & de Kleijn-de Vrankrijker, M. (2002). Work disability in the Netherlands: data, conceptual aspects, and perspectives. *Journal of Occupational and Environmental Medicine, 44,* 510–515.

Willer, B., Johnson, W., Rempel, R., & Linn, R. (1993). A note concerning misconceptions of the general public about brain injury. *Archives of Clinical Neuropsychology, 9,* 411–425.

Willer, B., Ottenbacher, K.J., & Coad, M.L. (1994). The Community Integration Questionnaire: A comparative examination. *American Journal of Physical Medicine and Rehabilitation, 73,* 103–111.

Willer, B., Rosenthal, M., Kreutzer, J.S., et al. (1993). Assessment of community integration following rehabilitation for traumatic brain injury. *Journal of Head Trauma Rehabilitation, 8,* 75–87.

Williams, D.H., Levin, H.S., & Eisenberg, H.M. (1990). Mild head injury classification. *Neurosurgery, 27,* 422–428.

Williams, J.D. & Klug, M.G. (1996). Aging and cognition: Methodological differences in outcome. *Experimental Aging Research, 22,* 219–244.

Williams, J.M. (1991). *Memory Assessment Scales.* Odessa, FL: Psychological Assessment Resources.

Williams, J.M. (1992). Neuropsychological assessment of traumatic brain injury in the intensive care and acute care environment. In C.E. Long & L.K. Ross (Eds.), *Handbook of head trauma.* New York: Plenum Press.

Williams, J.M. (1997). The prediction of premorbid memory ability. *Archives of Clinical Neuropsychology, 12,* 745–738.

Williams, J.M., Little, M.M., Scates, S., & Blockman, N. (1987). Memory complaints and abilities among depressed older adults. *Journal of Consulting and Clinical Psychology, 55,* 595–598.

Williams, J.R., Spencer, P.S., Stahl, S.M., et al. (1987). Interactions of aging and environmental agents: The toxicological perspective. In S.R. Baker & M. Rogul (Eds.), *Environmental toxicity and the aging process.* New York: Alan R. Liss.

Williams, M. (1965). *Mental testing in clinical practice.* Oxford, UK: Pergamon.

Williams, M. (1979). *Brain damage, behaviour, and the mind.* Chichester, UK: Wiley.

Williams, M.A., LaMarche, J.A., Alexander, R.W., et al. (1996). Serial 7s and alphabet backwards as brief measures of information processing speed. *Archives of Clinical Neuropsychology, 11,* 651–659.

Williams, M.A., Rich, M.A., Reed, L. K., et al. (1998). Visual Reproduction subtest of the Wechsler Memory Scale–Revised: Analysis of construct validity. *Journal of Clinical Psychology, 54,* 963–971.

Williams, S.M. (1991). Handedness inventories: Edinburgh versus Annett. *Neuropsychology, 5,* 43–48.

Williamson, D.J., Adair, J.C., Raymer, A.M., & Heilman, K.M. (1998). Object and action naming in Alzheimer's disease. *Cortex, 34,* 601–610.

Willingham, D.B., Nissen, M.J., & Bullemer, P. (1989). On the development of procedural knowledge. *Journal of Experimental Psychology: Learning, Memory, and Cognition, 15,* 1047–1060.

Willis, L., Behrens, M., Mack, W., & Chui, H. (1998). Ideomotor apraxia in early Alzheimer's disease: Time and accuracy measures. *Brain and Cognition, 38,* 220–233.

Willis, W.G. (1984). Reanalysis of an actuarial approach to neuropsychological diagnosis in consideration of base rates. *Journal of Consulting and Clinical Psychology, 52,* 567–569.

Wills, P., Clare, L., Shiel, A., & Wilson, B.A. (2000). Assessing subtle memory impairments in the everyday memory performance of brain injured people: Exploring the potential of the Extended Rivermead Behavioural Memory Test. *Brain Injury, 14,* 693–704.

Wilson, B.A. (1986). *Rehabilitation of memory.* New York: Guilford Press.

Wilson, B.A. (1988). Future directions in rehabilitation of brain injured people. In A.-L. Christensen & B.P. Uzzell (Eds.), *Neuropsychological rehabilitation.* Boston: Kluwer.

Wilson, B.A. (1993). Ecological validity of neuropsychological assessment: Do neuropsychological indexes predict performance in everyday activities? *Applied and Preventive Psychology, 2,* 209–215.

Wilson, B.A. (1998). Recovery of cognitive functions following nonprogressive brain injury. *Current Opinion in Neurobiology, 8,* 281–287.

Wilson, B.A. (2000). Compensating for cognitive deficits following brain injury. *Neuropsychology Review, 10,* 233–243.

Wilson, B.A., Alderman, N., Burgess, P.W., et al. (1996). *Behavioural Assessment of the Dysexecutive Syndrome.* Bury St. Edmunds, UK: Thames Valley Test.

Wilson, B.A., Clare, L., Baddeley, A.D., et al. (1999). *The Rivermead Behavioural Memory Test–Extended Version.* Bury St. Edmunds, UK: Thames Valley Test.

Wilson, B.A., Cockburn, J., & Baddeley, A. (1985). *The Rivermead Behavioral Memory Test.* Bury St. Edmunds, UK: Thames Valley Test.

Wilson, B.A., Cockburn, J., & Baddeley, A. (2003). *The Rivermead Behavioral Memory Test-II.* Bury St. Edmunds, UK: Thames Valley Test.

Wilson, B.(A.), Cockburn, J., Baddeley, A., & Hiorns, R. (1989). Development and validation of a test battery for detecting and monitoring everyday memory problems. *Journal of Clinical and Experimental Neuropsychology, 11,* 855–870.

Wilson, B.(A.), Cockburn, J., & Halligan, P. (1987a). *Behavioural Inattention Test.* Bury St. Edmunds, UK: Thames Valley Test Co.

Wilson, B.(A.), Cockburn, J., & Halligan, P. (1987b). Development of a behavioral test of visuospatial neglect. *Archives of Physical Medicine and Rehabilitation, 68,* 98–102.

Wilson, B.A., Emslie, H.C., Quirk, K., & Evans, J.J. (2001). Reducing everyday memory and planning problems by means of a paging system: A randomised control crossover study. *Journal of Neurology, Neurosurgery and Psychiatry, 70,* 477–482.

Wilson, B.A., Evans, J.J., Emslie, H., et al. (1998). The development of an ecologically valid test for assessing patients with a dysexecutive syndrome. *Neuropsychological Rehabilitation, 8,* 213–228.

Wilson, B.A. & McLellan, D.L. (1997). *Rehabilitation studies handbook.* Cambridge: Cambridge University Press.

Wilson, B.(A.), Vizor, A., & Bryant, T. (1991). Predicting severity of cognitive impairment after severe head injury. *Brain Injury, 5,* 189–197.

Wilson, B.A., Watson, P.C., Baddeley, A.D., et al. (2000). Improvement or simply practice? The effects of twenty repeated assessments on people with and without brain injury. *Journal of the International Neuropsychological Society, 6,* 469–479.

Wilson, J.T.L. (1990). Significance of MRI in clarifying whether neu-

ropsychological deficits after head injury are organically based. *Neuropsychology, 4,* 261–269.

Wilson, J.T.L., Edwards, P., Fiddes, H., et al. (2002). Reliability of postal questionnaires for the Glasgow Outcome Scale. *Journal of Neurotrauma, 19,* 999–1005.

Wilson, J.T.L., Hadley, D.M., Scott, L.C., & Harper, A. (1996). Neuropsychological significance of contusional lesions identified by MRI. In B.P. Uzzell & H.H. Stonnington (Eds.), *Recovery after brain injury.* Mahwah, NJ: Erlbaum.

Wilson, J.T.L., Pettigrew, L.E.L., & Teasdale, G.M. (2000). Emotional and cognitive consequences of head injury in relation to the Glasgow Outcome Scale. *Journal of Neurology, Neurosurgery and Psychiatry, 69,* 204–209.

Wilson, J.T.L., Wiedmann, K.D., Hadley, D.M., et al. (1988). Early and late magnetic resonance imaging and neuropsychological outcome after head injury. *Journal of Neurology, Neurosurgery and Psychiatry, 51,* 391–396.

Wilson, R.S., Bacon, L.D., Kaszniak, A.W., & Fox, J.H. (1982). The episodic-semantic memory distinction and paired associate learning. *Journal of Consulting and Clinical Psychology, 50,* 154–155.

Wilson, R.S., Beckett, L.A., Barnes, L.L., et al. (2002). Individual differences in rate of change in cognitive abilities of older persons. *Psychology and Aging, 17,* 179–193.

Wilson, R.S., Como, P.G., Garron, D.C., et al. (1987). Memory failure in Huntington's disease. *Journal of Clinical and Experimental Neuropsychology, 9,* 147–154.

Wilson, R.S., Gilley, D.W., Bennett, D.A., et al. (2000a). Hallucinations, delusions, and cognitive decline in Alzheimer's disease. *Journal of Neurology, Neurosurgery and Psychiatry, 69,* 172–177.

Wilson, R.S., Gilley, D.W., Bennett, D.A., et al. (2000b). Person-specific paths of cognitive decline in Alzheimer's disease and their relation to age. *Psychology and Aging, 15,* 18–28.

Wilson, R.S. & Kaszniak, A.W. (1986). Longitudinal changes: Progressive idiopathic dementia. In L.W. Poon (Ed.), *Handbook for clinical memory assessment of older adults.* Washington, D.C.: American Psychological Association.

Wilson, R.S., Kaszniak, A.W., & Fox, J.H. (1981). Remote memory in senile dementia. *Cortex, 17,* 41–48.

Wilson, R.S., Kaszniak, A.W., Klawans, H.L., Jr., & Garron, D.C. (1980). High speed memory scanning in parkinsonism. *Cortex, 16,* 67–72.

Wilson, R.S., Rosenbaum, G., & Brown, G. (1979). The problem of premorbid intelligence in neuropsychological assessment. *Journal of Clinical Neuropsychology, 1,* 49–54.

Winblad, B., Brodaty, H., Gauthier, S., et al. (2001). Pharmacotherapy of Alzheimer's disease: Is there a need to redefine treatment success? *International Journal of Geriatric Psychiatry, 16,* 653–666.

Winick, M. (1976). *Malnutrition and brain development.* New York: Oxford University Press.

Winogrond, I.R. & Fisk, A.A. (1983). Alzheimer's disease: Assessment of functional status. *Journal of the American Geriatrics Society, 31,* 780–785.

Winterling, D., Crook, T., Salama, M., & Gobert, J. (1986). A self-rating scale for assessing memory loss. In J. Cahn et al. (Eds.), *Senile dementia: Early detection.* London-Paris: John Libbey Eurotext.

Wiseman, O.J. & Fowler, C.J. (2002). Bladder and sexual dysfunction. In A.S. Asbury et al. (Eds.), *Diseases of the nervous system. Clinical neuroscience and therapeutic principles* (3rd ed.). Cambridge: Cambridge University Press.

Wishart, H. & Sharpe, D. (1997). Neuropsychological aspects of multiple sclerosis: A quantitative review. *Journal of Clinical and Experimental Neuropsychology, 19,* 810–824.

Wishart, H.A., Strauss, E., Hunter, M., & Moll, A. (1995). Interhemispheric transfer in multiple sclerosis. *Journal of Clinical and Experimental Neuropsychology, 17,* 937–940.

Witelson, S.F. (1976). Sex and the single hemisphere: Specialization of the right hemisphere for spatial processing. *Science, 193,* 425–427.

Witelson, S.F. (1980). Neuroanatomical asymmetry in left-handers: A review and implications for functional asymmetry. In J. Herron (Ed.), *Neuropsychology of left-handedness.* New York: Academic Press.

Witelson, S.F. (1985). The brain connection: The corpus callosum is larger in left-handers. *Science, 229,* 665–668.

Witelson, S.F. (1989). Hand and sex differences in the isthmus and genu of the human corpus callosum. *Brain, 112,* 799–835.

Witelson, S.F. (1991). Neural sexual mosaicism: Sexual differentiation of the human temporo-parietal region for functional asymmetry. *Psychoneuroendocrinology, 16,* 131–153.

Witelson, S.F. (1995). Neuroanatomical bases of hemispheric functional specialization in the human brain: Possible developmental factors. In F.L. Kitterle (Ed.), *Hemispheric communication: Mechanisms and models.* Hillsdale, NJ: Erlbaum.

Witelson, S.F., Glezer, I.I., & Kigar, D.L. (1995). Women have greater density of neurons in posterior temporal cortex. *Journal of Neuroscience, 15,* 3418–3428.

Witelson, S.F. & Goldsmith, C.H. (1991). The relationship of hand preference to anatomy of the corpus callosum in men. *Brain Research, 545,* 175–182.

Witelson, S.F. & Kigar, D.L. (1987). Individual differences in the anatomy of the corpus callosum: Sex, hand preference, schizophrenia and hemisphere specialization. In A. Glass (Ed.), *Individual differences in hemisphere specialization.* NATO ASI Series, Life Sciences. New York: Plenum Press.

Witelson, S.F. & Swallow, J.A. (1988). Neuropsychological study of the development of spatial cognition. In J. Stiles-Davis et al. (Eds.), *Spatial cognition. Brain bases and development.* Hillsdale, NJ: Erlbaum.

Witol, A.D. & Webbe, F.M. (2003). Soccer heading frequency predicts neuropsychological deficits. *Archives of Clinical Neuropsychology, 18,* 397–417.

Witt, E.D., Ryan, C., & Hsu, L.K.G. (1985). Learning deficits in adolescents with anorexia nervosa. *Journal of Nervous and Mental Disease, 173,* 182–184.

Wittenberg, W., Tremont, G., Zielinski, R.E., et al. (1996). Cognitive-behavioral prevention of postconcussion syndrome. *Archives of Clinical Neuropsychology, 11,* 139–145.

Woertgen, C., Rothoerl, R.D., & Brawanski, A. (2002). Early S-100B serum level correlates to quality of life in patients after severe head injury. *Brain Injury, 16,* 807–816.

Woertgen, C., Rothoerl, R.D., Holzchuh, M., et al. (1997). Comparison of serial S-100 and NSE serum measurements after severe head injury. *Acta Neurochirurgica, 139,* 1161–1164.

Wogar, M.A., Van den Broek, M.D., Bradshaw, C.M., & Szabadi, E. (1998). A new performance-curve method for the detection of simulated cognitive impairment. *British Journal of Psychology, 37,* 327–339.

Wolber, G. & Lira, F.T. (1981). Relationship between Bender designs and basic living skills of geriatric psychiatric patients. *Perceptual and Motor Skills, 52,* 16–18.

Wolber, G., Romaniuk, M., Eastman, E., & Robinson, C. (1984). Validity of the Short Portable Mental Status Questionnaire with elderly psychiatric patients. *Journal of Consulting and Clinical Psychology, 52,* 712–713.

Wolf, O.T., Preut, R., Hellhammer, D.H., et al. (2000). Testosterone and cognition in elderly men: A single testosterone injection blocks the practice effect in verbal fluency, but has no effect on spatial or verbal memory. *Biological Psychiatry, 47,* 650–654.

Wolf, P.A. (1997). Epidemiology and risk factor management. In K.M.A. Welch et al. (Eds.), *Primer on cerebrovascular diseases.* San Diego: Academic Press.

Wolf, P.A., Kannel, W.B., & McGee, D.L. (1986). Epidemiology of strokes in North America. In H.J.M. Bennett et al. (Eds.), *Stroke. Pathophysiology, diagnosis, and management.* New York: Churchill Livingstone.

Wolfe, N., Babikian, V.L., Linn, R.T., et al. (1994). Are multiple cerebral infarcts synergistic? *Archives of Neurology, 51,* 211–215.

Wolfe, N., Linn, R., Babikian, V.L., et al. (1990). Frontal systems impairment following multiple lacunar infarcts. *Archives of Neurology, 47,* 129–132.

Wolff, A.B., Radecke, D.D., Kammerer, B.L., & Gardner, J.K, (1989). Adaptation of the Stroop Color and Word Test for use with deaf adults. *The Clinical Neuropsychologist, 3,* 369–374.

Wolff, H.G. (1937). Personality features and reactions of subjects with migraine. *Archives of Neurology and Psychiatry, 37,* 895–921.

Wolff, P.H., Hurvitz, I., Imamura, S., & Lee, K.W. (1983). Sex differences and ethnic variations in speed of automatized naming. *Neuropsychologia, 21,* 283–288.

Wolf-Klein, G.P., Silverstone, F.A., Levy, A.P., et al. (1989). Screening for Alzheimer's disease by clock drawing. *Journal of the American Geriatrics Society, 37,* 730–734.

Wolkowitz, O.M. & Reus, V.I. (2001). Psychoneuroendocrine aspects of treatment-resistant mood disorders. In J.D. Amsterdam et al. (Eds.), *Treatment-resistant mood disorders.* Cambridge: Cambridge University Press.

Woloszyn, D.G., Murphy, S.G., Wetzel, L., & Fisher, W. (1993). Interrater agreement on the Wechsler Memory Scale–Revised in a mixed clinical population. *The Clinical Neuropsychologist, 7,* 467–471.

Wolters, E.C., Huang, C.C., Clark, C., et al. (1989). Positron emission tomography in manganese intoxication. *Annals of Neurology, 26,* 647–651.

Wong, E., Leong, M.K., Anantharaman, V., et al. (2002). Road traffic accident mortality in Singapore. *Journal of Emergency Medicine, 22,* 139–146.

Wong, J.L. & Gilpin, A.R. (1993). Verbal vs. visual categories on the Wechsler Memory Scale–Revised: How meaningful a distinction? *Journal of Clinical Psychology, 49,* 847–854.

Wong, J.L., Wetterneck, C., & Klein, A. (2000). Effects of depressed mood on verbal memory performance versus self-reports of cognitive difficulties. *International Journal of Rehabilitation and Health, 5,* 85–97.

Wong, T.M., Strickland, T.L., Fletcher-Janzen, E., et al. (2000). Theoretical and practical issues in neuropsychological assessment and treatment of culturally dissimilar patients. In E. Fletcher-Janzen et al. (Eds.), *Handbook of cross-cultural neuropsychology.* New York: Kluwer Academic/Plenum Press.

Wood, A.G., Saling, M.M., O'Shea, M.F., et al. (2000). Components of verbal learning and hippocampal damage assessed by T2 relaxometry. *Journal of the International Neuropsychological Society, 6,* 529–538.

Wood, F.B., McHenry, L.C., & Stump, D.A. (1981). *Memory and related neurobehavioral deficits in TIA patients: Behavioral, rCBF, and outcome measures.* NIH Research Protocol 188-18-8951. Durham, NC: Bowman Gray School of Medicine, unpublished manuscript.

Wood, R.L. (1984). Behaviour disorders following severe brain injury. Their presentation and psychological management. In N. Brooks (Ed.), *Closed head injury. Psychological, social, and family consequences.* Oxford: Oxford University Press.

Wood, R.L. (1986). Neuropsychological assessment in brain injury rehabilitation. In M.G. Eisenburg & R.C. Grzesiak (Eds.), *Advances in clinical rehabilitation*. New York: Springer.

Wood, R.L. (1990). Disorders of attention and their treatment in traumatic brain injury rehabilitation. In E.D. Bigler (Ed.), *Traumatic brain injury*. Austin, TX: Pro-Ed.

Woodard, J.L., Auchus, A.P., Godsall, R.E., & Green, R. C. (1998). An analysis of test bias and differential item functioning due to race on the Mattis Dementia Rating Scale. *Journals of Gerontology. Series B, Psychological Sciences and Social Sciences, 53,* P370–P374.

Woodard, J.L., & Axelrod, B.N. (1995). Parsimonious prediction of Wechsler Memory Scale–Revised indices. *Psychological Assessment, 7,* 445–449.

Woodard, J.L., Axelrod, B.N., & Henry, R.R. (1992). Interrater reliability of scoring parameters for the Design Fluency Test. *Neuropsychology, 6,* 173–178.

Woodard, J.L., Dunlosky, J.A., & Salthouse, T.A. (1999). Task decomposition analysis of intertrial free recall performance on the Rey Auditory Verbal Learning Test in normal aging and Alzheimer's disease. *Journal of Clinical and Experimental Neuropsychology, 21,* 666–676.

Woodard, J.L., Goldstein, F.C., Roberts, V.J., & McGuire, C. (1999). Convergent and discriminant validity of the CVLT (Dementia Version). *Journal of Clinical and Experimental Neuropsychology, 21,* 553–558.

Woodard, J., Salthouse, T., Godsall, R., & Green, R. (1996). Confirmatory factor analysis of Mattis Dementia Rating scale in patients with Alzheimer's disease. *Psychological Assessment, 8,* 85–91.

Woodcock, R.W. (1990). Theoretical foundations of the WJ-R measures of cognitive ability. *Journal of Psychoeducational Assessment, 8,* 231–258.

Woodcock, R.W. (1998). *The WJ-R and Batería-R in neuropsychological assessment. Research Report Number 1.* Itasca, IL: Riverside.

Woodcock, R.W. & Johnson, M.B. (1989). *Woodcock-Johnson Psycho-Educational Battery–Revised.* Itasca, IL: Riverside.

Woodcock, R.W., McGrew, K.W., & Mather, N. (2001a). *Woodcock-Johnson III.* Itasca, IL: Riverside.

Woodcock, R.W., McGrew, K.W., & Mather, N. (2001b). *Woodcock-Johnson III Tests of Achievement.* Itasca, IL: Riverside.

Woodcock, R.W., McGrew, K.W., & Mather, N. (2001c). *Woodcock-Johnson III Tests of Cognitive Abilities.* Itasca, IL: Riverside.

Woodcock, R.W. & Muñoz-Sandoval, A.F. (1996a). *Batería Woodcock-Muñoz: Pruebas de aprovechamiento–Revisada.* Itasca, IL: Riverside.

Woodcock, R.W. & Muñoz-Sandoval, A.F. (1996b). *Batería Woodcock-Muñoz: Pruebas de habilidad cognitiva-Revisada.* Itasca, IL: Riverside.

Woodcock, R.W. & Muñoz-Sandoval, A.F. (2001). The Batería-R in neuropsychological assessment. In M.O. Pónton & J. Léon-Carrion (Eds.), *Neuropsychology and the Hispanic patient.* Mahwah, NJ: Erlbaum.

Woodman, T. & Robertson, C.S. (1996). Jugular venous oxygen saturation monitoring. In R.K. Narayan et al. (Eds.), *Neurotrauma.* New York: McGraw-Hill.

Woodruff-Pak, D.S. (1997). *The neuropsychology of aging.* Malden, MA: Blackwell.

Woods, S.P. & Tröster, A.I. (2003). Prodromal frontal/executive dysfunction predicts incident dementia in Parkinson's disease. *Journal of the International Neuropsychological Society, 9,* 17–24.

Wooten, G.F. (1990). Parkinsonism. In A.L. Pearlman & R.C. Collins (Eds.), *Neurobiology of disease.* New York: Oxford University Press.

World Health Organization (1980). *International classification of impairments, disabilities, and handicaps.* Geneva: WHO.

World Health Organization (1997). *ICIDH-2: International classification of impairments, activities, and participation. A manual of dimensions for disablement and functioning.* Geneva: WHO.

World Health Organization (2001). *International classification of functioning, disability, and health.* Geneva: WHO.

Wragg, R.E. & Jeste, D.V. (1989). Overview of depression and psychosis in Alzheimer's disease. *American Journal of Psychiatry, 146,* 577–587.

Wright, L. (1970). The meaning of IQ scores among professional groups. *Professional Psychology, 1,* 265–269.

Wright, M.J., Burns, R.J., Geffen, G.M., & Geffen, L.B. (1990). Covert orientation of visual attention in Parkinson's disease: An impairment in the maintenance of attention. *Neuropsychologia, 28,* 151–159.

Wrightson, P. & Gronwall, D. (1999). *Mild head injury.* Oxford: Oxford University Press.

Wyller, T.B., Sodring, K.M., Sveen, U., et al. (1997). Are there gender differences in functional outcome after stroke? *Clinical Rehabilitation, 11,* 171–179.

Wyllie, E. & Lüders, H. (1997). Classification of the epilepsies. In E. Wyllie (Ed.), *The treatment of the epilepsies: Principles and practice* (2nd ed.). Baltimore, MD: Williams & Wilkins.

Xu, G., Meyer, J.S., Thornby, J., et al. (2002). Screening for mild cognitive impairment (MCI) utilizing combined mini-mental-cognitive capacity examinations for identifying dementia prodromes. *International Journal of Geriatric Psychiatry, 17,* 1027–1033.

Yaffe, K., Blackwell, T., Gore, R., et al. (1999). Depressive symptoms and cognitive decline in nondemented elderly women: A prospective study. *Archives of General Psychiatry, 56,* 425–430.

Yaffe, K., Sawaya, G., Lieberburg, I., & Grady, D. (1998). Estrogen therapy in postmenopausal women: Effects on cognitive function and dementia. *Journal of the American Medical Association, 279,* 688–695.

Yamadori, A., Mori, E., Tabuchi, M., et al. (1986). Hypergraphia: a right hemisphere syndrome. *Journal of Neurology, Neurosurgery and Psychiatry, 49,* 1160–1164.

Yamadori, A., Osumi, Y., Masuhara, S., & Okubo, M. (1977). Preservation of singing in Broca's aphasia. *Journal of Neurology, Neurosurgery and Psychiatry, 40,* 221–224.

Yamamoto, H., Matsumoto, M., Hashikawa, K., & Hori, M. (2001). Stroke onset and courses. In J. Bogousslavsky & L. Caplan (Eds.), *Stroke syndromes* (2nd ed.). Cambridge: Cambridge University Press.

Yamamoto, T. & Hirano, A. (1985). Nucleus raphe dorsalis in Alzheimer's disease: Neurofibrillary tangles and loss of large neurons. *Annals of Neurology, 17,* 573–577.

Yang, L. & Benardo, L.S. (2000). Valproate prevents epileptiform activity after trauma in an in vitro model in neocortical slices. *Epilepsia, 41,* 1507–1513.

Yarnell, P.R. & Rossie, G.V. (1988). Minor whiplash head injury with major debilitation. *Brain Injury, 2,* 255–258.

Yates, A.J. (1954). The validity of some psychological tests of brain damage. *Psychological Bulletin, 51,* 359–379.

Yeates, K.O., Ris, M.D., & Taylor, H.G. (Eds.) (2000). *Pediatric neuropsychology. Research, theory, and practice.* New York: Guilford Press.

Yeates, K.O., Taylor, H.G., Wade, S.L., et al. (2002). A prospective study of short- and long-term neuropsychological outcomes after traumatic brain injury in children. *Neuropsychology, 16,* 514–523.

Yedid, J. (2000a). The forensic neuropsychological evaluation. In G.J. Murrey (Ed.), *The forensic evaluation of traumatic brain injury.* Boca Raton, FL: CRC Press.

Yedid, J. (2000b). The forensic psychological evaluation of traumatic brain injury. In G.J. Murrey (Ed.), *The forensic evaluation of traumatic brain injury.* Boca Raton, FL: CRC Press.

Yehuda, R., Keefe, R.S.E., Harvey, P.D., et al. (1995). Learning and memory in combat veterans with posttraumatic stress disorder. *American Journal of Psychiatry, 152,* 137–139.

Yerkes, R.M. (Ed.) (1921). Psychological examining in the United States Army. *Memoirs of the National Academy of Sciences, 15,* Parts 1–3.

Yesavage, J.A. (1986). The use of self-rating depression scales in the elderly. In L.W. Poon (Ed.), *Handbook for clinical memory assessment of older adults.* Washington, D.C.: American Psychological Association.

Yesavage, J.A., Brink, T.L., Rose, T.L., et al. (1982). Development and validation of a geriatric depression screening scale: A preliminary report. *Journal of Psychiatric Research, 17,* 37–49.

Yeudall, L.T., Fromm, D., Reddon, J.R., & Stefanyk, W.O. (1986). Normative data stratified by age and sex for 12 neuropsychological tests. *Journal of Clinical Psychology, 42,* 918–946.

Yeudall, L.T., Reddon, J.R., Gill, D.M., & Stefanyk, W.O. (1987). Normative data for the Halstead-Reitan neuropsychological tests stratified by age and sex. *Journal of Clinical Psychology, 43,* 346–367.

Ylikoski, R., Ylikoski, A., Erkinjuntti, T., et al. (1993). White matter changes in healthy elderly persons correlate with attention and speed of mental processing. *Archives of Neurology, 50,* 818–824.

Ylikoski, R., Ylikoski, A., Erkinjuntti, T., et al. (1998). Differences in neuropsychological functioning associated with age, education, neurological status, and magnetic resonance imaging findings in neurological healthy elderly individuals. *Applied Neuropsychology, 5,* 1–14.

Yntema, D.B. & Trask, F.P. (1963). Recall as a search process. *Journal of Verbal Learning and Verbal Behavior, 2,* 65–74.

York, J.L. & Welte, J.W. (1994). Gender comparisons of alcohol consumption in alcoholic and nonalcoholic populations. *Journal of Studies on Alcohol, 55,* 743–750.

Young, A., Perrett, D., Calder, A., et al. (2002). *Facial Expressions of Emotion: Stimuli and Tests [FEEST].* Bury St. Edmunds, UK: Thames Valley Test.

Young, A.W., Hellawell, D.J., Van de Wal., C., & Johnson, M. (1996). Facial expression processing after amygdalotomy. *Neuropsychologia, 34,* 31–39.

Young, B., Ott, L., Phillips, R., & McClain, C. (1991). Metabolic management of the patient with head injury. *Neurosurgery Clinics of North America, 2,* 301–320.

Young, G.B. & Bolton, C.F. (2002). Renal disease and electrolyte disturbances. In A.K. Asbury et al. (Eds.), *Diseases of the nervous system* (3rd ed.). Cambridge: Cambridge University Press.

Young, H.A., Gleave, J. R. W., Schmidek, H. H., & Gregory, S. (1984). Delayed traumatic intracerebral hematoma: Report of 15 cases operatively treated. *Neurosurgery, 14,* 22–25.

Young, R.C., Manley, M.W., & Alexopoulos, G.S. (1985). "I don't know" responses in elderly depressives and in dementia. *Journal of the American Geriatrics Society, 33,* 253–257.

Youngjohn, J.R. (1995). Confirmed attorney coaching prior to neuropsychological evaluation. *Assessment, 2,* 279–283.

Youngjohn, J.R. & Crook, T.H. (1993a). Learning, forgetting, and retrieval of everyday material across the adult life span. *Journal of Clinical and Experimental Neuropsychology, 15,* 447–460.

Youngjohn, J.R. & Crook, T.H. (1993b). Stability of everyday mem-

ory in age-associated memory impairment: A longitudinal study. *Neuropsychology, 7,* 406–416.

Youngjohn, J.R., Larrabee, G.J., & Crook, T.H. (1992). Test–retest reliability of computerized everyday memory measures and traditional tests. *The Clinical Neuropsychologist, 6,* 276–286.

Youngjohn, J.R., Larrabee, G.J., & Crook, T.H. (1993). New adult age- and education-correction norms for the Benton Visual Retention Test. *The Clinical Neuropsychologist, 7,* 155–160.

Youngjohn, J.R., Lees-Haley, P.R., & Binder, L.M. (1999). Comment: Warning malingerers produces more sophisticated malingering. *Archives of Clinical Neuropsychology, 14,* 511–515.

Yousem, D.M., Geckle, R.J., Bilker, W.B., et al. (1999). Posttraumatic smell loss: Relationship of psychophysical tests and volumes of the olfactory bulbs and tracts and the temporal lobes. *Academic Radiology, 6,* 264–272.

Yuan, J. (2000). Apoptosis in the nervous system. *Nature, 407,* 802–809.

Yuan, J. & Yankner, B.A. (2000). Apoptosis in the nervous system. *Nature, 407,* 802–809.

Yucel, M., Stuart, G.W., Maruff, P., et al. (2001). Hemispheric and gender-related differences in the gross morphology of the anterior cingulated/paracingulate cortex in normal volunteers: An MRI morphometric study. *Cerebral Cortex, 11,* 17–25.

Yudofsky, S.C. & Hales, R.E. (Eds.) (2002). *The American Psychiatric Publishing textbook of neuropsychiatry and clinical neurosciences* (4th ed.). Washington, D.C.: American Psychiatric Publishing.

Yuspeh, R.L., Vanderploeg, R.D., & Kershaw, D.A.J. (1998). Normative data on a measure of estimated premorbid abilities as part of a dementia evaluation. *Applied Neuropsychology, 5,* 149–153.

Zachary, R.A. (1986). *Shipley Institute of Living Scale. Revised manual.* Los Angeles: Western Psychological Services.

Zafonte, R.D., Hammond, F.M., Mann, N.R., et al. (1996). Relationship between Glasgow Coma Scale and functional outcome. *American Journal of Physical Medicine and Rehabilitation, 75,* 364–369.

Zafonte, R.D., Mann, N.R., Millis, S.R., et al. (1997). Posttraumatic amnesia: its relation to functional outcome. *Archives of Physical Medicine and Rehabilitation, 78,* 1103–1106.

Zafonte, R.D., Watanabe, T., & Mann, N.R. (1998). Moving bullet syndrome: A complication of penetrating head injury. *Archives of Physical Medicine and Rehabilitation, 79,* 1469–1472.

Zafonte, R.D., Wood, D.L., Harrison-Felix, C.L., et al. (2001a). Penetrating head injury: A prospective study of outcomes. *Neurological Research, 23,* 219–226.

Zafonte, R.D., Wood, D.L., Harrison-Felix, C.L., et al. (2001b). Severe penetrating head injury: A study of outcomes. *Archives of Physical Medicine and Rehabilitation, 82,* 306–310.

Zagar, R., Arbit, J., Stuckey, M., & Wengel, W.W. (1984). Developmental analysis of the Wechsler Memory Scale. *Journal of Clinical Psychology, 40,* 1466–1473.

Zahn, T.P., Grafman, J., & Tranel, D. (1999). Frontal lobe lesions and electrodermal activity: Effects of significance. *Neuropsychologia, 37,* 1227–1241.

Zahn, T.P. & Mirsky, A.F. (1999). Reaction time indicators of attention deficits in closed head injury. *Journal of Clinical and Experimental Neuropsychology, 21,* 352–367.

Zaidel, E. (1978). Lexical organization in the right hemisphere. In P.A. Buser & A. Rougeul-Buser (Eds.), *Cerebral correlates of conscious experience.* INSERM Symposium 6. Amsterdam: Elsevier/North-Holland.

Zaidel, E. (1979). Performance on the ITPA following cerebral commissurotomy and hemispherectomy. *Neuropsychologia, 17,* 259–280.

Zaidel, E. (1990). Language functions in the two hemispheres following complete cerebral commissurotomy and hemispherectomy. In F. Boller & J. Grafman (Eds.), *Handbook of neuropsychology* (Vol. 4). Amsterdam: Elsevier.

Zaidel, E., Aboitiz, F., Clarke, J., et al. (1995). Sex differences in interhemispheric relations for language. In F.L. Kitterle (Ed.), *Hemispheric communication: Mechanisms and models.* Hillsdale, NJ: Erlbaum.

Zaidel, E., Clarke, J.M., & Suyenobu, B. (1990). Hemispheric independence: A paradigm case for cognitive neuroscience. In A. Scheibel & A. Wechsler (Eds.), *Neurobiological foundations of higher cognitive functions.* New York: Guilford Press.

Zaidel, E. & Iacoboni, M. (2003). *The parallel brain. The cognitive neuroscience of the corpus callosum.* Cambridge, MA: MIT Press.

Zaidel, E., Iacoboni, M., Zaidel, D.W., & Bogen, J.E. (2003). The callosal syndromes. In K.M. Heilman & E. Valenstein (Eds.), *Clinical neuropsychology* (4th ed.). New York: Oxford University Press.

Zaidel, E., Zaidel, D.W., & Bogen, J.E. (1990). Testing the commissurotomy patient. *Neuromethods, 17,* 147–201.

Zaidel, E., Zaidel, D.W., & Sperry, R.W. (1981). Left and right intelligence: Case studies of Raven's Progressive Matrices following brain bisection and hemidecortication. *Cortex, 17,* 167–186.

Zajano, M.J. & Gorman, A. (1986). Stroop interference as a function of percentage of congruent items. *Perceptual and Motor Skills, 63,* 1087–1096.

Zakzanis, K.K. (1998). Neurocognitive deficit in fronto-temporal dementia. *Neuropsychiatry, Neuropsychology, and Behavioral Neurology, 11,* 127–135.

Zalla, T., Plassiart, C., Pillon, B., et al. (2001). Action planning in a virtual context after prefrontal cortex damage. *Neuropsychologia, 39,* 759–70.

Zangwill, O.L. (1966). Psychological deficits associated with frontal lobe lesions. *International Journal of Neurology, 5,* 395–402.

Zappalá, G., Martini, E., Crook, T., & Amaducci, L. (1989). Ecological memory assessment in normal aging. In F.J. Pirozzola (Ed.), *Clinics in geriatric medicine* (Vol. 5, No. 3). Philadelphia: Saunders.

Zappoli, R. (1988). Event-related potentials' changes in the normal presenium and in patients with initial presenile idiopathic cognitive decline. In D. Giannitrapani & L. Murri (Eds.), *The EEG of mental activities.* Basel: Karger.

Zarit, S.H., Miller, N.E., & Kahn, R.L. (1978). Brain function, intellectual impairment and education in the aged. *Journal of the American Geriatrics Society, 26,* 58–67.

Zasler, N.D. (1991). Neuromedical aspects of alcohol use following traumatic brain injury. *Journal of Head Trauma Rehabilitation, 8,* 78–80.

Zasler, N.D. (1993). Sexuality issues after traumatic brain injury: Clinical and research perspectives. In F.P. Haseltine et al. (Eds.), *Reproductive issues for persons with physical disabilities.* Baltimore, MD: Paul H. Brooks.

Zatorre, R.J. (1984). Musical perception and cerebral functions: A critical review. *Music Perception, 2,* 196–221.

Zatorre, R.J. (1989). Effects of temporal neocortical excisions on musical processing. *Contemporary Music Review, 4,* 265–277.

Zatorre, R.J. & Jones-Gotman, M. (1990). Right-nostril advantage for discrimination of odors. *Perception and Psychophysics, 47,* 526–531.

Zatorre, R.J. & Jones-Gotman, M. (1991). Human olfactory discrimination after unilateral frontal or temporal lobectomy. *Brain, 114,* 71–84.

Zec, R.F. (1993). Neuropsychological functioning in Alzheimer's disease. In R.W. Parks et al. (Eds.), *Neuropsychology of Alzheimer's disease and other dementias.* New York: Oxford University Press.

Zec, R.F., Andrise, A., Vicari, S., et al. (1990). A comparison of phonemic and semantic word fluency in Alzheimer patients and elderly controls [abstract]. *Journal of Clinical and Experimental Neuropsychology, 12,* 18.

Zec, R.F., Landreth, E.S., Vicari, S.K., et al. (1992). Alzheimer Disease Assessment Scale: Useful for both early detection and staging of dementia of the Alzheimer type. *Alzheimer Disease and Associated Disorders, 6,* 89–102.

Zec, R.F., Zellers, D., Belman, J., et al. (2001). Long-term consequences of severe closed head injury on episodic memory. *Journal of Clinical and Experimental Neuropsychology, 23,* 671–691.

Zeitlin, C. & Oddy, M. (1984). Cognitive impairment in patients with severe migraine. *British Journal of Clinical Psychology, 23,* 27–35.

Zeki, S. (1997). Dynamism of a PET image: Studies of visual function. In R.S.J. Frackowiak, K.J. Friston, C.D. Frith, et al. (Eds.), *Human brain function.* San Diego: Academic Press.

Zelinski, E.M. & Burnight, K.P. (1997). Sixteen-year longitudinal and time lag changes in memory and cognition in older adults. *Psychology and Aging, 12,* 503–513.

Zelinski, E.M., Gilewski, M.J., & Thompson, L.W. (1980). Do laboratory tests relate to self-assessment of memory ability in the young and old? In L.W. Poon et al. (Eds.), *New directions in memory and aging.* Hillsdale, NJ: Erlbaum.

Zemlan, F.P., Jauch, E.C., Mulcahey, J.J., et al. (2002). C-tau biomarker of neuronal damage in severe brain injured patients: Association with elevated intracranial pressure and clinical outcome. *Brain Research, 947,* 131–139.

Zervas, I.M. & Jandorf, L. (1993). The Randt Memory test in electroconvulsive therapy: Relation to illness and treatment parameters. *Convulsive Therapy, 9,* 28–38.

Zetzsche, T., Meisenzahl, E.M., Preuss, U.W., et al. (2001). In-vivo analysis of the human planum temporale (PT): Does the definition of PT borders influence the results with regard to cerebral asymmetry and correlation with handedness? *Psychiatry Research, 107,* 99–115.

Zhang, L., Yang, K.H., & King, A.J. (2001a). Biomechanics of neurotrauma. *Neurological Research, 23,* 144–156.

Zhang, L., Yang, K.H., & King, A.I. (2001b). Comparison of brain responses between frontal and lateral impacts by finite element modeling. *Journal of Neurotrauma, 18,* 21–30.

Zhang, Q. & Sachdev, P.S. (2003). Psychotic disorder and traumatic brain injury. *Current Psychiatry Report, 5,* 197–201.

Zhu, J. & Tulsky, D.S. (2000). Co-norming the WAIS-III and WMS-III: Is there a test-order effect on IQ and memory scores? *The Clinical Neuropsychologist, 14,* 461–467.

Zhu, J., Tulsky, D.S., Price, L., & Chen, H.Y. (2001). WAIS-III reliability data for clinical groups. *Journal of the International Neuropsychological Society, 7,* 862–866.

Ziegler, D.K., Batnitzky, S., Barter, R., & McMillan, J.H. (1991). Magnetic resonance image abnormality in migraine with aura. *Cephalalgia, 11,* 147–150.

Zielinski, J.J. (1986). Selected psychiatric and psychosocial aspects of epilepsy as seen by an epidemiologist. In S. Whitman & B.P. Hermann (Eds.), *Psychopathology in epilepsy.* New York: Oxford University Press.

Zigmond, A.S. & Snaith, R.P. (1983). The Hospital Anxiety and Depression Scale. *Acta Psychiatrica Scandinavica, 67,* 361–370.

Zihl, J. (1989). Cerebral disturbances of elementary visual functions. In J.W. Brown (Ed.), *Neuropsychology of visual perception.* New York: IRBN Press.

Zihl, J., Von Cramon, D., & Mai, N. (1983). Selective disturbance of movement vision after bilateral brain damage. *Brain, 106,* 313–340.

Zillmer, E.A., Waechtler, C., Harris, B., et al. (1992). The effects of unilateral and multifocal lesions on the WAIS-R: A factor analytic study of stroke patients. *Archives of Clinical Neuropsychology, 7,* 29–40.

Zimatkin, S.M. & Zimatkina, T.I. (1996). Thiamine deficiency as predisposition to, and consequence of, increased alcohol consumption. *Alcohol and Alcoholism, 31,* 421–427.

Zimmerman, P. & Leclercq, M. (2002). Neuropsychological aspects of attentional functions and disturbances. In M. Leclercq & P. Zimmerman (Eds.), *Applied neuropsychology of attention. Theory, diagnosis and rehabilitation.* New York: Psychology Press.

Zipf-Williams, E.M., Shear, P.K., Strongin, D., et al. (2000). Qualitative Block Design performance in epilepsy patients. *Archives of Clinical Neuropsychology, 15,* 149–157.

Zivadinov, R., De Masi, R., Nasuelli, D., et al. (2001). MRI techniques and cognitive impairment in the early phase of relapsing-remitting multiple sclerosis. *Neuroradiology, 43,* 272–278.

Zivadinov, R., Sepcic, J., Nasuelli, D., et al. (2001). A longitudinal study of brain atrophy and cognitive disturbances in the early phase of relapsing-remitting multiple sclerosis. *Journal of Neurology, Neurosurgery and Psychiatry, 70,* 773–780.

Zola, S.M. & Squire, L.R. (2000). The medial temporal lobe and the hippocampus. In E. Tulving & F.I.M. Craik (Eds.), *The Oxford handbook of memory.* New York: Oxford University Press.

Zola-Morgan, S. (2003). Amnesia: Neuroanatomic and clinical aspects. In T.E. Feinberg & M.J. Farah (Eds.), *Behavioral neurology and neuropsychology* (2nd ed.). New York: McGraw-Hill.

Zorgdrager, A. & De Keyser, J. (1998). Premenstrual exacerbations of multiple sclerosis. *Journal of Neurology, Neurosurgery, and Psychiatry, 65,* 279–280.

Zorzon, M., Antonutti, L., Mase, G., et al. (1995). Transient global amnesia and transient ischemic attack : Natural history, vascular risk factors, and associated conditions. *Stroke, 26,* 1536–1542.

Zorzon, M., Zivadinov, R., Nasuelli, D., et al. (2002). Depressive symptoms and MRI changes in multiple sclerosis. *European Journal of Neurology, 9,* 491–496.

Zubair, M. & Besner, G.E. (1997). Pediatric electrical burns: Management strategies. *Burns, 23,* 413–420.

Zubenko, G.S. (1997). Molecular neurobiology of Alzheimer's disease (syndrome?). *Harvard Review of Psychiatry, 5,* 177–213.

Zubenko, G.S. (2000). Neurobiology of major depression in Alzheimer's disease. *International Psychogeriatrics, 12(Suppl. 1),* 217–230.

Zubenko, G.S., Sullivan, P., Nelson, J.P., et al. (1990). Brain imaging abnormalities in mental disorders of late life. *Archives of Neurology, 47,* 1107–1111.

Zuccala, G., Onder, G., Pedone, C., et al. (2001). Dose-related impact of alcohol consumption on cognitive function in advanced age: Results of a multicenter survey. *Alcoholism: Clinical and Experimental Research, 25,* 1743–1748.

Zuckerman, M. (1990). Some dubious premises in research and theory on racial differences. *American Psychologist, 45,* 1297–1303.

Zung, W.W.K. (1965). A Self-rating Depression Scale. *Archives of General Psychiatry, 12,* 63–70.

Zung, W.W.K. (1967). Factors influencing the Self-rating Depression Scale. *Archives of General Psychiatry, 16,* 543–547.

Test Index

Subject Index

Page numbers for definitions are in boldface.

Basal ganglia, **47**–48, 52, 281; *see also* Corpus striatum
aging, 295
aphasia and communication disorders, 48
assessments, 628
emotional disturbances, 49, 328, 329
frontal pathways, 46, 48, 76–77
hemispheric asymmetry, 48, 301
lesion effects, 48, 165, 339; *see also* Huntington's disease; Parkinson's disease; Progressive supranuclear palsy
memory and learning, 442
Baseline examination. *See* Longitudinal studies; Testing, baseline
Base rates. *See* Test interpretation
Batteries, test. *See* Test batteries; Batteries in The Test Index
Behavior–brain relationships. *See* Brain–behavior relationships
Behavioral disturbances. *See* Brain damaged patients; Emotional disturbances; *specific conditions, lesions, sites*
acute conditions, 290
chronic conditions, 291
Best performance method, 97–99, 654–654
Bilateral effects, unilateral lesions. *See* Lesions
Bilateral lesions, effects. *See* Brain damage, bilateral
Binswanger's disease. *See* Multi-infarct dementia
"Blackouts." *See* Alcohol-related disorders
psychogenic, 327
"Blind analysis." *See* Test interpretation
Blindness, 65, 66
cortical, 53, 54, **65–66**, 283
denial of. *See* Anton's syndrome
testing considerations, 119
Blindsight, **23**, 54, **65**
Blind spots, 65
Blood–brain barrier, **41**, 247
Body awareness. *See* Awareness, body; Orientation, personal
Body image distortions, 198
Body-part-as-object response, 639
Boredom. *See* Test-taking problems
Boxing. *See* Traumatic brain injury, risk factors
Bradykinesia, **225**; *see also* Alzheimer's disease; Manganese; Parkinson's disease; Progressive supranuclear palsy
Brain. *See also* Brain organization; Brain structure; Processing functions of the brain
Brain–behavior relationships, 3–4, 17, 31, 39–40, 87
clinical inference, 40, 65, 85, 101, 681
theories, 17, 30, 54–56, 62–63
variations from expected, 16, 40, 85, 467
Brain damage, 287; *see also* Brain damaged patients; Brain disorders

common symptoms, 35, 87, 123–126, 150
concept of, 17–18
as risk factor. *See* Risk factors
sex differences. *See* Sex differences
simulation. *See* Malingering
specificity of effects, 17, 24, 28–29, 30, 32, 54, 75, 76, 77, 78, 85, 135, 154–155
variables affecting expression, 56, 157–158; Chapter 8, *passim*
without apparent effects, 85, 86
Brain damage: behavioral effects
cognition, 20–21, 66, 87, 315
emotional disturbances. *See* Emotional disturbances
enhancements, 38, 59, 86
the experience of, 37
personality changes with, 62–63; *see also specific conditions*
sexual adjustment. *See* Sexual dysfunction
signs and symptoms, 150–151, 202
Brain damage: lesion characteristics
bilateral, 74, 635
bilateral, memory assessments, 419, 478
bilateral, orientation assessment, 338
bilateral, other functions, 515, 536
cortical symptoms (e.g., aphasia, apraxia, agnosia), 279, 281, 283, 639
diffuse. *See* Diffuse brain disorders; *specific brain disorders* (e.g., Multiple sclerosis; Toxic conditions; Traumatic brain injury)
disconnection effects. *See* Disconnection effects
focal, 40, 278–279, 286–287, 321
general versus specific effects, 19, 20–21, 54, 55, 375
ipsilateral effects. *See* Lesions, side, ipsilateral effects
lateralized impairment; *see* Lesions, side
nature of lesion. *See* Lesions, nature
pathophysiological considerations, 286, 289
severity. *See* Severity of brain damage
side, site, and size of lesion. *See* Lesions
subcortical. *See* Subcortical lesion effects; Subcortical structures
Brain damage and time
acute. *See* Acute brain conditions
chronic. *See* Chronic brain conditions
delayed defects, 158, 160, 163, 184, 271, 280, 283
depth of lesion. *See* Lesions, depth
dynamic aspects. *See* Lesions, dynamics
progressive. *See* Lesions, dynamics; Progressive disorders
time since onset. *See* Time since onset of condition
Brain damaged patients. *See also specific conditions*
common problems and complaints, 8, 35, 87, 169, 171–172, 254, 292, 324–325, 402
depression. *See* Depression

developmental disorders. *See* Developmental disorders
interindividual variability, 5, 15, 32, 74, 85, 87, 137; *see also specific conditions*
intraindividual performance discrepancies, 87, 97
intraindividual variability, 56, 64, 291
practical advice for, 8, 178, 291, 292
testing considerations, 105–106, 118–120, 127–128, 138, 147, 292, 471
Brain damaged patients: assessment findings (unspecified or mixed diagnoses). *See also specific conditions*
attentional functions, 359, 360, 369, 370, 372, 374
characteristics, 127, 291, 739, 742
executive functions, 474, 617, 623–624, 631
conceptual functions and reasoning, 596
construction, 564
lateralized effects. *See* Lateralized effects
memory, verbal, 418, 428
memory visual, 462, 476
memory, tactile, 471
motor abilities, 643, 644
personality, 748, 750
sensory and nonvisual perceptual functions, 406, 411
slowing, 387
verbal functions, 520, 522
visuoperception, 382, 387, 401
vulnerabilities, 130
Brain disorders. *See specific brain disorders in Chapter 7*; Epilepsy
etiology, 101, 292
evolving, 105–106, 138
identifying presence of, 86, 138, 157–158; *see also* Diagnosis
nonprogressive, 105
progressive, 21, 91, 101, 102, 105–106, 202, 203; *see also specific brain disorders*
Brain imaging. *See* Radiographic imaging techniques
Brain mapping. *See* Electrical stimulation of the brain
Brain organization
functional, 10, 24, 31, 39, 40, 42, 52–85, 316
structural, 42–52, 301, 315
vascular system, 42–43
Brain stem and nuclei, 42, 43, 44, 49
lesions, 44; *see also specific conditions*
Brain surgery, 9–10, 60–61, 234, 257, 277–278, 289
commissurotomy. *See* Commissurotomy
cortical stimulation, 75
epilepsy. *See* Epilepsy
psychiatric disorders (psychosurgery), 76, 291
psychiatric disorders, assessments, 353, 360, 367, 395, 403, 584, 585, 589, 617

[1]Note: unless otherwise specified, data in reports regarding dementia will be referenced under Alzheimer's disease

Left hemisphere: cognitive functions
  mathematical ability, 55, 57, 608
  memory functions, 432
  reasoning, 593
  spatial relationships, 57
Left hemisphere: noncognitive functions
  emotional functioning, 61
  musical capacities, 64
  nonverbal functions, 55
  sequencing activities, 55
  time sense, 55, 355
Left hemisphere lesions, 55, 56, 198; see
    also Frontal lobe lesions, left;
    Posterior lesions, left
  characteristic defects, 57–58, 531–532
  examination problems, 186
  outcome, 62
Left hemisphere lesions: assessment
    findings; see also Lateralized lesions,
    assessment findings
  academic skills, 526, 605, 662
  attentional functions, 353, 357, 360,
    366
  conceptual functions and reasoning,
    580, 581, 585, 598
  construction, 560
  inattention, 380
  memory and learning, 428, 442, 443,
    447, 465, 466, 474
  verbal functions, 92, 384, 506, 515,
    516, 529
  visual perception, 392, 393–394, 399
Left hemisphere lesions: cognitive
    deficits
  arithmetic, 58
  concept formation, 572
  construction, 58, 67
  memory and learning, 57, 58, 59–61
  spatial functions, 58
  verbal deficits. See Left hemisphere
    lesions: verbal deficits
  visuoperceptual abilities, 67
Left hemisphere lesions: noncognitive
    symptoms
  apraxia, 64, 71, 640
  auditory processesing defects, 407
  awareness of deficit, 61, 62, 63
  emotional functioning, 37, 61–63
  inattention, 72, 380, 407
  motor abilities, 58
  music. See Amusia
  personality characteristics, 62
  sequencing defects, 57, 58, 69, 633
  time-related functions, 55, 57
Left hemisphere lesions: verbal deficits
  aphasia, 48, 57, 70–71, 74–75, 198
  communication disorders, 48, 407
  naming disorder, 139, 511
  spelling, 526–527
  verbal fluency, 57, 518–519
  verbal memory, 60–61
  verbal skills, 58, 407
  writing defects, 58, 525–526
Left-right orientation defects. See
    Orientation defects, directional

Legal proceedings
  compensation claims, 129, 179, 187,
    325, 749, 756
  criminal proceedings, 129, 327, 756
  neuropsychological assessment, 4,
    10–11, 107, 128–130, 186
Lesions, **40**, 286–290; see also Brain
    damage
  depth, 287–288
  distance effects. See Diaschisis; Distance
    effects
  duration, 290
  dynamics, 40, 101, 102, 290
  focal. See Brain damage
  nature, 289, 292
  onset speed, 101, 286–290
  site, 198, 287, 291
  size, 20–21, 70, 72, 197, 198, 287,
    289–290, 291
  specificity of effects, 40, 61, 66, 68, 71,
    75, 76, 279, 287
  surgical. See Brain surgery
  unilateral, 55, 59, 160, 196, 287, 293; see
    also Cerebral hemispheres, asymmetry;
    Epilepsy; specific cerebral lobes
  unilateral, bilateral effects, 97, 411, 640
  unilateral, ipsilateral effects, 54, 197,
    288, 645
  white matter. See White matter lesions
  wide-ranging effects, 20–21, 79, 89
Lethargy and somnolence, 34, 44, 280
  diffuse brain damage, 270, 273, 282, 284
Leukoaraiosis, **202**; see also White matter
    lesions
Leukoencephalopathy, 266
Levodopa. See L-Dopa; Parkinson's
    disease, L-dopa
Lewy bodies, 227, 229
Lewy body dementia, 222–223
  assessments, 329, 404, 581, 705, 706, 709
Lhermitte's phenomenon, **250**
Lightning. See Electrical and lightning
    injuries
Limbic system, 46, 47, **49**, 75–76, 78; see
    also component structures, Amygdala;
    Gyrus Cingulate; Hippocampus;
    Mammillary bodies; Thalamus
  dementing disorders, 220, 242
  lesion effects, 50, 76, 79, 84, 289, 611
  lesion effects in brain disorders, 182,
    262, 275–276, 280, 328
  psychiatric disorders, 328, 330
Linear processing. See Left hemisphere,
    processing
Literacy, 562
Litigation. See Legal proceedings
Litigation effects, 127, 755, 758
Liver disease, 284, 493
Lobectomy. See Brain surgery,
    psychosurgery
Lobes. See specific lobes: Frontal;
    Occipital; Parietal; Temporal
Lobotomy. See Brain surgery,
    psychosurgery
LOC (loss of consciousness). See

Consciousness, impaired; Traumatic
    brain injury
Localization of (dys)function, 40, 65, 70,
    71, 76, 85, 287
Localization of lesions, 65, 74–75, 287, 560
  cautions, 85, 278, 589–590
Locus coeruleus, 209, 210, 227, 295
Logical reasoning. See Reasoning
Longitudinal organization. See Cerebral
    cortex
Longitudinal studies, 102, 214 (ex.); see
    also Aging; Testing, repeated
Long-term potentiation and depression, **41**
Long-term storage. See Learning
Luce, Clare Booth, 271

MA (mental age) score. See Test scores
Magnetic resonance imaging (MRI), **15**, 16,
    315; see also Radiographic imaging
    techniques; specific conditions (e.g.,
    Huntington's disease; Multiple
    sclerosis; Traumatic brain injury)
  fMRI, **16**, 306, 308
Magnetoencephalography, **15**, 17, 39
Malingering, 333–334, 755–759; see also
    Psychogenic disorders
  case examples, 333–334, 757, 776
  examining for, 11, 129, 333, 755,
    756–759, 770–771. See also Validity
    assessment
  research concerns, 756, 758–759
  signs and symptoms, 324, 325,
    756–757, 759
  specialized examination techniques,
    770–780
Mammillary bodies, **46**, 47
  lesion effects, 46, 209, 227, 262, 276
  mammillothalamic tract, **46**
Manganese, 273
Mania, 47, 182, 241, 275, 325
Manual dexterity. See Hand functions
Marijuana, 265–266; see also Drug effects
  cognition and test performance,
    265–266
  emotional and psychosocial effects, 265
Mathematical ability. See also Arithmetic;
    Calculations
  anatomic correlates, 56, 58, 608
  reasoning, 30, 68–69
  sex differences. See Sex differences
Mathematical defects, 71
  acalculia, 31, **67**, 71
  anarithmetria, 31, **71**
Mazes, 61
Medical status. See Health status
Medication. See Drugs and medications
Medulla oblongata, **43**
Memory, 20, 27, 46, 48, 49, 50, 70, 78,
    287, 414; see also Forgetting;
    Learning; Verbal memory and
    learning; Visual memory
  anatomic correlates, 26, 27, 46, 48, 49,
    50, 59–61, 70, 78, 287; see also
    Limbic system